Optum

Coders' Desk Reference for Procedures

Answers to your toughest CPT® coding questions

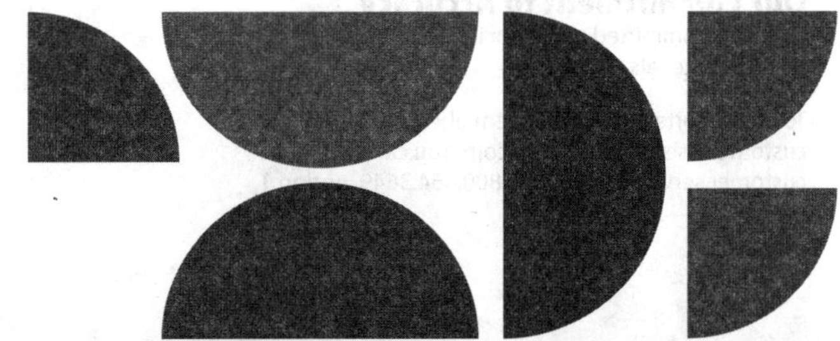

2025

optumcoding.com

Notice

Coders' Desk Reference for Procedures is designed to be an authoritative source of information about coding and reimbursement issues. Every effort has been made to verify accuracy and all information is believed reliable at the time of publication. Absolute accuracy cannot be guaranteed, however. This publication is made available with the understanding that the publisher is not engaged in rendering legal or other services that require a professional license. If you identify a correction or wish to share information, please email the Optum customer service department at customerservice@optum.com or fax us at 801.982.4033.

American Medical Association Notice

Copyright

Made in the USA.

ISBN 978-1-62254-915-3

Our Commitment to Accuracy

Optum is committed to producing accurate and reliable materials.

To report corrections, please email customerassistance@optum.com. You can also reach customer service by calling 1.800.464.3649, option 1.

Acknowledgments

The following staff contributed to the development and/or production of this book:

Marianne Randall, CPC, *Product Manager*
Stacy Perry, Manager, *Desktop Publishing*
Laura Anderson, RN, BSN, CCDS, *Subject Matter Expert*
LaJuana Green, RHIA, CCS, *Subject Matter Expert*
Nannette Orme, CCS-P, *Subject Matter Expert*
Tara N. Rose, CPC, CPC-I, CPMA, RHIA, CCS-P, *Subject Matter Expert*
Tracy Betzler, *Senior Desktop Publishing Specialist*
Hope M. Dunn, *Senior Desktop Publishing Specialist*
Katie Russell, *Desktop Publishing Specialist*
Kimberli Turner, *Editor*

Subject Matter Experts

LaJuana Green, RHIA, CCS

Ms. Green is a Registered Health Information Administrator with more than 35 years of experience in multiple areas of information management. She has proven expertise in the analysis of medical record documentation, assignment of ICD-10-CM and PCS codes, DRG validation, and CPT code assignment in ambulatory surgery units and the hospital outpatient setting. Her experience includes serving as a director of a health information management department, clinical technical editing, new technology research and writing, medical record management, utilization review activities, quality assurance, tumor registry, medical library services, and chargemaster maintenance. Ms. Green is an active member of the American Health Information Management Association (AHIMA).

Tara N. Rose, CPC, CPC-I, CPMA, RHIA, CCS-P

Ms. Rose has more than 15 years of experience in the health care profession. She has extensive experience in auditing, physician billing, and multi-specialty coding with assignment of CPT, HCPCS, and ICD-10-CM codes. She has served in roles as a coding consultant, trainer, clinical investigator, community college instructor, and coding lead. She has experience providing education to physicians and both new and experienced coders. Ms. Rose is a member of her local AAPC chapter and holds credentials from the American Health Information Management Association (AHIMA).

Contents

Introduction

Coding is a complicated business. It's not enough to have a current copy of a CPT® book. Medical coders also need dictionaries and specialty texts if they are to accurately translate physicians' operative reports or patient charts into CPT codes.

That's why Optum originally developed *Coders' Desk Reference*—now known as *Coders' Desk Reference for Procedures*—to provide a resource with answers to CPT coding questions. We polled the medical reimbursement community and our technical staff to determine the issues causing bottlenecks in a coder's workload.

We know that experienced coders are frustrated by limited definitions accompanying many CPT codes. Beginning coders need guidelines on the use of CPT codes and basic information about medical and reimbursement issues. Everyone requires up-to-date information about the anticipated changes in procedural coding.

Coders' Desk Reference for Procedures (CDR) answers the questions of both experienced and novice medical coders. Coders, physicians, registered nurses, physician assistants, and physical therapists contributed to the technical information contained in CDR. The result is a compendium of answers to a wide variety of CPT coding questions.

Since the first release of CDR in 1995, coders' corrections, suggestions, and tips have been incorporated into every printing, making this book as informative and useful as possible. Changes reflecting the dynamic world of coding are ongoing, and Optum encourages input for inclusion in future editions of the book. Information in CDR has been updated to reflect 2025 CPT codes.

Format

CDR is divided into convenient sections for easy use, with each section organized in alphabetic or numeric order. Simply access the section by thumbing through the convenient tabbing system to find the specific item of interest.

Using CPT Codes

For the new coder, and even for the veteran, this chapter provides an overview of the CPT book: what it is and how best to use this coding system for identifying procedures.

Using CPT Modifiers

Modifiers augment CPT codes to the satisfaction of private and government payers. Optum coding experts interpret CPT modifiers and identify their advantage in reimbursement.

Using E/M Codes

Although some of the most commonly used codes by physicians of all specialties, evaluation and management (E/M) codes are amongst the least understood. These codes, introduced in the 1992 CPT book, were designed to increase accuracy and consistency in the reporting of non-procedural encounters. This section contains the official 2025 guidelines.

Place of Service/Type of Service

This section contains place-of-service codes that should be used on professional claims and type-of-service codes used by the Medicare Common Working File.

Reimbursement Terms

In order to get reimbursed in a timely manner, it is important to have a clear understanding of the terminology used by major insurers and the federal government. This section includes up-to-date terminology that will help coders have a better understanding of the complex reimbursement climate.

Clinical Abbreviations, Prefixes, Suffixes, and Acronyms

The medical profession has its own shorthand for documentation. Here, acronyms, abbreviations, and symbols commonly seen on operative reports or medical charts are listed for easy reference.

The uniquely efficient language of medicine is based on prefixes and suffixes attached to root words to modify the meaning. Medical prefixes and suffixes evolved from the Greek and Latin used by pioneering physicians.

Procedural Eponyms

What is the Mitrofanoff operation? What is the Binet test? Eponyms honor the developer of a procedure or test, but do little to clarify what the procedure is. Subject matter experts have researched the procedural eponyms found in the index of the CPT book or used by surgeons and other medical personnel in medical reports, and provide simplified explanations of what the procedures are, along with applicable CPT codes.

Surgical and Laboratory Terms

Operative reports contain words and phrases that not only communicate the importance and urgency of surgery, but the techniques as well. Laboratory reports contain specialized terminology that reflect the various testing methods employed as well as diverse techniques for specimen collection. The glossary of surgical and laboratory terms in *Coders' Desk Reference for Procedures* includes terms most used in operative reports to describe techniques and tools, as well as those often seen on laboratory reports and requisitions that identify collection technique and methodology.

Anatomical Illustrations

Illustrations are included by body system with additional plates showing the planes of the body and Rule of Nines for burns.

CPT Lay Descriptions

The lay descriptions contained in the *Coders' Desk Reference for Procedures* are written to provide a common or generally accepted method of accomplishing the service indicated by the CPT code description. In cases where more than one procedure or method is reported by a single code, one example of those methods or procedures may be given in the lay description. No lay description in this product is intended to give an absolute, required method of performing the service described in the CPT code. Reflecting the full spectrum of variations in technology and of professional techniques would be impossible in a book this size. Each CPT code is followed by a detailed description of the procedure that code represents.

Coders' Desk Reference for Procedures was developed to help providers comply with the emerging standards by which medical services are coded, reported, and paid. Remember that *Coders' Desk Reference for Procedures* is a post-treatment medical reference and, as such, it is inappropriate to use this manual to select medical treatment.

Using CPT® Codes

The codes of the *Current Procedural Terminology* (CPT®) book constitute procedural and medical service components. The CPT book is in its fourth edition with revisions occurring every year.

The CPT coding system was selected as one of the National Code Sets mandatory for use to facilitate electronic transactions, including health claims, enrollments, eligibility, payment/remittance, and referral authorization. CPT codes are divided into three categories to enhance the use of the CPT system by practicing physicians, managed care and other payer organizations, and researchers. Category I codes refer to the current five-digit numerical system. Category II codes are a set of optional tracking codes, developed principally for performance measurement. The CPT Category III codes are temporary codes to identify new and emerging technologies.

The CPT Book Conventions

The CPT book is self-referencing. Its introductory material provides information about its rules, format, and guidelines. The introduction to the CPT book should be carefully studied at least once by medical coders and reviewed annually for changes. Classes and correspondence courses teach medical coding and several introductory coding books convey the CPT book fundamentals. Additionally, the AMA and private consultants sponsor coding seminars to discuss changes and methods to implement these changes into regular coding practice.

The heart of this chapter is a glossary of the CPT book terminology. Consult these listings as needed to solve procedural coding problems. However, a brief primer to conventions, rules, and anomalies is presented below.

The six major sections of Category 1 codes in the CPT book are:

- Evaluation and Management (E/M)
- Anesthesiology
- Surgery
- Radiology (including nuclear medicine and diagnostic ultrasound)
- Pathology and Laboratory
- Medicine

The CPT book instructions for use indicate that as medical techniques have continued to evolve so have the distinctions between surgery and medical procedures. As a result, when a service or procedure is identified within a certain area of the book, the user should not take this to mean that the service is limited to that specific section, whether it is for insurance or other purposes such as limiting that service to use by only a particular specialty. Many times codes are placed in a particular section for historical or other reasons; for example, peripheral vascular endovascular intervention codes are listed in the Cardiovascular subsection in the surgery section, while other coronary interventions are placed in the Cardiovascular subsection in the medicine section. Additionally, the procedures and services listed throughout the book are for use by any qualified physician or other qualified health care professional or entity (e.g., hospitals, laboratories, or home health agencies).

The use of the phrase "physician or other qualified health care professional" was adopted to identify other health care providers in addition to physicians. This type of provider is further described in CPT as an individual "qualified by education, training, licensure/regulation (when applicable), and facility privileging (when applicable)." State licensure guidelines determine the scope of practice and a qualified health care professional must practice within these guidelines, even if more restrictive than the CPT guidelines. The qualified health care professional may report services independently or under incident-to guidelines. The professionals within this definition are separate from "clinical staff" and are able to practice independently. CPT defines clinical staff as "a person who works under the supervision of a physician or other qualified health care professional and who is allowed, by law, regulation, and facility policy to perform or assist in the performance of a specified professional service, but who does not individually report that professional service." Keep in mind that there may be other policies or guidance that can also affect who may report a specific service.

Note that the use of the terms "physician,""other qualified health care professional," or "individual" in a code descriptor or guidelines within CPT does not preclude other entities from the reporting of that particular service or procedure.

Although required by almost all third-party payers, the existence of a CPT procedure code does not in any way guarantee payment when the work is performed. Insurance plans vary widely in reimbursement.

Format

The printed format is designed to save space while still making a great deal of sense. A key to interpreting this space-saving scheme involves the use of the semicolon (;).

A main code is typically a single-sentence description, constructed so that pertinent adjunct information follows the semicolon. The following indented codes appear only as brief adjunct information. An important coding axiom is that an indented code always includes the common portion of the preceding main code description as it appears up to and including the semicolon.

25500 Closed treatment of radial shaft fracture; without manipulation

25505 with manipulation

The complete description of code 25505 is: Closed treatment of radial shaft fracture; with manipulation. Although 25505 appears under 25500, it stands alone to describe a treatment requiring manipulation.

Resequencing of CPT Codes

The American Medical Association (AMA) employs a five-character numbering methodology. According to the AMA, there are instances where a new code is needed within an existing grouping of codes, but an unused code number is not available to keep the range sequential. In the case where the existing codes were not changed or had only minimal changes, the AMA assigns a code out of numeric sequence with the other related codes being grouped together. The resequenced codes and their descriptions have been placed with their related codes, out of numeric sequence. The AMA provides a summary of resequenced codes in Appendix N of the CPT book.

CPT codes within *Coders' Desk Reference for Procedures* are most often displayed in the resequenced order found in the CPT book, although there are slight differences in cases where more than one code applies to a given lay description or when the CPT book resequenced code follows an unlisted code, which this book does not include. Resequenced codes are enclosed in brackets for easy identification.

32998 [32994]
In 32998, the physician uses the heat created from high-frequency radio waves to destroy one or more tumors in the lung, pleura, or chest wall. A small incision is made in the skin of the chest and the lesion is accessed by inserting an ablation probe connected to a radiofrequency generator between the ribs. Under imaging guidance, the ablation probe is advanced into the lesion of the lung, pleura, or chest wall. Treatment with the heat probe usually takes several minutes and may include repositioning the probe within the lesion so that overlapping ablations treat the entire tumor. The incision is closed with sutures. This process may be repeated for multiple lesions within the same lung. Report 32994 when the procedure is performed using cryoablation. Imaging guidance is included in these procedures, when performed.

The following table identifies CPT codes that are not found in numerical order in *Coders' Desk Reference for Procedures*. The code that precedes the resequenced code is given to help find the correct placement in this book. **Note:** *Coders' Desk Reference* contains new codes that have been approved by the CPT Editorial Panel but are not included in the 2025 CPT book. Their placement coincides with that provided by the CPT Editorial Panel at the time this book was published.

Code	Follows Code
10004	10021
10005	10004
10006	10005
10007	10006
10008	10007
10009	10008
10010	10009
10011	10010
10012	10011
11045	11042
11046	11043
15769	15770
15853	15851
15854	15853
20560	20553

Code	Follows Code
20561	20560
21552	21556
21554	21552
22836	22847
22837	22836
22838	22837
22858	22860
22859	22854
23071	23076
23073	23071
24071	24076
24073	24071
25071	25076
25073	25071
26111	26116

Code	Follows Code
26113	26111
27043	27048
27045	27043
27059	27049
27329	27364
27337	27328
27339	27337
27632	27619
27634	27632
28039	28045
28041	28039
28295	28296
29914	29863
29915	29914
29916	29915

Code	Follows Code
95983	95977
95984	95983
96125	96105
96127	96113
96164	96159
96165	96164
96167	96165
96168	96167
96170	96168
96171	96170
96380	96377
96381	96380
97037	97032
97151	96041
97152	97151
97153	97152
97154	97153
97155	97154
97156	97155
97157	97156
97158	97157
97161	96936
97162	97161
97163	97162
97164	97163
97165	97164
97166	97165
97167	97166
97168	97167
97169	97168
97170	97169
97171	97170
97172	97171
98000	99215
98001	98000
98002	98001
98003	98002
98004	98003
98005	98004
98006	98005
98007	98006
98008	98007
98009	98008
98010	98009
98011	98010
98012	98011
98013	98012
98014	98013

Code	Follows Code
98015	98014
98016	98015
99091	99454
99177	99174
99415	99359
99416	99415
99417	99416
99418	99417
99421	99412
99422	99421
99423	99422
99424	99489
99425	99424
99426	99425
99427	99426
99437	99483
99439	99437
99451	99449
99452	99451
99453	99452
99454	99453
99457	99474
99458	99457
99459	99484
99473	99091
99474	99473
99484	99498
99485	99467
99486	99485
99490	99439
99491	99490
0253T	0184T
0464T	0333T
0488T	0403T
0510T	0335T
0511T	0510T
0512T	0102T
0513T	0512T
0523T	0626T
0563T	0207T
0614T	0580T
0620T	0505T
0623T	0496T
0624T	0623T
0625T	0624T
0626T	0625T
0640T	0490T
0643T	0545T

Code	Follows Code
0646T	0570T
0671T	0253T
0697T	0649T
0698T	0697T
0714T	0420T
0749T	0743T
0750T	0749T
0790T	0657T
0827T	0763T
0828T	0827T
0829T	0828T
0830T	0829T
0831T	0830T
0832T	0831T
0833T	0832T
0834T	0833T
0835T	0834T
0836T	0835T
0837T	0836T
0838T	0837T
0839T	0838T
0840T	0839T
0841T	0840T
0842T	0841T
0843T	0842T
0844T	0843T
0845T	0844T
0846T	0845T
0847T	0846T
0848T	0847T
0849T	0848T
0850T	0849T
0851T	0850T
0852T	0851T
0853T	0852T
0854T	0853T
0855T	0854T
0856T	0855T
0859T	0640T
0860T	0859T
0861T	0520T
0862T	0861T
0863T	0862T
0867T	0714T
0901T	0232T

Symbols

Symbols alert users to changes or other attributes of a code. The symbols appear in the left margin, just in front of the code number, as shown here:

●	A closed circle designates a new code.
▲	A closed triangle indicates a code description has been changed or altered.
+	A + symbol indicates an add-on code, which is reported secondarily in addition to the primary procedure.
⚡	A lightning bolt denotes codes for vaccines that are pending FDA approval.
★	The star icon identifies codes from Appendix P that may be reported as telemedicine services when modifier 95 is appended.
🔈	The speaker icon identifies codes from Appendix T that may be reported as audio only telemedicine services when modifier 93 is appended.
#	A number symbol identifies codes that have been resequenced and do not appear in numeric order.
⊘	An open circle with a slash denotes codes that are exempt from modifier 51.
▶◀	The "bow tie" symbol represents CPT Editorial Panel actions and identify new and revised text other than the procedure descriptors, including notification of deleted codes.
➲	The arrow within a circle symbol identifies *CPT Changes*, *CPT Assistant*, and *Clinical Examples in Radiology* references that the coder may refer to for additional information regarding that specific code.
♓	The ♓ symbol designates duplicate proprietary laboratory analyses (PLA) tests to indicate when a PLA code contains an identical code descriptor with the only difference being the inclusion of a proprietary name. A PLA code represents proprietary tests that are provided by a single laboratory or may be licensed to or marketed by many different providing laboratories signifying FDA approval. A listing of all PLA codes is located in Appendix O of the CPT book as well as in the PLA subsection within the main laboratory section.

These symbols may have a bearing on assignment of codes for a practice. In addition, deleted language within code descriptors that have revised text appears with a ~~strikethrough~~, while new text will be underlined. Consult Appendix B for a summary of the additions, deletions, and revisions made to the current CPT edition.

Modifiers

Code modifiers were introduced to the CPT book more than 40 years ago to flag a service that is altered in some way from the stated description. The basic definition of the coded service remains intact. Modifiers more precisely convey the nature of the service or procedure. Modifiers are two-digit codes and those commonly used in a practice become second nature. They may or may not affect the level of reimbursement.

Modifiers can indicate:

- A service or procedure represents only a professional or a technical component
- A service or procedure was performed by more than one physician or other qualified health care professional
- Only part of a service was performed
- An adjunct service was performed
- A bilateral service was performed
- A service or procedure was provided more than once
- Unusual events occurred
- A procedure or service was more difficult or took longer or was less involved or required less time

Consult Appendix A of the CPT book for a listing with full descriptions of modifiers. Additionally, individual sections of the CPT book may contain special instructions for the use of modifiers to codes in that particular section. See the Modifiers chapter of this book for further discussion.

Glossary of Terms

Use the following glossary of terms to troubleshoot and solve CPT code-related claims problems. Other chapters of this book will be useful for modifier-related and E/M problems. And, as stated earlier, the CPT book introduction and introductory material at the section heads can help coders sort out problem areas.

Add-on Code—CPT code representing a procedure performed in addition to the primary procedure and designated with a + in the CPT book. Add-on codes are never reported as stand-alone services but are reported secondarily in addition to the primary procedure. A summary listing of CPT add-on codes can be found in appendix D of the CPT book.

Alphabetic Index—The coding process begins with a careful examination of the medical record to determine primary and secondary procedures, as well as any modifying or extenuating circumstances. The alphabetic index is the starting point of all CPT coding. Do not select codes solely on the basis of information in the index—it is only a reference to the full listing of codes. The alphabetic index is not a substitute for the main text. The main text must be referenced to ensure appropriate code selection.

Anesthesia 00100–01999, 99100–99140, 99151–99153, 99155–99157—The Anesthesia section includes codes to report "general, regional, supplementation of local anesthesia, or other supportive services." For moderate (conscious) sedation, refer to code range 99151–99157, found in the Medicine section.

Appendixes—The CPT book contains several appendixes, including Appendix A, which is a complete list of Modifiers, and Appendix B, a listing of additions, deletions, and revisions made to the current CPT Edition. The appendixes provide clarity and definitions for using CPT codes. Refer to the current CPT book for a listing of all the current appendixes and their content.

Bilateral Procedure—Modifier 50 is used in those instances where a bilateral code for the same operative session is unavailable. The bilateral procedure is identified by the primary procedure code along with the modifier. An anatomical counterpart must exist for the procedure. See the Modifiers chapter of this book for more information.

Category Codes—The main section of CPT codes are considered Category I. Category I CPT codes describe a procedure or service identified with a five-digit CPT code and descriptor nomenclature.

Category II CPT codes are a set of codes used for supplemental tracking and performance measurements. Primarily these codes are used to report quality measures when participating in Medicare's Quality Payment Program (QPP). For more information about QPP, visit the CMS website at https://QPP.cms.gov.

Category III codes facilitate data collection for new services and procedures to substantiate usage and clinical efficacy. These codes are used to track new and emerging technologies.

Code Changes—To keep up with the dynamic nature of medicine, the AMA revises and publishes the CPT book on an annual basis. Appendix B consists of a summary of additions, deletions, and revisions to the current edition. These changes are indicated in the CPT book by the symbols discussed on the previous page.

Examples of the use of these symbols are shown below:

● 15011 **Harvest of skin for skin cell suspension autograft; first 25 sq cm or less**

▲ 25447 **Arthroplasty, ~~interposition,~~ intercarpal or carpometacarpal joints; <u>interposition (eg, tendon)</u>**

▶◀ ▶(Do not report 55881 in conjunction with 55882)◀

Code Ranges Listed in Index—Whenever more than one code applies to a given entry in the index, all applicable codes are listed. If two sequential codes or two or more nonsequential codes apply, they are separated by a comma. For example:

Laser Interstitial Thermal Therapy (LITT)
Intracranial 61736, 61737

Repair
Abdominal Wall 15830, 15847

If three or more sequential codes apply, a hyphen is used. For example:

Angiography
Renal Artery 36251-36254

Consultations—This term defines times when a treating physician, other qualified health care professional (QHP), or other appropriate source asks the advice or opinion of another physician or QHP. A consulting physician has a wide degree of latitude in providing services, but does not assume care or provide treatment plans. The E/M code range 99242–99245 and 99252–99255 reports consultation services and the E/M chapter of this book should be consulted for more information.

Correct Coding Initiative—Centers for Medicare and Medicaid Services (CMS) correct coding initiative (CCI) provides edits that determine the appropriateness of CPT code combinations in billing for Medicare claims. The edits are designed to detect "unbundling," or separate coding of the component parts of a procedure.

Cross-reference—The following reference appears in CPT to direct coders to additional material:

- See—this directs the user to refer to the term listed after the word "see."

Evaluation and Management (E/M) —This series of codes provides a means to classify and report the extent of a physician's involvement for a full range of common physician/patient encounters.

E/M codes describe the intensity of a medical encounter as measured by the risks and complexities associated with the diagnosis and medical decision making. The more detailed the components and the more complex the diagnosis and treatment plan, the more valuable the E/M service. New E/M guidelines for 2025 are found in the Using E/M Codes chapter of this book.

The simplest, most basic treatment constitutes what many refer to as level 1 in treatment. Higher levels are assigned consequential to the complexity of services and diagnoses. See the E/M chapter in this book for more information about this series of codes. Lay descriptions have been created for all E/M services and can be located following the medicine section in the back of this book.

Global Surgery Package—This denotes a normal surgical procedure with no complications that includes all of the elements needed to perform the procedure. Fragmentation, or "unbundling," refers to providers who may intentionally or accidentally charge separately for procedures included in the global package for that given surgical procedure. See also Surgical Package Procedures.

Guidelines—Guidelines appear at the beginning of each of the six major sections of CPT Category I codes. The guidelines define items that are necessary to interpret and report the procedures and services contained in that section.

Incidental Procedures—An incidental procedure is generally minor and considered an integral part of the primary procedure. Incidental procedures are not separately reimbursable and are included in the primary charge.

Indented Code Description—Indented code descriptions include all words up to the semicolon of the main description preceding it. See also Format.

Main Terms, Listing in Index—Procedures are listed in the CPT book index by:

- Procedure or service (endoscopy or splint)
- Organ or other anatomic site (tibia or colon)
- Condition (abscess or entropion)
- Key synonyms
- Key eponyms (disease or procedure named after a person, e.g., Mohs micrographic surgery)
- Abbreviations such as MRI for magnetic resonance imaging

Medicine Services—The CPT book's Medicine section is found at the end of the Category I section. Among the many diagnostic and therapeutic services included under medicine are immunizations, injections, specialty-specific codes, and special services. The guidelines begin with instructions on billing multiple procedures. Coders are instructed to report each procedure separately. Note that the word "procedures" may include procedural, medical, and/or evaluation and management services.

Modifiers, CPT—CPT modifiers show that a service was altered from the stated description without actually changing the basic definition of the service. The CPT Modifiers chapter of this book explains how modifiers are used and which modifiers affect reimbursement. For example, modifier 27 Multiple Outpatient Hospital E/M Encounters on the Same Date, identifies hospital resources used in relation to separate and distinct E/M encounters performed by physicians in multiple outpatient settings on the same date.

Outpatient Services—This term usually refers to physician office, clinical, and hospital outpatient department settings. See the Using E/M Codes chapter of this book for more information.

Parenthetical—A parenthetical phrase is one enclosed by parentheses ( ). Information specific to a given code may be included as a parenthetical phrase following the code. These constitute directions to the coder and should be followed. Read all of the rules, guidelines, and general information in each section and subsection.

Pathology and Laboratory—The Pathology and Laboratory section of the CPT book is divided into subsections. Many procedures are performed by various methods and coders must know the methodology used. In many instances, identification of method is the key to appropriate coding.

Pathology and Laboratory services are provided by pathologists or technologists under the supervision of a physician. If the pathologist must review a test result and/or render an opinion, the appropriate code should be selected and modifier 26 attached to indicate that only a professional component was provided.

Proprietary Laboratory Analyses—Proprietary Laboratory Analyses (PLA) codes. New PLA codes are released quarterly and are effective in the quarter following approval and publication.

A PLA is an alphanumeric CPT code and corresponding descriptor that labs or manufacturers use to identify their particular test with greater specificity. Any test assigned a PLA code is required to be performed on human specimens and must be requested by the clinical laboratory/manufacturer that offers the test.

The PLA section within CPT includes, but is not limited to, Advanced Diagnostic Laboratory Tests (ADLT) and Clinical Diagnostic Laboratory Tests (CDLT) as defined under the Protecting Access to Medicare Act of 2014 (PAMA). Analyses may include a range of medical laboratory tests that can include Multianalyte Assays with Algorithmic Analyses (MAAA) and Genomic Sequencing Procedures (GSP) to name a few. The PLA code descriptors, to the extent possible, follow existing coding conventions (e.g., MAAA, GSP). These codes represent proprietary clinical laboratory analyses and can be provided by a single laboratory or licensed or marketed to multiple laboratories cleared and/or approved by the Food and Drug Administration (FDA).

Radiology—Reporting radiological procedures involves two components: the technical and the professional. The technical component is that part of the procedure specific to the equipment, including the services of a technician. The professional component is specific to the physician's evaluation of the images. CPT coding and nomenclature in the radiology section is under constant review in an effort to reflect current standards of service for this broad specialty.

Separate Procedures—Separate procedures are defined in the CPT book as services that are "commonly carried out as an integral component of a total service or procedure." These services are noted in the CPT book with the parenthetical phrase (separate procedure) at the end of the description. When this phrase appears before the semicolon, all indented descriptions that follow are covered by it.

To reduce fragmented billing, review pertinent surgical codes that include the notation (separate procedure), and apply these guidelines:

- Code separate procedures only when the procedure is performed alone rather than in conjunction with related procedures.
- When a procedure that is ordinarily a component of a larger procedure is performed alone for a specific purpose, you can list it by itself or as a multiple procedure with modifier 51 and/or 59 attached. In other words, it is unrelated to the other procedure performed in a multiple setting. The operative report and associated ICD-10-CM code must be clear and specific to substantiate a separate procedure in conjunction with another major surgical procedure.

Subterms—A main term may be followed by a series of indented terms that modify the main term. Subterms affect the selection of appropriate codes.

Surgery—The Surgery section of CPT includes two types of procedures: therapeutic and diagnostic. To select CPT surgical codes that accurately reflect the service performed, read surgical code descriptions carefully and remember that modifiers may have a significant impact on reimbursement. See the lay description chapter of the *Coders' Desk Reference* for general explanations of procedures.

Surgical Package Procedures—The CPT book defines a surgical package in terms of a normal, uncomplicated performance of specific surgical services, with the assumption that on average, all surgical procedures of a given type are similar with respect to skill level, duration, and length of normal follow-up care. The majority of CPT surgical codes are package services; they include related minor procedures and normal follow-up. Reimbursement for package procedures includes the actual surgical service, local infiltration, metacarpal, metatarsal, and digital block or local anesthesia (when used), and an allowance for normal postoperative care. One related E/M encounter provided after the decision for surgery has been made is also normally included. See also Unbundling, Separate Procedures, and Global Surgical Package.

Unbundling—Unbundling a code is similar to coding an incidental procedure but usually involves less subtle fragmenting of a bill. Never divide the components of a procedure when one code covers all of the components. Examples of minor procedures always included in the primary surgical package include the following:

- Local infiltration of medication
- Closure of surgically created wounds, minor debridement, and wound culture
- Exploration of operative area
- Lysis of moderate amounts of adhesion and fulguration of bleeding points
- Application of dressings
- Application of splints with musculoskeletal procedures

Unlisted Procedure or Service—Codes have been designated to report services or procedures that are not found in the CPT book. These codes usually end in the number 99. When an unlisted procedure code is used, a manual review by the payer is necessary. Documentation, such as operative notes and a cover letter, should be submitted with the claim. The provider should establish the fee for an unlisted procedure. It may help the payer if the provider relates the service's value to a procedure of similar value and worth.

Using CPT® Modifiers

Modifiers allow coders to indicate that a service was altered in some way from the stated CPT® description without actually changing the basic definition of the service. Modifiers are considered an essential component of accurate coding. Some modifiers impact reimbursement and others identify special circumstances. Modifiers can indicate the following:

- A service or procedure represents only a professional or technical component
- A service or procedure was performed by more than one physician
- Only part of a service was performed
- An adjunctive service was performed
- A bilateral procedure was performed
- A service or procedure was provided more than once
- Unusual events occurred
- A procedure or service was more difficult or took longer or was less involved or required less time

Physical status modifiers, P1-P6, specifically used for anesthesia services, are not discussed in this chapter. HCPCS modifiers, beginning with an alpha character, may be appended to CPT codes in specific circumstances and are also not discussed in this chapter.

22 Increased Procedural Services

Modifier 22 is not appropriate for CPT codes with the term "simple" as part of the code description, nor should it be appended to a code for an E/M service. Rather, modifier 22 is used to indicate that a procedure was complicated, complex, difficult, or took significantly more time than usually required by the provider to complete the procedure. Documentation, including notations to the amount of time involved, should be provided with the billing and kept in the medical record when this modifier is used. Time notations in the documentation should include start and stop times, as well as the total amount of additional time required to complete the procedure. The provider should clearly state *specifically*, and in detail, what issues made the procedure more complex rather than simply using vague statements such as, "The patient had a lot of adhesions." When modifier 22 is used, an operative report should always be attached to the claim.

The fee reported for modifier 22 should be the usual and customary amount for the procedure plus an additional amount for the unusual circumstances. If modifier 22 is appended to a code that is not the primary code, and modifier 51 has been appended, modifier 22 should be paid in addition to the cut contract rate paid for the code.

Modifier 22 often produces an automatic review or audit by payers. If the operative report attached to the claim does not indicate appropriate use of the modifier, the increase in payment will be denied. Periodic training for all involved in the coding process is important from both a legal and reimbursement perspective.

Because modifier 22 is often used when complications are encountered during surgical procedures, medical necessity is substantiated by additional diagnostic codes that identify the complication. These diagnostic codes should reflect the operative condition and the complication(s) encountered during the surgery.

23 Unusual Anesthesia

This modifier is used by anesthesiologists to indicate that this procedure is normally performed under local anesthesia or regional block but due to unusual circumstances, general anesthesia is needed. This modifier is not appropriate for use with codes that include the term "without anesthesia" in the descriptor, or for procedures normally performed under general anesthesia.

24 Unrelated Evaluation and Management Service by the Same Physician or Other Qualified Health Care Professional During a Postoperative Period

This modifier reports that an unrelated E/M service was provided by the surgeon within the global period. Use of this modifier needs to be correlated to a diagnosis code that is unrelated to the surgical diagnosis code.

25 Significant, Separately Identifiable Evaluation and Management Service by the Same Physician or Other Qualified Health Care Professional on the Same Day of the Procedure or Other Service

This modifier indicates that on the same day a procedure or service identified by a CPT code is performed, the patient's condition required a significant, separately identifiable E/M code beyond the usual level of service required for the procedure. In addition, the modifier denotes that the patient's condition required services that were over and above the usual preoperative and postoperative care associated with the actual procedure performed.

This modifier is not appropriate with an E/M code that has a minimum level of service. Assign the proper E/M code and amount as appropriate for service rendered. Most payers will allow payment for significant E/M services on the day of a procedure. Performance of a procedure includes an evaluation of the patient as it relates to that procedure or service code. When the patient's condition causes the evaluation to exceed that usual level of service, the appropriate E/M code is listed and appended with modifier 25.

Paper documentation does not need to accompany the claim, but the medical record must clearly identify relevant criteria for separate reporting of an E/M service in addition to the procedure/service code.

Note: Modifier 25 has been approved for hospital outpatient use.

26 Professional Component

Modifier 26 identifies the physician's or other qualified healthcare professional's component of a two-component service. Do not use this modifier with procedures that are either 100 percent technical or 100 percent professional. It is only used on procedures comprised of both components, such as x-rays or pathology codes that result in payment being made for only the professional component of the service. Using modifier 26 also alerts payers to expect a separate claim from the facility for the technical component.

27 Multiple Outpatient Hospital E/M Encounters on the Same Date

Modifier 27 gives physicians the means for reporting the use of hospital resources when providing E/M services in multiple facility outpatient settings on the same date.

Note: Modifier 27 has been approved for hospital outpatient use.

32 Mandated Services

Modifier 32 identifies services that are mandated by Medicare, a peer review organization, a state, local, or government agency, and private payers. Reimbursement may be made at 100 percent of the allowable amount for the service or procedure (such as consultations and related diagnostic services). Deductibles or co-payments may also be waived by the payer. Keep in mind, however, that not all payers cover services when they are mandated, and often expect the government or requesting agency to pay for the service (e.g., an examination to determine abuse, disability, paternity, or confirm rape).

33 Preventive Services

Modifier 33 indicates that the service provided is covered as a preventive service and not subject to co-pays, coinsurance, or deductibles ("cost sharing") in accordance with the Patient Protection and Affordable Care Act (PPACA). Preventive services covered under this act fall into four categories:

- Services rated "A" or "B" by the U.S. Preventive Services Task Force updated annually at www.uspreventiveservicestaskforce.org/
- Routine immunizations for children, adolescents, and adults as outlined by the Centers for Disease Control and Prevention (CDC)
- Preventive care and screenings for children and infants
- Women's preventive care and screenings

Modifier 33 should not be appended to codes that are inherently preventive, for example screening mammography. If multiple preventive procedures are performed per day, the modifier can be applied to each of the codes representing those services.

Note: Modifier 33 has been approved for hospital outpatient use.

47 Anesthesia By Surgeon

Modifier 47 identifies that the surgeon administered regional or general anesthesia. The most common use of this modifier is for a Bier block, which is not identified with its own code. The claim should identify the time spent administering the block. The charge for anesthesia by a surgeon is usually based on time increments instead of a percentage of the total charge for the surgical service. Reimbursement policies for these situations vary dramatically. The predominant attitude of most payers is that a physician should perform the role of the operating surgeon or the anesthesiologist, but not both. Contact payers for specific instructions.

50 Bilateral Procedure

Modifier 50 identifies an identical procedure performed bilaterally during a single operative session.

Do not use modifier 50 when a code description specifically states that the procedure is bilateral, such as code 58700 *Salpingectomy, complete or partial, unilateral or bilateral (separate procedure)*. Also, modifier 50 should not be used on procedures where the organ is considered to be midline, such as the bladder, uterus, esophagus, or nasal septum. Modifier 50 is not reported in conjunction with add-on codes, which are exempt from the multiple procedure concept.

Note: Medicare and many national payers are moving toward the single line entry to identify a bilateral situation. However, careful monitoring will ensure correct reimbursement for both sides. Some payers allow 100 percent for each side if a separate incision is involved. Payers that do not allow 100 percent for the second side usually allow from 50 to 75 percent.

Because of the varying allowances, monitor your reimbursement to determine the percentage allowed for the second side.

Note: Modifier 50 has been approved for hospital outpatient use.

51 Multiple Procedures

Modifier 51 designates multiple procedures that are rendered at the same operative session or on the same day. CPT states that modifier 51 should be used when a combination of surgical services, medical services, or surgical and medical services are provided. Modifier 51 is not used with E/M services, physical medicine and rehabilitation services, or the provision of supplies (vaccines, etc.). It is applicable when multiple related procedures are performed and there is no single inclusive code available. List the primary procedure first on the electronic billing format or claim form, then attach modifier 51 to each secondary procedure code.

The following guidelines represent good billing and coding practices for modifier 51:

- List the procedure code with the highest value first when billing Medicare and commercial payers.
- List additional procedures by descending value.
- Clearly state in your operative reports which procedures were accomplished through separate incisions and which were done through the same incision.
- Do not combine charges when coding multiple, unrelated procedures. List each procedure separately on the claim form and indicate each charge.
- If a comprehensive procedure has a single CPT code, report that code rather than "unbundling" or listing the individual components.

Note: This modifier should not be appended to designated "add-on" codes.

52 Reduced Services

Modifier 52 identifies situations where the physician elects to reduce or eliminate a portion of a service or procedure. Cover letters or operative reports are not necessary when modifier 52 is used since these claims are not usually sent to medical review. Cover letters and operative reports may even impede claims processing. However, physicians may find it helpful to provide the payer with an explanation of the reduced fee compared to the usual fee. The reduction in charge reflects the reduction or elimination of a portion of the service.

Note: For hospital outpatient reporting of a previously scheduled procedure or service that is reduced or canceled due to extenuating circumstances or those that threaten the well being of the patient prior to or after administration of anesthesia, see modifiers 73 and 74, respectively.

Note: Modifier 52 has been approved for hospital outpatient use.

53 Discontinued Procedure

Modifier 53 is used to denote a surgical or diagnostic procedure terminated by the physician because of concerns about the procedure's impact on the patient's well being. Append modifier 53 to the code for the discontinued procedure. This code can only be used if the procedure was discontinued after anesthesia was administered and/or the patient was prepped in the operating suite.

Note: This modifier is not used to report the elective cancellation of a procedure prior to the patient's anesthesia induction and/or surgical preparation in the operating suite. For outpatient hospital/ambulatory surgery center (ASC) reporting of a previously scheduled procedure or service that is reduced or canceled due to extenuating circumstances or those that threaten the well being of the patient prior to or after anesthesia, see modifiers 73 and 74, respectively.

54 Surgical Care Only

Modifier 54 is used when one physician performs a surgical procedure and another provides preoperative and/or postoperative management. The surgeon who performs the procedure reports modifier 54. Both physicians need to determine what percentage of the overall fee each will bill for their individual services (e.g., 70 percent for the surgery and 30 percent for the postoperative care). Do not bill more than 100 percent for the service provided.

55 Postoperative Management Only

Modifier 55 is used when one physician provides postoperative management after another physician has performed the surgical procedure. The physician providing postoperative management bills the surgical procedure code at the percentage agreed upon (see modifier 54) with modifier 55 attached.

56 Preoperative Management Only

Modifier 56 identifies the physician providing preoperative care during the preoperative time clause established by the payer but not performed in the actual surgery. Append this modifier only with codes from the Surgery and Medicine sections of the CPT book. It does not appear in guidelines of the E/M codes.

57 Decision for Surgery

Modifier 57 identifies an E/M service that resulted in the initial decision to perform surgery. Because the CPT book does not designate whether the surgery decided upon is major or minor, diagnostic or therapeutic, use modifier 57 to identify when the decision for any surgery is made.

The prevailing industry standard is to use modifier 25 for minor procedures and modifier 57 on major procedures. CMS defines a minor procedure as having 10 or less follow-up days and defines a major procedure as having 90 follow-up days assigned. Providers are more likely to use modifier 25 to identify that a significant, separately reportable E/M service was provided on the same day a minor procedure was performed.

58 Staged or Related Procedure or Service by the Same Physician or Other Qualified Health Care Professional During the Postoperative Period

When reporting modifier 58, the physician may need to indicate that the procedure or service was one of the following: 1) Planned prospectively at the time of the primary procedure or planned as a staged procedure; 2) more difficult, problematic, or involved than the primary procedure; or 3) for therapeutic treatment following a prior procedure. Do not use this modifier to report the treatment of a problem that requires a return to the operating room (see modifier 78). Modifier 58 is included in the guidelines for Surgery services.

Note the following about modifier 58:

- The existence of CPT modifier 58 does not negate the global fee concept; therefore, services that are included in CPT as multiple sessions or are otherwise defined as including multiple services or events may not be reported with this modifier.
- Modifier 58 should not alter the amount charged or paid for subsequent unrelated or staged procedures that are performed during the postoperative period of a previous procedure.

Note: Modifier 58 has been approved for hospital outpatient use.

59 Distinct Procedural Service

Sometimes, a physician is required to report modifier 59 to indicate that a procedure or service is distinct from other services performed on the same day. Modifier 59 is used to identify procedures that are not usually reported together, but under the circumstances may be separately reported. According to the CPT book, this may represent "a different session, different procedure or surgery, different site or organ system, separate incision/excision, separate lesion, or separate injury (or area of injury in extensive injuries) not ordinarily encountered or performed on the same day by the same individual."

Note: Modifier 59 has been approved for hospital outpatient use.

62 Two Surgeons

Modifier 62 indicates that the skills of two or more surgeons (sometimes with different skills) are required to manage a specific surgical procedure. Multiple-surgeon procedures may be related or unrelated. When the procedures are unrelated, identify the separate services performed by each surgeon. List multiple related procedures as though one physician performed all procedures and add modifier 62. The surgeons should agree on charges, procedure codes, and reimbursement percentage splits prior to submission. Because of many variables, it is imperative that the physicians' billing is coordinated, and to submit complete and detailed documentation.

Note: If a co-surgeon assists in performing additional procedures during the same surgical session, those are reported using separate procedure codes with modifier 80 or 82, as appropriate.

63 Procedure Performed on Infants less than 4 kg

Modifier 63 is only appended to codes in the 20100–69990 range and 92920, 92928, 92953, 92960, 92986-92990, 92997-92998, 93312-93318, 93452, 93505, 93563-93564, 93568-93569, 93573-93575, 93580-93582, 93590-93598, and 93615-93616 from the Medicine/Cardiovascular section, unless specifically designated otherwise, to denote procedures performed on infants and neonates presently weighing up to 4 kg. The patient's small size increases the complexity and physician work for these procedures.

66 Surgical Team

Modifier 66 identifies complex procedures that require multiple concurrent services. Physicians from the same or different specialties, other personnel with experience and training specific to the procedures, and/or equipment required to complete the surgical procedures may be used in the surgery. Team surgery is usually used for organ transplants and re-transplants. Identify a team surgery by listing all procedures as though performed by one physician and add modifier 66 to each procedure code used. The surgeons should agree on charges, procedure codes, and reimbursement splits prior to claims submission. Because of many variables, carefully coordinate the physicians' billing and submit complete and detailed documentation. Also, include a cover letter explaining the reimbursement distribution for each member of the team. The total of charges for all procedures performed may be increased up to 50 percent for team surgery. The reimbursement is divided among the surgeons, contingent upon actual fees, complexity of procedures, and medical review.

73 Discontinued Out-Patient Hospital/ Ambulatory Surgery Center (ASC) Procedure Prior to the Administration of Anesthesia

Modifier 73 identifies those situations when a physician may cancel a surgical or diagnostic procedure subsequent to the patient's surgical prep (including sedation — when provided — and being taken to the room where the procedure is to be performed) but prior to the administration of anesthesia (local, regional block(s) or general). The physician may cancel a surgical or diagnostic procedure due to extenuating circumstances or those that threaten the well being of the patient. Under these circumstances, the intended service that is prepared for but canceled may be reported by its usual procedure number and the addition of modifier 73.

Note: The elective cancellation of a service prior to the administration of anesthesia and/or surgical preparation of the patient should not be reported. For physician reporting of a discontinued procedure, see modifier 53.

Note: Modifier 73 has been approved for hospital outpatient use.

74 Discontinued Out-Patient Hospital/ Ambulatory Surgery Center (ASC) Procedure After Administration of Anesthesia

Modifier 74 identifies those situations when a physician may terminate a surgical or diagnostic procedure after the administration of anesthesia (local, regional block(s) or general) or after the procedure was started (incision made, intubation started, scope inserted, etc.) due to extenuating circumstances or those that threaten the well being of the patient. Under these circumstances, the procedure started but terminated can be reported by its usual procedure number and the addition of modifier 74.

Note: The elective cancellation of a service prior to the administration of anesthesia and/or surgical prep of the patient should not be reported. For physicians reporting a discontinued procedure, see modifier 53.

Note: Modifier 74 has been approved for hospital outpatient use.

76 Repeat Procedure or Service By Same Physician or Other Qualified Health Care Professional

Modifier 76 indicates that the exact procedure had to be repeated by the same physician/health care professional. Append this modifier to identify a procedure or service that was repeated subsequent to the original procedure or service. This distinguishes the procedure or service from either a duplicate service or billing error. Payers may require additional documentation to establish medical necessity.

Modifier 76 is easily misused, so note the following applications of other modifiers:

- A staged or related procedure or service by the same physician during the postoperative period is reported with modifier 58.
- A return to the operating room for a related procedure or service during the postoperative period is reported with modifier 78.
- An unrelated procedure or service by the same physician during the postoperative period is reported with modifier 79.

Note: Modifier 76 has been approved for hospital outpatient use.

77 Repeat Procedure by Another Physician or Other Qualified Health Care Professional

Modifier 77 indicates that a service or procedure performed by one physician/health care professional was repeated by another physician/health care professional. This modifier is usually used during the postoperative period of the procedure or service. The second physician/health care professional appends the modifier to the procedure or service code used by the first physician/health care professional.

It is also appropriate to append modifier 22 when the repeat procedure is unusually complicated, or modifier 52 when only a portion of the procedure or service is repeated. The ICD-10-CM diagnostic codes must substantiate the medical necessity of repeating the procedure. Because payers often require additional documentation to establish medical necessity, it is advisable to submit the operative report with a cover letter.

Note: Modifier 77 has been approved for hospital outpatient use.

78 Unplanned Return to the Operating/ Procedure Room by the Same Physician or Other Qualified Health Care Professional Following Initial Procedure for a Related Procedure During the Postoperative Period

Modifier 78 is used to report related procedures performed in the operating room within the assigned postoperative period of a surgical procedure. Do not use modifier 78 for repeat procedures performed on the same day, rather, append modifier 76.

Note: Modifier 78 has been approved for hospital outpatient use.

79 Unrelated Procedure or Service by the Same Physician or Other Qualified Health Care Professional During the Postoperative Period

Modifier 79 was added to notify payers that the procedure was performed during a postoperative period of another procedure but is not related to that surgery. The diagnostic codes must document the medical necessity of the service, meaning the ICD-10-CM codes are usually different for this service from those reported with the initial procedure. Do not use modifier 79 to report staged or related procedures or services performed by the same physician during the assigned postoperative period of a procedure.

Note: Modifier 79 has been approved for hospital outpatient use.

80 Assistant Surgeon

Modifier 80 identifies surgical assistant services and is applied to the surgical procedure code. Assisting physicians usually charge 16 to 30 percent of their normal fee for performing the surgery alone. Be advised that payers may use the surgeon's contract rate to calculate the assistant's percentage, and usually will not pay a resident for an assistant surgeon fee.

81 Minimum Assistant Surgeon

Modifier 81 identifies minimal surgical assistant services when assistance is required for a short time. Minimal assistant surgeons usually charge from 10 to 15 percent for their services. Be advised that not all payers will allow this modifier to be used for that purpose. Always bill for non-physician assistants at surgery as instructed by the payer.

82 Assistant Surgeon (when qualified resident surgeon not available)

Modifier 82 identifies situations when a qualified resident is unavailable to assist in surgery in a facility with a teaching physician or residency program and another physician must be brought in to assist. The documentation should indicate why a qualified resident was unable to assist in surgery. Assisting physicians usually charge 16 to 30 percent of their normal fee. Be advised that modifier 80 is used more frequently than modifier 82 by surgeon assistants. Bill according to the payer rules for assistant surgery modifiers.

90 Reference (Outside) Laboratory

Modifier 90 identifies laboratory procedures performed by a party other than the treating or reporting physician. HMOs and private payers may allow a fee for a blood draw (arterial and/or venous) and a fee for transport to an outside facility. Code 99000 should be used to report this type of service—not modifier 90.

91 Repeat Clinical Diagnostic Laboratory Test

Modifier 91 identifies tests repeated on the same day for the same patient to obtain multiple results. However, do not report this modifier for tests rerun to confirm initial results or due to testing problems.

Note: Modifier 91 has been approved for hospital outpatient use.

92 Alternative Laboratory Platform Testing

Modifier 92 identifies testing that is performed utilizing a kit or transportable instrument that consists in part or entirely of a one-time use, disposable analytical chamber. The test is designed to be hand-carried or transported to the patient's location for immediate test administration at that site; it does not require permanent dedicated space. Examples of codes that might be appropriate for submission with modifier 92 include those for HIV testing (86701–86703 and 87389).

93 Synchronous Telemedicine Service Rendered Via Telephone or Other Real-Time Interactive Audio-Only Telecommunications System

Modifier 93 indicates audio only telemedicine service and is identified in CPT by a speaker icon. These services are most frequently reported in a traditional face-to-face setting but are also reportable when performed in a telemedicine setting, where the patient is located off-site from the location of the provider. These telemedicine services are provided using synchronous or "real-time" interactive audio only communications systems. The totality of the communication of information exchanged between the physician or other qualified health care professional and the patient during the course of the synchronous telemedicine service must be of an amount and nature that is sufficient to meet the key components and/or requirements of the same service when rendered via a face-to-face interaction.

This modifier should be used only for services with a corresponding code listed in appendix T of the CPT® manual.

Note: Report codes 98008-98015 for synchronous audio-only E/M services.

95 Synchronous Telemedicine Service Rendered Via a Real-Time Interactive Audio and Video Telecommunications System

Modifier 95 is appended to certain CPT codes as telemedicine services. CPT identifies these particular codes with a star icon. A complete listing of all CPT codes that may be reported as real-time telemedicine services can be found in CPT Appendix P. All of the services within this Appendix involve the provider and patient interacting and communicating in real-time through the use of telecommunications equipment involving, at a minimum, audio and video.

Additionally, the total degree of communication and information exchanged between the patient and clinician must equate to the amount and type to sufficiently meet the key components/requirements of the same service as when rendered face-to-face.

Medicare has a separate list of codes they have approved for telehealth services. During the public health emergency (PHE) they have included additional codes on a temporary basis. Medicare has also temporarily allowed greater latitude in the requirements of an acceptable audio or audiovisual communication device and the location of patient and/or provider.

It is recommended that you contact your payer for current guidelines.

Note: Report codes 98000-98007 for synchronous audio-video E/M services.

96 Habilitative Services

Modifier 96 should be appended to services or procedures that are considered to be habilitative. Habilitative services describe medically needed services and/or devices that assist a patient in part or fully, to learn, keep, and improve new skills or functioning required to perform daily living activities or manage a health condition. Habilitative services are provided to assist a patient in acquiring a skill for the first time.

97 Rehabilitative Services

Modifier 97 should be appended to services or procedures that are considered to be rehabilitative. Rehabilitative services describe a diverse range of services from complete specialized medically based inpatient programs to outpatient therapy in a variety of settings such as nursing homes or ambulatory centers designed to encourage the best possible level of total well-being (physical, mental, emotional, psychological, social and economic) of the patient to ensure they can function at the highest degree possible Rehabilitative services are provided to assist a patient in reacquiring a skill that was lost or impaired due to an acquired condition.

99 Multiple Modifiers

Modifier 99 identifies circumstances when two or more modifiers are necessary to delineate a service. Append modifier 99 to the procedure code and list all appropriate modifiers as subsequent line items.

Evaluation and Management (E/M) Services Guidelines

E/M Guidelines Overview

The E/M guidelines have sections that are common to all E/M categories and sections that are category specific. Most of the categories and many of the subcategories of service have special guidelines or instructions unique to that category or subcategory. Where these are indicated, eg, "Hospital Inpatient and Observation Care," special instructions are presented before the listing of the specific E/M services codes. It is important to review the instructions for each category or subcategory. These guidelines are to be used by the reporting physician or other qualified health care professional to select the appropriate level of service. These guidelines do not establish documentation requirements or standards of care. The main purpose of documentation is to support care of the patient by current and future health care team(s). These guidelines are for services that require a face-to-face encounter with the patient and/or family/caregiver. (For 99211 and 99281, the face-to-face services may be performed by clinical staff.)

▶In the **Evaluation and Management** section (98000-98016, 99202-99499), there are many code categories. Each category may have specific guidelines, or the codes may include specific details. These E/M guidelines are written for the following categories:

- Office or Other Outpatient Services
- Telemedicine Services
- Hospital Inpatient and Observation Care Services
- Consultations
- Emergency Department Services
- Nursing Facility Services
- Home or Residence Services
- Prolonged Service With or Without Direct Patient Contact on the Date of an Evaluation and Management Service◀

Classification of Evaluation and Management (E/M) Services

The E/M section is divided into broad categories, such as office visits, hospital inpatient or observation care visits, and consultations. Most of the categories are further divided into two or more subcategories of E/M services. For example, there are two subcategories of office visits (new patient and established patient) and there are two subcategories of hospital inpatient and observation care visits (initial and subsequent). The subcategories of E/M services are further classified into levels of E/M services that are identified by specific codes.

The basic format of codes with levels of E/M services based on medical decision making (MDM) or time is the same. First, a unique code number is listed. Second, the place and/or type of service is specified (eg, office or other outpatient visit). Third, the content of the service is defined. Fourth, time is specified. (A detailed discussion of time is provided in the Guidelines for Selecting Level of Service Based on Time.)

The place of service and service type are defined by the location where the face-to-face encounter with the patient and/or family/caregiver occurs. For example, service provided to a nursing facility resident brought to the office is reported with an office or other outpatient code.

New and Established Patients

Solely for the purposes of distinguishing between new and established patients, **professional services** are those face-to-face services rendered by physicians and other qualified health care professionals who may report evaluation and management services. A new patient is one who has not received any professional services from the physician or other qualified health care professional or another physician or other qualified health care professional of the **exact** same specialty **and subspecialty** who belongs to the same group practice, within the past three years.

An established patient is one who has received professional services from the physician or other qualified health care professional or another physician or other qualified health care professional of the **exact** same specialty **and subspecialty** who belongs to the same group practice, within the past three years. See Decision Tree for New vs Established Patients.

▶ ◀ = Contains new or revised text

In the instance where a physician or other qualified health care professional is on call for or covering for another physician or other qualified health care professional, the patient's encounter will be classified as it would have been by the physician or other qualified health care professional who is not available. When advanced practice nurses and physician assistants are working with physicians, they are considered as working in the **exact** same specialty **and subspecialty** as the physician.

No distinction is made between new and established patients in the emergency department. E/M services in the emergency department category may be reported for any new or established patient who presents for treatment in the emergency department.

The Decision Tree for New vs Established Patients is provided to aid in determining whether to report the E/M service provided as a new or an established patient encounter.

Decision Tree for New vs Established Patients

Received any professional service from the physician or other qualified health care professional in the same group of same specialty within past three years?

- YES → Exact same specialty?
  - YES → Exact same subspecialty?
    - YES → Established
    - NO → New patient
  - NO → New patient
- NO → New patient

Initial and Subsequent Services

Some categories apply to both new and established patients (eg, hospital inpatient or observation care). These categories differentiate services by whether the service is the initial service or a subsequent service. For the purpose of distinguishing between initial or subsequent visits, professional services are those face-to-face services rendered by physicians and other qualified health care professionals who may report evaluation and management services. An initial service is when the patient has not received any professional services from the physician or other qualified health care professional or another physician or other qualified health care professional of the exact same specialty and subspecialty who belongs to the same group practice, during the inpatient, observation, or nursing facility admission and stay.

Coding Tip

Instructions for Use of the CPT Codebook

When advanced practice nurses and physician assistants are working with physicians, they are considered as working in the exact same specialty and subspecialty as the physician. A "physician or other qualified health care professional" is an individual who is qualified by education, training, licensure/regulation (when applicable), and facility privileging (when applicable) who performs a professional service within his or her scope of practice and independently reports that professional service. These professionals are distinct from "clinical staff." A clinical staff member is a person who works under the supervision of a physician or other qualified health care professional, and who is allowed by law, regulation and facility policy to perform or assist in the performance of a specific professional service but does not individually report that professional service. Other policies may also affect who may report specific services.

CPT Coding Guidelines, Introduction, Instructions for Use of the CPT Codebook

A subsequent service is when the patient has received professional service(s) from the physician or other qualified health care professional or another physician or other qualified health care professional of the exact same specialty and subspecialty who belongs to the same group practice, during the admission and stay.

In the instance when a physician or other qualified health care professional is on call for or covering for another physician or other qualified health care professional, the patient's encounter will be classified as it would have been by the physician or other qualified health care professional who is not available. When advanced practice nurses and physician assistants are working with physicians, they are considered as working in the exact same specialty and subspecialty as the physician.

For reporting hospital inpatient or observation care services, a stay that includes a transition from observation to inpatient is a single stay. For reporting nursing facility services, a stay that includes transition(s) between skilled nursing facility and nursing facility level of care is the same stay.

Split or Shared Visits

Physician(s) and other qualified health care professional(s) (QHP[s]) may act as a team in providing care for the patient, working together during a single E/M service. The split or shared visits guidelines are applied to determine which professional may report the service. If the physician or other QHP performs a substantive portion of the encounter, the physician or other QHP may report the service. If code selection is based on total time on the date of the encounter, the service is reported by the professional who spent the majority of the face-to-face or non-face-to-face time performing the service. For the purpose of reporting E/M services within the context of team-based care, performance of a substantive part of the MDM requires that the physician(s) or other QHP(s) made or approved the management plan for the ***number and complexity of problems addressed at the encounter*** and takes responsibility for that plan with its inherent ***risk of complications and/or morbidity or mortality of patient management***. By doing so, a physician or other QHP has performed two of the three elements used in the selection of the code level based on MDM. If ***the amount and/or complexity of data to be reviewed and analyzed*** is used by the physician or other QHP to determine the reported code level, assessing an independent historian's narrative and the ordering or review of tests or documents do not have to be personally performed by the physician or other QHP, because the relevant items would be considered in formulating the management plan. Independent interpretation of tests and discussion of management plan or test interpretation must be personally performed by the physician or other QHP if these are used to determine the reported code level by the physician or other QHP.

Multiple Evaluation and Management Services on the Same Date

The following guidelines apply to services that a patient may receive for hospital inpatient care, observation care, or nursing facility care. For instructions regarding transitions to these settings from the office or outpatient, home or residence, or emergency department setting, see guidelines for **Hospital Inpatient and Observation Care Services or Nursing Facility Services**.

A patient may receive E/M services in more than one setting on a calendar date. A patient may also have more than one visit in the same setting on a calendar date. The guidelines for multiple E/M services on the same date address circumstances in which the patient has received multiple visits or services from the same physician or other QHP or another physician or other QHP of the exact same specialty and subspecialty who belongs to the same group practice.

Per day: The hospital inpatient and observation care services and the nursing facility services are "per day" services. When multiple visits occur over the course of a single calendar date in the same setting, a single service is reported. When using MDM for code level selection, use the aggregated MDM over the course of the calendar date. When using time for code level selection, sum the time over the course of the day using the guidelines for reporting time.

Multiple encounters in different settings or facilities: A patient may be seen and treated in different facilities (eg, a hospital-to-hospital transfer). When more than one primary E/M service is reported and time is used to select the code level for either service, only the time spent providing that individual service may be allocated to the code level selected for reporting that service. No time may be counted twice when reporting more than one E/M service. Prolonged services are also based on the same allocation and their relationship to the primary service. The designation of the facility may be defined by licensure or regulation. Transfer from a hospital bed to a nursing facility bed in a hospital with nursing facility beds is considered as two services in two facilities because there is a discharge from one type of designation to another. An intra-facility transfer for a different level of care (eg, from a routine unit to a critical care unit) does not constitute a new stay, nor does it constitute a transfer to a different facility.

Emergency department (ED) and services in other settings (same or different facilities): Time spent in an ED by a physician or other QHP who provides subsequent E/M services may be included in calculating total time on the date of the encounter when ED services are not reported and another E/M service is reported (eg, hospital inpatient and observation care services).

Discharge services and services in other facilities: Each service may be reported separately as long as any time spent on the discharge service is not counted towards the total time of a subsequent service in which code level selection for the subsequent service is based on time. This includes any hospital inpatient or observation care services (including admission and discharge services) time (99234, 99235, 99236) because these services may be selected based on MDM or time. When these services are reported with another E/M service on the same calendar date, time related to the hospital inpatient or observation care service (including admission and discharge services) may not be used for code selection of the subsequent service.

Discharge services and services in the same facility: If the patient is discharged and readmitted to the same facility on the same calendar date, report a subsequent care service instead of a discharge or initial service. For the purpose of E/M reporting, this is a single stay.

Discharge services and services in a different facility: If the patient is admitted to another facility, for the purpose of E/M reporting this is considered a different stay. Discharge and initial services may be reported as long as time spent on the discharge service is not counted towards the total time of the subsequent service reported when code level selection is based on time.

Critical care services (including neonatal intensive care services and pediatric and neonatal critical care): Reporting guidelines for intensive and critical care services that are performed on the same calendar date as another E/M service are described in the service specific section guidelines.

Transitions between office or other outpatient, home or residence, or emergency department and hospital inpatient or observation or nursing facility: See the guidelines for **Hospital Inpatient and Observation Care Services** or **Nursing Facility Services**. If the patient is seen in two settings and only one service is reported, the total time on the date of the encounter or the aggregated MDM is used for determining the level of the single reported service. If prolonged services are reported, use the prolonged services code that is appropriate for the primary service reported, regardless of where the patient was located when the prolonged services time threshold was met. The choice of the primary service is at the discretion of the reporting physician or other QHP.

Services Reported Separately

Any specifically identifiable procedure or service (ie, identified with a specific CPT code) performed on the date of E/M services may be reported separately.

The ordering and actual performance and/or interpretation of diagnostic tests/studies during a patient encounter are not included in determining the levels of E/M services when the professional interpretation of those tests/studies is reported separately by the physician or other qualified health care professional reporting the E/M service. Tests that do not require separate interpretation (eg, tests that are results only) and are analyzed as part of MDM do not count as an independent interpretation, but may be counted as ordered or reviewed for selecting an MDM level. The performance of diagnostic tests/studies for which specific CPT codes are available may be reported separately, in addition to the appropriate E/M code. The interpretation of the results of diagnostic tests/studies (ie, professional component) with preparation of a separate distinctly identifiable signed written report may also be reported separately, using the appropriate CPT code and, if required, with modifier 26 appended.

The physician or other qualified health care professional may need to indicate that on the day a procedure or service identified by a CPT code was performed, the patient's condition required a significant separately identifiable E/M service. The E/M service may be caused or prompted by the symptoms or condition for which the procedure and/or service was provided. This circumstance may be reported by adding modifier 25 to the appropriate level of E/M service. As such, different diagnoses are not required for reporting of the procedure and the E/M services on the same date.

History and/or Examination

E/M codes that have levels of services include a medically appropriate history and/or physical examination, when performed. The nature and extent of the history and/or physical examination are determined by the treating physician or other qualified health care professional reporting the service. The care team may collect information, and the patient or caregiver may supply information directly (eg, by electronic health record [EHR] portal or questionnaire) that is reviewed by the reporting physician or other qualified health care professional. The extent of history and physical examination is not an element in selection of the level of these E/M service codes.

Levels of E/M Services

Select the appropriate level of E/M services based on the following:

1. The level of the MDM as defined for each service, **or**
2. The total time for E/M services performed on the date of the encounter.

Within each category or subcategory of E/M service based on MDM or time, there are three to five levels of E/M services available for reporting purposes. Levels of E/M services are **not** interchangeable among the different categories or subcategories of service. For example, the first level of E/M services in the subcategory of office visit, new patient, does not have the same definition as the first level of E/M services in the subcategory of office visit, established patient. Each level of E/M services may be used by all physicians or other qualified health care professionals.

Guidelines for Selecting Level of Service Based on Medical Decision Making

Four types of MDM are recognized: straightforward, low, moderate, and high. The concept of the level of MDM does not apply to 99211, 99281.

MDM includes establishing diagnoses, assessing the status of a condition, and/or selecting a management option. MDM is defined by three elements. The elements are:

- ***The number and complexity of problem(s) that are addressed during the encounter.***

Evaluation and Management (E/M) Services Guidelines

- ***The amount and/or complexity of data to be reviewed and analyzed.*** These data include medical records, tests, and/or other information that must be obtained, ordered, reviewed, and analyzed for the encounter. This includes information obtained from multiple sources or interprofessional communications that are not reported separately and interpretation of tests that are not reported separately. Ordering a test is included in the category of test result(s) and the review of the test result is part of the encounter and not a subsequent encounter. Ordering a test may include those considered but not selected after shared decision making. For example, a patient may request diagnostic imaging that is not necessary for their condition and discussion of the lack of benefit may be required. Alternatively, a test may normally be performed, but due to the risk for a specific patient it is not ordered. These considerations must be documented. Data are divided into three categories:
  - Tests, documents, orders, or independent historian(s). (Each unique test, order, or document is counted to meet a threshold number.)
  - Independent interpretation of tests (not separately reported).
  - Discussion of management or test interpretation with external physician or other qualified health care professional or appropriate source (not separately reported).
- ***The risk of complications and/or morbidity or mortality of patient management***. This includes decisions made at the encounter associated with diagnostic procedure(s) and treatment(s). This includes the possible management options selected and those considered but not selected after shared decision making with the patient and/or family. For example, a decision about hospitalization includes consideration of alternative levels of care. Examples may include a psychiatric patient with a sufficient degree of support in the outpatient setting or the decision to not hospitalize a patient with advanced dementia with an acute condition that would generally warrant inpatient care, but for whom the goal is palliative treatment.

Shared decision making involves eliciting patient and/or family preferences, patient and/or family education, and explaining risks and benefits of management options.

MDM may be impacted by role and management responsibility.

When the physician or other qualified health care professional is reporting a separate CPT code that includes interpretation and/or report, the interpretation and/or report is not counted toward the MDM when selecting a level of E/M services. When the physician or other qualified health care professional is reporting a separate service for discussion of management with a physician or another qualified health care professional, the discussion is not counted toward the MDM when selecting a level of E/M services.

The Levels of Medical Decision Making (MDM) table (Table 1) is a guide to assist in selecting the level of MDM for reporting an E/M services code. The table includes the four levels of MDM (ie, straightforward, low, moderate, high) and the three elements of MDM (ie, number and complexity of problems addressed at the encounter, amount and/or complexity of data reviewed and analyzed, and risk of complications and/or morbidity or mortality of patient management). To qualify for a particular level of MDM, two of the three elements for that level of MDM must be met or exceeded.

Examples in the table may be more or less applicable to specific settings of care. For example, the decision to hospitalize applies to the outpatient or nursing facility encounters, whereas the decision to escalate hospital level of care (eg, transfer to ICU) applies to the hospitalized or observation care patient. See also the introductory guidelines of each code family section.

The elements listed in Table 1, Levels of Medical Decision Making, are defined in the guidelines for number and complexity of problems addressed at the encounter, amount and/or complexity of data to be reviewed and analyzed, and risk of complications and/or morbidity or mortality of patient management.

Table 1: Levels of Medical Decision Making (MDM)

Elements of Medical Decision Making			
Level of MDM (Based on 2 out of 3 Elements of MDM)	**Number and Complexity of Problems Addressed at the Encounter**	**Amount and/or Complexity of Data to Be Reviewed and Analyzed** ***Each unique test, order, or document contributes to the combination of 2 or combination of 3 in Category 1 below.***	**Risk of Complications and/or Morbidity or Mortality of Patient Management**
Straight-forward	**Minimal** • **1** self-limited or minor problem	**Minimal or none**	**Minimal risk of morbidity from additional diagnostic testing or treatment**
Low	**Low** • **2** or more self-limited or minor problems; **or** • **1** stable, chronic illness; **or** • **1** acute, uncomplicated illness or injury; **or** • **1** stable, acute illness; **or** • **1** acute, uncomplicated illness or injury requiring hospital inpatient or observation level of care	**Limited** *(Must meet the requirements of at least 1 out of 2 categories)* **Category 1: Tests and documents** • **Any combination of 2 from the following:** – Review of prior external note(s) from each unique source*; – Review of the result(s) of each unique test*; – Ordering of each unique test* **or** **Category 2: Assessment requiring an independent historian(s)** *(For the categories of independent interpretation of tests and discussion of management or test interpretation, see moderate or high)*	**Low risk of morbidity from additional diagnostic testing or treatment**
Moderate	**Moderate** • **1** or more chronic illnesses with exacerbation, progression, or side effects of treatment; **or** • **2** or more stable, chronic illnesses; **or** • **1** undiagnosed new problem with uncertain prognosis; **or** • **1** acute illness with systemic symptoms; **or** • **1** acute, complicated injury	**Moderate** *(Must meet the requirements of at least 1 out of 3 categories)* **Category 1: Tests, documents, or independent historian(s)** • **Any combination of 3 from the following:** – Review of prior external note(s) from each unique source*; – Review of the result(s) of each unique test*; – Ordering of each unique test*; – Assessment requiring an independent historian(s) **or** **Category 2: Independent interpretation of tests** • Independent interpretation of a test performed by another physician/other qualified health care professional (not separately reported); **or** **Category 3: Discussion of management or test interpretation** • Discussion of management or test interpretation with external physician/other qualified health care professional/appropriate source (not separately reported)	**Moderate risk of morbidity from additional diagnostic testing or treatment** *Examples only:* • Prescription drug management • Decision regarding minor surgery with identified patient or procedure risk factors • Decision regarding elective major surgery without identified patient or procedure risk factors • Diagnosis or treatment significantly limited by social determinants of health

Elements of Medical Decision Making			
Level of MDM (Based on 2 out of 3 Elements of MDM)	**Number and Complexity of Problems Addressed at the Encounter**	**Amount and/or Complexity of Data to Be Reviewed and Analyzed** ***Each unique test, order, or document contributes to the combination of 2 or combination of 3 in Category 1 below.***	**Risk of Complications and/or Morbidity or Mortality of Patient Management**
High	**High** • **1** or more chronic illnesses with severe exacerbation, progression, or side effects of treatment; **or** • **1** acute or chronic illness or injury that poses a threat to life or bodily function	**Extensive** *(Must meet the requirements of at least 2 out of 3 categories)* **Category 1: Tests, documents, or independent historian(s)** • **Any combination of 3 from the following:** – Review of prior external note(s) from each unique source*; – Review of the result(s) of each unique test*; – Ordering of each unique test*; – Assessment requiring an independent historian(s) **or** **Category 2: Independent interpretation of tests** • Independent interpretation of a test performed by another physician/other qualified health care professional (not separately reported); **or** **Category 3: Discussion of management or test interpretation** • Discussion of management or test interpretation with external physician/other qualified health care professional/appropriate source (not separately reported)	**High risk of morbidity from additional diagnostic testing or treatment** *Examples only:* • Drug therapy requiring intensive monitoring for toxicity • Decision regarding elective major surgery with identified patient or procedure risk factors • Decision regarding emergency major surgery • Decision regarding hospitalization or escalation of hospital-level care • Decision not to resuscitate or to de-escalate care because of poor prognosis • Decision regarding parenteral controlled substances

Number and Complexity of Problems Addressed at the Encounter

One element used in selecting the level of service is the number and complexity of the problems that are addressed at the encounter. Multiple new or established conditions may be addressed at the same time and may affect MDM. Symptoms may cluster around a specific diagnosis and each symptom is not necessarily a unique condition. Comorbidities and underlying diseases, in and of themselves, are not considered in selecting a level of E/M services **unless** they are addressed, and their presence increases the amount and/or complexity of data to be reviewed and analyzed or the risk of complications and/or morbidity or mortality of patient management. The final diagnosis for a condition does not, in and of itself, determine the complexity or risk, as extensive evaluation may be required to reach the conclusion that the signs or symptoms do not represent a highly morbid condition. Therefore, presenting symptoms that are likely to represent a highly morbid condition may "drive" MDM even when the ultimate diagnosis is not highly morbid. The evaluation and/or treatment should be consistent with the likely nature of the condition. Multiple problems of a lower severity may, in the aggregate, create higher risk due to interaction.

The term "risk" as used in the definition of this element relates to risk from the condition. While condition risk and management risk may often correlate, the risk from the condition is distinct from the risk of the management.

Problem: A problem is a disease, condition, illness, injury, symptom, sign, finding, complaint, or other matter addressed at the encounter, with or without a diagnosis being established at the time of the encounter.

Problem addressed: A problem is addressed or managed when it is evaluated or treated at the encounter by the physician or other qualified health care professional reporting the service. This includes consideration of further testing or treatment that may not be elected by virtue of risk/benefit analysis or patient/parent/guardian/surrogate choice. Notation in the patient's medical record that another professional is managing the problem without additional assessment or care coordination documented does not qualify as being addressed or managed by the physician or other qualified health care professional reporting the service. Referral without evaluation (by history, examination, or diagnostic study[ies]) or consideration of treatment does not qualify as being addressed or managed by the physician or other qualified health care professional reporting the service. For hospital inpatient and observation care services, the problem addressed is the problem status on the date of the encounter, which may be significantly different than on admission. It is the problem being managed or co-managed by the reporting physician or other qualified health care professional and may not be the cause of admission or continued stay.

Minimal problem: A problem that may not require the presence of the physician or other qualified health care professional, but the service is provided under the physician's or other qualified health care professional's supervision (see 99211, 99281).

Self-limited or minor problem: A problem that runs a definite and prescribed course, is transient in nature, and is not likely to permanently alter health status.

Stable, chronic illness: A problem with an expected duration of at least one year or until the death of the patient. For the purpose of defining chronicity, conditions are treated as chronic whether or not stage or severity changes (eg, uncontrolled diabetes and controlled diabetes are a single chronic condition). "Stable" for the purposes of categorizing MDM is defined by the specific treatment goals for an individual patient. A patient who is not at his or her treatment goal is not stable, even if the condition has not changed and there is no short-term threat to life or function. For example, a patient with persistently poorly controlled blood pressure for whom better control is a goal is not stable, even if the pressures are not changing and the patient is asymptomatic. The risk of morbidity **without** treatment is significant.

Acute, uncomplicated illness or injury: A recent or new short-term problem with low risk of morbidity for which treatment is considered. There is little to no risk of mortality with treatment, and full recovery without functional impairment is expected. A problem that is normally self-limited or minor but is not resolving consistent with a definite and prescribed course is an acute, uncomplicated illness.

Acute, uncomplicated illness or injury requiring hospital inpatient or observation level care: A recent or new short-term problem with low risk of morbidity for which treatment is required. There is little to no risk of mortality with treatment, and full recovery without functional impairment is expected. The treatment required is delivered in a hospital inpatient or observation level setting.

Stable, acute illness: A problem that is new or recent for which treatment has been initiated. The patient is improved and, while resolution may not be complete, is stable with respect to this condition.

Chronic illness with exacerbation, progression, or side effects of treatment: A chronic illness that is acutely worsening, poorly controlled, or progressing with an intent to control progression and requiring additional supportive care or requiring attention to treatment for side effects.

Undiagnosed new problem with uncertain prognosis: A problem in the differential diagnosis that represents a condition likely to result in a high risk of morbidity without treatment.

Acute illness with systemic symptoms: An illness that causes systemic symptoms and has a high risk of morbidity without treatment. For systemic general symptoms, such as fever, body aches, or fatigue in a minor illness that may be treated to alleviate symptoms, see the definitions for ***self-limited or minor problem*** or ***acute, uncomplicated illness or injury.*** Systemic symptoms may not be general but may be single system.

Acute, complicated injury: An injury which requires treatment that includes evaluation of body systems that are not directly part of the injured organ, the injury is extensive, or the treatment options are multiple and/or associated with risk of morbidity.

Chronic illness with severe exacerbation, progression, or side effects of treatment: The severe exacerbation or progression of a chronic illness or severe side effects of treatment that have significant risk of morbidity and may require escalation in level of care.

Acute or chronic illness or injury that poses a threat to life or bodily function: An acute illness with systemic symptoms, an acute complicated injury, or a chronic illness or injury with exacerbation and/or progression or side effects of treatment, that poses a threat to life or bodily function in the near term without treatment. Some symptoms may represent a condition that is significantly probable and poses a potential threat to life or bodily function. These may be included in this category when the evaluation and treatment are consistent with this degree of potential severity.

Amount and/or Complexity of Data to Be Reviewed and Analyzed

One element used in selecting the level of services is the amount and/or complexity of data to be reviewed or analyzed at an encounter.

Analyzed: The process of using the data as part of the MDM. The data element itself may not be subject to analysis (eg, glucose), but it is instead included in the thought processes for diagnosis, evaluation, or treatment. Tests ordered are presumed to be analyzed when the results are reported. Therefore, when they are ordered during an encounter, they are counted in that encounter. Tests that are ordered outside of an encounter may be counted in the encounter in which they are analyzed. In the case of a recurring order, each new result may be counted in the encounter in which it is analyzed. For example, an encounter that includes an order for monthly prothrombin times would count for one prothrombin time ordered and reviewed. Additional future results, if analyzed in a subsequent encounter, may be counted as a single test in that subsequent encounter. Any service for which the professional component is separately reported by the physician or other qualified health care professional reporting the E/M services is not counted as a data element ordered, reviewed, analyzed, or independently interpreted for the purposes of determining the level of MDM.

Test: Tests are imaging, laboratory, psychometric, or physiologic data. A clinical laboratory panel (eg, basic metabolic panel [80047]) is a single test. The differentiation between single or multiple tests is defined in accordance with the CPT code set. For the purpose of data reviewed and analyzed, pulse oximetry is not a test.

Unique: A unique test is defined by the CPT code set. When multiple results of the same unique test (eg, serial blood glucose values) are compared during an E/M service, count it as one unique test. Tests that have overlapping elements are not unique, even if they are identified with distinct CPT codes. For example, a CBC with differential would incorporate the set of hemoglobin, CBC without differential, and platelet count. A unique source is defined as a physician or other qualified health care professional in a distinct group or different specialty or subspecialty, or a unique entity. Review of all materials from any unique source counts as one element toward MDM.

Combination of data elements: A combination of different data elements, for example, a combination of notes reviewed, tests ordered, tests reviewed, or independent historian, allows these elements to be summed. It does not require each item type or category to be represented. A unique test ordered, plus a note reviewed and an independent historian would be a combination of three elements.

External: External records, communications and/or test results are from an external physician, other qualified health care professional, facility, or health care organization.

External physician or other qualified health care professional: An external physician or other qualified health care professional who is not in the same group practice or is of a different specialty or subspecialty. This includes licensed professionals who are practicing independently. The individual may also be a facility or organizational provider such as from a hospital, nursing facility, or home health care agency.

Discussion: Discussion requires an interactive exchange. The exchange must be direct and not through intermediaries (eg, clinical staff or trainees). Sending chart notes or written exchanges that are within progress notes does not qualify as an interactive exchange. The discussion does not need to be on the date of the encounter, but it is counted only once and only when it is used in the decision making of the encounter. It may be asynchronous (ie, does not need to be in person), but it must be initiated and completed within a short time period (eg, within a day or two).

Independent historian(s): An individual (eg, parent, guardian, surrogate, spouse, witness) who provides a history in addition to a history provided by the patient who is unable to provide a complete or reliable history (eg, due to developmental stage, dementia, or psychosis) or because a confirmatory history is judged to be necessary. In the case where there may be conflict or poor communication between multiple historians and more than one historian is needed, the independent historian requirement is met. It does not include translation services. The independent history does not need to be obtained in person but does need to be obtained directly from the historian providing the independent information.

Independent interpretation: The interpretation of a test for which there is a CPT code, and an interpretation or report is customary. This does not apply when the physician or other qualified health care professional who reports the E/M service is reporting or has previously reported the test. A form of interpretation should be documented but need not conform to the usual standards of a complete report for the test. A test that is ordered and independently interpreted may count both as a test ordered and interpreted.

Appropriate source: For the purpose of the **discussion of management** data element (see Table 1, Levels of Medical Decision Making), an appropriate source includes professionals who are not health care professionals but may be involved in the management of the patient (eg, lawyer, parole officer, case manager, teacher). It does not include discussion with family or informal caregivers. For the purpose of ***documents reviewed,*** documents from an appropriate source may be counted.

Risk of Complications and/or Morbidity or Mortality of Patient Management

One element used in selecting the level of service is the risk of complications and/or morbidity or mortality of patient management at an encounter. This is distinct from the risk of the condition itself.

Risk: The probability and/or consequences of an event. The assessment of the level of risk is affected by the nature of the event under consideration. For example, a low probability of death may be high risk, whereas a high chance of a minor, self-limited adverse effect of treatment may be low risk. Definitions of risk are based upon the usual behavior and thought processes of a physician or other qualified health care professional in the same specialty. Trained clinicians apply common language usage meanings to terms such as *high, medium, low,* or *minimal* risk and do not require quantification for these definitions (though quantification may be provided when evidence-based medicine has established probabilities). For the purpose of MDM, level of risk is based upon consequences of the problem(s) addressed at the encounter when appropriately treated. Risk also includes MDM related to the need to initiate or forego further testing, treatment, and/or hospitalization. The risk of patient management criteria applies to the patient management decisions made by the reporting physician or other qualified health care professional as part of the reported encounter.

Morbidity: A state of illness or functional impairment that is expected to be of substantial duration during which function is limited, quality of life is impaired, or there is organ damage that may not be transient despite treatment.

Social determinants of health: Economic and social conditions that influence the health of people and communities. Examples may include food or housing insecurity.

Surgery (minor or major, elective, emergency, procedure or patient risk):

> ***Surgery—Minor or Major:*** The classification of surgery into minor or major is based on the common meaning of such terms when used by trained clinicians, similar to the use of the term "risk." These terms are not defined by a surgical package classification.
>
> ***Surgery—Elective or Emergency:*** Elective procedures and emergent or urgent procedures describe the timing of a procedure when the timing is related to the patient's condition. An elective procedure is typically planned in advance (eg, scheduled for weeks later), while an emergent procedure is typically performed immediately or with minimal delay to allow for patient stabilization. Both elective and emergent procedures may be minor or major procedures.
>
> ***Surgery—Risk Factors, Patient or Procedure:*** Risk factors are those that are relevant to the patient and procedure. Evidence-based risk calculators may be used, but are not required, in assessing patient and procedure risk.

Drug therapy requiring intensive monitoring for toxicity: A drug that requires intensive monitoring is a therapeutic agent that has the potential to cause serious morbidity or death. The monitoring is performed for assessment of these adverse effects and not primarily for assessment of therapeutic efficacy. The monitoring should be that which is generally accepted practice for the agent but may be patient-specific in some cases. Intensive monitoring may be long-term or short-term. Long-term intensive monitoring is not performed less than quarterly. The monitoring may be performed with a laboratory test, a physiologic test, or imaging. Monitoring by history or examination does not qualify. The monitoring affects the level of MDM in an encounter in which it is considered in the management of the patient. An example may be monitoring for cytopenia in the use of an antineoplastic agent between dose cycles. Examples of monitoring that do not qualify include monitoring glucose levels during insulin therapy, as the primary reason is the therapeutic effect (unless severe hypoglycemia is a current, significant concern); or annual electrolytes and renal function for a patient on a diuretic, as the frequency does not meet the threshold.

Parenteral controlled substances: The level of risk is based on the usual behavior and thought processes of a physician or other qualified health care professional in the same specialty and subspecialty and not simply based on the presence of an order for parenteral controlled substances.

Guidelines for Selecting Level of Service Based on Time

Certain categories of time-based E/M codes that do not have levels of services based on MDM (eg, Critical Care Services) in the E/M section use time differently. It is important to review the instructions for each category.

Time is **not** a descriptive component for the emergency department levels of E/M services because emergency department services are typically provided on a variable intensity basis, often involving multiple encounters with several patients over an extended period of time.

When time is used for reporting E/M services codes, the time defined in the service descriptors is used for selecting the appropriate level of services. The E/M services for which these guidelines apply require a face-to-face encounter with the physician or other qualified health care professional and the patient and/or family/caregiver. For office or other outpatient services, if the physician's or other qualified health care professional's time is spent in the supervision of clinical staff who perform the face-to-face services of the encounter, use 99211.

For coding purposes, time for these services is the total time on the date of the encounter. It includes both the face-to-face time with the patient and/or family/caregiver and non-face-to-face time personally spent by the physician and/or other qualified health care professional(s) on the day of the encounter (includes time in activities that require the physician or other qualified health care professional and does not include time in activities normally performed by clinical staff). It includes time regardless of the location of the physician or other qualified health care professional (eg, whether on or off the inpatient unit or in or out of the outpatient office). It does not include any time spent in the performance of other separately reported service(s).

Each service that may be reported using time for code level selection has a required time threshold. The concept of attaining a mid-point between levels does not apply. A full 15 minutes is required to report any unit of prolonged services codes 99417, 99418.

Physician(s) and other qualified health care professional(s) may each provide a portion of the face-to-face and non-face-to-face work related to the service. When time is being used to select the appropriate level of services for which time-based reporting is allowed, the time personally spent by the physician(s) and other qualified health care professional(s) assessing and managing the patient and/or counseling, educating, communicating results to the patient/family/caregiver on the date of the encounter is summed to define total time. Only distinct time should be summed (ie, when two or more individuals jointly meet with or discuss the patient, only the time of one individual should be counted).

When prolonged time occurs, the appropriate prolonged services code may be reported. The total time on the date of the encounter spent caring for the patient should be documented in the medical record when it is used as the basis for code selection.

Physician or other qualified health care professional time includes the following activities, when performed:

- preparing to see the patient (eg, review of tests)
- obtaining and/or reviewing separately obtained history
- performing a medically appropriate examination and/or evaluation
- counseling and educating the patient/family/caregiver
- ordering medications, tests, or procedures
- referring and communicating with other health care professionals (when not separately reported)
- documenting clinical information in the electronic or other health record
- independently interpreting results (not separately reported) and communicating results to the patient/family/caregiver
- care coordination (not separately reported)

Do not count time spent on the following:

- the performance of other services that are reported separately
- travel
- teaching that is general and not limited to discussion that is required for the management of a specific patient

For split or shared visits, see the split or shared visits guidelines.

Unlisted Service

An E/M service may be provided that is not listed in this section of the CPT codebook. When reporting such a service, the appropriate unlisted code may be used to indicate the service, identifying it by "Special Report," as discussed in the following paragraph. The "Unlisted Services" and accompanying codes for the E/M section are as follows:

99429 **Unlisted preventive** medicine service

99499 **Unlisted evaluation and management** service

Special Report

An unlisted service or one that is unusual, variable, or new may require a special report demonstrating the medical appropriateness of the service. Pertinent information should include an adequate definition or description of the nature, extent, and need for the procedure and the time, effort, and equipment necessary to provide the service. Additional items that may be included are complexity of symptoms, final diagnosis, pertinent physical findings, diagnostic and therapeutic procedures, concurrent problems, and follow-up care.

Place of Service/Type of Service

Place-of-Service Codes for Professional Claims

Listed below are place of service codes and descriptions. These codes should be used on professional claims to specify the entity where service(s) were rendered. Check with individual payers (e.g., Medicare, Medicaid, other private insurance) for reimbursement policies regarding these codes. Comments or questions regarding place-of-service codes or descriptions should be directed to your Medicare administrative contractor (MAC).

01	Pharmacy	A facility or location where drugs and other medically related items and services are sold, dispensed, or otherwise provided directly to patients.
02	Telehealth Provided Other than in Patient's Home	The location where health services and health related services are provided or received, through telecommunication technology. Patient is not located in their home when receiving health services or health related services through telecommunication technology.
03	School	A facility whose primary purpose is education.
04	Homeless Shelter	A facility or location whose primary purpose is to provide temporary housing to homeless individuals (e.g., emergency shelters, individual or family shelters).
05	Indian Health Service Free-standing Facility	A facility or location, owned and operated by the Indian Health Service, which provides diagnostic, therapeutic (surgical and non-surgical), and rehabilitation services to American Indians and Alaska Natives who do not require hospitalization.
06	Indian Health Service Provider-based Facility	A facility or location, owned and operated by the Indian Health Service, which provides diagnostic, therapeutic (surgical and non-surgical), and rehabilitation services rendered by, or under the supervision of, physicians to American Indians and Alaska Natives admitted as inpatients or outpatients.
07	Tribal 638 Free-standing Facility	A facility or location owned and operated by a federally recognized American Indian or Alaska Native tribe or tribal organization under a 638 agreement, which provides diagnostic, therapeutic (surgical and non-surgical), and rehabilitation services to tribal members who do not require hospitalization.
08	Tribal 638 Provider-based Facility	A facility or location owned and operated by a federally recognized American Indian or Alaska Native tribe or tribal organization under a 638 agreement, which provides diagnostic, therapeutic (surgical and non-surgical), and rehabilitation services to tribal members admitted as inpatients or outpatients.
09	Prison/Correctional Facility	A prison, jail, reformatory, work farm, detention center, or any other similar facility maintained by either Federal, State or local authorities for the purpose of confinement or rehabilitation of adult or juvenile criminal offenders.
10	Telehealth Provided in Patient's Home	The location where health services and health related services are provided or received, through telecommunication technology. Patient is located in their home (which is a location other than a hospital or other facility where the patient receives care in a private residence) when receiving health services or health related services through telecommunication technology.

11	Office	Location, other than a hospital, skilled nursing facility (SNF), military treatment facility, community health center, State or local public health clinic, or intermediate care facility (ICF), where the health professional routinely provides health examinations, diagnosis, and treatment of illness or injury on an ambulatory basis.
12	Home	Location, other than a hospital or other facility, where the patient receives care in a private residence.
13	Assisted Living Facility	Congregate residential facility with self-contained living units providing assessment of each resident's needs and on-site support 24 hours a day, 7 days a week, with the capacity to deliver or arrange for services including some health care and other services.
14	Group Home	A residence, with shared living areas, where clients receive supervision and other services such as social and/or behavioral services, custodial service, and minimal services (e.g., medication administration).
15	Mobile Unit	A facility/unit that moves from place-to-place equipped to provide preventive, screening, diagnostic, and/or treatment services.
16	Temporary Lodging	A short term accommodation such as a hotel, campground, hostel, cruise ship or resort where the patient receives care, and which is not identified by any other POS code.
17	Walk-in Retail Health Clinic	A walk-in health clinic, other than an office, urgent care facility, pharmacy or independent clinic and not described by any other Place of Service code, that is located within a retail operation and provides, on an ambulatory basis, preventive and primary care services.
18	Place of Employment-Worksite	A location, not described by any other POS code, owned or operated by a public or private entity where the patient is employed, and where a health professional provides on-going or episodic occupational medical, therapeutic or rehabilitative services to the individual.
19	Off Campus-Outpatient Hospital	A portion of an off-campus hospital provider based department which provides diagnostic, therapeutic (both surgical and nonsurgical), and rehabilitation services to sick or injured persons who do not require hospitalization or institutionalization.
20	Urgent Care Facility	Location, distinct from a hospital emergency room, an office, or a clinic, whose purpose is to diagnose and treat illness or injury for unscheduled, ambulatory patients seeking immediate medical attention.
21	Inpatient Hospital	A facility, other than psychiatric, which primarily provides diagnostic, therapeutic (both surgical and nonsurgical), and rehabilitation services by, or under, the supervision of physicians to patients admitted for a variety of medical conditions.
22	On Campus-Outpatient Hospital	A portion of a hospital's main campus which provides diagnostic, therapeutic (both surgical and nonsurgical), and rehabilitation services to sick or injured persons who do not require hospitalization or institutionalization.
23	Emergency Room-Hospital	A portion of a hospital where emergency diagnosis and treatment of illness or injury is provided.
24	Ambulatory Surgical Center	A freestanding facility, other than a physician's office, where surgical and diagnostic services are provided on an ambulatory basis.
25	Birthing Center	A facility, other than a hospital's maternity facilities or a physician's office, which provides a setting for labor, delivery, and immediate post-partum care as well as immediate care of new born infants.
26	Military Treatment Facility	A medical facility operated by one or more of the Uniformed Services. Military Treatment Facility (MTF) also refers to certain former U.S. Public Health Service (USPHS) facilities now designated as Uniformed Service Treatment Facilities (USTF).

27	Outreach Site/Street	A non-permanent location on the street or found environment, not described by any other POS code, where health professionals provide preventive, screening, diagnostic, and/or treatment services to unsheltered homeless individuals.
28-30	Unassigned	N/A
31	Skilled Nursing Facility	A facility which primarily provides inpatient skilled nursing care and related services to patients who require medical, nursing, or rehabilitative services but does not provide the level of care or treatment available in a hospital.
32	Nursing Facility	A facility which primarily provides to residents skilled nursing care and related services for the rehabilitation of injured, disabled, or sick persons, or, on a regular basis, health-related care services above the level of custodial care to other than individuals with intellectual disabilities.
33	Custodial Care Facility	A facility which provides room, board and other personal assistance services, generally on a long-term basis, and which does not include a medical component.
34	Hospice	A facility, other than a patient's home, in which palliative and supportive care for terminally ill patients and their families are provided.
35-40	Unassigned	N/A
41	Ambulance-Land	A land vehicle specifically designed, equipped and staffed for lifesaving and transporting the sick or injured.
42	Ambulance—Air or Water	An air or water vehicle specifically designed, equipped and staffed for lifesaving and transporting the sick or injured.
43-48	Unassigned	N/A
49	Independent Clinic	A location, not part of a hospital and not described by any other Place of Service code, that is organized and operated to provide preventive, diagnostic, therapeutic, rehabilitative, or palliative services to outpatients only.
50	Federally Qualified Health Center	A facility located in a medically underserved area that provides Medicare beneficiaries with preventive primary medical care under the general direction of a physician.
51	Inpatient Psychiatric Facility	A facility that provides inpatient psychiatric services for the diagnosis and treatment of mental illness on a 24-hour basis, by or under the supervision of a physician.
52	Psychiatric Facility-Partial Hospitalization	A facility for the diagnosis and treatment of mental illness that provides a planned therapeutic program for patients who do not require full time hospitalization, but who need broader programs than are possible from outpatient visits to a hospital-based or hospital-affiliated facility.
53	Community Mental Health Center	A facility that provides the following services: outpatient services, including specialized outpatient services for children, the elderly, individuals who are chronically ill, and residents of the CMHC's mental health services area who have been discharged from inpatient treatment at a mental health facility; 24 hour a day emergency care services; day treatment, other partial hospitalization services, or psychosocial rehabilitation services; screening for patients being considered for admission to State mental health facilities to determine the appropriateness of such admission; and consultation and education services.
54	Intermediate Care Facility/Individuals with Intellectual Disabilities	A facility which primarily provides health-related care and services above the level of custodial care to individuals but does not provide the level of care or treatment available in a hospital or SNF.

55	Residential Substance Abuse Treatment Facility	A facility which provides treatment for substance (alcohol and drug) abuse to live-in residents who do not require acute medical care. Services include individual and group therapy and counseling, family counseling, laboratory tests, drugs and supplies, psychological testing, and room and board.
56	Psychiatric Residential Treatment Center	A facility or distinct part of a facility for psychiatric care which provides a total 24-hour therapeutically planned and professionally staffed group living and learning environment.
57	Non-residential Substance Abuse Treatment Facility	A location which provides treatment for substance (alcohol and drug) abuse on an ambulatory basis. Services include individual and group therapy and counseling, family counseling, laboratory tests, drugs and supplies, and psychological testing.
58	Non-residential Opioid Treatment Facility	A location that provides treatment for opioid use disorder on an ambulatory basis. Services include methadone and other forms of Medication Assisted Treatment (MAT).
59	Unassigned	N/A
60	Mass Immunization Center	A location where providers administer pneumococcal pneumonia and influenza virus vaccinations and submit these services as electronic media claims, paper claims, or using the roster billing method. This generally takes place in a mass immunization setting, such as, a public health center, pharmacy, or mall but may include a physician office setting.
61	Comprehensive Inpatient Rehabilitation Facility	A facility that provides comprehensive rehabilitation services under the supervision of a physician to inpatients with physical disabilities. Services include physical therapy, occupational therapy, speech pathology, social or psychological services, and orthotics and prosthetics services.
62	Comprehensive Outpatient Rehabilitation Facility	A facility that provides comprehensive rehabilitation services under the supervision of a physician to outpatients with physical disabilities. Services include physical therapy, occupational therapy, and speech pathology services.
63-64	Unassigned	N/A
65	End-Stage Renal Disease Treatment Facility	A facility other than a hospital, which provides dialysis treatment, maintenance, and/or training to patients or caregivers on an ambulatory or home-care basis.
66	Programs of All-Inclusive Care for the Elderly (PACE) Center	A facility or location providing comprehensive medical and social services as part of the Programs of All-Inclusive Care for the Elderly (PACE). This includes, but is not limited to, primary care; social work services; restorative therapies, including physical and occupational therapy; personal care and supportive services; nutritional counseling; recreational therapy; and meals when the individual is enrolled in PACE.
67-70	Unassigned	N/A
71	Public Health Clinic	A facility maintained by either State or local health departments that provides ambulatory primary medical care under the general direction of a physician.
72	Rural Health Clinic	A certified facility which is located in a rural medically underserved area that provides ambulatory primary medical care under the general direction of a physician.
73-80	Unassigned	N/A
81	Independent Laboratory	A laboratory certified to perform diagnostic and/or clinical tests independent of an institution or a physician's office.
82-98	Unassigned	N/A
99	Other Place of Service	Other place of service not identified above.

Type of Service

Common Working File Type of Service (TOS) Indicators

For submitting a claim to the Common Working File (CWF), use the following table to assign the proper TOS. Some procedures may have more than one applicable TOS. CWF will reject codes with incorrect TOS designations. CWF will produce alerts on codes with incorrect TOS designations.

The only exceptions to this annual update are:

- Surgical services billed for dates of service through December 31, 2007, containing the ASC facility service modifier SG must be reported as TOS F. Effective for services on or after January 1, 2008, the SG modifier is no longer applicable for Medicare services. ASC providers should discontinue applying the SG modifier on ASC facility claims. The indicator F does not appear in the TOS table because its use depends upon claims submitted with POS 24 (ASC facility) from an ASC (specialty 49). This became effective for dates of service January 1, 2008, or after.
- Surgical services billed with an assistant-at-surgery modifier (80-82, AS) must be reported with TOS 8. The 8 indicator does not appear on the TOS table because its use is dependent upon the use of the appropriate modifier. (See Pub. 100-4 *Medicare Claims Processing Manual,* chapter 12, "Physician/Nonphysician Practitioner," for instructions on when assistant-at-surgery is allowable.)
- TOS H appears in the list of descriptors. However, it does not appear in the table. In CWF, "H" is used only as an indicator for hospice. The contractor should not submit TOS H to CWF at this time.
- For outpatient services, when a transfusion medicine code appears on a claim that also contains a blood product, the service is paid under reasonable charge at 80 percent; coinsurance and deductible apply. When transfusion medicine codes are paid under the clinical laboratory fee schedule they are paid at 100 percent; coinsurance and deductible do not apply.

Note: For injection codes with more than one possible TOS designation, use the following guidelines when assigning the TOS:

When the choice is L or 1:

- Use TOS L when the drug is used related to ESRD; or
- Use TOS 1 when the drug is not related to ESRD and is administered in the office.

When the choice is G or 1:

- Use TOS G when the drug is an immunosuppressive drug; or
- Use TOS 1 when the drug is used for other than immunosuppression.

When the choice is P or 1:

- Use TOS P if the drug is administered through durable medical equipment (DME); or
- Use TOS 1 if the drug is administered in the office.

The place of service or diagnosis may be considered when determining the appropriate TOS. The descriptors for each of the TOS codes listed in the annual HCPCS update are:

0	Whole blood only
1	Medical care
2	Surgery
3	Consultation
4	Diagnostic radiology
5	Diagnostic laboratory
6	Therapeutic radiology
7	Anesthesia
8	Assistant at surgery
9	Other medical items or services
A	Used durable medical equipment (DME)
D	Ambulance
E	Enteral/parenteral nutrients/supplies
F	Ambulatory surgical center (facility usage for surgical services)
G	Immunosuppressive drugs
J	Diabetic shoes
K	Hearing items and services
L	ESRD supplies
M	Monthly capitation payment for dialysis
N	Kidney donor
P	Lump sum purchase of DME, prosthetics, orthotics
Q	Vision items or services
R	Rental of DME
S	Surgical dressings or other medical supplies
T	Outpatient mental health limitation
U	Occupational therapy
V	Pneumococcal/flu vaccine
W	Physical therapy

Reimbursement Terms

AAPC. National organization for coders and billers offering certification examinations based on physician-, facility-, or payer-specific guidelines or coding documentation. Upon successful completion of the selected examination, the credential for that examination is obtained.

AAPCC. Adjusted average per capita cost. Estimated average cost of Medicare benefits for an individual based upon criteria such as age, sex, institutional status, Medicaid, disability, and end-stage renal failure.

abstractor. Person who selects and extracts specific data from the medical record and enters the information into computer files.

accountable care organization. Recognized legal entity under state law comprised of providers of services and suppliers with an established mechanism for shared governance who work together to coordinate care for Medicare fee-for-service beneficiaries. Section 3022 of the Affordable Care Act required CMS to develop a shared savings program to promote coordination and cooperation among providers for the purposes of improving the quality of care for Medicare fee-for-service beneficiaries and minimize costs.

accreditation. Evaluative process in which a health care organization undergoes an examination of its policies, procedures, and performance by an external organization to ensure it is meeting predetermined criteria. It usually involves both on- and off-site surveys.

Accredited Standards Committee. Organization accredited by the American National Standards Institute (ANSI) for the development of American national standards.

accrual. Amount of money set aside to cover a health care benefit plan's expenses based upon estimates using a combination of data, including the claims system and the plan's prior history. In facility accounting, accrual accounting records the expenses as they are incurred and the revenue as it is generated. This contrasts with cash accounting where expenses are recorded only when payment is made or revenues are recorded only when payment is received.

ACH. Automated clearinghouse. Entity that processes or facilitates the processing of information received from another entity in a nonstandard format or containing nonstandard data content into standard data elements or a standard transaction, or that receives a standard transaction from another entity and processes or facilitates the processing of that information into nonstandard format or nonstandard data content for a receiving entity.

ACO. Accountable Care Organization.

ACR. ***1)*** Adjusted community rate. Calculation of what premium the plan charges to provide Medicare-covered benefits for greater frequency of use by participants. ***2)*** American College of Radiology. ***3)*** American College of Rheumatology.

activities of daily living. Self-care activities often used to determine a patient's level of function, such as bathing, dressing, using a toilet, transferring in and out of bed or a chair, continence, eating, and walking.

actual charge. Charge a physician or supplier bills for a service rendered or a supply item.

actuarial assumptions. Characteristics used in calculating the risks and costs of a plan, including age, sex, and occupation of enrollees; location; utilization rates; and service costs.

acute care facility. Health care institution primarily engaged in providing treatment to inpatients and diagnostic and therapeutic services for medical diagnosis, treatment, and care of injured, disabled, or sick persons who are in an acute phase of illness.

add-on code. Code representing a procedure performed in addition to the primary procedure and is represented with a + in the CPT book. Add-on codes are never reported for stand-alone services but are reported secondarily in addition to the primary procedure.

additional development request. Formal request from a Medicare contractor for additional information needed to determine if a claim is covered and/or payable

additional documentation request. When contractors cannot make a coverage or coding determination based upon the information on the claim and its attachments, the contractors may solicit additional documentation from the provider by issuing an ADR. Contractors must ensure that all records requested are from the period under review. Contractors must specify in the ADR the specific pieces of documentation needed (and ONLY those pieces needed) to make a coverage or coding determination.

ADG. Ambulatory diagnostic group.

adjudication. Processing and review of a submitted claim resulting in payment, partial payment, or denial. In relationship to judicial hearings, it is the process of hearing and settling a case through an objective, judicial procedure.

adjusted average per capita cost. Estimated average cost of Medicare benefits for an individual, based upon criteria including age, sex, institutional status, Medicaid, disability, and end-stage renal failure.

administrative code sets. Code sets that characterize a general business situation, rather than a medical condition or service. Under HIPAA, these are sometimes referred to as nonclinical or nonmedical code sets.

administrative services only. Contractual agreement between a self-funded plan and an insurance company in which the insurance company assumes no risk and provides administrative services only.

administrative simplification. Title II, subtitle of HIPAA, that gives HHS the authority to mandate the use of standards for the electronic exchange of health care data; to specify what medical and administrative code sets should be used within those standards; to require the use of national identification systems for health care patients, providers, payers (or plans), and employers (or sponsors); and to specify the types of measures required to protect the security and privacy of personally identifiable health care information. This is also the name of Title II, subtitle F, part C of HIPAA.

admission. Formal acceptance of a patient by a health care facility.

admission date. Date the patient was admitted to the health care facility for inpatient care, outpatient service, or the start of care.

ADS. Alternative delivery system. Any health care delivery system other than traditional fee-for-service.

advanced alternative payment models. Subset of Alternative Payment Models that gives added incentive payments to clinicians who provide high-quality, cost-efficient care. Advanced APMs encourage participants to earn even more rewards in exchange for taking on greater risk relative to their patients' outcomes. Advanced APMs must meet three specific criteria: require CEHRT use, base payment on MIPS-comparable quality measures, and be a Medicare Medical Home OR require participants to bear more than a nominal amount of risk.

Advanced Beneficiary Notice of Noncoverage. Written communication with a Medicare beneficiary given before Part B services are rendered informing the patient that the provider (including independent laboratories, imaging centers, physicians, practitioners, and/or suppliers) believes Medicare will not pay for some or all of the services to be rendered. Form CMS-R-131 may be used for all situations where Medicare payment is expected to be denied.
Synonym(s): *ABN.*

advanced determination of Medicare coverage. Request by a supplier or beneficiary that a determination be made in advance of delivery of an item as to whether or not it is a covered item. ADMC requests are limited to items that are customized or items that have been specified as not inexpensive by the secretary. This is a voluntary program. Suppliers and beneficiaries are not required to obtain an ADMC prior to delivery of supplies, but may wish to request an ADMC when the item is customized or when the item is on the not inexpensive list.

adverse selection. In health care contracting, the risk of enrolling members who are sicker than assumed and who will utilize expensive services more frequently.

age restriction. In health care contracting, limitation of benefits when a patient reaches a certain age.

age/sex rating. Health care contracting term meaning structuring capitation payments based on members' ages and genders.

aggregate amount. Contracted maximum for which a member is insured for any single event in a health plan.

AHA. American Hospital Association. Health care industry association that represents the concerns of institutional providers. The AHA hosts the National Uniform Billing Committee (NUBC), which has a formal consultative role under HIPAA. The AHA also publishes *Coding Clinic* for ICD-10 and HCPCS.

ALOS. Average length of stay. Utilization benchmark average compiled from the actual number of inpatient days calculated using factors such as geographical location and diagnosis.

ambulatory surgery. Surgical procedure in which the patient is admitted, treated, and released on the same day.

American Association of Payers, Administrators and Networks. Organization that functions to unify payers, administrators, and networks to support private group, government health, and workers' compensation plans in a single and cooperative effort to support and advance the cause of patient access to appropriate quality health care. The former American Association of Preferred Provider Organizations (AAPPO) and the Third Party Administrators Association of America (TPAAA) memberships dissolved their individual organizations and integrated under the AAPAN brand in early 2017 in order to ensure a stronger presence and public policy voice.

American Health Information Management Association. Association of health information management professionals offering various certification examinations for physician and facility based coders, clinical documentation improvement practitioners, and other technology and health informatics specialists.

AMLOS. Arithmetic mean length of stay. Average number of days patients within a given DRG stay in the hospital. The AMLOS is used to determine payment for outlier cases and to predict occupancy rates.

AP-DRG. All patient diagnosis-related group. 3M HIS made revisions and adjustments to the DRG system, now referred to as the All Patient DRGs. Early features of AP-DRGs included MDC 24, specifically devoted to HIV, and restructuring of the major diagnostic categories governing newborns.

APC. Ambulatory payment classification. Cost-containment tool developed by CMS and the basis for the outpatient prospective payment system (OPPS). Outpatient services are grouped by CPT code into multiple payment classifications based on resource utilization. Facilities are paid a fixed rate dependent on the service classification.

APG. Ambulatory patient group. Reimbursement methodology for outpatient services developed for CMS.

APM. Alternative Payment Model. Payment approach that gives added incentive payments to reward clinicians who provide high-quality, cost-efficient care. An APM can apply to a specific clinical condition, a care episode, or a population; for example, an APM with clinicians who focus on patients with cancer or those with end-stage renal disease.

appeal. Specific request made to a payer for reconsideration of a denial or adverse coverage or payment decision and potential restriction of benefit reimbursement.

appropriateness of care. Proper setting of medical care that best meets the patient's care or diagnosis, as defined by a health care plan or other legal entity.

APR. Average payment rate. Amount of money CMS could pay an HMO for services provided to Medicare recipients under a risk contract.

APR-DRG. All Patient Refined Diagnosis Related Group. Grouping system developed by 3M HIS that takes into account the severity of inpatient illness and the risk of mortality.

ART. Accredited record technician. Former AHIMA certification describing medical records practitioners; now known as a registered health information technician (RHIT).

ASO. Administrative services only. Contractual agreement between a self-funded plan and an insurance company in which the insurance company assumes no risk and provides administrative services only.

assignment. In medical reimbursement, the arrangement in which the provider submits the claim on behalf of the patient and is reimbursed directly by the patient's plan. By doing so, the provider agrees to accept what the plan pays.

assignment of benefits. Authorization from the patient allowing the third-party payer to pay the provider directly for medical services. Under Medicare, an assignment is an agreement by the hospital or physician to accept Medicare's payment as the full payment and not to bill the patient for any amounts over the allowance amount, except for deductible and/or coinsurance amounts or noncovered services.

at risk. In medical reimbursement, a type of contract between Medicare and a payer or a payer and a provider in which the payer (in the case of Medicare) and the provider (in the case of the payer contracts) gets paid a set amount for care of a patient base. If costs exceed the amount the payer or provider were paid, the patients still receive care during the term of the contract.

attained age. In medical reimbursement, the age of the member as of the last birthday.

auditor. Professional who evaluates a provider's utilization, quality of care, or level of reimbursement.

automated clearinghouse. Entity that processes or facilitates the processing of information received from another entity in a nonstandard format or containing nonstandard data content into standard data elements or a standard transaction, or that receives a standard transaction from another entity and processes or facilitates the processing of that information into nonstandard format or nonstandard data content for a receiving entity.

AWP. ***1)*** Any willing provider. Describing statutes requiring a provider network to accept any provider who meets the network's usual selection criteria. ***2)*** Average wholesale price. Pharmaceutical price based on common data that is included in a pharmacy provider contract.

backlog. In medical reimbursement, the queue of claims that have not been adjudicated.

balance billing. Arrangement prohibited in Medicare regulations and some payer contracts whereby a provider bills the patient for charges in excess of the contracted allowable rate or medical necessity denials not reimbursed by the payer. Insurance plan exclusions may still be billable.

basic coverage. Insurance providing coverage for hospital care.

basic health services. Defined set of benefits all federally qualified HMOs must offer enrollees.

board certification. Certification in a particular specialty based on the physician's demonstration of expertise and experience.

boarder. Individual who receives lodging, such as a parent, caregiver, or other family member, who is not a patient but may wish or need to be near the patient.

boarder baby. ***1)*** Newborn that remains in the nursery following discharge because the mother is still hospitalized. ***2)*** Premature infant who no longer needs intensive care but who remains for observation or to reach developmental milestones.

book of business. Payer's list of clients and contracts.

bundled. ***1)*** Gathering of several types of health insurance policies under a single payer. ***2)*** Inclusive grouping of codes related to a procedure when submitting a claim.

bundled payment. Inclusive grouping of codes related to a procedure resulting in a single payment for services.

business coalition. Employers who form a cooperative to purchase health care less expensively.

cafeteria plan. Employer's offer of various services of many payers as separate elements in a health care plan.

CAH. Critical Access Hospital. Designation assigned by CMS to rural facilities that meet certain criteria and are reimbursed on a cost basis. The designation was created in 1997 by Congress under the Balanced Budget Act due to a number of hospital closures during the 80s and early 90s.

Cap. ***1)*** Capitation. ***2)*** Contract maximum.

capitation. Contractual agreement whereby the provider is paid a fixed amount for treating enrolled patients regardless of utilization.

care unit. Specific department or facility within a hospital or long-term care facility designed and staffed for treating a particular type of patient.

carrier. Insurer or health plan that may underwrite, administer, or sell a range of health benefit programs.

carve-out. Medical benefits for a specific type of care considered covered by separate guidelines or not covered by the payer.

case management. Ongoing review of cases by professionals to assure the most appropriate utilization of services.

case manager. Medical professional (usually a nurse or social worker) who reviews cases every few days to determine necessity of care and to advise providers on payers' utilization restrictions. Certifies ongoing care.

case mix index. Sum of all DRG relative weights for cases over a given period of time, divided by the number of Medicare cases.

catastrophic case management. Method of reviewing ongoing cases in which the patient sustains catastrophic or extremely costly medical problems.

catchment area. Geographical area from which a health care organization draws its members.

Category III codes. Alphanumeric codes (four digits followed by the letter T) used to report new and emerging technology services or procedures. Released on January 1 and July 1 of each year, they supersede the use of unlisted codes.

CC. Complication, comorbid condition, or chief complaint.

CCI. Correct Coding Initiative. Official list of codes from the Centers for Medicare and Medicaid Services' (CMS) National Correct Coding Policy Manual that identifies services considered an integral part of a comprehensive code or mutually exclusive of it.

CCR. Cost-to-charge ratio.

CCU. Coronary care unit. Facility dedicated to patients suffering from heart attack, stroke, or other serious cardiopulmonary problems.

CDC. Centers for Disease Control and Prevention.

CDI. Clinical documentation improvement. Program designed to provide more specific and complete chart documentation in order to assure the proper use of resources, correct assessment of the patient's severity of illness, and compliance with regulatory requirements.

census. Medical reimbursement term referring to the quantity and demographics of patients or members.

certification. Approval by a payer's case manager to continue care for a given number of days or visits.

charge-based relative value scale. Value scale based on the relationship between current charges for various services.

chargemaster. File, usually in an electronic billing system, where charge amounts are kept for all procedures, services, and supplies in a hospital for use with billing software in claims submission.

charges. Dollar amount assigned to a service or procedure by a provider and reported to a payer.

cherry picking. Term used in medical reimbursement to describe the practice of enrolling only healthy individuals and excluding those with existing problems.

chief complaint. Term used in evaluation and management documentation and coding that identifies the reason or presenting problem that necessitated the patient's encounter for treatment. Typically, this is documented in the medical record using the patient's own words; for example, My head hurts.

CHIP. Children's Health Insurance Program. Provides health coverage to children meeting eligibility requirements through Medicaid and other CHIP programs. It is provided and managed by the states based on federal regulations with matching funds from the federal level to the states providing the coverage. Eligibility is based on family income that may be too high to apply for Medicaid but not sufficient to purchase private health care coverage.

church plan. Health plan established by and offered to employees of a church or other religious organization.

churning. *1)* Performance-based reimbursement system emphasizing provider productivity. *2)* When a provider sees a patient more than medically necessary with the intent of generating more revenue.

claim. Statement of services rendered requesting payment from an insurance company or a government entity.

claim adjustment reason code. Codes that are appended to a remittance advice or EOB in order to explain why a payment adjustment was applied to a particular service billed. If payment reflected equal billed amounts, no CARC would be indicated.

claim attachment. Any of a variety of hard copy documents or electronic records needed to process a claim in addition to the claim itself.

claim lag. Time elapsed between the date of a claim and its submission for payment.

claim manual. Administrative guidelines used by claims processors to adjudicate claims according to company policy and procedure.

claim rejection. Rejection of the entire claim. The provider may correct and resubmit the claim but may not appeal the claim.

claim status codes. National administrative code set that identifies the status of health care claims. This code set is used in the X12 277 claim status notification transaction and is maintained by the Health Care Code Maintenance Committee.

claims manager. Payer's manager who oversees the employee who processes routine claims.

claims review. Examination of a submitted demand for payment by a Medicare contractor, insurer, or other group to determine payment liability, eligibility, reasonableness, or necessity of care provided.

claims reviewer. Payer employee who reviews claims like an auditor, looking at coding, prior authority, contract violations, etc.

clean claim. Submitted bill for services rendered that does not need to be investigated by the payer, passes all internal billing edits and payer specific edits, and is paid without the need for further information.

CLIA. Clinical Laboratory Improvement Amendments. Requirements set in 1988, CLIA imposes varying levels of federal regulations on clinical procedures. Few laboratories, including those in physician offices, are exempt. Adopted by Medicare and Medicaid, CLIA regulations redefine laboratory testing in regard to laboratory certification and accreditation, proficiency testing, quality assurance, personnel standards, and program administration.

closed claim. Claim for which all apparent benefits have been paid.

closed panel. Arrangement in which a managed care organization contracts providers on an exclusive basis, restricting the providers from seeing patients enrolled in other payers' plans.

CMI. Case mix index. Sum of all DRG relative weights, divided by the number of Medicare cases. A low CMI may denote DRG assignments that do not adequately reflect the resources used to treat Medicare patients.

CMP. Competitive medical plan. Federal designation allowing plans to obtain eligibility to receive a Medicare risk contract without having to qualify as an HMO.

CMS. Centers for Medicare and Medicaid Services. Federal agency that administers the public health programs.

CMS-1500. Universal claim form used to file professional claims. Current version (02/12) ensures appropriate reporting of ICD-10-CM codes and revised format allows for additional diagnosis codes to be reported, as needed.

COA. Certificate of authority. State license to operate as an HMO.

COB. Coordination of benefits. In health care contracting, method of integrating benefits payable when there is more than one group insurance plan so that the insured's benefits and the payment of insurance benefits from all sources do not exceed 100 percent of the allowed medical expenses.

COBRA. Consolidated Omnibus Reconciliation Act. Federal law that allows and requires past employees to be covered under company health insurance plans for a set premium, allowing individuals to remain insured when their current plan or position has been terminated.

COC. Certificate of coverage. Legal document between the insurance company and the enrolling group to provide benefits to covered persons. It outlines the terms, conditions, exclusions, and limitations of the policy.

coder. Professional who translates documented, written diagnoses and procedures into numeric and alphanumeric codes.

coding conventions. Each space, typeface, indentation, and punctuation mark determining how ICD-10-CM codes are interpreted. These conventions were developed to help match correct codes to the diagnoses documented.

coding guidelines. Criteria that specifies how procedure, diagnosis, or supply codes are to be translated and used in various situations. Coding guidelines are issued by the AHA, AMA, CMS, NCHVS, and various other groups. Guidelines may vary by payer, type of coding system, and intended use.

coding specificity. Selection of classification codes (e.g., ICD-10-CM) that provides the highest degree of accuracy and completeness based on clinical documentation. For example, a six-character ICD-10-CM code cannot be reported when the specific code requires a 7th character.

coinsurance. Percentage of the allowed charges paid by a beneficiary toward the cost of care.

commercial carriers. For-profit insurance companies issuing health coverage.

common working file. System of local databases containing total beneficiary histories developed by CMS to improve Medicare claims processing. Medicare fiscal intermediaries, and/or carriers, interact with these databases to obtain data on eligibility, utilization, Medicare secondary payer (MSP), and other detailed claims information.

community rating. Methodology of state and federal governments that require qualified HMOs to request the same amount of money for each member in a plan.

comorbidity. Preexisting condition that causes an increase in length of stay by at least one day in approximately 75 percent of cases. Used in DRG reimbursement.

comparative performance report. Report that provides an annual comparison of a physician's services and procedures with those of another physician in the same specialty and geographic area.

complication. Condition arising after the beginning of observation and treatment that modifies the course of the patient's illness or the medical care required, or an undesired result or misadventure in medical care.

component code. In the National Correct Coding Initiative (NCCI), the column II code that cannot be charged to Medicare when the column I code is reported.

component coding. Coding a service that represents only a portion of the entire service provided, meant to standardize the reporting of interventional radiology services. Component coding allows a physician, regardless of specialty, to specifically identify and report those aspects of the service he or she provided, whether the procedural component, the radiological component, or both.

comprehensive codes. In the National Correct Coding Initiative (NCCI), the column I code that is reported to Medicare and precludes reporting column II codes.

condition code. Two-character alphanumeric code that is entered on the UB-04 claim form to indicate the conditions that affect processing and payment of the claim. Condition codes indicate such things as whether coverage exists under another insurance, whether the injury or illness is related to employment, whether the bill is an outlier, or if medical necessity affects room assignment among other things.

conditional payment. Medicare reimbursement requested by the provider or supplier when worker's compensation, no-fault, or liability insurance will not pay or will not pay promptly. Such payments are conditioned upon reimbursement to Medicare if the other insurer has or had the responsibility to make primary payment. Promptly is defined as within 120 days after the claim was filed with an insurer or a lien is filed against a potential liability settlement.

consultation. Advice or opinion regarding diagnosis and treatment or determination to accept transfer of care of a patient rendered by a medical professional at the request of the primary care provider.

continuity of coverage. In health care contracting, transfer of benefits from one plan to another without a lapse in coverage.

conversion. In health care contracting, shifting a member under a group contract to an individual contract in accordance with contract terms and occurring with a change in employer benefits or when the covered person leaves the group.

conversion factor. ***1)*** Dollar value for each relative value unit. When this dollar amount is multiplied by the total relative value units, it yields the reimbursement rate for the service. ***2)*** National multiplier that converts the geographically adjusted relative value units into Medicare fee schedule dollar amounts that applies to all services paid under the MPFS.

coordinated care. In health care contracting, system of health care delivery that influences utilization, quality of care, and cost of services. Managed care integrates financing and management with an employed or contracted organized provider network that delivers services to an enrolled population.

copayment. Cost-sharing arrangement in which a covered person pays a specified portion of allowed charges. In relation to Medicare, the copayment designates the specific dollar amount that the patient must pay and coinsurance designates the percentage of allowed charges.

Correct Coding Initiative. Official list of codes from the Centers for Medicare and Medicaid Services' (CMS) National Correct Coding Policy Manual for Medicare Services that identifies services considered an integral part of a comprehensive code or mutually exclusive of it.

corridor deductible. Fixed out-of-pocket amount the member must pay before benefits are available.

COT. ***1)*** Certified ophthalmic technician. ***2)*** Chain of trust. In health care contracting, pattern of agreements that extend protection of health care data. Each covered entity that shares health care data with a second entity must require the second entity to provide protections comparable to those provided by the covered entity. The second entity, in turn, must require any other entities with which it shares the data to satisfy the same requirements.

COTA. Certified occupational therapy assistant.

counseling. Discussion with a patient and/or family concerning one or more of the following areas: diagnostic results, impressions, and/or recommended diagnostic studies; prognosis; risks and benefits of management (treatment) options; instructions for management (treatment) and/or follow-up; importance of compliance with chosen management (treatment) options; risk factor reduction; and patient and family education.

covered charges. Charges for medical care and supplies that are medically necessary and met coverage and program guidelines.

covered person. Any person entitled to benefits under the policy, whether a member or dependent.

COVID-19. First diagnosed in December 2019 in China, coronavirus disease 2019 (COVID-19) is a respiratory infection caused by a newly identified (novel) virus not previously seen in humans, known as severe acute respiratory syndrome coronavirus 2 (SARS-CoV-2). Symptoms of this lower respiratory illness include fever, dry cough, loss of taste and/or smell, skin lesions of toes, gastrointestinal disturbances, and tiredness that may progress to include difficulty breathing and ventilator assistance. Older patients and those with high blood pressure, heart problems, diabetes, and obesity are more likely to develop serious symptoms of the illness and may result in death of the patient.

CPR. Computerized patient record. Computer application that allows all or most elements of a patient's medical record to be stored in a computerized database.

CPT. Current Procedural Terminology. Definitive procedural coding system developed by the American Medical Association that lists descriptive terms and identifying codes to provide a uniform language that describes medical, surgical, and diagnostic services for nationwide communication among physicians, patients, and third parties, used to report professional and outpatient services.

credentialing. ***1)*** Reviewing the medical degrees, licensure, malpractice, and any disciplinary record of medical providers for panel and quality assurance purposes and to grant hospital privileges. ***2)*** Coding certification.

critical access hospital. Participating Medicare facility located in a rural area of a state or in a Metropolitan Statistical Area (MSA) treated as a rural area and located more than a 35-mile drive from any other hospital or critical access hospital (CAH). In mountainous terrain or in areas with only secondary roads, the mileage criterion is 15 miles. CAHs must make available 24-hour emergency care services, and provide not more than 25 beds for acute (hospital-level) inpatient care or, in the case of a CAH with a swing bed agreement, swing beds used for SNF-level care. The CAH's length of stay cannot be longer than 96 hours. Inpatient CAH services are reported similarly to any inpatient claim with type of bill 011X. Outpatient services are billed under type of bill code 085X. Reimbursement is based on 101 percent of reasonable cost.

critical care. Treatment of critically ill patients in a variety of medical emergencies that requires the constant attendance of the physician (e.g., cardiac arrest, shock, bleeding, respiratory failure, postoperative complications, critically ill neonate).

crosswalk. Cross-referencing of CPT codes with ICD-10-CM, anesthesia, dental, or HCPCS Level II codes.

CSO. Clinical service organization. Health care organization developed by academic medical centers to integrate medical school, faculty practice plan, and hospital.

cutback. Reduction of the amount or type of insurance for a member who attains a specified age or condition (e.g., age 65, retirement).

daily benefit. Specified maximum benefit payable for room and board charges at a hospital.

database. Electronic store of utilization information used by payers to pay claims, negotiate contracts, and track utilization and cost of services.

date of service. Day the encounter or procedure is performed or the day a supply is issued.

DAW. Dispense as written. Notation from a physician to a pharmacist requesting that the brand name medication be given in lieu of a generic medication.

days per thousand. Standard unit of measurement of utilization determined by calculating the number of hospital days used in a year for each 1,000 covered lives.

decapitation. Inadequate capitation.

deductible. Predetermined dollar amount of covered billed charges that the patient must pay toward the cost of care.

diagnostic services. Examination or procedure performed on a patient to obtain information to assess the medical condition of the patient or to identify a disease and to determine the nature and severity of an illness or injury.

direct claim payment. Method where members deal directly with the payer rather than submitting claims through the employer.

direct contract model. Plan that contracts directly with individual private practice physicians rather than through an intermediary.

direct costs. Costs that are directly associated with a specific item or service, including such things as nonphysician labor, medical equipment, and medical supplies.

discharge plan. Treatment plan by the provider for continued patient care after discharge that may include home care, the services of case managers or other health care providers, or transfer to another facility.

discharge status. Disposition of the patient at discharge (e.g., left against medical advice, discharged home, transferred to an acute care hospital, expired).

discharge transfer. Discharge of a patient from one facility to another.

disposition of patient. Description of the patient's status and destination at discharge (e.g., discharged to home) used for data and quality assurance purposes.

DME. Durable medical equipment. Medical equipment that can withstand repeated use, is not disposable, is used to serve a medical purpose, is generally not useful to a person in the absence of a sickness or injury, and is appropriate for use in the home. Examples of durable medical equipment include hospital beds, wheelchairs, and oxygen equipment.

DMPAG. Digital Medicine Payment Advisory Group.

DOS. Date of service. Day the encounter or procedure is performed or the day a supply is issued.

DRG. Diagnosis related group. Method CMS uses to pay hospitals for Medicare recipients based on a statistical system of classifying any inpatient stay into one of several hundred groups. It is a classification scheme whose patient types are defined by patients' diagnoses or procedures and, in some cases, by the patient's age or discharge status. Each DRG is intended to be medically meaningful and would ordinarily require approximately equal resource consumption as measured by length of stay and cost.

drug formulary. List of prescription medications preferred for use by a health plan and dispensed through participating pharmacies to covered persons.

DSM-5. Manual used by health care providers to assist in determining the diagnosis and treatment of mental health disorders including, but not limited to, depression, schizophrenia, and substance abuse disorders.

dual option. Offering of an HMO and traditional plan by one carrier.

DUR. Drug utilization review. Review to assure prescribed medications are medically necessary and appropriate.

E/M. Evaluation and management services. Assessment, counseling, and other services provided to a patient and reported through CPT codes.

EAP. Employee assistance program. Services designed to help employees, their family members, and employers find solutions for workplace and personal problems that affect morale, productivity, or financial issues such as workplace stress, family/marital concerns, legal or financial problems, elder care, child care, substance abuse, emotional/stress issues, and other daily living concerns.

EDI. Electronic data interchange. Transference of claims, certifications, quality assurance reviews, and utilization data via computer in X12 format. May refer to any electronic exchange of formatted data.

EHO. Emerging healthcare organizations. Hospitals and other providers that are emerging or affiliating.

EHR. Electronic health record. Electronic version of patient medical history, maintained over time just like a paper chart, including all relevant information to that patient by specific provider including all demographics, progress notes, complaints, medication, vitals, history, vaccinations, and lab and radiology results. The EHR allows for immediate access to the patient information, improving patient care and streamlining communication between staff, as well as improving quality of care and reporting of patient outcomes.

elective admission. Admission made at the discretion of the patient and facility based on available resources.

ELOS. Estimated length of stay. Average number of days of hospitalization required for a given illness or procedure, based on prior histories of patients who have been hospitalized for the same illness or procedure.

emergency admission. Admission in which the patient requires immediate medical or psychiatric attention because of life-threatening, severe, and potentially disabling conditions.

emergency department. Organized hospital-based facility for the provision of unscheduled episodic services to patients who present for immediate medical attention. The facility must be available 24 hours a day.

emergency outpatient. Patient admitted for diagnosis and treatment of a condition requiring immediate attention but who will not stay at that facility or be transferred to another.

encoder. Computer application that assists in the assignment of a diagnosis or procedure code and may also assign reimbursement categories and values.

encounter. Direct personal contact between a patient and a physician, or other person who is authorized by state licensure law and, if applicable, by hospital staff bylaws, to order or furnish hospital services for diagnosis or treatment of the patient.

enrollee. In medical reimbursement, person who subscribes to a specific health plan.

enrollment. Number of lives covered by the plan.

EOB. Explanation of benefits. Statement mailed to the member and provider explaining claim adjudication and payment.

episode of care. One or more health care services received during a period of relatively continuous care by a hospital or health care provider.

EPO. Exclusive provider organization. In health care contracting, an organization similar to an HMO, but the member must remain within the provider network to receive benefits. EPOs are regulated under insurance statutes rather than HMO legislation.

ERA. Electronic remittance advice. Any of several electronic formats for explaining the payments of health care claims.

ERISA. Employee Retirement Income Security Act of 1974, Public Law 93-406. Mandates reporting, disclosure of grievance and appeals requirements, fiduciary standards for private group life and health plans, and preempts state benefit mandates and premium tax laws for self-funded group health plans.

established patient. ***1)*** Patient who has received professional services in a face-to-face setting within the last three years from the same physician/qualified health care professional or another physician/qualified health care professional of the exact same specialty and subspecialty who belongs to the same group practice. ***2)*** For OPPS hospitals, patient who has been registered as an inpatient or outpatient in a hospital's provider-based clinic or emergency department within the past three years.

exclusions. Services excluded from a plan's coverage by the employer or payer because of risk or cost.

experience rating. In medical reimbursement, designation of a group's previous claims history to help determine premium rates.

facility. Place of patient care, including inpatient and outpatient, acute or long term.

facility component. Contributions to the charge or cost of an item or service that are attributable to the physical location, including all services not performed by the physician or nonphysician practitioner.

facility of payment. Contractual relationship that permits the payer to pay someone other than the member or provider.

facility practice expense. One of the components used to determine the relative value of physician services paid under the resource-based relative value scale (RBRVS). Facility practice expense represents the physician's direct and indirect costs related to each service provided in a hospital, ambulatory surgery center (ASC), or skilled nursing facility (SNF).

facility services. Services furnished in a medical facility building such as a hospital, nursing home, or ASC.

FAR. Federal acquisition regulations. Regulations of the federal government's acquisition of services.

FDA. Food and Drug Administration. Federal agency responsible for protecting public health by substantiating the safety, efficacy, and security of human and veterinary drugs, biological products, medical devices, national food supply, cosmetics, and items that give off radiation.

Federal Register. Government publication listing changes in regulations and federally mandated standards, including coding standards such as HCPCS Level II and ICD-10-CM.

federally qualified HMO. HMO that meets CMS guidelines for Medicare reimbursement.

fee for service. Payment model where each service performed is individually paid. Fee-for-service arrangements may be discounted or undiscounted rates.

fee schedule. List of codes and related services with pre-established payment amounts by a provider that could be percentages of billed charges, flat rates, or maximum allowable amounts established by third-party payers. Medicare fee schedules apply to clinical laboratory, radiology, and durable medical equipment services.

FEHB. Federal Employee Health Benefits Program. Provides health plans to federal workers.

FEHBAR. Federal Employee Health Benefits Acquisition Regulations. Federal regulations for acquisition of health services used by government agencies and subcontractors.

FFS. Fee for service. ***1)*** Payment for services, usually physician services, on a service-by-service basis rather than an alternative payment system like capitation. Fee-for-service arrangements may be discounted or undiscounted rates. ***2)*** Situation in which the payer pays full charges for medical services.

formulary. List of prescription medications preferred for use by the health plan and dispensed through participating pharmacies to covered persons.

FPP. Faculty practice plan. Group practice developed around a teaching program or medical school.

fraternal insurance. Cooperative plan provided to members of an association or fraternal group.

FTE. Full time employee. Accounting equivalent of one full time employee that includes wages, benefits, and other costs.

gatekeeper. Primary care physician in a health care system in which a member's care must be provided by a primary care physician unless the physician refers the member to a specialist or approves the care provided by a specialist.

global surgery package. Services included in a surgical procedure that include all of the elements needed to perform the procedure and routine follow-up care.

GMLOS. Geometric mean length of stay. Statistically adjusted value for all cases for a given diagnosis-related group, allowing for the outliers, transfer cases, and negative outlier cases that would normally skew the data. The GMLOS is used to determine payment only for transfer cases (i.e., the per diem rate).

government mandates. Services mandated by state or federal law.

grace period. Set number of days past the due date of a premium payment during which medical coverage may not be canceled and the premium payment may be made, or after employment termination. It varies by health plan contract and state law but is generally 30 to 60 days.

group model. HMO that contracts with a group of providers.

group practice. Group of providers that shares facilities, resources, and staff, and who may represent a single unit in a managed care network.

grouper. Software program that assigns diagnosis-related groups (DRGs).

HCC model. Hierarchical condition categories model. Centers for Medicare and Medicaid Services risk adjustment payment model for Medicare managed care organizations (MCO) and other capitated programs. The CMS-HCC model is a prospective payment system that uses a hierarchical diagnosis classification system, as well as other demographic adjusters, to predict costs and set the payment rates for managed care services.

HCPCS. Healthcare Common Procedure Coding System.

HCPCS Level I. Healthcare Common Procedure Coding System Level I. Numeric coding system used by physicians, facility outpatient departments, and ambulatory surgery centers (ASC) to code ambulatory, laboratory, radiology, and other diagnostic services for Medicare billing. This coding system contains only the American Medical Association's Current Procedural Terminology (CPT) codes. The AMA updates codes annually.

HCPCS Level II. Healthcare Common Procedure Coding System Level II. National coding system, developed by CMS, that contains alphanumeric codes for physician and nonphysician services not included in the CPT coding system. HCPCS Level II covers such things as ambulance services, durable medical equipment, and orthotic and prosthetic devices.

HCPCS modifiers. Two-character code that identifies circumstances that alter or enhance the description of a service or supply. They are recognized by carriers nationally and are updated annually by CMS.

health plan ID. System for uniquely identifying all organizations that pay for health care services. Formerly referred to as the payer ID.

HHS. Health and Human Services. Cabinet department that oversees the operating divisions of the federal government responsible for health and welfare. HHS oversees the Centers for Medicare and Medicaid Services, Food and Drug Administration, Public Health Service, and other such entities.

hierarchy. Rank or order of codes. Hierarchy plays a key role in ICD-10-CM coding because each character beyond three adds more detail.

HIPAA. Health Insurance Portability and Accountability Act of 1996. Federal law that includes the provision allowing persons to qualify immediately for comparable health insurance coverage when they change their employment relationships.

HMO. Health maintenance organization. Medical health insurance coverage that pays claims based on a provider cost, per diem, or charge basis. Hospitals contract with an HMO to provide care at a contractually reduced price. HMO members pay a set monthly amount for coverage and are treated without additional cost, except for a copayment or deductible amount, payable by the patient. Like all managed care organizations, HMOs use a variety of mechanisms to control costs, including utilization management, discounted provider fee schedules, and financial incentives. HMOs use primary care physicians as gatekeepers and tend to emphasize preventive care.

hold harmless. Contractual clause stating that if either party is held liable for malpractice, the other party is absolved.

home health. Palliative and therapeutic care and assistance in the activities of daily life to home bound Medicare and private plan members.

hospice. Organization that furnishes inpatient, outpatient, and home health care for the terminally ill. Hospices emphasize support and counseling services for terminally ill people and their families, pain relief, and symptom management. When the Medicare beneficiary chooses hospice benefits, all other Medicare benefits are discontinued, except physician services and treatment of conditions not related to the terminal illness.

hospital admission plan. Used to facilitate admission to the hospital and to assure prompt payment to the hospital.

hospital issued notice of noncoverage. Notice issued by a hospital to a beneficiary when the hospital determines that the care the beneficiary is receiving or is about to receive is not covered because it is not medically necessary, is not being delivered in the most appropriate setting, or is custodial in nature. The HINN may be given prior to admission, at admission, or at any point during the inpatient stay.

hospital laboratory. Laboratory located in or operated by a hospital or its organized medical staff.

hospital outpatient. Person who has not been admitted as an inpatient but who is registered on the hospital or CAH records as an outpatient and receives services (rather than supplies alone) directly from the hospital or CAH. (Code of Federal Regulations, section 410.2.)

IBNR. Incurred but not reported. Amount of money the payer's plan accrues to forestall unknown medical expenses.

ICD-10. International Classification of Diseases, 10th Revision. Classification of diseases by alphanumeric code, used by the World Health Organization.

ICD-10-CM. International Classification of Diseases, 10th Revision, Clinical Modification. Clinical modification of the alphanumeric classification of diseases used by the World Health Organization, already in use in much of the world, and used for mortality reporting in the United States.

ICF. ***1)*** Intermediate care facility. Health care facility that furnishes services to patients who do not require the degree of care provided by a hospital or skilled nursing facility or a step-down facility for patients who are leaving the hospital but who cannot be discharged to home because of continuing medical needs. ***2)*** International Classification of Functioning, Disability, and Health. World Health Organization coding system for reporting an individual's capacity to cope in situations that are the consequence of disease. The classification identifies functional limits set by the severity of the disease, without identifying the disease itself. Code examples include d550, to report the ability to open bottles and cans, use eating implements, and consume meals in a culturally accepted way; or the ability to walk, reported for different distances with codes in the d450 category of ICF. The United States has not adopted ICF for use. However, it is under investigation at the National Center for Health Statistics as a reporting mechanism for the future.

immediate maternity. Coverage provided for pregnancies that began prior to the date the member became insured.

in plan. Services chosen from a network provider.

incontestable clause. Provision in a policy that prohibits the plan from disputing coverage for certain conditions after a specified period of time.

inpatient ancillary services. Inpatient services, other than accommodations or other inclusive routine services, usually provided in a specialized department such as radiology, laboratory, drugs, or other similar professional services.

inpatient hospitalization. Period in which a patient is housed in a single hospital usually without interruption.

inpatient reimbursement. Payment to hospital for the costs incurred to treat a patient.

inpatient services. Items and services furnished to a person staying at least overnight and usually longer in a specific institutional setting, including room and board, nursing care and related services, and diagnostic and therapeutic medical and surgical services.

insurance carrier. Insurer or health plan that may underwrite, administer, or sell a range of health benefit programs.

IPA. Individual practice association. Organization made up of providers who, along with the rest of a group, contract with payers at a discounted fee-for-service or capitated rate.

IPO. Individual practice organization. Organization made up of providers who, along with the rest of a group, contract with payers at a discounted fee-for-service or capitated rate.

IS. Information services. Administrators of the computer systems used by payers and providers.

Joint Commission. Organization that accredits health care organizations. In the future, the Joint Commission may play a role in certifying these organizations' compliance with the HIPAA A/S requirements. Previously known as the Joint Commission for the Accreditation of Hospitals or JCAHO.

lag study. Report used by plan managers to determine how long claims are pending and how much is paid out each month.

lapse. Terminated policy.

late charge. In relation to facility billing, a charge posted to an account after the final bill has been produced.

late effect. Abnormality, dysfunction, or other residual condition produced after the acute phase of an illness, injury, or disease is over. There is no time limit on when late effects can appear.

LCD. Published decision of coverage and related usage specific to a Medicare administrative contractor (MAC), fiscal intermediary or carrier, or in a designated geographic area.

liability insurance. Insurance that protects against claims for negligence or inappropriate action or inaction that resulted in injury to a person or damage to property.

lifetime maximum. Maximum amount an insurance plan pays on behalf of the insured for covered services received while enrolled.

limiting charge. Maximum amount a nonparticipating physician or provider can charge for services rendered to a Medicare patient.

limits. In medical reimbursement, the ceiling for benefits payable under a plan.

line item. Specific service or item detail of claim.

line item denial. Fiscal intermediary's denial of a specific line item on a claim that may be otherwise processable. Rejected line items cannot be corrected by the provider but may be appealed.

line of business. Different health plans offered by a larger insurer or insurance broker as a product line.

lives. Unit of measurement used by plans to determine the number of people covered. Calculated by multiplying the number of members by 2.5.

local coverage determination. Published decision of coverage and related usage specific to a Medicare administrative contractor (MAC), fiscal intermediary or carrier, or in a designated geographic area.

local medical review policy. Carrier-specific policy applied in the absence of a national coverage policy to make local Medicare coverage decisions, including the development of a draft policy based on a review of medical literature, an understanding of local practice, and the solicitation of comments from the medical community and Carrier Advisory Committee.

long-term care facility. Nursing home or, more specifically, a facility offering extended, nonacute care to a resident patient whose illness does not require acute care.

loss ratio. Ratio between the cost to deliver medical care and the amount of money taken in by the plan.

MAC. Medicare administrative contractor. Jurisdictional entity that contracts with CMS to adjudicate professional claims under Part A, Part B, and DME and is responsible for daily claims processing, utilization review, record maintenance, dissemination of information based on CMS regulations, and whether services are covered and payments are appropriate.

major complication/comorbidity (MCC). Diagnosis codes that reflect the highest level of severity and have the potential to increase DRG reimbursement. See also complication/comorbidity.

malingering. Feigning of illness, as the result of intentional deceit or as the result of mental illness.

managed health care. ***1)*** Managing active cases to ensure care is the most appropriate, efficient, and effective. ***2)*** Method of health care whereby contracted physicians participate in managing health care costs. ***3)*** System of health care meant to manage overall cost.

mandated benefits. Services mandated by state or federal law such as child abuse or rape, not necessarily covered by insurers.

maximum allowable charge. Amount set by the insurer as the highest amount that can be charged for a particular medical service or by a pharmacy vendor.

maximum out-of-pocket costs. Limit on total patient payments including copayments, deductibles, and coinsurance under a benefit contract in a specified time period.

MCE. ***1)*** Medical care evaluation. ***2)*** Medicare code editor.

MCO. Managed care organization. Generic term for various health benefit plans that provide coverage for health care services in conjunction with management and review of services provided to ensure that services are medically necessary and appropriate.

MDC. Major diagnostic category. Dividing all possible principal diagnoses into mutually exclusive categories. These broad classifications of diagnoses are typically grouped by body system.

Medicaid. Joint federal and state program that covers medical expenses for people with low incomes and limited resources who meet the criteria. The benefits for recipients vary from state to state.

medical consultation. Advice or an opinion rendered by a physician at the request of the primary care provider.

medical meaningfulness. Patients in the same DRG can be expected to evoke a set of clinical responses that result in a similar pattern of resource use.

medical necessity. Medically appropriate and necessary to meet basic health needs; consistent with the diagnosis or condition and national medical practice guidelines regarding type, frequency, and duration of treatment; rendered in a cost-effective manner.

Medicare. Federally funded program authorized as part of the Social Security Act that provides for health care services for people age 65 or older, people with disabilities, and people with end-stage renal disease (ESRD).

Medicare Beneficiary Identifier. Randomly generated number issued by CMS that replaces the Health Insurance Claim Number or HICN (beneficiary's social security number) as required by the Medicare Access and CHIP and Reauthorization Act of 2015 (MACRA). The identifier number uses the numbers 0 to 9 and all uppercase letters with the exception of S, L, O, I, B, and Z in order to eliminate any confusion when differentiating between some letters and numbers (e.g., the letter O and the number 0). The MBI card provides the beneficiary information necessary for processing Medicare claims. ***Synonym(s):*** *MBI, Medicare ID, Medicare number.*

Medicare fee schedule. Fee schedule based upon physician work, expense, and malpractice designed to slow the rise in cost for services and standardize payment to physicians regardless of specialty or location of service with geographic adjustments.

Medicare Part A. Hospital insurance coverage that includes hospital, nursing home, hospice, home health, and other inpatient care. Claims are submitted to intermediaries for reimbursement.

Medicare Part B. Supplemental medical insurance that includes outpatient hospital care and physician and other qualified professional care. Claims from providers or suppliers other than a hospital are submitted to carriers for reimbursement. Hospital outpatient claims are submitted to their FI/MAC.

Medicare secondary payer. Specified circumstance when other third-party payers have the primary responsibility for payment of services and Medicare is the secondary payer. Medicare is secondary to workers' compensation, automobile, medical no-fault and liability insurance, EGHPs, LGHPs, and certain employer health plans covering aged and disabled beneficiaries. The MSP program prohibits Medicare payment for items or services if payment has been made or can reasonably be expected to be made by another payer, as described above.

Medicare supplement. Private insurance coverage that pays the Medicare deductible and copayments and may also pay the costs of services not covered by Medicare.

Medigap policy. Health insurance or other health benefit plan offered by a private company to those entitled to Medicare benefits. The policy covers charges not payable by Medicare because of deductibles, coinsurance amounts, or other Medicare-imposed limitations.

member. Subscriber of a health plan.

member months. In medical reimbursement, total of months each member was covered.

member services. In health care contracting, the payer department that works as a patient advocate to solve problems and may take claims appeals to a final committee after all other processes have been exhausted.

mental health substance abuse. Payer term for services rendered to members for emotional problems or chemical dependency.

MET. Multiple employer trust. Group of employers that join together to purchase health insurance using a self-funded approach to lower costs by the broadening membership pool to prevent an adverse selection.

MEWA. Multiple employer welfare association. Group of employers that join together to purchase health insurance using a self-funded approach to lower costs by the broadening membership pool to prevent an adverse selection.

minor procedure. Self-limited procedure, usually with an assignment of 0 or 10 follow-up days by payers. A minor procedure may be considered by many payers to be part of the global package for a primary surgical service and cannot be billed separately from the primary procedure.

MIS. Management information system. Hardware and software facilitating claims management.

mixed model. HMO that includes both an open panel and closed panel option.

MLP. Midlevel practitioners. Professionals such as nurse practitioners, nurse midwives, physical therapists, physician assistants, and others who provide medical care but do so with physician input.

modifier. Two characters that can be appended to a HCPCS code as a means of identifying circumstances that alter or enhance the description of a service or supply.

morbidity rate. In health care contracting, an actuarial term describing predicted medical expense rate.

MSN. ***1)*** Master of science in nursing. ***2)*** Medicare summary notice.

multiple birth. Two or more infants delivered at the same time.

multiple employer group. Group of employers who contract together to subscribe to a plan, broadening the risk pool and saving money. Different from a multiple employer trust.

NAHMOR. National Association of HMO Regulators.

NAIC. National Association of Insurance Commissioners. Organization of state insurance regulators.

national coverage determination. National policy statement regarding the circumstances under which a service, item, or test is considered reasonable and necessary or otherwise not covered for Medicare purposes.

national coverage policy. Statement of Medicare coverage decisions that applies to all practitioners in states and regions. These policies indicate whether and under what circumstances procedures, services, and supplies are covered.

NCD. National coverage determinations. National policy statements granting, eliminating, or excluding Medicare coverage for a service, item, or test and indicate CMS policy regarding the circumstances under which the service, item, or test is considered reasonable and necessary or otherwise not covered for Medicare purposes.

NCHS. National Center for Health Statistics. Division of the Centers for Disease Control and Prevention that compiles statistical information used to guide actions and policies to improve the public health of U.S. citizens. The NCHS maintains the ICD-10-CM coding system.

NCQA. National Committee for Quality Assurance. Organization that accredits managed care plans, or HMOs. In the future, the NCQA may play a role in certifying these organizations' compliance with the HIPAA A/S requirements.

NEC. Not elsewhere classifiable. Condition or diagnosis that is not provided with its own specified code in ICD-10-CM, but included in a more broadly defined code for other specified conditions.

neonatal period. Period of an infant's life from birth to the age of 27 days, 23 hours, and 59 minutes.

network model. Plan that contracts with multiple groups of providers, or networks, to provide care.

new patient. Patient who is receiving face-to-face care from a provider/qualified health care professional or another physician/qualified health care professional of the exact same specialty and subspecialty who belongs to the same group practice for the first time in three years. For OPPS hospitals, a patient who has not been registered as an inpatient or outpatient, including off-campus provider based clinic or emergency department, within the past three years.

newborn admission. Infant born in the facility.

NICU. Neonatal intensive care unit. Special care unit for premature and seriously ill infants.

noncovered services. Health care services that are not reimbursable according to provisions of a given insurance policy.

normal delivery. Spontaneous vaginal delivery of a single live infant after completion of 38 to 42 weeks of gestation, with cephalic presentation, without instrumentation, and with no antepartum or postpartum conditions or complications. A normal delivery may also include the performance of an episiotomy, artificial rupture of membranes, or fetal monitoring.

NOS. Not otherwise specified. Condition or diagnosis remains ill-defined and is unspecified without the necessary information for selecting a more specific code.

observation patient. Patient who needs to be monitored and assessed for inpatient admission or referral to another site for care.

observation services. Services furnished on a hospital's premises, including use of a bed and periodic monitoring by a hospital's nursing or other staff, that are reasonable and necessary to evaluate an outpatient's condition or determine the need for a possible admission to the hospital as an inpatient.

occupational therapy. Training, education, and assistance intended to assist a person who is recovering from a serious illness or injury perform the activities of daily life.

Office of Inspector General. Agency within the Department of Justice that is ultimately responsible for investigating instances of fraud and abuse in the Medicare and Medicaid and other government health care programs and other governmental agencies.

OL. Outlier threshold. Component that figures in the reimbursement calculation for a DRG.

OOPs. Out-of-pocket costs/expenses.

open enrollment period. Time period during which subscribers in a health benefit program have the opportunity to re-enroll or select an alternative health plan being offered to them, usually without evidence of insurability or waiting periods.

open panel. Arrangement in which a managed care organization that contracts with providers on an exclusive basis is still seeking providers.

OPL. Other party liability. In coordination of benefits, the decision that the other plan is the primary plan.

orthotic. Associated with the making and fitting of an orthosis(es).

other qualified health care professional. Individual who is qualified by education, training, licensure/regulation, and facility privileging to perform a professional service within his or her scope of practice and independently (or as incident-to) report the professional service without requiring physician supervision. Payers may state exemptions in writing or state and local regulations may not follow this definition for performance of some services. Always refer to any relevant plan policies and federal and/or state laws to determine who may perform and report services.

out of plan. In health care contracting, services of a provider who is not a member of the preferred provider network.

out of service area. Medical care received out of the geographic area that may or may not be covered, depending on the plan.

outlier. Case classified to a specific MS-DRG but with exceptionally high costs compared with other cases classified to the same MS-DRG. The fiscal intermediary or MAC makes a payment in addition to the original MS-DRG amount for these situations. A cost outlier is paid an amount in excess of the cut-off threshold for a given MS-DRG. The day outlier no longer applies.

outpatient. Person who has not been admitted as an inpatient but who is registered on the hospital or CAH records as an outpatient and receives services (rather than supplies alone) directly from the hospital or CAH. (Code of Federal Regulations, section 410.2.)

outpatient code editor. Centers for Medicare and Medicaid Services' outpatient software program that analyzes hospital outpatient claims to detect incorrect billing and coding data, assign an ambulatory payment classification for covered services, and determine the appropriate payment. Medicare contractors use the OCE to test the validity of ICD-10-CM and HCPCS coding and to conduct compatibility edits. The OCE performs editing functions related to HCPCS codes, HCPCS modifiers, and ICD-10-CM diagnosis codes. It identifies individual errors and indicates the action to take with the claim (e.g., return to provider [RTP], suspend, deny).

outpatient pricer. Software used to determine the reimbursement amount including the line-item price, outlier payment, and other associated payments due (e.g., TOPS payment), such as the deductible and coinsurance amounts.

outpatient services. Medical and other services, diagnostic or therapeutic, provided to a person who has not been admitted to the hospital as an inpatient but is registered on the hospital records as an outpatient. Outpatient services usually require a stay of less than 24 hours.

outpatient surgery list. List of surgical procedures identified by CMS that can be performed on an outpatient basis without adversely affecting the quality of care.

outpatient visit. Encounter in a recognized outpatient facility.

overutilization. Services rendered by providers more frequently than usual.

PA. Physician assistant. Medical professional with additional training that can assess, treat, and prescribe medications under a physician's review.

paneled. In health care contracting, provider contracted with an HMO.

par provider. Participating provider. In health care contracting, provider who has contracted with the health plan to deliver medical services to covered persons.

partial disability. Congenital or acquired inability to perform part of one's job.

partial hospitalization. Situation in which the patient only stays part of each day over a long period. Cardiac, rehabilitation, and chronic pain patients, for example, could use this service.

partial payment. Payment to a provider or member with the expectation that other payments will be forthcoming before the claim is closed.

PAS norms. Based on a professional activity study performed regularly by the Commission on Professional and Hospital Activities and broken out by average length of stay (ALOS) by region.

PBM. Prescription benefit managers. HMO staff who monitor amount and use of drugs prescribed.

PCP. Primary care physician. Physician who makes an initial diagnosis and referral and retains control over the patient and utilization of services both in and outside of the plan.

pediatric patient. Patient usually younger than 14 years of age.

peer review. Evaluation of the quality of the total health care provided by medical staff with equivalent training, such as a physician-to-physician or nurse-to-nurse evaluation.

PEPM. Per employee per month.

PEPP. Payment error prevention program. Program to help reduce Medicare PPS inpatient hospital payment errors.

per diem reimbursement. In health care contracting, reimbursement to an institution based on a set rate per day rather than on a charge-by-charge basis.

perinatal death. Stillborn births and neonatal deaths.

physician services. Professional services performed by physicians, including surgery, consultations, and home, office, and institutional calls.

PIN. Physician identification number.

PLA codes. Services performed by a single "sole source" laboratory or for laboratory services that are cleared or approved by the Food and Drug Administration (FDA) and licensed and/or marketed to multiple providing laboratories. These services are often referred to as Proprietary Laboratory Analyses or PLA services.

plan manager. Payer employee managing all of the contracts and contract negotiations for one or more specific plans.

PMPM. Per member per month.

PMPY. Per member per year.

pooling. Health payers' practice of combining risk.

POS. Point of service. Health benefit plan allowing the covered person to choose to receive a service from a participating or nonparticipating provider, with different benefit levels associated with the use of participating providers.

posting date. Date a charge is posted to a patient account by the provider, frequently not the same as the actual date of service, but usually within five days of the actual date of service.

PPA. Preferred provider arrangement. Similar to a PPO.

PPO. Preferred provider organization. Program that establishes contracts with providers of medical care. Usually the benefit contract provides significantly better benefits and lower member cost for services received from preferred providers, encouraging covered persons to use these providers, who may be reimbursed on a discounted basis.

PPS. Prospective payment system. Reimbursement methodology that uses predetermined rates for each type of discharge, procedure, service, or item based on a standard type of case. For hospital inpatients, the Medicare PPS system of DRGs was implemented in 1983 to hold down the rising cost of healthcare. For hospital outpatients, OPPS has been based on ambulatory payment classifications effective August 1, 2000. For skilled nursing facilities, it is based on the patient-driven payment model (PDPM). For home health, it is based on the patient-driven groupings model (PDGM).

precertification. Confirmation that a payer covers a given procedure for a given patient, including admission or continued stay.

preexisting condition. Symptom that causes a person to seek diagnosis, care, or treatment for which medical advice or treatment was recommended or received by a physician within a certain time period before the effective date of medical insurance coverage. The preexisting condition waiting period is the time the beneficiary must wait after buying health insurance before coverage begins for a condition that existed before coverage was obtained.

premature delivery. Infant delivered with time of gestation less than 37 weeks.

presenting problem. Disease, condition, illness, injury, symptom, sign, finding, complaint, or other reason for the patient encounter.

primary care. Basic or general health care, traditionally provided by family practice, pediatrics, and internal medicine practitioners.

primary diagnosis. Current, most significant reason for the services or procedures provided.

principal diagnosis. Condition established after study to be chiefly responsible for occasioning the admission of the patient to the hospital for care.

principal procedure. Procedure performed for definitive treatment rather than for diagnostic or exploratory purposes, or that was necessary to treat a complication. Usually related to the principal diagnosis.

PRO. Peer review organization. Organization that contracts with CMS to conduct preadmission, preprocedure, and postdischarge medical reviews and determine medical necessity, appropriateness, and quality of certain inpatient and outpatient surgical procedures for which payment may be made in whole or in part under the Medicare program.

professional association plans. Plan provided by a professional association that affords self-employed professionals (e.g., physicians, CPAs, lawyers) less expensive coverage.

professional service. Service rendered face-to-face by a physician or other qualified health care provider with the patient and for which there is a specific CPT code reported.

provider. All-inclusive, generic term for people or institutions that provide health care. The provider may be a physician, hospital, pharmacy, other facility, or other health care provider.

PTMPY. Per thousand members per year.

public health emergency. Declaration by the Secretary of Health and Human Services (HHS) to promote, protect, and improve the health of individuals and communities specifically as a result of a disaster, outbreak of disease, catastrophic events, or other threats to public health and wellbeing. ***Synonym(s):*** *PHE.*

QA. ***1)*** Quality assurance. Monitoring and maintenance of established standards of quality for patient care. ***2)*** HCPCS Level II modifier used to identify when prescribed amounts of stationary oxygen for daytime use while at rest and nighttime use differ and the average of the two amounts is less than 1 liter per minute (lpm).

QIO. Quality Improvement Organization. Entity established under the Tax Equity and Fiscal Responsibility Act of 1982 (TEFRA) to review, monitor, educate, and improve the care given to patients. Primarily performed for Medicare, but may also review data for Medicaid and private insurers under separate contracts.

QM. Quality management. Monitoring and maintenance of established standards of quality.

RBRVS. Resource-based relative value scale. Fee schedule introduced by CMS to reimburse physician Medicare fees based on the amount of time and resources expended in treating patients with adjustments for overhead costs and geographical differences.

reasonable and customary. Fees charged for medical services that are considered normal, common, and in line with the prevailing fees in the provider's geographical area.

referral. Approval from the primary care physician to see a specialist or receive certain services. May be required for coverage purposes before a patient receives care from anyone except the primary physician.

regional medical center. Hospital that provides comprehensive services to a large regional area but that may not be a tertiary care facility. Largely used in the west where facilities may serve hundreds of square miles.

rehabilitation. Restoration of physical and mental functions to allow the usual daily activities of life.

reimbursement. Payment of actual charges or allowable incurred as a result of accident or illness.

reinsurance. Insurance purchased by an HMO, insurance company, or self-funded employer from another insurance company to protect itself against all or part of the losses that may be incurred in the process of honoring the claims of its participating providers, policy holders, or employees and covered dependents.

relative weight. Assigned weight that is intended to reflect the relative resource consumption associated with each MS-DRG. The higher the relative weight, the greater the payment to the hospital. The relative weights are calculated by CMS and published in the final prospective payment system rule.

remittance advice. Statement, voucher, or notice received by the service provider from a payer reflecting the status of adjudicated claims, either paid or denied.

review committee. Multidisciplinary committee that considers denied cases being appealed, catastrophic cases, or fee-for-service cases.

RHIA. Registered health information administrator. Accreditation for medical record administrators, previously known as a registered records administrator (RRA), through AHIMA.

RHIT. Registered health information technician. Accreditation for medical records practitioners, previously known as accredited records technician (ART), through AHIMA.

risk adjustment. Method of predicting and adjusting payment for expenditures related to health care services based upon patient diagnoses and certain demographic adjusters.

risk contract. Contract between Medicare and a payer or a payer and a provider in which the payer (in the case of Medicare) and the provider (in the case of the payer contracts) receive a set amount for care of a patient base. If costs exceed the amount the payer or provider was paid, the patients still receive care during the term of the contract.

risk factor reduction. Reduction of risk in the pool of health plan members.

risk manager. Person charged with keeping financial risk low, including malpractice cases.

risk pool. Pool of people who will be in the insured group, their medical and mental histories, other factors such as age, and their predicted health.

rush charge. Charge for expeditious test results.

RVS. Relative value study. Guide that shows the relationship between the time, resources, competency, experience, severity, and other factors necessary to perform procedures that is multiplied by a dollar conversion factor to determine a monetary value for the procedure.

RVU. Relative value unit. Measure of value assigned to a procedure based on difficulty and time consumed. Used for computing reimbursement under a relative value study.

sanction. Imposition of penalties or exclusion of a provider for fraud or infractions such as an inappropriate use of services, providing procedures that may harm the patient, or applying inferior techniques.

schedule. Listing of amounts payable for specific procedures.

SCHIP. State Children's Health Insurance Program. Referred to as Children's Health Insurance Program or CHIP.

screening test. Exam or study used by a physician to identify abnormalities, regardless of whether the patient exhibits symptoms.

SDOH. Social determinants of health.

second opinion. Medical opinion obtained from another health care professional, relevant to clinical evaluation, before the performance of a medical service or surgical procedure. Includes patient education regarding treatment alternatives and/or to determine medical necessity.

secondary insurer. In a COB arrangement, the insurer that reimburses for benefits pending after payment by the primary insurer.

self-funded plan. Plan where the risk is assumed by the employer rather than the insurer. The employer generally pays claims directly from a general fund account that may be managed by a third party.

self-insured. Individual or organization that assumes the financial risk of paying for health care.

self-pay patients. Patients who pay for medical care out-of-pocket.

separate procedures. Services commonly carried out as a fundamental part of a total service and, as such, do not usually warrant separate identification. These services are identified in CPT with the parenthetical phrase (separate procedure) at the end of the description and are payable only when performed alone.

service date. Date a charge is incurred for a service.

service plan. ***1)*** Another name for Blue Cross/Blue Shield plans. ***2)*** Plan that has contracts with providers but is not a managed care plan.

shadow pricing. Setting rates just below a competitor's rates. Maximizes profits but raises medical costs.

short-stay patients. Inpatients admitted for 48 hours or less, or outpatients who stay 24 hours or less.

sick baby. Infant with medical complications not resulting from premature birth.

small subscriber group aggregate. Aggregate of professional associations, small business, or other entities formed to be considered a single, large subscriber group.

SNF. Skilled nursing facility. Institution or a distinct part of an institution that is primarily engaged in providing skilled nursing care and related services for residents who require medical or nursing care; or rehabilitation services for the rehabilitation of injured, disabled, or sick persons. A SNF may be a part of a hospital or a separate entity, such as a nursing home. In order for a patient to be transferred between a hospital and a SNF, the transferring facility must complete a written transfer statement. A swing-bed hospital provides skilled nursing care and related services similar to those of a SNF.

social determinants of health. Socioeconomic factors that can affect a person's health, including both environmental and societal conditions such as education and literacy, employment, health behaviors, housing, lack of adequate food or water, occupational exposure to risk factors, social support, transportation, and violence. Tracking social needs that impact patients allows providers to identify population health trends and to promote the personalized care that addresses the medical and social needs of individual patients.

SSN. Social security number.

staff model. HMO that employs its own providers.

standard anesthesia formula. Reimbursement formula that consists of base units plus time units plus modifying units (e.g., physical status and qualifying circumstances) plus other allowed unit/charges that is multiplied by a conversion factor.

stat charge. Charge for expeditious test results.

state insurance commission. State group that approves insurance certificates for each state and regulates the industry based on statutes.

status indicator. One-letter code used in the outpatient prospective payment system (OPPS) and the Medicare physician fee schedule (MPFS) to signify how a specific code is treated under that payment system.

steering. Providing financial incentives to plan members to use the managed care provider panel.

stop loss. In health care contracting, a form of reinsurance that protects health insurance above a certain limit and minimizes risks for providers.

subrogation. Recovery of monies or benefits from a third party who is liable for the payment.

subsidiary codes. Services that are not included as part of the primary procedure but that are not performed alone and may be identified as each additional, or list-in-addition-to services. Phrases that help identify subsidiary codes include, but are not limited to: each additional, list in addition to, and done at time of other major procedure.

substantial comorbidity. Preexisting condition that will, because of its presence with a specific principal diagnosis, cause an increase in the length of stay by at least one day in approximately 75 percent of the cases.

substantial complication. Condition that arises during the hospital stay that prolongs the length of stay by at least one day in approximately 75 percent of the cases.

supplemental health services. Optional services that a health plan may cover or provide.

surgical package. Normal, uncomplicated performance of specific surgical services, with the assumption that, on average, all surgical procedures of a given type are similar with respect to skill level, duration, and length of normal follow-up care.

swing bed. Bed used for acute or long-term care, depending on the patient's need and the hospital's level of occupancy. Swing beds typically are available in small and rural hospitals. A swing-bed patient may be admitted and discharged from acute care and readmitted to a swing bed to receive skilled or intermediate levels of care. At times, the patient may remain in the same bed while changes occur in his or her care, charges, and payment.

TCC. Transitional care center. Facility used in lieu of an extended care facility or before discharge to an extended care facility.

technical component. Portion of a health care service that identifies the provision of the equipment, supplies, technical personnel, and costs attendant to the performance of the procedure other than the professional services.

TEFRA. Tax Equity and Fiscal Responsibility Act. Protects the rights of full-time employees to remain on the company's health plan to age 69.

telehealth service. Care by a provider with the patient at a remote site, usually rural, utilizing electronic communication to evaluate, monitor, and treat a patient.

telemedicine. Medical information exchanged from site to site via electronic communication. Examples include patient evaluation and consultation, monitoring, education and other clinical services.

tertiary care facility. Hospital providing specialty care to patients referred from other hospitals because of the severity of their injuries or illnesses.

therapeutic. Act meant to alleviate a medical or mental condition.

therapeutic procedure. Manner of effecting change through the application of clinical skills and/or services that attempt to improve function.

third-party payer. Public or private organization that pays for or underwrites coverage for health care expenses for another entity, usually an employer (e.g., Blue Cross Blue Shield, Medicare, Medicaid, commercial insurers).

time limit. In health care contracting, a set number of days in which a claim can be filed according to the payer or state insurance commission.

TPA. ***1)*** Third-party administrator. Firm that performs administrative functions for a self-funded plan but assumes no risk. ***2)*** Trading partner agreement. Agreement between the provider and the receiver of the claim transmission detailing the electronic data interchange requirements between the parties. For purposes of HIPAA, a trading partner agreement may not include any agreement to use the codes, segments, or transactions published in an implementation guide in a manner different from that prescribed in the applicable guide. The agreement does not need to be formal. It may take the form of a manual, bulletin, or memorandum.

TPL. Third party liability. Payer liable for the cost of an illness or injury, such as auto or homeowner insurer.

TQM. Total quality management. Concept that quality is an organic part of a plan's service and a provider's care and can be quantified and constantly improved.

transfer. Situation in which the patient is transferred to another acute care hospital for related care.

transitional pass-through payment. Certain drugs, biologicals, and devices that are eligible for payments in addition to the ambulatory payment classification payment under the outpatient prospective payment system.

treatment plan. Plan of care established by the provider outlining specific deficits and planned treatment that may be submitted to the case manager when seeking certification for a plan member.

triage. Medical screening of patients to determine priority of treatment based on severity of illness or injury and resources at hand.

TRICARE. Federal program that covers the health benefits for families of all uniformed service employees. Formerly called CHAMPUS.

triple option. Offering of an HMO, indemnity plan, and preferred provider organization by one insurance firm.

U.S. Preventive Services Task Force. Independent, volunteer panel of national experts in prevention and evidence-based medicine formed in 1984 that works to improve the health of all U.S. citizens by making evidence-based recommendations about clinical preventive services such as screenings, counseling services, and preventive medications. Task Force recommendations are published on the organization's website and/or in a peer-reviewed journal. Members include experts in various fields such as preventive medicine and primary care, including internal medicine, family medicine, pediatrics, behavioral health, obstetrics and gynecology, and nursing. All of the expert recommendations go through rigorous reviews of existing peer-reviewed evidence with the goal and objective of assisting primary care clinicians and patients in determining whether a preventive service is right for the patient's needs. Recommendations from the organization receive a letter grade (e.g., A, B, C, or D) or an I statement that is assigned on the strength of the evidence and the balance of benefits and harms of a preventive service. The Task Force does not factor in costs when determining a recommendation grade. All Task Force recommendations are applicable only to patients who present without signs or symptoms of the specific disease or condition under evaluation, and the recommendations address only services offered in the primary care setting or services referred by a primary care clinician.

UB-04. Uniform institutional claim form developed by the NUBC that was implemented in May 2007.

UCR. Usual, customary, and reasonable. Fees charged for medical services that are considered normal, common, and in line with the prevailing fees in a given geographical area. May also be referred to as customary, prevailing, and reasonable charges.

unbundling. Separately packaging costs or services that might otherwise be billed together including billing separately for health care services that should be combined according to the industry standards or commonly accepted coding practices.

underwriting. Evaluating and determining the financial risk a member or member group has on an insurer.

unlisted procedure. Procedural descriptions used when the overall procedure and outcome of the procedure are not adequately described by an existing procedure code. Such codes are used as a last resort and only when there is not a more appropriate procedure code.

unspecified. Codes for use when documentation is insufficient to assign a more specific code.

upcoding. Practice of billing a code that represents a higher reimbursement than the code for the procedure actually performed.

URAC. Utilization Review Accreditation Commission. Accrediting body of case management.

urgent admission. Admission in which the patient requires immediate attention for treatment of a physical or psychiatric problem.

utilization review. Formal assessment of the medical necessity, efficiency, and/or appropriateness of health care services and treatment plans on a prospective, concurrent, or retrospective basis.

utilization review nurse. Nurse who evaluates cases for appropriateness of care and length of service and can plan discharge and services needed after discharge.

value-added network. Vendor of electronic data interchange data communications and translation services.

verification of eligibility. Process by which the payer or provider determines that the beneficiary is currently enrolled in a plan and that the requested services are covered by the plan.

violation. Disregard or abuse of the laws, rules, or guidelines, knowingly or unknowingly resulting in receipt of inappropriate reimbursement.

waived test. Laboratory test defined by CLIA standards that can be conducted in a minimal laboratory setting with minimal chance of error.

waiver of liability. Provision established by Medicare to protect beneficiaries and physicians from liability when services are denied as inappropriate or medically unnecessary. Under the provision, if the Medicare beneficiary knew or should have known that the services billed for were not covered, the beneficiary is liable for paying for the services. If neither the beneficiary nor the hospital knew or reasonably could have been expected to know that the services were not covered, Medicare is liable for paying the claim. If the provider should have known and the beneficiary is protected from liability, then liability falls with the provider, and the hospital cannot bill the beneficiary for services other than deductibles and coinsurance amounts, even though no Medicare payment has been made. Beneficiaries who do not know that services were noncovered are protected from liability when the services are not reasonable and/or necessary (including adverse level of care determinations) and when custodial care is involved.

waste. Spend or use federal funds carelessly.

weighting. Assigning more worth to a fee based on the number of times it is charged, weighting the resource-based relative value fees for an area.

well-baby care. Medical services, immunizations, and regular provider visits considered routine for an infant.

whistleblower. Individual who discloses misconduct by a provider and may be eligible for monetary returns if the misconduct involves financial misconduct as determined on a case-by-case basis.

withhold. Percentage of payment to providers held by an HMO until the cost of referral or services has been determined. If the provider goes over the amount determined appropriate, the HMO keeps that amount.

workers' compensation. State-governed system designated to administer and regulate the provision and cost of medical treatment and wage losses arising from a worker's job-related injury or disease, regardless of who is at fault. In exchange, the employer is protected from being sued.

working aged. Patient or spouse, older than age 65, eligible for group health insurance through employment or the employment of his or her spouse. Under these circumstances, Medicare would be the secondary payer.

wraparound plan. Insurance or health plan coverage for copays and deductibles not covered under a member's base plan.

YTD. Year to date.

Clinical Abbreviations, Prefixes, Suffixes, and Acronyms

The acronyms, abbreviations, prefixes, suffixes, and symbols used by health care providers speed communications. The following list includes the most often seen acronyms, abbreviations, and symbols. In some cases, abbreviations have more than one meaning. Multiple interpretations are numbered. Abbreviations of Latin phrases are punctuated.

Prefixes/Suffixes

a- Without, away from, not.
ab- From, away from, absent.
acanth(o)- Thorny, spine.
acr(o)- Extremity, top, highest point.
ad- Toward, adherence to, or increase.
aden(o)- Relating to a gland.
adip(o)- Relating to fat.
aer(o)- Relating to gas or air.
all(o)- Difference or divergence from the norm.
all- Another, other, or different.
alge(si)- Awareness to pain.
ambi- ***1)*** About or around.
2) Both sides.
an- Without, away from, not.
angi- Relating to a vessel.
anis(o)- Dissimilar, unequal, or asymmetrical.
ankyl(o)- Bent, crooked, or two parts growing together.
ante- In front of, before.
anter(o)- Before, front, anterior.
anti- In opposition to, against.
antr(o)- Relating to a chamber or cavity.
aphth(o)- Ulcer.
arch(o)- Relating to the rectum or anus.
arch- Beginning, first, principal.
arteri(o)- Relating to an artery.
arthr(o)- Relating to a joint.
astr(o)- Star-like or shaped.
atel(o)- Incomplete or imperfect.
aut(o)- Relating to the self.
axi(o)- Relating to an axis.
balan(o)- Relating to the glans penis or glans clitoridis.
bar(o)- Relating to weight or heaviness.
basi(o)- Relating to the base or foundation.
bi- Double, twice, two.
blast(o)- Relating to an early, formative, or primitive stage of a cell or embryonic element or layer.
blenn(o)- Relating to mucus.
blephar(o)- Relating to the eyelid.
brachi(o)- Relating to the arm.
brachy- Short.
brady- Slow or prolonged.
bronch(o)- Relating to the trachea.
bucc(o)- Relating to the cheek.
cac- Diseased or bad.
cardi(o)- Relating to the heart.
cari(o)- Rot, decay.
carp(o)- Relating to the wrist.
cata- Down from, down, according to.
cathar(o)- Purging, cleansing.
caud(o)- Lower part of body.
cec(o)- Having to do with the cecum.
cel(o)- ***1)*** Cavity.
2) Tumor or hernia.
cerebr(o)- Relating to the brain.
cervic(o)- Relating to the neck or neck of an organ.
cheil(o)- Relating to the lip.
cheir(o)- Relating to the hand.
chil(o)- Relating to the lip.
chole- Relating to the gallbladder.
chondr(o)- Relating to or denoting cartilage.
circum- Encircling or around.
cleid(o)- Relating to the clavicle.
coen(o)- Common, shared.
cole(o)- Sheath.
colp(o)- Relating to the vagina.
cycl(o)- Round or recurring. May refer to shape or to a sequence of events occurring at repeated intervals.

cyst(o)-	Relating to the urinary bladder or a cyst.
cyt(o)-	In relation to a cell.
dacry-	Pertaining to the lacrimal glands.
dactyl-	Relating to the fingers or toes.
demi-	Half the amount.
desmo-	Relating to ligaments.
dextro-	Meaning on or to the right.
diplo-	Double.
dorsi-	Relating to the back.
dys-	Painful, bad, disordered, difficult.
echo-	Reverberating sound.
ecto-	External, outside.
ectro-	Congenital absence of something.
endo-	Within, internal.
entero-	Relating to the intestines.
epi-	On, upon, in addition to.
erythr(o)-	Red in color.
eu-	Well, healthy, good, normal.
exo-	Outside of, without.
fibro-	Relating to fibers or fibrous tissue.
galact(o)-	Relating to milk.
gastr(o)-	Relating to the stomach and abdominal region.
genit(o)-	Relating to reproduction.
gloss(o)-	Relating to the tongue.
gnath(o)-	Relating to the jaw.
gon(o)-	Relating to the genitals, offspring, origination.
gyn-	Relating to the female gender.
hema(to)-	Relating to blood.
hemi-	Half.
hepat(o)-	Relating to the liver.
heter(o)-	Different.
hex-	Six.
hidr(o)-	Sweat.
hist(o)-	Relating to tissue.
hom(eo)/(o)-	Indicates resemblance or likeness.
homo-	Same.
hydro-	Relating to fluid, water, or hydrogen.
hyper-	Excessive, above, exaggerated.
hypo-	Below, less than, under.
hyster(o)-	Relating to either the womb or hysteria.
idio-	Distinct or individual characteristics.
ileo-	Relating to the ileum (part of the small intestine).
ilio-	Relating to the pelvis.
infra-	Inferior to, beneath, under.
ipsi-	Same, similar.
irid-	Relating to the iris.
ischio-	Relating to the hip.
iso-	Equal.
jejuno-	Relating to the jejunum (part of the small intestine).
juxta-	Next to, near.
karyo-	Relating to the nucleus of a cell.
kerato-	Relating to the cornea or horny tissue.
laparo-	***1)*** Flank, loins. ***2)*** Operations through the abdominal wall.
laryngo-	Relating to the larynx.
leuk(o)-	White in color.
lien-	Relating to the spleen.
lip-	Relating to fat.
lith(o)-	Relating to a hard or calcified substance.
lumbo-	Relating to the loin region.
macro-	Oversized, large.
mal-	Bad, poor, ill.
medull(o)-	Middle, inner section.
megalo-	Large.
melano-	Dark or black in color.
meningo-	Relating to membranes covering the brain and spine.
mer(o)-	Relating to the thigh; part or portion.
mes(io)-	***1)*** Secondary. ***2)*** Toward the middle.
meta-	Indicates a change.
mis-	Bad, improper.
mono-	Single, once, one.
my(o)-	Relating to muscle.
myc(o)-	Relating to fungus.
myelo-	Relating to bone marrow or the spinal cord.
narco-	Indicates insensate condition or numbness.
necro-	Indicates death or dead tissue.
nephr(o)-	Relating to the kidney.
noci-	Relating to injury or pain.
nycto-	Relating to darkness or night.
odont-	Relating to the teeth.
oligo-	Indicates few or small.
omo-	Relating to the shoulder.
omphalo-	Relating to the navel.
onco-	Relating to a mass, tumor, or swelling.
onycho-	Relating to the finger- or toenails.
oophor-	Relating to the ovaries.
opistho-	Indicates behind or backwards.
orchi(o)-	Relating to the testicles.
orrhea-	Flow, discharge.
oscheo-	Relating to the scrotum.
osphresi(o)-	Sense of smell.
osteo-	Having to do with bone.
oto-	Relating to the ear.
pachy-	Indicates heavy, large, or thick.

pali(n)- Repetition, back again, recurring.
panto- Indicates the whole or all.
para- Indicates near, similar, beside, or past.
patho- Indicates sensitivity, feeling, or suffering.
ped(i)- Relating to the foot.
peri- About, around, or in the vicinity.
pero- Indicates being maimed or deformed.
phaco- Relating to the lens of the eye.
phago- Relating to eating and ingestion.
pharyngo- Relating to the pharynx.
phlebo- Relating to the vein.
phreno- ***1)*** Head or mind. ***2)*** Relating to the diaphragm.
pimel- Relating to fat.
platy- Indicates wide or broad.
pleio- More, additional.
pleur- Relating to the side or ribs.
pneum- Relating to respiration, air, the lungs.
pod(o)- Relating to the feet.
poly- Indicates much or many.
procto- Relating to the rectum and/or anus.
proso- Indicates toward the front, anterior, forward.
pseudo- Indicates false or imagined.
ptyal(o)- Saliva.
pulmo- Relating to the lungs and respiration.
pyelo- Relating to the pelvis.
pygo- Relating to the buttocks or rump.
pyle- Relating to an opening/orifice of the portal vein.
pyloro- Relating to the pylorus (the stomach opening into the duodenum).
pyo- Relating to pus.
pyreto- Indicates a fever, heat.
rachi(o)- Relating to the spine.
recto- Meaning straight or relating to the rectum.
retro- Indicates behind, backward, in a reverse direction.
rhabd(o)- Rod, stick.
rheo- Indicates a flow or stream of fluid.
rhino- Relating to the nose.
sacro- Relating to the sacrum (base of the vertebral column).
salpingo- Relating to the fallopian or eustachian tubes.
sarco- Relating to flesh.
scapho- Indicates deformed condition, shaped like a boat.
scapulo- Relating to the shoulder.
schisto- ***1)*** Fissure. ***2)*** Indicates cleft or split.
scoto- ***1)*** Relating to darkness. ***2)*** Visual field gap.
sex- Six.
sial- Relating to saliva.
sinistro- On or to the left.
somato- Relating to the body.
spheno- Relating to the sphenoid bone at the base of the skull.
sphygm(o)- Relating to the pulse.
splanch- ***1)*** Relating to the intestines. ***2)*** Viscera.
spondyl(o)- Relating to the vertebra.
staphyl(o)- Clusters.
steato- Relating to fat.
stetho- Relating to the chest.
stomato- Relating to the mouth.
strept(o)- Twisted chains.
sym- Indicates together with, along with, beside.
syn- Indicates being joined together.
tachy- Indicates swift or fast.
tarso- ***1)*** Relating to the foot. ***2)*** Margin of the eyelid.
teleo- Indicates complete or perfectly formed.
teno- Relating to tendons.
terato- Indicates being seriously deformed, especially a fetus.
thalamo- Relating to the thalamus (origin of nerves in the brain).
thanato- Relating to death.
thoraco- Relating to the chest.
thrombo- Relating to blood clots.
thymo- Relating to the thymus.
toco- Relating to birth.
trachelo- Relating to the neck.
trichi- ***1)*** Hair-like shape. ***2)*** Relating to hair.
tympano- Relating to the eardrum.
typhlo- ***1)*** Relating to blindness. ***2)*** Relating to the cecum.
uni- Single, once, one.
vaso- Relating to blood vessels.
ventro- ***1)*** Anterior surface of the body. ***2)*** Relating to the abdomen.
vesico- Relating to the bladder.
viscero- Relating to the abdominal organs.
xeno- Relating to a foreign substance.
xero- Indicates a dry condition.
-agra Severe pain.
-algia Pain.
-ase Denoting an enzyme.
-asthenia Weakness.

-atresia	Closure, occlusion.
-blast	Incomplete cellular development.
-centesis	Puncture.
-cephal	Relating to the head.
-cle	Small or little.
-cyte	Having to do with cells.
-dactyl	Relating to the fingers or toes.
-desis	Binding or fusion.
-ectomy	Excision, removal.
-emia	Blood.
-ferous	Produces, causes, or brings about.
-fuge	Drive out or expel.
-genic	Production, causation, generation.
-gram	Drawn, written, and recorded.
-graphic	Written or drawn.
-ia	State of being, condition (abnormal).
-iasis	Condition.
-itis	Inflammation.
-lysis	Release, free, reduction of.
-lytic	Destroy, breakdown.
-metry	Scientific measurement.
-odynia	Indicates pain or discomfort.
-oid	Indicates likeness or resemblance.
-ology	Study of.
-oma	Tumor.
-opathy	Relating to disease.
-opexy	Surgical fixation.
-oplasty	Surgical repair.
-orraphy	Suturing.
-orrhagia	Hemorrhage.
-orrhaphy	Suturing.
-oscopy	To examine.
-osis	Condition, process.
-ostomy	Indicates a surgically created artificial opening.
-otomy	Indicates a cutting.
-otripsy	Crushing, destroying.
-pagus	Indicates fixed or joined together.
-paraesis	Indicates weakness.
-pathic	Indicates a feeling, diseased condition, or therapy.
-penia	Indicates a deficiency, less than normal.
-pexy	Fixation.
-philia	Inordinate love of or craving for something.
-phobia	Abnormal fear of or aversion to.
-plasia	Indicates growth, growing.
-plasty	Indicates surgically formed or molded.
-plegia	Indicates a stroke or paralysis.
-pnea	Relating to breath, breathing.
-poietic	Indicates producing or making.
-praxis	Indicates activity, action, condition, or use.
-rhage	Indicates bleeding or other fluid discharge.
-rhaphy	Indicates a suture or seam joining two structures.
-rrhagia	Indicates an abnormal or excessive fluid discharge.
-rrhexis	Splitting or breaking.
-sarcoma	Malignant tumor of flesh or connective tissue.
-spasm	Contraction.
-taxy	Arrangement, grouping.
-tomy	Incision.
-trophy	Relating to food or nutrition.
-tropic	Indicates an affinity for or turning toward.
-tropism	Responding to an external stimulus.
-tumesc(o)	Swelling.

Abbreviations/Acronyms/Symbols

2019-nCoV	COVID-19.
<	Less than.
≤	Less than or equal to.
>	Greater than.
≥	Greater than or equal to.
@	At.
A	***1)*** Absorbance. ***2)*** Adenosine. ***3)*** Artery. ***4)*** Assessment. ***5)*** Blood type.
a fib	Atrial fibrillation.
a flutter	Atrial flutter.
A&O	Alert and oriented.
A&Ox3	Alert and oriented to person, place, and time.
A&P	Auscultation and percussion.
A-P	Anterior posterior.
A-V	***1)*** Arteriovenous. ***2)*** Atrioventricular.
a.a.	Of each.
a.c.	Before meals.
a.d.	***1)*** Right ear. ***2)*** To, up to.
a.m.	Morning.
a.p.	After meals.
a.s.	Left ear.
a.u.	Each ear, both ears.
A/G	Albumin-globulin ratio.

A/S, A.S., or AS	Administrative simplification.
A2	Aortic second sound.
AA	***1)*** Alcoholics Anonymous. ***2)*** Amino acid. ***3)*** Anaplastic astrocytoma. ***4)*** Anesthesiology assistant. ***5)*** Arytenoid adduction.
AAA	Abdominal aortic aneurysm.
AAASF	American Association for the Accreditation of Ambulatory Surgery Facilities.
AABB	American Association of Blood Banks.
AAC	American Academy of Cardiology.
AACD	Aging-associated cognitive decline.
AACG	Acute angle-closure glaucoma.
AACR	American Association for Cancer Research.
AAFP	American Academy of Family Physicians.
AAHomecare	American Association for Homecare.
AAHP	American Association of Health Plans.
AAI	Acute alcohol intoxication.
AAL	Anterior axillary line.
AAMT	American Association for Medical Transcription.
AAN	American Academy of Neurology.
AAO	American Academy of Ophthalmology.
AAO-HNS	American Academy of Otolaryngology—Head and Neck Surgery.
AAOA	American Academy of Otolaryngic Allergy.
AAOS	American Academy of Orthopaedic Surgeons.
AAOMS	American Association of Oral and Maxillofacial Surgeons
AAP	American Academy of Pediatrics.
AAPA	American Academy of Physician Assistants.
AAPAN	American Association of Payers, Administrators, and Networks.
AAPM	Advanced Alternative Payment Models.
AAPM&R	American Academy of Physical Medicine and Rehabilitation.
AAROM	Active assistive range of motion.
AAT	Alpha-1 antitrypsin.
AAV	***1)*** Adeno associated virus. ***2)*** AIDS-associated virus.
AAW	Anterior aortic wall.
AB	***1)*** Abortion. ***2)*** Antibiotic. ***3)*** Antibody. ***4)*** Blood type.
ABA	Allergic bronchopulmonary aspergillosis.
ABBI	Advanced breast biopsy instrumentation.
ABC™	Achievable Benchmark of Care™.
abd	Abdomen.
ABE	Acute bacterial endocarditis.
ABG	Arterial blood gas.
ABI	***1)*** Acquired brain injury. ***2)*** Ankle-brachial index. ***3)*** Auditory brainstem implant.
ABLB test	Alternate binaural loudness balance test.
ABN	Advance beneficiary notice of noncoverage.
abn.	Abnormal.
ABO	***1)*** Blood group system. ***2)*** Referring to ABO incompatibility.
ABPM	Ambulatory blood pressure monitoring.
ABR	Auditory brainstem response.
ABS	Agitated Behavior Scale.
abs. fev.	Absent fever, without fever.
ABVD	Adriamycin, bleomycin, vinblastine, and dacarbazine.
AC	***1)*** Acetate. ***2)*** Acromioclavicular. ***3)*** Adrenal cortex. ***4)*** Air conduction. ***5)*** Alternating current. ***6)*** Antecubital. ***7)*** Anterior cephalic. ***8)*** Anticoagulant. ***9)*** Atriocarotid. ***10)*** Autologous cell.
Ac	***1)*** Acetyl. ***2)*** Actinium.
aC	Arabinosylcytosine.
ac	Acetyl.
ACA	Affordable Care Act.
ACB	Albumin cobalt binding.
ACBE	Air contrast barium enema.
ACBG	Aortocoronary bypass graft.
ACC	***1)*** Adenoid cystic carcinoma. ***2)*** American College of Cardiology.
ACCORD	Action to Control Cardiovascular Risk in Diabetes.
ACD	Absolute cardiac dullness.
ACE	***1)*** Adrenal cortical extract. ***2)*** Angiotensin converting enzyme.
ACEI	Angiotensin-converting enzyme inhibitor.
ACEP	American College of Emergency Physicians.

ACG	***1)*** Ambulatory care group. ***2)*** American College of Gastroenterologists.
ACH	Automated clearinghouse.
ACI	Autologous chondrocyte implantation.
ACL	Anterior cruciate ligament.
ACLE	Acute cutaneous lupus erythematosus.
ACLF	Adult congregate living facility.
ACLS	Advanced cardiac life support.
ACMI	Age-consistent memory impairment.
ACOG	American College of Obstetricians and Gynecologists.
ACP	Acid phosphatase.
ACPO	Acute colonic pseudo-obstruction.
acq.	Acquired.
ACR	***1)*** Adjusted community rating. ***2)*** American College of Radiology. ***3)*** American College of Rheumatology.
ACRF	Acute-on-chronic respiratory failure.
ACS	American College of Surgeons.
ACSV	Aortocoronary saphenous vein.
ACSW	Academy of Certified Social Workers.
ACTH	Adrenocorticotropic hormone.
Acthar	Adrenocorticotropic hormone.
ACTHREL	Corticorelin ovine triflutate.
ACTSEB	Anterior chamber tube shunt to encircling band.
ACVB	Aortocoronary venous bypass.
ACVD	Acute cardiovascular disease.
AD	***1)*** Advance directive. ***2)*** Alzheimer's disease.
ad	To; up to.
ad lib	As desired, at pleasure.
ad part. dolent.	To the aching parts.
ad-hoc	Identification of specific information for a particular instance.
ad. hib.	To be administered.
ad. us. ext.	For external use.
ADA	***1)*** American Dental Association. ***2)*** American Diabetes Association. ***3)*** Americans with Disabilities Act.
ADAM	Androgen deficiency/decline in aging male.
ADAS-L	Alzheimer's Disease Assessment Scale - Late.
ADD	Attention deficit disorder.
ADE	Acute disseminated encephalomyelitis.
ADEM	Acute disseminated encephalomyelitis.
ADG	Ambulatory diagnostic group.
ADH	Antidiuretic hormone.
ADHD	Attention-deficit hyperactivity disorder.
ADKC	Atopic dermatitis with keratoconjunctivitis.
ADL	Activities of daily living.
adm	Admission, admit.
ADM	Alcohol, drug, or mental disorder.
ADMX	Adrenal medullectomy.
ADP	***1)*** Adenosine diphosphate. ***2)*** ALAD porphyria.
ADPKD	Autosomal dominant polycystic kidney disease.
ADR	***1)*** Additional development request. ***2)*** Adverse drug reaction.
ADS	Alternative delivery system.
adst. feb.	Fever is present.
ADT	Adaptation test.
ADT system	Admission/discharge/transfer system.
AE	Above the elbow (amputation).
AED	***1)*** Antiepilepsy drug. ***2)*** Automated external defibrillator.
AERS	Adverse event reporting system.
AESOP	Automated Endoscopic System for Optimal Positioning.
AF	Atrial fibrillation.
AFB	Acid fast bacilli.
AFDC	Aid to families with dependent children.
AFEHCT	Association for Electronic Health Care Transactions.
AFH	Angiofollicular lymph node hyperplasia.
AFI	Amniotic fluid index.
AFO	Ankle foot orthosis.
AFP	Alpha-fetoprotein.
AFT	Autologous fat transfer.
Ag	Silver.
ag. feb.	Increase in fever.
AGA	***1)*** American Gastroenterological Association. ***2)*** Appropriate (average) for gestational age.
AGB	Adjustable gastric banding.
AgNO3	Silver nitrate.
AGV	Ahmed glaucoma valve.
AHA	American Hospital Association.
AHC	Alternative health care.
AHF	Antihemophilic factor.
AHIMA	American Health Information Management Association.
AHIP	America's Health Insurance Plans.
AHRQ	Agency for Healthcare Research and Quality.
AI	***1)*** Aortic insufficiency. ***2)*** Artificial intelligence.

AICC Anti-inhibitor coagulant complex.
AICD Automatic implantable cardioverter-defibrillator.
AID ***1)*** Acute infectious disease.
2) Artificial insemination donor.
AIDS Acquired immunodeficiency syndrome.
AIED Autoimmune inner ear disease.
AIH ***1)*** Artificial insemination by husband.
2) Artificial insemination homologous.
AIHA Autoimmune hemolytic anemia.
AIN Anal intraepithelial neoplasia.
AION Anterior ischemic optic neuropathy.
AIP Acute intermittent porphyria.
AIS Androgen insensitivity syndrome.
AK ***1)*** Above the knee (amputation).
2) Actinic keratosis(es).
AKA ***1)*** Above knee amputation.
2) Also known as.
3) Antikeratin antibodies.
AKI Acute kidney injury.
Al Aluminum.
Ala ***1)*** Alanine.
2) Alpha-linolenic acid.
3) Aminolevulinic acid.
ALARA As low as reasonably achievable.
Alb Albumin.
alb. (albus) White.
ALD Assistive listening device.
ALIF Anterior lumbar interbody fusion.
ALJ Administrative law judge.
ALK Automated lamellar keratoplasty.
alk. phos. Alkaline phosphatase.
ALL Acute lymphocytic leukemia.
ALOS Average length of stay.
ALP Alkaline phosphatase.
ALS ***1)*** Advanced life support.
2) Amyotrophic lateral sclerosis.
ALT Alanine aminotransferase.
alt. dieb. Every other day.
alt. hor. Every other hour.
alt. noc. Every other night.
AMA ***1)*** Against medical advice.
2) American Medical Association.
amb Ambulate.
AMD Age-related macular degeneration.
AMH Anti-mullerian hormone.
AMI Acute myocardial infarction.
AMIA American Medical Informatics Association.
AML Acute myelogenous or myelocytic leukemia.
AMLOS Arithmetic mean length of stay.
AMLS Advanced medical life support.
AMML Acute myelomonocytic leukemia.
AMP ***1)*** Adenosine monophosphate.
2) Ampule.
AMT Amniotic membrane transplant.
ANA ***1)*** American Nursing Association.
2) Antinuclear antibodies.
ANC Absolute neutrophil count.
ANDI Aberrations of normal development and involution.
ANF Antinuclear factor.
ANP Atrial natriuretic peptide.
ANS ***1)*** American National Standards.
2) Autonomic nervous system.
ANSI American National Standards Institute.
ANSI/HISB American National Standards Institute Health Information Standards Board.
ant Anterior.
ANUG Acute necrotizing ulcerative gingivitis.
Ao Aorta.
AOA American Osteopathic Association.
AOD Arterial occlusive disease.
AODM Adult onset diabetes mellitus.
AOSD Adult onset Still's disease.
AP ***1)*** Angina pectoris.
2) Antepartum.
3) Anterior pituitary.
4) Anteroposterior.
5) Apical.
6) Arterial pressure.
AP-DRG All patient diagnosis-related group.
APA ***1)*** American Psychiatric Association.
2) Antipernicious anemia factor.
3) Antiphospholipid (antibody) syndrome.
APACHE II Acute physiology and chronic health evaluation score.
APAP ***1)*** Acetaminophen.
2) Autotitrating continuous positive airway pressure.
APB Abductor pollicis brevis.
APBI Accelerated partial breast irradiation.
APC ***1)*** Adenoidal pharyngeal conjunctival virus.
2) Ambulatory payment classification.
3) Antigen presenting cell.
APEC Asymmetrical periflexural exanthem of childhood.
APG Ambulatory patient group.
APL Abductor pollicis longus.
APLAS Antiphospholipid syndrome or antiphospholipid antibody syndrome.
APLS Antiphospholipid antibody syndrome.
APM ***1)*** Alternative Payment Model.
2) Arterial pressure monitoring.

Abbreviations

approx	Approximately.
appy	Appendectomy.
APR	Average payment rate.
APR-DRG	All Patient Refined Diagnosis Related Group.
APRN	Advanced Practice Registered Nurse.
APT	Admissions per thousand.
APTT	Activated partial thromboplastin time.
aq.	Water (aqua).
AQA	Ambulatory Care Quality Alliance.
AQMBF	Absolute quantitation of myocardial blood flow.
Ar	Periodic table chemical element symbol for argon.
AR	Acoustic reflex.
araC	Arabinosylcytosine.
ARB	Angiotensin receptor blocker.
ARC	AIDS-related complex.
ARD	Acute respiratory disease.
ARDS	Acute respiratory distress syndrome.
ARF	***1)*** Acute renal failure. ***2)*** Acute respiratory failure. ***3)*** Acute rheumatic fever.
ARMD	Age-related macular degeneration.
AROM	***1)*** Active range of motion. ***2)*** Artificial rupture of membranes.
ARPKD	Autosomal recessive polycystic kidney disease.
ARRA	American recovery and reinvestment act of 2009.
ART	***1)*** Accredited record technician. ***2)*** Arterial.
art.	Artery, arterial.
AS	***1)*** Aortic stenosis. ***2)*** Arteriosclerosis. ***3)*** Associate of Science.
ASA	Acetylsalicylic acid.
ASAP	As soon as possible.
ASC	Ambulatory surgery center.
asc.	Ascending.
ASCO	American Society of Clinical Oncology.
ASCP	***1)*** American Society for Clinical Pathology. ***2)*** American Society for Consultant Pharmacists.
ASCUS	Atypical squamous cells of undetermined significance.
ASCVD	Arteriosclerotic cardiovascular disease.
ASCX12N	American Standard Committee standard for claims and reimbursement.
ASD	***1)*** Atrial septal defect. ***2)*** Autism spectrum disorder.
ASH	Asymmetric septal hypertrophy.
ASHD	Arteriosclerotic heart disease.
ASIS	Anterosuperior iliac spine.
ASN	Associate of Science, Nursing.
Asn	Asparagine.
ASO	***1)*** Administrative services only. ***2)*** Antistreptolysin O.
Asp	Aspartic acid.
ASPE	Assistant Secretary for Planning and Evaluation.
ASPIRE	AFEHCT's Administrative Simplification Print Image Research Effort work group.
ASR	Age/sex rate.
Asst	Assistance (min= minimal; mod= moderate).
ASST	***1)*** Autologous serum skin test. ***2)*** Assistance (min = minimal; mod = moderate).
AST	Aspartate aminotransferase.
Ast	Astigmatism.
ASTM	American Society for Testing and Materials.
ASTRO	American Society for Radiation Oncology.
At	Periodic table chemical element symbol for astatine.
ATCB	Authorized Testing and Certification Body.
ATFL	Anterior talofibular ligament.
ATL	***1)*** Adult T-cell leukemia. ***2)*** Adult T-cell lymphoma.
ATLL	Adult T-cell leukemia/lymphoma.
ATP	Adenosine triphosphate.
ATT	Attached.
AUA	American Urological Association.
AUDIT	Alcohol use disorder identification test.
AUR	Ambulatory utilization review.
AuSCT	Autologous stem cell transplantation.
AV	***1)*** Arteriovenous. ***2)*** Atrioventricular.
AVF	Arteriovenous fistula.
AVM	Arteriovenous malformation.
AVN	Atrioventricular node.
AVP	Antiviral protein.
AW	Atomic weight.
AWP	***1)*** Any willing provider. ***2)*** Average wholesale price.
AWV	Annual wellness visit.
ax	***1)*** Axillary. ***2)*** Axis.
AZH	Assisted zonal hatching.
AZT	Azidothymidine.

b	Bone.
B&B	Bowel and bladder.
B-PLL	B-cell prolymphocytic leukemia.
b.i.d.	Two times a day.
b.i.n.	Twice a night.
b.i.s.	Twice.
BA	Business associate.
Ba	Barium.
BAC	Blood alcohol content or concentration.
BADL	Basic activities of daily living.
BAE	Bi-atrial enlargement.
BAEP	Brainstem auditory evoked potential.
BAER	Brainstem auditory evoked response.
BAHA	Bone anchored hearing aid.
BAL	Bronchoalveolar lavage.
bal.	Bath.
BALB	Binaural alternate loudness balance.
BAT	Brightness acuity test.
BB	Blow bottles.
BBA	Balanced Budget Act of 1997.
BBB	***1)*** Blood brain barrier. ***2)*** Bundle branch block.
BBRA	Balanced Budget Refinement Act of 1999.
BBT	Basal body temperature.
BCBS	Blue Cross Blue Shield.
BCBSA	Blue Cross and Blue Shield Association.
BCC	Basal cell carcinoma.
BCG live intravesical vaccine	Bacillus Calmette-Guerin bladder vaccine.
BCI	Bone conduction implant.
BCLS	Basic cardiac life support.
BCP	Birth control pill.
BCT	Breast-conservation therapy.
BDAE	Boston Diagnostic Aphasia Examination.
BE	***1)*** Barium enema. ***2)*** Below the elbow.
Be	Periodic table chemical element symbol for beryllium.
BFLS	Borjeson-Forssman-Lehmann syndrome.
BHR	Birmingham Hip Resurfacing system.
BI	Brain injury.
BIA-ALCL	Breast Implant Associated Anaplastic Large Cell Lymphoma.
BIB	Brought in by.
bib.	Drink.
BIBA	Brought in by ambulance.
BICROS	Bilateral routing of signals.
BID/b.i.d.	Twice daily.
BIID	Body integrity identity disorder.
BIPA	Benefits Improvement and Protection Act of 2000.
BiPap	Bilevel positive airway pressure.
BIS	Bioimpedance spectroscopy.
BK	Below the knee.
BKA	Below-the-knee amputation.
BLDS	Brachmann-de Lange syndrome.
BLS	***1)*** Basic life support. ***2)*** Bureau of Labor Statistics.
BM	Bowel movement.
BMA	Bone marrow aspiration.
BMAC	Breath methylated alkane contour.
BMD	Bone mineral density.
BMI	Body mass index.
BMP	Bone morphogenetic protein.
BMR	Basal metabolic rate.
BMS	Burning mouth syndrome.
BMT	***1)*** Bilateral myringotomy and tubes. ***2)*** Bone marrow transplant.
BNEd	Bachelor of Nursing Education.
BNO	Bladder neck obstruction.
BO	Body odor.
Bol.	Bolus.
BOOP	Bronchiolitis obliterans with organizing pneumonia.
BOW	Bag of waters.
BP	***1)*** Blood pressure. ***2)*** Business partner.
BPCI	Bundled Payments for Care Improvement.
BPD	***1)*** Biliopancreatic diversion. ***2)*** Bronchopulmonary dysplasia.
BPF	Bronchopleural fistula.
BPH	***1)*** Bachelor of Public Health. ***2)*** Benign prostatic hyperplasia. ***3)*** Benign prostatic hypertrophy.
bpm	Beats per minute.
BPPV	Benign positional paroxysmal vertigo.
Br	Bromine.
BRAO	Branch retinal artery occlusion.
BRAT	Bananas, rice cereal, applesauce or juice, and toast.
BRBPR	Bright red blood per rectum.
BrC	Breast care.
BRM	Biological response modifier.
BRP	***1)*** Bathroom, private. ***2)*** Bathroom privileges.
BS	***1)*** Bachelor of Science. ***2)*** Bowel sounds. ***3)*** Breath sounds.
BSA	Body surface area.

BSC Bedside commode.
BSD Bedside drainage.
BSE ***1)*** Bovine spongiform encephalopathy.
2) Breast self-examination.
BSER Brainstem evoked response.
BSN Bachelor of Science, Nursing.
BSO Bilateral salpingo-oophorectomy.
BSS Balanced salt solution.
BT Bleeding time.
BTE Behind the ear.
BTPS Body temperature, ambient pressure, saturated.
BTT Bridge to transplant.
BTX Botulinum toxin.
BUN Blood urea nitrogen.
BUR Back-up rate (ventilator).
BUS Bartholin urethra Skene's.
BW Body or birth weight.
bx Biopsy.
C ***1)*** Calorie.
2) Carbon.
3) Celsius.
4) Centigrade.
5) Cervical vertebrae.
6) Complements.
c With.
C&S Culture and sensitivity.
C-collar Cervical collar.
c.m. Tomorrow morning.
c.n. Tomorrow night.
C/A/Ox3 Conscious, alert, and oriented to person, place, and time.
c/m Counts per minute.
c/o Complains of.
C/S Cesarean section.
ca About or approximately.
CA ***1)*** Calcium.
2) Cancer or carcinoma.
3) Cardiac arrest.
4) Contrast angiography.
CABG Coronary artery bypass graft.
CAC Certified alcoholism counselor.
CACI Computer-assisted continuous infusion.
CAD ***1)*** Cold agglutinin disease.
2) Computer aided detection.
3) Coronary artery disease.
CAH Critical Access Hospital.
CAHPS Consumer Assessment of Healthcare Providers and Systems.
CAM ***1)*** Complementary and alternative medicine.
2) Continuous active motion.
CAO Conscious, alert, oriented.
Cap Capitation.
cap Capsule.
CAP ***1)*** Capitation.
2) Catabolite activator-protein.
3) College of American Pathologists.
4) Community-acquired pneumonia.
5) Contract maximum.
CAPD ***1)*** Central auditory processing disorder.
2) Continuous ambulatory peritoneal dialysis.
caps. Capsule.
CAPSO Cautery-assisted palatal stiffening operation.
Carb Carbohydrate.
CARC Claim adjustment reason code.
CART CMS Abstraction and Reporting Tool.
CAR-T Chimeric antigen receptor T-cell.
CAS Computer-assisted surgery.
CAT Computerized axial tomography.
cath Catheterize.
CBC Complete blood count.
CBG ***1)*** Capillary blood glucose.
2) Corticosteroid binding globulin.
CBGCD Closed-loop blood glucose control device.
CBI Continuous bladder irrigation.
CBN Chronic benign neutropenia.
CBO Congressional Budget Office or Cost Budget Office.
CBR Complete bedrest.
CBSA Core-based statistical area.
CBT Cognitive-behavioral therapy.
cc ***1)*** Chief complaint.
2) Complication or comorbid condition.
3) Cubic centimeter.
CCHD Critical Congenital Heart Defect/Disease.
CCI Correct Coding Initiative.
CCK Cholecystokinin.
CCM Cardiac contractility modulation.
CCM-D Cardiac contractility modulation-defibrillation.
CCNU Chloroethyl-cyclohexyl-nitrosourea.
CCP Cyclic citrullinated peptide.
CCPD Continuous cycling peritoneal dialysis.
CCU Coronary care unit.
CDA Certified dental assistant.
CDC Centers for Disease Control and Prevention.
CDD CDKL5 deficiency disorder.
CDGS Carbohydrate-deficient glycoprotein syndrome.

CDH	Congenital dislocation of hip.
CDI	Clinical documentation improvement.
CDKL5	Cyclin-dependent kinase-like 5.
CDP	Complex decongestive physiotherapy.
CDP-SOT	Computerized dynamic posturography sensory organization test.
CDS	Clinical Decision Support.
CDSM	Clinical Decision Support Mechanism.
CDT	Current Dental Terminology.
CE	***1)*** Cardiac enlargement. ***2)*** Covered entity.
CEA	***1)*** Carcinoembryonic antigen. ***2)*** Carotid endarterectomy.
CEC	Comprehensive ESRD care.
CEHRT	Certified electronic health record technology.
CEN	European Center for Standardization, or Comite Europeen de Normalisation.
CEPD	Cerebral embolic protective device.
CERT	Comprehensive Error Rate Testing.
CEU	Continuing education unit.
CF	Cystic fibrosis.
CFR	Code of Federal Regulations.
CGF	Congenital generalized fibromatosis.
CGM	Continuous glucose monitoring.
CGMS	Continuous glucose monitoring system.
CH	Cholesterol.
CH, Chol	Cholesterol.
CHAMPUS	Civilian Health and Medical Program of the Uniformed Services.
CHAMPVA	Civilian Health and Medical Program of the Department of Veterans Affairs.
CHCT	Caffeine halothane contracture test.
CHD	***1)*** Congenital heart disease. ***2)*** Congestive heart disease.
CHF	Congestive heart failure.
chgd	Changed.
CHIM	Center for Healthcare Information Management.
CHIME	College of Healthcare Information Management Executives.
CHIP	Children's Health Insurance Program.
CHL	Conductive hearing loss.
chr.	Chronic.
CHS	Cannabinoid hyperemesis syndrome.
CI	***1)*** Cardiac index. ***2)*** Chloride. ***3)*** Confidence interval.
CIC	Completely in the canal (hearing aid).
CIDP	Chronic inflammatory demyelinating polyradiculoneuropathy.
CIG	Cardiointegram.
CIM	Coverage Issues Manual.
CIN	***1)*** Cervical intraepithelial neoplasia. ***2)*** Contrast-induced nephropathy. See also nephrotoxicity, contrast-induced.
CIS	Carcinoma in situ.
CIU	Chronic idiopathic urticaria.
CJD	Creutzfeldt-Jakob disease.
CJR	Comprehensive care for joint replacement.
CK	Conductive keratoplasty.
CKD	Chronic kidney disease.
CL	Chloride.
cl liqs	Clear liquids.
CLA	Certified laboratory assistant.
CLC	Creative living center.
CLD	***1)*** Chronic liver disease. ***2)*** Chronic lung disease.
CLEAR	Clear lens extraction and replacement.
CLI	Critical limb ischemia.
CLIA	Clinical Laboratory Improvement Amendments.
CLL	Chronic lymphatic leukemia.
Clsd	Closed.
CLT	Complex lymphedema therapy.
cm	Centimeter.
cm2	Square centimeters.
CMA	Certified medical assistant.
CMC	Carpometacarpal.
CME	***1)*** Continuing medical education. ***2)*** Cystoid macular edema.
CMG	Cystometrogram.
CMHC	Community mental health center.
CMI	Case mix index.
CML	Chronic myelogenous leukemia.
CMMI	Centers for Medicare and Medicaid Innovation (CMS Innovation Center).
CMML	Chronic myelomonocytic leukemia.
CMN	Certificate of medical necessity.
CMO	Chief medical officer.
CMP	Competitive medical plan.
CMRI	Cardiac magnetic resonance imaging.
CMS	***1)*** Centers for Medicare and Medicaid Services. ***2)*** Circulation motion sensation.
CMS-1450	Universal form used to file institutional claims.
CMS-1500	Universal paper billing form developed by CMS.
CMSA	Consolidated Metropolitan Statistical Area.
CMT	Certified medical transcriptionist.
CMV	***1)*** Controlled mechanical ventilation. ***2)*** Cytomegalovirus.

Abbreviations

cn Cranial nerves.
CNA Certified nursing assistant.
CNM Certified nurse midwife.
CNP ***1)*** Community nurse practitioner.
2) Continuous negative airway pressure.
CNS Central nervous system.
co Cardiac output.
Co Periodic table chemical element symbol for cobalt.
CO2 Carbon dioxide.
COA Certificate of authority.
CoA Coenzyme A.
COB Coordination of benefits.
COBRA Consolidated Omnibus Reconciliation Act.
COC Certificate of coverage.
COH Controlled ovarian hyperstimulation.
COI Collection of information.
COLD Chronic obstructive lung disease.
COLST Clinician order for life-sustaining treatment.
COMP Compounded.
COMS Concurrent optical and magnetic stimulation.
CON Certificate of need.
conc Concentrate.
cont. Continue.
COPD Chronic obstructive pulmonary disease.
CORF Comprehensive outpatient rehabilitation facility.
COT ***1)*** Certified ophthalmic technician.
2) Chain of trust.
COTA Certified occupational therapy assistant.
COTD Cardiac output thermodilution.
COVID-19 Coronavirus disease 2019.
CP ***1)*** Cerebral palsy.
2) Clinical psychologist.
CPAP Continuous positive airway pressure.
CPB Cardiopulmonary bypass.
CPC+ Comprehensive Primary Care Plus.
CPCI Comprehensive Primary Care Initiative.
CPD Cephalopelvic disproportion.
CPHA Commission on Professional and Hospital Activities.
CPI Consumer price index.
CPK Creatine phosphokinase.
CPM Continuous passive motion.
CPOE Computerized provider order entry.
CPR ***1)*** Cardiopulmonary resuscitation.
2) Comparative performance report.
3) Computerized patient record.
4) Customary, prevailing, and reasonable.
CPRI-HOST Computer-based Patient Record Institute-Healthcare Open Systems and Trials.
CPS ***1)*** Chronic pain syndrome.
2) Composite performance score.
CPT ***1)*** Chest physical therapy.
2) Cold pressor test.
3) Current Procedural Terminology.
CPT-4 Current Procedural Terminology, Fourth Edition.
CPTA CPT® Assistant.
CQI Continuous quality improvement.
CQM Clinical quality measure.
CR ***1)*** Carrier replacement.
2) Creatine.
CRAO Central retinal artery occlusion.
CRBSI Catheter-related blood stream infection.
CRC Community rating by class.
CRF Chronic renal failure.
CRH Corticotropic releasing hormone.
crit. Hematocrit.
CRM Cardiac rhythm management.
CRNA Certified registered nurse anesthetist.
CROS Contralateral routing of signals.
CRP C-reactive protein.
CRPS Complex regional pain syndrome.
CRS Cytokine release syndrome.
CRT Certified respiratory therapist.
CS ***1)*** Cardiogenic shock.
2) Central service.
3) Cesarean section.
4) Culture and sensitivity.
CSAC Consensus Standards Approval Committee.
CSC Cancer stem cells.
CSE Convulsive status epilepticus.
CSF Cerebrospinal fluid.
CSO Clinical service organization.
CSR Coronary sinus reduction.
CST Certified surgical technologist.
CSV CMS-certified survey vendor.
CSW Clinical social worker.
CT ***1)*** Carpal tunnel syndrome.
2) Computed tomography.
3) Corneal thickness.
CTA Computed tomographic angiography.
CTLSO Cervical-thoracic-lumbar-sacral orthosis.

CTPN Central total parenteral nutrition.
CTR ***1)*** Capsular tension ring.
2) Cardiothoracic ratio.
CTZ Chemoreceptor trigger zone.
cu ***1)*** Chronic urticaria.
2) Cubic.
CUPS Cancer of unknown primary site.
CV Cardiovascular.
CVA ***1)*** Cerebrovascular accident.
2) Costovertebral accident.
3) Costovertebral angle.
4) Cough variant asthma.
CVC Central venous catheter.
CVD ***1)*** Cardiovascular disease.
2) Cerebrovascular disease.
cVEMP Cervical vestibular evoked myogenic potential.
CVI Chronic venous insufficiency.
CVL Central venous line.
CVMS Clean voided midstream urine.
CVP Central venous pressure.
CVS ***1)*** Cardiovascular system.
2) Chorionic villus sampling.
CVU Cerebrovascular unit.
CW Closed ward.
CWF Common working file.
CXR Chest x-ray.
CXy Chest x-ray.
CY Calendar year.
cysto Cystoscopy.
D ***1)*** Day.
2) Diopter.
D&C Dilation and curettage.
D.H.E. 45 Dihydroergotamine mesylate.
D/C ***1)*** Discharge.
2) Discontinue.
D/R Dayroom.
D/W Dextrose in water.
D5W Dextrose, 5 percent in water.
DAE Distal acinar emphysema.
DAFO Dynamic ankle foot orthoses.
DAST Drug abuse screening test.
DAW Dispense as written.
DBP Diastolic blood pressure.
DBS Deep brain stimulation.
DC ***1)*** Direct current.
2) Discontinue.
3) Doctor of chiropractic medicine.
DCA Diabetic cheiroarthropathy.
DCC Data Content Committee.
DCCT Diabetes control and complications trial.
DCd ***1)*** Discharged.
2) Discontinued.
DCP Dynamic compression plate.
DCR Dacryocystorhinostomy.
DD ***1)*** Data dictionary.
2) Down drain.
DDD Degenerative disc disease.
DDE Direct data entry.
DDH Developmental dysplasia of the hip.
DDKT Deceased donor kidney transplant.
DDST Denver developmental screening test.
DE Dose equivalent.
DeCC Dental Content Committee.
decem Ten.
decub. ***1)*** Decubitus ulcer.
2) Lying down.
def. Deficient, deficiency.
del Delivery.
dep. Dependent.
DEXA Dual energy x-ray absorptiometry.
dexter Right.
dextra Right.
DFSP Dermatofibrosarcoma protuberans.
DHEA Dehydroepiandrosterone.
DHHS Department of Health and Human Services.
DHS Dynamic hip screw.
DHT Dihydrotestosterone.
DI ***1)*** Diabetes insipidus.
2) Dorsal interossei.
DIC Disseminated intravascular coagulopathy.
DICOM Digital imaging and communications in medicine.
DIEP flap Deep inferior epigastric perforator flap.
DIF Direct immunofluorescence.
dil. Dilute, diluted.
DILE Drug-induced lupus erythematosus.
dim. Divide in half.
DIOS Distal intestinal obstruction syndrome.
DISA Data Interchange Standards Association.
DISH Diffuse idiopathic skeletal hyperostosis.
DISI Dorsal intercalated segment instability.
disp Disposition.
DJD Degenerative joint disease.
DKA Diabetic ketoacidosis.
dL Deciliter.
DLI Donor leukocyte infusion.
DM Diabetes mellitus.
DMAA Distal metatarsal articular angle.

DMARDS	Disease-modifying antirheumatic drugs.
DMD	Duchenne muscular dystrophy.
DME	Durable medical equipment.
DME MAC	Durable medical equipment Medicare administrative contractor.
DME PDAC	Durable Medical Equipment Pricing Data Analysis and Coding.
DMEPOS	Durable medical equipment, prosthetics, orthotics, and supplies.
DMERC	Durable medical equipment regional carrier.
DMPA	Depot medroxyprogesterone acetate.
DNA	Deoxyribonucleic acid.
DNET	Desembryoplastic neuroepithelial tumor.
DNH	Do not hospitalize.
DNP	Do not publish.
DNR	Do not resuscitate.
DNS	***1)*** Deviated nasal septum. ***2)*** Do not show. ***3)*** Dysplastic nevus syndrome.
DO	Doctor of osteopathy.
DOA	Dead on arrival.
DOAC	Direct oral anticoagulant.
DOB	Date of birth.
doc.	Doctor.
DOE	Dyspnea on exertion.
DOJ	Department of Justice.
DOMS	Delayed onset muscle soreness.
DOR	Diminished ovarian reserve.
DOS	Date of service.
DPM	***1)*** Doctor of podiatric medicine. ***2)*** Double-plated Molteno.
DPNP	Diabetic peripheral neuropathy pain.
DPOW	Dilated Pore of Winer.
DPR	Drug price review.
DPT	***1)*** Days per thousand. ***2)*** Diphtheria-pertussis-tetanus.
DPU	Delayed pressure urticaria.
Dr	Doctor.
DR	***1)*** Delivery room. ***2)*** Diagnostic radiology. ***3)*** Diurnal rhythm.
dr.	Dram.
DRE	Digital rectal exam.
DRG	Diagnosis related group.
DRS	Duane's retraction syndrome.
Dsg	Dressing.
DSH	Disproportionate share hospital, as designated by CMS.
DSI	Dysfunction of sensory integration.
DSM-5	Diagnostic and Statistical Manual of Mental Disorders, Fifth Edition.
DSM-IV-TR	Diagnostic and Statistical Manual of Mental Disorders, Fourth Edition,
DSMO	Designated Standard Maintenance Organization.
DSMT	Diabetes self-management training.
DSS	***1)*** Dioctyl sulfosuccinate. ***2)*** Double simultaneous stimulation.
DSTU	Draft standard for trial use.
DT	Delirium tremens.
DTI	Diffusion tensor imaging.
DTPI	Deep tissue pressure injury.
DTR	Deep tendon reflexes.
DUE	Drug use evaluation.
duo	Two.
duodecim.	Twelve.
DUR	Drug utilization review.
dur. dolor.	While pain lasts.
DVD	Developmental verbal dyspraxia.
DVM	Doctor of Veterinary Medicine.
DVT	Deep vein thrombosis.
Dx	Diagnosis.
DX	Diagnosis code.
DXA	Dual energy x-ray absorptiometry.
dz	Disease.
e.g.	For example.
e.m.p.	As directed.
E/M	Evaluation and management services.
E/M codes	Evaluation and management service codes.
E2	Estradiol.
Ea	Each.
EAC	***1)*** Esophageal adenocarcinoma. ***2)*** External auditory canal.
ead.	Same.
EAP	Employee assistance program.
EBL	Estimated blood loss.
EBUS	Endobronchial ultrasound.
EBV	Epstein-Barr virus.
EC	***1)*** Electronic commerce. ***2)*** Eligible clinician.
ECCE	Extracapsular cataract extraction.
ECF	***1)*** Extended care facility. ***2)*** Extracellular fluid.
ECG	Electrocardiogram.
eCGI	Electronic clinical quality improvement.
ECHO	***1)*** Echocardiogram. ***2)*** Enterocytopathogenic human orphan virus.
ECLS	Extracorporeal life support.

ECMO	Extracorporeal membrane oxygenation.
ECOG	Electrocochleography.
ECP	Endoscopic cyclophotocoagulation.
eCQM	Electronic Clinical Quality Measure.
ECT	***1)*** Electroconvulsive therapy. ***2)*** Emission computerized tomography.
ectopic	Ectopic pregnancy (OB).
ED	***1)*** Effective dose. ***2)*** Egg donation. ***3)*** Emergency department.
Ed.D	Doctor of education.
EDC	***1)*** Estimated date of confinement. ***2)*** Expected date of confinement.
EDI	Electronic data interchange.
EDIFACT	Electronic Data Interchange for Administration, Commerce, and Transport.
EDR	Extreme drug resistance.
EDS	Ehlers-Danlos syndrome.
EEG	Electroencephalogram.
EENT	Eye, ear, nose, and throat.
EES	Everolimus-eluting stent.
EF	Ejection fraction.
EFAST	Extended focused assessment with sonography in trauma.
EFT	Electronic funds transfer.
EGA	Estimated gestational age.
EGD	Esophagus, stomach, and duodenum.
EGFR	Epidermal growth factor receptor.
EGHP	Employer group health plan.
EGIDs	Eosinophilic gastrointestinal disorders.
EGPA	Eosinophilic granulomatosis with polyangiitis.
EHBF	Estimated hepatic blood flow.
EHNAC	Electronic Healthcare Network Accreditation Commission.
EHO	Emerging healthcare organizations.
EHR	Electronic health record.
EI	Electrical impedance.
EIA	Enzyme immunoassay.
EIB	Exercise induced bronchospasm.
EIN	Employer identification number.
EIS	Electrical impedance spectroscopy.
EKG	Electrocardiogram.
ELBW	Extremely low birth weight.
ELISA	Enzyme-linked immunosorbent assay.
ELOS	Estimated length of stay.
ELT	Excimer laser trabeculostomy.
EMC	Electronic media claims.
EMG	Electromyogram.
EMI	Electromagnetic interference.
EMR	Electronic medical record.
EMS	Emergency medical service.
EMT	Emergency medical technician.
EMT-P	Paramedic.
EMTALA	Emergency Medical Treatment and Active Labor Act.
en	***1)*** Clyster. ***2)*** Enema.
en bloc	In total.
ENG	Electronystagmogram.
eng.	Engorged.
ENOG	Electroneuronography.
ENT	Ear, nose, and throat.
EO	Elbow orthosis.
EOB	Explanation of benefits.
EOG	Electrooculography.
EOI	Evidence of insurability.
EOM	***1)*** End of month. ***2)*** Extraocular motion. ***3)*** Extraocular muscles.
EOMB	Explanation of Medicare benefits.
EOMI	Extraocular motion intact.
EOP	External occipital protuberance.
EOTTS	Extra osseous talotarsal stabilization.
EOY	End of year.
EP	***1)*** Electrophysiologic. ***2)*** Eligible professional.
EPB	Extensor pollicis brevis.
EPCA	Early prostate cancer antigen.
EPF	Endoscopic plantar fasciotomy.
Epis.	Episiotomy.
EPO	***1)*** Epoetin alpha. ***2)*** Exclusive provider organization.
EPP	Erythropoietic protoporphyria.
EPS	***1)*** Electrophysiological stimulation. ***2)*** Electrophysiological study.
EPSDT	Early and Periodic Screening, Diagnosis and Treatment Program.
ER	Emergency room.
ER+	Estrogen receptor positive status.
ER-	Estrogen receptor negative status.
ERA	Electronic remittance advice.
ERC	Endoscopic retrograde cholangiography.
ERCP	Endoscopic retrograde cholangiopancreatography.
ERG	Electroretinogram.
ESR	Erythrocyte sedimentation rate.
ESRD	End stage renal disease.
EST	Electroshock therapy.
ESW	Extracorporeal shockwave.
ESWL	Extracorporeal shockwave lithotripsy.

Abbreviations

et	And.
ET	Endotracheal.
ETD	Eustachian tube dysfunction.
ETG	Episode treatment group.
ETOH	Alcohol.
ETS	Endoscopic thoracic sympathectomy.
EVALI	E-cigarette or vaping product use-associated lung injury.
EVAR	***1)*** Endovascular aneurysm repair. ***2)*** Endovascular aortic repair.
EVD	Ebola virus disease.
EVR	Evoked visual response.
Ex	***1)*** Examination. ***2)*** Extended.
exc	Excise.
Ext	External.
ext.	Extremity.
extr.	Extract.
F	***1)*** Fahrenheit. ***2)*** Female. ***3)*** Firm. ***4)*** French.
F (on OB)	Firm.
f.m.	Make a mixture.
F/U	Follow-up.
FA	***1)*** Fatty acid. ***2)*** Fractional anisotropy.
FACS	Fluorescence-activated cell sorting.
FAP	Familial adenomatous polyposis.
FAQ	Frequently asked question.
FAR	Federal acquisition regulations.
FAS	Fetal alcohol syndrome.
FAST	***1)*** Focused aspiration of scar tissue. ***2)*** Functional assessment staging. ***3)*** Focused assessment with sonography in trauma.
FB	***1)*** Finger breadths. ***2)*** Foreign body.
FBR	Foreign body removal.
FBS	Fasting blood sugar.
FCE	Functional capacity evaluation.
FCMS	Foix-Chavany-Marie syndrome.
FCR	Flexor carpi radialis.
FDA	Food and Drug Administration.
FDG	2-(Flourine-18)-fluoro-2-dexoy-D-glucose.
FDG-PET	Positron emission with tomography with 18 fluorodeoxyglucose.
FDH syndrome	Focal dermal hypoplasia syndrome.
FDP	***1)*** Fibrin degradation products. ***2)*** Flexor digitorum profundus tendon.
FDS	Functional dementia scale.
Fe	***1)*** Female. ***2)*** Iron.
FEF	Frontal eye field.
FEHB	Federal Employee Health Benefits Program.
FEHBAR	Federal Employee Health Benefits Acquisition Regulations.
Fem	Female.
FERPA	Family Educational Rights and Privacy Act.
FES	Functional electrical stimulation.
FESS	Functional endoscopic sinus surgery.
FET	Frozen embryo transfer.
FEV	Forced expiratory volume.
FFDM	Full field digital mammography.
FFL	Flexible fiberoptic laryngoscopy.
FFP	Fresh frozen plasma.
FFR	Fractional flow reserve.
FFS	Fee for service.
FGM	Female genital mutilation.
FH	Family history.
FHI	Fuchs' heterochromic iridocyclitis.
FHR	Fetal heart rate.
FHT	Fetal heart tone.
FI	***1)*** Firm one finger down from umbilicus. ***2)*** Fiscal intermediary.
FIA	FIA
FiO2	Fraction of inspired oxygen.
FIPS	Federal information processing standards.
FLA	Focal laser ablation.
Fld.	Fluid(s).
fluoro	Fluoroscopy.
FM	Face mask.
FMD	Fibromuscular dysplasia.
FME	Full-mouth extraction.
FMG	Fine mesh gauze.
FMP	Final menstrual period.
FMPA	Focused microwave phased array.
FMR	Focused medical review.
FMR1	Fragile x messenger ribonucleoprotein 1.
fMRI	Functional magnetic resonance imaging.
FMT	Focused microwave therapy.
FNP	Family nurse practitioner.
FO	Finger orthosis.
FOBT	Fecal occult blood test.
FOD	Free of disease.
fort.	Strong (fortis).
FOTO	Focus on therapeutic outcomes.

FP	***1)*** Family planning. ***2)*** Family practitioner.
FPD	Fixed partial denture.
FPL	Flexor pollicis longus.
FPP	Faculty practice plan.
FQHC	Federally qualified health center.
FR	***1)*** Family relationship. ***2)*** Federal Register.
FRAT	Free radical assay test.
FREDI	Fallopian replacement of egg with delayed intrauterine insemination.
FSA	Flexible spending account.
FSE	Fetal scalp electrode.
FSF	Frontal sinus fracture.
FSH	Follicle stimulating hormone.
ft	Foot.
FTE	Full time employee.
FTND	***1)*** Fagerstrom Test for Nicotine Dependence. ***2)*** Full-term normal delivery.
FTQ	Fagerstrom Tolerance Questionnaire.
FTSG	Full thickness skin graft.
FTT	Failure to thrive.
FUO	Fever of unknown origin.
FVC	Forced vital capacity.
fx	Fracture.
fxBB	Fracture, both bones.
FY	Fiscal year.
G	Gram.
G-CSF	Filgrastim (granulocyte colony-stimulating factor).
g-tube	Gastrostomy tube.
GA	Gastric analysis.
GAO	***1)*** General accounting office. ***2)*** Government Accountability Office.
GAP	Gluteal artery perforator.
gav.	Gavage.
GAVE	Gastric antral vascular ectasia.
GB	Gallbladder.
GBM	Glioblastoma multiforme.
GBS	Group B Streptococcus.
GCA	Giant cell arteritis.
GCS	Glasgow Coma Score.
GDD	Glaucoma drainage device.
GDM	Gestational diabetes mellitus.
GDS	Geriatric depression scale.
GEA	Global endometrial ablation.
GEM	General equivalence mapping.
GERD	Gastroesophageal reflux disease.
GES	Gastric electric stimulation.
GFR	Glomerular filtration rate.
GGO	Ground glass opacity.
GH	Growth hormone.
GHP	Group health plan.
GI	Gastrointestinal.
GID	Gender identity disorder.
GIFT	Gamete intrafallopian transfer.
GLBA	Gramm-Leach-Bliley Act.
GLC	Gas liquid chromatography.
GLM	General linear modeling.
Gly. supp.	Glycerin suppository.
gm	Gram.
GME	Graduate medical education.
GMLOS	Geometric mean length of stay.
GMP	Guanosine monophosphate.
GNID	Gram-negative intracellular diplococci.
GnRH	Gonadotropin-releasing hormone.
GP	General practitioner.
GPCI	Geographic practice cost indexes.
gr.	Grain.
grad	Gradually; by degrees.
grav	Number of pregnancies.
GS	General surgeon.
GSR	Galvanic skin response.
GSS syndrome	Gerstmann-Straussler-Scheinker syndrome.
GSW	Gunshot wound.
gt.	Drop.
GTD	Gestational trophoblastic disease.
GTF	Gunther Tulip filter.
GTT	Glucose tolerance test.
gtt.	Drops.
Gu	Guaiac.
GU	Genitourinary.
GVHD	Graft-versus-host disease.
GXT	Graded exercise test.
gyn	Gynecology.
H	Hertel measurement.
h (hora)	Hour.
H&H	Hemoglobin and hematocrit.
H&P	History and physical.
h.d.	At bedtime.
H.O.	House officer.
h.s.	At bedtime.
h/o	History of.
H1N1	Swine flu, swine influenza, pandemic swine flu, or pandemic swine influenza.
H2O	Water.
H2O2	Hydrogen peroxide.
H2	Histamine.
HA	***1)*** Headache. ***2)*** Hearing aid.
HAA	Hepatitis antigen.

HAAb	Hepatitis antibody A.
HaAg	Hepatitis antigen A.
HAART	Highly active antiretroviral therapy.
HAASC	Hospital affiliated ambulatory surgical center.
HAC	Hospital acquired conditions.
HAGMA	High anion gap metabolic acidosis.
HAI	***1)*** Hemagglutination test. ***2)*** Hospital acquired infection.
HALS	Hand-assisted laparoscopic surgery.
HAPE	High altitude pulmonary edema.
HAV	Hepatitis A virus.
HBcAg	Hepatitis antigen B.
HBD	Hydroxybutyric dehydrogenase.
HBIG	Hepatitis B immune globulin.
HBO	Hyperbaric oxygen.
HbO2	Oxyhemoglobin.
HBOC	Hereditary breast and ovarian cancer.
HBP	***1)*** High blood pressure. ***2)*** Hospital based physician.
HBS	***1)*** Hepatobiliary scintigraphy. ***2)*** Hungry bone syndrome.
HBsAb	Hepatitis surface antibody B.
HBsAg	Hepatitis antigen B.
HBV	***1)*** Hepatitis B vaccine. ***2)*** Hepatitis B virus.
HCAHPS	Hospital Consumer Assessment of Healthcare Providers and Systems.
HCC	***1)*** Hepatocellular carcinoma. ***2)*** Hierarchical condition category.
HCC model	Hierarchical condition categories model.
HCG	Human chorionic gonadotropin.
HCl	Hydrochloric acid.
HCM	Hypertrophic cardiomyopathy.
HCP	Hereditary coproporphyria.
HCPCS	Healthcare Common Procedure Coding System.
Hct	Hematocrit.
Hctz	Hydrochlorothiazide.
HCVD	Hypertensive cardiovascular disease.
HD	***1)*** Hepatogenous diabetes. ***2)*** Hip disarticulation.
HDE	Humanitarian device exemption.
HDL	High-density lipoproteins.
HDM	House dust mite.
HDS	***1)*** Hasegawa Dementia Screening. ***2)*** Healthcare documentation specialist.
HDV	Hepatitis D virus.
HEDIC	Healthcare EDI Coalition.
HEDIS	Health plan employer data and information set.
HEENT	Head, eyes, ears, nose, and throat.
HEV	Hepatitis E virus.
HF	Heart failure.
HFMA	Healthcare Financial Management Association.
HFO	Hand-finger orthosis.
Hgb	Hemoglobin.
HGH	Human growth hormone.
HGNC	HUGO gene nomenclature committee.
HGSIL	High-grade squamous intraepithelial lesion.
HGVS	Human genome variation society.
HHIC	Hawaii Health Information Corporation.
HHNS	Hyperosmolar hyperglycemic nonketotic syndrome.
HHRG	Home health resource groups.
HHS	Health and Human Services.
HHT	Hereditary hemorrhagic telangiectasia.
HHV	Human herpes virus.
HI-LO	High-low.
HIAA	Hydroxyindoleacetic acid.
Hib	Hemophilus influenzae vaccine.
HIBCC	Health Industry Business Communications Council.
HIC number	Health insurance claim number.
HICN	Health insurance claim number.
HIE	***1)*** Health information exchange. ***2)*** Hypoxic-ischemic encephalopathy.
HIFU	High-intensity focused ultrasound.
HIM	Health information management.
HIMSS	Healthcare Information Management Systems Society.
HIO	Health information organization.
HIPAA	Health Insurance Portability and Accountability Act of 1996.
HIPC	Health Information Policy Council.
HIPEC	Hyperthermic intraperitoneal chemotherapy.
HIPPS	Health insurance prospective payment system.
HISB	Health Informatics Standards Board.
HIT	***1)*** Health information technology. ***2)*** Heparin-induced thrombocytopenia. ***3)*** Home infusion therapy.
HITECH	Health information technology for economic and clinical health.
HIV	Human immunodeficiency virus.
HKAFO	Hip-knee-ankle foot orthosis.
HL7	Health Level Seven.
HLA	Human leukocyte antigen.
HLV	Herpes-like virus.
HMD	Hyaline membrane disease.
HMES	Heat and moisture exchange system.

HMO	Health maintenance organization.
HMS	Haim-Munk syndrome.
HNAD	Hyperosmolar nonacidotic diabetes.
HNP	Herniated nucleus pulposus.
HNPCC	Hereditary nonpolyposis colorectal cancer.
HNS	Hyperosmolar nonketotic syndrome.
HOB	Head of bed.
HOH	Hard of hearing.
hor. decub.	At bedtime.
HORF	High output renal failure.
HPC	Hematopoietic progenitor cell.
HPF	High power field.
HPG	Human pituitary gonadotropin.
HPI	History of present illness.
HPID	Health plan identifier.
HPL	Human placental lactogen.
HPOA	Hypertrophic pulmonary osteoarthropathy.
HPOES	Health Plan and Other Entity Enumeration System.
HPS	***1)*** Hantavirus pulmonary syndrome. ***2)*** Hot packs.
HPSA	Health professional shortage area.
HPV	Human papilloma virus.
HR	***1)*** Harrington rod. ***2)*** Heart rate. ***3)*** Hour.
HRA	Health reimbursement account.
HRS	Heart Rhythm Society.
HRSA	Health Resources and Services Administration.
HRT	Hormone replacement therapy.
hrt.	Heart.
HS	Heelstick.
HSA	***1)*** Health savings account. ***2)*** Health service agreement.
HSBG	Heelstick blood gas.
HSG	Hysterosalpingogram.
HSM	Hepatosplenomegaly.
HSP	Health service plan.
HSRV	Hospital-specific relative value.
HSV	Herpes simplex virus.
ht.	Height.
HTA system	Hydro Term Ablator System.
HTLV/III	Human T-cell lymphotropic.
HTN	Hypertension.
HUD	Humanitarian use device.
HUGO	Human genome organization
HVA	Homovanillic acid.
Hx	History.
hypo	Hypodermic injection.
I&D	Incision and drainage.
I&O	Intake and output.
IA	***1)*** Improvement activities. ***2)*** Intra-arterial.
IAB	Intra-aortic balloon.
IABC	Intra-aortic balloon counterpulsation.
IABP	Intra-aortic balloon pump or intra-arterial blood pressure.
iADL	Instrumental activities of daily living.
IAIABC	International Association of Industrial Accident Boards and Commissions.
IBM	Inclusion body myositis.
IBNR	Incurred but not reported.
IBS	Irritable bowel syndrome.
IBW	Ideal body weight.
IC	Infant care.
ICAT	Indirect Coombs test.
ICBG	Iliac crest bone graft.
ICCE	Intracapsular cataract extraction.
ICD	***1)*** Implantable cardioverter defibrillator. ***2)*** International Classification of Disease.
ICD-10	International Classification of Diseases, 10th Revision.
ICD-10-CM	International Classification of Diseases, 10th Revision, Clinical Modification.
ICD-10-PCS	International Classification of Diseases, 10th Revision, Procedure Coding System.
ICE syndrome	Iridocorneal endothelial syndrome.
ICF	***1)*** Intermediate care facility. ***2)*** International Classification of Functioning, Disability, and Health.
ICF syndrome	Intravascular coagulation-fibrinolysis.
ICH	Intracranial/cerebral hemorrhage.
ICHI	International Classification of Health Interventions.
ICHT	***1)*** Intermittent combined hormone therapy. ***2)*** Intracellular hyperthermia therapy.
ICM	Implantable cardiovascular monitor.
ICN	Internal control number.
ICP	Intracranial pressure.
ICRS	Intrastromal corneal ring segments.
ICS	Intercostal space.
ICSH	Interstitial cell-stimulating hormone.
ICSI	Intracytoplasmic sperm injection.
ICU	Intensive care unit.
ID	Infective dose.
Id31	Radioactive iodine.
IDDM	Insulin dependent diabetes mellitus.
IDE	Investigational device exemption.

IDET Intradiscal electrothermal therapy.
IDH Isocitric dehydrogenase.
IDK Internal derangement of the knee.
IDM Infant of diabetic mother.
IDN Integrated delivery network.
IDSA Infectious Diseases Society of America.
IG ***1)*** Immunoglobulin.
2) Implementation guide.
IGS Implantable gastric stimulator.
IH Infectious hepatitis.
IHC Internet Healthcare Coalition.
IHS Indian Health Service.
IHSS Idiopathic hypertrophic subaortic stenosis.
IHT ***1)*** Induced hypothermic therapy.
2) Intermittent hormone therapy.
IIHI Individually identifiable health information.
ILC Interstitial laser coagulation.
ILD Interstitial lung disease.
ILP ***1)*** Interstitial laser photocoagulation.
2) Isolated link perfusion.
ILR Implantable loop recorder.
IM ***1)*** Infectious mononucleosis.
2) Internal medicine.
3) Intramuscular.
IMC ***1)*** In my care.
2) Intermediate care.
IMCA Immunochemiluminometric assay.
IME ***1)*** Independent medical evaluation.
2) Indirect medical evaluation.
IMO Integrated multiple option.
IMPACT Act Improving Medicare Post-Acute Care Transformation Act of 2014.
IMRT Intensity modulated radiation therapy.
IMS Intramuscular stimulation.
IMT Intima-media thickness.
IMV Intermittent mandatory ventilation.
in Inch.
inc. Incision.
IND Investigation of new drug.
indep Independent.
INF ***1)*** Inferior.
2) Infusion.
INFH Ischemic necrosis of femoral head.
INH Inhalation solution.
INJ Injection.
INPH Idiopathic normal pressure hydrocephalus.
instill Instillation.
Int. Internal.
intra Within.
IOL Intraocular lens.
IOM Institute of Medicine.
IONM Intraoperative neurophysiological monitoring.
IOP Intraocular pressure.
IP ***1)*** Interphalangeal.
2) Intraperitoneal.
IPA Individual practice association.
IPD Intermittent peritoneal dialysis.
IPF ***1)*** Inpatient psychiatric facility.
2) Interstitial pulmonary fibrosis.
IPO Individual practice organization.
IPOC Infection Prevention (Management of) Outcomes.
IPPB Intermittent positive pressure breathing.
IPPE Initial preventive physical examination.
IPPS Inpatient short-term acute-care prospective payment system.
IPS Idiopathic postprandial syndrome.
IPT Insulin potentiation therapy.
IPV ***1)*** Intrapulmonary percussive ventilator.
2) Poliovirus vaccine, inactivated.
IQ Intelligence quotient.
IRB Institutional review board.
IRDS Idiopathic respiratory distress syndrome.
IRF Inpatient rehabilitation facility.
IS Information services.
Isa Interchange control header segment.
ISC Infant servo-control.
ISD Intrinsic (urethral) sphincter deficiency.
ISG Immune serum globulin.
ISHLT International Society for Heart and Lung Transplantation.
ISMM In situ malignant melanoma.
ISO International Organization for Standardization.
IT ***1)*** Information technology.
2) Intrathecal administration.
ITC In the canal, as seen in ENT documentation.
ITE In the ear, as seen in ENT documentation.
ITP Idiopathic thrombocytopenia purpura.
IU International units.
IUD Intrauterine device.
IUGR Intrauterine growth restriction.
IUI Intrauterine insemination.
IUUS Intrauterine ultrasound.
IV Intravenous.
IVC ***1)*** Inferior vena cava.
2) Intravenous cholangiogram.

IVF In vitro fertilization.

IVH Intraventricular hemorrhage.

IVP Intravenous pyelogram.

IVUS Intravascular ultrasound.

JCAHO Joint Commission for the Accreditation of Hospitals.

JD Doctor of jurisprudence.

JHITA Joint Healthcare Information Technology Alliance.

JNA Juvenile nasopharyngeal angiofibroma.

JODM Juvenile onset diabetes mellitus.

JPA Juvenile pilocytic astrocytoma.

Jt. Joint.

JVD Jugular venous distention.

JVP Jugular venous pressure.

K Potassium.

KAFO Knee-ankle-foot orthosis.

Kcal Kilocalorie.

KCL Potassium chloride.

kg Kilogram.

KI Potassium iodine.

KJ Knee jerk.

KO ***1)*** Keep open.
2) Knee orthosis.

KOH Potassium hydroxide.

KPS Karnofsky Performance Scale.

KSPT Kaufman Speech Praxis Test.

KSS Kearns-Sayre syndrome.

KTS Klippel-Trenaunay syndrome.

KUB Kidneys, ureters, bladder.

KVO Keep vein open.

L ***1)*** Left vertebrae.
2) Lumbar vertebrae.

L&A Light and accommodation.

L&D Labor and delivery.

L&W Living and well.

LA ***1)*** Left atrium.
2) Long-acting.

LAA Left atrial appendage.

LAC Long arm cast.

LAD Left anterior descending.

LADA Latent autoimmune diabetes in adults.

LAE Left atrial enlargement.

LAH Left atrial hemodynamic.

LAIS Lateral internal anal sphincterotomy.

LAP ***1)*** Left atrial pressure.
2) Leucine aminopeptidase.

lap. ***1)*** Laparoscopy.
2) Laparotomy.

LASEK Laser-assisted subepithelial keratomileusis.

LAT Lateral.

LAUP Laser-assisted uvulopalatoplasty.

LAV Lymphadenopathy-associated virus.

LAVH Laparoscopically assisted vaginal hysterectomy.

LAW Left atrial wall.

LB ***1)*** Large bowel.
2) Leg bag.

LBB Left bundle branch.

LBBB Left bundle branch block.

LBD Lewy body disease.

LBP Lower back pain.

lbs Pounds.

LBW Low birth weight.

LCCA Left common carotid artery.

LCH Langerhans cell histiocytosis.

LCIS Lobular carcinoma in situ.

LCNB Large core needle biopsy.

LCSW Licensed clinical social worker.

LD Lethal dose.

LDH Lactic dehydrogenase.

LDKT Living donor kidney transplant.

LDL Low density lipoprotein.

LDO Large Dialysis Organization.

LDS Lipodystrophy syndrome.

LDT Lymph drainage therapy.

LE ***1)*** Lower extremity.
2) Lupus erythematosus.

LEAT Least expensive alternative treatment.

LEEP Loop electrode excision procedure.

LFH Left femoral hernia.

LFT Liver function test.

LGA Large for gestational age.

LGHP Large group health plan.

LGL Large granular lymphoma.

LGSIL Low-grade squamous intraepithelial lesion.

LGV Lymphogranuloma venereum.

LH Luteinizing hormone.

LHC Left heart catheterization.

LHF Left heart failure.

LHR Leukocyte histamine release.

Li Lithium.

LICA Left internal carotid artery.

LIDO Lidocaine.

LIDS Latex induced disease system.

Li-ESWT Low-intensity extracorporeal shock wave therapy.

lig. Ligament.

LIMA Left internal mammary artery.

LIP Lymphocytic interstitial pneumonia.

liq. Solution (liquor).
LIT Leukocyte immune therapy.
LITT Laser interstitial thermotherapy or laser-induced interstitial thermotherapy.
LKS Liver, kidneys, spleen.
LLB Long leg brace.
LLD Language-based learning disability.
LLE Left, lower extremity.
LLETZ Large loop excision of transformation zone of cervix of uterus.
LLL Left lower lobe.
LLQ Left lower quadrant.
LLWC Long leg walking cast.
LMA Laryngeal mask airway.
LMD Local medical doctor.
LML Left mediolateral position.
LMM Lentigo malignant melanoma.
LMN Lower motor neuron.
LMP Last menstrual period.
LMRP Local medical review policy.
LMS ***1)*** Lateral medullary syndrome.
2) Left main stem.
3) Left mentum anterior position (chin).
4)Leiomyosarcoma.
LMT Left mentum transverse position.
LNE Lymph node enlargement.
LNMP Last known menstrual period.
LNP Lipid nanoparticle.
LNTX Long chain neurotoxin.
Lo Low.
LOA Leave of absence.
LOC ***1)*** Level of consciousness.
2) Loss of consciousness.
LOINC Logical observation identifiers names and codes.
LOM Limitation of motion.
LOP Left occiputoposterior position.
LOPS Loss of protective sensation.
LOS Length of stay.
LOT Left occiput transverse position.
LOX Liquid oxygen.
LP Lumbar puncture.
LPF Low powered field.
LPM Liters per minute.
LPN Licensed practical nurse.
LR ***1)*** Lactated Ringer's.
2) Log roll.
LRD Living related donor.
LRSA Linezolid and methicillin resistant Staphylococcus aureus.
LRTI ***1)*** Ligament reconstruction and tendon interposition.
2) Lower respiratory tract infection.
LS fusion Lumbar sacral fusion.
LSA Left sacrum anterior position.
LSB Left sternal border.
LSC Left subclavian.
LSO Lumbar sacral orthosis.
LT Left.
LTBI Latent tuberculosis infection.
LTC Long-term care.
LTC-DRG Inpatient long-term acute-care diagnosis-related group.
LTCH Long-term care hospital.
LTD Lowest tolerated dose.
LTK ***1)*** Laser thermal keratoplasty.
2) Left total knee (replacement).
LTOT Long-term oxygen therapy.
LUE Left upper extremity.
LUL Left upper lobe.
LULA Laparoscopy under local anesthesia.
LUPA Low utilization payment adjustment.
LUQ Left upper quadrant.
LUSCS Lower uterine segment cesarean section.
LUSS Liver ultrasound scan.
LUTO Lower urinary tract obstruction.
LUTS Lower urinary tract symptoms.
LV Left ventricle.
LVAD Left ventricular assist device.
LVEDP Left ventricular end diastolic pressure.
LVN ***1)*** Licensed visiting nurse.
2) Licensed vocational nurse.
LVRS Lung volume reduction surgery.
lymphs Lymphocytes.
lytes Electrolytes.
M ***1)*** Male.
2) Manifest refraction.
M.Ed Master of education.
M1 Mitral first sound.
M2 Mitral second sound.
MA ***1)*** Master of arts degree.
2) Medical assistant.
3) Mental age.
MA1 Volume respirator.
MAAC Maximum allowable actual charge.
MAC ***1)*** Maximum allowable charge.
2) Medicare Administrative Contractor.
3) Monitored anesthesia care.
MACE Major adverse cardiac event.
MACRA Medicare Access and CHIP Reauthorization Act of 2015.
MACs Medicare administrative contractors.

MAE Major arrhythmic event.
MAHA Microangiopathic hemolytic anemia.
MALT Mucosa-associated lymphoid tissue.
man. prim. First thing in the morning.
MAO Monoamine oxidase (inhibitor).
MAP Mean arterial pressure.
MAR Medication administration record.
MARSI Medical adhesive-related skin injury.
MASER Microwave amplification by stimulated emission of radiation.
MAST Military antishock trousers.
MAT Multifocal atrial tachycardia.
MAV Measure applicability validation.
MBC ***1)*** Male breast cancer.
2) Maximum breathing capacity.
3) Metastatic breast cancer.
MBD Minimal brain dysfunction.
MBI Medicare Beneficiary Identifier.
MCCE Magnetically-controlled capsule endoscopy.
MCD Macular corneal dystrophy.
MCE ***1)*** Medical care evaluation.
2) Medicare code editor.
mcg Microgram.
MCH Mean corpuscular hemoglobin.
MCHC Mean corpuscular hemoglobin concentration.
mCi Millicurie.
MCKD Multicystic kidney disease.
MCL ***1)*** Midclavicular line.
2) Modified chest lead.
MCLS Mucocutaneous lymph node syndrome.
MCM Medicare Carriers Manual.
MCO Managed care organization.
MCP ***1)*** Metacarpophalangeal.
2) Monthly capitation payment.
MCR Modified community rating.
MCS Minimally conscious state.
MCT ***1)*** Mediastinal chest tube.
2) Motor control test.
MCTD Mixed connective tissue disease.
MCV ***1)*** Major cardiovascular condition.
2) Mean corpuscular volume.
MD ***1)*** Manic depression.
2) Medical doctor.
3) Muscular dystrophy.
4) Myocardial disease.
MDC Major diagnostic category,
MDCT Multi-slice detector computed tomography.
MDD Manic-depressive disorder.
MDH Medicare dependent hospital.
MDI Metered-dose inhaler.
MDM Medical decision making.
MDMA Methylenedioxymethamphetamine.
MDR Multidrug resistance.
MDS ***1)*** Minimum data set.
2) Myelodysplastic syndrome.
MDUFMA Medical Device User Fee and Modernization Act of 2002.
ME Medical examiner.
MEA Microwave endometrial ablation.
Mec Meconium.
MED Minimal effective dose.
med-surg Medical, surgical.
MedPAC Medicare Payment Advisory Commission.
MedPAR Medicare provider analysis and review file.
meds Medications.
MEG Magnetoencephalography.
MEI Medicare economic index.
MELAS Mitochondrial myopathy, encephalopathy, lactic acidosis, stroke.
mEq Milliequivalent.
mEq/1 Milliequivalent per liter.
MERRF Myoclonus epilepsy associated with ragged-red fibers.
MESA Micro-epididymal sperm aspiration.
MET Multiple employer trust.
MEWA Multiple employer welfare association.
MFD Minimum fatal dose.
MFS Medicare fee schedule.
MFT Muscle function test.
mg Milligram.
MG Myasthenia gravis.
Mg Magnesium.
MGCRB Medicare Geographic Classification Review Board.
MGMA Medical Group Management Association.
mgs Milligrams.
MH/CD Mental health/chemical dependency.
MH/SA Mental health/substance abuse.
MHA Master of health administration.
MHC Mental health clinic.
MHDC Massachusetts Health Data Consortium.
MHDI Minnesota Health Data Institute.
MHT Megahertz.
MI ***1)*** Microwave imaging.
2) Myocardial infarct.
MIC Minimum inhibitory concentration.
MID Minimum infective dose.

MIDAS	Migraine disability assessment scale.
MIE	Meconium ileus equivalent.
MIF	Migration inhibitory factor.
min	Minimum, minimal, minute.
MIP	Medicare Integrity Program.
MIPPA	Medicare Improvements for Patients and Providers Act of 2008.
MIPS	Merit-Based Incentive Payment System.
MIPS APM	Merit-based Incentive Payment System Alternative Payment Model.
MIS	***1)*** Management information system. ***2)*** Memory impairment screen. ***3)*** Minimally invasive surgery.
MIS-C	Multisystem inflammatory syndrome in children.
misc.	Miscellaneous.
ml	Milliliter.
ML	Midline.
MLB test	Monaural loudness balance test.
MLC	Midline catheter.
MLD	***1)*** Manual lymph drainage. ***2)*** Minimum lethal dose.
MLM	Manual lymphatic mapping.
MLN	Medicare Learning Network.
MLNS	Mucocutaneous lymph node syndrome.
MLP	Midlevel practitioners.
MLR	Minimum Loss Rate (Medical Loss Ratio).
MLT	Medical laboratory technician.
MLV	Modified live vaccine.
MM	***1)*** Malignant melanoma. ***2)*** Millimeter. ***3)*** Mucous membrane.
mmHg	Millimeters of mercury.
MMPI	Minnesota Multiphasic Personality Inventory.
MMR	Measles, mumps, and rubella.
MMRV	Measles, mumps, rubella vaccine.
MMSEA	Medicare, Medicaid, and State Children's Health Insurance Program (SCHIP) Extension Act of 2007.
MNK	Menkes syndrome.
MNS	Microcurrent nerve stimulator.
MNT	Medical nutrition therapy.
MoAbs	Monoclonal antibodies.
MoCA	Montreal Cognitive Assessment.
MOD	Multiple organ dysfunction.
MODY	Maturity-onset diabetes of the young.
MOLST	Medical orders for life-sustaining treatment.
MOM	Milk of magnesia.
mono	***1)*** Monocyte. ***2)*** Mononucleosis.
mor. dict.	In the manner directed.
MOST	Medical orders for scope of treatment.
MOU	Memorandum of understanding.
MP	Metacarpal phalangeal.
MPA	Microscopic polyangiitis.
MPAP	Mean pulmonary artery pressure.
MPD	Maximum permissible dose.
MPFS	Medicare physician fee schedule.
MPH	Master of public health.
MPNST	Malignant peripheral nerve sheath tumor.
MPR	Multifetal pregnancy reduction.
MR	***1)*** Magnetic resonance. ***2)*** Medical review. ***3)*** Mitral regurgitation.
MRA	Magnetic resonance angiography.
MRCP	Magnetic resonance cholangiopancreatography.
MRDD	Mentally retarded/developmentally disabled.
MRE	Medical Reference Engine.
MRG	Murmurs, rubs, or gallops.
MRgFUS	MR-guided, focused ultrasound system.
MRHFP	Medicare Rural Hospital Flexibility Program, a CMS designation.
MRI	***1)*** Magnetic resonance imaging. ***2)*** Medical Records Institute.
MRM	Modified radical mastectomy.
MRN	***1)*** Magnetic resonance neurography. ***2)*** Medical record number.
mRNA	Messenger RNA.
MRND	Modified radical neck dissection.
MRS	Magnetic resonance spectroscopy.
MRSA	Methicillin resistant staphylococcus aureus.
MRSE	Magnetic Resonance Safety Expert.
MS	***1)*** Mitral stenosis. ***2)*** Morphine sulfate. ***3)*** Multiple sclerosis.
MS-DRG	Medicare severity-adjusted diagnosis related group.
MSA	***1)*** Medical savings account. ***2)*** Metropolitan statistical area.
MSHJ	Medical staff hospital joint venture.
MSLT	Multiple sleep latency testing.
MSN	***1)*** Master of science in nursing. ***2)*** Medicare summary notice.
MSO	Management service organization.
MSPB	Medicare Spending per Beneficiary.
MSR	Minimum savings rate.

MSS	Medical social services.
MSSA	Methicillin-susceptible Staphylococcus aureus.
MSSP	Medicare Shared Savings Program.
MSSU	Midstream specimen urine.
MSW	Master's in social work.
MT	***1)*** Medical technologist. ***2)*** Medical transcriptionist.
MTC	Medullary thyroid carcinoma.
MTD	Right eardrum.
MTM	Metamucil.
MTP	Metatarsophalangeal.
MTS	Left eardrum.
MTWA	Microvolt T-wave alternans.
MTX	Methotrexate.
MU	Meaningful use.
MUA	Medically underserved area.
MUGA scan	Multiple gated acquisition scan.
multip.	Multipara.
MuSK	Muscle-specific kinase.
MV	Mitral valve.
MVA	***1)*** Manual vacuum aspiration. ***2)*** Motor vehicle accident.
MVD	Microvascular decompression.
MVP	Mitral valve prolapse.
MVPS	Medicare volume performance standard.
MWA	Microwave ablation.
MWS	Mickey-Wilson syndrome.
N	Nitrogen.
N&V	Nausea and vomiting.
n.p.o.	Nothing by mouth.
N/T	Not tender.
N0M0	Lymph node, zero; metastases, zero.
N2O	Nitrous oxide.
NA	Nurse assistant.
Na	Sodium.
NAAT	Nucleic acid amplification test.
NaCl	Sodium chloride (salt).
NAD	No acute distress.
NAFLD	Nonalcoholic fatty liver disease.
NAHDO	National Association of Health Data Organizations.
NAHMOR	National Association of HMO Regulators.
NAIC	National Association of Insurance Commissioners.
NAION	Nonarteritic anterior ischemic optic neuropathy.
NANDA	North American Nursing Diagnoses Association.
NARP syndrome	Neuropathy-ataxia-retinitis pigmentosa syndrome.
NAS	Neonatal abstinence syndrome.
NASMD	National Association of State Medicaid Directors.
NAT	Nonaccidental trauma.
NAW	Nasoantral window.
NB	Newborn.
NBICU	Newborn intensive care unit.
NBT	Nitroblue tetrazolium.
NCA	***1)*** National coverage analyses. ***2)*** Neurocirculatory asthenia.
NCAP	Nasal continuous airway pressure.
NCCI	National correct coding initiative.
NCD	National coverage determinations.
NCHICA	North Carolina Healthcare Information and Communications Alliance.
NCHS	National Center for Health Statistics.
NCHVS	National Committee on Health and Vital Statistics.
NCI	National Cancer Institute.
NCPDP	National Council of Prescription Drug Programs.
NCPR	No cardiopulmonary resuscitation.
NCQA	National Committee for Quality Assurance.
NCR	No cardiac resuscitation.
NCS	Nerve conduction study.
NCV	Nerve conduction velocity.
NCVHS	National Committee on Vital and Health Statistics.
ND	Doctor of naturopathy.
NDC	National drug code.
NEC	***1)*** Necrotizing enterocolitis. ***2)*** Not elsewhere classified.
NECMA	New England county metropolitan areas.
NED	No evidence of disease.
neg.	Negative.
NETT	National Emphysema Treatment Trial.
NF	National formulary.
NfL	Neurofilament light chain.
NFL	Nerve fiber layer.
NG	***1)*** Nasogastric. ***2)*** Next generation.
NGACO	Next Generation Accountable Care Organization Model.
NGU	Nongonococcal urethritis.
NH	Nursing home.
NHCS	National Health Care Survey.
NHII	National Health Information Infrastructure.
NHK	Normal human keratinocytes.

NHL Non-Hodgkin's lymphoma.
NIBP Non-invasive blood pressure.
NICE National Institute for Clinical Excellence.
NICO Neuralgia-inducing cavitational osteonecrosis.
NICU Neonatal intensive care unit.
NIDDM Non-insulin dependent diabetes mellitus.
NIHL Noise induced hearing loss.
NINDS National Institute of Neurological Disorders and Stroke.
NIPD Nocturnal intermittent peritoneal dialysis.
NIPS ***1)*** Neonatal infant pain scale.
2) Noninvasive programmed electrical stimulation.
NIRS Near infrared spectroscopy.
NJ Nasojejunal.
NKA No known allergies.
NKDA ***1)*** No known drug allergies.
2) Non-ketotic diabetic acidosis.
NKHC Non-ketotic hyperglycemic coma.
NKHHC Nonketotic hyperglycemic-hyperosmolar coma.
NKMA No known medical allergies.
NM Nodular melanoma.
NMES Neuromuscular electrical stimulation.
NMM Nodular malignant melanoma.
NMO Neuromyelitis optica.
NMSC Nonmelanoma skin cancer.
NNR New and nonofficial remedies.
NOC ***1)*** Not otherwise classified.
2) Nursing outcomes classification.
noc. Night.
NOI Notice of intent.
non-par Non-participating provider.
NOS Not otherwise specified.
novem. Nine.
NP ***1)*** Neuropsychiatry.
2) Nurse practitioner.
NP-CPAP Nasopharyngeal continuous positive airway pressure.
NPA ***1)*** Nasopharyngeal airway.
2) National prescription audit.
3) Non-par approved.
NPC Nasopharyngeal carcinoma.
NPD Nightly peritoneal dialysis.
NPEP Non-occupational post exposure prophylaxis.
NPF National provider file.
NPI National provider identifier.
NPN ***1)*** Non-par not approved.
2) Nonprotein nitrogen.
NPO Nothing by mouth.
NPPES National Plan and Provider Enumeration System.
NPQ Not physically qualified.
NPRM Notice of proposed rulemaking.
NPS National provider system.
npt Normal pressure and temperature.
NPWT Negative pressure wound therapy.
NQF National Quality Forum.
NQS National Quality Strategy.
NS ***1)*** Normal saline.
2) Not significant.
NSAID Nonsteroidal anti-inflammatory drug.
NSC Non-service connected.
NSD Nominal standard dose.
NSF National standard format.
NSR Normal sinus rhythm.
NST Nonstress test.
NSTEMI Non-ST elevation myocardial infarction.
NSU Nonspecific urethritis.
NSV Nonspecific vaginitis.
NSVB Normal spontaneous vaginal bleeding.
NSVD Normal spontaneous vaginal delivery.
NT ***1)*** Nasotracheal.
2) Nontender.
NTD Nitroblue tetrazolium dye test.
NTE Neutral thermal environment.
NTL Near total laryngectomy.
NTP Normal temperature and pressure.
NTT Near total thyroidectomy.
NUBC National Uniform Billing Committee.
NUBC EDI TAG National Uniform Billing Committee's Electronic Data Interchange Technical Advisory Group.
NUCC National Uniform Claim Committee.
NV Nausea and vomiting.
NVHRI National Voluntary Hospital Reporting Initiative, a CMS designation.
NVP Nausea and vomiting of pregnancy.
NYD Not yet diagnosed.
o No information.
O ***1)*** Blood type.
2) Oxygen.
O&P Ova and parasites.
O.D. Oculus dexter. Right eye.
o.m. ***1)*** Every morning.
2) Otitis media.
o.n. Every night.
O.S. Oculus sinister. Left eye.
O.U. Oculus uterque. Each eye.

O2	Oxygen.
OA	***1)*** Open access. ***2)*** Osteoarthritis.
OAB	Overactive bladder.
OAE	Otoacoustic emissions.
OAG	Open angle glaucoma.
OASIS	Outcome and assessment information set.
OAV syndrome	Oculoauriculovertebral dysplasia.
OB	Obstetrician.
OB-GYN	Obstetrics and gynecology.
OBRA	Omnibus Budget Reconciliation Act.
OC	***1)*** Office call. ***2)*** Open crib. ***3)*** Oral contraceptive.
OCD	Obsessive-compulsive disorder.
OCE	Outpatient code editor.
OCM	Oncology Care Model.
OCR	***1)*** Oculocephalic response. ***2)*** Office for Civil Rights.
OCT	***1)*** Optical coherence tomography. ***2)*** Ornithine carbamyl transferase. ***3)*** Oxytocin challenge.
octo	Eight.
ODM	Ophthalmodynamometry.
OEID	Other entity identifier.
OESS	Office of E-Health Standards and Services.
OFC	Occipitofrontal circumference.
OGT	Orogastric tube.
OHS	Obesity hypoventilation syndrome.
OHSS	Ovarian hyperstimulation syndrome.
OIC	Osteogenesis imperfecta congenital.
OIG	Office of Inspector General.
oint	Ointment.
OIT	Osteogenesis imperfecta tarda.
OJ	Orange juice.
OL	Outlier threshold.
OMB	Office of Management and Budget.
omn. hor.	Every hour.
OMS	Oromaxillofacial surgery.
OMT	Osteopathic manipulation therapy.
ONB	Olfactory neuroblastoma.
ONH	***1)*** Optic nerve head. ***2)*** Optic nerve hypoplasia.
OOA	Out-of-area.
OOB	Out of bed.
OOPs	Out-of-pocket costs/expenses.
OOX	Oophorectomy.
OPA	Oropharyngeal airway.
OPD	Outpatient department.
OPG	Oculoplethysmography.
ophth	Ophthalmology.
OPL	Other party liability.
OPPS	Outpatient prospective payment system.
OPS	Objective pain scale.
OPV	Oral polio vaccine.
OQHCP	Other qualified health care professional.
OR	Operating room.
ORAL	Oral administration.
ORIF	Open reduction internal fixation.
oris	Mouth.
ORT	Oral rehydration therapy.
ortho	Orthopedics.
os	Mouth.
OSA	Obstructive sleep apnea.
OSAS	Obstructive sleep apnea syndrome.
OSCAR	Online Survey Certification and Reporting, a CMS designation.
OSI	Open systems interconnection.
Ost	Ostomy.
OST	Oxytocin stress test.
OT	***1)*** Occupational therapy. ***2)*** Outlier threshold.
OTC	Over-the-counter.
OTD	Organ tolerance dose.
OTH	Other routes of administration.
OTR	Occupational therapist registered.
OTW	Over the wire.
OUD	Opioid use disorder.
ov.	***1)*** Office visit. ***2)*** Ovum.
OVC	Ovarian cancer.
oVEMP	Ocular vestibular evoked myogenic potential.
OVR	Oculovestibular response.
OW	Open ward.
OXY	Oxytocin.
oz	Ounce.
P	***1)*** After. ***2)*** Phosphorus. ***3)*** Plan. ***4)*** Pulse.
P&A	Percussion and auscultation.
P&T	Pharmacy and therapeutics.
P+PD	Percussion and postural drainage.
p.c.	After eating.
p.m.	After noon.
p.p.	Near point of visual accommodation.

p.r.	***1)*** Pulsefar point of visual accommodation. ***2)*** Through the rectum.
p.r.n.	As needed for.
p/o	By mouth.
p/w	Present with.
P2	Pulmonic 2nd sound.
P4	Progesterone.
PA	***1)*** Physician assistant. ***2)*** Posteroanterior. ***3)*** Pulmonary artery.
PAB	Premature atrial beats.
PAC	***1)*** Preadmission certification. ***2)*** Premature atrial contraction. ***3)*** Pulmonary apical cap.
PACE	Programs of all-inclusive care for the elderly.
PACU	Postanesthesia care unit.
PAD	***1)*** Peripheral artery disease. ***2)*** Pulmonary artery diastolic.
PAF	Platelet activating factor.
PAG	Policy advisory group.
PAH	Para-aminohippurate.
PAL	***1)*** Probe for aspiration/lavage. ***2)*** Progressive addition lens.
palp	Touch gently, feel.
PAMI	Primary angioplasty in acute myocardial infarction.
PAN	Polyarteritis nodosa.
PANDAS	Pediatric autoimmune neuropsychiatric disorder associated with streptococcal infections.
PAP	***1)*** Papanicolaou test or smear. ***2)*** Pulmonary artery pressure.
PAPP-A	Plasma protein-A, pregnancy associated.
PAPVR	Partial anomalous pulmonary venous return.
par	Participating provider.
PAR	***1)*** Parenteral. ***2)*** Postanesthesia recovery.
para	***1)*** Alongside of. ***2)*** Number of pregnancies, as para 1, 2, 3, etc.
PARK	Photorefractive astigmatic keratectomy.
PARR	Postanesthesia recovery room
part. vic.	Divided doses.
PASA	Proximal articular set angle.
PASG	Pneumatic antishock garment.
PAT	***1)*** Paroxysmal atrial tachycardia. ***2)*** Peripheral arterial tone.
path	***1)*** Pathology. ***2)*** Physicians at teaching hospitals.
PATIO	Present at the time of the inpatient order.
PATOS	Payment (received) at the time of service.
PB	Pulmonary barotrauma.
PBD	Provider-based outpatient department.
PBI	Protein-bound iodine.
PBM	***1)*** Photobiomodulation. ***2)*** Prescription benefit managers.
PBO	Pharmacy benefit optimizer.
PBSC	Peripheral blood stem cell.
PBSCT	Peripheral blood stem cell transplant.
PC	***1)*** Packed cells. ***2)*** Prostate cancer.
PCA	***1)*** Patient-controlled analgesia. ***2)*** Posterior communicating artery.
PCD	Polycystic disease.
PCG	Phonocardiogram.
PCH	Pouch.
PCI in AMI	Percutaneous coronary intervention in acute myocardial infarction.
PCL	Posterior cruciate ligament.
PCMH	Patient-centered medical home.
PCN	***1)*** Penicillin. ***2)*** Primary care nurse.
PCNSL	Primary central nervous system lymphoma.
PCOS	Polycystic ovarian syndrome.
PCP	***1)*** Phencyclidine. ***2)*** Pneumocystis pneumonia. ***3)*** Primary care physician.
PCPI	Physician Consortium for Performance Improvement.
PCPM	Per contract per month.
PCR	***1)*** Physician contingency reserve. ***2)*** Polymerase chain reaction.
PCT	***1)*** Porphyria cutanea tarda. ***2)*** Postcoital test.
PCTA	Percutaneous transluminal angioplasty.
PCV	Packed cell volume.
PCV13	Pneumococcal conjugate vaccine.
PCW	Pulmonary capillary wedge.
PCWP	Pulmonary capillary wedge pressure.
PD	***1)*** Parkinson's disease. ***2)*** Peritoneal dialysis. ***3)*** Postural drainage.
PDA	***1)*** Patent ductus arteriosus. ***2)*** Posterior descending artery.
PDD	Pervasive development disorder.
PDR	Physicians' Desk Reference.
PDT	Percutaneous dilatational tracheostomy.
PDxCC	Principal Diagnosis as CC.

PDxMCC Principal Diagnosis as MCC.

PE ***1)*** Physical examination.
2) Practice expense.
3) Pulmonary edema.
4) Pulmonary embolism.

PE tube Pressure equalization tube.

PEARLA Pupils equal and react to light and accommodation.

PEC Pre-existing condition.

PECOS Provider Enrollment, Chain & Ownership System.

Peds Pediatrics.

PEG Percutaneous endoscopic gastrostomy.

PEGJJ Percutaneous endoscopic gastrojejunostomy.

PEJ Percutaneous endoscopic jejunostomy.

PEN Parenteral and enteral nutrition.

PENS Percutaneous electrical nerve stimulation.

PEP Post-exposure prophylaxis.

PEPM Per employee per month.

PEPP Payment error prevention program.

PERRLA Pupils equal, round, reactive to light and accommodation.

PERT Pancreatic enzyme replacement therapy.

PESA Percutaneous epididymal sperm aspiration.

PET ***1)*** Positron emission tomography.
2) Pressure equalizing tube.

PEU Protein-energy undernutrition.

PFC Persistent fetal circulation.

PFG Percutaneous fluoroscopic gastrostomy.

PFPM Physician-Focused Payment Models.

PFROM Pain-free range of motion.

PFS Physician Fee Schedule.

PFT Pulmonary function test.

PFX Pseudoexfoliation.

PG Prostaglandin.

PGD Preimplantation genetic diagnosis.

Pgraph Penile plethysmograph.

PGS Persian Gulf syndrome.

PGU Postgonococcal urethritis.

PH Patient history.

pH Potential of hydrogen.

PharmD Doctor of pharmacy.

PHB Pharmacy benefits manager.

PHCA Profound hypothermic cardiac arrest.

PhD Doctor of philosophy.

PHE Public health emergency.

PHI Protected health information.

PHN Postherpetic neuralgia.

PHO Physician-hospital organization.

PHP ***1)*** Partial hospitalization program.
2) Physician hospital plan.
3) Pre-paid health plan.

PHPT Primary hypoparathyroidism.

PHS Public Health Service.

PI ***1)*** Patient information.
2) Present illness.

PICA Porch Index of Communicative Abilities.

PICC Peripherally inserted central catheter.

PICD Primary irritant contact dermatitis.

PICHI Pulse-inversion contrast harmonic imaging.

PICT Pancreatic islet cell transplantation.

PID Pelvic inflammatory disease.

PIE ***1)*** Post irradiation examination.
2) Pulmonary infiltration with eosinophilia.
3) Pulmonary interstitial emphysema.

PIE syndrome Pulmonary infiltration with eosinophilia.

PIFG Poor intrauterine fetal growth.

PIH Pregnancy-induced hypertension.

PILO Pilocarpine.

PIOL Phakic intraocular lens.

PION Posterior ischemic optic neuropathy.

PIP ***1)*** Periodic interim payment.
2) Proximal interphalangeal joint.

PIP-DCG Model Principal inpatient diagnostic cost group.

PJRT Permanent junctional reciprocating tachycardia.

pk. Pack.

PKD Polycystic kidney disease.

PKP Penetrating keratoplasty.

PKR Photorefractive therapy.

PKU Phenylketonuria.

PL Public Law, as in PL 104-191 (HIPAA).

PLED Periodic lateralized epileptiform discharge.

PLEVA Pityriasis lichenoides et varioliformis acuta.

PLGA Polymorphous low-grade adenocarcinoma.

PLIF Posterior lumbar interbody fusion.

PLMS Periodic limb movement in sleep.

PM ***1)*** Paramedic.
2) Program Memorandum.

PMD Progressive muscular dystrophy.

PMDC Pre-major diagnostic category.

PMEI Polymorphic epilepsy in infancy.

PMG Primary medical group.

PMHx	Prior medical history.
PMI	Point of maximum intensity.
PML	Progressive multifocal leukoencephalopathy.
PMMA	Polymethylmethacrylate.
PMN	Polymorphonuclear neutrophil leukocytes.
PMP	Previous menstrual period.
PMPM	Per member per month.
PMPY	Per member per year.
PMR	Polymyalgia rheumatica.
PMS	Premenstrual syndrome.
PNB	Pulseless, not breathing.
PNC	Premature nodal contraction.
PND	***1)*** Paroxysmal nocturnal dyspnea. ***2)*** Post nasal drip.
PNE	Peripheral neuroepithelioma.
PNES	Psychogenic nonepileptic seizures.
PNET	Primitive neuroectodermal tumor.
PNH	Paroxysmal nocturnal hemoglobinuria.
PNS	Peripheral nervous system.
PO	***1)*** By mouth; per oral. ***2)*** Postoperative.
POA	Present on admission.
POAG	Primary open angle glaucoma.
POD	Postoperative day.
POEM	Peroral endoscopic myotomy.
POLST	Physicians orders for life-sustaining treatment.
polys	Polymorphonuclear neutrophil leukocytes.
PONV	Postoperative nausea and vomiting.
POP	Progestin-only pill.
POR	***1)*** Postoperative recovery. ***2)*** Problem oriented record.
PORN	Progressive outer retinal necrosis.
POS	Point of service.
POS codes	Place of service codes.
pos.	Positive.
POST	Physicians orders for scope of treatment.
post or PM	Postmortem exam or autopsy.
post. cib.	After meals.
POTS	Postural orthostatic tachycardia syndrome.
Pow	Powder.
POX	Point of exit.
PP	Postprandial.
PPA	Preferred provider arrangement.
PPACA	Patient Protection and Affordable Care Act.
PPBS	Postprandial blood sugar.
PPD	***1)*** Percussion and postural drainage. ***2)*** Purified protein derivative.
PPE	Palmar-plantar erythrodysesthesia.
PPH	Postpartum hemorrhage.
PPK	Palmoplantar keratoderma.
Ppl	Pleural pressure.
PPO	Preferred provider organization.
PPP	***1)*** Preperitoneal pelvic packing. ***2)*** Protamine paracoagulation.
PPPD	Pylorus-preserving pancreaticoduodenectomy.
PPS	Prospective payment system.
PPV	Pneumococcal polysaccharide vaccine.
ppx/pphx	Prophylaxis/history of prophylaxis.
PQ	Partial qualifying participant.
PQRI	Physician Quality Reporting Initiative.
PR	Per rectum.
PRA	***1)*** Paperwork Reduction Act. ***2)*** Per resident amount.
PRBC	Packed red blood cells.
PRC	Patient Relationship Categories and Codes.
preg	Pregnant.
PRES	***1)*** Posterior reversible encephalopathy syndrome. ***2)*** Progressive resistive exercises.
previa	Placenta previa.
PRG	Procedure-related group.
primip	Primipara.
PRITS	Partial resection inferior turbinates.
PRK	Photoreactive keratectomy.
PRN	Pro re nata. Latin for whenever necessary or as needed.
PRO	Peer review organization.
PROM	Premature rupture of membranes.
ProPAC	Prospective Payment Assessment Commission.
PROST	Pronuclear stage tube transfer.
PROSTALAC	Prosthesis with antibiotic-loaded acrylic cement.
PRRB	Provider Reimbursement Review Board.
PRS	Pierre Robin syndrome.
PS	***1)*** Pulmonary stenosis. ***2)*** Pyloric stenosis.
PS&R	Provider statistical and reimbursement report.
PSA	***1)*** Primary service area. ***2)*** Prostate specific antigen.
PSAD	PSA density.
PSAV	PSA velocity.
PSC	Program safeguard coordinators.
PSM	Presystolic murmur.

PSMS Physical Self Maintenance Scale.

PSP *1)* Phenolsulfonphthalein.
2) Progressive supranuclear palsy.

PSVT Paroxysmal supraventricular tachycardia.

PsyD Doctor of psychology.

PT *1)* Physical therapy.
2) Prothrombin time.

Pt Patient.

PTA *1)* Percutaneous transluminal angioplasty.
2) Physical therapy assistant.
3) Prior to admission.

PTAC Physician-Focused Payment Model Technical Advisory Committee.

PTB Patellar tendon bearing.

PTCA Percutaneous transluminal coronary angioplasty.

PTFE Polytetrafluoroethylene.

PTH Parathyroid hormone.

PTHC Percutaneous transhepatic cholangiography.

PTK Phototherapeutic keratectomy.

PTLD Post-transplant lymphoproliferative disorder.

PTMPY Per thousand members per year.

PTPN Peripheral total parenteral nutrition.

PTSD Post traumatic stress disorder.

PTT Partial thromboplastin time.

PUBS Percutaneous umbilical blood sampling.

PUD *1)* Peptic ulcer disease.
2) Periurethral diathermy.

PUG Percutaneous ultrasound gastrostomy.

pulv. Powder.

PUNL Percutaneous ultrasonic nephrolithotripsy.

PUO Pyrexia of unknown origin.

PUS Percutaneous ureteral stent.

PUV Posterior urethral valves.

PV Percutaneous vertebroplasty.

PVA Percutaneous vertebral augmentation.

PVC *1)* Polyvinyl chloride.
2) Premature ventricular contraction.

PVD *1)* Peripheral vascular disease.
2) Premature ventricular depolarization.

PVDA Prednisone, vincristine, daunorubicin, and asparaginase.

PVL Periventricular leukomalacia.

PVP Prime Vendor Program.

PVS *1)* Peripheral vascular system.
2) Persistent vegetative state.

PWA Person with AIDS (autoimmune deficiency syndrome).

PWI Posterior wall infarct.

Px *1)* Pneumothorax.
2) Prognosis.

PXA Pleomorphic xanthoastrocytoma.

PY Performance year.

PZI Protamine zinc insulin.

Q. Every.

q.2h Every two hours.

q.a.m. Every morning.

q.d. Every day.

q.h. Every hour.

q.h.s. Every night.

q.i.d. Four times daily.

q.n. Every night.

q.o.d. Every other day.

q.q.h. Every four hours.

QA Quality assurance.

QCDR Qualified Clinical Data Registry.

QCT Quantitative computed tomography.

QDC Quality data code.

QHP Qualified healthcare professional.

QIC Qualified independent contractor.

QID Quarter in die. Latin for four times a day.

QIN Quality Innovation Network.

QIO Quality Improvement Organization.

QM Quality management.

qns Quantity not sufficient.

QOD Every other day.

qoh Every other hour.

QOL Quality of life.

QP Qualifying Advanced APM Participant.

qPCR Quantitative polymerase chain reaction.

QPIT Quantitative pilocarpine iontophoresis test.

QPP Quality Payment Program.

QRDA Quality Reporting Document Architecture.

QRUR Quality Resource and Use Report.

qs Quantity sufficient.

QST Quantitative sensory testing.

QTc Corrected QT interval.

quad Fourth, four.

quattour Four.

quicdecem Fifteen.

quinque Five.

quotid Daily.

R	***1)*** Respiration. ***2)*** Right. ***3)*** Right atrium.
R&C	Reasonable and customary.
R*	Roentgen units (x-rays).
R,R,& E	Round, regular, and equal.
R/O	Rule out.
RA	***1)*** Remittance advice. ***2)*** Rheumatoid arthritis. ***3)*** Risk assessment.
RAC	Recovery Audit Contractor.
RAD	Reactive airway disease.
RAE	Right atrial enlargement.
RAEB	Refractory anemia with excessive blasts.
RAEBT	Refractory anemia with excessive blasts in transformation.
RAI	***1)*** Radioactive iodine. ***2)*** Resident assessment instrument.
RAIU	Radioactive iodine uptake.
RAO	Retinal artery occlusion.
RAP	Resident assessment protocol.
RARS	Refractory anemia with ringed sideroblasts.
RAST	Radioallergosorbent test.
RATx	Radiation therapy.
RAW	Relativity Assessment Workgroup of the American Medical Association (AMA).
RBB	Right branch bundle or right bundle branch.
RBBB	Right bundle branch block.
RBC	Red blood cell.
RBL	Rubber band ligation.
RBN	Retrobulbar neuritis.
RBOW	Ruptured bag of water.
RBRVS	Resource based relative value scale.
RCA	Right coronary artery.
RCC	Renal cell carcinoma.
RCCA	Right common carotid artery.
RCD	Relative cardiac dullness.
RCE	Reasonable compensation equivalent.
RCL	Renal clearance.
RCM	Radiocontrast media.
RCT	Randomized controlled trials.
RDI	Respiratory disturbance index.
RDS	Respiratory distress syndrome.
RDW	Red cell distribution width.
REEDA	Redness, edema, ecchymosis, drainage, approximation.
REM	Rapid eye movement.
REMS	Radiofrequency echographic multi-spectrometry.
Repl	Replace.
RESA	Radial cryosurgical ablation.
resp	Respiration, respiratory.
Retro	Retrospective rate derivation.
rev.	Revise, revision.
RFA	***1)*** Radiofrequency ablation. ***2)*** Regulatory Flexibility Act.
RFI	Request for information.
RFT	Renal function test.
RGO	Reciprocating gait orthosis.
Rh	Rhesus.
Rh neg	Rhesus factor negative.
RHB	Right heart bypass.
RHC	***1)*** Right heart catheterization. ***2)*** Rural health clinic.
RHD	***1)*** Relative hepatic dullness. ***2)*** Rheumatic heart disease.
RHF	Right heart failure.
RHHI	Regional home health intermediary.
RHIA	Registered health information administrator.
RHIO	Regional health information organization.
RHIT	Registered health information technician.
RIA	***1)*** Radioimmunoassay. ***2)*** Regulatory Impact Analysis.
RICA	Right internal carotid artery.
RIG	Rabies immune globulin.
RIH	Right inguinal hernia.
RIJ	Right internal jugular.
RIND	Reversible ischemic neurologic event.
RIST	Radioimmunosorbent test.
RITE	Rapid intraoperative tissue expansion.
RL	Ringer's lactate.
RLE	Right lower extremity.
RLF	Retrolental fibroplasia.
RLL	Right lower lobe.
rlq	Right lower quadrant.
RLS	Restless legs syndrome.
RM	Respiratory movement.
RMA	Right mentum anterior position.
RMC	Rating method code.
RML	Right middle lobe.
RMP	Right mentum posterior position.
RMS	Rhabdomyosarcoma.
RMT	Right mentum transverse position.
RN	Registered nurse.
RNA	Ribonucleic acid.
RNFL	Retinal nerve fiber layer.
RNV	Radionuclide ventriculography.
ROA	Right occiput anterior position.

ROM	Range of motion.
ROP	***1)*** Retinopathy of prematurity. ***2)*** Right occiput posterior position.
ROS	Review of systems.
ROSC	Return of spontaneous circulation.
ROSE	Rapid onsite cytology.
RP	Radical prostatectomy.
RPG	Retrograde pyelogram.
RPh	Registered pharmacist.
RPP	Radical perineal prostatectomy.
RPR	Venereal disease report.
RPT	Registered physical therapist.
RR	Recovery room.
RRA	Registered records administrator.
RRB	Railroad Retirement Board.
RRC	Rural referral center.
RRP	Radical retropubic prostatectomy.
RRR	Regular rate and rhythm.
RRT	Registered respiratory therapist.
rRT-PCR	Real-time reverse transcription-polymerase chain reaction.
RS	Reducing substances.
RSA	Radiostereometric analysis.
RSB	Recurrent sinus barotrauma.
RSC	Right subclavian.
RSR	Regular sinus rhythm.
RSS	Russell Silver syndrome.
RSV	Respiratory syncytial virus.
RSV-IGIV	Respiratory syncytial virus immune globulin intravenous.
RT	***1)*** Recreational therapist. ***2)*** Respiratory therapist. ***3)*** Resting tracing. ***4)*** Right.
RTA	Renal tubular acidosis.
RTC	Return to clinic.
RTI	Reproductive tract infection.
rTMS	Repetitive transcranial magnetic stimulation.
RTP	Return to provider.
RTPCR	Reverse transcriptase polymerase chain reaction.
RUCA	Rural-urban commuting area, a CMS designation.
RUG	Resource utilization group.
RUL	Right upper lobe.
ruq	Right upper quadrant.
RV	Right ventricle.
RVS	Relative value study.
RVT	Renal vein thrombosis.
RVU	Relative value unit.
RW	Relative weight.
Rx	Take (prescription; treatment).
RxN	Reaction.
RYGBP-E	Roux-en-Y gastric bypass—extended.
s	Without.
S tach	Sinus tachycardia.
S&A	Sugar and acetone.
S-C disease	Sickle cell hemoglobin-c disease.
s-JIA	Systemic onset juvenile idiopathic arthritis.
s.c.	Subcutaneous.
s.l.	Under the tongue, sublingual.
S.O.S.	If necessary (si opus sit).
S/P	Status post.
S/S	Signs and symptoms.
SA node	Sinoatrial node.
SAANDS	Selective apoptotic antineoplastic drugs.
SAARD	Slow-acting anti-rheumatic drug.
SAB	Spontaneous abortion.
SABA	Supplied air-breathing apparatus.
SAC	Short arm cast.
SACH	Solid ankle, cushion heel.
SACS	Sleep and circadian study.
SAD	Seasonal affective disorder.
SADMERC	Statistical Analysis Durable Medical Equipment Regional Carrier.
SAED	Semiautomatic external defibrillator.
SAFHS	Sonic accelerated fracture healing system.
SAGES	Society of American Gastrointestinal Endoscopic Surgeons.
SAH	Subarachnoid hemorrhage.
SAL	Suction assisted lipectomy.
SALT	***1)*** Sequential aggressive local therapy. ***2)*** Serum alanine aminotransferase. ***3)*** Skin associated lymphoid tissue.
SAMHSA	Substance Abuse and Mental Health Services Administration.
SANS	Stoller afferent nerve stimulation.
SARS	Severe acute respiratory syndrome.
SARS-CoV-2	COVID-19, COVID, COVID19, coronavirus.
SAS	Signs and symptoms.
SAST	Serum aspartate aminotransferase.
SAVER	Surgical anterior ventricular endocardial restoration.
SB	***1)*** Sinus bradycardia. ***2)*** Small bowel. ***3)*** Spina bifida.
SBA	Standby assist.
SBE	Subacute bacterial endocarditis.
SBFT	Small bowel follow-through.

SBGM	Self blood glucose monitoring.
SBO	***1)*** Side branch occlusion. ***2)*** Small bowel obstruction.
SBP	Systolic blood pressure.
SBRT	Stereotactic body radiation therapy.
SC	***1)*** Subcommittee. ***2)*** Subcutaneous.
SCA	Sickle cell anemia.
SCBE	Single contrast barium enema.
SCC	Squamous cell carcinoma.
SCCHN	Squamous cell carcinoma of the head and neck.
SCD	***1)*** Sickle cell disease. ***2)*** Sudden cardiac death. ***3)*** Systemic carnitine deficiency.
SCFE	Slipped capital femoral epiphysis.
SCH	Sole community hospital.
SCI	Spinal cord injury.
SCID	Severe combined immunodeficiency disorder.
SCIWORA	Spinal cord injury without radiologic (neuroimaging) abnormality.
SCORE	Simple calculated osteoporosis risk estimation.
SCR	Standard class rate.
SCSA	Skin cell suspension autograft.
SCT	Specialty care transport.
SD	Still's disease.
SDO	Standards development organization.
SDOH	Social determinants of health.
SEB	Scleral expansion band.
sed rate	Sedimentation rate of erythrocytes.
SEER	Surveillance, epidemiology, and end results.
SEM	Systolic ejection murmur.
Seno supp	Senokot suppository.
SEO	Shoulder-elbow orthosis.
SEP	Somatosensory evoked potentials.
SEPS	Subfascial endoscopic perforator surgery.
septem	Seven.
SERM	Selective estrogen receptor modulator.
SETTLE	Spindle epithelial tumor with thymus-like element.
SEWHO	Shoulder-elbow-wrist-hand orthosis.
SEXA	Single energy x-ray absorptiometry.
SFMS	Smith-Fineman-Myers syndrome.
SG	Swan-Ganz.
SGA	***1)*** Small for gestational age. ***2)*** Substantial gainful activity.
SGAP	Superior gluteal artery perforator.
SGC	Swan-Ganz catheter.
SGD	Speech generating device.
SGOT	Serum glutamic oxaloacetic acid.
SGR	Sustainable growth rate.
SH	Social history.
SHBG	Sex hormone binding globulin.
SHM	Society of Hospital Medicine.
SHP	Schonlein-Henoch purpura.
SIADH	Syndrome of inappropriate antidiuretic hormone.
SIB	Severe Impairment Battery.
SIC	Standard industry code.
SICD	Subcutaneous implantable cardio-defibrillator.
SID	Sensory integration dysfunction.
SIDS	Sudden infant death syndrome.
SIEA	Superficial inferior epigastric artery.
Sig.	Write on label (Rx) or let it be labeled.
Sig. S. (Signa)	Mark or write.
sine	Without.
SIR	Society of Interventional Radiology.
SIRF	Severely impaired renal function.
SIRS	Systemic inflammatory response syndrome.
SIRT	Selective internal radiation therapy.
SISI	Short increment sensitivity index.
SJS	Schwartz-Jampel syndrome.
SK	Seborrheic keratosis(es).
SLAP	Superior labral anteroposterior (lesion).
SLB	Short leg brace.
SLC	Short leg cast.
SLE	Systemic lupus erythematosus.
SLI	Speech language impairment.
SLP	Speech-language pathology.
SLR	Straight-leg raising.
SLUD	Salivation, lacrimation, urination, defecation.
SLWC	Short leg walking cast.
SM	Samarium.
SMAS	Superficial musculoaponeurotic system.
SMBG	Self-monitored blood glucose.
SMBP	Self-measured blood pressure monitoring.
SMEI	Severe myoclonic epilepsy in infancy.
SMM	Smoldering multiple myeloma.
SMO	***1)*** Slip made out. ***2)*** Supra-malleolar orthotic.
SMRR	Submucosal resection and rhinoplasty.
SNCT	Sensory nerve conduction test.
SNF	Skilled nursing facility.
SNIP	Strategic national implementation process.
SNOMED	Systemized nomenclature of medicine.

SNOMED-CT Systemized nomenclature of medicine, clinical terms.
SNS *1)* Sacral nerve stimulation. *2)* Somatic nervous system. *3)* Sympathetic nervous system.
SO *1)* Sacroiliac orthosis. *2)* Shoulder orthosis.
SOAP Subjective objective assessment plan.
SOB Shortness of breath.
SOF Signature on file.
SOI Severity of illness.
Sol Solution.
SOP Standard operation procedure.
SOW Scope of work.
SPA Subperiosteal abscess of the orbit.
SPAP Systolic pulmonary artery pressure.
SPD Summary plan description.
SPECT Single photon emission computerized tomography.
SpGr Specific gravity.
SPJ Saphenopopliteal junction.
SPKT Simultaneous pancreas-kidney transplant.
SpO2 Peripheral capillary oxygen saturation or blood oxygen saturation.
SPR Selective posterior rhizotomy.
SQ *1)* Status quo. *2)* Subcutaneous.
SR *1)* Seclusion room. *2)* Sedimentation rate. *3)* Superior rectus muscle.
SROM Spontaneous rupture of membrane.
SRP Surgical reversal of presbyopia.
SRS Stereotactic radiosurgery.
SRT Speech reception threshold.
SRUS Solitary rectal ulcer syndrome.
SRVs Small round viruses.
SS *1)* Half. *2)* Social Security. *3)* Social services. *4)* Somatostatin.
SSA Social Security Act.
SSE Soap suds enema.
SSEP Sensory evoked potential.
SSM Superficial spreading melanoma.
SSN Social security number.
SSO Standard-setting organization.
SSOP Second Surgical Opinion Program.
SSPE Subacute sclerosing panencephalitis.
SSSGS Similarly sized subscriber groups.
ST *1)* Schiotz tonometry. *2)* Sinus tachycardia.
staph Staphylococcus.
stat Immediately.
STB Stillborn.
STD Sexually transmitted disease.
STE *1)* Speckle tracking echocardiography. *2)* Subperiosteal tissue expander.
STEMI ST elevation myocardial infarction.
STFCS Standard transaction format compliance system.
STH Somatotrophic hormone.
STJ Subtalar joint.
STM Short-term memory.
strep Streptococcus.
STS *1)* Serology test for syphilis. *2)* Society of Thoracic Surgeons.
STSG Split thickness skin graft.
STU Skin test unit.
STWS Stuve Wiedemann syndrome.
STX Stricture.
sub Below.
sub q Subcutaneous.
SUBC State Uniform Billing Committee.
subcu Subcutaneous.
subind. Immediately after.
SUD Single use device.
SUDEP Sudden unexpected death in epilepsy.
SUI Stress urinary incontinence.
SUNCT Short-lasting, unilateral, neuralgiform headaches with conjunctival injection and tearing.
supp Suppository.
SUZI Subzonal insemination.
Sv Scalp vein.
SVC Service.
SVCS Superior vena cava syndrome.
SVD Spontaneous vaginal delivery.
SVG Saphenous vein graft.
SVR Surgical ventricular restoration.
SVRS Statistically valid random sample.
SVS Society for Vascular Surgery.
SVT Supraventricular tachycardia.
SWG Sub-workgroup.
SWISS Siblings with Ischemic Stroke Study.
Sx *1)* Sign. *2)* Symptom.
Syr Syrup.
Sz Seizure.
SZZ Sézary syndrome.
T *1)* Temperature. *2)* Tender. *3)* Thoracic vertebrae.
T&A Tonsillectomy and adenoidectomy.
T&C Type and crossmatch.

Abbreviations

T&CM	Type and cross match.
T(O)	Oral temperature.
t.d.s.	Three times a day.
t.i.d.	Three times a day.
T/O	Time out.
T3	***1)*** Free triiodothyronine. ***2)*** Triiodothyronine.
T4	Thyroxine.
TA	***1)*** Tension by applanation. ***2)*** Transactional analysis.
tab.	Tablet (tabella).
TABS	Tablets.
TACT	Trial to Assess Chelation Therapy.
TAG	Technical advisory group.
TAH	Total abdominal hysterectomy.
TAHBSO	Total abdominal hysterectomy, bilateral salpingo-oophorectomy.
Tap/H2O/E	Tap water enema.
TAPVR	Total anomalous pulmonary venous return.
TAS	Transcatheter atrial septostomy.
TAT	***1)*** Tetanus antitoxin. ***2)*** Turnaround time.
TAVI	Transcatheter aortic valve implantation.
TAVR	Transcatheter aortic valve replacement.
Tb	Tubercule bacillus.
TB	Tuberculosis.
TBA	***1)*** To be arranged. ***2)*** Transluminal balloon angioplasty.
TBE	Tick-borne encephalitis.
TBF	***1)*** Total body failure. ***2)*** Total body fat.
TBG	***1)*** Thyroid binding globulin. ***2)*** Thyroxine.
TBI	***1)*** Total body irradiation. ***2)*** Traumatic brain injury.
TBNA	Transbronchial needle aspiration.
TBSA	Total body surface area.
TBV	Total blood volume.
TC	Technetium.
Tc 99m	Technetium isotope.
TC&DB	Turn, cough, and deep breathe.
TCC	***1)*** Transitional care center. ***2)*** Transitional cell carcinoma.
TCD	Transcranial doppler.
TCDB	Turn, cough, deep breathe.
TCF	Transciliary filtration.
TCMI	T cell mediated immunity.
TCPI	Transforming Clinical Practice Initiative.
TCR	T-cell receptor.
Td	Tetanus.
TDD	Thoracic duct drainage.
TDF	Time dose fractionation factor.
TEB	Thoracic electrical bioimpedance.
TED	Thrombo-embolism deterrent.
TEDS	Anti-embolism stockings.
TEE	Transesophageal echocardiography.
TEFRA	Tax Equity and Fiscal Responsibility Act.
temp	Temperature.
TEMS	Transanal endoscopic microsurgical excision of rectal tumor.
TENS	Transcutaneous electrical nerve stimulation/stimulator.
TEP	Tracheoesophageal puncture.
TES	Threshold (or therapeutic) electrical stimulation.
TESA	Testicular sperm aspiration.
TEST	Tubal embryo stage transfer.
TEVAP	Transurethral electrovaporization of prostrate.
TFT	***1)*** Tectonic fallopian tunnel. ***2)*** Transfer factor test.
TG	Task group.
TGA	Transient global amnesia.
TGF	Tumor growth factor.
TGV	Transposition of great vessels.
THA	Total hip arthroplasty.
THAD	Transient hepatic attenuation differences.
Thal	Thalassemia.
THBR	Thyroid hormone binding ratio.
THC	Tetrahydrocannabinol.
THD	***1)*** Total hospice days. ***2)*** Transanal hemorrhoidal dearterialization.
THKAO	Thoracic-hip-knee-ankle orthosis.
THR	Total hip replacement.
TI	Tricuspid insufficiency.
TIA	Transient ischemic attack.
TIBC	Total iron binding capacity.
TIG	Tetanus immune globulin vaccine.
TIL	Tumor infiltrating lymphocytes.
TIM	Topical immunomodulator.
TIMI	Thrombolysis in myocardial infarction.
TIMP-1	Tissue inhibitor of metalloproteinase 1.
TIN	Tax identification number.
tinct	Tincture.
TIPPS	Test for intermediary prospective payment system.
TIPS	Transvenous intrahepatic portosystemic shunt.
TIS	***1)*** Thoracic insufficiency syndrome. ***2)*** Transcatheter intracardiac shunt.

TKA	Total knee arthroplasty.
TKE	Terminal knee extension.
TKO	To keep open.
TKR	Total knee replacement.
TL	***1)*** Triple lumen. ***2)*** Tubal ligation.
TLE	Temporal lobe epilepsy.
TLH	Total laparoscopic hysterectomy.
TLIF	Transforaminal lumbar interbody fusion.
TLM	Torn lateral meniscus.
TLP	Transitional living program.
TLS	Tumor lysis syndrome.
TLSO	Thoracolumbosacral orthosis.
TLT	Tonsillectomy.
TM	***1)*** Transcendental meditation. ***2)*** Tympanic membrane.
TME	Total mesorectal excision.
TMJ	Temporomandibular joint.
TML	Tongue midline.
TMR	Transmyocardial revascularization.
TMS	Transcranial magnetic stimulation.
TMTJ	Tarsometatarsal joint.
TMX	Tamoxifen.
TNA	Total nail avulsion.
TNB	Transthoracic needle biopsy.
TND	Term normal delivery.
TNE	Transnasal esophagoscopy.
TN-EGD	Transnasal esophagogastroduodenoscopy.
TNF	Tumor necrosis factor.
TNM	Tumor, node, metastases.
TNR	Tonic neck reflex.
TNS	Transcutaneous nerve stimulator or stimulation.
TNTC	Too numerous to count.
TNU	Tobacco nonuser.
TO	Telephone order.
TOA	***1)*** Time of arrival. ***2)*** Tubo-ovarian abscess.
ToF	Tetralogy of Fallot.
TORCH	Toxoplasma, other (includes syphilis), rubella, cytomegalovirus, and herpes virus.
TOS	Thoracic outlet syndrome.
TP	***1)*** Total protein. ***2)*** Tuberculin precipitation.
TPA	***1)*** Third-party administrator. ***2)*** Tissue plasminogen activator. ***3)*** Trading partner agreement.
TPAL	Term pregnancies, premature infants, abortions, living children.
TPBF	Total pulmonary blood flow.
TPC	Treatment planning conference.
TPL	Third party liability.
TPLA	Transperineal laser ablation.
TPN	Total parenteral nutrition.
TPOPP	Transportable physician orders for patient preferences.
TPPV	Total pars plana vitrectomy.
TPR	Temperature, pulse, respirations.
TQM	Total quality management.
Tr	***1)*** Tinctura, tincture. ***2)*** Trace.
TRALI	Transfusion related acute lung injury.
TRAM	Transverse rectus abdominis musculocutaneous.
trans	***1)*** Across, through. ***2)*** Transverse.
TRCV	Total red cell volume.
TRD	Treatment-resistant depression.
tres	Three.
TRF	Thyrotropin releasing factor.
TRH	Thyrotropin releasing hormone.
tri	Triple, three.
TRISS	Trauma and injury severity score.
tRNA	Transfer ribonucleic acid.
TRUSP	Transrectal ultrasound of prostate.
TS	***1)*** Tension by Schiotz. ***2)*** Tourette's syndrome.
TSA	***1)*** Thermal sensory analysis. ***2)*** Tumor specific antigen.
TSD	Tay-Sachs disease.
TSE	Testicular self-exam.
TSEB	Total skin electron beam.
TSH	Thyroid stimulating hormone.
TSS	Toxic shock syndrome.
TT	Thrombin time.
TTB	Third trimester bleeding.
TTD	Temporary total disability.
TTE	Transthoracic echocardiography.
tTG	Tissue transglutaminase.
TTN	Transient tachypnea of newborn.
TTP	Thrombotic thrombocytopenia purpura.
TTS	Transdermal therapeutic system.
TTT	Tibial tubercle transfer.
TTTS	Twin-to-twin transfusion syndrome.
TTVI	Transcatheter tricuspid valve implantation.
TTVR	Transcatheter tricuspid valve replacement.
TTWB	Toe-touch weight bearing.
TULIP	Transurethral ultrasound guided laser induced prostatectomy.

TUMT	Transurethral microwave thermotherapy.
TUNA	Transurethral needle ablation of prostate.
TUOD	Transurethral occlusive device.
TUR	Transurethral resection.
TURBT	Transurethral resection of bladder tumor.
TURP	Transurethral resection of the prostate.
TVCVB	Transvaginal chorionic villus biopsy.
TVH	Total vaginal hysterectomy.
TVS	Transvaginal sonography.
TWB	Touch weight bar.
TWE	Tap water enema.
TWI	T wave inversion on EKG, ECG.
Tx	Treatment.
U	***1)*** Unit. ***2)*** Uranium.
U&C	Usual and customary.
U-arm	Upper arm.
U/A	Urinalysis.
UAC	Umbilical artery catheter or catheterization.
UAE	Uterine artery embolization.
UAMCDS	Uniform ambulatory medical care data set.
UAO	Upper airway obstruction.
UAP	Upper abdominal pain.
UARS	Upper airway resistance syndrome.
UAS	Upper airway stimulation.
UASA	Upper airway sleep apnea.
UAVC	Univentricular atrioventricular connection.
UBF	Uterine blood flow.
UBO	Unidentified bright object.
UBW	Usual body weight.
UC	***1)*** Ulcerative colitis. ***2)*** Unit clerk.
UCBT	Unrelated cord-blood transplant.
UCD	Urine collection device.
UCDSS	Uniform Clinical Data Set System.
UCF	Uniform claim form, as in UCF-1500.
UCHD	Usual childhood diseases.
uCi	Microcurie.
UCR	Usual, customary, and reasonable.
UCTF	Uniform claim task force.
UCX	Urine culture.
UE	Upper extremity.
UES	Upper esophageal sphincter.
UFE	Uterine fibroid embolization.
UFR	Uroflowmetry.
UGI	Upper gastrointestinal.
UGS	Urogenital sinus.
UHDDS	Uniform hospital discharge data set.
UHIN	Utah Health Information Network.
UIP	Usual interstitial pneumonitis.
ULN	Upper limits of normal.
ULO	Ultra low oxygen.
ULV	Ultra low volume.
UM	***1)*** Unit manager. ***2)*** Utilization management.
UMN	Upper motor neuron.
UMO	Utilization management organization.
UN/CEFACT	United Nations Centre for Facilitation of Procedures and Practices for Administration, Commerce, and Transport.
UN/EDIFACT	United Nations Rules for Electronic Data Interchange for Administration, Commerce, and Transport.
ung.	Ointment.
UNSM	United Nations Standard Messages.
unus.	One.
UPJ	Ureteropelvic junction.
UPL	Upper payment limit, in Medicaid.
UPLIFT	Uterine positioning via ligament investment fixation and truncation.
UPP	Urethral pressure profile.
UPPP	Uvulopalatopharyngoplasty.
UR	Utilization review.
ur.	Urine.
URAC	Utilization Review Accreditation Commission.
URI	Upper respiratory infection.
URN	Utilization review nurse.
URT	Upper respiratory tract.
US	***1)*** Ultrasound. ***2)*** Unstable spine.
USC	United States Code.
USDHHS	United States Department of Health and Human Services.
USG	Ultrasonography.
USP	United States pharmacopoeia.
USPHS	United States Public Health Service.
USPSTF	U.S. Preventive Services Task Force.
USRDS	United States renal data system.
ut dict.	As directed.
UTI	Urinary tract infection.
UV	Ultraviolet light.
UVC	Umbilical vein catheter.
UVR	Ultraviolet radiation.
UW	Unilateral weakness.
V fib	Ventricular fibrillation.
V tach	Ventricular tachycardia.

Va	Visual acuity.
VA	Veterans Administration.
VACTERL	Vertebral, anal, cardiac, tracheal, esophageal, renal, and limb.
VAD	Ventricular assist device.
VADCS	Ventricular atrial distal coronary sinus.
VAIN	Vaginal intraepithelial neoplasia.
VALE	Visual acuity, left eye.
VAN	Value-added network.
VAP	Ventilator-associated pneumonia.
VAR	Various routes of administration.
VARE	Visual acuity, right eye.
VASS	Vacuum assisted sock system.
VAT	Vestibular autorotation test.
VATER	Vertebral, anal, tracheal, esophageal, and renal anomalies.
VATS	Video assisted thoracic surgery.
VAX-D	Vertebral axial decompression.
VBAC	Vaginal birth after cesarean section.
VBG	Vertical banding gastroplasty.
VBS	Vertebrobasilar artery syndrome.
VBT	Vertebral body tethering.
VC	Vena cava.
VCF	Vertebral compression fracture.
VCG	Vectorcardiogram.
vCJD	Variant Creutzfeldt-Jakob disease.
VCU	Voiding cystourethrogram.
VCUG	Voiding cystourethrogram.
VD	Venereal disease.
VDH	Valvular disease of the heart.
VDO	Varus derotational osteotomy.
VDRL	Venereal disease report.
VDRR	Vitamin D resistant rickets.
VE	Voluntary effort.
VEF	Ventricular ejection fraction.
VEGF	Vascular endothelial growth factor.
VEMP	Vestibular evoked myogenic potential.
VEP	Visual evoked potentials.
VF	***1)*** Ventricular fibrillation. ***2)*** Visual field.
VFL	Vinflunine.
VFR	Voiding flow rate.
VGH	Very good health.
VGM	Vein graft myringoplasty.
VH-IVUS	Virtual histology intravascular ultrasound.
ViCPs	Vi capsular polysaccharide, a type of typhoid vaccine.
VIN	Vulvar intraepithelial neoplasia.
VIP	Vasoactive intestinal peptide.
VISION	Vital information system to improve outcomes in nephrology.
vit	Vitamin (followed by specific letter).
VKA	Vitamin K antagonist.
VLAT	Visual laser ablation of trigone.
VLB	Vincaleukoblastine.
VLBW	Very low birth weight.
VLCD	Very low calorie diet.
VLDL	Very low density lipoprotein.
VM	Value-based payment modifier.
VM-26	Teniposide.
VMA	Vanillylmandelic acid.
VMD	Vitelliform macular dystrophy.
VML	Very malignant leanings.
VMPAC	Verbal Motor Production Assessment for Children.
VMST	Visual motor sequencing test.
VNS	Vagus nerve stimulator.
VO	Verbal order.
VO2	Maximum oxygen consumption.
VOR	Vestibulo-ocular response.
VOSS	Visual observation shivering score.
VP	***1)*** Variegate porphyria. ***2)*** Vasopressin. ***3)*** Voiding pressure.
VP-16	Etoposide.
VPB	Ventricular premature beat.
VPC	Ventricular premature contraction.
VPL	Ventro-posterolateral.
VPN	Virtual private network.
VPRC	Volume of packed red cells.
VPS	Volume Performance Standard.
VPT	Vibration perception threshold.
VRA	Visual reinforcement audiometry.
VS	***1)*** Vesicular sound. ***2)*** Visual snow. ***3)*** Vital signs.
VSA	Vital signs absent.
VSD	Ventricular septal defect.
VSW	Ventricular stroke work.
VT	Ventricular tachycardia.
VTG	Volume thoracic gas.
vv	Veins.
VW	Vessel wall.
VZIG	Varicella-zoster immune globulin.
VZV	Varicella zoster virus.
w	With.
W-D	Wet to dry (dressings).
w/	With.
W/C	Wheelchair.
w/HSBH	Warmed heelstick blood gas.
w/o	Without.
WAK	Wearable artificial kidney.

WB	Whole blood.
WBC	White blood count.
WBRT	Whole brain radiation therapy.
wc	Wheelchair.
WCC	Well child care.
WD	Well-developed.
WEDI	Work group on electronic data interchange.
WG	Work group.
WHFO	Wrist-hand-finger orthotic.
WHO	World Health Organization.
WHZ	Wheeze.
WIFC	Widely invasive follicular carcinoma.
WIHS	Women's Interagency HIV Study.
WISC	Wechsler Intelligence Scale for Children.
WIT	Water-induced thermotherapy.
WJG	Widers-Jongsma-van Ginneken (pacemaker model).
Wk	Week.
WKD	Wilson-Kimmelstiel disease.
WKI	Wakefield Inventory.
WKS	Wernicke-Korsakoff syndrome.
WLQ	Work limitation questionnaire.
WLS	Wet lung syndrome.
WM	Waldenström's macroglobulinemia.
WMFT	Wolf Motor Function Test.
WMP	Warm moist packs.
WMT	Word Memory Test.
WMX	Whirlpool, massage, and exercise.
WN	Well-nourished.
WNE	West Nile encephalitis.
WNL	Within normal limits.
WOCN	Wound, Ostomy and Continence Nursing.
WOP	Without pain.
WOPN	Walled off pancreatic necrosis.
WPC	Washington Publishing Company.
WPFM	Wright peak flow meter.
WPPSI	Wechsler Preschool and Primary Scale of Intelligence.
WPW	Wolff-Parkinson-White syndrome.
WR	***1)*** Wasserman reaction. ***2)*** Wrist.
WRAT	Wide Range Achievement Test.
WRUED	Work-related upper extremity disorder.
WSEP	Williams syndrome in early puberty.
Wt	Weight.
WT1	Wilms tumor 1 protein.
WT2	Wilms tumor 2 protein.
WTHD	Wish to hasten death.
x	Except.
XC	Cross clamp.
Xe	Xenon (isotope mass of xenon 133).
XFS	Exfoliation syndrome.
XLID	X-linked intellectual disability.
XLS	Excimer laser system.
XM	Cross match.
XML	Extensible Markup Language.
XR	Extremely rare.
XRBT	External beam radiotherapy.
XRT	External radiotherapy.
y-o	Year-old.
YDV	Yeast-derived hepatitis B vaccine.
YOB	Year of birth.
YOD	Year of death.
YPLL	Years of potential life lost before age 65.
YTD	Year to date.
ZEEP	Zero end-expiratory pressure.
ZHC	Zajdela hepatoma cell.
ZIFT	Zygote intrafallopian transfer.
Zn	Zinc.
ZPIC	Zone Program Integrity Contractor.
ZSRDS	Zung Self-Rating Depression Scale.

Procedural Eponyms

The medical custom of honoring a popular procedure's originator by name may prove to be problematic for the coder, who may have no trouble coding a Marshall-Marchetti but be faced with choosing one of the many Maze procedures.

The following list includes many of the procedures described by eponym in operative notes or other medical documentation; several are also included in the CPT® book.

Abbe-Estlander procedure

40527 Excision of lip; full thickness, reconstruction with cross lip flap (Abbe-Estlander)

40761 Plastic repair of cleft lip/nasal deformity; with cross lip pedicle flap (Abbe-Estlander type), including sectioning and inserting of pedicle

Surgical technique for a lip repair.

Adson test

95870 Needle electromyography; limited study of muscles in 1 extremity or non-limb (axial) muscles (unilateral or bilateral), other than thoracic paraspinal, cranial nerve supplied muscles, or sphincters

Physiological assessment for thoracic outlet syndrome.

Altemeier procedure

45130 Excision of rectal procidentia, with anastomosis; perineal approach

45135 Excision of rectal procidentia, with anastomosis; abdominal and perineal approach

Removal of a rectal prolapse through a perineal approach or through a combined abdominal and perineal approach.

Anderson's method of tibial lengthening

27715 Osteoplasty, tibia and fibula, lengthening or shortening

Technique in which the tibia is severed and screws are affixed to plates supporting the bone across the gap to lengthen the patient's leg.

Aries-Pitanguy mammaplasty

19318 Breast reduction

Procedure to reduce breast size.

Babcock's operation

37700 Ligation and division of long saphenous vein at saphenofemoral junction, or distal interruptions

Varicose veins are eliminated using a long probe and tying the end of the vein to it to draw out the vein by invagination.

Baker tube

44021 Enterotomy, small intestine, other than duodenum; for decompression (eg, Baker tube)

Tube placed into the jejunum or small bowel for decompression or extensive adhesions.

Bankart procedure

23455 Capsulorrhaphy, anterior; with labral repair (eg, Bankart procedure)

Procedure used to treat recurrent dislocation of the shoulder requiring reconstruction of the avulsed capsule and labrum at the glenoid lip.

Barany caloric test

92533 Caloric vestibular test, each irrigation (binaural, bithermal stimulation constitutes 4 tests)

Extent of nystagmus is determined by irrigating the external auditory meatus with hot or cold water.

Barkan operation

65820 Goniotomy

Technique corrects glaucoma by opening Schlemm's canal.

Barsky's operation

26580 Repair cleft hand

Cleft hand repaired by closing the cleft, bringing the ring and index fingers closer together, and correcting webbing between the fingers.

Batch-Spittler-McFaddin operation

27598 Disarticulation at knee

Leg is severed at the knee joint, which offers an alternative to severing a long bone.

Belsey procedure

43328 Esophagogastric fundoplasty partial or complete; thoracotomy

43334 Repair, paraesophageal hiatal hernia (including fundoplication), via thoracotomy, except neonatal; without implantation of mesh or other prosthesis

43335 Repair, paraesophageal hiatal hernia (including fundoplication), via thoracotomy, except neonatal; with implantation of mesh or other prosthesis

Open surgical procedure using a thoracic incision to resolve reflux.

Bender-Gestalt test

96130 Psychological testing evaluation services by physician or other qualified health care professional, including integration of patient data, interpretation of standardized test results and clinical data, clinical decision making, treatment planning and report, and interactive feedback to the patient, family member(s) or caregiver(s), when performed; first hour

96131 Psychological testing evaluation services by physician or other qualified health care professional, including integration of patient data, interpretation of standardized test results and clinical data, clinical decision making, treatment planning and report, and interactive feedback to the patient, family member(s) or caregiver(s), when performed; each additional hour (List separately in addition to code for primary procedure)

96136 Psychological or neuropsychological test administration and scoring by physician or other qualified health care professional, two or more tests, any method; first 30 minutes

96137 Psychological or neuropsychological test administration and scoring by physician or other qualified health care professional, two or more tests, any method; each additional 30 minutes (List separately in addition to code for primary procedure)

96138 Psychological or neuropsychological test administration and scoring by technician, two or more tests, any method; first 30 minutes

96139 Psychological or neuropsychological test administration and scoring by technician, two or more tests, any method; each additional 30 minutes (List separately in addition to code for primary procedure)

96146 Psychological or neuropsychological test administration, with single automated, standardized instrument via electronic platform, with automated result only

Psychological test gauges perceptual-motor coordination to assess personality dynamics, review organic brain impairment, and measure neurological maturity.

Benedict test

81005 Urinalysis; qualitative or semiquantitative, except immunoassays

Test using sodium or potassium citrate and sodium carbonate in a reagent to determine dextrose content of urine.

Bennett procedure

27430 Quadricepsplasty (eg, Bennett or Thompson type)

Correction of a shortened or fibrotic quadriceps muscle.

Bernstein test

91013 Esophageal motility (manometric study of the esophagus and/or gastroesophageal junction) study with interpretation and report; with stimulation or perfusion (eg, stimulant, acid or alkali perfusion) (List separately in addition to code for primary procedure)

91030 Esophagus, acid perfusion (Bernstein) test for esophagitis

Acid perfusion test used to differentiate substernal chest pain due to gastroesophageal reflux disease (GERD).

Betke-Kleihauer test

85460 Hemoglobin or RBCs, fetal, for fetomaternal hemorrhage; differential lysis (Kleihauer-Betke)

Venipuncture blood test taken to determine the amount of Rh immune globulin an Rh-negative woman should receive in order to prevent formation of antibodies against her fetus.

Bevan's operation

54640 Orchiopexy, inguinal or scrotal approach

Relocation of an undescended testicle down into the scrotum.

Biesenberger mammaplasty

19318 Breast reduction

Reduction procedure for transposition of the nipple with excision of the side of the mammary gland and rotation of the remaining glandular pedicle to form a skin brassiere.

Billroth I or II

43631 Gastrectomy, partial, distal; with gastroduodenostomy

43632 Gastrectomy, partial, distal; with gastrojejunostomy

43633 Gastrectomy, partial, distal; with Roux-en-Y reconstruction

43634 Gastrectomy, partial, distal; with formation of intestinal pouch

Anastomosis of the stomach to the duodenum or jejunum.

Binet test

96130 Psychological testing evaluation services by physician or other qualified health care professional, including integration of patient data, interpretation of standardized test results and clinical data, clinical decision making, treatment planning and report, and interactive feedback to the patient, family member(s) or caregiver(s), when performed; first hour

96131 Psychological testing evaluation services by physician or other qualified health care professional, including integration of patient data, interpretation of standardized test results and clinical data, clinical decision making, treatment planning and report, and interactive feedback to the patient, family member(s) or caregiver(s), when performed; each additional hour (List separately in addition to code for primary procedure)

96136 Psychological or neuropsychological test administration and scoring by physician or other qualified health care professional, two or more tests, any method; first 30 minutes

96137 Psychological or neuropsychological test administration and scoring by physician or other qualified health care professional, two or more tests, any method; each additional 30 minutes (List separately in addition to code for primary procedure)

96138 Psychological or neuropsychological test administration and scoring by technician, two or more tests, any method; first 30 minutes

96139 Psychological or neuropsychological test administration and scoring by technician, two or more tests, any method; each additional 30 minutes (List separately in addition to code for primary procedure)

96146 Psychological or neuropsychological test administration, with single automated, standardized instrument via electronic platform, with automated result only

Test that gauges mental capacity among children and youth using a standard series of questions based on the capacity of normal intellect among the same age groups.

Bischof myelotomy

63170 Laminectomy with myelotomy (eg, Bischof or DREZ type), cervical, thoracic, or thoracolumbar

Incision of the spinal cord longitudinally for relief of peripheral pain or spasticity.

Blalock-Hanlon procedure

33735 Atrial septectomy or septostomy; closed heart (Blalock-Hanlon type operation)

33736 Atrial septectomy or septostomy; open heart with cardiopulmonary bypass

Atrial septectomy procedure to allow free mixing of the blood from the right and left atria.

Blalock-Taussig procedure

33750 Shunt; subclavian to pulmonary artery (Blalock-Taussig type operation)

Surgical anastomosis between the subclavian artery and pulmonary artery in order to increase blood flow to the lungs in infants with pulmonary blood flow obstruction.

Bricker operation

50820 Ureteroileal conduit (ileal bladder), including intestine anastomosis (Bricker operation)

Surgical procedure to connect the ureters to a segment of the ileal colon to divert urine flow through the bowel.

Bristow procedure

23460 Capsulorrhaphy, anterior, any type; with bone block

Anterior capsulorrhaphy prevents chronic separation of the shoulder. In this procedure, the bone block is affixed to the anterior glenoid rim with a screw.

Brock's operation

33474 Valvotomy, pulmonary valve, open heart, with cardiopulmonary bypass

Surgical relief of pulmonary valvular stenosis by passing a valvulotome through the wall of the right ventricle into the pulmonary artery.

Browne's operation

54324 1-stage distal hypospadias repair (with or without chordee or circumcision); with urethroplasty by local skin flaps (eg, flip-flap, prepucial flap)

Hypospadias is repaired with a strip of epithelium left on the top of the penis to form a top of the urethra. Margins of the incision are used to form the bottom.

Burrow's operation (triangle)

14000 Adjacent tissue transfer or rearrangement, trunk; defect 10 sq cm or less

14001 Adjacent tissue transfer or rearrangement, trunk; defect 10.1 sq cm to 30.0 sq cm

14020 Adjacent tissue transfer or rearrangement, scalp, arms and/or legs; defect 10 sq cm or less

14021 Adjacent tissue transfer or rearrangement, scalp, arms and/or legs; defect 10.1 sq cm to 30.0 sq cm

14040 Adjacent tissue transfer or rearrangement, forehead, cheeks, chin, mouth, neck, axillae, genitalia, hands and/or feet; defect 10 sq cm or less
14041 Adjacent tissue transfer or rearrangement, forehead, cheeks, chin, mouth, neck, axillae, genitalia, hands and/or feet; defect 10.1 sq cm to 30.0 sq cm
14060 Adjacent tissue transfer or rearrangement, eyelids, nose, ears and/or lips; defect 10 sq cm or less
14061 Adjacent tissue transfer or rearrangement, eyelids, nose, ears and/or lips; defect 10.1 sq cm to 30.0 sq cm
14301 Adjacent tissue transfer or rearrangement, any area; defect 30.1 sq cm to 60.0 sq cm
14302 Adjacent tissue transfer or rearrangement, any area; each additional 30.0 sq cm, or part thereof (List separately in addition to code for primary procedure)

Triangles of skin at the base of the pedicle of a skin flap are excised to achieve advancement.

Caldwell-Luc operation

21385 Open treatment of orbital floor blowout fracture; transantral approach (Caldwell-Luc type operation)

Intraoral antrostomy approach into the maxillary sinus for the removal of tooth roots or tissue, or for packing the sinus to reduce zygomatic fractures by creating a window above the teeth in the canine fossa area.

Callander knee disarticulation

27598 Disarticulation at knee

Patella is removed and the long anterior and posterior skin flaps of the tibia are retained to enhance healing.

Campbell arthrodesis

27870 Arthrodesis, ankle, open

Extra-articular fusion of the ankle and subtalar joint, done to treat arthritic conditions, infection, or a failed prior surgery on the joint.

Carpue's operation

30400 Rhinoplasty, primary; lateral and alar cartilages and/or elevation of nasal tip

Repair of the nose by folding a flap from the forehead and pedicle at the root of the nose around the area to be repaired.

Chiari osteotomy

27151 Osteotomy, iliac, acetabular or innominate bone; with femoral osteotomy
27156 Osteotomy, iliac, acetabular or innominate bone; with femoral osteotomy and with open reduction of hip
27158 Osteotomy, pelvis, bilateral (eg, congenital malformation)

Top of the femur is altered to correct a dislocated hip caused by congenital conditions or cerebral palsy. Plate and screws are often used.

Coffey operation

58400 Uterine suspension, with or without shortening of round ligaments, with or without shortening of sacrouterine ligaments; (separate procedure)

Surgical technique in which the uterus is suspended by suturing over the cornual wound using the broad and round ligaments.

Cotte's operation

58410 Uterine suspension, with or without shortening of round ligaments, with or without shortening of sacrouterine ligaments; with presacral sympathectomy

Presacral neurectomy to relieve severe dysmenorrhea.

Cotting's operation

11765 Wedge excision of skin of nail fold (eg, for ingrown toenail)

Excisional treatment for ingrowing toenail.

Damus-Kaye-Stansel procedure

33606 Anastomosis of pulmonary artery to aorta (Damus-Kaye-Stansel procedure)

Corrective procedure done for transposition of the great vessels, in which the pulmonary artery is cut just before it divides into the right and left branches and anastomosed to the side of the ascending aorta.

Dana rhizotomy

63185 Laminectomy with rhizotomy; 1 or 2 segments
63190 Laminectomy with rhizotomy; more than 2 segments

Posterior nerve roots of the spine are severed to relieve chronic pain or spasms.

Dandy ventriculocisternostomy

62200 Ventriculocisternostomy, third ventricle;
62201 Ventriculocisternostomy, third ventricle; stereotactic, neuroendoscopic method

Operation in which an opening from the third ventricle to the interpeduncular cistern is established.

Darrach resection

25240 Excision distal ulna partial or complete (eg, Darrach type or matched resection)

Operation relieves pain and stiffness in the radioulnar joint.

David procedure

33864 Ascending aorta graft, with cardiopulmonary bypass with valve suspension, with coronary reconstruction and valve-sparing aortic root remodeling (eg, David Procedure, Yacoub Procedure)

Surgical procedure that involves replacement of the aortic root and ascending aorta. The valve is connected to the new section of the aorta inside the Dacron graft with implantation of the coronary arteries. While the valve itself is not replaced, it may require repair/reimplantation.

Day test

82270 Blood, occult, by peroxidase activity (eg, guaiac), qualitative; feces, consecutive collected specimens with single determination, for colorectal neoplasm screening (ie, patient was provided 3 cards or single triple card for consecutive collection)

Test determines presence of blood in the feces.

Delorme pericardiectomy

33030 Pericardiectomy, subtotal or complete; without cardiopulmonary bypass

33031 Pericardiectomy, subtotal or complete; with cardiopulmonary bypass

Method for excising a diseased pericardium constricting the ventricle.

Dor procedure

33548 Surgical ventricular restoration procedure, includes prosthetic patch, when performed (eg, ventricular remodeling, SVR, SAVER, Dor procedures)

Therapeutic procedure to treat congestive heart failure by restoring the heart to a more normal size and shape. The ventricular muscle and chamber are resized with the aid of a plastic model, in hopes of improving heart function. This procedure is often performed with bypass or valve repair, which is reported separately.

Dupuy-Dutemps reconstruction

67971 Reconstruction of eyelid, full thickness by transfer of tarsoconjunctival flap from opposing eyelid; up to two-thirds of eyelid, 1 stage or first stage

67973 Reconstruction of eyelid, full thickness by transfer of tarsoconjunctival flap from opposing eyelid; total eyelid, lower, 1 stage or first stage

67974 Reconstruction of eyelid, full thickness by transfer of tarsoconjunctival flap from opposing eyelid; total eyelid, upper, 1 stage or first stage

Eyelid reconstruction involving the skin from the opposing lid.

Dwyer osteotomy

28300 Osteotomy; calcaneus (eg, Dwyer or Chambers type procedure), with or without internal fixation

Operation to correct a frontal plane deformity of the varus in the cavus foot.

Eggers procedure

27100 Transfer external oblique muscle to greater trochanter including fascial or tendon extension (graft)

Hamstring muscles of the knee and thigh area are transferred to a new position on the femoral condyle.

Emmet operation

57720 Trachelorrhaphy, plastic repair of uterine cervix, vaginal approach

Repair of the perineum and the cervix uteri.

Farr test

82784 Gammaglobulin (immunoglobulin); IgA, IgD, IgG, IgM, each

82785 Gammaglobulin (immunoglobulin); IgE

82787 Gammaglobulin (immunoglobulin); immunoglobulin subclasses (eg, IgG1, 2, 3, or 4), each

Antibody reacts to radioactive antigen and precipitates, leaving a free antigen in solution. Radio markers tag the suspected antigen.

Foley Y-pyeloplasty

50400 Pyeloplasty (Foley Y-pyeloplasty), plastic operation on renal pelvis, with or without plastic operation on ureter, nephropexy, nephrostomy, pyelostomy, or ureteral splinting; simple

50405 Pyeloplasty (Foley Y-pyeloplasty), plastic operation on renal pelvis, with or without plastic operation on ureter, nephropexy, nephrostomy, pyelostomy, or ureteral splinting; complicated (congenital kidney abnormality, secondary pyeloplasty, solitary kidney, calycoplasty)

Y-shaped flap prepared from the renal pelvis of the kidney and advanced into the ureter to correct a defect.

Fontan procedure

33615 Repair of complex cardiac anomalies (eg, tricuspid atresia) by closure of atrial septal defect and anastomosis of atria or vena cava to pulmonary artery (simple Fontan procedure)

33617 Repair of complex cardiac anomalies (eg, single ventricle) by modified Fontan procedure

Surgical bypass procedure that corrects tricuspid atresia and other selected congenital conditions by connecting the right atrium directly to the pulmonary artery by anastomosis or by inserting a closed prosthesis between

Procedural Eponyms

the right atrium and the pulmonary artery and closing the interatrial communication.

Frazier-Spiller operation

61450 Craniectomy, subtemporal, for section, compression, or decompression of sensory root of gasserian ganglion

Sensory root of the gasserian ganglion is compressed or decompressed to relieve trigeminal neuralgia.

Frickman operation

45550 Proctopexy (eg, for prolapse); with sigmoid resection, abdominal approach

To correct rectal prolapse, rectum is sutured to the anterior presacral fascia and attached to the sigmoid colon, which has been shortened to help suspend the rectum.

Frost suture

67875 Temporary closure of eyelids by suture (eg, Frost suture)

Temporary sutures of the eyelid.

Gil-Vernet pyelotomy

50120 Pyelotomy; with exploration

Exploration of the calyces and renal pelvis of the kidney.

Glenn procedure

33766 Shunt; superior vena cava to pulmonary artery for flow to 1 lung (classical Glenn procedure)

33767 Shunt; superior vena cava to pulmonary artery for flow to both lungs (bidirectional Glenn procedure)

Creation of a shunt by anastomosing the superior vena cava to the pulmonary artery to increase perfusion to both lungs.

Graefe's operation

66830 Removal of secondary membranous cataract (opacified posterior lens capsule and/or anterior hyaloid) with corneo-scleral section, with or without iridectomy (iridocapsulotomy, iridocapsulectomy)

Cataracts are corrected by removing the lens, lacerating the capsule, and performing an iridectomy via the sclera.

Grice arthrodesis

28725 Arthrodesis; subtalar

Bone graft is planted in the lateral part of the subtalar joint.

Gritti operation

27590 Amputation, thigh, through femur, any level;

27591 Amputation, thigh, through femur, any level; immediate fitting technique including first cast

27592 Amputation, thigh, through femur, any level; open, circular (guillotine)

Supracondylar amputation of the femur is performed with the patella placed as a cap on the amputated end.

Gundersen flap

68362 Conjunctival flap; total (such as Gunderson thin flap or purse string flap)

Procedure in which a damaged section of cornea is replaced using part of the conjunctiva.

Guthrie test

84030 Phenylalanine (PKU), blood

Bacterial inhibition assay measures serum phenylalanine. It is in widespread use for detection of phenylketonuria in newborns.

Halsted mastectomy

19305 Mastectomy, radical, including pectoral muscles, axillary lymph nodes

Radical mastectomy, which includes removal of the breast along with the pectoral minor muscle.

Ham test

85475 Hemolysin, acid

Laboratory test that checks for acidified serum.

Harrington rod technique

22840 Posterior non-segmental instrumentation (eg, Harrington rod technique, pedicle fixation across 1 interspace, atlantoaxial transarticular screw fixation, sublaminar wiring at C1, facet screw fixation) (List separately in addition to code for primary procedure)

22850 Removal of posterior nonsegmental instrumentation (eg, Harrington rod)

Device used in nonsegmental spinal instrumentation that affixes at the ends and may span several vertebral segments without attaching to the segments in between. The Harrington rod is placed to correct spinal curvature problems and occasionally fractures.

Hartley-Krause operation

61450 Craniectomy, subtemporal, for section, compression, or decompression of sensory root of gasserian ganglion

Gasserian ganglion is removed to relieve trigeminal neuralgia.

Hartmann procedure

44143 Colectomy, partial; with end colostomy and closure of distal segment (Hartmann type procedure)

44206 Laparoscopy, surgical; colectomy, partial, with end colostomy and closure of distal segment (Hartmann type procedure)

The lower part of the sigmoid colon and/or the upper part of the rectum is excised. The descending colon is

manipulated and sutured to the skin to create a colostomy. The proximal end of the descending colon is oversewn and a pouch is formed.

Heaf test

86580 Skin test; tuberculosis, intradermal

Laboratory test that checks for tuberculin antibodies.

Heller myotomy

32665 Thoracoscopy, surgical; with esophagomyotomy (Heller type)

43279 Laparoscopy, surgical, esophagomyotomy (Heller type), with fundoplasty, when performed

43330 Esophagomyotomy (Heller type); abdominal approach

43331 Esophagomyotomy (Heller type); thoracic approach

Longitudinal division of the distal esophageal muscle down to the submucosal layer. Cardia muscle fibers may also be divided. This procedure is used to treat achalasia.

Hicks-Pitney test

85730 Thromboplastin time, partial (PTT); plasma or whole blood

Thromboplastin generation test that measures the efficiency of plasma in forming thromboplastin.

Holten test

82575 Creatinine; clearance

Creatines are used to test renal efficiency.

Holter monitor procedure

93224 External electrocardiographic recording up to 48 hours by continuous rhythm recording and storage; includes recording, scanning analysis with report, review and interpretation by a physician or other qualified health care professional

93225 External electrocardiographic recording up to 48 hours by continuous rhythm recording and storage; recording (includes connection, recording, and disconnection)

93226 External electrocardiographic recording up to 48 hours by continuous rhythm recording and storage; scanning analysis with report

93227 External electrocardiographic recording up to 48 hours by continuous rhythm recording and storage; review and interpretation by a physician or other qualified health care professional

Patient wears a portable instrument to chart long-term behavior of the heart.

Hori procedure

25430 Insertion of vascular pedicle into carpal bone (eg, Hori procedure)

Procedure involves complex repair of an injury that affects the dorsal skin, subcutaneous fat, including the nerves and blood vessels, and the covering immediately adjacent to the tendon.

Howard test

52005 Cystourethroscopy, with ureteral catheterization, with or without irrigation, instillation, or ureteropyelography, exclusive of radiologic service;

Both ureters are catheterized and urine is collected from each kidney to test renal function.

Huggin operation

54520 Orchiectomy, simple (including subcapsular), with or without testicular prosthesis, scrotal or inguinal approach

Testes removed due to prostate cancer, among other diagnoses.

Hummelsheim operation

67340 Strabismus surgery involving exploration and/or repair of detached extraocular muscle(s) (List separately in addition to code for primary procedure)

Correction of strabismus by adjusting the eye muscles.

Jannetta decompression

61458 Craniectomy, suboccipital; for exploration or decompression of cranial nerves

Microsurgery relieving pressure on the cranial nerves.

Jatene procedure

33770 Repair of transposition of the great arteries with ventricular septal defect and subpulmonary stenosis; without surgical enlargement of ventricular septal defect

33771 Repair of transposition of the great arteries with ventricular septal defect and subpulmonary stenosis; with surgical enlargement of ventricular septal defect

33774 Repair of transposition of the great arteries, atrial baffle procedure (eg, Mustard or Senning type) with cardiopulmonary bypass;

33775 Repair of transposition of the great arteries, atrial baffle procedure (eg, Mustard or Senning type) with cardiopulmonary bypass; with removal of pulmonary band

33776 Repair of transposition of the great arteries, atrial baffle procedure (eg, Mustard or Senning type) with cardiopulmonary bypass; with closure of ventricular septal defect

33777 Repair of transposition of the great arteries, atrial baffle procedure (eg, Mustard or Senning type) with cardiopulmonary bypass; with repair of subpulmonic obstruction

33778 Repair of transposition of the great arteries, aortic pulmonary artery reconstruction (eg, Jatene type);

33779 Repair of transposition of the great arteries, aortic pulmonary artery reconstruction (eg, Jatene type); with removal of pulmonary band

33780 Repair of transposition of the great arteries, aortic pulmonary artery reconstruction (eg, Jatene type); with closure of ventricular septal defect

33781 Repair of transposition of the great arteries, aortic pulmonary artery reconstruction (eg, Jatene type); with repair of subpulmonic obstruction

Corrective measure performed for transposition of the great vessels when there is subaortic stenosis and narrowing of the left aortic ventricular junction, requiring reconstruction of these sites as well as surgical correction of the transposed aortic and pulmonary arteries.

Johannsen procedure

53400 Urethroplasty; first stage, for fistula, diverticulum, or stricture (eg, Johannsen type)

First stage of a two-phase surgical procedure in which the urethra is reconstructed.

Jones and Cantarow test

84545 Urea nitrogen, clearance

Laboratory test to determine renal efficiency by testing collected urine for urea concentration.

Kasai procedure

47701 Portoenterostomy (eg, Kasai procedure)

Surgical procedure in which the jejunum is connected to the bile ducts and other portal structures of the liver and gallbladder.

Kelikian procedure

28280 Syndactylization, toes (eg, webbing or Kelikian type procedure)

Surgical procedure performed to correct a deformity of the foot when toes are missing and a large gap exists between the toes present. Osteotomies and bone alignments are performed to approximate the toes and eliminate the gap, producing an artificial syndactylism or webbing of the toes.

Killian operation

31070 Sinusotomy frontal; external, simple (trephine operation)

Surgical procedure in which the anterior wall of the frontal sinus is excised, the diseased tissue removed, and a permanent opening is created between the nasal cavity and the maxillary sinus in order to facilitate sinus drainage.

Kock procedure

44316 Continent ileostomy (Kock procedure) (separate procedure)

Surgical procedure in which the physician forms a reservoir of distal ileum (Kock pouch) and brings it through the abdominal wall onto the skin as a continent ileostomy.

Koyanagi procedure

54332 1-stage proximal penile or penoscrotal hypospadias repair requiring extensive dissection to correct chordee and urethroplasty by use of skin graft tube and/or island flap

Proximal hypospadias is corrected using lateral flaps of penile skin to create a tube.

Kraske procedure

45116 Proctectomy, partial, with anastomosis; transsacral approach only (Kraske type)

Surgical procedure in which a portion of the rectum is removed through a transsacral approach.

Kroenlein procedure

67420 Orbitotomy with bone flap or window, lateral approach (eg, Kroenlein); with removal of lesion

Lateral orbital decompression to relieve forward pressure on the eye when the orbital contents have increased in size (e.g., Graves's disease, thyroid eye disease).

Krupin-Denver valve implant

66180 Aqueous shunt to extraocular equatorial plate reservoir, external approach; with graft

66185 Revision of aqueous shunt to extraocular equatorial plate reservoir; with graft

67120 Removal of implanted material, posterior segment; extraocular

Eponym for an eye implant used to mitigate glaucoma.

Lambrinudi arthrodesis

28715 Arthrodesis; triple

Triple fusion prevents the foot drop that may result from polio.

Laroyenne operation

57010 Colpotomy; with drainage of pelvic abscess

Douglas pouch is punctured to evacuate pus and to facilitate drainage.

Linton procedure (ligation)

37760 Ligation of perforator veins, subfascial, radical (Linton type), including skin graft, when performed, open,1 leg

Radical subfascial ligation of the tributaries of the great saphenous vein, called perforator veins, connecting it to other veins of the lower leg. They are tied off to separate the communication of deep and superficial veins along the course of the leg.

Lisfranc operation

28600 Closed treatment of tarsometatarsal joint dislocation; without anesthesia

28605 Closed treatment of tarsometatarsal joint dislocation; requiring anesthesia

28606 Percutaneous skeletal fixation of tarsometatarsal joint dislocation, with manipulation

28615 Open treatment of tarsometatarsal joint dislocation, includes internal fixation, when performed

Eponym describing the treatment of a fracture-dislocation injury in the ball of the foot or distal to it, named for Napoleon's field surgeon who treated frostbite on the Russian front. The tarsometatarsal joint is also known as Lisfranc joint.

Longmire anastomosis

47765 Anastomosis, of intrahepatic ducts and gastrointestinal tract

Biliary obstruction is corrected with an intrahepatic cholangiojejunostomy and partial hepatectomy.

Lorenz's operation

27258 Open treatment of spontaneous hip dislocation (developmental, including congenital or pathological), replacement of femoral head in acetabulum (including tenotomy, etc);

Chronic dislocation of the hip is corrected by tying the head of the femur to the acetabulum to develop a socket.

Lowsley's operation

54380 Plastic operation on penis for epispadias distal to external sphincter;

Simple epispadias is corrected by closing the glandular cleft urethra, splitting the glans, and burying the repaired urethra deep into the soft tissue.

Magnuson-Stack procedure

23450 Capsulorrhaphy, anterior; Putti-Platt procedure or Magnuson type operation

Treatment for recurrent anterior dislocation of the shoulder that involves tightening and realigning the subscapularis tendon.

Magpi procedure

54322 1-stage distal hypospadias repair (with or without chordee or circumcision); with simple meatal advancement (eg, Magpi, V-flap)

Surgical procedure involving reconstruction of the meatus and glans, performed in order to correct hypospadias with chordee.

Mallory-Weiss procedure

43502 Gastrotomy; with suture repair of pre-existing esophagogastric laceration (eg, Mallory-Weiss)

Gastrotomy with repair of a tear in the esophagus in which the patient has experienced several hours or days of vomiting, marked by vomiting of blood.

Manchester operation

58400 Uterine suspension, with or without shortening of round ligaments, with or without shortening of sacrouterine ligaments; (separate procedure)

Preservation of the uterus following prolapse by amputating the vaginal portion of the cervix, shortening the cardinal ligaments, and performing a colpoperineorrhaphy posteriorly.

Mantoux test

86580 Skin test; tuberculosis, intradermal

Standard test checks for tuberculosis.

Maquet procedure

27418 Anterior tibial tubercleplasty (eg, Maquet type procedure)

Surgical procedure performed for treatment of patellofemoral joint pain entailing anterior displacement of the tibial tubercle and insertion of a bony block. The result is decreased force on the patella as it crosses the femoral condyles and an alteration in its weight-bearing position.

Marshall-Marchetti-Krantz

51840 Anterior vesicourethropexy, or urethropexy (eg, Marshall-Marchetti-Krantz, Burch); simple

51841 Anterior vesicourethropexy, or urethropexy (eg, Marshall-Marchetti-Krantz, Burch); complicated (eg, secondary repair)

58152 Total abdominal hysterectomy (corpus and cervix), with or without removal of tube(s), with or without removal of ovary(s); with colpo-urethrocystopexy (eg, Marshall-Marchetti-Krantz, Burch)

58267 Vaginal hysterectomy, for uterus 250 g or less; with colpo-urethrocystopexy (Marshall-Marchetti-Krantz type, Pereyra type) with or without endoscopic control

Surgical procedure to correct urinary stress incontinence in which the bladder is suspended by placing several sutures through the tissue surrounding the urethra and into the vaginal wall. The sutures are pulled tight so that the tissues are tacked up to the symphysis pubis and the urethra is moved forward.

Mathieu procedure

54324 1-stage distal hypospadias repair (with or without chordee or circumcision); with urethroplasty by local skin flaps (eg, flip-flap, prepucial flap)

Distal hypospadias repair and urethroplasty using local skin flaps.

Maze procedure

33254 Operative tissue ablation and reconstruction of atria, limited (eg, modified maze procedure)

33255 Operative tissue ablation and reconstruction of atria, extensive (eg, maze procedure); without cardiopulmonary bypass

33256 Operative tissue ablation and reconstruction of atria, extensive (eg, maze procedure); with cardiopulmonary bypass

33265 Endoscopy, surgical; operative tissue ablation and reconstruction of atria, limited (eg, modified maze procedure), without cardiopulmonary bypass

33266 Endoscopy, surgical; operative tissue ablation and reconstruction of atria, extensive (eg, maze procedure), without cardiopulmonary bypass

Creation of multiple incisions in the left atria through the endocardium to obliterate aberrant atrial conduction pathways and allow a normal impulse to activate the atrium, thereby stopping atrial fibrillation or flutter.

McCannel suture

66682 Suture of iris, ciliary body (separate procedure) with retrieval of suture through small incision (eg, McCannel suture)

Securing the haptic loop of an intraocular lens to the iris by threading the suture through the cornea without opening the eye.

McDonald cerclage

57700 Cerclage of uterine cervix, nonobstetrical

Opening of cervix is decreased via sutures around the bottom of the cervix.

McIndoe vaginal construction

57291 Construction of artificial vagina; without graft

Construction of an artificial vagina without using a graft.

Mikulicz resection

44320 Colostomy or skin level cecostomy;

44322 Colostomy or skin level cecostomy; with multiple biopsies (eg, for congenital megacolon) (separate procedure)

Procedure is done in stages and includes exteriorizing a section of intestine, usually the colon, resecting the exteriorized loop, and eliminating the fecal fistula by crushing the spur between the two barrels of the anastomosis. The fecal fistula is closed.

Miles procedure

44155 Colectomy, total, abdominal, with proctectomy; with ileostomy

44212 Laparoscopy, surgical; colectomy, total, abdominal, with proctectomy, with ileostomy

Lower sigmoid colon and rectum are removed for treatment of cancer. Physician removes the pelvic colon, mesocolon, and adjacent lymph nodes and establishes a permanent colostomy.

Millin-Read operation

57288 Sling operation for stress incontinence (eg, fascia or synthetic)

Suprapubic approach is used in the procedure to remedy stress incontinence.

Mitrofanoff procedure

50845 Cutaneous appendico-vesicostomy

Treatment of urinary incontinence in which the appendix is used as a conduit between the bladder and the surface of the abdomen as an opening for urine.

Mosenthal test

81002 Urinalysis, by dip stick or tablet reagent for bilirubin, glucose, hemoglobin, ketones, leukocytes, nitrite, pH, protein, specific gravity, urobilinogen, any number of these constituents; non-automated, without microscopy

Urine test for kidney function that is taken while the patient prescribes to a general diet.

Mustard procedure

33774 Repair of transposition of the great arteries, atrial baffle procedure (eg, Mustard or Senning type) with cardiopulmonary bypass;

33775 Repair of transposition of the great arteries, atrial baffle procedure (eg, Mustard or Senning type) with cardiopulmonary bypass; with removal of pulmonary band

33776 Repair of transposition of the great arteries, atrial baffle procedure (eg, Mustard or Senning type) with cardiopulmonary bypass; with closure of ventricular septal defect

33777 Repair of transposition of the great arteries, atrial baffle procedure (eg, Mustard or Senning type) with cardiopulmonary bypass; with repair of subpulmonic obstruction

Corrective measure for transposition of great vessels involves an intra-atrial baffle made of pericardial tissue or synthetic material. The baffle is secured between pulmonary veins and mitral valve and between mitral and tricuspid valves. The baffle directs systemic venous flow into the left ventricle and lungs and pulmonary venous flow into the right ventricle and aorta.

Naffziger operation

67414 Orbitotomy without bone flap (frontal or transconjunctival approach); with removal of bone for decompression

Removal of the lateral and superior orbital walls to decompress the orbit in cases of severe malignant exophthalmos.

Nagel test

92283 Color vision examination, extended, eg, anomaloscope or equivalent

Extended color vision examination involving an anomaloscope or equivalent, which is an instrument used to diagnose abnormalities of color perception in which one half of a field of color is matched by mixing two other colors.

Nissen procedure (fundoplasty)

43327 Esophagogastric fundoplasty partial or complete; laparotomy

43328 Esophagogastric fundoplasty partial or complete; thoracotomy

Surgical repair technique that involves the fundus of the stomach being wrapped around the lower end of the esophagus to treat reflux esophagitis.

Norwood procedure

33619 Repair of single ventricle with aortic outflow obstruction and aortic arch hypoplasia (hypoplastic left heart syndrome) (eg, Norwood procedure)

Surgical correction to widen the diameter of the aorta and repair single ventricle with aortic outflow obstruction. The pulmonary valve is transformed into the systemic arterial heart valve by means of encircling it with the application of a large pericardial patch, used to enlarge the aorta and sewn as a tube along the sides of the hypoplastic ascending aorta and aortic arch.

Park septostomy

33741 Transcatheter atrial septostomy (TAS) for congenital cardiac anomalies to create effective atrial flow, including all imaging guidance by the proceduralist, when performed, any method (eg, Rashkind, Sang-Park, balloon, cutting balloon, blade)

Increases blood flow across the atrial septum in children with certain forms of cyanotic congenital heart disease.

Patey's operation

19307 Mastectomy, modified radical, including axillary lymph nodes, with or without pectoralis minor muscle, but excluding pectoralis major muscle

Modified radical mastectomy, which includes removal of the breast and axillary lymph nodes with preservation of the pectoralis major muscle.

Pean's amputation

27290 Interpelviabdominal amputation (hindquarter amputation)

Arteries and veins are ligated during each step to amputate the hip joint.

Pemberton osteotomy

27158 Osteotomy, pelvis, bilateral (eg, congenital malformation)

Osteotomy is performed to position triradiate cartilage as a hinge for rotating the acetabular roof in cases of dysplasia of the hip in children.

Polya anastomosis

43632 Gastrectomy, partial, distal; with gastrojejunostomy

Anastomosis of the transected stomach to the side of the jejunum following gastrectomy.

Potts-Smith operation

33762 Shunt; descending aorta to pulmonary artery (Potts-Smith type operation)

Side-to-side anastomosis of the descending aorta to the left pulmonary artery creating a shunt that enlarges as the child grows.

Prentiss orchiopexy

54640 Orchiopexy, inguinal or scrotal approach

Inguinal incision is made to move undescended testicles to the scrotum.

Putti-Platt procedure

23450 Capsulorrhaphy, anterior; Putti-Platt procedure or Magnuson type operation

The subscapularis is tightened by altering the insertion point, creating a "sling" for the humeral head.

Rashkind procedure

33741 Transcatheter atrial septostomy (TAS) for congenital cardiac anomalies to create effective atrial flow, including all imaging guidance by the proceduralist, when performed, any method (eg, Rashkind, Sang-Park, balloon, cutting balloon, blade)

Transvenous balloon atrial septectomy or septostomy performed by cardiac catheterization. A balloon catheter is inserted into the heart either to create or enlarge an opening in the interatrial septal wall.

Rastelli operation

33786 Total repair, truncus arteriosus (Rastelli type operation)

Correction of persistent truncus arteriosus in which the pulmonary artery is separated from the primitive truncus to create a right ventricle-to-pulmonary artery conduit.

Reinsch test

83015 Heavy metal (eg, arsenic, barium, beryllium, bismuth, antimony, mercury); qualitative, any number of analytes

Laboratory test that determines the level of heavy metals in body tissue.

Roux-en-Y anastomosis

43621 Gastrectomy, total; with Roux-en-Y reconstruction

43633 Gastrectomy, partial, distal; with Roux-en-Y reconstruction

43634 Gastrectomy, partial, distal; with formation of intestinal pouch

43644 Laparoscopy, surgical, gastric restrictive procedure; with gastric bypass and Roux-en-Y gastroenterostomy (roux limb 150 cm or less)

43846 Gastric restrictive procedure, with gastric bypass for morbid obesity; with short limb (150 cm or less) Roux-en-Y gastroenterostomy

47740 Cholecystoenterostomy; Roux-en-Y

47741 Cholecystoenterostomy; Roux-en-Y with gastroenterostomy

47780 Anastomosis, Roux-en-Y, of extrahepatic biliary ducts and gastrointestinal tract

47785 Anastomosis, Roux-en-Y, of intrahepatic biliary ducts and gastrointestinal tract

48540 Internal anastomosis of pancreatic cyst to gastrointestinal tract; Roux-en-Y

Y-shaped attachment of the distal end of a divided small intestine segment to the stomach, esophagus, biliary tract, or other structure with anastomosis of the proximal end to the side of the small intestine further down for reflux-free drainage.

Salter osteotomy

27158 Osteotomy, pelvis, bilateral (eg, congenital malformation)

Innominate bone of the hip is cut, removed, and repositioned to repair a congenital dislocation, subluxation, or deformity.

Shirodkar procedure

59325 Cerclage of cervix, during pregnancy; abdominal

Treatment of an incompetent cervical os by placing nonabsorbent suture material in purse-string sutures as a cerclage to support the cervix.

Snodgrass procedure

54326 1-stage distal hypospadias repair (with or without chordee or circumcision); with urethroplasty by local skin flaps and mobilization of urethra

Midline incision made in the penis, which is then rolled around a catheter and secured with the intent of the tissue epithelializing and healing.

Stoffel rhizotomy

63185 Laminectomy with rhizotomy; 1 or 2 segments

63190 Laminectomy with rhizotomy; more than 2 segments

Nerve roots are sectioned to relieve pain or spastic paralysis.

Taarnhoj procedure

61450 Craniectomy, subtemporal, for section, compression, or decompression of sensory root of gasserian ganglion

The skull is opened at the temporal region and the gasserian ganglion nerve root is sectioned, decompressed, or compressed, depending on the patient's complaint.

Thompson procedure

27430 Quadricepsplasty (eg, Bennett or Thompson type)

Correction of a shortened or fibrotic quadriceps muscle.

Token test

96105 Assessment of aphasia (includes assessment of expressive and receptive speech and language function, language comprehension, speech production ability, reading, spelling, writing, eg, by Boston Diagnostic Aphasia Examination) with interpretation and report, per hour

Standardized evaluation of subtle language dysfunction like that seen in Broca's aphasia.

Torkildsen procedure

62180 Ventriculocisternostomy (Torkildsen type operation)

Creation of a shunt from the lateral ventricle to the cisterna magna to treat noncommunicating hydrocephalus.

Tzank smear

88160 Cytopathology, smears, any other source; screening and interpretation

88161 Cytopathology, smears, any other source; preparation, screening and interpretation

Laboratory test that determines if there are altered epithelial cells (Tzank cells) in the fluid of the bullae of pemphigus vulgaris.

Van Den Bergh test

82247 Bilirubin; total

Laboratory test comparing serum or plasma to bilirubin.

Van Slyke method

82131 Amino acids; single, quantitative, each specimen

Laboratory test that checks for amino-acid nitrogen.

Walsh modified radical prostatectomy

55810 Prostatectomy, perineal radical;

Radical prostatectomy resects the rectum and surrounding tissue.

Waterston procedure

33755 Shunt; ascending aorta to pulmonary artery (Waterston type operation)

Type of aortopulmonary shunting done to increase pulmonary blood flow. The ascending aorta is anastomosed to the right pulmonary artery.

Wertheim hysterectomy

58210 Radical abdominal hysterectomy, with bilateral total pelvic lymphadenectomy and para-aortic lymph node sampling (biopsy), with or without removal of tube(s), with or without removal of ovary(s)

Radical operation for uterine carcinoma that includes excising a portion of the vagina and lymph nodes.

Westergren test

85651 Sedimentation rate, erythrocyte; non-automated

85652 Sedimentation rate, erythrocyte; automated

Laboratory test that determines the sedimentation rate of red blood cells in fluid blood by mixing venous blood with an aqueous solution of sodium citrate and allowing it to stand for measured periods of time.

Wheeler procedure

66820 Discission of secondary membranous cataract (opacified posterior lens capsule and/or anterior hyaloid); stab incision technique (Ziegler or Wheeler knife)

Procedure is to correct entropion with secondary membranous cataract.

Whipple procedure

48150 Pancreatectomy, proximal subtotal with total duodenectomy, partial gastrectomy, choledochoenterostomy and gastrojejunostomy (Whipple-type procedure); with pancreatojejunostomy

48152 Pancreatectomy, proximal subtotal with total duodenectomy, partial gastrectomy, choledochoenterostomy and gastrojejunostomy (Whipple-type procedure); without pancreatojejunostomy

Pancreaticoduodenectomy (removal of gallbladder, part of the duodenum, and the head of the pancreas) performed to treat pancreatic cancer or chronic pancreatitis.

Whitehead hemorrhoidectomy

46260 Hemorrhoidectomy, internal and external, 2 or more columns/groups;

Two circular incisions above and below hemorrhoidal veins pull down normal mucosa for suturing to anal skin.

Whitman astragalectomy

28130 Talectomy (astragalectomy)

Removal of cartilage of the talus.

Yacoub procedure

33864 Ascending aorta graft, with cardiopulmonary bypass with valve suspension, with coronary reconstruction and valve-sparing aortic root remodeling (eg, David Procedure, Yacoub Procedure)

Remodeling procedure that establishes a new Dacron aortic root. Its shape has been designed to add to the life and efficiency of the prosthesis.

Surgical and Laboratory Terms

A special language is spoken in both the surgical suite and the laboratory. That language is then written into the medical charts documenting procedures and tests performed. The following list includes many of the medical terms heard most often in the operating room or seen on laboratory reports.

abdominoplasty. Excision of excess skin, fat, and subcutaneous tissue in the abdominal area, with8 repair.

ablation. Removal or destruction of tissue by cutting, electrical energy, chemical substances, or excessive heat application.

abrasion. Removal of layers of the skin occurring as a superficial injury, or a procedure for removal of problematic skin or skin lesions.

absorbable sutures. Strands used for suture or repair of tissue prepared from collagen or a synthetic polymer and capable of being absorbed by tissue over time.

acetabuloplasty. Surgical repair or reconstruction of the large, cup-shaped socket in the hipbone (acetabulum) that articulates with the head of the femur.

achalasia. Failure of the smooth muscles within the gastrointestinal tract to relax at points of junction; most commonly referring to the esophagogastric sphincter's failure to relax when swallowing.

acromionectomy. Surgical treatment for acromioclavicular arthritis, degeneration, or injury where the distal portion of the acromion process is removed.

acromioplasty. Repair of the part of the shoulder blade that connects to the deltoid muscles and clavicle.

acute myocardial infarction. Sudden, severe death of heart muscle due to decreased coronary blood flow. Classification is based on the location of the affected tissue, when known.

adduction. Pulling toward a central reference line, such as toward the midline of the body.

adenoidectomy. Surgical procedure in which the adenoids (the lymphoid tissue in the back wall and roof of the nasopharynx) are removed, often in conjunction with other procedures such as tonsillectomy or placement of tympanostomy tubes, most often performed in pediatric patients.

adipectomy. Surgical excision of fatty tissue. Adipectomy can be performed with or without suction assistance. ***Synonym(s):*** *lipectomy.*

adjacent tissue transfer. Rotation or advancement of skin from an adjacent area to repair or fill in a defect while maintaining attachment to original blood supply.

advance. Move away from the starting point.

allograft. Graft from one individual to another of the same species.

amputation. Removal of all or part of a limb or digit through the shaft or body of a bone.

analysis. Study of body fluid, tissue, section, or parts.

anastomosis. Surgically created connection between ducts, blood vessels, or bowel segments to allow flow from one to the other.

aneurysm. Circumscribed dilation or outpouching of an artery wall, often containing blood clots and connecting directly with the lumen of the artery.

angioplasty. Reconstruction or repair of a diseased or damaged blood vessel.

anterior. Situated in the front area or toward the belly surface of the body.

antibody. Immunoglobulin or protective protein encoded within its building block sequence to interact only with its specific antigen.

antigen. Substance inducing sensitivity or triggering an immune response and the production of antibodies.

antrum. Chamber or cavity, typically with a small opening.

appliance. Device providing function to a body part.

approach. Method or anatomical location used to gain access to a body organ or specific area for procedures. The approach is not coded separately although it may be a specified component of the procedure, such as laparoscopic versus incisional, or spinal procedures in which the amount of dissection required to expose the spine significantly alters with the site of approach.

arteriovenous fistula. Connecting passage between an artery and a vein.

arthrocentesis. Puncture and aspiration of fluid from a joint for diagnostic or therapeutic purposes or injection of anesthetics or corticosteroids.

arthrodesis. Surgical fixation or fusion of a joint to reduce pain and improve stability, performed openly or arthroscopically.

arthroplasty. Surgical reconstruction of a joint to improve function and reduce pain; may involve partial or total joint replacement.

arthroscopy. Use of an endoscope to examine the interior of a joint (diagnostic) or to perform surgery on joint structures (therapeutic).

arthrotomy. Surgical incision into a joint that may include exploration, drainage, or removal of a foreign body.

articulate. Comprised of separate segments joined together, allowing for movement of each part on the other.

aspiration. Drawing fluid out by suction.

assay. Test of purity or the amount of any particular constituent of a mixture.

astragalectomy. Surgical removal of the astragalus (talus), the bone that forms the ankle joint by articulating with the tibia and fibula.

augmentation. Add to or increase the substance of a body site, usually performed as plastic reconstructive measures. Augmentation may involve the use of an implant or prosthesis, especially within soft tissue or grafting procedures, such as bone tissue.

autograft. Any tissue harvested from one anatomical site of a person and grafted to another anatomical site of the same person. Most commonly, blood vessels, skin, tendons, fascia, and bone are used as autografts.

avulse. Tear away from, whether in an accidental injury or as a surgical procedure.

Baker tube. Tube placed into the jejunum or small bowel for decompression or extensive adhesions.

Baker's cannula. Flexible cannula used on the trachea.

benign. Mild or nonmalignant in nature.

biofeedback. Process by which a person learns to influence autonomic or involuntary nervous system responses and physiologic responses normally regulated voluntarily, but whose control has been affected by trauma or disease.

biometry. Statistical analysis of biological data.

biopsy. Tissue or fluid removed for diagnostic purposes through analysis of the cells in the biopsy material.

blood type. Classification of blood by group.

bougie. Probe used to dilate or calibrate a body part.

boutonniere deformity. Finger deformity with hyperextension of the distal joint and flexion of the interphalangeal joint.

brachytherapy. Form of radiation therapy in which radioactive pellets or seeds are implanted directly into the tissue being treated to deliver their dose of radiation in a more directed fashion. Brachytherapy provides radiation to the prescribed body area while minimizing exposure to normal tissue.

bridge. Connection between two parts of an organ or body part.

brush. Tool used to gather cell samples or clean a body part.

burr. Specialized surgical drill used to shape or make holes in bones or gain access into the cranium.

bursa. Cavity or sac containing fluid that occurs between articulating surfaces and serves to reduce friction from moving parts.

bypass. Auxiliary or diverted route to maintain continuous flow.

C-arm. Portable x-ray fluoroscopy machine often used in surgery.

calculus. Abnormal, stone-like concretion of calcium, cholesterol, mineral salts, or other substances that forms in any part of the body.

cannula. Tube inserted into a blood vessel, duct, or body cavity to facilitate passage.

capsulorrhaphy. Suturing or repair of a joint capsule.

capsulotomy. Incision of a joint capsule.

carcinoma in situ. Malignancy that arises from the cells of the vessel, gland, or organ of origin that remains confined to that site or has not invaded neighboring tissue.

cast. Rigid encasement or dressing molded to the body from a substance that hardens upon drying to hold a body part immobile during the healing period; a model or reproduction made from an impression or mold.

catheter. Flexible tube inserted into an area of the body for introducing or withdrawing fluid.

cauterize. Heat or chemicals used to burn or cut.

celiotomy. Incision into the abdominal cavity.

cement. Any substance that solidly bonds two objects or surfaces together.

centesis. Puncture.

cephalad. Toward the head.

cerclage. Looping or encircling an organ or tissue with wire or ligature for positional support.

chemodenervation. Chemical destruction of nerves. A substance, for example, Botox, is used to temporarily inhibit the transfer of chemicals at the presynaptic membrane, blocking the neuromuscular junctions.

chemosurgery. Application of chemical agents to destroy tissue, originally referring to the in situ chemical fixation of premalignant or malignant lesions to facilitate surgical excision.

chemotherapy. Treatment of disease, especially cancerous conditions, using chemical agents.

chisel. Instrument for cutting or planing bone.

chondral. Relating to cartilage.

chromotubation. Injection of a medication or saline solution into the uterine cavity and fallopian tubes to verify patency of the tubes.

cicatricial. Of or relating to scarring.

cicatricial entropion. Scarring that results in inversion of the eyelid, causing the lid margin to rest against and irritate the eyeball.

cicatricial lagophthalmos. Scarring that results in an eye that cannot be completely closed.

cicatricial pemphigoid. Autoimmune disease causing blisters on the skin often accompanied by itching and/or burning and resulting in scarring.

ciliary. Pertaining to the eyelid, eyelashes, or specific structures of the eyeball.

ciliary block. Increase in intraocular pressure that is accompanied by a shallow anterior chamber and forward displacement of the iris and lens.

ciliary body. Structure of the eye that produces the aqueous humor within the anterior chamber that nourishes the lens and cornea. The ciliary body is part of the uvea and connects anteriorly to the root of the iris and posteriorly to the choroid at the ora serrata retinae. It is divided into the pars plana and the pars plicata.

circumcise. Circular cutting around the genitals to remove the prepuce or foreskin.

clamp. Tool used to grip, compress, join, or fasten body parts.

closed treatment. Realignment of a fracture or dislocation without surgically opening the skin to reach the site. Treatment methods employed include with or without manipulation and with or without traction.

closure. Repairing an incision or wound by suture or other means.

clysis. Fluids injected into the body.

coctolabile. Capable of being destroyed or altered when boiled.

Colles' fracture. Fracture of the radius at the wrist in which the distal fragment is pushed posteriorly. The dorsal angulation of the fragment results in the wrist cocking up.

comminuted. Fracture type in which the bone is splintered or crushed.

commissure. Juncture where two corresponding parts come together, especially referring to the union site of adjacent heart valve cusps.

comorbid condition. Condition present that is not the primary reason for treating the patient, but one that affects the patient's care.

complex. Composite or collection of related things, such as symptoms, anatomical parts, or surgical procedures.

complex repair. Surgical closure of a wound requiring more than layered closure of the deeper subcutaneous tissue and fascia (i.e., debridement, scar excision, placement of stents or retention sutures, and sometimes site preparation or undermining that creates the defect requiring complex closure).

condyle. Rounded end of a bone that forms an articulation.

conization. Excision of a cone-shaped piece of tissue.

constriction. Narrowed or squeezed portion of a tubular or luminal structure, such as a duct, vessel, or tube (e.g., esophagus). The narrowing can be a defect that is occurring naturally, or one that is surgically induced for therapeutic reasons.

contour. Act of shaping along desired lines.

contralateral. Located on, or affecting, the opposite side of the body, usually as it relates to a bilateral body part.

coronal. Relating to the top of a tooth or the crown of the head.

corpectomy. Removal of the body of a bone, such as a vertebra.

correct. Body part modification.

craterization. Excision of a portion of bone creating a crater-like depression to facilitate drainage from infected areas of bone.

cross match. Test used to match the compatibility of a donor's blood or organ to the recipient.

crus. ***1)*** Any body part resembling a leg. ***2)*** Lower part of the leg.

cryotherapy. Any surgical procedure that uses intense cold for treatment.

culture. Growth of microorganisms in a medium conducive to their development.

curettage. Removal of tissue by scraping.

cutaneous. Relating to the skin.

cystotomy. Surgical incision into the gallbladder or urinary bladder.

debridement. Removal of dead or contaminated tissue and foreign matter from a wound.

decompress. To relieve pressure.

decubitus. Patient lying on the side.

dehiscence. Complication of healing in which the surgical wound ruptures or bursts open, superficially or through multiple layers.

deligation. Closure by tying up; sutures, ligatures.

depressor. Tool used to push body tissue out of the way.

dermabrasion. Cosmetic procedure that smooths out flaws and disfigured skin and promotes the growth of a new layer of skin cells by removing the outer layer of skin by mechanical or chemical means such as fine sandpaper, wire brushes, and caustic substances.

destruction. Ablation or eradication of a structure or tissue.

detection. Search for presence of a tissue or material.

diagnostic. Examination or procedure to which the patient is subjected, or which is performed on materials derived from a hospital outpatient, to obtain information to aid in the assessment of a medical condition or the identification of a disease. Among these examinations and tests are diagnostic laboratory services such as hematology and chemistry, diagnostic x-rays, isotope studies, EKGs, pulmonary function studies, thyroid function tests, psychological tests, and other tests given to determine the nature and severity of an ailment or injury.

dialysis. Artificial filtering of the blood to remove contaminating waste elements and restore normal balance.

diaphysis. Central shaft of a long bone.

diathermy. Applying heat to body tissues by various methods for therapeutic treatment or surgical purposes to coagulate and seal tissue.

dilation. Artificial increase in the diameter of an opening or lumen made by medication or by instrumentation.

dilution. Concentration reduction of a mixture or solution by adding more fluid.

disarticulation. Removal of a limb through a joint.

discectomy. Surgical excision of an intervertebral disk.

dislocation. Displacement of a bone in relation to its neighboring tissue, especially a joint.

dissection. Separating by cutting tissue or body structures apart.

distal. Located farther away from a specified reference point or the trunk.

distention. Enlarged or expanded due to pressure from inside.

diversion. Rechanneling of body fluid through another conduit.

diverticulum. Pouch or sac in the walls of an organ or canal.

division. Separating into two or more parts.

donor. Person from whom tissues or organs are removed for transplantation.

dorsal. Pertaining to the back or posterior aspect.

dorsum. Back side or back part of the body or individual anatomical structure.

dosimetry. Component in the administration of radiation oncology therapy in which a radiation dose is calculated to a specific site, including implant or beam orientation and exposure, isodose strengths, tissue inhomogeneities, and volume.

drain. Device that creates a channel to allow fluid from a cavity, wound, or infected area to exit the body.

drill. Making a hole in a bone or hard tissue.

Dwyer instrumentation technique. Anterior procedure using rods and attachments to straighten the spine as in treatment of adolescent idiopathic scoliosis.

dynamic. Manifesting motion in response to force.

echography. Radiographic imaging that uses sound waves reflected off the different densities of anatomic structures to create images.

ectopic. ***1)*** Fertilized ovum that implants and develops outside the uterus. The ovum may implant itself in different sites, such as the fallopian tube, the ovary, the abdomen, or the cervix. ***2)*** Organ or other structure that is aberrant or out of place.

edentulous. Loss of all or some of the natural teeth.

electrocautery. Division or cutting of tissue using high-frequency electrical current to produce heat, which destroys cells.

elevator. Tool for lifting tissues or bone.

elution. Separation of one solid from another, usually by washing.

embolism. Obstruction of a blood vessel resulting from a clot or foreign substance.

endoscopy. Visual inspection of the body using a fiberoptic scope.

enterostomy. Surgically created opening into the intestine through the abdominal wall.

enzyme. Complex proteins produced by cells that provide specific chemical functions within the body.

enzyme immunoassay. Any of several diagnostic immunoassay methods in which an enzyme is bound to an antigen or antibody and acts as a label; it is one of the primary diagnostic tests for many infectious diseases.

enzyme-linked immunosorbent assay. Laboratory immunoassay technique used in the diagnosis of certain diseases in which antibodies bound to enzymes reveal and quantify the amount of a substance in a solution, such as serum. It is performed using a solid surface to which the antibodies and other molecules adhere. In the last step, an enzymatic reaction occurs that results in a color change that can be read using a specialized instrument.

epiphysis. Proximal and distal rounded ends of a long bone; communicates with the joint.

episiotomy. Deliberate incision in the perineal tissue to facilitate delivery of the fetus and avoid traumatic tearing. In a midline or median episiotomy, the incision is made from the vagina straight down toward the anus. In a mediolateral episiotomy, the incision slants to one side.

epithelize. Formation of epithelial cells over a surface.

escharotomy. Surgical incision into the scab or crust resulting from a severe burn in order to relieve constriction and allow blood flow to the distal unburned tissue.

esophagoscopy. Internal visual inspection of the esophagus through the use of an endoscope placed down the throat.

evacuation. Removal or purging of waste material.

evisceration. Removal of contents of a cavity.

examination. Comprehensive visual and tactile screening and specific testing leading to diagnosis or, as appropriate, to a referral to another practitioner.

exchange. Substitution of one thing for another.

excise. Remove or cut out.

exenteration. Surgical removal of the entire contents of a body cavity, such as the pelvis or orbit.

exfoliate. Skin falling off in layers.

exploration. Examination for diagnostic purposes.

exposure. In surgery, to display, reveal, or make accessible.

expression. In surgery, the squeezing out of tissue.

exteriorize. In surgery, to expose an organ temporarily for observation.

external fixation. Rods and pins connected in a lattice to secure bone.

extract. Condensed medication.

fascia. Fibrous sheet or band of tissue that envelops organs, muscles, and groupings of muscles.

fasciotomy. Incision or transection of fascial tissue.

fenestration. Presence of small openings from piercing or perforations.

fibrosis. Formation of fibrous tissue as part of the restorative process.

filiform. Probe with woven-thread end.

fissure. Deep furrow, groove, or cleft in tissue structures.

fistula. Abnormal tube-like passage between two body cavities or organs or from an organ to the outside surface.

fistulization. Creation of a communication between two structures that were not previously connected.

fit. Attack of acute symptoms.

fixate. Hold, secure, or fasten in position.

fixation. Act or condition of being attached, secured, fastened, or held in position.

flap. Mass of flesh and skin partially excised from its location but retaining its blood supply that is moved to another site to repair adjacent or distant defects.

fluorescence immunoassay. Form of immunoassay that uses a fluorescent compound as the detection reagent. This compound absorbs light or energy at a particular wavelength and then emits light or energy at a different wavelength.

fluoroscopy. Radiology technique that allows visual examination of part of the body or a function of an organ using a device that projects an x-ray image on a fluorescent screen.

follow-up. Visits or treatment following a procedure.

forceps. Tool used for grasping or compressing tissue.

fossa. Indentation or shallow depression.

Fowler's position. Position assumed by patient when the head of the bed is raised 18 or 20 inches and the individual's knees are elevated.

fragment. Small piece broken off a larger whole; to divide into pieces.

free graft. Unattached piece of skin and tissue moved to another part of the body and sutured into place to repair a defect.

frozen section. Group of similar cells that have been frozen and thinly sliced according to specifications to preserve the tissue for diagnostic or histochemistry studies.

fulgurate. Destruction by electric current.

furuncle. Inflamed, painful abscess, cyst, or nodule on the skin caused by bacteria, often Staphylococcus, entering along the hair follicle.

fusion. Union of adjacent tissues, especially bone.

Gardner Wells tongs. Immobilizing device used for cervical spine injuries. Two sharp metal pins are screwed into the superficial layer of the skull and then connected to traction devices for stabilization of the spine.

gene expression profiling. Measurement of messenger RNA (mRNA) levels that show the genes expressed by a cell. Understanding how a cell is functioning at a specific time can aid in the diagnosis or treatment of a condition.

Gigli saw. Saw made of thin, flexible wire with teeth along the edge used for cutting bones (e.g., craniotomy).

graft. Tissue implant from another part of the body or another person.

Greenfield filter. Permanent umbrella-shaped filter implanted in the vena cava and designed to trap small clots of blood or plaque before they reach the lungs and cause pulmonary embolism. The filter is inserted intraluminally, usually through the femoral or jugular veins.

guillotine. Instrument used for severing tonsils from their attachments.

halo. Tool for stabilizing the head and spine.

harvest. Removal of cells or tissue from their native site to be used as a graft or transplant to another part of the donor's body or placed into another person.

hematoma. Tumor-like collection of blood in some part of the body caused by a break in a blood vessel wall, usually as a result of trauma.

hemilaminectomy. Excision of a portion of the vertebral lamina.

hemiphalangectomy. Excision of part of the phalanx.

hemoperitoneum. Effusion of blood into the peritoneal cavity, the space between the continuous membrane lining the abdominopelvic walls and encasing the visceral organs.

hemostasis. Interruption of blood flow or the cessation or arrest of bleeding.

hemostat. Tool for clamping vessels and arresting hemorrhaging.

hernia. Protrusion of a body structure through tissue.

hidradenitis. Infection or inflammation of a sweat gland, usually treated by incision and drainage.

Hoffman device. External fixation device.

homograft. Graft from one individual to another of the same species.

hyperthermia. Body temperature rising above 99 degrees Fahrenheit. This elevated temperature can be the result of illness or artificially created as a therapy.

hypertrophic. Enlarged or overgrown from an increase in cell size of the affected tissue.

hypophysectomy. Destruction of the pituitary gland.

hypothermia. Therapeutic lack of heat or decrease in body temperature.

identification. Recognition of body part or tissue.

imaging. Radiologic means of producing pictures for clinical study of the internal structures and functions of the body, such as x-ray, ultrasound, magnetic resonance, or positron emission tomography.

imbrication. Overlapping of tissues during closure.

immunoassay. Method that uses binding between an antigen and antibody for determination of the presence of certain chemical substances.

immunochemiluminometric assay. Form of immunoassay in which the antigen-antibody complex is measured using light emission produced from a chemical reaction.

immunotherapy. Therapeutic use of serum or gamma globulin.

implant. Material or device inserted or placed within the body for therapeutic, reconstructive, or diagnostic purposes.

impression. Mold of a body part to be used as a pattern in making a replacement part, prosthesis, or stabilizing device for that area of the body.

in situ. Located in the natural position or contained within the origin site, not spread into neighboring tissue.

incise. To cut open or into.

incubation. Culture cultivation under controlled conditions.

inferior. Located toward the feet or lower part of the body.

infusion. Introduction of a therapeutic fluid, other than blood, into the bloodstream.

inguinal. Within the groin region.

inject. Introduction into body tissues.

innervate. Supplying a stimulus or energy to nerve fibers connected to a part.

inseminate. Inject with semen.

instillation. Administering a liquid slowly over time, drop by drop.

instrumentation. Use of a tool for therapeutic reasons.

insufflation. Blowing air or gas into a body cavity.

intermediate repair. *1)* Surgical closure of a wound requiring closure of one or more of the deeper subcutaneous tissue and non-muscle fascia layers in addition to the skin. *2)* Contaminated wounds with single layer closure that need extensive cleaning or foreign body removal.

internal skeletal fixation. Repair involving wires, pins, screws, and/or plates placed through or within the fractured area to stabilize and immobilize the injury.

interpretation. Professional health care provider's review of data with a written or verbal opinion.

interstitial. Within the small spaces or gaps occurring in tissue or organs.

intracavitary. Within a body cavity.

intubate. Insertion of a tube into a body canal or organ.

inversion. Turning inward, inside out, or upside down.

ipsilateral. Located on, or affecting, the same side of the body, usually as it relates to a bilateral body part.

irrigate. Washing out, lavage.

keratotomy. Surgical incision of the cornea.

kinetics. Motion or movement.

laminectomy. Removal or excision of the posterior arch of a vertebra to provide additional space for the nerves and widen the spinal canal.

lance. Incise with a lancet.

lancet. Pointed surgical knife.

laparoscopy. Direct visualization of the peritoneal cavity, outer fallopian tubes, uterus, and ovaries utilizing a laparoscope, a thin, flexible fiberoptic tube.

laparotomy. Incision through the flank or abdomen for therapeutic or diagnostic purposes.

laryngoscopy. Examination of the hypopharynx, larynx, and tongue base with an endoscope.

laser. Concentrated light used to cut or seal tissue.

lateral. On/to the side.

lavage. Washing.

lesion. Area of damaged tissue that has lost continuity or function, due to disease or trauma. Lesions may be located on internal structures such as the brain, nerves, or kidneys, or visible on the skin.

ligation. Tying off a blood vessel or duct with a suture or a soft, thin wire.

light chains. Proteins produced by plasma (immune) cells; also called kappa and lambda light chains.

limited. Bounded.

lingual. Surface of the tooth closest to the tongue or relating to the tongue and its surrounding areas.

lithotomy position. Common position patients may be placed in for some surgical procedures and examinations involving the pelvis and/or lower abdomen. The patient is placed supine (on their back), hips and knees flexed, thighs apart, with feet supported in raised stirrups.

lithotripsy. Destruction of calcified substances in the gallbladder or urinary system by smashing the concretion into small particles to be washed out. This may be done by surgical or noninvasive methods, such as ultrasound.

localization. Limitation to one area.

lysis. Destruction, breakdown, dissolution, or decomposition of cells or substances by a specific catalyzing agent.

malignant. Any condition tending to progress toward death, specifically an invasive tumor with a loss of cellular differentiation that has the ability to spread or metastasize to other body areas.

manipulate. Treatment by hand.

manometric. Pertaining to pressure, as measured in a meter.

marsupialization. Creation of a pouch in surgical treatment of a cyst in which one wall is resected and the remaining cut edges are sutured to adjacent tissue creating an open pouch of the previously enclosed cyst.

mastectomy. Surgical removal of one or both breasts.

mastotomy. Incision of the breast, often performed for exploration of suspicious tissue or for drainage of an abscess.

meatus. Opening or passage into the body.

medial. Middle or midline.

metastasize. Spread, invade, or extend to a new location.

metatarsectomy. Excision or resection of a metatarsal bone in the foot between the tarsal and phalangeal bones.

microdissection. Dissection of tissue using a microscope.

microrepair. Repair of tissue at a level that requires using a microscope.

middle cranial fossa. Support for the temporal lobes of the brain comprising the greater wings of the sphenoid (anteriorly), the squamous portions of temporal bone (laterally), and the petrous portions of the temporal bones (posteriorly).

modality. ***1)*** Form of imaging (e.g., x-ray, fluoroscopy, ultrasound, nuclear medicine, duplex Doppler, CT, and MRI). ***2)*** Any physical agent applied to produce therapeutic changes to biologic tissue including, but not limited to, thermal, acoustic, light, mechanical, or electric energy.

modification. Changing of tissues.

monitoring. Recording of events; keep track, regulate, or control patient activities and record findings.

morbidity. Diseased condition or state.

mortality. Condition of being mortal (subject to death).

motility. Capability of independent, spontaneous movement.

myocutaneous flap. Skin, subcutaneous tissue, and intact muscle tissue that are transferred to a recipient site while retaining sufficient blood supply from its own vascular bed.

myotomy. Surgical cutting of a muscle to gain access to underlying tissues or for therapeutic reasons.

necropsy. Autopsy or postmortem examination performed in order to ascertain the cause of death or the changes caused by disease.

necrosis. Death of cells or tissue within a living organ or structure.

nephrotic. Degeneration of renal epithelium.

neurectomy. Excision of all or a portion of a nerve.

neurotomy. Dissection of a nerve.

obliterate. Get rid or do away with completely.

observation. Perception of events.

obturate. To occlude or close off an opening.

obturator. Prosthesis used to close an acquired or congenital opening in the palate that aids in speech and chewing.

occlusion. Constriction, closure, or blockage of a passage.

oophorectomy. Surgical removal of all or part of one or both ovaries, either as open procedure or laparoscopically. Menstruation and childbearing ability continues when one ovary is removed.

open fracture. Exposed break in a bone, always considered compound due to its high risk of infection from the open wound leading to the fracture. Broken bone ends may protrude through the skin and contaminants or foreign bodies are often embedded in the tissues.

open wound. Opening or break of the skin.

operating microscope. Compound microscope with two or more lens systems or several grouped lenses in one unit that provides magnifying power to the surgeon up to 40X.

operating room (OR) procedure. Defined group of procedures that normally require the use of an operating room.

orchiectomy. Surgical removal of one or both testicles via a scrotal or groin incision, indicated in cases of cancer, traumatic injury, and sex reassignment surgery.

ostectomy. Excision of bone.

osteomyelitis. Inflammation of bone that may remain localized or spread to the marrow, cortex, or periosteum, in response to an infecting organism, usually bacterial and pyogenic.

osteophytes. Bony outgrowth.

osteoplasty. Plastic surgery of a bone.

osteoporotic. Porous condition of bones from a loss of bone mass or density.

osteotome. Tool used for cutting bone.

osteotomy. Surgical cutting of a bone.

oversew. Suture technique to reinforce primary repair, control a bleed or leak, repair an injury, or to close an ulcer, a cardiac valve, a cyst, or a left atrial appendage (LAA). Various suture patterns can be used.

packing. Material placed into a cavity or wound, such as gels, gauze, pads, and sponges.

palpate. Examination by feeling with the hand.

paring. Cutting away an edge or a surface.

paronychia. Infection or cellulitis of nail structures.

pathology. Medical science, and specialty practice, regarding all aspects of disease, with special reference to the essential nature, causes, and development of abnormal conditions, as well as the structural and functional changes that result from the disease processes.

pedicle. Stem-like, narrow base or stalk attached to a new growth.

peduncle. Connecting structures of the brain.

penetrate. Pierce.

percutaneous. Through the skin.

percutaneous skeletal fixation. Treatment that is neither open nor closed and the injury site is not directly visualized. Fixation devices (pins, screws) are placed through the skin to stabilize the dislocation using x-ray guidance.

periosteum. Double-layered connective membrane on the outer surface of bone.

phacoemulsification. Cataract extraction in which the lens is fragmented by ultrasonic vibrations and simultaneously irrigated and aspirated.

photocoagulation. Application of an intense laser beam of light to disrupt tissue and condense protein material to a residual mass, used especially for treating ocular conditions.

pilonidal. Containing a tuft of hair.

pinning. Bone fastening.

plasma. Liquid portion of normal unclotted blood that contains red cells, white cells, and platelets.

plethysmography. Recording of the volume changes in an organ or body part, particularly related to the amount of blood circulating through it.

pleurodesis. Injection of a sclerosing agent into the pleural space for creating adhesions between the parietal and the visceral pleura to treat a collapsed lung caused by air trapped in the pleural cavity, or severe cases of pleural effusion.

plication. Surgical technique involving folding, tucking, or pleating to reduce the size of a hollow structure or organ.

portable. Movable.

posterior. Located in the back part or caudal end of the body.

probing. Exploration using a slender, often flexible rod.

procedure. Diagnostic or therapeutic service provided for the care and treatment of a patient, usually conforming to a specific set of steps or instructions.

process. Anatomical projection or prominence on a bone.

prognosis. Forecast of the probable outcome of a condition or disease and the prospects of recovery and disease residual, dependent on the nature of the disease and the patient's response to treatment.

prone. Lying face downward.

prophylaxis. Intervention or protective therapy intended to prevent a disease.

prostate. Male gland surrounding the bladder neck and urethra that secretes a substance into the seminal fluid.

prosthesis. Man-made substitute for a missing body part.

prostrate. Recline on one's front.

proximal. Located closest to a specified reference point, usually the midline or trunk.

pump. Forcing gas or liquid from a body part.

puncture. Creating a hole.

pyelotomy. Incision or opening made into the renal pelvis.

qualitative. To determine the nature or characteristics of the components of a substance.

quantitative. To determine the number or amount of the components of a substance.

radical. Extensive surgery.

radiograph. Image made by an x-ray.

radiopaque dye. Medium injected into the body that is impenetrable by x-rays.

ream. Shape or enlarge a hole.

recess. Small empty cavity in a body part.

reconstruct. Tissue rebuilding.

reduce. Restoration to normal position or alignment.

reduction. Correction of a fracture, dislocation, or hernia to the correct place and alignment, manually or by surgery.

refer. Recommendation to another source.

regulation. Directive, order, ruling, or law put forth by an executive authority granted such powers by law.

reimplant. Reinsert or reattach tissue.

reinforce. Enhancement of strength.

reinnervation. Restoration of nerve function.

release. Disconnection of a tendon or ligament.

reoperation. Repeat performance of operation.

repair. Surgical closure of a wound. The wound may be a result of injury/trauma or it may be a surgically created defect. Repairs are divided into three categories: simple, intermediate, and complex.

replacement. Insertion of new tissue or material in place of old one.

reposition. Placement of an organ or structure into another position or return of an organ or structure to its original position.

resect. Cutting out or removing a portion or all of a bone, organ, or other structure.

reservoir. Space or body cavity for storage of liquid.

response. Reaction to stimulus.

retraction. Act of holding tissue or a structure back away from its normal position or the field of interest.

revascularize. Restoring blood flow or blood supply to a body part.

revision. Reordering or rearrangement of tissue to suit a particular need or function.

rhinoplasty. Reconstructive, restorative, or cosmetic plastic surgery of the nose.

rod. Straight, slim, cylindrical metal instrument for therapeutics.

rongeur. Sharp-edged instrument with a scoop-tip used to cut through tissue and bone.

routine. Normal activity.

sagittal. Up and down along the length of the body, as opposed to across it (transverse).

sagittal plane. Imaginary plane in the human body that travels from the top to the bottom of the body, dividing it into left and right portions.

sclerose. To become hard or firm and indurated from increased formation of connective tissue or disease.

section. Process of cutting a division or segment out of a part.

selective. Separation.

sequestrectomy. Surgical excision of a nonviable piece of bone that has become walled off, or sequestered, away from living bone during necrosis.

serum. Clear liquid portion of the blood that remains after the clotting proteins and blood cells have been removed.

seton. Finely spun thread or other fine material for leading the passage of wider instruments through a fistula, canal, or sinus tract.

sever. Separate completely.

shunt. Surgically created passage between blood vessels or other natural passages, such as an arteriovenous anastomosis, to divert or bypass blood flow from the normal channel.

sialolith. Calculus, stone, or concretion within the salivary ducts or glands.

sigmoidoscopy. Endoscopic examination of the entire rectum and sigmoid colon, often including a portion of the descending colon and usually performed with a flexible fiberoptic scope in conjunction with a surgical procedure.

simple repair. Surgical closure of a superficial wound requiring single layer suturing of the skin (epidermis, dermis, or subcutaneous tissue).

skeletal traction. Applying direct pulling force on the long axis of bones by inserted wires or pins and using weights and pulleys to keep the bone in proper alignment.

skin traction. Application of a pulling force to a limb accomplished by a device fixed to felt dressings or strappings applied to the body surface.

smear. Specimen for study that is spread out across a glass slide.

snare. Wire used as a loop to excise a polyp or lesion.

sound. Long, slender tool with a type of curved, flat probe at the end for dilating strictures or detecting foreign bodies.

spatulate. Cut the open end of a tubular structure with a lengthwise incision and open the end out further for greater opening size in an anastomosis.

specimen. Tissue cells or sample of fluid taken for analysis, pathologic examination, and diagnosis.

speculum. Tool used to enlarge the opening of any canal or cavity.

spiculum. Small, needle-like body or spike.

splint. Brace or support for an anatomical structure after surgery or injury.

steal. Diversion of blood to another channel.

stenosis. Narrowing or constriction of a passage.

stent. Tube to provide support in a body cavity or lumen.

stereotaxis. Three-dimensional method for precisely locating structures.

stoma. Opening created in the abdominal wall from an internal organ or structure for diversion of waste elimination, drainage, and access.

strapping. Application of overlapping strips of tape or bandaging to put pressure on and immobilize the affected area.

stricture. Narrowing of an anatomical structure.

subluxation. Partial or incomplete dislocation (separation) of a joint with misalignment but maintenance of some contact between the bones.

subtraction. Process of using an image to remove an overlying structure in another image to better visualize the area underneath the overlying structure.

suction. Vacuum evacuation of fluid or tissue.

superior. Located toward the head or top of the body.

supine. Lying on the back.

suppression. Holding back, putting in check, or inhibiting an act, function, thought, or desire.

suppurative. Forming pus.

survival. Continued life.

suspension. Fixation of an organ for support; temporary state of cessation of an activity, process, or experience.

suture. Stitching technique employed in wound closure.

symphysis. Joint that unifies two opposed bones by a junction of bony surfaces to a plate of fibrocartilage.

synchondrosis. Two bones joined by hyaline cartilage or fibrocartilage. Typically, the bones fuse as they mature.

synovia. Clear fluid lubricant of joints, bursae, and tendon sheaths, secreted by the synovial membrane.

talectomy. Surgical removal of the astragalus (talus), the bone that forms the ankle joint by articulating with the tibia and fibula. Indications include trauma, congenital abnormalities, severe fractures, chronic infection, or tumors.

tap. Withdraw fluid through a needle or trocar.

technique. Manner of performance.

teletherapy. External beam radiotherapy or other treatment applied from a source maintained at a distance away from the body.

tenodesis. Stabilization of a joint by anchoring tendons.

tenolysis. Release of a tendon from adhesions.

therapeutic. Act meant to alleviate a medical or mental condition.

thoracentesis. Surgical puncture of the chest cavity with a specialized needle or hollow tubing to aspirate fluid from within the pleural space for diagnostic or therapeutic reasons.

thoracotomy. Surgical procedure for opening the chest wall in order to access the lungs, esophagus, trachea, aorta, heart, and diaphragm.

thrombectomy. Removal of a clot (thrombus) from a blood vessel utilizing various methods.

tomograph. Method of precise x-ray.

tomosynthesis. Digital breast tomosynthesis (DBT), also referred to as three-dimensional (3D) mammography, creates a three-dimensional picture of the breast from many angles using low-dose x-rays. Several images, usually between 10 and 15, are taken over approximately seven seconds. Once the images have been taken, computer programs produce clear and highly-focused 3D representations of the breast that the radiologist can view as thin layers of breast tissue, similar to CT scan images.

tracheostomy. Formation of a tracheal opening on the neck surface with tube insertion to allow for respiration in cases of obstruction or decreased patency. A tracheostomy may be planned or performed on an emergency basis for temporary or long-term use.

traction. Drawing out or holding tension on an area by applying a direct therapeutic pulling force.

tractor. Instrument for pulling an organ.

transcatheter. Procedure or treatment performed via a catheter.

transection. Transverse dissection; to cut across a long axis; cross section.

transfer. Situation in which the patient is transferred to another acute care hospital for related care.

transplant. Insertion of an organ or tissue from one person or site into another.

transposition. Removal or exchange from one side to another; change of position from one place to another.

transverse. Crosswise at right angles to the long axis of a structure or part.

treatment. Management of patient.

Trendelenburg position. Lying on a flat back with the supporting structure angled to lower the patient's head downward 15 to 30 degrees.

trephine. ***1)*** Instrument that removes small disc-shaped buttons of corneal tissue for transplanting. ***2)*** Specialized round saw for cutting circular holes in bone, especially the skull.

trocar. Cannula or a sharp pointed instrument used to puncture and aspirate fluid from cavities.

tube. Long, hollow cylindrical instrument or body structure.

ulcer. Open sore or excavating lesion of skin or the tissue on the surface of an organ from the sloughing of chronically inflamed and necrosing tissue.

ultrasound. Imaging using ultra-high sound frequency bounced off body structures.

undiversion. Restoration of continuity, flow, or passage through the normal channel.

urachus. Embryonic tube connecting the urinary bladder to the umbilicus during development of the fetus that normally closes before birth, generally in the fourth or fifth month of gestation.

ureostomy. Connection of the ureter to a stoma on the abdominal skin.

ureterocele. Saccular formation of the lower part of the ureter, protruding into the bladder.

ureteropyelogram. Radiologic study of the renal pelvis and the ureter.

V-Y operation. Plastic surgery technique that is used to cover defects or wounds on surface areas of the body and also to lengthen some anatomic structures. Incision or wound shape is in a V pattern and the flap is approximated to cover the defect area as a Y shape. V-Y operation is used in many types of repairs and reconstructions, such as injuries, skin defects, nasal deformities, perianal or perineal areas after tumor resection or necrotizing fasciitis, fingertip amputations, and penile elongation in cases of hidden penis.

valve. Fold or membrane within a body canal or passageway that prevents backflow of fluids running through it.

varices. Enlarged, dilated, or twisted turning veins.

vascular family. Group of vessels (family) that branch from the aorta or vena cava. At each branching, the vascular order increases by one. The first order vessel is the primary branch off the aorta or vena cava. The second order vessel branches from the first order, the third order branches from the second order, and any further branching is beyond the third order. For example, for the inferior vena cava, the common iliac artery is a first order vessel. The internal and external iliac arteries are second order vessels, as they each originate from the first order common iliac artery. The external iliac artery extends directly from the common iliac artery and the internal iliac artery bifurcates from the common iliac artery. A third order vessel from the external iliac artery is the inferior epigastric artery and a third order vessel from the internal iliac artery is the obturator artery.

vasectomy. Surgical procedure involving the removal of all or part of the vas deferens, usually performed for sterilization or in conjunction with a prostatectomy.

ventral. Pertaining or relating on, to, or toward the lower abdominal plane of the body; located on, near, or toward the front area of the body.

vermilion border. Red margin of the upper and lower lip that commences at the exterior edge of the intraoral labial mucosa, and extends outward, terminating at the extraoral labial cutaneous junction.

vestibuloplasty. Surgical procedure in which the vestibule of the mouth is deepened for the purpose of increasing the height of the alveolar ridge.

vestigial. Remains or remnant of a structure occurring in the fetal stage of growth.

vomer. Flat bone that forms the lower, posterior portion of the nasal septum.

vulvectomy. Surgical removal of all or part of the vulva, often performed to treat malignant or premalignant lesions. Lymph nodes may be removed at the same surgical session.

W-D. Wet to dry (dressings).

Walsh modified radical prostatectomy. Radical prostatectomy resects the rectum and surrounding tissue trying to save sexual function of the patient.

wedge excision. Surgical removal of a section of tissue that is thick at one edge and tapers to a thin edge.

whistle tip catheter. Catheter design with a lateral and terminal opening.

wick catheter. Device used to monitor interstitial fluid pressure, and sometimes used intraoperatively during fasciotomy procedures to evaluate the effectiveness of the decompression.

wound. Injury to living tissue often involving a cut or break in the skin.

wound closure. Closure or repair of a wound created surgically or due to trauma (e.g., laceration). Closure technique depends on the type, site, and depth of the defect, as well as cosmetic and functional outcome. Single layer closure involves approximation of the edges of the wound. Other types of closure involve closing one or more deeper layers of tissue prior to skin closure. Complex closure may include techniques such as debridement or undermining, which involves manipulation of tissue around the wound to allow the skin to cover the wound. AMA CPT® book defines these as simple, intermediate, and complex repair.

wound repair. Closure of a wound created surgically or due to trauma (e.g., laceration). Closure technique depends on the type, site, and depth of the defect, as well as cosmetic and functional outcome. Primary (simple) closure involves approximation of the edges of the wound. Intermediate closure involves closing the deeper layers of tissue prior to skin closure. Complex closure may include techniques such as debridement or undermining, which involves manipulation of tissue around the wound to allow the skin to cover the wound.

xenograft. Tissue that is harvested from one species and grafted to another. Pigskin is the most common xenograft for human skin and is applied to a wound as a temporary closure until a permanent option is performed.

xenotransplantation. Use of live, nonhuman animal cells, tissues, and organs grafted into humans, such as porcine skin grafts derived from pigs.

z-plasty. Plastic surgery technique used primarily to release tension or elongate contractured scar tissue in which a Z-shaped incision is made with the middle line of the Z crossing the area of greatest tension. The triangular flaps are then rotated so that they cross the incision line in the opposite direction, creating a reversed Z.

ZEEP. Zero end-expiratory pressure.

zygoma. Zygomatic process of the temporal bone that creates the cheekbone.

zygomatic arch. Part of the temporal bone of the skull that forms the prominence of the cheek.

Anatomical Illustrations

Body Planes and Movements

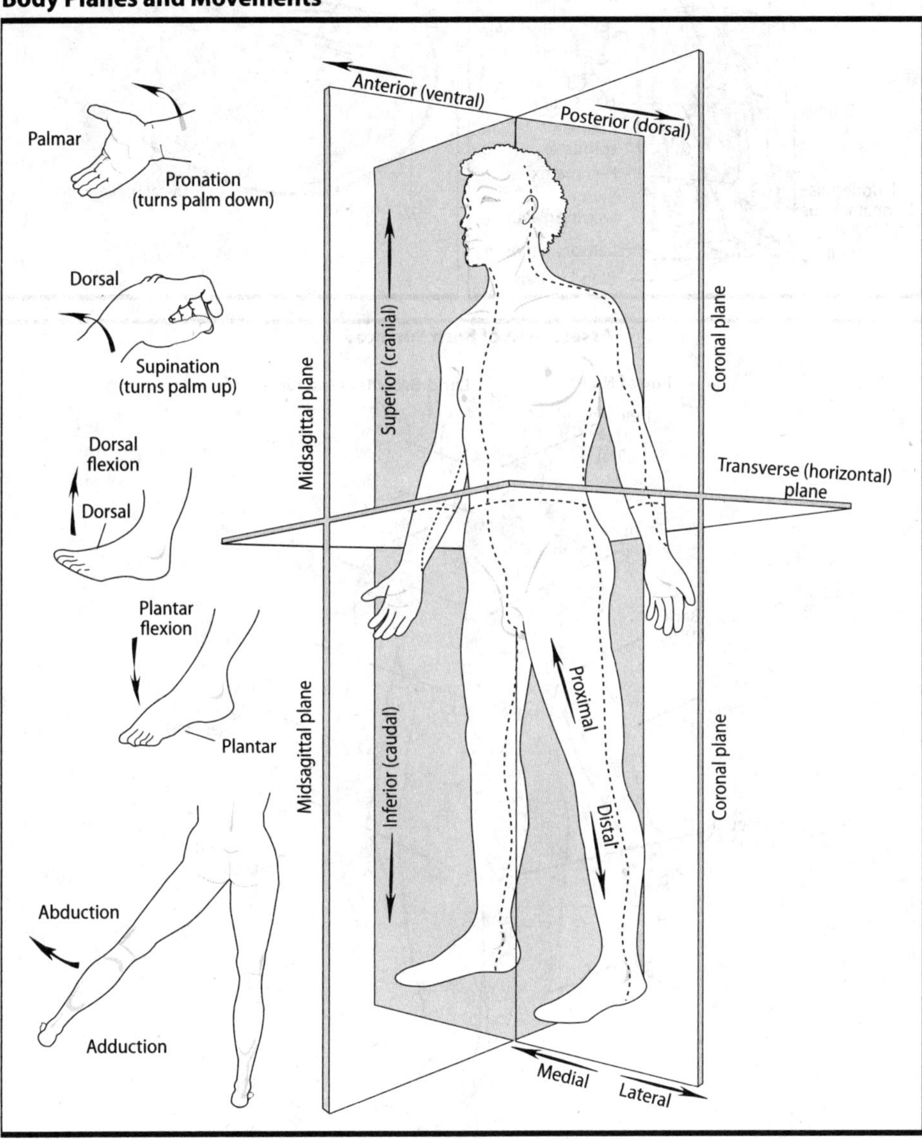

Integumentary System

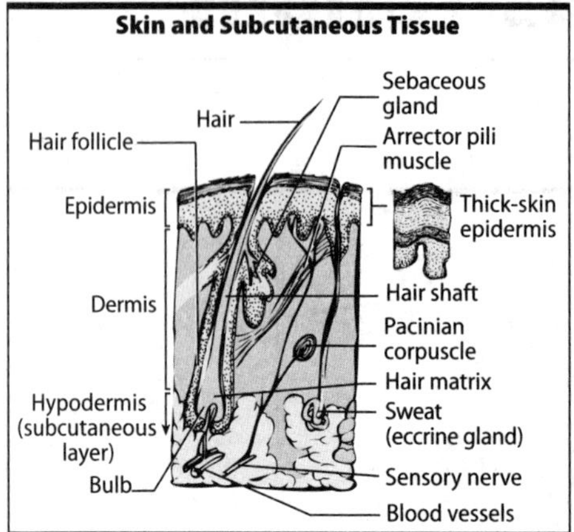

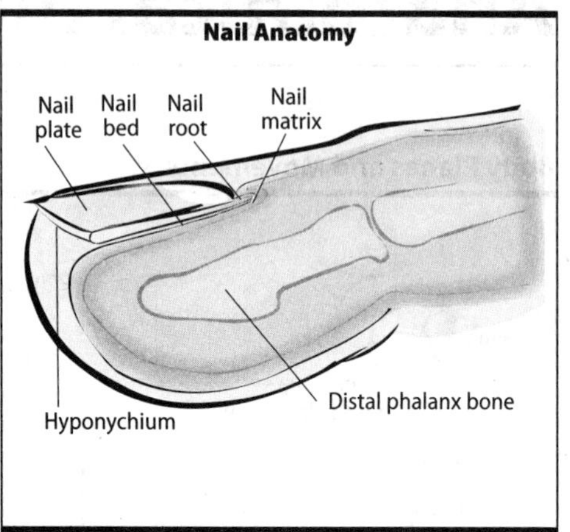

Assessment of Burn Surface Area

Rule of Nines

Head and neck (9%)
Front (18%)
Back (18%)
Arm (9%)
Perineum (1%)
Leg (18%)

Lund-Browder Classification

Head (7%)
Neck (2%)
Front (13%)
Back (13%)
Each arm/left/right
Upper (4%)
Lower (3%)
Perineum (1%)
Each hand (2.5%)
Each leg/left/right
Upper (9.5%)
Lower (7%)

Musculoskeletal System

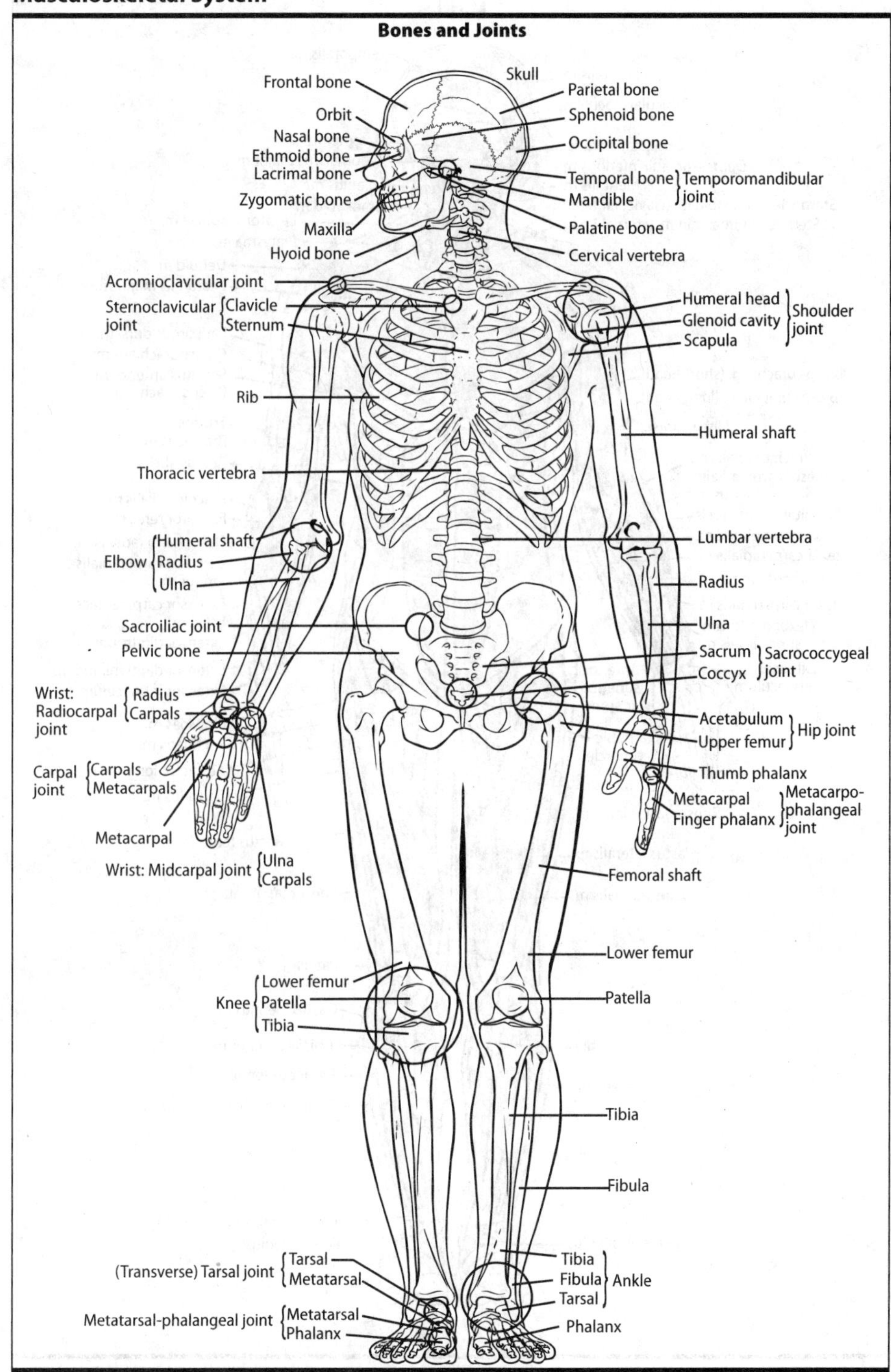

Muscles

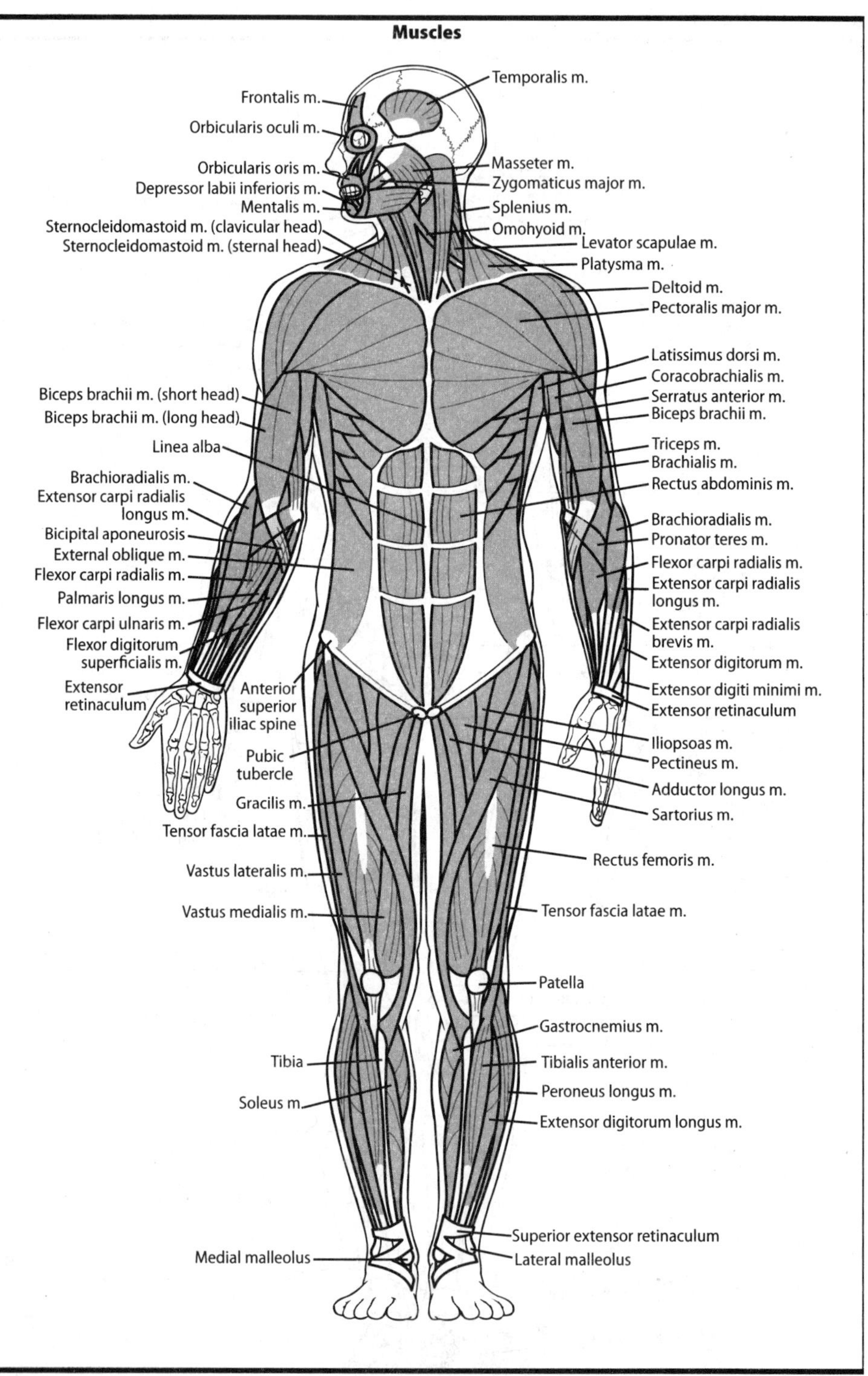

Temporalis m.
Frontalis m.
Orbicularis oculi m.
Orbicularis oris m.
Depressor labii inferioris m.
Mentalis m.
Sternocleidomastoid m. (clavicular head)
Sternocleidomastoid m. (sternal head)
Masseter m.
Zygomaticus major m.
Splenius m.
Omohyoid m.
Levator scapulae m.
Platysma m.
Deltoid m.
Pectoralis major m.
Latissimus dorsi m.
Coracobrachialis m.
Serratus anterior m.
Biceps brachii m.
Biceps brachii m. (short head)
Biceps brachii m. (long head)
Linea alba
Triceps m.
Brachialis m.
Rectus abdominis m.
Brachioradialis m.
Extensor carpi radialis
longus m.
Bicipital aponeurosis
External oblique m.
Flexor carpi radialis m.
Palmaris longus m.
Flexor carpi ulnaris m.
Flexor digitorum
superficialis m.
Extensor
retinaculum
Anterior
superior
iliac spine
Pubic
tubercle
Brachioradialis m.
Pronator teres m.
Flexor carpi radialis m.
Extensor carpi radialis
longus m.
Extensor carpi radialis
brevis m.
Extensor digitorum m.
Extensor digiti minimi m.
Extensor retinaculum
Iliopsoas m.
Pectineus m.
Adductor longus m.
Sartorius m.
Gracilis m.
Tensor fascia latae m.
Vastus lateralis m.
Vastus medialis m.
Rectus femoris m.
Tensor fascia latae m.
Patella
Gastrocnemius m.
Tibia
Tibialis anterior m.
Soleus m.
Peroneus longus m.
Extensor digitorum longus m.
Superior extensor retinaculum
Medial malleolus
Lateral malleolus

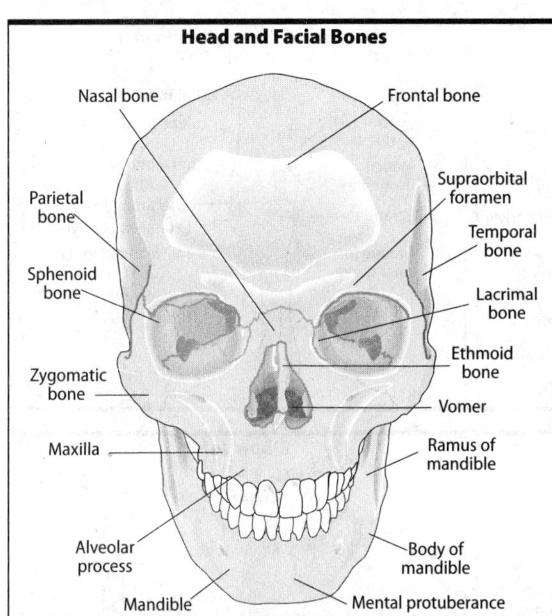
Head and Facial Bones
Nasal bone
Frontal bone
Supraorbital foramen
Parietal bone
Temporal bone
Sphenoid bone
Lacrimal bone
Ethmoid bone
Zygomatic bone
Vomer
Maxilla
Ramus of mandible
Alveolar process
Body of mandible
Mandible
Mental protuberance

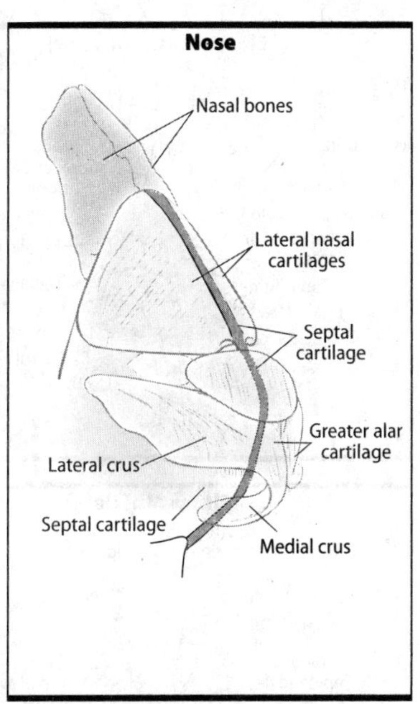
Nose
Nasal bones
Lateral nasal cartilages
Septal cartilage
Greater alar cartilage
Lateral crus
Septal cartilage
Medial crus

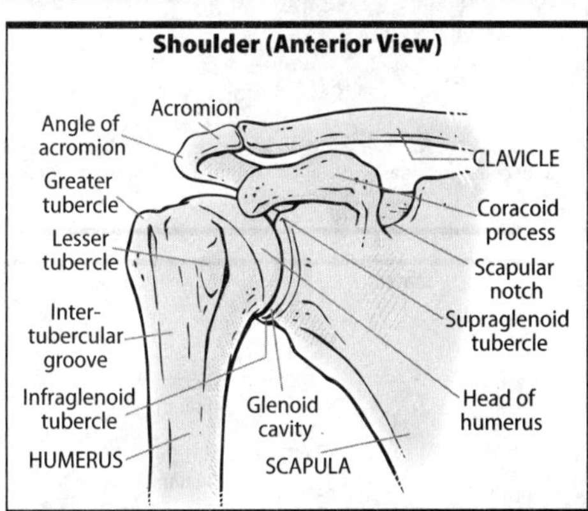
Shoulder (Anterior View)
Acromion
Angle of acromion
CLAVICLE
Greater tubercle
Coracoid process
Lesser tubercle
Scapular notch
Inter-tubercular groove
Supraglenoid tubercle
Infraglenoid tubercle
Glenoid cavity
Head of humerus
HUMERUS
SCAPULA

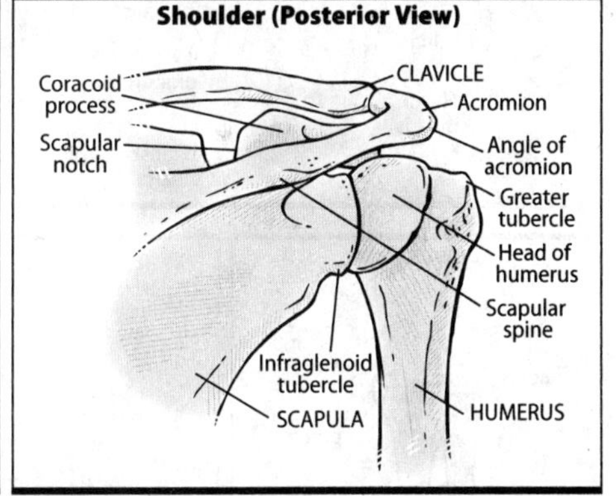
Shoulder (Posterior View)
Coracoid process
CLAVICLE
Acromion
Scapular notch
Angle of acromion
Greater tubercle
Head of humerus
Scapular spine
Infraglenoid tubercle
SCAPULA
HUMERUS

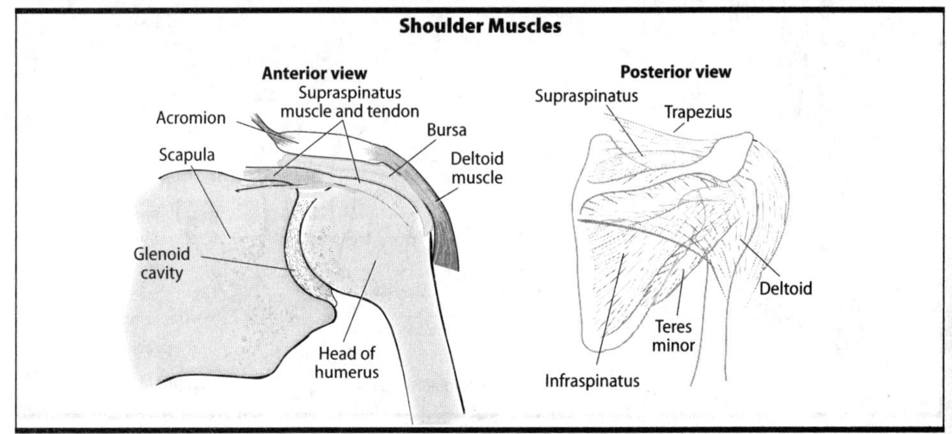
Shoulder Muscles
Anterior view
Supraspinatus muscle and tendon
Acromion
Bursa
Scapula
Deltoid muscle
Glenoid cavity
Head of humerus
Posterior view
Supraspinatus
Trapezius
Deltoid
Teres minor
Infraspinatus

Elbow (Anterior View)

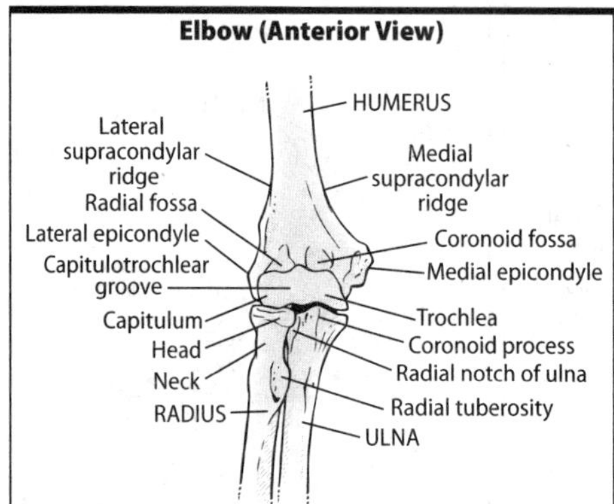

Elbow (Posterior View)

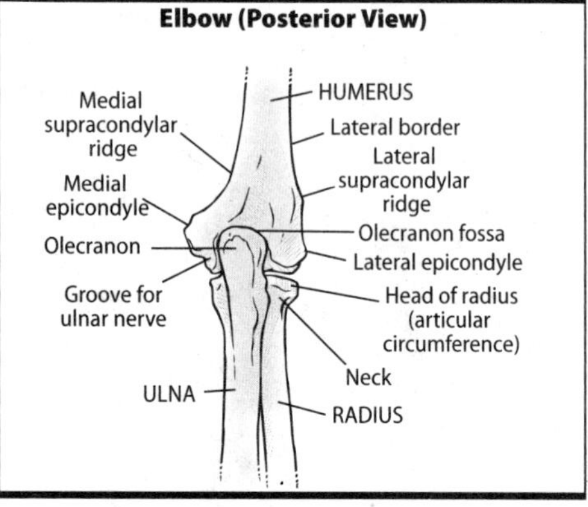

Elbow Muscles

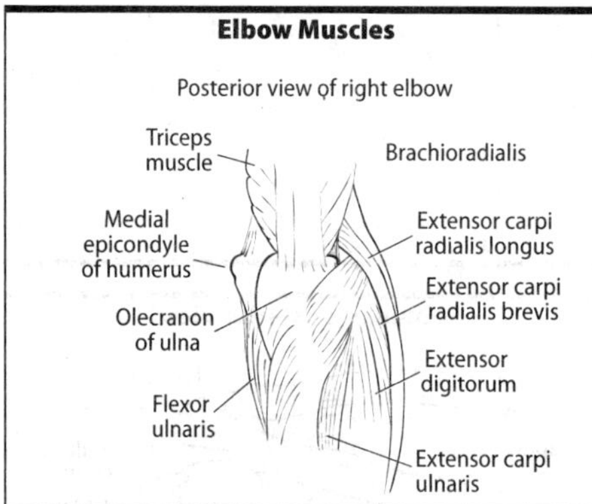

Elbow Joint

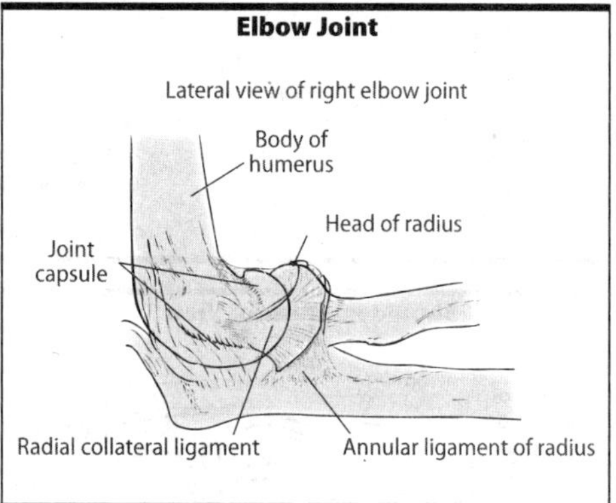

Lower Arm

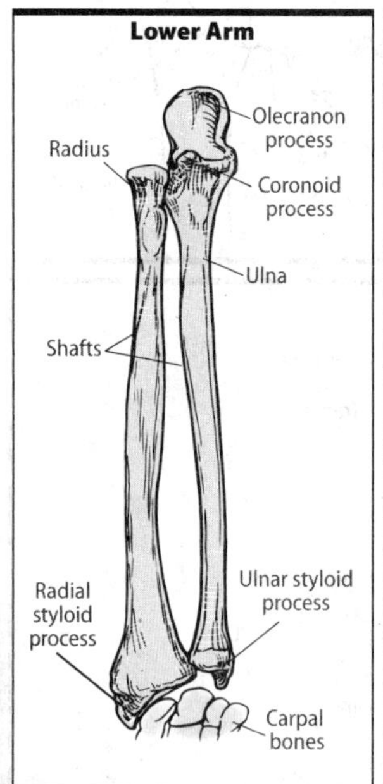

Hand

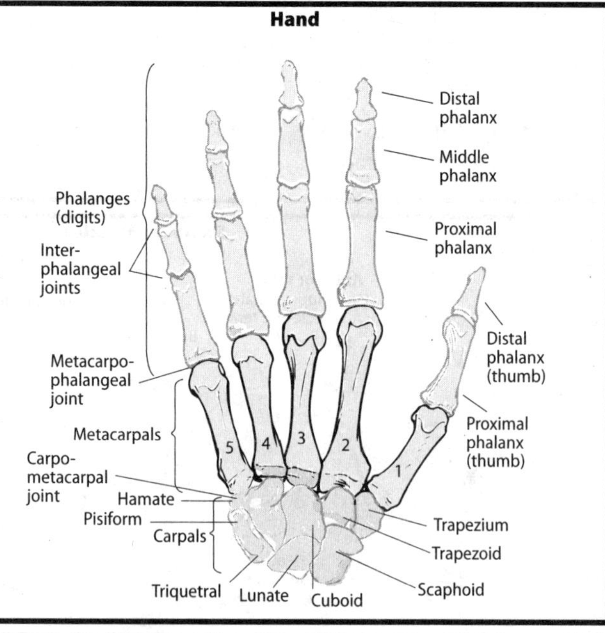

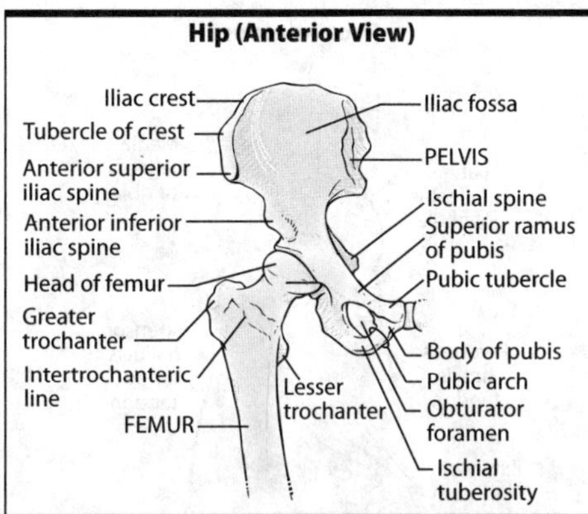
Hip (Anterior View)
Iliac crest
Tubercle of crest
Anterior superior iliac spine
Anterior inferior iliac spine
Head of femur
Greater trochanter
Intertrochanteric line
FEMUR
Lesser trochanter
Iliac fossa
PELVIS
Ischial spine
Superior ramus of pubis
Pubic tubercle
Body of pubis
Pubic arch
Obturator foramen
Ischial tuberosity

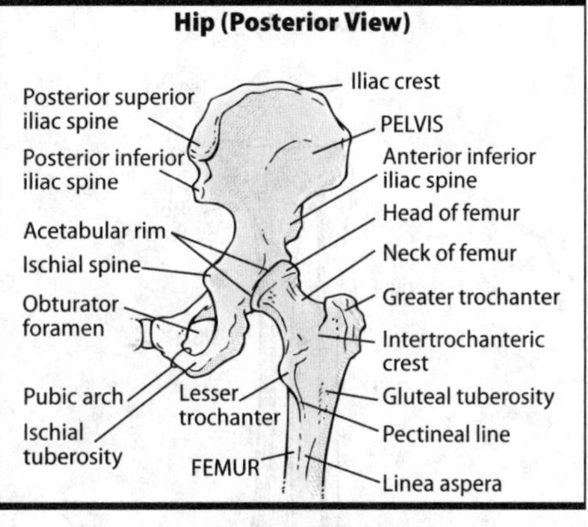
Hip (Posterior View)
Posterior superior iliac spine
Posterior inferior iliac spine
Acetabular rim
Ischial spine
Obturator foramen
Pubic arch
Ischial tuberosity
Lesser trochanter
FEMUR
Iliac crest
PELVIS
Anterior inferior iliac spine
Head of femur
Neck of femur
Greater trochanter
Intertrochanteric crest
Gluteal tuberosity
Pectineal line
Linea aspera

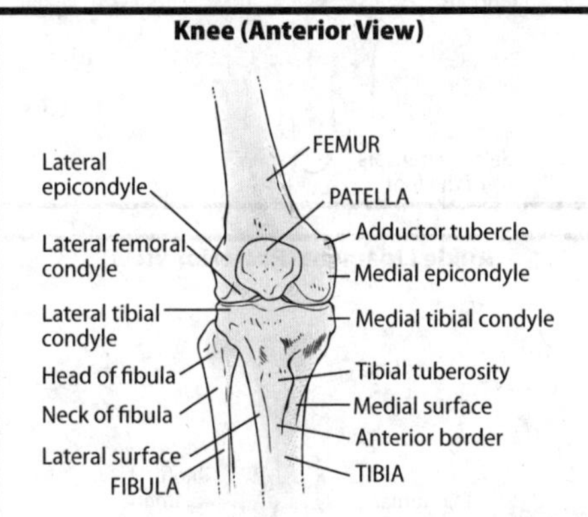
Knee (Anterior View)
Lateral epicondyle
Lateral femoral condyle
Lateral tibial condyle
Head of fibula
Neck of fibula
Lateral surface
FIBULA
FEMUR
PATELLA
Adductor tubercle
Medial epicondyle
Medial tibial condyle
Tibial tuberosity
Medial surface
Anterior border
TIBIA

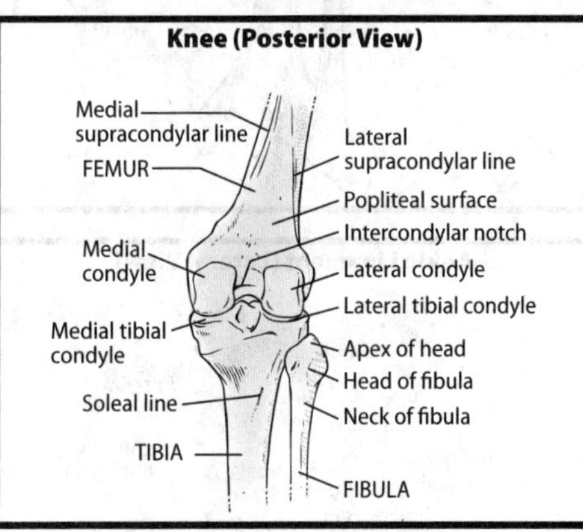
Knee (Posterior View)
Medial supracondylar line
FEMUR
Medial condyle
Medial tibial condyle
Soleal line
TIBIA
Lateral supracondylar line
Popliteal surface
Intercondylar notch
Lateral condyle
Lateral tibial condyle
Apex of head
Head of fibula
Neck of fibula
FIBULA

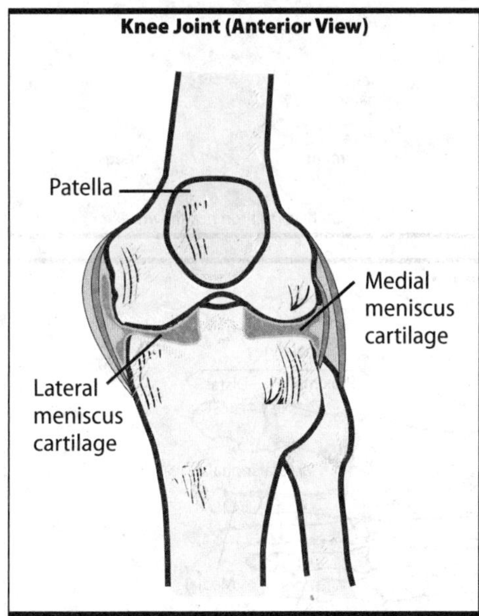
Knee Joint (Anterior View)
Patella
Medial meniscus cartilage
Lateral meniscus cartilage

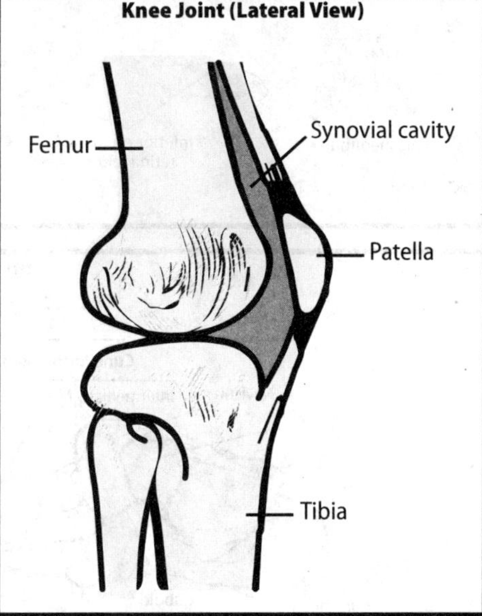
Knee Joint (Lateral View)
Femur
Synovial cavity
Patella
Tibia

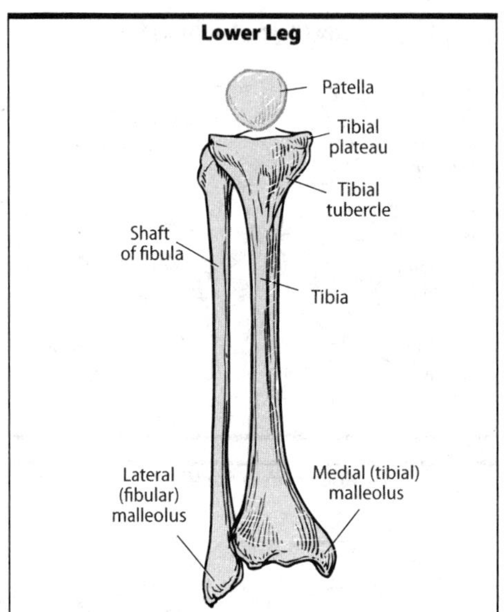

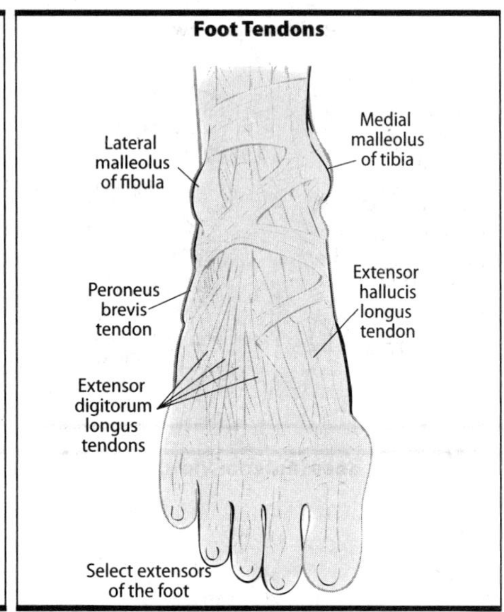

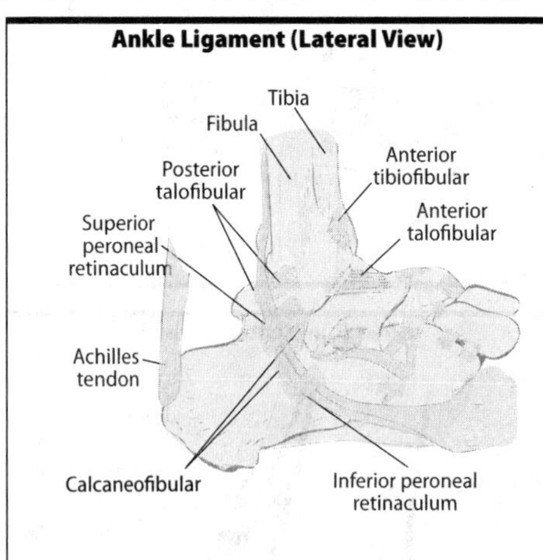

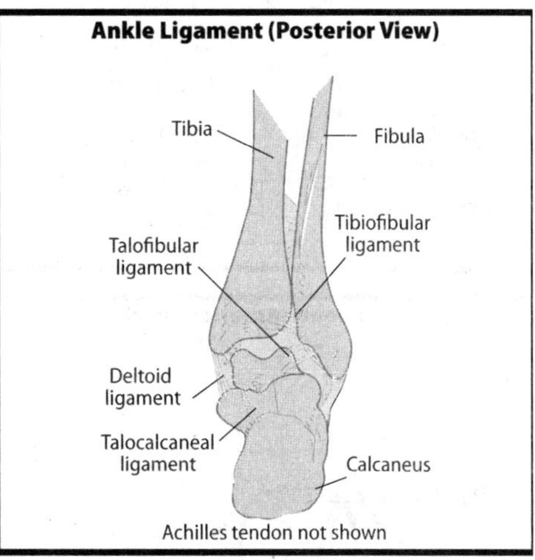

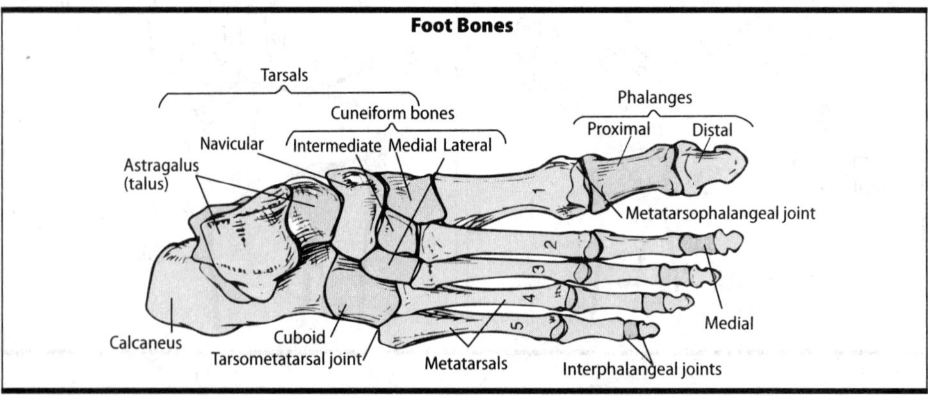

Anatomical Illustrations

Respiratory System

Nasal cavity and paranasal sinuses
Nostril
Oral cavity
Pharynx
Larynx
Trachea
Right lung
Right main / primary bronchus
Diaphragm
Pleura
Left lung
Carina of trachea
Left main/primary bronchus
Secondary (lobar) bronchi
Tertiary (segmental) bronchi
Bronchioles
Alveoli

Upper Respiratory System

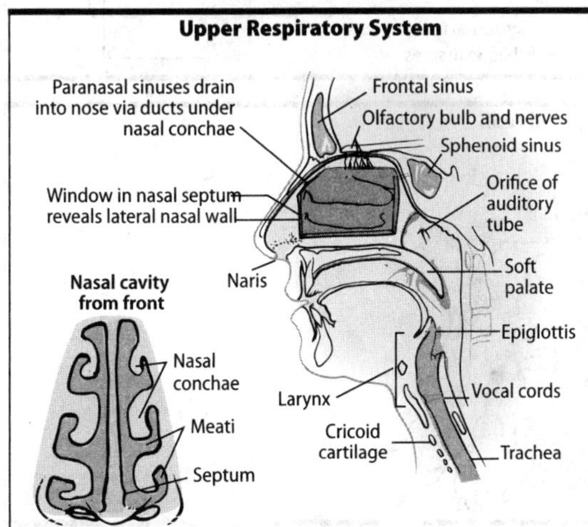

Nasal Turbinates

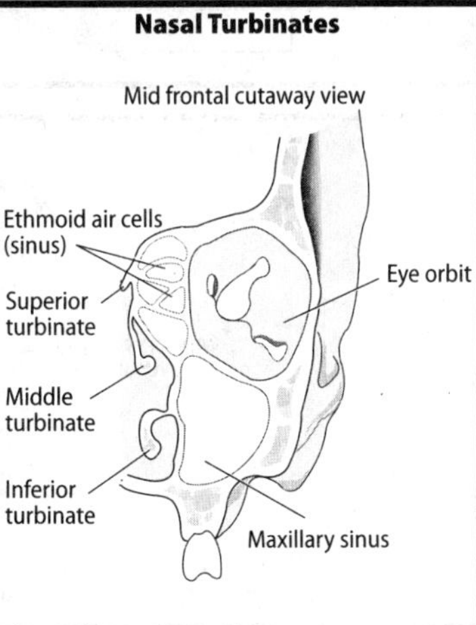

Paranasal Sinuses

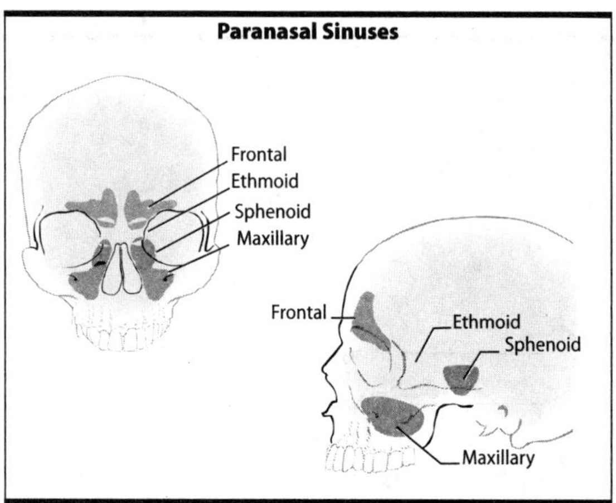

Lower Respiratory System

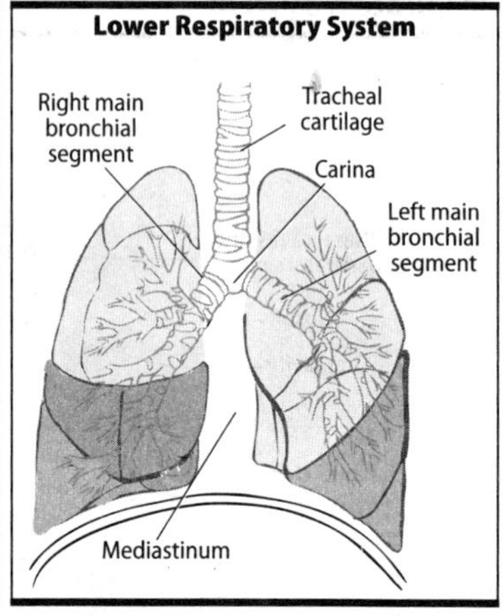

Lung Segments

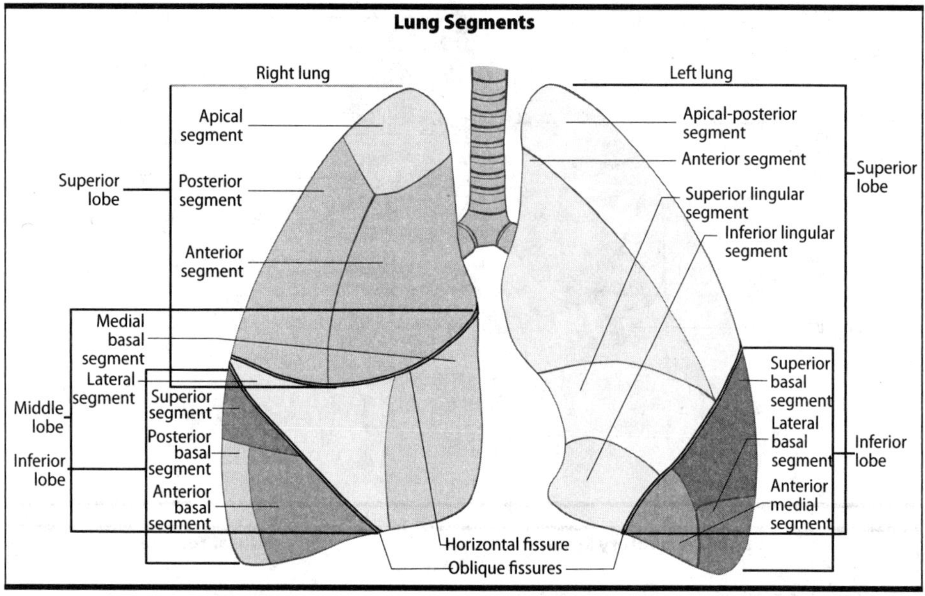

Alveoli

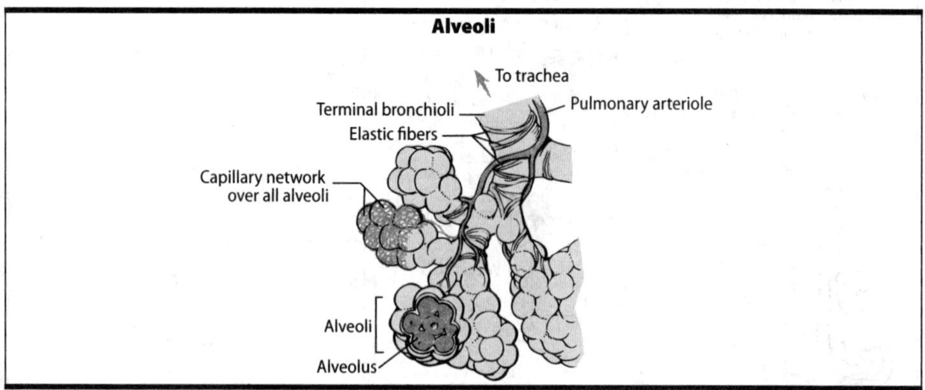

Arterial System

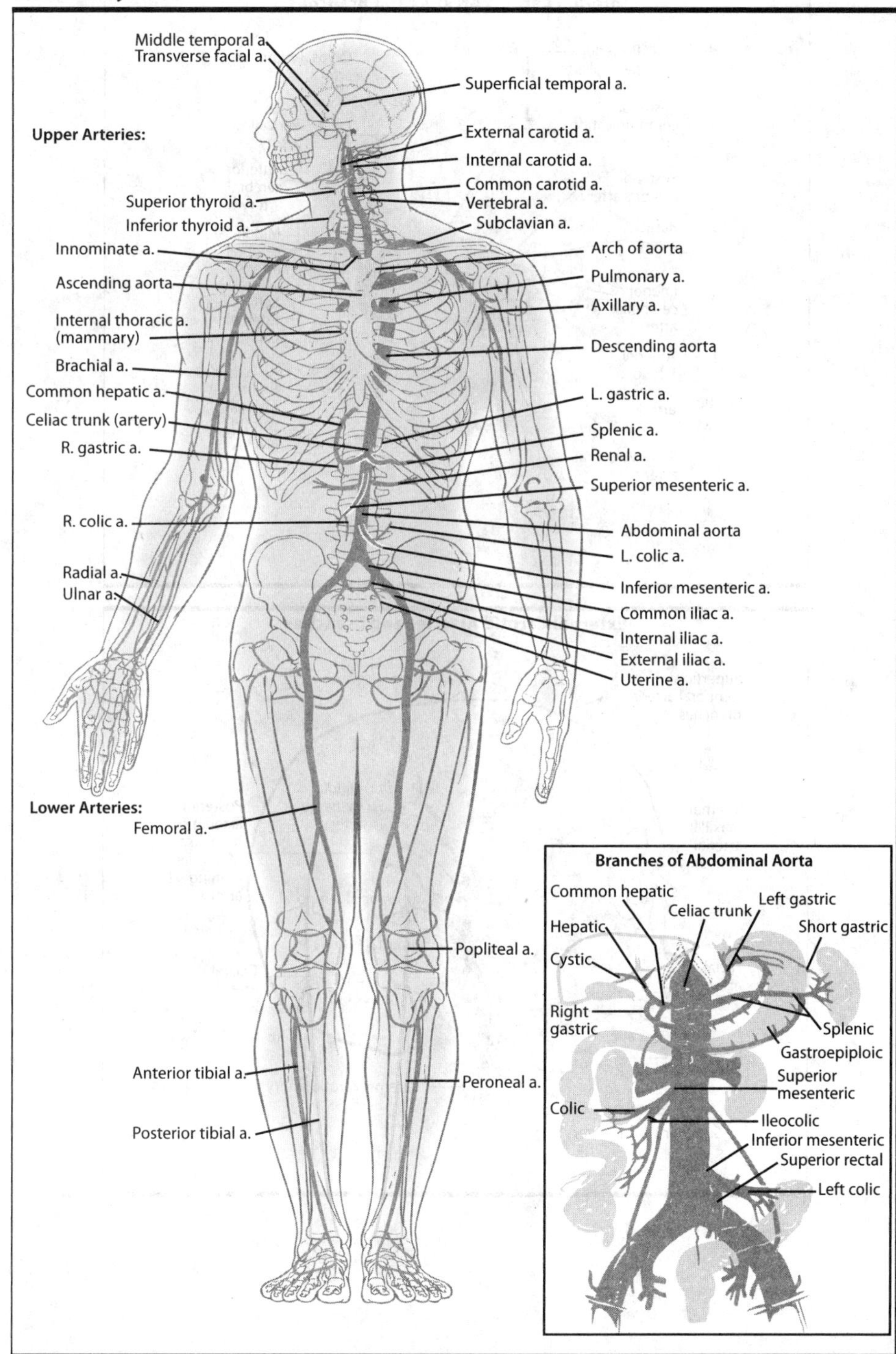

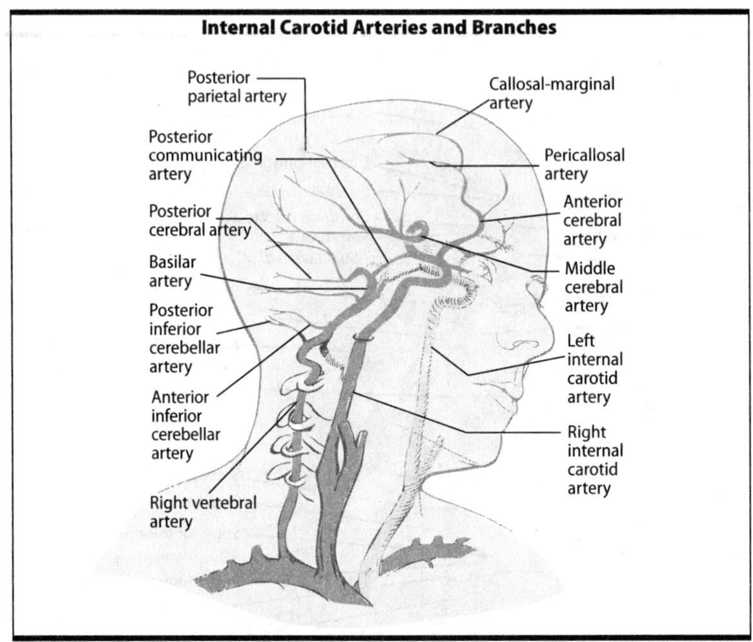
Internal Carotid Arteries and Branches
Posterior parietal artery
Callosal-marginal artery
Posterior communicating artery
Pericallosal artery
Posterior cerebral artery
Anterior cerebral artery
Basilar artery
Middle cerebral artery
Posterior inferior cerebellar artery
Left internal carotid artery
Anterior inferior cerebellar artery
Right internal carotid artery
Right vertebral artery

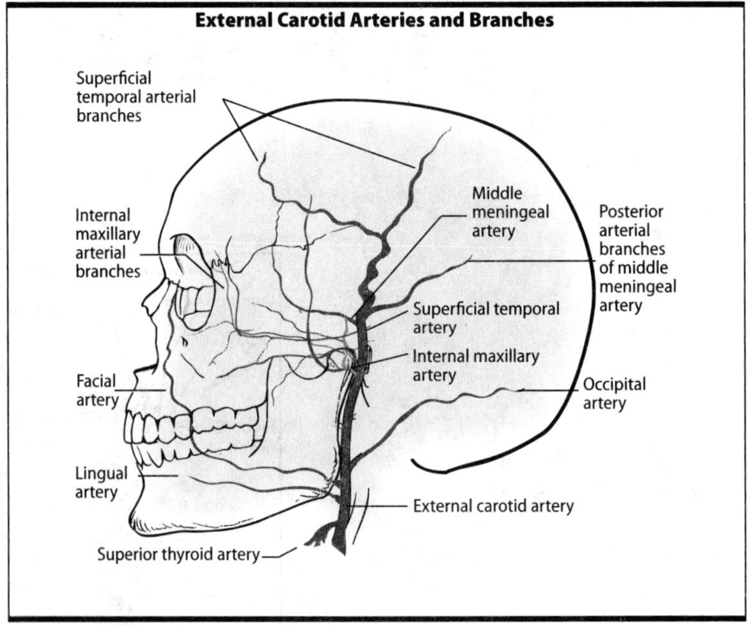
External Carotid Arteries and Branches
Superficial temporal arterial branches
Middle meningeal artery
Internal maxillary arterial branches
Posterior arterial branches of middle meningeal artery
Superficial temporal artery
Internal maxillary artery
Facial artery
Occipital artery
Lingual artery
External carotid artery
Superior thyroid artery

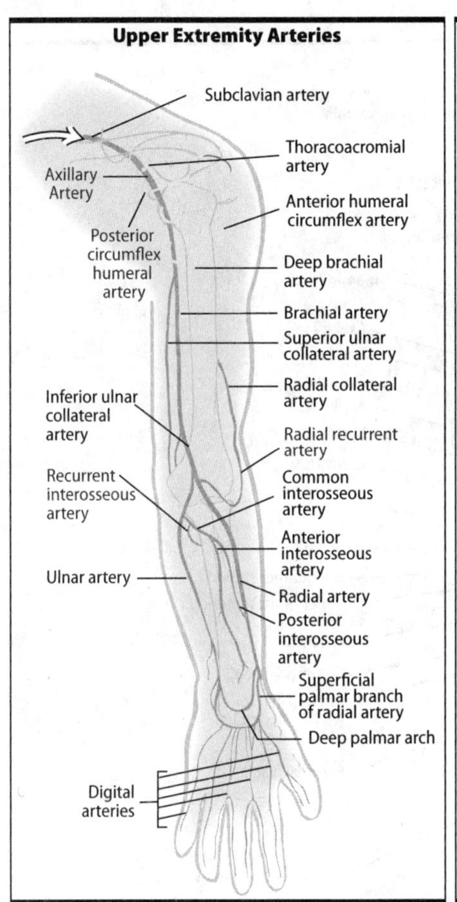
Upper Extremity Arteries
Subclavian artery
Thoracoacromial artery
Axillary Artery
Anterior humeral circumflex artery
Posterior circumflex humeral artery
Deep brachial artery
Brachial artery
Superior ulnar collateral artery
Radial collateral artery
Inferior ulnar collateral artery
Radial recurrent artery
Recurrent interosseous artery
Common interosseous artery
Anterior interosseous artery
Ulnar artery
Radial artery
Posterior interosseous artery
Superficial palmar branch of radial artery
Deep palmar arch
Digital arteries

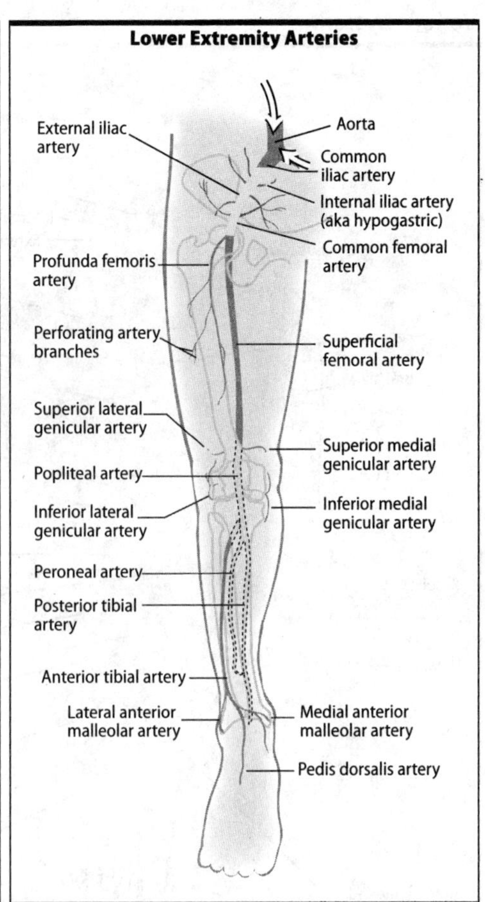
Lower Extremity Arteries
External iliac artery
Aorta
Common iliac artery
Internal iliac artery (aka hypogastric)
Common femoral artery
Profunda femoris artery
Perforating artery branches
Superficial femoral artery
Superior lateral genicular artery
Superior medial genicular artery
Popliteal artery
Inferior lateral genicular artery
Inferior medial genicular artery
Peroneal artery
Posterior tibial artery
Anterior tibial artery
Lateral anterior malleolar artery
Medial anterior malleolar artery
Pedis dorsalis artery

Venous System

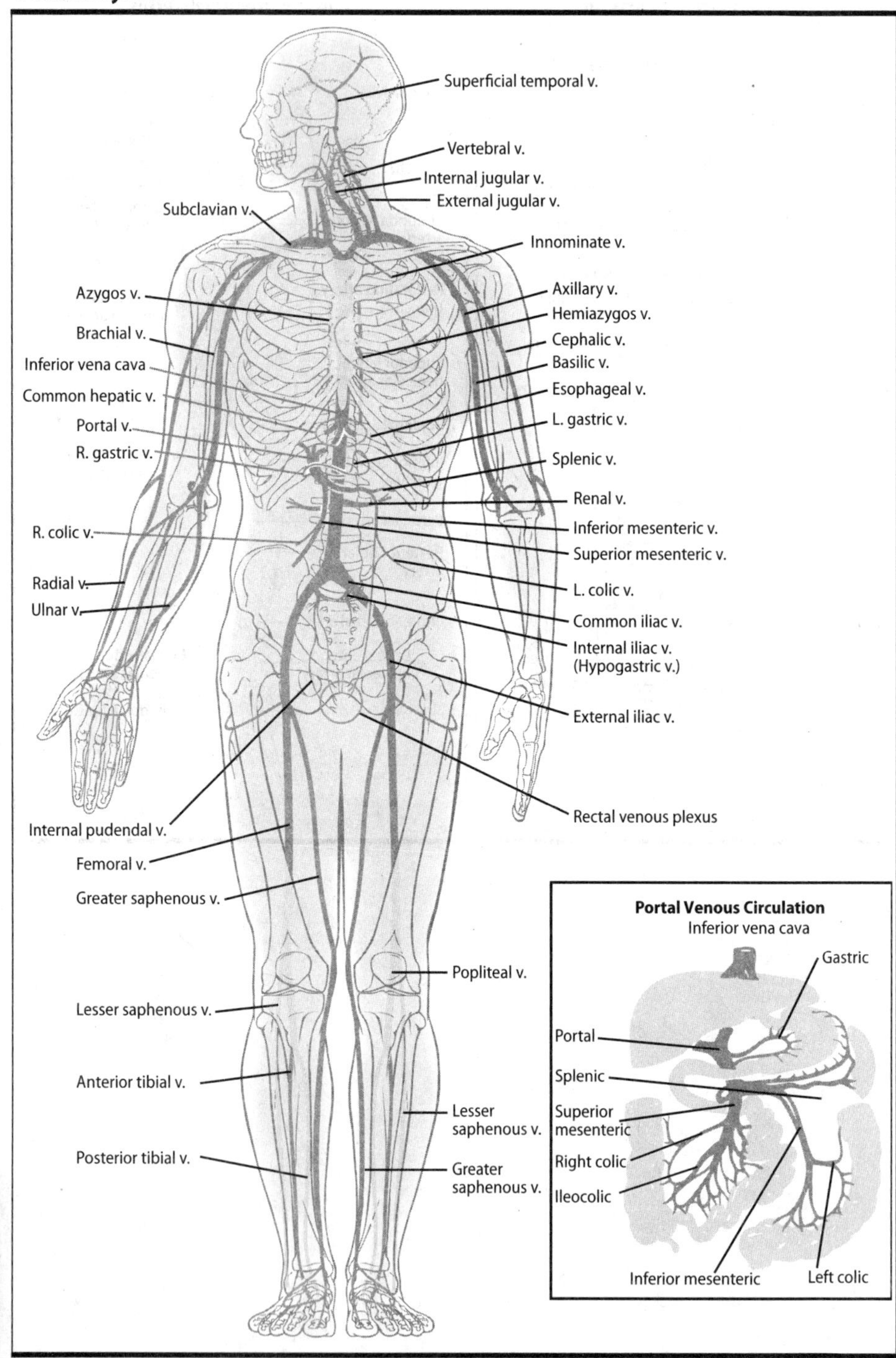

Head and Neck Veins

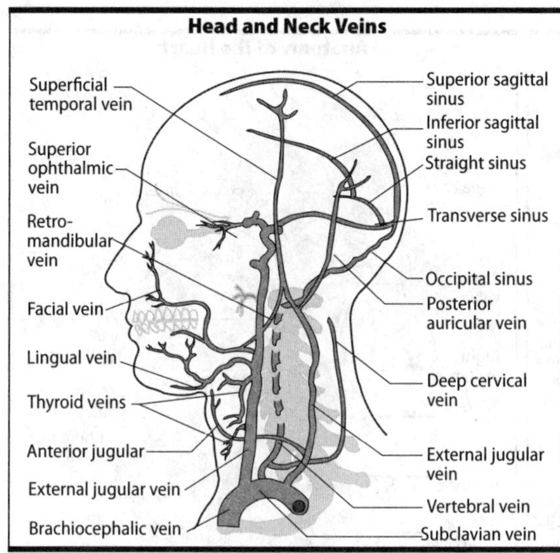

Upper Extremity Veins

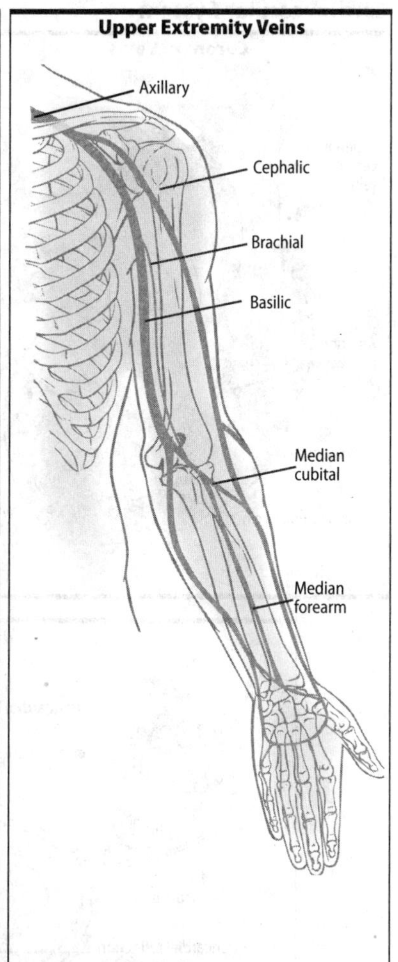

Venae Comitantes

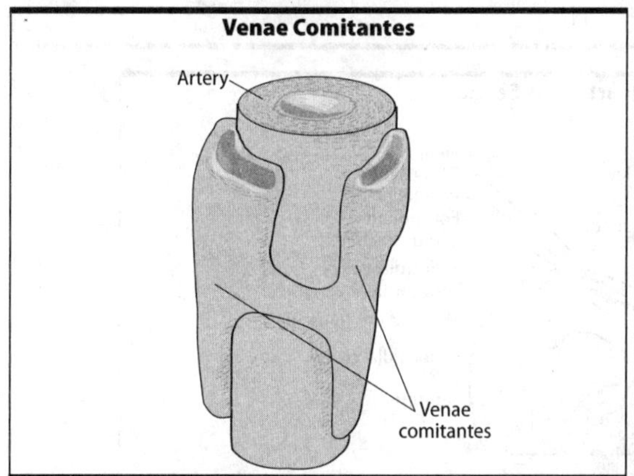

Venous Blood Flow

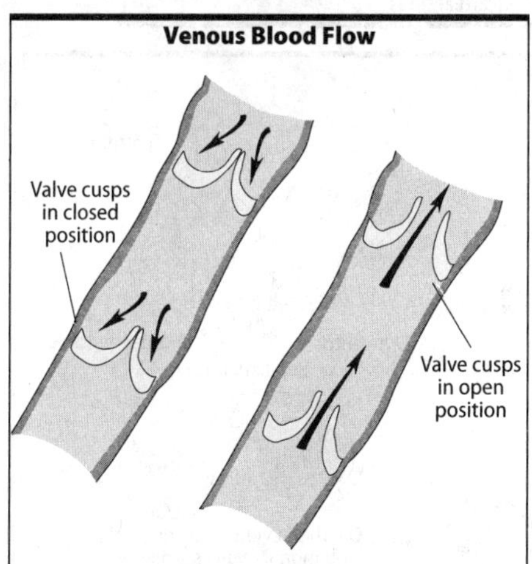

Abdominal Veins

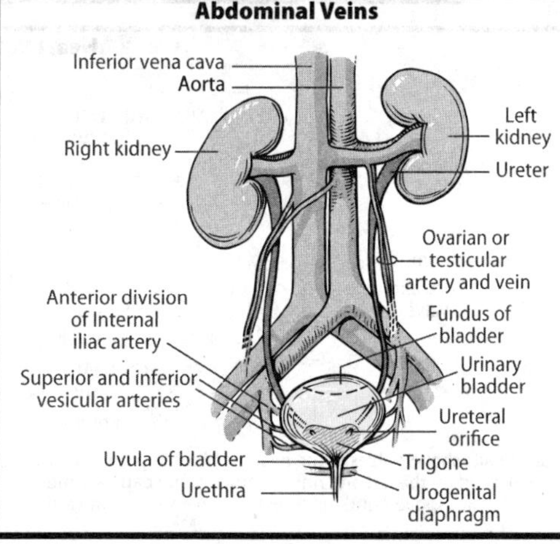

Cardiovascular System

Coronary Veins

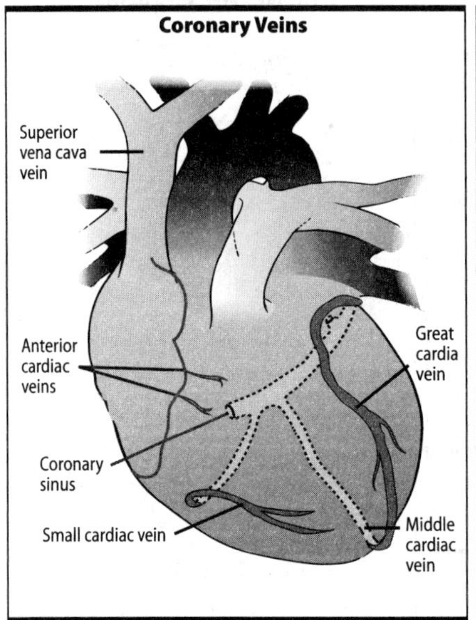

Anatomy of the Heart

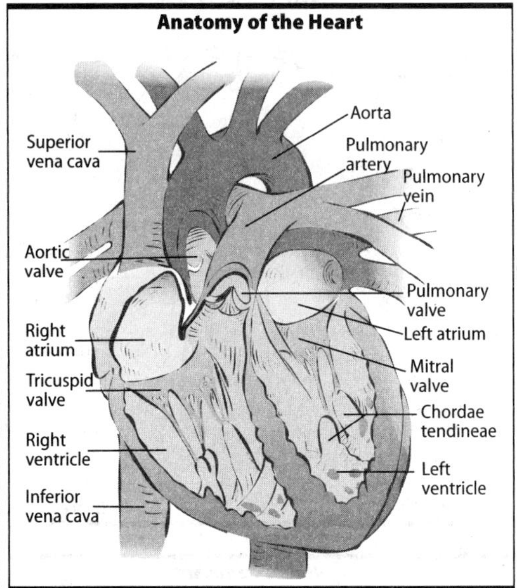

Heart Cross Section

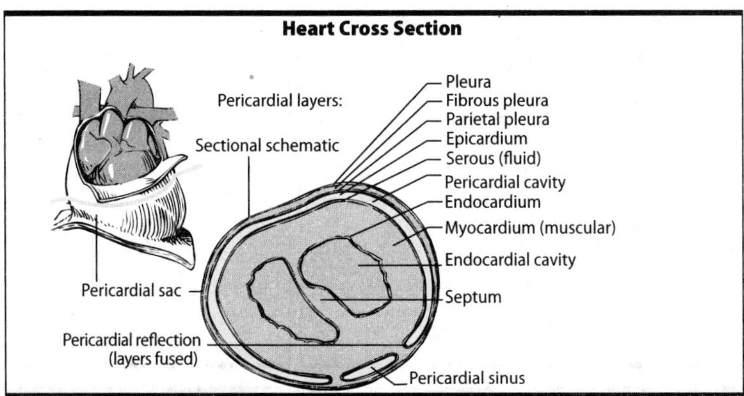

Heart Valves

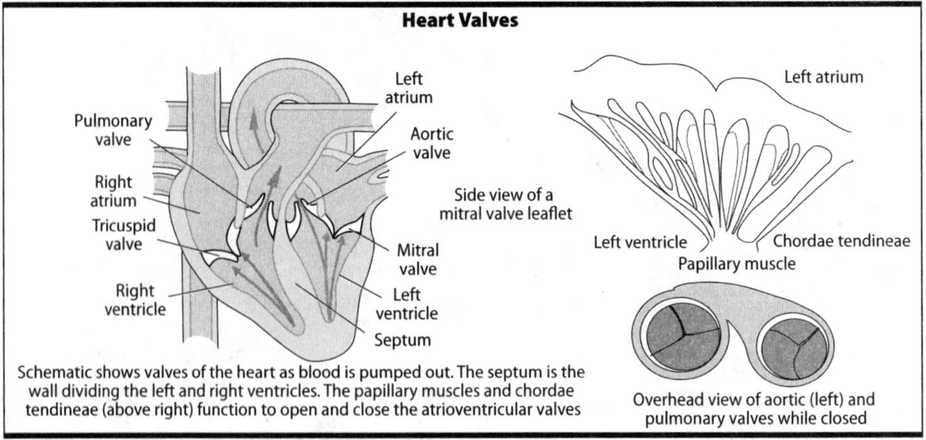

Schematic shows valves of the heart as blood is pumped out. The septum is the wall dividing the left and right ventricles. The papillary muscles and chordae tendineae (above right) function to open and close the atrioventricular valves

Overhead view of aortic (left) and pulmonary valves while closed

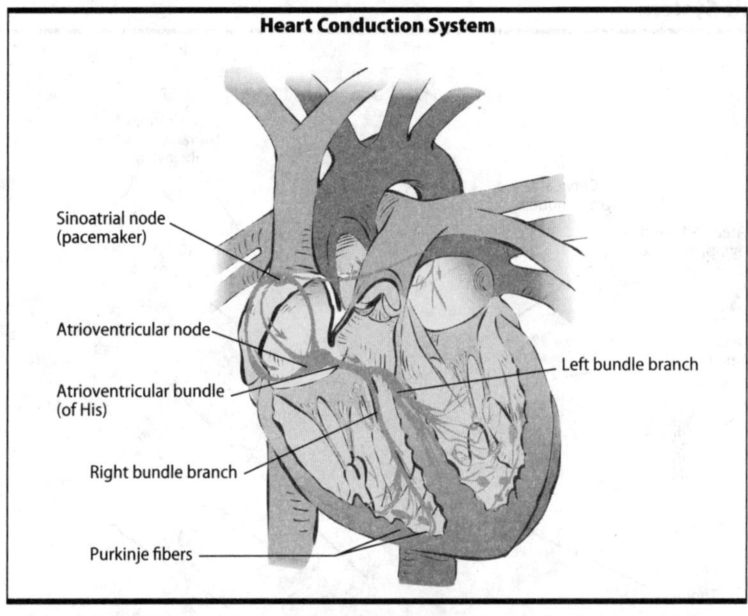
Heart Conduction System
Sinoatrial node (pacemaker)
Atrioventricular node
Atrioventricular bundle (of His)
Right bundle branch
Purkinje fibers
Left bundle branch

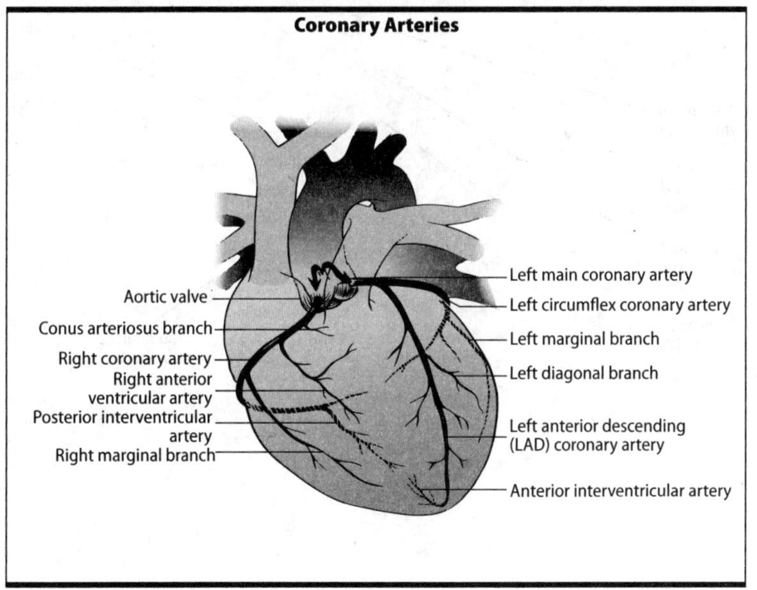
Coronary Arteries
Aortic valve
Conus arteriosus branch
Right coronary artery
Right anterior ventricular artery
Posterior interventricular artery
Right marginal branch
Left main coronary artery
Left circumflex coronary artery
Left marginal branch
Left diagonal branch
Left anterior descending (LAD) coronary artery
Anterior interventricular artery

Lymphatic System

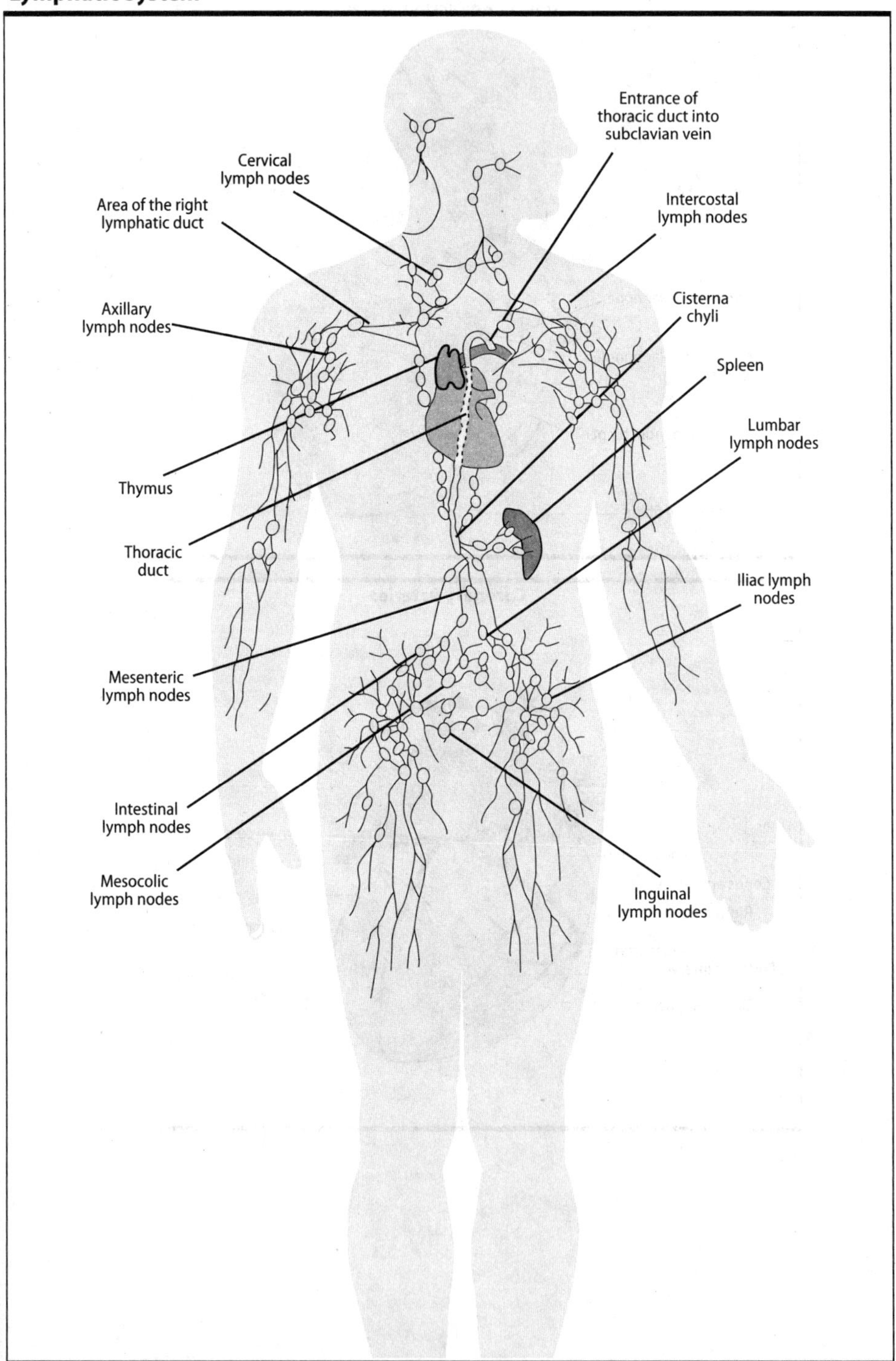

Axillary Lymph Nodes

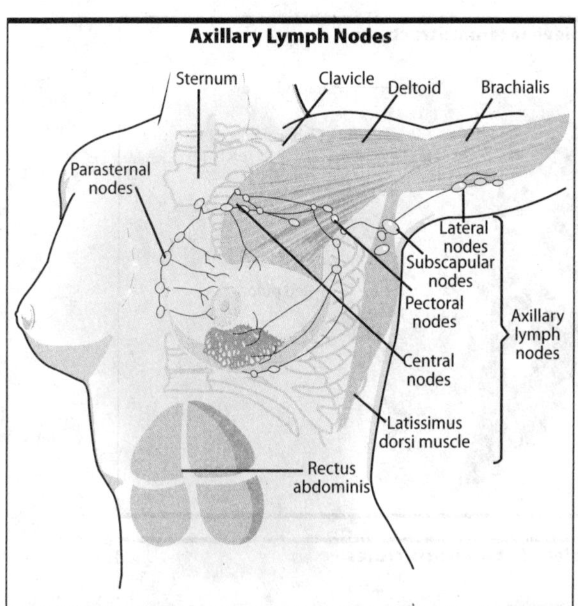

Lymphatic Capillaries

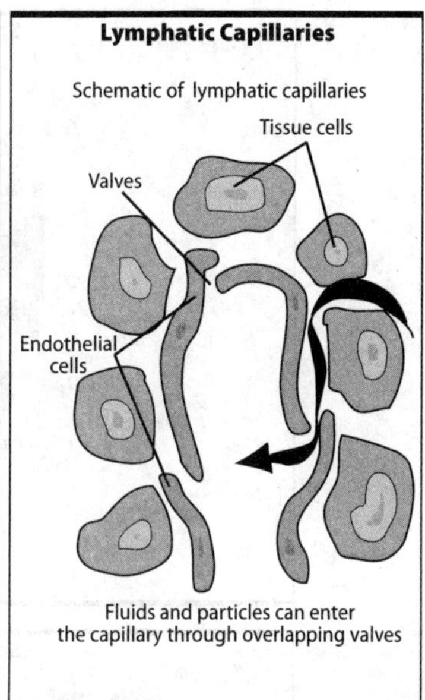

Lymphatic System of Head and Neck

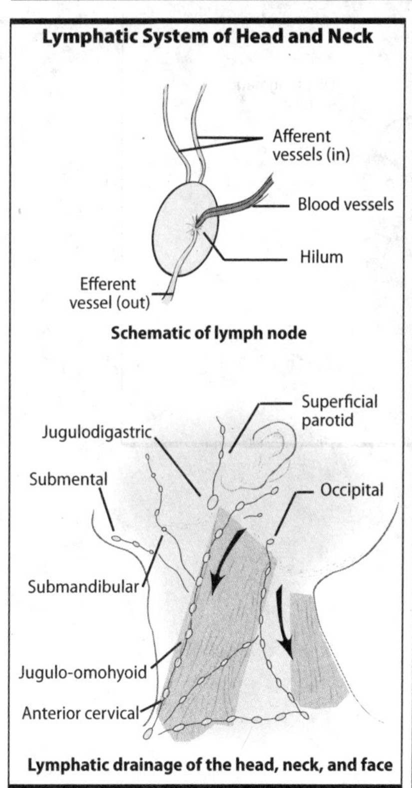

Lymphatic Drainage

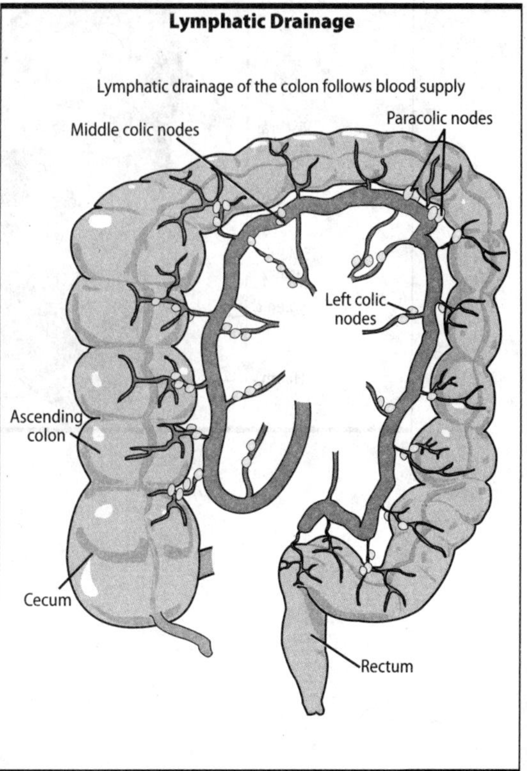

Spleen Internal Structures

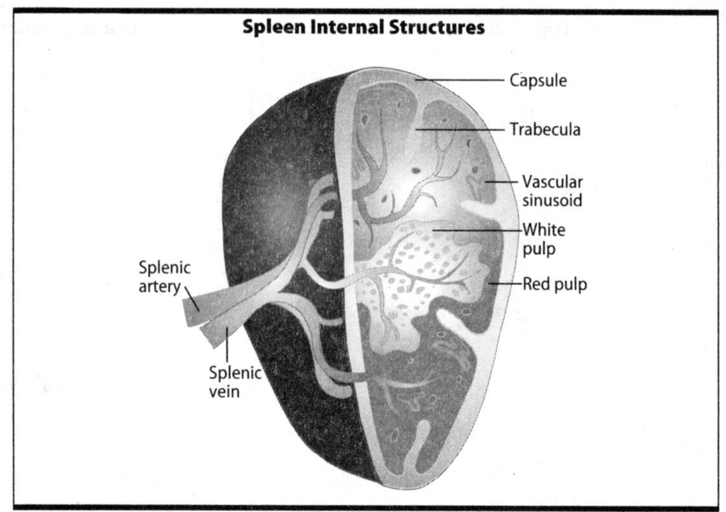

Spleen External Structures

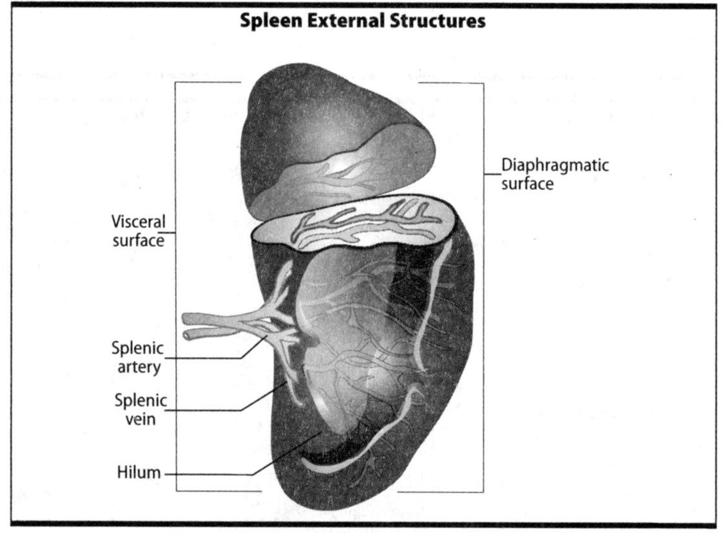

Digestive System

Pharynx
Salivary glands
Parotid
Sublingual
Submandibular
Oral cavity
Uvula
Tongue
Wharton duct
Esophagus
Stomach
Splenic flexure
Liver
Pancreas
Gallbladder
Common bile duct
Hepatic flexure
Duodenum
Jejunum
Ileum
Small intestine
Mesentery
Transverse colon
Ascending colon
Descending colon
Ileocecal valve
Cecum
Appendix
Rectum
Sigmoid colon
Anus

Gallbladder

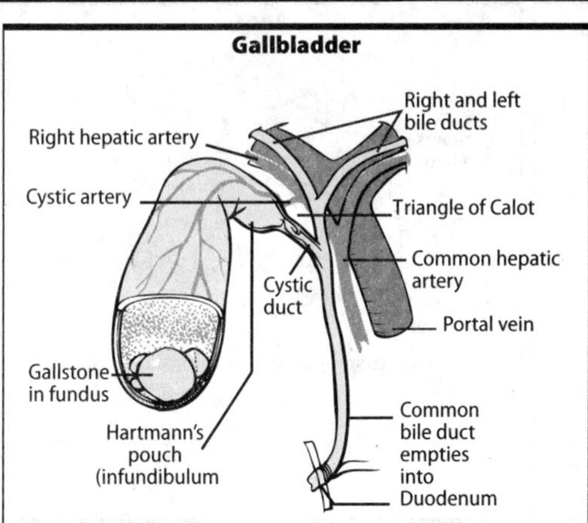

Stomach

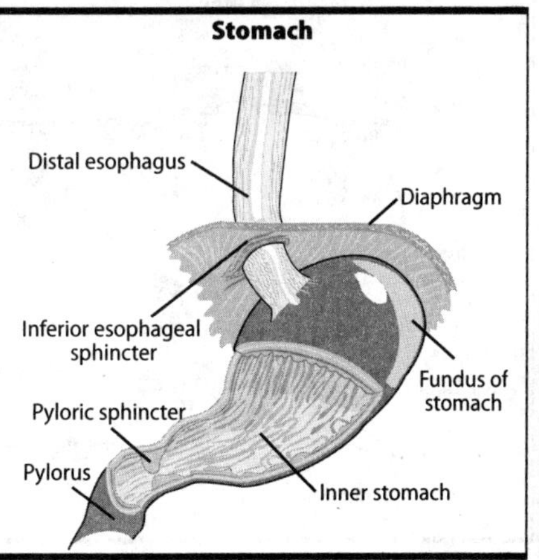

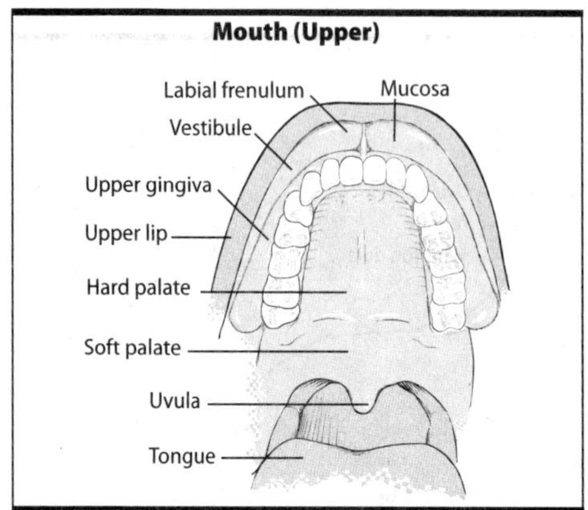
Mouth (Upper)
Labial frenulum
Mucosa
Vestibule
Upper gingiva
Upper lip
Hard palate
Soft palate
Uvula
Tongue

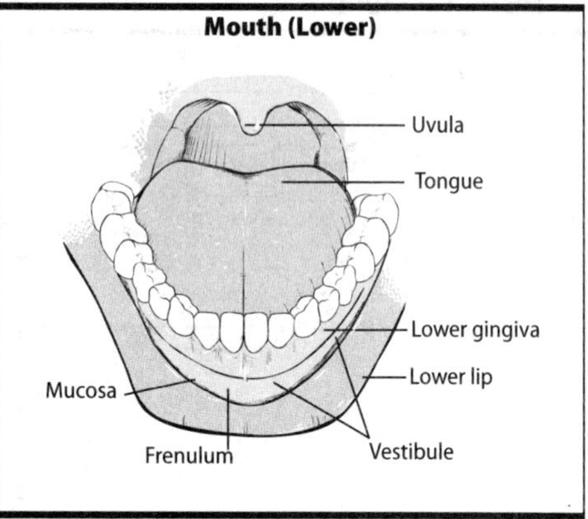
Mouth (Lower)
Uvula
Tongue
Lower gingiva
Lower lip
Mucosa
Frenulum
Vestibule

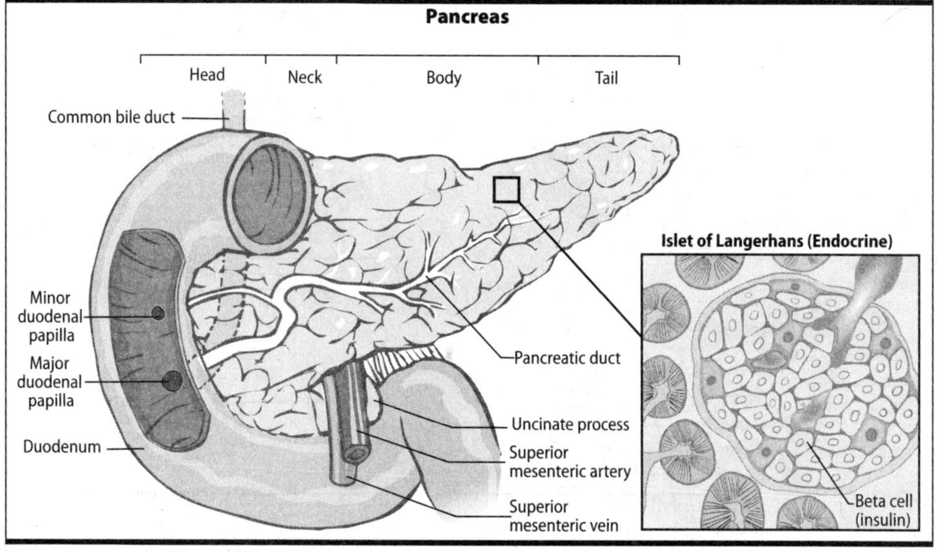
Pancreas
Head
Neck
Body
Tail
Common bile duct
Islet of Langerhans (Endocrine)
Minor duodenal papilla
Major duodenal papilla
Duodenum
Pancreatic duct
Uncinate process
Superior mesenteric artery
Superior mesenteric vein
Beta cell (insulin)

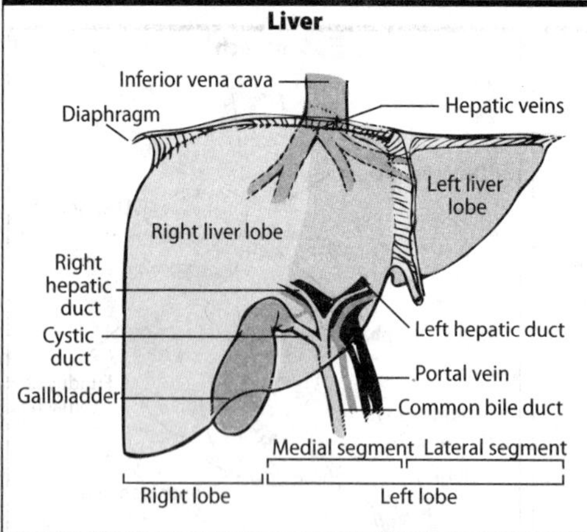
Liver
Inferior vena cava
Diaphragm
Hepatic veins
Left liver lobe
Right liver lobe
Right hepatic duct
Cystic duct
Gallbladder
Left hepatic duct
Portal vein
Common bile duct
Medial segment
Lateral segment
Right lobe
Left lobe

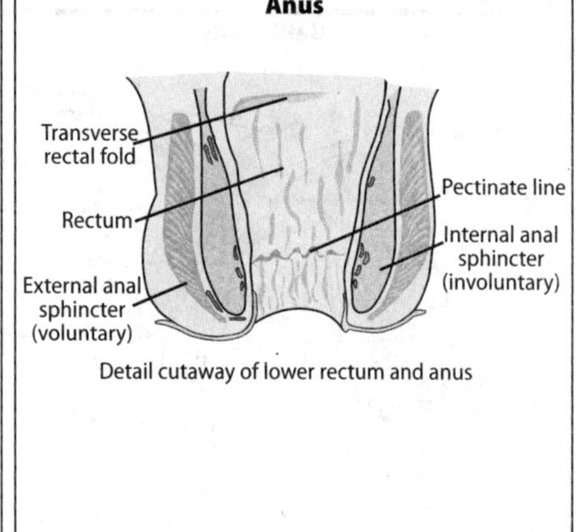
Anus
Transverse rectal fold
Rectum
External anal sphincter (voluntary)
Pectinate line
Internal anal sphincter (involuntary)
Detail cutaway of lower rectum and anus

Genitourinary System

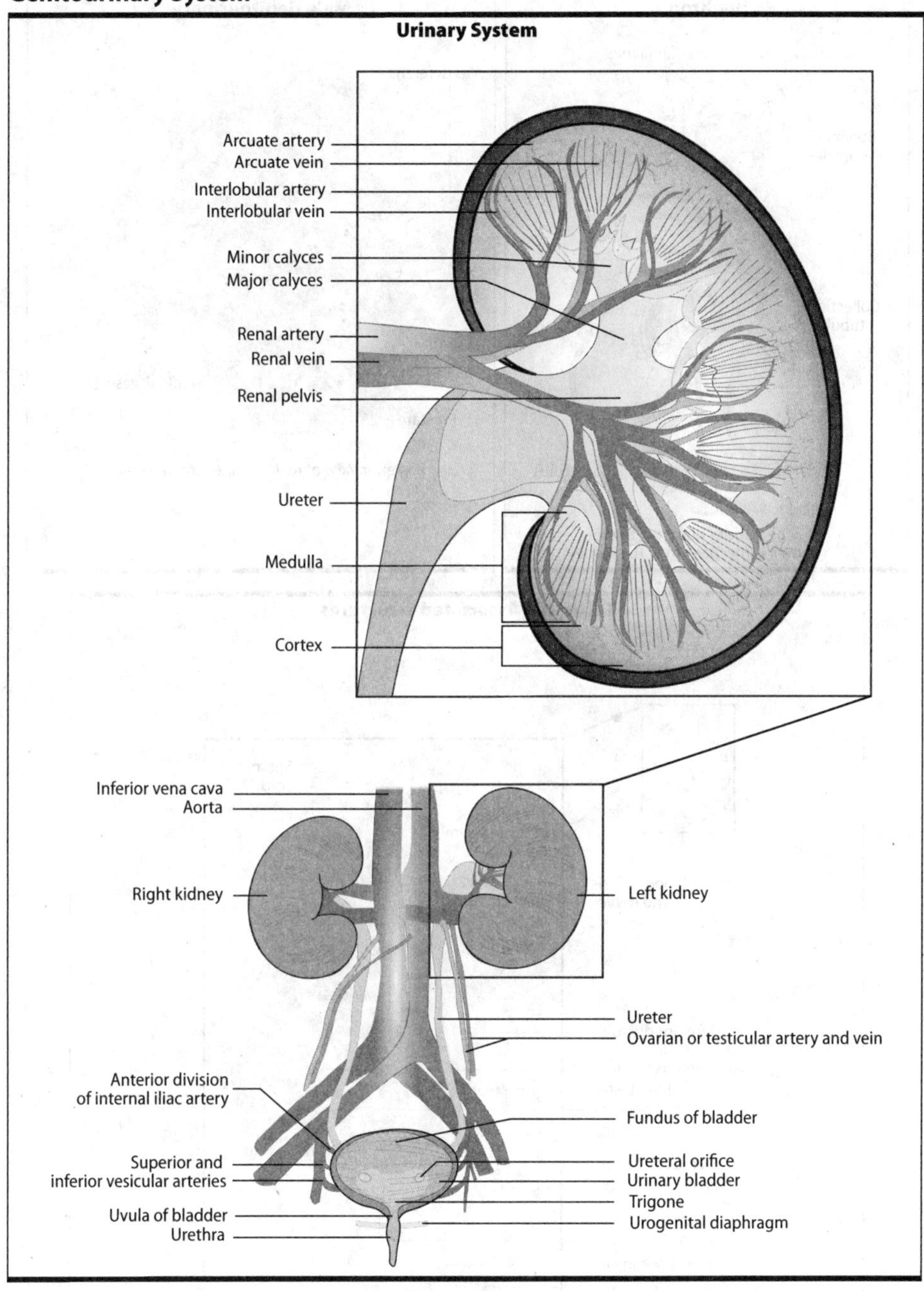

Nephron

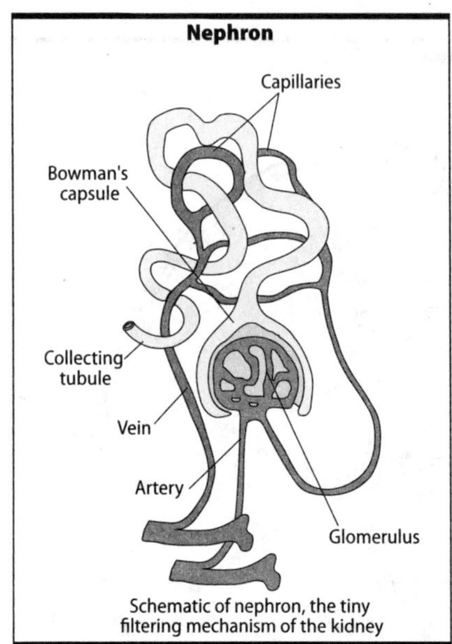

Schematic of nephron, the tiny filtering mechanism of the kidney

Male Genitourinary

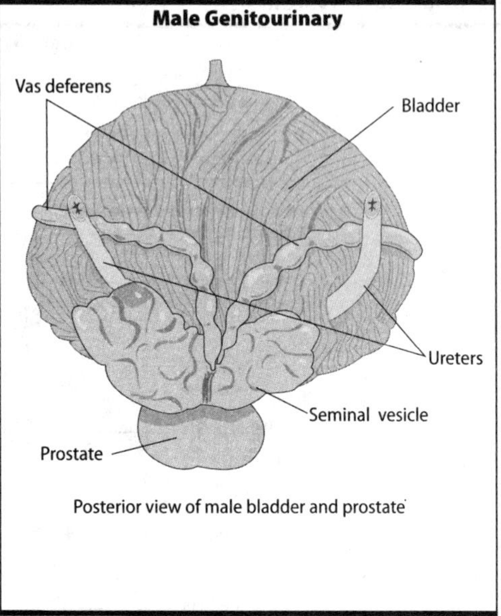

Posterior view of male bladder and prostate

Testis and Associated Structures

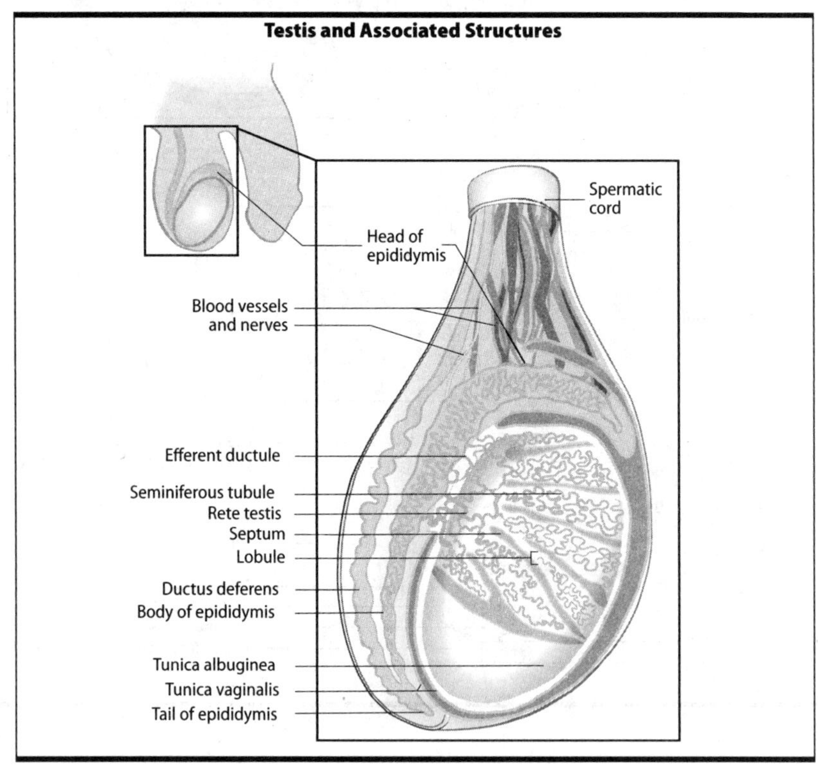

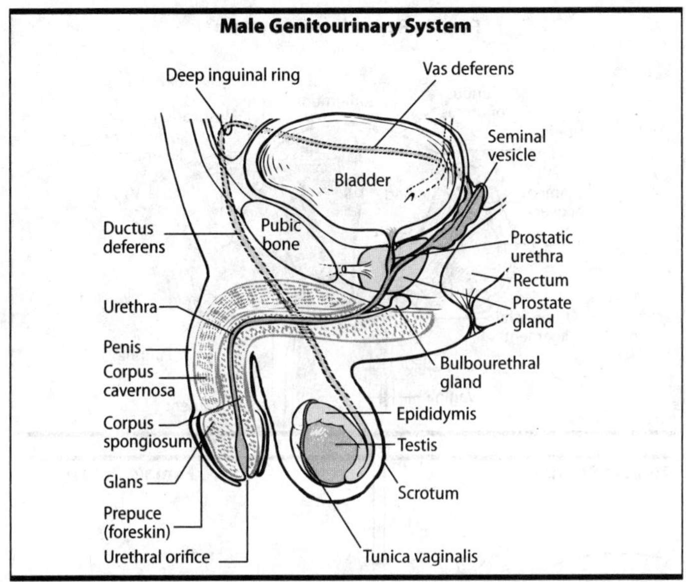
Male Genitourinary System
Deep inguinal ring
Vas deferens
Seminal vesicle
Bladder
Ductus deferens
Pubic bone
Prostatic urethra
Rectum
Urethra
Prostate gland
Penis
Corpus cavernosa
Bulbourethral gland
Epididymis
Corpus spongiosum
Testis
Glans
Scrotum
Prepuce (foreskin)
Urethral orifice
Tunica vaginalis

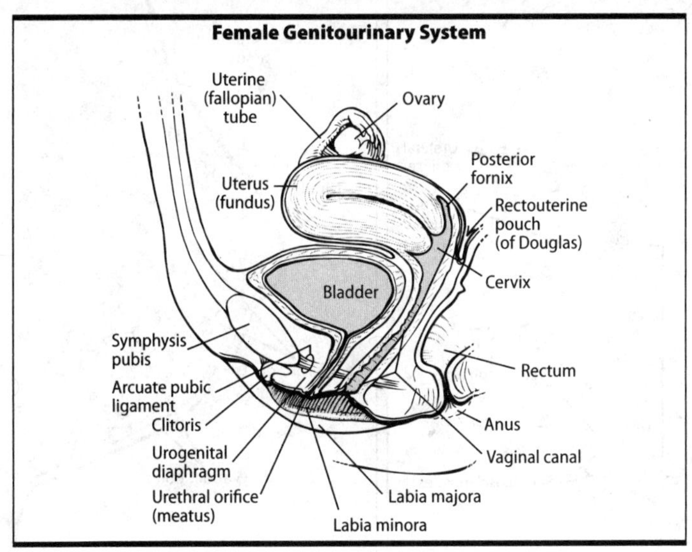
Female Genitourinary System
Uterine (fallopian) tube
Ovary
Posterior fornix
Uterus (fundus)
Rectouterine pouch (of Douglas)
Cervix
Bladder
Symphysis pubis
Rectum
Arcuate pubic ligament
Clitoris
Anus
Urogenital diaphragm
Vaginal canal
Urethral orifice (meatus)
Labia majora
Labia minora

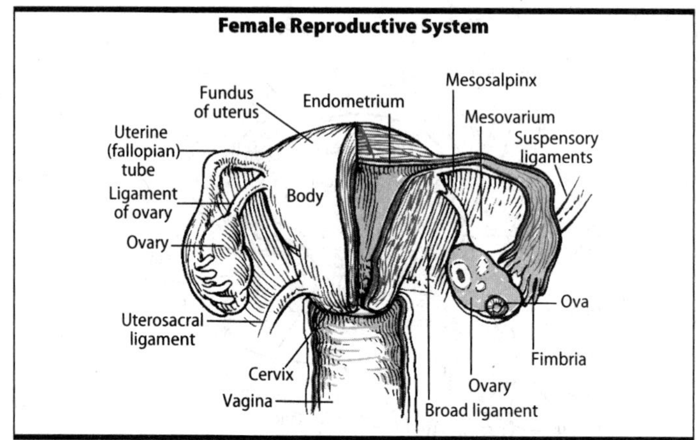
Female Reproductive System
Fundus of uterus
Endometrium
Mesosalpinx
Mesovarium
Suspensory ligaments
Uterine (fallopian) tube
Ligament of ovary
Body
Ovary
Uterosacral ligament
Cervix
Vagina
Ova
Fimbria
Ovary
Broad ligament

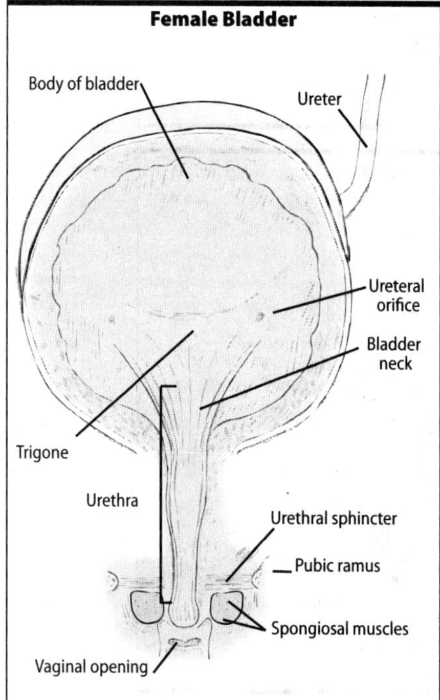
Female Bladder
Body of bladder
Ureter
Ureteral orifice
Bladder neck
Trigone
Urethra
Urethral sphincter
Pubic ramus
Spongiosal muscles
Vaginal opening

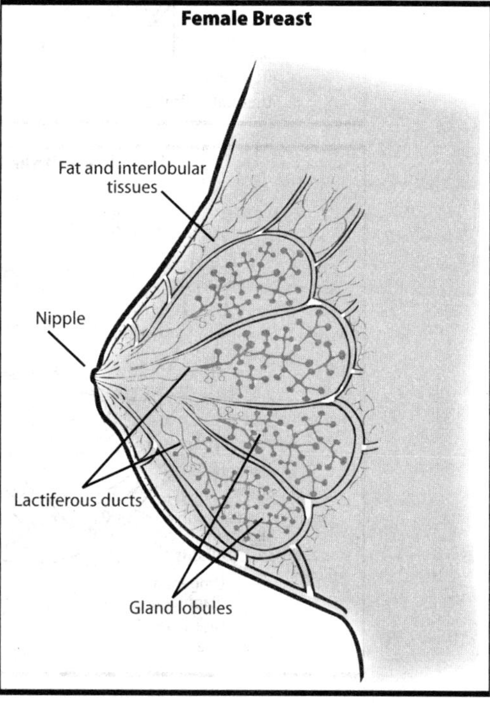
Female Breast
Fat and interlobular tissues
Nipple
Lactiferous ducts
Gland lobules

Endocrine System

Pineal gland
Hypothalamus
Pituitary gland
Thyroid
Parathyroid gland
Adrenal gland
Pancreas
Ovaries

Structure of an Ovary

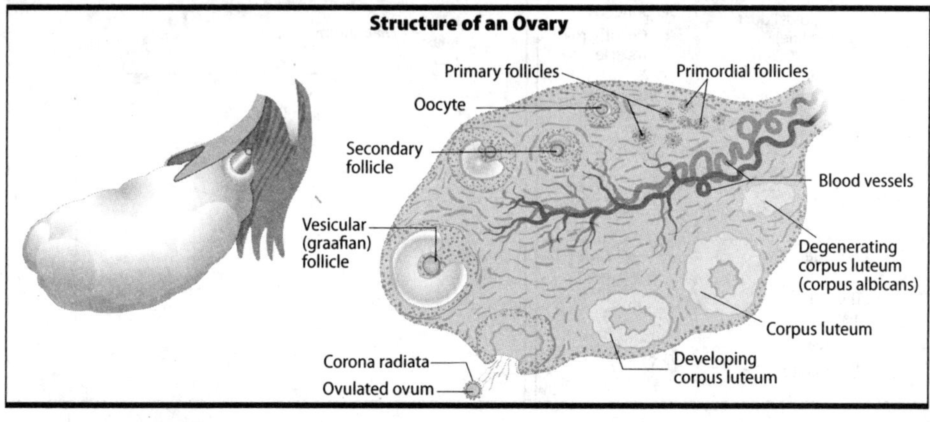

Thyroid and Parathyroid Glands

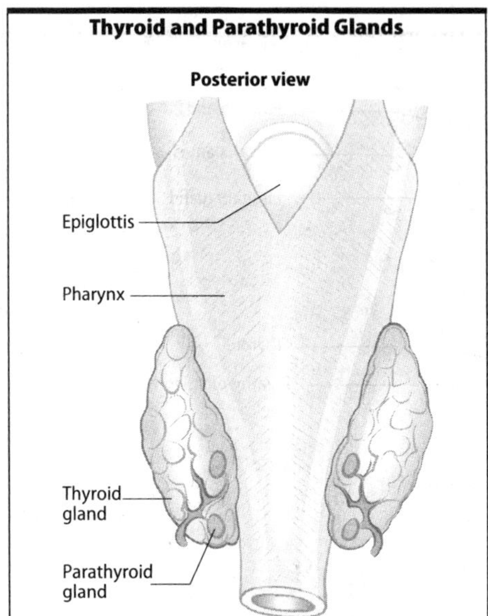

Adrenal Gland

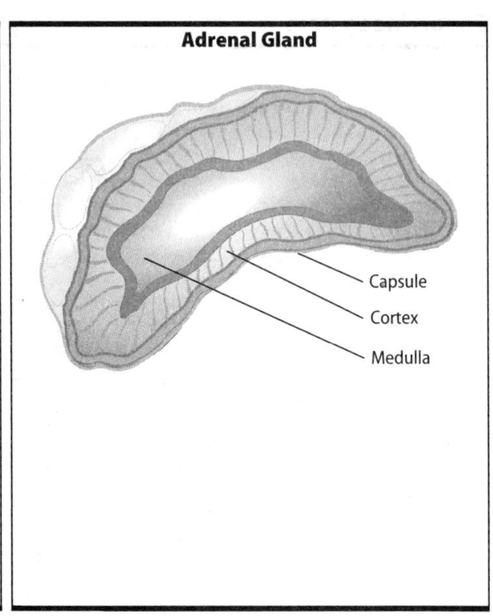

Thyroid

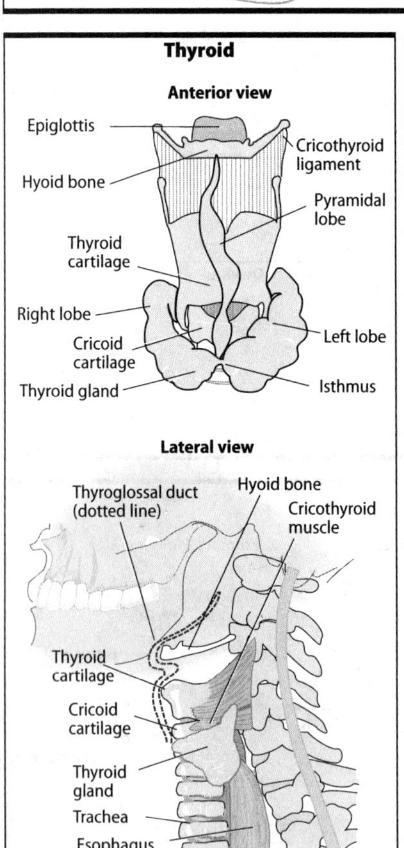

Thymus

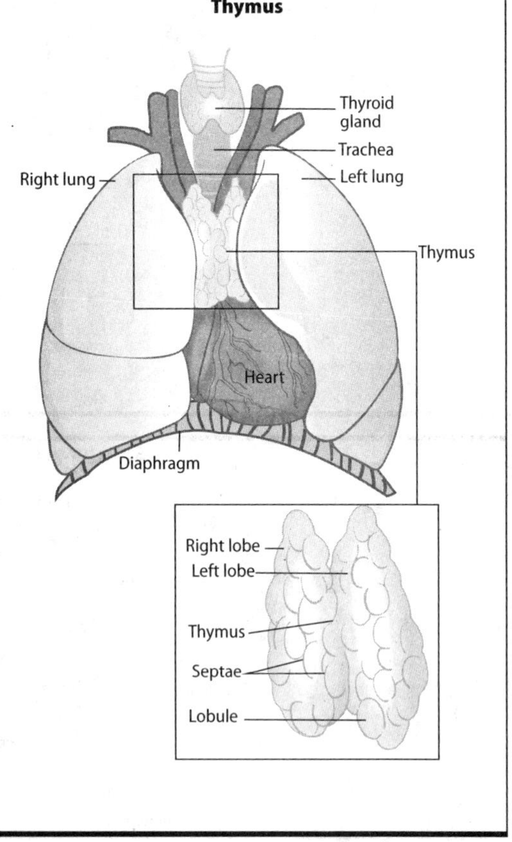

Nervous System

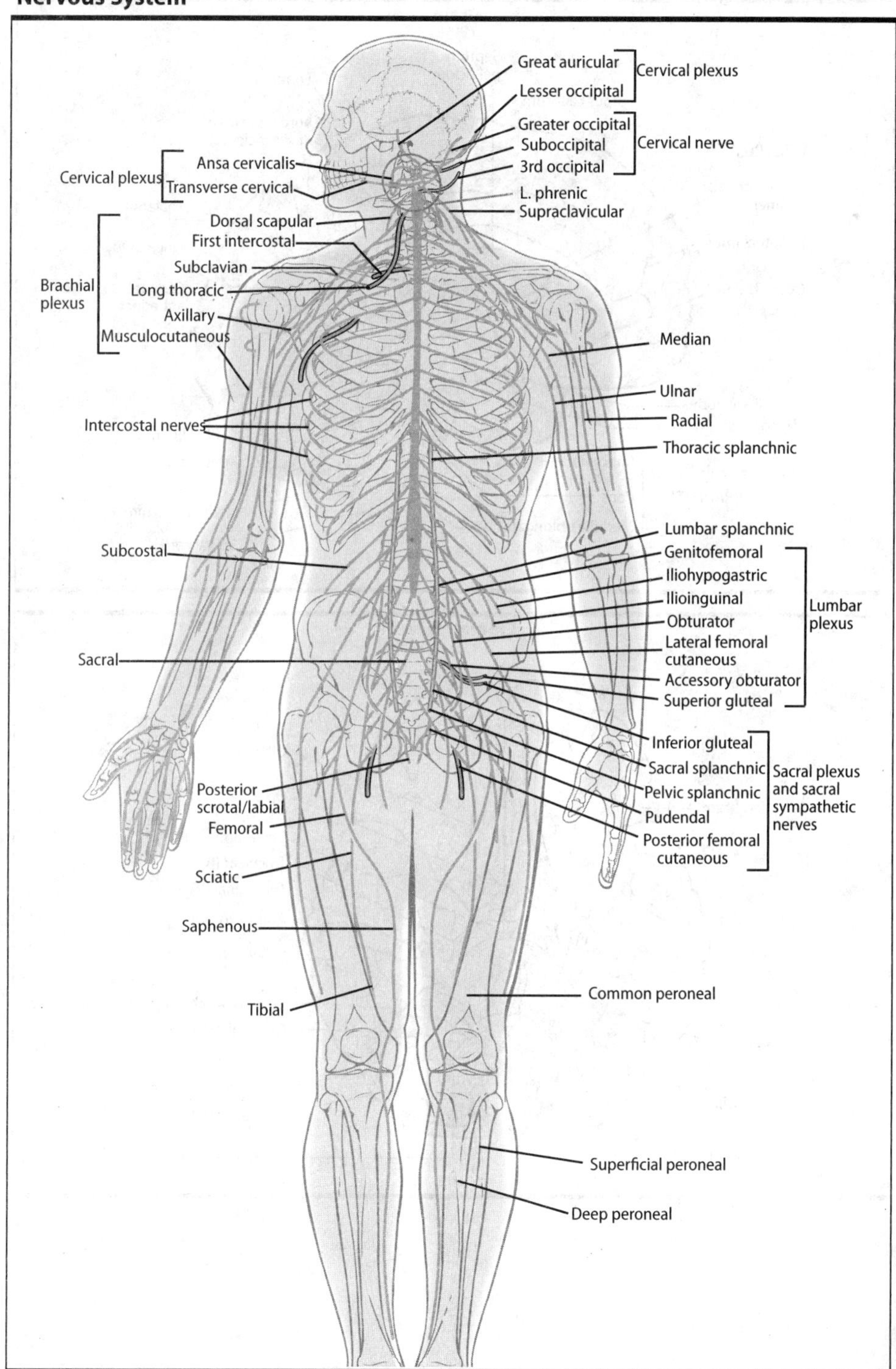

Brain

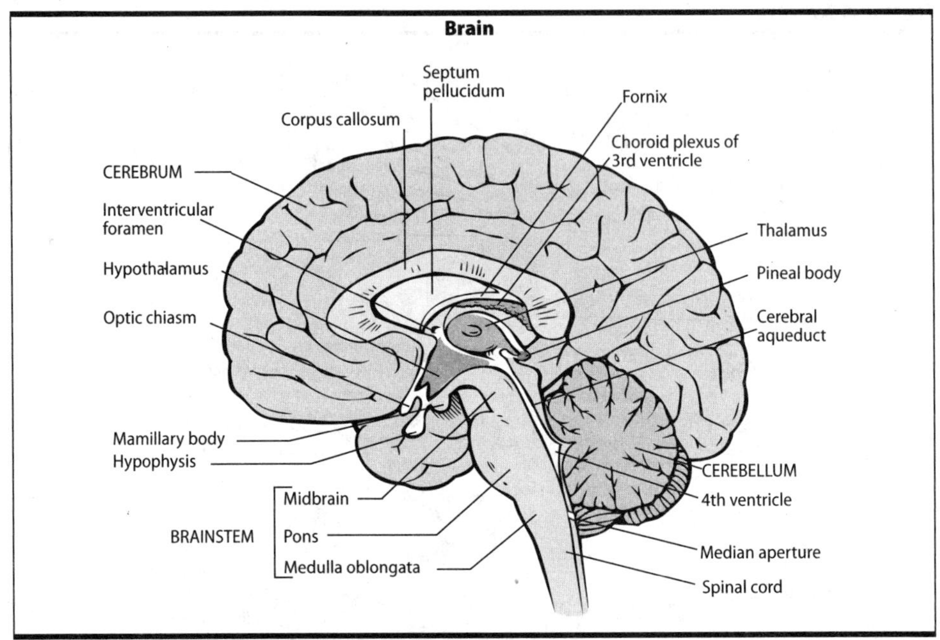

Cranial Nerves

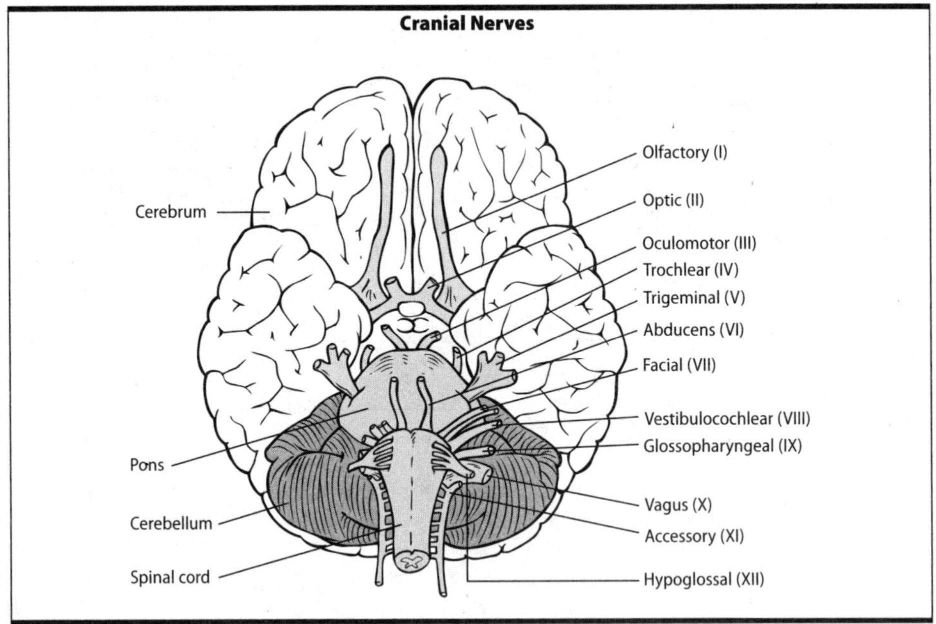

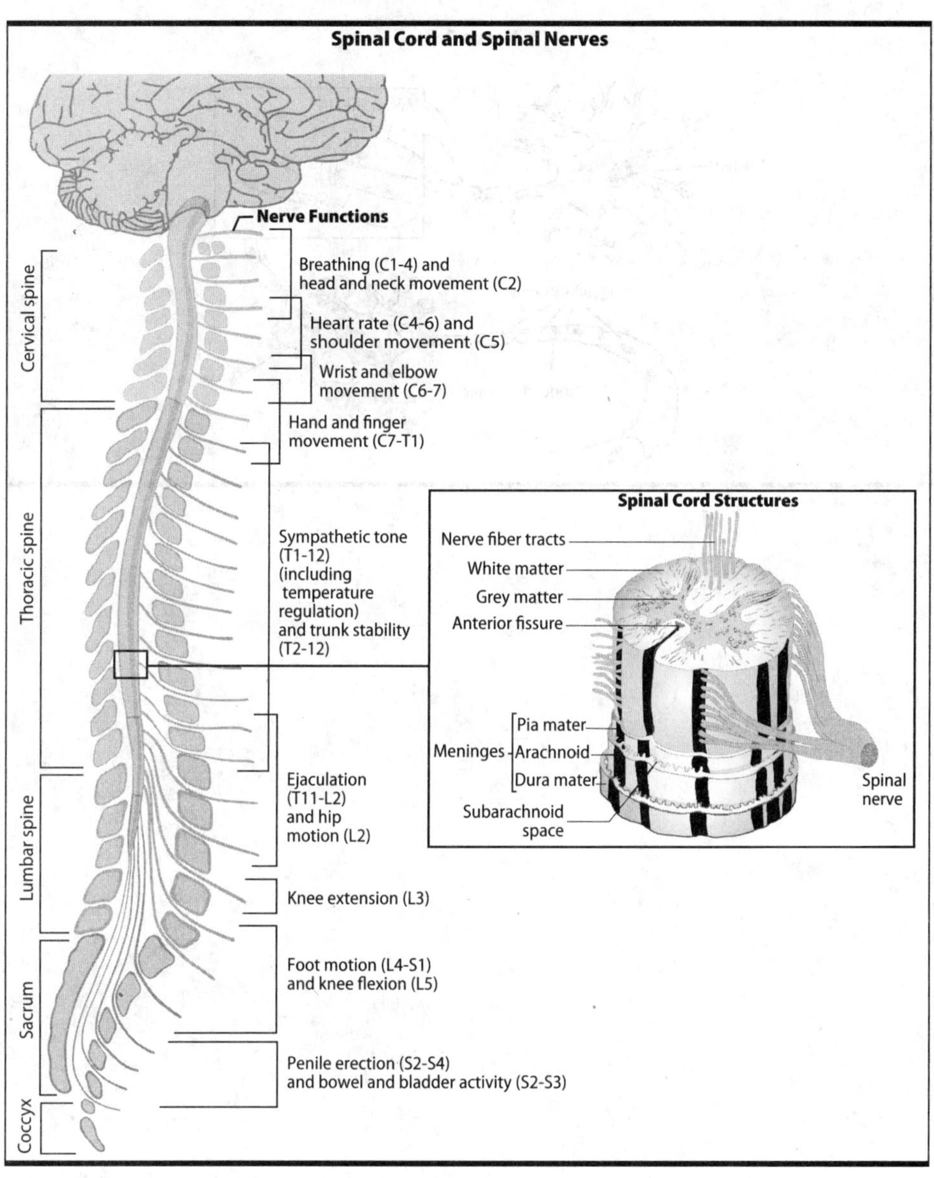
Spinal Cord and Spinal Nerves
Nerve Functions
Breathing (C1-4) and head and neck movement (C2)
Heart rate (C4-6) and shoulder movement (C5)
Wrist and elbow movement (C6-7)
Hand and finger movement (C7-T1)
Sympathetic tone (T1-12) (including temperature regulation) and trunk stability (T2-12)
Ejaculation (T11-L2) and hip motion (L2)
Knee extension (L3)
Foot motion (L4-S1) and knee flexion (L5)
Penile erection (S2-S4) and bowel and bladder activity (S2-S3)
Cervical spine
Thoracic spine
Lumbar spine
Sacrum
Coccyx
Spinal Cord Structures
Nerve fiber tracts
White matter
Grey matter
Anterior fissure
Meninges
Pia mater
Arachnoid
Dura mater
Subarachnoid space
Spinal nerve

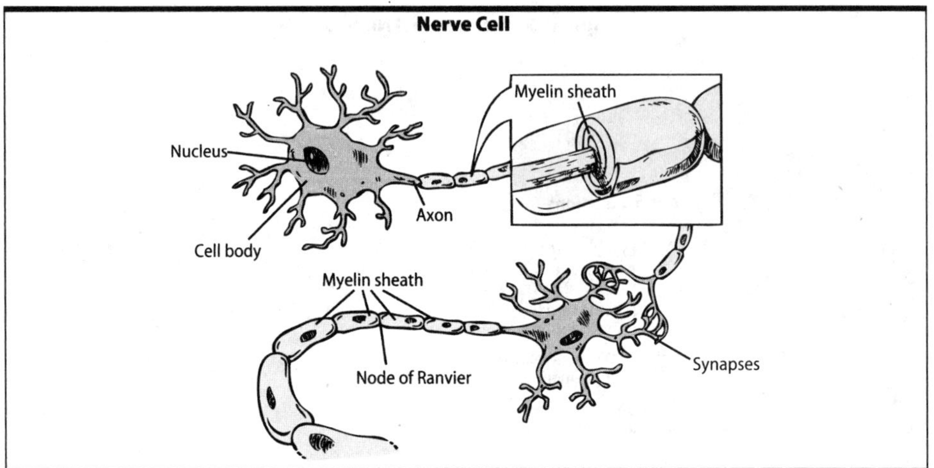
Nerve Cell
Myelin sheath
Nucleus
Axon
Cell body
Myelin sheath
Node of Ranvier
Synapses

Eye

Eye Structure

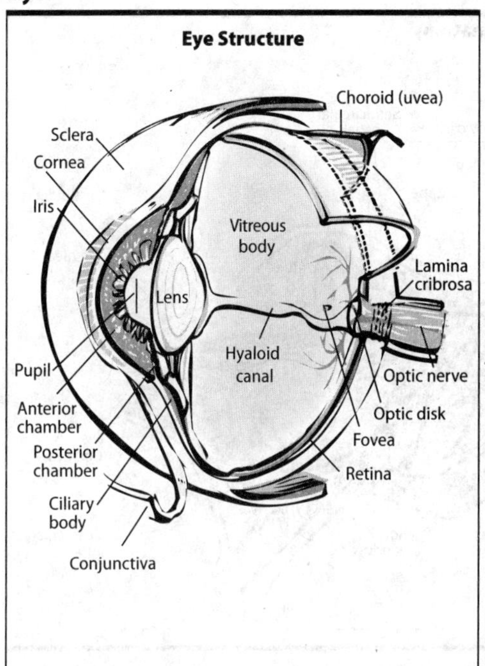

Posterior Pole of Globe/Flow of Aqueous Humor

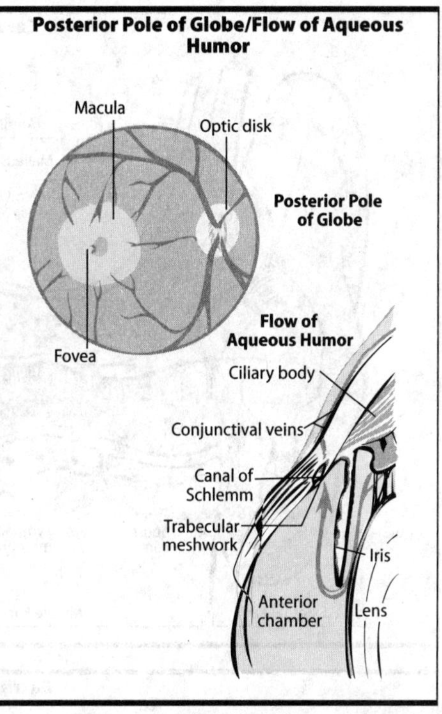

Eye Musculature

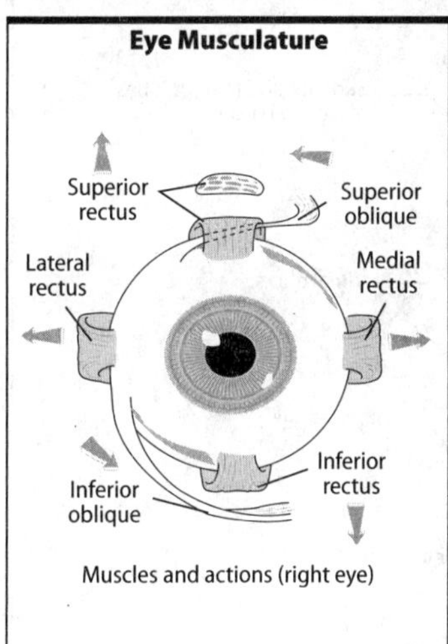

Muscles and actions (right eye)

Eyelid Structures

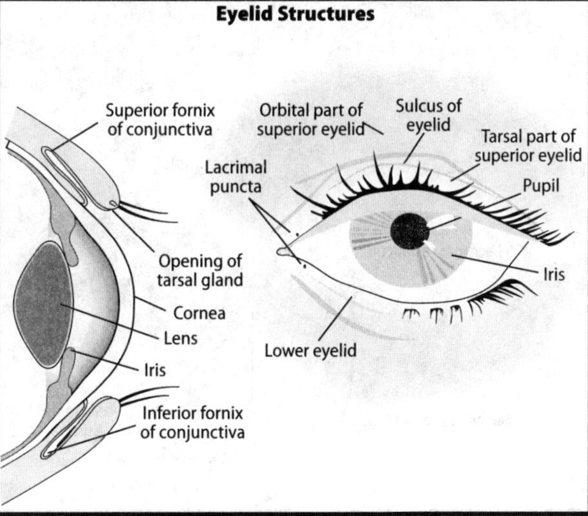

Ear and Lacrimal System

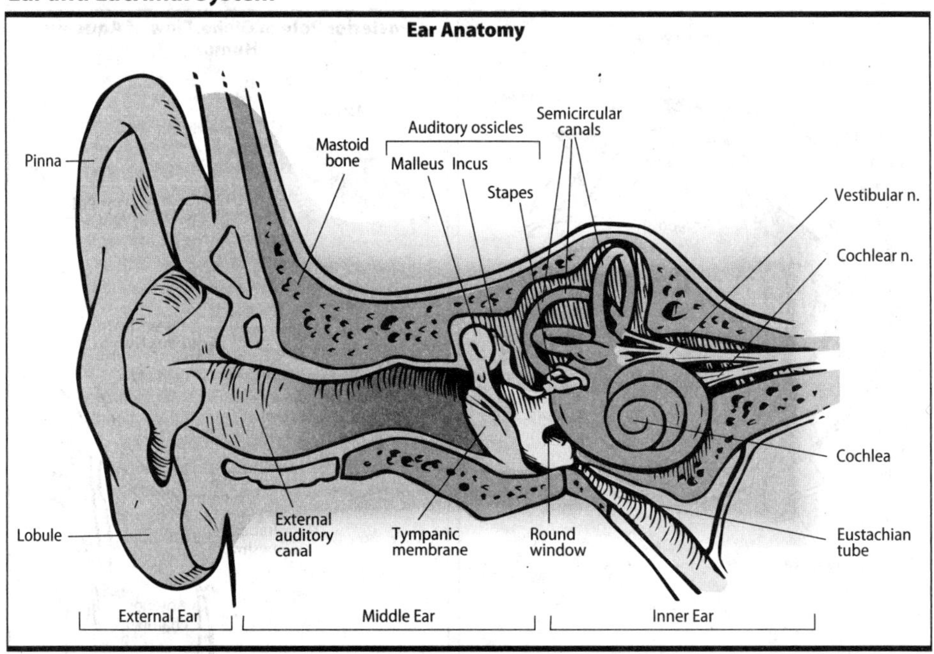

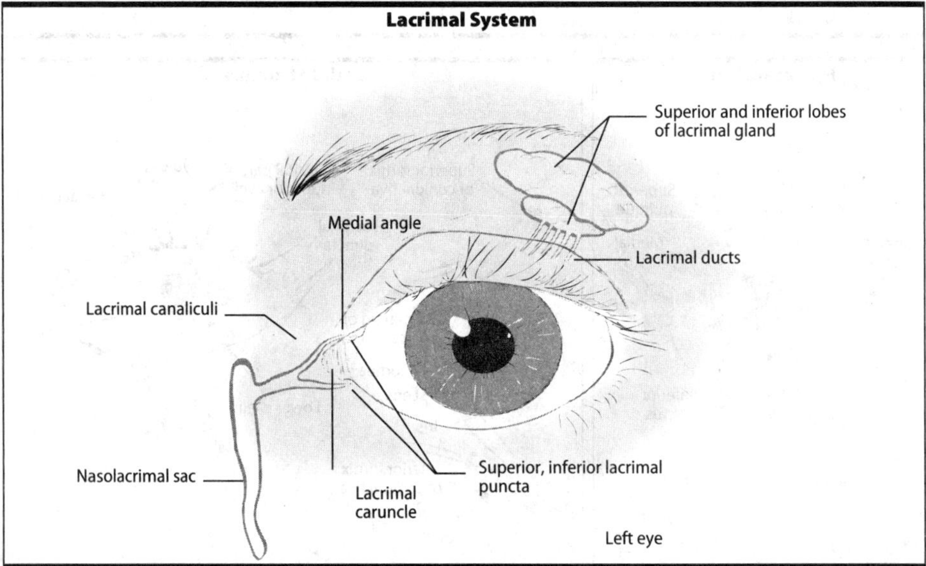

CPT® Lay Descriptions

CPT® descriptions are written for people with medical training but may not offer the details needed to choose a code based on a patient's chart or an operative report. The following overview of the procedures listed in CPT describes the most common methods of each in general terms. Where possible, descriptions are in lay terms for coders' use. Key words used in the operative report are included to facilitate coding.

Unlisted procedures are excluded from this chapter. Be aware insurance payers usually review unlisted procedure codes manually, increasing processing time and the need for documentation.

Because some consecutive codes describe similar procedures, their descriptions have been combined under one heading, which indicates the range of codes described. If a satisfactory code description cannot be matched with the patient's chart, consult the physician.

Integumentary

10021 [10004, 10005, 10006, 10007, 10008, 10009, 10010, 10011, 10012]

Fine needle aspiration (FNA) is a diagnostic percutaneous procedure that uses a fine gauge needle (often 22 or 25 gauge) and a syringe to sample fluid from a cyst or remove clusters of cells from a solid mass. The skin is cleansed. If a lump can be felt, the radiologist or surgeon guides a needle into the area by palpating the lump. If the lump is non-palpable, the FNA procedure is performed using ultrasound, fluoroscopy, computed tomography (CT), or MR imaging with the patient positioned according to the area of concern. Ultrasonography-guided aspiration biopsy involves inserting an aspiration catheter needle device through the accessory channel port of the echoendoscope; the needle is placed into the area to be sampled under endoscopic ultrasonographic guidance. After the needle is placed into the region of the lesion, a vacuum is created and multiple in and out needle motions are performed. Several needle insertions are usually required to ensure that an adequate tissue sample is taken. In fluoroscopic guidance, intermittent fluoroscopy guides the advancement of the needle. CT image guidance allows computer-assisted targeting of the area to be sampled. At the completion of the procedure, the needle is withdrawn and a small bandage is placed over the area. MR image guidance involves the use of a magnetic field, radiowaves, and computer-assisted targeting to identify the area for biopsy without the use of ionizing radiation. Report 10021 for fine needle aspiration of the initial lesion performed without imaging guidance; for each subsequent lesion, report 10004. Report 10005 for FNA of the first lesion using ultrasound guidance; for each additional lesion, report 10006. Report 10007 for FNA of the first lesion using fluoroscopy; for each additional lesion, report 10008. Report 10009 for FNA of the first lesion utilizing CT imaging; for each subsequent lesion, report 10010. Report 10011 when MR imaging is used for the initial lesion; for each additional lesion, report 10012.

10030

A fluid collection in the soft tissue, such as a hematoma, seroma, abscess, lymphocele, or cyst, is drained using a catheter. The area over the abnormal tissue is cleansed and local anesthesia is administered. Imaging is performed to assist in the insertion of a needle or guidewire into the fluid collection. Small tissue samples may be collected from the site for pathological examination. A catheter is inserted to drain and collect the fluid for analysis. More imaging may be performed to ensure hemostasis. In some cases, the catheter may be attached to a drainage system to allow for further drainage over the course of days. Once the fluid has completely drained, the catheter is removed. A bandage is applied. Report 10030 for each fluid collection drained using a separate catheter.

10035-10036

The physician places a soft tissue localization device prior to a biopsy. Using image guidance, the physician places a metallic clip, pellet, wire, needle, or radioactive seed adjacent to a soft tissue lesion to mark the site for an open soft tissue procedure or a percutaneous soft tissue biopsy to be performed during the same or a different encounter. Report 10035 for the first lesion and 10036 for each additional lesion, whether on the same or the contralateral side, marked using imaging guidance.

10040

The physician makes a small incision through the skin overlying a lesion, or multiple lesions, such as comedones (blackheads), cysts, or pustules for acne surgery. The skin over the lesion is removed. The lesion is opened with a surgical instrument and the fluid is drained for secondary healing. The lesion may be removed or marsupialized by exteriorizing the cyst and making a pouch where it used to be enclosed. No sutures are needed. Do not report a benign lesion excision code (11400-11446) and chemical exfoliation for acne (17360) on same date of service with 10040.

10060-10061

The physician makes a small incision through the skin overlying an abscess for incision and drainage (e.g., carbuncle, cyst, furuncle, paronychia, hidradenitis). The abscess or cyst is opened with a surgical instrument, allowing the contents to drain. The lesion may be curetted and irrigated. The physician leaves the surgical wound open to allow for continued drainage or the physician may place a Penrose latex drain or gauze strip packing to allow continued drainage. Report 10060 for incision and drainage of a simple or single abscess. Report 10061 for complex or multiple cysts. Complex or multiple cysts may require surgical closure at a later date.

10080-10081
The physician incises and drains a pilonidal cyst. A pilonidal cyst is an abnormal pocket in the skin and subcutaneous tissue that may contain hair follicles, skin debris, fluid, and exudate. The cyst is usually located in the sacrococcygeal region near the tailbone and cleft of the buttocks. An incision overlying the pocket is made to allow drainage of the contents. The wound may be left open and packed until the cyst heals. Report 10081 if the procedure is more complicated and requires marsupialization, approximation of the wound's edges, and/or primary closure.

10120-10121
The physician removes a foreign body embedded in subcutaneous tissue. The physician makes a simple incision in the skin overlying the foreign body. The foreign body is retrieved using hemostats or forceps. The skin may be sutured or allowed to heal secondarily. Report 10121 if the procedure is more complicated, requiring dissection of underlying tissues.

10140
The physician makes an incision in the skin to decompress and drain a hematoma, seroma, or other collection of fluid. A hemostat bluntly penetrates the fluid pockets, allowing the fluid to evacuate. A latex drain or gauze packing may be placed into the incision site. This will allow the escape of any fluids that may continue to enter the pocket. A pressure dressing may be placed over the region. Any drain or packing is removed within 48 hours. The incision can be closed primarily or may be left to granulate without closure.

10160
The physician performs a puncture aspiration of an abscess, hematoma, bulla, or cyst. The palpable collection of fluid is located subcutaneously. The physician cleanses the overlying skin and introduces a large bore needle on a syringe into the fluid space. The fluid is aspirated into the syringe, decompressing the fluid space. A pressure dressing may be placed over the site.

10180
This procedure treats an infected postoperative wound. A more complex than usual incision and drainage procedure is necessary to remove the fluid and allow the surgical wound to heal. The physician first removes the surgical sutures or staples and/or makes additional incisions into the skin. The wound is drained of infected fluid. Any necrotic tissue is removed from the surgical site and the wound is irrigated. The wound may be sutured closed or packed open with gauze to allow additional drainage. If closed, the surgical site may have suction or latex drains placed into the wound. If packed open, the wound may be sutured again during a later procedure.

11000-11001
The physician surgically removes extensive diseased or infected skin. The skin may be of an eczematous nature possessing erythema, vesicles, and scales. Bacteria or fungus may be causing the skin infection. Wet compresses are used initially to remove scaly skin. Abrasive techniques may be employed to remove remaining scales. A scalpel may be used to decompress vesicles and excise dead skin. After debridement, topical lubricants and antibiotic preparations are placed on the skin. Report 11000 for up to 10 percent of the body surface. Report 11001 once for each additional 10 percent of the body surface, or part thereof, in addition to the primary procedure.

11004-11006
Debridement is carried out for a severe type of tissue infection that causes gangrenous changes, systemic disease, and tissue death. These types of infections are caused by virulent strains of bacteria, such as "flesh-eating" *Streptococcus*, and affect the skin, subcutaneous fat, fascia, and muscle tissue. Surgery is performed immediately upon diagnosis to open and drain the infected area and excise the dead or necrotic tissue. Report 11004 for surgical debridement of necrotic soft tissue of the external genitalia and perineum; 11005 for the abdominal wall, with or without repair of the abdominal fascia; and 11006 for both areas, with or without repair of the abdominal fascia.

11008
The physician removes prosthetic material or mesh previously placed in the abdominal wall. This may be done due to the presence of a chronic infection, a necrotizing soft tissue infection, or a recurrent mesh infection. Surgery is performed immediately after diagnosis and usually under general anesthesia. The skin is incised and the tissue dissected exposing the prosthetic material. Debridement of the tissue adjacent to or incorporated in the mesh may be performed with instruments or irrigation. Unincorporated or infected areas of the mesh are excised and removed with any remaining areas of infection or necrotic tissue. Incorporated mesh that is not infected may be left in the wound. The area is irrigated and the wound is sutured. Note that 11008 is reported in addition to the code for the primary procedure of complex incision and drainage of a postoperative wound infection or debridement of a necrotizing soft tissue infection.

11010-11012
The physician surgically removes foreign matter and contaminated or devitalized skin and other tissue in and around the site of an open fracture or open dislocation. Debridement reported with this service includes prolonged cleansing of the wound; removal of all foreign or dead tissue or material using forceps,

scissors, scalpel, or other instruments; exploration of all injured soft tissue, including tendons, ligaments, and nerves; and irrigation of all tissue layers. Contamination of a wound by foreign matter is typically associated with open fractures; this excisional debridement is done in preparation for treating the fracture, to reduce swelling and bleeding, and to leave behind viable tissue. Report 11010 for debridement of skin and subcutaneous tissue; 11011 for debridement of skin, subcutaneous tissue, muscle fascia, and muscle; and 11012 for debridement of skin, subcutaneous tissue, muscle fascia, muscle, and bone.

11042 [11045]

The physician surgically removes foreign matter and contaminated or devitalized subcutaneous tissue (including epidermis and dermis, if performed) caused by injury, infection, wounds (excluding burn wounds), or chronic ulcers. Using the appropriate surgical instrument, the physician excises the affected subcutaneous tissue until viable, bleeding tissue is encountered. A topical antibiotic is placed on the wound. A gauze dressing or an occlusive dressing may be placed over the surgical site. Report 11042 for the first 20 sq cm or less and 11045 for each additional 20 sq cm or part thereof.

11043 [11046]

The physician surgically removes necrotic muscle and/or fascia, including epidermis, dermis, and subcutaneous tissue, if performed. The physician uses the appropriate surgical instrument (i.e., scalpel) to excise the affected tissue into the muscle layer. The dissection is continued until viable, bleeding tissue is encountered. Depending on wound size, closure may be immediate or delayed. The wound may be packed open with gauze and require immediate or delayed reconstruction. Report 11043 for the first 20 sq cm or less and 11046 for each additional 20 sq cm or part thereof.

11044, 11047

The physician surgically removes foreign matter and contaminated or devitalized bone (including epidermis, dermis, subcutaneous tissue, muscle, and/or fascia, if performed) caused by injury, infection, wounds (excluding burn wounds), or chronic ulcers. The physician uses the appropriate surgical instrument (i.e., scalpel) to excise the affected tissues into the bone. Depending on wound size, closure may be immediate or delayed. The wound may be packed open with gauze and require immediate or delayed reconstruction. Report 11044 for the first 20 sq cm or less and 11047 for each additional 20 sq cm or part thereof.

11055-11057

The physician removes a benign hyperkeratotic skin lesion such as a corn or callus by cutting, clipping, or paring. Report 11055 when one lesion is removed; 11056 when two to four lesions are removed; and 11057 when more than four lesions are removed.

11102-11107

The physician removes a biopsy sample of skin or subcutaneous tissue for the purpose of performing a diagnostic histopathologic study under a microscope. Skin biopsies are reported based on one of three techniques used: tangential, punch, or incisional. Tangential technique describes a biopsy performed via a sharp blade to obtain a superficial, epidermal tissue specimen that may or may not include sections of underlying dermis and does not involve a full-thickness biopsy. Punch technique involves the use of a specific punch tool to obtain a full-thickness, barrel-shaped, or columnar-shaped specimen. Simple closure, including any manipulation of the biopsy defect, is included in the performance of a punch biopsy. The incisional biopsy technique describes a biopsy utilizing a sharp blade (no punch tool) to obtain a full-thickness specimen via a wedge or vertical incision. This technique type may involve specimens of subcutaneous fat. Closure of an incisional biopsy, other than simple closure, is reported separately. Report 11102 for a tangential biopsy, initial lesion; each additional lesion, report 11103. Report 11104 for a punch biopsy, initial lesion; each additional lesion, report 11105. Report 11106 for an incisional biopsy, initial lesion; each additional lesion, report 11107.

11200-11201

The physician removes skin tag lesions. Skin tags are common benign tumors found on many body regions, most frequently around the axillae, inguinal area, head, and neck. The physician uses sharp excision with scissors or scalpel, chemical cautery, electrical cautery, ligature strangulation, or any combination of these methods. Report 11200 for up to 15 lesions and 11201 for each additional 10 lesions, or part thereof, beyond the initial 15.

11300-11303

The physician removes a single, elevated epidermal or dermal lesion from the trunk, arm, or legs by shave excision. Local anesthesia is injected beneath the lesion. A scalpel blade is placed against the skin adjacent to the lesion and the physician uses a horizontal slicing motion to excise the lesion from its base. The wound does not require suturing and bleeding is controlled by chemical or electrical cauterization. Report 11300 for a lesion diameter 0.5 cm or less; 11301 for 0.6 cm to 1 cm; 11302 for 1.1 cm to 2 cm; and 11303 for lesions greater than 2 cm.

11305-11308

The physician removes a single, elevated epidermal or dermal lesion from the scalp, neck, hands, feet, or genitalia by shave excision. Local anesthesia is injected beneath the lesion. A scalpel blade is placed against the skin adjacent to the lesion and the physician uses a horizontal slicing motion to excise the lesion from its base. The wound does not require suturing and bleeding is controlled by chemical or electrical cauterization. Report 11305 for a lesion diameter 0.5 cm or less; 11306 for 0.6 cm to 1 cm; 11307 for 1.1 cm to 2 cm; and 11308 for lesions greater than 2 cm.

11310-11313
The physician removes a single, elevated epidermal or dermal lesion from the face, ears, eyelids, lips, nose, or mucous membrane by shave excision. Local anesthesia is injected beneath the lesion. A scalpel blade is placed against the skin adjacent to the lesion and the physician uses a horizontal slicing motion to excise the lesion from its base. The wound does not require suturing and bleeding is controlled by chemical or electrical cauterization. Report 11310 for a lesion diameter 0.5 cm or less; 11311 for 0.6 cm to 1 cm; 11312 for 1.1 cm to 2 cm; and 11313 for lesions greater than 2 cm.

11400-11406
The physician removes a benign skin lesion located on the trunk, arms, or legs. After administering a local anesthetic, the physician makes a full thickness incision through the dermis with a scalpel, usually in an elliptical shape around and under the lesion. The lesion and a margin of normal tissue are removed. The wound is repaired using a single layer of sutures, chemical or electrocauterization. Complex or layered closure is reported separately, if required. Each lesion removed is reported separately. Report 11400 for an excised diameter 0.5 cm or less; 11401 for 0.6 cm to 1 cm; 11402 for 1.1 cm to 2 cm; 11403 for 2.1 cm to 3 cm; 11404 for 3.1 cm to 4 cm; and 11406 if the excised diameter is greater than 4 cm.

11420-11426
The physician removes a benign skin lesion located on the scalp, neck, hands, feet, or genitalia. After administering a local anesthetic, the physician makes a full thickness incision through the dermis with a scalpel, usually in an elliptical shape around and under the lesion. The lesion and a margin of normal tissue are removed. The wound is repaired using a single layer of sutures, chemical or electrocauterization. Complex or layered closure is reported separately, if required. Each lesion removed is reported separately. Report 11420 for an excised diameter 0.5 cm or less; 11421 for 0.6 cm to 1 cm; 11422 for 1.1 cm to 2 cm; 11423 for 2.1 cm to 3 cm; 11424 for 3.1 cm to 4 cm; and 11426 if the excised diameter is greater than 4 cm.

11440-11446
The physician removes a benign skin lesion located on the face, ears, eyelids, nose, lips, or mucous membranes. After administering a local anesthetic, the physician makes a full thickness incision through the dermis with a scalpel, usually in an elliptical shape around and under the lesion. The lesion and a margin of normal tissue are removed. The wound is repaired using a single layer of sutures, chemical or electrocauterization. Complex or layered closure is reported separately, if required. Each lesion removed is reported separately. Report 11440 for an excised diameter 0.5 cm or less; 11441 for 0.6 cm to 1 cm; 11442 for 1.1 cm to 2 cm; 11443 for 2.1 cm to 3 cm; 11444 for 3.1 cm to 4 cm; and 11446 if the excised diameter is greater than 4 cm.

11450-11451
Hidradenitis is a chronic, relapsing disease that occurs in tissue where apocrine glands are found. Localized nodules develop from occlusion of the apocrine ducts. Recurrence of the lesions may produce superimposed infections, recurrent abscesses with or without sinus formation, and scarring. The physician performs an excision of the affected skin and subcutaneous tissue of the axilla including margins. Intraoperative mapping of any existing sinus tracts may be performed to ensure complete removal. In 11450, the wound is left open to heal by granulation or is repaired using single or multiple layers of sutures. Report 11451 if more than layered closure (complex repair) is required.

11462-11463
Hidradenitis is a chronic, relapsing disease that occurs in tissue where apocrine glands are found. Localized nodules develop from occlusion of the apocrine ducts. Recurrence of the lesions may produce superimposed infections, recurrent abscesses with or without sinus formation, and scarring. The physician performs a wide excision of the affected skin and subcutaneous tissue of the groin (inguinal) region including margins. Intraoperative mapping of any existing sinus tracts may be performed to ensure complete removal. In 11462, the wound is left open to heal by granulation or is repaired using single or multiple layers of sutures. Report 11463 if more than layered closure (complex repair) is required.

11470-11471
Hidradenitis is a chronic, relapsing disease that occurs in tissue where apocrine glands are found. Localized nodules develop from occlusion of the apocrine ducts. Recurrence of the lesions may produce superimposed infections, recurrent abscesses with or without sinus formation, and scarring. The physician performs a wide excision of the affected skin and subcutaneous tissue of the perianal, perineal, or umbilical region including margins. Intraoperative mapping of any existing sinus tracts may be performed to ensure complete removal. In 11470, the wound is left open to heal by granulation or is repaired using single or multiple layers of sutures. Report 11471 if more than layered closure (complex repair) is required.

11600-11606
The physician removes a malignant lesion located on the trunk, arms, or legs. After administering a local anesthetic, the physician makes a full-thickness incision through the dermis, usually in an elliptical shape around and under the lesion. The lesion and a margin of normal tissue are removed. The wound is repaired using a single layer of sutures, chemical or electrocauterization. Complex, layered, or reconstructive (excluding adjacent tissue transfer) wound repair is reported separately, if required. Each lesion removed is reported separately. Report 11600 for an excised diameter 0.5 cm or less; 11601 for 0.6 cm to 1 cm; 11602 for 1.1 cm to 2 cm; 11603 for 2.1 cm to 3 cm; 11604 for 3.1 cm to 4 cm; and 11606 if the excised diameter is greater than 4 cm.

11620-11626

The physician removes a malignant lesion located on the scalp, neck, hands, feet, or genitalia. After administering a local anesthetic, the physician makes a full-thickness incision through the dermis, usually in an elliptical shape around and under the lesion. The lesion and a margin of normal tissue are removed. The wound is repaired using a single layer of sutures, chemical or electrocauterization. Complex, layered, or reconstructive (excluding adjacent tissue transfer) wound repair is reported separately, if required. Each lesion removed is reported separately. Report 11620 for an excised diameter 0.5 cm or less; 11621 for 0.6 cm to 1 cm; 11622 for 1.1 cm to 2 cm; 11623 for 2.1 cm to 3 cm; 11624 for 3.1 cm to 4 cm; and 11626 if the excised diameter is greater than 4 cm.

11640-11646

The physician removes a malignant lesion located on the face, ears, eyelids, nose, or lips. After administering a local anesthetic, the physician makes a full-thickness incision through the dermis, usually in an elliptical shape around and under the lesion. The lesion and a margin of normal tissue are removed. The wound is repaired using a single layer of sutures, chemical or electrocauterization. Complex, layered, or reconstructive (excluding adjacent tissue transfer) wound repair is reported separately, if required. Each lesion removed is reported separately. Report 11640 for an excised diameter 0.5 cm or less; 11641 for 0.6 cm to 1 cm; 11642 for 1.1 cm to 2 cm; 11643 for 2.1 cm to 3 cm; 11644 for 3.1 cm to 4 cm; and 11646 if the excised diameter is greater than 4 cm.

11719

A physician trims a fingernail or toenail, usually with scissors, nail cutters, or other instruments. This code is reported when the nails are not defective from nutritional or metabolic abnormalities. It is reported for one or more nails.

11720-11721

The physician debrides fingernails or toenails, including tops and exposed undersides, by any method. The cleaning is performed manually with cleaning solutions, abrasive materials, and tools. The nails are shortened and shaped. Report 11720 for one to five nails and 11721 for six or more.

11730-11732

The physician avulses a nail plate partially or completely. A digital nerve block is used to numb the top of the digit. The physician bluntly dissects the nail plate from the nail bed. Any bleeding is cauterized. The digit is bandaged. Report 11730 if only one nail plate is removed. Report 11732 for each additional nail plate removed.

11740

Blood from a hematoma located beneath a fingernail or toenail is drained. The nail plate is pierced using an electrocautery tool or large gauged needle creating a large enough opening to allow the hematoma to drain. Pressure may be applied to the nail bed to force the blood from beneath the nail plate. Gauze, a bandage, or a splint may be applied to allow for continued drainage.

11750

The physician removes all or part of a fingernail or toenail, including the nail plate and matrix permanently. The nail plate is bluntly dissected and lifted away from the nail bed. The nail plate is detached from the matrix using a scalpel. The matrix is destroyed using chemical ablation, CO2 laser, or electrocautery. The wound is dressed loosely.

11755

The physician removes a portion of the nail unit for a biopsy sample. Sections may be taken from the hard nail itself, the nail bed, lateral skin, or underlying soft tissue. The specimen is excised by clippers or with a scalpel.

11760

The physician repairs a damaged nail bed. The physician removes the damaged and surrounding nail from the nail bed. The nail bed is sutured into correct position. Bleeding is controlled through electrocautery and the wound is dressed.

11762

A damaged nail bed inhibits nail adherence and promotes nail deformities. The physician cleans the nail bed and prepares it for grafting. Using a scalpel, a nail bed graft is obtained from the nail bed of an adjacent phalange or from the great toe's nail bed and sutured into place covering the defect. Hemostasis is achieved and a dressing is applied.

11765

The physician excises a wedge of restrictive skin in the nail fold to free an ingrown nail. The physician performs a wedge excision of the skin overlapping the lateral nail. The nail is examined and trimmed to encourage straight growth. The wound is dressed.

11770-11772

A pilonidal cyst or sinus is entrapped epithelial tissue located in the sacrococcygeal region above the buttocks. These lesions are usually associated with ingrown hair. A sinus cavity is present and may have a fluid-producing cystic lining. With a small or simple sinus in 11770, the physician uses a scalpel to completely excise the involved tissue. The wound is sutured in a single layer. In 11771, an extensive sinus is present superficial to the fascia overlying the sacrum but with subcutaneous extensions. The physician uses a scalpel to completely excise the cystic tissue. The wound may be sutured in several layers. In 11772, the sinus involves many subcutaneous extensions superficial to the fascia overlying the sacrum. The physician uses a scalpel to completely excise the cystic tissue. Local soft tissue flaps (i.e., Z-plasty, Y-V plasty, myofasciocutaneous flap) may be required for closure of a large defect or the wound may be left open to heal by granulation.

11900-11901
The physician uses a syringe to inject a pharmacologic agent underneath or into any diagnosed skin lesion. Steroids, anesthetics (excluding preoperative local anesthesia), or any non-chemotherapy pharmacological agent may be injected. Report 11900 for injection of seven or fewer lesions. Report 11901 when more than seven lesions are treated.

11920-11922
The physician introduces insoluble opaque pigment into color defects of the skin. A marking pen is used first to outline the area to be tattooed. The dye is injected into the skin with a pneumatic tattooing instrument to create an artificially pigmented area that approximates the appearance of normal skin tissue. Report 11920 for a tattoo area of 6 sq cm or less, 11921 for 6.1 sq cm to 20 sq cm, and 11922 for each additional 20 sq cm or part thereof.

11950-11954
The physician uses an injectable dermal implant to correct small soft tissue deformities. This technique is used to treat facial wrinkles, post-surgical defects, and acne scars. The injectable filling material can be autologous fat, synthetic surgical compound, or a commercially produced collagen preparation. The physician uses a syringe to inject the selected material into the subcutaneous tissue. The injection will augment the dermal layer and alleviate the soft tissue depression. Report 11950 for an injection of 1 cc or less; 11951 for 1.1 cc to 5 cc; 11952 for 5.1 cc to 10 cc; and 11954 for an injection of more than 10 cc.

11960
The physician uses a tissue expander to stretch skin and soft tissue prior to definitive reconstruction of tissue other than breast. These expanders are balloon-type devices that stretch the skin and enhance epithelial and collagen expansion and reduce or eliminate the need for skin grafts during reconstruction. The physician makes an incision into the skin. The subcutaneous layer is identified. Blunt dissection is used to separate the skin and subcutaneous layers. The tissue expander is placed into the prepared site. The wound is sutured. The expander is inflated. During the postoperative visits, greater volume is placed into the expander stretching the skin. The expander remains in place until the final reconstruction is performed.

11970
The physician removes a subcutaneous tissue expander and places a permanent implant for final reconstruction. The tissue expander is deflated. The physician uses a scalpel to make an incision. Blunt dissection is used to remove the tissue expander. The permanent implant is placed into the recipient bed. The implant may be an autologous graft or a commercially prepared synthetic material. The graft implant may require stabilization with sutures, wires, or screws. The incision is closed with sutures.

11971
The physician removes a subcutaneous tissue expander without placing an implant or performing final reconstruction. Initially, the tissue expander is deflated. The physician uses a scalpel to make an incision. Blunt dissection is used to remove the tissue expander. A surgical drain may be placed in the wound. The incision is closed with sutures.

11976
The physician makes a small incision in the skin on the inside of the upper arm of a female patient and removes contraceptive capsules previously implanted subdermally. The incision is closed.

11980
Biodegradable time-release medication pellets are implanted subcutaneously for the slow delivery of hormones. The physician makes a small incision in the skin with a scalpel. A trocar and cannula are inserted into the incised area. Hormone pellets are inserted through the cannula and the cannula is withdrawn. Pressure is applied to the incised area until any bleeding is stopped, and the incision is closed with Steri-strips. The time-release medication is typically used for women who require hormone replacement therapy during menopause. One method is to implant pellets of testosterone and/or estradiol (taken in conjunction with progesterone) into the fatty tissue of the buttocks. New pellets may be inserted whenever symptoms recur, usually in six to nine months.

11981-11983
A drug delivery implant, which may be nonbiodegradable or biodegradable/bioresorbable, is inserted to deliver a therapeutic dose of a drug continuously at a predetermined rate of release. One such system works via a semipermeable membrane at one end of the subcutaneous cylinder that permits the entrance of fluid; the drug is delivered from a port at the other end of the cylinder at a controlled rate appropriate to the specific therapeutic agent. The physician injects local anesthesia and makes a small incision in the skin with a scalpel to insert the miniature drug-containing cylinder, which is held in place with sutures tied by a knot or secured by a single running stitch. Various types of medications for different indications may be administered via drug delivery implants. In 11982, the physician removes a previously placed nonbiodegradable drug delivery implant, such as a miniature drug-containing titanium cylinder, through a small incision. In 11983, the physician removes the previously placed nonbiodegradable implant through a small incision and reinserts a new one. The wounds are sutured closed.

12001-12007
The physician performs wound closure of superficial lacerations of the scalp, neck, axillae, external genitalia, trunk, or extremities using sutures, staples, tissue adhesives, or a combination of these materials. A local anesthetic is injected around the wound and it is cleansed, explored, and often irrigated with a saline

solution. The physician performs a simple, one-layer repair of the epidermis, dermis, or subcutaneous tissues. For multiple wounds of the same complexity and in the same anatomical area, the length of all wounds sutured is summed and reported as one total length. Report 12001 for a total length of 2.5 cm or less; 12002 for 2.6 cm to 7.5 cm; 12004 for 7.6 cm to 12.5 cm; 12005 for 12.6 cm to 20 cm; 12006 for 20.1 cm to 30 cm; and 12007 if the total length is greater than 30 cm.

12011-12018

Superficial wounds located on the face, ears, eyelids, nose, lips, and/or mucous membranes are repaired. A local anesthetic is injected around the laceration and the wound is cleansed, explored, and often irrigated with a saline solution. The physician performs a simple, one-layer repair of the epidermis, dermis, or subcutaneous tissue with sutures. With multiple wounds of the same complexity and in the same anatomical area, the length of all wounds sutured is summed and reported as one total length. Report 12011 for a total length of 2.5 cm or less; 12013 for 2.6 cm to 5 cm; 12014 for 5.1 cm to 7.5 cm; 12015 for 7.6 cm to 12.5 cm; 12016 for 12.6 cm to 20 cm; 12017 for 20.1 cm to 30 cm; and 12018 if the total length is greater than 30 cm.

12020-12021

There has been a breakdown of the healing skin either before or after suture removal. The skin margins have opened. The physician cleanses the wound with irrigation and antimicrobial solutions. The skin margins may be trimmed to initiate bleeding surfaces. Report 12020 if the wound is sutured in a single layer. Report 12021 if the wound is left open and packed with gauze strips due to the presence of infection. This allows infection to drain from the wound and the skin closure will be delayed until the infection is resolved.

12031-12037

The physician performs a repair of a wound of the scalp, axillae, trunk, and/or extremities (except hands and feet) using sutures, staples, tissue adhesives, or a combination of these materials to perform a layered closure. Due to deeper or more complex lacerations, deep subcutaneous or layered repair techniques are required. A local anesthetic is injected around the laceration, and the wound is cleansed, explored, and often irrigated with a saline solution. Extensive cleaning or removal of foreign matter from a heavily contaminated wound that is closed with a single layer may also be reported as an intermediate repair. For multiple wounds of the same complexity and in the same anatomical area, the length of all wounds repaired is summed and reported as one total length. Report 12031 for a total length of 2.5 cm or less; 12032 for 2.6 cm to 7.5 cm; 12034 for 7.6 cm to 12.5 cm; 12035 for 12.6 cm to 20 cm; 12036 for 20.1 cm to 30 cm; and 12037 if the total length is greater than 30 cm.

12041-12047

The physician performs a repair of a wound located on the neck, hands, feet, and/or external genitalia. A local anesthetic is injected around the laceration, and the wound is cleansed, explored, and often irrigated with a saline solution. Due to deeper or more complex lacerations, deep subcutaneous or layered suturing techniques are required. The physician closes tissue layers under the skin with dissolvable sutures before suturing the skin. Extensive cleaning or removal of foreign matter from a heavily contaminated wound that is closed with a single layer may also be reported as an intermediate repair. With multiple wounds of the same complexity and in the same anatomical area, the length of all wounds sutured is summed and reported as one total length. Report 12041 for a total length of 2.5 cm or less; 12042 for 2.6 cm to 7.5 cm; 12044 for 7.6 cm to 12.5 cm; 12045 for 12.6 cm to 20 cm; 12046 for 20.1 cm to 30 cm; and 12047 if the total length is greater than 30 cm.

12051-12057

The physician performs a repair of a wound located on the face, ears, eyelids, nose, lips, and/or mucous membranes. A local anesthetic is injected around the laceration, and the wound is cleansed, explored, and often irrigated with a saline solution. Due to deeper or more complex lacerations, deep layered suturing techniques are required. The physician closes tissue layers under the skin with dissolvable sutures before suturing the skin. Extensive cleaning or removal of foreign matter from a heavily contaminated wound that is closed with a single layer may also be reported as an intermediate repair. With multiple wounds of the same complexity and in the same anatomical area, the length of all wounds sutured is summed and reported as one total length. Report 12051 for a total length of 2.5 cm or less; 12052 for 2.6 cm to 5 cm; 12053 for 5.1 cm to 7.5 cm; 12054 for 7.6 cm to 12.5 cm; 12055 for 12.6 cm to 20 cm; 12056 for 20.1 cm to 30 cm; and 12057 if the total length is greater than 30 cm.

13100-13102

The physician repairs complex wounds of the trunk. The physician performs complex, layered suturing of torn, crushed, or deeply lacerated tissue. The physician debrides the wound by removing foreign material or damaged tissue. Irrigation of the wound is performed and antimicrobial solutions are used to decontaminate and cleanse the wound. The physician may trim skin margins with a scalpel or scissors to allow for proper closure. The wound is closed in layers. The physician may perform scar revision, which creates a complex defect requiring repair. Stents or retention sutures may also be used in complex repair of a wound. Reconstructive procedures, such as utilization of local flaps, may be required and are reported separately. Report 13100 for wounds 1.1 cm to 2.5 cm; 13101 for 2.6 cm to 7.5 cm; and 13102 for each additional 5 cm or less.

13120-13122

The physician repairs wounds located on the scalp, arms, and/or legs. The physician performs complex, layered suturing of torn, crushed, or deeply lacerated tissue. The physician debrides the wound by removing foreign material or damaged tissue. Irrigation of the wound is performed and antimicrobial solutions are used to decontaminate and cleanse the wound. The physician may trim skin margins with a scalpel or scissors to allow for proper closure. The wound is closed in layers. The physician may perform scar revision, which creates a complex defect requiring repair. Stents or retention sutures may also be used in a complex repair of a wound. Reconstructive procedures, such as utilization of local flaps, may be required and are reported separately. Report 13120 for wounds 1.1 cm to 2.5 cm; 13121 for 2.6 cm to 7.5 cm; and 13122 for each additional 5 cm or less.

13131-13133

The physician repairs wounds located on the forehead, cheeks, chin, mouth, neck, axillae, genitalia, hands, and/or feet. The physician performs complex, layered suturing of torn, crushed, or deeply lacerated tissue. The physician debrides the wound by removing foreign material or damaged tissue. Irrigation of the wound is performed and antimicrobial solutions are used to decontaminate and cleanse the wound. The physician may trim skin margins with a scalpel or scissors to allow for proper closure. The wound is closed in layers. The physician may perform scar revision, which creates a complex defect requiring repair. Stents or retention sutures may also be used in complex repair of a wound. Reconstructive procedures, such as utilization of local flaps, may be required and are reported separately. Report 13131 for wounds 1.1 cm to 2.5 cm; 13132 for 2.6 cm to 7.5 cm; and 13133 for each additional 5 cm or less.

13151-13153

The physician repairs complex wounds of the eyelids, nose, ears, and/or lips. The physician performs complex, layered suturing of torn, crushed, or deeply lacerated tissue. The physician debrides the wound by removing foreign material or damaged tissue. Wound irrigation is performed with an antimicrobial solution to decontaminate and cleanse the wound. The physician may trim skin margins to allow for proper closure. The wound is closed in layers. The physician may perform scar revision, which creates a complex defect requiring repair. Stents or retention sutures may also be used in complex repair. Reconstructive procedures, such as local flaps, may be required and are reported separately. Report 13151 for wounds 1.1 cm to 2.5 cm; 13152 for 2.6 cm to 7.5 cm; and 13153 for each additional 5 cm or less. A code for simple or intermediate repair is reported for wounds that are 1 cm or less.

13160

The physician secondarily repairs a surgical skin closure after an infectious breakdown of the healing skin. After resolution of the infection, the wound is now ready for closure. The physician uses a scalpel to excise granulation and scar tissue. Skin margins are trimmed to bleeding edges. The wound is sutured in several layers.

14000-14001

The physician transfers or rearranges adjacent tissue to repair traumatic or surgical wounds of the trunk. This includes, but is not limited to, such rearrangement procedures as Z-plasty, W-plasty, ZY-plasty, or tissue transfers such as rotational or advancement flaps. Report 14000 for defects that are 10 sq cm or less and 14001 for defects that are 10.1 sq cm to 30 sq cm.

14020-14021

The physician transfers or rearranges adjacent tissue to repair traumatic or surgical wounds of the scalp, arms, and/or legs. This includes, but is not limited to, such rearrangement procedures as Z-plasty, W-plasty, ZY-plasty, or tissue transfers such as rotational or advancement flaps. Report 14020 for defects that are 10 sq cm or less and 14021 for defects that are 10.1 sq cm to 30 sq cm.

14040-14041

The physician transfers or rearranges adjacent tissue to repair traumatic or surgical wounds on the forehead, cheeks, chin, mouth, neck, axillae, genitalia, hands, and/or feet. This includes, but is not limited to, such rearrangement procedures as Z-plasty, W-plasty, ZY-plasty, or tissue transfers such as rotational flaps or advancement flaps. Report 14040 for defects that are 10 sq cm or less and 14041 for defects that are 10.1 sq cm to 30 sq cm.

14060-14061

The physician transfers or rearranges adjacent tissue to repair traumatic or surgical wounds of the eyelids, nose, ears, and/or lips. This includes, but is not limited to, such rearrangement procedures as Z-plasty, W-plasty, ZY-plasty, or tissue transfers such as rotational flaps or advancement flaps. Report 14060 for defects that are 10 sq cm or less and 14061 for defects that are 10.1 sq cm to 30 sq cm.

14301-14302

The physician transfers or rearranges adjacent tissue of any area to repair traumatic or surgical wounds. This includes, but is not limited to, such rearrangement procedures as Z-plasty, W-plasty, ZY-plasty, or tissue transfers such as rotational flaps or advancement flaps. Report 14301 for defects 30.1 sq cm to 60 sq cm. Report 14302 for each additional 30 sq cm or part thereof.

14350

The physician creates a filleted finger or toe flap to repair a large defect on the hand or foot. The physician makes a bilateral longitudinal incision and dissects the tissue away from the donor site. Bone and necrotic tissue are removed while blood vessels and nerves are preserved. The recipient site is prepared and the flap is rotated into place. Excess tissue is excised and the wound is sutured in layers.

15002-15003

The physician prepares tissue to receive a free skin graft needed to close or repair a defect. Skin, subcutaneous tissue, scars, burn eschar, and lesions are excised to provide a healthy, vascular tissue bed (where new vessels have been formed) onto which a skin graft will be placed. Alternatively, the physician may prepare tissue by incising or excising a scar contracture that is causing excessive tightening of the skin. Simple debridement of granulations or of recent avulsion is included. Report 15002 for the first 100 sq cm or 1 percent of body area of infants and children for grafts of the trunk arms and legs. Report 15003 for each additional 100 sq cm (or part thereof) of graft area or each additional 1 percent of surface body area in infants and children within the same areas.

15004-15005

The physician prepares tissue to receive a free skin graft needed to close or repair a defect. Skin, subcutaneous tissue, scars, burn eschar, and lesions are excised to provide a healthy, vascular tissue bed (where new vessels have been formed) onto which a skin graft will be placed. Alternatively, the physician may prepare tissue by incising or excising a scar contracture that is causing excessive tightening of the skin. Simple debridement of granulations or of recent avulsion is included. Report 15004 for the first 100 sq cm or 1 percent of body area in infants and children of the face, scalp, eyelids, mouth, neck, ears, orbits, genitalia, hands, and/or feet. Report 15005 for each additional 100 sq cm (or part thereof) or each additional 1 percent of body area in infants and children.

15011-15012

The physician harvests skin for a skin cell suspension autograft (SCSA) for another area of the body needing repair. Autologous skin cell suspension is a technique that uses isolated skin cells for the treatment of thermal burn and full-thickness skin wounds. A dermatome is used to obtain a thin, split-thickness sample of epidermal and dermal skin, typically at a depth of 0.006-0.008 inches, which can be processed to create a skin cell suspension for application to the recipient site wound. One sq cm of harvested skin can treat a wound up to 80 sq cm. Multiple skin samples may be obtained depending on the volume of skin cells required to fully cover the wound. The skin may be segmented into smaller parts for processing. Report 15011 for the first 25 sq cm or less of harvested skin and 15012 for each additional 25 sq cm or part thereof. Preparation and application of the autograft are reported separately.

15013-15014

The physician or other qualified health care professional prepares a skin cell suspension autograft (SCSA). Autologous skin cell suspension is a technique that uses isolated skin cells for the treatment of thermal burn and full-thickness skin wounds. Harvested skin is incubated in an enzyme solution that breaks down skin cell adhesions and the extracellular matrix. The skin is rinsed with a buffer solution and cells are separated by scraping the dermal and epidermal layers. The remaining cells include keratinocytes, fibroblasts, and melanocytes, which can aid in healing of wounds and repigmentation. The skin cells and buffer solution are drawn into a syringe for application. Report 15013 for the first 25 sq cm or less of harvested skin and 15014 for each additional 25 sq cm or part thereof. Harvesting of the skin and application of the autograft are reported separately.

15015-15016

The physician applies a skin cell suspension autograft (SCSA) to recipient and donor wound sites. Autologous skin cell suspension is a technique that uses isolated skin cells for the treatment of thermal burn and full-thickness skin wounds. Skin is harvested and a skin cell suspension is prepared and drawn into a syringe prior to application. The suspension is sprayed evenly across the wound and donor sites to promote epidermal regeneration on the trunk, arms, or legs. A dressing is applied over each wound and secured in place with glue, sutures, or staples. Report 15015 for the first 480 sq cm or less and 15016 for each additional 480 sq or part thereof. Harvesting of the skin and preparation of the skin cell suspension are reported separately.

15017-15018

The physician applies a skin cell suspension autograft (SCSA) to recipient and donor wound sites. Autologous skin cell suspension is a technique that uses isolated skin cells for the treatment of thermal burn and full-thickness skin wounds. Skin is harvested and a skin cell suspension is prepared and drawn into a syringe prior to application. The suspension is sprayed evenly across the wound and donor sites to promote epidermal regeneration on the face, scalp, eyelids, mouth, neck, ears, orbits, genitalia, hands, feet, and/or multiple digits. A dressing is applied over each wound and secured in place with glue, sutures, or staples. Report 15017 for the first 480 sq cm or less and 15018 for each additional 480 sq or part thereof. Harvesting of the skin and preparation of the skin cell suspension are reported separately.

15040

The physician harvests skin (keratinocytes and dermal tissue), 100 sq cm or less, to use for a tissue cultured skin autograft. The donor site is first injected with epinephrine solution to control blood loss and aid the skin harvesting technique. Skin is harvested by taking a split-thickness graft with a dermatome, up to 100 sq cm, and the donor site is dressed. This code reports only the skin harvesting to be used for tissue-cultured autograft. Later, skin cells will be isolated from the outer layer (epidermis) and inner layer (dermis) and placed in a nutrient solution that stimulates exponential division of the harvested skin cells. Using this tissue culture technique, even a smaller biopsy of skin will provide large populations of skin cells that are stored in liquid nitrogen until needed for grafting. The cells are combined with a fabric made from collagen and the outer surface is exposed to the air to stimulate development of an epidermal barrier. Once the epidermal barrier has developed, the cultured skin autograft may be used for grafting.

Integumentary

15050
The physician obtains one or more pinch grafts to cover a 2 cm or less open area, such as an ulcer of the toe or fingertip. The physician incises the skin to obtain a split thickness skin graft. The donor site is closed. The recipient site is cleaned and prepared. The graft is sewn into place.

15100-15101
The physician takes a split-thickness skin autograft from one area of the body and grafts it to an area needing repair. This procedure is performed when direct wound closure or adjacent tissue transfer is not possible. The physician harvests a split-thickness skin graft with a dermatome. The epidermis or top layer of skin is taken, along with a small portion of the dermis or bottom layer of the skin. This graft is applied to the recipient area on the trunk, arms, or legs. Report 15100 for the first 100 sq cm or less in adults or 1 percent of the total body area of infants and children. Report 15101 for each additional 100 sq cm or each additional 1 percent of the total body area in infants and children.

15110-15111
The physician takes an epidermal autograft from one area of the body and grafts it to an area needing repair. This procedure is performed when direct wound closure or adjacent tissue transfer is not possible. The physician harvests an epidermal skin graft with a dermatome. The epidermal autograft should be as thin as possible: 0.05 mm (0.002 inches) to 0.13 mm (0.005 inches). Only the epidermis or top layer of skin is taken. The dermis or bottom layer of the skin is left behind and will regenerate new skin. The epidermal autograft is sutured or stapled to the recipient area on the trunk, arms, or legs. Report 15110 for the first 100 sq cm or less in adults or children age 10 or older or 1 percent of the total body surface area of infants and children younger than age 10. Report 15111 for each additional 100 sq cm or part thereof in adults or each additional 1 percent of the total body area or part thereof in infants and children.

15115-15116
The physician takes an epidermal autograft from one area of the body and grafts it to an area needing repair. This procedure is performed when direct wound closure or adjacent tissue transfer is not possible. The physician harvests an epidermal skin graft with a dermatome. The epidermal autograft should be as thin as possible: 0.05 mm (0.002 inches) to 0.13 mm (0.005 inches). Only the epidermis or top layer of skin is taken. The dermis or bottom layer of the skin is left behind and will regenerate new skin. The epidermal autograft is sutured or stapled onto the recipient area on the face, scalp, eyelids, neck, ears, orbits, mouth, genitalia, hands, feet, and/or multiple digits. Report 15115 for the first 100 sq cm or less in adults or children age 10 or older or 1 percent of the total body surface area in infants and children younger than age 10. Report 15116 for each additional 100 sq cm or part thereof in adults or each additional 1 percent of the total body area or part thereof in infants and children.

15120-15121
The physician takes a split-thickness skin autograft from one area of the body and grafts it to an area needing repair. This procedure is performed when direct wound closure or adjacent tissue transfer is not possible. The physician harvests a split-thickness skin graft with a dermatome. The epidermis or top layer of skin is taken, along with a small portion of the dermis or bottom layer of the skin. This graft is sutured or stapled onto the recipient area of the face, scalp, eyelids, neck, ears, orbits, mouth, genitalia, hands, feet, and/or multiple digits. Report 15120 for the first 100 sq cm or less in adults or children age 10 or over or 1 percent of the total body area of infants and children younger than age 10. Report 15121 for each additional 100 sq cm and each additional 1 percent of total body area of infants and children.

15130-15131
The physician takes a dermal autograft from one area of the body and grafts it to an area needing repair. This procedure is performed when direct wound closure or adjacent tissue transfer is not possible. A dermal skin graft is harvested by first raising a split-thickness skin graft 0.010 to 0.015 inches in depth with a dermatome, but not removing it. The dermatome is adjusted to remove the desired graft and a second pass is made over the newly created donor site at that depth to remove a dermal layer autograft. The dermal autograft is sutured or stapled onto the recipient area on the trunk, arms, or legs. Report 15130 for the first 100 sq cm or less in adults or children age 10 or older or 1 percent of the total body surface area in infants and children younger than age 10. Report 15131 for each additional 100 sq cm or part thereof in adults or each additional 1 percent of the total body area or part thereof in infants and children.

15135-15136
The physician takes a dermal autograft from one area of the body and grafts it to an area needing repair. This procedure is performed when direct wound closure or adjacent tissue transfer is not possible. A dermal skin graft is harvested by first raising a split-thickness skin graft 0.010 to 0.015 inches in depth with a dermatome, but not removing it. The dermatome is adjusted to remove the desired graft and a second pass is made over the newly created donor site at that depth to remove a dermal layer autograft. The dermal autograft is sutured or stapled onto the recipient area on the face, scalp, eyelids, neck, ears, orbits, mouth, genitalia, hands, feet, and/or multiple digits. Report 15135 for the first 100 sq cm or less in adults or children age 10 or older or 1 percent of the total body surface area in infants and children younger than age 10. Report 15136 for each additional 100 sq cm or part thereof in adults or each additional 1 percent of the total body area or part thereof in infants and children.

15150-15152
The physician takes a previously prepared, tissue-cultured skin autograft from the transport medium and grafts it to an area needing repair on the

trunk, arms, or legs. The autograft is applied and secured to the recipient bed with sutures, staples, or fibrin sealant, and a dressing is applied to the site. The tissue-cultured autograft was previously prepared, in a separate procedure, by harvesting skin (epidermal keratinocytes and autologous fibroblasts) from the patient and placing the cells in a nutrient solution to stimulate exponential division of the harvested skin cells. The cells are combined with a fabric made from collagen, and once the tissues have reached the acceptable size, the cultured skin autograft is used for grafting. The cultured skin cells are stored in liquid nitrogen until needed for grafting. These codes report the grafting procedure. Report 15150 for the first 25 sq cm or less of graft area on the trunk, arms, or legs. Report 15151 for an additional 1 sq cm to 75 sq cm of graft area. Report 15152 for each additional 100 sq cm of graft area in adults and children age 10 or older or each additional 1 percent of total body surface area or part thereof in infants and children younger than age 10.

15155-15157

The physician takes a previously prepared, tissue-cultured skin autograft from the transport medium and grafts it to an area needing repair on the face, scalp, eyelids, mouth, neck, ears, orbits, genitalia, hands, feet, and/or multiple digits. The autograft is applied and secured to the recipient bed with sutures, staples, or fibrin sealant, and a dressing is applied to the site. The tissue-cultured autograft was previously prepared, in a separate procedure, by harvesting skin (epidermal keratinocytes and autologous fibroblasts) from the patient and placing the cells in a nutrient solution to stimulate exponential division of the harvested skin cells. The cells are combined with a fabric made from collagen, and once the tissues have reached the acceptable size, the cultured skin autograft is used for grafting. The cultured skin cells are stored in liquid nitrogen until needed for grafting. These codes report the grafting procedure. Report 15155 for the first 25 sq cm or less of graft area. Report 15156 for an additional 1 sq cm to 75 sq cm of graft area. Report 15157 for each additional 100 sq cm of graft area in adults and children age 10 or older or each additional 1 percent of total body surface area or part thereof in infants and children younger than age 10.

15200-15201

The physician harvests a full-thickness skin graft from one area of the body and grafts it to an area on the trunk needing repair. A full-thickness skin graft consists of the superficial and deeper layers of skin (epidermis and dermis). The resulting surgical wound at the donor site is closed by lifting the remaining skin edges and placing sutures to close directly. Residual adipose tissue is removed from the underside of the graft. The graft is sutured onto the wound bed to cover a defect of no more than 20 sq cm. Report 15201 for each additional 20 sq cm or part thereof.

15220-15221

The physician harvests a full-thickness skin graft from one area of the body and grafts it to an area on the scalp, arms, and/or legs needing repair. A full-thickness skin graft consists of the superficial and deeper layers of skin (epidermis and dermis). The resulting surgical wound at the donor site is closed by lifting the remaining skin edges and placing sutures to close directly. Residual adipose tissue is removed from the underside of the graft. The graft is sutured onto the wound bed to cover a defect of no more than 20 sq cm. Report 15221 for each additional 20 sq cm or part thereof.

15240-15241

The physician harvests a full-thickness skin graft from one area of the body and grafts it to an area on the forehead, cheeks, chin, mouth, neck, axillae, genitalia, hands, and/or feet needing repair. A full-thickness skin graft consists of the superficial and deeper layers of skin (epidermis and dermis). The resulting surgical wound at the donor site is closed by lifting the remaining skin edges and placing sutures to close directly. Residual adipose tissue is removed from the underside of the graft. The graft is sutured onto the wound bed to cover a defect of no more than 20 sq cm. Report 15241 for each additional 20 sq cm or part thereof.

15260-15261

The physician harvests a full-thickness skin graft from one area of the body and grafts it to an area on the nose, ears, eyelids, and/or lips needing repair. A full-thickness skin graft consists of both the superficial and deeper layers of skin (epidermis and dermis). The resulting surgical wound at the donor site is closed by lifting the remaining skin edges and placing sutures to close directly. Residual adipose tissue is removed from the underside of the graft. The graft is sutured onto the wound bed to cover a defect of the nose, ears, eyelids, and/or lips of no more than 20 sq cm. Report 15261 for each additional 20 sq cm or part thereof.

15271-15272

The physician applies a skin substitute for temporary wound closure to a wound on the trunk, arms, or legs. Skin substitutes are used as a temporary measure to close wounds and provide a barrier against infection and fluid loss, reduce pain, and promote healing of underlying tissues until a permanent graft can be applied. Common skin substitutes include acellular dermal replacement, temporary allograft, acellular dermal allograft, tissue cultured allogenic skin substitute, and xenografts. The skin substitute is fashioned to fit the size and contours of the previously prepared wound bed on the trunk, arms, or legs. It is then placed over the wound and sutured or stapled into place. These codes are reported for a total wound surface area of less than 100 sq cm. Report 15271 for the first 25 sq cm or less. Report 15272 for each additional 25 sq cm or less.

15273-15274

The physician applies a skin substitute for temporary wound closure to a wound on the trunk, arms, or legs. Skin substitutes are used as a temporary measure to close wounds and provide a barrier against infection and fluid loss, reduce pain, and promote healing of underlying tissues until a permanent graft can be applied. Common skin substitutes include acellular dermal replacement, temporary allograft, acellular dermal allograft, tissue cultured allogenic skin substitute, and xenografts. The skin substitute is fashioned to fit the size and contours of the previously prepared wound bed on the trunk, arms, or legs. It is then placed over the wound and sutured or stapled into place. These codes are reported for a total wound surface area 100 sq cm or larger in adults or children age 10 or older or 1 percent of the total body surface area in infants and children younger than age 10. Report 15273 for the first 100 sq cm in adults or 1 percent of the total body surface area in infants and children. Report 15274 for each additional 100 sq cm in adults or 1 percent of the total body surface area in infants and children.

15275-15276

The physician applies a skin substitute for temporary wound closure to a wound on the face, scalp, eyelids, mouth, neck, ears, orbits, genitalia, hands, feet, and/or multiple digits. Skin substitutes are used as a temporary measure to close wounds and provide a barrier against infection and fluid loss, reduce pain, and promote healing of underlying tissues until a permanent graft can be applied. Common skin substitutes include acellular dermal replacement, temporary allograft, acellular dermal allograft, tissue cultured allogenic skin substitute, and xenografts. The skin substitute is fashioned to fit the size and contours of the previously prepared wound bed. It is then placed over the wound and sutured or stapled into place. These codes are reported for a total wound surface area of less than 100 sq cm. Report 15275 for the first 25 sq cm or less. Report 15276 for each additional 25 sq cm or less.

15277-15278

The physician applies a skin substitute for temporary wound closure to a wound on the face, scalp, eyelids, mouth, neck, ears, orbits, genitalia, hands, feet, and/or multiple digits. Skin substitutes are used as a temporary measure to close wounds and provide a barrier against infection and fluid loss, reduce pain, and promote healing of underlying tissues until a permanent graft can be applied. Common skin substitutes include acellular dermal replacement, temporary allograft, acellular dermal allograft, tissue cultured allogenic skin substitute, and xenografts. The skin substitute is fashioned to fit the size and contours of the previously prepared wound bed. It is then placed over the wound and sutured or stapled into place. These codes are reported for a total wound surface area 100 sq cm or larger in adults or children age 10 or older or 1 percent of the total body surface area in infants and children younger than age 10. Report 15277 for the first 100 sq cm in adults or 1 percent of the total body surface area in infants and children. Report 15278 for each additional 100 sq cm in adults or 1 percent of the total body surface area in infants and children.

15570-15576

The physician forms a direct or tubed pedicle flap to reconstruct traumatic defects. A pedicle flap of full-thickness skin and subcutaneous tissue that retains its supporting blood vessels is developed in the donor area. A tubed pedicle flap maintains two vascular ends and the cut edges of the raised flap are sutured together to form a tube. The flap may be rotated or transferred to the defect area and sutured to the recipient bed in layers. The physician closes the harvest region in layers or covers it with a split-thickness skin graft. Repairs to the donor area using skin grafts or flaps are reported separately. Other exposed regions, including portions of the pedicle, may also be covered with a split-thickness skin graft. Once the recipient site has healed, a second surgery will detach the pedicle and return the unused flap to its anatomic location. Report 15570 for a pedicle flap on the trunk; 15572 for the scalp, arms, or legs; 15574 for the forehead, cheeks, chin, mouth, neck, axillae, genitalia, hands, or feet; and 15576 if the pedicle flap is applied to the eyelids, nose, ears, lips, or intraoral area.

15600-15630

The physician sections the direct or tubed pedicle flap several weeks following reconstruction of traumatic defects. Blood flow is now established in the recipient area. The unused portion of the flap is detached and prepared for reinsertion into its original anatomic site. Previous skin grafts are removed from the donor beds. The returned flap is sutured in layers to the harvest site. Any exposed subcutaneous tissue is closed primarily or covered with a split-thickness skin graft. Report 15600 if performed at the trunk; 15610 for the scalp, arms, or legs; 15620 for the forehead, cheeks, chin, neck, axillae, genitalia, hands, or feet; and 15630 if performed on the eyelids, nose, ears, or lips.

15650

A previously placed pedicle flap has been in position long enough to receive a good blood supply from the recipient area. As an intermediate step, the physician releases the flap from its donor attachment and moves it completely to a new location. This same tissue may be moved further along the body in a similar manner at a later date. This is known as walking the flap or walk up procedure.

15730

The physician creates a midface flap to correct a defect while preserving the vascular pedicle, the zygomaticofacial vessels. The physician determines the best site for creation of the flap, marks the area, and verifies the location of the pertinent arteries via Doppler where appropriate. Facial nerve branches may be identified with a nerve stimulator and marked. The physician cuts and undermines the skin and subcutaneous tissue, taking care to preserve vascular flow to the flap tissue by ensuring that no kinking or excessive twisting of the pedicle occurs. The dissection continues in the subperiosteal plane. The thickness of the flap is tailored, depending on the thickness of the defect at the recipient site. The flap is carefully evaluated for viability, then rotated or advanced to the defect site, where it is inset and secured with fixation screws or sutures. The donor site is closed in a layered fashion.

15731

The paramedian forehead flap (PFF) is a two-stage procedure that employs a forehead-based pedicle flap most often utilizing the supratrochlear artery. It is commonly used in nasal tip reconstructive surgery and is typically chosen when the nasal defect cannot be adequately treated with adjacent tissue transfer, free skin graft, or primary closure. A template of the defect is made, and the necessary pedicle length is determined. Doppler ultrasound may be used to mark the course of the supratrochlear artery. With the patient under appropriate anesthesia, the physician cuts and undermines the skin and subcutaneous tissue of the forehead, taking care to preserve vascular flow to the flap tissue by ensuring that no kinking or excessive twisting of the pedicle occurs. The flap is carefully evaluated for viability and mobilized, thinned distally, and secured in the nasal defect with interrupted sutures. Hemostasis in the exposed pedicle stalk is controlled and the pedicle is loosely wrapped in a nonadherent dressing and secured. The forehead donor site is often closed primarily.

15733-15738

The physician repairs a defect area using a muscle, muscle and skin, or a fasciocutaneous flap. The physician rotates the prepared flap from the donor area to the site needing repair, suturing the flap in place. The donor area is closed primarily with sutures. If a skin graft or flap is used to repair the donor site, it is considered an additional procedure and is reported separately. Report 15733 for a muscle, myocutaneous, or fasciocutaneous flap obtained from the head and neck with named vascular pedicle such as temporalis or sternocleidomastoid; 15734 if obtained from the trunk; 15736 if obtained from an upper extremity; and 15738 if obtained from a lower extremity.

15740-15750

Skin and subcutaneous tissue containing a neurovascular link is trimmed for use as an island pedicle flap. The extra tissue is removed from the pedicle so that the connection to the donor site is little more than an innervated artery and vein. A defect is covered by elevation of a flap of skin and subcutaneous tissue from a nearby but not immediately adjacent donor site. The flap involves an anatomically named blood vessel in its creation. Often this tissue is transferred through a tunnel underneath the skin and sutured into its new position. The donor site is closed directly. Report 15750 if the pedicle is neurovascular, containing nerve and blood vessel elements.

15756

The physician implants a free muscle or myocutaneous flap with microvascular anastomosis. With the patient under general anesthesia, the physician prepares and irrigates the wound. The muscle or myocutaneous flap is removed from the donor site and prepared. The physician inserts the flap and uses half-mattress sutures to secure the section. Using microscopy, the physician joins the vessels, uniting the flap tissue to the site. Before all are joined, the physician may inject fluorescein dye in the vascular system and check the area for fluorescence under an ultraviolet light. Adjustments and corrections to the vascular connections are made and the physician sutures the skin. A light dressing is applied and, in many cases, the flap is splinted to help prevent shrinkage. The donor site is sutured and covered with a light dressing.

15757

The physician implants a free skin flap with microvascular anastomosis. With the patient under general anesthesia, the physician prepares and irrigates the wound. The new skin is removed from the donor site and prepared. The physician inserts the new skin and uses half-mattress sutures to secure the section. Using microscopy, the physician joins the vessels and nerves uniting the new skin to the site. Before all are joined, the physician may inject fluorescein dye in the vascular system and check the area for fluorescence under an ultraviolet light. Adjustments and corrections to the vascular connections are made, and the physician sutures the skin. Light dressing is applied; and, in many cases, the flap is splinted to help prevent shrinkage. The donor site is sutured and covered with a light dressing.

15758

The physician implants a free fascial flap with microvascular anastomosis. With the patient under general anesthesia, the physician prepares and irrigates the wound. The new fascia is removed from the donor site and prepared. The physician inserts the new fascia and uses sutures to secure the section. Using microscopy, the physician joins the vessels and nerves uniting the new fascia to the site. Before all are joined, the physician may inject fluorescein dye in the vascular system and check the area for fluorescence under an ultraviolet light. Adjustments and corrections to the vascular connections are made and the physician sutures the skin. A light dressing is applied and, in many cases, the flap is splinted to help prevent shrinkage. The donor site is sutured and covered with a light dressing.

15760

The physician takes a full-thickness composite graft of more than one tissue type, such as a mixture of cartilage, from the external ear or nasal ala area, with a scalpel. This type of graft is used on defects that need both skin and structural support to ensure survival of the graft with minimal scarring and contraction, and to maintain the continuity of the local flesh. The graft tissue is "assembled" into the recipient bed and primary closure is done on the donor area with layered sutures.

15770

The physician takes a graft composed of derma, fat, and fascia to repair and blend in defects left behind by atrophy, surgical excisions, or other fleshy defects, much like a composite graft. The derma-fat-fascia graft may be a continuous piece of all three of these layers, individual sections done layer by layer, or graft pieces laid in the recipient bed as combinations, such as a fascia-fat layer, followed by a dermal layer. The graft is used on defects much like a composite graft to maintain support for the continuity of the local flesh. The graft is laid in the recipient area so as to fill and blend in pockets of defects to restore the surrounding area to normal positioning and to maintain the continuity of the local flesh.

[15769]

In a facility setting, the physician performs an autologous graft comprised of fat, dermis, fascia, or other soft tissue. With the patient under appropriate anesthesia, the physician incises, dissects, and prepares the recipient bed, taking care to identify adjacent nerves. The necessary graft size is measured and planned. The physician measures and marks the intended donor site, then makes an incision and dissects through the epithelium, dermis, and subcutaneous tissues to the required layer. The graft is removed and placed in saline while the physician undermines and closes the donor site wound, typically using layered closure. The tissue from the donor site is trimmed to fit the recipient defect site, placed, and secured with absorbable sutures during the same operative episode. A drain may be placed through a separate stab incision. The wound is closed in a layered manner.

15771-15774

Autologous fat grafting may be utilized in many areas of soft tissue augmentation or reconstruction, including congenital defects, contouring of face or breasts, and scarring as a result of burns, radiation, surgical procedures, or trauma. The physician obtains an autologous fat graft by liposuction technique. After identifying the most suitable area of fat harvesting (commonly the abdomen, trochanteric region, or the insides of the thighs and/or knees), the physician makes small incisions in the skin overlying the harvest area. A liposuction cannula is inserted through the incision. The physician moves the cannula through the fat deposits, collecting parcels of fat. The fat graft is processed using a variety of techniques, most commonly sedimentation, filtering, washing, and centrifugation. The physician inserts the fat graft at the chosen anatomical region. A small incision is made, a cannula is inserted, and the fat graft is typically distributed in small portions at varying depths into the soft tissues. Donor and recipient incisions are closed. Report 15771 once per session for grafting of 50 cc or less of the fat injectate to the trunk, breasts, scalp, arms, and/or legs, and 15772 for each additional 50 cc. Report 15773 once per session for grafting of 25 cc or less of the fat injectate to the face, eyelids, mouth, neck, ears, orbits, genitalia, hands, and/or feet, and 15774 for each additional 25 cc.

15775-15776

The physician performs a punch graft for hair transplant. The physician uses a punch tool to remove a small segment of scalp containing hair and hair follicles. This is transferred and inset into a non-hair bearing area. Report 15775 for one to 15 punch grafts and 15776 for more than 15 punch grafts.

15777

The physician inserts a biologic implant to correct a soft tissue defect of the trunk or breast caused by trauma or surgery. Biologic implants are usually porcine or allogenic grafts that have been decellularized. When tissue is decellularized, the cells, cell debris, DNA, and RNA are removed in a way that is not damaging to the collagen matrix, reducing the probability of rejection.

15778

The physician implants absorbable mesh or other prosthetic material for delayed closure of defects caused by trauma or soft tissue infection to sites such as the abdominal wall, external genitalia, or perineum. The exact placement of the mesh is determined by the type of defect. Typically, mesh or prosthetic material is placed over the defect and fixated circumferentially around the defect using absorbable sutures. The incision is closed in a standard fashion.

15780-15783

The physician performs dermabrasion of the total face in 15780 for conditions such as acne scarring, fine wrinkling, rhytids, and general keratoses. The physician uses a powered rotary instrument to sand down or smooth scarred or wrinkled areas. The physician lowers raised lesions or thins thickened tissue to regenerate skin with a smoother appearance. Report 15781 for a dermabrasion performed on one segment of the face; 15782 for regional dermabrasion, other than the face; and 15783 for a superficial dermabrasion on any site.

15786-15787

The physician uses abrasive techniques to smooth down or remove an isolated lesion such as a scar or skin thickening secondary to sun damage. Report 15786 for a single lesion and 15787 for each additional four lesions or less.

15788-15793

The physician performs a chemical peel of the epidermal or dermal layers of the skin. The physician uses chemical agents, such as glycolic acid or phenol, to remove fine wrinkles or areas of abnormal pigmentation. The treatment is localized to surface layers of facial skin only in 15788. Report 15789 for a chemical facial peel of the deeper dermal layer; 15792 for an epidermal chemical peel other than facial; and 15793 for a dermal chemical peel other than facial.

15820-15821

The physician performs a blepharoplasty of the lower eyelid. Through an incision beneath the eyelash line, the physician dissects the skin of the lower eyelid to the subcutaneous/muscle fascial layers. The skin is pulled tight and excess skin is excised. Muscle fascia may be sutured to support sagging muscles. In 15821, orbital fat, or an extensive herniated fat pad, is removed from the tissues. The incision is closed with layers.

15822-15823
The physician performs a blepharoplasty of the upper eyelid. Through an incision usually in the crease of the upper eyelid, the physician dissects the skin of the upper eyelid to the subcutaneous/muscle fascial layers. The skin is pulled tight and redundant skin is excised. Muscle fascia may be sutured to support sagging muscles. In 15823, orbital fat may be removed from the tissues as well as excessive redundant skin that mechanically weighs down the eyelid, obstructing the visual field. The incision is closed with layers.

15824, 15826
The physician performs a rhytidectomy of the forehead. The physician excises a portion of skin in order to eliminate wrinkles in the forehead. Most commonly an incision is made in the hairline and a subcutaneous dissection is carried down to the level of the eyebrow. The excess skin is removed and the forehead is elevated and sutured into the new position. Incisions are repaired in layers. Report 15826 if the rhytidectomy is done to reduce glabellar frown lines, the vertical furrows in the forehead area between the eyebrows caused by the corrugator and procerus muscles that may be debulked before incisions in the eyebrows are closed.

15825
The physician performs a rhytidectomy of the neck. The physician makes an incision usually in front of the ear. Tension is increased in the facial muscles by freeing the superficial musculoaponeurotic system (SMAS) (facial muscles are interlinked by the SMAS). The physician trims and tightens the SMAS by securing it with sutures to tissues in front of the ear. An additional incision below the chin is necessary to correct the platysma muscle. The physician makes an incision through the platysma muscle, creating a flap, which is moved up and back. The muscle is tightened, trimmed, and secured with layered sutures. The skin incisions are closed with layered sutures.

15828-15829
The physician makes an incision in a crease or wrinkle of the cheek, chin, or neck to perform a rhytidectomy. Tension is increased by removing excess skin and fat. An additional incision in front of the ear may be necessary. Tension is increased in the facial muscles by freeing the superficial musculoaponeurotic system (SMAS) (facial muscles are interlinked by the SMAS). The physician trims and tightens the SMAS by securing it with sutures to tissues in front of the ear. Report 15829 for a SMAS flap.

15830-15839
The physician removes excessive skin and subcutaneous tissue (including lipectomy). In 15830, the physician makes an incision traversing the abdomen below the belly button in a horizontal fashion. Excessive skin and subcutaneous tissue are elevated off the abdominal wall and excess tissue and fat are excised. The flaps are brought together and sutured in at least three layers. The physician may also suture the rectus abdominis muscles together in the midline to reinforce the area. Report 15832 for removal of excess skin and subcutaneous tissue on the thigh; 15833 for the leg; 15834 for the hip; 15835 for the buttock; 15836 for the arm; 15837 for the forearm or hand; 15838 for the submental fat pad (inferior to the chin); and 15839 for any other area.

15840-15845
The physician harvests a graft for facial nerve paralysis. The physician removes connective tissue (fascia) from a predetermined location of the body (often fascia lata from the leg). This graft is transplanted to the face and sutured into place underneath the skin in order to partially suspend or reanimate previously paralyzed areas of the face. Report 15841 if a free muscle graft is used; 15842 if a free muscle flap by microsurgical technique is used; and 15845 if a regional muscle transfer is performed.

15847
The physician excises excess skin, usually the result of significant weight loss in the patient, while preserving the position of the umbilicus. A wide transverse incision is made in the lower abdomen. The physician dissects fat and skin free from underlying muscle and fascia from the site of the incision to the ribs. The umbilicus is dissected free from the skin but remains attached by a stalk to the abdomen. The physician uses sutures or staples to plicate and tighten the rectus sheath. The dissected skin is stretched back over the abdomen and excess skin and fat are excised. An incision is made in the skin to accommodate the umbilicus, which is sutured in place. The skin is closed in layers and a temporary drain may be placed. Note that 15847 is reported in addition to the code for the primary procedure of infraumbilical panniculectomy.

15851 [15853, 15854]
The physician removes sutures or staples with or without the aid of sedation or general anesthesia. The area around the wound is cleaned with normal saline or is sometimes soaked if crusting prohibits access to sutures or staples. The sutures/staples are removed while the wound lines are observed for separation during the procedure. Hemostasis is obtained and adhesive strips and sterile dressings applied as needed. Report 15851 for removal of sutures or staples under general anesthesia or moderate sedation; removal with local anesthesia is not reported with this code. Report 15853 for removal of sutures or staples and 15854 when both sutures and staples are removed. Codes 15853 and 15854 do not require anesthesia.

15852
The physician changes a dressing on a wound other than a burn while the patient is under sedation or general anesthesia. This is commonly done for severe

crush injuries where serial tissue debridement is required and also for certain types of infection.

15860
The physician injects a dye such as fluorescein or methylene blue to test the viability of blood vessels in a flap or graft. The agent is injected intravenously.

15876
The physician performs a lipectomy of the head and neck. The physician makes small incisions inside the mouth or in the skin of the chin overlying an area of fat deposits. A liposuction cannula is inserted through the incision and the physician moves the cannula through the fat deposits, creating tunnels and removing excess deposits. A separate incision behind the ear may be necessary to remove additional fat deposits. The incisions are closed simply.

15877
The physician performs a lipectomy of the trunk. The physician makes incisions on the trunk overlying an area of fat deposits. A liposuction cannula is inserted through the incision. The physician moves the cannula through the fat deposits, creating tunnels and removing excess deposits. The incisions are closed with sutures.

15878-15879
The physician performs a lipectomy of the upper or lower extremity. The physician makes small incisions in the skin overlying an area of fat deposits on the upper or lower extremity. A liposuction cannula is inserted through the incision. The physician moves the cannula through the fat deposits, creating tunnels and removing excess deposits. The incisions are closed with sutures.

15920-15922
The physician excises a coccygeal pressure ulcer with coccygectomy. The patient is positioned prone (face down) and the physician makes an elliptical incision over the coccyx (tailbone), removing the strip of skin that contains the pressure sore. After freeing the coccyx from the surrounding soft tissues, it is separated from the sacrum and removed. The soft tissue is brought back together and the wound is closed with sutures. Report 15922 if the wound is closed using a skin flap from the groin or other donor site. The flap is sutured in place and covered with mesh petroleum gauze and loose bandages.

15931-15933
The physician excises a sacral pressure ulcer. The patient is positioned prone (face down) and the physician makes an elliptical incision over the sacrum, removing the strip of skin that contains the pressure sore. The wound is irrigated and the soft tissue is brought back together and closed with sutures. Report 15933 if bone below the wound is removed before the soft tissue is brought back together and closed.

15934-15935
The physician excises a sacral pressure ulcer. The patient is positioned prone (face down) and the physician makes an elliptical incision over the sacrum, removing the strip of skin that contains the pressure sore. The wound is irrigated and closed using a skin flap from the groin or other donor site. The flap is sutured in place and covered with mesh petroleum gauze and loose bandages. Report 15935 if bone below the wound is removed before the wound is repaired with a skin flap.

15936-15937
The physician excises a sacral ulcer to prepare for muscle or myocutaneous flap or skin graft closure. The physician makes an incision around the pressure sore that lies over the sacrum. The infected wound is removed and the area is irrigated. The space that remains is filled with a muscle flap graft, usually taken from the latissimus dorsi muscle and the overlying skin. The donor site is prepared and the incision is made for the appropriate size of graft to be taken. Once the portion of the muscle is removed, the overlying skin is removed and the wound is sutured closed. The graft is sutured in place and a soft dressing is applied. Report 15937 if the underlying bone is removed before the wound is repaired with the flap or graft.

15940-15941
The physician excises an ischial pressure ulcer. An incision is made around the wound over the ischial tuberosity to remove the infected pressure sore. The remaining healthy tissues are irrigated, the wound is closed with sutures, and a soft dressing is applied. Report 15941 if a portion of bone from the ischium is removed before the wound is sutured closed.

15944-15945
The physician excises an ischial pressure ulcer, with skin flap closure. An incision is made around the wound over the ischial tuberosity in order to remove the infected pressure sore. The infected tissue is removed; however, the wound is large enough to require a flap of skin from another part of the body, such as the groin area at the front of the hip, to completely close the area. The physician makes an appropriate size flap from the donor area and sutures it in place following the removal of the infected tissue. The donor site is sutured closed and soft dressings are used to cover the wounds. Report 15945 if a portion of bone from the ischium is removed before the wound is closed with the flap.

15946
The physician excises an ischial pressure ulcer and part of the ischial bone underlying the ulcer. The defect that remains is prepared for a graft that is reported separately, most commonly a gluteal thigh rotation flap, but it may also be a myocutaneous or muscle graft involving the gluteus maximus muscle. The graft is sutured in place and a soft dressing is applied.

15950-15951
The physician excises a trochanteric pressure ulcer, with primary suture closure. The physician makes an elliptical shaped incision around the wound, which is

located over the outer hip bone. The infected pressure ulcer is removed and the wound is irrigated. The soft tissues are brought back together and closed with sutures. A soft dressing is applied. Report 15951 if a portion of the underlying bone is also removed because of the extent of the infection.

15952-15953
The physician excises a trochanteric pressure ulcer with skin flap closure. An incision is made around the wound over the trochanter (outer hip bone) in order to remove the infected pressure sore. The remaining defect requires skin flap closure. The most common skin flap donor sites are the groin area at the front of the hip, gluteal thigh, or anterior thigh. The physician takes an appropriate size graft from the donor area and sutures it in place covering the defect. The donor site is also sutured closed. Soft dressings are used to cover the wounds. Report 15953 if a portion or all of the trochanter is removed during the ulcer excision.

15956-15958
The physician excises a trochanteric pressure ulcer. The defect that remains is prepared for a myocutaneous or muscle graft that is reported separately, most commonly harvested from the tensor fasciae latae (AFT) muscle. The graft is sutured in place and a soft dressing is applied. Report 15958 if a portion or all of the trochanter is removed during the ulcer excision.

16000
The physician treats a first-degree burn. The physician performs a simple cleaning and applies an ointment or a dressing.

16020-16030
The physician applies dressing material(s) and/or debrides a partial-thickness burn of blisters and nonviable or nonadherent tissue, initial or subsequent. The physician removes devitalized tissue or tissue that is contaminated by bacteria, foreign material, dead cells, or a crust. The wound is cleansed and a dressing is applied. Report 16020 for treatment of a small burn area, less than 5 percent of total body surface area; 16025 for a medium-sized area, 5 to 10 percent of total body surface area, such as the whole face or a whole extremity; and 16030 for a large burn area, greater than 10 percent of total body surface area, such as more than one extremity.

16035-16036
The physician performs an escharotomy. Eschar is a leathery slough produced by thermal burns. The physician makes an incision through the area of eschar and undermines it. With adequate incision of the eschar, the physician achieves release of movement for the underlying tissue. Report 16035 for the initial incision and 16036 for each additional incision.

17000-17003
The physician destroys or excises premalignant lesions using a laser, electrosurgery, cryosurgery, chemical treatment, or surgical curettement. Local anesthesia is included. Report 17000 when one lesion is destroyed and 17003 when two to 14 lesions are destroyed.

17004
The physician excises or destroys premalignant lesions using a laser, electrosurgery, cryosurgery, chemical treatment, or surgical curettement. Local anesthesia is included. This code reports destruction of 15 or more lesions during the same surgical session.

17106-17108
The physician destroys a collection of abnormal proliferative blood vessels within the skin; various methods may be utilized. In one, the physician applies a laser treatment in a technique similar to painting the skin. This destroys the vessels, creating scar tissue that eventually fades. No incision is made, and no tissue is removed. Report 17106 if the treated area totals less than 10 sq cm; 17107 for 10 sq cm to 50 sq cm; and 17108 for more than 50 sq cm.

17110-17111
The physician uses a laser, electrosurgery, cryosurgery, chemical treatment, or surgical curettement to obliterate or vaporize benign lesions other than skin tags or lesions such as cutaneous vascular proliferative lesions. Examples of lesions that may be removed under this code description include, but are not limited to, molluscum contagiosum or melanocytic nevi. Report 17110 when one to 14 lesions are removed and 17111 when 15 or more lesions are removed.

17250
The physician destroys a form of exuberant or excessive healing tissue known as granulation tissue or proud flesh. The physician destroys the tissue by applying chemicals such as silver nitrate.

17260-17266
The physician destroys a malignant lesion of the trunk, arms, and legs. Destruction may be accomplished by using a laser or electrocautery to burn the lesion, cryotherapy to freeze the lesion, chemicals to destroy the lesion, or surgical curettement to remove the lesion. Report 17260 for a lesion diameter 0.5 cm or less; 17261 for 0.6 cm to 1 cm; 17262 for 1.1 cm to 2 cm; 17263 for 2.1 cm to 3 cm; 17264 for 3.1 cm to 4 cm; and 17266 if the lesion diameter is greater than 4 cm.

17270-17276
The physician destroys a malignant lesion of the scalp, neck, hands, feet, or genitalia. Destruction may be accomplished by using a laser or electrocautery to burn the lesion, cryotherapy to freeze the lesion, chemicals to destroy the lesion, or surgical curettement to remove the lesion. Report 17270 for a lesion diameter 0.5 cm or less; 17271 for 0.6 cm to 1 cm; 17272 for 1.1 cm to 2 cm; 17273 for 2.1 cm to 3 cm; 17274 for 3.1 cm to 4 cm; and 17276 if the lesion diameter is greater than 4 cm.

17280-17286
The physician destroys a malignant lesion of the face, ears, eyelids, nose, lips, or mucous membranes. Destruction may be accomplished by using a laser or electrocautery to burn the lesion, cryotherapy to freeze the lesion, chemicals to destroy the lesion, or surgical curettement to remove the lesion. Report 17280 for a

lesion diameter 0.5 cm or less; 17281 for 0.6 cm to 1 cm; 17282 for 1.1 cm to 2 cm; 17283 for 2.1 cm to 3 cm; 17284 for 3.1 cm to 4 cm; and 17286 if the lesion diameter is greater than 4 cm.

17311-17315

The physician uses Mohs micrographic technique to excise skin cancer that is complex or not well defined. The physician acts as both the surgeon and pathologist, performing both the excision and histologic examination of the surgical margins. An incision is made around the area of the planned excision. Debulking of the tissue is performed to remove visible cancer without attention to margins or normal tissue. Hatch marks are made for orientation of the specimen to the defect. For the first stage, a thin layer of tissue, usually 1 mm to 3 mm thick, is removed. One or more pieces of the tissue are placed on a plate (block) and embedded in a mounting medium for sectioning. More than one tissue block may be necessary, depending on how many tissue pieces fit on one plate (block). The tissue is color coded with dye around the edges, and a map is created that corresponds to the surgical wound. The tissue pieces are processed by frozen section pathology, including routine stains. The physician examines the frozen sections of tissue with a microscope to determine if additional stages are needed. The process is repeated as necessary until all margins are free of cancer. Report 17311 for the first stage, up to five tissue blocks of the head, neck, hands, feet, genitalia, or any location with surgery directly involving muscle, cartilage, bone, tendon, major nerves, or vessels and 17312 for each additional stage, up to five tissue blocks. Report 17313 for the first stage, up to five tissue blocks of the trunk, arms, or legs and 17314 for each additional stage, up to five tissue blocks. Report 17315 in addition to the code for the primary procedure for each additional block after the first five tissue blocks, any stage.

17340

The physician performs cryotherapy for acne. The physician freezes the area of acne with a chemical such as liquid nitrogen by applying a soaked cotton tip to the lesion for a short period of time. This leads to scabbing and healing.

17360

The physician destroys the area of acne with a chemical exfoliator such as acne paste or acid by touching a soaked cotton tip applicator to the lesion for a short period of time (commonly 30 seconds). This leads to formation of eschar and healing.

17380

The physician uses electrolysis to remove hair. This code is used to report a 30-minute session. The physician inserts the electroneedle into the hair follicle and applies electrical current, killing the follicle. The electroneedle is removed.

19000-19001

The physician punctures with a syringe needle the skin of the breast overlying a cyst. The needle is inserted into the cyst and fluid is evacuated into the syringe, thus reducing the size of the cyst. The physician withdraws the needle and applies pressure to the puncture wound to stop the bleeding. Report 19001 for aspiration of each additional cyst of the breast.

19020

The physician makes an incision in the skin of the breast over the site of an abscess or suspicious tissue for exploration or drainage. The infected cavity is accessed and specimens for culture are taken before the cavity is irrigated with warm saline solution. Bleeding vessels may be tied or cauterized. If no abscess or suspicious tissue is found, the wound is closed with sutures. In the case of an abscess, the wound is usually loosely packed with gauze to promote free drainage rather than being closed with sutures.

19030

The physician performs an injection procedure for mammary ductogram or galactogram. A cannula or needle is inserted into the duct of the breast. Contrast media is introduced into the breast duct for the purpose of radiographic study. A dissecting microscope may be used to aid in placing the cannula. The needle or cannula is removed once the study has been completed.

19081-19082

The physician performs a breast biopsy with image guidance using a percutaneous needle core or automated vacuum assisted or rotating biopsy device and insertion of a localization device. Using image guidance, the physician places a metallic clip or pellet adjacent to a breast lesion to mark the site. A large gauge (e.g., 14 gauge), hollow core biopsy needle or the biopsy device is inserted through the skin of the breast and into the suspicious breast tissue. The physician takes multiple core tissue samples from a single lesion to obtain a sufficient amount of tissue for diagnosis. The needle or automated vacuum assisted or rotating biopsy device is withdrawn. Pressure and bandages are applied to the puncture site. Report 19081 for the first lesion and 19082 for each additional lesion removed using stereotactic guidance.

19083-19084

The physician performs a breast biopsy with image guidance using a percutaneous needle core or automated vacuum assisted or rotating biopsy device and insertion of a localization device. Using image guidance, the physician places a metallic clip or pellet adjacent to a breast lesion to mark the site. A large gauge (e.g., 14 gauge), hollow core biopsy needle or the biopsy device is inserted through the skin of the breast and into the suspicious breast tissue. The physician takes multiple core tissue samples from a single lesion to obtain a sufficient amount of tissue for diagnosis. The needle or automated vacuum assisted or rotating biopsy device is withdrawn. Pressure and bandages are applied to the puncture site. Report 19083 for the first lesion and 19084 for each additional lesion using ultrasound guidance.

19085-19086
The physician performs a breast biopsy with image guidance using a percutaneous needle core or automated vacuum assisted or rotating biopsy device and insertion of a localization device. Using image guidance, the physician places a metallic clip or pellet adjacent to a breast lesion to mark the site. A large gauge (e.g., 14 gauge), hollow core biopsy needle or the biopsy device is inserted through the skin of the breast and into the suspicious breast tissue. The physician takes multiple core tissue samples from a single lesion to obtain a sufficient amount of tissue for diagnosis. The needle or automated vacuum assisted or rotating biopsy device is withdrawn. Pressure and bandages are applied to the puncture site. Report 19085 for the first lesion and 19086 for each additional lesion using magnetic resonance imaging (MRI).

19100
The physician inserts a large gauge needle through the skin of the breast and into the suspect breast tissue. The needle is removed along with a core of breast tissue. Pressure is applied to the puncture site to stop any bleeding.

19101
The physician removes tissue for biopsy. The physician makes an incision in the skin of the breast near the site of the suspect mass. The mass is identified and a sample of the lesion is removed. This specimen is often examined immediately. If the lesion is benign, the incision is repaired with layered closure. If malignant, the incision may be closed pending a separate, more extensive surgical session, or a more extensive surgery may occur immediately, in which case this code would not be reported.

19105
The physician uses cryotherapy to obliterate a fibroadenoma of the breast. The patient's skin is cleansed and the ablation site is anesthetized. Ultrasound is used to locate the tumor. A cryoprobe is inserted through a small incision and placed within the fibroadenoma under ultrasound. The device initiates ice ball formation. The cryoprobe is warmed before removal from the breast. This code reports treatment of one fibroadenoma.

19110
The physician makes an incision at the edge of the areola near the site of a suspect duct for nipple exploration, with or without excision of a solitary lactiferous duct or a papilloma lactiferous duct. The duct is dissected from surrounding tissue and examined. Surrounding ducts and tissue are also examined. The suspect duct may be excised. Bleeding vessels are controlled with electrocautery or ligated with sutures. The incision is sutured in layered closure and a light pressure dressing is applied.

19112
The physician makes an incision around the abnormal opening of a lactiferous duct fistula on the skin. The fistula is dissected down to the duct. The duct, fistula, and skin opening are all excised. The remaining portion of the duct may be ligated. The wound is irrigated with warm sterile saline and closed in layers.

19120
The physician excises breast tissue for biopsy. The physician makes an incision in the skin of the breast overlying the site of the mass. Skin and tissue are dissected from the abnormality. The lesion is removed. Bleeding vessels are controlled with electrocautery or ligated with sutures. A drain may be inserted into the wound. The incision is sutured in layered closure and a light pressure dressing is applied.

19125-19126
The physician uses radiologic markers to identify breast tissue to be excised for biopsy. The physician makes an incision in the skin of the breast over the site of the lesion marked for excision by preoperative placement of a radiological marker. The lesion and marker are excised. Bleeding vessels are controlled with electrocautery or ligated with sutures. A drain may be inserted into the wound. The incision is sutured in layered closure and a light dressing is applied. Report 19126 for each additional lesion identified by a preoperative marker and removed during the same surgical session.

19281-19282
The physician places a breast localization device prior to a breast biopsy. Using image guidance, the physician places a metallic clip, pellet, wire, needle, or radioactive seed adjacent to a breast lesion to mark the site for an open breast procedure or a percutaneous breast biopsy to be performed during the same or a different encounter. Report 19281 for the first lesion and 19282 for each additional lesion marked using mammographic guidance.

19283-19284
The physician places a breast localization device prior to a breast biopsy. Using image guidance, the physician places a metallic clip, pellet, wire, needle, or radioactive seed adjacent to a breast lesion to mark the site for an open breast procedure or a percutaneous breast biopsy to be performed during the same or a different encounter. Report 19283 for the first lesion and 19284 for each additional lesion marked using stereotactic guidance.

19285-19286
The physician places a breast localization device prior to a breast biopsy. Using image guidance, the physician places a metallic clip, pellet, wire, needle, or radioactive seed adjacent to a breast lesion to mark the site for an open breast procedure or a percutaneous breast biopsy to be performed during the same or a different encounter. Report 19285 for the first lesion and 19286 for each additional lesion marked using ultrasound guidance.

19287-19288
The physician places a breast localization device prior to a breast biopsy. Using image guidance, the physician places a metallic clip, pellet, wire, needle, or

radioactive seed adjacent to a breast lesion to mark the site for an open breast procedure or a percutaneous breast biopsy to be performed during the same or a different encounter. Report 19287 for the first lesion and 19288 for each additional lesion using magnetic resonance imaging (MRI).

19294

The radiation oncologist delivers intraoperative radiation therapy (IORT) at the same time as the patient is undergoing a lumpectomy or partial mastectomy. A miniature, low energy, isotope-free x-ray source is brought into the operating room at the time the lumpectomy is performed to deliver a precise and targeted dose of radiation directly to the lumpectomy cavity. The surgeon removes the malignant tumor and awaits the initial pathology report. Once the malignancy is confirmed, the physician prepares the tumor cavity for temporary insertion of a flexible balloon applicator. The radiation oncologist inserts the miniature x-ray source inside a balloon-shaped catheter device and a single dose of radiation is directed at the tumor cavity while medical personnel remain behind a rolling shield. The process takes eight to 12 minutes. Once the treatment is complete, the catheter is withdrawn and the applicator is removed. The incision is closed.

19296-19297

A remote single or multichannel afterloading expandable catheter for interstitial radiotherapy treatment is placed in the breast following partial mastectomy. A catheter is placed at a later date, separate from the lumpectomy surgery in 19296, and concurrently with the lumpectomy in 19297. This is a single catheter with an expandable balloon tip that holds the radioactive seed or treatment source, which is loaded and removed for each session. The catheter can be single or multichannel, depending on the treatment delivery requirements. During the lumpectomy surgery, an uninflated balloon catheter is inserted into the recently created tumor cavity and positioned under imaging with a portion of the catheter remaining outside of the body. If a separate procedure is done after surgery, a small incision is first made and the uninflated balloon catheter is guided into position under imaging. After correct placement is determined, the balloon is inflated with saline to fit snugly into the lumpectomy cavity, and the breast is bandaged. The catheter remains until radiotherapy treatment sessions are complete.

19298

Using imaging guidance, at the time of a partial mastectomy, or subsequent to a partial mastectomy having been performed, remote afterloading catheters are placed into the breast for interstitial radiotherapy application. The lumpectomy site is identified. A template with pre-drilled holes that function as coordinates for catheter placement around the surgical area may be applied for imaging. Brachytherapy needles are first inserted into the chosen coordinates. The brachytherapy catheters are fed into position through the needles, which are removed. A catheter button is positioned to hold each catheter in place and imaging confirms their position. These remain in place until the actual loading of the radioactive material for treatment. This code reports only the placement of the catheters.

19300

The physician performs a mastectomy for gynecomastia on a male patient. The physician makes a circular incision in the skin of the breast at the edge of the areola or in the inframammary fold. Extraneous fat and breast tissue are dissected from the pectoral fascia and removed. Bleeding vessels are ligated with sutures or cauterized. The incision is sutured in layered closure and a dressing is applied.

19301-19302

The physician excises a breast tumor and a margin of normal tissue by performing a partial mastectomy by making an incision through the skin and fascia over a breast malignancy and clamping any lymphatic and blood vessels. The physician excises the mass along with a margin or rim of healthy tissue. This procedure is often referred to as a segmental mastectomy or a quadrantectomy, but is also called a lumpectomy. In 19302, an axillary lymphadenectomy is also performed. The lymph nodes between the pectoralis major and the pectoralis minor muscles and the nodes in the axilla are removed through a separate incision. A drainage tube may be placed through a separate stab incision to enhance drainage from the wound or lymphatic system. The incision is repaired with layered closure and a dressing is applied.

19303

The physician removes all subcutaneous breast tissue, with or without nipple and skin. The physician makes an elliptical incision around the breast that includes the tail of Spence, the extension of mammary tissue into the axillary region. The breast tissue is dissected from the pectoral fascia and sternum. The breast tissue is removed, along with a portion of skin, including the nipple. In a modification of the simple mastectomy, skin and nipple may be spared, but all subcutaneous breast tissue is removed. The physician ligates any bleeding vessels. A closed wound drainage catheter may be inserted and the edges of skin are approximated, sutured, and a dressing is applied.

19305

The physician performs a radical mastectomy. The physician makes an elliptical incision that includes the nipple and the tail of Spence, the extension of mammary tissue into the axillary region. The breast, along with the overlying skin, the pectoralis major and minor muscles, and the lymph nodes in the axilla, are removed as a single specimen. Bleeding vessels are ligated or electrocauterized. In large-breasted patients, adequate skin may be available for primary closure. Patients with insufficient skin for coverage may require skin grafts or myocutaneous flaps. If no implant is to be inserted, a closed wound suction catheter may be inserted. The wound is closed and a pressure dressing is applied.

19306

The physician performs a radical Urban-type mastectomy. The physician makes an elliptical incision that includes the nipple and the tail of Spence, the extension of mammary tissue into the axillary region. The breast tissue, skin, and pectoral muscles are removed. All tissue within the parameters of the sternum, the rectus fascia, the latissimus dorsi muscle, and the clavicle are removed, including the axillary and internal mammary lymph nodes. Bleeding vessels are ligated or electrocauterized. In large-breasted patients, adequate skin may be available for primary closure. Patients with insufficient skin for coverage may require skin grafts or myocutaneous flaps. If no implant is to be inserted, a closed wound suction catheter may be inserted. The wound is closed and a pressure dressing is applied.

19307

The physician performs a modified radical mastectomy. The physician makes an elliptical incision that includes the nipple and the tail of Spence, the extension of mammary tissue into the axillary region. The breast tissue and skin are dissected from the pectoral fascia and removed from the pectoral muscle. The pectoralis minor muscle may also be resected to facilitate the axillary dissection, but the pectoralis major muscle is left intact. Bleeding vessels are ligated or electrocauterized. The breast tissue and axillary tissue, including lymph nodes, are removed en bloc and the wound is irrigated. Adequate skin is usually available for primary closure. Patients with insufficient skin for coverage may require skin grafts or myocutaneous flaps. If no implant is to be inserted, a closed wound suction catheter may be inserted. The wound is closed and a pressure dressing is applied.

19316

The physician performs a breast lift, or mastopexy, relocating the nipple and areola to a higher position and removing excess skin below the nipple and above the lower breast crease. The physician makes a skin incision above the nipple, in the location to which the nipple will be elevated. Another skin incision is made around the circumference of the nipple. Two skin incisions are made from the circular cut above the nipple to the fold beneath the breast, one on either side of the nipple, forming a keyhole shaped skin incision. This skin is cut away from the breast tissue and removed. The physician elevates the breast to its new position and closes the incision, excising any redundant skin in the fold beneath the breast. The incision is repaired with layered closure.

19318

The physician reduces the size of the breast, removing wedges of skin and breast tissue from a female patient. The physician makes a circular skin incision above the nipple, in the position to which the nipple will be elevated. Another skin incision is made around the circumference of the nipple. Two incisions are made from the circular cut above the nipple to the fold beneath the breast, one on either side of the nipple, creating a keyhole shaped skin and breast incision. Wedges of skin and breast tissue are removed until the desired size is achieved. Bleeding vessels may be ligated or cauterized. The physician elevates the nipple and its pedicle of subcutaneous tissue to its new position and sutures the nipple pedicle with layered closure. The remaining incision is repaired with layered closure.

19325

The physician increases the size of the breast by inserting an implant. The physician makes an incision in the fold under the breast and dissects the breast tissue and muscle layer free from the chest wall to accommodate an implant positioned under the muscle. As an alternative, the implant may also be positioned between the muscle and the existing breast tissue or skin. If fat grafting obtained by liposuction is performed in addition to the implant insertion, this is reported separately. The incision is repaired with layered closure.

19328

A breast implant that is still intact is removed. The physician makes an incision in the fold under the breast, around the nipple, or at the site of an existing mastectomy incision and dissects muscle, fat, and breast tissue from the existing implant. The intact implant is removed. Any infection is irrigated. The physician repairs the incision with layered closure.

19330

A breast implant that is leaking, ruptured, or defective is removed. The physician makes an incision in the fold under the breast or around the nipple and dissects muscle, fat, and breast tissue from the existing implant. The implant material is removed, including all implant contents such as saline or silicone gel. The surrounding tissue is checked closely for adhesions or deposits of the material that have infiltrated beyond the capsule. The implant material and any affected tissue are excised. If a new implant is placed during the same operative session, it is reported separately. The physician repairs the incision with layered closure.

19340

The physician performs an immediate breast implant insertion following mastectomy. The physician dissects the breast tissue and muscle layer free from the chest wall to accommodate an implant positioned under the muscle in a patient who has just undergone a mastectomy during this same surgical session. The same surgical skin incisions are most often used. As an alternative, the implant may also be positioned between the muscle and the existing breast tissue or skin. The incision is repaired with layered closure.

19342

The physician inserts or replaces a silicone gel- or saline-filled breast implant after a patient has had previous breast surgery. This procedure is performed on a separate day from the mastectomy, typically after the wound has healed, and may be several months after the original surgery. The physician makes an incision in the fold under the breast or along a previous surgical incision and removes an existing implant, if present. The physician dissects the tissue and muscle layer free from the chest wall to accommodate an implant positioned under the muscle. As an alternative, the implant may also be positioned between the muscle and the existing breast tissue or skin. The incision is repaired with layered closure.

19350
The nipple and areola are reconstructed. The physician excises graft skin, usually from the inner thigh, behind the ear, or a section excised from the patient's existing areola. The donor site is repaired with sutures. To create a new nipple, the physician excises the lower section of tissue from the patient's existing nipple or removes tissue from the ear or labia. This donor site is repaired with sutures. A thin, circular layer of surface skin is removed from the breast at the site of the graft. The areola skin graft is positioned and sutured to the breast and the nipple graft is sutured to a small, circular incision in the areola's center.

19355
Inverted nipples are corrected by making two or more radial incisions in the areola and elevating the inverted nipple into an everted position. Ductal channels and fibrous bands may be transected to accomplish this. Tissue may be removed. The nipple is secured with sutures and incisions in the areola are closed.

19357
The physician performs breast reconstruction with a tissue expander; this code reports the initial expander placement as well as subsequent expansions. The physician makes an incision in the skin of a patient who has undergone a mastectomy. A pocket is created using an existing chest wall muscle and an expandable implant is placed into it at the site of the mastectomy. In some cases, the implant's button-shaped portal may be brought out through the skin so it is accessible by needle. Typically, however, the portal remains beneath the surface of the skin. The physician injects saline into the access portal to expand the implant until it has stretched the surrounding tissue to a size slightly larger than the patient's existing breast. In some cases, the expander remains a permanent prosthesis and a small amount of fluid is aspirated until it duplicates the size of the existing breast. In other cases, a second surgery (reported separately) excises the implant and replaces it with a permanent breast implant.

19361
The physician performs breast reconstruction with a latissimus dorsi flap. The physician transfers skin and muscle from the patient's back to the breast area to correct defects created from a previous modified radical or radical mastectomy. The physician makes a skin incision in the back and dissects a portion of the latissimus muscle and the overlying skin from surrounding structures. The muscle-skin flap remains attached to a main artery. In preparation for the transfer, the mastectomy scar is excised. The muscle flap is rotated to the front of the chest through a tunnel under the armpit so that it extends through to the mastectomy incision. The incision in the back is repaired with layered closure. The physician adjusts the flap for the most aesthetic appearance and secures it with sutures to the chest wall, adjacent muscles, and skin. The incision is repaired with sutures. This code includes flap harvesting, donor site closure, and flap insetting and shaping. If placement of a breast implant or a tissue expander is performed with flap reconstruction, it is reported separately.

19364
The physician excises a free flap of skin, fat, and muscle from another site on the patient for use in the reconstruction of the breast following a modified radical or radical mastectomy. The free flap is excised with careful dissection of vascular channels, commonly from the thigh or buttocks, and the operative wound is sutured in a layered repair. In preparation for the graft, the mastectomy scar is excised with blood vessels preserved. The free flap is transferred to the mastectomy site and microvascular anastomosis is done to provide the graft with a viable blood supply. The physician adjusts the flap for the most aesthetic appearance and secures it with sutures to the chest wall, adjacent muscles, and skin. If the free flap does not have enough fat, a breast implant may be required. The chest incision is repaired with sutures. This code includes flap harvesting, donor site closure, and flap insetting and shaping. If placement of a breast implant or a tissue expander is performed with flap reconstruction, it is reported separately.

19367-19369
The physician performs a transverse rectus abdominis myocutaneous flap (TRAM) procedure for breast reconstruction. The physician first designs and then cuts a skin island flap on the lower abdominal wall. A superior skin and fat flap is elevated off the rectus abdominis muscle. A transverse incision is made in the rectus sheath and the muscle is divided and elevated, keeping the superior epigastric arteries intact for blood supply. Once the muscle is elevated, the physician makes an incision through the chest skin. This is also elevated, creating a pocket for the muscle flap. A connecting tunnel is made between the elevated chest skin and the inferiorly positioned flap. The flap is passed superiorly under the tunnel of tissue, placed into its new position, and sutured, after contouring a breast. The abdominal wall is closed by reapproximating the remaining anterior rectus muscle to the remaining lateral muscle and sheath. Skin edges are brought together and sutured in layers. Suction drains are also placed. Report 19368 if microvascular anastomosis for connecting blood vessels is used. Report 19369 if the muscle/skin complex has two pedicles or both sides of the rectus abdominis are elevated (bilateral or hemiflaps). These codes include flap harvesting, donor site closure, and flap insetting and shaping. If placement of a breast implant or a tissue expander is performed with flap reconstruction, it is reported separately.

19370
The physician revises a peri-implant capsule of the breast by making an incision in the skin of the breast, at the site of a mastectomy scar, in the skin fold beneath the breast, or around the nipple. In a capsulotomy, the physician uses a cautery knife to cut into the area of fibrous scarring associated with a breast implant. Incisions are made into the scar (contracted capsule) to cut around its circumference and enlarge the pocket in which the implant is placed. Loosening the capsule relieves pain and tightness caused by the contracture. No tissue is removed. The incision is repaired with layered closure. A capsulorrhaphy reshapes or recontours the capsule while tightening and repositioning the capsule pocket so that the capsule fits back within the sutures surrounding the implant, while the capsulectomy described by this code removes a portion of the capsule.

19371
The physician performs a peri-implant capsulectomy on the breast. An incision is made in the skin of the breast at the site of a mastectomy scar, in the skin fold beneath the breast, or around the nipple. The physician uses a cautery knife to cut into the area of fibrous scarring associated with a breast implant. The contracted capsule is excised from the breast tissue and the implant, along with all intracapsular contents. If the removal of extracapsular silicone in cases of a ruptured silicone implant is performed during the same operative session, this is reported separately. The incision is repaired with layered closure.

19380
Revision is done on a reconstructed breast, usually to correct a problem with asymmetry. This may require substantial tissue removal, reinsertion or readvancement of flaps in autologous reconstruction, or, in implant-based reconstruction, significant revision of the capsule in conjunction with soft tissue excision. The physician makes an incision in the breast skin along the areola or at the fold under the breast or in prior surgical incisions. Tissue therein may be rearranged or secured with sutures to revise the shape of the reconstructed breast. An existing breast implant may be replaced with an implant of a different configuration. Excess skin or tissue from the reconstructed breast may be removed. Once the breast has been revised to its desired shape, the physician repairs the incision with layered closure.

19396
The physician creates a custom breast implant model or moulage that closely resembles the remaining breast configuration of a mastectomy patient. From this a custom breast implant will be created.

Musculoskeletal

20100-20103
The physician explores a penetrating wound in the operating room, such as a gunshot or stab wound, to help identify damaged structures. Nerve, organ, and blood vessel integrity is assessed. The wound may be enlarged to help assess the damage. Debridement, removal of foreign bodies, and ligation or coagulation of minor blood vessels in the subcutaneous tissues, fascia, and muscle are also included in this range of codes. Damaged tissues are debrided and repaired when possible. The wound is closed (if clean) or packed open if contaminated by the penetrating body. Report 20100 for exploration of a neck wound. Report 20101 for exploration of a chest wound. Report 20102 for exploration of an abdomen, flank, or back wound. Report 20103 for exploration of a wound to an extremity.

20150
Excision of the epiphyseal bar is a procedure performed to treat a partial epiphyseal arrest in a patient with significant remaining growth in a long bone, such as the femur, tibia, or fibula. This is caused, in many cases, by an injury or infection involving the epiphyseal plate (growth plate). The patient is placed in the supine position and a tourniquet is applied to the proximal thigh and raised to the appropriate pressure. For excision of the distal femur or proximal tibia, the knee is extended on a radiolucent operating table with the intention of resecting two rectangular areas, one on the medial side and one on the lateral side of the bone. Under fluoroscopic image intensification, a stab wound incision is made laterally or medially at the level of the growth plate. On one side at a time, an osteotome is driven to a depth of 1 cm into the growth plate and rotated 180 degrees to create an opening in the epiphysis. An oval curette is directed through the hole to a depth of about one-third the width of the growth plate. The physician sweeps the curette across the growth plate to remove the rectangular area. If an excision of the epiphyseal bar of the proximal tibia or fibula is performed, the peroneal nerve must be protected. The proximal growth plate of the fibula is approached through an incision anterior to the fibula and exposed anteriorly by subcutaneous blunt dissection. The growth plate is identified by subperiosteal elevation and a rectangular area is removed with a curette. The tourniquet is released and hemostasis is achieved. A piece of autogenous fat from the subcutaneous tissue (though the same incision) or an inert substance may be interpositioned in the cavity allowing growth to continue in the epiphysis. The wound is closed with sutures and the wound is wrapped with a compressive dressing to reduce the formation of a hematoma. The limb is placed in a knee immobilizer.

20200-20205
The physician secures a sample of tissue from a muscle for biopsy. The physician incises the overlying skin and bluntly dissects to the suspect muscle. The muscle tissue is obtained. Bleeding is controlled and the wound is sutured in layers. Report 20200 if the muscle site sampled is superficial and 20205 if the muscle site sampled is deep.

20206
The physician removes a sample of muscle tissue using a percutaneous needle. The physician applies a local anesthetic to the skin. The physician uses a bore needle to pierce the skin, fascia, and muscle, obtaining a sample of muscle tissue. The needle is withdrawn. No repair is usually necessary. Radiologic supervision, if necessary, is reported separately.

20220-20225
The physician usually performs a biopsy on bone to confirm a suspected growth, disease, or infection. The physician normally uses local anesthesia; however, general anesthesia may be used. The physician places a large needle into the spinous process or other superficial bone to obtain the sample in 20220. For sampling a deeper lying bone, such as a vertebra in 20225, an exploring needle is passed through a larger needle to the desired depth and a piece of tissue is removed for testing. Different approaches are taken for vertebral biopsies, based on differing levels of vertebrae. The top three cervical vertebrae are approached from a pharyngeal or anterior approach. The lower four cervical vertebrae are approached from a lateral direction. Thoracic and lumbar vertebra are approached from behind and to the right to avoid major arteries. Radiographs are sometimes used to confirm the placement of the needle.

20240-20245
The physician performs an open biopsy on bone to confirm a suspected growth, disease, or infection. With the patient under general anesthesia, and placed in the appropriate position, the physician makes an incision overlying the biopsy site and carries it down through the tissue to the level of the bone. A piece of bone tissue is removed and sent for examination. The wound is sutured closed and the patient is moved to the recovery area. Report 20240 for a superficial bone biopsy (rib, sternum, spinous or olecranon process, patella, calcaneus, tarsal or metatarsal, carpal or metacarpal, and phalanx). Report 20245 if the bone biopsied lies deep, such as the femoral or humeral shaft and ischium.

20250-20251
This procedure is used to confirm a suspected growth, disease, or infection of a vertebral body. The patient is placed in a prone position. A midline incision is made overlying the vertebra to be biopsied. The incision is carried down and the fascia is incised. Paravertebral muscles are retracted and the vertebral area to be biopsied is identified. A piece of tissue is excised or a needle is used to extract a sample of tissue for evaluation. The paravertebral muscles are replaced in their anatomical position and the incision is closed in layers. Report 20250 for thoracic vertebral biopsy and 20251 for lumbar or cervical vertebral biopsy.

20500
A physician injects a sinus tract (a canal or passage leading to an abscess) with a therapeutic agent such as Betadine, to act as a chemical irritant or antibiotic to clear the infection in an abscess or a cyst. X-rays are reported separately.

20501
The physician injects a sinus tract (a canal or passage leading to an abscess) with a radiopaque agent, to determine the existence, nature, or size of an abscess or a cyst. X-rays are reported separately.

20520-20525
The physician removes a foreign body in a muscle or tendon sheath. The physician incises the skin and dissects to the muscle or sheath. The foreign body is isolated by palpation or radiographic imagery (separately reported) and removed. The incision may be closed if clean or packed if contaminated by the object. Report 20520 if the removal is simple; report 20525 if the foreign object lies deep or requires a complicated procedure to remove it.

20526
A physician administers a single therapeutic injection of corticosteroid or anesthetic, 4 cm proximal to the wrist crease between the tendons of the radial flexor and the long palmar muscles on the lateral side of the forearm. This procedure is performed for therapeutic relief of the persistent symptoms of carpal tunnel syndrome.

20527
This physician corrects connective tissue shortening and thickening in the hand causing "bent finger" or Dupuytren's contracture. Local anesthesia is applied to the hand. An enzyme (clostridial collagenase) is injected directly into the contracted tissues. The enzyme weakens and dissolves the connective tissue in preparation for manipulation to break the connective tissue loose and straighten the finger(s). This procedure is typically followed by manipulation one or more days after the injection, which is reported separately.

20550-20551
The physician injects a therapeutic agent into a single tendon sheath, or ligament, aponeurosis such as the plantar fascia in 20550 and into a single tendon origin/insertion site in 20551. The physician identifies the injection site by palpation or radiographs (reported separately) and marks the injection site. The needle is inserted and the medicine is injected. After withdrawing the needle, the patient is monitored for reactions to the therapeutic agent.

20552-20553
The physician injects a therapeutic agent into a single or multiple trigger point of one or two muscles in 20552 and into a single or multiple trigger point for three or more muscles in 20553. Trigger points are focal, discrete spots of hypersensitive irritability identified within bands of muscle. These points cause local or referred pain. Trigger points may be formed by acute or repetitive trauma to the muscle tissue, which puts too much stress on the fibers. The physician identifies the trigger point injection site by palpation or radiographic imaging and marks the injection site.

The needle is inserted, and the medicine is injected into the trigger point. The injection may be done using image guidance, which is reported separately. After withdrawing the needle, the patient is monitored for reactions to the therapeutic agent. The injection procedure is repeated at the other trigger points for multiple sites.

[20560, 20561]

The physician inserts a dry solid filament needle through the skin and into one or two muscles in 20560 and into three or more muscles in 20561. Indicated for myofascial pain relief and movement impairments, trigger points (focal, discrete spots of hypersensitive irritability identified within bands of muscle) are often the target of insertion. These points cause local or referred pain and may be formed by acute or repetitive trauma to the muscle tissue. This procedure, also known as dry needling or trigger-point acupuncture, does not involve the administration of injectable therapeutic agents.

20555

Interstitial radioelement application is a form of brachytherapy (treatment involving the placement of radioactive isotopes for internal radiation) in which the applicators are placed directly within the tissues of the body. The physician places needles or catheters into muscle and/or soft tissue close to the tumor bed for subsequent interstitial radioelement application to treat such tumors as soft tissue sarcoma. If the tumor bed is close to bone or neurovascular structures, materials such as gel-foam may be inserted between the catheters and the critical structures. Catheters may be secured to muscle with absorbable sutures. The radioactive isotopes, such as iridium-192, may be introduced directly after the needle or catheter insertion or on a subsequent visit. The isotopes are contained within tiny seeds (sources) that are left in place to deliver radiation over a period of weeks or months. They do not cause any harm after becoming inert. This method provides radiation to the prescribed body area while minimizing exposure to normal tissue.

20600-20611

After administering a local anesthetic, the physician inserts a needle through the skin and into a joint or bursa. A fluid sample may be removed from the joint for examination or a fluid may be injected for lavage or drug therapy. The needle is then withdrawn and pressure is applied to stop any bleeding. Report 20600 for arthrocentesis of a small joint or bursa, such as the fingers or toes, without ultrasound guidance; 20604 for arthrocentesis of a small joint or bursa, with ultrasound guidance, including permanent record and report; 20605 for an intermediate joint or bursa, such as the wrist, elbow, ankle, olecranon bursa, or temporomandibular or acromioclavicular area, without ultrasound guidance; 20606 for intermediate joint or bursa, with ultrasound guidance, including permanent record and report; 20610 for a major joint or bursa injection or aspiration, such as of the shoulder, hip, knee joint, or subacromial bursa, without ultrasound guidance; 20611 for a major joint or bursa, with ultrasound guidance, including permanent record and report.

20612

The physician aspirates and/or injects a ganglion cyst. After administering a local anesthetic, the physician inserts a needle through the skin and into the ganglion cyst. A ganglion cyst is a benign mass consisting of a thin capsule containing clear, mucinous fluid arising from an aponeurosis or tendon sheath, such as on the back of the wrist or foot. A fluid sample may be withdrawn from the cyst or a medicinal substance may be injected for therapy. The needle is withdrawn and pressure is applied to stop any bleeding.

20615

After administering a local anesthetic, the physician inserts a needle through the skin and into a bone cyst. A fluid sample is removed from the cyst and medication injected for lavage or drug therapy. The needle is withdrawn and pressure is applied to stop any bleeding.

20650

The physician makes a small skin incision laterally or medially over the affected bone. A Steinmann pin is drilled transversely through the bone so that an end protrudes through the skin from either side. An apparatus with a weight is attached to the pin, providing a traction force to reduce (reposition) and align the fracture as a temporary measure to stabilize it until the fracture itself can be addressed.

20660

The physician applies cranial tongs, a caliper, or a stereotactic frame to stabilize an injured cervical spine for radiography, a stretch test, surgery, or spinal realignment. The physician places the patient supine with the head supported just over the end of the table. The physician applies Betadine solution with sponges to the hair above the ears. The physician separates or removes hair 1 cm above the ears slightly posterior to the midlateral line. A local anesthetic is injected into the areas selected for pin insertion. Tongs are held in the appropriate position while both skull pins are inserted simultaneously, keeping the tongs equidistant from the skull on either side. The pins are advanced until the indicator button on one pin protrudes 2 to 3 mm. Lock nuts are applied and the pins are checked every two to three hours for proper tightness.

20661-20663

The physician applies a cranial halo to stabilize an injured cervical spine for radiography, traction, or to facilitate surgery in 20661. The physician places the patient supine (lying on the back) with the head supported just over the end of the stretcher. Skin and scalp are sterilized with a povidone-iodine solution. The halo is positioned about the patient's head below the area of greatest skull diameter. A local anesthetic is injected into the areas selected for frame pin insertion. The anterior pins are inserted first, followed by the posterior pins. Two diagonally opposed pins are tightened simultaneously until all four engage the skin and bone. Using a torque screwdriver, all are tightened and secured with nuts or set screws before attachment to a traction setup or to a halo vest or cast. Report 20662 for application of a pelvic halo and 20663 for a femoral halo. These procedures include removal of the halo.

20664

The physician places a cranial halo on the skull of a child whose skull is unusually thin because of a congenital or developmental problem. The physician sterilizes the skin and scalp with a povidone-iodine solution. The halo is positioned on the patient's head with six or more pins, which are advanced until firm, but not to the tension allowed by a normal skull. Diagonally opposed pins are tightened simultaneously. All are secured with nuts. This code includes the removal of the halo.

20665

A health care professional removes tongs or a halo applied by another professional. Maintaining alignment of the cervical spine, the provider unscrews the frame pins from the skull and removes the tongs or halo. Bone wax may be applied to the wounds to promote healing of the skull. Dressing may be applied to the skin wounds and the skin may be sutured.

20670

The physician makes a small incision overlying the site of the implant. The implant is located. The physician removes the implant by pulling or unscrewing it. The incision is closed with sutures and/or Steri-strips.

20680

The physician makes an incision overlying the site of the implant. Deep dissection is carried down to visualize the implant, which is usually below the muscle level and within bone. The physician uses instruments to remove the implant from the bone. The incision is repaired in layers using sutures, staples, and/or Steri-strips.

20690-20692

The physician applies an external fixation system to help a fracture or joint injury heal. This procedure is performed in addition to a coded treatment of fracture or joint injury unless listed as part of the basic procedure. This procedure uses an external fixator to stabilize an injury such as a simple fracture. One or more pins or wires may be used. Small stab incisions are made in the skin and a drill is used to make a hole into the bone. Each pin or wire is inserted into the bone through the drill holes and secured to an external fixation device. This holds the fracture or joint in a stable position. Report 20690 if uniplane fixation is applied and 20692 if multiplane fixation is applied.

20693

The physician performs adjustment or revision of external fixation to allow for healing that may be hindered due to the development of neurovascular problems, infections, loosening of pins, or failure of the bone fracture to heal. The physician places the patient under anesthesia. Additional pins, wires, rings, or bars may be needed or existing ones moved. The physician drills a hole through the bone and inserts the pin or other fixation instrument, which is attached to external frame devices.

20694

The physician removes the external fixation frame and pulls pins out manually while the patient is under anesthesia. Incisions are closed with sutures and Steri-strips.

20696-20697

Using stereotactic computer-assisted adjustment, such as a spatial frame, the physician applies a unilateral external fixation system with pins or wires in more than one plane (multiplane) to help a fracture or joint injury heal. This procedure is performed in addition to a reported treatment of fracture or joint injury unless listed as part of the basic procedure. This procedure uses an external fixator to stabilize an injury such as a simple fracture. Small stab incisions are made in the skin, and a drill is used to make a hole into the bone. Each pin or wire is inserted into the bone through the drill holes and secured to an external fixation device. This holds the fracture or joint in a stable position. Report 20696 for the application, including imaging, initial and subsequent alignments, assessments, and computations of adjustment schedules. Report 20697 for the removal and replacement of each strut.

20700-20701

In conjunction with open procedures (excluding those in which placement of a spacer is a component of the surgery) in which infection may be anticipated, suspected, or present, the physician or other qualified health care professional manually prepares and inserts a drug-delivery device that is not prefabricated into the deep tissues in 20700. Antibiotics or other therapeutic agents are mixed with a carrier substance, shaped into drug-delivery devices such as beads, nails, or spacers, and placed into the subfascial tissues. The associated procedures, such as arthrotomy, excisional debridement, open bone biopsies/excisions, sequestrectomy, or incision and drainage of abscesses or hematomas of deep tissues, are reported separately. Removal of a subfascial device, performed in conjunction with procedures such as excisional debridement, complex repairs, tissue transfers, or other wound reconstruction procedures, is reported with 20701.

20702-20703

In conjunction with open procedures (excluding those in which placement of a spacer is a component of the surgery) in which infection may be anticipated, suspected, or present, the physician or other qualified health care professional manually prepares and inserts a drug-delivery device that is not prefabricated into intramedullary spaces in 20702. Antibiotics or other therapeutic agents are mixed with a carrier substance, shaped into a drug-delivery device, and placed into the intramedullary space. The associated procedures, such as removal of deep implants, application or removal of external fixation systems, reimplantation procedures, bone incision/excision, open treatment of fractures/dislocations, malunion/nonunion repairs, and intramedullary implant insertions, are reported separately. One example includes the preparation of an antibiotic nail to insert into the intramedullary canal in the treatment of a proximal humeral fracture. Removal of an intramedullary device, performed in conjunction with procedures such as bone grafts or nonunion/malunion repair, is reported with 20703.

20704-20705

In conjunction with open procedures (excluding those in which placement of a spacer is a component of the surgery) in which infection may be anticipated, suspected, or present, the physician or other qualified health care professional manually prepares and inserts a drug-delivery device that is not prefabricated into intra-articular spaces in 20704. Antibiotics or other therapeutic agents are mixed with a carrier substance, shaped into a drug-delivery device, and placed into the intra-articular space. The associated procedures, such as joint arthrotomy, artificial disc removal, incision and drainage of deep abscess or hematoma of joint regions, and removal or revision of joint prostheses, are reported separately. In one example, antibiotic cement is placed into a silicone mold. After hardening, it is placed within the affected joint. Removal of an intra-articular device, performed in conjunction with procedures such as removal of artificial discs, arthrotomy, incision and drainage of a deep abscess or hematoma, or removal or revision of joint prostheses, is reported with 20705.

20802

The physician replants an arm following a complete amputation. The physician reattaches the upper extremity at a level between the elbow and shoulder. With the patient under anesthesia, the physician identifies the severed neurovascular structures, muscles, bone, and tendons. Each tissue is systematically reattached using sutures, wires, plates, or other fixation devices. Dead tissue is debrided. The skin is joined and closed with sutures after thorough cleaning and irrigation.

20805

The physician reattaches a severed forearm at a level between the wrist and the elbow. With the patient under anesthesia, the physician identifies each structure that has been cut or separated. The nerves, blood vessels, tendons, and bone are each reattached using sutures, wires, plates, or other fixation devices. Dead tissue is debrided. The skin is joined and closed with sutures after thorough cleaning and irrigation.

20808

The physician reattaches a hand that has been completely severed from the forearm between the wrist and the fingers. With the patient under anesthesia, the physician identifies the nerves, blood vessels, tendons, and bones. Each structure is reattached in a systematic fashion with debridement of dead tissue. Sutures, wires, plates, or other devices may be used. Copious irrigation is required. The overlying soft tissues and skin are joined with sutures in layers.

20816

The physician reattaches one of the four fingers, excluding the thumb, which has been completely severed from the hand at or near its articulation with its specific metacarpal bone. With the patient under anesthesia, the physician identifies the nerves, tendons, blood vessels, and bones. Dead tissue is debrided and the wound is irrigated. Each tissue is systematically reattached using sutures, wires, plates, or other devices. Skin is joined and sutured closed.

20822

The physician reattaches one of the four fingers, excluding the thumb, which has been completely severed from the hand at a level between the fingertip and the attachment of the finger to the hand itself. With the patient under anesthesia, the physician identifies severed structures, including nerves, blood vessels, tendons, and bones. Dead tissue is debrided and the wound is irrigated. Each tissue is systematically reattached using sutures, wires, plates, or other devices. Skin is joined in layers with sutures.

20824

The physician reattaches the thumb that has been completely severed from the hand at the attachment of the thumb to the hand itself. With the patient under anesthesia, the physician identifies severed structures, including nerves, blood vessels, tendons, and bones. Dead tissue is debrided and the wound is irrigated. Each tissue is systematically reattached using sutures, wires, plates, or other devices. Skin is joined in layers with sutures.

20827

The physician reattaches a thumb that has been completely severed from the hand at a point distal to where the thumb attaches to the hand. With the patient under anesthesia, the physician identifies severed tissues, including nerves, blood vessels, tendons, and bones. Dead tissue is debrided and the wound is irrigated. Each tissue is systematically reattached using sutures, wires, plates, or other devices. Skin is joined in layers with sutures.

20838

The physician reattaches a foot that has been completely amputated at or near the ankle. With the patient under anesthesia, the physician identifies severed structures, including blood vessels, nerves, tendons, and bones. Dead tissue is debrided and the wound is irrigated. Each tissue is reattached using sutures, wires, plates, pins, or other devices. Skin is joined in layers with sutures.

20900-20902

Bone grafts offer physicians excellent building blocks when repairing skeletal problems. The physician makes an incision overlying the rib, ilium, fibula, or other site from which the autograft will be harvested. Fascia and muscles are incised and retracted. A knife, chisel, cutter, or saw may be used to obtain the bone graft, which will be prepared as needed for implantation. Cancellous bone chips may be obtained, as well. The incision is closed with sutures. Report 20900 if the graft is small. Report 20902 if the graft is larger than a dowel or a button.

20910

The physician takes a cartilage graft from the rib for later use in reconstructing areas of the lower face such as the temporomandibular joint (TMJ). The physician makes a small incision in the skin through the pectoralis muscle and dissects adjacent tissues away near the sternum. The rib is exposed where the bone and cartilage meet. The cartilage is removed. After the cartilage is harvested, the donor site is closed with layered sutures.

20912

The physician takes a cartilage graft from the nasal septum for later use in an autologous reconstructive procedure. For instance, harvested nasal cartilage is often used as a spreader graft or as a nasal alar batten graft to repair a dysfunctional or collapsed internal nasal valve. Usually under local anesthesia and through a small internal incision (6-8 mm), the physician harvests a piece of septal cartilage from within the nose for later grafting. Graft sizes vary and can be 1-3 mm thick, from 4-8 mm wide, and up to 35 mm in length. A generous amount of cartilage must be maintained to continue functioning as nasal support.

20920

The physician harvests fascia lata by making a small incision over the lateral aspect of the lower thigh. A stripper instrument is advanced upward underneath the fascia as the physician maintains downward pressure on the cut end of fascia lata. Once the desired graft length is obtained, the cutting mechanism on the stripper is used to release the fascia from above. The stripper and graft are removed together and the wound is sutured. A compressive dressing is also applied.

20922

Fascia lata is a thick band of connective tissue lying underneath the skin of the thigh. It is also called the external investing fascia. To obtain a portion to use for a graft, the physician incises skin and subcutaneous tissue, elevates the flap off the fascia lata. The amount of connective tissue is acquired by incising and elevating the fascia of the thigh musculature. A small strip or patch may be obtained in this manner. The wound is closed primarily.

20924

The physician decides on a donor site and makes a cut down to the desired tendon. The tendon is severed and one end held with a hemostat. Dissection is carried to the muscular origin and the tendon is removed. A pressure dressing is applied.

20930-20931

In 20930, the physician inserts an osteopromotive material, such as bone morphogenetic protein (BMP), autogenous growth factor concentrate, bovine bone-derived osteoinductive protein, or recombinant human MP52, to promote bone healing and enhance fusion rates in patients undergoing spinal surgery. Alternately, the physician may use an allograft (a graft from the same species) that has been prepared as cancellous chips (morselized). The physician obtains a bone graft from a cadaver donor that is frozen or freeze dried until used. The physician prepares and inserts the allograft in a spinal procedure that is reported separately. In 20931, the physician inserts an allograft that has been prepared in a bicortical or tricortical shape for structural use.

20932-20934

These codes describe bone transplanted from the same species (person to person) after processing. These types of allografts function as an option for reconstruction related to large bone defects, particularly those due to bone tumors. The physician obtains a bone graft from a cadaver donor that is frozen or freeze dried until used. The physician prepares and inserts the allograft in a procedure that is reported separately. When performed, these procedures include templating, cutting, placement, and internal fixation. Osteoarticular (bone-containing joint surface) allografts are reported with 20932. Report 20933 for a partial cylindrical (hemicylindrical) allograft and 20934 for a complete cylindrical allograft.

20936

During a vertebral fusion or other spinal procedure that is reported separately, the physician may use bone fragments taken from the vertebral bodies adjacent to the affected disc, from the spinous process, or laminar fragment. Some of these may have been removed during the surgery or as part of the surgical approach. Local grafts prevent extra morbidity caused by obtaining an iliac or a tibial graft and lessen the possibility of cadaver-borne transmittable diseases. When grafts are harvested, they are obtained through the use of power tools or chisels. The grafts may be morselized, carved into pegs, or shaped as bars.

20937-20938

Bone grafts offer physicians excellent building blocks when repairing vertebral problems. The physician makes an incision over the ilium, fibula, or other site from which the autograft will be obtained. Fascia and muscles are incised and retracted. A knife, chisel, cutter, or saw may be used to obtain the autograft, which will be prepared as needed for implantation in the spine. In 20937, cancellous bone chips (morselized) are obtained. In 20938, structural bicortical or tricortical grafts are obtained. The incision is closed with sutures. Note that these codes are reported in addition to those for the primary procedure.

20939

During spinal surgery that is reported separately, the physician performs bone marrow aspiration (BMA) for bone grafting. The physician inserts a BMA needle containing a number of distal holes. A small volume of bone marrow is collected, usually no more than 2 cc's of aspirate, from various anatomic sites at the same time. Using a proprietary system designed to concentrate platelets and white blood cells from a combination of BMA and whole blood, the physician moistens the allograft or autograft with the platelet-rich plasma (PRP).

20950

The physician inserts an interstitial fluid pressure monitoring device into one or more muscle compartments of an extremity using a wick catheter, needle, or other method. The physician checks the monitoring device for escalation of pressure, which indicates developing compartment syndrome and tissue ischemia. Once the data has been gathered, the catheter or needle is removed.

20955-20962

The physician takes a bone graft from the fibula in 20955 for later reconstruction of another area. The physician makes an incision in the skin overlying the fibula. The bone is isolated and dissected away from adjacent structures with the small blood vessels that supply blood to the bone attached. The bone is grafted to the recipient area to eliminate a defect. The small blood vessels are sutured to blood vessels at the recipient site to provide blood flow to the grafted bone. After the graft is complete, the skin incision is closed with layered sutures. Report 20956 if the iliac crest bone is removed; 20957 if metatarsal bone is removed; and 20962 if other than fibula, iliac crest, or metatarsal bone is used for the graft.

20969

The physician makes an incision in the skin overlying the area of harvest from a bone other than the iliac crest, metatarsal, or great toe. The physician includes a portion of the overlying skin to be removed along with bone. The skin remains viable by being supplied with blood from vessels coming from the bone. The bone is isolated and dissected away from adjacent structures with the small blood vessels that supply blood to the bone still attached. This allows the surgeon to reconstruct a defect of bone and skin using a grafted osteocutaneous flap.

20970-20973

The physician harvests a portion of the iliac crest along with overlying skin in 20970. The physician makes an incision in the skin overlying the iliac crest. The bone is isolated and dissected away from adjacent structures with the small blood vessels that supply blood to the bone still attached. In this case, the surgeon usually includes the deep circumflex iliac artery. The wound is closed, suction drains placed, and a pressure dressing is applied. Report 20972 if the procedure is performed at the metatarsal. Report 20973 if the procedure is performed on the great toe with web space.

20974

The physician performs electrical stimulation of bone to promote fracture or defect healing. The physician places electrodes over the skin surface on opposite sides of a fracture or defect and administers a low voltage current. This is a nonsurgical technique used to stimulate bone healing.

20975

The physician performs electrical stimulation of bone to promote fracture or defect healing. An incision over the site of the fracture or defect is made. The physician places an electrode, known as a cathode, into the site of a fracture or defect and a second electrode, known as an anode, in the nearby soft tissue. The cathode and anode are connected to power generating units, which may be implanted or worn externally. The generator administers a low voltage current to the site through the cathode for several months.

20979

A rehabilitation specialist or physical therapist applies low-intensity ultrasound to a bone by placing a transducer on the skin to stimulate bone healing.

20982-20983

Percutaneous radiofrequency ablation of bone tumors is a minimally invasive procedure that may be done as a safe and effective alternative or adjunct to radiation/chemotherapy for metastatic bone cancer lesions or as an effective alternative/adjunct to surgical treatment for benign, but painful, osteoid osteomas. Tumors are destroyed using heat energy, in which a needle or probe is inserted into the tumor and the tumor is heated and destroyed, or by extreme cold/freezing the tumors. These procedures are performed with the patient under conscious sedation or general anesthesia. The patient is connected to an electrical circuit by placing grounding pads on the thighs. A tiny needle-electrode with an insulated shaft and an uninsulated tip is inserted through the skin, directly into the tumor. Ultrasound, CT scan, or MRI may be used to guide the needle. These procedures include imaging guidance when performed. The electrode is connected to a radiofrequency generator. The appropriate amount of wattage and current are sent through the needle from the generator. Active ablation is done for about 10 to 15 minutes. The energy leads to cell death and coagulation, resulting in a sphere of dead tissue after every treatment session. A small margin of normal tissue next to the tumors is also burned in order to try to leave no single tumor cell behind. Report 20982 for radiofrequency ablation and 20983 for cryoablation.

20985

Imageless computer-assisted surgery (CAS) is an adjunct process used in conjunction with certain orthopaedic procedures. Using such tools as markers, reference frames, intraoperative sensing, and computer workstations, imageless computer-assisted navigational procedures increase visualization of the surgical field and aid in precise navigation with minimally invasive approaches. Imageless navigation uses angles and measurements (kinematics) for anatomy determination. Through direct imageless applications, landmarks are established on a universal limb model. This application requires touch-pointing the anatomic landmarks, which are then registered in the computer for use in accurate navigation and measurement in relation to any bone or instrument movement as the surgery is performed. This application provides a way to establish coordinates as an aid for precisely locating anatomical structures in open or percutaneous procedures without the use of preoperative or intraoperative images. Code 20985 is reported in addition to the procedure code when the physician uses an imageless system to help determine coordinates.

21010
The physician makes an incision into the temporomandibular joint (TMJ). The physician may use several incisional patterns, including the preauricular approach, making an incision through the skin anterior to the contour of the ear. The physician may also approach the TMJ through an incision inside or behind the ear. The physician dissects the tissue layers away until the TMJ is exposed and the joint can be incised. The skin incision is closed with sutures.

21011-21014
The physician removes a soft tissue tumor from the subcutaneous tissues (21011-21012) or the subfascial tissues (21013-21014) of the face or scalp, not involving bone. An incision is made over the tumor and dissection exposes it. The tumor and any adjacent tissue that may be affected are excised. Large resections may be needed. The type of tumor determines the extent of the tumor margin resection area. Muscle or fascia may need to be repaired and drains may be placed. The surgical wound may be repaired with layers of sutures, staples, or Steri-strips. Report 21011 (subcutaneous) or 21013 (subfascial) for excision of tumors whose resected area is less than 2 cm; report 21012 (subcutaneous) or 21014 (subfascial) for excision of tumors 2 cm or greater.

21015-21016
The physician performs a radical resection of a malignant soft tissue tumor (i.e., sarcoma) from the face or scalp, not involving bone. An incision is made over the tumor and dissection exposes it. The tumor and any adjacent tissue that may be affected by the spread of the neoplasm are excised. Large resections may be needed. The type and stage of the lesion determines the extent of the tumor margin resection area. Muscle or fascia may need to be repaired and drains may be placed. The surgical wound may be closed using simple or intermediate repair. Alternately, complex closure, adjacent tissue transfer, or graft may be required; these would be reported separately. Report 21015 for excision of tumors whose resected area is less than 2 cm and 21016 for excision of tumors 2 cm or greater.

21025
The physician removes infected or dead bone tissue from the mandible. This procedure can be performed intraorally through the mucosa or extraorally through a skin incision. If only a small amount of bone is affected, the physician may saucerize the area by grinding the dead bone away with drills or osteotomes. Healthy bone and the continuity of the mandible are left intact. Antibiotic-impregnated acrylic beads may be implanted into the surgical site to stop infection after the removal of bone. These beads are removed at a later time. Extensive bone removal in large sections or blocks may require a separate bone harvesting/grafting procedure to repair continuity defects. The incisions are closed simply.

21026
The physician removes dead or infected bone from facial bones. A transoral incision in the maxillary buccal vestibule is the most frequent approach. Facial incisions would only be used for large lesions or for additional surgical access. The physician reflects the overlying mucosa, exposing the dead bone. Drills, saws, and osteotomes are used to remove the bone. The transoral incisions are closed in a single layer. Any cutaneous incision is closed in layers.

21029
The physician removes a benign tumor from a facial bone by contouring the excess bone down to the appropriate structure. A transoral incision is made in the maxillary buccal vestibule. The physician reflects the overlying mucosa, exposing the excessive bone. Rotary burrs, files, and osteotomes are used to remove this bone. The transoral incision is closed in a single layer.

21030
The physician removes a cyst or benign tumor from the maxilla (upper jaw) or the zygoma (arched cheekbone) by enucleation and/or curettage, not requiring osteotomy. Using an intraoral approach, the physician incises and reflects a mucosal flap of tissue inside the mouth overlying the tumor. In an extraoral approach, the physician approaches the defect through an external skin incision. The tumor is identified and removed from the maxilla or zygoma by scraping with a curette or by cutting the tumor out in such a way as to leave it intact and remove it whole. The mucosal flap is sutured primarily or the subcutaneous tissues and skin incisions on the face are closed with layered sutures.

21031
The physician removes a benign outgrowth of bone (torus mandibularis) most commonly from the lingual (tongue) side of the mandible. Using an intraoral approach, the physician makes an incision in the mucosa overlying the outgrowth of bone and reflects the tissue. The excess bone is removed with a drill or osteotome. The mucosal incision is closed with sutures.

21032
The physician excises a torus palatinus (a bony protuberance), usually found at the junction of the intermaxillary and transverse palatine structures, by making an incision through the mucosa overlying the protuberance. The torus is exposed. Drills, osteotomes, or files are used to remove and contour the bone. The tissue is sutured directly over the bone. Some soft

tissue may be excised prior to closure for adaptation over the newly contoured bone.

21034
The physician excises a malignant tumor from the maxilla (upper jaw) or the zygoma (arched cheekbone). Incisions include transoral (e.g., maxillary buccal vestibular) and facial (e.g., Weber-Ferguson). The bony mass is excised with the use of drills, saws, and osteotomes. The tumor is removed to "free margins" as determined with intraoperative tissue specimens sent to the pathologist for immediate microscopic examination. The physician may remove teeth and overlying mucosa. Some surgical defects may require immediate soft tissue reconstruction (e.g., myocutaneous flaps). Transoral incisions are closed in a single layer and facial incisions are closed in layers. Intraoral surgical splints may be used.

21040
The physician removes a cyst or benign tumor from the mandible by enucleation and/or curettage, not requiring osteotomy. Using an intraoral approach, the physician incises and reflects a mucosal flap of tissue inside the mouth overlying the tumor. In an extraoral approach, the physician approaches the defect through an external skin incision. The tumor is identified and removed from the mandible by scraping with a curette or by cutting the tumor out in such a way as to leave it intact and remove it whole. The mucosal flap is sutured primarily or subcutaneous tissue and skin incisions on the face are closed with layered sutures.

21044
The physician removes a malignant tumor from the mandible. Through an intraoral and/or extraoral approach, the physician isolates and dissects the mandibular tumor. The tumor and surrounding tissues are removed. The tissues are closed with layered sutures or may be packed and left open. A reconstructive procedure, such as bone harvesting, may be necessary and is reported separately.

21045
The physician removes a malignant tumor from the mandible in a radical resection. An intraoral and/or extraoral approach is used to reach the site of the tumor. The tumor and surrounding tissues are removed. Resection or removal of a part or all of the mandible is performed. Immediate or delayed reconstruction with bone grafts, tissue rearrangement, flaps, or prosthetic devices is sometimes required. The skin incisions are closed with layered sutures.

21046-21047
The physician excises a cyst or benign tumor from the mandible (lower jaw) by intraoral osteotomy in 21046 and by extraoral osteotomy and partial mandibulectomy in 21047. For the intraoral approach, the physician incises and reflects a mucosal flap of tissue inside the mouth overlying the tumor to reach the bone. In an extraoral approach, the physician approaches the defect through an external skin incision and dissects down through the tissue layers to reach the tumor. The tumor is identified and removed along with overlying bone by cutting into the mandible using a drill or osteotome. Additional bone removal from the mandible is done in 21047 to excise the tumor fully. With large tumors, the surgical wounds may be packed and sutured or reconstructive procedures such as harvesting of bone for grafting may be needed, depending on the size of the surgical wound. The mucosal flap is sutured primarily or the subcutaneous tissues and skin incisions on the face are closed with layered sutures.

21048-21049
The physician excises a cyst or benign tumor from the maxilla (upper jaw) by intraoral osteotomy in 21048 and by extraoral osteotomy and partial maxillectomy in 21049. For the intraoral approach, the physician incises and reflects a mucosal flap of tissue inside the mouth overlying the tumor to reach the bone. In an extraoral approach, the physician approaches the defect through an external skin incision and dissects down through the tissue layers to reach the tumor. The tumor is identified and removed along with overlying bone by cutting into the maxilla using a drill or osteotome. Additional bone removal from the maxilla is done in 21049 to excise the tumor fully. With large tumors, the surgical wounds may be packed and sutured or reconstructive procedures, such as harvesting of bone for grafting, may be needed, depending on the size of the surgical wound. The mucosal flap is sutured primarily or the subcutaneous tissues and skin incisions on the face are closed with layered sutures.

21050
The physician removes the condyle of the mandible, the posterior, rounded projection on the angled branch of the jaw that articulates with the temporal bone. An incision is usually made in the skin anterior to the contour of the ear. The physician dissects the tissue layers until the condyle is exposed. The condyle is cut with drills or saws from the mandible and removed. An additional incision just under the angle of the mandible may be required. The area can be reconstructed with bone and cartilage, or a prosthetic condyle may be inserted. The skin incision is closed with layered sutures and a pressure dressing may be applied.

21060
The physician removes part or all of the meniscus (articular disc) of the temporomandibular joint. An incision is usually made in the skin anterior to the contour of the ear. The physician dissects the tissue layers until the meniscus is exposed. The meniscus is clamped and removed. The joint may be left without a disc or the disc may be replaced with tissue grafted from other areas of the body or with an artificial disc. The skin incision is closed with layered sutures and a pressure dressing may be applied.

Musculoskeletal

21070
The physician removes the diseased or fractured coronoid process of the mandible, the anterior projection on the angled branch of the jaw to which the temporal muscle is attached. The physician makes an incision intraorally along the external oblique ridge of the mandible. The tissue is reflected from the bone, exposing the coronoid process. Using drills and/or osteotomes, the coronoid process is clamped and sectioned from the mandible. The muscle attachments are cut from the coronoid process and will retract, forming scar tissue. The coronoid process is removed. The mucosal incision is closed primarily.

21073
With the patient under general anesthesia or monitored anesthesia care (MAC), the physician applies a downward pressure on the posterior teeth while pushing the mandible back over the articular eminence and returning it to its correct position. No incisions are made and no intermaxillary fixation is used.

21076
The physician or other qualified health care provider fabricates a custom obturator prosthesis to separate the mouth from other structures of the face and skull while performing surgery or allowing facial injuries to heal. The provider identifies the extent of the patient's injuries and determines the type of prosthesis that is required. Impressions of the mouth are taken to make models. A custom obturator prosthesis for a particular patient is prepared from the models.

21077
The physician or other qualified health care provider fabricates a custom orbital prosthesis for the orbit of the eye for the purpose of protecting surrounding structures while surgery is performed or for the healing of facial and skull injuries. The provider identifies the extent of the patient's injuries or disease to determine the exact nature of the required prosthesis. Impressions of the orbit of the eye are taken and used to make models. A custom prosthesis for a particular patient is made from the models.

21079-21080
The physician or other qualified health care provider fabricates an obturator prosthesis to provide a separation between the mouth and the surgical site and/or protect the surgical site while assisting the patient's ability to talk and chew. Impressions are made of the mouth. The impressions are used to make models from which a custom obturator prosthesis is fabricated. The provider makes an interim or temporary obturator prosthesis in 21079 and a definitive obturator prosthesis in 21080, which separates the nasal and sinus complex from the mouth.

21081
The physician or other qualified health care provider fabricates a prosthesis used in a mandibular resection procedure. Impressions are made of the mandible. The impression is fashioned into a cast model, which the provider uses to construct an external prosthetic device.

21082
The physician or other qualified health care provider fabricates a prosthesis used to augment the palate. Impressions are made of the maxilla and palate. The impression is fashioned into a cast model. The prosthesis is fabricated from this cast.

21083
The physician or other qualified health care provider fabricates a palatal lift prosthesis for a patient who requires the prosthesis to maintain velopharyngeal competence. Impressions are made of the maxilla and palate. The impression is fashioned into a cast model. A customized prosthesis is fabricated from this cast.

21084
The physician or other qualified health care provider fabricates a prosthesis used to aid speech. An impression is made of the affected area and the provider customizes a prosthetic device from a cast model of the impression.

21085
The physician or other qualified health care provider fabricates a splint used in an oral surgical procedure. An impression is made of the area and the physician customizes the splint from the cast model of the impression. These splints may be used in orthognathic reconstructive jaw surgery (repositioning of jaws), for repair of traumatic injuries, or in ablative tumor surgery with or without jaw resection.

21086
The physician or other qualified health care provider designs and prepares a prosthesis for the auricle (pinna or external ear). An impression is taken, from which a cast is made, and the prosthesis is fabricated from this mold. The mold is shaped and honed to fit.

21087
The physician or other qualified health care provider makes a nasal prosthesis after resection of part or all of the nose. A full-face impression or moulage is taken before or after removal of the nose. A stone cast of the patient's face is made from the moulage. Presurgical photographs of the patient are also used as a guide. A customized nasal prosthesis is fabricated on the face cast. The prosthesis is made of latex and is painted to match the color of the patient's skin. This artificial nose is placed and maintained with skin adhesive glue.

21088
The physician or other qualified health care provider makes a facial prosthesis after resection of part or all of the face. A full-face impression or moulage is taken before or after removal of the affected facial area. A stone cast of the patient's face is made from the moulage. Presurgical photographs of the patient are also used as a guide. A customized prosthesis is fabricated on the face cast. The prosthesis is made of latex and is painted to match the color of the patient's

skin. This artificial face is placed and maintained with skin adhesive glue.

21100

The physician places the halo for maxillofacial fixation over the patient's head and tightens four screws into place. The halo is connected to interdental fixation, which has the jaws wired together. Arch bars, ivy loops, or other wires are attached to the teeth and wired together. For edentulous patients (without teeth), or partially edentulous patients, dentures or splints may be wired to the jaws first and wired together to provide intermaxillary fixation. Orthodontic appliances may also be used.

21110

The physician applies interdental fixation to wire the jaws together for conditions other than a fracture or dislocation. Arch bars, ivy loops, or other wires are attached to the teeth and wired together. For edentulous patients (without teeth), or partially edentulous patients, dentures or splints may be wired to the jaws first and wired together to provide intermaxillary fixation. Orthodontic appliances may also be used.

21116

The physician injects a radiopaque dye into the temporomandibular joint. The physician or radiologist threads a small catheter into the temporomandibular joint by inserting a needle through the skin and into the superior and/or inferior joint spaces. Dye is injected. Separately reported radiographs are taken to study the soft tissue anatomy of the joint, such as the articular disc or ligaments.

21120-21123

The physician places an implant or a graft onto the chin to augment or enlarge it. Various materials can be used, including tissue grafted from the patient's own body or taken from a tissue bank. Prosthetic devices may also be used. This procedure is most commonly performed from an intraoral approach. The physician makes an incision in the mandibular labial vestibule inside the lower lip. The mucosa is reflected from the chin and the implanted material placed between the mucosa and the bone. A skin incision may also be made under the chin. The implant may be secured to the bone using wires or screws or may be left to be held in place by the surrounding tissue. The mucosa is sutured simply. Report 21121 if a sliding osteotomy is performed to correct the chin; 21122 if two or more osteotomies are performed; and 21123 if interpositional bone grafts are used for the genioplasty.

21125

The physician uses prosthetic material to augment the body or angle of the mandible. The physician may use an intraoral approach or may make skin incisions extraorally below the body or angle of the mandible. The physician dissects tissues away and the bone of the body or angle is exposed. A synthetic material is placed on the mandible to augment the contours. The material is secured with screws or wires. The incisions are sutured simply.

21127

The physician uses a bone graft to augment the body or angle of the mandible. The physician harvests bone from another site on the patient's body, most commonly the rib, hip, or skull, and repairs the surgically created wound of the harvest site. The physician may use an intraoral approach or skin incisions. The physician dissects adjacent structures away and the body or angle of the mandible is exposed. The graft is placed on an area of the body or angle to augment the contours. The graft may also be placed between portions of bone of the body or angle (interpositional grafting). The graft is secured with screws or wires. The intraoral incisions are sutured simply. The extraoral incisions are closed with layered sutures.

21137

The physician performs surgery on the forehead to correct a skeletal deformity. With the patient under anesthesia, the physician makes an incision in the hairline to expose the forehead of the skull. The deformity in the bone is identified and fully exposed. The physician uses a variety of surgical instruments to reshape the bone to make it follow a more normal contour. The wound is irrigated and closed in layers.

21138

The physician performs surgery on the forehead to correct a skeletal deformity using the application of prostheses or bone grafts to obtain a more normal contour. With the patient under anesthesia, the physician makes an incision in the hairline to expose the forehead of the skull. The deformity in the bone is identified and fully exposed. The physician uses a variety of surgical instruments to reshape the bone to make it follow a more normal contour. Prostheses may be applied and/or autografts may be harvested and applied as part of the procedure. The wounds are irrigated and closed in layers.

21139

The physician corrects a skeletal deformity of the frontal sinus or repairs the anterior frontal sinus wall. An incision is made at the forehead hairline or the eyebrows. The forehead is exposed directly over the frontal sinus wall. The deformity or deficit is identified. Soft tissue is debrided. The physician reshapes the anterior wall of the sinus. If the wall is prominent or badly misshapen, the physician elevates it from the forehead and resets it in the appropriate anatomic and cosmetic position. Fixation devices such as wires may be required to maintain the repaired wall. The wound is irrigated and closed in layers. A soft dressing is applied.

21141-21143

The physician performs a LeFort I osteotomy to repair congenital malformations or acquired deformities of the facial bones, without using a bone graft. With the patient under anesthesia, the physician makes a

Musculoskeletal

horizontal cut through the maxillary sinuses and nasal septum through an intraoral incision, and into the pterygoid fissure. Surgical instruments are used to complete the separation of the maxilla from the skull base. The maxilla is down-fractured to mobilize it and can be moved into the proper predetermined position. If segmental surgery in the maxilla was necessary, the mobilized segments are held in position by a template secured to the upper teeth. Maxillary malpositioning is corrected and the maxilla is wired to the mandible, which is positioned as a whole unit. Rigid fixation of the maxilla is achieved with miniplates or intermaxillary wires. The operative site is irrigated with antibiotic solution and the oral mucosa is closed as needed. Report 21141 if a single piece segment if repositioned; 21142 for lower maxillary midface reconstruction with two piece segmental movement; and 21143 if multiple piece (three or more) osteotomies are performed.

21145-21147

The physician performs a LeFort I osteotomy and bone grafts to repair congenital malformations or acquired deformities of the facial bones. With the patient under anesthesia, the physician makes a horizontal cut through the maxillary sinuses and nasal septum through an intraoral incision and into the pterygoid fissure. Surgical instruments are used to complete the separation of the maxilla from the skull base. The maxilla is down-fractured to mobilize it for movement into the proper predetermined position. If segmental surgery in the maxilla was necessary, the mobilized segments are held in position by a template secured to the upper teeth. Maxillary malpositioning is corrected. Cranial or iliac bone grafts are placed and the donor site repaired. The maxilla is wired to the mandible, which is positioned as a whole unit. Rigid fixation of the maxilla is achieved with miniplates or intermaxillary wires. The operative site is irrigated with antibiotic solution and the oral mucosa is closed as needed. Report 21145 if a single piece segment is repositioned; 21146 for lower maxillary midface reconstruction with two piece segmental movement; and 21147 if multiple piece (three or more) segmental osteotomies are performed.

21150

The physician reconstructs the midface to correct developmental or acquired skeletal deformities. The physician may use a variety of incisions, including a bicoronal scalp flap, lower eyelid, and transoral incisions. Through these incisions, the nasofrontal junction, inferior orbital rims, and maxilla are exposed. Osteotomies of the pyramidal naso-orbitomaxillary midface (LeFort II) are performed with saws, burrs, or osteotomes. The midface is down-fractured from the stable bone. The physician removes excess bone at fracture sites to accommodate anterior intrusion (superior repositioning) of the midface. The midface is reduced in the desired position with wires, plates, and/or screws. The transoral incision is closed in a single layer. Lower eyelid and scalp incisions are closed in layers. Intermaxillary fixation may be applied.

21151

The physician reconstructs the midface to correct developmental or acquired skeletal deformities. The physician may use a variety of incisions, including a bicoronal scalp flap, lower eyelid, and transoral incisions. Through these incisions, the physician exposes the nasofrontal junction, inferior orbital rims, and maxilla. Osteotomies of the pyramidal midface (LeFort II) are performed with saws, burrs, or osteotomes. The midfacial segment is down-fractured from the stable bone and rotated or advanced with precise measurement into a new position. The physician reduces the midface with wires, plates, and/or screws. The physician harvests bone grafts from the patient's hip, rib, or skull and closes the surgically created wound. The interpositional bone grafts are placed between the bony interfaces of the repositioned naso-orbitomaxillary midface. The transoral incisions are closed in a single layer. Lower eyelid and scalp incisions are closed in layers. Intermaxillary fixation may be applied.

21154

The physician reconstructs the midface to correct developmental or acquired skeletal deformities. The physician uses a variety of incisions, including a bicoronal scalp flap, lower eyelid, and transoral incisions. Complete separation of the midface from the cranial base is necessary. Surgical fractures are made through the zygomas, orbits, and bones of the nasofrontal region. Osteotomies of the complete midface (LeFort III) are performed with saws, burrs, or osteotomes. The midface is down-fractured from the stable cranial bone and placed with precise measurement into presurgically determined position. The physician reduces the midface with wires, plates, and/or screws. The physician harvests bone grafts from the patient's hip, rib, or skull, and closes the surgically created wound. The interpositional bone grafts are placed between the bony interfaces of the midface. The transoral incisions are closed in a single layer. Lower eyelid and scalp incisions are closed in layers. Intermaxillary fixation may be applied.

21155

The physician reconstructs both the midface and the maxilla to correct developmental or acquired skeletal deformities. The physician uses a variety of incisions, including a bicoronal scalp flap, lower eyelid, and transoral incisions. Complete separation of the midface (LeFort III) from the cranial base is necessary. Additionally, horizontal down-fracture of the maxilla is necessary to correct alignment of the teeth. Surgical fractures are made through the zygomas, orbits, and bones of the nasofrontal region with saws, burrs, or osteotomes. The physician also makes a horizontal osteotomy, separating the maxilla from the midface. The midface is down-fractured from the stable cranial base and the maxilla is down-fractured from the midface segment. Both the midface and the maxilla are placed into new positions and reduced with wires, plates, and/or screws. The physician harvests bone grafts from the patient's hip, rib, or skull, and closes the surgically created wound. The interpositional bone grafts are placed between the bony interfaces of the maxilla and the midface. The transoral incisions are closed in a single layer. Lower eyelid and scalp incisions are closed in layers. Intermaxillary fixation may be applied.

21159

The physician reconstructs the midface with the forehead to correct developmental or acquired skeletal deformities. Surgical fractures are made through the zygomas, frontal bone, and orbits. Complete separation of the midface with the frontal bone from the cranial base is necessary. The physician uses a variety of incisions, including a bicoronal scalp flap, eyelid, and transoral incisions. Osteotomies of the complete midface (LeFort III) together with the frontal bone are performed with saws, burrs, or osteotomes. The midface with the frontal bone is down-fractured from the stable cranial base. The midface and frontal bone are placed with precise measurement into new positions and reduced with wires, plates, and/or screws. The physician harvests bone grafts from the patient's hip, rib, or skull and closes the surgically created wound. The interpositional bone grafts are placed between the bony interfaces of the newly positioned midface and forehead segment. The transoral incisions are closed in a single layer. Eyelid and scalp incisions are closed in layers. Intermaxillary fixation may be applied.

21160

The physician reconstructs both the midface with the forehead and the maxilla to correct developmental or acquired skeletal deformities. Complete separation of the midface with the frontal bone from the cranial base is necessary along with horizontal down-fracture of the maxilla from the midface. Surgical fractures are made through the zygomas, frontal bone, and orbits. The physician uses a variety of incisions, including a bicoronal scalp flap, eyelid, and transoral incisions. Osteotomies of the complete midface (LeFort III) together with the frontal bone and the lower maxilla from the midface are performed with saws, burrs, or osteotomes. The midface and frontal bones are down-fractured from the stable cranial base and the maxilla is horizontally down-fractured from the midface. The midface with the frontal bone and the maxilla are placed into new positions and reduced with wires, plates, and/or screws. The physician harvests bone grafts from the patient's hip, rib, or skull and closes the surgically created wound. The interpositional bone grafts are placed between the bony interfaces of the maxilla and the midface segment. The transoral incisions are closed in a single layer. Eyelid and scalp incisions are closed in layers. Intermaxillary fixation may be applied.

21172

The physician performs reconstructive surgery on the lower forehead and superior-lateral orbit of the eye to correct skeletal abnormalities, with or without grafts. The physician may use a variety of incisions, including through the eyelids and scalp, to obtain access to the site. The soft tissues are dissected as needed to expose the bones. The physician performs osteotomies of the forehead and orbit as needed. The bones are manipulated and realigned to the desired position. The physician may obtain bone grafts from the patient's hip, rib, or skull that can be placed to augment the forehead and orbit reconstruction. The bones are held in place with the use of wires, plates, or screws. The wounds are irrigated and each closed in layers.

21175

The physician performs reconstructive surgery on the lower forehead and both superior lateral orbital rims to correct skeletal abnormalities of the cranium, with or without grafts. The physician utilizes a variety of incisions about the eyes, forehead, and scalp to gain access to these bones. The soft tissues are dissected as needed to expose the bones. Several osteotomies of the forehead and orbits are made so that the deformity can be corrected. The bones are manipulated, contoured, and shifted as needed to place them in the desired positions. The physician may obtain bone grafts from the patient's hip, rib, or skull that can be placed to augment the reconstruction. Various internal fixation devices are employed to hold the reduction rigidly in place, such as wires, pins, plates, or screws. The wounds are irrigated and closed in layers.

21179-21180

The physician performs reconstructive surgery of the forehead and the supraorbital rims of both eyes to correct skeletal deformities of the cranium. With the patient under anesthesia, the physician uses any of a variety of incisions about the eyes, forehead, and scalp to gain access to these bones. The soft tissues are dissected as needed to expose the bones. Osteotomies of the bones are performed in multiple places to facilitate manipulating the bones into the desired position. The bones are shaped as needed. In 21179, the physician utilizes allografts or synthetic prosthetic material to augment the reconstruction. In 21180, the physician employs autografts, harvested from the patient's hip, rib, or skull. Pins, wires, plates, and screws are used to hold the bones and graft in rigid reduction. The wounds are irrigated and closed in layers.

21181

The physician performs surgery to correct distortion expansion or deformity of a cranial bone caused by a benign extracranial lesion. The physician utilizes any of a variety of incisions to access the site. The incisions are carried deep to the bone and the tumor is identified and exposed. The physician uses surgical instruments to debride, reshape, and contour the cranial bone to conform to its normal anatomic position and profile. The bone and wounds are irrigated and closed in layers.

21182-21184

The physician performs reconstructive surgery of the cranial bones including the orbit walls and rims, forehead, and nasoethmoid complex following the excision of benign tumors from within and without the cranium. The physician utilizes a variety of incisions through the mouth, eyelids, and scalp to gain access to these bones. The incisions are carried deep, soft tissues are reflected, and the bones are individually identified and exposed. Osteotomies are performed as needed to surgically fracture and manipulate the bones into their desired and acceptable positions. This may require advancement of the forehead. Bone grafts are harvested from a site such as the hip, skull, or ribs. Multiple grafts may be required to augment and stabilize the reconstructed cranial bones following tumor removal. Internal fixation devices such as wires, plates, and screws are used to hold the reduction securely in place. The incisions are all irrigated and closed in layers. Report 21182 if the total area of bone grafting is less than 40 sq cm; 21183 if the total area of bone grafting is greater than 40 sq cm but less than 80 sq cm; and 21184 if the total area of bone grafting is greater than 80 sq cm.

21188

The physician reconstructs the midface to correct developmental or traumatic skeletal deformities. Reconstruction includes both osteotomies and bone grafts. The physician may use a variety of incisions, including a bicoronal scalp flap, eyelid, and transoral incisions. Through the incisions, the physician performs osteotomies as necessary of the midface with saws, burrs, or osteotomes. The osteotomies performed here do not follow the standard LeFort surgical fracture lines. The midfacial bones are down-fractured from the stable cranial base. The midface is placed with precise measurement into a new position. Bone grafts are harvested from the patient's hip, rib, or skull and the surgically created wound is closed. The interpositional bone grafts are placed between the bony interfaces of the repositioned maxilla and midface. Internal fixation devices such as wires, plates, and screws are used to hold the reduction securely in place. The transoral incisions are closed in a single layer. Eyelid and scalp incisions are closed in layers. Intermaxillary fixation may be applied.

21193-21194

The physician reconstructs the ramus of the mandible using various osteotomies (bone cuts) to correct mandibular deformities. Vertical, horizontal, L, inverted L, and C osteotomies are used. The type of osteotomy refers to the shape and direction of the bone cuts. The physician makes a skin incision below the angle of the mandible. Vertical ramus and horizontal osteotomies may also be accomplished from an intraoral approach. The tissue is dissected to the mandible and the bone of the mandibular ramus is exposed. Bone cuts are made in various shapes according to necessity using drills, saws, or osteotomes. The physician moves part of the separated mandible into a new position. The osteotomy cuts are securely reduced with wires, screws, or plates. The incision is sutured. No bone grafts are used in 21193. Report 21194 if bone grafts are taken from another site on the patient's body, such as the rib, hip, or skull, and used to aid reconstruction and healing of the mandible.

21195-21196

The physician reconstructs the mandibular ramus to lengthen, set back, or rotate the mandible. Using an intraoral approach, the physician makes an incision overlying the external oblique ridge, through the mucosa near the second mandibular molars. The mandibular ramus is exposed by reflecting the tissue from both sides of the ramus. Drills, saws, and/or osteotomes are used to cut the mandible along the inside, top, and outside surfaces of the bone, but not completely through. The physician uses osteotomes and/or other instruments to pry the mandible apart along the bone cuts in a sagittal plane. Once separated, the physician moves the mandible into the desired position and holds the bone in reduction using wires. No rigid internal fixation devices are used in 21195. In 21196, screws or plates are placed in or on the bone. The physician may also make small 0.5 cm skin incisions near the mandibular angle, through which instruments place the plates or screws. The mucosal and skin incisions are sutured closed.

21198-21199

The physician performs an osteotomy on a segment of the mandible to correct a localized deformity. The teeth are moved within a segment or block of bone. Using an intraoral approach, the physician makes an incision in the mucosa to expose the segment of bone to be moved. Drills, saws, and/or osteotomes are used to cut a section of the alveolar bone. These cuts do not extend through the mandible, but include only a segment above the inferior border. The segment is moved into the desired position and held in reduction with wires, screws, or plates. The segment may also be held in place by a preformed acrylic interocclusal splint. The mucosa is sutured simply. Report 21198 when a segmental osteotomy of the mandible is performed. Report 21199 when a segmental osteotomy of the mandible is performed and the genioglossus (primary tongue muscle) is advanced.

21206

The physician performs an osteotomy on a segment of the maxilla to correct a localized deformity. The teeth are moved within a segment or block of bone. Using a circumvestibular incision, the physician exposes the segment of bone to be moved. Drills, saws, and/or osteotomes are used to cut a section of the alveolar bone. These cuts do not extend through the maxilla, but include only a segment. The segment is moved into the desired position and held in reduction with wires, screws, or plates. The segment may also be held in place by a preformed acrylic interocclusal splint. The mucosa is sutured simply and intermaxillary fixation may be placed.

21208

The physician augments the facial bones with implanted grafts or prosthetic devices, altering the contours of the face. The physician may use an intraoral approach or other incisions to access the operative site. The tissue is dissected, exposing the bone for augmentation. A bone graft is taken from another part of the body, such as the hip, rib, or skull, and grafted onto the facial bone to contour the face. Other materials such as prosthetic implants or donor bone may also be used. The implant is secured to the bone using screws, wires, or plates. The mucosa is sutured simply.

21209

The physician removes protrusions of excess or misshaped facial bone to reduce the contours of the face. The physician may use an intraoral approach or other incisions to access the operative site. The tissue is dissected, exposing the bone for reduction. A reciprocation saw or drill is used to cut and remove the bone, reducing its contours. The mucosal incision is sutured simply.

21210

The physician reconstructs the nasal, maxillary, or malar area bones with a bone graft to correct defects due to injury, infection, or tumor resection. The procedure may also be performed to augment atrophic or thin bone, or to aid in healing fractures. The physician harvests bone from the patient's hip, rib, or skull. Incisions are made overlying the harvest site. Tissues are dissected away to the desired bone. The physician removes the bone as needed for grafting to the defect area. After the bone is harvested, the donor site is repaired in layers. Access incisions are made to the recipient site and the area of bony defect is exposed. The graft is placed to repair the defect and may be held in place with wires, plates, or screws. The access sites are irrigated and sutured closed.

21215

The physician reconstructs the mandible with a bone graft to correct defects due to injury, infection, or tumor resection. The procedure may also be performed to augment atrophic or thin mandibles, or to aid in healing fractures. The physician harvests bone from another site on the patient's body, most commonly the rib, hip, or skull, and repairs the surgically created wound. The physician makes facial skin incisions to expose the mandible and place the graft from the donor site. Occasionally, intraoral incisions are used. The graft is held firmly positioned with wires, plates, or screws. The incisions are sutured with a layered closure.

21230

The physician reconstructs an area of the face, chin, nose, or ear with a cartilage graft harvested from the ribs. The physician makes a small incision near the sternum through the pectoralis muscle exposing the rib where the bone and cartilage meet. Cartilage is removed from the area and the donor site is closed directly. The physician may make lower eyelid incisions to expose the defect area of the face or nose. Recipient sites of the chin or the ear may also be prepared for the rib cartilage graft. The graft is placed and held in place with wires, plates, sutures, or screws. The incisions are sutured with a layered closure.

21235

The physician reconstructs an area of the nose or ear with a cartilage graft harvested from the ear. The physician makes a small incision of the posterior portion or other identified inconspicuous area of the ear. Cartilage is removed from the area and the donor site is closed directly. The physician may make lower eyelid incisions to expose the defect area of the nose. Recipient sites of the ear may also be prepared for the cartilage graft. The graft is secured in place with wires, plates, sutures, or screws. The incisions are sutured with a layered closure.

21240

The physician repairs or reconstructs the temporomandibular joint. An incision is made through the skin anterior to the contour of the ear or within the ear. The tissues are dissected and the joint is exposed. Once the joint is exposed, a variety of repairs may be performed. The articular disc may be repositioned or the ligaments may be repaired or shortened. The condylar head may be smoothed or recontoured, or the articular disc may be removed. If removed, tissue may be taken from another part of the body to replace the articular disc. The tissue may be fascia from nearby muscles such as the temporalis muscle, cartilage from the ear, dermis, or other tissues. The incisions are closed directly.

21242

The physician repairs or reconstructs the temporomandibular joint with a donor graft. An incision is made through the skin anterior to the contour of the ear or within the ear. The tissues are dissected and the joint is exposed. Once the joint is exposed, a variety of repairs may be performed. Donor tissue (allograft material) is used to replace the articular disc or other parts of the joint. The incisions are closed directly.

21243

The physician partially or totally replaces the diseased or injured temporomandibular joint with a prosthetic joint. An incision is made through the skin anterior to the contour of the ear or within the ear. An additional skin incision just beneath the angle of the mandible may also be necessary. An artificial fossa can be placed above the condyle and secured with screws. If the condyle needs replacement, it is removed and a prosthetic condyle is secured to the remaining condylar neck, typically using screws. Both the fossa and the condyle may need to be replaced. The incisions are closed directly.

21244

The physician reconstructs the mandible by inserting a bone plate with posts that extend through the lower border of the mandible and into the mouth. The posts can be used to retain dentures in an atrophic or thin mandible. The physician makes an incision through the skin under the chin and dissects the tissues to the bone. Holes are drilled upward through the bone and into the mouth. The posts of the plate are placed through the holes and into the mouth. The plate is secured extraorally to the mandible with screws and the incision is closed with layered sutures.

21245-21246

The physician places a metal framework between the mucosa and the bone of the maxilla or mandible. The metal framework has posts that extend vertically and protrude through the mucosa into the mouth. The posts are used to retain an upper denture in the maxilla or lower denture in the mandible when teeth are missing. Intraoral surgery is performed in one or two sessions. The physician makes an incision along the crest of the edentulous area (without teeth) and exposes as much of the bone as possible. If performed in two sessions, the physician makes impressions of the exposed bone and sutures the mucosa closed. The impression is used to make models for custom framework. At the second surgical session, the physician removes the sutures and again exposes the bone. The metal framework, with the attached posts, is placed on the bone. The mucosa and periosteum are sutured over the framework and around the protruding posts. Scarring, which occurs with healing, keeps the framework in place. If performed in one session, a CT scan is used to make a plastic model of the mandible or maxilla from which the framework and posts are fabricated. A single surgical session is used to insert the framework as described above. Incisions are closed simply with sutures. Report 21245 for partial reconstruction. Report 21246 for complete reconstruction.

21247

The physician reconstructs the mandibular condyle of the temporomandibular joint (TMJ) using bone and cartilage taken from the rib. The physician harvests the rib by making a small incision through the pectoralis major muscle and dissecting through the tissue to the rib. Part of the rib and the cartilage near the sternum are removed. The donor site is closed with layered sutures. The physician makes incisions through the skin anterior to the contour of the ear and dissects tissue to the TMJ site. Another incision is often made beneath the angle of the mandible and the tissue is dissected to the bone. The bone is exposed superiorly as far as possible. The rib graft is inserted through the lower incision with the cartilaginous end placed upward into the joint, replacing the condyle. Through both incisions, the rib is manipulated into the proper position and secured to the mandible using plates, screws, or wires. The incisions are closed with layered sutures.

21248-21249

The physician places metal implants into the bone of the maxilla or mandible. Metal posts attached to the implants protrude through the mucosa into the mouth. Artificial teeth or dentures are attached to the roots to replace missing teeth. These implants may be cylindrical or thin blades. The physician makes incisions through the mucosa to expose the bone using an intraoral approach. Precision holes are drilled in the bone where the implants are to be placed. With blade style implants, the posts are already attached to the implant and the mucosa is sutured simply around the post. With cylindrical implants, the mucosa is sutured over the top of the implant and is allowed to heal while buried under the mucosa. The incisions are closed simply. A second procedure is performed three to eight months later. The implant is exposed again and the abutment connectors are attached. Report 21248 for partial reconstruction. Report 21249 for complete reconstruction.

21255

The physician reconstructs the zygomatic arch and glenoid fossa. Bone and cartilage grafts are used in reconstruction. The physician harvests bone grafts from the patient's hip, rib, or skull and closes the surgically created wound. Costal cartilage grafts are most frequently used. The physician makes a hemicoronal incision with a preauricular (in front of the ear) extension. The tissues are reflected to access the zygomatic arch of the cheekbone and the glenoid fossa (depression of the temporal bone at the base of the arch where the mandible articulates). The grafts are placed and the reconstructed arch and fossa are stabilized with internal fixation of sutures, wires, plates, and/or screws. The incision is closed in layers.

21256

The physician increases both the size of the bone structure and outline of the bony orbit. The physician uses a variety of incisions to access the surgical site including bicoronal, lower eyelid, eyebrow, and maxillary vestibular incisions. Cuts are made in the orbital rims using drills or saws. The bone is advanced to desired positions and secured with wires, plates, and/or screws. The physician harvests bone from the patient's hip, rib, or skull and closes the surgically created graft donor site. These bone grafts are fashioned by the physician to augment bone or replace congenitally absent bone. The grafts are secured with wires, plates, and/or screws. Incisions through skin are repaired with a layered closure. Intraoral incisions are closed in a single layer.

21260

The physician moves the orbits closer to one another. The physician uses a variety of incisions to access the surgical sites including bicoronal, lower eyelid, eyebrow, and maxillary vestibular incisions. The reconstruction techniques for repositioning of the orbits center around the naso-orbital area and include reconstruction of the nose and the maxilla. Strategic cuts are made around the orbits with drills or saws. Bony cuts are made in the nasal and ethmoid bones and portions of these bones are removed. The bony orbits are realigned to desired positions and secured with wires, plates, and/or screws. The physician harvests bone from the patient's hip, rib, or skull and closes the surgically created graft donor site. These bone grafts are fashioned by the physician to augment bone, filling in the spaces left by the repositioning, and to maintain the medial positions of the orbits. Small, separate bone grafts may be placed directly on bony step defects. Large grafts are secured with wires, plates, and/or screws. Incisions through skin are repaired with a layered closure. Intraoral incisions are closed in a single layer.

21261

The physician moves the orbits closer to one another. For severe cases, a combined intra- and extracranial approach is used. The physician uses a variety of incisions to access the surgical site including bicoronal, lower eyelid, eyebrow, and maxillary vestibular incisions. To gain complete access to the orbits, a frontal craniotomy is performed, temporarily removing a portion of the frontal bone, retracting the brain, and making orbital osteotomy cuts from the inside of the skull. Cuts are made to release the bony orbits of the eye so they may be positioned closer together, using drills or saws. Bony cuts are made in the nasal and ethmoid bones and portions of these bones are removed. The bony orbits are realigned to desired positions and secured with wires, plates, and/or screws. The physician harvests bone from the patient's hip, rib, or skull and closes the surgically created graft donor site. These bone grafts are fashioned by the physician to augment bone, filling in the spaces left by the repositioning, and to maintain the medial positions of the orbits. Small, separate bone grafts may be fashioned by the physician and placed directly on bony step defects. Large grafts are secured with wires, plates, and/or screws. The frontal bone is again placed in its anatomic location and secured with wires, plates, and/or screws. Incisions through skin are repaired with a layered closure. Intraoral incisions are closed in a single layer.

21263

The physician moves the orbits closer to one another and advances the frontal bone to increase forehead contours. The physician uses a variety of incisions to access the surgical site including bicoronal, lower eyelid, eyebrow, and maxillary vestibular incisions. To gain complete access to the orbits, a frontal craniotomy is performed, temporarily removing a portion of the frontal bone, retracting the brain, and making orbital cuts from the inside of the skull. Cuts are made to release the bony orbits of the eye so they may be positioned closer together, using drills or saws. Bony cuts are made in the nasal and ethmoidal bones and portions of these bones are removed. The bony orbits are realigned and the frontal bone of the forehead is advanced and repositioned into the desired location and secured with wires, plates, and/or screws. The physician harvests bone from the patient's hip, rib, or skull and closes the surgically created graft donor site. These bone grafts are fashioned by the physician to augment bone, filling in the spaces left by the repositioning, and to maintain the medial positions of the orbits. Small, separate bone grafts may be placed directly on bony step defects. Large grafts are fixated with wires, plates, and/or screws. Incisions through skin are repaired with a layered closure. Intraoral incisions are closed in a single layer.

21267

The physician moves the positioning of an orbit on one side. The physician uses a variety of incisions to access the surgical site including coronal, lower eyelid, eyebrow, and maxillary vestibular incisions. Cuts are made in the orbital rims using drills or saws. The bony orbit is realigned to the desired position and secured with wires, plates, and/or screws. The physician harvests bone from the patient's hip, rib, or skull and closes the surgically created graft donor site. These bone grafts are fashioned by the physician to augment bone, replace congenitally absent bone, and recontour facial shapes while maintaining the new position of the orbit. Small separate bone grafts may be placed directly on bony step defects. Large grafts are fashioned and secured with wires, plates, and/or screws. Incisions through skin are repaired with a layered closure. Intraoral incisions are closed in a single layer.

21268

The physician moves the positioning of an orbit on one side. The physician uses a variety of incisions to access the surgical site including coronal, lower eyelid, eyebrow, and maxillary vestibular incisions. To gain complete access to the orbit, a frontal craniotomy is performed, temporarily removing a portion of the frontal bone, retracting the brain, and making cuts from the inside of the skull. Cuts are made in the orbital rims using drills and saws. The bony orbit is realigned to the desired position and secured with wires, plates, and/or screws. The physician harvests bone from the patient's hip, rib, or skull and closes the surgically created graft donor site. These bone grafts are fashioned by the physician to augment bone, replace congenitally absent bone, and recontour facial shapes while maintaining the new position of the orbit. Small, separate bone grafts may be placed directly on bony step defects. Large grafts are secured with wires, plates, and/or screws. The frontal bone is replaced in its anatomic location and secured with wires, plates, and/or screws. Incisions through skin are repaired with a layered closure. Intraoral incisions are closed in a single layer.

21270

The physician augments the malar (cheek) prominence with prosthetic material. Incisions are made through the lower eyelids and maxillary buccal vestibule to expose the malar defect. The prosthetic implant is positioned and fixated on the malar prominence with wires, plates, and/or screws. The eyelid incisions are closed in layers. The oral vestibular incision is closed in a single layer.

21275

The physician performs a second procedure to continue corrections of skeletal deformities of the orbits and face. The physician uses a variety of incisions to access the surgical site including bicoronal, lower eyelid, eyebrow, and maxillary vestibular incisions. Revision cuts are made using drills and saws. Bone is realigned to the desired positions and secured again with wires, plates, and/or screws. The physician may harvest bone from the patient's hip, rib, or skull and close the surgically created graft donor site. Bone grafts are fashioned by the physician and secured with wires, plates, and/or screws, if necessary. Incisions through skin are repaired with a layered closure. Intraoral incisions are closed in a single layer.

21280

The physician reattaches the medial canthal ligament. The medial canthal ligament is attached medially to nasal-orbital bones and laterally to the orbital fascia, the upper eyelid, and the lower eyelid. The ligament is isolated through a bicoronal incision or through skin incisions placed beside the ligament. After locating the ligament, stainless steel suture or wire is placed through the ligament. A hole is made in the nasal bones on the opposite side with a drill or awl. The suture or wire is passed under the nasal complex to the opposite side through the bony hole. The suture or wire is ligated to the bone. Any incisions are repaired with a layered closure.

21282

The physician reattaches the lateral canthal ligament to correct soft tissue structures of the lateral aspect of the eye and eyelids. The lateral canthal ligament is attached laterally to the orbital aspect of the zygoma and medially to the orbital fascia, the upper eyelid, and the lower eyelid. The ligament is isolated through a horizontal skin incision placed beside the ligament. After locating the ligament, the physician places stainless steel suture or wire through the ligament. A hole is made in the zygoma with a drill. The physician passes the suture or wire through the bony hole. The suture or wire is ligated to the bone. Skin incisions are repaired with a layered closure.

21295-21296

The physician reduces the size of the masseter muscle and bone when the muscle has become hypertrophic (overly enlarged). The physician makes skin incisions in the neck just beneath the angle of the mandible. The tissues are dissected to expose the masseter muscle and mandible. The physician removes appropriate amounts of muscle and may use drills, saws, or osteotomes to remove bone in the area of the angle to produce the desired contour. The incision is repaired with a layered closure and pressure dressings are placed on the site. Report 21295 for an extraoral approach. Report 21296 for an intraoral approach.

21315-21320

The physician treats a displaced nasal fracture by manipulating the fractured bones. The physician places nasal elevators or forceps into the nose and realigns the nasal bones. Report 21315 if no additional stabilization is required following realignment. If the bones remain slightly mobile following manipulation and realignment, additional stabilization with splints may be required. External splinting may consist of a cast taped to the reduced nose, while internal splinting consists of supporting the nasal septum by splints or packing with gauze strips. Report stabilization with 21320.

21325

The physician treats a displaced nasal fracture. After unsatisfactory results with closed manipulation of the fractured bones, the physician performs open treatment. Open reduction allows the physician to visualize the fracture. Lacerations may be present, allowing direct visualization. Incisions are made inside the nose to expose the nasal septum and portions of the nasal bones. The physician realigns the fractured bones using nasal elevators and forceps. It may be necessary to remove small segments of bone for adequate realignment. Intranasal incisions are closed in a single layer. Any lacerated skin areas are closed in layers. After the bones are realigned, they remain slightly mobile and require additional stabilization with splints. External splinting may consist of a cast taped to the reduced nose. Internal splinting consists of supporting the nasal septum by splints or packing with gauze strips.

21330

The physician treats a displaced nasal fracture. After unsatisfactory results with closed manipulation of the fractured bones, the physician performs open treatment. Open reduction allows the physician to visualize the fracture. Lacerations may be present, allowing direct visualization. Incisions are made inside the nose to expose the nasal septum and portions of the nasal bones. Additionally, bicoronal or other local skin incisions may be used to expose the fractured nasal bones. The physician realigns the fractured bones using nasal elevators and forceps. The bones are fixed in reduction with wires, plates, and/or screws. Intranasal incisions are closed in a single layer. Lacerations and other skin incisions are repaired with layered closure.

21335

The physician makes an incision to treat a displaced nasal fracture and also repair the fractured nasal septum. Open treatment is necessary after unsatisfactory results with closed manipulation of the fractured bones and allows the physician to visualize the fractures. Lacerations overlying the fractures may allow direct visualization. Incisions may be made inside the nose to expose the nasal septum and portions of the nasal bones. Additionally, bicoronal and other local skin incisions may be used to expose the fractured nasal bones. The nasal septum is exposed and portions of the fractured cartilaginous and bony septum are removed. The physician realigns the nasal bones using nasal elevators and forceps. Transseptal sutures are placed to prevent formation of a septal hematoma. Intranasal incisions are closed in a single layer. Lacerations and other skin incisions are repaired with layered closure. After the bones are realigned, they remain slightly mobile and require additional stabilization with splints. External splinting may consist of a cast taped to the reduced nose. Internal splinting consists of supporting the nasal septum by splints or packing with gauze strips.

21336

The physician makes an incision to repair a nasal septal fracture. Open treatment is necessary after unsatisfactory results with closed manipulation of the fractured septum and allows the physician to visualize the septal fracture. Incisions are made inside the nose. The nasal septum is exposed and portions of the fractured cartilaginous and bony septum are removed. Transseptal sutures are placed to prevent formation of a septal hematoma. Intranasal incisions are closed in single layers. Stabilization such as internal splinting may be used to support the septum during healing. Internal splinting consists of supporting the nasal septum by splints or packing with gauze strips.

21337

The physician repairs a fracture of the nasal septum. No intranasal incisions are made. The physician uses nasal elevators and forceps to realign the septal fracture. Transseptal sutures are placed to prevent formation of a septal hematoma. Internal splints or packing with gauze strips may be used for stabilization to support the septum during healing.

21338-21339

The physician repairs fractures of the nasoethmoid region, which includes nasal and ethmoid bones and the medial wall of the orbit. Lacerations may be present allowing direct visualization. The physician may use bicoronal, local skin, and lower eyelid incisions to expose the fractured bones. The medial canthal ligaments are examined and, if detached, are repaired in a separately reportable procedure with transnasal stainless steel sutures or wire. The physician realigns the fractured bones and holds them in rigid reduction with internal wires, plates, and/or screws. Any lacerated skin areas are repaired and other skin incisions are closed in layers. No external fixation is employed in 21338. Report 21339 if external pin fixation is used to support grossly depressed fractures.

21340

The physician repairs fractures of the nasoethmoid region with percutaneous (through the skin) approaches. Percutaneous pins or screws are placed into stable bone and attached to external support such as splints, headcaps, or wire fixation to aid in reduction of the fractures. If the medial canthal ligaments are detached, they are repaired through a percutaneous approach with awls or K-wires and transnasal stainless steel sutures or wire. Injuries of the nasolacrimal complex are repaired using non-resorbable sutures and polyethylene tubing.

21343

The physician realigns a depressed frontal bone fracture overlying the frontal sinus. This fracture does not involve injury to the nasofrontal duct drainage of the frontal sinus. The physician may access the frontal bone with a bicoronal incision or local skin incisions overlying the fracture. Sinus mucosa may be removed. The bone is realigned and stabilized with wires, plates, and/or screws. The incisions are repaired with a layered closure.

21344

The physician realigns a complicated frontal bone fracture and obliterates the frontal sinus. This fracture injures the duct drainage of the frontal sinus and requires obliteration of the nasofrontal duct to prevent postoperative sinus complications. The physician may access the frontal bone with a bicoronal incision or local skin incisions overlying the fracture. Sinus mucosa is removed from the frontal sinus. If the posterior wall of the sinus is fractured, the bony wall may be removed, thus cranializing the sinus. The nasofrontal duct is plugged (i.e., bone) and obliterating material (i.e., fat, muscle) is placed into the sinus cavity. The frontal bone is realigned and stabilized with wires, plates, and/or screws. The incisions are repaired with a layered closure.

21345

The physician realigns a pyramidal fracture (LeFort II type) of the nasal and maxillary complex without making incisions. The fractured bones are realigned without internal fixation. Intermaxillary fixation is used to realign the fracture. Arch bars are placed onto the patient's upper and lower dental arches with individual wire ligatures around the teeth to provide interdental fixation. The proper occlusion is maintained by securing the maxillary and mandibular arch bars together. For edentulous patients, a splint or the patient's dentures can be modified to provide the necessary fixation.

21346

The physician realigns a pyramidal (LeFort II type) midface fracture of the nasomaxillary complex. An incision is made through the maxillary buccal vestibule (cheek side) to expose the bony maxilla. The nasomaxillary complex is manipulated, realigning the fracture. The physician uses wires, plates, and/or screws to stabilize the fracture. The mucosal incision is closed in a single layer. Intermaxillary fixation may be applied.

21347

The physician realigns a complex pyramidal (LeFort II type) midface fracture of the nasomaxillary complex using more than one site of open access. Multiple incisions are made to expose the fracture sites. These incisions include the bicoronal scalp flap, lower eyelid, and transoral incisions. The nasomaxillary complex is manipulated, realigning the fractured bones. The fracture is stabilized with wires, plates, and/or screws. The transoral incision is closed in a single layer. The scalp and lower eyelid incisions are repaired with a layered closure. Intermaxillary fixation may be applied.

21348

The physician realigns a complex pyramidal (LeFort II type) midface fracture of the nasomaxillary complex with bone grafting. Access incisions may include the bicoronal scalp flap, lower eyelid, and/or transoral incisions. The pyramidal fracture is exposed and the complex is manipulated, realigning the fractured bones. Comminution of bone (e.g., nasofrontal region, orbital floors) requires bone grafting of these areas.

The physician uses wires, plates, and/or screws to stabilize the fracture. Through a separate incision, the physician may harvest a bone graft from the patient's hip, rib, or skull and close the surgically created wound. The physician reconstructs areas of bony defect. The transoral incision is closed in a single layer. The scalp and lower eyelid incisions are repaired with a layered closure. Intermaxillary fixation may be used to additionally stabilize the fracture.

21355
The physician percutaneously reduces a fracture of the malar or cheek area, including the zygomatic arch. A stab incision is made through the skin overlying the fracture area. Without soft tissue dissection, an instrument (e.g., bone hook, Carroll-Girard screw) is inserted and used to lift, manipulate, and reduce the fracture. The stab incision is closed in a single layer.

21356
The physician reduces a depressed fracture of the zygomatic arch through an indirect approach. No internal fixation is used. A facial incision (e.g., Gillies approach) is made in the scalp extending beneath the temporalis fascia. An instrument is inserted through the incision, following underneath the fascia, and taken to the middle surface of the zygomatic arch. The instrument is swept along the arch upwardly and outwardly to reduce the fracture back into proper position. A transoral incision (e.g., Keen approach) may also be used, made in the posterior buccal sulcus. An elevator instrument is inserted through the incision and taken to the medial surface of the zygomatic arch, avoiding damage to branches of the facial nerve passing beside the arch. The arch is lifted laterally to its correct anatomic position. The facial incision is closed in layers. The transoral incision is closed in a single layer.

21360
The physician reduces a fracture of the malar complex. No internal fixation is used. The physician makes facial incisions through the scalp, eyebrow, and/or lower eyelid. A transoral incision is also made through the maxillary buccal vestibule. The fracture sites are exposed. Instruments may be inserted into the bone (e.g., Carroll-Girard screw) or beneath the complex to lift the fracture. The fractured malar complex is reduced manually. The facial incisions are closed in layers. The transoral incision is closed in a single layer.

21365
The physician reduces a complicated fracture of the malar area. Internal fixation is necessary for fracture stability. The physician makes multiple incisions to expose and explore the fracture. Facial incisions are made through the scalp, eyebrow, and/or lower eyelid. A transoral incision is made though the maxillary buccal vestibule. Instruments may be inserted into the bone (e.g., Carroll-Girard screw) or beneath the complex to lift the fracture. The fractured malar complex is reduced and fixated with wires, plates, and/ or screws. The facial incisions are closed in layers. The transoral incision is closed in a single layer.

21366
The physician reduces a complicated fracture of the malar area. Bone grafting is necessary to reconstruct bony defects (e.g., orbital floor, anterior maxillary wall) and internal fixation is necessary for fracture stability. The physician makes multiple incisions to expose and explore the fracture. Facial incisions are made through the scalp, eyebrow, and/or lower eyelid. A transoral incision is made though the maxillary buccal vestibule. Instruments may be inserted into the bone (e.g., Carroll-Girard screw) or beneath the malar complex to lift the fracture. The fractured complex is reduced and fixated with wires, plates, and/or screws. Through a separate incision, the physician harvests a bone graft from the patient's hip, rib, or skull and closes the surgically created wound. The graft is placed on the malar defect area and may be stabilized with sutures, wires, plates, and/or screws. The facial incisions are closed in layers. The transoral incision is closed in a single layer.

21385
The physician repairs a blowout fracture of the orbital floor. A maxillary vestibular incision is made on the side of the orbital fracture. In the maxillary bone, a window opening is made into the maxillary sinus, using a drill and bone forceps. The orbital floor is visualized from inside the maxillary sinus. The fractured orbital floor is realigned and supported from inside the maxillary sinus with lubricated gauze packing or a ballooned catheter. The physician sutures the end portion of the gauze or catheter to the maxillary mucosa. Most of the intraoral incision is sutured in a single layer. The exposed gauze or catheter remains in place and is removed after adequate healing.

21386
The physician repairs a blowout fracture of the orbital floor. Lower eyelid incisions are made in the subtarsal skin crease along the inferior orbital margin with a lateral extension to expose and explore this fracture. This allows the physician to inspect the floor, infraorbital rim, and medial/lateral orbital walls. The physician realigns the fractured orbital floor by gentle manipulation. The realigned orbital floor is stable or the fracture is very small, not requiring an implant or bone graft. The lower eyelid incision is closed in layers.

21387
The physician repairs a blowout fracture of the orbital floor with a combined periorbital and maxillary sinus approach. The physician makes both lower eyelid skin incisions and intraoral incisions to expose and explore this fracture. A lower eyelid incision allows the physician to inspect the infraorbital rim and floor. Additionally, the orbital floor is visualized from inside the maxillary sinus by a maxillary vestibular incision above the tooth apices on the side of the fracture. The physician realigns the fractured orbital floor by manipulation from either access. The realigned orbital floor may be supported from inside the maxillary sinus with lubricated gauze packing or a ballooned catheter.

The physician sutures the end portion of the gauze or catheter to the maxillary mucosa. Most of the intraoral incision is sutured in a single layer. The lower eyelid incision is closed in layers. The exposed gauze or catheter remains in place intraorally and is removed after adequate healing.

21390
The physician repairs a blowout fracture of the orbital floor using lower eyelid incisions made in the subtarsal skin crease along the inferior orbital margin with a lateral extension. This allows the physician to inspect the floor, infraorbital rim, and medial/lateral orbital walls. The physician elevates the orbital soft tissue from the bone, exposing the fracture. Small fragments of fractured bone may be removed and the remaining fractured bone is realigned by gentle manipulation. A bony hole remains in the orbital floor, requiring an implant to prevent orbital soft tissue from entering the maxillary sinus below. The physician fashions an alloplastic implant material to cover the hole. The physician places the implant over the bony hole. The lower eyelid incision is closed in layers.

21395
The physician repairs a blowout fracture of the orbital floor using lower eyelid incisions made in the subtarsal skin crease along the inferior orbital margin with a lateral extension. This allows the physician to inspect the floor, infraorbital rim, and medial/lateral orbital walls. The physician elevates the orbital soft tissue from the bone, exposing the fracture. Small fragments of fractured bone may be removed and the remaining fractured bone is realigned by gentle manipulation. A bony hole remains in the orbital floor and will require a graft to prevent orbital soft tissue from entering the maxillary sinus below. The physician harvests bone from the patient's hip, rib, or skull, and closes the surgically created graft donor site. The harvested bone is fashioned to cover the hole. The physician places the bone graft over the bony hole and may secure it to the infraorbital rim with wire or sutures. The lower eyelid incision is repaired with a layered closure.

21400
The physician treats a fracture of the orbit, other than a floor blowout fracture. Incisions and bony manipulation are not necessary. This is a non-displaced or minimally displaced fracture of the orbital rims or walls that can be identified on x-ray.

21401
The physician treats a fracture of the orbit, other than a floor blowout fracture. No incisions are necessary. This is a minimally displaced fracture of the orbital rims or walls that can be identified on x-ray. The physician realigns the fracture bones by using manual manipulation or with bone hooks and Carroll-Girard screws. The realigned bones are stable and no internal fixation is necessary.

21406
The physician openly treats a fracture of the orbit, other than a floor blowout fracture. This is a displaced fracture of the orbital rims or walls that can be identified on x-ray. The physician makes periorbital incisions to expose the fracture site. The fractured bones are realigned and may be stabilized with wires, plates, and/or screws. No sizable bony holes that would require coverage remain in the orbit. The incisions are closed in layers.

21407
The physician openly treats a fracture of the orbit, other than a floor blowout fracture. This is a displaced fracture of the orbital rims or walls that can be identified on x-ray. The physician makes periorbital incisions to expose the fracture site. The fractured bones are realigned and may be stabilized with wires, plates, and/or screws. After realignment, bony holes remain in the orbit that require coverage to prevent orbital soft tissue from entering into these holes. These holes are usually found in the medial or lateral walls of the orbit. An alloplastic implant is selected, shaped, and placed over the bony hole. The incisions are closed in layers.

21408
The physician openly treats a fracture of the orbit, other than a floor blowout fracture. This is a displaced fracture of the orbital rims or walls that can be identified on x-ray. The physician makes periorbital incisions to expose the fracture site. The fractured bones are realigned and may be stabilized with wires, plates, and/or screws. After realignment, bony holes remain in the orbit, requiring coverage to prevent orbital soft tissue from entering these holes. The holes are usually found in the medial or lateral walls of the orbit. The physician harvests bone from the patient's hip, rib, or skull, and closes the surgically created graft donor site. The bone graft is shaped and placed over the bony hole. The incisions are closed in layers.

21421
The physician treats a palatal or maxillary fracture (LeFort I type) by applying interdental (intermaxillary) fixation for stabilization. No incisions are made with this technique. Intermaxillary fixation is used to realign the fracture. Arch bars are placed onto the patient's upper and lower dental arches with individual wire ligatures around the teeth. The fracture reduction is maintained in proper occlusion by securing the maxillary and mandibular arch bars together. For edentulous patients, a custom-made acrylic splint or the patient's dentures can be modified to provide the necessary interdental fixation.

21422
The physician uses open treatment to reposition and stabilize a palatal or maxillary fracture (LeFort I type). Transoral incisions are made in the maxillary buccal (cheek) vestibule to expose the maxillary fracture. The fracture is repositioned and stabilized with plates, screws, and/or wires. The transoral mucosal incision is closed in a single layer. A customized acrylic palatal splint may be wired to the maxillary teeth to stabilize the palatal fracture. Intermaxillary fixation may be applied.

21423

The physician repositions and stabilizes a complicated palatal or maxillary fracture (LeFort I type). Transoral incisions are made in the maxillary buccal vestibule to expose the maxillary fracture. Additional lower eyelid or other skin incisions may be necessary to assist in repair of the fracture. The maxilla is repositioned and stabilized with plates, screws, and/or wires. The infraorbital nerve may need to be repositioned. The anterior maxillary walls may need bone grafting to support the infraorbital nerve. The transoral mucosal incision is closed in a single layer. Any skin or eyelid incisions are closed in layers. A customized acrylic palatal splint may be wired to the maxillary teeth to stabilize a palatal fracture. Intermaxillary fixation may be applied.

21431

The physician treats a craniofacial separation (LeFort III type) without surgically opening the fracture but with the use of interdental wiring of denture or splint. The physician uses surgical instruments intranasally and intraorally to reduce the separation. Intermaxillary (interdental) wire fixation is used to realign the fracture. A custom-made acrylic splint or the patient's dentures are wired to the jaw to provide for the necessary fixation. Arch bars are placed onto the patient's upper and lower dental arches with individual wire ligatures around the teeth. The fracture reduction is maintained in proper occlusion by securing the maxillary and mandibular arch bars together for immobilization until healing is complete.

21432-21436

The physician performs surgery to openly treat a craniofacial separation (LeFort III type). The physician uses any of a variety of incisions, including intraoral and lateral eyebrow incisions. Surgical instruments are utilized to reduce the separation. The physician uses wire, plates, and screws to hold the bones in their acceptable anatomic positions for healing. The wounds are irrigated and closed in layers. Report 21433 if the procedure is complicated (comminuted or involving the cranial nerve), requiring multiple incisions to be made for more than one site of open access. Report 21435 if the procedure is complicated, utilizing internal and/or external fixation techniques such as transosseous wiring, pins, or miniplates at the fracture site, or cranial vault fixation such as head caps or halo frames with suspension wires. Report 21436 if the procedure is complicated, using multiple surgical approaches and internal fixation of the fracture bones, together with bone grafts, taken from a separate donor site on the patient.

21440

The physician stabilizes and repairs a fracture of the mandibular or maxillary alveolar bone without making incisions. The physician moves the fractured bone into the desired position manually. The fracture is stabilized by wiring both the involved teeth and adjacent stable teeth to an arch bar. Another technique utilizes dental composite bonding of both involved and stable teeth to a heavy, stainless steel wire. A customized acrylic splint may be used to stabilize the teeth. Intermaxillary fixation may also be applied.

21445

The physician stabilizes and reduces a fracture of the mandibular or maxillary alveolar bone from an incisional access site. Intraoral incisions are made in the buccal vestibule to expose the fracture. The physician moves the fractured bone into the desired position manually. The fracture is stabilized by wiring both the involved teeth and adjacent stable teeth to an arch bar. A customized acrylic splint may be used to stabilize the teeth. The fractured alveolar bone may be reduced by wires, plates, and/or screws. Intermaxillary fixation may also be applied. The intraoral incision is closed in a single layer.

21450-21451

The physician treats a mandibular fracture with no direct manipulation or stabilization in 21450. Close observation, a soft diet, or other restrictions of activity are examples of treatment. The physician repositions a mandibular fracture with some manipulation in 21451. The physician moves the fractured bone back into the desired position manually. No incisions are made with this technique.

21452

The physician treats a mandibular fracture percutaneously by applying external fixation. The physician makes 0.5 cm stab incisions in the skin at several points near the inferior border of the mandible on both sides of the fracture. Without soft tissue dissection, holes are drilled and threaded rods or pins are screwed into the holes and used to manipulate and reduce the fracture. A metal or acrylic bar is connected to the protruding posts in a horizontal fashion, stabilizing the fracture.

21453

The physician treats a mandibular fracture by applying interdental or intermaxillary fixation (wiring the jaws together) for stabilization. No incisions are made with this technique. The physician wires arch bars to the upper and lower dental arches with individual wire ligatures around the teeth or uses other wiring techniques to provide the intermaxillary fixation. Edentulous patients (without teeth) may have dentures or custom-made acrylic splints wired to the jaws first. The jaws are wired together to provide intermaxillary fixation.

21454

The physician treats a mandibular fracture through incisions and by applying external fixation. An intraoral approach may be used or a skin incision may be made overlying the area. The tissue is dissected to the bone and the fracture is exposed and repositioned directly. The fracture may also be approached through traumatic lacerations. Once the fracture is moved to the desired position, the physician makes 0.5 cm incisions in the skin at several points near the inferior border of the mandible on both sides of the fracture.

Holes are drilled into the mandible and threaded rods or pins are screwed into the holes. A metal or acrylic bar is connected to the protruding posts in a horizontal fashion, stabilizing the fracture. Intermaxillary fixation may be placed.

21461-21462

The physician repositions and stabilizes a mandibular fracture. Incisions are made in the skin overlying the fractured area or intraorally through the mucosa. The tissue is dissected to the bone and the fracture exposed. The fracture is repositioned and the bones stabilized with plates, screws, or wires. The incisions are closed with sutures. Intermaxillary fixation is not applied in 21461. In 21462, intermaxillary or interdental fixation is applied. Arch bars are placed onto the patient's upper and lower dental arches with individual wire ligatures around the teeth and the jaws are wired together.

21465

The physician openly repositions and/or stabilizes a fracture of the mandibular condyle. An incision is made through the skin anterior to the contour of the ear or through the ear. An intraoral approach is used on occasion. The tissues are dissected to the temporomandibular joint and the fractured condyle is exposed. Depending on the location of the fracture, a second skin incision below the angle of the mandible may be necessary to move the fracture to the desired position. The fractured condyle is repositioned, manually or with instruments. The fracture is stabilized with wires, screws, or plates, or may be left without internal fixation. The incision is closed with layered sutures. Intermaxillary fixation may be placed.

21470

The physician openly repositions and/or stabilizes a complicated fracture of the mandible. Multiple incisions are made through the skin and/or the intraoral mucosa to approach and treat the fracture. Once in proper position, the fractured bones are held in rigid reduction with internal fixation of wires, screws, or plates, and the mandible is immobilized with interdental (intermaxillary) fixation. The mucosal incisions are sutured simply and the skin incisions are closed with layered sutures. The physician wires arch bars to the upper and lower dental arches with individual wire ligatures around the teeth or uses other wiring techniques. Edentulous patients (without teeth) may have dentures or custom-made acrylic splints wired to the jaws first. The jaws are wired together to provide interdental fixation.

21480

The physician repositions a dislocation of the temporomandibular joint. No incisions are made and no intermaxillary fixation is used. The physician corrects the dislocation manually to rearticulate the joint.

21485

The physician repositions a dislocation of the temporomandibular joint. This is a complicated dislocation that may be recurrent and requires immobilization. The physician corrects the dislocation manually to rearticulate the joint. Intermaxillary fixation is applied. The physician wires arch bars to the upper and lower dental arches with individual wire ligatures around the teeth or uses other wiring and splinting techniques and the jaws are wired together.

21490

The physician surgically repositions a dislocation of the temporomandibular joint. The physician exposes the joint by making an incision anterior to the contour of the ear or through the ear. Tissues are dissected to expose the joint. The condyle and disc are moved into normal position using instruments. The ligaments may be repaired. The incision is closed with layered sutures.

21497

The physician treats conditions other than fractures, such as temporomandibular dislocations, by applying intermaxillary fixation (wiring the jaws together) for immobilization. No incisions are made with this technique; however, the physician may have already surgically reduced the dislocation. The physician may wire arch bars to the teeth or use other wiring techniques to provide the interdental fixation. For edentulous patients (without teeth), dentures or custom made acrylic splints are wired to the jaws. The jaws are wired together.

21501-21502

The physician performs surgery to remove or drain an abscess or hematoma from the deep soft tissues of the neck or thorax. With proper anesthesia administered, the physician makes an incision overlying the site of the abscess or hematoma of the neck or thorax. Dissection is carried down through the deep subcutaneous tissues and may be continued into the fascia or muscle to expose the abscess or hematoma. The incision may be extended if the mass is larger than expected. The abscess or hematoma is incised and the contents are drained. The area is irrigated and the incision is repaired in layers with sutures, staples, and/or Steri-strips; closed with drains in place; or simply left open to further facilitate drainage of infection. Report 21502 if a partial rib ostectomy is performed during this procedure.

21510

The physician incises the bone cortex of infected bone in the thorax to treat an abscess or osteomyelitis. The physician makes an incision over the affected area. Dissection is carried down through the soft tissues to expose the bone. The periosteum is split and reflected from the bone overlying the infected area. A curette may be used to scrape away the abscess or infected portion down to healthy bony tissue or drill holes may be made through the cortex into the medullary canal in a window outline around the infected or abscessed bone. The area is drained and debrided of infected bony and soft tissue. The physician irrigates the area with antibiotic solution, the periosteum is closed over the bone, and the soft tissues are sutured closed; or the wound is packed and left open, allowing the area to drain. Secondary closure is performed approximately three weeks later. Dressings are changed daily.

21550
The physician performs a biopsy of the soft tissues of the neck or thorax. With proper anesthesia administered, the physician identifies the mass through palpation and x-ray (reported separately), if needed. An incision is made over the site and dissection is taken down to the subcutaneous fat or further into the fascia or muscle to reach the lesion. A portion of the tissue mass is excised and submitted for pathology. The area is irrigated and the incision is closed with layered sutures.

21555-21556 [21552, 21554]
The physician removes a tumor from the soft tissue of the neck or anterior thorax (chest) that is located in the subcutaneous tissue in 21552 or 21555 and in the deep soft tissue, below the fascial plane or within the muscle, in 21554 or 21556. With the proper anesthesia administered, the physician makes an incision in the skin overlying the mass and dissects down to the tumor. The extent of the tumor is identified and a dissection is undertaken all the way around the tumor. A portion of neighboring soft tissue may also be removed to ensure adequate removal of all tumor tissue. A drain may be inserted and the incision is repaired with layers of sutures, staples, or Steri-strips. Report 21555 for excision of subcutaneous tumors whose resected area is less than 3 cm and 21552 for excision of subcutaneous tumors 3 cm or greater. Report 21556 for excision of subfascial or intramuscular tumors whose resected area is less than 5 cm and 21554 for excision of subfascial or intramuscular tumors 5 cm or greater.

21557-21558
The physician performs a radical resection of a soft tissue tumor (i.e., sarcoma) from the neck or anterior thorax, not involving bone. The tumor may be malignant or an aggressive benign tumor of the connective tissue. An incision is made over the tumor and dissection exposes it. The tumor and any adjacent tissue that may be affected by the spread of the neoplasm are excised. Large resections may be needed. The type and stage of the lesion determines the extent of the tumor margin resection area. Muscle or fascia may need to be repaired and drains may be placed. The surgical wound may be closed using simple or intermediate repair or separately reportable complex closure, adjacent tissue transfer, or graft. Report 21557 for excision of tumors whose resected area is less than 5 cm and 21558 for excision of tumors 5 cm or greater.

21600
The physician removes part of one rib. With the patient under anesthesia, the physician makes an incision in the skin of the chest overlying the rib. The tissues are dissected deep to the rib itself. The rib is identified. The physician removes the desired part of the rib using a saw and other instruments. The remaining pieces of the rib and the wound itself are irrigated and debrided. The incision is sutured in layers.

21601
The physician excises a chest wall tumor, including ribs. An incision in the skin of the chest overlying the site of the tumor is made. The tumor and surrounding tissue are excised. The tissue removed includes at least one adjacent rib above or below the tumor site and any associated intercostal muscles. It may also include rib cage resection and/or an en bloc resection of muscles, including the pectoralis minor or major, the serratus anterior, or the latissimus dorsi. The physician ligates or cauterizes bleeding vessels. A chest tube may be placed to re-expand the lung. The incision is repaired with layered closure and a pressure dressing is applied to the wound.

21602-21603
The physician excises a chest wall tumor, involving ribs, with plastic reconstruction. The physician makes an incision in the skin of the chest overlying the tumor. The tumor and surrounding tissue are excised and includes at least one adjacent rib above and below the tumor site and all intervening intercostal muscles. It may also include an en bloc resection of muscles, including the pectoralis minor or major, the serratus anterior, or the latissimus dorsi. In 21603, lymphatic tissue lying within the mediastinum is also removed. The physician ligates or cauterizes bleeding vessels. A chest tube may be placed to re-expand the lung. Plastic reconstruction is done and may involve rib grafts and/or a myocutaneous flap. A pressure dressing is applied to the wound.

21610
The physician resects the costovertebral joint. The physician makes a posterior incision overlying the joint. The tissues are dissected from the joint and the transverse process is cut from the vertebral body. The physician removes all or a portion of the adjacent rib. The incision is sutured in layers.

21615-21616
The physician performs surgery to remove the first rib and/or an extraneous cervical rib. With the patient under anesthesia, an incision is made in the skin just above the clavicle on the affected side and carried deep to the rib. The rib is identified and the attached soft tissues are dissected from the bone. The physician excises the rib using a saw and other surgical instruments. The rib is freed from its articulation and removed. The wound is irrigated and closed in layers. A dressing is applied. Report 21616 if a sympathetic nerve pathway is cut during the procedure.

21620
The physician removes a portion of the sternum from the chest. With the patient under anesthesia, the physician makes an incision in the skin overlying the sternum. This is carried deep through the subcutaneous tissues to the bone. The sternum is identified and the attached soft tissues are dissected from the bone. The physician marks the portion of the

sternum to be removed. The bone is cut in the appropriate places using a saw and other surgical instruments. The remaining portion of the bone is irrigated and smoothed as needed. The wound is closed in layers and a dressing is applied.

21627

The physician performs a debridement of the sternum. With the patient under anesthesia, the physician makes an incision in the skin overlying the sternum. The incision is carried deep to the bone. The sternum is debrided as warranted using any of a variety of hand or powered surgical instruments. Irrigation is used so that debridement can be completed as extensively as indicated. The wound may be loosely packed and a dressing applied or it may be closed in layers and a dressing applied.

21630

The physician removes most or all of the sternum from the chest. With the patient under anesthesia, the physician makes a long incision overlying the sternum and anterior chest. This is carried deep to the bone. Dissection is performed around the sternum. Ribs are disarticulated as needed and thorough debridement is accomplished. Using saws and other surgical instruments, the physician removes the bone. Internal fixation devices (reported separately) are often needed to support the ribs and chest wall. The wound is irrigated and closed in layers.

21685

The hyoid bone is a small C-shaped bone in the neck above the Adam's apple, or thyroid cartilage, with muscles of the tongue and throat attached to it. Hyoid myotomy and suspension is done to open the orohypopharyngeal airway for correcting breathing in sleep apnea. It involves repositioning and fixating the hyoid bone to improve the airway. A submental incision is made to expose the hyoid bone in the neck. The muscles below the hyoid are transected and separated to expose a small, isolated, mid-portion of the hyoid bone. Strips of fascia lata (bands of fibrous tissue), nonresorbable suture, or other strong materials are wrapped around the body of the hyoid and used to pull it forward and secure it to the inferior mandibular border. An alternative method pulls the hyoid downward to the voicebox cartilage for thyro-hyoid suspension, and secures it there.

21700-21705

The physician performs a surgical procedure where the scalenus anticus muscle is divided, usually for the purpose of treating thoracic outlet syndrome. With the patient under anesthesia, the physician makes an incision overlying the scalene muscle. This incision is carried deep to the muscle. The muscle is exposed and identified. A discission of the muscle is performed in line of the fibers. This relieves the pressure on the neurovascular structures. The wound is irrigated and closed in layers. Report 21700 if the procedure does not include resection of the cervical rib. Report 21705 if resection of the cervical rib is performed during the procedure.

21720-21725

Torticollis is a dysfunction of the neck with congenital or traumatic onset. The head becomes inclined toward the affected side and the face toward the opposite side. The physician makes an incision 5 cm long above and parallel to the medial end of the collarbone to access the tendons of the sternocleidomastoid muscle. A blunt instrument is placed behind the tendons to protect vital structures in the neck. The muscle's tendons attach just behind the ear and to the collarbone. The physician splits the tendons further up the muscle to release the restriction. The physician probes the wound to identify remaining tight muscles or fascia, which are cut until full motion is obtained. The physician closes the incision with sutures and Steri-strips. A cervical collar is applied for six weeks in 21720 and a cast is applied to hold the neck in place in 21725.

21740

The physician performs surgery on the anterior chest to correct pectus excavatum (a depression in the chest wall) or pectus carinatum (a forward projection of the chest wall). With the patient under anesthesia, the physician makes an incision overlying the anterior sternum. This is carried deep to the bone. The costal cartilages are exposed and deformed rib ends are freed from their sternal attachments. The sternum is mobilized and restored to its normal position. Internal fixation devices are employed to hold the sternum in corrected alignment. The physician irrigates the wound and closes it in layers with sutures.

21742-21743

The physician performs a Nuss procedure, also known as minimally invasive repair of pectus excavatum (MIRPE), without thoracoscopy in 21742 and with thoracoscopy in 21743. Pectus excavatum is a depression of the sternum and chest, giving a sunken appearance. The chest is first marked at strategic points and the length of a curved steel bar, called the Lorenz pectus bar, to be inserted into the sternum is measured and shaped to fit the individual's chest. Midaxillary line incisions are made on the right and left side aligned with the deepest depression point. A skin tunnel is raised from the incisions and another small lateral incision is made for insertion of a thoracoscope. The skin incisions are elevated and a long introducer instrument is inserted through the right intercostal space at the top of the pectus ridge and slowly advanced across the anterior mediastinal space with videoscopic guidance. The sternum is forcefully lifted as the introducer is passed to the other side. Once behind the sternum, the tip is pushed through the intercostal space at the top of the pectus ridge on the left side and brought out through that skin incision. Umbilical tape is pulled through the tunnel and used to guide the prepared bar. The bar is inserted with the convex curve facing posteriorly and rotated with a flipping instrument until the convex curve faces anteriorly. The bar can be pulled back out and bent in a more ideal curvature for correction as many times as needed. Usually only one bar is placed. With the bar in position, a stabilizing bar is sutured around the pectus bar and to the muscle. Sutures are placed in the lateral chest wall musculature as well as one other fixation point to the side of the sternum around one rib and the pectus bar. Wounds are closed and the patient is extubated while deeply anesthetized and kept well sedated for a few days with pain management therapy.

21750
The physician performs surgery on the sternum bone to put the bone back together following previous surgical separation. With the patient under anesthesia, the physician makes an incision overlying the sternum. The incision is carried deep to the bone and the separated pieces are identified. The physician may debride soft tissue or bone. The bony fragments are manipulated back together and held in place. The physician uses wire or other internal fixation devices to maintain the bone in appropriate position. The wound is irrigated and closed in layers.

21811-21813
The physician performs surgery on one or more unilateral rib fractures requiring internal fixation. With the patient under anesthesia, the physician makes an incision overlying the fractured rib. This is carried deep to the bone. The fracture is found, the pieces are identified, and dead tissue is debrided as needed. The physician manipulates and aligns the fracture fragments into an acceptable position and stabilizes the fragments using devices such as pins, rods, screws, or wires. The wound is irrigated and closed in layers. Report 21811 for treatment of one to three ribs; 21812 for four to six ribs; and 21813 for seven or more ribs. This includes thoracoscopic visualization when utilized.

21820
Separately reportable x-rays are used to identify if a fracture of the sternum is present. If the fracture is nondisplaced and stable, closed treatment is initiated. Braces or splints are not used. The patient's activity is modified while the fracture heals.

21825
The physician performs an open surgical reduction of a sternum fracture. The patient is positioned supine on the operating table. A longitudinal incision is made along the midportion of the sternum. Dissection exposes the fractured sternum. The surgeon reduces the fracture. If fixation is needed to keep the fracture stable, the physician drills holes on either side of the fracture. Wire is passed through the holes and around the fracture and the wire ends are twisted together to immobilize the fracture. The incision is repaired in layers with sutures, staples, or Steri-strips.

21920-21925
The physician performs a biopsy of the soft tissues of the back or flank. The patient is positioned lying on the side or prone. With proper anesthesia administered, an incision is made over the biopsy area. Dissection is carried down within the superficial soft tissue layers in 21920, usually the subcutaneous fat to the uppermost fascial layer. In 21925, dissection is taken down deep within the soft tissue, such as into the fascial layer or within the muscle. A portion of the tissue is excised and submitted for pathology. The area is irrigated and the incision is closed with layered sutures, staples, or Steri-strips.

21930-21933
The physician removes a tumor from the soft tissue of the back or flank that is located in the subcutaneous tissue in 21930-21931 and in the deep soft tissue, below the fascial plane or within the muscle, in 21932-21933. The patient is positioned lying on the side or prone. With the proper anesthesia administered, the physician makes an incision in the skin overlying the mass and dissects down to the tumor. The extent of the tumor is identified and a dissection is undertaken all the way around the tumor. A portion of neighboring soft tissue may also be removed to ensure adequate removal of all tumor tissue. A drain may be inserted and the incision is repaired with layers of sutures, staples, or Steri-strips. Report 21930 for excision of subcutaneous tumors whose resected area is less than 3 cm and 21931 for excision of subcutaneous tumors 3 cm or greater. Report 21932 for excision of subfascial or intramuscular tumors whose resected area is less than 5 cm and 21933 for excision of subfascial or intramuscular tumors 5 cm or greater.

21935-21936
The physician performs a radical resection of a soft tissue tumor (i.e., sarcoma) from the back or flank, not involving bone. The tumor may be malignant or an aggressive benign tumor of the connective tissue. An incision is made over the tumor and dissection exposes it. The tumor and any adjacent tissue that may be affected by the spread of the neoplasm are excised. Large resections may be needed. The type and stage of the lesion determines the extent of the tumor margin resection area. Muscle or fascia may need to be repaired and drains may be placed. The surgical wound is closed using single or intermediate repair or separately reportable complex closure, adjacent tissue transfer, or graft. Report 21935 for excision of tumors whose resected area is less than 5 cm and 21936 for excision of tumors 5 cm or greater.

22010-22015
The physician performs an open incision and drainage of a deep abscess of the posterior spine. Once a paraspinal soft tissue abscess or a lumbar psoas muscle abscess is identified by MRI or CT scan, an aspiration biopsy may be performed prior to open surgical drainage. The extent of the surgery depends on the size of the abscess and the area affected. The deep fascia is incised and the wound opened, irrigated, and debrided. Necrotic tissue and debris are removed and the cavity is irrigated with antibiotic solution. The wound is closed in layers and a drain or wound vacuum device may be placed. Report 22010 for incision and drainage of a deep abscess in the cervical, thoracic, or cervicothoracic region of the posterior spine and 22015 for the lumbar, sacral, or lumbosacral region.

22100-22103

The physician removes spurs, other growths, or bone disease by partial resection of a posterior vertebral component such as the spinous process, lamina, or facet. The patient is placed prone and an incision is made overlying the affected vertebra and taken down to the level of the fascia. The fascia is incised and the paravertebral muscles are retracted. The physician removes the affected part of the spinous process, lamina, or facet. Paravertebral muscles are repositioned and the tissue and skin is closed with layered sutures. Report 22100 for a cervical vertebral segment; 22101 for a thoracic vertebral segment; and 22102 for a lumbar vertebral segment. Report 22103 for each additional segment in conjunction with the code for the primary procedure.

22110-22116

The physician removes spurs, other growths, or bone disease by partial resection of a vertebral body. With the patient stabilized by a halo or cranial tongs, the physician makes an anterior incision to reach the vertebral body. Lower cervical vertebrae are approached above the clavicle, dividing the superficial muscles and fascia and retracting the trachea, esophagus, and thyroid medially. After blunt division of the deep fascia and paravertebral muscles, the anterior aspect of the cervical spine is exposed. The bony lesion is identified and excised from the affected vertebral body. Once the lesion is removed, a drain is placed and the incision is closed in layered sutures. The halo or tongs are attached to a body jacket to assure stabilization of the spine. Report 22110 for a cervical segment; 22112 for a thoracic segment; and 22114 for a lumbar vertebral segment. Report 22116 for each additional segment in conjunction with the code for the primary procedure.

22206-22208

Three-column spinal osteotomy is performed to correct moderate to severe spinal deformities that result in limited flexibility. Also known as pedicle subtraction osteotomy, it involves cutting and removing one or more portions of the vertebral segment in order to prepare for spinal realignment. The three columns consist of the anterior (anterior two-thirds of the vertebral body), the middle (posterior third of the vertebral body and the pedicle), and the posterior (articular facets, lamina, and spinous process). Using a posterior or posterolateral approach, the surgeon excises all posterior elements at the site of the correction, including the pedicles and the adjacent facet joints (inferior and superior). The physician then removes a posterior wedge of cancellous bone from the vertebral body to achieve the desired correction. The entire posterior and lateral vertebral body walls may also be removed. The osteotomy is closed by extending the patient's position on the operative frame or through instrumentation compression. Report 22206 if the procedure is performed on a thoracic vertebral segment and 22207 if the segment is lumbar. Report 22208 for each additional vertebral segment in conjunction with the code for the primary procedure.

22210-22216

Spinal osteotomy is performed to correct spinal deformities, such as severe cervical kyphosis occurring with rheumatoid arthritis that makes it difficult to properly elevate the chin off the chest. For a cervical posterior osteotomy, the patient is placed in the prone position with a supporting chest pad and the head resting on a frame or in a sitting position with the head supported by a halo and traction with the arms resting on the table. A posterior midline incision is made over the cervicothoracic junction. The physician exposes the spinous processes from C5 to T1. The muscles and ligamentous attachments are stripped from the spinous process at the desired level and dissection continues subperiosteally. The posterior elements of C7, the spinous process and laminae, are removed as are the articulating inferior half of C6 and upper portion of T1. The osteotomy continues with lateral resections of bone that are beveled toward each other so the opposing surfaces are parallel after extension. Assuring the absence of any nerve root compression, the forward parts of the vertebrae are fractured. The gap closes posteriorly as the lateral masses meet. The muscles are reattached and the wound is closed with layered sutures over a suction drain. The angle of the neck is adjusted and stabilized using the halo and a halo vest. Report 22212 if a similar osteotomy procedure is performed on a thoracic vertebral segment and 22214 if the segment is lumbar. Report 22216 for each additional vertebral segment in conjunction with the code for the primary procedure. If bone grafts and/or spinal instrumentation are needed to maintain the spine in the straightened position, report them separately in addition to the definitive procedure.

22220-22226

Spinal osteotomy is performed to correct spinal deformities. In this procedure, the physician uses an anterior approach to reach the involved vertebrae. For a cervical vertebral segment in 22220, an incision is made through the neck, avoiding the esophagus, trachea, and thyroid. For a thoracic vertebral segment in 22222, an incision is made through the chest, with possible detachment of the clavicle, costal cartilage, and manubrium. For a lumbar vertebral segment in 22224, an incision is made through the tenth rib, into the chest cavity with rib spreaders, and dissection of abdominal contents away from the diaphragm. Retractors separate the intervertebral muscles. A marker is inserted in the affected vertebral segment and the location is confirmed by separately reportable x-ray. With a rongeur, the physician cleans out the intervertebral disc space between the concerned vertebral bone and its neighboring vertebrae. An osteotomy of the single vertebral segment is carried out by removing a wedge of bone from the middle portion of the vertebral body. The spine is extended to achieve correction and separately reportable bone grafts and/or spinal instrumentation may need to be

Musculoskeletal

placed to maintain the spine in the straightened position. The muscles are reattached and the wound is closed with layered sutures. Report 22226 for each additional vertebral segment in conjunction with the code for the primary procedure.

22310

The physician performs closed treatment of a vertebral body fracture and applies casting or bracing without any prerequisite manipulation.

22315

Following dislocation or traumatic or pathological fracture of the vertebrae, the physician decompresses the spine into proper alignment and immobilizes the vertebrae. The fracture or dislocation may be realigned by manual manipulation of the spine. If traction is employed, the patient is placed supine with a halo or tongs affixed to the skull. Traction is applied to the feet and to the halo or tongs, decompressing the vertebrae. As the traction is increased in stages, the physician assures that there is no additional neurological deficit. Traction is removed when the desired correction of the spine is accomplished. The patient is immobilized with bracing or casting, such as a halo cast.

22318-22319

The physician performs open treatment and/or reduction of an odontoid fracture and/or dislocation, including the os odontoideum. The os odontoideum (dens) is the tooth-like process located on the second cervical vertebra in the neck. The patient is placed in a supine position and the fracture or dislocation is reduced with skeletal traction. The physician makes an anterior 6 to 7 cm transverse skin incision at the level of the C5-6 disc space. Dissection is carried down to the odontoid process by longitudinally splitting the muscle and by blunt careful dissection of the space between the carotid, trachea, and esophagus. A retractor is placed and the anterior longitudinal ligament is incised. The superior thyroid artery may be ligated. Using imaging intensification, internal fixation is applied to hold the fracture in proper reduction. Guidewires are inserted into an area of the dens and screws are placed over the wires. No grafting is done in 22318. In 22319, bone grafts are placed to stabilize the fracture or dislocation. When the procedure is completed, a drain may be placed and the wound is closed with layered sutures.

22325-22328

The physician performs open treatment and/or reduction of a vertebral fracture or dislocation from a posterior approach. The patient is placed prone and the skin, fascia, and paravertebral muscles are incised and retracted to expose the fractured vertebra or dislocated segment. The proper rod (e.g., Harrington, Edwards) is selected and anatomic or C-shaped hooks are placed on vertebrae above and below the injury. The rod is inserted in the hooks and the spine is aligned. If fusion is desired, the physician may place separately reportable grafts between the vertebrae or place sleeves on the rod and position them to stabilize the injured vertebrae. The incision is closed by layered sutures. Report 22325 if the site is lumbar; 22326 if the site is cervical; and 22327 if the site is thoracic. Report 22328 for each additional fractured vertebra or dislocated segment in conjunction with the code for the primary procedure.

22505

Spinal manipulation under anesthesia (SMUA) is performed mostly by osteopaths although orthopedists may also use it to treat spinal dysfunction and alleviate neck and back pain. The induction of anesthesia reduces muscle tone and the natural reflex actions so that the spine can be manipulated more effectively to restore joint function and reduce pain. The manipulations are carried out so as to break up fibrotic adhesions of the soft tissues in and around to the spinal joints. SMUA is usually followed by a week of daily rehabilitative manipulation to maintain joint mobility and prevent re-adhesion of the fibrotic tissue.

22510-22512

Percutaneous vertebroplasty is a minimally invasive, image-guided procedure performed by a one- or two-sided injection of a vertebral body. A local anesthetic is administered. A needle is guided into the fractured vertebra under imaging guidance through a small puncture in the patient's skin. Sterile biomaterial such as methyl methacrylate is injected from one or both sides into the damaged vertebral body and acts as a bone cement to reinforce the fractured or collapsed vertebra. The procedure does not restore the original shape to the vertebra, but it does stabilize the bone, preventing further fracture or collapse. Following the procedure, the patient may experience significant, almost immediate pain relief. These codes include a vertebral bone biopsy, if performed, during the same operative session. Report 22510 for percutaneous vertebroplasty of one vertebral body at the cervicothoracic level; 22511 for percutaneous vertebroplasty of one vertebral body at the lumbosacral level; and 22512 for each additional cervicothoracic or lumbosacral vertebral body treated. All imaging guidance is included in these procedures.

22513-22515

The physician performs a minimally invasive percutaneous kyphoplasty, a modification of the percutaneous vertebroplasty, to reduce the pain associated with osteoporotic vertebral compression fractures. This procedure has the added advantage of restoring vertebral body. The patient is placed in a prone, slightly flexed position. A 5 mm to 7 mm incision is made and small cannulae are inserted into the vertebral body from one or both sides. Balloon catheters, called "tamps," are inserted into the vertebra and inflated. Tamps create a void in the soft trabecular bone and restore vertebral alignment. Balloons are then deflated and high viscosity cement under direct image control is injected into the void previously created by bone tamps. Report 22513 when the procedure is performed in the thoracic spine; 22514 when the procedure is performed in the lumbar spine; and 22515 for each additional vertebral body. These codes include all imaging guidance performed.

22526-22527

Percutaneous intradiscal annuloplasty is a minimally invasive technique performed under fluoroscopic guidance to treat small tears in the annulus without an associated disc protrusion. The most common technique is intradiscal electrothermal therapy (IDET). In IDET, the physician advances a needle into the disc using x-ray image guidance. The appropriate treatment catheter is selected and inserted through the needle. Once the catheter is in position, the temperature of the heating portion of the catheter is increased gradually, raising the temperature of the affected site. The increased heat contracts and thickens the collagen disc wall, which may result in contracture and closure of the tears in the annulus. The physician may perform the procedure on one (unilateral) or both sides of the disc. Report 22526 when a single disc is treated and 22527 for one or more additional discs.

22532-22534

Arthrodesis is performed by lateral extracavitary approach. A midline incision is made in the area of the fractured segment and inferiorly curved out to the lateral plane. The paraspinous muscles are exposed, lifted off the spinous processes, and divided and lifted off the ribs. Imaging must be used to identify the targeted interspace. The corresponding rib is dissected from the intercostal muscles and resected in one piece from the curve to the costovertebral connection. The appropriate transverse process and part of the facet and pedicle are removed with a drill from the lateral aspect. The dura and the vertebral body are exposed from the dorsolateral view. Further posterior and lateral access to the vertebral body is gained by gently retracting the nerve root and surrounding structures. A minimal discectomy is now done to prepare the interspace by removing the damaged tissue with curettes and rongeurs. Cartilage is scraped, bone is decorticated, and the arthrodesis is accomplished by tapping bone graft material into the vertebral endplates. A drain is placed and closure is done in layers. Report 22532 for thoracic arthrodesis; 22533 for lumbar arthrodesis; and 22534 for each additional thoracic or lumbar vertebral segment done by lateral extracavitary approach.

22548

Spinal arthrodesis, or fusion, may be done for conditions of herniated disc, degenerative, traumatic, and/or congenital lesions, or to stabilize fractures or dislocations of the spine. Skull tong traction is applied. Avoiding the esophagus, pharynx, or esophageal nerve, the physician may incise the back of the throat, but most often enters from the outside of the neck, left of the throat to reach the C1-C2 (atlas-axis) vertebrae. Retractors separate the intervertebral muscles. A drill is inserted in the affected vertebrae and the location confirmed by x-ray. The physician incises a trough in the front of the vertebrae with a drill or saw. The physician cleans out the intervertebral disc spaces with a rongeur and removes the cartilaginous plates above and below the vertebrae to be fused. The odontoid process (dens), the tooth-like projection located on the second cervical vertebra in the neck, may be excised. The physician obtains and packs separately reportable grafts of iliac or other donor bone into the spaces and trims them. Traction is gradually decreased to maintain the graft in its bed. The fascia is sutured. A drain is placed in the incision and the incision is sutured.

22551-22552

The physician performs spinal fusion (arthrodesis) for indications such as herniated disc; degenerative, traumatic, and/or congenital lesions; or to stabilize fractures or dislocations of the spine. Skull tong traction is applied. The physician uses an anterior approach to reach the damaged vertebrae. An incision is made through the neck, avoiding the esophagus, trachea, and thyroid. Retractors separate the intervertebral muscles. The physician cleans out the intervertebral disc space with a rongeur, removing the cartilaginous material above and below the vertebra to be fused. Preparation includes discectomy and osteophytectomy for nerve root or spinal cord decompression. The physician obtains and packs separately reportable graft material of iliac or other donor bone into the spaces. Traction is gradually decreased to maintain the graft in its bed. The fascia is sutured. A drain is placed and the incision is sutured. Report 22551 for a single cervical interspace below C2. Report 22552 for each additional interspace below C2.

22554-22585

Spinal arthrodesis, or fusion, may be done for conditions of herniated disc, degenerative, traumatic, and/or congenital lesions, or to stabilize fractures or dislocations of the spine. Skull tong traction is applied. The physician uses an anterior approach to reach the damaged vertebrae. For cervical vertebrae in 22554, an incision is made through the neck, avoiding the esophagus, trachea, and thyroid. Retractors separate the intervertebral muscles. A drill is inserted in the affected vertebrae and the location is confirmed by separately reportable x-ray. The physician incises a trough in the front of the vertebrae with a drill or saw. The physician cleans out the intervertebral disc spaces with a rongeur and removes the cartilaginous plates above and below the vertebrae to be fused. The physician obtains and packs separately reportable grafts of iliac or other donor bone into the spaces and trims them. Traction is gradually decreased to maintain the graft in its bed. The fascia is sutured. A drain is placed and the incision is sutured. Report 22556 if the spinal arthrodesis site is thoracic. Report 22558 if the spinal arthrodesis site is lumbar. Report 22585 for each additional interspace treated in conjunction with the code for the primary procedure.

22586

A fusion involving the L5-S1 interspace is performed. This procedure is sometimes referred to as the transsacral interbody fusion or axial lumbar interbody fusion. A small incision is made near the patient's sacrum. Under imaging guidance, a tube is placed into the L5-S1 disc space. Using suction, the disc is removed. An implant or cage is inserted into the disc space and filled with bone growth material (bone graft) to restore height to the intravertebral space. Using additional incisions, pedicle screws are placed in the L5 and S1 vertebrae. Rods are connected to these screws. All surgical instruments are removed and the incisions are closed.

22590

Spinal arthrodesis, or fusion, may be done for conditions of herniated disc, degenerative, traumatic, and/or congenital lesions, or to stabilize fractures or dislocations of the spine. The patient is placed in a Stryker frame with a previously applied halo vest. The physician incises the skin from the occiput to the C3 vertebra, opens the fascia, and retracts the paravertebral muscles. A horizontal hole is drilled in the occiput using a burr. A second hole is drilled in the base of C2. The physician places wires through these holes. A third wire is placed around the ring of C1. Separately reportable bone grafts are obtained from the iliac crest or other donor bone. They are prepared, positioned, and tied in place using the wires. The retractors are removed and the incision is closed over a drain.

22595

Spinal arthrodesis, or fusion, may be done for conditions of herniated disc, degenerative, traumatic, and/or congenital lesions, or to stabilize fractures or dislocations of the spine. The patient is placed in a Stryker frame with a previously applied halo vest. The physician makes an incision from the occiput to the fourth or fifth vertebra. The physician exposes the posterior arch of the atlas (C1) and laminae of the axis (C2) and removes all soft tissue from bony surfaces. The upper arch of C1 is exposed and a wire loop is brought from below upward under the arch of the atlas and sutured. The physician passes the free ends through the loop, grasping the arch of C1. A graft taken from the iliac crest or other donor bone is placed against the lamina of the C2 and the arch of C1 beneath the wire. The physician passes one end of the wire through the spinous process of C2 and twists it securely into place. The retractors are removed and the incision is closed over a drain.

22600-22614

Spinal arthrodesis, or fusion, may be done for conditions of herniated disc; degenerative, traumatic, and/or congenital lesions; or to stabilize fractures or dislocations of the spine. These codes represent arthrodesis (or fusion) using a posterior or posterolateral technique. The physician makes an incision overlying the vertebrae and separates the fascia and the supraspinous ligaments in line with the incision. The physician prepares the vertebrae and lifts ligaments and muscles out of the way. A chisel elevator is used to strip away the capsules of the lateral articulations, and the articular cartilage and cortical bone are excised. Separately reportable bone chips are cut from the fossa below the lateral articulations and from the laminae, or fragments of the spinous process are taken for grafting. The graft is placed alongside (lateral) the vertebrae to be fused to fill the interlaminar space and the gap left by the articular cartilage removal. Also reported separately are additional bone grafts that may be taken from the ilium or other donor bone through a separate incision and used to join the laminae, as well as spinal fusion instrumentation placed to stabilize the graft. The periosteum, ligaments, and paravertebral muscles are sutured to secure the bone grafting. The skin and subcutaneous tissues are closed in layers with sutures. Report 22600 for cervical arthrodesis; 22610 for thoracic arthrodesis; 22612 for lumbar arthrodesis; and 22614 for each additional vertebral interspace.

22630-22632

Spinal arthrodesis, or fusion, may be done for conditions of herniated disc; degenerative, traumatic, and/or congenital lesions; or to stabilize fractures or dislocations of the spine. These codes represent arthrodesis (or fusion) using a posterior interbody technique. The physician makes an incision overlying the lumbar vertebrae and separates the fascia and the supraspinous ligaments in line with the incision. The physician prepares the vertebrae and lifts ligaments and muscles out of the way. A chisel elevator is used to strip away the capsules of the lateral articulations and the articular cartilage and cortical bone are excised. Bone fragments taken from the vertebral bodies adjacent to the affected disc, from the spinous process, or laminar fragments may be taken for grafting and are reported separately. Laminectomies and partial facetectomies are performed to facilitate preparation of the interspace for fusion. The intervertebral disc is removed using rongeurs or curettes. The disc space is measured, and a bone spacer (graft, metal, or plastic) is inserted between the vertebrae. Additional bone grafts, which are reported separately, may be taken from the ilium or other donor bone used to fill the disc space. Spinal fusion instrumentation, also reported separately, may be placed to stabilize the graft. The periosteum, ligaments, and paravertebral muscles are sutured to secure the bone grafting. The skin and subcutaneous tissues are closed in layers with sutures. Report 22630 for the first interspace and 22632 for each additional interspace.

22633-22634

Spinal arthrodesis, or fusion, may be done for conditions of herniated disc; degenerative, traumatic, and/or congenital lesions; or to stabilize fractures or dislocations of the spine. These codes represent arthrodesis (or fusion) using a combination of posterior/posterolateral and posterior interbody techniques. The physician makes an incision overlying the lumbar vertebrae and separates the fascia and the supraspinous ligaments in line with the incision. The physician prepares the vertebrae and lifts ligaments and muscles out of the way. A chisel elevator is used to strip away the capsules of the lateral articulations and the articular cartilage and cortical bone are excised. Separately reportable chips are cut from the fossa below the lateral articulations and from the laminae, or fragments of the spinous process are taken for grafting. Laminectomies and partial facetectomies are performed to facilitate preparation of the interspace for fusion. The intervertebral disc is removed using rongeurs or curettes. The disc space is measured, and a bone spacer (graft, metal, or plastic) is inserted between the vertebrae. A bone graft is placed alongside (lateral to) the vertebrae to be fused and is used to fill the interlaminar space and the gap left by the articular cartilage removal. Also reported separately are additional bone grafts that may be taken from the ilium or other donor bone through a separate incision and used to join the laminae, as well as spinal fusion instrumentation placed to stabilize the graft. The periosteum, ligaments, and paravertebral muscles are sutured to secure the bone grafting. The skin and subcutaneous tissues are closed in layers with sutures. Report 22633 for the first interspace and 22634 for each additional interspace.

22800-22804

Spinal arthrodesis, or fusion, is done here to correct a spinal deformity. The patient is placed prone. A midline posterior incision is made overlying the affected vertebrae. The fascia and the paravertebral muscles are incised and retracted. The physician uses a curette and rongeur to clean interspinous ligaments. One of several techniques may be used. In one, the spinous processes are split and removed and a curette is used to cut into the lateral articulations. Thin pieces of separately reportable iliac or other donor bone graft are placed in these slots. Grafts are obtained, prepared, and packed on both sides of the spinal curve, with more bone chips on the concave sides. Separately reportable instrumentation may be affixed to the spine. The incision is closed with layered sutures. A cast may be applied to stabilize the spine. Report 22800 for fusion of up to six vertebral segments; 22802 for fusion of seven to 12 vertebral segments; and 22804 for 13 or more vertebral segments.

22808-22812

Spinal arthrodesis, or fusion, is done here to correct a spinal deformity. An anterior approach is used. In the case of affected thoracolumbar vertebrae, the dissection is carried out through the abdominal muscles to the tenth rib, which is resected to allow access to the vertebrae in back. Dissection continues until the vertebral bodies are exposed. The physician cleans out the intervertebral disc spaces and removes the cartilaginous plates above and below the vertebrae to be fused. The physician obtains and packs separately reportable grafts of iliac or other donor bone into the spaces. Separately reportable instrumentation may be affixed to the spine. A drainage tube may be placed and the surgical wound is sutured closed. A cast may be applied to stabilize the spine. Report 22808 if two to three vertebral segments are fused; 22810 if four to seven vertebral segments are fused; and 22812 if eight or more vertebral segments are fused.

22818-22819

The physician performs this procedure for spinal deformities of kyphosis, a hunchback type increase in the convex curvature of the thoracic spine. The patient is placed prone. The physician makes a posterior midline incision, superior to the spinal abnormality, and dissects the periosteum of the normal vertebrae above and down into the lamina of the affected vertebrae, until the foramina are exposed on both sides of the spine. The nerve, artery, and vein within the foramina are divided, exposing the dural sac. The sac is dissected and the dura is closed with suture, leaving the sac remnant. Dissection is continued around the affected vertebral bodies and the intervertebral disc of the vertebra at the apex of the kyphosis is removed first, followed by the vertebra. Just enough vertebrae are removed to correct the kyphosis. The sac remnant that was left is used to cover the site of the resected vertebrae. Removed vertebral bodies are morselized and used for bone grafting. Rod instrumentation is applied and segmental wires are used to hold the rod in place. The wound is irrigated and closed with layered sutures over suction drains. A body jacket is applied. Report 22818 if a single or two-segment kyphectomy is performed. Report 22819 if a three or more segments kyphectomy is performed.

22830

The physician explores an existing fusion to diagnose and correct problems. The patient is placed in various positions depending on how the original fusion was performed (e.g., anterior, posterior, posterolateral). The physician makes an incision overlying the fused vertebrae. Fascia and paravertebral muscles are incised and retracted. The physician explores previous instrumentation, grafts, and wires; any or all may be partially replaced or adjusted during the exploration. When the exploration is complete, the fascia and vertebral muscles are repaired and returned to their anatomical positions. The incision is closed with layered sutures.

22840

The physician uses spinal instrumentation to correct a defect of the spine caused by disease, trauma, or congenital anomaly and to stabilize the spine to reduce risks of neurological damage or nonfusion after arthrodesis. Non-segmental instrumentation is a construct placed with fixation at either end only and not in the intervening levels. The physician makes a midline incision in the skin, fascia, and paravertebral muscles over the affected vertebrae. Upper and lower hooks or screws are introduced into the vertebral pedicles. A rod fashioned to fit the spinal contours is anchored to the screws or hooks. To achieve correction, distraction is applied with an instrument to increase the distance between the hooks at each end of the rod, which is secured in position. Another method of securing the rod is to use wires passed under prepared lamina and tightened around the rods. The wound is closed with layered sutures. These Harrington rod instrumentation techniques have become outdated and are being replaced by more rigid, segmental fixation methods. Report this code in addition to the code for the primary procedure.

22841

Internal spinal fixation by wiring the spinous processes, also called Drummond wiring, is done with

Musculoskeletal

wires attached to a button that gives the needed purchase at the base of the spinous process and has a hole in its surface for the wire coming from the opposite direction to pass through. The spine is exposed in the standard manner and a hook is used to grasp the upper and lower pedicle of the selected fusion levels. Using an awl or a clamp, the physician makes a hole in the base of each involved spinous process and passes two button wire implants in opposite directions through the bony hole, making sure that each wire also passes through the hole in the opposite button, and pulls the buttons snugly to the base of the spinous process. The buttons are tamped into place. In some cases, only one button wire is passed from the convex to the concave side. A contoured distraction rod is inserted into the open loops of the wire implants and the hooks at the top and bottom and secured. Distraction is applied for correction, which is maintained by tightening the wires. Further distraction may be applied to the rod and a clamp placed to prevent loss of the correction. The laminae and transverse processes lateral to the buttons may be decorticated before closure of the wound. Report this code in addition to the code for the primary procedure.

22842-22844

Segmental instrumentation is a construct placed with fixation not only at either end but also with at least one attachment in between. The physician makes a midline incision in the skin, fascia, and paravertebral muscles over the affected vertebrae. Multiple hooks or screws are introduced into the vertebral pedicles where fixation is needed. Dual rods, such as Harrington distraction and compression rods, are anchored to the screws or hooks. Distraction is the force that produces kyphosis and compression corrects kyphosis, the abnormal hunchback curvature of the spine. To achieve correction, the compression assembly is tightened in place before distraction is applied and secured in position. The wound is closed with layered sutures. The Harrington rod instrumentation techniques are being replaced by three-dimensional correction techniques where rods can be bent along the length and applied at any level, in rotation, with distraction and compression applied between segments. Report 22842 for fixation of three to six vertebral segments; 22843 for seven to 12 vertebral segments; and 22844 for 13 or more vertebral segments. These codes are reported in addition to codes for the primary procedure.

22845-22847

Several methods and types of anterior instrumentation are available (e.g., Dwyer, Zielke, Scottish Rite) but all are based on a rod or cable fixated through large-headed, slotted, or cannulated screws. Anterior exposure for thoracic or lumbar spinal procedures may require a thoracic or general surgeon to assist for the intraoperative exposure, mainly thoracoabdominal or abdominal retroperitoneal. A hole is made in the cervical, thoracic, or lumbar vertebral body on the lateral side as posteriorly as possible. The screw is inserted across the midportion of the vertebra to the opposite cortex in a slight posteroanterior angle. A flexible threaded rod or cable is inserted in the angled screw heads. The spine is derotated and the rod is locked into its straighter position with nuts. The wound is closed in a routine manner. Report 22845 for two to three vertebral segments; 22846 for four to seven vertebral segments; and 22847 for eight or more vertebral segments. These codes are reported in addition to codes for the primary procedure.

[22836, 22837, 22838]

The physician performs anterior vertebral body tethering of the thoracic spine, a non-fusion, minimally invasive surgical procedure intended to correct idiopathic scoliosis. Under general anesthesia, the patient is placed in the lateral decubitus (side) position with the spinal convexity side up and the concavity side down. Typically using a percutaneous endoscopic approach, a video-assisted thoracoscopy is performed through four to five small portal incisions in the hemithorax. A lung may need to be collapsed during the procedure for visualization. Under endoscopic visualization, with CT scan or fluoroscopic guidance, titanium screws and anchors are placed in the vertebral bodies on the convexity side. The screws are then connected to the tether device, usually a polyethylene terephthalate flexible cord that secures the instrumentation under the appropriate tension as controlled by the surgeon. When the tether cord is tightened, it compresses the convex side of the spine to help straighten the spine. The scoliotic curve shows an immediate improvement after surgery and continuous improvement as the patient's spine grows, creating a straighter spine. Alternately, the procedure may be carried out with an open approach via anterior thoracotomy. During the surgery, one or both lungs are collapsed, and the parietal pleura is opened over the spine. Screws and anchors are placed in the vertebral bodies and the polyethylene tether is attached and tightened. A chest drainage tube may be placed and set to suction. Report 22836 if up to seven thoracic vertebral segments are treated, and 22837 if treatment involves eight or more segments. Report 22838 for replacement, removal, or revision (including augmentation or division of tether). These codes include thoracoscopy when performed.

22848

The physician joins axial connectors, such as the tail end of spinal instrumentation devices, to a rod configured to fit along the flat of the sacrum and impacted longitudinally between the cornices of the ilium just above the greater sciatic notch. The rod is driven through the ilium and negates the need for anterior instrumentation. This procedure, usually called the "Galveston technique," often accompanies a procedure for scoliosis, myelomeningocele, or paralytic spinal defects where sacral fixation is not desirable. Report this code in addition to the code for the primary procedure.

22849
This code describes the procedures used following failure of devices such as wires, screws, cables, plates, or rods used in spinal fixation. The patient is placed in the position dictated by the failure. The physician makes a midline incision overlying the damaged section. The fascia, paravertebral muscles, and ligaments are retracted. A number of reparative techniques may be used, depending on the device and point of failure. In most cases, the device must be replaced. The physician closes the muscles, fascia, and skin with layered sutures.

22850
Previously applied posterior spinal nonsegmental instrumentation is removed. Instrumentation is sometimes removed when correction is complete and stable, when the patient is a growing juvenile, or when the instrumentation causes complications, such as infection or pain. The patient is placed prone. The physician makes an incision overlying the affected area through the skin, fascia, and paravertebral muscles. Collagen is removed. The instrumentation is exposed and the superior hook or screw is loosened. Using forceps, the upper and lower hooks are disconnected from the vertebra and the hardware is removed.

22852
Previously applied posterior spinal segmental instrumentation is removed. Instrumentation is sometimes removed when correction is complete and stable, when the patient is a growing juvenile, or when the instrumentation causes complications, such as infection or pain. The patient is placed prone. The physician makes a midline incision overlying the affected area through the skin, fascia, and paravertebral muscles. Collagen is removed. The instrumentation is exposed. Using forceps, the superior hook is loosened. The superior, inferior, and all segmental hooks between are disconnected from the vertebrae. The hardware is removed. The incision is closed with layered sutures.

22853
The physician replaces an intervertebral disc resected due to destruction by disease, trauma, or other processes. Once the vertebral disc has been removed by a separately identifiable procedure, a hole is cored out of the vertebral bodies above and below the removed vertebrae to secure a biomechanical device (synthetic cage or mesh) into the resulting intervertebral disc space. The physician selects the biomechanical device best suited to the location and type of deformity being corrected. Screws, wires, or plates may be used to secure the device. Muscles are allowed to fall back into place and the wound is closed over a drain with layered sutures.

22854
The physician replaces a vertebral body or partial vertebral body resected due to destruction by disease, trauma, or other processes. Once the vertebral body has been removed by a separately identifiable procedure, a hole is cored out of the vertebral bodies above and below the removed vertebrae to secure a biomechanical device (synthetic cage or mesh) into the resulting intervertebral defect. The physician selects the biomechanical device best suited to the location and type of deformity being corrected. Screws, wires, or plates may be used to secure the device. Muscles are allowed to fall back into place and the wound is closed over a drain with layered sutures.

[22859]
The physician replaces a vertebral body or partial vertebral body resected due to destruction by disease, trauma, or other processes. Once the vertebral body has been removed by a separately identifiable procedure, a hole is cored out of the vertebral bodies above and below the removed vertebrae to secure a biomechanical device (metal/synthetic cage, mesh, or methylmethacrylate) into the resulting vertebral body defect or intervertebral disc space without the use of interbody arthrodesis. The physician selects the biomechanical device best suited to the location and type of deformity being corrected. For example, to correct a deformity caused by a malignancy, the physician may elect to inject methylmethacrylate into the area and allow it to dry to replace the excised vertebral body. Screws, wires, or plates may be used to secure the device. Muscles are allowed to fall back into place and the wound is closed over a drain with layered sutures. Report this code for each contiguous defect.

22855
Previously applied anterior spinal instrumentation is removed. Instrumentation is sometimes removed when correction is complete and stable, when the patient is a growing juvenile, or when the instrumentation causes complications, such as infection or pain. The patient is placed supine for the removal of anterior spinal fixation devices. The physician makes an abdominal retroperitoneal or thoracic incision to reach the affected area. Collagen is removed. The instrumentation is exposed and the superior hook or screw is loosened. Using forceps, the superior hook or screw is disconnected from the vertebra, as are the inferior and all segmental hooks or screws. The hardware is removed. The incision is closed with layered sutures.

22856-22857, 22860 [22858]
Total disc arthroplasty is performed to replace a severely damaged or diseased intervertebral disc, most often caused by degenerative disc disease. The physician uses an anterior approach to reach the damaged cervical vertebrae in 22856 by making an incision through the neck, avoiding the esophagus, trachea, and thyroid. In 22857, the physician uses an anterior approach to reach the damaged lumbar vertebrae by making an incision through the abdomen. Some implants require only minimal access, approximately 7 cm long, for a mini-retroperitoneal approach. Retractors separate the intervertebral muscles. The affected intervertebral disc location is confirmed by separately reportable x-ray. The physician cleans out the intervertebral disc space with

Musculoskeletal

a rongeur, removing the cartilaginous material to be replaced in preparation for inserting the implant. Preparation may include discectomy, osteophytectomy for nerve root or spinal cord decompression, and/or microdissection. One type of implant for total disc replacement has two endplates made of a metal alloy and a convex weight-bearing surface made of ultra-high molecular weight polyethylene. The endplates are inserted in a collapsed form and seated into the vertebral bodies above and below the interspace. Minimal distraction is applied to open the intervertebral space, and the polyethylene disc material is snap-fitted into the lower endplate. With the disc assembly complete, the wound is closed and a drain may be placed. Each of these codes reports a single interspace and includes fluoroscopy when performed. Report 22858 for a second level, cervical vertebra. Report 22860 for a second level, lumbar vertebra.

22861-22862

The physician revises an artificial disc prosthesis placed during a previous disc arthroplasty through anterior approach. The prosthesis may be migrating from a lack of fixation and require components to be replaced or adjusted. The physician approaches the cervical vertebrae in 22861 by making an incision through the neck, avoiding the esophagus, trachea, and thyroid. The lumbar vertebrae (22862) are approached by making an incision through the abdomen. Retractors separate the intervertebral muscles. The implant is located, the area is explored, and any adhesions are freed. Distraction is applied to open the intervertebral space. The arthroplastic disc is removed, and the endplates of the vertebral body are reshaped and prepped for reinsertion. New height, depth, and width dimensions may also be taken with the vertebral body distracted in cases where another, more appropriately sized disc prosthesis is required. The components are reinserted, and the fascia and vertebral muscles are repaired and returned to their anatomical positions. The incision is closed. Each of these codes reports a single interspace and includes fluoroscopy when performed.

22864-22865

The physician removes an artificial disc prosthesis placed during a previous disc arthroplasty by anterior approach. The physician approaches the cervical vertebrae in 22864 by making an incision through the neck, avoiding the esophagus, trachea, and thyroid. The lumbar vertebrae (22865) are approached by making an incision through the abdomen. Retractors separate the intervertebral muscles. The implant is located and any adhesions are freed. Distraction is applied to open the intervertebral space, and the implant is removed. The area is explored and debrided. When the procedure is complete, the fascia and vertebral muscles are repaired and returned to their anatomical positions, drains are placed, and the wound is closed. Each of these codes reports a single vertebral interspace and includes fluoroscopy when performed.

22867-22868

Insertion of interspinous/interlaminar process stabilization/distraction devices is performed to increase the space within the neural foramen and release nerve pressure thereby decreasing pain. Interspinous devices are inserted within the vertebral spinous processes and interlaminar devices are inserted between adjoining lamina and spinous processes to create effective stabilization with wings enclosing the inferior and superior spinous processes. The device opens the space while maintaining the spine's ability to bend in that area. This procedure secures the supraspinous ligament, which helps keep the device intact. Some devices may necessitate extraction of the interspinous ligament with enclosure of the upper and lower spinous processes. This may be done after decompression surgery or as a substitute for decompression surgery. The devices are inserted via a small incision (4 cm to 8 cm) among the spinous processes with the patient mildly anesthetized or utilizing a local anesthesia. In 22867, an open decompression (laminectomy) is also performed. During this procedure, the lamina of the affected area is removed to release pressure on the spinal cord and nerves. The foramen may be expanded by an anterior approach and by creating an opening within the disc space at the front of the spine or between two pedicle screws inserted posteriorly. At this point, the interspinous/interlaminar devices are inserted. Report 22867 for insertion of these devices in addition to open decompression of a lumbar vertebra, without fusion. Report 22868 when the same procedure is performed at a second vertebral level. Imaging guidance, when performed, is included.

22869-22870

Insertion of interspinous/interlaminar process stabilization/distraction devices is performed to increase the space within the neural foramen and release nerve pressure thereby decreasing pain. Interspinous devices are inserted within the vertebral spinous processes and interlaminar devices are inserted between adjoining lamina and spinous processes to create effective stabilization with wings enclosing the inferior and superior spinous processes. The device opens the space while maintaining the spine's ability to bend in that area. This procedure secures the supraspinous ligament, which helps keep the device intact. Some devices may necessitate extraction of the interspinous ligament with enclosure of the upper and lower spinous processes. This may be done after decompression surgery or as a substitute for decompression surgery. The devices are inserted via a small incision (4 cm to 8 cm) among the spinous processes with the patient mildly anesthetized or utilizing a local anesthesia. Report 22869 for insertion of these devices at a single lumbar vertebral level, without fusion or open decompression. Report 22870 when the same procedure is performed at a second vertebral level. Imaging guidance, when performed, is included.

22900-22903
The physician removes a tumor from the soft tissue of the abdominal wall that is located in the subcutaneous tissue in 22902-22903 and in the deep soft tissue, below the fascial plane or within the muscle, in 22900-22901. The patient is positioned supine on the operating table. With the proper anesthesia administered, the physician makes an incision in the skin overlying the mass and dissects down to the tumor. The extent of the tumor is identified and a dissection is undertaken all the way around the tumor. A portion of neighboring soft tissue may also be removed to ensure adequate removal of all tumor tissue. A drain may be inserted and the incision is repaired with layers of sutures, staples, or Steri-strips. Report 22902 for excision of subcutaneous tumors whose resected area is less than 3 cm and 22903 for excision of subcutaneous tumors 3 cm or greater. Report 22900 for excision of subfascial or intramuscular tumors whose resected area is less than 5 cm and 22901 for excision of subfascial or intramuscular tumors 5 cm or greater.

22904-22905
The physician performs a radical resection of a soft tissue tumor (i.e., sarcoma) from the abdominal wall, not involving bone. The tumor may be malignant or an aggressive benign tumor of the connective tissue. An incision is made over the tumor and dissection exposes it. The tumor and any adjacent tissue that may be affected by the spread of the neoplasm are excised. Large resections may be needed. The type and stage of the lesion determines the extent of the tumor margin resection area. Muscle or fascia may need to be repaired and drains may be placed. The surgical wound is closed using simple or intermediate repair or separately reportable complex closure, adjacent tissue transfer, or graft. Report 22904 for excision of tumors whose resected area is less than 5 cm and 22905 for excision of tumors 5 cm or greater.

23000
The physician removes subdeltoid calcareous deposits by making a small incision over the deltoid muscle to expose the rotator cuff tendons. The raised area over the calcium deposits is incised in line with the axis of the fibers and the calcareous deposits are removed. A large cavity is made in the tendon with a curette to remove all damaged tissue. The opening is closed with side-to-side sutures. Once the tendon is repaired, the skin incision is closed and a soft dressing is applied.

23020
Capsular contracture release is not commonly performed unless the shoulder is fixed in marked internal rotation and adduction. In this position, the arm is unable to move away from the body. The physician makes an incision at the front of the shoulder where the deltoid meets the pectoral muscle. The subscapularis tendon is removed from the glenoid rim. The anterior capsule is left intact. The pectoralis major tendon is severed from its attachment on the humerus. The skin incision is closed and a soft dressing is applied. The arm is positioned in abduction (arm elevated out to the side of the body).

23030-23031
The physician drains a deep abscess or hematoma in 23030 or an infected bursa in 23031 from the shoulder area. The physician makes an incision in the shoulder overlying the site of the abscess, hematoma, or bursa to be incised. Dissection is carried down through the deep subcutaneous tissues and may be continued into the fascia or muscle to expose the abscess or hematoma. The incision may be extended if the mass is larger than expected. When the infected bursa, abscess, or hematoma is identified, it is incised and the contents are drained. The area is irrigated and the incision is repaired in layers with sutures, staples, and/or Steri-strips; closed with drains in place; or simply left open to further facilitate drainage of infection.

23035
The physician incises bone cortex in the shoulder area to treat a bone abscess or osteomyelitis. The physician makes an incision over the affected area of the shoulder. Dissection is carried down through the soft tissues to expose the bone. The periosteum is split and reflected from the bone overlying the infected area. A curette may be used to scrape away the abscess or infected portion down to healthy bony tissue or drill holes may be made through the cortex into the medullary canal in a window outline around the infected or abscessed bone. The area is drained and debrided of infected bony and soft tissue. The physician irrigates the area with antibiotic solution, the periosteum is closed over the bone, and the soft tissues are sutured closed; or the wound is packed and left open, allowing the area to drain. Secondary closure is performed approximately three weeks later. Dressings are changed daily. A splint may be applied to limit shoulder movement.

23040-23044
The physician performs an arthrotomy of the glenohumeral joint in 23040 or the acromioclavicular or sternoclavicular joint in 23044 that includes exploration, drainage, or removal of any foreign body. An incision is made over the joint to be exposed. The soft tissues are dissected away and the joint capsule is exposed and incised. The joint space is explored, any necrotic tissue is removed, and infection or abnormal fluid is drained. If a foreign body is present (e.g., bullet, nail, gravel), it is exposed and removed. The wound is irrigated with antibiotic solution. The physician may leave the wound packed open with daily dressing changes to allow for further drainage and secondary healing by granulation. If the incision is repaired, drain tubes may be inserted and the incision is repaired in layers with sutures, staples, and/or Steri-strips. A splint may be applied to limit shoulder motion.

23065-23066
The physician performs a biopsy of the soft tissues of the shoulder area. With proper anesthesia administered, an incision is made over the biopsy area. Dissection is carried down within the superficial soft

Musculoskeletal

tissue layers in 23065, usually the subcutaneous fat to the uppermost fascial layer. In 23066, dissection is taken down deep within the soft tissue, such as into the fascial layer or within the muscle. A portion of the tissue is excised and submitted for pathology. The area is irrigated and the incision is closed with layered sutures, staples, or Steri-strips.

23075-23076 [23071, 23073]

The physician removes a tumor from the soft tissue of the shoulder area that is located in the subcutaneous tissue in 23071 and 23075 and in the deep soft tissue, below the fascial plane or within the muscle, in 23073 and 23076. With the proper anesthesia administered, the physician makes an incision in the skin overlying the mass and dissects down to the tumor. The extent of the tumor is identified and a dissection is undertaken all the way around the tumor. A portion of neighboring soft tissue may also be removed to ensure adequate removal of all tumor tissue. A drain may be inserted and the incision is repaired with layers of sutures, staples, or Steri-strips. Report 23075 for excision of subcutaneous tumors whose resected area is less than 3 cm and 23071 for excision of subcutaneous tumors 3 cm or greater. Report 23076 for excision of subfascial or intramuscular tumors whose resected area is less than 5 cm and 23073 for excision of subfascial or intramuscular tumors 5 cm or greater.

23077-23078

The physician performs a radical resection of a soft tissue tumor (i.e., sarcoma) from the shoulder area, not involving bone. The tumor may be malignant or an aggressive benign tumor of the connective tissue. An incision is made over the tumor and dissection exposes it. The tumor and any adjacent tissue that may be affected by the spread of the neoplasm are excised. Large resections may be needed. The type and stage of the lesion determines the extent of the tumor margin resection area. Muscle or fascia may need to be repaired and drains may be placed. The surgical wound is closed using simple or intermediate repair or separately reportable complex closure, adjacent tissue transfer, or graft. Report 23077 for excision of tumors whose resected area is less than 5 cm and 23078 for excision of tumors 5 cm or greater.

23100

The physician performs an arthrotomy and biopsy of the glenohumeral joint. An incision is made over the shoulder joint and carried down through the soft tissues to gain access into the glenohumeral joint. A biopsy sample of the joint tissue is removed and saved for testing. The wound is repaired in layered sutures.

23101

The physician makes an incision into the acromioclavicular or sternoclavicular joint to remove torn cartilage and take a tissue sample. An incision is made through the skin and the underlying muscle is divided to gain access to the joint capsule. Once the capsule is penetrated, any torn cartilage is identified and removed. A tissue specimen is removed for biopsy. The joint is irrigated, the capsule is closed, and the soft tissues are sutured in layers. A soft dressing is applied.

23105-23106

The physician performs an arthrotomy and synovectomy of the glenohumeral joint, with or without biopsy. With the patient lying on one side and the arm suspended in traction, the physician makes an incision overlying the shoulder. The joint capsule is exposed by dissecting down through the soft tissues and freeing and reflecting the muscles. The joint capsule is incised to expose the synovium. Motorized resectors are used to remove the synovium, the inner membrane of the articular capsule that lines the joint cavity. A sample of the tissue for biopsy may also be removed. Following completion of the synovectomy, the shoulder is irrigated, a drain tube may be placed, and the incision is closed in layers with sutures, staples, or Steri-strips. Report 23106 if the procedure is done on the sternoclavicular joint.

23107

The physician performs an arthrotomy of the glenohumeral joint with joint exploration and removal of any loose or foreign bodies. An incision is made over the glenohumeral joint. The soft tissues are dissected away and the joint capsule is exposed and incised. The joint space is explored and any loose or foreign body (e.g., free cartilage, bone fragments, gravel) is exposed and removed. The wound is irrigated with antibiotic solution. The physician may leave the wound packed open with daily dressing changes to allow for further drainage and secondary healing by granulation. If the incision is repaired, drain tubes may be inserted and the incision is repaired in layers with sutures, staples, and/or Steri-strips. A splint may be applied to limit shoulder motion.

23120-23125

Removal of the clavicle (collar bone) is successfully performed without significant loss of function to the upper extremity for such problems as old, chronic, or acute unreduced dislocations. An incision is made horizontally along the portion of the bone to be removed. The skin is reflected, the bone is cleared of soft tissue attachments, and divided with an osteotome or bone-cutting rongeurs. For a partial resection, the remaining end of the clavicle is rounded and smoothed to eliminate the rough edge. If the medial end of the clavicle is removed, the clavicle may be stabilized to the first rib and the sternocleidomastoid may be detached. The periosteum and soft tissues are plicated and sutured over the raw end of the clavicle. The wound is closed and a soft dressing is applied. Report 23120 for a partial claviculectomy and 23125 for total claviculectomy.

23130

A partial acromioplasty or acromionectomy, with or without coracoacromial ligament release, is done. This procedure is also commonly performed during repair to the rotator cuff in an effort to increase the space below the acromion where the cuff tendons traverse toward their insertion on the humerus. An incision is made overlying the area. Dissection is carried down to the acromion. Acromioplasty involves the division of the acromioclavicular ligament followed by the use of a burr to cut away the under surface of the acromion. During acromionectomy, the distal portion of the acromion is removed. The coracoacromial ligament, a wide, strong band spanning between the acromion and the coracoid process of the scapula, may also be released. The joint is irrigated and the incisions are closed with sutures or Steri-strips.

23140-23146

A bone cyst or benign tumor of the clavicle or scapula is removed. The physician makes an incision overlying the cyst or tumor. The skin and underlying soft tissues are reflected to expose the periosteum, which is separated from the bone. Curettes or osteotomes are used to scrape or cut the lesion from the bone. Once the benign tumor or cyst is removed and healthy bone tissue is present, the periosteum is repositioned and the incision is repaired in layers. If the bone defect created requires a graft for repair, the physician obtains the necessary size bone graft from a separate donor site on the patient and packs it into the site where the tumor or bone cyst was removed or uses a bone bank allograft. Report 23145 if an autograft is obtained and 23146 if an allograft is used.

23150-23156

A bone cyst or benign tumor of the proximal humerus is removed. The physician makes an incision in the upper arm overlying the cyst or tumor. The skin and underlying soft tissues are reflected to expose the periosteum, which is separated from the bone. Curettes or osteotomes are used to scrape or cut the lesion from the bone. Once the benign tumor or cyst is removed and healthy bone tissue is present, the periosteum is repositioned and the incision is repaired in layers. If the bone defect created requires a graft for repair, the physician obtains the necessary size bone graft from a separate donor site on the patient and packs it into the site where the tumor or bone cyst was removed or uses a bone bank allograft. Report 23155 if the procedure is done with an autograft and 23156 if an allograft is used.

23170-23174

The physician removes infected portions of the clavicle in 23170 due to a bone abscess or osteomyelitis. This infection often leaves open sinus tracts in the bone that require removal. The physician makes an incision overlying the sequestered area of bone in the clavicle. Once the skin and soft tissues are reflected, a small window is cut into the bone to gain access to the sequestrum, or necrosed piece of bone that has become separated from sound bone. All purulent material and scarred or necrotic tissue are removed. The remaining space is filled with surrounding soft tissues or free tissue transfer. The area is irrigated and an antibiotic solution is used to prevent further infection. The wound is closed loosely over drains if possible. The arm is positioned in a sling or splint and protected to prevent fracture of the clavicle. Report 23172 if the sequestrectomy is performed on the scapula and 23174 if this procedure is performed on the humeral head to the surgical neck.

23180-23184

The physician performs a partial excision of the clavicle in 23180 to remove infected bone. An incision is made over the infected part of the clavicle and the underlying soft tissues are divided to expose the bone. The periosteum is reflected and the infected portion of bone is removed and irrigated. The excavation of bone may excise a crater-like piece, leave a small saucer-like shelf depression in the bone, or may remove a portion of the shaft (diaphysis) of a long bone. If a significant portion of bone is removed, the physician may use bone graft material to fill the cavity left in the bone. The periosteum is closed over the bone, the soft tissues are sutured closed, and a soft dressing is applied. Report 23182 for partial excision of the scapula and 23184 for partial excision of the proximal humerus.

23190

The physician removes a portion of the scapula (shoulder blade). An oblique skin incision is made across the scapula and the underlying trapezius muscle is reflected to expose the superior medial angle. The portion of the scapula is removed and the remaining border is smoothed to prevent trauma to the surrounding tissues. A portion of the supraspinatus and levator scapulae tendons are resected and sutured to the trapezius muscle and remaining border of the scapula. The wound is irrigated and the incision is sutured. A soft dressing is applied.

23195

The physician performs a resection of the humeral head. An incision is made over the joint in the upper arm and the underlying muscles are divided to expose the bone. The joint capsule is incised and tendons are removed from the bone. The physician makes a horizontal cut through the humerus just distal to the head and removes the bone. Separately reportable hemiarthroplasty to replace the proximal humeral bone with an implant for attaching the tendons and reconstructing the joint usually follows.

23200-23210

The physician performs a radical resection of a tumor of the clavicle bone in 23200. Either end may be resected or the bone may be excised. An incision is made horizontally along the portion of the bone with the tumor to be removed. The skin and soft tissues are reflected. The acromioclavicular and/or sternoclavicular ligaments may need to be divided to free the bone from the joint at either respective end. The bone is cleared of soft tissue attachments, such as the platysma and pectoral muscles, and the diseased bone is resected with an osteotome or bone-cutting rongeurs, along with any soft tissues involved with the tumor. If the tumor is removed from one end, the remaining end of the clavicle is rounded and smoothed to eliminate the rough edge. The periosteum and soft tissues are plicated and sutured over the raw end of the clavicle. The wound is closed and a soft dressing is applied. Report 23210 if a similar procedure is performed on the scapula.

23220
The physician performs a radical resection of a tumor of the proximal humerus. Removal of the proximal portion of the humerus is often performed for aggressive benign lesions and low-grade malignancies. A longitudinal incision is made from the acromioclavicular joint to the lateral border of the biceps tendon. The underlying muscles are divided to expose the bone. The joint capsule is incised and tendons are removed from the bone at the level of the proximal joint. The humerus is divided by a horizontal cut a few centimeters distal to the tumor site. A portion of the remaining medullary bone is taken for testing. The proximal portion of the bone is removed, along with any soft tissues involved with the tumor. Reconstructive alternatives following resection include reconstruction with flail shoulder, with passive spacer, with arthrodesis, and with arthroplasty.

23330-23333
The physician removes a foreign body of the shoulder. In 23330, a subcutaneous foreign body is removed. The physician makes a small incision over the foreign body and reflects the skin to expose it. The foreign body is removed, the wound is irrigated, and the skin is closed with sutures or Steri-strips. In 23333, a deep foreign body is removed. The physician removes a foreign body from deep within the shoulder. A long incision is made overlying the shoulder. The physician dissects through each layer down to the subfascial or intramuscular tissue. The physician may debride any inflamed or other scar tissues. The foreign body is removed from within the shoulder tissue. The physician may irrigate the joint with antibiotic solution. The wound is closed in layers unless there is infection present. If infection is present, the wound is left open to drain.

23334-23335
The physician removes an artificial joint component from deep within the shoulder. A long incision is made overlying the shoulder. The physician dissects through each layer of tissue down to the bones in the shoulder exposing the shoulder joint. The physician may debride any inflamed synovial or other scar tissues. The prosthesis is removed from within the joint and/or from inside the humerus bone. The physician irrigates the joint with antibiotic solution. The wound is closed in layers unless there is infection present. If infection is present, the wound is left open to drain. Report 23334 if the glenoid or humeral prosthesis is removed. Report 23335 if both components are removed.

23350
This procedure is commonly used in the diagnosis of a rotator cuff tear. The patient is positioned supine on the x-ray table. The skin and deep tissues lateral to the coracoid process are injected with a local anesthetic. A no. 20 spinal needle 7.5 cm long is inserted into the joint at the same location and the position is checked by separately reportable x-ray. From 15 ml to 20 ml of a suitable contrast medium is injected; resistance is felt when the joint is full. The shoulder is taken through a full range of motion and separately reportable x-rays are taken to see if there is leakage of the substance to other parts of the joint and a proper diagnosis is made.

23395-23397
In the case of bicipital syndrome with rotator cuff pathology, the biceps tendon has become detached from the shoulder. The physician makes an anterior superior approach to the shoulder and splits and reflects the deltoid muscle. An acromioplasty is performed and the coracoacromial ligament is excised. The long head of the biceps tendon is identified and reattached to the humerus by tenodesis procedure. The rotator cuff is repaired prior to closure of the incisions. A soft dressing and sling are applied for two weeks. If the rotator cuff is repaired, an abduction pillow is used for four to six weeks. Report 23397 if multiple muscle transfers are performed during the procedure.

23400
Sprengel's deformity is a congenital deformity where the scapula is positioned higher in the thoracic region than normal. The physician makes an incision beginning 1 cm superior to the middle of the scapular spine continuing medially along the spine to the medial portion of the bone and inferiorly to the inferior angle of the scapula. The deep fascia is reflected to expose the insertion of the trapezius on the scapular spine. It is reflected along with the supraspinatus muscle. The rhomboid major and minor and levator scapula muscles are also reflected to release the scapula from its abnormal position. If the upper portion of the bone is abnormally shaped, a portion of it may be removed. Once the scapula is normally positioned to match the opposite side, the muscles are reattached to the bone in their new orientation. A portion of the trapezius may now form a flap or may require a portion to be excised in order to take up slack in the muscle. The incision is closed with sutures and a Velpeau bandage is applied for two weeks.

23405-23406
This procedure may be performed if closed manipulation under anesthesia is unsuccessful to gain adequate motion of the shoulder. An incision along the anterior deltoid and pectoral region is made and the skin is reflected to expose the underlying muscles. The subscapularis tendon is removed from the glenoid rim of the scapula. The physician may also release portions of the pectoral muscle fibers to gain further motion of the shoulder. The incision is closed with sutures and the arm is passively placed in abduction. Report 23406 if a tenotomy is performed on multiple tendons through the same incision.

23410-23412
The physician repairs a ruptured rotator cuff. A longitudinal incision is made along the anterior portion of the shoulder and the skin is reflected. The deltoid fibers and the underlying tissues are divided. The coracoacromial ligament is divided and the

supraspinatus tendon is detached by a transverse incision along the greater tuberosity. The distal frayed edges of the tendon are removed. A trench is chiseled into the humeral bone along the level of the anatomical neck of the humerus. The supraspinatus tendon flap is buried in it. The flap is fixed with sutures tied to the tendon and passed through holes drilled in the bone. The repair is completed with side-to-side sutures of the supraspinatus to the adjacent subscapularis and infraspinatus tendons. The incision is closed, and a soft dressing is applied. Protected motion in a specific progression of exercises is followed. Report 23410 if the repair is done for an acute rupture of the musculotendinous cuff and 23412 if chronic. If the procedure begins arthroscopically and minimal work is performed, such as debridement of tendon edges and subacromial decompression, and then an open incision is made to complete the repair, report 23410 or 23412 as appropriate. If most of either procedure is completed arthroscopically and minimal work is performed through an additional open incision, report 29827.

23415
The physician performs a coracoacromial ligament release, with or without acromioplasty. The patient is positioned on the side with the affected side up. The physician makes an incision centered over the acromioclavicular joint. The soft tissues are reflected and the ligament between the coracoid and the acromion is released. The physician may perform an acromioplasty where the underside of the acromion is reduced to allow more room for the rotator cuff tendons. Acromioplasty involves the division of the acromioclavicular ligament followed by the use of a burr to cut away the under surface of the acromion. During acromionectomy, the distal portion of the acromion is removed. Following completion, the joint is irrigated and the incisions are closed with sutures or Steri-strips.

23420
The most common approach to reconstruct a complete rotator cuff avulsion tear of the shoulder is an anterior approach through an incision over the acromioclavicular joint. If the infraspinatus is to be shifted, a second incision is made along the scapular spine posteriorly, detaching a portion of the posterior deltoid if necessary. The margins of the tear are freshened and a non-absorbable suture closes the longitudinal portion of the tear. A portion of the articular cartilage on the underside of the humeral head is removed. The raw edges of the torn tendon are brought into contact with raw bone and the ends of the sutures are passed through holes drilled through the greater tuberosity and tied over its lateral aspect. The physician performs an acromioplasty. Acromioplasty involves the division of the acromioclavicular ligament followed by the use of a burr to cut away the under surface of the acromion. During acromionectomy, the distal portion of the acromion is removed. Once the reconstruction is complete, the incision is closed and the arm may be positioned in an abduction splint or pillow for protection.

23430
Open tenodesis is performed on the long tendon of the biceps. The long head of the biceps tendon may become frayed and ruptured in chronic impingement syndrome, bicipital tenosynovitis, or degenerative conditions of the shoulder. Complete ruptures may leave a frayed proximal segment attached to the supraglenoid tubercle, which may become trapped between the humeral head and glenoid. In this case, the remaining stump of the tendon can be removed by a motorized shaver. The tendon end is cleaned of frayed fragments. Sutures are placed within the tendon and pulled into a humeral socket that has been drilled at the top of the bicipital groove. The end of the tendon is fixed into the bicipital groove using a bioabsorbable interference anchor or screw. A simultaneous subacromial decompression may be performed.

23440
The long tendon of the biceps is resected or transplanted. The long head of the biceps tendon is an important stabilizer of the humeral head. When the proximal end of the tendon is detached from the glenoid, it is rolled or knotted, sutured, and inserted through a keyhole-shaped opening in the cortex of the humerus in the floor of the bicipital groove. This is performed through a longitudinal incision at the anterior aspect of the shoulder. Once proper fixation is obtained, the incision is closed and the arm is supported in a sling. Active elbow flexion and shoulder elevation are limited until proper fixation and healing are complete.

23450-23455
An anterior capsulorrhaphy is performed on the shoulder in a Putti-Platt or Magnuson type operation. An anterior incision is made at the deltopectoral-pectoral interval. The coracoid process is identified and the tendon of the biceps (short head) is at times incised distal to the coracoid for exposure. The anterior capsule is visualized through a small transverse incision of the subscapularis tendon, which is tagged for identification and removed from its attachment on the capsule. The quality and laxity of the capsule are assessed and the joint is explored for damage to the labrum or glenoid. The joint is irrigated to remove any loose bodies. If there is no other abnormal laxity, the capsule is advanced superiorly and attached to the labrum with sutures. An appropriate amount of slack is taken up to provide stability within the joint. Once the capsule is reattached, the subscapularis tendon is reapproximated but not tightened and repaired. A subcutaneous drain is placed and the wound is closed. Report 23455 if a Bankart type operation with labral repair is done.

23460-23462
An anterior capsulorrhaphy of any type with bone block is performed on the shoulder. If there is

Musculoskeletal

significant damage to the glenoid where more than one third of the glenoid is deficient, a bone block procedure is performed to increase the surface area of the glenoid. The patient is placed in a lateral position or modified beach chair position. A horizontal or vertical incision is placed inferior to the scapular spine, allowing a bone graft to be taken from the scapular spine if necessary. An additional incision is made at the lateral border of the acromion and carried posteriorly to the axillary crease. The deltoid is split to expose the infraspinatus and teres minor tendons. The capsule is exposed and incised with a T-shaped cut. The capsule is reattached to the glenoid through drill holes or by means of suture anchors taking up slack on the inferior portion of the capsule. The capsular repair may be reinforced using the infraspinatus tendon if the local tissue is felt to be insufficient. The bone block is placed on the posterior inferior portion of the glenoid fossa and fixated with a screw. This bone fragment is usually obtained from the spine of the scapula through a posterior incision. Report 23462 if the procedure is performed with coracoid process transfer.

23465

A posterior capsulorrhaphy of the glenohumeral joint is done with or without bone block. The patient is placed in a lateral position or modified beach chair position. A horizontal or vertical incision is placed inferior to the scapular spine, allowing a bone graft to be taken from the scapular spine if necessary. An additional incision is made at the lateral border of the acromion and carried posteriorly to the axillary crease. The deltoid is split to expose the infraspinatus and teres minor tendons. The capsule is exposed and incised with a T-shaped cut. The capsule is reattached to the glenohumeral joint through drill holes or by means of suture anchors taking up slack on the inferior portion of the capsule. The capsular repair may be reinforced using the infraspinatus tendon if the local tissue is felt to be insufficient. When a bone block is used, it is placed at the posterior inferior quadrant of the glenohumeral joint to increase the articulation surface of the glenoid. This technique is rarely used. Once the incision is closed, the arm is placed in an Orthoplast splint with the arm in external rotation for the first six weeks. Motion is protected.

23466

A capsulorrhaphy of the glenohumeral joint for any type of multidirectional instability is done. The surgical approach may differ from patient to patient depending upon the patient's history. The incision is determined by the side of most significant instability. A separately reportable arthroscopic examination of the shoulder should be performed first to fully determine the extent of damage to the joint and the appropriate surgical approach. An anterior H-plasty is commonly used to tighten the capsule. In some cases, both medial and lateral capsular incisions may be required to provide sufficient capsular tension.

23470

Hemiarthroplasty is performed on the glenohumeral joint. A long curved incision is made from the superior aspect of the acromion along the deltopectoral interval to the deltoid insertion. The deltoid is retracted laterally and the pectoralis medially. The fascia between the pectoralis and the clavicle is divided and the subacromial space is freed with a gloved finger or periosteal elevator. The coracoacromial ligament is freed and often an acromioplasty is performed to allow for freedom of movement after surgery. The subscapularis tendon is tagged and removed from the capsule. The anterior joint capsule is divided and the glenohumeral joint is dislocated by further external rotation and extension of the arm. The joint is explored and all loose bodies are removed. The humeral head is removed with a reciprocating saw or osteotome. A trial prosthesis is placed along the proximal humerus as a guide for proper inclination of the osteotomy. A horizontal cut (osteotomy) is made as previously determined and a large curette is used to open the medullary canal for placement of the stem of the prosthesis. The canal is enlarged with a reamer to the appropriate size. The prosthesis is positioned in proper rotational alignment to articulate with the glenoid. Any remaining osteophytes (bone spurs) are removed. The joint is irrigated. The prosthesis is reduced into the glenoid and the subscapularis tendon is sutured in place with multiple interrupted non-absorbable sutures with the shoulder in neutral position. The deltopectoral interval is closed loosely over drainage tubes. The arm is placed in a sling and swathe bandage.

23472

A total shoulder replacement is done for the glenohumeral joint. A long, curved incision is made from the superior aspect of the acromion along the deltopectoral interval to the deltoid insertion. The deltoid is retracted laterally and pectoralis medially. The fascia between the pectoralis and the clavicle is divided and the subacromial space is freed with a gloved finger or periosteal elevator. The coracoacromial ligament is freed and often an acromioplasty is performed to allow for freedom of movement after surgery. The subscapularis tendon is tagged and removed from the capsule. The anterior joint capsule is divided and the glenohumeral joint is dislocated by further external rotation and extension of the arm. The joint is explored and all loose bodies are removed. The humeral head is removed with a reciprocating saw or osteotome. In addition, a prosthetic device is placed proximally at the glenoid to articulate with the prosthetic humeral head. Prior to placement of the humeral prosthesis, the joint is opened to fully expose the glenoid surface. The surface cartilage of the glenoid is removed. A power drill is used to cut a slot into the glenoid the exact size of the holding device of the glenoid component. Small curettes are used to remove cancellous bone from the base of the coracoid bone. With a burr, articular cartilage is removed from the surface of the glenoid. A trial glenoid component is used to properly prepare the bone and fit the prosthesis. Once the glenoid preparation is complete, the glenoid vault is drilled and filled with polymethylmethacrylate (bone cement). The glenoid component is pushed into place and held until the cement is cured. Prior to final insertion of the humeral component, an anterior acromioplasty and acromioclavicular arthroplasty are performed, if necessary. If large rotator cuff tears are found, they are repaired at this time. The joint is brought through a full range of motion and fully irrigated. The subscapularis tendon is repaired to stabilize the joint; however, the joint capsule is not usually resutured. Drains are placed and the deltopectoral interval is sutured closed. The arm is placed in a sling and swathe.

23473-23474

The physician revises a total shoulder arthroplasty. The physician may access the shoulder joint through the previous incision. Muscles are reflected and the joint capsule is incised. Any scar tissue is removed. The physician manually dislocates the shoulder. Cement is removed from around the glenoid component with a motorized or hand instrument and the component is removed. Once prepared properly, the glenoid vault is filled with polymethylmethacrylate (bone cement) and the new glenoid component is pushed into place and held until the cement cures. The physician removes scar tissue and cement from around the humeral component with chisels and gouges. The humeral component is removed from its bed. The physician reconstructs the humerus with instrumentation and/or bone graft. A new humeral component is inserted. The physician may augment the area with an autograft or allograft. The physician reduces the shoulder and closes the capsule. Suction drains may be placed in the wound. The incision is repaired in layers with sutures, staples, and/or Steri-strips.

23480

The physician performs an osteotomy (bone cut) of the clavicle. The physician makes an incision in the skin overlying the clavicle. Tissue is dissected down to the bone. Using a surgical saw or other sharp instrument, the physician cuts through the bone. Surgical screws, a metal plate, or wires may secure the cut bone in the correct position. The wound is irrigated and the skin is closed in layers.

23485

The physician performs an osteotomy (bone cut) of the clavicle that is not healing or has healed in an unacceptable position. The physician makes an incision in the skin overlying the clavicle. Tissue is dissected down to the bone. Using a surgical saw or other sharp instrument, the physician cuts through the bone. Surgical screws, a metal plate, or wires may secure the cut bone in the correct position. The physician harvests a bone graft from the patient through a separate incision. The physician repairs the surgically created graft donor site. The graft is placed in the clavicle. Surgical screws, plates, or other hardware secure the bone graft. The incision is closed in layers.

23490-23491

The physician performs a preventative nailing, plating, pinning, or wiring of the clavicle to the coracoid process in order to gain better fixation and prevent further dislocation of the acromioclavicular joint. Access to the joint is obtained through a lateral incision over the acromion process. The skin and soft tissues are reflected. The screw or other fixation device of choice is positioned and may be checked by separately reportable x-ray. The procedure may be accomplished with the use of methylmethacrylate, which can be injected into a weak or defective bone area and hardens to act like a bone cement. The incision is closed with sutures and movement is restricted for four to six weeks. The hardware is removed when stability is determined. Report 23491 for similar prophylactic treatment of the proximal humerus.

23500-23505

The physician treats a fracture of the clavicle bone without surgery or manipulation. Separately reportable x-rays confirm the stable position of the fractured pieces. No manipulation is required. The physician may apply a clavicle brace, tape, or splint until the fracture heals. In 23505, the fracture is displaced and manipulation is required. A local anesthetic may be given. The physician pushes or pulls on the bony pieces or manipulates the shoulder in such a way to properly align the fracture. The physician may apply a clavicle brace, tape, or splint until the fracture heals.

23515

The physician treats a fracture of the clavicle with open surgery. The physician makes an incision overlying the fractured area of the clavicle. Tissue is dissected down to the bone and the fracture is identified. The physician debrides any nonviable tissues. Any tissue that has become lodged between the fracture pieces is removed. The physician may apply screws, wires, or plates to secure the fracture. The wound is irrigated and the incision is closed. A splint or brace may also be applied on the outside of the clavicle or shoulder.

23520-23525

The physician treats a dislocation of the joint between the sternum and the clavicle (sternoclavicular) without making incisions and without any manipulation in 23520. The physician applies a splint or brace to hold the joint in place until it has healed. In 23525, manipulation is required. Anesthesia may be necessary. The physician pushes, pulls, or moves the arm and chest to restore the joint to correct position and alignment. After manipulation, the patient is placed in a brace or splint.

23530-23532

The physician treats a chronic or acute dislocation of the sternoclavicular joint. The physician makes an incision overlying the joint between the clavicle and sternum where the dislocation has occurred. The tissues are dissected down to the joint and the dislocation is visualized. The physician may debride the area before realigning the joint back to proper position. In 23532, the physician harvests a fascial graft from the patient through a separate incision. The physician repairs the surgically created graft donor site.

The fascial graft is attached to the bones in the sternoclavicular joint, preventing recurrent dislocation. Fixation may be applied. The joint is irrigated and the incision is closed in layers. A splint or brace may be applied to the outside of the body.

23540-23545
The physician treats a dislocation of the acromioclavicular joint (between the acromion process of the scapula and the clavicle). In 23540, no manipulation is required and the physician places the affected shoulder and arm in a sling or other brace. In 23545, manipulation is necessary to correct the dislocation. Anesthesia may be needed. The physician manipulates the joint by pushing or pulling on the shoulder and arm to align the bones. The physician applies a sling or other brace.

23550-23552
The physician treats an acute or chronic dislocation of the acromioclavicular joint (between the acromion process of the scapula and the clavicle). An incision is made overlying the shoulder at the articulation of the acromion of the scapula and the end of the clavicle. Dissection is carried through the tissues to the joint. Any nonviable tissue is removed. The bones are identified and the dislocation is visualized. The physician uses a heavy nonabsorbable suture, a wire, or screws to secure the two bones in their proper joint alignment. In 23552, the physician harvests a fascial graft from the patient through a separate incision. The physician repairs the surgically created graft donor site. The fascial graft is a strong piece of connective tissue that is attached to the bones in the acromioclavicular joint, preventing recurrent dislocation. When the joint is restored, the wound is irrigated and the incision is closed in layers. A dressing is applied. A sling or brace is applied to the shoulder and arm.

23570
The physician treats a fracture of the scapula bone without surgery or any type of manipulation. Separately reportable x-rays confirm the stable position of the fractured pieces. The physician places the shoulder in a sling or other brace until the fracture heals.

23575
The physician treats a fracture of the scapula bone without any incisions. Separately reportable x-rays confirm the nature of the fracture and the displacement of the pieces. The physician manipulates (pushes, pulls, or moves) the scapula and arm to align the fractured pieces. Separately reportable serial x-rays may be necessary while the manipulation is performed to confirm alignment. The physician may apply traction devices to the body to maintain satisfactory fracture reduction. A brace, splint, or cast may be applied to hold the bones in the correct position until they are healed.

23585
The physician treats a fracture of the scapula with open surgery. The physician makes an incision overlying the area of the fractured scapula and dissects the tissues down to the bone to visualize the fracture. Nonviable tissues or those between the fragments are debrided. The physician places the fragments back together in their correct anatomic position manually or with instruments. Internal fixation devices such as screws, metal plates, sutures, or wire may be applied to secure the bones. The wound is irrigated and the incisions are closed in layers with sutures.

23600-23605
Separately reportable x-rays confirm a stable, non-displaced proximal humeral fracture. No manipulation or open reduction is required in 23600. The arm is positioned in a sling and protected from movement to allow adequate healing. In 23605, the physician manipulates (pushes, pulls, or moves) the upper arm in the shoulder area to align the fractured pieces. Separately reportable serial x-rays may be necessary while the manipulation is performed to confirm alignment. The physician may apply traction devices to the body to maintain satisfactory fracture reduction. A brace, splint, or cast may be applied to hold the bones in the correct position until they are healed.

23615-23616
The physician performs open treatment of a proximal humeral (surgical or anatomical neck) fracture. An incision is made anteromedially extending posteriorly along the acromion to the lateral half of the spine of the scapula. The deltoid is detached from the exposed portion of the spine of the scapula. The deltoid is reflected down to expose the joint capsule and the humerus. The fractured portion of the proximal humerus (surgical or anatomical neck) is identified and the fracture is aligned. If the tuberosity is involved, it may also be repaired. Internal fixation may be used to stabilize the fracture site. Once the fracture is stabilized, the wound is irrigated. The deltoid is repositioned and sutured in place. The skin is sutured and the wound is covered with a soft dressing. The arm is positioned in a sling and movement is restricted to allow for proper healing. Report 23616 when the fracture cannot be repaired and a prosthetic proximal humeral replacement is necessary.

23620-23625
Separately reportable x-rays determine a stable, non-displaced greater humeral tuberosity fracture. The arm is positioned in a sling and motion of the shoulder is protected to prevent pull of the muscles that attach to the bone of the upper arm. Report 23625 if the fracture is displaced and manipulation is required. A local anesthetic may be given. The physician pushes or pulls on the bony pieces or manipulates them in such a way to properly align the fracture.

23630
The physician performs open treatment of a greater humeral tuberosity fracture. An anterior longitudinal incision is made and the underlying deltoid fibers are divided to expose the fracture site. Often this injury will include damage to the rotator cuff tendons

requiring repair of the soft tissues in addition to the fracture site. The soft tissues are reflected to expose the bone and any loose bodies are removed. The fracture may be stabilized by internal fixation and the soft tissues are reattached by suture. The skin incision is closed and a soft dressing is applied. The arm is placed in a sling and movement is restricted to allow for adequate healing.

23650-23655
The physician performs closed treatment of a shoulder dislocation by manipulation. The most common form of shoulder dislocation is the traumatic anterior inferior dislocation. A closed manipulation requires the patient to be positioned to allow the arm to hang forward. The physician applies gentle traction to distract the joint and manually relocates the glenohumeral joint back into position. Report 23655 if the manipulation treatment requires anesthesia.

23660
The physician performs open treatment of an acute shoulder dislocation. A posterior dislocation would be more likely to require an open reduction procedure than an anterior dislocation. The shoulder is approached through a deltopectoral incision. The joint is inspected and the head of the humerus is reduced into its proper position. The subscapularis tendon is attached to the head of the humerus with sutures or screws. If there is significant posterior translation, the posterior capsule is tightened. The incision is closed and the arm is immobilized in 20 degrees of external rotation.

23665
The physician performs closed reduction of a shoulder dislocation with greater humeral tuberosity fracture. With the patient positioned prone and the arm hanging toward the floor, manual distraction is attempted. If not successful, the physician may hang a five-pound weight from the arm in an attempt to reduce the shoulder into place. Once shoulder reduction is obtained, a neurovascular examination is performed and treatment of the humeral tuberosity fracture is addressed. The arm is immobilized for three to six weeks.

23670
The physician performs open reduction of a shoulder dislocation with greater humeral tuberosity fracture. The physician may enter the shoulder anteriorly through a deltopectoral approach or superiorly through a deltoid splitting approach. The soft tissues are reflected and the fracture is observed. Once the dislocated joint is reduced into proper position, the repair of the humeral tuberosity fracture is addressed. Larger fragments may be stabilized with screws, wire sutures, staples, or other internal fixation measures. These fragments usually require later removal of the fixation device to allow full motion of the shoulder. If the fragment is small, it can be removed and the tendons of the rotator cuff advanced and attached to the defect in the bone. Once the fracture is stable, the incision is closed and the arm is protected in a sling for four to six weeks.

23675
The physician performs closed reduction of a shoulder dislocation with surgical or anatomical neck fracture. With the patient positioned prone and the arm hanging toward the floor, manual distraction is attempted. If not successful, the physician may hang a five-pound weight from the arm in an attempt to reduce the shoulder into place. Once shoulder reduction is obtained, a neurovascular examination is performed and treatment of the humeral surgical or anatomical neck fracture is addressed. The arm is immobilized for three to six weeks.

23680
The physician performs open reduction of a shoulder dislocation with surgical or anatomical neck fracture. The physician may enter the shoulder anteriorly through a deltopectoral approach or superiorly through a deltoid splitting approach. The soft tissues are reflected and the fracture is observed. Once the dislocated joint is reduced into proper position, the repair of the humeral surgical or anatomical neck fracture is addressed. Larger fragments may be stabilized with screws, wire sutures, staples, or other internal fixation measures. These fragments usually require later removal of the fixation device to allow full motion of the shoulder. An intramedullary rod may be placed through the shaft of the bone as well. Once the fracture is stable, the incision is closed and the arm is protected in a sling for four to six weeks.

23700
Manipulation of the shoulder under anesthesia may be necessary to regain the loss of motion that occurs in the case of frozen shoulder or following a surgical procedure. The patient is positioned supine and given general anesthesia. Following full evaluation, the physician manipulates the shoulder to achieve the appropriate range of motion. A fixation apparatus may also be applied.

23800-23802
The physician performs arthrodesis of the glenohumeral joint. The shoulder is positioned in what is considered the most functional position, slightly abducted to the side with forward elevation. A dorsolateral semicircular incision is made across the glenohumeral joint and carried distally at the midpoint. The articular cartilage is removed from the head of the humerus (ball) and the glenoid cavity (socket). The head is split and a wedge of bone is removed. This wedge is where the acromion will rest when the arm is positioned in abduction. At this point, bone grafting or plate fixation may be added to the procedure to stabilize the glenohumeral joint. If a plate is used, a second procedure will be needed to remove the hardware. Cast application or external fixation may be used in a number of ways. Report 23802 if an autogenous graft is used.

23900
This radical procedure reflects removal of the upper extremity along with the scapula and a portion of the clavicle. The physician incises the skin overlying the shoulder and dissects the disease-free soft tissue away from the bone to create a skin flap to cover the wound. The clavicle is disarticulated from the sternum and the chest wall is freed from muscular attachments to the arm. The subclavian and brachial vessels are located and clamps are placed. The quarter section is removed and the wound is sutured in layers. If enough disease-free tissue is not available for primary closure, the wound is packed closed with gauze possibly leading to skin graft. Given the current therapies and optimal responses for high-grade sarcomas, this procedure is rarely performed.

23920-23921
The physician disarticulates the shoulder. The physician incises the skin overlying the shoulder. The rotator cuff is incised, freeing the arm of ligamentous and muscular attachments. The arm is removed and the wound is sutured in layers. Report 23920 for the first amputation. Report 23921 for a secondary closure of the wound or scar revision.

23930-23931
The physician drains a deep abscess or hematoma in 23930 or an infected bursa in 23931 from within the upper arm or elbow area. With proper anesthesia administered, the physician makes an incision in the upper arm or elbow overlying the site of the abscess, hematoma, or bursa to be incised. Dissection is carried down through the deep subcutaneous tissues and may be continued into the fascia or muscle to expose the abscess or hematoma. The incision may be extended if the mass is larger than expected. When the infected bursa, abscess, or hematoma is identified, it is incised and the contents are drained. The area is irrigated and the incision is repaired in layers with sutures, staples, and/or Steri-strips; closed with drains in place; or simply left open to further facilitate drainage of infection.

23935
The physician incises the bone cortex of infected bone in the humerus or elbow to treat an abscess or osteomyelitis. The physician makes an incision over the affected area. Dissection is carried down through the soft tissues to expose the bone. The periosteum is split and reflected from the bone overlying the infected area. A curette may be used to scrape away the abscess or infected portion down to healthy bony tissue or drill holes may be made through the cortex into the medullary canal in a window outline around the infected or abscessed bone. The area is drained and debrided of infected bony and soft tissue. The physician irrigates the area with antibiotic solution, the periosteum is closed over the bone, and the soft tissues are sutured closed; or the wound is packed and left open, allowing the area to drain. Secondary closure is performed approximately three weeks later. Dressings are changed daily. A splint may be applied to limit elbow movement.

24000
The physician performs an arthrotomy on the elbow that includes exploration, drainage, or removal of any foreign body. A longitudinal incision over the part of the elbow to be exposed (e.g., the anterior, posterior, medial, or lateral aspect) is made. The soft tissues are dissected away and the joint capsule is exposed and incised. The joint is explored, any necrotic tissue is removed, and infection or abnormal fluid is drained. If a foreign body is present (e.g., bullet, nail, gravel), it is exposed and removed. The wound is irrigated with antibiotic solution. The physician may leave the wound packed open with daily dressing changes to allow for further drainage and secondary healing by granulation. If the incision is repaired, drain tubes may be inserted and the incision is repaired in layers with sutures, staples, and/or Steri-strips. A splint may be applied to limit elbow motion.

24006
The physician performs an arthrotomy of the elbow with capsular excision for release. The physician makes an incision over the anterior part of the elbow. Dissection exposes the joint capsule. The radial nerve is identified and protected. The anterior elbow joint capsule is incised and portions of it are removed. By excising the capsule, any scarring limiting elbow motion is minimal. Additional incisions (e.g., medial elbow incision) are made if other parts of the capsule are also to be excised. The physician repairs the incision in layers with sutures, staples, and/or Steri-strips. The elbow is placed in a posterior splint.

24065-24066
The physician performs a biopsy of the soft tissues of the upper arm or elbow area. With proper anesthesia administered, an incision is made over the biopsy area. Dissection is carried down within the superficial soft tissue layers in 24065, usually the subcutaneous fat to the uppermost fascial layer. In 24066, dissection is taken down deep within the soft tissue, such as into the fascial layer or within the muscle. A portion of the tissue is excised and submitted for pathology. The area is irrigated and the incision is closed with layered sutures, staples, or Steri-strips.

24075-24076 [24071, 24073]
The physician removes a tumor from the soft tissue of the upper arm or elbow area that is located in the subcutaneous tissue in 24071 and 24075 and in the deep soft tissue, below the fascial plane or within the muscle, in 24073 and 24076. With the proper anesthesia administered, the physician makes an incision in the skin overlying the mass and dissects down to the tumor. The extent of the tumor is identified and a dissection is undertaken all the way around the tumor. A portion of neighboring soft tissue may also be removed to ensure adequate removal of all tumor tissue. A drain may be inserted and the incision is repaired with layers of sutures, staples, or Steri-strips. Report 24075 for excision of subcutaneous

tumors whose resected area is less than 3 cm and 24071 for excision of subcutaneous tumors 3 cm or greater. Report 24076 for excision of subfascial or intramuscular tumors whose resected area is less than 5 cm and 24073 for excision of subfascial or intramuscular tumors 5 cm or greater.

24077-24079

The physician performs a radical resection of a soft tissue tumor (i.e., sarcoma) from the upper arm or elbow area, not involving bone. The tumor may be malignant or an aggressive benign tumor of the connective tissue. An incision is made over the tumor and dissection exposes it. The tumor and any adjacent tissue that may be affected by the spread of the neoplasm are excised. Large resections may be needed. The type and stage of the lesion determines the extent of the tumor margin resection area. Muscle or fascia may need to be repaired and drains may be placed. The surgical wound is closed using simple or intermediate repair or separately reportable complex closure, adjacent tissue transfer, or graft. The arm may be placed in a posterior splint. Report 24077 for excision of tumors whose resected area is less than 5 cm and 24079 for excision of tumors 5 cm or greater.

24100-24101

The physician makes a long, straight, lateral incision to access the elbow joint and perform an arthrotomy. The physician may also use a medial, anterior, or posterior approach. The joint capsule is exposed by dissecting down through the soft tissues and freeing and reflecting the common origin of the extensor muscles. The joint capsule is incised to expose the synovium, which lies within the joint capsule. A small portion of the synovium is excised for biopsy in 24100. In 24101, additional dissection is carried out to further explore the joint cavity. Any loose or foreign bodies (e.g., free cartilage, bone chips, gravel) are removed and a biopsy may be taken. The physician irrigates the joint. The physician may leave the wound packed open with daily dressing changes to allow for further drainage and secondary healing by granulation. A drain tube may be placed and the incision repaired in layers with sutures, staples, and/or Steri-strips. A splint may be applied to limit elbow movement.

24102

The physician makes a long, straight, lateral incision over the elbow to perform an arthrotomy and remove the synovium. The physician may also use a medial, anterior, or posterior approach. The joint capsule is exposed by dissecting down through the soft tissues and freeing and reflecting the common origin of the extensor muscles. The joint capsule is incised to expose the synovium, the inner membrane of the articular capsule that lines the joint cavity. The inflamed or enlarged synovium is dissected away from the capsule and the bones and removed. Motorized shavers may be used. A drain tube may be placed and the incision is repaired in layers with sutures, staples, and/or Steri-strips. A splint may be applied to limit elbow movement.

24105

The physician excises the olecranon bursa by making a longitudinal incision along the posteromedial border of the elbow and dissecting down to expose the bursa, the fluid filled sac that lubricates the joint against friction. The bursa is excised. The surrounding tissue is examined for any sign of infection. The wound is irrigated and the incision is repaired in layers with sutures, staples, and/or Steri-strips.

24110-24116

A bone cyst or benign tumor of the humerus is removed. The physician makes an incision in the upper arm overlying the cyst or tumor. The skin and underlying soft tissues are reflected to expose the periosteum, which is separated from the bone. Curettes or osteotomes are used to scrape or cut the lesion from the bone. Once the benign tumor or cyst is removed and healthy bone tissue is present, the periosteum is repositioned and the incision is repaired in layers. If the bone defect created requires a graft for repair, the physician obtains the necessary size bone graft from a separate donor site on the patient and packs it into the site where the tumor or bone cyst was removed, or uses a bone bank allograft. Report 24115 if the procedure is done with an autograft and 24116 if an allograft is used.

24120-24126

The physician uses excision or curettage to remove a bone cyst or benign tumor of the head or neck of the radius or olecranon process in 24120. The physician makes a longitudinal incision along the lateral aspect of the elbow. A posterior incision may also be made to access the olecranon process. To expose the radial head and/or neck, the common origin of the extensor muscles is reflected and the joint capsule is incised. The bone cyst or tumor is identified and the periosteum is separated from the bone. Curettes or osteotomes are used to scrape or cut the lesion from the bone. Once the benign tumor or cyst is removed and healthy bone tissue is present, the periosteum is repositioned and the incision is repaired in layers, including the joint capsule, if incised. If the bone defect created requires a graft for repair, the physician obtains the necessary size bone graft from a separate donor site on the patient and packs it into the site where the tumor or bone cyst was removed or uses a bone bank allograft. Report 24125 if an autograft is obtained and 24126 if an allograft is used.

24130

The radial head is excised in this procedure. The physician makes a longitudinal incision along the lateral aspect of the elbow. The elbow joint is exposed by freeing and reflecting the common origin of the extensor muscles. The joint capsule is incised and the radial head is exposed. The physician uses a bone-cutting saw to excise the radial head. The capsule is closed with sutures and the incision is repaired in layers with sutures, staples, and/or Steri-strips.

24134-24138
The physician removes infected portions of bone, due to a bone abscess or osteomyelitis, from the shaft or distal humerus in 24134, from the radial head or neck in 24136, and from the olecranon process in 24138. This infection often leaves open sinus tracts in the bone that require removal. The physician makes an incision overlying the sequestered area of bone, which includes incising the capsule if the elbow joint is involved. Once the skin and soft tissues are reflected, a small window is cut into the bone to gain access to the sequestrum, or necrosed piece of bone that has become separated from sound bone. All purulent material and scarred or necrotic tissue are removed. The remaining space is filled with surrounding soft tissues or free tissue transfer. The area is irrigated and an antibiotic solution is used to prevent further infection. The wound is closed loosely over drains if possible or may be packed open with dressings. The patient may be placed in a splint to limit elbow motion.

24140-24147
The physician performs a partial excision of the humerus in 24140, the radial head or neck in 24145, or the olecranon process in 24147 to remove infected bone. An incision is made over the infected part of the bone and the underlying soft tissues are divided to expose the bone. The elbow joint capsule may be incised if necessary. The periosteum is reflected and the infected portion of bone is removed and irrigated. The excavation of bone may excise a crater-like piece, leave a small saucer-like shelf depression in the bone, or may remove a portion of the shaft (diaphysis) of a long bone. If a significant portion of bone is removed, the physician may use bone graft material to fill the cavity left in the bone. The periosteum is closed over the bone, the soft tissues are sutured closed, and a soft dressing is applied. A long splint may be applied to limit elbow motion.

24149
The physician radically resects the elbow joint capsule, undesirable soft tissue and bone, and releases a contracture of a muscle or tendon. With the patient under anesthesia, the physician makes a long longitudinal incision overlying the elbow. Depending on the extent of the excess bone to be removed or the severity of the contracture, additional incisions may be required. The incision is continued deep to the elbow joint capsule itself. Nerves, vessels, and tendons are retracted. The capsule is fully exposed. A thorough debridement is undertaken to excise unwanted soft tissue. The overgrown and excess bone is isolated and excised. The capsule is resected. The contracture of the elbow involving muscle, tendon, scar tissue, or soft tissue is identified and explored. The physician releases the offending tissue to allow full elbow range of motion. The wound or wounds are irrigated and closed in layers. A dressing is applied.

24150
The physician performs a radical resection of a tumor of the shaft or distal humerus. The physician makes an incision overlying the involved area of bone, dissecting down to expose the tumor site. The involved vessels and nerves are protected. Proximate muscles are detached extraperiosteally by sharp dissection, and the tumor is excised, including the immediately surrounding bone and any involved soft tissue. The wound is closed with layered sutures.

24152
The physician performs a radical resection of a tumor of the radial head or neck. The physician makes an anterolateral incision overlying the elbow or forearm. Dissection exposes the radial head or neck. The radial vessels and nerve are protected. The tumor is excised, including the radial head or neck. The physician selects the level of the radius to be divided. The physician uses a bone saw to divide the bone at the appropriate level. The muscles are detached by sharp dissection. Radical resection may also include removal of surrounding soft tissues such as muscles, fascia, and vessels. The wound is closed with layered sutures.

24155
An elbow joint arthrectomy is performed to remove the joint by resection of the distal humerus and the proximal radius and ulna. The physician makes a longitudinal incision along the lateral elbow. Dissection is carried down through the joint capsule to expose the distal humerus and the proximal radius and ulna. The physician selects the level at which the bones are to be resected. The physician uses a bone saw to divide the bones at the appropriate level. The physician preserves the surrounding muscle attachments to maintain some support and function for moving the elbow. However, gross instability of the elbow is present. The incision is repaired in layers using staples, sutures, and/or Steri-strips.

24160-24164
The physician removes an artificial joint from the elbow. An incision is made overlying the prosthesis. The incision may be made on the medial, lateral, or posterior portion of the elbow dependent on the component being removed. Dissection exposes the prosthesis. The physician uses instruments to remove the implant from the bone. The incision is repaired with sutures and/or Steri-strips. Report 24160 if the humeral and ulnar components of the prosthesis are removed. Report 24164 if the prosthesis is removed from the radial head.

24200-24201
The physician removes a foreign body of the upper arm or elbow area. If the foreign body is a result of trauma, an open wound may already exist. The physician may make a separate incision or access the foreign body through the open wound. Location of the foreign body may be determined prior to surgery by separately reportable x-rays. A subcutaneous foreign body is located between the skin and muscle layer in 24200. The foreign body is deep and may be within muscle in

24201. More extensive dissection and a larger incision may be necessary for a deep foreign body. Once the foreign body is visualized, it is removed. The physician may also debride any surrounding damaged soft tissue. The wound is irrigated. Drains may be placed in the wound and the incision repaired in layers with sutures, staples, and/or Steri-strips. A splint may be applied to limit elbow motion.

24220
Elbow arthrography provides information about the capsule size, the synovial lining, the articular surfaces of the joints, and detects loose bodies and capsular leaks. The patient is positioned sitting or supine (lying face up) with the elbow flexed at 90 degrees. One of two injection sites may be used, a lateral or posterior approach. The contrast medium is injected. A fluoroscope is used to study the elbow. No incisions are made. This code reports the injection only. The radiological exam is reported separately.

24300
Manipulation of the elbow under anesthesia may be necessary to gain the loss of motion following a surgical procedure or due to scar tissue. Following the induction of general anesthesia, the physician evaluates the elbow. The elbow is manipulated by stretching, rotation, and other maneuvers to gain the appropriate range of motion.

24301
The physician performs a muscle or tendon transfer of the upper arm or elbow. An example is transfer of the latissimus dorsi muscle. This transfer restores active elbow flexion by transferring the origin and belly of the latissimus dorsi to the arm and anchoring the origin near the radial head. The patient is placed side lying with the affected side up. An incision is made starting at the loin and extending up to the axilla and distally along the medial aspect of the arm to the anterior elbow. The physician cuts free the origin of the latissimus dorsi. The muscle itself is cut free from the underlying abdominal muscles. The origin of the latissimus dorsi muscle is sutured to the biceps tendon and the periosteal tissues about the radial tuberosity. The incision is repaired in layers with sutures, staples, and/or Steri-strips.

24305
The physician lengthens a tendon of the upper arm or elbow. An anterior curvilinear incision is made, for example, over the anterior elbow to lengthen the biceps tendon. Dissection exposes the distal biceps tendon. The biceps tendon is divided by Z-plasty and stretched into extension, causing it to stretch and release to a lengthened position. If the elbow joint capsule is thickened, the physician may elect to excise this part of the capsule and any fibrous bands or bone spurs in the anterior part of the elbow joint. A drain is inserted into the wound and the incision is repaired in layers using sutures, staples, and/or Steri-strips. The elbow is placed in a splint or cast in an extended position.

24310
For tenotomy of the distal biceps tendon, an incision is made over the anterior elbow to expose the biceps tendon. The tendon is cut all the way through so as to release the flexion contracture. No repair of the tendon is made. The incision is repaired with sutures. The elbow may be placed in a splint to keep it in as much extension as possible.

24320
A Seddon-Brookes type upper arm tenoplasty with muscle transfer restores elbow flexion by prolonging the tendon of the pectoralis major muscle with the long head of the biceps brachii. The physician makes an incision from the deltopectoral groove to the midportion of the upper arm. The pectoralis major tendon is exposed through dissection, detached from its insertion, and mobilized from the chest wall toward the clavicle. The tendon of the long head of the biceps is exposed and severed from its origin and withdrawn into the wound. The long head of the biceps is dissected from the short head. An L-shaped incision is made over the anterior aspect of the elbow. The long head of the biceps is divided and freed distally to its attachment on the radius. The biceps tendon and muscle are withdrawn through the distal L-shaped incision. Through the proximal incision, the tendon and muscle belly of the long head of the biceps is passed through two slits in the tendon of the pectoralis major and looped on itself so that its proximal tendon is brought into the distal L-shaped incision. The end of the proximal tendon is sutured through a slit in the distal tendon and the tendon of the pectoralis major is sutured to the long head of the biceps at their junction. The incisions are repaired in layers using sutures, staples, and/or Steri-strips. A posterior plaster splint is applied with the elbow in flexion.

24330-24331
To perform a Steindler-type advancement for flexor-plasty of the elbow, the physician transfers the common origin of the pronator teres, flexor carpi radialis, palmaris longus, flexor digitorum sublimis, and flexor carpi ulnaris from the medial epicondyle of the humerus proximally and laterally onto the anterior surface of the humerus so that it performs elbow flexion rather than forearm pronation. This is done when the biceps brachii and brachialis are paralyzed. The physician makes a curved longitudinal incision over the medial side of the elbow extending over the medial condyle area and along the pronator teres. The ulnar nerve is identified and retracted for protection. The common origin of the pronator teres, flexor carpi radialis, palmaris longus, flexor digitorum sublimis, and flexor carpi ulnaris is detached as a whole from the medial epicondyle. These muscles are freed up for about 4 cm. A fascia lata graft is taken from the lateral thigh and one end is sutured to the common origin to extend it, while the other end is advanced and attached 5 cm up the lateral side of the humerus. A cast is applied with the elbow in flexion. In 24331, an anterior transfer of the triceps (extensor advancement)

is performed in conjunction with elbow flexor-plasty. A posterolateral incision is made over the lower upper arm. The triceps tendon is exposed and divided at its insertion, dissected from the back of the lower humerus, and brought around to the lateral side. An anterolateral curvilinear incision is made to expose the radial tuberosity. Another 4 cm long fascia lata graft is harvested and attached to the triceps tendon to extend it for advancement. The other end of the fascia lata graft is attached to the tuberosity of the radius. This creates added elbow flexibility. A cast is applied with the elbow in flexion.

24332
Tenolysis involves transection of adhesions that have formed between the tendon and its surrounding tissues. Beginning proximally along the supracondylar ridge and ending near the subcutaneous border of the ulna, the physician makes a deep dissection to the anterior aspect of the capsule. The triceps tendon is retracted posteriorly to expose the olecranon fossa and tenolysis of the triceps and posterior capsulectomy is performed. Tenolysis should be performed under a local anesthetic so that full release can be confirmed. If, however, general or regional anesthesia is used, the physician may check the adequacy of the removal of all adhesions by manually pulling the tendons.

24340
The physician treats a rupture of a distal biceps tendon by reattachment of the biceps tendon to the radius, direct reimplantation, or inserting a loop of fascia lata graft around the proximal radius. Reattachment of the biceps tendon to the radius is described. The patient is placed supine. The physician makes an anterior lateral incision on the lower upper arm, extending transversely across the antecubital fossa. The torn biceps tendon is identified and the tear is minimally debrided. Two Bunnell sutures are placed in the torn end. A second incision is made over the dorsal aspect of the proximal forearm to expose the radial tuberosity. The physician uses a high-speed burr to evacuate a 5 mm to 7 mm defect in the radial tuberosity. Three holes are drilled through this window to the opposite side of the tuberosity. The physician places sutures through the holes and places the tendon into the window in the tuberosity. The sutures are pulled tight and secured. The incisions are repaired in layers with drains inserted. The elbow is placed in a splint in 90 degrees of flexion and full supination.

24341
The physician repairs one of the muscles or tendons in the upper arm or elbow, not including those of the rotator cuff. With the patient under general anesthesia, the physician makes an incision directly overlying the torn muscles or tendon. The incision is carried deep through the subcutaneous tissue. The extent of the tear is ascertained through debridement and exploration. The physician repairs the tissue using appropriate fixation devices such as sutures, wires, or screws. Additional incisions are often required when a tendon is completely ruptured. When the repair is complete, the incision is closed in layers. Use this code to report both the initial, primary repair done near the time of injury or a secondary repair, done sometime after the incident of injury or following a previous surgical repair.

24342
The physician performs reinsertion of a distal ruptured biceps or triceps tendon. For the triceps tendon, a posterior longitudinal incision is made to expose the tendinous portion of the triceps. Drill holes are made in the olecranon. Sutures from the triceps tendon are passed through the drill holes, pulled tight, and secured. The physician may harvest a fascia graft from the forearm. The proximal attachment of the fascia graft is left attached to the epicondyle. The distal part is detached, raised, and sutured to the distal triceps for reinforcement. The incision is repaired in layers with sutures, staples, and/or Steri-strips. The arm is immobilized in less than 90 degrees of flexion.

24343
The lateral collateral ligament (LCL) is the ligament of the elbow along the outer aspect that connects the distal end of the humerus to the proximal end of the radius and provides lateral stability to the joint. Injury to the LCL can lead to elbow dislocation. Anterior-posterior and lateral x-rays of the elbow are taken and reported separately. The physician administers a local anesthetic block, makes an incision, and dissects down to the damaged lateral collateral ligament. If the ligament has been pulled from its attachment on the bone, the ligament is reattached with large sutures or a metal bone staple. More than one incision may be necessary. The damaged collateral ligament is repaired with local tissue that can be used to restore its functionality. For mid-ligament tears, the ends of the ligament are sewed together to repair ligament continuity.

24344
The lateral collateral ligament (LCL) of the elbow is reconstructed with a tendon graft. The LCL is the ligament along the outer aspect of the elbow that connects the distal end of the humerus to the proximal end of the radius. It provides lateral stability to the joint and injury to the LCL can lead to elbow dislocation. Anterior-posterior and lateral x-rays of the elbow are taken and reported separately. The physician administers a local anesthetic block, makes an incision, and dissects to the damaged lateral collateral ligament. The palmaris longus tendon is usually used for the graft. The physician makes a transverse proximal wrist crease incision directly over the tendon, divides it, and holds it taut. A second transverse incision is made about 8 cm above the first incision on the forearm to again identify the tendon. The graft segment is divided and withdrawn. Alternatively, a tendon stripper can be used. The tendon is grafted to the lateral collateral ligament to restore functionality. The wound is closed and a dressing applied. The hand and wrist may be put in a plaster cast, splint, or bandage, depending on which tendons were involved.

24345

The medial collateral ligament (MCL) is posterior to the axis of elbow flexion and primarily serves as the medial stabilizer of the flexed elbow joint. X-rays (reported separately) are taken to identify abnormally wide joint space on the medial side. An MRI (reported separately) may be taken to show focal discontinuity of the ligament and joint fluid extravasation. Repair of a freshly torn medial collateral ligament usually requires the surgeon to make an incision through the skin over the area where the tear in the ligament has occurred. If the ligament has been pulled from its attachment on the bone, the ligament is reattached with large sutures or a metal bone staple. More than one incision may be necessary. The damaged ligament is repaired with local tissue that can be used to restore its functionality. For mid-ligament tears, the ends of the ligament are sewed together to repair ligament continuity. The procedure is normally performed under general anesthesia or with a local block.

24346

The medial collateral ligament (MCL) is posterior to the axis of elbow flexion and primarily serves as the medial stabilizer of the flexed elbow joint. X-rays (reported separately) are taken to identify abnormally wide joint space on the medial side. An MRI (reported separately) may be taken to show focal discontinuity of the ligament and joint fluid extravasation. The palmaris longus tendon is the most commonly used tendon graft for the elbow. The procedure is normally performed under general anesthesia. The physician makes a transverse proximal wrist crease incision directly over the tendon, divides it, and holds it taut. A second transverse incision is made about 8 cm above the first incision on the forearm to again identify the tendon. The graft segment is divided and withdrawn. Alternatively, a tendon stripper can be used. The tendon is grafted to the medial collateral ligament to restore functionality. The wound is closed and a dressing applied. The hand and wrist may be put in a plaster cast, splint, or bandage, depending on which tendons were involved.

24357

The physician performs a percutaneous (through the skin) procedure to treat lateral epicondylitis (tennis elbow) or medial epicondylitis (golfer's elbow). Following administration of a local anesthetic, the physician advances an 18- or 20-guage needle through the abnormal region of the tendon. The tip of the needle is drawn back and forth to repeatedly perforate (fenestrate) the tendinotic tissue in multiple locations. Any calcifications or spurs are mechanically fragmented and the bony surface of the apex and epicondylar face is abraded to stimulate new blood vessels. The fenestrated tendon is infiltrated with a corticosteroid/bupivacaine solution.

24358-24359

The physician performs an open tenotomy (cutting or release) to treat lateral epicondylitis (tennis elbow) or medial epicondylitis (golfer's elbow). An incision is made over the affected epicondyle of the humerus. In 24358, the physician removes (debrides) damaged soft tissue or bone. In 24359, the physician also repairs or reattaches the affected tendon. The incision is repaired in layers with sutures, staples, and/or Steri-strips. The arm is placed in a sling.

24360

The physician performs a membrane arthroplasty of the elbow. A longitudinal incision is made over the lateral elbow. All soft tissue is dissected from the distal humerus. The elbow is dislocated. Osteophytes and articular cartilage are removed from the distal humerus so that a smooth, rounded surface remains. Articular cartilage is left intact on the proximal ulna and radius. The physician uses a motorized dermatome to remove a thin split-thickness skin graft from the patient's lower abdomen. Small drill holes are made in the distal end of the humerus. The graft is sutured into place over the distal end of the humerus with the dermal surface placed against the bone and the fat facing the new joint space. The elbow joint is reduced (realigned). The physician repairs the incision in layers using sutures, staples, and/or Steri-strips. The elbow is placed in a posterior splint in 90 degrees of flexion.

24361

The physician performs an arthroplasty of the elbow with distal humeral prosthetic replacement. The physician makes a 10 cm longitudinal incision over the medial aspect of the elbow. The ulnar nerve is identified and retracted to protect it from injury. The joint capsule is excised and the radius and ulna are separated from the humerus. A Kirschner wire is drilled into the trochlea (distal humerus) along the axis of the joint. Using an osteotome, high speed burr, or saw, the physician trims and remodels the distal end of the humerus. A prosthesis is fitted to the distal humerus and hammered into place. The ulna and radius are reduced to the prosthesis. If the radial head is severely deformed or arthritic, the physician may resect (remove) it. Other adjustments may be made, such as sculpting the semilunar notch or olecranon. Sculpting allows better articulation with the prosthesis and better elbow motion. The flexor origins are reattached to the epicondyle. The physician repairs the incision in layers with sutures, staples, and/or Steri-strips. A long arm cast or splint is applied with the elbow in 90 degrees of flexion.

24362

The physician performs an arthroplasty of the elbow with an implant and fascia lata ligament reconstruction. The physician makes a 10 cm longitudinal incision over the medial aspect of the elbow. The ulnar nerve is identified and retracted to protect it from injury. The joint capsule is excised and the radius and ulna are separated from the humerus. A Kirschner wire is drilled into the trochlea (distal humerus) along the axis of the joint. Using an osteotome, high speed burr, or saw, the physician trims and remodels the distal end of the humerus. A prosthesis is fitted to the distal humerus and hammered into place. The ulna and radius are reduced to the prosthesis. If the radial head is severely deformed or arthritic, the physician may resect (remove) it. Other adjustments may be made, such as sculpting the semilunar notch or olecranon. Sculpting allows better articulation with the prosthesis and better elbow motion. The flexor origins are reattached to the epicondyle. For the fascia lata ligament reconstruction, an additional incision may be necessary on the posterior aspect of the elbow and forearm. The radial head and olecranon are exposed. Through an incision on the lateral side of the thigh, a long rectangle of fascia lata is removed. The fascia is folded in half crosswise and the folded edge is anchored to the anterior part of the capsule with sutures. The distal half is sutured in place over the trochlear notch. A fold of the same fascia is inserted between the radial head and ulna and fixed with sutures. The capsule is sutured closed. The incisions are repaired in layers with sutures, staples, and/or Steri-strips. A long arm cast or splint immobilizes the elbow at 90 degrees of flexion.

24363

The physician performs a total elbow arthroplasty with distal humerus and proximal ulnar prosthetic replacement. The patient is placed supine with the affected arm on the chest and a sandbag beneath the shoulder. Different types of prosthetic implants are available. Selection depends on capsuloligamentous structures, muscular integrity, and the amount of bone remaining at the elbow joint. A technique for a semiconstrained (two to three part) hinged prosthesis is described. The physician makes a straight, midline, posterior incision. The ulnar nerve is identified and retracted for protection. The triceps mechanism is elevated from the olecranon. The collateral ligaments are preserved. A portion of the olecranon is cut and removed to allow implantation of the ulnar stem. The distal humerus is prepared by removing cancellous bone with a curette. The physician uses a rasp to open and contour the humeral and ulnar medullary canals for insertion of the prosthetic stems. Cement is inserted into the ulnar and humeral medullary canals with a cement gun or syringe. The elbow is flexed and the prosthesis is inserted into the humeral and ulnar medullary canals at the same time. The elbow joint is fully extended while the cement hardens. The triceps mechanism is sutured back to fascia. The ulnar nerve is positioned anterior to the elbow. The physician inserts drain tubes. The incision is repaired in layers with sutures, staples, and/or Steri-strips. A posterior splint is applied to the elbow in 90 degrees of flexion.

24365

The physician performs an arthroplasty on the radial head by making a 5 cm to 6 cm longitudinal incision along the lateral aspect of the elbow. The elbow joint is exposed by freeing and reflecting the common origin of the extensor muscles. The joint capsule is incised and the radial head is exposed. The physician uses a bone cutting saw to excise the radial head. The capsule is closed with sutures and the incision is repaired in layers with sutures, staples, and/or Steri-strips.

24366

The physician performs an arthroplasty on the radial head with an implant. The patient is positioned supine or lateral (lying on one side) with the affected elbow up. The physician makes an incision beginning just above the lateral epicondyle and extending distally approximately 6 cm across the joint. Dissection exposes the capsule, which is incised. The annular ligament is incised transversely so that the neck of the radius can be osteotomized. A burr or rasp is used to prepare the medullary canal of the radius to accept the implant. The implant is inserted into the medullary canal of the radius and positioned into contact with the capitellum. The annular ligament is reattached. A suction drain is inserted. The physician repairs the incision in layers using sutures, staples, and/or Steri-strips. The arm may be placed in a posterior elbow splint at 90 degrees of flexion.

24370-24371

The physician revises a total elbow arthroplasty. Different types of prosthetic implants may be revised. Initial selection depends on capsuloligamentous structures, muscular integrity, and the amount of bone remaining at the elbow joint. The physician may access the elbow joint through the previous incision. Nerves, muscles, and ligaments are reflected and the joint capsule is incised. Any scar tissue is removed. The physician manually dislocates the elbow prosthesis. Cement is removed from the humeral and/or ulnar components with a motorized or hand instrument and the component(s) needing revision is removed. The physician uses a rasp to revise and contour the humeral and/or ulnar medullary canals for insertion of the prosthetic stems. Cement is inserted into the ulnar and/or humeral medullary canals with a cement gun or syringe. The elbow is flexed and the prosthesis is inserted. The elbow joint is fully extended while the cement hardens. The triceps mechanism is sutured back to fascia. The ulnar nerve is positioned anterior to the elbow. The physician inserts drain tubes. The incision is repaired in layers with sutures, staples, and/or Steri-strips. A posterior splint is applied to the elbow in 90 degrees of flexion.

24400

The physician performs an osteotomy of the humerus with or without internal fixation. The physician makes a longitudinal incision overlying the involved portion of the shaft of the humerus to expose the affected part of the bone. An osteotomy is made through the humerus, usually in a wedge shape. This allows the bone to be realigned. The physician may apply plates and screws to hold the bone together in the correct position (internal fixation). The incision is repaired in layers with sutures, staples, and/or Steri-strips. The arm may be placed in a cast or splint for immobilization.

24410

The physician performs multiple osteotomies with realignment on an intramedullary rod of the humeral shaft. This is done to treat the deformities of osteogenesis imperfecta. The physician makes a longitudinal incision through the skin, fascia, and muscle to expose the shaft of the bone subperiosteally. Osteotomies are made through the proximal and distal metaphyses; the shaft is removed and studied to determine how many osteotomies must be made to thread the segments onto the intramedullary rod. Additional osteotomies, usually three or four, are performed to correct the alignment. The fragments are shifted and rotated to facilitate aligning them end to end on the straight nail. Autografts may be added if the cortex is thin. The intramedullary nail is inserted so that the ends extend into the canals at the distal and proximal ends. The periosteum is sutured over the bone and the wound is closed and dressed.

24420
The physician performs osteoplasty of the humerus for shortening or lengthening. An incision is made through the skin, fascia, and muscle in the upper arm over the humeral shaft. Vessels and nerves are exposed and retracted. Dissection continues to expose the shaft of the humerus. An osteotomy is made at the determined point on the humerus. The physician removes a wedge of bone. To shorten the humeral shaft, a plate is attached to the distal segment with screws. Reduction forceps are used to hold and compress the osteotomy while the plate is attached to the proximal fragment with screws. To lengthen the bone, the segments are retracted, usually 2 mm to 3 mm, and fixed at that distance with plates and screws. X-rays (reported separately) are used to check rotational alignment of the segments. Drain tubes are inserted, the incision is repaired in layers with sutures, staples, and/or Steri-strips, and the arm is immobilized.

24430-24435
The physician repairs a nonunion or malunion of the humerus without using a graft in 24430 and with an iliac or other autograft in 24435. The physician exposes the nonunion or malunion of the humerus by making a 10 cm to 15 cm longitudinal incision through the skin, fascia, and muscle over the fracture site. With a reciprocating saw, the bone is divided through the nonunion. The fragments are aligned. A compression plate is centered over the fracture and screws are inserted. In 24435, a bone graft is needed to help heal the fracture due to bone loss. Autogenous iliac bone is typically used, but proximal tibia grafts may also be used. Both require a separate incision and wound closure of the harvest site. The physician uses an osteotome to harvest strips of bone, which are placed around the ends of the humeral fracture in addition to the compression plate for internal fixation. The incision is repaired in layers with sutures, staples, and/or Steri-strips. The limb is immobilized.

24470
The physician performs a hemiepiphyseal arrest. Angular deformities are typically a complication of fractures of the lateral condylar physis. The most common deformity is cubitus valgus. To treat cubitus valgus, the physician makes a longitudinal posterior incision along the distal humerus. The humerus is exposed. If a nonunion exists from a previous condylar physeal fracture, it may be approached from the same incision and the ends are denuded and a local bone graft is applied. The physician applies a cancellous screw to provide fixation and compression across the nonunion. An osteotomy is performed across the distal humerus, correcting both the angulation and realigning the longitudinal axis of the humerus with that of the forearm. The osteotomy is secured with screws. The physician repairs the incision in layers with sutures, staples, and/or Steri-strips. The elbow is immobilized in a splint or brace.

24495
The physician performs a decompression fasciotomy in the forearm with exploration of the brachial artery. The physician makes a longitudinal incision on the anterior forearm, from just lateral and proximal to the biceps tendon distal toward the radial styloid, excising the deep fascia, and exposing the brachioradialis laterally and the biceps and brachialis medially, to decompress the compartment. The brachial artery is explored proximally to identify the origin of decreased circulation. The fascial incision remains open. The skin incision may be left open or closed.

24498
The physician applies prophylactic treatment to prevent fracture. A longitudinal incision is made through the skin, fascia, and muscle along the humerus to expose the worrisome area. Pins or a plate and screws are used to stabilize the bone. If defects in the bone do not allow for good internal fixation, methylmethacrylate, a bone cementing substance when hard, may be used to fill in the gaps. Wiring may also be wrapped around the bone to provide additional fixation. An intramedullary nail may also be inserted through the canal of the humerus to provide internal stabilization. The incisions are repaired in layers with sutures, staples, and/or Steri-strips.

24500-24505
The physician performs closed treatment of a humeral shaft fracture. In 24500, the segments are determined to be aligned and stable and no manipulation of the bone fragments is necessary. Treatment involves immobilization, using one of several methods, of the elbow and possibly of the glenohumeral joint for several weeks until union is established. In 24505, the physician must first manually coerce the fractured bone into alignment. Skeletal traction may also be applied in 24505.

24515
The physician repairs a humeral shaft fracture openly with a plate or screws, with or without cerclage. A lateral or anterolateral incision is made overlying the fracture site. The fracture is reduced by manipulation and bone reduction forceps. A compression plate with screws secures and compresses the fragments. Cerclage wiring might be used to facilitate fixation of the fracture. One or more wires may be placed around the humerus, over the fracture site. The incision is closed with sutures, staples, and/or Steri-strips.

24516
The physician repairs a humeral shaft fracture with insertion of an intramedullary implant, with or without cerclage and/or locking screws. A straight lateral incision is made through the skin, fascia, and muscles to expose the fracture site. If there are multiple fragments or if there is a long spiral fracture, cerclage wires may be wrapped around the bone to hold the fragments in place. Using a guide rod to direct a reamer and rod, an intramedullary nail is placed within the humeral shaft. The nail may be locked in place proximally and distally with locking screws. The wound is irrigated, a drain may be inserted, and the wound is closed in layers.

24530-24535
Closed treatment of a supracondylar or transcondylar fracture, which may have an extending fracture line between the condyles, is indicated when the fragments are not separated and appear stable. No manipulation is required in 24530. Supracondylar fractures in the adult are usually treated with a caption splint or hanging arm cast. Transcondylar fractures may be treated conservatively with a hanging arm cast and elbow immobilization. In 24535, manipulation is necessary to realign the fracture into proper reduction. Skin or skeletal traction may also be applied. Pins, wires, or tongs are inserted into the bone for skeletal traction through a small incision without opening the fracture. A weight and pulley system is attached to exert a constant force of traction and keep the fractured bones in alignment.

24538
The physician performs percutaneous skeletal fixation of a supracondylar or transcondylar humeral fracture, which may have an extending fracture line between the condyles. The elbow is prepared and draped. The fracture is reduced by applying longitudinal traction and manipulating the fracture into alignment. Pins are inserted through the condyles and metaphysis diagonally, avoiding the ulnar nerve to hold the fractured pieces stable. The pins are clipped and bent beneath the skin. The incision is closed with layered sutures and the arm is immobilized.

24545-24546
In 24545, the physician performs open treatment of a supracondylar or transcondylar humeral fracture that does not have an extending fracture line present between the condyles. In 24546, the humeral condylar fracture has an extending fracture line between the condyles that may create a third fracture piece. The physician makes a posterior incision from midline of the arm to just distal to the olecranon, exposing the olecranon, triceps tendon, and distal humerus. The ulnar nerve is isolated and retracted. Preserving as much soft tissue attachment as possible, the physician exposes and assembles the fragments, reducing the condyles and fixing the fragments with screws, pins, or plates as may be needed to hold the condyles firmly reduced to the metaphysis. The joint is irrigated and the wounds are closed with drain placement if needed.

24560-24565
The physician repairs a humeral medial or lateral epicondylar fracture without incision or manipulation in 24560. Closed treatment of a humeral epicondylar fracture is indicated when the fragments are not separated and appear stable. No manipulation is required. No incisions are made. The arm is placed in a posterior elbow splint at 90 degrees of flexion. Report 24565 if manipulation is required to reduce the fracture into position.

24566
The physician fixates a humeral medial or lateral epicondylar fracture percutaneously. The physician uses separately reportable fluoroscopy to realign the fracture by manipulation first. Once the bone is realigned, the physician fixates the pieces to the humeral shaft by driving percutaneous wires through the pieces and into the shaft.

24575
The physician openly treats a fracture of the medial or lateral epicondyle of the humerus. The physician makes an incision in the skin overlying the fractured epicondyle. This is carried deep through the fascia to the bone. Fracture fragments are identified and manipulated into the appropriate anatomic position. The epicondyle may be immobilized in place using internal fixation devices such as plates, screws, or wires if needed. The wound is irrigated and closed in layers.

24576-24577
The physician repairs a humeral medial or lateral condylar fracture without incision or manipulation in 24576. Closed treatment of a humeral condylar fracture is indicated when the fragments are not separated and appear stable. No manipulation is required. No incisions are made. The arm is placed in a posterior elbow splint at 90 degrees of flexion. Report 24577 if manipulation is required to reduce the fracture into position.

24579
The physician openly repairs a humeral condylar fracture, medial or lateral. The physician makes an incision exposing the posterior elbow. Skin and subcutaneous tissue are reflected to expose the olecranon and triceps tendon. The ulnar nerve is retracted. The condyles are reduced and may be temporarily fixed with internal fixation devices such as wires, or screws may be placed across the major fragments. Small fragments may require excision. The incision is closed with sutures and the elbow is immobilized in a posterior elbow splint.

24582
The physician fixates a humeral medial or lateral condylar fracture percutaneously by manipulating the fracture in a closed fashion and inserting pins through the skin and bones to maintain appropriate position. Separately reportable x-rays, including fluoroscopic views, are obtained to ascertain the extent of the fracture. The physician manipulates the arm, elbow, and forearm in such a way to restore the fractured

pieces to the acceptable position. The physician places pins through the skin and into the bones to immobilize the reduction until healing is complete.

24586-24587

The physician openly treats a periarticular fracture (distal humerus and proximal ulna and/or proximal radius) and/or dislocation of the elbow. The physician may make more than one incision depending on the extent of the fractures and/or dislocation. If there is a dislocation, it is reduced (realigned) first. The fractures are reduced and secured with plates, screws, pins, wires, or a combination of these. The physician may place a pin through the olecranon for skeletal traction in a patient with multiple injuries to temporarily stabilize the fracture and/or dislocation. In 24587, if joint surface congruity cannot be restored, the physician performs a total elbow arthroplasty. For elbow arthroplasty, the physician makes a straight, midline, posterior incision. The ulnar nerve is identified and retracted for protection. The triceps mechanism is elevated from the olecranon. The collateral ligaments are preserved. A portion of the olecranon is cut and removed to allow implantation of the ulnar stem. The distal humerus is prepared by removing cancellous bone with a curette. The physician uses a rasp to open and contour the humeral and ulnar medullary canals for insertion of the prosthetic stems. Cement is inserted into the ulnar and humeral medullary canals with a cement gun or syringe. The elbow is flexed and the prosthesis is inserted into the humeral and ulnar medullary canals at the same time. The elbow joint is fully extended while the cement hardens. The triceps mechanism is sutured back to fascia. The ulnar nerve is positioned anterior to the elbow. Arthroplasty may be performed in conjunction with some internal fixation for fracture reduction and stabilization.

24600-24605

The physician performs closed treatment of an elbow dislocation when there are no fractures. The forearm typically dislocates posteriorly. The physician manually reduces (realigns) the dislocation with pressure to the area. The elbow is placed in a posterior elbow splint or elbow brace at 90 degrees of flexion with the forearm supinated. The procedure is performed without anesthesia in 24600 or with anesthesia in 24605.

24615

To openly treat an acute or chronic elbow dislocation, the physician may use the Osborne-Cotterill technique of dislocation treatment. The physician makes a longitudinal incision over the lateral aspect of the elbow. The physician dissects the elbow posterior to the lateral collateral ligament. Any bone fragments are removed. The physician roughens the bone at the lateral epicondyle and lateral side of the capitellum. The physician uses an awl to make one or two transverse holes through the lateral condyle close to the articular surface of the humerus. Sutures are passed through these holes and through the posterolateral part of the capsule. The capsule is fixed to the bone as tightly as possible. The incision is repaired in layers. A long arm cast or splint is applied with the elbow in 40 degrees of flexion for approximately four weeks.

24620

The physician treats a Monteggia type fracture dislocation at the elbow (fracture of the proximal end of the ulna with dislocation of the radial head) by manipulation. No incisions are made. The physician manually realigns the radial head back into position. If alignment of the ulnar fracture is not adequate, the physician may also manually align this fracture. Once satisfactory and stable reduction (realignment) is achieved, the elbow is placed in a posterior splint or cast. The elbow is immobilized at 120 degrees of flexion to prevent recurrent dislocation of the radial head.

24635

The physician openly treats a Monteggia type fracture dislocation at the elbow (fracture of the proximal end of the ulna with dislocation of the radial head), with or without internal fixation. The physician makes a longitudinal incision along the lateral aspect of the elbow. Dissection exposes the radial head and proximal ulna. The physician determines the status of the annular ligament. If the ligament is intact, the physician incises it so the radial head can be reduced. The ligament is repaired with nonabsorbable sutures. More commonly, the ligament is torn or avulsed, requiring reconstruction. If so, a strip of fascia 1.3 cm wide and 11 cm long is dissected from the muscles of the forearm. If the ulnar fracture is stable, no internal fixation is required. If the fracture is unstable, internal fixation is typically applied. A compression plate or an intramedullary nail may be utilized for internal fixation. The new annular ligament (fascial strip) is sutured about the radial neck. The incision is repaired in layers with sutures, staples, and/or Steri-strips. The elbow is placed in a posterior splint or cast at 120 degrees of flexion, preventing redislocation of the radial head.

24640

The physician performs closed treatment of nursemaid elbow in a child with manipulation. To realign a subluxated (partially dislocated) radial head, the physician supinates the forearm (palm upward) while flexing the elbow. No incisions are made. If stability of the radial head is questionable, a cast or splint is applied with the elbow in 90 degrees of flexion.

24650-24655

The physician performs closed treatment of a radial head or neck fracture without manipulation in 24650 and with manipulation in 24655. In 24650, the radial fracture is determined to be stable and nondisplaced and can be splinted or braced without requiring manipulation. In 24655, the physician performs manual manipulation to realign the fractured bone by applying pressure. No incisions are made. The arm is placed in a posterior elbow splint or brace.

24665-24666

The physician performs open treatment of a radial head or neck fracture, with or without internal fixation or radial head excision in 24665 and with radial head prosthetic replacement in 24666. The physician makes an incision along the posterolateral aspect of the elbow. The common origin of the extensor muscles is reflected and the joint capsule is incised, exposing the radial head and neck. All loose particles of bone are removed, the elbow joint is irrigated, and the fractured fragments are reduced. In 24665, the physician may need to remove the radial head to achieve good reduction and screws or other internal fixation devices may be employed to stabilize the fracture. In 24666, the physician uses a bone cutting saw to excise the radial head and replaces it with a prosthesis before repairing the capsule and the incision in layers with sutures, staples, and/or Steri-strips. A posterior elbow splint is applied with the elbow at 90 degrees of flexion.

24670-24675

The physician performs closed treatment of an olecranon or coronoid process fracture. No manipulation is required in 24670. In 24675, mild or slight separation of the fragments requires manipulation. The physician manually manipulates the area, reducing the proximal end ulnar fracture. No incisions are made. The arm may be placed in a posterior elbow splint at 90 degrees of flexion.

24685

The physician openly treats a fracture of the olecranon or coronoid process (proximal end of the ulna). The physician makes a 10 cm incision along the posterolateral border of the elbow. Dissection exposes the fracture. If the fracture is not comminuted, a figure-of-eight wire loop stabilizes the fracture. The physician drills a hole from side to side in the distal fragment. Wire is passed through the drill hole in the distal fragment and through the triceps aponeurosis. This creates a figure-of-eight loop. The wire is pulled tight and twisted. If the fracture is more distal, a medullary pin or screw may be used as well. If medullary fixation is used, the pin or screw is inserted through the olecranon and into the medullary canal of the ulna. The physician repairs the incision in layers with sutures, staples, and/or Steri-strips.

24800-24802

The physician performs an arthrodesis of the elbow joint and makes a posterior longitudinal or posterolateral incision. If the physician does not use a bone graft, the triceps tendon is split and released from the olecranon. The joint capsule is incised to expose the radial head and neck and the radial head is excised. A posterior and anterior synovectomy is performed. The physician trims the olecranon into a triangular shape with a saw. A triangular hole is created through the lower end of the humerus and the olecranon is inserted through this triangular hole. The physician places a bone screw obliquely through the humerus and into the ulna. The triceps tendon is repaired with sutures. The physician repairs the incision in layers and the elbow is immobilized in a long arm cast. If a bone graft is used, the physician prepares a bed for the graft in the posterior surface of the lower humerus. A cleft is formed in the upper part of the tip of the olecranon. If local autograft bone is used, it is harvested from the surrounding healthy bone and no separate incision is required. The autograft is fitted into the olecranon cleft and humeral bed. If allograft (donor) bone is used, it is fitted in the same manner. In 24802, an autogenous graft is harvested from the patient's upper tibia or iliac crest with an osteotome. The physician repairs the surgically created graft donor site. One or two screws are inserted through the graft and into the humerus to make it secure. Bone chips are packed into the humeral-ulnar joint. The physician repairs the incision in layers with sutures. A long arm cast is applied with the elbow in approximately 90 degrees of flexion.

24900

The physician amputates the arm through the humerus. The physician makes an incision distal to the intended level of bone section, and fashions anterior and posterior skin flaps. The brachial artery and vein are identified, double ligated, and divided just proximal to the level of bone section. Nerves are also divided proximal to the site to ensure retraction to the end of the stump. Muscles are sectioned slightly distal to the stump. The humerus is divided and the end is smoothed. The triceps muscle is flapped over the end of the bone and sutured into the anterior fascia. The wound is closed over a drain tube with suction and the fascia and skin flaps are closed.

24920

The physician amputates the arm through the humerus using an open, circular technique. The physician makes an incision distal to the intended level of bone section in a circular manner to the fascia and fashions anterior and posterior skin flaps. The brachial artery and vein are identified, double ligated, and divided just proximal to the level of bone section. Nerves are also divided proximal to the site to ensure retraction to the end of the stump. Muscles are sectioned slightly distal to the stump. The humerus is divided and the end is smoothed. The triceps muscle is flapped over the end of the bone and sutured into the anterior fascia. The wound is closed over a drain tube with suction and the fascia and skin flaps are closed.

24925

The physician performs a secondary closure or scar revision of an existing amputation. The physician excises the granulation and scar tissues and remodels the soft tissues to close over the amputation again. In this procedure, no additional bone is sectioned. Arteries and veins are identified, ligated, and divided, as necessary, as well as nerves. The wound is closed over a drain tube with suction and the fascia and skin flaps are closed. When closing the wound, opposing tissue layers are sewn under physiologic tension, and care must be taken so that the final closure is neither too tight nor too loose.

24930

The physician re-amputates the arm through the humerus. The physician makes an incision distal to the intended level of bone section and fashions anterior and posterior skin flaps. The brachial artery and vein are identified, double ligated, and divided just proximal to the level of bone section. Nerves are also divided proximal to the site to ensure retraction to the end of the stump. Muscles are sectioned slightly distal to the stump. The humerus is divided again and the end is smoothed. The triceps muscle is flapped over the end of the bone and sutured into the anterior fascia. The wound is closed over a drain tube with suction and the fascia and skin flaps are closed.

24931

The physician amputates the arm through the humerus bone and places a surgical implant in the arm. The physician makes an incision in a circular fashion around the arm distal to the level of the planned amputation of the humerus. The vessels and nerves are identified, divided, and ligated. The humerus bone is divided in two, completing the amputation. The physician spares the skin, soft tissue, and muscle needed to close the amputation incision. Any of a variety of implants, such as rods, are utilized to maintain the length of the arm or to replace a portion of the amputated humerus. Fixation devices are used. The incision is irrigated. Retained muscle flaps are closed over exposed bone. The wound is closed in layers and a soft dressing is applied.

24935

The physician elongates a stump of an upper extremity. First, the physician obtains the bone graft. The physician incises the skin over the area where the bone graft is to be obtained (usually the iliac crest). The tissue is dissected away from the bone and the graft is harvested. The wound is sutured in layers. The skin overlying the stump is incised to expose the bony stump. The graft is pinned or plated to the existing bone. The tissues are replaced around the bone and the wound is sutured in layers.

24940

Cineplasty is an outdated procedure performed for upper arm amputation to create a muscle motor that acts on an inserted pin to provide the energy for prosthetic action or movement. A muscle tunnel is created into a muscle such as the flexors and extensors of the forearm biceps, the triceps, and pectoralis major. The muscle must be one that functions voluntarily, delicately, and forcibly enough to exert energy over a good range. A skin-lined tube is created within the muscle tunnel that can, after healing, accept a pin for prosthesis being inserted and removed at will. Contraction of the muscle causes displacement of the tunnel and the pin and provides the motor energy for prosthetic action. This has been replaced by technological advances that use myoelectrical sensors attached to the skin.

25000

The physician incises the extensor tendon sheath over the wrist. The physician incises the skin just proximal to the anatomic snuffbox. The tissues are dissected and the extensor retinaculum of the first extensor compartment is identified and incised. The incision is sutured in layers.

25001

The physician incises the flexor tendon sheath over the wrist. The physician makes a radial incision. The tissues are dissected to the tendon sheath. The compartment is identified and incised. When incising the flexor carpi radialis (FCR), the tendon sheath is opened proximal to distal. The fibro-osseous tunnel is released along the ulnar border of the trapezium. The incision is closed with layered sutures.

25020-25023

The physician performs a decompression fasciotomy of the forearm and/or wrist extensor or flexor compartment without debridement in 25020 and with debridement of any nonviable tissue, including muscles and nerves in 25023. The physician makes an incision over the flexor or extensor compartment of the forearm. This is carried deep to the fascia and the fascia itself is incised and released. In 25020, the skin is sutured closed, if possible. In 25023, the physician explores the compartment and debrides any nonviable tissue that may include muscle, nerve, or fascia. The wound is irrigated and typically left open. Closure is accomplished during a later, separately reportable procedure.

25024-25025

The physician performs a decompression fasciotomy of the forearm and/or wrist extensor and flexor compartment without debridement in 25024 and with debridement of any nonviable tissue, including muscles and nerves in 25025. A decompression fasciotomy of the forearm for compartment syndrome is described here. An anterior curvilinear incision for volar fasciotomy is made beginning on the ulnar side of the forearm, crossing the elbow crease at an angle to reach the radial side, curving back to the ulnar side, and while continuing toward the palm, the incision is centered where it crosses the wrist flexion crease, and extends into the palm medially along the crease. The superficial volar compartment is released along its length, to free the fascia over the compartment muscles. Muscles and nerves are retracted to expose the flexor digitorum profundus in the deep compartment. If its overlying fascia is tight, it too is incised. Report 25025 if any nonviable tissue that may include muscle, nerve, or fascia is found and requires debridement. The dorsal compartments are checked and/or pressure measurements are taken. The volar fasciotomy usually sufficiently decompresses the dorsal musculature also. If the dorsal compartments still require release, an incision is made beginning distal to the lateral epicondyle and extending about 10 cm distally. The subcutaneous tissue is undermined and the fascia is released over the extensor retinaculum. A dressing and a long arm splint are applied to hold the elbow in flexion. The arm is elevated and wound closure is usually done at five days.

25028-25031
The physician drains a deep abscess or hematoma in 25028 or an infected bursa in 25031 from the forearm and/or wrist. The physician makes an incision in the forearm or wrist overlying the site of the abscess, hematoma, or bursa. Dissection is carried down through the deep subcutaneous tissues and may be continued into the fascia or muscle to expose the abscess or hematoma. The incision may be extended if the mass is larger than expected. When the infected bursa, abscess, or hematoma is identified, it is incised and the contents are drained. The area is irrigated and the incision is repaired in layers with sutures, staples, and/or Steri-strips; closed with drains in place; or simply left open to further facilitate drainage of infection.

25035
The physician incises the bone cortex of infected bone in the forearm and/or wrist to treat an abscess or osteomyelitis. The physician makes an incision over the affected area. Dissection is carried down through the soft tissues to expose the bone. The periosteum is split and reflected from the bone overlying the infected area. A curette may be used to scrape away the abscess or infected portion down to healthy bony tissue or drill holes may be made through the cortex into the medullary canal in a window outline around the infected or abscessed bone. The area is drained and debrided of infected bony and soft tissue. The physician irrigates the area with antibiotic solution, the periosteum is closed over the bone, and the soft tissues are sutured closed; or the wound is packed and left open, allowing the area to drain. Secondary closure is performed approximately three weeks later. Dressings are changed daily. A splint may be applied to limit wrist motion.

25040
The physician performs an arthrotomy of a radiocarpal or midcarpal joint that includes exploration, drainage, or removal of any foreign body. An incision is made over the joint to be exposed. The soft tissues are dissected away and the joint capsule is exposed and incised. The joint space is explored, any necrotic tissue is removed, and infection or abnormal fluid is drained. If a foreign body is present (e.g., bullet, nail, gravel), it is exposed and removed. The wound is irrigated with antibiotic solution. The physician may leave the wound packed open with daily dressing changes to allow for further drainage and secondary healing by granulation. If the incision is repaired, drain tubes may be inserted and the incision is repaired in layers with sutures, staples, and/or Steri-strips.

25065-25066
The physician performs a biopsy of the soft tissues of the forearm and/or wrist. With proper anesthesia administered, an incision is made over the biopsy area. Dissection is carried down within the superficial soft tissue layers in 25065, usually the subcutaneous fat to the uppermost fascial layer. In 25066, dissection is taken down deep within the soft tissue, such as into the fascial layer or within the muscle. A portion of the tissue is excised and submitted for pathology. The area is irrigated and the incision is closed with layered sutures, staples, or Steri-strips. If the wrist is involved, a splint may be applied to limit motion.

25075-25076 [25071, 25073]
The physician removes a tumor from the soft tissue of the forearm and/or wrist area that is located in the subcutaneous tissue in 25071 and 25075 and in the deep soft tissue, below the fascial plane or within the muscle, in 25073 and 25076. With the proper anesthesia administered, the physician makes an incision in the skin overlying the mass and dissects down to the tumor. The extent of the tumor is identified and a dissection is undertaken all the way around the tumor. A portion of neighboring soft tissue may also be removed to ensure adequate removal of all tumor tissue. A drain may be inserted and the incision is repaired with layers of sutures, staples, or Steri-strips. Report 25075 for excision of subcutaneous tumors whose resected area is less than 3 cm and 25071 for excision of subcutaneous tumors 3 cm or greater. Report 25076 for excision of subfascial or intramuscular tumors whose resected area is less than 3 cm and 25073 for excision of subfascial or intramuscular tumors 3 cm or greater.

25077-25078
The physician performs a radical resection of a soft tissue tumor (i.e., sarcoma) from the forearm and/or wrist area, not involving bone. The tumor may be malignant or an aggressive benign tumor of the connective tissue. An incision is made over the tumor and dissection exposes it. The tumor and any adjacent tissue that may be affected by the spread of the neoplasm are excised. Large resections may be needed. The type and stage of the lesion determine the extent of the tumor margin resection area. Muscle or fascia may need to be repaired and drains may be placed. The surgical wound is closed using simple or intermediate repair or separately reportable complex closure, adjacent tissue transfer, or graft. If the wrist is involved, a splint may be applied to limit motion. Report 25077 for excision of tumors whose resected area is less than 3 cm and 25078 for excision of tumors 3 cm or greater.

25085
The physician performs a capsulotomy of the wrist. The physician makes an incision overlying the wrist joint. The tissues are dissected to the joint capsule. The physician makes an incision in the capsule, allowing better joint movement. The incision is closed in layers with sutures.

25100-25101
The physician makes a longitudinal incision over the part of the wrist to be exposed (e.g., anterior, posterior, medial, or lateral aspect) to access the wrist joint and perform an arthrotomy. The soft tissues are dissected away to expose the joint capsule, which is incised to expose the synovium lying within the capsule. A small portion of the synovium is excised for biopsy in 25100.

In 25101, additional dissection is carried out to further explore the joint cavity. Any loose or foreign bodies (e.g., free cartilage, bone chips, gravel) are removed and a biopsy may be taken. The physician irrigates the joint. The physician may leave the wound packed open with daily dressing changes to allow for further drainage and secondary healing by granulation. A drain tube may be placed and the incision repaired in layers with sutures, staples, and/or Steri-strips. A splint may be applied to limit wrist movement.

25105

The physician makes a longitudinal incision over the part of the wrist to be exposed (e.g., anterior, posterior, medial, or lateral aspect) to perform an arthrotomy and remove the synovium. The joint capsule is exposed by dissecting down through the soft tissues and freeing and reflecting the muscles. The joint capsule is incised to expose the synovium, the inner membrane of the articular capsule that lines the joint cavity. The inflamed or enlarged synovium is dissected away from the capsule and the bones and removed. A drain tube may be placed and the incision is repaired in layers with sutures, staples, and/or Steri-strips. A splint may be applied to limit wrist movement.

25107

The physician performs a distal radioulnar arthrotomy for repair of a triangular cartilage complex. The physician incises the skin over the wrist and dissects down through the soft tissues to expose the joint and locate the triangular cartilage complex. The defect is identified and debrided or sutured to return to a correct anatomic state. The wound is repaired in layers with sutures, staples, and/or Steri-strips. A splint may be applied to limit wrist movement.

25109

The physician excises a flexor or extensor tendon of the wrist or forearm. The physician incises the overlying skin and dissects the tendon. The tendon is freed and resected. The operative incision is closed in sutured layers.

25110

The physician makes an incision overlying the affected tendon in the volar or dorsal aspect (flexor or extensor tendons) of the forearm and/or wrist. Dissection exposes the affected tendon. The lesion is excised or shelled out, leaving normal tissue intact. If incised, the tendon sheath is closed. The incision is repaired in layers with sutures, staples, and/or Steri-strips.

25111-25112

The physician removes a ganglion from the wrist in 25111 or a recurrent ganglion in 25112. An incision is made overlying the ganglion. The tissues are dissected around the ganglion, freeing it from surrounding tissue. (Scar tissue may be removed in 25112.) The physician may dissect deep within the wrist joint in order to excise all of the ganglion. The ganglion is removed. The joint or muscle tissue may be repaired in 25112. The physician irrigates the wound with antibiotic solution and closes the wound in layers.

25115-25116

Radical excision is removal of all diseased and/or inflamed tissue and may include removal of a portion of surrounding normal tissue. The physician excises the bursa, synovia of the wrist, or forearm tendon sheaths of the flexors in 25115 and extensors in 25116. The physician makes a longitudinal incision over the volar aspect of the distal forearm and wrist. Dissection exposes the flexor tendons of the wrist. The physician excises the bursa and any inflamed and hypertrophied tissues from around the tendons. The tendons are left intact, allowing them to glide better during wrist movement. In 25116, the physician may perform a transposition of the dorsal retinaculum if enough tissue is removed from the wrist extensors. A transposition makes a smooth gliding surface no longer present between the extensor tendons and carpal bones of the wrist. The dorsal retinaculum is incised in the mid-line, tucked underneath the extensor tendons, and closed with sutures. The incisions are repaired in layers with sutures, staples, and/or Steri-strips. The wrist may be placed in a splint.

25118-25119

The physician performs a synovectomy of the extensor tendon sheath in the wrist. The physician makes a curved, longitudinal incision over the back of the wrist, radial to the ulna. A longitudinal incision is made through the deep fascia and the extensor retinaculum, entering the involved compartment. Hypertrophic synovium is removed from each extensor tendon sheath. If an area of a tendon appears frayed to the point of possible rupture, it may be sutured to an adjacent extensor tendon above and below the damaged area. After completing the tenosynovectomy, the physician evaluates the wrist. If synovitis is present, the joint is opened and a wrist synovectomy is performed. The dorsal retinaculum is sutured back into place, deep to the exterior tendons. Closure is performed after a drain is placed. The wrist is held in a neutral position, the fingers in extension. Report 25119 if resection of the distal ulna is performed as part of the procedure.

25120-25126

A bone cyst or benign tumor of the radius or ulna, excluding the head, neck, or olecranon process, is removed. The physician makes an incision in the forearm overlying the cyst or tumor. The skin and underlying soft tissues are reflected to expose the periosteum, which is separated from the bone. Curettes or osteotomes are used to scrape or cut the lesion from the bone. Once the benign tumor or cyst is removed and healthy bone tissue is present, the periosteum is repositioned and the incision is repaired in layers. If the bone defect created requires a graft for repair, the physician obtains the necessary size bone graft from a separate donor site on the patient and packs it into the site where the tumor or bone cyst was removed or uses a bone bank allograft. Report 25125 if the procedure is done with an autograft and 25126 if an allograft is used.

25130-25136
A bone cyst or benign tumor of the carpal bones is removed. The physician makes an incision in the wrist overlying the cyst or tumor. The skin and underlying soft tissues are reflected to expose the periosteum, which is separated from the bone. Curettes or osteotomes are used to scrape or cut the lesion from the bone. Once the benign tumor or cyst is removed and healthy bone tissue is present, the periosteum is repositioned and the incision is repaired in layers. If the bone defect created requires a graft for repair, the physician obtains the necessary size bone graft from a separate donor site on the patient and packs it into the site where the tumor or bone cyst was removed or uses a bone bank allograft. Report 25135 if the procedure is done with an autograft and 25136 if an allograft is used.

25145
The physician removes infected portions of bone from the forearm and/or wrist. The physician makes an incision overlying the sequestered area of bone, which includes incising the capsule if the wrist joint is involved. Once the skin and soft tissues are reflected, a small window is cut into the bone to gain access to the sequestrum, or necrosed piece of bone that has become separated from sound bone. All purulent material and scarred or necrotic tissue are removed. The remaining space is filled with surrounding soft tissues or free tissue transfer. The area is irrigated and an antibiotic solution is applied. The wound is closed loosely over drains or may be packed open with dressings. The patient may be placed in a posterior elbow splint or wrist splint to limit motion.

25150-25151
The physician performs a partial excision of the ulna in 25150 or the radius in 25151 to remove infected bone. An incision is made over the infected part of the bone and the underlying soft tissues are divided to expose the bone. The periosteum is reflected and the infected portion of bone is removed and irrigated. The excavation of bone may excise a crater-like piece, leave a small saucer-like shelf depression in the bone, or may remove a portion of the shaft (diaphysis) of a long bone. If a significant portion of bone is removed, the physician may fill the cavity in a separately reported grafting procedure The periosteum is closed over the bone, the soft tissues are sutured closed, and a soft dressing is applied to the elbow or a wrist splint may be used to limit elbow and/or wrist motion.

25170
The physician performs a radical resection of a tumor of the radius or ulna. The physician makes a skin incision along the lateral, anterior, or dorsal aspect of the forearm, depending on the area of resection. Resection of the proximal ulna is described. The physician makes a longitudinal posterior incision, dissecting down to expose the tumor site. The triceps insertion is detached from the ulna. The physician uses a bone saw to make an osteotomy cut in the ulna and the tumor is excised, including the immediate surrounding bone and any involved soft tissue. If much of the proximal ulna is removed, the radius may be dislocated posteriorly so that the radial neck articulates with the trochlea and the triceps tendon is sutured to the radial head. Drains are inserted and the incision is repaired in layers. A posterior splint is applied. No bone graft is used. Similar technique may be used for the radius.

25210
The physician removes one of the eight carpal bones of the wrist. An incision is made in the wrist overlying the carpal bone to be removed. The tissues are dissected down to the bone. The physician identifies the bone visually and dissects it free of the surrounding structures. Some ligaments may be reattached to other bones. The carpal bone is excised. The physician cleans the wound with antibiotic solution. The wound is repaired in layers.

25215
The physician removes all four bones in the proximal row of the carpal bones of the wrist. An incision is made overlying the wrist. The physician carries the incision down to the carpal bone. The physician identifies the two rows of carpal bones. The physician removes all four bones in the proximal row one by one while preserving tendons, nerves, and blood vessels. Each of the bones is dissected free and removed. Ligaments may need to be reattached to other bones. The physician irrigates the wound with antibiotic solution. The wound is closed in layers.

25230
The physician performs a radial styloidectomy by making a bayonet-shaped incision along the radial aspect of the wrist. The radial artery and nerve are exposed. The joint capsule is incised to expose the radial styloid. The physician uses a thin osteotome or thin oscillating saw blade to cut the radial styloid perpendicular to the long axis of the radius. The incision is repaired in layers with sutures, staples, and/or Steri-strips. The wrist is placed in an anterior splint.

25240
The distal ulna is partially or completely excised. The physician makes a medial longitudinal incision to expose the distal ulna. The ulna is located subcutaneously and does not require much dissection. The periosteum is incised and reflected to expose the distal ulna. Drill holes are made through the ulna 2.5 cm above the distal head. The physician uses bone-biting forceps to complete the division of the bone and remove the fragment. To stabilize the free end of the ulna, the physician reefs (overlaps) the periosteal envelope and ligament. The incision is repaired in layers with sutures, staples, and/or Steri-strips. Immobilization of the wrist is usually not necessary.

25246
The physician injects contrast material into the wrist joint for arthrography. The physician inserts a needle into the wrist and aspirates joint fluid for culture.

Contrast material is injected into the wrist and the wrist is manipulated to distribute the dye. As the dye fades, a second injection may be made.

25248

The physician removes a deeply implanted foreign body from the forearm or wrist. The physician incises the site and dissects down to reach the area where the foreign object is embedded. Exploration of the site is done. Separately reportable x-rays may be taken to locate the object. All parts of the object are removed. The wound is sutured in layers.

25250

The physician removes a prosthesis from the wrist. An incision is made overlying the wrist. The physician extends the incision deep to the wrist joint, opening the joint. The physician identifies the artificial joint piece that has failed. Using hand and powered instruments, the physician removes the prosthesis. The joint and incision both are irrigated with antibiotic solution and repaired in layers. If infection is present, the incision is left open to drain temporarily.

25251

The physician performs a complicated removal of all of the parts of a wrist joint prosthesis, including total wrist. An incision is made overlying the wrist. The physician may use the previous wrist surgery incision. The physician extends the incision down to the wrist joint by dividing and dissecting tissues. Some tissue may require debridement. The joint is entered through an arthrotomy cut. The physician identifies the pieces of artificial joint. Each piece is dissected free from the bone. Any loose pieces are removed. The joint is explored. The physician may smooth or debride the ends of the exposed bone. Any nonviable soft tissue and synovium is removed. The joint is irrigated with antibiotic solution. If infection is present, the joint and incision are left open for temporary drainage. Otherwise, the incisions are repaired in layers.

25259

Manipulation of the wrist under anesthesia may be necessary to gain the loss of motion following a surgical procedure or due to scar tissue. Following the induction of general anesthesia, the physician evaluates the wrist. The wrist is manipulated by stretching, rotation, and other maneuvers to gain the appropriate range of motion.

25260-25263

The physician repairs a flexor tendon or muscle of the forearm and/or wrist. The repair is done to restore continuity for normal function by reapproximating the severed ends. Primary tendon repairs can be performed when a clean wound is presented close to the time of injury that can be satisfactorily stabilized for a good end result-such as wounds inflicted with a sharp edge. Secondary tendon repairs are those that must wait because of complicated wounds or those that are performed again after an unsatisfactory first repair. The physician identifies the tendon or muscle by extending the original laceration or making new incisions. The ends of the severed tendon are identified and repaired at the level of separation. The ends are reapproximated using the suture configuration of choice from several different stitching techniques. If the injury occurs in the area of carpal tunnel, at the wrist flexion crease, complete or partial release of the transverse carpal ligament may be necessary. The flexor profundus and sublimis tendons are repaired with attention to proper orientation and location in the carpal tunnel. After the ends are properly matched and sutured, nerves and vessels are repaired as needed. The wound is closed and the limb is immobilized in a posterior splint at approximately 45 degrees of flexion. Involved fingers are held in passive flexion by an elastic band attached at the wrist level and at the fingernail by a wire. Report 25260 for a primary repair, one performed within the first 12-24 hours of injury where tendons are involved. Report 25263 for a secondary repair, one performed 10 or more days out from the injury or a subsequent repair done when the first procedure failed to restore function. Use these codes once for each tendon or muscle repaired.

25265

The physician performs a secondary repair of a flexor tendon or muscle of the forearm and/or wrist with a free graft. A secondary tendon repair is one performed 10 or more days out from the injury because of complicated wounds that would compromise immediate repair or one performed again after the first procedure failed to restore function. When the flexor tendons in the forearm and wrist area have become tightly contracted, a graft is necessary to bring the ends together. The palmaris longus is the graft of choice. The physician first approaches the involved flexor muscle or tendon through a zigzag incision on the palmar surface of the wrist or forearm, depending on the area of the tendon in need of grafting. The possibly scarred flexor tendon is freed and brought out through the incision, preserving as much healthy sheath as possible. The free graft is obtained by making a transverse incision in the volar wrist, dividing the palmaris longus tendon at its insertion, and while holding tension on the graft at its distal end with a clamp, advancing a tendon stripper into the proximal forearm. The proximal end is mobilized and the graft is withdrawn. Likewise, another incision may be made more proximally in the forearm, the tendon divided, and the segment withdrawn. The transverse skin incision is closed. The tendon graft is threaded through the forearm using a tendon passer. The tendon ends must be attached to the graft under the right tension. The junctures are secured using a monofilament wire and several possible suturing techniques. The wound is closed and dressed. A dorsal splint is applied maintaining wrist flexion to protect repair.

25270-25272

The physician repairs an extensor tendon or muscle of the forearm and/or wrist. The repair is done to restore continuity for normal function by reapproximating the severed ends. Primary tendon repairs can be performed when a clean wound is presented close to the time of injury that can be satisfactorily stabilized for a good end result, such as wounds inflicted with a sharp edge. Secondary tendon repairs are those that must wait because of complicated wounds or those that are performed again after an unsatisfactory first repair. The physician identifies the tendon or muscle by extending the original laceration or making new incisions. The ends of the severed tendon are identified and repaired at the level of separation. The ends are reapproximated using the suture configuration of choice from several different stitching techniques. Tendons in the dorsal wrist area are retained by the dorsal carpal ligament (extensor retinaculum) and are encased in fibro-osseous canals. They tend to get stuck in their canals as they heal; therefore, release of the sutured area may be necessary by excising a portion of the overlying carpal ligament. Many extensor tendons in the dorsal forearm are covered by their respective muscles and must be sutured, since sutures placed in muscle tend to pull out of the tissue. The wound is closed and the wrist is immobilized with a volar splint, in moderate or full extension. Report 25270 for a primary repair, one performed within the first 12-24 hours of injury. Report 25272 for a secondary repair, one performed 10 or more days out from the injury or a subsequent repair done when the first procedure failed to restore function. Use these codes once for each tendon or muscle repaired.

25274

The physician performs a secondary repair of an extensor tendon or muscle of the forearm and/or wrist with a free graft. A secondary tendon repair is one performed 10 or more days out from the injury because of complicated wounds that would compromise immediate repair or one performed again after the first procedure failed to restore function. When the extensor tendons in the forearm and wrist area have become tightly contracted or a segment of tendon has been lost, a graft is necessary to bring the ends together. The palmaris longus is the graft of choice. The physician first approaches the involved extensor muscle or tendon through an incision on the dorsal surface of the wrist or forearm, depending on the area of the tendon in need of grafting. The possibly scarred tendon is freed and the ends brought out through the incision for repair. The free graft is obtained by making a transverse incision in the volar wrist, dividing the palmaris longus tendon at its insertion, and while holding tension on the graft at its distal end with a clamp, advancing a tendon stripper into the proximal forearm. The proximal end is mobilized and the graft is withdrawn. Likewise, another incision may be made more proximally in the forearm, the tendon divided, and the segment withdrawn. The transverse skin incision is closed. The tendon graft is threaded through the forearm using a tendon passer. The tendon ends must be attached to the graft under the right tension. The junctures are secured using a monofilament wire and several possible suturing techniques. The wound is closed and the wrist is immobilized with a volar splint, in moderate or full extension.

25275

The physician repairs an extensor tendon sheath of the forearm and/or wrist with a free graft. This is done for extensor carpi ulnaris (ECU) subluxation. The ECU passes through a groove at the distal end of the ulna and is covered by a ligament. The ECU is the only wrist extensor that lies in its own retaining fibro-osseous sheath tunnel. Disruption of this compartment sheath is what allows the extensor carpi ulnaris to sublux. An incision is made and the underlying tissues are dissected to reach the sheath disruption of the ECU tendon. If the fibro-osseous sheath has ruptured so that the sheath lies under the ECU tendon on its ulnar groove, the sheath is sutured together directly over the tendon. When the fibro-osseous sheath has ruptured so that the sheath lies superficial to the tendon, the sheath is reconstructed with a piece of the extensor retinaculum, the fibrous sheet, or band of fascia overlying the extensor tendons. The subcutaneous tissues and skin are closed and a dressing is applied.

25280

The physician lengthens or shortens a flexor or extensor tendon of the forearm and/or wrist. For lengthening, the physician makes an incision in the forearm and down through the tissues to identify the affected tendon. The physician may make a series of small, equal-depth cuts spaced on opposite sides of the tendon to allow it to stretch without tearing through. An elongated Z incision may be cut in the tendon and the ends of the long half of each section are sewn together or an oblique incision is made across the tendon and the ends are slid apart until the pointed tips meet, which are sutured together. Several methods are also used to shorten a tendon that has become too long to function properly. A Z incision may be made in the tendon and the two short sides of the Z brought together and reapproximated. The tendon can be doubled over on itself with a small fold and sutured. A wedge-shaped piece may be excised and the two ends sutured. The soft tissue is closed in layers and a bandage is applied.

25290

The physician performs an open tenotomy on a flexor or extensor tendon of the forearm and/or wrist. An incision is made in the wrist or forearm over the site where the tendon to be cut may be accessed. The subcutaneous tissues and fascia are dissected to reach the target tendon. The usual method is to cut into the tendon so as to allow it to expand and heal as a longer tendon, thereby releasing a contracture caused by the tendon. The tissue layers and skin are closed and a dressing is applied.

25295

Tenolysis of a flexor or extensor tendon is indicated in the case of extrinsic extensor or flexor tendon tightness. In the case of flexor tightness, the physician approaches the involved flexor system through a zigzag incision that is long enough to uncover the length of the flexor. The physician excises all limiting adhesions, whether the excess scarring is located proximally in the forearm and/or distally in the wrist. The tendon involved is released of motion-limiting adhesions. The retinacular pulley system is preserved. During the procedure, the patient's active motion is re-evaluated. To achieve this, a local anesthesia is supplemented by an intravenous analgesic-tranquilizer combination drug. After tissue closure, the physician applies a splint over the dressing. These must be applied in a manner that allows continued flexion to maintain the tendon's gliding action through the lysed scars. The above techniques are the same for extrinsic extensors, except there is no critical annular pulley system to preserve, although the sagittal bands must be protected.

25300-25301

The physician performs a tenodesis at the wrist. In 25300, the physician exposes the flexor tendons of the fingers at the wrist level. The terminal phalangeal flexors to be fixated (usually all four) are identified in the depths of the wound. A window is made in the anterior surface of the distal radius proximal to the wrist. A similar second window is made more proximally. A crisscross type of suture is passed through all four flexor digitorum profundi tendons side-by-side. The tendons are transected proximal to this suture. The tendons are drawn into the more distal window in the radius, through the medullary canal, out the proximal window, and sutured back to themselves. The tension on the tenodesis is adjusted so that with the wrist in extension, the fingers naturally flex into the palm, closing the hand as desired. Tenodesis of the finger flexors can give an enhanced natural grip action using wrist extension for those with impaired control of movement. All open soft tissues are sutured in layers. The wrist is immobilized in five to 10 degrees of extension with the metacarpophalangeal joints flexed and the interphalangeal joints extended. Report 25301 if the extensors of the fingers are fixated to bone at the wrist.

25310-25312

The physician performs a flexor or extensor tendon transplantation or transfer in the forearm and wrist. The physician exposes the tendon to be transferred by making a longitudinal incision near its insertion. The insertion is released from near its bony attachment for transfer to the involved tendon. The tendon may not be released, but rather only the central portion. Through a separate incision, the physician exposes the involved tendon. A tunnel is prepared around or through the arm between the transferred and involved tendon. This tunnel must permit a straight line of pull between the two tendons. The transferred tendon is passed through the tunnel. A small, longitudinal hole is created in the involved tendon. The distal end of the transferred tendon is passed through the involved tendon and sutured to that tendon. After these procedures are complete, all wounds are closed with sutures. Report 25312 if the procedure is performed with tendon grafts, each tendon.

25315-25316

The physician performs a flexor origin slide in the forearm or wrist for conditions such as cerebral palsy. The physician makes a longitudinal incision from within a few centimeters proximal to the medial epicondyle, distally through the middle of the forearm. The ulnar nerve, median nerve, and brachial artery are identified and tagged. A periosteal elevator is inserted between the brachialis and the common flexor-pronator origin from the medial epicondyle. The elevator is brought out between the numeral and ulnar heads of the flexor carpi ulnaris on the anterior side of the elbow. The origin of the flexors is dissected using a scalpel to detach the muscle subperiosteally. The origins of the pronator teres, flexor carpi radialis, palmaris longus, and the numeral head of the flexor carpi ulnaris are released. The physician dissects the origins of the flexor digitorum superficialis. The ulnar head of the flexor carpi ulnaris is detached subperiosteally. The physician brings together the detached muscles from the proximal and ulnar sides at the interosseous space on the proximal side. Neurolysis of the median and ulnar nerves is performed. The muscles are slid distally the desired amount and are fixed in several places to periosteum and subcutaneous tissue. The ulnar nerve is transposed over the medial epicondyle. The wound is closed in layers. The elbow joint is maintained at 90 degrees, the wrist and fingers in extension, the forearm in supination. Report 25316 if this procedure is performed with a tendon transfer.

25320

The physician performs an open capsulorrhaphy or reconstruction of the wrist by any method (capsulodesis, ligament repair, tendon transfer, or graft), including synovectomy, capsulotomy, and open reduction to stem carpal instability. The wrist and finger extensors are retracted laterally and medially. The capsule is longitudinally cut over the involved carpus for exposure. If dislocation was present prior to surgery, this is reduced. The necessary fixation is carried out (i.e., Kirchner wires, screws). Carpal instability may result from dislocation of carpal bones and any number of ligamentous injuries that require reduction and repair, involving the joint capsule. Scapholunate dissociation and instability is one of the most common injuries. Dorsal intercarpal ligament capsulodesis may be performed to reduce the scapholunate gap. A flap of dorsal intercarpal ligament is elevated off the trapezoid and left attached to the triquetrum. The scaphoid inherently tends to sublux in the palmar direction in a flexed posture with dorsal rotational subluxation of the posterior pole. The scaphoid is brought out of its flexed position by applying dorsal pressure to the posterior pole and the scapholunate gap is reduced. The ligamentous flap is rotated down, stretched, and attached to the distal pole of the scaphoid. A flap of wrist capsule may also be created that is left attached to the radius and inserted into the distal pole of the scaphoid to tether it in chronic conditions.

25332
The physician performs an arthroplasty of the wrist. The physician makes a straight, dorsal, longitudinal incision centered over the wrist from the middle of the third metacarpal proximally. Skin and subcutaneous tissues are elevated off the fascia and retinaculum. The retinaculum over the fourth dorsal compartment is incised longitudinally and elevated medially and laterally. The extensor pollicis longus is freed, retracted radially, and left in the rerouted position at the end of the procedure. A longitudinal incision is made in the capsule. A capsular periosteal flap is elevated through the dorsal radioulnar ligaments. The distal radius is excised, as is the distal ulna if it is dislocated or severely involved. A cut is made through the hamate, capitate, trapezoid, and distal scapho-trapezoid area. The carpus is removed. The medullary canal of the radius is reamed. A fine awl is used to penetrate the base of the capitate and the shaft of the third metacarpal. The medullary canal of this bone is reamed. If using a double-stemmed component, an additional canal is prepared in the second metacarpal. Appropriate short canals are prepared in the carpal bones. With the wrist in 10 to 20 degree extension, the capsular-periosteal sleeves are repaired over the prosthesis. The extensor retinaculum may be used to reinforce the capsule, or may be repaired anatomically. The skin is closed over a deep and a superficial suction drain.

25335
The physician performs a centralization of the wrist on the ulna for conditions including radial club hand. The physician makes two incisions. A transverse incision is made over the end of the ulna to remove excess skin and fatty tissue and to expose the distal ulna. A Z-plasty incision may be needed on the radial surface of the distal forearm and wrist to give extra length to the tight skin on this side. The physician next incises the capsule, flexes the elbow, and reduces the carpus over the ulna. Insertions of the flexor carpi radialis and brachioradialis are cut. The distal end of the ulna is shaved to flatten its surface, and a Kirschner wire is drilled through the capitate and through the base of the third metacarpal. The second wire is removed and the ulnar wire is driven through the hole it created. The distal ulnocarpal capsule is pulled proximally over the ulna and sutured with nonabsorbable suture. The extensor carpi ulnaris is advanced distally over the fifth metacarpal tightly. The flexor carpi ulnaris is sutured with the extensor carpi ulnaris. The two incisions are closed. The wrist is placed in a neutral position, and a bulky dressing is applied.

25337
Restoring stability to a wrist with an unstable distal ulna or distal radioulnar joint may require just a few procedures, or it may dictate many procedures. In all cases, the physician must expose the distal radioulnar joint by making a curvilinear incision on the dorsal wrist starting proximal to the ulnar styloid and extending it dorsally, over the ulnar styloid to the carpus. The proximal and ulnar half of the extensor retinaculum is reflected radially. The extensor digiti minimi is retracted, revealing the styloid notch of the radius and the triangular fibrocartilage complex (TFC). The capsule is sharply detached from the radius exposing the ulnar head. If a styloid fracture is found, two drill holes are made proximally from the fracture to exit facing the radius. A wire is passed around or through the styloid using similar drill holes, and the two free ends of the wire are passed proximally through the fracture site into the previously drilled holes in the proximal shaft. The wire is twisted, compressing the styloid to the shaft. If the triangular fibrocartilaginous complex is avulsed from styloid, an intraosseous wiring as described above may be used to restore distal radioulnar stability. If the TFC is not avulsed, an intraosseous wire with a 24-gauge, or larger, should be used. The capsule is sutured closed, and the skin is closed in layers. Over the dressing, a long-arm cast is applied with the elbow flexed, the forearm in zero degree extension, and the wrist in neutral.

25350-25355
The physician performs an osteotomy (bone cut) of the radius. An incision is made in the forearm overlying the distal third area of the radius in 25350 or the middle or proximal third in 25355. The physician performs dissection through the tissue layers and down to the bone. The periosteum is removed from the bone site where the osteotomy will be made. The physician cuts through the radius. The physician realigns the bone to the desired position. Metal plates and screws are typically applied to stabilize the bone. The wound is irrigated with antibiotic solution and repaired in layers. A cast or splint may be applied to further stabilize and support the bone.

25360-25365
The physician performs an osteotomy of the ulna in 25360 or of both the ulna and radius in 25365. The physician makes a longitudinal incision along the medial border of the forearm to expose the affected part of the ulna. Two separate incisions may be necessary in 25365. An osteotomy (bone cut) is made through the ulna, usually in a wedge shape. This allows the bone to be realigned. The physician applies plates and screws to hold the osteotomy together in the correct position. The incisions are repaired in layers with sutures, staples and/or Steri-strips. The arm may be placed in a splint for immobilization.

25370-25375
The physician treats the radius or ulna in 25370 or both in 25375. A longitudinal incision is made to expose the shaft of the bone. Two separate incisions may be necessary in 25375. The physician makes an osteotomy (bone cut) through the proximal and distal ends of the bone shaft. The bone shaft is removed from the wound. The physician studies the bone shaft to determine how many times it must be osteotomized so that its segments can be threaded onto a medullary nail. The osteotomies are made, and each fragment placed end to end on the medullary nail. Because the cortex of the ulna and radius are very thin, a bone graft is usually added. This may be harvested from the

surrounding area, or a separate incision may be needed. A separate incision would be made over the iliac crest, bone harvested, and the incision closed. The medullary nail is inserted into place. The periosteum is sutured into place. The physician repairs the incision in layers with sutures, staples, and/or Steri-strips. The arm is immobilized in a cast.

25390, 25392

The physician shortens the radius or ulna in 25390 and shortens both in 25392. An incision is made on the anterior aspect of the distal forearm. Any exposed arteries are retracted. The physician continues dissection to expose the distal shaft of the radius and/or ulna. Based on preoperative x-rays, an osteotomy is made at the distal end of the radius and/or ulna. A more proximal osteotomy is made which shortens the radius and/or ulna usually by 2 mm to 3 mm. The physician removes the bone fragment. A plate is attached to the distal segment with screws. Reduction forceps hold and compress the osteotomy while the plate is attached to the proximal fragment with screws. Separately reportable x-rays are used to check radioulnar length. Drain tubes are inserted. The physician repairs the incision in layers with sutures, staples, and/or Steri-strips. However, the forearm fascia is left open to minimize the chances of compartment syndrome. The forearm is placed in a splint.

25391, 25393

The radius or ulna of the forearm is lengthened with an autograft in 25391 and both are lengthened with an autograft in 25393. One bone is often bowed due to the shortened and hypoplastic development of the other, as in congenital pseudoarthrosis. The forearm is incised and the overlying tissue is dissected to reach the bone. A few centimeters of bone may need to be resected to remove the deformity, taking care to preserve the epiphysis is the case of growing children. Surrounding abnormal tissues are also resected. The newly created defect is bridged with a vascularized bone graft from the patient, often taken from the fibula. The autograft is fixed to the bone of the radius and/or ulna with an intramedullary K-wire and may be proximally supported by placing another K-wire. Vascular anastomosis is completed between the artery of the graft and the ulnar or radial artery and the graft vein and the basilic vein. The wound is closed. A skin island that was preserved with the vascularized autograft may also be incorporated in the wound closure. A cast is applied to the forearm.

25394

The physician shortens a carpal bone. The physician makes the incision over the area of the carpal bone. Dissection is carried down to the level of the carpal bone and an osteotomy is done. The bone is shortened. The amount of bone removed is dependent on the condition treated. The incision is closed with sutures.

25400-25405

The physician exposes a nonunion or malunion of the radius or ulna by making a 10 cm to 15 cm longitudinal incision over the fracture site. With a reciprocating saw, each bone is divided through the nonunion. The fragments are aligned. A compression plate is centered over the fracture and screws are inserted. In 25405, a bone graft is needed to help heal the nonunion due to loss of bone. For example, if the nonunion is old, approximately 0.6 cm to 1.3 cm of bone is resected from the ends of the fragments. Autogenous iliac bone is typically used. Bone from the upper tibia may also be used. This requires an incision over the site of harvest. The physician uses an osteotome to harvest strips of bone. These strips are placed around the ends of the fracture along with the compression plate for internal fixation. The incision is repaired in layers with sutures, staples, and/or Steri-strips. However, the deep fascial layer is not closed because of the potential to develop compartment syndrome. A long arm cast is applied with the elbow at 90 degrees of flexion.

25415-25420

The physician exposes the nonunions through two 10 cm to 15 cm longitudinal incisions One incision is made on the lateral aspect and one on the medial aspect of the forearm. With a reciprocating saw, the physician divides each bone through the nonunion. The fragments are aligned. The physician centers a compression plate over the fracture and inserts screws. In 25420, a bone graft is needed to help bone healing of the nonunion due to loss of bone. For example, if the nonunion is old, approximately 0.6 cm to 1.3 cm of bone is resected from the ends of the fragments. Autogenous iliac bone graft is typically used. The physician makes an incision over the iliac crest. Once the bone is exposed, an osteotome is used to harvest strips of bone. These strips are placed around the ends of the fracture. Internal fixation with a compression plate is the same as for 25415. The incision are repaired in layers with sutures, staples, and/or Steri-strips. However, the deep fascial layer is not closed because of the potential to develop compartment syndrome. A long arm cast is applied with the elbow in 90 degrees of flexion.

25425-25426

The physician repairs a defect of the radius or ulna in 25425 or of both the radius and ulna in 25426. The physician makes a longitudinal incision along the forearm. An anterior approach is made for the radius, medial for the ulna, or two incision for both. The defect is exposed through dissection. To harvest the bone graft, the physician makes a separate incision over the iliac crest. Bone from the upper tibia may also be used. The bone is exposed, and the physician uses an osteotome to harvest strips of bone. These bone strips are used to fill the defect. A screw or wire wrapped around the defect holds the bone graft in place. The incision is repaired in layers with sutures, staples, and/or Steri-strips. However, the deep fascial layer is not closed because of the potential to develop compartment syndrome. The arm may be placed in a long arm cast with the elbow at 90 degrees of flexion.

25430

The physician makes an incision over the dorsal aspect of the distal forearm and wrist. The dorsal tendons that cover the fourth compartment are identified and the anterior interosseous artery and vein are identified and isolated. Using magnification the distal artery and vein are ligated. After radiological confirmation the skin over the lunate is incised. Dissection is completed through the lunate capsule. A small hole is drilled into the cancellous portion of the lunate bone. The distal ends of the ligated artery and vein are inserted into the lunate opening and secured with nylon sutures. The capsule is closed and the skin is closed in layers.

25431

Nonunion of the carpal bone refers to fractures that still allow free movement of bone ends more than six months after the injury and the start of treatment. In the case of a complex nonunion, the physician may take a graft from the medial aspect of the ulna and reinsert it into the prepared carpal site. Intravenous anesthesia is administered. An autogenous iliac bone graft is typically used for repair, which is obtained through an incision over the iliac crest. Once the bone is exposed, an osteotome is used to harvest strips of bone. These strips are placed between the carpal bones of the fracture through a 2 centimeter incision made at the base of the involved metacarpus. The physician centers a compression plate over the fracture and inserts screws. Lunate fractures require a short-arm spica cast or splint with thumb immobilization. Fractures of the pisiform can be immobilized with a volar splint. Injuries to the triquetrum are best treated with a sugar tong splint. Treatment of a hamate fracture involves a short-arm cast with the fourth and fifth metacarpophalangeal joints held in flexion.

25440

The physician performs this procedure when a scaphoid fracture has not healed and particularly if nonunion is accompanied by displacement of the fracture. The physician makes a 4 cm to 5 cm longitudinal incision along the radial border of the flexor carpi radialis tendon to expose the fracture site. The capsule is divided longitudinally, and the underlying ligaments are retracted. An egg-shaped cavity is created in the fracture fragments. A cancellous bone graft is obtained and the graft is jammed between the fragments as they are distracted. The physician uses internal fixation such as a Kirschner wires to affix the bones if instability exists. If a radial styloidectomy is performed, the physician makes an incision on the radial wrist at the base of the thumb. Radial styloid bone is removed. The physician closes the incision(s) with sutures.

25441

The physician performs an arthroplasty on the wrist to relieve function-limiting wrist pain. The physician makes a T-shaped incision overlying the dorsal wrist. The capsule and synovium are incised and elevated. The distal end of the radius and the proximal carpal row are excised to accommodate the implant. The medullary canal of the third metacarpal is exposed and an awl is placed into the canal for reaming. The awl is removed and the prosthetic awl is impacted into the base of the carpus and third metacarpal shaft. The medullary canal of the radius is reamed and implanted with the prosthesis. Cement is injected into the medullary canal of the third metacarpal after previously inserting a small cancellous bone plug. The distal component is impacted home first. The proximal component is generally not cemented and is impacted only. The capsule is repaired over the prosthesis with strong sutures. A suction drain is placed beneath the capsule. The retinaculum is repaired over all of the extensor tendons. The skin is sutured closed, and the wrist is immobilized.

25442

The physician performs this arthroplasty to decrease ulnar bone overgrowth following resection of the distal ulna. The physician makes a dorsal ulnar longitudinal incision overlying the ulnar head. The extensor retinaculum is incised. The neck of the ulna is subperiosteally exposed and the ulnar head is resected at the neck. The cut edge of the ulna is smoothed and medullary canal reamed to accept the stem of the implant. The implant is tested and two drill holes are made 2 cm from the resected bone. The physician stabilizes the distal ulna by attaching the base of the sixth dorsal compartment retinaculum to the interosseous membrane with sutures. The distal end of the ulna is pressed volarly and is sutured tightly into the soft tissue on the radial side with the radial itself. The wound is closed with sutures over a drain. A conforming dressing is applied.

25443

The physician performs an arthroplasty with prosthetic replacement of the scaphoid. The physician makes a straight, longitudinal, or curvilinear incision over the anatomic snuff-box (superficial to the scaphoid), the "V" between the thumb and index finger. The capsule is incised longitudinally. The scaphoid is removed maintaining ligament stability. If a defect is found in the distal capsule, this is closed with a nonabsorbable suture. A hole is made in the proximal joint surface of the trapezium for insertion of the prosthetic stem. An implant is inserted. The implant is stabilized with sutures through drill holes in the lunate and radial styloid. The implant is also stabilized with a K-wire passed through the implant into an adjacent carpal bone or the radius. The capsule is closed, followed by skin closure. A compression dressing is applied.

25444

The physician performs an arthroplasty with prosthetic replacement of the lunate. The physician makes a straight, longitudinal or transverse incision over the dorsum of the wrist ulnar to Lister's tubercle of the radius. The fourth dorsal compartment is opened and the radiocarpal joint capsule is transversely cut. The scapholunate and lunate-triquetral interosseous ligaments are cut. The lunate is removed. If a defect in the volar ligamentous capsule is found, it is repaired. A hole is made in the middle of the triquetrum to accept the prosthetic stem. The implant is fixed to the carpus and radius with a K-wire. An absorbable suture may be placed through the scaphoid and prosthesis to increase stability. The distal capsule flap is sutured to the radius with nonabsorbable sutures. The wounds are closed and a bulky compression dressing is applied.

25445

The physician performs an arthroplasty with prosthetic replacement of the trapezium. The physician makes a straight, longitudinal cut from the middle of the thumb metacarpal to the radial styloid. The capsule is split longitudinally from the metacarpal to the scaphoid. The capsule and periosteum are elevated off the trapezium. The radial portion of the trapezoid is removed. The base of the first metacarpal is squared off. A triangular hole is made in the base of the metacarpal, and the canal is made to accept the implant stem. The size of the implant should be slightly smaller than a tight fit. The capsule is repaired and reinforced by suturing slips of the abductor pollicis and flexor carpi radialis muscles to the capsule. A K-wire is placed through the implant and into the trapezoid or capitate to stabilize the position for six weeks. The skin is closed, leaving the wire protruding through incision, and a bulky dressing is applied to keep the thumb abducted.

25446

The physician performs a total wrist arthroplasty. The physician makes a straight, dorsal, longitudinal incision centered over the wrist from the middle of the third metacarpal proximally. The skin and subcutaneous tissues are elevated off the underlying fascia and retinaculum. The retinaculum over the fourth dorsal compartment is incised longitudinally and elevated. The extensor pollicis longus is freed and retracted radically. A longitudinal incision is made in the capsule overlying the distal radius. Ulnarly, a capsular periosteal flap is elevated through the dorsal radioulnar ligaments. Radially, the subperiosteal dissection continues to the radial styloid beneath the first dorsal compartment. The distal radius is excised, as is the distal ulna if it is dislocated or severely involved. A cut, made to match the shape of the prosthesis of choice, is made through the hamate, capitate, trapezoid, and distal scaphotrapezoid area. The carpus is removed. The medullary canal of the radius is reamed. A fine awl is used to penetrate the base of the capitate and the shaft of the third metacarpal. The medullary canal of this bone is reamed. If using a double-stemmed component, an additional canal is prepared in the second metacarpal. The component is inserted into the canals. Appropriate short canals are prepared in the carpal bases. The metallic components are inserted. The prosthetic polyethylene ball is placed on the trunnion and motion is tested. When desired motion is achieved, cement is mixed and injected into the medullary canals. The capsular-periosteal tissues are repaired over the prosthesis. The extensor retinaculum may be used to reinforce the capsule. The skin is closed over a deep and a superficial suction drain.

25447-25448

The physician performs interposition or suspension arthroplasty of the intercarpal or carpometacarpal joints. In 25447, for interposition arthroplasty performed on a non-thumb joint, the physician makes an incision over the carpometacarpal joint. The joint is vertically incised to release the capsule. The joint is completely dislocated to expose the proximal metacarpal or distal carpal bone surface. The physician resects the proximal metacarpal or the distal carpal. The base is shaped to allow the insertion of a metacarpal prosthesis. Soft tissue, usually a piece of harvested tendon or fascia, is inserted in place of the excised bone. A Kirschner wire may be inserted for temporary stabilization of the joint. The capsule and wounds are sutured closed. When interposition arthroplasty is performed on a thumb joint, the physician makes an incision over the proximal one third of the first metacarpal and extends over the trapezioscaphoid joint. The muscles covering the first metacarpal, trapezium, first carpometacarpal joint capsule, and scaphoid trapezial joint capsule are incised. The trapezium and possibly the base of the first metacarpal are excised and the interposition material, usually a piece of harvested tendon or fascia, is inserted in the defect. A Kirschner wire may be inserted for temporary stabilization of the joint. The capsule and wounds are sutured closed. This procedure may be referred to as a ligament reconstruction and tendon interposition (LRTI). In 25448, the physician performs a modified technique called suspension arthroplasty. A bone tunnel is created in the base of the first metacarpal. The flexor carpi radialis tendon is dissected or split at the base of the second metacarpal, pulled through the drill hole in the base of the first metacarpal, and the ends are secured in place with sutures. The capsule and wounds are sutured closed. This code includes transfer or transplant of the tendon, with interposition, when performed.

25449

The physician revises an arthroplasty, including removal of an implant in the wrist joint. The physician makes an incision over the wrist, reduces the joint if it is not already dislocated, and removes the device from the radius and the one or two metacarpals in which it was implanted. If necessary, a new device is placed into the wrist. The skin is closed in layers and a bulky dressing is applied.

25450-25455

The physician makes an incision overlying the distal forearm and along the medial (ulna) or lateral (radius) aspect in 25450 or both in 25455. The distal epiphyseal plate is located here. Dissection exposes the epiphyseal plate. The physician may elect to use a curette to scrape out the epiphysis (growth plate). A staple may be placed through the epiphyseal plate instead. Either procedure arrests further growth of that particular bone. The physician repairs the incision in layers with sutures, staples, and/or Steri-strips.

25490-25492
The physician applies prophylactic treatment. The physician treats the radius in 25490. A longitudinal incision is made along the forearm. Dissection exposes the affected part of the radius. In 25491, the ulna is treated. A longitudinal incision is required along the medial aspect of the ulna. In 25492, both the radius and ulna are treated, which may require two separate incisions. Pins or a plate with screws are used to stabilize the bone. If there are defects in the bone, such that the internal fixation does not provide good purchase with the bone, methyl methacrylate (cement) is used to fill in the gaps. Wiring (cerclage) may also be wrapped around the bone to provide additional fixation. The physician may also insert an intramedullary nail through the canal of the radius to provide internal stabilization. This is usually inserted through the distal end of the radius. The incisions are repaired in layers with sutures, staples, and/or Steri-strips.

25500-25505
The physician treats a radial shaft fracture without manipulation in 25500 or with manipulation in 25505. No incisions are made. If manipulation is required (25505), anesthesia may be necessary to relax the muscles. With the elbow at 90 degrees of flexion, the physician uses a combination of traction and countertraction while the radius is reduced. The patient may be placed in a long arm cast. The cast is removed after approximately 18 days and a functional brace is applied, allowing wrist and elbow movement, but limited pronation and supination.

25515
The physician treats a radial shaft fracture. If internal fixation is required, the physician may use plate and screw fixation or a medullary nail. A plate and screw fixation is described. If the fracture is in the lower half of the radius, an anterior forearm incision is made. If the fracture is in the upper half of the radius, a posterior forearm incision is made. Dissection exposes the fractured fragments. The physician uses bone-holding forceps to reduce the fracture. A plate of appropriate length is selected and centered over the fracture. Plates with five or six holes are usually required. The screws are inserted. The incision is repaired in layers. The deep fascia is not closed because of the potential of developing compartment syndrome. Depending on the rigidity of the fixation, a cast or splint may be applied.

25520
The physician treats a radial shaft fracture and a dislocation of the distal radio-ulnar joint. No incisions are made. The physician may reduce the fracture and dislocation by manipulation with traction force. A long arm cast is applied to immobilize the elbow and wrist.

25525
The physician makes a 5 to 6 inch longitudinal incision over the anterior aspect of the forearm and centered over the fracture. Dissection exposes the pronator quadratus muscle, which is freed from the radius. The physician reduces the fracture with bone-holding forceps. A plate of appropriate length may be selected and centered over the fracture. The screws are inserted. The pronator quadratus muscle is reattached. The incision is repaired in layers with sutures, staples, and/or Steri-strips. The deep fascia is not closed. The physician places the arm in a cast. The physician may also apply percutaneous skeletal fixation. Kirschner wires are inserted through small stab incisions through the radius and into the ulna to stabilize the radius.

25526
The physician treats a radial shaft fracture via an open approach, using internal fixation when required. This procedure includes repair of the triangular fibrocartilage complex. After the affected hand is suspended in finger traps, the physician reduces the fracture and confirms the reduction radiographically. Under separately reportable radiographic guidance, a Kirschner wire is inserted from the tip of the radial styloid obliquely across the fracture site. A second pin is inserted in a slightly more longitudinal direction. Finger traps are removed and the pins are cut off approximately 2 cm above the skin and bent at right angles. If tears are present in the fibrocartilage complex, they are repaired with sutures. Skin incisions may be made to prevent skin tethering. A dressing and splint are applied.

25530-25535
The physician treats an ulnar shaft fracture without manipulation in 25530 or with manipulation in 25535. No incisions are made. If manipulation is required, the physician uses a combination of traction and countertraction with manual manipulation of the fracture. The patient is placed in a long arm cast with the elbow at 90 degrees of flexion. A functional splint or brace is applied.

25545
The physician makes an incision along the subcutaneous border of the ulna, exposing the shaft fracture. The physician reduces the fracture with bone-holding forceps. If internal fixation is required, a plate of appropriate length is selected and centered over the fracture. The screws are inserted. Only the subcutaneous tissue is closed. The skin incision is repaired with sutures, staples, and/or Steri-strips. Depending on the rigidity of the fixation, a cast or splint may be applied.

25560-25565
For nondisplaced and stable fractures, the physician immobilizes the elbow and wrist with a long arm cast in 25560. Separately reportable x-rays are taken to confirm that displacement does not occur. In 25565, the fractures are displaced and manual reduction is required. Analgesia or a certain degree of sedation may be necessary. The physician uses a combination of

traction and manual manipulation to reduce the fractures. A long arm cast immobilizes the elbow and wrist.

25574-25575

When both the radius and ulna are fractured, the physician exposes and reduces both fractures prior to fixation. Separate incisions along the forearm may be needed to expose the fracture. In 25574, only one fracture is stabilized, requiring only one incision. The other fracture is stable and does not require fixation. In 25575, both radial and ulnar fractures require fixation, usually requiring separate incisions. Once the fracture site is exposed and reduced, internal fixation is applied. A plate of appropriate length is selected and centered over the fracture. The physician inserts the screws. The incisions are repaired in layers with sutures, staples, and/or Steri-strips. The deep fascia is not closed, preventing the development of compartment syndrome. Depending upon the rigidity of the fixation, a cast or splint may be applied.

25600-25605

The physician treats a distal radial fracture. A Colles' fracture is a fracture of the distal radius with dorsal displacement. A Smith fracture is palmar displacement of the distal radius. The ulnar styloid is usually fractured. If good alignment and correct angulation of the distal radial articular surface is present, the physician immobilizes the wrist and forearm in a cast or splint until the fracture or epiphyseal separation is stable. In 25605, manipulation is required to reduce an unstable and/or displaced fracture or epiphyseal separation. For either 25600 or 25605, closed treatment of the ulnar styloid may be performed. Analgesia or sedation may be necessary to achieve reduction. The physician uses a combination of longitudinal distraction of the fracture and manipulation of the distal fragment to achieve reduction. The wrist and forearm are placed in a cast or splint until the fracture or epiphyseal separation is stable.

25606

The physician treats a fracture of the distal radius. The physician first manipulates the area to reduce the fracture. The physician applies a combination of traction on the wrist and manipulation of the distal radius to reduce the fracture. An assistant maintains the reduction. Using a drill, the physician inserts two Kirschner wires percutaneously (directly through the skin) through the radial styloid, across the fracture, and into the opposite metaphyseal cortex of the ulna. The Kirschner wires are cut off just beneath the skin. The arm is immobilized in a cast. The wires are removed in six weeks. If there is a severely comminuted fracture of the distal radius that is not suitable for percutaneous Kirschner wire stabilization alone, the physician may apply a traction cast or an Ace-Colles external fixator. For application of a traction cast, the fracture or separation is first reduced and a Steinmann pin is inserted transversely through the proximal elbow. A second pin is inserted transversely through the bases of the second and third metacarpals. A plaster cast is applied above and below the elbow and incorporates the two pins. The pins and cast are left in place for approximately eight weeks. With an external fixator, the fracture or separation is first reduced by manipulation and traction. The external fixator is applied to the forearm and wrist to stabilize the fracture or separation.

25607-25609

The physician makes a 7.5 cm longitudinal incision along the anterolateral aspect of the distal forearm. The physician exposes the fracture by dissecting between the planes of muscles and tendons of the lateral wrist area while protecting the median nerve. The pronator quadratus muscle is severed from the radius. The physician reduces the fracture or separation. A small T-plate is fixed to the proximal fragment with one or two screws. Usually no screw is inserted through the distal part of the plate since it acts as a buttress and helps hold the fracture in reduction. Direct visualization and separately reportable x-rays are used to confirm correct reduction and restoration of the joint surface. The pronator quadratus is replaced at its origin on the radius. The incision is repaired in layers using sutures, staples, and/or Steri-strips. The arm is immobilized in a cast. Report 25607 for open treatment of the fracture with internal fixation; 25608 for fracture repair in which two fragments of bone in the joint receive internal fixation; and 25609 for fracture repair in which three or more fragments of bone in the joint receive internal fixation.

25622-25624

The physician treats a scaphoid fracture of the wrist without open surgery or manual manipulation in 25622. Separately reportable x-rays confirm the position and alignment of the bone. In 25624, manipulation of the bone is required. The patient may require anesthesia. The physician manipulates the area by pushing on the wrist bones, particularly the scaphoid. The physician also pulls on the fingers and forearm, moving the fractured area back into position. Separately reportable x-rays confirm alignment. In both 25622 and 25624, a cast is placed on the wrist and forearm with a thumb spica to hold the fracture in position.

25628

The physician treats a fracture of the wrist scaphoid bone. An incision is made over the scaphoid bone. The physician extends the incision down to the bone and the fracture is identified. Soft tissue is debrided as necessary. The physician places the bone fragments in their correct anatomical position. Typically, screws are applied to hold the pieces together. The physician irrigates the wound and closes it in layers. A cast or splint is applied to provide additional support of the area.

25630-25635

The physician performs closed treatment of a fracture of the carpal bone, reported for each bone treated. Triquetrum fractures are usually nondisplaced and respond well to casting or splinting for six weeks.

Capitate fractures are generally treated by conservative casting, immobilizing the wrist and thumb. Hamate fractures are accompanied by fractures at the base of the ulnar metacarpal, and become asymptomatic after a four to six week-period of immobilization. Lunate fractures are similarly treated by immobilization. Report 25630 if no manipulation is performed; report 25635 if manipulation is performed, each bone.

25645
The physician performs open treatment of a fracture of the carpal bone. Only some carpal bones are treated with open procedures. For hook of the hamate fractures, the physician makes an incision over the ulnar aspect of the wrist. The fracture is reduced and fixed with Kirschner wires, or the hook is excised. The tissue is closed in layers and a compression dressing is applied. Trapezium fractures are often treated with open surgery and may require secondary surgery to treat symptoms of pain. Capitate fractures—especially if associated with scaphoid fractures—are often treated with reduction and internal fixation via Kirschner wires. In cases in which lunate fractures do not respond well to immobilization, the physician may elect open treatment. An incision is made over the lunate to excise avulsed fragments. The soft tissue is closed in layers and a compression dressing is applied.

25650
The physician treats an ulnar styloid fracture with a cast or splint. No manual manipulation and no incisions are required.

25651
The physician performs percutaneous skeletal fixation of an ulnar styloid fracture. Following fixation of the ulnar styloid fragment, the remaining depressed articular fragments are elevated and reduced with traction, direct pressure, or with use of a small incision and application of pointed reduction clamps.

25652
If closed reduction of the ulnar styloid fracture is not possible, the physician extends an incision down to the bone and identifies the fracture. Soft tissue is debrided as necessary. The physician places the bone fragments in their correct anatomical position. The wound is irrigated and closed in layers. A cast or splint is applied to provide additional support.

25660
The physician repairs the dislocation of radiocarpal or intercarpal bones with manipulation. Sustained traction is held while the physician applies force to reduce the dislocated bone(s) into the proper anatomical position. Immobilization post-reduction depends on the physician's preference.

25670
The physician performs an open treatment of radiocarpal or intercarpal dislocation, one or more bones. The physician makes a dorsal incision overlying the wrist, and the dislocation is reduced. If involved ligaments are torn, they are repaired to stabilize the reduction. The physician may use the overlying capsule to reinforce the stabilization. The soft tissue is closed in layers and a compression dressing is applied.

25671
Percutaneous pinning is commonly performed at 10 days from injury. The physician may use fluoroscopic guidance to perform an initial closed reduction and to insert pins from the radial styloid to the ulnar cortex of the radius for percutaneous fixation.

25675
The physician performs a closed treatment of distal radioulnar dislocation with manipulation. The physician reduces the dislocation by pronation (if the ulna is volar) and supination (if the ulna is dorsal). The arm is immobilized.

25676
The physician performs an open treatment of a distal radioulnar dislocation, acute or chronic. For a locked dislocation or incongruous reduction, the physician opens the joint for reduction and repairs the triangular fibrocartilage (TFC)/ulnar collateral ligament complex (UCLC), stabilizing the repair with Kirschner wires. The physician incises the dorsum of the wrist on the ulnar side. The proximal and ulnar half of the extensor retinaculum is raised radially. The extensor digiti minimi is retracted to reveal the TFC. The capsule is detached from the radius and reflected ulnar. After the dislocated joint is reduced, the TFC lesion may be repaired or reconstructed using a local or grafted tissue from the retinaculum, extensor carpi ulnaris, or flexor carpi ulnaris. Kirschner wires may be used to stabilize the repair, after which the overlying soft tissue is sutured closed and a bulky dressing is applied.

25680
The physician performs closed treatment of a trans-scaphoperilunar type of fracture dislocation using manipulation. After being placed in continual traction for five to 10 minutes, the patient's hand is dorsiflexed while maintaining traction. While stabilizing the lunate volar, gradual palmar flexion reduces the capitate. The wrist is immobilized in a dorsal plaster thumb spica splint at 30 degrees volar flexion. Usually, if the scaphoid is properly reduced (visualized via separately reportable radiographs), the midcarpal joint is adequately reduced as well.

25685
The physician performs open treatment of trans-scaphoperilunar type of fracture dislocation. The physician makes a longitudinal, volar incision overlying the wrist, radial to the flexor carpi radialis tendon. This muscle is retracted toward the ulnar side, and the wrist joint is opened exposing the scaphoid fracture. After the fracture is reduced, Kirschner wires are drilled into the scaphoid to hold the reduction. If fixation of the scaphoid adequately stabilizes the midcarpal joint, no further fixation is required. If separately reportable radiographs visualize even the slightest tendency of volar subluxation, or rotary instability of the lunate, the volar incision must be extended and occasionally, a

dorsal incision must be made. In such cases, additional Kirschner wires should be introduced to stabilize the capitate-lunate joint. If this operation is performed within two to three weeks of injury, bone grafting is not used. If open reduction is delayed for more than three weeks post-surgery, bone grafting (reported separately) may be used. Capsular and skin closure is performed.

25690
The physician treats a lunate dislocation with manipulation. During sustained traction, the physician applies force to reduce the dislocated lunate. Immobilization post reduction depends on the physician's preference.

25695
The physician performs an open lunate dislocation. The physician makes both dorsal and volar incisions over the wrist. Through the dorsal longitudinal incision, the extensor tendons are retracted. The proximal pole of the scaphoid is retracted to expose the capitate. Through the volar longitudinal incision, the flexor tendons and median nerve are retracted to the radial side exposing a tear in the volar capsule and ligaments. The dislocated lunate is reduced through the volar approach by manually pushing it back between the capitate and radius while an assistant applies axial traction through the hand. The physician repairs the capsular-ligamentous complex tear with nonabsorbable sutures. On the dorsal side, the physician reduces the proximal pole of the capitate into the distal concavity of the lunate. The proximal pole of the scaphoid is reduced. Kirschner wires are drilled into the scaphoid, lunate, and capitate for stabilization. The physician repairs the dorsal ligamentous complex. The skin is closed.

25800-25810
The physician performs fusion of the wrist joint, including the radiocarpal, intercarpal and/or carpometacarpal joints. The physician exposes the wrist through a dorsal, longitudinal incision. A dorsal tenosynovectomy is performed, and the wrist capsule is elevated exposing the radiocarpal joint. The physician excises the distal ulna and performs a synovectomy of the radiocarpal joint. The radial collateral ligament is released from the radial styloid. The cartilage and sclerotic bond is removed from the distal radius and proximal carpal row. Using an awl, the physician makes a channel in the medullary canal of the radius, through which a Steinmann pin is used for internal fixation. The pin is drilled through the carpus to exit between the second and third, or between the third and fourth metacarpal, depending on alignment between the carpus and the radius. One or two small staples, or an obliquely-placed Kirschner, may be used to provide additional fixation on the radiocarpal joint. The position of the wrist can be varied only five to 10 degrees by adjusting the direction of the pin as it is driven into the radius. A drain is placed in the subcutaneous and prior to skin closure. A milky compression dressing is applied, and the wrist is splinted in the desired position of fusion. Report 25800 if performed without bone graft. Report 25805 if performed with sliding graft. Report 25810 if performed with iliac or other autograft.

25820-25825
The physician performs intercarpal or radiocarpal fusion. The physician makes a curved dorsal incision from the bases of the second and third metacarpal to the tubercle. The wrist joint capsule is opened via a longitudinal incision centered over the capitate-lunate joint. The dorsal three-quarters of the capitate, lunate, and scaphoid bones are removed. Approximately 25 degrees of wrist dorsiflexion will lock the graft in place. If the graft needs further stabilization, crossed Kirschner wires may be used for fixation. The skin is closed in layers. A long-arm cast is placed for six weeks followed by a short-arm gauntlet for an additional six weeks. Report 25820 if a graft is not used. Report 25825 if a fitted circular or rectangular corticocancellous graft from the iliac crest is removed and precisely shaped to fit the recipient. This graft is fit into the proximal row carpal area that has been removed.

25830
The physician performs fusion of the distal radioulnar joint and resection of the ulna, sometimes using a bone graft. The physician makes a dorsal, curvilinear incision over the distal radioulnar joint. The extensor retinaculum is reflected, uncovering the extensor carpi ulnaris and extensor digiti minimi tendons. The capsule is cut and reflected, exposing the ulnar head. A small lamina spreader may be used to view the sigmoid notch of the radius. The periosteum is stripped from the ulna just proximal to the articular surface. The dorsal radioulnar ligaments are stripped sharply. If the distal ulna has been removed, or part of the distal ulna is missing, the remaining portion is decorticated. The radius is prepared by making a notch in the ulnar aspect where the distal ulna can be slotted. The ulna is manually compressed into the notch, holding the forearm in 10-15 degree pronation. The physician drives a Kirschner wire from the ulna into the radius and two compression screws from the outer aspect of the ulna through both cortices of the radius. The extensor retinaculum is reconstructed and the skin is closed.

25900
In elective below-elbow amputations, the physician cuts the soft tissue flaps distal to the intended level of bone amputation. The physician dissects the superficial veins and cuts them at the level of the amputation. Cutaneous nerves are cut proximal to the level of the amputation. The dorsal and volar antebrachial fascia is cut, and, depending on the level of amputation, the tendons or muscle bellies are divided after the radial and ulnar vessels are severed. Muscle bellies are incised just distal to the planned level of bony resection. Nerves are cut through a separate incision, and brought under the muscle. The anterior and posterior interosseous vessels should be ligated or coagulated with electrocautery. An incision in the periosteum is carried out sharply and

Musculoskeletal

circumferentially. The bone is transected at the desired level at this time and the specimen is removed. The bone ends are smoothed with a rasp. Closure is accomplished after hemostasis is obtained following tourniquet release. The skin flaps can be fashioned, and subcutaneous tissue and skin are closed in separate layers. A drain is sometimes placed. The stump is dressed and wrapped with an elastic bandage applied more firmly distally than proximally.

25905
The physician performs a guillotine amputation. Just distal to the level of intended bone section, the physician incises the skin in a circular manner down to the deep fascia and allows it to retract. The muscles at the edge of the retracted skin are divided. All vessels encountered are ligated and divided. All major nerves are divided at a proximal level so that they retract proximal to the end of the stump. The physician sections the bone at the ends of the retracted muscles. The bone end is covered by the distal muscle bulk, and the skin is stretched over the stump and sutured closed. The stump is covered with a compressive dressing to control post-surgical edema.

25907
The physician performs secondary closure or scar revision after the stump has granulated or healed by a scar. In this procedure, no additional bone is sectioned. The physician resects the scar and granulation tissue from the end of the stump. Skin flaps are fashioned as close as possible to the thick scar surrounding the granulating wound. The dense layer of scar tissue is excised from over the end of the bone. Additional muscle may be removed as well. The skin flaps are pulled over the end of the stump and connected with nonabsorbable sutures. A temporary drain or suction tubes may also be used.

25909
The physician performs a reamputation. A reamputation may be necessary at a proximal level to reach healthy tissue. The physician cuts the soft tissue flaps distal to the intended level of bone amputation. The physician dissects the superficial veins and cuts them at the level of the amputation. Cutaneous nerves are cut proximal to the level of the amputation. The dorsal and volar antebrachial fascia is cut, and, depending on the level of amputation, the tendons or muscle bellies are divided after the radial and ulnar vessels are severed. Muscle bellies are incised just distal to the planned level of bony resection. Nerves are cut through a separate incision, and brought under the muscle. The anterior and posterior interosseous vessels should be ligated or coagulated with electrocautery. An incision in the periosteum is carried out sharply and circumferentially. The bone is transected at the desired level at this time and the specimen is removed. The bone ends are smoothed with a rasp. Closure is accomplished after hemostasis is obtained following tourniquet release. The skin flaps can be fashioned and subcutaneous tissue and skin are closed.

25915
The physician performs the Krukenberg procedure, a forearm amputation. The physician longitudinally splits the stump into radial and ulnar rays by making a dorsal, longitudinal incision toward the ulnar aspect of the forearm. Also, a volar, longitudinal incision is made toward the radial aspect of the forearm. The muscles left or transferred to the radial side of the forearm are the radial wrist extensors and flexors, the flexors of the index and long fingers, the index and long finger extensors, the pronator teres, the palmaris longus, and the brachioradialis. The remaining muscles are left or inserted on the ulnar side of the forearm. On occasion, some muscles need resection to reduce bulk, but the pronator teres must be preserved. The interosseous membrane is freed along its ulnar border. Skin closure is performed, ensuring the tactile skin is placed over the contact surfaces between the radius and ulna.

25920-25924
The physician disarticulates (amputates) the hand from the forearm through the wrist. The physician makes a long, palmar flap and a short, dorsal flap at a level distal to the radioulnar joint. These flaps are pulled back proximally and all veins are ligated. The physician cuts the superficial branch of the radial nerve and the dorsal sensory branch of the ulnar nerve. The lateral and medial antebrachial cutaneous nerves are cut. The radial and ulnar blood vessels are severed proximate to the wrist. The median nerve is cut while traction is applied. The flexor and extensor tendons are pulled distally and cut. The physician makes a transverse, dorsal incision of the dorsal radiocarpal ligament to view the radiocarpal joint. Circumferential dissection of the radiocarpal capsular and ligamentous attachments are carried out. The amputated specimen is removed. The styloid processes are rounded off, and the skin flaps are closed in two layers of subcutaneous tissue and skin. A soft dressing is applied distal to proximal. Report 25920 if an amputation through the wrist is performed. Report 25922 if a secondary closure or scar revision is performed on the stump. Report 25924 if a re-amputation is performed. All use a similar technique.

25927-25931
The physician amputates the fingers. The physician makes circumferential incisions around each digit excluding the thumb. These incisions are carried out at the mid-proximophalangeal level. The extensor digitorum communis of each digit (also the extensor indicis proprius of the index and the extensor digiti minimi of the little) are transected at the metacarpal bases. Individually, each metacarpal bone is transected and elevated from its soft tissue bed. The lumbricals and dorsal interossei are sectioned. Identified blood vessels are ligated. Nerves are ligated and transected. The flexor tendons are transected and allowed to retract in the palm. The volar plate, ligaments, and palmar fascia at this level are all cut and amputated digits are removed. The open periosteal tubes are closed. The soft tissue flaps are drawn over the end of the stump, and interrupted sutures are used. A soft

dressing is applied. Report 25927 if an amputation is performed. Report 25929 if a secondary closure or scar revision is performed. Report 25931 if a re-amputation is performed. All use a similar technique.

26010-26011
The physician drains an abscess located in a finger. In 26010, the physician lances an abscess located in the cutaneous tissue of a finger. In 26011, the abscess just reaches deep subcutaneous tissue and requires debridement and irrigation. The wound may be left open to drain.

26020
The physician drains fluid located in a tendon sheath located in a finger or in the palm. The physician incises the skin above the affected sheath and dissects to the tendon sheath. The sheath is lanced and drained. An irrigation catheter may be placed and the wound is irrigated for up to 48 hours. The incision is sutured in layers.

26025-26030
The physician drains a palmar bursa or multiple bursas located on the ulnar or radial side of the palm. The physician incises the skin over the bursa and dissects to the bursa. The bursa is lanced and irrigated with a catheter. The catheter is removed and the incision is sutured in layers. Report 26025 for a single bursa, report 26030 for multiple and/or complicated bursas.

26034
The physician incises the bone cortex of infected bone in the hand or finger to treat an abscess or osteomyelitis. The physician makes an incision over the affected area. Dissection is carried down through the soft tissues to expose the bone. The periosteum is split and reflected from the bone overlying the infected area. A curette may be used to scrape away the abscess or infected portion down to healthy bony tissue or drill holes may be made through the cortex into the medullary canal in a window outline around the infected or abscessed bone. The area is drained and debrided of infected bony and soft tissue. The physician irrigates the area with antibiotic solution, the periosteum is closed over the bone, and the soft tissues are sutured closed; or the wound is packed and left open, allowing the area to drain. Secondary closure is performed approximately three weeks later. Dressings are changed daily. A splint may be applied to limit movement.

26035
The physician decompresses fingers and/or a hand damaged due to an injection injury. The physician incises the skin overlying the entry point of the injection injury. The tissue is dissected to the fascial or periosteal layers and injected material is removed. If the injected material has followed the periosteum or fascia proximally, the incision length is increased until all the injected material is removed. The wound is irrigated and sutured in layers.

26037
The physician decompresses the hand fascia. The physician incises the skin overlying the affected fascia. The fascia is incised and the underlying tissues are irrigated. The incision is sutured in layers.

26040-26045
The physician incises the palmar fascia to release a Dupuytren's contracture. A Dupuytren's contracture is a shortening of the palmar fascia resulting in flexion deformity of a finger. In 26040, the physician makes a stab wound through the subcutaneous to the palmar fascia, which is incised. In 26045, the subcutaneous tissue is incised and retracted to expose the palmar fascia. The palmar fascia is incised to relieve tension and allow the hand to extend correctly. The operative wound is sutured in layers.

26055
The physician repairs a trigger finger, a condition caused by irritation and thickening of the flexor tendon along the palm's distal aspect. The affected tendon catches at the edge of the first annular (A1) pulley, causing abnormal movement and locking of the tendon within the tendon sheath of the affected digit. In a procedure also referred to as an A1 pulley release, the physician first administers a local anesthetic. A small incision is made in the palm of the hand, the tendon sheath is located, and the physician incises the band of tissue (the A1 pulley) along the sheath to allow more space for the flexor tendon to move freely. The incision is closed.

26060
The physician incises a tendon at the subcutaneous level. The physician incises the overlying skin. The tendon is severed through the subcutaneous tissue. The incision is sutured in layers. Report each digit separately.

26070-26080
The physician performs an arthrotomy of a carpometacarpal joint in 26070, a metacarpophalangeal joint in 26075, or an interphalangeal joint in 26080 that includes exploration, drainage, or removal of any loose or foreign body. An incision is made over the joint to be exposed. The soft tissues are dissected away and the joint capsule is exposed and incised. The joint space is explored, any necrotic tissue is removed, and infection or abnormal fluid is drained. If a foreign body is present (e.g., bullet, nail, gravel), it is exposed and removed. The wound is irrigated with antibiotic solution. The physician may leave the wound packed open with daily dressing changes to allow for drainage and secondary healing by granulation. If the incision is repaired, drain tubes may be inserted and the incision closed in layers with sutures, staples, and/or Steri-strips. Report 26075 and 26080 once for each specified joint.

26100-26110
The physician performs an arthrotomy of a carpometacarpal joint in 26100, a

metacarpophalangeal joint in 26105, or an interphalangeal joint in 26110 with biopsy. An incision is made over the joint to be exposed. The soft tissues are dissected away and the joint capsule is exposed and incised. The joint space is explored and a biopsy sample, such as from the synovial membrane, or fluid is removed. The wound is irrigated and may be left open with daily dressing changes to allow for secondary healing. If the incision is repaired, drain tubes may be inserted and the incision closed in layers with sutures, staples, and/or Steri-strips. Report codes 26100-26110 once for each specified joint.

26115-26116 [26111, 26113]
The physician removes a tumor or vascular malformation from the soft tissue of the hand or finger that is located in the subcutaneous tissue in 26111 and 26115 and in the deep soft tissue below the fascial plane, or within the muscle, in 26113 or 26116. With the proper anesthesia administered, the physician makes an incision in the skin overlying the mass and dissects down to the tumor or malformation. The extent of the tumor is identified and a dissection is undertaken all the way around the tumor. The blood vessels are ligated and the defective tissue of the vascular malformation is excised. A portion of neighboring soft tissue may also be removed to ensure adequate removal of all tumor tissue. A drain may be inserted, and the incision is repaired with layers of sutures, staples, or Steri-strips. Report 26115 for excision of subcutaneous tumors whose resected area is less than 1.5 cm and 26111 for excision of subcutaneous tumors 1.5 cm or greater. Report 26116 for excision of subfascial or intramuscular tumors whose resected area is less than 1.5 cm and 26113 for excision of subfascial or intramuscular tumors 1.5 cm or greater.

26117-26118
The physician removes a malignant soft tissue tumor (i.e., sarcoma) from the hand or finger, not involving bone. An incision is made over the tumor and dissection exposes it. The tumor and any adjacent tissue that may be affected by the spread of the neoplasm are excised. Large resections may be needed. The type and stage of the lesion determine the extent of the tumor margin resection area. Muscle or fascia may need to be repaired and drains may be placed. The surgical wound is closed using simple or intermediate repair or separately reportable complex closure, adjacent tissue transfer, or graft. Report 26117 for excision of tumors whose resected area is less than 3 cm and 26118 for excision of tumors 3 cm or greater.

26121-26125
The physician removes the palmar fascia. The physician incises the overlying skin and subcutaneous tissue. The palmar fascia is exposed and resected. Tendon sheaths are freed. The incision is sutured in layers if possible. Z-plasties are performed or skin grafts are obtained to close the wound if necessary. In 26121, the palmar fascia is removed. In 26123, part of the palmar fascia is removed and flexor tendons at proximal interphalangeal joints are released. Use 26125 to report additional digits.

26130
The physician removes the synovial membrane from the carpometacarpal joint. The physician incises the skin overlying the affected joint. The joint capsule is exposed by dissecting down through the soft tissues and freeing and reflecting the muscles. The joint capsule is incised to expose the synovium, the inner membrane of the articular capsule that lines the joint cavity. The inflamed or enlarged synovium is dissected away from the capsule and the bones and removed. A drain tube may be placed and the incision is repaired in layers with sutures, staples, and/or Steri-strips. A splint may be applied to limit movement.

26135
The physician removes the synovial membrane from the metacarpophalangeal joint, releases intrinsic musculature, and reconstructs the extensor hood. The physician incises the skin overlying the affected joint and dissects down through the soft tissues to the joint capsule. The joint capsule is incised and the synovium, the inner membrane of the articular capsule that lines the joint cavity, is removed. Intrinsic muscle contractions are released by exposing the extensor aponeurosis and incising the fibers at their insertion down into the tendon with a parallel incision, while preserving the transverse fibers. The adequacy of the dissection is tested and adjusted before the remaining flap part of the extensor hood is resected. The incision is closed with running sutures and a plaster splint is applied to hold the metacarpophalangeal joints in extension but allow full movement of the interphalangeal joints. Report each finger separately.

26140
The physician removes the synovial membrane from the proximal interphalangeal joint and reconstructs the extensor tendon. The physician makes a midlateral incision overlying the proximal interphalangeal joint, severs the attachment of the transverse retinacular ligament, and elevates the extensor hood. The collateral ligament and central tendon are identified and the joint is entered. The synovium, the inner membrane of the articular capsule that lines the joint cavity, is removed. The transverse retinacular ligament is relocated and the extensor tendons over the dorsum of the finger are repaired as needed and reattached to the joint. The incision is sutured in layers. Report each finger separately.

26145
The physician removes the synovial membrane from a flexor tendon sheath (tenosynovectomy) at the palm or finger. The physician incises the skin of the affected finger on the palmar side in a zigzag fashion and exposes the flexor tendon sheath. Taking care not to damage neurovascular bundles, the sheath is excised, except for a small area in the middle of the phalanx sections. The synovium is removed as much as possible and the incision is closed with interrupted sutures. A

compression dressing and supportive wrist splint are applied.

26160

The physician excises a lesion of the tendon sheath or joint capsule in the hand or finger, such as a cyst or ganglion. The physician incises the overlying skin and dissects to locate the affected area. The lesion, cyst, or ganglion is identified and excised from the tendon sheath or joint capsule. The incision is sutured in layers.

26170-26180

The physician excises a flexor or extensor tendon in the hand or finger. Included in these codes are flexor tendons extending from the palm of the hand to the fingertips, essential to grasping motion, and extensor tendons stretching from the wrist along the back of the hand to the fingertips, essential to opening the hand. The physician incises the overlying skin and dissects to the flexor or extensor tendon. The tendon is freed and resected. The incision is sutured in layers. Report 26170 for each flexor or extensor tendon of the hand and 26180 for each flexor or extensor tendon of the finger.

26185

This procedure is rarely performed, but may be necessary in cases of sesamoid fracture or when performing a metacarpal-sesamoid synostosis. The physician makes a midlateral incision over the metacarpophalangeal joint of the thumb on the radial side. The radial side of the extensor apparatus is opened, and the radial carpal ligament is dissected. The opponens pollicis muscle is separated from its attachment to the metacarpal neck. The metacarpophalangeal joint is opened through incision. In the case of a fracture, the fractured bone is exposed and removed. In a synostosis, the lateral sesamoid bone is exposed, its cartilage is removed along with the cortex of the first metacarpal neck. Drill holes are placed in the metacarpal neck and a wire suture is passed around the sesamoid bone. The capsule and overlying tissue are sutured closed.

26200-26205

A bone cyst or benign tumor of the metacarpal bones is removed. The physician makes an incision in the hand overlying the cyst or tumor. The skin and underlying soft tissues are reflected to expose the periosteum, which is separated from the bone. Curettes or osteotomes are used to scrape or cut the lesion from the bone. Once the benign tumor or cyst is removed and healthy bone tissue is present, the periosteum is repositioned and the incision is repaired in layers. If the bone defect created requires a graft for repair, the physician may obtain the necessary size bone graft from a separate donor site on the patient and pack it into the site where the tumor or bone cyst was removed. Report 26205 if an autograft is obtained.

26210-26215

A bone cyst or benign tumor of the proximal, middle, or distal phalanx of the finger is removed. The physician makes an incision in the finger overlying the cyst or tumor. The skin and underlying soft tissues are reflected to expose the periosteum, which is separated from the bone. Curettes or osteotomes are used to scrape or cut the lesion from the bone. Once the benign tumor or cyst is removed and healthy bone tissue is present, the periosteum is repositioned and the incision is repaired in layers. If the bone defect created requires a graft for repair, the physician may obtain the necessary size bone graft from a separate donor site on the patient and pack it into the site where the tumor or bone cyst was removed. Report 26215 if an autograph is obtained.

26230-26236

The physician performs a partial excision of a metacarpal bone in 26230, the proximal or middle phalanx of a finger in 26235, or the distal phalanx of a finger in 26236 to remove infected bone. An incision is made over the infected part of the hand or finger and the underlying soft tissues are divided to expose the bone. The periosteum is reflected and the infected portion of bone is removed and irrigated. The excavation of bone may excise a crater-like piece, leave a small saucer-like shelf depression in the bone, or may remove a portion of the shaft (diaphysis) of a long bone. If a significant portion of bone is removed, the physician may use bone graft material to fill the cavity left in the bone. The periosteum is closed over the bone, the soft tissues are sutured closed, and a soft dressing is applied.

26250-26262

The physician performs a radical resection of a tumor. The physician incises the overlying skin and dissects to determine the extent of invasion. The bone and surrounding tissues are resected. If a graft is needed for reconstruction, it is obtained from the distal radius or iliac crest. Skin is approximated over the surgical defect and sutured in layers. In 26250, a tumor of the metacarpal bone is excised. In 26260, a tumor of the proximal or middle phalanx of a finger is excised. In 26262, a tumor of the distal phalanx of a finger is excised.

26320

The physician removes a previously placed implant from a finger or hand. The physician incises the overlying skin and dissects to the implant. The implant is removed and the incision is sutured in layers.

26340

Manipulation of the finger joint under anesthesia may be necessary to regain the loss of motion following a surgical procedure or due to scar tissue. Following the induction of general anesthesia, the physician evaluates the finger. The finger is manipulated by stretching, rotation, and other maneuvers to gain the appropriate range of motion.

26341

Manipulation is the second half of a noninvasive procedure performed to correct connective tissue shortening and thickening in the hand causing "bent finger" or Dupuytren's contracture. This procedure is usually preceded by a separately reported injection of an enzyme (clostridial collagenase) into contracted connective tissue in the hand. The enzymes weaken and dissolve the tissue to facilitate the release of the contracture that occurs during this manipulation.

26350-26352
The physician repairs or advances a single tendon not located in "no man's land." "No man's land" is located between the A1 pulley and the insertion of the superficialis tendon. The physician incises the skin overlying the proximal or distal phalanx and dissects to the tendon. The tendon is repaired with sutures or advanced to improve joint function. Primary repair is done immediately after injury. Secondary repair is done sometime after the incident of injury or following a previous surgical repair. If a graft is needed for secondary repair, it is obtained from the palmaris longus tendon or from the foot. The incision is sutured in layers. Report 26350 for each primary or secondary tendon repair without autograft. Report 26352 for each secondary tendon repair with autograft.

26356-26358
The physician repairs or advances a single flexor tendon located in "no man's land." "No man's land" is located between the A1 pulley and the insertion of the superficialis tendon. The physician incises the skin overlying the medial phalanx and dissects to the tendon. The tendon is repaired with sutures or advanced and sutured to improve joint function. Primary repair is done immediately after injury. Secondary repair is done sometime after the incident of injury or following a previous surgical repair. If a graft is needed for secondary repair, it is obtained from the palmaris longus tendon or from the foot. The incision is sutured in layers. Report 26356 for each primary flexor tendon repair or advancement without a free graft. Report 26357 for each secondary flexor tendon repair or advancement without a free graft and 26358 for each secondary tendon repair with a free graft (includes harvesting the graft).

26370-26373
The physician repairs or advances the profundus flexor tendon; the superficialis tendon is intact. The physician incises the skin overlying the damaged tendon. The tendon is repaired with sutures or advanced to improve joint function. Primary repair is done immediately after injury. Secondary repair is done sometime after the incident of injury or following a previous surgical repair. If a graft is needed for secondary repair, it is obtained from the palmaris longus tendon or from the foot. The incision is sutured in layers. Report 26370 for each primary tendon repair without graft. Report 26372 for each secondary tendon repair with free graft. Report 26373 for each secondary tendon repair without free graft.

26390
The physician excises a flexor tendon in a finger or hand and implants a synthetic rod for delayed tendon graft. The physician incises the overlying skin and dissects to the tendon. The tendon is freed. The proximal and distal ends are severed and the tendon is removed. The physician implants a synthetic rod so the surrounding tissue will form a natural tube for a tendon graft. The incision is closed. This code is reported once for each rod that is implanted.

26392
The physician removes a synthetic rod used to create a natural location for a tube graft and inserts a flexor tendon graft. The physician incises the overlying skin and dissects to the rod. The rod is removed. A graft is obtained from the palmaris longus tendon or from the foot and inserted in the new position. The proximal and distal ends are sutured into place and the incision is sutured in layers. This code is reported once for each rod that is removed and replaced by a tendon graft.

26410-26412
The physician repairs or advances a single extensor tendon located in the hand. The physician incises the skin overlying the tendon. The tendon is repaired with sutures or advanced to improve joint function. Primary repair is done immediately after injury. Secondary repair is done sometime after the incident of injury or following a previous surgical repair. If a graft is needed for secondary repair, it is obtained from the palmaris longus tendon or from the foot. The incision is sutured in layers. Report 26410 for each primary or secondary tendon repair without free graft. Report 26412 for each secondary tendon repair with free graft.

26415
The physician excises an extensor tendon in a finger or hand and implants a synthetic rod for delayed tendon graft. The physician incises the overlying skin and dissects to the tendon. The tendon is freed. The proximal and distal ends are severed and the tendon is removed. The physician implants a synthetic rod so the surrounding tissue will form a natural tube for a tendon graft. The incision is closed. This code is reported once for each rod that is implanted.

26416
The physician removes a synthetic rod used to create a natural location for a tube graft and inserts an extensor tendon graft. The physician incises the overlying skin and dissects to the rod. The rod is removed. A graft is obtained from the palmaris longus tendon or from the foot and inserted in the new position. The proximal and distal ends are sutured into place and the incision is sutured in layers. This code is reported once for each rod that is removed and replaced by a tendon graft.

26418-26420
The physician repairs or advances a single extensor tendon located in the finger. The physician incises the skin overlying the tendon. The tendon is repaired with sutures or advanced to improve joint function. Primary repair is done immediately after injury. Secondary repair is done sometime after the incident of injury or following a previous surgical repair. If a graft is needed for secondary repair, it is obtained from the palmaris longus tendon or from the foot. The incision is sutured in layers. Report 26418 for each primary or secondary

tendon repair without free graft. Report 26420 for each secondary tendon repair with free graft.

26426-26428
The physician repairs a Boutonniere, or buttonhole, deformity of the central slip extensor tendon with a soft tissue procedure that reconstructs the central slip using the lateral band in 26426 or a free tendon graft in 26428. In this deformity, the tendons are imbalanced due to synovitis in the proximal interphalangeal (PIP) joint that causes a stretching of the central slip and subluxation of the lateral bands, which become tight from the swollen joint pressure and act as flexors to the PIP joint. This causes hyperextension deformities in the distal interphalangeal and metacarpophalangeal joints. The physician makes a dorsal, longitudinal incision over the proximal interphalangeal joint to the distal IP joint. The displaced lateral bands are mobilized and a tenotomy is done on the two lateral tendons next to the distal IP joint. The functionality of the central tendon must be restored. The lateral bands are aligned with the central tendon and used as local tissue to reconstruct the central slip. Report 26428 if a separate free tendon graft must be harvested to repair the central slip. A synovectomy is done. Tendon balance must be assured before the proximal IP joint is fixed in extension. The finger is later placed in a dynamic extension splint after removal of the fixation wire.

26432
The physician repairs the distal insertion extensor tendon without incising the skin. The physician uses a splint to pin the finger in an extended position. If extensive damage occurred during injury, pins may be used to stabilize the joint.

26433-26434
The physician repairs the distal insertion of an extensor tendon (mallet finger), using a graft if necessary. The physician incises the overlying skin and dissects to the damaged tendon. The tendon is repaired with sutures to improve joint function. If a graft is needed for repair, it is obtained from the palmaris longus tendon or from the foot. The incision is sutured in layers. Primary repair is done immediately after injury. Secondary repair is done sometime after the incident of injury or following a previous surgical repair. Report 26433 for primary or secondary repair without a graft and 26434 for primary or secondary repair requiring a graft.

26437
The physician realigns an extensor tendon in the hand. The physician incises the overlying skin and dissects to the damaged tendon. The tendon is realigned to correct finger position. The incision is sutured in layers. Report each tendon separately.

26440-26442
The physician removes scar tissue to release a flexor tendon in a finger or the palm. The physician incises the overlying tissue and dissects to the affected tendon. The scar tissue is debrided and removed, freeing the tendon. The incision is sutured in layers. In 26440 repair is limited to the palm or finger. In 26442, repair extends to the hand and finger. Report each tendon separately.

26445-26449
The physician removes scar tissue to release an extensor tendon in a finger or the dorsum of hand. The physician incises the overlying tissue and dissects to the affected tendon. The scar tissue is debrided and removed, freeing the tendon. The incision is sutured in layers. In 26445 repair is limited to the hand or finger. In 26449, repair extends to the finger, including forearm. Report each tendon separately.

26450-26455
The physician incises a flexor tendon. The physician incises the overlying skin and dissects to the flexor tendon. The tendon is incised. The incision is sutured in layers. In 26450, the tendon is located in the palm. In 26455, the tendon is located in a finger. Report each tendon separately.

26460
The physician incises an extensor tendon in a hand or finger. The physician incises the overlying skin and dissects to the extensor tendon. The tendon is incised. The incision is sutured in layers. Report each tendon separately.

26471-26474
The physician sutures the tendon to the proximal or distal interphalangeal joint for stabilization. The physician incises the overlying skin and dissects to the joint. The tendon is incised and sutured over the joint space, providing joint stabilization. The incision is sutured in layers. In 26471, the proximal joint is stabilized. In 26474, the distal joint is stabilized. Report each joint separately.

26476
The physician lengthens an extensor tendon in a hand or a finger. The physician incises the overlying skin and dissects to the tendon. The physician performs step cuts to lengthen the tendon. The incision is sutured in layers. Report each tendon separately.

26477
The physician shortens an extensor tendon in a hand or a finger. The physician incises the overlying skin and dissects to the tendon. The physician removes a section of the tendon and sutures the ends back together, shortening the tendon. The incision is sutured in layers. Report each tendon separately.

26478
The physician lengthens a flexor tendon in a hand or a finger. The physician incises the overlying skin and dissects to the tendon. The physician performs step cuts to lengthen the tendon. The incision is sutured in layers. Report each tendon separately.

26479
The physician shortens a flexor tendon in the hand or finger. The physician incises the overlying skin and dissects to the tendon. The physician removes a section of the tendon and sutures the ends back

together, shortening the tendon. The incision is sutured in layers. Report each tendon separately.

26480-26489
The physician transfers or transplants a tendon; a free tendon graft may be used if necessary. The physician incises the overlying skin and dissects to the tendon to be moved. The tendon is freed, transferred and sutured into place. If a free tendon graft is used, it is obtained from the palmaris longus tendon or from the foot. The incision is sutured in layers. For transfer or transplant of a carpometacarpal or dorsum of hand tendon without a free graft report 26480 for each tendon; report 26483 if a free graft is used. For transfer or transplant of a palmar tendon without a free graft, report 26485 for each tendon; report 26489 if a free tendon graft is used.

26490-26494
The physician transfers the superficialis tendon to restore palmar abduction to the thumb. The physician incises the overlying skin and dissects to the superficialis tendon. The tendon is freed and transferred to restore function. If a graft is used, the graft is obtained from the palmaris longus or the abductor digiti minimi. The graft is approximated and sutured into place. The incision is sutured in layers. Report 26490 if no graft is used. Report 26492 if a graft is used. Report each tendon separately. In 26494 the hypothenar muscle is transferred. The muscle tendon is resected from its distal attachment, transferred to the site and sutured into place.

26496
The physician performs this procedure when opposition of the thumb is lost because of median nerve paralysis. Methods described using this code include (1) attaching the extensor pollicis brevis to the extensor carpi ulnaris around the ulnar border of the wrist; (2) attaching the extensor carpi radialis longus to the extensor pollicis longus around the ulnar border of the wrist; (3) attaching the extensor indicis proprius tendon, with a small portion of the extensor hood, to the flexor pollicis longus tendon just distal to the metacarpophalangeal (MP) joint; (4) attachment of the extensor digiti minimi around the ulnar border of the wrist to the thumb MP joint; (5) attachment of the extensor indicis proprius with a small portion of the extensor hood around the ulnar border of the wrist to the thumb MP joint; (6) transfer of the adductor pollicis to the tendon of the superficial head of the flexor pollicis brevis; (7) attachment of the flexor pollicis longus around the ulnar aspect of the flexor carpi ulnaris into the abductor pollicis brevis of the interphalangeal joint.

26497-26498
The physician transfers a tendon to restore intrinsic function to the fingers. The physician incises the overlying skin and dissects to the affected tendon. The tendon is freed, transferred and sutured into place to restore function to the flexor digitorum profundus. The incision is sutured in layers. In 26497, intrinsic function is restored to the ring and small finger. In 26498, intrinsic function is restored to all four fingers.

26499
The physician corrects a claw finger. The superficialis technique involves splitting the flexor digitorum superficialis of the long finger into four slips. One slip is passed through the lumbrical canal of each finger to be inserted into the radial lateral band of the dorsal apparatus. This slip is sutured with the wrist in 30 degrees palmar flexion, the MP joints in 80 to 90 degree flexion, and the interphalangeal joints in full extension. In the dorsal approach, the tendon slips of the extensor carpi radialis brevis are passed superficial to the dorsal carpal ligament, through the intermetacarpal spaces, through the lumbrical canal volar to the deep transverse metacarpal ligament. The tendon is attached to the radial lateral bands of the long, ring and little fingers, and the ulnar lateral band of the index finger. A modification of the latter procedure involves detaching the extensor carpi radialis longus at its insertion and passing it deep to the brachioradialis to the volar sides of the forearm proximate to the wrist. The grafts of the plantaris or palmaris tendons are used. The lateral bands are identified through dorsoradial incisions over the proximal phalanx (except the index finger, which has the ulnar lateral band exposed). The tendon slips are directed through the carpal tunnel volar to the deep transverse metacarpal ligament and into the lateral bands. The tendons are sutured with the wrist dorsiflexed 45 degrees, the MP joints are flexed 70 degrees, and the interphalangeal joints are fixed at zero degrees. Incisions are closed.

26500-26502
The physician reconstructs a tendon pulley. The physician incises the overlying skin and dissects to the damaged pulley located in the A1 position or the distal interphalangeal joint position. In 26500, the tendon pulley is reconstructed using neighboring tissue. In 26502, the physician obtains a fascial graft for reconstruction.

26508
The physician incises the thenar muscle to release, for example, thumb contracture. The physician incises the overlying skin and dissects to the thenar muscle. The scarred muscle tissue is incised to release contracture. The incision is sutured in layers.

26510
The physician performs a cross intrinsic transfer to restore anatomic position and intrinsic function to the fingers. The physician incises the overlying skin and dissects to the affected tendons. The ulnar tendon is resected and transferred to the radial side of the joint, where it is sutured into place. The incision is sutured in layers.

26516-26518
The physician performs a capsulodesis to stabilize the metacarpophalangeal joint. The physician incises the overlying the skin and dissects to the MP joint. The

capsule of the joint is sutured to the proximal and distal bones to stabilize the joint. The incision is sutured in layers. In 26516 one digit is repaired. In 26517 two digits are repaired. In 26518 three or four digits are repaired.

26520-26525

The physician removes or incises the joint capsule to release contracture and restore function. The physician incises the overlying the skin and dissects to the metacarpophalangeal joint. The capsule of the joint is incised or resected and removed. The incision is sutured in layers. In 26520, the capsulectomy or capsulotomy is performed on the metacarpophalangeal joint. In 26525 the capsulectomy or capsulotomy is performed on the interphalangeal joint. Report each joint separately.

26530-26531

The physician performs an arthroplasty on the metacarpophalangeal joint. The physician incises the overlying the skin and dissects to the MP joint. In 26530 the joint is reconstructed using neighboring tissue. In 26531, a prosthetic joint is used to replace the diseased joint. Report each joint separately. Report each tendon separately.

26535-26536

The physician performs an arthroplasty on the interphalangeal joint. The physician incises the overlying skin at the back of the interphalangeal joint. Debridement of the joint is performed to remove aggravating bone and/or tissue. In 26535, the joint is reconstructed using neighboring tissue. This procedure typically requires only local anesthesia. In 26536, a prosthetic joint is used to replace the diseased joint, which requires regional or general anesthesia. In both cases, report each joint separately. At the conclusion of the procedure, deep tissues are closed and the skin is sutured. A dressing or cast may be applied depending upon the extent of the procedure.

26540-26542

The physician performs a primary repair on a collateral ligament of a metacarpophalangeal joint, possibly using a graft or advancement. The physician incises the overlying the skin and dissects to the MP joint. In 26540, the ligament is repaired with sutures. In 26541, a palmaris longus tendon or fascial graft is obtained. The graft is sutured into place. In 26542, an adductor tendon is advanced and sutured into place to stabilize the joint. The incision is sutured in layers.

26545

The physician uses a graft to repair a collateral ligament of an interphalangeal joint. The physician incises the overlying the skin and dissects to the I-P joint. A palmaris longus tendon or fascial graft is obtained and sutured into place. to stabilize the joint. The incision is sutured in layers. Report each joint separately.

26546

The physician performs this procedure to promote healing of a fractured phalanx or metacarpal that fails to heal. The physician makes an incision overlying the dorsal aspect of the fracture of the digit. The extensor mechanism is retracted and the fracture is exposed. Surgical resection of the nonunion itself may be performed. If this resection takes place, fibrous tissue must be removed until there are freshened fracture ends. If a resultant gap produces unacceptable shortening. Fixation such as Kirschner wires or pins, or AO plates is applied. The physician closes the incision with sutures.

26548

The physician repairs a volar plate of an interphalangeal joint. The physician incises the overlying the skin and dissects to the I-P joint. The plate of the joint is sutured to the proximal and distal bones to stabilize the joint. The incision is sutured in layers.

26550

The physician replaces all or part of a thumb with the index finger. The extent of an index finger used is determined by the size of the defect. The physician harvests the index finger with its tendons, blood vessels, and nerves intact and transfers the digit to the thenar eminence. If the thenar eminence must be created, the physician will transfer the index metacarpal along with the digit. If the index metacarpal is not needed, it is removed to provide space for function. The tendons are sutured to the new digit to provide abduction function. The skin is reapproximated and sutured in layers.

26551

The physician performs this procedure to provide functional thumb reconstruction in cases of traumatic thumb amputation and congenital absence of the thumb. Two surgical teams are employed, one at the hand and the other at the foot. One physician makes a linear incision over the dorsal aspect of the foot, traveling from proximal to distal, aiming toward the great toe. This incision stops at the base of the toe and a circular incision is made around the toe. The medial and lateral dorsal foot flaps are raised. The first dorsal metatarsal artery (FDMA) and deep peroneal nerve (DPN) are identified and exposed proximally to the dorsalis pedis artery (DPA). The portion of the DPA that passes to the plantar side of the foot is ligated. On the plantar surface, the flexor hallucis longus (FHL) is identified along with the plantar digital nerves and arteries on either side. The physician dissects into the web space between the great and second toes where the first plantar metatarsal artery (FPMA) is divided, as are vessels to the second toe. The DPN is split and the fibers to the great toe are divided. On the plantar surface, the digital nerves are divided. The FHL is divided through a separate incision in the midfoot, and is pulled into the distal wound. The tourniquet is released and adequate circulation is confirmed. The great toe is perfused for 20 minutes prior to completion of the dissection and transfer to the hand. The second surgical team begins preparing the hand soon after toe dissection begins. The physician on this team makes a radially-based palmar thumb skin flap.

The dorsal incision extends into the wrist area where the cephalic vein, superficial radial nerve, dorsal dominant branch of the radial artery, and extensor tendons are identified. A transverse incision is made over the volar wrist to allow identification of the flexor pollicis longus (FPL). The thumb metacarpal or phalanx is cut squarely at a right angle to two vertically placed interosseous compression wires and longitudinally placed K-wire, which helps hold the digit in extension. Extensor tendon and flexor tendon repairs are performed. The abductor and adductor tendons are repaired to the extensor mechanism. The vascular repairs are completed using standard microvascular techniques. The superficial radial nerve and DPN are joined dorsally, and the digital nerve repairs are completed volarly. The skin is closed with drains. If a skin graft is necessary, it is placed dorsally over the area of the dorsal veins. The donor site is closed by removal of the metatarsal condyles and suturing of the volar plate and sesamoids to the distal metatarsal.

26553-26554

The physician sometimes uses this procedure in cases of traumatic thumb amputation or congenital absence. Two surgical teams are used to complete the transfer. The first team makes a linear incision over the dorsal aspect of the foot, lateral to the dorsalis pedis artery (DPA), traveling from proximal to distal, aiming toward the second toe. Depending on the joint used, the physician may save skin for a graft. The physician harvests two veins in the foot, the dorsalis pedis and metatarsal arteries, the deep peroneal nerve branch, and the extensor tendon to the second toe, and performs an osteotomy at the joint needed. Digital nerves are harvested from the plantar surface. The second team prepares for the toe by making an incision over the wrists where the cephalic vein, superficial radial nerve, dorsal dominant branch of the radial artery, and the flexor pollicis longus (FPL). The thumb metacarpal or phalanx is cut squarely at a right angle to its long axis after appropriate measurement. If the toe is being transferred to a different finger position, the vein, superficial nerve, digital artery, and extensor tendon are all dissected. To attach the toes to the needed position, the physician affixes the bones by crossed Kirschner wires. The flexor muscles are attached to those of the toe. The digital nerves are repaired, and the palmar wounds are closed. The extensor tendons are attached, followed by the approximation of the dorsal sensory nerves, followed by vascular anastomoses. Incisions are closed using sutures. Report 26554 if more than one toe must be transferred because of finger/thumb deficit.

26555

The physician removes a digit, including the metacarpal bone, to improve hand function following trauma or disease. The physician incises the skin overlying the damaged bone. The bone, tendons, nerves, and muscles are removed. The remaining fingers are reapproximated and sutured to provide correct positioning. The skin is reapproximated and sutured in layers.

26556

The physician performs this procedure if finger joint function is absent, disturbed, or destroyed because of congenital malformation, trauma, or disease. The graft may be an autograft or allograft. Techniques include (1) toe proximal interphalangeal joint (PIPJ) transfer for finger metacarpophalangeal joint (MPJ) and PIPJ reconstruction; (2) metatarsophalangeal (MTPJ) transfer for MPJ or trapeziometacarpal (TMJ) reconstruction; (3) PIPJ or digital interphalangeal joint (DIPJ) "finger bank" transfer. If performing the toe PIPJ transfer for finger PIPJ reconstruction, the physician will engage two teams to prepare the donor and recipient sites simultaneously. One physician makes a longitudinal dorsal incision overlying the toe. The dorsalis pedis and first dorsal metatarsal arteries are dissected, as are dorsal veins. The tibial-side digital artery is divided distally at the level of the DIPJ. The fibular side artery is ligated. The extensor mechanism is cut proximally and distally and the joint is isolated by distal disarticulation through the DIPJ and proximal osteotomy through the first phalanx. The second team prepares the hand by excising the involved PIPJ and dissecting a suitable artery. The toe joint is transferred and stabilized with an intraosseous wire and longitudinal Kirschner wire. The extensor mechanism from the toe is attached to that of the finger. The artery from the toe is attached to that of the finger. At least two veins from the foot are sutured to veins of the hand. The foot wound is closed. The hand wound is also sutured closed. If performing the toe MTPJ transfer for MPJ reconstruction, the physician makes a curved incision to expose the finger joint. The ulnar side of the extensor hood is incised and retracted, and the joint is resected. The radial artery and the cephalic vein are identified through a separate incision. A small branch of the superficial radial nerve is dissected at the wrist level to be sutured to the nerve of the transplanted joint. The donor site is prepared by dissection of the great saphenous vein and first dorsal metatarsal artery. The terminal branch of the deep peroneal nerve is dissected. The toe graft is turned 180 degrees around its longitudinal axis, from dorsal to volar, and attached to the finger. The physician uses a Kirschner wire and anastomoses the vessels. The extensor mechanism is sutured and the skin is closed. The donor site is filled with the finger joint or by bone graft.

26560-26562

The physician repairs a syndactyly (web finger) using skin flaps and grafts. The physician incises the skin of the web for digital release and the underlying tissues are freed. In 26560, the repair is accomplished with skin flaps from the incision area. In 26561, the physician obtains grafts to provide skin coverage. In 26562, the syndactyly is complex and involves the phalangeal bones and fingernails. When possible, the bones are separated. Bone grafts are obtained when necessary for reconstruction. When reconstruction is complete, the skin is reapproximated and sutured in layers.

26565-26567
The physician performs an osteotomy to correct the metacarpal or phalanx. The physician incises the skin and dissects to the bone. The bone is incised and removed. The incision is sutured in layers. In 26565 a metacarpal is corrected, in 26567, a phalanx of the finger is corrected.

26568
The physician performs an osteoplasty to lengthen a metacarpal or phalanx. The patient is given brachial anesthesia and the physician incises the skin and dissects to the defective bone. The periosteum is incised and pulled away from the bone. The bone is cut and the proximal and distal ends are distanced. A wire may be inserted within the metacarpal for alignment. The periosteum is laid over the bone, and the incision is sutured in layers. The hand is splinted in anatomic position until bone callous is formed. Two K-wires inserted into the proximal and distal areas of the osteotomy site may be utilized when a distractor device is required. The distractor is connected to the wires, allowing for gradual lengthening (distraction) of the area. This distraction method generally begins on postop day five at a predetermined rate with radiological evaluation every week for the first three weeks, and every three weeks after until the optimal length is reached and cohesion of three cortices is achieved.

26580
The physician repairs a cleft hand. A cleft hand is a malformation where the division between the fingers extends into the metacarpus. The middle digits may be absent and remaining digits are abnormally large. The physician incises the overlying skin and dissects to the deformity. The tissues are brought together with sutures, and the tendons are approximated to produce tensor and extensor function. Following correction of the metacarpus, the skin is reapproximated, reduced, and sutured in layers.

26587
The physician reconstructs the hand by removing a polydactylous (extra) digit where the digit contains both soft tissue and bone. Excision of a digit containing soft tissue only is reported using 11200. The physician incises the skin at the base of the supernumerary digit. The bone is cut and the digit is resected. The skin is reapproximated, reduced, and sutured in layers.

26590
The physician corrects macrodactylia, which is an abnormal largeness of the fingers. The physician incises and retracts the skin to expose the underlying tissue. Reduction is accomplished by removing excess connective tissue and bone if necessary. The tissues are reanastomosed and secured with sutures. The incisions are sutured in layers.

26591
The physician repairs the intrinsic muscles of the hand to restore intrinsic function. The physician incises the overlying skin and dissects to the damaged muscle. The integrity of the tendons and muscles are tested. Defects are corrected to restore function. The incision is sutured in layers. When reporting this procedure, indicate which intrinsic muscle was repaired (interossei or lumbricales). Report each muscle separately.

26593
The physician releases the intrinsic muscles of the hand to restore intrinsic function. The physician incises the overlying skin and dissects to the contracted muscle. The intrinsic muscle is incised to release contracture. The incision is sutured in layers. When reporting this procedure, indicate which intrinsic muscle was released (interossei or lumbricals). Report each muscle separately.

26596
The physician excises a constricting ring of finger using multiple Z-plasties. The physician cuts the restricted skin in z shaped incisions. The Z flaps are reapproximated, increasing skin surface area without using grafts. The flaps are sutured closed.

26600-26605
The physician treats a metacarpal fracture with or without manipulation. The physician uses an x-ray to determine the location and severity of the fracture. In 26600, the fracture does not require realignment. In 26605, the proximal and distal ends of the fracture are not in correct anatomical position, and the physician reduces the fracture to correct alignment. The bones are splinted in anatomic position. Report each bone separately.

26607
The physician treats a metacarpal fracture with manipulation and external fixation. The physician uses a separately reportable x-ray to determine the location and severity of the fracture. The physician reduces the fracture to correct alignment of the proximal and distal ends of the bone. External fixation is placed to stabilize the fracture. The bones are splinted in anatomic position. Report each bone separately.

26608
The physician fixates a metacarpal fracture using a percutaneously placed wire. The physician uses an x-ray to determine the location and severity of the fracture. The physician reduces the fracture to correct alignment of the proximal and distal ends of the bone. The physician drills a wire through the metacarpophalangeal joint, through the fracture, and into the proximal bone. The drill entry point dressed and the hand is splinted.

26615
The physician performs open correction of a metacarpal fracture. Internal fixation may be used. The physician uses an x-ray to determine the location and severity of the fracture. The physician incises the overlying skin to expose the fracture. A wire or plate may be placed for internal fixation. The incision is sutured in layers and the hand is splinted.

Musculoskeletal

26641-26645
The physician manipulates a carpometacarpal dislocation or fracture dislocation of the thumb to restore anatomical position. The physician determines the dislocated position of the bone. The bone is relocated to correct anatomical position using external manipulation, and the hand is splinted. Report 26641 for dislocation without fracture, report 26645 for dislocation including fracture (Bennett fracture).

26650
The physician manipulates a carpometacarpal fracture dislocation of the thumb to restore anatomical position and secures the bone with a wire. The physician determines the dislocated position of the bone. The bone is relocated to correct anatomical position using external manipulation. The physician drills a wire through the metacarpophalangeal joint, through the fracture, and into the proximal bone. The drill entry point is dressed and the hand is splinted.

26665
The physician performs open reduction of a carpometacarpal fracture dislocation of the thumb. The physician uses an x-ray to determine the position and severity of the defect. The physician incises the overlying skin to expose the fracture and the bones are reapproximated. A wire or plate may be placed for internal fixation. The incision is sutured in layers and the hand is splinted.

26670-26675
The physician treats a carpometacarpal (other than the thumb) dislocation using manipulation; anesthesia may be used if necessary. The physician determines the dislocated position of the bone. The physician uses external manipulation to relocate the bone. In 26670, dislocation is minor and no anesthesia is needed. In 26675, dislocation is major and anesthesia is required.

26676
The physician manipulates a carpometacarpal dislocation (other than the thumb) to restore anatomical position and secures the bone with a wire. The physician determines the dislocated position of the bone. The bone is relocated to the correct anatomical position using external manipulation. The physician drills a wire through the carpometacarpal joint. The drill entry point is dressed and the hand is splinted.

26685-26686
The physician performs open reduction of a carpometacarpal dislocation on a joint other than the thumb. The physician uses a separately reportable x-ray to determine the position and severity of the defect. The physician incises the overlying skin to expose the dislocation. A wire or plates may be placed for internal fixation. The incision is sutured in layers and the hand is splinted. Report 26685 for each joint that is repaired simply. Report 26686 for complex or multiple dislocations, or when delayed treatment of the dislocation is performed.

26700-26705
The physician treats a metacarpophalangeal dislocation using manipulation; anesthesia may be used if necessary. The physician determines the dislocated position of the bone. The physician uses external manipulation to relocate the bone. In 26700, dislocation is minor and no anesthesia is needed. In 26705, dislocation is major and anesthesia is required.

26706
The physician manipulates a metacarpophalangeal dislocation to restore anatomical position and secures the bone with a wire. The physician determines the dislocated position of the bone. The bone is relocated to correct anatomical position using external manipulation. The physician drills a wire into the metacarpophalangeal joint, through the fracture, and into the proximal bone. The drill entry point dressed and the hand is splinted.

26715
The physician performs open reduction of a metacarpophalangeal fracture dislocation. The physician uses an x-ray to determine the position and severity of the defect. An incision is made on the overlying skin to expose the fracture and the bones are reapproximated. A wire or plate may be placed for internal fixation. The incision is sutured in layers and the hand is splinted.

26720-26725
The physician treats a phalangeal shaft fracture of the proximal or middle phalanx, finger, or thumb with or without manipulation. In 26720, no manipulation is necessary. In 26725, the physician manipulates the bones to restore anatomical position. The hand is splinted for stabilization.

26727
The physician treats a phalangeal shaft fracture of the proximal or middle phalanx, finger, or thumb with manipulation and secures it with a wire. The physician drills a wire into the tip of the finger bone, through the fracture, and into the proximal bone. The drill entry point dressed and the hand is splinted.

26735
The physician performs open correction of a phalangeal shaft fracture. The physician uses an x-ray to determine the position and severity of the defect. The physician incises the overlying skin to expose the fracture and the bones are reapproximated. A wire or plate may be placed for internal fixation. The incision is sutured in layers and the hand is splinted.

26740-26742
The physician treats an articular fracture involving a metacarpophalangeal or interphalangeal joint with or without manipulation. In 26740, no manipulation is necessary. In 26742, the physician manipulates the bones to restore anatomical position. The hand is splinted for stabilization.

26746
The physician performs open reduction of an articular fracture involving a metacarpophalangeal or interphalangeal joint. The physician uses an x-ray to determine the position and severity of the defect. An incision is made on the overlying skin to expose the fracture and the bones are reapproximated. A wire or plate may be placed for internal fixation. The incision is sutured in layers and the hand is splinted.

26750-26755
The physician treats distal phalangeal fracture of the finger or thumb with or without manipulation. In 26750, no manipulation is necessary. In 26755, the physician manipulates the bones to restore anatomical position. The hand is splinted for stabilization.

26756
The physician treats a distal phalangeal fracture of the finger or thumb with manipulation and secures it with a wire. The physician drills a wire into the tip of the finger bone, through the fracture, and into the proximal bone. The drill entry point dressed and the hand is splinted.

26765
The physician performs open reduction of a distal phalangeal fracture of the finger or thumb. The physician uses an x-ray to determine the position and severity of the defect. An incision is made on the overlying skin to expose the fracture and the bones are reapproximated. A wire or plate may be placed for internal fixation. The incision is sutured in layers and the hand is splinted.

26770-26775
The physician treats an interphalangeal joint dislocation using manipulation; anesthesia may be used if necessary. The physician determines the dislocated position of the bone and uses external manipulation to relocate the bone. In 26770, dislocation is minor and no anesthesia is needed. In 26775, dislocation is major and anesthesia is required.

26776
The physician manipulates an interphalangeal joint dislocation to restore anatomical position and secures the bone with a wire. The physician determines the dislocated position of the bone. The bone is relocated to correct anatomical position using external manipulation. The physician drills a wire through the interphalangeal joint for stabilization and the hand is splinted.

26785
The physician performs open correction of an interphalangeal joint dislocation. The physician uses an x-ray to determine the position and severity of the defect. An incision is made on the overlying skin to expose the dislocated joint and the bones are reapproximated. A wire may be placed for internal fixation. The incision is sutured in layers and the hand is splinted.

26820
The physician fuses the thumb in opposition. The physician incises the overlying skin and dissects to the metacarpophalangeal joint. A bone graft is obtained from the distal radius or iliac crest and placed to secure the joint. A wire is placed through the joint until fusion is complete. The incision is sutured in layers and the thumb is splinted for stabilization.

26841-26844
The physician fuses the carpometacarpal joint of a finger or the thumb. Internal or external fixation may be used. The physician incises the overlying skin and dissects to the carpometacarpal joint. The joint is fixated with a wire, screws, or plates. The incision is sutured in layers and the hand is splinted. If a graft is obtained, the physician harvests bone from the distal radius or iliac crest. The graft is interposed between the two bones to prevent movement and a wire is placed through the joint until fusion is complete. In 26841, the thumb is treated; report 26842 if an autograft is obtained and used. In 26843, a finger joint is treated; report 26844 if an autograft is obtained and used. The incision is sutured in layers and the hand is splinted.

26850-26852
The physician fuses a metacarpophalangeal joint. Internal or external fixation may be used. The physician incises the overlying skin and dissects to the metacarpophalangeal joint. The physician may use a wire to stabilize the joint until fusion is complete. Report 26852 if an autograft is obtained and used. Bone is harvested from the distal radius or iliac crest and interposed between the two bones to prevent movement. The incision is sutured in layers and the hand is splinted.

26860-26863
The physician fuses an interphalangeal joint. Internal or external fixation may be used. The physician incises the overlying skin and dissects to the interphalangeal joint. The physician may use a wire to stabilize the joint until fusion is complete. Report 26861 for each additional interphalangeal joint. Report 26862 if an autograft is obtained and used. A graft is harvested from the distal radius or iliac crest and interposed between the bones to prevent movement. Report 26863 for autografts on each additional interphalangeal joints. The incision is sutured in layers and the hand is splinted.

26910
The physician amputates a metacarpal bone including a finger or the thumb. An interosseous transfer may be performed. The physician incises the overlying skin and dissects to the defective metacarpal bone. The bone is freed of all muscular and vascular attachments and removed. Tissues that are no longer necessary for anatomical function are removed. Interossei muscles may be transferred to adjacent metacarpals to retain intrinsic muscle function. Soft tissue structures are returned to anatomic position; the skin is reapproximated, reduced and sutured in layers.

26951-26952
The physician amputates a finger or thumb, primary or secondary to injury. Neurectomies are performed. The overlying skin is incised and the tissues are dissected to the bone. The bone is removed. The vessels and nerves are ligated using microsurgical techniques. Primary amputation is removal of the digit following an acute injury or infection. Secondary amputation occurs when earlier attempts to preserve the digit have failed. In 26951, the wound is approximated, reduced, and sutured in layers. In 26952, local advancement flaps are necessary for closure.

26990-26991
The physician drains a deep abscess or hematoma in 26990 or an infected bursa in 26991 from the pelvis or hip joint area. The physician makes an incision overlying the site of the abscess, hematoma, or bursa. Dissection is carried through the deep subcutaneous tissues and may be continued into the fascia or muscle to expose the abscess or hematoma. The incision may be extended if the mass is larger than expected. When the infected bursa, abscess, or hematoma is identified, it is incised and the contents are drained. The area is irrigated and the incision is repaired in layers with sutures, staples, and/or Steri-strips; closed with drains in place; or simply left open to further facilitate drainage of infection.

26992
The physician incises the bone cortex of infected bone in the pelvis and/or hip joint to treat an abscess or osteomyelitis. The physician makes an incision over the affected area. Dissection is carried through the soft tissues to expose the bone. The periosteum is split and reflected from the bone overlying the infected area. A curette may be used to scrape away the abscess or infected portion to healthy bony tissue or drill holes may be made through the cortex into the medullary canal in a window outline around the infected or abscessed bone. The area is drained and debrided of infected bony and soft tissue. The physician irrigates the area with antibiotic solution, the periosteum is closed over the bone, and the soft tissues are sutured closed; or the wound is packed and left open, allowing the area to drain. Secondary closure is performed approximately three weeks later. Dressings are changed daily.

27000
The physician makes a small incision approximately 0.5 inches long over the origin of the adductor muscles. Dissection is carried to the adductor tendon. The physician uses a small blade to release (free by incision) the tendon. The incision is repaired in layers with sutures and Steri-strips. A spica cast is applied for three to four weeks to keep the hip in abduction.

27001-27003
The physician performs a tenotomy of the adductor of the hip. An incision is made starting at the pubis and extending approximately 5 cm along the inner thigh, in line with the V adductor longus muscle. The tendinous origins of the adductor muscles are identified and separated to allow lengthening. In 27003, the adductor muscles are separated from each other and the obturator nerve is located. The anterior and posterior branches of the nerve are removed. To perform a tenotomy, the tendinous origins of the adductor muscles are divided. The physician repairs the incision in layers. A cast may be applied for three to six weeks to hold the hip in abduction.

27005
The physician makes a 10 cm to 15 cm incision overlying the anterior iliofemoral area. The iliacus muscle and femoral nerve are identified and separated. The iliacus muscle and psoas tendon are separated. The psoas tendon is transferred superiorly and sutured to the anterior capsule of the hip joint. The iliacus muscle is also sutured to the capsule. The incision is repaired in layers.

27006
The patient is placed in a lateral position. A transverse incision is made starting just below the anterosuperior iliac spine and extending to just above the greater trochanter. The gluteus medius and minimus are tenotomized. To perform a tenotomy, the tendinous origins of the abductor muscles are separated. The incision is repaired in layers over a suction drain.

27025-27027
The physician performs a fasciotomy of any type in 27025, treating a swollen area of the hip or thigh. In 27027, the physician performs a unilateral decompression fasciotomy of the pelvic compartments (including gluteus medius-minimus, gluteus maximus, iliopsoas, and/or tensor fascia lata muscle) to treat compartment syndrome. Swelling applies pressure to the neurovascular tissues and muscles and may result in tissue death and loss of limb. One or more incisions are made over the affected area. The fascial planes are dissected out and separated to release pressure caused by swelling. The wounds are left open for approximately 72 hours and repaired in layers with sutures and/or staples.

27030
The physician performs an arthrotomy of the hip to drain infection. An incision is made over the hip. The soft tissues are dissected away, the joint capsule is exposed and incised, and the infection or abnormal fluid is drained. The wound is irrigated with antibiotic solution. The physician may pack the wound and leave it open with daily dressing changes to allow for further drainage and secondary healing by granulation tissue. If the incision is repaired, drain tubes may be inserted and the incision closed in layers with sutures, staples, and/or Steri-strips.

27033
The physician performs an arthrotomy of the hip that includes exploration or removal of any loose or foreign body. An incision is made over the hip, the soft tissues are dissected away, and the joint capsule is exposed and incised. The joint space is explored and any necrotic tissue is removed. If a loose or foreign body is

present (e.g., bone fragment, free cartilage, bullet, gravel), it is exposed and removed. The wound is irrigated with antibiotic solution. The physician may leave the wound open with daily dressing changes to allow for secondary healing or drainage. If the incision is repaired, drain tubes may be inserted and the incision closed in layers with sutures, staples, and/or Steri-strips.

27035
The physician makes an incision overlying a nerve of the hip joint. The physician uses a posterior approach to the sciatic or an anterior approach to its branches (the femoral or obturator nerves). The physician dissects the tissue to locate and isolate the nerve. The nerve is cut and the incision repaired in layers.

27036
The physician performs surgery on the hip joint capsule. An incision is made over the hip. Sharp and blunt dissection is utilized to continue deep through the fascia to the hip capsule. The capsule itself is incised. The physician removes all or part of the capsule. Excess bone in and around the capsule is identified, exposed, and removed. To accomplish this, the physician releases some or all of the hip flexor muscle. After the capsule and the excess bone have been removed, the muscles are repaired as warranted. The wound is closed in layers. A drain may be left in the hip joint.

27040-27041
The physician performs a biopsy to evaluate soft tissue. The area for biopsy is in the subcutaneous tissue between the muscle and skin layers in 27040. The suspect area is deeper and may be within muscle in 27041. An incision is made to expose the area. A tumor is typically surrounded by a capsule. The physician makes an incision through the capsule, removing a portion of the tumor for biopsy. The incision is repaired in layers using sutures, staples, and/or Steri-strips.

27047-27048 [27043, 27045]
The physician removes a tumor from the soft tissue of the pelvis and hip area that is located in the subcutaneous tissue in 27043 and 27047 and in the deep soft tissue, below the fascial plane, or within the muscle in 27045 and 27048. With the proper anesthesia administered, the physician makes an incision in the skin overlying the mass and dissects to the tumor. The extent of the tumor is identified and a dissection is undertaken all the way around the tumor. A portion of neighboring soft tissue may also be removed to ensure adequate removal of all tumor tissue. A drain may be inserted and the incision is repaired with layers of sutures, staples, or Steri-strips. Report 27047 for excision of a subcutaneous tumor whose resected area is less than 3 cm and 27043 for excision of a subcutaneous tumor 3 cm or greater. Report 27048 for excision of a subfascial or intramuscular tumor whose resected area is less than 5 cm and 27045 for excision of a subfascial or intramuscular tumor 5 cm or greater.

27049 [27059]
The physician removes a malignant soft tissue tumor (i.e., sarcoma) from the pelvis and hip area, not involving bone. An incision is made over the tumor and dissection exposes it. The tumor and any adjacent tissue that may be affected by the spread of the neoplasm are excised. Large resections may be needed. The type and stage of the lesion determine the extent of the tumor margin resection area. Muscle or fascia may need to be repaired and drains may be placed. The surgical wound is closed using simple or intermediate repair or separately reportable complex closure, adjacent tissue transfer, or graft. Report 27049 if the resection area is less than 5 cm. Report 27059 if the resection area is 5 cm or greater.

27050-27052
The physician performs an arthrotomy of the sacroiliac joint in 27050 and the hip joint in 27052 with a biopsy. An incision is made over the joint to be incised. The soft tissues are dissected away and the joint capsule is exposed and incised. A tissue sample is removed for biopsy and the wound is irrigated. The incision is closed in layers with sutures, staples, and/or Steri-strips.

27054
The physician makes an incision over the hip joint to be exposed and performs an arthrotomy to remove the synovium. The joint capsule is exposed by dissecting through the soft tissues and freeing and reflecting the muscles. The joint capsule is incised to expose the synovium, the inner membrane of the articular capsule that lines the joint cavity. The inflamed or enlarged synovium is dissected away from the capsule and the bones and removed. A drain tube may be placed and the incision is repaired in layers with sutures, staples, and/or Steri-strips.

27057
The physician performs a unilateral decompression fasciotomy of the pelvic compartments (including gluteus medius-minimus, gluteus maximus, iliopsoas, and/or tensor fascia lata muscle) to treat compartment syndrome. Swelling applies pressure to the neurovascular tissues and muscles and may result in tissue death and loss of limb. One or more incisions are made over the affected area. The fascial planes are dissected out and separated to release pressure caused by swelling, and nonviable muscle is debrided. The wounds are left open for approximately 72 hours and repaired in layers with sutures and/or staples.

27060-27062
The physician makes an incision overlying the ischial tuberosity at the base of the buttock. Dissection exposes the ischial bursa in 27060. For excision of a trochanteric bursa in 27062, an incision is made over the lateral aspect of the hip. The infected or calcified bursa is dissected out from the surrounding tissue and removed. The incision is repaired in layers using sutures, staples, and/or Steri-strips.

Musculoskeletal

27065-27067

The physician excises a superficial (27065) or subfascial (27066) bone cyst or benign tumor from the iliac wing, the symphysis pubis, or the greater trochanter of the femur. The physician makes an incision overlying the area, exposing the bone cyst or tumor. Further soft tissue dissection may be required. The lining of the bone (periosteum) may also be incised to further expose the cyst or tumor. The physician may make a few cuts above and below the area for removal or may remove it with a curette, depending on the position and location of the cyst or tumor. If the cyst or tumor was large enough to weaken the integrity of the bone, a bone autograft may be necessary and is included in these codes, when performed. Bone chips are harvested from the surrounding cancellous (spongy) bone and are packed into place where the cyst or tumor was removed. In 27067, a separate incision is required to harvest bone from the patient's iliac crest or other donor site. Both cortical and cancellous bone is acquired for bone grafting and the donor site is repaired. The bone graft is placed and the incision is repaired in layers using sutures, staples, and/or Steri-strips.

27070-27071

The physician performs a superficial (27070) or subfascial or intramuscular (27071) partial excision of the iliac wing, symphysis pubis, or greater trochanter of the femur, often to treat osteomyelitis or a bone abscess. An incision is made over the infected area and the underlying soft tissues are divided to expose it. The periosteum is reflected and the infected portion of bone is removed and irrigated. The excavation of bone may excise a crater-like piece or leave a small saucer-like shelf depression in the bone. If a significant portion of bone is removed, the physician may use bone graft material to fill the cavity left in the bone. The periosteum is closed over the bone, the soft tissues are sutured closed, and a soft dressing is applied.

27075

The physician performs a radical resection (excision) of a tumor. The patient is positioned for a lithotomy with the buttock elevated. For resection of a tumor of the pubis and/or ischium, an incision is made from the pubic tubercle to the ischial tuberosity. The adductor and obturator muscles are detached from the pubis and ischium. Additional dissection is carried down to better expose the pubis and ischium. The remaining muscles and ligaments are released (freed by incision) while the pudendal and genital nerves and vessels are protected. The bone(s) is separated and cut with bone-cutting forceps and an osteotome or saw. The bone segments are removed. A separate incision is made to resect the ilium. The portion of the ilium needing resection is dissected out by releasing muscles, tendons, and ligaments. The incisions are repaired in layers.

27076

The physician performs a radical resection (excision) of a tumor. The patient is placed in a lateral decubitus (lying on the side) position. The physician makes an incision from the posterior crest of the ilium to the symphysis pubis. A vertical extension of this incision is made, extending into the proximal thigh. The physician carries dissection down, while protecting the femoral artery, vein, and nerve. The physician uses a saw to divide (separate) the ilium and the pubic bone. Any remaining soft tissue is released (freed by incision) from the segment of bone to be removed. The inguinal ligament is reattached to the iliopsoas tendon to prevent a hernia. The incision is repaired in layers over a suction drain.

27077

The physician performs a radical resection (excision) of a tumor of the innominate bone in which the bone is removed in total. The patient is placed in a supine position with the involved side elevated. The physician makes an incision extending from the posterosuperior iliac spine, along the iliac crest, to the symphysis pubis. A vertical incision is made extending into the upper thigh. The abdominal muscles are detached. All muscles that attach to the innominate bone are divided and detached. Vessels and nerves are also separated and/or ligated. The hip joint capsule is incised. The sacroiliac joint is exposed and divided with an osteotome. The innominate bone is removed. The incision is repaired in layers.

27078

The physician performs a radical resection (excision) of a tumor of the ischial tuberosity and greater trochanter of the femur. The patient is positioned prone to access the ischial tuberosity and a lateral decubitus position to access the greater trochanter. The physician makes an incision overlying the involved bone and dissects through the deep layers. The ischial tuberosity or greater trochanter is exposed and resected. The wound is closed in layers with sutures.

27080

The physician makes a 15 cm vertical incision over the coccyx. The coccyx is freed from surrounding soft tissue and disarticulated from the sacrum (separated from the joint). The incision is repaired in layers using sutures, staples, and/or Steri-strips. If infection is present, the physician may pack the wound with gauze, allowing the wound to heal by granulation tissue from within.

27086-27087

The physician makes an incision overlying the site of the foreign body in the pelvis or hip. The foreign body is removed from the subcutaneous tissue in 27086. Deeper dissection is required in 27087 and more attention may be given to possibly damaged vessels and/or nerves. The physician irrigates the wound. The incision is repaired with sutures, staples, and/or Steri-strips.

27090

The patient is placed in a lateral decubitus position (lying on the side). The physician may access the prosthesis through the previous hip surgery incision.

The physician exposes and incises the hip joint capsule. The hip is manually dislocated. Any scar tissue is removed. The physician disimpacts the femoral prosthesis, removing cement as needed. The physician repairs the incision in layers with sutures.

27091

The patient is placed in a lateral decubitus position (lying on the side). The physician may access the prosthesis through the previous hip surgery incision. Any scar tissue is resected. The physician exposes and incises the hip joint capsule. The hip is manually dislocated. Methylmethacrylate (cement) is removed from the upper portion of the stem. The physician removes the stem with forceful blows. The physician removes any cement. The physician may make a bone window in the femoral cortex to remove additional cement. If there is bony ingrowth, flexible osteotomes may be used to remove the bone, allowing further stem retraction. The physician removes cement from the border of the implant with chisels and gouges. The physician removes the acetabular components with instruments. Any remaining loose cement is removed with a large curette or other instrument. A spacer of methylmethacrylate formed into a cube shape may be inserted into the space between the femur and tibia. The spacer prevents the soft tissues from compressing the joint space. The spacer is secured until another prosthesis is inserted. Drains may be placed. The wound may be left open for healing or the incision is repaired in layers.

27093-27095

The physician may apply skin traction to increase the space between the femoral head and acetabulum. Using a fluoroscope, the physician places a metallic marker over the femoral neck. The point is marked on the skin with ink. The femoral artery is palpated and marked on the skin as well, avoiding inadvertent puncture. The physician inserts a needle (1 1/2" for children, 3 1/2" for adults) and passes it into the capsule (located by fluoroscope). The synovial fluid is aspirated for a culture check. After aspiration, a contrast agent is injected into the hip joint and the needle is removed. X-rays are taken with the hip in neutral, external, and internal rotation for children and adults. The frog leg position is also taken for children. A second set of x-rays may be taken following the hip movements. The procedure is performed without anesthesia in 27093 and with anesthesia in 27095.

27096

The physician injects the sacroiliac joint, the articulation between the sacrum and the ilium in the pelvis. The physician draws contrast, an anesthetic, and/or steroid into a syringe. Through a posterior approach, a needle (syringe attached) is inserted into the sacroiliac joint. Arthrography, CT, or fluoroscopic guidance may be used to guide the needle placement. The physician pushes on the syringe to deliver its content into the joint. The needle is withdrawn.

27097

The hamstring tendon is a fibrous connective tissue extension that attaches the (hamstrings) muscles to bone. The hamstrings include the semitendinosus, semimembranosus, and biceps femoris; they flex and extend the thigh. The hamstrings origins are in the ischium or femur and the insertions are in the tibia and fibula. The physician makes an incision overlying the hamstring origin. Muscle and fascia is exposed. The physician makes multiple cuts in muscle fascia. The incision is repaired in layers.

27098

The patient is placed in the lithotomy position with the buttocks at the end of the operating table, and the legs in pelvic stirrups. The physician makes an incision starting just superior to the adductor longus tendon, and extending posteriorly in a straight line to the ischial tuberosity. The adductor longus tendon is severed from its origin on the pubic ramus. Next, the physician releases by incision the origins of the pubic adductor brevis, gracilis, and adductor magnus tendons. The physician grasps the freed ends of the tendons with a clamp, holding them along the side of the ischial tuberosity. The ends of the tendons are sutured to the tuberosity with nonabsorbable sutures. The incision is repaired in layers. A spica cast may also be applied for three weeks.

27100

The physician performs a muscle transfer, substituting the external oblique muscle for a paralyzed abductor of the hip. An incision is made starting at the pubic tubercle and extending along the crest of the ilium to its mid-point. Two incisions are made in the aponeurosis of the external oblique, freeing it from its medial and lateral origins. An aponeurosis connects a muscle with the parts it moves. The cut edges of the external oblique are folded under and sutured together to form a cone-shaped structure. The physician makes a 6 cm lateral incision over the greater trochanter. Two holes are drilled through the greater trochanter, 1 cm in diameter. A subcutaneous tunnel is made extending proximally across the ilium. The cone-shaped external oblique muscle is passed distally through the tunnel. While the hip is held in wide abduction, the end of the muscle (which serves as a tendon) is passed through the holes in the trochanter, and sutured firmly to itself. When desired, a strong tensor fascia latae tendon may be transferred posteriorly on the iliac crest as well. The incision is repaired in layers. A spica cast is applied for four weeks.

27105

The physician makes an incision overlying the paraspinal muscle. The muscle is detached from its insertion point. The muscle is transferred and reattached to the hip. The incision is repaired in layers with sutures.

27110

The physician performs a transfer of the iliopsoas for weakened or paralyzed gluteus minimus and medius muscles. An incision is made along the anterior

Musculoskeletal

two-thirds of the iliac crest and extending distally along the inner border of the sartorius muscle to the middle of the thigh. Dissection is carried down to the deep fascia. The iliac crest is exposed. If there is a hip flexion contracture, the physician may release both of these at the same time by incision. Next, the femoral nerve is identified and moved from the surgical area. The abdominal muscles are detached from the anterior two-thirds of the iliac crest. The lesser trochanter is identified and detached from the femur along with the insertion portion of the iliopsoas tendon. Using blunt and sharp dissection, the iliacus muscle is detached from the pelvis. The physician makes an oval hole through the iliac wing and passes the iliopsoas tendon and the iliacus muscle through the hole. The greater trochanter is exposed through dissection. Using an awl and burr, a hole is made through the greater trochanter, through which the iliopsoas tendon is passed. Several strong sutures are used to anchor the tendon securely to the greater trochanter. The iliacus muscle is sutured to the ilium, and the abdominal muscles to the iliac crest. The incision is repaired in layers. A spica cast is applied for three to four weeks, holding the hip in full abduction, extension, and neutral rotation.

27111

The physician makes an incision beginning lateral and posterior to the anterosuperior iliac spine. The incision extends anteriorly and distally, crossing the tensor fascia latae. The periosteum along the crest of the ilium is incised, reflecting the tensor fascia latae and gluteal muscles. The physician also reflects the attachment of the abdominal muscles until the iliacus is exposed. The anterosuperior iliac spine is resected along with the origin of the sartorius muscle. This muscle is reflected distally. The physician identifies the femoral nerve and vessels. The nerve and vessels are retracted to identify the apex of the lesser trochanter. The physician uses an osteotome to divide or separate the trochanter. The tensor fascia latae is divided halfway between its origin and insertion, so that a trough can be cut in the wing of the ilium. The physician will lay the iliopsoas in the trough. The iliopsoas is transferred laterally, determining its position on the femur. The thigh is held in full abduction during the transfer so that the iliopsoas has powerful tension. A small window is cut on the femur at this site, and the lesser trochanter is anchored to it. The vastus lateralis is sutured to the edge of the iliopsoas tendon and the iliacus muscle to the psoas. The tensor fascia latae is repaired and the anterosuperior spine is anchored back to the ilium. The incision is repaired in layers. A spica cast is applied with the hip in internal rotation, slight flexion, and full abduction for four weeks.

27120

Acetabuloplasty redirects the inclination of the acetabular roof by an osteotomy of the ilium. The Pemberton acetabuloplasty is described as follows: The patient is placed in a supine position. Using an anterior iliofemoral approach, the physician carries dissection down to expose the hip joint capsule and sciatic notch. The capsule is incised. Using a curved osteotome, a bone cut is made through the lateral cortex of the ilium. Another cut is made through the medial cortex of the ilium. After completing the osteotomy, a wide, curved osteotome is inserted into the front part of the osteotomy and used to lever the distal fragment distally, until the front edges are 2.5 cm to 3 cm apart. A wedge of bone is removed from the iliac crest and placed in the osteotomy made earlier in the ilium. The wedge is driven firmly into place. If necessary, the graft may be secured with pins. The hip is repositioned and the capsule is tightened with sutures. The incision is repaired in layers. A spica cast is applied from the nipple line to the toes on the affected side and to above the knee on the opposite side. The cast is worn for approximately three months.

27122

The physician incises the hip joint capsule to expose the femoral head, neck, and acetabular rim. These components are removed. The physician uses a curette to remove any remaining necrotic or infected bone. The physician drains any intrapelvic abscesses. Drains are inserted. The incision is repaired in layers with sutures, staples, and/or Steri-strips. The hip is immobilized in a cast or with traction.

27125

The physician makes a posterolateral incision over the hip with the patient in a lateral decubitus position. The fascia lata is incised and the muscles around the hip joint are retracted to visualize the capsule. The physician incises the capsule, exposing the femoral neck. The femoral neck is removed with a reciprocating saw. The excised femoral head is measured with a caliper to determine the appropriate size for replacement. The physician prepares the femoral by enlarging the canal with a rasp. The stem is secured into the femoral shaft. The stem is inserted and pounded into place with an impactor. The physician repositions the femoral stem prosthesis. Hip motion and stability are evaluated. The capsule is closed and the incision repaired in layers.

27130

The physician makes an incision along the posterior aspect of the hip with the patient in a lateral decubitus position. The short external rotator muscles are released by incision from their insertion on the femur, exposing the joint capsule. The physician incises the capsule. The hip is dislocated posteriorly. The physician removes the femoral head with a reciprocating saw. The physician removes any osteophytes around the rim of the acetabulum with an osteotome. The acetabulum is reamed out with a power reamer, exposing both subchondral and cancellous bone. The acetabular component is inserted. The femoral canal is prepared using a hand or power reamer. The physician prepares the femoral shaft by enlarging the canal with a rasp. The stem is secured into the femoral shaft. The stem is inserted and pounded into place with an impactor. The physician repositions the femoral stem prosthesis. The physician may augment the area with an autograft or allograft. The graft may be donor bone or harvested from the removed femoral head. The physician places the bone graft into the canal and/or acetabulum. The hip is repositioned. The external rotator muscles are reattached. The incision is repaired in layers with suction drains.

27132

The physician performs a conversion of a previous hip surgery to total hip replacement. Total hip replacement is replacement of both the femoral head and acetabulum. The physician may access the area through the previous hip surgery incision, extending it to allow adequate exposure of the hip joint. Muscles are reflected as well. The physician removes any hardware (internal fixation). The physician incises the capsule. The hip is dislocated. The physician removes the femoral head with a reciprocating saw. Next, the acetabulum is prepared. The physician removes any osteophytes around the rim of the acetabulum with an osteotome. The acetabulum is reamed out with a power reamer, exposing both subchondral and cancellous bone. The acetabular component is inserted. The femoral canal is prepared using a hand or power reamer. The excised femoral head is measured with a caliper to determine the appropriate size for replacement. The physician prepares the femoral shaft by enlarging the canal with a rasp. The physician selects the type of stem to be used. The stem is secured into the femoral shaft. The stem is inserted and pounded into place with an impactor. The physician reduces the femoral stem prosthesis. The physician may augment the area with an autograft or allograft. The graft may be harvested from the resected femoral head (autograft). Donor bone (allograft) may be used instead. The hip is reduced. Any reflected muscles are reattached. The incision is repaired in layers with suction drains.

27134

The physician revises a total hip arthroplasty. With the patient in a lateral decubitus position, the physician may access the hip through the previous hip surgery incision. Muscles are reflected. A trochanteric osteotomy may be performed with an oscillating saw. The physician incises the hip joint capsule. Any scar tissue is removed. The physician manually dislocates the hip. Cement is removed from the upper portion of the femoral stem with a motorized or hand instrument. The stem may be removed. If the stem has fractured, the physician may drill a hole in the femoral shaft so that an instrument may remove the broken portion. The physician removes scar tissue and cement from around the acetabular component with chisels and gouges. The acetabular component is removed from its bed. The physician reconstructs the acetabulum with cement or screws and bone graft. The new femoral stem is inserted into the femoral shaft. The physician may augment the area with an autograft or allograft. The physician reduces the hip and closes the capsule. The greater trochanter is wired into place. Suction drains may be placed in the wound. The incision is repaired in layers with sutures, staples, and/or Steri-strips.

27137

The physician revises a total hip arthroplasty. With the patient in a lateral decubitus position, the physician accesses the acetabular component through a previous hip surgery incision. Muscles are reflected. The physician may perform an osteotomy of the greater trochanter with an oscillating saw. The capsule is incised and the hip manually dislocated. Any scar tissue is removed from around the acetabulum. The physician removes cement from around the acetabular component with chisels and gouges. The acetabulum is levered out from its bed. The acetabulum may need to be reamed out in preparation for the new component. The physician reconstructs the acetabulum with or without cement. If the acetabulum is reconstructed without cement, the component is usually inserted and fixed with screws. Prior to the acetabulum placement, the physician may harvest a bone graft from the patient's iliac crest and close the surgically created graft donor site. Donor bone (allograft) may be used instead. If cement is used, it secures the new component in the acetabular bed. Once the cement has dried, the hip is reduced and the capsule closed. The physician may place suction drains in the wound. The incision is repaired in layers with sutures, staples, and/or Steri-strips.

27138

With the patient in a lateral decubitus position, the physician may access the femoral component through the previous hip surgery incision. Muscles are reflected. The physician may perform an osteotomy of the greater trochanter. The hip joint capsule is exposed and incised. The physician dislocates the hip joint. If cement was used on the previous arthroplasty, the physician uses a motorized or hand instrument to remove it from around the upper portion of the femoral stem. If loose enough, the stem is removed with forceful blows. If the stem cannot be removed, additional cement may need to be removed from the femoral shaft, so the stem can be extracted. The physician may place cement in the femoral shaft and insert the new femoral component. If the revision is cementless, donor bone (allograft) may be inserted as needed into the femoral shaft between the cortex and femoral component. The hip is reduced. The physician reattaches the greater trochanter with wires. The incision is repaired in layers with sutures, staples, and/or Steri-strips.

27140

The physician makes a longitudinal incision over the greater trochanter with the patient in a lateral decubitus position. The physician detaches the greater trochanter with a Gigli saw or osteotome. The physician may reposition the trochanter more lateral, or more distal and lateral. Repositioning increases the abductor lever arm and/or tightens the abductor musculature. The physician drills holes to secure the trochanter to the femur with wire. The incision is repaired in layers.

Musculoskeletal

27146

For a Salter innominate osteotomy, the patient is placed supine. The adductor muscles are released by a subcutaneous tenotomy. The physician makes a small incision approximately 0.5 inch long over the origin of the adductor muscles. Dissection is carried down to the adductor tendon. The physician uses a small blade to release (free by incision) the tendon. The physician makes an incision from the middle of the iliac crest to the inguinal area. The rectus femoris is released from its attachment by incision. The physician exposes and incises the joint capsule. If the ligamentous teres is hypertrophied, it is excised. If the femoral head remains unstable, an osteotomy of the innominate bone is performed. The hip is allowed to dislocate. The physician makes an osteotomy cut on the innominate bone using a Gigli saw. The osteotomy extends from the sciatic notch to the anteroinferior spine. The physician may harvest a separately reportable full thickness bone graft from the anterior part of the iliac crest and close the surgically created graft donor site. The graft is trimmed to the shape of the wedge and inserted into the osteotomy. A Kirschner wire is drilled through the ilium, bone graft, and into the lower fragment. Another wire is placed parallel to the first. Joint stability is reevaluated. Any released muscles are reattached. The capsule is closed with sutures, giving added stability to the reduction. The incision is repaired in layers. A single spica cast is applied.

27147

For a Salter innominate osteotomy, the patient is placed supine. The adductor muscles are released by a subcutaneous tenotomy. The physician makes a small incision approximately 0.5 inch long over the origin of the adductor muscles. Dissection is carried down to the adductor tendon. The physician uses a small blade to release the tendon. The physician makes an incision from the middle of the iliac crest to the inguinal area. The rectus femoris is released from its attachment by incision. The physician exposes and incises the joint capsule. If the ligamentous teres is hypertrophied, it is excised. The physician reduces the femoral head into the acetabulum. If the femoral head remains unstable, an osteotomy of the innominate bone is performed. The hip is allowed to dislocate. The physician makes an osteotomy cut on the innominate bone using a Gigli saw. The osteotomy extends from the sciatic notch to the anteroinferior spine. The physician may harvest a separately reportable full thickness bone graft from the anterior part of the iliac crest and close the surgically created graft donor site. The graft is trimmed to the shape of the wedge and inserted into the osteotomy. A Kirschner wire is drilled through the ilium, bone graft, and into the lower fragment. Another wire is placed parallel to the first. The femoral head is reduced again into the acetabulum. Any released muscles are reattached. The capsule is closed with sutures, giving added stability to the reduction. The incision is repaired in layers. A single spica cast is applied for eight to 10 weeks.

27151-27156

The patient is placed in a supine position. The physician makes an incision from the middle of the iliac crest to the inguinal area. The rectus femoris is released from its attachment by incision. The physician exposes and incises the joint capsule. If the ligamentous teres is hypertrophied, it is excised. The physician reduces the femoral head into the acetabulum. If the femoral head remains unstable, an osteotomy of the innominate bone is performed. The hip is allowed to dislocate. The physician makes an osteotomy cut on the innominate bone using a Gigli saw. The osteotomy extends from the sciatic notch to the anteroinferior spine. The physician harvests a separately reportable full thickness bone graft from the anterior part of the iliac crest and closes the surgically created graft donor site. The graft is trimmed to the shape of the wedge and inserted into the osteotomy. A Kirschner wire is drilled through the ilium, bone graft, and into the lower fragment. Another wire is placed parallel to the first. For femoral osteotomy, a lateral incision is made from the greater trochanter, extending down the leg 8 cm to 12 cm. Dissection exposes the lateral femur. Transverse and longitudinal orientation lines are made on the femoral cortex with an osteotome. The physician makes an osteotomy cut at the transverse line in a transverse or oblique direction. Another cut is made at an angle so that a wedge of bone can be removed to complete the correction. The rectus femoris is reattached to its insertion point. In 27156, the hip is reduced as well. A side plate is secured to the femur with bone screws. The incision is repaired in layers. A one and one-half spica cast is applied for eight to 12 weeks.

27158

The patient is placed in a supine position. The physician releases the adductor muscles by subcutaneous tenotomy. The physician makes a small incision over the origin of the adductor muscles. Dissection is carried down to the adductor tendon. The physician uses a small blade to release (free by incision) the tendon. The physician makes an incision from the middle of the iliac crest to the middle of the inguinal ligament. The head of the rectus femoris muscle is released. Dissection exposes the hip joint capsule, which is incised in a T-shaped fashion. The periosteum is stripped from the medial surface of the ilium to the sciatic notch. The ilium is divided or cut with a Gigli saw in a straight line from the sciatic notch to the anteroinferior spine. A full-thickness bone graft is removed from the iliac crest and trimmed to the shape of a wedge. The physician closes the surgically created graft donor site. This allows the acetabulum together with the pubis and ischium to be rotated as a unit. The bone graft is inserted into the osteotomy. Two Kirschner wires are drilled parallel to each other through the ilium and bone graft for fixation. The femoral head is reduced into the acetabulum. The capsule is repaired and tightened with sutures to add stability to the joint. The incision is repaired in layers. The same procedure is performed on the other side. Both hips are placed in spica casts.

27161
With the patient in a lateral position, the physician makes an incision extending from the anterosuperior iliac spine, over and to a point 10 cm below the greater trochanter. The fascia lata and gluteal muscles are divided or separated. Dissection exposes the hip joint. The physician incises the capsule. The physician makes two osteotomy cuts in the femoral neck. The size of the osteotomies is determined by separately reportable x-ray prior to surgery. A Steinmann pin may be drilled into the femoral neck before the osteotomy is completed to control the position of the proximal femur. The cut wedge of bone is removed. The physician inserts several 5 mm Steinmann pins through the femoral neck and across the osteotomy site and epiphyseal plate to prevent further slipping. The capsule is closed. The incision is repaired in layers.

27165
The physician exposes the lateral aspect of the proximal femur by making a lateral longitudinal incision. The femur is divided or separated with an osteotome at a level slightly above the lesser trochanter. The physician places the extremity in the corrected position. A rigid internal fixation device, such as a plate and screws, may stabilize the area. External fixation may be applied instead. The incision is repaired in layers with sutures, staples, and/or Steri-strips. A spica cast is applied for eight to 12 weeks.

27170
The physician harvests autologous bone for grafting, usually from the iliac crest. The physician makes an incision over the affected area of the femur (femoral head, neck, intertrochanteric or subtrochanteric area). The harvested bone chips are packed around the affected site of the femur. Occasionally, an allograft (donor bone) may be used. The incisions are repaired in layers with sutures, staples, and/or Steri-strips.

27175-27176
Separately reportable x-rays are taken to determine the position of the slipped femoral epiphysis. The physician may apply skin traction in 27175 with the limb in internal rotation for three to four days. Gradual improvement is accomplished without reduction. In 27176, the physician makes a small stab incision. Use of a fluoroscope determines the correct site for inserting pins through the lateral femoral cortex, femoral neck, and into the epiphysis to stabilize the slip. The small stab incision is closed with sutures. The patient is placed on crutches for four to six weeks.

27177
The physician makes an anterior iliofemoral incision with the patient in a supine position. Dissection exposes the capsule of the hip. The physician incises the capsule, retracting it to expose the femoral neck and epiphysis. A square window is made in the anterior surface of the femoral neck. Under separately reportable x-ray, the physician inserts a hollow mill through the window and drills across the epiphyseal plate and into the epiphysis. The tunnel is enlarged with a curette. The physician makes a separate incision over the ilium and removes sections of bone from the outer surface of the ilium. The bone sections are sandwiched together, placed in the tunnel, and driven across the epiphyseal plate into the epiphysis. If the physician uses single or multiple pinning rather than a bone graft, an incision is made overlying the greater trochanter and upper femur. The physician exposes the intertrochanteric area. Under separately reportable x-ray, the physician inserts a guide pin through the femur, femoral neck, and into the femoral head. One or two pins are inserted parallel to the guide pin. The guide pin is removed and the incision repaired in layers. The physician may place the limb in skin traction.

27178
The physician treats a slipped femoral epiphysis by manipulating the area. Following manipulation by the physician, the reduction is confirmed with separately reportable x-ray. The epiphysis is secured with Knowles pins or cannulated hip screws. An incision is made overlying the greater trochanter and upper femur. The physician exposes the intertrochanteric area. Under separately reportable x-ray, the physician inserts a guide pin through the femur, femoral neck, and into the femoral head. One or two 3/16 inch Knowles pins are inserted parallel to the guide pin. The guide pin is removed and the incision repaired in layers. The physician may place the limb in skin traction.

27179
With the patient in a supine position, the physician makes an anterior iliofemoral incision. Dissection exposes the capsule, which is incised and retracted. Retraction of the capsule exposes the femoral neck and the slipped epiphysis. To correct the deformity, the physician resects a wedge of bone from the anterosuperior aspect of the femoral neck with an osteotome. A single Knowles pin is drilled into the epiphysis. The physician uses the pin to rotate the epiphysis into its normal position and to hold it into place as well. The edges of the osteotomy are brought together. The physician makes a short, lateral skin incision just below the greater trochanter. Under separately reportable x-ray, the physician inserts three Knowles pins through the incision, the trochanter, and into the neck and epiphysis. The single Knowles pin is removed from the epiphysis and the incision repaired in layers. If fixation is secure, the limb may be placed in balanced suspension. Otherwise, a cast is applied from the nipple line to the toes on the affected side.

27181
With the patient in a supine position, the physician makes an anterior iliofemoral incision. Dissection is carried down to the hip joint capsule. The capsule is incised and retracted, exposing the femoral neck and epiphysis. A single Knowles pin is drilled into the epiphysis to control its position later. The physician resects a wedge of bone (osteotomy) from the anterosuperior part of the femoral neck. The physician fractures the posterior cortex of the femoral neck. The Knowles pin is used to rotate the epiphysis into its

Musculoskeletal

normal position in the acetabulum. The physician rotates the thigh internally to oppose the osteotomy surfaces. A short, lateral skin incision is made just below the greater trochanter. Under separately reportable x-ray, the physician inserts three Knowles pins through the incision, the trochanter, and into the femoral neck and epiphysis. The single Knowles pin is removed and the incision repaired in layers. Depending on how secure the fixation is, the physician may place the extremity in a balanced suspension or apply a cast from the nipple line to the toes on the affected side.

27185

Epiphyseal arrest is performed to arrest or stop growth of the greater trochanter growth plate. The patient is placed in a side-lying position. The physician makes a straight incision over the greater trochanter. Dissection exposes the area. The physician uses a curette to scrape out the growth plate. Screw(s) or staples are placed through the greater trochanter, across the growth plate, and into the femur. The incision is repaired in layers.

27187

The patient is placed supine or in a side-lying position, depending on the area for treatment. The physician may make tiny incisions to insert pins under roentgenographic control. The physician may need to perform an open procedure. In an open procedure an incision is made and dissection carried down to the femoral neck or proximal femur. The internal fixation (nailing, plating with screws, or cerclage with wires wrapped around the femur) is applied. The physician may use cement (methylmethacrylate) as needed to secure the fixation or strengthen the bone. The incision is repaired in layers.

27197

The physician treats a unilateral or bilateral posterior (toward the rear position-wise) pelvic ring fracture, dislocation, diastasis, or subluxation of the ilium, sacroiliac joint, and/or the sacrum. This code includes treatment of an anterior fracture or dislocations of the pubic symphysis and/or above or below the rami, when performed at the same time. The displacement or dislocation is less than 1 cm. No manipulation is required. Treatment typically is bed rest and crutches.

27198

The physician performs unilateral or bilateral manual manipulation to reduce a posterior (toward the rear position-wise) pelvic ring fracture, dislocation, diastasis, or subluxation of the ilium, sacroiliac joint, and/or the sacrum and includes treatment of an anterior fracture or dislocations of the pubic symphysis and/or above or below the rami, when performed at the same time. Vigorous manipulation may be necessary and requires a greater level of sedation (general, moderate conscious sedation, epidural) for pain control and for placement of skeletal traction through the distal femur or proximal tibia, when necessary. Separately reportable x-rays may be used to verify position of the reduced fracture, dislocation, diastasis, or subluxation.

27200

For closed treatment of a coccygeal fracture, the physician will prescribe bed rest to alleviate symptoms. Sitting on a rubber ring may also lessen symptoms. Closed manual manipulation may be performed as well.

27202

The patient is positioned prone. The physician makes a vertical incision in the gluteal fold. Dissection is carried down to the coccyx. The fractured portion is removed or internal fixation is applied. The incision is repaired in layers.

27215

The physician performs open treatment of iliac spine(s), tuberosity avulsion, or iliac wing fracture(s) by making an incision overlying the site of injury. Dissection exposes the avulsion and/or fracture. For an avulsion, a screw(s) is drilled through the bone fragment, reattaching the tendon and bone fragment to the original positions. The physician stabilizes an iliac wing fracture with a plate and screws across the fracture. The incision is repaired in layers. Suction drains may be applied. This code reports unilateral treatment for fracture patterns of the pelvic bone that do not disrupt the pelvic ring and includes internal fixation when performed.

27216

The physician performs unilateral percutaneous skeletal fixation of a posterior pelvic bone fracture (including ipsilateral ilium, sacroiliac joint, and/or sacrum) for fracture patterns that disrupt the pelvic ring. With the patient in a supine position, the physician inserts two to three pins through the skin and into the iliac crest. The pins are directed at specific angles. The physician attaches pin holders to each ring and curved ring segments to pin holders. The physician uses the rings to gently reduce (reposition) an unstable pelvic fracture or dislocation, if needed. Frame clamps are attached to the rings and tightened to secure fixation. The frame is left in place for approximately eight to 12 weeks.

27217

The physician performs unilateral open treatment of an anterior pelvic bone fracture or dislocation (includes the pubic symphysis and/or ipsilateral superior/inferior rami). With the patient in a supine position, the physician makes a curvilinear, transverse incision above the superior pubic ramus. Dissection exposes the pubic symphysis and/or rami. The separation (fracture and/or dislocation) may be reduced by the physician by applying manual ilium-to-ilium compression. For internal fixation, a plate is applied with screws directed into the bone. The incision is repaired in layers with suction drains. This code is reported for fracture patterns that disrupt the pelvic ring and includes internal fixation when performed.

27218

The physician performs unilateral open treatment of a posterior pelvic bone fracture or dislocation (includes ipsilateral ilium, sacroiliac joint, and/or sacrum). With the patient in a supine position, the physician makes an incision along the anterior iliac crest. The iliacus muscle is dissected and reflected medially with the abdominal contents to expose the injury. If needed, the physician manipulates the pelvis and leg to reduce (reposition) the fracture or dislocation. Compression plates and screws achieve internal fixation. In other approaches, reconstruction plates, transiliac rod fixators, or screws alone may be used for internal fixation of the ilium, sacroiliac joint, and/or sacrum. The incision is repaired in layers with suction drains. This code reports treatment for fracture patterns that disrupt the pelvic ring and include internal fixation when performed.

27220-27222

Closed treatment of an acetabulum fracture may be indicated when a fracture is non-displaced, bone is osteoporotic, or when only a minor portion of the acetabulum is involved. The patient may be placed in skin (Bucks) traction for eight to 12 weeks. The physician performs closed reduction (repositioning) with manipulation in 27222. General anesthesia is usually required. The physician may apply skeletal traction, placing a Kirschner wire or Steinmann pin through the tibia by the tibial tuberosity. Weight is attached to provide a traction force. While traction force is applied along the axis of the leg, a lateral traction force is applied to the proximal thigh. The physician manipulates the leg through abduction and internal rotation, and adduction. Typically, skeletal traction is continued for eight to 12 weeks.

27226

For a posterior wall fracture, the patient is placed in a lateral position. The incision extends from the greater trochanter to within 6 cm of the posterosuperior iliac spine. For an anterior wall fracture, the physician approaches the fracture through the ilioinguinal area. The patient is positioned supine. The physician makes an incision just above the symphysis pubis and extends it laterally to the iliac crest. For an anterior wall fracture, skeletal traction may be applied during the procedure. In both cases, extensive dissection of muscles and fascia is required to expose the fracture site. The joint is debrided of any free fragments. The fractured fragments are reduced. For a posterior wall fracture, internal fixation is achieved by using screws and a plate across the posterior wall to buttress the fragments. For an anterior wall fracture, internal fixation is usually achieved with the use of a two screw technique. The incision is repaired in layers using sutures, staples, and/or Steri-strips. Closed suction drainage is used.

27227

A transverse fracture involves both the anterior column and posterior column of the acetabulum. For transverse fractures, an approach as for a posterior wall fracture (see 27226) can often be used. If the fracture is more complex, different approaches may be used, providing exposure to both the anterior and posterior columns without making two separate incisions. Internal fixation is accomplished using screws and plate(s) techniques (see 27226). The incision is repaired in layers using sutures, staples, and/or Steri-strips. Closed suction drainage is used.

27228

The patient is placed supine. The physician makes an incision beginning at the upper portion of the symphysis pubis, extending upwards along the iliac crest, and ending at its most superior aspect. The origins of the abdominal muscles and iliacus are elevated from the iliac crest. Dissection is carried down through the inguinal canal, protecting vessels and nerves. The physician treats the anterior column fracture first by reducing the fragments and securing fixation with lag screws. The physician uses pointed reduction forceps to reduce (reposition) the fracture. The fracture is stabilized with a combination of lag screw and plate fixation. There may be an associated T-fracture which has a transverse pattern with a vertical split extending through the obturator ring. For a T-fracture, the physician makes a posterior incision with the patient in a prone (face down) position. At times, the two column fracture and T-fracture can be treated from a posterior approach. An anterior approach may be necessary, in which the patient is turned from prone to supine. All incisions are repaired in layers. Postoperative immobilization or traction is only necessary if satisfactory reduction and fixation are not achieved.

27230-27232

The physician treats a non-displaced, stable fracture of the femur. No manual manipulation is necessary in 27230. Manipulation is required in 27232 to treat a displaced fracture. The physician manually flexes the hip while applying manual traction force and internally rotating and abducting the hip. The patient may be placed in a supine position and Buck's (skin) traction applied. A splint may be applied to stabilize the fracture for three to six weeks. Skeletal traction may be necessary as well. A Steinmann pin or Kirschner wire is inserted through the tibia near the tibial tuberosity. A weight is attached. Traction may be continued for approximately six weeks.

27235

The physician performs percutaneous skeletal fixation of the proximal end of a femoral neck fracture. The physician makes a small stab incision (1 cm to 2 cm) overlying the lateral aspect of the thigh and just below the greater trochanter. A pin is drilled at approximately a 45 degree angle through the cortex and neck and into the femoral head. Two to five additional pins are inserted parallel to the first pin. Final x-rays are taken to confirm positions. The physician may close the stab incision made for each pin with a single suture.

Musculoskeletal

27236

The physician directly exposes the femoral fracture for treatment. The patient is placed in a supine position or slightly rolled up onto the other side. A 15 cm incision is made over the lateral hip. The fascia lata is split and the vastus lateralis muscle is detached from the femur. The physician exposes the femoral neck and head. A small periosteal elevator or Kirschner wire is used to reduce (reposition) the fracture. The physician places guide pins through the bone and across the fracture. The guide pins help determine correct screw length. The physician may use cannulated screws or compression hip screws and a plate to achieve internal fixation. In some cases due to the risk of subsequent non-union or avascular necrosis, the physician may replace the femoral head with a femoral prosthesis. The femoral canal is reamed out. A prosthesis of the proper size and length is selected and inserted into the femoral canal. The physician reduces the prosthesis into the acetabulum. The incision is repaired in layers with sutures, staples, and/or Steri-strips.

27238-27240

For a non-displaced, stable fracture in 27238, the physician applies a spica cast or brace. Manual manipulation is necessary to align fragments in 27240. The physician applies skeletal traction using a tibial pin. A Steinmann pin is inserted transversely across the upper tibia. With the thigh supported in slings, weight is applied to create the traction force. Traction remains in place for approximately 12 weeks, after which a spica cast may be applied. If skeletal traction is not necessary, a form of Russell's skin traction is placed on the lower leg. This type of traction is a foam boot with an attached weight providing the traction force.

27244

The physician makes an incision over the upper lateral thigh, exposing the fracture area through tissue dissection. The patient is in a lateral decubitus (lying on the side) position or may be placed in traction on a table. The fracture is reduced. Placement of an interfragmentary screw may achieve initial stability. A plate is inserted and screws stabilize the fragments. If additional fixation is needed, the physician may apply cerclage wiring, placing a wire around the fractured bones. The incision is repaired in layers with sutures, staples, and/or Steri-strips.

27245

The patient is placed in a supine position, or slightly rolled up onto the opposite side. The physician makes an incision over the posterolateral aspect of the hip. The fascia lata is divided or separated. The vastus lateralis muscle is detached from its origin site. The physician will place the intramedullary nail into the canal medial to the tip of the greater trochanter. Both the proximal and distal canals are reamed in preparation for placement of the intramedullary nail. The physician reduces the fracture with bone-holding forceps or cerclage wires (wires wrapped around the fragments), or both. The intramedullary nail, is placed through the proximal fragment, into the canal, and driven into the shaft of the femur. The physician inserts a nail or screw into the femoral head by drilling a tunnel from the lateral cortex, passing through a hole in the intramedullary nail, and into the femoral head. The triflange nail is driven through the tunnel, through the hole in the intramedullary nail and into the femoral head. The physician may elect to place cerclage wires for added stability. The vastus lateralis muscle is reattached and the fascia lata repaired as well. The incision is repaired in layers with sutures, staples, and/or Steri-strips.

27246-27248

In 27246, the physician treats a greater trochanteric fracture without manipulation. The fracture is not displaced and may be treated with skin traction while in wide abduction. Other treatments include a spica cast applied for six weeks or protected weight bearing with crutches for four to six weeks. In 27248, the fracture may be displaced and may require internal fixation. The physician makes a straight, lateral skin incision overlying the greater trochanter. Dissection is carried to visualize the fragment. The physician may apply bone screws, pegs, or wire loops to secure the fragment. The incision is repaired in layers with sutures, staples, and/or Steri-strips. Toe touch weight bearing with crutches is allowed for three to four weeks, followed by partial weight bearing for another three to four weeks.

27250-27252

The physician treats a traumatic hip dislocation without anesthesia in 27250 or with anesthesia in 27252. Two types of closed reduction techniques are used depending on the type of dislocation: the Stimson maneuver and the Allis maneuver. General or spinal anesthesia is applied. The Stimson maneuver is a procedure for posterior dislocations. The patient is positioned prone (face down) with the lower limbs hanging from the end of the table. Stabilizing pressure is placed on the sacrum. The physician holds the knee and ankle flexed to 90 degrees and applies gentle downward pressure to the leg, just below the knee. The Allis maneuver is a procedure for anterior dislocations. The patient is positioned supine. The pelvis is stabilized, and lateral traction force is applied to the inside of the thigh. The physician applies longitudinal traction in line with the axis of the femur, and gently abducts and internally rotates the femur to achieve reduction. Other techniques like those described above may also be used. After reduction, light skin traction may be applied.

27253

The physician performs open treatment of a traumatic hip dislocation. The physician makes an incision along the posterior aspect of the hip. The gluteus maximus muscle is split. The physician exposes the hip joint, allowing manual reduction of the dislocated hip. Reduction is accomplished without traumatizing the articular cartilage. The incision is repaired in layers with sutures, staples, and/or Steri-strips.

27254

The physician treats a traumatic hip dislocation. The physician makes an incision along the posterior aspect of the hip. The gluteus maximus muscle is split and the hip joint exposed. Fractures of the acetabulum and femoral head are visualized. If the fractures remain stable and the joint surface congruent when reduced, no internal fixation is required. If the fractures are not stable after reduction of the dislocation, internal fixation is applied. Cancellous bone screws or Kirschner wires may stabilize the fractures. The incision is repaired in layers with sutures, staples, and/or Steri-strips. The limb may be placed in skeletal or skin traction following the reduction. External fixation is applied if there is significant soft tissue trauma around the hip.

27256-27257

The physician treats a spontaneous hip dislocation. For an infant patient (age birth to six months) a Pavlik harness is applied. The harness is a dynamic flexion abduction orthosis. The harness consists of a chest strap, two shoulder straps, and two stirrups. The physician applies the harness with the child in a supine position. The harness holds the hip in 90 to 110 degrees of flexion, and moderate abduction. Skin traction may also be applied to infants of six to 18 months of age. A mechanical pulley is attached to the patient's leg with ace wraps securing the material to the skin. Weight is attached to the other end of the pulley to apply the traction force to the hip, allowing a gentle reduction of the hip dislocation. The hip is maintained in approximately 30 to 40 degrees of flexion. Traction time varies from two to six weeks. A splint or hip spica cast is applied to hold the hips in abduction. In an older patient, reduction may be possible by applying skin traction to the affected lower extremity. The procedure is performed without anesthesia in 27256 or with anesthesia in 27257.

27258

The physician performs open treatment of a spontaneous hip dislocation. The physician first performs an adductor tenotomy. The physician makes a small incision approximately 0.5 inch long over the origin of the adductor muscles. Dissection is carried down to the adductor tendon. The physician uses a small blade to release (free by incision) the tendon. The physician makes an incision from the middle of the iliac crest to a point midway between the anterosuperior iliac spine and the midline of the pelvis. Dissection exposes the capsule. The iliac epiphysis is detached from the ilium. The sartorius and rectus femoris tendons are divided or separated. The physician makes a T-shaped incision in the capsule. The entrance to the acetabulum is enlarged with sequential incisions in the labrum, which surrounds the acetabulum. This allows the femoral head to be reduced. Once the reduction is concentric and stable, the capsule is tightened and closed with sutures, stabilizing the hip joint. The rectus femoris and sartorius tendons are sutured to their origins. The iliac epiphysis is also reattached. The incision is repaired in layers. A double hip spica cast is applied with the hip in 90 degrees of flexion and 40 to 55 degrees of abduction.

27259

The physician performs open treatment of a spontaneous hip dislocation. The physician first performs an adductor tenotomy. The physician makes an incision from the middle of the iliac crest to a point midway between the anterosuperior iliac spine and the midline of the pelvis. Dissection exposes the capsule. The iliac epiphysis is detached from the ilium. The sartorius and rectus femoris tendons are separated. The physician makes a T-shaped incision in the capsule. The entrance to the acetabulum is enlarged with sequential incisions in the labrum, which surrounds the acetabulum. This allows the femoral head to be reduced. Once the reduction is concentric and stable, the capsule is tightened and closed with sutures, stabilizing the hip joint. The rectus femoris and sartorius tendons are sutured to their origins. The iliac epiphysis is also reattached. Femoral shaft shortening is performed as well. The physician makes both an anterior ilioinguinal and a straight lateral incision from the tip of the greater trochanter to the distal third of the femoral shaft. Open reduction is performed through the ilioinguinal incision. The femoral shaft is exposed through the lateral incision. A lag screw is inserted into the femoral neck. Once the bone cut is made at the appropriate distance below the first cut and angled to allow varus and derotation of the femur, the cut segment is removed. A side plate with screws secures the two segments. The incisions are repaired in layers. A spica cast is applied with the extremity in neutral rotation and slight flexion and abduction.

27265-27266

The physician treats a post hip arthroplasty dislocation with manual manipulation. Distal manipulative traction is applied to the leg, reducing the dislocation. No anesthesia is necessary in 27265. Regional or general anesthesia is required in 27266.

27267-27268

The physician treats a closed fracture of the femoral head. No incision is made and the surgeon does not expose the bone. No manual manipulation is necessary in 27267. In 27268, manipulation, or manual correction of the bone to its correct anatomical position, is required. General anesthesia may be necessary and Buck's (skin) or other forms of traction may be utilized.

27269

The physician directly exposes the femoral head fracture for treatment. After determining the position and severity of the defect by x-ray, the physician incises the overlying skin and muscle to expose the hip joint. Fractures of the femoral head are visualized. If the fractures remain stable and the joint surface congruent when reduced, no internal fixation is required. If the fractures are not stable after reduction of the dislocation, internal fixation is applied. The incision is repaired in layers with sutures, staples, and/

or Steri-strips. The limb may be placed in skeletal or skin traction.

27275
The patient is administered general anesthesia. If manipulation is performed to increase motion, the physician applies gradual pressure in the desired direction. The gradual pressure releases adhesions or scar tissue, increasing motion. Manipulation of the hip joint is a closed procedure, requiring no incision.

27278
The physician performs a sacroiliac (SI) joint fusion using a percutaneous approach and the placement of one or more intra-articular stabilization devices such as structural bone allografts or synthetic devices. This procedure does not transfix the SI joint; rather, it distracts the joint by placing a standalone allograft into the ligamentous portion of the joint. In one method, the patient is given appropriate anesthesia and placed in a prone position. Using imaging guidance, the physician identifies both the inferior and superior poles of the SI joint and places a guide pin at each location via a 2 cm incision. A joint finder is placed over each of the guide pins and tapped until slight separation of the joint is achieved. Through a working cannula, the physician inserts a drill and creates a hole in each section of the SI joint. The joint finder is inserted again and advanced to the appropriate depth by tapping. Once a cavity is created, demineralized bone matrix (DBM) is placed into each of the openings; this allows for growth of bony union and provides mechanical stabilization of the joint. This is followed by insertion of the bone allograft, which provides immediate joint stabilization.
Instrumentation is removed, hemostasis is achieved, and the small incisions are closed in standard fashion. Placement of the intra-articular implants are included in this code.

27279
A unilateral sacroiliac (SI) joint fusion using a percutaneous or minimally invasive method is performed, in which one or more internal fixation devices are passed through the ilium, across the SI joint, and into the sacrum, thereby transfixing the SI joint. The procedure is performed under general anesthesia with the patient in the prone position. The buttock and pelvis are prepped and draped. A small incision is made through the gluteal fascia and muscle to reach the ilium. In one method, a pin is placed from the ilium through the sacroiliac joint to the lateral portion of the sacrum under fluoroscopic or CT guidance. A soft tissue protector is inserted over the pin, and a drill is used to create a pathway and to decorticate bone through the ilium to the sacrum. A depth gauge is used to determine implant length. One or more transfixation implants may be inserted; these are typically metal devices that are threaded or impacted into place. The incision is irrigated and closed in layers. Placement of the transfixation device and bone grafting (if performed) are included in this service.

27280
The physician performs a unilateral open arthrodesis of the sacroiliac joint, including obtaining a bone graft. The physician makes an open incision along the posterior two-thirds of the iliac crest, continuing the curve around the posterosuperior spine. The soft tissues are reflected to expose the ilium. A rectangular bone window is cut and removed from the ilium. The physician removes cartilage from the sacral surface of the joint, as well as from the joint surface of the block of bone. The physician replaces the block of bone and countersinks it so that its cancellous surface contacts the cancellous bone of the sacrum. The edges of the bone window are osteotomized and the fragments turned inward to secure the block and promote bone formation. The incision is repaired in layers using sutures. The physician may place the patient in a trunk and pelvic cast or brace. Instrumentation is included in this service, when performed.

27282
The physician makes an incision overlying the symphysis pubis. Dissection is carried down to the joint. Soft tissue between bone is excised. The physician may harvest a bone graft from the patient through a separate incision or from surrounding bone. The physician closes the surgically created graft donor site. Internal fixation is applied to the fusion with screws and/or plates. The incision is repaired in layers.

27284
To perform an intra-articular arthrodesis, the physician makes an anterior iliofemoral incision. The sartorius and rectus femoris muscles are detached from their origins. The iliopsoas is reflected from the front of the hip joint. The physician dislocates the hip anteriorly. Cartilage is removed from the femoral head and acetabulum down to bleeding cancellous bone. The physician packs the space between the surfaces of the femoral head and acetabulum with cancellous autogenous bone grafts. An example of the position in which the hip may be fused is: 30 degrees of flexion, 0 to 5 degrees of adduction, and 10 degrees of external rotation. The physician may use compression screws to increase the stability of the fusion. The sartorius and rectus femoris muscles are reattached. The screws are placed through the femoral head and into the supra-acetabular area of the ilium. The incision is repaired in layers with suction drains. The limb may be placed in a single spica cast or in balanced suspension.

27286
To perform an intra-articular arthrodesis, the physician makes an anterior iliofemoral incision. The sartorius and rectus femoris muscles are detached from their origins. The iliopsoas is reflected from the front of the hip joint. The physician dislocates the hip anteriorly. Cartilage is removed from the femoral head and acetabulum down to bleeding cancellous bone. The physician packs the space between the surfaces of the femoral head and acetabulum with cancellous autogenous bone grafts. The physician harvests a bone graft from the patient's iliac wing and crest and closes

Musculoskeletal

the surgically created graft donor site. The graft is positioned so it spans the anterior aspect of the hip from the pubic ramus to the femoral neck. The graft is secured with cancellous lag screws. The arthrodesis is performed so that the hip is in 10 degrees of external rotation, 0 to 5 degrees of adduction, and 30 degrees of flexion. A subtrochanteric osteotomy (bone cut) is made just below the lesser trochanter. The sartorius and rectus femoris muscles are reattached and the iliopsoas muscle is repositioned. The incision is repaired in layers with suction drains. A one and one-half spica cast is applied.

27290

The patient is placed in a lateral (on the side) position with the operative side up. There are three parts to this procedure including, anterior, perineal, and posterior. Each part requires a separate incision for exposure, dissection, and development of skin flaps. The physician separates the nerves and ligates the vessels. Vessels are ligated anteriorly and posteriorly; the sciatic nerve is cut high and tied. The pelvic ring, extending from the symphysis pubis to the attachment of the ilium to the sacrum, is sectioned and removed. Some muscle is retained, such as the gluteus maximus part of the skin flaps. The flaps are closed with interrupted sutures over drains. The drains are removed in 48 to 72 hours.

27295

The physician makes an anterior racquet-shaped incision beginning at the anterosuperior iliac spine and curving distally and medially. The incision extends to a point on the medial aspect of the thigh, 5 cm below the origin of the adductor muscles. The femoral artery and vein are ligated. The femoral nerve is divided. The physician continues the incision around the posterior aspect of the thigh to 5 cm below the ischial tuberosity and laterally to the base of the greater trochanter. All muscles around the hip are detached. The physician detaches the gluteal muscles, reflecting the muscle mass proximally for later use as a flap. The sciatic nerve is ligated and separated. The physician incises the hip joint capsule and ligamentum teres to complete the disarticulation. The gluteal flap is brought around the wound and sutured. The physician places a drain in the inferior part of the incision. The edges of skin are closed with nonabsorbable sutures.

27301

The physician drains an abscess, a hematoma, or a bursa from deep within the thigh or knee region. The physician makes an incision in the thigh or knee overlying the site of the abscess, hematoma, or bursa to be incised. Dissection is carried through the deep subcutaneous tissues and may be continued into the fascia or muscle to expose the abscess, hematoma, or bursa. The incision may be extended if the mass is larger than expected. When the bursa, abscess, or hematoma is identified, it is incised and the contents are drained. The area is irrigated and the incision is repaired in layers with sutures, staples, and/or Steri-strips; closed with drains in place; or simply left open to further facilitate drainage of infection.

27303

The physician incises the bone cortex of infected bone in the femur or knee to treat an abscess or osteomyelitis. The physician makes an incision over the affected area. Dissection is carried through the soft tissues to expose the bone. The periosteum is split and reflected from the bone overlying the infected area. A curette may be used to scrape away the abscess or infected portion down to healthy bony tissue or drill holes may be made through the cortex into the medullary canal in a window outline around the infected or abscessed bone. The area is drained and debrided of infected bony and soft tissue. The physician irrigates the area with antibiotic solution, the periosteum is closed over the bone, and the soft tissues are sutured closed; or the wound is packed and left open, allowing the area to drain. Secondary closure is performed approximately three weeks later. Dressings are changed daily. A splint may be applied to limit knee movement.

27305

For release of the iliotibial band, the patient is placed in a lateral decubitus position. The physician exposes the iliotibial tract through a 4 cm lateral, longitudinal incision just above the femoral condyle. The physician incises the iliotibial tract, fascia lata, and intramuscular septum transversely 2.5 cm above the patella. In severe contractures, the physician may remove a segment of the iliotibial tract and septum. The incision is closed in layers with sutures, staples, and/or Steri-strips.

27306-27307

The physician performs a percutaneous tenotomy (cut) of the adductor or hamstring muscle. The physician palpates the tendon to be released. A small incision is made to access the tendon. The physician's thumb presses on the tendon to create tension. The physician uses an 11-blade to make a cut through the tendon, releasing it. More than one tendon is released in 27307. The incision is closed with sutures.

27310

The physician performs an arthrotomy on the knee that includes exploration, drainage, or removal of any foreign body. An incision is made over the knee. The soft tissues are dissected away and the joint capsule is exposed and incised. The patella may be moved laterally for better exposure. The compartments are explored, any necrotic tissue is removed, and infection or abnormal fluid is drained. If a foreign body is present (e.g., bullet, nail, gravel), it is exposed and removed. The wound is irrigated with antibiotic solution. The physician may leave the wound packed open temporarily to allow for drainage in the case of any purulent exudate. If the incision is repaired, drain tubes may be inserted and the incision is closed in layers with sutures, staples, and/or Steri-strips.

27323-27324

The physician performs a biopsy of the soft tissues of the thigh or knee area. With proper anesthesia administered, an incision is made over the biopsy area. Dissection is carried down within the superficial soft

Musculoskeletal

tissue layers in 27323, usually the subcutaneous fat to the uppermost fascial layer. In 27324, dissection is taken deep within the soft tissue, such as into the fascial layer or within the muscle. A portion of the tissue is excised and submitted for pathology. The area is irrigated and the incision is closed with layered sutures, staples, or Steri-strips.

27325
The physician performs an incisional resection of a segment of a nerve. The physician makes a transverse incision over the hamstring muscle. The fascia is divided to expose the nerves that supply the muscle. The appropriate nerve branch is identified by stimulating it with an electrical current or gently pressing it with forceps. Once this is accomplished, the nerve is divided and removed from the muscle, resolving the clonus or spasm. The incision is repaired in layers.

27326
The physician performs an incisional resection of a segment of a nerve. The physician makes a transverse incision over the distal portion of the popliteal (back of the knee) fossa. The fascia is divided to expose the tibial nerve. The appropriate nerve branch is identified by stimulating it with an electrical current or gently pressing it with forceps. Once this is accomplished, the nerve is divided and removed from the muscle, resolving the clonus or spasm. The incision is repaired in layers.

27327-27328 [27337, 27339]
The physician removes a tumor from the soft tissue of the thigh or knee area that is located in the subcutaneous tissue in 27327 and 27337 and in the deep soft tissue, below the fascial plane, or within the muscle in 27328 and 27339. With the proper anesthesia administered, the physician makes an incision in the skin overlying the mass and dissects to the tumor. The extent of the tumor is identified and a dissection is undertaken all the way around the tumor. A portion of neighboring soft tissue may also be removed to ensure adequate removal of all tumor tissue. A drain may be inserted and the incision is repaired with layers of sutures, staples, or Steri-strips. Report 27327 for excision of a subcutaneous tumor whose resected area is less than 3 cm, and 27337 for excision of a subcutaneous tumor that is 3 cm or greater. Report 27328 for excision of a subfascial or intramuscular tumor whose resected area is less than 5 cm, and 27339 for excision of a subfascial or intramuscular tumor that is 5 cm or greater.

27330-27331
The physician usually makes an anteromedial incision to gain adequate exposure of the knee joint. The patella is shifted to the side to examine the area. Each compartment of the knee joint is visually examined. The physician may need to make an additional incision to further explore other areas of the knee joint. If there is suspicion that synovium may be diseased, a tissue biopsy is taken. Any loose bodies or foreign bodies are removed in 27331. Incisions are closed with sutures, staples, and/or Steri-strips. A temporary drain may be placed.

27332-27333
The physician makes an incision along the anteromedial or anterolateral aspect of the knee, depending on which cartilage is torn (medial or lateral in 27332 or both in 27333). Dissection is carried down to the cartilage. The patella is shifted aside and the knee joint exposed. The torn cartilage is removed and the roughened edges are smoothed. A partial synovectomy and release or excision (partial or total) of plica may be performed. Plica is a fold, pleat, band, or shelf of synovial tissue (e.g., transverse suprapatellar, medial suprapatellar, mediopatellar and infrapatellar). The chondral surface of the patella may be debrided as well. A temporary drain may be applied. The incision is repaired in layers with sutures, staples, and/or Steri-strips.

27334-27335
The physician makes an anteromedial incision for anterior synovectomy. Once the knee joint is accessed, proliferative, diseased synovium is removed. If posterior synovectomy is required, the physician will position the patient prone and make an "s" shaped incision along the popliteal (back of the knee) area. Both anterior and posterior synovectomy is performed in 27335. Dissection exposes the knee joint. Diseased synovium is removed. Incisions are closed with sutures, staples, and/or Steri-strips. A temporary drain may be applied.

27340
The physician makes a small incision over the upper portion of the patella. The bursal sac is located in fat in front of the patella. Dissection is carried down to the area of infection or inflammation. The bursa is removed. The incision is repaired in layers with sutures and Steri-strips.

27345
A Bakers cyst is located in the popliteal space (back of the knee). The physician makes a popliteal incision, carrying dissection to expose the semimembranosus tendon. The cyst is typically located around this tendon. The cyst is excised from the tendon. The incision is repaired in layers with sutures.

27347
The physician excises a lesion of the meniscus or capsule of the knee. Types of lesions treated include a cyst or ganglion (fluid-filled sac). Lesions may be located in the meniscus—the cartilage between the knee joint—(following an injury), or on the capsule, the fibrous covering over the joint space. Through an incision over the knee the physician dissects the tissues to the level of the cyst or ganglion. The lesion is excised, and the wound is closed with layered sutures.

27350
Patellectomy is removal of the patella. A hemipatellectomy or partial patellectomy is removal of cartilage from the patella or removal of a portion of the bone. A transverse "u" shaped incision is made over the

anterior aspect of the knee joint just below the patella. The patella is excised from the tissue surrounding it (capsule, quadriceps, and patellar tendons). The physician takes the upper part of the capsule and quadriceps tendon medially and distally so that they overlap the lower part of the capsule. The physician sutures the capsule and tendon in place. Incisions are repaired with sutures, staples, and/or Steri-strips.

27355-27358

A bone cyst or benign tumor of the femur is removed. The physician makes an incision in the thigh overlying the cyst or tumor. The skin and underlying soft tissues are reflected to expose the periosteum, which is separated from the bone. Curettes or osteotomes are used to scrape or cut the lesion from the bone. Once the benign tumor or cyst is removed and healthy bone tissue is present, the periosteum is repositioned and the incision is repaired in layers. If the bone defect created requires a graft for repair, the physician obtains the necessary size bone graft from a separate donor site on the patient and packs it into the site where the tumor or bone cyst was removed or uses a bone bank allograft. Report 27356 if an allograft is used and 27357 if an autograft is obtained. Report 27358 as an additional code if internal fixation is applied for more stability, such as bone screws, compression plates, or an intramedullary nail.

27360

The physician performs a partial excision of the femur, proximal tibia, and/or fibula to remove infected bone. An incision is made over the infected part of the bone and the underlying soft tissues are divided to expose it. The periosteum is reflected and the infected portion of bone is removed and irrigated. The excavation of bone may excise a crater-like piece, leave a small saucer-like shelf depression in the bone, or may remove a portion of the shaft (diaphysis) of a long bone. If a significant portion of bone is removed, the physician may use bone graft material to fill the cavity left in the bone. The periosteum is closed over the bone, the soft tissues are sutured closed, and a soft dressing is applied.

27364 [27329]

The physician performs a radical resection (excision) of a malignant soft tissue tumor (i.e., sarcoma) from the thigh or knee area, not involving bone. An incision is made over the tumor and dissection exposes it. The tumor and any adjacent tissue that may be affected by the spread of the neoplasm are excised. Large resections may be needed. The type and stage of the lesion determines the extent of the tumor margin resection area. Muscle or fascia may need to be repaired and drains may be placed. The surgical wound is closed using simple or intermediate repair or separately reportable complex closure, adjacent tissue transfer, or graft. Report 27329 for a resection area of less than 5 cm and 27364 for a resection area 5 cm or greater.

27365

The physician makes an incision overlying a tumor of the femur or knee. Adequate exposure is accomplished. Resection is performed including adjacent periosteum and muscle, a cuff of normal bone both proximal and distal to the lesion, and skin and soft tissues as necessary. For a malignant neoplasm of the femur or knee, additional bone and/or soft tissue may need to be removed, thus compromising the stability or integrity of the femur or knee joint. Separately reportable procedures, such as reconstruction of ligaments and/or tendons, reattachment of muscles, placement of donor bone graft, and use of an external fixator may be necessary as well. The incision is repaired in layers.

27369

The physician injects contrast for knee arthrography or contrast enhanced CT/MRI knee arthrography. Arthrography is radiological imaging for evaluation of joints. Typical arthrography involves the use of fluoroscopy as well as contrast containing iodine. In arthrography, utilizing magnetic resonance imaging (MRI), a different type of contrast material containing gadolinium, a material that affects the local magnetic field of the MRI, is injected into the joint outlining the structures within the joint. For CT arthrography, the contrast material is the same as that used for standard arthrography. The patient is placed supine (lying on the back) on an x-ray table with the knee flexed over a small pillow. A skin anesthetic may be applied. The physician passes a 20-gauge needle into the femoropatellar space. Air and/or a single or double contrast agent are injected into the space in preparation for the procedure. After the injection is complete, the patient is asked to move the knee to ensure adequate distribution of the contrast material in the joint structures. Multiple roentgenographic views are taken of the knee.

27372

The physician removes a foreign body (i.e., nail, piece of wood) in the thigh or knee. For a foreign body in the thigh, an incision is made overlying the object. Tissue is dissected around the object. The physician may need to suture damaged muscle or other soft tissues. The wound is irrigated with antibiotic solution. The incision will typically be closed, unless an infection is present, in which case it will be left open temporarily to drain.

27380-27381

An incision is made from the upper portion of the patella and extending to a point just medial to the lower part of the tibial tuberosity. The patellar tendon is exposed, and all scar tissue removed. The ruptured ends of the tendon are debrided. Sutures are passed through the ruptured ends to bring them together. A fascia lata graft may be used for reinforcement of the suture line by being incorporated in both ends of the ruptures in a figure "8" fashion. Another technique for reinforcement is to sever the semitendinosus tendon, and make transverse drill holes through the distal third of the patella and transversely through the tibial tuberosity. The semitendinosus tendon is looped through the drill holes and sewn back onto itself at the tibial tubercle. In 27381, the repair is augmented with tissues (tendon or fascia) from surrounding areas or

Musculoskeletal

allograft tissue. The incision is closed with sutures and staples or Steri-strips.

27385-27386
The physician makes an incision over the site of injury. Dissection is carried down to the ruptured muscle. The torn ends are debrided so that healthy muscle tissue can be accurately opposed. Nonabsorbable sutures are placed close together around the circumference of the muscle. In 27386, the repair may be reinforced by using strips of fascia lata tissue. The physician makes an incision over the fascia lata in order to obtain the needed tissue. The fascia lata strips are interwoven with sutures around the ruptured muscle. Incisions are repaired with sutures and staples or Steri-strips.

27390-27392
The patient is positioned prone (lying face down). The physician makes a 7 to 10 cm, longitudinal incision beginning just above the popliteal crease and extending upward. Dissection exposes the hamstring tendons. The tendon sheath is divided and the tendon is incised transversely at two levels, 3 cm apart. The physician flexes the hip while the knee remains extended, causing the tendon to lengthen. The tendon sheath is closed. In 27391, two or three tendons are lengthened on the same leg. In 27392, the same technique is performed on both legs. The incision is repaired in layers.

27393-27395
The patient is positioned prone (lying face down). The physician makes a 7 to 10 cm, longitudinal incision beginning just above the popliteal crease and extending upward. Dissection exposes the hamstring tendons. The tendon sheath is divided and the tendon is incised transversely at two levels, 3 cm apart. The physician flexes the hip while the knee remains extended, causing the tendon to lengthen. The tendon sheath is closed. In 27394, two or three tendons are lengthened on the same leg. In 27395, the same technique is performed on both legs. The incision is repaired in layers.

27396-27397
The physician performs a transplant or transfer of a single thigh tendon in 27396 and performs multiple transplants or transfers in 27397, using redirection or rerouting of muscle. The incisions are closed in layers.

27400
The physician makes a curvilinear incision over the biceps femoris tendon, extending just above the fibular head. The peroneal nerve is retracted so that the biceps tendon is exposed. This tendon is divided and repositioned on the lateral femoral condyle where it is anchored firmly. A similar incision is made on the medial side of the knee to expose the semimembranosus, semitendinosus, and gracilis tendons. The tendons are each divided and anchored firmly to the medial femoral condyle. The incisions are repaired in layers.

27403
With the knee in 60 degrees of flexion, the physician makes a vertical incision on the medial or lateral joint line area, depending on which meniscus needs repair. The meniscus is exposed and the edges of the tear are debrided with a small curette or scalpel. A rasp abrades the debrided edges of the tear, creating an increased inflammatory healing response. Sutures are placed through the tear in the meniscus every 3 mm to 4 mm. The incision is repaired with sutures and Steri-strips.

27405-27409
For a primary collateral repair (27405), the physician makes an incision on the lateral or medial aspect of the knee, depending on which ligament is torn (medial collateral or lateral collateral). Sutures may be used to tie the torn ends together. If the attachment of the ligament to the bone is torn away, a screw may be used for fixation. For a cruciate ligament primary repair (27407), an incision is made to gain access into the knee joint (the physician may use the arthroscope for part of the procedure). Screws and/or sutures are used to reattach the torn end to the bone. Both collateral and cruciate ligaments are repaired in 27409. Incisions are closed with sutures, staples, and/or Steri-strips. A temporary drain may be applied.

27412
Autologous chondrocyte implantation is performed to treat knee defects caused by damage to the hyaline cartilage. Some of the patient's own cartilage is collected and placed in an ex vivo culture to produce more articular cartilage cells. An initial arthroscopy with biopsy (reported separately) is performed to harvest normal cartilage from a minor load-bearing area within the knee approximately four to six weeks prior to implantation. The chondrocytes are sent to the laboratory where they are isolated from the cartilage matrix and cultured to increase the number of viable cells. The cells are returned in suspension for surgical implantation. The physician performs a knee arthrotomy or mini-arthrotomy to place the autologous cultured chondrocyte implant. An incision is made over the knee joint and carried down through the soft tissues to gain access into the area of the chondral or osteochondral defect. The defect bed is prepared with debridement of any damaged or fibrous tissue to create stable borders. Using a template created to match the defect, the chondrocyte implant is trimmed and sized. Fibrin sealant is placed in the base of the defect, followed by the implant with the cell-side facing down. Additional sutures or fibrin sealant may be applied to ensure fixation of the implant. The incision is closed in layers by suturing.

27415
An osteochondral allograft is a type of bone/cartilage transplant that treats defects of the knee from disabling cartilage injury or disease, such as osteochondritis dissecans. Arthroscopic imaging, x-rays, and/or MRI is done to determine the size and type of lesion. Donor tissue from a tissue bank is used fresh. For open transplantation, the surgeon exposes

the defect area by cutting to the bone and retracting the soft tissue. The defect is excised, and the margins are squared off and abraded to reach healthy, bleeding, subchondral bone. Using coring reamers, the graft is sized out of the donor material and press-fit into the defect like a type of bone plug. Supplementary fixation may be used by inserting biodegradable pins. The incision is closed. When a mosaic technique is used, cylindrical grafts are taken from the donor material and placed in corresponding cylindrical holes of the same depth and diameter made in the recipient area.

27416
The physician performs a mosaicplasty of the knee, in which cylindrical "plugs" of cartilage and underlying bone are taken from non-weightbearing areas and repositioned to damaged areas. Each plug is a few millimeters in diameter; when multiple cartilage plugs are positioned into the defective area the result is a mosaic-tile appearance. The physician makes an incision over the area of cartilage damage. A coring tool is utilized to form a round hole, sized to fit the plug, in the bone at the damaged area. The physician harvests the plug of normal cartilage, along with the underlying bone. The harvested plugs are implanted into the hole created in the damaged area.

27418
A lateral parapatellar incision is made extending from the top of the patella to the tibial tubercle. Small osteotomes or an oscillating saw is used to free a 6 cm to 8 cm block of bone, which includes the tibial tubercle near its upper end. A small bony platform is made on the medial side of the long bone block. The block is elevated anteriorly and its upper end is swung up onto the platform, while the lower end pivots. Cancellous bone is removed from the lower end of the block in order to improve the cosmetic appearance. Two bone screws secure the block. Incisions are closed with sutures, staples, or Steri-strips. By elevating the tibial tubercle, forces are decreased on the underneath surface of the patella.

27420
An incision is made on the anteromedial aspect of the knee beginning above the patella and ending 1.3 cm below the tibial tuberosity. The area where the patellar tendon inserts into the tibial tuberosity is resected, including a thin piece of bone 1.3 cm square. The patellar tendon is pulled medially and distally on the tibia and a site is selected for reattachment. At the site, an "I" shaped incision is made and the patellar tendon is secured here temporarily with sutures. Next, the insertion of the vastus medialis muscle is transformed laterally and distally and sutured in place. After the alignment of the patella has been checked, the patellar tendon is anchored into the tibia with a staple. The incision is closed with sutures, staples, or Steri-strips.

27422
An anteromedial incision is made parallel to the quadriceps tendon and the patella. Dissection is carried down to the vastus medialis muscle/tendon to the site where it attaches to the patella. An incision is made along the vastus medialis tendon parallel to the patella. The tendon is overlapped and sutured, pulling the patella more medially and allowing for improved patellar alignment. Tissue layers are closed with sutures. The incision is closed with sutures and Steri-strips.

27424
Patellectomy is removal of the patella. A transverse U-shaped incision is made over the anterior aspect of the knee just below the patella. The skin edges are retracted, and the incision is carried through the quadriceps expansion at the level of the distal third of the patella. The patella is excised from the capsule, quadriceps, and patellar tendons. The proximal part of the capsule and quadriceps tendon are taken medially and distally so that they overlap the distal part of the capsule by 1.3 cm and sutured in place. The insertion of the vastus medialis is freed and transferred distally and laterally. Incisions are closed in layers with sutures.

27425
The physician performs an open lateral retinacular release. Lateral retinacular release is done when too much lateral tension on the patella from tightness of the lateral retinaculum causes patellar misalignment, not allowing correct movement. This can be associated with articular cartilage lesions and idiopathic chondromalacia. The physician makes an incision to access the lateral patellofemoral and the lateral patellotibial ligaments. These tight lateral ligaments that are holding the patella out of alignment, are released, detaching the patella from the soft tissue structures, including the lateral retinaculum, muscle fibers, and joint capsule.

27427-27429
The physician performs an extra-articular and/or an intra-articular ligamentous reconstruction procedure of the knee. In 27427, an extra-articular augmentation is performed on one or more of the stabilizing ligaments external to the knee joint that are damaged or torn. The physician makes an incision over the affected ligament. The torn end may be attached to the bone using anchors, staples, or a screw and washer or the tear may be repaired and attached to the bone using a graft. Commonly, the patient's own tendon is harvested to be used as the graft material. In 27428, the physician makes an incision to access the knee joint and the ligaments within the joint. The injured ligament is identified and reattached at its torn end. If reattachment is not possible, the physician obtains a graft (such as a tendon) harvested from the patient or a donor graft, and attaches it to the original location of the ligament. In 27429, both extra- and intra-articular ligamentous reconstruction are performed. In all three methods, a temporary drain is inserted and incisions are repaired in layers with sutures, staples, and/or Steri-strips.

27430
The physician corrects a shortened or fibrotic quadriceps muscle. An anterior longitudinal incision is

Musculoskeletal

made from the upper one third of the thigh to the lower part of the patella. Deep fascia is divided and the rectus femoris muscle is separated from the vastus medialis and lateralis muscles. The vastus intermedius muscle is excised because it is usually scarred and is binding the posterior surface of the rectus femoris and patella to the femur. If the vastus medialis and lateralis muscles are badly scarred, subcutaneous tissue and fat are interposed between them and the rectus. If these muscles are relatively normal, they are sutured to the rectus at the lower one third of the thigh. Layers and incisions are closed with sutures and staples or Steri-strips.

27435

The physician corrects severe flexion contractures of the knee that cannot be corrected by more conservative means. The patient is positioned prone and a curvilinear incision (approximately 15 cm long) is made over the popliteal (back of the knee) space. The medial and lateral aspects of the joint capsule are exposed by dissecting through subcutaneous tissue and deep fascia. The common peroneal nerve and popliteal vessels and nerves are retracted. The medial and lateral portions of the capsule are divided, allowing the knee to be completely extended. The subcutaneous tissue and skin incisions are repaired in layers.

27437-27438

The physician makes a medial patellar incision, exposing the underneath surface (subchondral bone) of the patella. Abrasion arthroplasty or a smoothing of the bone surface is performed to encourage growth of new cartilage. If cancellous bone is exposed and abrasion arthroplasty would not be effective, the physician may place a prosthesis (also called hemiarthroplasty) on the back side of the patella in 27438. The underneath side of the patella is smoothed to make room for the prosthesis. The physician secures the prosthesis with screws or glue. The prosthesis sits in the trochlear groove in the position where the patella slides up and down when the knee bends and straightens. The incision is repaired in layers with sutures, staples, and/or Steri-strips.

27440

The physician replaces the damaged or degenerated tibial portion of the knee joint. The physician makes a medial incision along the patella. Dissection exposes the knee joint and tibial plateau. The menisci and anterior cruciate ligament are removed. The physician may also need to release other soft tissues around the knee to correct contractures and restore range of motion. The physician makes a bone cut through the tibial plateau using a cutting-alignment jig. Peg holes are made on the remaining tibial plateau and the tibial component is placed into position. Screws and/or glue secure the component. The incision is repaired in layers with sutures, staples, and/or Steri-strips.

27441

The physician replaces the damaged or degenerated cartilage of the tibial component of the knee joint. The physician makes a medial incision along the patella. Dissection exposes the knee joint and tibial plateau. The menisci and anterior cruciate ligament are removed. The physician may also need to release other soft tissues around the knee to correct contractures and restore range of motion. If the synovium around the knee joint is diseased, the physician may remove it as well. Any osteophytes (bony outgrowths) interfering with motion may be removed. The physician makes a bone cut through the tibial plateau using a cutting-alignment jig to achieve correct alignment. Peg holes are made on the remaining tibial plateau and the tibial component is placed into position. Screws and/or glue secure the tibial component. The incision is repaired in layers with sutures, staples, and/or Steri-strips.

27442-27443

The physician replaces the damaged or degenerated cartilage of the femoral condyles or tibial plateau. The physician makes a medial incision along the patella and carries dissection to expose the knee joint. If the femoral condyles are replaced, the physician uses a cutting-alignment jig to determine proper alignment of the bone cut and resects or cuts the distal femur. Additional smaller cuts may be made on the femur for rotational alignment. The physician may need to release soft tissues around the knee to correct contractures and restore range of motion. If the tibial plateau is replaced, the physician first removes the menisci and other soft tissue as needed. A cutting alignment jig is used to determine proper alignment of the tibial bone cut. Once the bone cuts are made, peg holes are also made into the bone. The prosthesis is placed into position and secured with screws and/or glue. In 27443, debridement and synovectomy are also performed. Any osteophytes interfering with range of motion are debrided and removed. The physician will also remove any diseased synovium present around the knee joint. The incision is repaired in layers with sutures, staples, and/or Steri-strips.

27445

The physician exposes the knee joint by making a straight longitudinal incision directly over the knee. Bone cuts are made to resect the anterior and posterior femoral condyles. A tibial cutting guide is used to remove a minimal amount of bone from the proximal tibia. A template is placed on the cut tibial surface and an osteotome is used to remove a square of bone from the tibial surface as outlined by the hole in the tibial template. The stem of the tibial component is placed into the hole and the femoral component is placed on the distal femur. Two polyethylene bushings are inserted into the femoral component and joined to the tibial component with the metal axle. The patellar component is applied by making a cut along the articular surface, making a peg hole, and inserting the component. If the patella does not track properly, a separately reportable lateral retinacular release is performed. All components are cemented into place. The joint is irrigated. The incision is closed in layers and placement of temporary suction drainage tubes.

27446
The physician replaces one diseased or damaged compartment of the knee, including the femoral condyle and tibial plateau on the same side. A medial incision is made along the patella and dissection exposes the knee joint. The physician prepares the selected compartment for arthroplasty by removing the meniscus. Other soft tissue around the compartment may also need to be released. Using a cutting-alignment jig, the physician makes bone cuts on the femoral condyle and tibial plateau of the compartment being replaced. The other compartment is left intact. Peg holes are made into the bone and the femoral and tibial components are placed into position. The components are secured with screws and/or glue. The incision is repaired in layers with sutures, staples, and/or Steri-strips.

27447
The physician replaces severely damaged or worn cartilage of the knee joint. A midline incision is made over the knee. Dissection exposes the knee joint. The physician may release soft tissues and/or ligaments in order to correct deformities and improve range of motion. The physician uses a cutting-alignment jig placed on the upper tibia to remove the tibial joint surface (both medial and lateral compartments) by making a bone cut. A cutting-alignment jig is also used on the femoral condyles to make the appropriate bone cut. Depending on the integrity of the joint surface of the patella, the physician may also make a bone cut to remove damaged cartilage. If the joint surface is healthy, it is left intact. Peg holes are usually made, and the components of the prosthesis are placed into position on the tibia, femur, and, if needed, the patella. The components are secured with glue and/or bone screws. The incision is repaired in layers with sutures, staples, and/or Steri-strips.

27448-27450
The physician performs an osteotomy of the femur. A medial or lateral incision is made to approach the femur. After the femur is exposed, a Kirschner wire is placed where a blade-plate is to be inserted. The physician inserts the blade of the plate at the determined angle an osteotomy (bone cut) that is performed transversely. The physician may use a nail plate and screws for internal fixation in 27450. Alignment of the knee now allows weight bearing to occur on the healthier compartment of the knee joint. The incision is repaired in layers with sutures, staples, and/or Steri-strips.

27454
The physician exposes the shaft of the femur with a long, longitudinal, lateral incision. An osteotomy (bone cut) is made through the proximal and distal ends of the femur. The femoral shaft is removed. Osteotomies are made (three or four) on the shaft, and the fragments are threaded end-to-end and aligned on a nail. If the cortex of the bone is very thin, the physician may need to add a separately reportable bone graft. The nail is inserted into the proximal and distal ends of the femur. The periosteum (bone lining) is sutured over the bone and the incision is repaired in layers.

27455
The physician removes a wedge of bone from the upper tibia below the growth plate. To correct the tibial varum (bow-legs) in an eight-year-old child, for example, a 3 cm to 4 cm lateral incision is made over the fibula. An oblique osteotomy of the fibula is performed. An anterolateral incision is made to gain access to the upper tibia. A Steinmann pin is inserted through the midshaft of the tibia, parallel to the ankle joint, and another pin is inserted through the upper tibia parallel to the knee joint. The pins are used as guides to make a bony wedge cut (osteotomy) using a bone saw and chisel. The bone ends are approximated, correcting the deformity. The physician may use an AO five-hole compression plate or staples for internal fixation. The excised bone wedge may be used as a bone graft to fill in any defects. The incisions are closed, and the leg placed in a cast with the knee in 30 to 45 degrees of flexion.

27457
The physician performs an osteotomy of the proximal tibia to remove loading forces from damaged cartilage and bone. The load is transferred to normal cartilage and bone of the opposite knee compartment. For a valgus osteotomy (bone cut), the physician makes an incision over the lateral proximal tibia. For a varus osteotomy, the incision is made medially. Dissection is carried down to the bone. For a valgus osteotomy, the fibular head is removed with an oscillating saw. The osteotomy is made approximately 2 cm below the joint line. The degree of correction has been calculated before surgery with x-ray films. The physician uses an oscillating saw to cut a wedge of bone at the determined angle, three-quarters of the width through the tibia. The cut wedge is removed and an osteotome completes the bone cut. The cut edges of the osteotomy are brought together and secured with a staple. The incision is repaired in layers with sutures, staples, and/or Steri-strips.

27465-27468
Femoral shortening or lengthening techniques equalize leg lengths or treat malunions of the femur. The physician shortens the femur in 27465. An incision is made to expose the tip of the greater trochanter. The femoral canal is reamed and prepared for the insertion of an intramedullary nail. Next the femur is exposed through a lateral longitudinal incision at the middle third of the thigh. Two bone cuts are made to remove a length of bone. After the cut segment is removed, the bone ends are approximated, and the intramedullary nail is inserted into the femoral canal. Plates and screws may be used for fixation if the intramedullary nail is contraindicated, as in osteomyelitis or a deformity that precludes the use of a nail. The leg is placed in a Thomas splint. For femoral lengthening in 27466, two puncture wounds are made laterally in the distal and proximal femur. Two holes at each end are drilled in the bone, and a screw is inserted in each drill hole. The physician makes a lateral longitudinal

Musculoskeletal

incision 6 cm to 8 cm long to expose the femur. At the osteotomy site, an oscillating saw cuts through the femur. The Wagner distraction apparatus is attached to the two sets of screws, so that the apparatus is 1 cm to 2 cm lateral to the thigh. The incision is repaired in layers. The device is distracted up to 5 mm to 6 mm immediately. The apparatus is operated by a knob. Lengthening is about 1.5 mm or 1 cm per week. Both lengthening and shortening are performed in 27468. When the appearance of the femur is normal and the medullary has been reestablished, the plate and screws are removed.

27470-27472

The physician repairs a nonunion or malunion of the femur. The physician makes a lateral incision to expose the femur. If there is no distortion of the intramedullary canal, intramedullary nailing is performed for fixation of the nonunion. If failed internal fixation is present, the physician removes the plates and screws. If there is malalignment of the medullary canal, a compression plate and screws are used for repair. In 27472, there is a loss of bone. The physician harvests bone with an osteotome from the iliac crest or from the femur itself and closes the surgically created donor site. Copious amounts of bone are placed around the nonunion site. The incision is repaired in layers and a temporary drain is applied.

27475-27479

The physician performs epiphysiodesis to achieve complete arrest of the longitudinal growth at the physis (growth plate) of the longer limb. A 5 cm to 7 cm longitudinal incision is made along the lower femur, beginning just above the joint line. The distal femur physis is exposed. Osteotomes excise a rectangular piece of bone from the epiphyseal plate. The growth plate is drilled in anterior, posterior, and distal directions. A curette is used to remove the growth plate. The physician harvests bone from the patient's hip or femur and closes the surgically created graft donor site. The separately reportable cancellous bone graft is packed into the defect created by the removal of the growth plate. The rectangular piece of bone is reinserted into its original bed and securely seated with a mallet. The arrest procedure is the same whether performed on the medial or lateral side. The periosteum and incision are repaired in layers. In 27477, the same procedure is performed for the proximal tibial and fibular epiphyseal growth plates. In 27479, a combination of distal femur and proximal tibia and fibula epiphyseal arrest is performed.

27485

The physician performs hemiepiphyseal arrest on the distal femur or proximal tibia or fibula. For genu valgus, arrest of the medial femoral physis and/or proximal tibia is performed to realign the knee joint. A 5 cm to 7 cm, longitudinal incision is made along the lower femur, beginning just above the joint line. The distal femur physis is exposed. Osteotomes excise a rectangular piece of bone from the epiphyseal plate. The growth plate is drilled in anterior, posterior, and distal directions. A curette is used to remove the growth plate. The physician harvests bone from the patient's hip or femur and closes the surgically created graft donor site. The separately reportable cancellous bone graft is packed into the defect created by the removal of the growth plate. The rectangular piece of bone is reinserted into its original bed and securely seated with a mallet. The periosteum and incision are repaired in layers.

27486-27487

The physician performs a revision of a total knee arthroplasty. Typically, previous skin incisions are incorporated to expose the knee. In 27486, one of the femoral or tibial components or the polyethylene liner is removed as determined by the physician. In order to remove the components, an osteotome or saw may be used to loosen the cement or bone so that the prosthesis can be popped out with a mallet. If any cement is present, it is removed in order to protect and preserve as much bone as possible. Bone cuts are made to accommodate the new prosthesis. If significant bone defects are present on the femur, tibia, or both, a bone graft may be needed. An allograft (donor bone) may be packed into the defect. The components of the new prosthesis are placed into position and may be cemented for fixation. In 27487, the femoral and tibial components are both revised. The incision is repaired with sutures, staples, and/or Steri-strips.

27488

The physician inserts a temporary spacer into the knee joint. To remove the knee prosthesis, the physician makes an incision directly over the original incision line. The prosthesis is exposed. An osteotome or saw may loosen the cement or bone around the components, so that they may be tapped out with a mallet. The cement is removed a piece at a time to protect and preserve as much bone as possible. Once the prosthesis is removed, there is an open space where the knee prosthesis was between the femur and tibia. A spacer of methylmethacrylate formed into a cube shape may be inserted into the space between the femur and tibia. The spacer prevents the soft tissues from compressing the joint space. The spacer is secured until another prosthesis is inserted. The incision is repaired in layers.

27495

The physician applies a prophylactic treatment to the femur. Methylmethacrylate may be applied to an area of resection because of malignancy. Fixation (nailing, pinning, plating, or wiring) and a prophylactic treatment may be an alternative to bone grafting.

27496-27497

The physician performs a decompression fasciotomy on one compartment of the thigh and/or knee. A longitudinal incision is made over the affected compartment. Dissection is carried through the fascial layers to the muscle compartments. An incision may also be made through the intramuscular septum to release pressure. If any necrotic tissue is present, it is debrided. Debridement of nonviable muscle and/or nerve is performed in addition in 27497. The incision may be left open for two to five days and repaired in layers with sutures.

27498

The physician performs a decompression fasciotomy on multiple compartments of the thigh and/or knee. One incision may be used to gain access to one or two compartments of the thigh. If not, a longitudinal incision is made over each compartment. Once the incision is made, dissection is carried through the fascial layers to the muscle compartments. An incision may also be made through the intramuscular septum to release pressure. The incision may be left open for two to five days and repaired in layers with sutures.

27499

The physician performs a decompression fasciotomy of multiple compartments of the thigh and/or knee, and debrides any nonviable tissue. The physician makes one or more extensive longitudinal incisions over the involved compartments. The incisions are carried deep to the fascia of each compartment. These fascia are incised to expose the compartments and relieve the pressures. A thorough exploration is undertaken and the physician debrides any nonviable tissue. This would typically be muscle, but it may also include other tissues within the compartment. The incisions are normally left open for several days before secondary closure is accomplished.

27500

The physician treats a femoral shaft fracture without manipulation. The fractured segments are aligned and stable. Treatment may be with a molded long leg cast, cast brace, or spica cast for several weeks until union is established.

27501

The physician treats a supracondylar or transcondylar femoral fracture without manipulation. The fractured segments are aligned and stable and no manipulation is required. If there is an intercondylar extension of the fracture such as a "T" or "Y" fracture extending into the joint, the intra-articular relationships of the knee must be reestablished. Treatment may be with a molded long leg cast, cast brace, or spica cast for several weeks until union is established.

27502

Closed reduction of the fracture is required by manual reduction by the physician or in conjunction with skin or skeletal traction. If skin traction is used, the leg is placed in full extension and bandages and straps are encircled around the leg starting at the foot and extending to the thigh. Weight is added to provide the traction force. The best application of skin traction is to temporarily provide comfort and support to the fractured limb until a definitive form of therapy is available. For skeletal traction, a pin is placed transversely through the proximal tibia with the knee in slight flexion. Traction weight is 15 to 20 pounds, and thereafter may be reduced gradually. If the physician is concerned about accurate reduction, a second pin may be placed through the distal femur, permitting early movement of the knee. Traction can maintain position until bone healing is well established. If traction is not needed, the extremity is placed in a spica cast or cast brace.

27503

The physician may reduce a displaced fracture manually without the use of skin or skeletal traction. If the intra-articular relationships of the knee cannot be reestablished manually, traction is generally not as effective as skeletal traction, but can be used by wrapping circular wraps around the lower extremity and attaching weight. Skeletal traction is more commonly used by placing a pin through the proximal tibia with the thigh, knee, and leg supported in suspension with some knee flexion. Traction weight of 15 to 20 pounds is applied and thereafter reduced gradually. The physician may need to perform manipulative reduction while in traction if accurate reduction cannot be obtained by traction alone. Traction is used to maintain position until bone healing is well established, or a cast or cast brace may be applied after the fracture becomes stable.

27506

With the patient in a lateral or supine (lying on the back) position, the physician makes a straight lateral incision to expose the fracture site. If there are large butterfly-type fragments or there is a long spiral fracture, cerclage wires may be wrapped around the bone to hold the fragments in place. The intramedullary nail is put into place by making a 4 cm to 6 cm incision over the tip of the greater trochanter. The trochanteric fossa is exposed. A drill hole is made into the center of the femoral canal. A reaming guide is used to ream out the intramedullary canal to the desired length, making room for the implant or nail. A nail-driving guide is inserted, and the nail is driven into place with a hammer. If it is a comminuted fracture, the physician may use interlocking screws to provide better fixation. One or two screws are placed proximally and/or distally through the femur and intramedullary implant. This technique helps secure rotator stability. The interlocking screws may be removed after six to eight weeks.

27507

With the patient in a supine (lying on the back) or lateral decubitus (lying on the side) position, the physician makes a lateral or anterolateral incision. The fracture is reduced by manipulation and bone reduction forceps. A compression plate with screws and/or leg screws secure and compress the fragments. The physician may elect to use cerclage wiring in conjunction with plates or screws in order to facilitate fixation of the fracture. The wire is placed around the femur, over the fracture site. One or more wires may be used. The incision is closed with sutures, staples, and/or Steri-strips.

27508

Closed treatment of a femoral fracture of the distal end of the medial or lateral condyle is indicated if the

Musculoskeletal

intra-articular relationships of the knee are intact and stable, as found upon x-ray. If the fracture does not need reduction, skeletal traction is not required. A spica cast brace is used until bony union is secure.

27509
Percutaneous skeletal fixation can be used for internal fixation in nonunions, malunions, and open or closed fractures of the distal femur area. Fixation pins are introduced through stab wounds (small incision over the bone). A small hole is drilled and a pin placed across the fracture line to hold it in place. Two, three, or more pins may be used. The ends of the pins are cut off beneath the skin, and the small incision closed with suture or Steri-strips. The pins are left in place approximately three to six weeks, and removed.

27510
Closed treatment of femoral fracture of the distal end of the medial or lateral condyle is indicated if the intra-articular relationships of the knee are intact and stable upon x-ray. If reduction of the fracture is required, skeletal traction is most commonly used. A pin is placed through the proximal tibia and the leg is supported in suspension with some knee flexion. Traction weight is 15 to 20 pounds initially, and thereafter may be reduced gradually. If reduction cannot be obtained by traction alone, the physician may manually reduce the fracture under anesthesia. The physician may use a second pin through the distal femur to aid in accurate reduction and permit early movement in the knee. Traction can be used to maintain position until bone healing is well established.

27511
The physician performs open treatment of a femoral supracondylar or transcondylar fracture. An incision is made along the medial or lateral femoral condyle area to expose the fracture site. The fragments are manually reduced and internal fixation is typically accomplished using a buttress blade plate or screw-plate with screws. The incision is closed.

27513
The physician performs open treatment of a femoral supracondylar or transcondylar fracture with intercondylar extension. Since this type of fracture includes a fracture line extending into the joint, it is important to secure accurate articular surface restoration and to retain the reduction. An incision is made over the medial or lateral femoral condyle to expose the fracture site. The fracture is reduced. Cancellous bone screws or bolts may be used to secure the condyle fracture, and a blade-plate with screws for the supracondylar fracture. The physician may repair only the condyles, leaving the patient in skeletal traction for treatment of the supracondylar portion of the fracture.

27514
The physician performs open treatment of a fracture of the lateral or medial distal end of the femur. A curvilinear incision is made along the lateral or medial distal end of the femur, exposing the fracture site. The physician reduces the fracture, ensuring restoration of the articular surface of the knee joint and of the patellofemoral groove. After reduction, if the fracture is stable, no internal fixation is used. However, with this type of fracture internal fixation is typically used. A dynamic condylar screw system or an angled blade-plate with screws may achieve internal fixation of the fracture. The incision is closed with sutures, staples, and/or Steri-strips, or left open for secondary closure.

27516-27517
An abduction type separation is caused by a blow to the lateral side of the distal femur. There may typically be a fracture in conjunction with the epiphyseal separation. If alignment and stability are adequate, a single hip spica cast is used with the knee immobilized in extension. In 27517, closed reduction is attempted first in a more problematic fracture or separation such as in a hyperextension injury. If this is unsuccessful, the physician may insert a Steinmann pin in the femur above the fracture or separation, and another pin in the proximal third of the tibia. Gentle skeletal traction is applied to disengage the fragments while the physician reduces the displacement. A hip spica cast is applied with the knee in 45 to 60 degrees of flexion. In three to four weeks, the cast and pins are removed and an above-knee cast is applied.

27519
The physician performs open treatment of a distal femoral epiphyseal separation. The physician makes an anteromedial or anterolateral, longitudinal incision to expose the epiphysis on the distal femoral condyle area. The articular surface of the epiphysis is examined. The physician may use a Knowles pin placed into the displaced epiphyseal fragment, and use it as a handle to guide the displaced fragment back into position. Additional threaded pins or screws are directed transversely across the epiphysis or across the metaphysis as needed to complete fixation. The incision is closed with sutures and placed in a splint or long leg brace. If there is an open wound associated with the injury, the wound is irrigated and debrided.

27520
Closed treatment of a patellar fracture is indicated when there is 2 mm or less displacement, separation, or step off. X-ray determines any displacement. The leg is placed in a long leg cast or splint to keep the knee immobilized for three to six weeks.

27524
A vertical midline incision is made beginning 5 cm above the patella and ending at the midportion of the patellar tendon. The patellar fracture is identified and the knee joint is irrigated and inspected for any loose fragments. Clotted blood is removed from the fracture surfaces. The physician may use two types of treatment, depending on the type of fracture. The physician may place tension band wiring through drill holes made in the fragments to hold them together. Other fractures require screw fixation placed

perpendicular to the fractured surfaces. If the patellar fracture is so severely fragmented that internal fixation or tension band wiring cannot be used, partial or complete removal of the patella is performed by the physician. If only a partial patellectomy is performed, the patellar tendon is reattached to the remaining patella with sutures and wire. Dissection and/or soft tissue repair of surrounding tissues may be necessary. Incisions are closed with sutures, staples, and/or Steri-strips.

27530-27532

Closed treatment of a tibial plateau fracture is indicated when the fractured segments are stable, in good alignment, and the tibial joint surface is congruent. The physician may need to perform a manual reduction in 27532 to realign the fractured segments. The physician may also use skeletal traction such as Kirschner wire. A wire is placed through the tibia and a traction bow is applied, reducing or realigning the fractured segments.

27535-27536

The physician makes a vertical incision on the side of the patella overlying the medial or lateral tibial plateau to correct a unicondylar (27535) fracture. A bicondylar fracture (27536) is treated by making both a medial and a lateral parapatellar incision. The incision extends downward to the upper portion of the tibia. If reduction is needed to realign the joint surfaces, the physician may use an AO distracter, an external device anchored with screws in the tibia and medial femoral condyle to distract the fractured fragments, allowing them to realign. Instead of a distracter, the physician may use a bone punch to raise fragments. Kirschner wires may be applied to provide provisional fixation of the fragments. A plate, such as a "T" or "L" plate, is fitted to the contour of the bone. Screws are inserted to secure fixation and to compress the fragments so that healing may occur. The incision is closed with sutures, staples, and/or Steri-strips.

27538

There are three types of fractures of the intercondylar spine and tibial tuberosity. Types I and II of the intercondylar spine and Type I of the tibial tuberosity are typically treated in a closed reduction. If the fragment appears stable and is not displaced, no manipulation for reduction is needed. If the fragment is displaced, reduction may be achieved by extending the knee. The knee may also be aspirated. A splint or a locked, long-leg knee brace may be used for four to six weeks.

27540

The physician performs open treatment of an intercondylar spine and/or tuberosity fracture of the knee. If adequate closed reduction of the fragment cannot be achieved, an open procedure is needed to ensure normal knee range of motion and function. Open treatment is typically performed for Type III intercondylar spine fracture and Types II and III tibial tuberosity fracture. The physician makes an anteromedial incision to expose the knee, and the fragments are identified. For the intercondylar spine fracture, the fragment is reduced by placing the knee in full extension. Two holes are drilled through the tibial epiphysis. A wire or nonabsorbable suture is passed through the lowest portion of the anterior cruciate ligament and through the drill holes and tied together. The knee is flexed and extended so the reduction is stable. For a tibial tuberosity fracture, the fragment is reduced by extending the knee. Two small pins or a bone screw are placed through the fragment to hold it in place. The incision is closed. A splint or brace is applied for four to six weeks.

27550-27552

Radiographic evaluation is performed to help determine the direction of knee dislocation. Minor instabilities can be reduced without anesthesia by applying manual longitudinal traction (27550). If secondary restraints (ligaments) were damaged, anesthesia may be required in order to reduce the dislocation (27552). The knee is usually aspirated, and placed in a posterior splint for support. The physician may do further tests to evaluate ligamentous, capsular, meniscal, and vascular integrity. The knee is usually placed in a splint or immobilizer.

27556-27557

In an open knee dislocation there is considerable soft tissue trauma. The physician may debride the injury and explore the popliteal space for arterial evaluation and/or repair. If the joint is unstable after the dislocation is reduced, the physician may decide to use internal fixation for a period of time. Two transfixion pins drilled across the joint can provide good stability against recurrent dislocation. The wound may be left open to allow for drainage and treatment of infection. In 27557, primary ligamentous repair is performed at the same time, or at a later date after certification of popliteal artery flow, or after artery repair. The torn ligaments are reattached with screws, staples, and/or sutures. The incision or wound is closed or left open temporarily depending on the size of the wound, or if an infection is present.

27558

In an open knee dislocation, there will be considerable soft tissue trauma. The physician may need to debride the injury and explore the popliteal space for arterial evaluation and/or repair. If the joint is unstable after the dislocation is reduced, the physician may apply internal fixation for a period of time. Two transfixion pins drilled across the joint can provide good stability against recurrent dislocation. Those ligaments not able to be repaired directly may need augmentation or reconstruction. Typically the posterior cruciate ligament and sometimes the anterior cruciate ligament will be reconstructed by drilling bone tunnels in the tibia and femur, and passing donor ligament grafts through the tunnels and into the knee joint to take the place of the torn ligaments. The incision or wound is closed or left open temporarily depending on the size of the wound, or if an infection is present.

27560-27562
When the patella dislocates, it typically moves to the lateral side of the knee and off of the femoral condyles. Frequently the physician is able to gently extend the knee, causing the patella to move back into its normal position without administering anesthesia (27560). If the patient is in pain and guarding excessively, the physician may use anesthesia (27562) to relax the patient so the patella can be realigned. An x-ray may be taken to check the position of the patella. A splint or brace may be applied to give the patella additional support.

27566
If there is significant damage to the patella, such as an osteochondral fracture, or severe cartilage breakdown associated with a patellar dislocation, a partial or total patellectomy may need to be performed with this procedure. A medial longitudinal patellar incision is made to expose the patella and medial retinaculum. If the patella is still dislocated, it is reduced at this time. If significant damage has occurred to the patella as noted above, the physician may remove a portion or all of it. This is done by incising the tendon that encases the patella and using a saw and osteotome to resect the damaged portion of the patella. The tendon sheath is closed with sutures. To repair the patellar dislocation, the physician places the sutures in the medial retinaculum to tighten it down, which in turn keeps the patella or the tendon sheath from moving out from the trochlear groove. The incision is closed with sutures, staples, and/or Steri-strips.

27570
The physician increases range of knee motion limited by adhesions or scar tissue. After general anesthesia is administered, the physician bends the knee and applies gradual pressure until the desired range of motion for the knee is achieved. Traction or other fixation devices may be applied.

27580
The physician makes a long incision along the inside of the patella. The patella is reflected laterally to expose the knee joint. Bone cuts are made to flatten out the joint surfaces of the femur and tibia. A U-shaped groove is made on the underneath side of the patella and a corresponding one on the femur. The patella is placed into the femoral groove and secured with screws. The physician makes an incision overlying the iliac crest, harvests a graft, and closes the surgically created graft donor site. The bone graft is placed between the joint surfaces. An external fixator compresses the joint surfaces. The knee is typically fused in 10 to 15 degrees of flexion. The incision is closed with sutures, staples, and/or Steri-strips.

27590-27591
The physician makes incisions so that equal anterior and posterior flaps are fashioned. Dissection is carried down to the femur. Arteries and veins are doubly ligated and transected. The sciatic nerve is divided. A Gigli saw is used to section the femur and bevel the cut ends. The anterior and posterior myofascial flaps are sutured together and secured to the lower end of the femur through drill holes. Incisions are closed in layers and a temporary drain is applied. For fitting (27591) an immediate postoperative prosthesis (IPOP), a rigid dressing is applied at the time of amputation. A closed-end stump sock is placed over the dressings. Felt pads are used over bony prominences to evenly distribute the pressure. An elastic, plaster cast is applied over the amputation site. A belt suspension apparatus may be incorporated into the cast. If immediate weight bearing is planned, an end-plate is wrapped into the lower portion of the cast to allow attachment of a temporary prosthesis.

27592
An open amputation is one in which the skin is not closed over the end of the stump, but is rather followed by a secondary closure (reamputation, scar revision) at a later date. The purpose of this type of amputation is to prevent or eliminate infection so that final closure of the stump may be carried out without breakdown of the wound. This procedure is usually used in severe traumatic wounds with extensive destruction of tissue. Just below the intended bone section, the physician makes a circular incision to the deep fascia. Muscles and nerves are divided and all vessels ligated. The bone is sectioned, and the wound is dressed. Skin traction is applied by covering the stump with a stockinette which is glued to the skin. The free end of the stockinette is split into 4 tails and tied together over the stump. A rope is attached to the stockinette and traction of 3 to 5 pounds is applied in order to gradually stretch the skin over the stump, while the stump is healed by a sear. This may take two to three weeks or more. The stump is dressed at intervals while continuing the traction.

27594
The physician performs a secondary closure or scar revision after the stump has granulated or healed by a scar. In this procedure, no additional bone is sectioned. The physician resects the scar and granulation tissue from the end of the stump. Skin flaps are fashioned as close as possible to the thick scar surrounding the granulating wound. The dense layer of scar tissue is excised from over the end of the bone. Additional muscle may be removed as well. The skin flaps are pulled over the end of the stump and connected with nonabsorbable sutures. When closing the wound, opposing tissue layers are sewn under physiologic tension, and care must be taken so that the final closure is neither too tight nor too loose. A temporary drain or suction tubes may also be used.

27596
After the stump has granulated or healed by scar, the physician performs secondary closure or scar revision. This procedure is usually performed two to three weeks or more after the initial open amputation was completed. Additional bone is sectioned, usually at a more proximal or higher level. Skin flaps are fashioned and pulled over the stump and closed with nonabsorbable sutures. A temporary drain or suction tubes are used as well.

27598
The physician performs disarticulation at the knee, which is a disjoining but not removal of bone above the knee. Equal anterior and posterior incisions are made around the knee. The patellar tendon is sectioned close to where it attaches to the tibial tubercle. The tendons surrounding the knee are divided from their insertions on the tibia. The same is done with the cruciate ligaments. Arteries and veins are ligated and nerves are divided. The patella is removed. A saw is used to remove the femoral condyles 1.5 cm above the level of the knee joint. The patellar tendon is pulled into the intercondylar notch and sutured to the remaining portions of the cruciate ligaments. The hamstring tendons are sutured to the patellar tendon. A temporary drain is placed in the knee joint and the incision is closed in layers.

27600-27602
The physician performs a decompression fasciotomy on the compartments of the leg to reduce high pressure within those compartments. The physician treats the anterior or lateral compartments of the leg in 27600, the posterior compartments in 27601, or the anterior and/or lateral and posterior compartments in 27602. The physician makes incisions overlying the compartments measured at dangerous levels. The incisions are carried deep to the respective fascia. The physician makes long incisions in the fascia to relieve the pressure. The fascial and skin incisions are left open. Any nonviable tissue is removed.

27603-27604
The physician drains an abscess or hematoma in 27603 or an infected bursa in 27604 from deep within the leg or ankle. The physician makes an incision in the leg or ankle overlying the site of the abscess, hematoma, or bursa to be incised. Dissection is carried through the deep subcutaneous tissues and may be continued into the fascia or muscle to expose the abscess or hematoma. The incision may be extended if the mass is larger than expected. When the infected bursa, abscess, or hematoma is identified, it is incised and the contents are drained. The area is irrigated and the incision is repaired in layers with sutures, staples, and/or Steri-strips; closed with drains in place; or simply left open to further facilitate drainage of infection.

27605-27606
The physician performs a percutaneous tenotomy of the Achilles tendon. A knife blade or tenotome held vertically is inserted through the skin and subcutaneous tissue into the Achilles tendon. The blade is turned medially and laterally and swept back and forth, creating a nick in the tendon, until the foot can be dorsiflexed at the ankle. Pressure is applied over the incision for about five minutes. A dressing and long leg cast is applied with the ankle in 10-degree dorsiflexion and the knee in maximal extension. Report 27605 when local anesthesia is infiltrated through the skin and into the Achilles tendon, usually 1 cm above insertion into the calcaneus. When general anesthesia is required, report 27606.

27607
The physician incises infected bone in the tibia, fibula, or ankle to treat a bone abscess or osteomyelitis. The physician makes an incision over the affected area. Dissection is carried through the soft tissues to expose the bone. The periosteum is split and reflected from the bone overlying the infected area. A curette may be used to scrape away the abscess or infected portion to healthy bony tissue or drill holes may be made through the cortex into the medullary canal in a window outline around the infected or abscessed bone. The area is drained and debrided of infected bony and soft tissue. The physician irrigates the area with antibiotic solution, the periosteum is closed over the bone, and the soft tissues are sutured closed; or the wound is packed and left open, allowing the area to drain. Secondary closure is performed approximately three weeks later. Dressings are changed daily. A splint may be applied to limit ankle movement.

27610
The physician performs an arthrotomy of the ankle that includes exploration, drainage, or removal of any foreign body. An incision is made over the ankle area to be exposed. The soft tissues are dissected away and the joint capsule is exposed and incised. The joint space is explored, any necrotic tissue is removed, and infection or abnormal fluid is drained. If a foreign body is present (e.g., bullet, nail, gravel), it is exposed and removed. The wound is irrigated with antibiotic solution. The physician may leave the wound packed open with daily dressing changes to allow for further drainage or secondary healing by granulation. If the incision is repaired, drain tubes may be inserted and the incision is closed in layers with sutures, staples, and/or Steri-strips.

27612
The physician performs an arthrotomy on the ankle for posterior capsular release, with or without Achilles tendon lengthening by making an incision along the Achilles tendon and retracting the muscles to expose the posterior ankle capsule. The capsule is incised to increase dorsiflexion. If the Achilles tendon is lengthened, the physician notches the tendon at the medial and lateral aspects to release contracture. The wound is sutured in layers.

27613-27614
The physician performs a biopsy of the soft tissues of the leg or ankle area. With proper anesthesia administered, an incision is made over the biopsy area. Dissection is carried down within the superficial soft tissue layers in 27613, usually the subcutaneous fat to the uppermost fascial layer. In 27614, dissection is taken deep within the soft tissue, such as into the fascial layer or within the muscle. A portion of the tissue is excised and submitted for pathology. The area is irrigated and the incision is closed with layered sutures, staples, or Steri-strips.

27615-27616
The physician performs a radical resection (excision) of a soft tissue tumor (i.e., sarcoma) from the leg or ankle

Musculoskeletal

area, not involving bone. The tumor may be malignant or an aggressive benign tumor of the connective tissue. An incision is made over the tumor and dissection exposes it. The tumor and any adjacent tissue that may be affected by the spread of the neoplasm are excised. Large resections may be needed. The type and stage of the lesion determine the extent of the tumor margin resection area. Muscle or fascia may need to be repaired and drains may be placed. The surgical wound is closed using simple or intermediate repair or separately reportable complex closure, adjacent tissue transfer, or graft. Report 27615 for a resected area that is less than 5 cm and 27616 for a resected area that is 5 cm or greater.

27618-27619 [27632, 27634]
The physician removes a tumor from the soft tissue of the leg or ankle area that is located in the subcutaneous tissue in 27618 and 27632 and in the deep soft tissue, below the fascial plane, or within the muscle in 27619 and 27634. With the proper anesthesia administered, the physician makes an incision in the skin overlying the mass and dissects to the tumor. The extent of the tumor is identified and a dissection is undertaken all the way around the tumor. A portion of neighboring soft tissue may also be removed to ensure adequate removal of all tumor tissue. A drain may be inserted and the incision is repaired with layers of sutures, staples, or Steri-strips. Report 27618 for excision of a subcutaneous tumor whose resected area is less than 3 cm, and 27632 for a resected area 3 cm or greater. Report 27619 for excision of a subfascial or intramuscular tumor whose resected area is less than 5 cm, and 27634 for a resected area 5 cm or greater.

27620
The physician performs an arthrotomy of the ankle that includes exploration, drainage, or removal of any foreign body. An incision is made over the ankle area to be exposed. The soft tissues are dissected away and the joint capsule is exposed and incised. The joint space is explored, any necrotic tissue is removed, and infection or abnormal fluid is drained. If a foreign body is present (e.g., bullet, nail, gravel), it is exposed and removed. The wound is irrigated with antibiotic solution. The physician may leave the wound packed open with daily dressing changes to allow for further drainage or secondary healing by granulation. If the incision is repaired, drain tubes may be inserted and the incision is closed in layers with sutures, staples, and/or Steri-strips.

27625
The physician performs an arthrotomy of the ankle and removes the synovium. An incision is made over the ankle. The soft tissues are dissected away and the joint capsule is exposed. An incision is made through the capsule and into the joint. The synovium is removed through the incision. The wound is irrigated with antibiotic solution the incision is closed in layers with sutures, staples, and/or Steri-strips.

27626
To correct thickening of the synovium, the physician makes an incision over the tendon and exposes the tendon sheath. The synovium is the lining that bathes the joint in fluid. The physician removes the affected sheath from the tendon and the joint space is opened and the synovium is removed. The wound is irrigated and closed with sutures.

27630
The physician makes an incision over the site of the lesion on the tendon sheath or capsule. Dissection exposes the tendon or capsule. The tissues are dissected around the lesion, freeing it from surrounding tissue and the lesion is excised. The operative site is irrigated with antibiotic solution and the wound closed with layered sutures.

27635-27638
A bone cyst or benign tumor of the tibia or fibula is removed. The physician makes an incision in the lower leg overlying the cyst or tumor. The skin and underlying soft tissues are reflected to expose the periosteum, which is separated from the bone. Curettes or osteotomes are used to scrape or cut the lesion from the bone. Once the benign tumor or cyst is removed and healthy bone tissue is present, the periosteum is repositioned and the incision is repaired in layers. If the bone defect created requires a graft for repair, the physician obtains the necessary size bone graft from a separate donor site on the patient and packs it into the site where the tumor or bone cyst was removed or uses a bone bank allograft. Report 27637 if an autograft is obtained and 27638 if an allograft is used.

27640-27641
The physician performs a partial excision of the tibia in 27640 or the fibula in 27641 to remove infected bone. An incision is made over the affected part of the bone and the underlying soft tissues are divided to expose it. The periosteum is reflected and the infected portion of bone is removed and irrigated. The excavation of bone may excise a crater-like piece, leave a small saucer-like shelf depression in the bone, or may remove a portion of the shaft (diaphysis) of a long bone. If a significant portion of bone is removed, the physician may use bone graft material to fill the cavity left in the bone. The periosteum is closed over the bone, the soft tissues are sutured closed, and a soft dressing is applied.

27645-27647
The physician removes a tumor with radical resection. The physician incises the overlying skin and dissects to the bone, freeing the involved bone from muscular attachments and the tissue bed. The area affected by tumor is removed, and the wound is sutured in layers. The surgical wound is repaired by simple, intermediate, or complex closure; adjacent tissue transfer; or graft. Report 27645 if the tumor is located in the tibia; 27646 if located in the fibula; and 27647 if located on the talus or calcaneus.

27648
The physician injects radiopaque fluid into the ankle for arthrography. The physician inserts a needle into the ankle joint and aspirates if necessary. Opaque contrast solution is injected into the ankle, and the needle is removed. A separately reportable arthrogram is taken of the ankle.

27650-27652
The physician repairs a ruptured Achilles tendon. An incision is made overlying the tendon. The physician extends the incision through the tissues to the tendon. The physician identifies the tear and debrides any rough edges. In 27652, the physician harvests a fascial graft from the patient through a separate incision. The physician repairs the surgically created graft donor site. The graft is incorporated into the repair of the tendon and secured to the area with fixation (e.g., screw). The tendon is repaired, typically with a heavy nonabsorbable suture. The wound is irrigated with antibiotic solution and closed in layers. A cast, splint, or brace may be applied.

27654
The physician repairs a secondarily torn Achilles tendon. An incision is made overlying the tendon. The physician extends the incision deep to the tendon. The tear or rupture is identified. Because the repair is secondary, significant scar tissue may be debrided. Any nonviable tissue is also removed. A graft may be harvested from the patient through a separate incision. The physician repairs the surgically created graft donor site and the tendon with a suture or with both the graft and suture. The graft may be secured to the area of repair with a screw. The physician irrigates the wound with antibiotic solution. The wound is closed in layers. A cast or splint may be applied.

27656
The physician repairs a fascial defect of the leg. The physician incises the skin overlying the defect. If underlying muscles are herniated through the fascial defect, they are pulled to their correct anatomical position and secured with sutures. The wound is sutured in layers.

27658-27659
An incision is made overlying the damaged flexor tendon in the leg. The physician extends the incision deep to the tendon. The tear or rupture is identified. If the repair is secondary, significant scar tissue may be debrided, and a graft may be necessary. Any nonviable tissue is also removed. The physician repairs the tendon with sutures or by placing a graft and suturing. The graft may be secured to the area of repair with a screw. The physician irrigates the wound with antibiotic solution. The wound is closed in layers. A cast or splint may be applied. Primary repair is done immediately after injury. Secondary repair is done sometime after the incident of injury or following a previous surgical repair. Report 27658 for a primary repair without graft and 27659 for a secondary repair, with or without a graft.

27664-27665
The physician makes a midline, longitudinal incision to expose the damaged extensor tendon in the leg. The surgical site is irrigated and the torn ends of the tendon are realigned to provide for better attachment and brought together and sutured. The tendon may be attached to the retinaculum around the knee. If the repair is secondary, significant scar tissue may be debrided, and a graft may be necessary. Any nonviable tissue is also removed. The physician repairs the tendon with sutures or by placing a graft and suturing. The graft may be secured to the area of repair with a screw. The physician irrigates the wound with antibiotic solution. The wound is closed in layers. A cast or splint may be applied. Primary repair is done immediately after injury. Secondary repair is done sometime after the incident of injury or following a previous surgical repair. Report 27664 for a primary repair without graft and 27665 for a secondary repair, with or without a graft.

27675
The physician makes a longitudinal curved incision that extends from the distal end of the fibula, over the lateral border of the foot to the cuboid bone. A posterior skin flap is elevated at the lateral malleolus, using the deep fascia with its base attached to the tip of the lateral malleolus. The peroneal tendons and sheaths are identified and placed in their appropriate anatomic position and secured in place with sutures or drill holes and suture anchors. The incision is sutured in layers.

27676
A longitudinal lateral ankle incision is made and a groove created in the posterior aspect of the fibular malleolus (fibular osteotomy). The peroneal tendons are placed in the groove and held in place with a thick osteoperiosteal flap from the surface of the malleolus that is swung posteriorly over the tendons or with a wedge of bone cut from the lateral malleolus that is displaced posteriorly over the tendons. The wound is irrigated and sutured in layers. A short leg cast is usually applied and modified to a walking cast once the stitches are removed.

27680-27681
The physician corrects a tightened or adhesed tendon sheath in the leg or ankle by making a longitudinal incision over the restricted tendon. Skin is retracted and scar tissue is removed. The physician dissects the tendon with a sharp instrument to free it from the bone. The wound is sutured and dressed with compression bandages. Report 27680 if the procedure is performed on a single tendon. Report 27681 if multiple tendons, requiring separate incisions, are freed from tightened or adhesed tendon sheaths.

27685-27686
The physician makes three incisions on the lateral side of the foot centered over the sinus tarsi. The physician exposes the extensor digitorum brevis tendon, and reflects it distally to expose the anterior part of the talocalcaneal joint. The calcaneocuboid joint is

identified and all tight surrounding structures are released. A second incision is made on the medial side of the foot centered over the prominent head of the talus. The physician releases all tight structures on the medial and dorsal aspects of the head of the talus and the navicular. The anterior part of the talus is freed from its attachments to the navicular and calcaneus. If the peroneal, and extensor hallucis longus and extensor digitorum longus tendons remain contracted the physician lengthens them by Z-plasty. A third incision is made on the medial side of the Achilles tendon, lengthened by Z-plasty. The physician inserts a Steinmann pin through the navicular and into the neck of the talus to maintain the reduction. The wound is closed in layers and a long-leg cast with the knee flexed and the foot in proper position. The Steinmann pins are removed in eight weeks.

27687

The physician performs a gastrocnemius recession. To lengthen the gastrocnemius muscle using the Strayer procedure, the physician makes a posterior longitudinal incision 10 cm to 15 cm long overlying the middle of the calf. The medial sural nerve is retracted and the incision is deepened to the fascia to expose the gastrocnemius. This muscle is dissected bluntly from the underlying soleus muscle to their common tendon at the calcaneus. A probe or clamp is inserted deep to the gastrocnemius and its tendon is severed. The physician dorsiflexes the foot until there is a 2 cm to 2.5 cm gap between the two tendon segments. The two muscle bellies are dissected from their fascial attachments proximally to the popliteal fossa. The physician passes a finger from side-to-side beneath the muscle to completely separate the gastrocnemius from the soleus. The proximal part of the tendon is sutured to the soleus with fine interrupted silk sutures. The wound is closed.

27690-27692

Because these procedures involve transfer or transplant of a single tendon from a number of different sites on the foot, the exact procedure will differ depending on the specific tendon involved. When transfer of the anterior tibial tendon is performed, an anterior lower-leg incision is made and the tendon extracted and passed posteriorly through the interosseous membrane to the calcaneus. A posterior heel incision is made and the tendon end is fixed to the calcaneus and/or Achilles tendon. The wound is closed in layers over a drain with a subcutaneous layer closed so that the skin can be brought together under minimal tension. The patient is placed into a dressing incorporating plaster splints. Report 27690 for superficial transfer or transplant of a single tendon. Report 27691 for deep transfer or transplant of a single tendon. Report 27692 for each additional tendon.

27695-27696

The physician repairs a disruption or tear of the medial or lateral collateral ligament. There are two groups of ligaments that make up the collateral ligaments of the ankle. These groups are referred to as the lateral collateral and medial collateral ligaments. The physician makes a curved incision over the affected ligament. The skin is reflected to expose the tear. Holes are drilled diagonally across the talus or the medial malleolus, depending upon the site of the injury, and nonabsorbable sutures are placed to secure the ligament. The wound is closed and dressed. The leg is immobilized in a long leg cast with the knee flexed to 30 to 45 degrees for four weeks followed by a walking cast for four weeks. Report 27695 if the medial or lateral collateral ligaments are repaired. Report 27696 if both of the collateral ligaments are repaired during the same operative episode.

27698

This procedure reports a secondary repair of a disrupted collateral ligament of the ankle. Secondary repair is done sometime after the incident of injury or following a previous surgical repair. There are several techniques, including Watson-Jones, Evan and Chrisman-Snook. In a Watson-Jones repair, an ankle incision is made and the peroneus brevis tendon divided and mobilized. It is passed through drill holes in the talus and fibular malleolus to reconstruct both the calcaneofibular and anterior talofibular ligaments (lateral collateral ligament). An Evans procedure involves mobilizing the peroneus brevis tendon and passing it through a drill hole in the lateral fibular malleolus to reconstruct the collateral ligament. A Chrisman-Snook procedure involves dividing the peroneus brevis tendon and using it in the repair of the collateral ligament.

27700-27703

The physician performs arthroplasty to correct joint problems caused by arthritis. Three portal incisions are made at the front and sides of the ankle. Joint surfaces are smoothed and scar tissues are removed from the joint. Loose cartilage fragments may be removed along with other debridement. The articular surface may be abraded to initiate reparative cartilage growth. If excessive damage is noted, the physician replaces damaged parts of the ankle with a prosthesis and reports 27702. Report 27703 if a loose component must be revised.

27704

The physician removes an implant. The preexisting skin incision is opened and the tibial and talus components are removed with accompanying cement. Bone grafts are placed in the resulting defect and the ankle is secured with compression or screws. The wound is sutured and a cast is applied for up to 12 weeks.

27705-27709

The physician performs an osteotomy (bone cut) of the tibia in 27705, of the fibula in 27707, or of both in 27709. An incision is made in the skin overlying the osteotomy site. Separate incisions may be necessary to access both tibia and fibula in 27709. The physician dissects the tissues down to the bone. The bone is exposed. The physician makes a cut through the tibia, fibula, or both in the desired location and plane. The bone is aligned to the proper position. Fixation, such as screws or plates may be applied to maintain position. The physician irrigates the area with antibiotic solution and closes it in layers. A splint, cast, or brace may be applied.

27712
The physician makes an incision along the shaft of the limb, exposing the bone. Another incision is made through the periosteum to expose the entire shaft. The physician cuts through the proximal and distal ends of the bone, temporarily removes the shaft, and makes three or four cuts through the shaft. These segments are threaded onto a medullary nail and shifted as necessary to alignment. Bone grafts are added if the cortex is extremely thin. The shaft is placed back into position with the medullary nail extending into the bone at either end. The periosteum is sutured over the bone and the wound is closed with sutures. The extremity is immobilized by cast until healed.

27715
The patient is placed prone and an incision is made over the distal lateral fibula. The physician places two screws 1.5 cm apart through fibula to the tibia, securing the fibula during the procedure. The fibula is cut above the screws. Incisions are made at the top and bottom of the tibia, and Schanz screws are placed parallel to the plane of the knee outside the leg. Another incision is made at the front of the tibia, making a transverse cut through the bone. The Achilles tendon may be lengthened. An external distraction device is attached to the screws and the distance increased by 1.5 cm per day or 10 cm per week. After the desired length is achieved, a shortened or lengthened metal plate and screws are attached, with possible bone grafting. The wound is closed.

27720-27722
To correct nonunion of the tibia in 27720, the physician makes an incision on the medial aspect of the tibia through the periosteum. The bone is divided by transverse cuts and the pieces are manually rotated into position and stabilized with a metal plate and screws. In 27722, the physician makes an anteromedial incision and fibrous tissue is removed from the site. The ends of the fragments are roughened and the distal segment is hollowed out. A rectangular window is cut into the bone just above the site, cancellous bone is removed, and placed around the fixation site. A sliding graft is applied to the site at both ends of the fracture allowing for equal compression when tightened. The wound is closed, dressed, and a cast is applied.

27724
The physician repairs a tibia fracture that has not healed or has healed in malalignment. An incision is made in the skin overlying the tibial fracture site. The incision is extended to the bone. The physician identifies the fracture or malunion. Any scar tissue is debrided from around and between the fracture pieces so that the clean edges of bone can be approximated. A bone graft is harvested through a separate incision from the patient's ilium or from another bone. The physician repairs the surgically created graft donor site. The graft is placed at the fracture site and the fracture is manipulated into the desired position and alignment. The physician applies fixation, such as screws, plates, wires, or rods to stabilize the fracture. The wound is irrigated with antibiotic solution and closed in layers. A splint, brace, or cast may be applied.

27725
The physician repairs a fracture of the tibia that has not healed or has healed in malalignment. An incision is made in the skin overlying the fracture site. The physician extends the incision deep to the bone. The fracture or malunion is identified. Any scar tissue is debrided from around and between the fracture pieces. An osteotomy of the bone is performed if needed to correct the malalignment. Using the adjacent fibula as a strut, the fibula is attached to the tibia with fixation, such as plates, screws, or wires. This attachment allows the fibula to heal to the tibia in a synostosis. The physician irrigates the wound with antibiotic solution and closes it in layers. A brace, cast, or splint may be applied.

27726
Nonunion of a fracture is the absence of healing between fractured bone parts, while in malunion some healing occurs but the fracture fragments are in poor alignment. The physician repairs a nonunion or malunion of the fibula utilizing internal fixation. The physician exposes the nonunion or malunion by making an incision through the skin, fascia, and muscle over the fracture site. Intervening scar tissue may be removed and the bone is divided. The fragments are aligned and an internal fixation device is inserted. The incision is repaired in layers with sutures, staples, and/or Steri-strips. The limb is immobilized.

27727
Congenital anterolateral bowing of the tibia is a rare condition that is present in one in 250,000 live births. The affected leg is bowed forward and usually shortened. By age 2, the bowed tibia fractures spontaneously and does not heal. However, before the fracture occurs, the physician may place the affected leg in a thermoplastic brace to protect it. Once the fracture occurs, it does not heal, and forms a pseudarthrosis (nonunion). Surgical repair using fibula graft or using the Ilizarov technique of repair is often used.

27730-27742
The physician performs epiphyseal arrest on the distal tibia (lower leg toward the ankle). The physician makes a 2 cm incision over the physis on the deformed side of the bone. A 1 square cm bone block is removed from the physeal line. A curette is used to roughen the remaining walls of the block site. The block is rotated and replaced in its original space. The wound is closed with sutures. Report 27732 if performed on the distal fibula; report 27734 if performed on both the distal tibia and fibula (two bones of the lower leg); report 27740 if performed on both ends of the bones; and report 27742 if performed on the distal femur.

Musculoskeletal

27745
Preventive nailing of a bone may be performed if a surgeon feels that a bone is not stable on its own despite the lack of a true fracture site. An incision is made to reflect the soft tissues and the periosteum is divided to expose the bone. The bone is plated or pinned as necessary. the soft tissues are repositioned and skin is closed with sutures. Often weight-bearing is progressed as with normal fractures or internal fixation procedures.

27750
The physician treats a fracture of the tibial shaft without open surgery or any manipulation of the bones. Separately reportable x-rays confirm a fracture of the tibial shaft with or without a simultaneous fibular fracture. The position and alignment of the fracture fragments are stable. The physician applies a cast or brace to maintain the stability of the fragments.

27752
The physician treats a tibial shaft fracture without surgery but with manipulation of the bones. Separately reportable x-rays confirm a fracture of the tibial shaft with or without a simultaneous fibular fracture. Using anesthesia, and with the use of skeletal traction as required, the physician manipulates the fracture. Manipulation is accomplished by pushing, pulling, rotating, or otherwise maneuvering the bones so they are properly aligned. Separately reportable x-rays confirm proper alignment. Skeletal traction may not be removed and a cast or brace may be applied to the leg to maintain stability of the bone.

27756
The physician treats a fracture of the tibia shaft by placing pins or screws through the skin and into the bone. Separately reportable x-rays confirm that the fracture, with or without an associated fibular fracture, can be treated without any long incisions or exposure of the bone. The physician makes small stab wounds in the skin overlying the fracture. Using separately reportable fluoroscopic x-ray as needed, the physician inserts the pins or screws through the small incisions and through the fractured pieces. The pins or screws hold the fractured pieces together. The wounds are irrigated with antibiotic solution and the skin is closed. A dressing is applied. The leg is placed in a cast, splint, or brace.

27758
The physician repairs a fracture of the shaft of the tibia using internal fixation devices. An incision is made overlying the fracture area of the tibia. The physician extends the incision deep to the bone, identifying and exposing the fracture. Tissue is debrided as needed. The physician manipulates the pieces of bone together under direct visualization. Fixation devices, such as plates and screws or cerclage wires, are applied to hold the fracture in the desired position. The wound is irrigated with antibiotic solution. The physician may close the wound in layers or the wound may be left open to drain.

27759
The physician makes an incision over the proximal tibia. The tissue is dissected. The physician carries the incision to the bone. Separately reportable fluoroscopic x-ray may be used throughout the rest of the procedure to confirm stabilization of the fracture. The physician drills a hole in the proximal tibia and places a long guidewire into the marrow canal of the bone. This guide wire is threaded distally in the canal and across the fracture site to the distal tibia. Bone reamers are sequentially placed over the guide wire in even larger sizes to ream the inside of the bone. Reaming is continued until the desired size is reached. The physician chooses the correct size rod to be implanted in the canal. The physician inserts the rod into the proximal tibia over the guide wire and drives it through the intramedullary canal to the distal tibia. The guide wire is removed. The incision is irrigated with antibiotic solution and the skin is closed in layers. A splint or brace may be applied to the leg.

27760
The physician treats a fracture of the medial malleolus of the ankle without surgery or any manipulation of the bones. Separately reportable x-rays confirm the fracture is in an acceptable position. A cast or brace is placed on the leg to hold the fragments in place.

27762
The physician treats a fractured medial malleolus without open surgery but with manipulation of the fracture. Separately reportable x-rays confirm the fracture is in an unacceptable position. Using anesthesia as needed, the physician manipulates the fracture by pushing, pulling, or maneuvering the fracture into the desired position. Traction may be used to aid in the manipulation or for stabilization. A cast or brace is applied to the leg.

27766
The physician makes an incision overlying the medial malleolus near the ankle. The incision is extended through the tissue and deep to the bone. The fractured medial malleolus is identified. The physician places the fractured pieces of bone into proper position and alignment. The physician applies bone fixation devices, such as screws or pins, to secure the fractured pieces. The wound is irrigated with antibiotic solution and closed in layers. A splint, cast, or brace is applied to the leg.

27767-27768
In 27767, the physician treats a fracture of the posterior malleolus of the ankle without open surgery or any manipulation of the bones. Separately reportable x-rays confirm the fracture is in an acceptable position. A cast or brace is placed on the leg to hold the fragments in place. In 27768, the physician treats a fractured posterior malleolus without open surgery but with manipulation of the fracture. Using anesthesia as needed, the physician manipulates the fracture by pushing, pulling, or maneuvering the fracture into the desired position. Traction may be

used to aid in the manipulation or for stabilization. A cast or brace is applied to the leg.

27769
The physician performs open treatment of a posterior malleolus fracture. The physician makes an incision overlying the posterior malleolus near the ankle. The incision is extended through the tissue and deep to the bone. The fractured posterior malleolus is identified. The physician places the fractured pieces of bone into proper position and alignment. The physician may apply bone fixation devices, such as screws or pins, to secure the fractured pieces. The wound is irrigated with antibiotic solution and closed in layers. A splint, cast, or brace is applied to the leg.

27780-27781
The physician treats a fracture of the fibula without open surgery or any manipulation of the bony fragments in 27780. Separately reportable x-rays are obtained that confirm a stable fracture of the proximal fibula or shaft. The physician applies a cast or brace to the leg to secure the fracture while it heals. In 27781, separately reportable x-rays confirm a fracture that is unstable and requires manipulation. Using anesthesia as needed, the physician pushes, pulls, or maneuvers the leg until the fracture is in the proper position and alignment. A cast or brace is placed on the leg to hold the fracture in place while it heals.

27784
The physician makes an incision in the skin of the leg overlying the fractured area of the fibula. The tissues are dissected deep to the bone and the fracture is identified. Any nonviable tissue is debrided. The physician places the bony fragments into their correct position and alignment. Fixation devices, such as plates, screws, or wires may be applied to maintain the fracture reduction. With the fracture stabilized, the physician irrigates the wound with antibiotic solution. The wound is closed in layers. A cast, splint, or brace may be applied to the leg.

27786-27788
The physician treats a fracture of the distal fibula (also known as the lateral malleolus) without open surgery or any manipulation of the bones in 27786. Separately reportable x-rays confirm the fracture of the distal fibula with the bony fragments in stable position. The physician applies a cast or brace to hold the fracture in place until it heals. In 27788, separately reportable x-rays confirm a fracture that is unstable and requires manipulation. Using anesthesia as needed, the physician pushes, pulls, or maneuvers the leg until the fracture is in the proper position and alignment. A cast or brace is placed on the leg to hold the fracture in place while it heals.

27792
The physician makes an incision in the skin of the leg overlying the fractured area of the distal fibula. The tissues are dissected deep to the bone and the fracture is identified. Any nonviable tissue is debrided. The physician places the bony fragments into their correct position and alignment. Fixation devices, such as plates, screws, or wires, may be applied to maintain the fracture reduction. With the fracture stabilized, the physician irrigates the wound with antibiotic solution. The wound is closed in layers. A cast, splint, or brace may be applied to the leg.

27808-27810
The physician treats a bimalleolar fracture of the ankle without open surgery or any manipulation of the fractured pieces in 27808. A bimalleolar fracture may include the lateral and medial malleoli, the lateral and posterior malleoli, or the medial and posterior malleoli. Separately reportable x-rays confirm the fracture of the malleoli with the bony fragments in stable position. The physician applies a cast or brace to hold the fracture in place until it heals. In 27810, separately reportable x-rays confirm fractures of the malleoli that are unstable and require manipulation. Using anesthesia as needed, the physician pushes, pulls, or maneuvers the foot, ankle, and leg until the fracture is in the proper position and alignment. A cast or brace is placed on the leg to hold the fracture in place while it heals.

27814
The physician performs open treatment of a bimalleolar ankle fracture. The fracture may consist of the lateral and medial malleoli, the lateral and posterior malleoli, or the medial and posterior malleoli. The physician makes incisions on each side of the ankle overlying the fractures. Each incision is carried deep through the soft tissues and to the bone. The fractures are identified by exposing the fragments. Nonviable tissue and any intervening tissue between the ends of the fractured pieces are debrided. Each malleolus fracture is placed into its correct position one at a time. Bony fixation devices, such as metal plates, screws, wires, or pins, may be applied to stabilize the fractures. When the fractures are stabilized, the skin incisions are irrigated with antibiotic solution and closed in layers. A cast or brace may be applied to the leg.

27816-27818
The physician treats a fracture of the ankle involving all three of the malleoli (medial, lateral, and posterior) without open surgery or any manipulation of the fractured pieces in 27816. Separately reportable x-rays confirm the fracture of the malleolus of the ankle with the bony fragments in stable position. The physician applies a cast or brace to hold the fracture in place until it heals. In 27818, separately reportable x-rays confirm trimalleolar ankle fracture that is unstable and requires manipulation. Using anesthesia as needed, the physician pushes, pulls, or maneuvers the foot, ankle, and leg until the fracture is in the proper position and alignment. A cast or brace is placed on the leg to hold the fracture in place while it heals.

27822-27823
The physician makes at least two separate incisions in the skin overlying the trimalleolar fracture. This fracture involves all three malleoli: medial, lateral, and posterior. The incisions are carried deep to the bones

and the extent of each fracture is identified. Any nonviable or intervening tissue is dissected and debrided as needed. One at a time, the physician restores the fractured pieces to their correct positions. Using bony fixation devices, such as pins, plates, or screws, the physician repairs the fractures of the lateral and medial malleolus. The posterior malleolus (lip) fracture is left in position without applying fixation devices in 27822. In 27823, the posterior malleolus (lip) fracture is also repositioned to its correct position and secured similarly. Another incision may be required to obtain adequate fixation of all three fractures. The wounds are irrigated with antibiotic solution and closed in layers. A cast or brace is applied to the foot and leg.

27824-27825

The physician treats a fracture of the distal tibia extending into the ankle joint without open surgery or any manipulation of the fractured pieces. Separately reportable x-rays confirm the fracture of the distal tibia extending into the ankle joint (e.g., pilon or tibial plafond) with the bony fragments in stable position. Using anesthesia as needed, the physician applies a cast or brace to the foot and leg to hold the fracture in place until it heals. In 27825, separately reportable x-rays confirm a distal tibia fracture (e.g., pilon or tibial plafond) that is unstable and requires manipulation. Using anesthesia as needed, the physician pushes, pulls, or maneuvers the foot, ankle, and leg until the fracture is in the proper position and alignment. Traction may be applied. A cast or brace is applied to the foot and leg.

27826-27828

The physician treats a fracture of the distal tibia with fixation of the fibula only in 27826, the tibia only in 27827, or both in 27828. The physician makes an incision overlying the ankle to treat a fracture of the distal tibia, extending into the ankle joint (pilon or tibial plafond fracture). The incision is carried to the bone. Often, two or more incisions are necessary in 27828. Any nonviable tissues are dissected and debrided. The fracture pieces are placed in appropriate position. Using the fibula bone as a strut or splint, the physician may apply fixation devices such as screws or plates to stabilize the fracture. No fixation devices are applied to the tibia in 27826. In 27827, the physician applies fixation to the tibia to stabilize the fractured pieces. In 27828, fixation is applied to both the tibia and fibula. The wound is irrigated with antibiotic solution and closed in layers. A cast, brace, or splint is applied.

27829

The physician makes an incision in the skin overlying the ankle. The tissues are dissected to the distal joint between the tibia and fibula. Nonviable tissues are debrided as needed. The physician places the tibia and fibula in the correct position to reduce or realign the disruption. Fixation devices, such as screws, are applied as needed to hold the joint (also known as a syndesmosis) in the correct position. The wound is irrigated and closed in layers. A cast or brace may be applied to the leg.

27830-27831

The physician treats a dislocation of the proximal joint (near the knee) between the tibia and fibula without the use of anesthesia in 27830 or with anesthesia in 27831. Separately reportable x-rays are obtained that confirm the dislocation. No open surgery or extensive manipulation is necessary in 27830. Anesthesia is necessary in 27831 to perform manipulation of the leg and correctly aligning the bones. The physician applies a brace or splint to the leg and knee to hold the bones in appropriate position while healing takes place.

27832

The physician makes an incision overlying the joint between the tibia and fibula and near the knee to reposition a dislocation of these two bones. Tissue is dissected to the joint and the joint is exposed. The physician identifies the dislocation and treats it one of several ways. The area may be treated by holding the joint together with fixation devices such as screws, pins, or wires. The physician may excise or remove a piece of the proximal fibula. The physician irrigates the wound and closes it in layers. A brace or splint may be applied to protect the joint and maintain its position until it heals.

27840-27842

The physician treats a dislocation of the ankle joint without anesthesia in 27840. A cast or brace is applied to stabilize the dislocation. In 27842, anesthesia is required and manipulation of the dislocated ankle joint may be performed. Percutaneous skeletal fixation, such as pins, may also be applied. The physician makes small incisions in the skin and inserts the pins through the skin and into the bones of the ankle joint. No open incisions are necessary. When the ankle joint is stabilized, the physician applies a cast or brace.

27846-27848

The physician treats a dislocation of the ankle joint with open surgery. An incision is made overlying the ankle joint and is extended deep to the joint. More than one incision may be necessary in 27848. Tissues are dissected around the joint. The joint may need to be surgically opened to restore it in the appropriate position. Percutaneous skeletal fixation may be applied to stabilize the dislocation. If applied, the physician makes small incisions in the skin and inserts the pins through the skin and into the bones. No repair or internal fixation is necessary in 27846. In 27848, bony fixation devices, such as screws, plates, or wires are necessary. External fixation devices may also be applied on the outside of the ankle to maintain joint position. The physician irrigates the joint and wound and closes the wound in layers. A brace, splint, or cast is applied to maintain the relocated joint.

27860

The physician performs manipulation of the ankle with the patient under general anesthesia. The physician pushes, pulls, and maneuvers the foot, ankle, and leg to treat a stiff ankle. The physician may apply traction devices to the ankle to help perform the manipulations. Traction is removed.

27870
The physician performs surgery on the ankle to fuse the ankle joint. The physician makes two or more incisions overlying the ankle joint, exposing the joint. The incisions are individually extended deep to the joint. The physician opens the joint through an arthrotomy incision. Tissue is dissected and debrided as necessary. The surfaces of the joint are prepared so that they can be fused together. Preparation includes debriding and smoothing so that an intimate fit can be accomplished. Numerous methods can be used to fuse the joint, including screws, plates, or external fixation devices. The physician irrigates the joint and closes the arthrotomy. The incisions are irrigated and closed in layers. A cast or brace is applied to hold the newly fused joint in place until the bones heal together.

27871
The periosteum is stripped from the anteroposterior fibula, the lateral talus, and the calcaneus. The distal portion of the fibula is removed about 1.5 centimeters above the level of the distal tibia and the dissection is carried over the anterior distal tibia to the medial malleolus. The physician makes an incision along the tibia and the periosteum is stripped distally to the level of the calcaneus. Using a saw, the physician cuts through the neck of talus to mobilize and remove the talus as one large fragment or morselized fragments. With the talus gone, the calcaneus can be seen. The distal end of the tibia is removed perpendicular to the long axis of the tibia. The physician uses a saw to remove the dorsal calcaneus and to create a flat surface for the arthrodesis. The two flat surfaces of the distal tibia and dorsal calcaneus are brought together to establish a varus/valgus and dorsiflexion/ plantar flexion alignment. A cut is made along the anterior tibia parallel to the cut made in the neck of the talus which creates a flat surface for apposing the neck of the talus. The bone surfaces are deeply scaled to prepare for internal fixation. Kirschner wires are used to place the tibia and calcaneus in apposition. Using an anterior cruciate guide, a pin is guided form the calcaneus across the fusion site to the anterior cortex of the tibia. Once satisfactory fixation has been achieved, cannulated screws are placed through the neck of the talus into the tibia. The wound is closed over a drain and a dressing incorporating plaster splints is applied. Marcaine is instilled through the drain tube into the wound.

27880
The physician performs an amputation of the leg below the knee. The physician makes an incision in the skin of the leg at the level where the amputation is to take place. The incision is carried completely around the leg. The tissue is dissected to the bones. The large arteries, veins, and nerves are identified and tied off prior to being cut. Tissue is further debrided as needed. The tibia and fibula are identified. The physician surgically cuts the bones, completing the amputation. The wound is irrigated and closed in layers, including the skin. A soft dressing is placed over the stump.

27881
The physician performs an amputation of the leg below the knee and the fitting technique for an artificial leg. The physician makes an incision in the skin of the leg at the level where the amputation will be performed. The incision is extended completely around the leg. The tissue is dissected to the bones. The large arteries, veins, and nerves are identified and tied off prior to being cut. Tissue is further debrided as needed. The physician surgically cuts the tibia and fibula individually to complete the amputation. The wound is irrigated with antibiotic solution. The wound and skin are closed in layers. The remaining stump is fitted with a cast to prepare it for eventual placement of an artificial leg.

27882
The physician places a pneumatic tourniquet on the thigh. The limb is measured for optimal stump length and marks are made for the optimal amputation site. Progressive incisions are made through soft tissues, and nerves and vessels are ligated. The tibia and fibula are bisected with a circular saw, rounded, and smoothed. Bleeding points are electrocoagulated and nerves are cut, allowing retraction. This type of amputation does not usually include wound closure; however, skin flaps may be tacked to prevent further retraction. The tourniquet is released and a soft dressing is applied. Debridement may be performed every couple of days until infection and necrotic tissues are removed.

27884
The physician performs a secondary closure of a wound or scar revision of an existing amputation. Open wounds are debrided as necessary and scars are excised. The physician dissects the tissue around the tibia and fibula. In this procedure, no additional bone is sectioned. The wounds are irrigated with antibiotic solution and closed in layers. Any previous wounds left open are also irrigated and closed. Any scars that may cause problems with the use of an artificial leg are excised and revised. When closing the wound, opposing tissue layers are sewn under physiologic tension, and care must be taken so that the final closure is neither too light nor too loose. The stump may be placed in a soft dressing.

27886
The physician performs an amputation on the leg below the knee in a patient who has already undergone amputation. The physician identifies the additional area of the remaining stump requiring amputation. An incision is made in the skin at the appropriate site and extended laterally and medially around the leg. The tissue is dissected to the bones. The large arteries, veins, and nerves are identified and tied off prior to being cut. Tissue is further debrided as needed. The physician surgically cuts the tibia and fibula individually to complete the reamputation. The

wound is irrigated with antibiotic solution. The wound and skin may be closed in layers. If infection is present, the incision may be temporarily left open to drain.

27888
The physician performs an amputation of the foot near the ankle while leaving much of the soft tissue of the heel intact. The physician makes a long incision in the skin overlying the ankle at about the level of the medial and lateral malleoli. The incision is carried deep to the ankle joint. The talus bone is removed from the joint and the incision is carried to the heel bone (calcaneus). The soft tissues of the bottom of the heel are kept with the leg. The skin on the bottom of the foot is cut to complete the amputation of the foot. The major arteries, veins, and nerves are identified and ligated. The wound is irrigated with antibiotic solution and may be closed in layers. If infection of the foot is present, this operation is performed in two stages. The amputation is performed and later the soft tissues and skin are repaired and closed. A soft dressing is applied.

27889
The physician performs an amputation of the ankle directly through the joint with removal of the foot. An incision is made overlying the ankle joint. The incision is carried around the ankle and deep to the joint. The tissues are dissected and the major arteries, veins, and nerves are identified and individually ligated. The ankle joint is opened through an arthrotomy incision and the foot is dislocated from the ankle joint and removed. Tissue is debrided as necessary. Muscles and tendons are attached to the remaining tibia and fibula bones as appropriate. The wound is irrigated with antibiotic solution and may be closed in layers. If infection is present, the incision is temporarily left open to drain. A soft dressing, cast, or splint may be applied.

27892
The physician performs surgery on the anterior and/or lateral compartments of the leg reducing high pressure within the compartments. The physician makes incisions in the skin overlying the respective compartments. Multiple incisions may be required. The incisions are extended deep to the muscle fascia. Long incisions are made in the fascia to relieve the pressure. The muscles are examined and any nonviable muscle or nerve tissue is debrided and removed. The physician may also debride and remove nonviable muscle tissue from within the compartments. The incisions in the fascia and skin are left open.

27893
The physician performs surgery on the posterior compartments of the leg to reduce high pressure within the compartments. The physician also removes muscle tissue from within the compartments that has become nonviable because of the high pressures. The physician makes incisions in the skin overlying the posterior compartments of the leg. Several incisions may be required. These are extended deep to the muscle fascia. Long incisions are made in the fascia the full length of the compartments. The underlying muscles are examined. Any and all nonviable muscle and nerve tissue is debrided and removed. The fascia and skin incisions are left open.

27894
The physician performs surgery on all the compartments of the leg to reduce high pressures within the compartments. Muscle and nerve tissue that has become nonviable because of the high pressures is debrided. The physician makes multiple incisions in the skin overlying the respective compartments of the leg. These incisions are carried deep to the muscle fascia. Long incisions are made in the fascia the full length of the muscles. The muscles in each compartment are examined. Any nonviable muscle or nerve tissue is debrided. The incisions in the skin and the fascia are left open.

28001
The physician performs this procedure to correct bursa, fluid-filled sacks that reduce friction. The physician makes an incision over the bursa. Soft tissues are retracted and an incision is made in the bursa to drain fluid. An antibiotic is often injected to clear the infection. The incision is sutured and dressed.

28002-28003
An incision is made through skin and fascia to expose the infection. The infected tissue is removed, and the bursal sac may be removed or simply incised and drained. If the wound is large, the physician may leave the incision open after irrigating the area, treating it with antibiotic, and packing it with petroleum gauze. The wound heals from inside. Report 28003 if more than one incision is necessary.

28005
The physician incises the bone cortex of infected bone in the foot to treat an abscess or osteomyelitis. The physician makes an incision over the affected area. Dissection is carried through the soft tissues to expose the bone. The periosteum is split and reflected from the bone overlying the infected area. A curette may be used to scrape away the abscess or infected portion to healthy bony tissue or drill holes may be made through the cortex into the medullary canal in a window outline around the infected or abscessed bone. The area is drained and debrided of infected bony and soft tissue. The physician irrigates the area with antibiotic solution, the periosteum is closed over the bone, and the soft tissues are sutured closed; or the wound is packed and left open, allowing the area to drain. Secondary closure is performed approximately three weeks later. Dressings are changed daily. A splint may be applied to limit movement.

28008
There are two common techniques used in fasciotomies of the foot and/or toes. For flexion contracture of the toe, a plantar incision is made. A transverse division of the fibrotic and contracted cord of plantar fascia in the foot and/or toe is performed through one or more incisions. A percutaneous procedure may be performed instead which involves

making a stab incision over the center of the plantar fascia where it attaches to the calcaneus. The plantar fascia is transversely divided.

28010-28011
This procedure is performed to correct mallet or hammer toe. The physician makes a small incision at the crease of the toe where the tendon is restricted. The tendon is released from the bone and the toe is straightened. The incision is sutured and dressing applied. Report 28011 if more than one tendon is being straightened.

28020-28024
The physician performs an arthrotomy of an intertarsal or tarsometatarsal joint in 28020, a metatarsophalangeal joint in 28022, or an interphalangeal joint in 28024 that includes exploration, drainage, or removal of any loose or foreign body. An incision is made over the joint to be exposed. The soft tissues are dissected away and the joint capsule is exposed and incised. The joint space is explored, any necrotic tissue is removed, and infection or abnormal fluid is drained. If a foreign body is present (e.g., bullet, nail, gravel), it is exposed and removed. The wound is irrigated with antibiotic solution. The physician may leave the wound packed open with daily dressing changes to allow for drainage and secondary healing by granulation. If the incision is repaired, drain tubes may be inserted and the incision is closed in layers with sutures, staples, and/or Steri-strips.

28035
The physician releases the tarsal tunnel, decompressing the posterior tibial nerve. The tarsal tunnel is located on the inside of the ankle. A curved incision is made along the inner ankle, behind the medial malleolus. Dissection exposes the flexor retinaculum. The retinaculum is released along the tunnel. The posterior tibial nerve is identified by blunt dissection and traced as it courses down through the tarsal tunnel. Three branches of the posterior tibial nerve are also traced at the point. Once the posterior tibial nerve and its terminal branches are released, the nerve is inspected to see if any other constrictions are present. The incision is closed layers without closing the retinaculum.

28043-28045 [28039, 28041]
The physician removes a tumor from the soft tissue of the foot or toe that is located in the subcutaneous tissue in 28039 and 28043 and in the deep soft tissue, below the fascial plane, or within the muscle in 28041 and 28045. With the proper anesthesia administered, the physician makes an incision in the skin overlying the mass and dissects down to the tumor. The extent of the tumor is identified and a dissection is undertaken all the way around the tumor. A portion of neighboring soft tissue may also be removed to ensure adequate removal of all tumor tissue. A drain may be inserted and the incision is repaired with layers of sutures, staples, or Steri-strips. Report 28043 for excision of a subcutaneous tumor whose resected area is less than 1.5 cm and 28039 for a resected area that is 1.5 cm or greater. Report 28045 for excision of a subfascial or intramuscular tumor whose resected area is less than 1.5 cm and 28041 for a resected area 1.5 cm or greater.

28046-28047
The physician performs a radical resection (excision) of a tumor (i.e., sarcoma) from the foot or toe, not involving bone. The tumor may be malignant or an aggressive benign tumor of the connective tissue. An incision is made over the tumor and dissection exposes it. The tumor and any adjacent tissue that may be affected by the spread of the neoplasm are excised. Large resections may be needed. The type and stage of the lesion determine the extent of the tumor margin resection area. Muscle or fascia may need to be repaired and drains may be placed. The surgical wound is closed using simple or intermediate repair or separately reportable complex closure, adjacent tissue transfer, or graft. Report 28046 for a resected area of less than 3 cm and 28047 for a resected area of 3 cm or greater.

28050-28054
Arthrotomy is performed to determine the type and extent of a growth. The physician makes the incision at the joint line and opens the skin to remove a part of the growth. The incision is often left open to allow for pathology confirmation of the growth's composition and allow for synovectomy if malignant. Once complete, the wound is sutured closed. Report 28050 for an intertarsal or tarsometatarsal joint; report 28052 for metatarsophalangeal joint; and report 28054 for an interphalangeal joint.

28055
The patient lies in the supine position and is placed under general anesthesia. A physician, using loupe magnification, marks the dorsal side of the affected web space, including both metatarsal heads and metatarsophalangeal joints. The physician makes a straight dorsal skin incision midline in the intermetatarsal space beginning at the metatarsal heads and extending to the terminal skin fold of the web space. A blade is used to deepen the incision through subcutaneous tissue to the level of the interosseous fascia. The layer is split to expose the transverse metatarsal ligament, which is also divided. The physician uses a laminar to spread the metatarsal heads and the nerve is dissected out in the web space to its bifurcation. The inflamed bursal tissue is removed, though the plantar fat pad generally is left intact. The physician dissects the nerve 3 cm and cleanly divides at its proximal point. The wound is irrigated. The subcutaneous tissue and skin are sutured and a compression dressing is used to protect the wound.

28060-28062
Heel pain originates deep within the foot, directly on the heel bone or within the foot's connective tissues, called the fascia. Pain can result when these tissues become irritated or inflamed, or when small spurs

Musculoskeletal

grow on the heel bone. Prior to surgery a tourniquet is applied to the ankle. The surgeon makes a longitudinal incision inside the heel and the fat that has filled the wound is separated with a key elevator. The medial third of the plantar fascia is identified using right angle retractors under direct vision. Report 28062 when the medial third of the plantar fascia is incised and a 1-centimeter segment is removed. The tourniquet is released and the skin closed with nonabsorbable sutures. A dressing and a removable walking boot are applied. The sutures are removed in about three weeks and weightbearing is increased; though the radical procedure increases postoperative recovery period.

28070-28072
The physician makes an incision on the top of the foot over the small bones of the foot in front of the ankle. The skin is reflected to expose the tendons. They are divided and the soft tissue reflected to expose the bones. The synovium is the lining between the bones that becomes thickened and inflamed with some disease processes. The synovium is removed by careful dissection. The bones are allowed back into their original position and the skin is closed with sutures. Report 28072 if the area of incision is further toward the toes, between the long bones of the foot and the phalanges (toes).

28080
Surgery for Morton's neuroma involves removal of the fibrous nerve growth from between the toes. The physician places a tourniquet at the ankle and a small incision is made on the top of the foot between the third and fourth metatarsal bones. The soft tissue is reflected in the web space and the bones are separated. Pressure is applied to the bottom of the foot under the web space causing the neuroma to protrude upward. The neuroma is removed and the nerve trunk is cut to prevent regrowth. The tourniquet is removed and the incision is closed with sutures.

28086-28088
A synovectomy is performed to relieve pain in the active stages of disease before joint destruction. For this procedure description the flexor hallucis longus (FHL) tendon was used as the example. The patient is placed in a supine position with a tourniquet placed around the ankle. The physician makes a 5-centimeter incision behind the medial malleolus and toward the navicular. The neurovascular bundle is retracted, revealing the FHL in its fibro-osseous sheath. The reticulum is released to the level of the sustentaculum tali and the tendon is inspected. A tenosynovectomy is performed and the tenosynovial tissue is debrided. Any nodules are excised and longitudinal tears are repaired. The FHL is released until the retinaculum no longer prohibits its motion. The distal soft tissue is approximated and the skin is sutured closed. A below-knee splint or cast is applied. This procedure varies depending upon which tendon is affected. Report 28088 when the affected tendon is the extensor tendon.

28090-28092
The physician makes an incision through the skin on the foot to expose a portion of the tendon requiring removal and suturing ends together, or a portion of the joint capsule or lining of the joint may be removed from the foot. The lesion, usually a cyst or benign ganglion growth, is excised or removed from the tissue surrounding the tendon. Every effort is made not to disrupt the tendon itself. The incision is closed and a soft dressing is applied. Report 28092 if the lesion is located in the toes. Report each toe separately.

28100-28103
A bone cyst or benign tumor of the talus or calcaneus is removed. The physician makes an incision in the ankle or heel overlying the cyst or tumor. The skin and underlying soft tissues are reflected to expose the periosteum, which is separated from the bone. Curettes or osteotomes are used to scrape or cut the lesion from the bone. Once the benign tumor or cyst is removed and healthy bone tissue is present, the periosteum is repositioned and the incision is repaired in layers. If the bone defect created requires a graft for repair, the physician obtains the necessary size bone graft from a separate donor site on the patient (usually the iliac crest) and packs it into the site where the tumor or bone cyst was removed or uses a bone bank allograft. Report 28102 if an autograft is obtained and 28103 if an allograft is used.

28104-28107
A bone cyst or benign tumor of the tarsal or metatarsal is removed. The physician makes an incision in the foot overlying the cyst or tumor. The skin and underlying soft tissues are reflected to expose the periosteum, which is separated from the bone. Curettes or osteotomes are used to scrape or cut the lesion from the bone. Once the benign tumor or cyst is removed and healthy bone tissue is present, the periosteum is repositioned and the incision is repaired in layers. If the bone defect created requires a graft for repair, the physician obtains the necessary size bone graft from a separate donor site on the patient (usually the iliac crest) and packs it into the site where the tumor or bone cyst was removed or uses a bone bank allograft. Report 28106 if an autograft is obtained and 28107 if an allograft is used.

28108
A bone cyst or benign tumor of the phalanges of the foot is removed. The physician makes an incision in the affected toe overlying the cyst or tumor. The skin and underlying soft tissues are reflected to expose the periosteum, which is separated from the bone. Curettes or osteotomes are used to scrape or cut the lesion from the bone. Once the benign tumor or cyst is removed and healthy bone tissue is present, the periosteum is repositioned and the incision is repaired in layers.

28110
The physician makes a lateral incision over the distal third of the fifth metatarsal bone to expose the metatarsal head. An osteotome is used to remove the

lateral extension of the bone (bunionette). The cut is made along the shaft of the bone. The wound is irrigated and the soft tissues are sutured. Soft dressing is applied and weight bearing is allowed as tolerated.

28111-28114

The patient is placed under regional anesthesia and an ankle tourniquet is applied. The physician incises the first metatarsophalangeal joint and inserts a Weitlaner retractor into the wound to remove the joint capsule as well as any proliferative synovial tissue. The physician detaches the adductor hallucis tendon from the base of the phalanx and cuts the metatarsal head and base with an osteotome. A longitudinal incision is made in the second and fourth dorsal web spaces, which exposes the base of the phalanx for excision with a bone cutter. The same is done for all the lesser toes. The physician uses blunt dissection to strip the plantar structures that are around the metatarsal head and places them on the plantar aspect of the foot. The fat pad is returned to its position under the metatarsal heads. If an arthrodesis is performed, the physician drives Steinmann pins through the tip of the toe and back across to the site of the arthrodesis. The skin is sutured closed and a dressing applied. Report 28111 for a complete excision of the first metatarsal head. Report 28112 for the excision of the second, third, or fourth metatarsal heads and 28113 for the fifth metatarsal head. Report 28114 when using a Clayton type procedure in the approach to the metatarsal heads. The physician makes an incision over the metatarsal heads that curves to overlie the first metatarsophalangeal joint. The exposed extensor tendons are retracted or, if contracted, cut in the line of the incision. The physician opens the incision by depressing the toes and the bases of the proximal phalanges, thus, delivering the heads into the wound. The metatarsal heads are dissected free with partial excision of the proximal phalanges, excluding the first metatarsal. Only the subcutaneous tissue and skin are sutured. If the extensor tendon has been cut, it is resutured.

28116

A tarsal coalition is an abnormal fusion of the tarsal bones or small bones of the foot near the ankle. A common procedure is for the physician to reproduce the division of the calcaneus and the navicular. An incision is made on the dorsal aspect of the foot. The soft tissues and tendons are reflected to expose the bones. An osteotome is used to divide the calcaneus and the navicular. The ends of the bones are smoothed for better articulation or movement of the joint. The wound is irrigated and sutured closed.

28118

The patient is placed supine and the physician makes a lateral or medial incision of the ankle dependent upon the location of the patient's complaint. The bursa and tendons are dissected to the insertion point of the Achilles tendon. The periosteum of the calcaneus is incised and resected. An osteotome is used to remove the prominence of the calcaneal tuber. The remaining periosteum is rasped and trimmed to remove any sharp edges. Bone anchors and/or sutures may be placed to augment the Achilles tendon insertion if it is thought to be compromised during surgery. Any procedures performed on the Achilles tendon, such as debridement, are reported separately. The incisions are closed and the patient is placed in a short leg cast with no weight bearing instructions.

28119

The physician applies a tourniquet to the ankle. The medial third of the plantar fascia is incised and, through the incision, the abductor hallucis muscle is elevated and a portion of the deep fascia of the abductor hallucis released, if required. To excise the spur, a key elevator is placed forward and back of the spur and the spur is transected with an osteotome. The cut spur is removed using a rongeur and the bone edges smoothed. Thrombin or bone wax can be packed at the cut edge of the bone. In some cases, part of the flexor digitorum brevis must be removed for a calcaneal spur that is deeply embedded. Once the spur is removed, the margins are smoothed with a bone rasp. The wound is irrigated and a dressing is applied.

28120-28124

The physician performs a partial excision of the talus or calcaneus in 28120, a tarsal or metatarsal bone in 28122, or the phalanx of a toe in 28124 to remove infected bone or bony prominence. An incision is made over the affected part of the foot, ankle, heel, or toe and the underlying soft tissues are divided to expose the bone. The periosteum is reflected and the infected portion of bone is removed and irrigated. The excavation of bone may excise a crater-like piece, leave a small saucer-like shelf depression in the bone, or may remove a portion of the shaft (diaphysis) of a long bone. If a significant portion of bone is removed, the physician may use bone graft material to fill the cavity left in the bone. The periosteum is closed over the bone, the soft tissues are sutured closed, and a soft dressing is applied. A short leg cast may be applied to keep the foot and ankle in position.

28126

This procedure is often performed in conjunction with other separately reportable procedures in an effort to correct alignment of the toes. A dorsal longitudinal incision is made on top of the foot where the toe joins the foot. The soft tissues are reflected to expose the bone. A wedge of bone is cut out of and removed from the proximal phalanx. The remaining portions of the bone are approximated to realign the toe. The bones are held in this position by a Kirschner wire that is drilled and placed through the end of the bone. The wound is sutured and the foot is elevated for 72 hours. After that time the patient is allowed to bear weight as tolerated in a wood soled shoe.

28130

The physician performs surgery on the astragalus, the bone that articulates with the fibula and tibia to form the ankle joint. The physician makes a curved incision overlying the lateral part of the ankle. The incision is carried down to the joint capsule of the subtalar and talonavicular joints. The capsule is excised and the surrounding ligaments are divided. The talus is removed. If further correction is needed, the physician may elect to excise the navicular bone in a procedure to be reported separately. The calcaneus is usually placed in the ankle mortise and held in place by inserting a Kirschner wire through the heel into the tibia. The incision is closed in layers.

28140
The physician makes an incision on the dorsal aspect of the foot over the affected metatarsal. With the patient under anesthesia, the physician dissects to the metatarsal bone. The affected part of the metatarsal is cut with a bone saw on either end and removed. The incision is closed in layers with sutures, staples, and Steri-strips.

28150
The physician removes a single phalanx of a toe. An incision is made over the involved toe. This is carried deep through the fascia to the bone. The specific phalanx is identified. Using blunt and sharp dissection, the phalanx is isolated and exposed. The physician removes the bone as indicated. The wound is irrigated and the tissues are closed in layers to include the skin. Code for each phalanx removed.

28153
The physician resects the condyle of the distal end of the phalanx, amputating the toe. The physician makes a curvilinear incision to fashion "fish-mouth" skin flaps side-to-side or dorsally to plantarly. The amputation can be done as a disarticulation or by resecting through the bone. If the head of the toe is disarticulated, the capsular ligaments are severed and the distal phalanx is removed. The capsule is approximated with sutures. If the bone is resected, a power saw is used to transect the proximal phalanx. A drain may be used. The skin flaps are approximated with sutures and a compression dressing is applied. Report each toe separately.

28160
The physician removes a part of the phalanges or interphalangeal joint for problems including trauma, infection, tumors, and gangrene resulting from diabetes. The physician makes an oblique incision over the toe and dissection exposes the affected bone. Using a small bone cutter, the physician excises the involved bone that may include the interphalangeal joint. Any angular areas of bone are rounded to relieve internal and external pressure. Sutures are used to close the incision and skin flaps without tension.

28171-28175
The physician performs a radical resection (excision) of a tumor. Radical tumor removal involves complete removal of the affected tarsal bone (28171), including the navicular, cuboid, or any of the three cuneiform bones, and the soft tissues that surround it. This is performed in order to prevent spreading of the tumor to adjacent tissues. If it is determined that the foot is going to be spared from amputation, the affected bone and soft tissues would be removed through a dorsal incision at the front of the ankle. The skin and tendons are reflected and the bone is identified. The capsule is released and the bone is removed in one piece. Tissue samples are taken to determine the extent of tumor growth and need of soft tissue removal. Once complete, the wound is closed with sutures and dressing and cast are applied. Report 28173 if the tumor resection is performed on the metatarsal bone(s) in which case an incision is made longitudinally over the affected metatarsal bone(s). Report 28175 if the tumor resection involves the phalanges of the toe (proximal, middle, or distal).

28190-28192
A foreign body located within the tissue of the foot is removed and the wound is irrigated and closed, if applicable. A dressing is applied and aftercare may include antibiotic injection into the wound and/or orally. Weight bearing is allowed as the wound heals. Report 28190 if the foreign body is located beneath the skin in the subcutaneous tissue. Report 28192 if the foreign body lies deeper in the foot below the subcutaneous layer.

28193
A foreign body located within the tissue of the foot is removed. An incision may be made to reach the foreign body and the wound is irrigated and closed. Repair of any torn tendons, nerves, and/or blood supply is performed during the foreign body removal. A dressing is applied and aftercare may include antibiotic injection into the wound and/or orally. Weight bearing is allowed as the wound heals.

28200-28202
If the tendon has ruptured, surgery may be required to repair the ruptured tendon or to replace it with a tendon graft. Usually, another tendon in the foot, such as the tendon that bends the four lesser toes is used as a tendon graft to replace the function of the posterior tibial tendon. In cases of a fixed flatfoot, the physician may perform a fusion (or arthrodesis) of the foot that requires the removal of a joint between two bones and the two bones on either side of the joint are allowed to grow together. This type of operation is used to stop pain from joints or to realign the bones. Several joints must be fused to control the flatfoot after a posterior tibial tendon rupture. Report 28202 if a free graft is used for the repair. The patient may be placed in a cast for six to eight weeks.

28208-28210
A dorsal incision is made on top of the foot over the injured extensor tendon. The skin is reflected and the ends of the tendon are exposed. They are cleaned for easier attachment. The ends are brought together and sutured. The wound is closed and a soft dressing and cast are applied for 3 weeks. Report 28210 if secondary with free graft, each tendon.

28220-28222
The patient is in a supine position and general anesthesia is administered. A tourniquet is placed on

the thigh to create a bloodless field desirable for the procedure. An incision is made over the flexor hallucis longus (FHL); a procedure often used to alleviate the pain associated with "dancer's tendonitis." The deep fascia is divided and the surgeon retracts the neurovascular bundle. The fascia is opened and the surgeon frees the tendon from any surrounding adhesions. The tendon is retracted and inspected for tears that should be debrided or repaired. The wound is irrigated and closed in layers with catgut. A plaster cast or splint is applied. Report 28222 when the procedure is performed on multiple tendons.

28225-28226

The patient is in a supine position and general anesthesia is administered. A tourniquet is placed on the thigh to create a bloodless field desirable for the procedure. The foot and great toe is placed in a dorsiflex position to simplify finding of the proximal and distal ends of the extensor hallucis longus. An incision is made over the dorsal aspect of the first metatarsal. The fascia is opened and the physician frees the tendon from the any surrounding adhesions. The tendon is retracted and inspected for tears that should be debrided or repaired. The wound is irrigated and closed in layers with catgut A short-leg compression dressing incorporating plaster splints is applied. Report 28226 when the procedure is performed on multiple tendons.

28230

A small incision is made on the back of the ankle and a sharp blade knife is inserted into the Achilles tendon and rotated medially and laterally. The foot is forced into dorsiflexion to stretch the tendon to the appropriate length. Direct pressure is applied to control bleeding. A suture is made in the incision and a dressing is applied.

28232-28234

This procedure is often done for repair of hammer toe. A small incision is made on the crease of the toe on the bottom of the foot. The skin is reflected and the tendon is exposed. The tendon is released from its attachment site, allowing the toe to extend. This is usually accompanied by other procedures. The incision is closed with sutures and a soft dressing is applied. Report 28234 if the incision is made on the dorsal toe and the extensor tendon is released.

28238

The physician advances the posterior tibial tendon with excision of the accessory navicular bone. The physician makes a longitudinal skin incision on the medial side of the foot from the tip of the medial malleolus to the medial cuneiform. Dissection exposes the posterior tibialis tendon. The accessory navicular is identified and removed with sharp dissection. The physician detaches the distal portion of the posterior tibialis tendon and drills a hole through the navicular. The tendon is passed through the drill hole and sutured back to itself or to surrounding periosteal tissue. Wounds are sutured closed.

28240

A dorsal incision is made over the first metatarsal bone extending to the middle of the big toe. The skin is reflected to expose the underlying soft tissues. The abductor hallucis muscle is identified and its distal insertion is removed from the bone of the big toe. This allows the toe to move back out into proper alignment. The incision is closed with sutures and a soft dressing is applied. The patient can bear weight while using a wood soled shoe.

28250

A longitudinal incision is made on the medial side of the heel and is carried distally to the other side of the heel in order to expose the underlying soft tissues. The superficial and deep layers of the plantar fascia are separated from the muscle and fat by blunt dissection. This allows for freedom of movement of the fascia and releases the scar tissue. Once sufficient movement is obtained, the incision is sutured and a soft dressing is applied. Weight bearing is allowed as the wound heals.

28260-28262

This procedure is often performed in an effort to correct club foot deformity. A medial incision is made on the inner ankle to expose the underlying tissues. The skin and tendons are reflected to expose the joint capsule of the talonavicular joint. The joint capsule is cut by sharp dissection to release the deformity of the mid foot. Several releases can be made from this approach. A particular order is followed in order to obtain the appropriate amount of release. The incision is closed with sutures and a cast is applied. Report 28261 if tendon lengthening is also performed. Report 28262 when posterior, medial, and subtalar soft tissue contractures are released to correct severe clubfoot deformity. The patient is placed supine and a posteromedial skin incision is made. The tibialis posterior, flexor digitorum longus, and flexor hallucis longus are identified and mobilized. The contracted tendons are lengthened. The talonavicular and talotibial joint capsules are incised. The joint capsules are cut by sharp dissection to release the deformity. Bones are placed in correct alignment and secured with a single Kirschner wire.

28264

Two straight incisions are made, one between the first and second metatarsals and the second in line with the fourth metatarsal. The tendons and nerve bundles are reflected to expose the intermetatarsal space. The ligament is divided by careful dissection. The dorsal capsule of the first tarsometatarsal joint is divided. The second tarsometatarsal joint is identified and divided. Similar incisions are made at the bases of other metatarsals. When sufficient motion is gained, the bleeding is controlled and the incisions are closed with sutures. A series of short leg casts are applied for eight to 12 weeks.

28270-28272

An incision is above the metatarsophalangeal or interphalangeal joint to expose the anatomy. The tendons and nerve bundles are reflected to expose the joint space. When sufficient motion is gained, the bleeding is controlled and the incisions are closed with sutures. In 28270, the capsule of a metatarsophalangeal joint is divided. This procedure may also include associated tendon lengthening or tenorrhaphy. In 28272, the capsule of an interphalangeal joint is divided.

28280

This procedure is performed when there is a deformity of the foot where toes are missing and a large gap exists between the toes present. A dorsal incision is made along the web space extending to the ends of both toes. The skin is reflected and the alignment of the bones are corrected with osteotomies of the base of the proximal phalanx. The toes are approximated and the incisions closed bringing the toes together and eliminating the gap between them. This produces an artificial syndactylism or webbing of the toes. A soft dressing is applied and weight bearing is allowed in two to three weeks.

28285

Hammertoe describes an abnormal flexion posture of the proximal interphalangeal joint of one of the lesser toes. Conservative treatment is usually unsuccessful. The physician makes an elliptical incision over the proximal interphalangeal joint 5 mm to 6 mm wide. A portion of the extensor tendon and joint capsule under the skin is removed. The collateral ligaments are cut to allow the toe to be flexed to 90 degrees. The head and neck of the proximal phalanx are removed with a small power blade saw and the ends of the bones are smoothed. The toe is checked for ROM and the extensor tendon is reattached and the incision is closed with sutures.

28286

An elliptical shaped incision is made in the skin under the fifth toe. The soft tissues are reflected to expose the underlying structures. The proximal phalanx is removed leaving a space between the base of the metatarsal and the distal phalanx. The deep tissues and skin incisions are closed with sutures.

28288

The physician surgically removes a portion of a metatarsal head of the foot. A separate incision is made for each involved bone in the dorsal aspect of the foot. The tendons are retracted and preserved. The incision is carried deep to the particular metatarsal head. The bony spurs or prominences are excised from the head using appropriate surgical instruments. The physician debrides and smooths the remaining bone. The wound is irrigated and closed in layers. Code for each metatarsal head removed.

28289-28291

The physician corrects a hallux rigidus deformity and performs a cheilectomy. Hallux rigidus is a condition caused by degenerative (DJD) arthritic changes at the first metatarsophalangeal joint, causing pain, limited range of motion, and dorsiflexion. In the context of this procedure, a cheilectomy refers to excision of part of the lip of the first metatarsophalangeal joint. The podiatrist makes a dorsal incision over the first metatarsophalangeal joint. The extensor hallucis longus tendon is retracted and the joint capsule is entered. Osteophytes and part of the metatarsal head are excised. Bony irregularities may be removed using a chisel and edges smoothed with a rasp. When adequate dorsiflexion (60 to 80 degrees) is obtained, the capsule is closed, the tendon is returned to its correct anatomical position, and the skin is closed with sutures. Report 28291 when the procedure includes an implant.

28292

The physician surgically corrects a bunion of the foot using various methods. In one, the physician makes an incision along the medial aspect (inside) of the big toe. The incision is carried deep to the metatarsophalangeal (MP) joint. The median eminence and one-third of the base of the proximal phalanx are resected. This is followed by repair of the plantar plate and stabilization with a longitudinal K-wire. In an alternate procedure, the adductor tendon and transverse metatarsal ligament are released through an incision made between the first and second toe. Following the release of the contractured lateral structures, the subluxated first MP joint is reduced and the median eminence is excised. The medial capsule of the first MP joint is imbricated through a medial arthrotomy incision. In yet another method, the first metatarsal head and its articular cartilage are removed, and the remaining bone is restructured. Excision of a medial exostosis is performed. The external joint capsule is configured so that it can be used as cartilage between the metatarsal bone and the base of the first proximal phalanx. Fixation devices may hold the bone fragments in position. The procedure includes a sesamoidectomy and resection of the proximal phalanx base, when performed. The wound is closed in layers after thorough irrigation.

28296

The physician treats a bunion of the foot by performing a distal metatarsal osteotomy, a cut in the first metatarsal bone, using various methods. In one, the physician makes an incision in the skin over the distal (furthest point of attachment) part of the foot and carries it deep to the bone. A "V" or chevron-shaped cut is made near the end of the bone. Tissue is dissected and debrided as needed. The bony eminence, or bunion, is removed from the first metatarsal head. The pieces of bone are realigned to their correct position. Fixation devices may hold the bone fragments in position. Removal of the sesamoid may also be included in this procedure. The wound is closed in layers after thorough irrigation.

[28295]

The physician performs a proximal metatarsal osteotomy, a cut in the first metatarsal bone, to treat a bunion of the foot. In one method, the physician makes an incision in the skin over the top of the foot from the medial cuneiform to the base of the proximal (nearer to the center) phalanx while identifying and protecting nearby neurovascular structures. Following release of the adductor hallucis tendon, the incision is carried distally down to the metatarsophalangeal joint capsule. The capsule is lifted from the metatarsal head and proximal phalanx base and the medial eminence excised. The long extensor tendon is then retracted and the base of the first metatarsal exposed, an osteotomy performed, and the metatarsal realigned and fixated. Removal of the sesamoid may also be included in this procedure. The wound is closed in layers after thorough irrigation.

28297

The physician treats a bunion of the foot using any method in which the joint between the first metatarsal bone and medial cuneiform bone is fused (arthrodesis). The physician makes an incision in the skin between the first and second toes on the top of the foot. The incision is extended deep to the first metatarsophalangeal joint. The physician releases the contractured structures of the lateral joint. The bony eminence, or bunion, is removed from the first metatarsal head. A second incision is made in the top of the foot over the medial metatarsocuneiform joint. The joint capsule is exposed and opened. The articular cartilage of the joint is removed. The ends of the bones are fashioned so they fit intimately together. The joint and bones of the big toe are manipulated into alignment. Fixation devices are needed to fuse the metatarsal and cuneiform bones. Prior to closing the incisions, the sesamoid bones are examined and removed as needed. The wounds are irrigated and closed in layers.

28298

The physician treats a bunion of the foot with proximal phalanx osteotomy by any method. This procedure consists of removal of a bony wedge from the base of the proximal phalanx. A medial based wedge (0.3 mm to 0.4 mm) is cut, allowing reorientation of bone while leaving the lateral cortex intact. The medial eminence is excised. Fixation is usually accomplished by crossed K-wires, pins, or screws. The wound is closed in layers after irrigation. Removal of the sesamoid bones, if performed, is included.

28299

The physician treats a severe hallux valgus (bunion) deformity of the foot by double osteotomy. The physician makes an incision over the first metatarsal. The bony eminence, or bunion, is removed from the first metatarsal head. Various methods of double osteotomy may be performed. In one method, the soft tissue is corrected, and a V-osteotomy is made through the metatarsal head and neck that is displaced laterally to replace the metatarsal head over sesamoids. K wire fixation is used, and a cast is applied. Removal of the sesamoid bones, if performed, is included.

28300-28302

The physician performs an osteotomy of the calcaneus with or without internal fixation in 28300. An incision is made on the lateral aspect of the foot. The sural nerve is exposed and retracted. The calcaneus is exposed by stripping off the peroneal sheath from the calcaneus. A saw blade is used to make an oblique cut in the calcaneus. Another cut is made to free a 4 mm to 8 mm wedge of bone. The physician gently manipulates and closes the osteotomy site, stabilizing the site with a screw, staple, or Steinmann pin, if necessary. The incision is closed in layers and a dressing is applied. Report 28302 if this procedure is performed on the talus.

28304-28305

The physician makes an incision over the base of the first metatarsal, and over the second and third metatarsals depending on the extent and type of repair. The physician retracts the tendons and incises the periosteum to expose the tarsal. A sagittal saw is used to remove a wedge of bone. Staples, screws, or Kirschner wires are used for fixation. After the immediate postoperative dressing, immobilization may be applied. Report 28305 when a bone graft is necessary. For this procedure, the physician debrides the intended graft recipient site of the tarsal and a bone graft from the iliac crest or other site is shaped and placed between the prepared surfaces. The physician uses a lamina spreader to place the bone graft. Staples, screws, or wires may be used to secure the bone graft. The tissue and skin are sutured closed. A dressing is applied and the area may be immobilized.

28306-28308

A dorsomedial incision is made over the big toe and the skin and soft tissues are reflected. In many cases this procedure is performed in an effort to correct the poor alignment of the big toe. In addition to removal of the medial eminence, a cut is made through the metatarsal shaft and a portion of the bone is removed in order to correct the alignment of the bone. Wires are used to reattach the bone in its corrected alignment. Sutures are used to close the incision. Weight bearing is protected for several weeks. Report 28307 if a bone graft is used to correct the alignment of the first metatarsal shaft and attached with wire or screws. Report 28308 if the procedure is performed on other metatarsal bones.

28309

The physician treats a patient with a high arch (pes cavus) by performing osteotomies (bone cuts) on the metatarsal bones of the foot. Two or more incisions are made on the dorsal surface (top) of the foot over the metatarsal bones. The incisions are carried deep to the bones. Tissue is dissected and debrided as needed. The physician makes cuts through the metatarsal bones one at a time. The bones are each manipulated in such a way that the angles are changed. The manipulation allows the high arch to be shifted to an appropriate position. Multiple fixation devices such as screws, plates, or pins are applied to hold the bones in their new positions. The incisions are irrigated and closed in layers.

28310-28312
A medial incision is made on the proximal phalanx or first digit of the big toe. The periosteum is divided from the bone and a wedge section of bone is removed. The toe is properly aligned and a screw is place through the bone to maintain alignment. The incision is closed with sutures. Weight bearing is allowed in six weeks at that time the screw is commonly removed. Report 28312 when procedure is performed on any other phalanges of any toe.

28313
In this procedure the correction of the toe deformity is made by releasing soft tissues and possibly involving tendon transfers. It does not include cutting or realigning the shafts of the bones. An incision is made on top of the toe to be operated on. The involved tendons are identified and released and reattached at another portion of the bone and the joint capsule may be released to decrease the abnormal pull on the joint. Once proper alignment is obtained, the incisions are closed and a soft dressing is applied. Weight bearing is protected and gradually progressed.

28315
The sesamoid bone is a small bone that lies under the metatarsal heads of each toe. This procedure involves the removal of that bone. A dorsal incision is made between the first and second metatarsal bones proximal to the web space. The soft tissues are reflected in order to separate the two metatarsal heads. The inter-sesamoid ligament is released and the sesamoid bone is removed with small Kocher clamp or forceps. The soft tissues are replaced and the incision is closed with sutures. Weight bearing is permitted as the wound heals.

28320
Nonunion or malunion of the talus may result from trauma. Fractures are rare but may unite in malposition. The treatment of choice depends upon the portion of bone involved. If the top if the talus (articular surface) is involved, the treatment of choice is to fuse the talus to the tibia with bone grafting and casting. The same can be done for malunion of the calcaneus. In this case the calcaneus may be fused to the talus.

28322
An incision is made on the dorsum of the foot parallel with the shaft of the affected bones. The old fracture is exposed and divided with an osteotome. A small portion of the bone must be removed to produce a nonunion or division between the bone surfaces. The bones alignment is corrected and stabilized with a medullary pin. The incision is closed with sutures and a cast is applied. At three weeks the medullary pin is removed and a walking boot is applied. A felt pad is placed under the metatarsal region to maintain proper alignment.

28340-28341
Macrodactyly is the overgrowth of one or several adjacent digits of a hand or foot. The physician generally stages the surgery to control blood supply. In the first stage, reported using 28340, the physician removes the distal half of the middle phalanx and the tip of the remaining shaft is shaped to a pencil point. The articular surface of the distal phalanx is reamed to create a receptacle, which is fitted over the end of the middle phalanx. Kirschner wires are used to hold the position. An incision is made across the digit at the mid phalanx level and carried down to the midsagittal line. The soft tissue (up to 20 percent) is excised over the dorsum. A hump is created with the plantar tissue. In the second stage, reported using 28341, the physician performs the underlying bony work following the excision of soft tissue over the dorsum. Kirschner wire is used to stabilize the digit and the extensor tendon is shortened while the flexor tendon is left alone. Epiphysiodesis of the bones is performed during growth.

28344
This is a congenital anomaly where an extra toe is present. Correction is obtained by surgical removal of the accessory digit. An oval shaped incision is made at the base of the toe to be removed. The underlying tendons are drawn distally and divided. The joint capsule of the metatarsophalangeal joint is incised, the joint is disarticulated, and the toe is removed. If x-rays reveal any development of an extra metatarsal bone, the incision is continued proximally, and the bone is also removed. The incision is closed, and a soft dressing is applied.

28345
The physician surgically corrects the congenital deformity of webbed skin between the toes of the foot. Separately reportable x-rays are obtained of the foot and toes to ensure that no extra bones are present. The physician operates on one web space at a time. The skin is incised between each toe and the excess tissue is removed. A thorough debridement is performed, including the removal of any extraneous subcutaneous or nonviable tissues. Skin grafts may be required depending on the extent of the webbing removed and the debridement performed. The incisions are individually closed in layers to ensure proper skin coverage of the toes. A soft dressing is typically applied.

28360
Cleft foot (lobster foot) is an anomaly in which a single cleft or division extends proximally into the foot, sometimes even as far as the midfoot. Generally one or more toes are missing and often their metatarsals are absent. The goal is to improve function of the foot. A V-shaped incision is made at the cleft and the skin of the opposing surfaces within the cleft is removed, but the dorsal and plantar skin flaps are left to close the cleft when sutured together. Any bone or joint deformity is corrected at the time of surgery. This may include capsulotomies and osteotomies of any retained metatarsals and phalanges. If pin fixation is required the pins and short leg cast are removed at six weeks.

28400
The physician treats a fracture of the calcaneus bone without open surgery or manipulation of the bone. Separately reportable x-rays confirm a fracture of the calcaneus bone with the fracture fragments in acceptable position. The physician places the foot and leg in a cast, brace, or splint to provide protection while the bone heels.

28405
The physician treats a fracture of the calcaneus without open surgery but with manipulation of the fracture pieces. Separately reportable x-rays confirm a fractured calcaneus with the fracture pieces in an unacceptable position. The physician pushes and otherwise maneuvers the fracture fragments into the proper position. No incisions are required.

28406
The physician treats a fracture of the calcaneus without open surgery but with the use of manipulation and pins placed through the skin and into the bone. With the patient under anesthesia, the physician pushes and otherwise maneuvers the fracture fragments into the proper position. Through small holes in the skin, the physician places pins that are driven into the pieces of the bone in appropriate places to hold the fracture in position for healing. X-rays (separately reported) are used to help guide the pins correctly. With the fracture reduced, the physician places the foot and leg in a cast, splint, or brace.

28415
The physician performs surgery on a fracture of the calcaneus bone. An incision is made in the skin overlying the fractured area of the calcaneus. The incision is extended deep to the bone. Tissues are dissected and debrided as required. The fracture fragments are identified. The physician places the bony pieces in their correct position. Fixation devices may be applied on the inside adjacent to the bone. The incision is irrigated and closed in layers.

28420
The physician treats a fracture of the calcaneus with open surgery and the use of bone graft. The physician makes an incision in the skin overlying the fractured calcaneus. Tissues are dissected and debrided as needed as the incision is carried down to the bone. The fracture is identified and exposed. Through a separate incision, the physician obtains a bone graft from the patient's ilium and closes the surgically created graft donor site. The fractured pieces are placed in appropriate position and the bone graft is placed in and around the fracture site. Fixation devices are applied to hold the fracture and graft in the correct position. The wound is irrigated and closed in layers.

28430
The physician treats a fracture of the talus bone in the ankle without performing open surgery or any manipulation of the fracture. X rays (reported separately) confirm a fracture of the talus bone with the fractured pieces in an acceptable position. The physician applies a cast, brace, or splint to protect the ankle and keep the fracture positioned correctly. No incisions are required.

28435
The physician treats a fracture of the talus bone of the ankle without performing open surgery but with manipulation of the fracture. X rays (separately reported) confirm a fracture of the talus bone with the fractured pieces in an unacceptable position. With the patient under anesthesia (separately reported), the physician pushes, pulls, or otherwise maneuvers the foot, ankle, and leg to restore the fracture to a satisfactory position.

28436
The physician treats a fracture of the talus bone of the ankle without open surgery but with the use of manipulation and pins placed through small holes in the skin and into the bone. With the patient under anesthesia, the physician pushes, pulls, or otherwise maneuvers the foot, ankle, and leg to restore the fracture to a satisfactory position. Surgical pins are placed through the skin and guided into the talus bone. The pins help manipulate the fracture pieces and hold them in the proper place. Screws may also be applied. X-rays (separately reported) are obtained to confirm the correct placement of the fixation and the fracture.

28445
The physician treats a fracture of the talus bone of the ankle with open surgery. An incision is made in the skin overlying the fractured talus. This is extended deep to the talus bone. Tissues are dissected and debrided as needed. The fracture is identified and exposed. Any intervening tissue between the fractured pieces is removed. The physician reduces (realigns) the fracture, placing the pieces back into satisfactory position. Fixation devices are applied as needed to hold the fragments in place internally. The wound is irrigated and closed.

28446
After the size and type of lesions are determined radiographically, the physician performs an open osteochondral autograft on the talus (ankle bone). The physician exposes the defect area by cutting to the bone and retracting the soft tissue. The defect is excised and the margins are squared off and abraded to reach healthy, bleeding, subchondral bone. Using coring reamers, an osteochondral graft is harvested from a non-load bearing region of articular cartilage and implanted into the damaged joint location. Supplementary fixation may be used by inserting biodegradable pins. The incision is closed.

28450
The physician treats a fracture of one of the tarsal bones, other than the calcaneus or the talus without performing open surgery or any manipulation. X-rays (separately reported) confirm a fracture of the navicular, cuboid, or one of the three cuneiforms, with the fragments in acceptable position. The physician

Musculoskeletal

applies a cast, brace, or splint to the foot and leg to protect the fracture and hold it in the appropriate position.

28455
The physician treats a fracture of one of the tarsal bones other than the talus or calcaneus without performing open surgery but with manipulation of the fracture. Separately reportable x-rays confirm a fracture of the navicular, cuboid, or one of the cuneiform bones with the fracture fragments in an unacceptable position. With the patient under anesthesia as needed, the physician pushes, pulls, or otherwise maneuvers the foot, ankle, or leg to restore the bony pieces to a satisfactory position.

28456
The physician treats a fracture of one of the tarsal bones other than the talus or calcaneus without open surgery but with the aid of manipulation and pins placed through skin and into the bone. The physician pushes, pulls, or otherwise maneuvers the foot, ankle, or leg to restore the fracture of the navicular, cuboid, or one of the cuneiforms to a satisfactory position. Pins or screws are placed through small holes in the skin and guided into the bone. X-rays (separately reported) are used to help manipulate the fracture as needed. A cast, brace or splint is applied.

28465
The physician treats a fracture of one of the tarsal bones, other than the talus or calcaneus, with open surgery. The physician makes an incision in the skin of the foot overlying the particular fracture of the navicular, cuboid, or one of the three cuneiform bones. Tissue is dissected and debrided deep to the bone. The fracture is identified and exposed. The physician places the fracture fragments in their correct position. Any intervening or nonviable tissue is removed. Fixation devices such as screws, plates, pins, or wires are applied as needed to hold the fracture properly. The incision is irrigated and closed in layers.

28470
The physician treats a fracture of one of the five metatarsal bones without open surgery or any manipulation of the fracture. X-rays (separately reported) confirm a fracture of a metatarsal bone of the foot with the fracture fragments in acceptable position and alignment. The physician places the foot, ankle, and leg in a cast, splint, or brace as needed.

28475
The physician treats a fracture of one of the five metatarsal bones in the foot without performing open surgery but with manipulation of the fracture. X-rays (separately reported) confirm a fracture of the metatarsal bone with the bony pieces in an unacceptable position. The physician pushes, pulls, or other maneuvers the foot to restore the fracture fragments to a satisfactory position and alignment. X-rays (separately reportable) confirm desired results. The foot and leg are placed in a cast or brace.

28476
The physician treats a fracture of one of the five metatarsal bones without performing open surgery but with the use of manipulation and fixation pins that are placed through skin and into the bone. The physician pushes, pulls, or otherwise maneuvers the foot, toes, or ankle to restore the fractured bone to its proper position. Fixation pins, wires, or screw are inserted through small holes in the skin and guided into the fracture pieces. X-rays (separately reported) are often used to aid in the proper placement of the fixation and to ensure that the fracture is in satisfactory position.

28485
The physician treats a fracture of one of the five metatarsals with open surgery. An incision is made overlying the particular metatarsal fracture. The tissues are dissected and debrided as needed. The fracture is identified and exposed. Any tissue between the fracture pieces is removed. The fracture fragments are reduced (realigned) to their correct position. Fixation devices are applied as needed to hold the fracture in place. The wound is irrigated and closed in layers.

28490
The physician treat as a fracture of the big toe involving one or both of the bones without any open surgery or manipulation of the bones. X-rays (separately reported) confirm a fracture or fractures of the bones in the big toe with the fragments in an acceptable position for healing. The physician places a cast, sling, or brace on the toe and foot as needed.

28495
The physician treats a fracture of the big toe involving one or both of the bones without open surgery, but with manipulation of the fracture. X-rays (reported separately) of the big toe confirm a fracture or fracture of the bones in the big toe in an unacceptable position. With the patient under anesthesia as required, the physician pulls or pushes on the toe and foot to restore the bony pieces to their proper place. X-rays (separately reported) are taken to ensure that the fracture is aligned correctly. A cast, splint, or brace is placed on the toe and foot.

28496
The physician treats a fracture of the big toe involving one or both of the bones without open surgery but with pin fixation through the skin and manipulation of the fractures. The physician pushes, pulls, or otherwise maneuvers the toe and foot to place the fracture pieces in their appropriate position. Fixation devices such as pins or wires are inserted through small holds in the skin and guided into the bone. The fixation is used to manipulate the fracture further into proper position and to hold bones in the right place. X-rays (separately reported) are used to confirm the desired placement and fracture alignment.

28505
The physician treats a fracture of the big toe involving one or both of the bones with open surgery. An

incision is made in the skin overlying the big toe. The tissues are dissected and debrided down to the bones. The fracture or fractures are identified and exposed. The physician places the fracture fragments into their proper position removing any intervening tissue. Fixation devices such as pins screws, wires, or plates are applied to hold the bony pieces together as required. The wound is irrigated and closed in layers. A cast, splint, or brace may be applied to the toe and foot.

28510

The physician treats a fracture of one of the four toes other than the big toe. No open surgery or manipulation of the toe or foot is required. X-rays (reported separately) of the toe confirm a fracture or fractures of the bones where the fragments are in an acceptable position. The physician applies a splint, brace, or cast to the toe and foot.

28515

The physician treats a fracture of one of the four toes other than the big toes involving one or more of the bones in the toe without performing open surgery but with manipulation of the toe and foot. X-rays (reported separately) confirm a fracture or fractures of the toe with the bony pieces in unacceptable positions for correct healing. The physician pulls or pushes on the toe or foot in such a way as to restore the bones to their correct alignment. X-rays (reported separately) are taken to confirm the desired result. A splint, cast or brace may be applied.

28525

The physician treats a fracture of one of the four toes, other than the big toe, with open surgery and fixation devices as needed. An incision is made in the skin overlying the fractured toe. The tissues are dissected to identify and expose the fracture or fractures. The physician places the fracture fragments into their correct position. Fixation devices are applied as needed to hold the bony pieces together. This may include pins, wires, or screws. The wound is irrigated and closed in layers.

28530

The physician treats a fracture of a sesamoid bone in the foot without performing any open surgery. X-rays (separately reported) confirm a fracture of the sesamoid bone. The physician places the foot and ankle in a splint, brace, or cast to protect the bone while it heals.

28531

The physician treats a fracture of a sesamoid bone in the foot by open surgery. An incision is made in the foot over the fractured sesamoid bone. The incision is carried deep to the bone, tissue is dissected, and tissue is debrided to expose the fracture. The physician may apply a fixation device to hold the fracture together. The bone may be excised if it is nonviable. The wound is irrigated and closed in layers.

28540

The physician reduces a tarsal bone dislocation, other than talotarsal, without requiring anesthesia. Separately reportable x-rays are obtained of the foot to demonstrate a tarsal bone dislocation in such a position that the physician can return it to the correct position without the need for anesthesia. The physician manipulates the involved bones to restore normal anatomy and function. Separately reportable x-rays are again obtained to note the desired outcome. A cast or brace is applied as indicated.

28545

The physician reduces a tarsal bone dislocation, other than talotarsal, with the use of anesthesia. Separately reportable x-rays are obtained of the foot to demonstrate a tarsal bone dislocation which will require anesthesia to reduce. General or regional anesthesia is employed. Without any surgical incision, the physician manipulates the involved bones so as to return them to the appropriate anatomic position. Separately reportable x-rays are obtained to confirm the adequacy of the reduction. A cast or brace is applied.

28546

The physician treats dislocation of a bone in the foot, other than talotarsal, with manipulation and percutaneous skeletal fixation. The physician performs this procedure on the joints of the mid-foot with the patient soothed by general anesthesia or a nerve block. The physician manually reduces the dislocation between the tarsal bones. Radiographs or fluoroscopy (reported separately) are typically used to confirm proper alignment and position. To stabilize the dislocation, small stab incisions are made, and holes are drilled through the bone. Pins are inserted through the drill holes and cross the affected joint(s) to maintain the reduction. The pins are cut just below the surface of the skin.

28555

The physician performs open treatment of a dislocation of the tarsal bone, sometimes using internal fixation. With the patient under anesthesia, the physician makes an incision and dissects down to the dislocated tarsal bones that are located in the mid-foot. The physician reduces the dislocation. To stabilize the dislocation, the physician may elect Kirschner wires placed through drill holes in the adjacent bone or bone screws. The incision is closed in layers with sutures and Steri-strips. A cast may be applied.

28570-28575

The physician treats talotarsal joint dislocation without surgery. The physician may use separately reportable x-rays to identify dislocation and congruency of joint surfaces. The physician manipulates the bones back into position. A short leg cast is applied with the foot in a plantar flexed position. Report 28570 if the manipulation is performed without anesthesia. Report 28575 if anesthesia is required to perform the procedure.

Musculoskeletal

28576
The physician repairs the dislocation of a joint of the foot with percutaneous skeletal fixation, with manipulation. The physician performs this procedure with the patient soothed by general anesthesia or a spinal block. The physician manually reduces the dislocation between the talus and tarsal bones and uses separately reportable x-ray or fluoroscopy to confirm alignment and position. To stabilize the dislocation, small stab incisions are made and holes are drilled through the bones. Pins are inserted through the drill holes that cross the affected joint(s) and maintain the reduction. The pins are cut just below the surface of the skin.

28585
The physician treats a talotarsal joint dislocation, in which the talus dislocates on the calcaneus and/or the navicular bone; internal fixation is sometimes used. In one scenario, the dislocation involves the talonavicular joint. Open treatment is required in cases where closed reduction was unsuccessful or where the dislocation is unstable. An incision is made over the dorsal part of the foot and dissection exposes the talonavicular joint dislocation. The physician reduces the dislocation. The physician may elect to use Kirschner wires or screws that are placed through drilled holes in the talus and navicular to hold them in place. The incision is closed in layers with sutures and Steri-strips.

28600-28605
The patient is positioned supine on the table. The physician manually manipulates the foot in an effort to reposition the tarsal and metatarsal bones into proper alignment. Report 28600 if no anesthesia is required; however, pain medication may be given orally if needed. Report 28605 if performed with patient under general or regional anesthesia.

28606
With the patient under anesthesia, the foot is manually manipulated to correct the dislocation of the tarsometatarsal joint. A small stab incision is made over the tarsal bone and a small pin or screw is inserted to stabilize the affected tarsal and metatarsal bones. The incision is closed with one to two sutures and a cast is applied.

28615
The physician performs open treatment of a tarsometatarsal joint dislocation. A dorsal incision is made over the dislocated bones. The soft tissues are reflected to expose the joint. The joint is properly aligned and stabilized with screws, plates, or wire fixation. The incision is closed with sutures and a cast is applied. Weight bearing is allowed at six weeks. At that time the physician may remove the metal fixation.

28630-28635
The patient is placed supine on the table. The physician manually manipulates the foot in order to reduce the dislocation of the metatarsophalangeal joint (joint between the long bone of the foot and the toe). Report 28630, if this is performed without anesthesia. Report 28635 if performed under general anesthesia.

28636
With the patient under anesthesia, the foot is manually manipulated to correct the dislocation of the long bone of the foot and the toe. A small stab incision is made over the metatarsal bone and a small pin or screw is inserted to stabilize the two bones. The incision is closed with one to two sutures and a cast is applied.

28645
The physician performs open treatment of a metatarsophalangeal joint dislocation. A dorsal incision is made over the dislocated bones. The soft tissues are reflected to expose the joint. The joint is properly aligned and stabilized with screws, plates, or wire fixation. The incision is closed with sutures and a cast is applied. Weight bearing is allowed at six weeks. At that time the physician removes the metal fixation.

28660
The physician reduces a dislocation of an interphalangeal joint of a toe without the need of anesthesia. Separately reportable x-rays are obtained which identify the specific dislocation. The physician manipulates the toe without performing surgery to reduce the dislocation. Post reduction x-rays are obtained.

28665
The physician reduces a dislocation of an interphalangeal joint of a toe with the use of anesthesia. Separately reportable x-rays are obtained to identify the specific dislocation. A local or regional anesthetic is employed. The physician manipulates the toe to reduce the dislocation. Separately reportable x-rays are obtained to confirm that appropriate position has been accomplished.

28666
The physician reduces the dislocation of an interphalangeal joint of a toe with the use of percutaneous fixation. Separately reportable x-rays are obtained to demonstrate the dislocated joint. Anesthesia is typically employed. The physician inserts metal pins or wires directly through the sterilized skin of the toe and into the affected phalanges. The toe is manipulated with the help of these fixation devices to reduce the dislocation. Separately reportable x-rays are obtained to ensure that the joint is again anatomically correct. The pins or wires may be removed or retained for later removal.

28675
The physician reduces a dislocation of the interphalangeal joint of a toe by surgically opening the joint. Separately reportable x-rays are obtained to determine the extent of the dislocation. The patient is taken to the operating room and anesthesia is utilized. The physician makes a longitudinal incision over the dislocated bones. The incision is continued deep to the joint. The capsule is identified and opened. The physician identifies the dislocation and reduces it. This

may require the use of internal fixation devices to complete the reduction and/or hold it in place. The wound is irrigated and closed in layers. A dressing is applied.

28705

The physician fuses several joints in and around the ankle. It can be performed in one operation or in two separate surgeries. In either case, the physician makes at least one incision around the ankle. Incisions are continued deep to the ankle mortise itself and to the following joints: the talocalcaneal, the talonavicular, and the calcaneocuboid. The capsule of each joint is opened, explored, and debrided. Osteotomies are performed so that viable bone is available on each side of the joints. The physician utilizes a variety of internal fixation devices such as pins, wires, plates, or screws to connect the bones together across each joint. This allows the bones to fuse together as they heal. Because of the extensive nature of the surgery, and the time required for healing, the surgery is frequently performed in two stages. Incisions are irrigated and closed as usual. A cast is applied until the fusion is solidly healed.

28715

The physician fuses the talonavicular, the calcaneocuboid, and the subtalar (talocalcaneal) joints. The physician makes incisions on each side of the foot. These are carried deep to the joints. Tendons are reflected and protected. Each joint is identified. Soft tissues are debrided. The capsules are opened and the joints visualized. Surgical curettes are used to remove the articular cartilage of the joints one at a time so that viable bone is exposed. The physician uses any of a variety of surgical fixation devices including screws, plates, or wires to connect the bones of each individual joint together. The incisions are irrigated and closed in layers. A cast is applied and continued until all three joints are solidly fused.

28725

The physician fuses the subtalar (talocalcaneal) joint. An incision is made over the lateral ankle and foot. The physician extends this incision deep to the subtalar joint. Tendons and nerves are retracted and protected. Soft tissues are debrided. The joint capsule is incised and the joint is debrided as necessary. Surgical instruments including curettes are utilized to remove the articular cartilage of the joint. Fixation devices such as screws, pins, or wires are employed to maintain fixation of the talus. The incision is closed in layers. A cast is typically applied.

28730

The physician performs surgery on the foot in which more than one of the midtarsal or tarsometatarsal joints are fused. The physician makes one or more incisions over the dorsal aspect of the foot in the skin overlying the affected joints. The incisions are continued deep through the subcutaneous tissue. Nerves and tendons are retracted. The physician identifies the specific problem joints of the tarsals and metatarsals, performing capsulotomies. The joints are entered, explored, and debrided. The physician utilizes any of a variety of friction devices to hold each joint in its fused position. The wounds are irrigated and closed in layers.

28735

The physician performs surgery on the foot in which more than one of the midtarsal or tarsometatarsal joints are fused. The metatarsals are also osteotomized to correct for a flat foot deformity. The physician makes one or more incisions in the dorsal skin of the foot overlying the affected joints and metatarsals. The incisions are continued deep to the particular joints. Nerves and tendons are retracted. The shafts of the metatarsals that will undergo osteotomy are isolated and debrided. The physician performs capsulotomy on each joint to be fused. The metatarsals are cut and realigned in a plantar flexion position to correct flatfoot deformity. The joints, debrided of their articular cartilage, are fashioned for a close fit. The physician utilizes any of a variety of fixation devices such as wires, plates, pins, or screws to hold the metatarsal and the joints in alignment. The incisions are irrigated and closed in layers.

28737

The physician fuses the navicular and cuneiform bones of the foot and advances distally with the posterior tibial tendon the calcaneonavicular, navicular cuneiform and cuneiform metatarsal ligaments. An incision is made over the medial aspect of the foot. This is carried to the tendon and ligaments. The physician creates an osteoperiosteal flap incorporating the tibial tendon and the ligaments. The navicular-cuneiform and metatarsal-cuneiform joints are opened. The surfaces of the joints are denuded of their articular cartilage. The physician utilizes fixation devices such as screws, pins, wires, or plates to hold the joints in position. The flap of ligaments and tendon together is passed forward beneath the anterior tibia and transplanted to the first cuneiform bone and the base of the first metatarsal bone. Friction devices are employed to hold the flap. The incision is irrigated and closed in layers.

28740

The physician fuses one of the midtarsal or tarsometatarsal joints of the foot. Separately reportable x-rays are used to determine the particular joint to be fused. The physician makes an incision in the skin directly overlying the joint. Tendons and nerves are retracted and a capsulotomy is performed. The physician removes the articular cartilage of the bones on both sides of the joint. The bony surfaces are fashioned for a close fit. Any of a variety of fixation devices are used to hold the bones in proper alignment. The wound is irrigated and debrided. The incision is closed in layers.

28750

The physician fuses the joint between the great toe and the first metatarsal bone. A longitudinal incision is made on the dorsal surface of the first toe. It is deepened through the subcutaneous tissue and fascia to the first metatarsophalangeal joint. The nerves and tendons are retracted. A capsulotomy is performed. The physician makes parallel cuts of the metatarsal with a saw or osteotome. The two cuts are placed together in the desired alignment and position. Fixation devices hold the bones in position. The wound is irrigated and closed in layers.

28755
The physician fuses the interphalangeal joint on the great toe. An incision is made over the dorsal aspect of the toe directly overlying the joint. The incision is continued deep to the joint. A capsulotomy is performed. Parallel cuts are made on the two phalanges that constitute the joint. The physician places the cut bones together. Pins or screws hold the bones in the correct alignment. The wound is irrigated and closed.

28760
The physician performs a Jones type procedure. The physician fuses the interphalangeal joint of the great toe and transfers the extensor hallucis longus tendon from its insertion on the phalanges to the first metatarsal bone. An incision is on the dorsal aspect of the great toe and distal first metatarsal. It is continued deep to the extensor hallucis longus tendon. The physician fuses the interphalangeal joint. Fixation devices hold the fusion in place for healing. The neck of the first metatarsal bone is identified dorsally. The extensor hallucis longus tendon is identified dorsally. The extensor hallucis longus tendon is attached to the metatarsal using any of a variety of fixation devices. The incision is irrigated and closed in layers.

28800
The physician amputates the foot across the midtarsal region. The physician makes the incision so that skin flaps are made dorsally and plantarly. The skin is refracted and the dissection is carried down through the soft tissue. The tendons are severed and allowed to retract. The dorsal and plantar ligaments of the calcaneocuboid and talonavicular joints are released so that the foot can be removed. The physician may also perform a percutaneous Achilles tenotomy (reported separately) to prevent flexion contracture. Skin flaps are closed and a soft compression dressing is applied.

28805
The physician amputates the foot across the transmetatarsal region. The physician makes the incision so that skin flaps are made dorsally and plantarly. The skin is refracted and the dissection is carried down through the soft tissue. The tendons are severed and allowed to retract. The dorsal and plantar ligaments are released so that the foot can be removed. The physician may also perform a percutaneous Achilles tenotomy (reported separately) to prevent flexion contracture. Skin flaps are closed and a soft compression dressing is applied.

28810
The physician performs an amputation of a metatarsal bone and its attached toe. An incision is made dorsally over the involved metatarsal and toe. This is carried deep to the tarsometatarsal joint. The joint and capsule are identified. A capsulotomy is performed and the metatarsal is disarticulated from the other toes. The incision is continued around the toe itself. Tendons are retracted or removed as indicated. The metatarsal bone and the toe are completely dissected free from the foot and removed. The wound is irrigated and debrided. It is closed in layers. A dressing and a cast or a brace are applied.

28820
The physician performs an amputation of a toe at the metatarsophalangeal joint. An incision is made over and around the affected toe where the toe joins the foot. The physician continues the incision deep to the metatarsophalangeal joint. The capsule is identified and a capsulotomy is performed. The proximal phalanx bone is disarticulated from the metatarsal bone. The joint is debrided. The tendon and soft tissues are excised for closure and skin coverage. The toe is excised free from the foot. The wound is irrigated and closed in layers. A dressing and firm-soled shoe are applied.

28825
The physician performs an amputation of a portion of a toe at the level of an interphalangeal joint. An incision is made over the involved toe. It is carried deep to the planned interphalangeal joint amputation site. Skin is preserved around the toe for closure. The physician extends the incision deep to the joint capsule. A capsulotomy is performed and the joint is disarticulated. Debridement is performed. The soft tissues are excised and prepared for the amputation. The desired portion of toe to include the disarticulated bone is excised free. The wound is irrigated and closed in layers. A dressing and post-operative shoe are applied.

28890
The physician or other qualified health care provider treats plantar fasciitis with extracorporeal shock wave therapy (ESWT). This condition is the result of inflammation of the connective tissue from the base of the toes, extending across the arch of the foot, and inserting into the heel bone. When associated with a heel spur, it may also be referred to as "heel spur syndrome." When the condition fails to respond to a more conservative treatment regimen, including exercise, anti-inflammatories, physical therapy modalities, and orthotic devices, ESWT may be indicated. ESWT is the administration of high intensity sound waves at the rate of two or three times per second, from outside of the body. Treatment is provided on an outpatient basis and takes about 30 minutes to perform. Local anesthesia may be provided.

29000
The physician constructs this body cast to provide a foundation for a halo in which the cervical spine must

be stabilized. This involves use of a torso body cast to which the halo is attached. Casting material is applied tightly, beginning at the pelvis and extending up the torso to the upper chest. Extenders from the halo (which is already inserted around the head) can be attached to the body cast. This holds the halo very securely. An alternative is to use a prefabricated torso/chest brace that is placed on the upper torso. The previously applied halo is attached.

29010-29015

The physician applies a Risser jacket, a method of correction for a scoliotic curve. The physician places the patient face up on a canvas strap tied to a rectangular frame. A stockinette is stretched over the patient from the head to the knees. A metallic half-circle carrying a moveable jack with a metal plate to be directed toward the apex of the angulation of the ribs is suspended beneath the frame. The rib angulation area is protected by a heave piece of felt covered with a contoured square piece of plaster that rests on the plate. The jack is turned so that it presses the plate in a direction on the rib angulation that corrects the scoliotic curvature. A second jack may be applied to correct a double primary curve or a secondary lumbar curve. The cast is applied in sections while traction is applied to the head with a hatter and the pelvis with a pelvic belt attached to the plaster girdle. The casting begins with a well-molded neck and shoulder section and finishes with incorporating the trunk. Separately reportable spinal instrumentation largely eliminates the use of the Risser jacket. Report 29015 if this jacket includes the head.

29035-29046

The physician applies a body cast, shoulder to hips. The physician applies two layers of stockinette to the patient's torso (armpits to hips), adding cotton and felt padding over bony prominences. Fiberglass or plaster cast is applied over the stockinette to create a rigid cast. Report 29035 for application of the cast. Report 29040 if the cast includes the head, Minerva type. Report 29044 if the cast includes one thigh. Report 29046 if the cast includes both thighs.

29049-29085

The physician applies a figure-of-eight cast to maintain shoulder retraction while a clavicle fracture heals. A cast method is seldom used; shoulder retraction is maintained with a figure-of-eight shoulder strap. Report 29049 for the cast itself. Report 29055 if the cast includes a shoulder spica. Report 29058 if the cast includes a plaster Velpeau. Report 29065 if the cast is constructed from shoulder to hand. Report 29075 if the cast is constructed from the elbow to finger. Report 29085 if the cast is constructed over the hand and lower forearm.

29086

The hand is placed in the functioning position, with the thumb opposed. The physician extends a synthetic stockinette from the proximal interphalangeal (PIP) joints of the hand to the wrist joint and cuts a hole for the thumb. The physician covers the gap at the thumb metacarpophalangeal (MCP) joint by splitting the thumb tube to extend it proximal to the MCP joint. Synthetic cast padding is wrapped to cover the cast area two to three layers thick, with extra layers at the proximal wrist to protect the wrist joint during flexion and extension. The physician uses 1-inch or 2-inch casting tape to wrap the hand and thumb in a thumb spica. The wrapping starts with one full around the metacarpals and wrapping the tape around the thumb and hand in a figure-eight pattern, alternating the direction of the wrap around the thumb. The free ends of the stockinette are tucked under the second layer of wrap.

29105

The physician applies a splint from the shoulder to the hand. A long arm posterior splint is used to immobilize a number of injuries around the elbow and forearm. A cotton bandage is wrapped around the forearm from the midpalm region to midarm. Plaster strips or fiberglass splints are applied along the back of the arm and forearm, maintain the elbows and wrist in the desired position.

29125-29126

The physician applies a splint from the forearm to the hand. A short arm splint is used to immobilize the wrist. Cotton padding is applied from midforearm to the midpalm region. Plaster strips or fiberglass splint material are applied along the palm side of the hand, extending to midforearm, maintain the wrist in the desired position. An Ace wrap is applied by the physician to hold the splint material in position. Report 29125 if the splint is static, keeping the wrist totally immobilized. Report 29126 if the splint is dynamic, allowing some movement.

29130-29131

The physician applies a finger splint. This type of splint is applied to immobilize the digits. A twin layer of cotton padding is applied by the physician to the digit, covering the last two joints of that digit. Plaster casting or fiberglass splint material is applied to the finger from just beyond the knuckle to the tip of the finger. Usually, the finger is immobilized in a straight position. Report 29130 if the splint applied is static for full immobilization. Report 29131 if the splint applied is dynamic for some movement.

29200-29280

The physician or a medical professional under the physician's direction performs strapping with tape on a patient of any age. In 29200, this technique was once more frequently used to compress the thorax offering some support and to limit deep inhalation following fracture. This support does not promote healing, but provides palliative relief. A thoracic elastic or canvas binder is more commonly used. Report 29240 if the strapping is applied to the shoulder; report 29260 if strapping is applied to the elbow or wrist; and report 29280 if strapping is applied to the hand or finger.

Musculoskeletal

29305-29325
The physician applies a hip spica cast. The hip spica cast is ideal for patients of all ages who may have hip problems ranging from fractures to dislocations. The physician applies cast padding to the lower torso and hips and extends this down the affected leg in 29305. It may extend below the knee depending on the physician's preference and the extent of hip immobilization desired. The hip is placed at the desired angle and casting material is placed over the padding material and allowed to dry. Report 29325 if the physician applies a one and one-half spica or a cast that envelopes both legs.

29345-29355
The physician applies a cast from the thigh to the toes. The physician places the ankle and knee at the desired angle. Cast padding is applied from the toes to the upper portion of the thigh. Casting material is moistened and applied in an overlapping pattern from the toes to the upper thigh and allowed to harden. Report 29355 if the cast is a walker or ambulatory type.

29358
The physician applies a long leg cast brace for a fracture. Code with caution: this cast is rarely applied, having been replaced by a pre-fabricated long leg brace. The physician places a metal or plastic support (with or without a hinge) on either side of the knee. Casting material is applied over the supports to hold them in place. The cast allows the knee to bend and straighten while stabilizing the knee during side-to-side movement.

29365
The physician applies a cylinder cast from thigh to ankle. This cast is used for fractures of the femur that extend into the knee joint. The knee is positioned at the desired angle. The cast and material are applied and allowed to dry.

29405-29425
The physician applies a cast below the knee to the toes. The physician positions the ankle at the desired angle. Cast padding is applied from the toes to just below the knees. Casting material is moistened and applied to the leg in an overlapping fashion and allowed to dry. Report 29425 if the cast is a walking or ambulatory type.

29435
The physician applies the patellar tendon bearing (PTB) cast for tibial shaft fractures. The cast is constructed to transfer weight to the upper tibia rather than the shaft of the tibia. The physician applies the casting material so that a shelf is formed under the tibial tuberosity/patellar tendon to bear the load of the cast. The foot is also included as part of the cast.

29440
The physician adds a walker to a previously applied cast. Lower extremity casts may be modified for walking with the addition of a walker. There are two types of walkers available: those made of hard rubber and incorporated into the cast and those applied over the cast like a shoe or boot. If the rubber walker is used, it must be secured to the cast with additional casting material.

29445
The physician applies a rigid total contact leg cast. The rigid total contact leg cast is applied to feet and legs demonstrating venous stasis ulcers. Of primary importance in applying this cast is even distribution of contact of the cast over the foot, ankle, and lower leg. The method and cast material used varies with the applicator. Sometimes wound dressing must be applied over the ulcers prior to application of the cast. The cast begins at the foot and extends to just below the knee.

29450
The physician applies a clubfoot cast with molding or manipulation. The cast may be long or short. If applying a cast to the right foot, the physician uses the left hand to grasp the right heel of the patient, placing the thumb over the talar prominence. The physician's right hand grasps the forefoot. The thumb and index finger hold the metatarsophalangeal joint of the great toe and longitudinal traction is exerted on the forefoot. At the same time, gentle pressure is exerted over the head of the talus. After one to two minutes of traction, the foot elongates. It is held in this corrected position while a cast made of fast-setting plaster is applied by a second person over layers of sheet cotton. The cast may be applied only to the foot and connected to the leg in separate parts or the cast may be applied at one time. If applied to the left foot, the physician uses the right hand to grasp the heel.

29505
The physician applies a long leg splint from thigh to the ankle or toes. A long leg posterior splint is used to immobilize a number of injuries around the knee or ankle. The physician wraps cotton bandaging around the involved leg from the upper thigh to the ankle or toes. Plaster strips or fiberglass splint material are applied along the posterior aspect of the leg from the upper thigh to the ankle or toes. After the splint material dries, it is secured into place by an Ace wrap.

29515
The physician applies a short leg splint from calf to foot. A short leg splint is used to immobilize the ankle. The physician wraps cotton bandaging from just below the knee to the toes. Plaster strips or fiberglass splinting material are applied to the posterior of the calf, around the heel, and along the bottom of the foot to the toes. The splint material is allowed to dry. The splint is secured into place with an Ace wrap.

29520-29550
The physician or medical professional uses tape to strap a lower extremity. Multiple strips are used to overlap and build support of the affected area. The strips are often placed from one area to another to construct temporary support to the tendons and muscles. Report 29520 if the site taped is the hip;

29530 for the knee; 29540 for the ankle and/or foot; and 29550 for the toes.

29580
The physician applies an Unna boot to the leg or foot of a patient. An Unna boot is typically used to treat or prevent venostasis dermatitis or ulcers of the lower leg or foot. It is also used to control postoperative edema like that resulting from an amputation. The physician prepares this semirigid dressing by first making a paste of zinc oxide, gelatin, and glycerin. This is applied to the skin of the leg. A spiral or figure eight bandage is wrapped evenly over the leg. Paste is reapplied and further bandages are applied in the same fashion until the desired rigidity is obtained. Elastic bandages are often added to the dressings for reinforcement. The dressing is typically replaced at least once a week or more often as needed.

29581-29584
A health care practitioner applies a multilayer compression device. Compression therapy is often used in the treatment of extensive venous ulcers. The device may consist of a multilayer bandaging system composed only of elastic bandages, or may be paired with a knitted, tubular compression garment. In one method, after wound debridement and dressing, cotton gauze and cotton crepe bandages are applied. A positioner is placed over the bandages and adjusted to the desired position. The compression device is slipped over the positioner, adjusted to assure appropriate placement, and the positioner removed. Report 29581 for application of the system below the knee (including ankle and foot). Report 29584 when it is applied to the upper arm, forearm, hand, and fingers.

29700-29710
The physician removes or bivalves a cast, which is to simply cut it in half for the purpose of using one half of the cast as a splint or for intermittent immobilization. Bivalve cast might be required in cases where frequent inspection is required. A manual cast saw is used to make two cuts in the cast. One cut is extended along the medial edge of the cast. The second cut is extended along the lateral edge of the cast. These cuts are started proximally and are extended distally. Once the cuts are made, the cast may be removed. The front and back portion of the cast may be applied and secured using an Ace bandage intermittently for immobilization. Only one half may be Ace wrapped for splinting purposes. Report 29700 if the cast is a gauntlet, boot, or body cast. Report 29705 if a full arm or full leg cast is removed. Report 29710 if a shoulder cast or hip spica, Minerva or Risser jacket, is removed.

29720
The physician repairs a spica, body cast, or jacket due to normal wear and tear, revision of the cast or jacket, or the cutting of a window to check the status of a wound, incision, or other area. Additional casting material is applied in the normal manner.

29730
The physician chooses this procedure to check the status of a wound that is underneath the cast or to visualize an area under the cast where infection may exist. A cast saw is used to cut a section in the cast. This is removed to create a window. Once the status is determined, the physician may reinsert the section and hold it in place with casting material.

29740-29750
The physician wedges a cast. X-rays (reported separately) of a casted, fractured extremity may show slight malalignment. Wedging of the cast may correct this malalignment without having to remove the cast. The bony deformities identified by the physician and the necessary direction and amount of correction is decided. The necessary cut is made in the cast using a cast saw. A wedge of plastic or wood is wedged into the cast cut to redirect the pressure of the cast on the fracture site to correct the bony deformity. Report 29740 if the wedge is placed in a cast. Report 29750 if the cast wedge is placed in a cast that has been applied for correction of clubfoot deformity.

29800
The physician inserts an arthroscope into the temporomandibular joint to examine the joint space(s). The physician may lavage or wash the joint. The physician makes a 0.5 cm vertical incision anterior to the contour of the ear. The arthroscope is inserted into the joint through the incision. A needle is placed into the joint in front of the arthroscope to allow the saline from the arthroscope to flow out of the joint. An instrument may also be inserted through the arthroscope for biopsy of the synovium (lining of the joint). The arthroscope and outflow needle are removed and the incision is closed with simple sutures.

29804
The physician inserts two arthroscopic cannulas into the temporomandibular joint. The physician introduces an arthroscope into one cannula to view the joint and operative field. Through the other arthroscopic cannula, small instruments are inserted and used to surgically repair the joint. The physician makes a 0.5 cm vertical incision anterior to the contour of the ear. The arthroscope is inserted through the incision into the joint. A second arthroscopic cannula is inserted into the joint through which instruments are inserted to repair the joint. A biopsy of the synovium (lining of the joint) may be performed. The arthroscopes are removed and the incisions are closed with layered sutures.

29805
A local or general anesthetic is commonly administered for shoulder arthroscopic procedures. Small percutaneous poke hole incisions are made above the joint and fluid is introduced into the joint space to provide a better view. A band may be placed to restrict blood flow for shoulder arthroscopy. A small incision, or percutaneous access, is made on one side of the joint and the arthroscope is inserted. The inside of the joint may be viewed through the eyepiece or the

Musculoskeletal

image can be reproduced on a screen. A cannula may be introduced to take a synovial biopsy. Once the biopsy is completed, the physician irrigates the joint until it is clear of blood and loose particles. A long-acting local anesthetic may be injected into the joint to help with postoperative pain. The joint is irrigated and sutures, a band-aid, or Steri-strips may be used to close the incisions. The area is covered with a dressing and a sling or shoulder immobilizer may be applied.

29806
The physician performs an arthroscopic capsulorrhaphy to repair and tighten the connective tissue surrounding the shoulder. The patient is placed in a lateral decubitus position, and the operative arm is suspended with traction. With the patient under general anesthesia, two to four percutaneous or small poke hole incisions are made to allow access to all areas of the shoulder joint. The arthroscope is inserted, allowing the physician to perform a diagnostic examination to determine the extent of damage to the joint. Through a cannula, a suture passer is used to loop a suture through the shoulder capsule and around the labrum. Any adhesions encountered are released. The inferior glenohumeral ligament may require tightening or relocation. One or more bone anchors are placed to stabilize the capsule. A drill guide is used to create a drill hole; the bone anchor is sutured into place. A long-acting local anesthetic may be injected into the joint to help with postoperative pain. The joint is irrigated, and all instruments are removed. The portal incisions are closed with sutures.

29807
SLAP lesions are injuries to the labrum that extend from anterior to the biceps tendon to posterior to the biceps tendon. For a SLAP lesion repair, the physician makes small percutaneous incisions for the arthroscope, the suture hook, and the cannula. The surgeon prepares the bony bed with a small ball burr and drills or punches a hole at the cartilage bone junction of the superior labrum. A hook is passed through the anterior superior portal and the inside limb is grasped with a suture retrieval forceps. The physician sets an anchor into the drill hole by mounting the suture anchor on the inserter and sliding it down the suture. The physician closes the loop with a slipknot that is tied and tightened outside the cannula. A knot pusher secures the knot under arthroscopic control. A long-acting local anesthetic may be injected into the joint to help with postoperative pain. The joint is irrigated and suture, band aid, or Steri-strips close the incisions. The area is covered with a dressing and a sling or shoulder immobilizer is applied.

29819
To remove loose bodies, such as floating cartilage, the physician visualizes the foreign bodies and removes them with instruments passed through the percutaneous portal holes. For a synovectomy, the physician uses the arthroscope to investigate any problems associated with the synovium. Through the arthroscope, the physician removes the synovium from inside the shoulder joint using cutting tools and arthroscopic suction equipment. A long-acting local anesthetic may be injected into the joint to help with postoperative pain. The joint is irrigated and suture, band aid, or Steri-strip closes the incisions. The area is covered with a dressing and a sling or shoulder immobilizer is applied.

29820-29821
The patient is positioned side-lying with arm suspended using a weight and a pulley system. An anesthetic is administered. Two to four small poke hole (port) incisions are made around the shoulder joint to allow access to all areas of the shoulder joint. A solution is pumped through one of these incisions and into the joint to expand the joint for better visualization and to cleanse the joint. The arthroscope is inserted percutaneously or through a small incision allowing the physician to perform a diagnostic arthroscopic exam by visualizing the shoulder joint. The synovium is removed with a motorized synovial resector inserted through a port. The instruments are removed and a long-acting local anesthetic may be injected into the joint to help with postoperative pain. The joint is irrigated and suture, band aid, or Steri-strips close the incisions. The area is covered with a dressing and a sling or shoulder immobilizer is applied. Report 29820 for a partial synovectomy and 29821 for a complete synovectomy.

29822-29823
The patient is positioned side-lying with arm suspended using a weight and a pulley system. An anesthetic is administered. Small percutaneous poke hole (port) incisions are made around the shoulder joint to allow access to all areas of the shoulder joint. A solution is pumped through one of these incisions and into the joint to expand the joint for better visualization and to cleanse the joint. The arthroscope is inserted allowing the physician to perform a diagnostic arthroscopic exam by visualizing the shoulder joint. A long-acting local anesthetic may be injected into the joint to help with postoperative pain. The joint is irrigated and sutures, band aids, or Steri-strips close the incisions. The area is covered with a dressing and a sling or shoulder immobilizer is applied. Report 29822 if the arthroscopic surgery is performed with limited debridement consisting of one or two discrete structures, including the articular capsule, the articular or bursal side of the rotator cuff, biceps anchor complex or tendon, glenoid or humeral bone or articular cartilage, labrum, subacromial bursa, or one or more foreign bodies. Report 29823 if the debridement is extensive and includes three or more of these structures.

29824
The physician makes small percutaneous poke hole incisions around the shoulder joint to allow access to all areas of the joint. A solution is pumped through one of these incisions and into the joint to expand the joint for better visualization and to cleanse the joint. The arthroscope is inserted allowing the physician to perform a diagnostic arthroscopic exam by visualizing

the shoulder joint. The physician may shell the bone out of its periosteal lining, including the distal articular surface, when using arthroscopic guidance. A long-acting local anesthetic may be injected into the joint to help with postoperative pain. The joint is irrigated and suture, band aid, or Steri-strips close the incisions. The area is covered with a dressing and a sling or shoulder immobilizer is applied.

29825

The physician makes small percutaneous poke hole incisions around the shoulder joint to allow access to all areas of the joint. A solution is pumped through one of these incisions and into the joint to expand the joint for better visualization and to cleanse the joint. The arthroscope is inserted allowing the physician to perform a diagnostic arthroscopic exam by visualizing the shoulder joint. The physician may shell the bone out of its periosteal lining, including the distal articular surface, when using arthroscopic guidance. The physician lyses and resects adhesions, with or without manipulation. A long-acting local anesthetic may be injected into the joint to help with postoperative pain. The joint is irrigated and suture, band aid, or Steri-strips close the incisions. The area is covered with a dressing and a sling or shoulder immobilizer is applied.

29826

The physician makes small percutaneous poke hole incisions around the shoulder joint to allow access to all areas of the joint. A solution is pumped through one of these incisions and into the joint to expand the joint for better visualization and to cleanse the joint. The subacromial space is decompressed and a partial acromioplasty, with or without coracoacromial release, is performed. The patient is seated with the torso raised and a sheet placed on the medial border of the affected scapula. Anterior, lateral, and posterior arthroscopic portals are established and a cannula is inserted through the anterior and lateral portals to accommodate the inflow and instrumentation. The arthroscope is inserted into the posterior portal, where it is driven into the subacromial space for visualization of the subacromial joint. A limited bursectomy is performed using a full radius shaver and, if necessary, the physician clears the undersurface of the anterolateral acromion of soft tissue using intra-articular cautery. The acromial ligament may be released. A long-acting local anesthetic may be injected into the joint to help with postoperative pain. The joint is irrigated and suture, band aid, or Steri-strips close the incisions. The area is covered with a dressing and a sling or shoulder immobilizer is applied.

29827

The physician performs a surgical arthroscopy of the shoulder to repair a torn rotator cuff. The patient is positioned side-lying with the arm suspended. Small percutaneous poke hole incisions are made around the shoulder through which the arthroscopic instruments are inserted. A solution is pumped through one of these incisions to cleanse and expand the joint for better visualization. The physician first performs a diagnostic arthroscopic exam to assess the joint. A limited bursectomy may be performed with a subacromial decompression in which the undersurface of the anterolateral acromion is cleared of soft tissue, if necessary. The deltoid muscle is split from its acromion attachment about 5 cm and the tendon edge is debrided and mobilized. A transverse bony trough 3 to 4 mm is made, and tunnels are drilled through the bone trough to the lateral cortex of the greater tuberosity. The tendon edge is brought into the trough with permanent sutures and anchor sutures are placed. Sutures are placed into the bone and brought through the tendon. A hemostat is placed on the cuff to retract the tendon and take tension off the sutures. The anchor sutures are tied down, followed by the sutures to the bony trough. The free ends of the sutures are passed through the tunnels and tied over a bony bridge. The longitudinal portions of the tear are closed with absorbable suture and a range of motion check is done on the arm. The deltoid splits, subcutaneous tissue, and skin are closed with suture, band aid, or Steri-strip, and the arm is placed in a sling to maintain abduction. If necessary, a small percutaneous incision may be made laterally, incorporating one of the portholes to facilitate the arthroscopic repair. When most of the procedure is performed arthroscopically, report 29827. When the arthroscopic work is minimal and most of the procedure is performed via open access, report 23412.

29828

The physician performs arthroscopic biceps tenodesis. With the patient under appropriate anesthesia, standard arthroscopic portals are established. A monofilament suture is passed through an 18-gauge needle placed into the biceps tendon, and an arthroscopic suture instrument is utilized to retrieve the suture. The physician uses an arthroscopic basket to release the tendon from its origin, and the arthroscopic equipment is transferred to the subacromial space. Using the arthroscopic basket, the physician identifies and opens the tendon sheath. Electrocautery may be used to clean the surrounding tissues. A probe is utilized to free the tendon, which is extracted through one of the arthroscopic portals. The tendon is pulled into a humeral socket that has been drilled at the top of the bicipital groove. Under arthroscopic control, it is fixed using a bioabsorbable interference screw. Instrumentation is removed and the arthroscopic portals are closed with sutures, band aids, or Steri-strips.

29830-29838

The physician performs elbow arthroscopy with the patient in a supine position. Appropriate anesthesia is administered. The physician makes 1 cm portal incisions, or percutaneous access, to insert the arthroscope into the elbow joint space. The five most commonly used portals are the lateral, anterolateral, anteromedial, posterolateral, and straight positions. Small percutaneous poke hole incisions above the joint and fluid are introduced into the joint space to provide

Musculoskeletal

a better view. The physician places the arthroscope into the elbow joint and examines the humeral-ulnar, humeral-radial, and/or radial-ulnar joints. The elbow is flexed and extended and pronated and supinated to allow visualization and examination of all joint spaces and surfaces. If there is evidence of synovial proliferation or inflammation indicating disease, the physician uses an instrument to obtain a small piece of synovium for biopsy, when performed. In 29830, the physician performs a diagnostic arthroscopy. In 29834, the physician examines all parts of the elbow joint with the arthroscope. Any loose bodies (e.g., small pieces of cartilage from chondral injuries) or foreign bodies (e.g., bullet or nail) are removed by identifying them through the arthroscope and using another portal incision to remove the object. In 29835, the physician may also perform a partial synovectomy; in 29836, the physician may perform a complete synovectomy. In 29837, the physician performs a limited debridement. In 29838, the physician uses the arthroscope to examine all parts of the elbow joint. Debridement is performed on proliferative cartilage, a degenerative joint, or roughened or frayed articular cartilage. The physician uses instruments through the arthroscope to cut and remove inflamed and proliferated synovium and to clean and smooth the articular joint surfaces of the elbow. Extensive debridement includes all joints of the elbow. The portal incisions are closed with sutures or Steri-strips.

29840-29845

The physician performs wrist arthroscopy. The joint is distended using finger traps on the index and long fingers that are attached to a 10-pound weight pulley. Counter traction is applied to the arm with a second 10-pound pulley. The joint may be injected with lidocaine and epinephrine to distend the capsule. A wrap may be applied to the forearm to prevent extravasation of fluid. Portal incisions are made. The scope is inserted. Irrigation fluid is directed into each compartment of the wrist joint using the arthroscope for visualization. The physician inspects the wrist joint. The wrist is manipulated to allow visualization of all joint spaces and surfaces. In 29840, a diagnostic arthroscopy is performed. A synovial biopsy may also be obtained. In 29843, an infection is treated using lavage and drainage. Lavage is continued until the fluid is clear. A motorized suction cutter may be used to remove encrusted fluid (exudate) and any fibrinous clots. Drains are placed as needed. The portal incisions are closed with sutures or Steri-strips. In 29844, the synovial membrane lining the joint capsule is partially removed. In 29845, it is completely removed by use of a motorized, suction cutting resector. The joint is irrigated and all instruments are removed. Drains are placed as needed. The portal incisions are closed with sutures or Steri-strips.

29846

The physician performs surgical wrist arthroscopy with excision and/or repair of the triangular fibrocartilage and/or joint debridement. The joint is distended using finger traps on the index and long fingers that are attached to a 10 lb weight pulley. Counter traction is applied to the arm with a second 10 lb pulley. The joint is injected with lidocaine and epinephrine to distend the capsule. A wrap is applied to the forearm to prevent extravasation of fluid. Portal incisions are made. The scope is inserted. The physician inspects the wrist joint. The wrist is manipulated to allow visualization of all joint spaces and surfaces. The joint is debrided, which involves removing any inflamed or devitalized tissue. The articular surfaces are cleaned and smoothed. Tears present in the triangular fibrocartilage are sutured or the cartilage is removed with instruments placed through the arthroscope. The joint is irrigated and all instruments are removed. The portal incisions are closed with sutures or Steri-strips.

29847

The physician performs surgical wrist arthroscopy with internal fixation for a fracture or joint instability. The joint is distended using finger traps on the index and long fingers that are attached to a 10 lb weight pulley. Counter traction is applied to the arm with a second 10 lb pulley. The joint is injected with lidocaine and epinephrine to distend the capsule. A wrap is applied to the forearm to prevent extravasation of fluid. Portal incisions are made. The scope is inserted. The physician inspects the wrist joint. The wrist is manipulated to allow visualization of all joint spaces and surfaces. The site of the fracture or instability is identified. The physician uses instruments placed through the arthroscope to manipulate the fracture or unstable area into proper alignment. Internal fixation, consisting of wires, pins, and/or screws, is applied. The joint is irrigated and all instruments are removed. The portal incisions are closed with sutures or Steri-strips.

29848

The patient is placed supine with the arm positioned on a hand table. Endoscopic release may be accomplished by a one or two portal technique. In a single portal technique, a small, 1 1/2 cm, horizontal incision is made at the wrist. Using a two portal technique, two small incisions are made, one in the palm and one at the wrist. The palmar skin, underlying cushioning fat, protective fascia, and muscle are not cut. The endoscope is introduced underneath the transverse carpal ligament. The endoscope allows the physician to view the procedure on a monitor. A blade attached to the arthroscope is used to incise the transverse carpal ligament from the inside of the carpal tunnel. The instruments are removed and the portal(s) closed with sutures or Steri-strips. A splint may be applied.

29850-29851

The physician makes 1 cm long portal incisions on either side of the patellar tendon for arthroscopic access into the knee joint. The knee joint is examined with the arthroscope and the fracture site is identified. Any loose bodies are removed and the physician may debride the knee joint. If the fracture is not displaced (29850) and appears stable, no fixation is needed. If the fracture is not stable (29851), the physician may reduce the fracture by manipulating it into place and applying one or more screws for adequate fixation. An additional incision may be made for better access in applying fixation. Incisions are closed with sutures and staples and/or Steri-strips. A temporary drain may be applied. A post-op brace or splint may be used.

29855-29856
The physician treats a unicondylar (29855) or bicondylar (29856) tibial fracture. The physician makes 1 cm long incisions on either side of the patellar tendon to access the knee joint and insert the arthroscope. The knee may be irrigated free of blood. The knee joint is examined with the arthroscope and, if possible, the fracture fragments are identified. A calibrated hole probe can be used to palpate the bone fragments and to measure their size and displacement. An osteotome or probe can sometimes be used in conjunction with the arthroscope to reduce the fracture fragments. If not, an additional incision is made 3 to 4 cm below the joint line. An impactor is used to elevate the fragment. The fracture may be stabilized with cancellous screws. Incisions are closed with sutures and Steri-strips.

29860
The physician performs an arthroscopy for diagnostic purposes with the patient supine or in a side-lying position. The hip is abducted and distracted with enough force to allow adequate visualization through the arthroscope. Once joint distraction has been verified, a needle is inserted into the joint using fluoroscopic guidance to create a portal just superior to the greater trochanter. Using the Seldinger technique, a wire is introduced through the needle. A small skin incision, or percutaneous access, is made, a trocar is placed over the wire, and it is advanced to the hip capsule where the sharpened end is used to break through the hip capsule and into the joint. Using the same technique, a second (anterolateral) port is established to aid in the examination of the joint structures and to pass instruments. Irrigation fluid is directed into each compartment of the joint using the arthroscope for visualization. The joint is examined and a portion of synovium may be removed for biopsy. The instruments are removed. A temporary drain may be placed, and the incisions are closed with Steri-strips and/or sutures.

29861
The physician performs an arthroscopy for removal of a loose or foreign body with the patient in a supine or lateral (side-lying) position. The hip is abducted and distracted with enough force to allow adequate visualization through the arthroscope. Once joint distraction has been verified radiologically, the hip is prepped and draped and a needle is inserted (avoiding neurovascular structures), by use of fluoroscopic guidance, into the joint to create a portal just superior to the greater trochanter. Using the Seldinger technique, a wire is introduced through the needle. A small skin incision is made, a trocar is placed over the wire, and it is advanced to the hip capsule where the sharpened end is used to break through the hip capsule and into the joint. A fiberoptic arthroscope especially designed for hip arthroscopy is placed over the trocar into the joint. Using the same technique, a second (anterolateral) port is established to aid in the examination of the joint structures and to pass instruments. Irrigation fluid is directed into each compartment of the joint using the arthroscope for visualization. The joint is examined. Small loose bodies can be suctioned or irrigated from the joint. Larger loose bodies are divided into smaller pieces, or shaved, and grasped by a clamp and removed. The instruments are removed. A temporary drain may be placed, and the incisions are closed with Steri-strips and/or sutures.

29862
The physician performs arthroscopy to remove a lesion of the articular cartilage and/or to resect the labrum with the patient in a supine or side-lying position. The hip is abducted and distracted with enough force to allow adequate visualization through the arthroscope. Once joint distraction has been verified radiologically, a needle is inserted with fluoroscopic guidance into the joint to create a portal just superior to the greater trochanter. Using the Seldinger technique, a wire is introduced through the needle. A small skin incision is made, a trocar is placed over the wire, and it is advanced to the hip capsule where the sharpened end is used to break through the hip capsule and into the joint. A fiberoptic arthroscope is placed over the trocar into the joint. Using the same technique, a second (anterolateral) port is established to aid in the examination of the joint structures and to pass instruments. If a third port is necessary, it is usually placed close to the anterolateral port. Irrigation fluid is directed into each compartment of the joint using the arthroscope for visualization. The joint is examined. The articular cartilage is debrided/shaved or an abrasion arthroplasty is performed until bleeding bone is reached. The joint is irrigated. A resection of the labrum (acetabular lip) may be performed. The instruments are removed. A temporary drain may be placed and the incisions are closed with Steri-strips and/or sutures.

29863
The physician performs arthroscopy with a synovectomy with the patient in a supine or side-lying position. The hip is abducted and distracted with enough force to allow adequate visualization through the arthroscope. Once joint distraction has been verified radiologically, a needle is inserted with fluoroscopic guidance into the joint to create a portal just superior to the greater trochanter. Using the Seldinger technique, a wire is introduced through the needle. A small skin incision is made, a trocar is placed over the wire, and it is advanced to the hip capsule where the sharpened end is used to break through the hip capsule and into the joint. An arthroscope is placed over the trocar into the joint. Using the same technique, a second (anterolateral) port is established to aid in the examination of the joint structures and to pass instruments. If a third port is necessary, it is usually placed close to the anterolateral port. Irrigation fluid is directed into each compartment of the joint

using the arthroscope for visualization. The joint is examined. Using an instrument passed through the anterolateral port, perilabial, ligamentum teres, and inferior capsule synovium may be excised and removed. The instruments are removed. A temporary drain may be placed, and the incisions are closed with Steri-strips and/or sutures.

[29914]
The physician performs an arthroscopic femoroplasty for the treatment of a cam lesion, a type of femoroacetabular impingement caused by a "bump" on the surface of the femoral head that abuts against the acetabulum rim; most common in young athletic males. With the patient under appropriate anesthesia, the hip is subluxed using leg traction to allow adequate visualization through the arthroscope. The physician creates portals through which an arthroscope and surgical instruments are inserted. Irrigation fluid is directed into each compartment of the joint using the arthroscope for visualization. Targeted sections of the femoral head and anterior femoral neck are removed to increase clearance in the joint. Range of motion (ROM) and any residual impingement are evaluated. The instruments are removed. A temporary drain may be placed, and the incisions are closed with Steri-strips and/or sutures.

[29915]
The physician performs an arthroscopic acetabuloplasty for the treatment of a pincer lesion, a type of femoroacetabular impingement caused by an abnormal overhand of the acetabular rim; most common in middle-aged women. With the patient under appropriate anesthesia, the hip is subluxed using leg traction to allow adequate visualization through the arthroscope. The physician creates portals through which an arthroscope and surgical instruments are inserted. Irrigation fluid is directed into each compartment of the joint using the arthroscope for visualization. If necessary, due to the size of the pincer lesion, the labrum may be detached using a curved blade. Using a motorized burr, the acetabuloplasty is performed, removing a portion of the acetabular rim. Suture repair is performed if detachment of the labrum is necessary. The instruments are removed. A temporary drain may be placed, and the incisions are closed with Steri-strips and/or sutures.

[29916]
The physician performs an arthroscopic repair of the labrum, the cartilage that lines the rim of the acetabulum. Labral tears are often associated with femoroacetabular impingement (FAI). A primary, or type 1, labral tear is one in which the labrum is detached from the acetabular rim, and is typically caused by a cam impingement. A type 2 labral tear is most often caused by the labrum being crushed against the neck of the femur by an overhanging rim of the acetabulum, also known as a pincer lesion. With the patient under appropriate anesthesia, the hip is subluxed using leg traction to allow adequate visualization through the arthroscope. The physician creates portals through which an arthroscope and surgical instruments are inserted. Irrigation fluid is directed into each compartment of the joint using the arthroscope for visualization. After determining the type of tear and assessing its severity, the surgeon may excise the torn piece of labrum or may debride, trim, and repair it. The instruments are removed. A temporary drain may be placed, and the incisions are closed with Steri-strips and/or sutures.

29866-29867
An osteochondral graft is a bone/cartilage transplant that treats defects of the knee from disabling cartilage injury or disease, such as osteochondritis dissecans. Arthroscopic osteochondral grafting using the mosaicplasty technique is described here. Multiple cylindrical grafts are placed in corresponding size cylindrical holes made in the recipient area, instead of using one larger bone plug. Portals for inserting the instruments are chosen to ensure perpendicular access to the recipient site. Irrigation fluid is directed into each compartment of the joint using the arthroscope for visualization. Detached cartilage is excised, the margins squared off, and the subchondral bone is abraded to healthy, bleeding tissue. The number and size of grafts needed is determined. In 29866, a tubular chisel is used to harvest cylindrical osteochondral grafts down to the desired level, perpendicular to the cartilage surface, from the patient. Grafts are harvested from the non-weight bearing patellofemoral area, medial or lateral femoral trochlear rim, or the intercondylar notch periphery. The grafts are ejected from the chisel. A guide tube is put in place and the recipient hole is drilled to the desired depth with a graduated bit, replaced with a tapered dilator, and the graft is inserted and tamped into place. This is repeated until all grafts have been placed. Report 29867 when fresh donor tissue from a tissue bank is used instead of harvested from the patient. A temporary drain may be placed, and the incisions are closed with Steri-strips and/or sutures.

29868
A previously removed meniscus, the fibrocartilaginous support of the knee joint, is replaced with a cadaver donor meniscus, medial or lateral. Imaging is done to size-match the graft to the recipient knee. The arthroscope and a tibial guide are placed through portal holes. Irrigation fluid is directed into each compartment of the joint using the arthroscope for visualization. The remaining native meniscal cartilage is removed, including resecting the native horns. Pins are placed at posterior and anterior horn locations, suture tunnels are drilled over the pins, and sutures are passed. The anterior portal is widened, and both the anterior and posterior sutures are brought out together. The graft is brought in through the widened incision, or a necessary arthrotomy, and sutures are placed through each horn of the implant. The posterior and anterior horn sutures are drawn out through the tibial tunnel and secured to the tibial bone. Meniscal repair techniques are used to suture the graft securely to the capsule placing knots directly over the capsule.

Routine closure is performed. Other techniques may employ separate bone plugs attached to the horns to insert the graft or a common bone attached to both horns on the graft inserted into a receiving slot in the tibia. A temporary drain may be placed, and the incisions are closed with Steri-strips and/or sutures.

29870
The physician performs a diagnostic arthroscopy of the knee. Portal incisions of 1 cm in length are made on either side of the patellar tendon for arthroscopic access into the knee joint. With the use of the arthroscope and a probe, each compartment of the knee is examined for pathology. This includes examination of the patellar-articular surface, medial and lateral meniscus, cruciate ligaments, and joint surfaces. Additional portal incisions may be made to better access some compartments. If there is suspicion of a primary disease of the synovium, a biopsy is performed. A temporary drain may be applied. Incisions are closed with sutures and Steri-strips.

29871
The physician makes 1 cm long portal incisions on either side of the patellar tendon to arthroscopically access the knee joint. Lavage is accomplished with a minimum of 4 liters of a physiologic solution. The irrigation solution is directed into each compartment while visualizing through the arthroscope. Lavage is continued until the outflow is clear. A motorized suction cutter is used to remove encrusted fluid (exudate) and any fibrinous clots. Drains are placed as needed and incisions are closed with sutures and Steri-strips. The drains are removed after 48 to 78 hours.

29873
The physician performs a knee arthroscopy with lateral release. Lateral retinacular release is done when too much lateral tension on the patella from tightness of the lateral retinaculum causes patellar misalignment, not allowing correct movement. This can be associated with articular cartilage lesions and idiopathic chondromalacia. The physician makes 1 cm long portal incisions on either side of the patellar tendon to arthroscopically access the knee joint. The instruments are inserted and the knee is assessed. The release is done at the end of the arthroscopy. The tight lateral ligaments, including the lateral patellofemoral and the lateral patellotibial ligament, are released detaching the patella from the soft tissue structures, including the lateral retinaculum, muscle fibers, and joint capsule.

29874
The physician makes 1 cm long portal incisions on either side of the patellar tendon for arthroscopic access into the knee joint. A thorough exam is made of each compartment in the knee. Additional portal incisions may be made to gain better access to the knee compartments. Any loose bodies (fragments of cartilage or bone) encountered are removed through the portal incisions. Small loose bodies can be suctioned or irrigated from the joint. Larger loose bodies are grasped by a clamp and removed. Very large loose bodies may require enlargement of a portal or division with an arthroscopic scissor before removal. A temporary drain may be applied and incisions are closed with sutures and Steri-strips.

29875-29876
The physician performs an arthroscopic synovectomy. The physician makes 1 cm long portal incisions on either side of the patellar tendon for arthroscopic access into the joint. Proliferative, diseased synovium is removed with a motorized, suction, cutting resector. If the plica located along the medial side of the patella is inflamed, it may require removal. Removal is accomplished by dividing and excising the plica. The synovectomy is limited in 29875. For a more extensive synovectomy (29876), up to six portal incisions may be made to access all of the involved compartments of the knee. A temporary drain may be applied and incisions are closed with sutures and Steri-strips.

29877
The physician makes 1 cm long portal incisions on either side of the patellar tendon for arthroscopic access into the knee joint. Lesions in the articular cartilage are identified by the arthroscope and the use of a probe. Additional portal incisions may be made to provide better access to the cartilage lesions. Debridement of the unstable hyaline cartilage or partially fragmented cartilage is accomplished with a motorized suction cutter. This smooths the roughened or damaged cartilage. Any loose bodies are removed. After debridement, the joint is flushed. A temporary drain may be applied, and incisions are closed with sutures and Steri-strips.

29879
The physician makes 1 cm long portal incisions on either side of the patellar tendon for arthroscopic access into the knee joint. Lesions of the articular cartilage are identified by the arthroscope and the use of a probe. Additional portal incisions may be made to provide better access to the lesions. Debridement of the unstable or fragmented cartilage is accomplished with a motorized suction cutter. The cartilage is smoothed down to the layer of subchondral bone which promotes bleeding and regeneration of cartilage. Any loose bodies are removed. The physician may also drill holes into the subchondral bone or create tiny fractures (microfractures) to further promote cartilage regeneration. The joint is flushed. A temporary drain may be applied. Incisions are closed with sutures and Steri-strips.

29880-29881
The physician makes 1 cm long portal incisions on either side of the patellar tendon for arthroscopic access into the knee joint. Once the meniscal tear is identified, additional portal incisions may be made to provide easier access to the area. There may be a tear on both the medial and lateral meniscus (29880) or only the medial or the lateral meniscus (29881). The procedure is the same for medial or lateral meniscal tears. Angled scissors, a motorized cutter, or punch

forceps remove torn fragments. The remaining intact meniscus is trimmed and contoured. Lesions in the articular cartilage in the same or a different compartment may be identified by the arthroscope and the use of a probe. Additional portal incisions may be made to provide better access to the cartilage lesions. Debridement of the unstable hyaline cartilage or partially fragmented cartilage is accomplished with a motorized suction cutter. This smooths the roughened or damaged cartilage. Any loose bodies are removed. After debridement, the joint is flushed. A temporary drain may be applied and the incisions closed with sutures and Steri-strips.

29882-29883

The physician makes 1 cm long portal incisions on either side of the patellar tendon for arthroscopic access into the knee joint. The meniscal tear(s) is identified through the arthroscope. There may be a tear on only the medial or the lateral meniscus (29882) or both may be torn (29883). Depending on the site of the tear, other portal incisions may be made to gain better access. Angled scissors, motorized cutters, and punch forceps are used to debride the tear margins and break the surface of the adjacent synovium in preparation for repair. A 3 cm to 4 cm incision is made along the medial or lateral joint line, depending on which meniscus is torn. A cannula passes sutures through the meniscal tear and out through the joint line incision. A temporary drain may be applied. Subcutaneous layers are sutured and skin closure is with Steri-strips. Typically, a hinged knee brace is applied after surgery.

29884

The physician makes 1 cm long portal incisions for arthroscopic access into and around the knee joint. A blunt trocar, a knife, scissors, or a mechanical shaver may remove any adhesions limiting range of knee motion. If a manipulation is performed, the physician will remove the arthroscope and apply gradual, progressive pressure to bend or straighten the knee. Manipulation helps the knee regain range of motion. A drain may be applied. Incisions are closed with sutures and Steri-strips.

29885

The physician makes a 1 cm long portal incision on either side of the patellar tendon. The defect is visualized through the arthroscope. Any loose bodies are removed with grasping instruments. A motorized suction cutter is used to debride the disrupted hyaline cartilage. Drill holes 2 cm in depth are made into the lesion, penetrating the vascular bone at the base of the defect. This promotes bleeding and subsequent healing of the lesion. Bone is harvested from the patient's hip, rib, or skull for grafting and the surgically created donor site is closed. The bone graft is sized to fit the defect. The physician determines if a screw is needed for internal fixation. If so, a screw is placed. A temporary drain may be applied. The incisions are closed with sutures and Steri-strips.

29886

The physician makes a 1 cm long portal incision on either side of the patellar tendon. The defect is visualized through the arthroscope. A motorized suction cutter is used to debride the disrupted hyaline cartilage. Drill holes 2 cm in depth are made into the lesion in order to penetrate the vascular bone at the base of the defect. This promotes bleeding and subsequent healing of the lesion. The incisions are closed with sutures and Steri-strips. A temporary drain may be applied.

29887

The physician makes a portal incision 1 cm long on either side of the patellar tendon. The defect is visualized through the arthroscope. A motorized suction cutter debrides the disrupted hyaline cartilage. Drill holes 2 cm in depth are made into the lesion in order to penetrate the vascular bone at the base of the defect. This promotes bleeding and subsequent healing of the lesion. Internal fixation is accomplished by placing a screw into the lesion. The incisions are closed with sutures and Steri-strips. A temporary drain may be applied.

29888-29889

The physician makes a portal incision 1 cm long on either side of the inferior patella for arthroscopic access into the knee joint. If the ligament is intact but torn away from its bony attachment, the physician may reattach the ligament with a screw. If the ligament is nonfunctional, it is removed with the arthroscope. For an anterior cruciate ligament reconstruction (29888), a 5 cm to 12 cm incision is made on the anterior lower patella and upper tibia. A tunnel is drilled through the tibia into the knee joint. A second tunnel is drilled from inside the knee joint, through the femur. With the aid of the arthroscope for visualization, a new ligament graft is placed in the tibial tunnel and positioned inside the knee joint. The bony ends of the ligament are placed in the tibial and femoral tunnels. The ligament is secured with interference screws in both tunnels. For a posterior cruciate ligament reconstruction (29889), an additional 3 cm to 5 cm incision is made along the medial aspect of the knee joint to allow for proper location of the femoral tunnel. Incisions are closed with staples or Steri-strips. A temporary drain may be inserted.

29891

The physician performs an arthroscopy to excise an osteochondral defect, including drilling of the talus and/or tibia. The patient is placed supine with the hip and upper part of the leg elevated, rotated slightly forward, and with the lower part of the leg, ankle, and foot resting on a cushioned platform. The ankle joint is distended to allow access for the first port. Distraction is usually not performed. The skin is superficially incised anterolaterally. The tissues and tendons are separated to the joint capsule by a clamp, and a blunt trocar is inserted into the joint. The arthroscope in placed over the trocar and advanced into the joint. A second anteromedial portal is established for further examination and for instrument passage. The joint is examined and any loose bodies are removed. The osteochondral defect of the talus and/or tibia is excised and the sides of the crater are contoured. Multiple holes may be drilled in the bone to promote vascularization. The joint is irrigated, and the instruments are removed. A temporary drain may be placed, and the incisions are closed with Steri-strips and/or sutures.

29892
The physician performs an arthroscopy to aid in the repair of a large osteochondritis dissecans lesion, talar dome fracture, or tibial plafond fracture. The patient is placed supine with the hip and upper part of the leg elevated, rotated slightly forward, and with the lower part of the leg, ankle, and foot resting on a cushioned platform. The ankle joint is distended to allow access for the first port. The skin is superficially incised. The tissues and tendons are separated to the joint capsule by a clamp, and a blunt trocar is inserted into the joint. The arthroscope is placed over the trocar and advanced into the joint. A second anteromedial portal is established for further examination and for instrument passage. The joint is examined, and any loose bodies are removed. A large osteochondritis dissecans lesion is excised, and the sides of the crater are contoured; a talar dome or tibial plafond fracture is treated. Internal fixation may be applied at the fracture site. A temporary drain may be placed, and the incisions are closed with Steri-strips and/or sutures.

29893
The physician performs a plantar fasciotomy using an endoscope. The patient is placed prone. After administering a local anesthetic, the physician makes a small incision to create a passage for the endoscope. Other incisions are made as needed for additional instruments. One or more transverse divisions of the contracted and fibrotic cord(s) of plantar fascia in the foot are performed for therapeutic release. The instruments are removed and the wound closed with simple or layered sutures.

29894
The physician performs arthroscopy on an ankle joint to remove a loose body or foreign body from the joint. After induction of anesthesia in the operating room, the physician makes two to four 0.5 cm incisions around the ankle. Using arthroscopic instruments, the physician enters the ankle through these small incisions. The offending loose body or foreign body is identified. Instruments are introduced through the portal incisions and utilized to remove the foreign body. The joint is examined through the arthroscope and irrigated. The skin portals are closed and a dressing is applied.

29895
The physician performs arthroscopy on an ankle joint to remove the synovial lining of the joint. With the patient soothed by general anesthesia, the physician makes two to four 0.5 cm skin incisions around the ankle. The physician introduces the arthroscope into the ankle and conducts an exam. The offending synovial tissue is identified. Additional instruments are placed through the incisions. Using the arthroscope, the physician uses these instruments to excise the synovium. The joint is irrigated and the skin portals are closed. A dressing is applied.

29897
The physician performs arthroscopy on the ankle joint to minimally debride the joint. With the patient under general anesthesia, the physician makes two to four 0.5 cm skin incisions around the ankle joint. The arthroscope is introduced into the ankle joint and an examination is performed. The physician identifies areas of the joint where debridement is required. Additional surgical instruments are placed through the skin portals and into the joint. These are used to debride frayed, nonviable, or extraneous tissue. The ankle is irrigated and the skin incisions are closed. A dressing is applied.

29898
The physician performs arthroscopy on the ankle joint to extensively debride the joint. With the patient under general anesthesia, the physician makes two to four 0.5 cm skin incisions around the ankle joint. The arthroscope is introduced into the joint and the physician conducts an examination. Frayed cartilage, redundant synovium, defects in the articular surfaces, or bony abnormalities are identified. Additional arthroscopic instruments are placed into the joint through the skin incisions. These are used to extensively debride, excise, smooth, and/or wash out the offending tissues. A thorough irrigation is undertaken. The skin incisions are closed and a dressing is applied.

29899
The physician performs an arthroscopic arthrodesis of the ankle to fuse the joint in cases of severe degenerative or inflammatory arthritis. The patient is supine of the table with the ankle hanging off the table and a leg holder applied for positioning. Traction is applied and three small poke hole incisions are made around the ankle for portals through which the arthroscopic instruments are inserted. In the medial compartment, a full-radius resector is used to remove the soft tissue and expose the medial malleolus, medial side of the talus, and the talar dome. The articular cartilage is removed from the medial malleolus and talus around to the side of the ankle and as far posteriorly as is visible. The avascular subchondral bone is removed the same way starting laterally. The posterior tissues are removed next. After debridement of the articular cartilage and subchondral bone, a guide pin is placed through the fibula at an angle and a similar guide pin is placed through the tibia. Pin position is confirmed. The pins are backed out slightly while the joint is reduced and traction is removed. Joint reduction is checked. Guide pins are advanced into the talus under fluoroscopy and cancellous screws are passed over the pins. The joint is held in position while the screws are secured. Parallel medial screws are placed, one in the talus dome apex

Musculoskeletal

and the other behind and parallel to the first. X-rays are taken to confirm adequate reduction and fixation. The incisions are closed and a drain is placed.

29900
The metacarpophalangeal joints consist of the convex heads of the metacarpals articulating with the concave bases of the proximal phalanges. The metacarpophalangeal joint of interest is placed for easy access and an injection of local anesthetic is administered. Incisions for portals are made in the respective metacarpal to allow the arthroscope and surgical instruments to be introduced into the joint. The arthroscope is inserted through a portal into the joint, and the surgical equipment is passed through a second portal. A third portal may have been made for pumping fluid in to expand the joint space for clearer visualization. A needle is inserted through the trocar and twisted to cut out the tissue segment for biopsy. The biopsy needle, trocar, and arthroscope are removed. The site is cleansed and a pressure bandage is applied.

29901
The metacarpophalangeal joints consist of the convex heads of the metacarpals articulating with the concave bases of the proximal phalanges. The metacarpophalangeal joint of interest is placed for easy access and an injection of local anesthetic is administered. Incisions for portals are made in the respective metacarpal to allow the arthroscope and surgical instruments to be introduced into the joint. The arthroscope is inserted through a portal into the joint, and the surgical equipment is passed through a second portal. A third portal may have been made for pumping fluid in to expand the joint space for clearer visualization. Arthroscopic debridement is carried out over the surface of the lesion. The physician must avoid debridement of the adjacent joint surface, so as to avoid possible ankylosis. Closure of the wound includes a re-approximation of the attachment of adductor tendon to the dorsal extensor hood.

29902
The physician makes an incision along the midlateral aspect of the thumb, curves the incision over the MP joint, and extends the incision to the EPL tendon. The Stener lesion can be seen as a mass of tissue proximal to the adductor aponeurosis. A Stener lesion occurs when a torn distal edge of ulnar collateral ligament displaces superficially and proximally to the adductor aponeurosis. The ruptured end of ligament is no longer in contact with its area of insertion of the phalanx. A longitudinal incision is made through the aponeurosis volar to the edge of the EPL, leaving a rim of tissue on the tendon to be used for later closure. The adductor tendon is retracted volarly and the dorsal capsule is reflected to permit a clear view of the joint and the inside portion of the collateral ligament. The physician assesses the injury (i.e., ligament rupture at the insertion into the phalanx). The ulnar collateral ligament flap is partially dissected and mobilized off the metacarpal and the volar edge of the proximal phalange is debrided of soft tissue. The physician drills two parallel holes distally and dorsally to exit on the far side of the cortex. Sutures are passed through the distal ligament and pulled through the drill holes and tied over a padded button. Closure of the wound includes a re-approximation of the attachment of adductor tendon to the dorsal extensor hood.

29904-29907
The physician performs arthroscopy on the subtalar joint (the joint of the foot located at the meeting point of the talus and the calcaneus, or heel bone). After induction of anesthesia, the physician makes two to four 0.5 cm incisions around the ankle. Using arthroscopic instruments, the physician enters the ankle through these small incisions. In 29904, instruments are introduced through the portal incisions and utilized to remove loose or foreign bodies. In 29905, the physician removes the synovial lining of the joint using arthroscopic tools. The offending synovial tissue is identified and additional instruments are placed through the portals. Using the arthroscope, the physician uses these instruments to excise the synovium. In 29906, the physician debrides the joint. The physician identifies areas of the joint where debridement is required. Additional surgical instruments are placed through the skin portals and into the joint. These are used to debride frayed, nonviable, or extraneous tissue. In 29907, the physician performs arthrodesis (fusion) of the subtalar joint using arthroscopic equipment. Morcellized bone grafting and internal screw fixation may be utilized. Following each of these procedures, the joint is examined through the arthroscope and irrigated. The skin portals are closed and a dressing is applied.

Respiratory

30000-30020
The physician makes an incision to decompress and drain a collection of pus or blood in the nasal mucosa for 30000 or septal mucosa for 30020. A hemostat bluntly penetrates the pockets and allows the fluid to evacuate. Once decompressed, a small latex drain may be placed into the incision site. This allows an escape for any fluids that may continue to enter the pocket. If a drain is used, it is removed within 48 hours. The nasal cavity may be packed with gauze or Telfa to provide pressure against the mucosa and assist decompression after drainage. The incision may be closed primarily or may be left to granulate without closure.

30100
The physician removes mucosa from inside the nose for biopsy. This biopsy is performed when the mucosa is suspicious for disease. Some normal tissue adjacent to the diseased mucosa is also removed during the biopsy. This allows the pathologist to compare diseased versus nondiseased tissues. The excision site may be closed primarily with sutures or may be allowed to granulate without closure.

30110
The physician removes a polyp from inside the nose. Nasal polyps may obstruct both the airway passages and sinus drainage ducts in the nose. The area is approached intranasally. Topical vasoconstrictive agents are applied to the nasal mucosa. Local anesthesia is injected underneath and around the polyp. A scalpel or biting forceps excise the polyp. Small polyps may leave mucosal defects that do not require closure. With larger defects, the mucosa is closed with sutures in a single layer. The physician may place Telfa to pack the nasal cavity during the first 24 hours.

30115
The physician removes complicated nasal polyps in a hospital setting. Nasal polyps may obstruct both the airway passages and sinus drainage ducts in the nose. The area is approached intranasally. Topical vasoconstrictive agents are applied to the nasal mucosa. Local anesthesia is injected underneath and around the polyp. Large polyps are removed with a wire snare stretching the polyp base; the snare or a scalpel can be used to detach the polyp from its mucosal base. A scalpel or biting forceps excise smaller polyps. Small polyps may leave mucosal defects that do not require closure. With larger defects, the mucosa is closed with sutures in a single layer. The physician may place Telfa to pack the nasal cavity during the first 24 hours.

30117-30118
The physician removes or destroys intranasal soft tissue lesions using techniques such as surgical excision, cryosurgery, chemical application, or laser surgery. The lesion is approached intranasally in 30117. The physician performs a lateral rhinotomy by retracting the lateral ala to expose the internal nose in 30118. Surgical excision can be utilized to remove the lesion. Cryosurgery freezes and kills soft tissue lesions. Laser surgery vaporizes and emulsifies the lesions. Chemical application of topical vasoconstrictive agents and local anesthesia cauterizes vessels and limits postsurgical hemorrhage. Postoperative wound closure or intranasal packing may not be necessary.

30120
Rhinophyma describes a chronic skin disorder categorized under part of an advanced staged rosacea called phymatous rosacea, identified with significant disfigurement from severe redness and a bulbous nose caused by hypertrophy and hyperplasia of the sebaceous nasal glands. The condition can also seriously impact the function of the nose and without surgery may produce a functional airway compromise (airway obstruction). The physician surgically removes diseased tissue caused by rhinophyma from the external nasal tip. Local anesthesia is injected into the nasal tip. The excess tissue is removed by carving and recontouring hyperplastic tissue from the area. Scalpels, dermabrasion (planing with fine sandpaper or wire brushes), and lasers are common methods of removing this excess tissue. A thin layer of epithelium is maintained over the nasal cartilages to ensure adequate healing. Separately reportable skin grafting may be necessary for very large lesions.

30124-30125
The physician removes a dermoid (developmental) cyst of the nose that may be associated with the soft tissue only in 30124 or may extend into bone and/or cartilage in 30125. If associated with the nasal bone, the usual location is at the bone-cartilage junction. Dependent on the size and location, the cyst may be removed using skin or intranasal incisions. A fistula opening may be present and its tract would be excised. Commonly, an incision is made overlying the cyst in the nasal skin. The cyst is removed from its cavity using curettes. The defect size dictates post-removal cavity packing and/or separately reportable reconstruction. Incisions may be closed in single and layers.

30130
The physician removes a part of or the entire inferior nasal turbinate located on the lateral wall of the nose. The turbinate is primarily removed in cases of hypertrophy that obstruct the nasal airway. The physician places topical vasoconstrictive drugs on the turbinate to shrink the blood vessels. A mucosal incision is made around the base of the turbinate. The physician fractures the bony turbinate from the lateral nasal wall with a chisel or drill. The turbinate is excised. Electrocautery may control bleeding. The nasal mucosa is sutured in single layers. The nasal cavity may be packed with gauze.

30140
The physician removes a part of or all of the inferior turbinate bone through a submucous incision. The physician places vasoconstrictive drugs on the turbinate to shrink the blood vessels. A full thickness incision is made over the anterior-inferior surface of the turbinate and continued deep to bone. The physician lifts the mucoperiosteum with an elevator to expose the bony turbinate. A chisel or forceps is used to remove portions of the bony turbinate. Electrocautery may control bleeding. The turbinate mucosa is closed in a single layer.

30150-30160
The physician resects a portion of the nose in 30150 or the total nose in 30160, leaving a surgical defect. The extent of the resection is determined by the extent of the tumor or trauma. A full thickness incision is made through the external nose. All diseased or damaged soft tissue is excised to clear margins. Underlying bone or cartilage may be removed. Exposed bone or cartilage is covered with mucosal flaps or separately reportable skin grafts.

30200
The physician injects a pharmacologic agent (i.e., steroids, sclerosing agents) into the submucosal tissue overlying the nasal turbinate. The inferior nasal turbinate is most commonly involved. Enlarged turbinates obstruct airflow through the nasal cavity. Turbinates with allergic hypertrophy or hypertrophy

Respiratory

compensating for septal deviation may benefit from therapy.

30210

The physician displaces mucopurulent secretions (pus and mucous) from sinuses by gravity replacement with a second liquid. This therapy is effective for the ethmoid and sphenoid sinuses. While lying supine, the patient's head is hyperextended. The nose is filled with isotonic saline solution. The physician closes one nostril and applies suction to the other nostril. The patient repeats vowels or words (phonates), elevating the soft palate and creating negative pressure. While the patient is phonating, the physician suctions the nostril. The saline solution enters the sinus, displacing the secretions of the sinuses. The secretions are suctioned from the nostril.

30220

The physician uses an alloplastic button to obturate (close) a nasal septal opening. This procedure is performed as an option to surgical reconstruction of the septum such as grafting. The commercially available alloplastic button is made of silicone rubber. The physician inserts the button into the septal perforation securing it with transseptal sutures.

30300-30310

The physician removes a foreign body from the inside of the nasal cavity, in the office for 30300 or under general anesthesia for 30310. Foreign bodies are defined as objects not normally found in the body. An object may be embedded in normal tissue as a result of some type of trauma. Topical vasoconstrictive agents and local anesthesia are applied to the nasal mucosa. A small incision may be necessary to access the foreign body. Blunt dissection and retrieval of the object is performed with hemostats or forceps. Sutures may close the mucosa in a single layer if the size of the dissection requires.

30320

The physician removes a foreign body from deep within the nasal cavity, accessing the area with a lateral rhinotomy surgical approach. This foreign body is located in an area of difficult access and requires complex surgery to remove it. Foreign bodies are defined as objects not normally found in the body. The object may be embedded in normal tissue as a result of some type of trauma. Topical vasoconstrictive agents and local anesthesia are applied to the nasal mucosa. A full-thickness skin incision is made from the nostril extending along the nasal alar rim and continuing superiorly. The incision can extend to the medial aspect of the eyebrow if necessary. The lateral aspect of the nose is retracted, exposing the bony structures beneath the soft tissue. Blunt dissection and retrieval of the object is performed with hemostats or forceps. The surgical wound is closed in layers.

30400

The physician performs surgery to reshape the external nose. No surgery to the nasal septum is necessary. The physician may perform surgery via an open (external skin incisions) or closed (intranasal incisions) approach. Topical vasoconstrictive agents are applied to shrink the blood vessels and local anesthesia is injected into the nasal mucosa. After incisions are made, dissections expose the external nasal cartilaginous and bony skeleton. The cartilages may be reshaped with files. Fat may be removed from the subcutaneous regions. Incisions are closed in single layers. Steri-strip tape is used to support cartilaginous surgery of the nasal tip.

30410

The physician performs surgery to reshape the external nose. No surgery to the nasal septum is necessary. This surgery can be performed open (external skin incisions) or closed (intranasal incisions). Topical vasoconstrictive agents are applied to shrink the blood vessels and local anesthesia is injected in the nasal mucosa. After incisions are made, dissections expose the external nasal cartilaginous and bony skeleton. The cartilages may be reshaped by trimming or may be augmented by grafting. Local grafts from adjacent nasal bones and cartilage are not reported separately. The physician may reshape the dorsum with files. The physician fractures the lateral nasal bones with chisels. Fat may be removed from the subcutaneous regions. Incisions are closed in single layers. Steri-strip tape is used to support cartilaginous surgery of the nasal tip. An external splint or cast supports changes in bone position.

30420

The physician performs surgery to reshape the external and internal nose. The nasal septum internally supports the shape of the external nasal appearance. The physician reshapes a fractured or deformed septum. Rhinoplasties can be performed open (external skin incisions) or closed (intranasal incisions). Topical vasoconstrictive agents are applied to shrink the blood vessels and local anesthesia is injected into the nasal mucosa. After incisions are made, dissections expose the external nasal cartilaginous and bony skeleton. The cartilages may be reshaped by trimming or may be augmented by grafting. Local grafts from adjacent nasal bones and cartilage are not reported separately. The physician may reshape the dorsum with files. Fat may be removed from the subcutaneous regions. A vertical incision is made in the septal mucosa and the mucoperichondrium is elevated from the septal cartilage. Septal cartilage may be removed or grafted. The physician fractures the lateral nasal bones with chisels and manually repositions them in the desired positions. Incisions are closed in single layers. Steri-strip tape is used to support cartilaginous surgery of the nasal tip. An external splint or cast supports changes in bone position.

30430

The physician performs a second surgery to reshape the external nose and correct unfavorable results from the initial rhinoplasty. Secondary rhinoplasties can be performed open (external skin incisions) or closed (intranasal incisions). Topical vasoconstrictive agents are applied to shrink the blood vessels and local anesthesia is injected in the nasal mucosa. After incisions are made, dissections expose the external nasal cartilaginous and bony skeleton. The cartilages and nasal tip may be reduced by trimming or may be augmented by grafting. The bony dorsum may receive grafts. Local grafts from adjacent nasal bones and cartilage are not reported separately. Incisions are closed in single layers. Steri-strip tape is used to support cartilaginous surgery of the nasal tip.

30435

The physician performs a second surgery to reshape the external nose and correct unfavorable results from the initial rhinoplasty. Secondary rhinoplasties can be performed open (external skin incisions) or closed (intranasal incisions). Topical vasoconstrictive agents are applied to shrink the blood vessels and local anesthesia is injected in the nasal mucosa. After incisions are made, dissections expose the external nasal cartilaginous and bony skeleton. The physician refractures the lateral nasal bones with chisels and manually repositions them in the desired positions. The bony dorsum may receive grafts. Local grafts from adjacent nasal bones and cartilage are not reported separately. Incisions are closed in single layers. Steri-strip tape is used to support cartilaginous surgery of the nasal tip. An external splint or cast supports changes in bone position.

30450

The physician performs a second surgery to reshape the external nose and correct unfavorable results from the initial rhinoplasty. Secondary rhinoplasties can be performed open (external skin incisions) or closed (intranasal incisions). Topical vasoconstrictive agents are applied to shrink the blood vessels and local anesthesia is injected in the nasal mucosa. After incisions are made, dissections expose the external nasal cartilaginous and bony skeleton. The cartilages and nasal tip may be reduced by trimming or augmented by grafting. The bony dorsum may receive grafts as well. Local grafts from adjacent nasal bones and cartilage are not reported separately. The physician refractures the lateral nasal bones with chisels and manually repositions them in the desired position. Incisions are closed in single layers. Steri-strip tape is used to support cartilaginous surgery of the nasal tip. An external splint or cast supports changes in bone position.

30460

The physician reshapes the external nose and corrects secondary developmental cleft lip and/or palate deformities. Rhinoplasties can be performed open (external skin incisions) or closed (intranasal incisions). Topical vasoconstrictive agents are applied to shrink the blood vessels and local anesthesia is injected in the nasal mucosa. After incisions are made, dissections expose the external nasal cartilaginous and bony skeleton. The cartilages and nasal tip may be reduced by trimming or may be augmented by grafting. Local grafts from adjacent nasal bones and cartilage are not reported separately. Incisions are closed in single layers. Steri-strip tape supports cartilaginous surgery of the nasal tip.

30462

The physician reshapes the external and internal nose and corrects developmental cleft lip and/or palate deformities. Deflection of the nasal septum can cause airway obstruction and affect both support and appearance of the external nasal cartilages. Rhinoplasties can be performed open (external skin incisions) or closed (intranasal incisions). Topical vasoconstrictive agents are applied to shrink the blood vessels and local anesthesia is injected in the nasal mucosa. After incisions are made, dissections expose the external nasal cartilaginous and bony skeleton. The cartilages and nasal tip may be reduced by trimming or may be augmented by grafting. The physician makes a vertical incision in the septal mucosa and elevates the mucoperichondrium from the septal cartilage. Septal cartilage may be removed or grafted. The nasal dorsum may be a graft recipient. Local grafts from adjacent nasal bones and cartilage are not reported separately. The physician fractures the lateral nasal bones with chisels and manipulates the bones into the desired positions. Incisions are closed in single layers. Steri-strip tape supports cartilaginous surgery of the nasal tip. An external splint or cast supports changes in bone position.

30465

The physician repairs a nasal vestibular stenosis using a variety of techniques. Separately reportable cartilage (e.g., auricular composite) graft may be used to support the cartilaginous skeleton and vestibular soft tissue scarring. In one external approach the physician makes an incision in the upper lateral cartilage, in another approach a "V" shaped cut may be made. In either case the incision is followed by an osteotomy of the medial aspect of the nasal bones. A spreader graft is placed to widen the nasal vestibule. The incision is closed or closed in a V-Y manner (lengthens the columella) with suture.

30468-30469

The physician repairs a bilateral nasal valve collapse in 30468 using one or more subcutaneous or submucosal lateral wall implants. In one method, a proprietary absorbable implant is used to support the upper and lower cartilage inside the side (lateral) wall of the nose in patients with airway obstruction. A small cannula is inserted just inside the nostril. Upon reaching the targeted area, a thin, clear absorbable implant is injected into the subcutaneous or submucosal tissue and the cannula is removed. Implant position is confirmed by palpation. In 30469, bilateral repair of the nasal valve collapse is performed by remodeling the subcutaneous or submucosal tissues using low energy, temperature-controlled methods such as radiofrequency (RF). In one method, the physician anesthetizes the nose and positions the patient into a reclined-seated or semi-supine position. A stylus, with the treatment tip covered in surgical gel for patient comfort and ease of movement, is inserted into the nasal passageway to deliver temperature-controlled RF energy treatment along the lateral wall of the posterior middle meatus. The stylus is gently pushed upwards into the middle turbinate. Multiple treatments may be delivered along the middle meatus and inferior turbinate during the procedure, with each treatment lasting a few seconds. This treatment remodels narrow or obstructive nasal anatomy, helping to improve airflow. Once treatment is complete, the stylus is removed from the nasal passage.

30520
The physician reshapes the nasal septum, correcting airway obstruction. Topical vasoconstrictive agents are applied to shrink the blood vessels and local anesthesia is injected in the nasal mucosa. The physician makes a vertical incision in the septal mucosa and elevates the mucoperichondrium from the septal cartilage. The deviated portion of the bony and cartilaginous septum is excised or augmented by grafting. Local grafts from adjacent nasal bones and cartilage are not reported separately. If the cartilaginous septum remains bowed, partial or full-thickness incisions are made in the cartilage to straighten the septum. Excess cartilage is excised from the bone-cartilage junction. Incisions are closed in single layers. Transseptal sutures are placed. Septal splints may support the septum during healing.

30540
The physician reconstructs the congenitally or acquired absent openings between the nasal cavity and the pharynx (throat). Topical vasoconstrictive agents are applied, and local anesthesia is injected in the nasal mucosa. A mastoid curette or scalpel is placed in the nose and passed to the closure along the floor of the nose. The physician gently punctures the closure to create an opening in the nasopharynx. Sequential rubber tubes of increasing size are placed through the new opening. Once the new opening is dilated to the desired diameter, the rubber tubes are sutured to the nasal columella. The tubes remain for a three- to eight-week healing period to ensure patency of the new posterior nares after removal.

30545
The physician reconstructs the congenitally or acquired absent openings between the nasal cavity and the pharynx (throat). Topical vasoconstrictive agents are applied to the nasal mucosa. Local anesthesia is injected in the nasal mucosa and maxilla. A midpalatal incision is made extending posterior to the nasopalatine foramen to the soft palate. The mucoperiosteum is elevated, exposing the hard palate. Using drills and chisels, the physician creates bony windows at the posterior hard palate, removing bony obstructions between the nasal floor and the pharynx. The physician places rubber tubes along the nasal floor through the new openings into the nasopharynx. The rubber tubes are sutured to the nasal columella. The palatal incision is closed in a single layer. The rubber tubes remain for a three- to eight-week healing period to ensure patency of the new posterior nares after removal.

30560
The physician removes mucosal scarring which blocks the passage of air in the nose. Nasal synechiae are formed when two bleeding mucosal surfaces contact forming scar tissue and eventual fibrosis. These patients are unable to breathe through the nose. The physician makes an intranasal approach to the synechia. Topical vasoconstrictive agents are applied and local anesthesia is injected in the nasal mucosa. An attempt to minimize intra- and postoperative mucosal bleeding is made. A scalpel is used to excise the mucosal tissue. Mucosal edges are sutured with resorbable sutures. Postoperative gauze packing or splints may be used to absorb hemorrhage until mucosal healing occurs. Long term splinting may be necessary to prevent reformation of the synechiae.

30580
The physician closes an opening between the mouth and the maxillary sinus. The communication is through the maxillary bone and this tract is lined with epithelium. Local anesthesia is injected into the mucosa. The physician uses a scalpel to excise the epithelized tract. An incision is made into the palatal mucosa and a local mucosal flap is developed. The flap is sutured in layers, covering the oromaxillary tract. Careful postoperative instructions are given to limit sinus pressure by not allowing nose blowing which would reopen the tract and impair healing.

30600
The physician closes an opening between the mouth and nasal cavity. The communication is through the maxillary hard palate and the tract is lined with epithelium. Local anesthesia is injected into the mucosa. The physician uses a scalpel to excise the epithelized tract. An incision is made into the palatal mucosa and a local mucosal flap is developed. The flap is sutured in layers, covering the oronasal tract.

30620
The physician removes diseased intranasal mucosa and replaces it with a separately reportable split thickness graft. The surgery is performed on one nasal side. A lateral rhinotomy is made to expose the intranasal mucosa. The diseased mucosal tissue is excised from the septum, nasal floor, and anterior aspect of the inferior turbinate. A split thickness graft is sutured to the recipient bed, covering the exposed cartilage and submucosal surfaces. Gauze packing and splints are placed in the grafted nasal cavity.

30630
The physician repairs perforations in the nasal septum. Topical vasoconstrictive agents are applied and local anesthesia is injected into the nasal mucosa. The physician creates local mucoperichondrial flaps on either side of the perforation with a scalpel. Each flap is designed only exposing one side of the septal cartilage while retaining mucosal coverage of the septal cartilage on the opposite side. The flaps are sutured in a single layer to cover the perforation. Larger defects may require the use of separately reportable autogenous grafts (i.e., muscle fascia) in addition to

local flaps. Transseptal sutures and septal stents support the septal mucosa and maintain the new position of the flaps.

30801-30802
The physician uses electrocautery, tissue volume reduction, and/or radiofrequency ablation to reduce inflammation or remove excessive mucosa from the soft tissue of the inferior nasal turbinates unilaterally or bilaterally. Ablation procedures may be performed superficially in 30801 or deep in the mucosa (intramural) in 30802. Topical vasoconstrictive agents are applied to the nasal mucosa. Excessive or hypertrophied mucosa is cauterized or ablated and may be excised. Postoperative bleeding is minimal and there is typically no need for intranasal packing.

30901-30903
To control a less serious nosebleed in 30901, the physician applies electrical or chemical coagulation or packing materials to the anterior (front) section of the nose. Only limited electrical or chemical coagulation is used. To control a less responsive nosebleed in 30903, the physician uses extensive electrical coagulation or extensive packing in the anterior (front) section of the nose.

30905-30906
To control bleeding that is coming from the posterior (back) of the nose (nasopharynx), the physician places extensive packing into the nasal cavity through the back of the throat. Extensive electrical coagulation may be required. The patient may return (e.g., 30906) if the bleeding recurs.

30915
When nasal packing fails to control nasal hemorrhage, the physician administers a local anesthetic and makes an incision along the side of the nose near the inner canthus of the eye to expose the ethmoid arteries. The periosteum (periorbitum) is elevated. The anterior ethmoid artery is identified in the suture line between the frontal and ethmoid bones. The posterior ethmoid artery is located entering the posterior medial wall near the orbital apex. A clip or suture completes the ligation. The incision is repaired with a layered closure.

30920
When nasal packing proves inadequate to stop nasal hemorrhage, the physician makes an incision in the mucous membrane under the upper lip. The incision above the canine tooth on the side of the hemorrhage is commonly referred to as a Caldwell-Luc approach. An opening is created through the bone into the normal maxillary sinus. Through an operating microscope, the physician locates and incises the posterior wall of the maxillary sinus. Through this incision, The maxillary artery is isolated and ligated with sutures or a clip. The posterior maxillary sinus wall is repaired. The incision is repaired with a layered closure.

30930
The physician fractures a portion of the inferior turbinate bone to reposition the nasal turbinate. This procedure is performed on a hypertrophied (enlarged) inferior turbinate obstructing the nasal airway. With repositioning, the hypertrophied turbinate should shrink in size, allowing normal airflow. Topical vasoconstrictive drugs are placed on the turbinate to shrink the blood vessels. Commonly, the physician uses a blunt instrument to out-fracture the turbinate. This can be performed with or without incisions. If visualization is necessary, the physician makes a full thickness incision over the anterior-inferior surface of the turbinate and continues it deep to bone. An elevator lifts the mucoperiosteum, exposing the bony turbinate. The physician fractures the bony turbinate with a chisel. Electrocautery may control bleeding. The turbinate mucosa is closed in a single layer.

31000-31002
The physician irrigates infected sinuses through cannulas. Topical vasoconstrictive agents are applied. The maxillary sinus is entered in 31000 through the natural ostium or opening in the middle meatus of the nasal cavity or through an antral puncture beneath the inferior nasal turbinate. The sphenoid sinus is entered in 31002 through the sphenoethmoidal recess in the superior nasal cavity. A flexible cannula is inserted into these openings and the sinuses are irrigated with saline solutions. These lavages will reduce inflammation and remove purulent (pus) discharge in the sinuses.

31020
The physician surgically creates an opening from the nasal cavity into the maxillary sinus to allow adequate sinus drainage. An antral "window" is made in the inferior meatus or by enlargement of the natural ostium in the middle meatus. Topical vasoconstrictive agents are applied to the nasal mucosa. Local anesthesia is injected into the nasal mucosa. A trocar is used to create an opening into the desired antral window location. The opening is enlarged with biting forceps. The maxillary sinus can be inspected and irrigated with direct visualization. A temporary irrigation catheter may be placed into the sinus and secured with sutures to the nose. The nasal cavity may be packed for 24 to 48 hours if excessive bleeding occurs during the procedure.

31030-31032
The physician creates several maxillary sinus openings to allow adequate sinus drainage for treatment of irreversible maxillary sinus disease. An intraoral incision is made in the labial mucosa, exposing the canine fossa. The canine fossa is perforated with a trocar and biting forceps increase the opening into the maxillary sinus. Sinus mucosa is removed with curettes. A second opening is made from the nasal cavity into the inferior meatus. Topical vasoconstrictive agents are applied to the nasal mucosa and local anesthesia is injected. A trocar perforates an opening into the inferior meatus. The opening is enlarged with biting forceps. An antrochoanal polyp is present in 31032 within both the maxillary sinus and nasal cavity. The mucosa adjacent to the natural ostium is removed

with the polyps. The intraoral incision is repaired in a single layer.

31040

The physician performs surgery by any approach in the pterygomaxillary fossa, a space between the bones of the maxilla, sphenoid, and palatine bones. The fossa includes layers of fat, blood vessels, and neural structures such as the vidian and maxillary nerves. In one technique, an endoscope is placed into the nose and advanced to the posterior maxillary sinus. An opening is created in the wall between the sinus and pterygomaxillary fossa using a burr drill or rongeur. Areas of concern are addressed with interventions such as biopsy, tumor removal, nerve block, or artery ligation. Electrocautery may be used for hemostasis. The nose may be packed if excessive bleeding occurs.

31050-31051

The physician enters the diseased sphenoid sinus. While open, biopsies may be taken of the sphenoidal masses. The sinus mucosa or mucosal polyps are removed in 31051. Due to its location deep within the skull, the sphenoid sinus surgery is accessed through structures overlying the sinus. Most commonly, an intraoral incision is made in the maxillary labial vestibule. The nasal septal cartilage is dissected from the nasal floor and is detached from the anterior nasal spine. The anterior cartilaginous septum is displaced and dissection continues to the bony nasal septum. The physician uses rongeurs to remove the bony septum, exposing the sphenoid region. The anterior wall of the sphenoid sinus is also removed with rongeurs. The physician uses an operating microscope to remove sinus contents. The nasal midline is reestablished and the cartilage is reattached to the nasal spine. Transseptal sutures are placed. The intraoral incision is closed in a single layer. The nose is packed and external nasal dressings may be placed.

31070

The physician uses a trephine to access the frontal sinus. The frontal sinus opening is obstructed by sinus disease, not allowing the sinus to drain into the nose. A small skin incision is made beneath the unshaven medial eyebrow. The dissection is carried to the frontal bone overlying the frontal sinus. The physician uses a round burr to make an opening into the sinus cavity. Tissue for culture may be taken at this time. The sinus is irrigated with saline solutions. Two irrigation catheters are placed into the sinus through the bony opening. The wound is closed in layers. The catheters are sutured to the skin. The exposed catheters are used to irrigate the sinus and are removed once the sinus inflammation subsides and the irrigation fluid starts to exit through the nose.

31075

The physician makes an external skin incision in the medial orbit to access the frontal sinus. The curvilinear incision is made beneath the eyebrow along the medial orbit extending to the superior aspect of the orbit. The dissection continues to the bone. The physician uses a drill and forceps to create an opening into the frontal sinus and, if needed, the ethmoid sinus. Pathologic and/or diseased tissue membrane is removed with curettes. The inferior wall of the sinus can be removed, increasing the drainage from the sinus into the nose. The wound is closed in layers.

31080-31081

The physician removes the frontal sinus mucosa and places material into the sinus cavity to prevent regrowth of the sinus mucosa. To access the frontal sinus through a brow incision in 31080, a full thickness incision is made from the superior aspect of one eyebrow, extending through the nasofrontal junction to the opposite eyebrow. A bicoronal flap may access the frontal sinus in 31081. After the physician exposes the sinus, the frontal bone overlying the frontal sinus is removed with drills, saws, and chisels. The contents of the exposed sinus are removed with curettes and burrs. The nasofrontal duct is obstructed with an alloplastic or autogenous material (bone). The sinus cavity is obliterated with autologous fat harvested from the abdomen or buttocks. The removed frontal bone is returned and secured with wires, plates, and/or screws. Incisions are repaired in layers.

31084-31085

The physician removes the frontal sinus mucosa and places material into the sinus cavity to prevent regrowth of the sinus mucosa. In the frontal sinus access, an osteoplastic flap is used. The periosteum of the excised frontal bone is preserved. When the frontal sinus is accessed by brow incision in 31084, an incision is made from the superior aspect of one eyebrow, extending through the nasofrontal junction to the opposite eyebrow. A bicoronal flap accesses the frontal sinus in 31085. Dissection is carried to the periosteal layer. A template is made from a radiograph outlining the frontal sinus. The template is placed over the frontal sinus and the periosteum is excised around the template. The physician removes the frontal bone, with attached periosteum overlying the frontal sinus, using drills, saws, and chisels. The contents of the exposed sinus are removed with curettes and burrs. The nasofrontal duct is obstructed with an alloplastic (synthetic) or autogenous material (i.e., bone). The sinus cavity is obliterated with autologous fat harvested from the abdomen or buttocks. The frontal bone flap is returned and secured with sutures, wires, plates, and/or screws. The incisions are repaired in layers.

31086-31087

The physician enters the frontal sinus to remove pathologic lesions and diseased sinus mucosa. In the frontal sinus access, an osteoplastic flap is used in which the periosteum of the excised frontal bone is preserved. When the frontal sinus is accessed by brow incision in 31086, an incision is made from the superior aspect of one eyebrow, extending through the nasofrontal junction to the opposite eyebrow. A bicoronal flap accesses the frontal sinus in 31087. Dissection is carried to the periosteal layer. A template is made from a radiograph outlining the frontal sinus. The template is placed over the frontal sinus and the periosteum is excised around the template. The physician removes the frontal bone with attached periosteum overlying the frontal sinus using drills, saws, and chisels. The contents of the exposed sinus are removed with curettes and burrs. No obliteration of the sinus is necessary. The frontal bone flap is returned and secured with sutures, wires, plates, and/or screws. The incisions are repaired in layers.

31090
The physician enters three or more sinuses to remove diseased sinus contents using multiple approaches. Sinus disease may involve any of the maxillary, ethmoid, sphenoid, and/or frontal sinuses. The physician uses multiple approaches to the sinus including, intraoral, intranasal, skin and/or bicoronal incisions. Once the sinus is accessed, the physician removes its contents with curettes. Incisions are repaired in both single and layers, depending on the access.

31200
The physician removes diseased tissue from the ethmoid sinuses. The physician accesses the ethmoid sinuses through the nose. Topical vasoconstrictive agents are placed on the nasal mucosa to shrink the blood vessels. Local anesthesia is injected into the nasal mucosa. The physician retracts the middle turbinate anteriorly, exposing the sinus opening. A small curette may be advanced into the anterior ethmoid cells. The physician uses the curette to remove any diseased tissue of the anterior sinus, and allows the sinus to drain.

31201
The physician removes diseased tissue from the anterior and posterior ethmoid sinuses. The physician accesses the ethmoid sinuses through the nose. Topical vasoconstrictive drugs are placed on the nasal mucosa. Local anesthesia is injected into the nasal mucosa. The physician retracts the middle turbinate anteriorly, exposing the sinus opening. A small curette is used to remove the uncinate process in the bone. The physician may advance the curette into the anterior ethmoid cells. The physician uses blunt forceps to open posterior bony cells. Curettes remove diseased tissue and allow postoperative drainage of both the anterior and posterior ethmoid sinuses.

31205
The physician removes diseased tissue of the ethmoid sinuses. A curvilinear incision is made between the nasal dorsum and the medial canthus of the eye. Dissection is carried to the medial orbital bone. A bony window is made through the lamina papyracea bone, exposing the lateral ethmoid sinus. The physician removes all diseased tissue. The nasal cavity is penetrated through the medial ethmoid region. Nasal gauze packing is placed through the extranasal incision. The external skin incision is repaired with a layered closure.

31225
The physician removes a portion of or all of the diseased maxilla. Incisions may be intraoral or may include skin incisions such as the Weber-Ferguson approach. Dissection is continued to expose and isolate the planned bony excision. The physician uses drills, saws, and chisels to fracture the maxilla from the midface. The fractured maxilla and adjacent tissue are loosened and removed to "free margins" as determined with intraoperative tissue specimens sent to the pathologist for immediate microscopic examination. All sinus mucosa is removed. Exposed bone may be covered with a separately reportable split thickness skin graft. A splint may be placed to obturate (block) the mouth from the surgical area. All skin incisions are repaired with a layered closure.

31230
The physician removes the maxilla, eye, and orbital soft tissue. Incisions may be intraoral or may include skin incisions such as a modified Weber-Ferguson incision that includes incision in the upper eyelid. Dissection is continued to expose and isolate the planned bony excision. The physician uses drills, saws, and chisels to fracture the maxilla from the midface. The fractured maxilla and adjacent tissue are loosened and removed to "free margins" as determined with intraoperative tissue specimens sent to the pathologist for immediate microscopic examination. The upper eyelid incision is dissected to the periosteum of the superior orbit. The maxilla is retracted downward, so the physician can visualize the optic nerve and blood vessels. The optic nerve is severed and the vessels are ligated. The maxilla, adjacent soft tissue, and orbital contents are removed in one specimen. All sinus mucosa is removed. Exposed bone is covered with a separately reportable split thickness skin graft. A splint may be placed to obturate (block) the mouth from the surgical area. All skin incisions are repaired with a layered closure.

31231
The physician uses an endoscope for a diagnostic evaluation of the nose. An endoscope has a rigid fiberoptic telescope that allows the physician both increased visualization and magnification of internal anatomy. Topical vasoconstrictive agents are applied to the nasal mucosa and nerve blocks with local anesthesia are performed. The endoscope is placed into the nose and a thorough inspection of internal nasal structures is accomplished. No surgical procedure is performed.

31233
The physician uses an endoscope for a diagnostic evaluation of the nose and the maxillary sinus. An endoscope has a rigid fiberoptic telescope that allows the physician both increased visualization and magnification of internal anatomy. Topical vasoconstrictive agents are applied to the nasal mucosa and nerve blocks with local anesthesia are performed. The endoscope is placed into the nose and a thorough inspection of the internal nasal structures is

accomplished. A trocar puncture is made directly into the inferior meatus area of the nose or after a mucosal incision into the canine fossa of the maxilla. The endoscope is placed into the maxillary sinus for evaluation. The intraoral mucosa may be closed in a single layer. The nasal puncture wound does not require closure. No other procedure is performed on the sinus at this time.

31235

The physician uses an endoscope for a diagnostic evaluation of the nose and the sphenoid sinus. An endoscope has a rigid fiberoptic telescope that allows the physician both increased visualization and magnification of internal anatomy. Topical vasoconstrictive agents are applied to the nasal mucosa and nerve blocks with local anesthesia are performed. The endoscope is placed into the nose and a thorough inspection of the internal nasal structures is accomplished. Access to the sphenoid sinus is accomplished by a trocar puncture made directly into the sphenoid sinus after negotiation through the ethmoids or by cannulation of the sphenoid drainage system that enters the sphenoethmoidal recess. The endoscope is placed into the sphenoid sinus for evaluation. The sphenoidal puncture wound does not require closure. No other procedure is performed on the sinus at this time.

31237

The physician performs endoscopic biopsy, debridement, or polypectomy of the nose. An endoscope has a rigid fiberoptic telescope that allows the physician both increased visualization and magnification of internal anatomy. Topical vasoconstrictive agents are applied to the nasal mucosa and nerve blocks with local anesthesia are performed. The endoscope is placed into the nose and a thorough diagnostic inspection of the internal nasal structures is accomplished. Any identified polyps or lesions are biopsied or removed by intranasal instruments placed parallel to the endoscope. Scalpels, forceps, snares, or other cutting and grasping instruments may be used to remove diseased or necrotic tissue from the internal nose, often in the form of postoperative debridement in cases of delayed healing or retained foreign material that interferes with the healing process. The nose may be packed if excessive bleeding occurs.

[31242, 31243]

The physician destroys the posterior nasal nerve using an endoscopic approach to treat chronic rhinitis. An endoscope has a rigid fiberoptic telescope that allows the physician both increased visualization and magnification of internal anatomy. Topical vasoconstrictive agents are applied to the nasal mucosa and nerve blocks with local anesthesia are performed. The endoscope is placed into the nose and a thorough inspection of the internal nasal structures is accomplished. The tip of the ablation device is advanced to the posterior nasal nerve via the middle meatus. In 31242, temperature-controlled radiofrequency is applied to the area to disrupt the posterior nasal nerve. Multiple cycles may be necessary to create lines of lesions that cross the path of the nerve. In 31243, cryoablation is performed to freeze the affected area for posterior nasal nerve disruption.

31238

The physician uses an endoscope for a diagnostic evaluation of the bleeding nose. An endoscope has a rigid fiberoptic telescope that allows the physician both increased visualization and magnification of internal anatomy. Topical vasoconstrictive agents are applied to the nasal mucosa and nerve blocks with local anesthesia are performed. The endoscope is placed into the nose and a thorough inspection of the internal nasal structures is accomplished. Any bleeding sources are identified. Electrocautery instruments or lasers are placed parallel to the endoscope and are used to stop internal nasal bleeding.

31239

The physician uses an endoscope to visually and surgically assist during a dacryocystorhinostomy. When the lacrimal system is obstructed and excessive tearing is a problem for the patient, a dacryocystorhinostomy is performed. In this procedure, the new lacrimal drainage system is surgically created from the lower eyelid into the nose. An endoscope allows the physician both increased visualization and magnification of the internal anatomy. Topical vasoconstrictive agents are applied to the nasal mucosa and nerve blocks with local anesthesia are performed. The endoscope is placed into the nose. The nasolacrimal duct and other lacrimal structures are visualized. Endoscopy may aid in location of structures or enhance intranasal procedures like osteotomies and internal splinting with Teflon tubes.

31240

The physician uses an endoscope for an intranasal evaluation and surgical resection of a concha bullosa, an intranasal cyst has caused distention (stretching or swelling) of the turbinate bone. This swelling is called a concha bullosa. An endoscope has a rigid fiberoptic telescope that allow the physician both increased visualization and magnification of internal anatomy. Topical vasoconstrictive agents are applied to the nasal mucosa and nerve blocks with local anesthesia are performed. The endoscope is placed into the nose and thorough inspection of internal nasal structures is accomplished. A scalpel or biting forceps are introduced parallel to the endoscope and are used to excise the concha bullosa. Electrocautery may be used for hemostasis. The nasal cavity may be packed with Telfa or gauze for 24 to 48 hours.

31241

Under general anesthesia, the physician uses an endoscope for a diagnostic evaluation of the nose. An endoscope has a rigid fiberoptic telescope that allows the physician increased visualization and magnification of internal anatomy. Any nasal packing placed prior to the surgery is removed. Topical vasoconstrictive agents are applied to the nasal mucosa and nerve blocks with local anesthesia are performed. The endoscope is placed into the nose and a thorough inspection of the internal nasal structures is accomplished. Ligation or cautery of the sphenopalatine artery (SPA) is performed for traumatic intractable epistaxis. The SPA, sphenopalatine vein, and the nasal palatine nerve are located in the neurovascular pedicle in the crista ethmoidalis of the palatine bone. The SPA is the main artery branch that supplies the main parts of the nasal mucosa. A middle meatal antrostomy with enlargement posteriorly may also be required to ensure access. A mucoperiosteal flap is made in order to create an opening under the sphenopalatine neurovascular bundle. Once the SPA is identified, it is ligated via clipping or high-frequency electric currents. The physician places the flap back into position and the nose is left unpacked.

31254-31255

The physician uses an endoscope to perform a partial surgical anterior ethmoidectomy. Disease of the anterior ethmoid sinus may block maxillary sinus drainage. An endoscope allows increased visualization and magnification of internal anatomy. Topical vasoconstrictive agents are applied to the nasal mucosa and nerve blocks with local anesthesia are performed. The endoscope is placed into the nose and a thorough inspection of internal nasal structures is accomplished. The middle turbinate is medialized to provide access. A scalpel or biting forceps is introduced parallel to the endoscope and is used to remove diseased tissues. Polyps may be excised. Electrocautery may be used for hemostasis. The nasal cavity may be packed with Telfa or gauze for 24 to 48 hours. Report 31255 if a total (anterior and posterior) ethmoidectomy is performed.

[31253, 31257, 31259]

The physician uses an endoscope to perform a total surgical anterior and posterior ethmoidectomy. Disease of the anterior ethmoid sinus may block maxillary sinus drainage. An endoscope allows increased visualization and magnification of internal anatomy. Topical vasoconstrictive agents are applied to the nasal mucosa and nerve blocks with local anesthesia are performed. The endoscope is placed into the nose and a thorough inspection of internal nasal structures is accomplished. The middle turbinate is medialized to provide access. A scalpel or biting forceps is introduced parallel to the endoscope and is used to remove diseased tissues. Polyps may be excised. Electrocautery may be used for hemostasis. The nasal cavity may be packed with Telfa or gauze for 24 to 48 hours. Report 31253 if a total (anterior and posterior) ethmoidectomy is performed, including frontal sinus exploration with tissue removal, when performed. Report 31257 if a total ethmoidectomy is performed, including incision of the sphenoid sinus (sphenoidotomy). Report 31259 if a total ethmoidectomy is performed, including sphenoidotomy with tissue removal.

31256, 31267

The physician uses an endoscope for surgical access to the maxillary sinus. Topical vasoconstrictive agents are applied to the nasal mucosa and nerve blocks with local anesthesia are performed. The endoscope is placed into the nose and a thorough inspection of internal nasal structures is accomplished. The middle turbinate is medialized to provide access. A scalpel or biting forceps is introduced parallel to the endoscope and is used to remove diseased tissues. Polyps may be excised. A maxillary antrostomy is performed in 31256, creating an opening for drainage from the maxillary sinus. Additionally, in 31267, the maxillary sinus may be opened, and the physician performs limited or extensive removal of maxillary sinus disease such as fungal debris/concretions, polyps, bony partitions, or mucous membranes. In either case, electrocautery may be used for hemostasis. The nasal cavity may be packed with Telfa or gauze for 24 to 48 hours.

31276

Topical vasoconstrictive agents are applied to the nasal mucosa and nerve blocks with local anesthesia. The physician inserts an endoscope into the nose and a thorough inspection of the internal nasal structures is accomplished. A sinusotomy of the frontal sinus ostium is performed. If diseased or abnormal tissue is present within the frontal sinus, a scalpel or biting forceps is introduced parallel to the endoscope and is used to remove the tissue. This procedure includes polypectomy, debridement, or biopsy of the frontal sinus tissue, when performed. Electrocautery may be used for hemostasis. The nasal cavity may be packed with Telfa or gauze for 24 to 48 hours.

31287-31288

The physician uses an endoscope for surgical access of the sphenoid sinus. The sphenoid can be explored with direct access or through the posterior ethmoid sinus. The isolated access to the sphenoid sinus is through dilation of the sphenoid ostium. The middle turbinate may be fractured or partially removed for access. The ostium is cannulated and dilated. The physician uses forceps or a sphenoid punch to open the sinus cavity. Additionally, diseased mucosa or tissue is removed in 31288. The nose may be packed if excessive bleeding occurs.

31290-31291

The physician uses an endoscope for surgical access and repair of cerebrospinal fluid leaks in ethmoid and sphenoid sinuses. Topical vasoconstrictive agents and local anesthesia are applied to the nasal mucosa. The endoscope is placed into the nose. The middle turbinate may be fractured to provide access. In 31290, the ethmoid sinus is entered through the ethmoid bulla. In 31291, the sphenoid sinus can be explored through the posterior ethmoid sinus or through direct access. If accessed through the ethmoid sinus, the sphenoid ostium is cannulated and dilated. The physician uses forceps or a sphenoid punch to open the sinus cavity. Once the sinus cavity is entered, the cerebrospinal fluid leak is isolated. Local mucosal or muscle flaps may be developed to plug the defect. Autologous fat, muscle or fascia lata may also be used to seal the leak.

31292-31293
The physician uses an endoscope for surgical access to decompress the orbit. Decompression may occur through one orbital wall (31292) or two orbital walls (31293). The inferior orbital wall (the roof of the maxillary sinus) is approached through a canine fossa puncture into the maxillary sinus. Forceps remove orbital bone while preserving the orbital periosteum. This allows orbital contents to herniate into the maxillary sinus. The medial orbital wall (the lateral wall of the ethmoids) can be approached through the ethmoid sinuses. The ethmoids may be opened through the maxillary sinus or by a separate intranasal ethmoid approach. Bone is removed from this region, also allowing orbital contents to herniate into the ethmoid regions. The nose may be packed if excessive bleeding occurs.

31294
The physician uses an endoscope for surgical access to decompress the optic nerve in the posterior orbit. The optic nerve sends transmissions that provide the sense of sight. This nerve enters the posterior cone through the optic foramen (orbital apex). The orbital apex may be approached through the sphenoid sinus. The sphenoid sinus may be explored through the posterior ethmoid sinus or directly. The middle turbinate may be fractured or partially removed to provide access. Isolated access to the sinus is through cannulation and dilation of the sphenoid ostium. The physician uses a forceps or a sphenoid punch to gain entry into the sinus cavity. Bone is removed from the lateral portion of the sinus, decompressing the optic nerve. The nose may be packed if excessive bleeding occurs.

31295-31298
The physician uses an endoscope for surgical access to perform balloon dilation of the maxillary (31295), frontal (31296), or sphenoid (31297) sinus ostium or frontal and sphenoid sinus ostia (31298). Following application of a vasoconstrictor and under appropriate anesthesia, the physician inserts a sinus guide cannula and positions it near the entrance of the involved sinus under endoscopic visualization. Using fluoroscopic guidance, the physician inserts a sinus guidewire through the cannula and into the sinus ostium. The physician advances a catheter with an attached balloon over the guidewire, through the cannula, and into the targeted sinus. Once correct placement is confirmed, the balloon is inflated using a radiopaque fluid. The balloon is left inflated for several seconds and then deflated. Repositioning and reinflation may be necessary. Following deflation and removal of the balloon, the endoscope is used to inspect the frontal recess or sinus ostium.

31300
A laryngocele is an air-filled dilation of the laryngeal ventricle that connects with the laryngeal cavity. The physician first performs a tracheostomy on the patient. Using a horizontal neck incision, the physician exposes the larynx and performs a thyrotomy and laryngofissure, opening the larynx at the midline of the thyroid cartilage. The laryngocele or tumor is isolated, dissected, and excised. A cordectomy, the excision of all or part of the vocal cord, may also be performed. The incision is repaired in sutured layers.

31360-31365
The physician removes the larynx in 31360, and removes the larynx and surrounding tissues in 31365. First, a tracheostomy is performed. The physician makes a low collar or midline cervical incision for 31360 or a horizontal neck incision for 31365. The strap muscles of the neck and thyroid isthmus are cut. Part or all of the hyoid bone is removed. The trachea and inferior pharyngeal constrictor muscles are transected. By cutting the hypopharyngeal walls, the larynx is freed and removed. Resected tissues may include part of the esophagus and base of the tongue for 31360. In 31365, an extensive dissection may include removal of the sternocleidomastoid muscle, the submandibular salivary gland, the internal jugular vein and the lymph nodes of the lateral neck, under the chin and mandible, and the supraclavicular nodes. Any reconstruction performed at this time is separately reported. When either excision is completed, the incision is sutured in layers.

31367-31368
The surgeon removes the larynx in 31367, and the larynx and surrounding tissues in 31368. First, a tracheostomy is performed. The physician approaches the larynx through the thyroid cartilage for 31367 or a horizontal neck incision for 31368. The epiglottis, false vocal cords, mucosal lining of the ventricles, part or all of the hyoid bone, and superior part of the laryngeal cartilage are removed in 31367. In 31368, an extensive dissection may include removal of the sternocleidomastoid muscle, the submandibular salivary gland, the internal jugular vein and the lymph nodes of the lateral neck, under the chin and mandible, and the supraclavicular nodes. Any reconstruction performed at this time is separately reported. When either excision is completed, the incision is sutured in layers.

31370-31382
The physician removes a portion of the larynx. A tracheostomy is performed. The physician makes a low collar or midline cervical incision. The strap muscles of the neck are retracted and a midline incision of the perichondrium is made, exposing the larynx. The laryngeal cartilage is incised. In 31370, a horizontal incision is made above or below the affected area, and the diseased tissue is excised. The airway is reconstructed above to the pharynx or below to the trachea. In 31375, the vocal cord and adjacent cartilage are resected. In 31380, incisions are made into both halves of the thyroid cartilage, and the anterior part of the thyroid cartilage and the affected portions of both vocal cords are excised. In 31382, the area of resection also includes part or all of the arytenoid. In each instance, the pharynx is closed by suturing the

perichondrium and strap muscles. The incision is sutured in layers.

31390
The physician removes the larynx and pharynx. First, a tracheostomy is performed. The physician approaches the pharynx and larynx through a horizontal neck incision. The epiglottis, false vocal cords, mucosal lining of the ventricles, part or all of the hyoid bone, pharynx, and superior part of the laryngeal cartilage are removed. Extensive dissection may include removal of the sternocleidomastoid muscle, the submandibular salivary gland, the internal jugular vein and the lymph nodes of the lateral neck, under the chin and mandible, and the supraclavicular nodes. When either excision is completed, the incision is sutured in layers.

31395
The physician removes the larynx and pharynx and performs reconstruction with available tissues. First, a tracheostomy is performed. The physician approaches the pharynx and larynx through a horizontal neck incision. The epiglottis, false vocal cords, mucosal lining of the ventricles, part or all of the hyoid bone, pharynx, and superior part of the laryngeal cartilage are removed. Extensive dissection may include removal of the sternocleidomastoid muscle, the submandibular salivary gland, the internal jugular vein and the lymph nodes of the lateral neck, under the chin and mandible, and the supraclavicular nodes. Reconstruction of the pharyngeal area can be achieved in a number of ways; one of the most common is the myocutaneous flap reconstruction using the pectoralis major muscle and its overlying skin. The flap is rotated and inserted through a previously created tunnel between the clavicle and overlying skin. The flap is sutured into place to reconstruct the pharynx. The incision is sutured in layers.

31400
The physician secures the arytenoid process. First, a tracheostomy is performed. The physician exposes and transects the inferior pharyngeal constrictor muscle and continues dissection to reach the arytenoid cartilage. In an arytenoidopexy, the arytenoid cartilage is tacked against the thyroid ala to lateralize the arytenoid. In an arytenoidectomy, the arytenoid cartilage is resected and removed. The incision is closed with layered sutures.

31420
The physician excises all or part of the epiglottis, the cartilage that protects the entrance to the larynx. The physician uses an intra-oral approach to access and remove the epiglottis or lesions involving the tip of the epiglottis. If the affected area is minor, no sutures are needed. If the area involve most or all of the epiglottis, the remaining tissues are sutured together.

31500
The physician places an endotracheal tube to provide air passage in emergency situations. The patient is ventilated with a mask and bag and positioned by extending the neck anteriorly and the head posteriorly. The physician places the laryngoscope into the patient's mouth and advances the blade toward the epiglottis until the vocal cords are visible. An endotracheal tube is inserted between the vocal cords and advanced to the proper position. The cuff of the endotracheal tube is inflated.

31502
The physician removes the indwelling tracheotomy tube and replaces it with a new one. The procedure is performed before healing sufficient to form a fistula tract has taken place; usually a few days within placement of the original tube.

31505-31513
The physician administers a topical anesthetic to the oral cavity, pharynx, and larynx and positions the patient's head and laryngoscopic mirror so as to view the larynx through the reflection. In 31505, the interior of the larynx is examined for diagnostic purposes. In 31510, suspect tissue or a lesion may be stained for identification and a biopsy of the tissue is taken. In 31511, a foreign body is identified and withdrawn by grasping it with forceps. In 31512, a lesion is identified and excised. In 31513, an injection is administered into the vocal cords.

31515
The physician uses an aspirator to remove excess saliva or semi-solid foreign material from the larynx. After applying topical anesthesia to the oral cavity and pharynx, the physician inserts the laryngoscope through the patient's mouth. An aspirator is fed through the laryngoscope and the larynx is cleared of saliva and semi-solid foreign material. If a tracheoscopy is performed, a bronchoscope is inserted through the laryngoscope for microscopic visualization of the trachea and bronchi. No other procedure is performed.

31520-31525
The physician places a rigid laryngoscope to examine the patient's larynx. The physician administers a topical anesthetic to the oral cavity, pharynx, and larynx and inserts the laryngoscope through the patient's mouth. The interior of the larynx of a newborn is examined in 31520 and of a patient other than a newborn in 31525. If a tracheoscopy is performed, a bronchoscope is inserted through the laryngoscope for visualization of the trachea and bronchi. No other procedure is performed at this time.

31526
The physician uses an operating microscope or telescope to examine the interior of the larynx. After administering a topical anesthetic to the oral cavity, pharynx, and larynx, the physician inserts the laryngoscope into the patient's mouth and examines the larynx. If a tracheoscopy is performed, a bronchoscope is inserted through the laryngoscope for microscopic visualization of the trachea and bronchi. No other procedure is performed at this time.

31527
The physician administers a topical anesthetic to the oral cavity, pharynx, and larynx and inserts the laryngoscope through the patient's mouth. The interior of the larynx is examined. An obturator is an object that is used to close an opening. A wire is threaded through a cannulated needle which has been placed into the larynx. The end of the wire is grasped with forceps and drawn out through the laryngoscope. The wire is drawn through the obturator and threaded through another needle in the supraglottic space. The external ends of the wire are knotted over a stent.

31528-31529
The physician dilates a tracheobronchial stenosis. A topical or general anesthetic is administered, and the laryngoscope is inserted into the patient's mouth. The interior of the larynx is examined. The physician manipulates the laryngoscope to dilate areas of the tracheobronchial stenosis. Report 31528 for initial dilations (i.e., when it is the first dilation of a new area or for a new clinical condition, it has been three years or longer since the last dilation, previous dilations were performed by a physician from a different group practice, or it is the first lifetime dilation for the patient) and 31529 for subsequent dilations. If a tracheoscopy is performed, a bronchoscope is inserted through the laryngoscope for visualization of the trachea and bronchi.

31530-31531
The physician performs a direct, operative laryngoscopy to remove a foreign body. A topical anesthetic is administered to the oral cavity, pharynx, and larynx and the laryngoscope is inserted into the patient's mouth. The interior of the larynx is examined. In 31530, the foreign body is located, grasped with biopsy forceps, and withdrawn. In 31531, the physician uses a microscope or telescope to locate and remove the foreign body.

31535-31536
The physician performs a direct, operative laryngoscopy with biopsy. A topical anesthetic is administered to the oral cavity, pharynx, and larynx and the laryngoscope is inserted into the patient's mouth. The interior of the larynx is examined. In 31535, a lesion is biopsied with a sharp basket or cup forceps. Sometimes staining with toluidine blue is used to delineate the biopsy site. In 31536, the physician uses an operating microscope or a telescope to isolate and biopsy the lesions. This is usually done for smaller lesions.

31540-31541
The physician performs a direct operative laryngoscopy with excision of tumor and/or stripping of the vocal cords or epiglottis. A topical anesthetic is administered to the oral cavity, pharynx, and larynx and the laryngoscope is inserted into the patient's mouth. The interior of the larynx is examined and a laryngeal tumor may be isolated, dissected, and excised. The vocal cords or epiglottis may also be removed using stripping forceps. An operating microscope or a telescope is used in 31541. This is usually done for smaller lesions.

31545-31546
The physician removes a non-neoplastic lesion(s) of the vocal cords. Non-neoplastic lesions include nodules, polyps, and cysts. The physician administers a topical anesthetic to the oral cavity, pharynx, and larynx and inserts the laryngoscope into the patient's mouth. The interior of the larynx is examined. A solution of saline and adrenaline is infused beneath the surface of the vocal fold to better define the lesion(s) and to protect the deeper vocal tissue from injury. The vocal lesion(s) is identified and isolated. Lesions are decorticated rather than excised using a submucosal (subepithelial) technique. This technique disturbs only the superficial tissue layers while preserving the surface membrane. Mucosal incisions are made on the superior (ventricular) surface of the lesion(s). The lesion(s) is removed with gentle dissection and or suction. If there is sufficient redundant mucosa following removal of the lesion(s), a local tissue flap is created by trimming and redraping the mucosa over the vocal fold (31545). If there is not sufficient mucosa to form a local flap, a mucosal tissue autograft is harvested and applied (31546). Since these procedures require the use of high magnification and specially designed micro-instruments, an operating microscope or telescope is included and should not be reported separately.

31560-31561
The physician performs a direct, operative laryngoscopy with removal of the arytenoid cartilage. A topical anesthetic is administered to the oral cavity, pharynx, and larynx and the laryngoscope is inserted into the patient's mouth. The interior of the larynx is examined and the arytenoid cartilage is exposed by excising the overlying mucosa. The arytenoid is dissected from its muscular attachments and removed. An operating microscope or a telescope is used in 31561.

31570-31571
The physician performs a direct laryngoscopy with therapeutic injection into the vocal cords. The physician injects the vocal cords with a therapeutic substance such as glycerin, sesame oil, Gelfoam, or Teflon paste (Polytef). Injury to the larynx may result in a permanently damaged voice. An injection with a therapeutic substance into an affected vocal cord can augment its size and help bring it into apposition with the other vocal cord, creating a more complete glottic closure. The injected material hardens and retains its shape for improvement in voice quality. A Teflon paste injection is used when a permanent augmentation is desired. A glycerin, sesame oil, or Gelfoam injection is used to create a temporary augmentation until a permanent solution to an incomplete glottic closure is found. The physician administers a topical anesthetic to the oral cavity, pharynx, and larynx and inserts the laryngoscope into the patient's mouth. The interior of the larynx is examined and the physician injects the vocal cord at one to three sites with the selected

therapeutic substance. No other procedure is performed. An operating microscope or a telescope is used in 31571.

31575-31576

The physician administers a topical anesthetic to the oral cavity, pharynx, and larynx and uses a nasal or oral approach to insert a flexible laryngoscope. The interior of the larynx is examined in 31575. In 31576, a lesion is also biopsied with a sharp basket or cup forceps. Sometimes staining with toluidine blue is used to delineate the biopsy site.

31577

The physician removes a foreign body from the larynx. The physician administers a topical anesthetic to the oral cavity, pharynx, and larynx and uses a nasal or intraoral approach to insert a flexible laryngoscope. The interior of the larynx is examined and the foreign body is located, grasped with forceps, and withdrawn.

31578 [31572]

The physician removes a lesion from the larynx. The physician administers a topical anesthetic to the oral cavity, pharynx, and larynx and uses a nasal or intraoral approach to insert a flexible laryngoscope. The interior of the larynx is examined. In 31578, the physician locates and excises the lesion. In 31572, a lesion on only one side is destroyed or ablated via the use of a laser.

[31573, 31574]

The physician administers a topical anesthetic to the oral cavity, pharynx, and larynx and uses a nasal or oral approach to insert a flexible laryngoscope and examine the interior of the larynx. In 31573, the physician administers a unilateral therapeutic injection, such as a corticosteroid or a botulinum toxin, by an injected percutaneous or transoral approach or through an endoscopic channel. In 31574, injection augmentation of the vocal cords is performed unilaterally to treat insufficiency of the vocal cord. The physician uses a substance including, but not limited to, autologous fat, collagen or a gel-based bulking agent, skin/tissue substitute, soft tissue fillers, or hyaluronic acid gel products.

31579

The physician examines the larynx and vocal cord function. The patient is prepared with a nasal spray containing topical decongestant and anesthetic. The physician passes a flexible or rigid telescopic laryngoscope through the patient's nose into the pharynx and larynx, which are examined. The stroboscope responds to the fundamental frequency of the vibrating vocal cords, allowing the physician to see vocal cord function. No other procedure is performed.

31580

The physician excises a laryngeal web, a congenital malformation of the larynx. The physician performs a laryngotomy on the patient. Using a horizontal neck incision, the physician exposes the laryngeal web. The web lies between the vocal cords. The physician excises the web and inserts a laryngeal indwelling keel, or stent, between the vocal cords. The laryngotomy incision is closed.

[31551, 31552, 31553, 31554]

The physician treats laryngeal stenosis. The physician performs a laryngotomy on the patient. Using a horizontal neck incision, the physician exposes the stenosis, in the affected area of the supraglottis, glottis, and/or subglottis. A cartilage graft is obtained and sewn to provide anterior and/or posterior stability to the larynx and adjacent trachea. The incision is sutured in layers. Report 31551 for procedures performed without placement of an indwelling stent on patients 12 years of age or younger and 31552 for patients older than age 12. Report 31553 for procedures that include placement of an indwelling stent on patients younger than 12 years of age and 31554 for patients over age 12.

31584

The physician performs an open reduction and fixation (plating) of a fractured larynx. Using a horizontal neck incision, the physician exposes the laryngeal cartilage fracture and repairs the mucosal defects. The cartilage is stabilized with wire stents or microplates. The procedure includes tracheostomy to secure the airway and prevent extravasation of air into the surrounding tissues, when performed. The incision is repaired in sutured layers.

31587

The physician restores a cricoid split, a break in the circular cartilage of the larynx. The physician performs a low tracheostomy on the patient. Using a horizontal neck incision, the physician exposes the cricoid split and restores it to its normal anatomical position (reduction). The cartilage is affixed with wire. A stent may be placed to maintain cricotracheal continuity. No graft is placed. The incision is repaired in sutured layers.

31590

The physician restores innervation to the larynx using a neuromuscular pedicle (flap). In one method, the physician utilizes an innervated omohyoid muscle pedicle, transferred onto the paralyzed posterior cricoarytenoid muscle. After making a horizontal neck incision, the physician identifies the anterior belly of the omohyoid, which is located in close proximity of the larynx, and a small muscle flap pedicled on the ansa cervicalis is made. The physician creates a thyroid cartilage window and transposes the nerve-muscle flap onto the fibers of the lateral cricoarytenoid muscle, securing it with sutures. The incision is then sutured in layers.

31591

The physician performs a medialization laryngoplasty. Through an incision in the neck, the physician exposes the larynx and makes a square or block-shaped opening in the cartilage. An implant is placed and the larynx is viewed with a flexible laryngoscope. Implants can be created using a variety of materials including, but not limited to, carved silastic or ceramic blocks, expanded polytetrafluoroethylene (ePTFE) strips, and silastic shims. Patients are typically sedated in such a manner to ensure pain tolerance during the procedure, though alert enough during the portion of the procedure where the implant is being placed to be able to respond to commands and speak enough that the size of the implant can be customized to the patient's specific anatomy. The incision is closed. Once properly placed and functioning, notable improvements in areas of loudness, maximum phonation time, and noise-to-harmonic ratio should be experienced by the patient, as well as other subjective areas.

31592

The physician removes a narrowed portion of the trachea usually below the larynx. A horizontal skin incision is made across the base of the neck or, in some cases, a sternotomy may be necessary. The prior tracheotomy stoma is removed when applicable. Flaps are lifted from the level of the hyoid bone to the suprasternal notch. The cricoid cartilage is split vertically and examined to be certain one intact ring between the area of resection and stoma is available in order for appropriate anastomosis between the trachea and larynx. Sutures are placed on both sides of the trachea just under the lowest level of the resection. Portions of the cricoid cartilage are removed from the anterior and lateral positions, avoiding the cricoarytenoid joint. The area of stenosis is removed with focus on avoiding the underlying esophagus. Upon removal of the narrowed portion, the ends are tied with absorbable sutures within the tracheal wall. Skin incisions are closed with sutures or staples. Sutures join the skin on the lower chin to the chest to prevent backward movement of the head or a neck brace may be utilized to keep sutures intact. This procedure may be performed as a single or double stage procedure depending on the exact location of the stenosis. In a single stage (SSCTR) procedure, a previously placed tracheotomy tube is removed and an endotracheal tube inserted. In a double stage (DSCTR) procedure, a stent may be inserted above the tracheotomy tube or a T-tube may be utilized instead of the tracheotomy tube. This allows the airway to remain open and is removed four to six weeks postop.

31600-31610

The physician creates a tracheostomy. The physician makes a horizontal neck incision and dissects the muscles to expose the trachea. The thyroid isthmus is cut if necessary. The trachea is incised and an airway is inserted. After bleeding is controlled, a stoma is created by suturing the skin to the tissue layers. In 31600, the tracheostomy is a planned procedure. In 31601, it is a planned procedure performed on patients younger than 2 years of age. In 31603, it is performed under emergency conditions by puncturing the trachea and inserting a cannula. In 31605, it is performed under emergency conditions by puncturing the cricothyroid membrane located just above the cricoid and inserting a cannula. This is not a true tracheostomy and is usually converted to a tracheostomy once the situation is no longer emergent. In 31610, skin flaps are used to create a more permanent stoma.

31611

The physician constructs a tracheal esophageal fistula for vocalization. The physician makes a horizontal neck incision and dissects the tissues between the tracheostoma and the esophagus. The esophagus is incised and a laryngeal speech prosthesis is inserted between the esophagus and the trachea, creating a fistula. The prosthesis, called a voice button or a Blom-Singer prosthesis, is a one-way valve enabling the patient to phonate. The physician closes the incision around the prosthesis.

31612

The physician punctures the trachea with a needle to aspirate secretions or inject a therapeutic agent. The physician palpates the site and inserts a hollow point needle. Secretions are aspirated or a therapeutic agent is injected. The needle is removed.

31613-31614

The physician revises a tracheal stoma. The physician incises the stoma area and resects redundant scar tissue or a poorly healing wound. The skin is re-anastomosed and sewn to the stoma in sutured layers. Report 31613 for performance of a simple revision and 31614 if a complex procedure is performed with flap rotation.

31615

The physician views the airway using a bronchoscope placed through an existing tracheostomy. The physician examines the conducting airways. The bronchoscope is removed.

31622-31624

The physician views the airway using a flexible fiberoptic or rigid bronchoscope that is introduced under appropriate anesthesia through the nasal or oral cavity. The bronchoscope is inserted and advanced past the larynx to inspect the bronchus. In 31622, after diagnostic visualization of the bronchus, cell washings may be obtained through the bronchoscope. In 31623, sample lung tissue is obtained with brushings or protected brushing through the scope. In 31624, the bronchoscopy includes bronchial alveolar lavage, which allows lung tissue to be sampled by irrigating with saline followed by suctioning the fluid. The bronchoscope is removed. These codes include fluoroscopic guidance, when performed.

31625

The physician views the airway using a flexible fiberoptic or rigid bronchoscope that is introduced under appropriate anesthesia through the nasal or oral cavity. The bronchoscope is inserted and advanced past the larynx to inspect the bronchus, including fluoroscopic guidance, if used. After diagnostic visualization of the bronchus, a sample of bronchial or endobronchial tissue is removed for study. More than one site may be biopsied. Bleeding is assessed and controlled, and the bronchoscope is removed.

31626

The physician views the airway using a flexible fiberoptic or rigid bronchoscope that is introduced under appropriate anesthesia through the nasal or oral cavity. The bronchoscope is inserted and advanced past the larynx to inspect the bronchus, including fluoroscopic guidance, if used. After diagnostic visualization of the bronchus, one or more fiducial markers are placed.

31627

The physician views the airway using a flexible fiberoptic or rigid bronchoscope that is introduced under appropriate anesthesia through the nasal or oral cavity. The bronchoscope is inserted and advanced past the larynx to inspect the bronchus, including fluoroscopic guidance, if used. This code reports the use of computer-assisted, image-guided navigation, includes 3D reconstruction, and is reported in addition to the code for the primary procedure.

31628-31629

The physician views the airway using a flexible fiberoptic or rigid bronchoscope that is introduced under appropriate anesthesia through the nasal or oral cavity. The bronchoscope is inserted and advanced past the larynx to inspect the bronchus, including fluoroscopic guidance, if used. After diagnostic visualization of the bronchus, the physician passes closed biopsy forceps (31628) through a channel in the bronchoscope and through the bronchial wall to obtain one or more lung tissue samples from a single lobe. Alternately, the physician passes a needle (31629) through a channel in the bronchoscope and through the bronchial wall to obtain one or more aspiration biopsies of the trachea, main stem, and/or lobar bronchi. Bleeding is assessed and controlled, and the bronchoscope is removed.

31630

The physician performs tracheal/bronchial dilation or closed fracture reduction using a flexible fiberoptic or rigid bronchoscope introduced under appropriate anesthesia through the nasal or oral cavity. The physician uses the views obtained through the bronchoscope to identify any narrowing or fracture of the trachea or bronchus. The physician introduces a wire through the narrowed or fractured part of the airway and removes the bronchoscope. A series of dilators or stents are passed over the wire to open the airway until sufficient dilation or closed reduction of the stricture or fracture is accomplished. This may be done with or without fluoroscopic guidance.

31631

The physician places a tracheal stent or stents using a flexible fiberoptic or rigid bronchoscope introduced under appropriate anesthesia through the nasal or oral cavity. The physician uses the views obtained through the bronchoscope to identify any narrowing or area of the trachea that requires stenting for support. The physician introduces a wire through the narrowed part of the trachea and removes the bronchoscope. If dilation is first required, a series of dilators are passed over the wire to open the airway until sufficient tracheal/bronchial dilation is accomplished. A stent is passed over the wire to the target area in the trachea and positioned in place to maintain an open airway. This may be done with or without fluoroscopic guidance.

31632-31633

The physician views the airway using a flexible fiberoptic or rigid bronchoscope that is introduced under appropriate anesthesia through the nasal or oral cavity. The bronchoscope is inserted. It is advanced through the larynx to the bronchus. Fluoroscopy (x-ray) may be used to assist with navigation of the bronchoscope tip to the abnormal tissue to be biopsied. In 31632, the physician passes closed biopsy forceps through a channel in the bronchoscope, through the bronchial wall, and obtains tissue samples in one lobe. Report 31632 for each additional lobe in which this is done. In 31633, a needle is passed through a channel in the bronchoscope, into the trachea, main stem, and/or a lobe of the bronchus, and an aspiration biopsy is obtained. Report 31633 for each additional lobe in which this is done.

31634

The physician treats a bronchopleural fistula (BPF) with bronchoscopic balloon occlusion. BPF is often a serious postoperative complication of thoracic surgery, although it can also occur as a complication in a diseased lung or a previously normal lung. The physician views the airway using a flexible fiberoptic or rigid bronchoscope that is introduced under appropriate anesthesia through the nasal or oral cavity. The bronchoscope is inserted. It is advanced through the larynx to the bronchus. Fluoroscopy (x-ray) may be used to assist with navigation of the bronchoscope tip to the area of the air leak, which is assessed. A balloon catheter is placed at the site of the leak and inflated until the leak is occluded. Keeping the inflated catheter in this position, an appropriate sealant (e.g., fibrin) may be injected. Once effective sealing is verified, the catheter and bronchoscope are removed.

31635

The physician views the airway using a flexible fiberoptic or rigid bronchoscope introduced under appropriate anesthesia through the nasal or oral cavity. The physician uses the views obtained through the bronchoscope to locate the foreign body within the airway. The physician passes a snare, basket, or biopsy forceps through a channel in the bronchoscope to grasp the foreign body. The bronchoscope and foreign body are removed. This may be done with or without fluoroscopic guidance.

31636-31638

A rigid or flexible bronchoscopy is performed under appropriate anesthesia, with or without fluoroscopic guidance, to place a bronchial stent. The type of stent used, as well as the level of patency versus obstruction in the airway, will vary the placement technique. Initial assessment with the bronchoscope is done to determine the lesion's size and location. If fluoroscopy is used, the distal target position for stent placement is marked with a radiopaque object, such as a treated paperclip taped to the chest. If the airway is near completely occluded, a flexible tipped guidewire is placed through the bronchoscope, a balloon catheter is fed over the guidewire, and initial dilation is done. With the bronchoscope removed and the wire still in place, the stent, such as woven mesh or a single wire stent with polyurethane covering, is passed over the guidewire by a stent catheter just past the obstruction. The stent is deployed by slowly sliding the plastic sheath covering back until it is snugly fitted. Report 31636 for the initial bronchial stent placement, 31637 for each additional major bronchus stented, and 31638 for the revision of a stent inserted in a previous session.

31640

The physician views the airway using a flexible fiberoptic or rigid bronchoscope introduced under appropriate anesthesia through the nasal or oral cavity. The physician uses the views obtained through the bronchoscope to identify the tumor from within the airway. The physician may use fluoroscopy (x-ray) to assist with navigation of the bronchoscope tip to the abnormal tissue. The physician passes forceps through channels in the bronchoscope to grasp and excise the tumor. The bronchoscope is removed. This may be done with or without fluoroscopic guidance.

31641

The physician views the airway using a bronchoscope introduced under appropriate anesthesia through the nasal or oral cavity. The physician uses the views obtained through the bronchoscope to identify the tumor and/or area of stenosis from within the airway. Fluoroscopy (x-ray) may be used to assist with navigation of the bronchoscope tip to the abnormal tissue and is included when performed. The physician passes a laser or freezing (cryo) probe through a channel in the bronchoscope to destroy the tumor or any areas of stenosis. The bronchoscope is removed.

31643

The physician views the airway using a bronchoscope with a fiberoptic camera and operating device. Under appropriate anesthesia, the bronchoscope is introduced through the nasal or oral cavity and advanced through the bronchus. A catheter is inserted through the bronchoscope into a lung cavity and is placed at the site where, in a separately reportable procedure, intracavitary radioelements will be applied. This code includes the use of fluoroscopic guidance, when performed.

31645-31646

The physician views the airway using a bronchoscope introduced under appropriate anesthesia through the nasal or oral cavity. The physician uses the views obtained through the bronchoscope to identify the closest approach to the fluid collection from within the airway. The physician may use fluoroscopy (x-ray) to assist with navigation of the bronchoscope tip to the fluid collection. The physician passes a catheter through a channel in the bronchoscope and aspirates the tracheobronchial tree. Alternately, the physician passes a needle through a channel in the bronchoscope into the fluid collection and aspirates fluid through the needle. The bronchoscope is removed. Report 31645 for the initial treatment only. Report 31646 for any subsequent aspiration procedures performed during the same hospital stay. These codes include the use of fluoroscopic guidance, when performed.

31647 [31651]

The physician inserts one or more bronchial valves using a bronchoscopic approach. Typically, a bronchial valve is inserted to control leaks within the bronchus due to lung disease (e.g., emphysema). This small, umbrella-shaped valve redirects airflow from damaged areas, while secretions and trapped air can pass through. Under appropriate anesthesia, the physician sizes the airway, often using a calibrated balloon, in order to determine the appropriate valve diameter size. A flexible fiberoptic bronchoscope is introduced through the nasal or oral cavity and advanced past the larynx and into the bronchus. The valve is housed in a catheter delivery system comprised of a flexible internal rod that stabilizes the valve and an outer sheath that is withdrawn to release the valve. The physician assures accurate placement of the valve in the tapering airways under direct vision. Once placement is confirmed, the valve is deployed, and the bronchoscope is removed.

31648-31649

The physician removes one or more previously placed bronchial valves using a bronchoscopic approach. Under appropriate anesthesia, the physician introduces a flexible fiberoptic or rigid bronchoscope through the nasal or oral cavity and advances it past the larynx and into the bronchus. The bronchial valve is visualized by fluoroscopy, if utilized, grasped with biopsy forceps, and removed.

31652-31654

Endobronchial ultrasound (EBUS) is a minimally invasive technique utilizing ultrasound in conjunction with bronchoscopy to view the airway wall and adjacent structures. Utilizing appropriate anesthesia, the physician performs a transbronchial needle aspiration (TBNA) biopsy on lymph nodes via a thin flexible instrument (bronchoscope) fitted with an ultrasound processor, as well as a fine-gauge aspiration needle guided through the patient's mouth and trachea permitting real-time imaging of the airways, blood vessels, lungs, and lymph nodes. The physician can view hard to reach areas and gain greater access to biopsy smaller lymph nodes than would be possible via conventional mediastinoscopy. A pathologist in the operating room with the physician can immediately process the biopsy samples and/or request additional samples as necessary, leading to a quicker diagnosis of cancer, infections, or other inflammatory diseases of the lungs, as well as to assist in staging lung cancer. There are two types of EBUS: radial probe EBUS and linear probe EBUS. The radial probe EBUS has a rotating mechanical transducer with very good image quality that permits the airway layers to be identified but TBNA is not possible with this device. The linear probe EBUS is a fixed array of electronic transducer aligned in a curvilinear pattern and permits real-time guidance for mediastinal lesion sampling. EBUS procedures may be performed under general anesthesia or with moderate conscious sedation and typically allow for patients to go home the same day as the procedure. Report 31652 for EBUS-guided biopsy for one or two mediastinal and/or hilar lymph node stations or structures and 31653 for three or more. Report 31654 when EBUS using a radial ultrasound probe is performed during diagnostic or therapeutic bronchoscopy for peripheral lesions.

31660-31661
Bronchial thermoplasty is performed to reduce the amount of smooth muscle in the airway walls in asthmatic patients. Under appropriate anesthesia, the bronchoscope is inserted and advanced through the nasal or oral cavity and past the larynx to inspect the bronchus. Fluoroscopic guidance is included if used. A catheter with an electrode array is introduced to the area of the lung that is to be treated. Radiofrequency energy is used to heat and reduce the amount of smooth muscle. Once the procedure is complete, the catheter and array are removed.

31717
The physician catheterizes the trachea to obtain a bronchial brush biopsy. The physician inserts a needle through the cricoid cartilage or the trachea. A catheter is passed over the needle and a brush is placed through the catheter to obtain bronchial tissue. A bronchoscope may be used to guide the brush. The brush is withdrawn through the catheter and both are removed. The incision may be closed with sutures.

31720-31725
The physician aspirates sputum from the lungs using a nasal tracheal catheter. The physician passes a suction catheter through the nose into the trachea. Saline may be used to liquefy secretions. The secretions are removed with suction and the catheter is removed. Report 31725 if a tracheobronchial approach with fiberscope is used at bedside.

31730
The physician introduces a needle wire dilator/stent into the trachea to relieve a subglottic stenosis. The physician places a needle through the cricoid membrane or trachea. A wire is passed through the needle and the needle is removed. A series of dilators or stents are passed over the wire to open the trachea. When sufficient dilation is gained, a stent or indwelling tube for oxygen therapy is left in place to maintain patency.

31750
The physician performs an anterior cervical incision and dissects surrounding tissues and muscles to expose the trachea. An airway is inserted and the trachea is incised. Surgical repair of the trachea is undertaken. End-to-end anastomosis of the trachea may be performed. For satisfactory reconstruction, it may be necessary for the physician to surgically repair the trachea using splints constructed from rib or costal cartilage to patch the length of the trachea. Once repair is achieved, the airway is removed and the incisions are closed.

31755
The physician performs an anterior cervical incision and dissects surrounding tissues and muscles to expose the trachea and pharynx. An airway may be inserted and the trachea and pharynx are incised. The physician incises the trachea and pharynx in such a way as to create an opening from the trachea to the pharynx. The physician may implant a device like the Singer-Blom prosthesis between the trachea and pharynx. The purpose of the prosthesis is to produce speech in a previously laryngectomized patient. Once repair is achieved, the airway, if inserted, is removed and the incisions are closed.

31760
The physician makes an incision in the thorax and approaches the trachea by opening the rib cage. An airway is inserted and the trachea is incised. Surgical repair of the trachea is undertaken. End-to-end anastomosis of the trachea may be performed. For satisfactory reconstruction, it may be necessary for the physician to surgically repair the trachea using splints constructed from rib or costal cartilage to patch the length of the trachea. Once repair is achieved, the airway is removed and the incisions are closed.

31766
The physician reconstructs the carina. The carina is the junction of the trachea and the bronchi. The physician uses a midline sternotomy or a lateral thoracotomy approach to access the carina. The carina is located and repaired primarily if possible. More extensive damage may be repaired with a Silastic stent or an autograft. A chest tube is inserted, and the wound is sutured in layers.

31770-31775
The physician repairs a bronchus. The physician makes a lateral thoracotomy incision to access the bronchus. An autograft or Silastic stent may be used to repair the bronchus in 31770. A chest tube is inserted and the wound is sutured in layers. Report 31775 if an excision stenosis and anastomosis are performed with this procedure.

31780
The physician excises a tracheal stenosis and re-anastomoses the trachea. The physician makes a horizontal neck incision to access the stenosis. The trachea is incised and the stenosis is resected. The proximal and distal portions of the trachea are brought together and closed with sutures. The wound is sutured in layers.

31781
The physician excises a tracheal stenosis and re-anastomoses the trachea. The physician makes a cervicothoracic incision to access the stenosis. The trachea is incised and the stenosis is resected. The proximal and distal portions of the trachea are brought together and closed with sutures. The wound is sutured in layers.

31785
The physician excises a tracheal tumor or carcinoma. The physician makes a horizontal neck incision to access the mass. The trachea is incised and the mass is resected. If necessary, the proximal and distal portions of the trachea are brought together and closed with sutures. The wound is sutured in layers.

31786
The physician excises a tracheal tumor or carcinoma. The physician makes a thoracic approach to access the mass. The trachea is incised and the mass is resected. If necessary, the proximal and distal portions of the trachea are brought together and closed with sutures. The wound is sutured in layers.

31800-31805
The physician closes a wound or injury of the cervical trachea in 31800 or the intrathoracic trachea in 31805. The physician debrides the wound and closes the trachea with sutures. The tissues are sutured in layers.

31820-31825
The physician closes a tracheostomy or fistula. The physician excises the scarred tissue forming the tracheostomy or fistula. If the trachea has healed, it is closed with sutures. The remaining tissues of the tracheostomy or fistula are pulled together and the wound is sutured in layers. Report 31820 if the tracheostomy or fistula is closed without plastic repair; report 31825 if the tracheostomy or fistula is closed with plastic repair of the skin made to hide the repair.

31830
The physician revises a tracheostomy scar. The physician incises the skin around the tracheostomy scar and removes the scarred tissues. The incision is sutured in layers, leaving a less noticeable scar.

32035
The physician removes the purulent fluid of an empyema by creating a drainage wound in the chest. Using a scalpel, an incision is made through the skin of the chest and the incision is deepened to expose a portion of a rib. To enter the chest cavity, a short segment of the exposed rib is removed using rib cutters. The resulting defect in the chest wall allows for the continuous release of pus from the empyema (abscess in the chest cavity).

32036
The physician removes the purulent fluid of an empyema (abscess in the chest cavity) by creating a drainage wound in the chest. Using a scalpel, an incision is made through the skin of the chest and the incision is deepened to expose a portion of a rib. To create a drainage site, a short segment of the rib is removed using rib cutters. The resulting defect in the chest wall allows for the continuous release of pus from the empyema. To ensure that the drainage wound stays open, a flap is created in the skin and subcutaneous tissues.

32096-32098
The physician removes a sample of tissue from the lung or the pleura. Using a scalpel, the skin between two ribs is incised and the tissues separated to expose the inside of the chest cavity. A representative sample of tissue is removed from the lung or pleura using a biopsy needle or by cutting with a scalpel or scissors. The surgical wound is closed by suturing. Report 32096 when the biopsy is performed to sample unilateral lung infiltrates. Report 32097 when the biopsy is of a unilateral lung nodule or mass. Report 32098 when the tissue biopsied is the pleura.

32100
The physician opens the chest cavity widely to directly visualize and assess the organs and structures in the chest. Using a scalpel, the surgeon makes a long incision around the side of the chest between two of the ribs. The incision is carried through all of the tissue layers into the chest cavity. Rib spreaders are inserted into the wound and the ribs are spread apart exposing the lung, heart, and other structures. Alternately, the chest cavity can be opened and the operation performed through a vertical incision in the center of the chest through the sternum. The skin incision is carried down to the sternum bone and a saw is used to split the sternum. With the sternum split in half, the chest is entered by spreading the sternum apart with a set of rib spreaders. The chest cavity is explored and the anatomy visualized using a gloved hand and large gauze sponges. The surgical instruments are removed. A chest tube(s) may be used to provide drainage for the chest cavity. When the procedure is complete, if applicable, the sternotomy is repaired using wires to bring the two halves of the sternum together, and the operative wound is closed by sutures or staples.

32110
The physician opens the chest cavity widely to directly visualize and assess the organs and structures in the chest. Using a scalpel, the surgeon makes a long incision around the side of the chest between two of the ribs. The incision is carried through all of the tissue layers into the chest cavity. Rib spreaders are inserted into the wound and the ribs are spread apart exposing the lung, heart, and other structures. Alternately, the chest cavity can be opened and the operation performed through a vertical incision in the center of the chest through the sternum. The skin incision is carried down to the sternum bone and a saw is used to split the sternum. With the sternum split in half, the chest is entered by spreading the sternum apart with a set of rib spreaders. The chest cavity is explored and the anatomy visualized using a gloved hand and large gauze sponges. The site of the hemorrhage or lung tear is identified and repaired. The surgical instruments are removed. A chest tube(s) may be used to provide

drainage for the chest cavity. When the procedure is complete, if applicable, the sternotomy is repaired using wires to bring the two halves of the sternum together, and the operative wound is closed by sutures or staples.

32120

The physician performs a thoracotomy to identify any thoracic postoperative complications. The physician opens the chest cavity widely to directly visualize and assess the organs and structures in the chest. Using a scalpel, the surgeon makes a long incision around the side of the chest between two of the ribs. The incision is carried through all of the tissue layers into the chest cavity. Rib spreaders are inserted into the wound and the ribs are spread apart exposing the lung, heart, and other structures. Alternately, the chest cavity can be opened and the operation performed through a vertical incision in the center of the chest through the sternum. The skin incision is carried down to the sternum bone and a saw is used to split the sternum. With the sternum split in half, the chest is entered by spreading the sternum apart with a set of rib spreaders. The chest cavity is explored and the anatomy visualized using a gloved hand and large gauze sponges. The surgical instruments are removed. A chest tube(s) may be used to provide drainage for the chest cavity. When the procedure is complete, if applicable, the sternotomy is repaired using wires to bring the two halves of the sternum together, and the operative wound is closed by sutures or staples.

32124

The physician opens the chest cavity widely to directly visualize and separate the surface of the lung, which has become adherent to the inside surface of the chest cavity. Using a scalpel, the surgeon makes a long incision around the side of the chest between two of the ribs. The incision is carried through all of the tissue layers into the chest cavity. Rib spreaders are inserted into the wound and the ribs are spread apart exposing the lung. Alternately, the chest cavity can be opened and the operation performed through a vertical incision in the center of the chest through the sternum. The skin incision is carried down to the sternum bone and a saw is used to split the sternum. With the sternum split in half, the chest is entered by spreading the sternum apart with a set of rib spreaders. Using a gloved hand and a large moist gauze sponge, the surgeon manually divides the tissues attaching the lung to the wall of the chest cavity. When the procedure is complete, the instruments and gauze sponges are removed. A chest tube(s) may be used to provide drainage for the chest cavity. If applicable, the sternotomy is repaired using wires to bring the two halves of the sternum together, and the operative wound is closed by sutures or staples.

32140

The physician opens the chest cavity widely to remove one or more lung cysts. Using a scalpel, the surgeon makes a long incision around the side of the chest between two of the ribs. The incision is carried through all of the tissue layers into the chest cavity. Rib spreaders are inserted into the wound and the ribs are spread apart exposing the lung. Alternately, the chest cavity can be opened and the operation performed through a vertical incision in the center of the chest through the sternum. The skin incision is carried down to the sternum bone and a saw is used to split the sternum. With the sternum split in half, the chest is entered by spreading the sternum apart with a set of rib spreaders. Space is made in the chest by packing the uninvolved lung away from the operative field by using large moist gauze sponges. In order to perform the procedure, the pleural surface may require an operative procedure such as pneumonolysis (separation of the surface of the lung that has become adherent to the inside surface of the chest cavity). The lung cyst is located and removed by sharp and blunt dissection of the tissues. When the procedure is complete, the instruments and gauze sponges are removed. A chest tube(s) may be used to provide drainage for the chest cavity. If applicable, the sternotomy is repaired using wires to bring the two halves of the sternum together, and the operative wound is closed by sutures or staples.

32141

The physician opens the chest cavity widely to remove one or more lung bullae (large nonfunctional air sacs). Using a scalpel, the surgeon makes a long incision around the side of the chest between two of the ribs. The incision is carried through all of the tissue layers into the chest cavity. Rib spreaders are inserted into the wound and the ribs are spread apart exposing the lung. Alternately, the chest cavity can be opened and the operation performed through a vertical incision in the center of the chest through the sternum. The skin incision is carried down to the sternum bone and a saw is used to split the sternum. With the sternum split in half, the chest is entered by spreading the sternum apart with a set of rib spreaders. Space is made in the chest by packing the uninvolved lung away from the operative field using large moist gauze sponges. In order to perform the procedure, the pleural surface may require an operative procedure such as pneumonolysis (separation of the surface of the lung that has become adherent to the inside surface of the chest cavity). The lung bullae is located and removed by sharp and blunt dissection of the tissues and often by folding and suturing of the tissues (plication). When the procedure is complete, the instruments and gauze sponges are removed. A chest tube(s) may be used to provide drainage for the chest cavity. If applicable, the sternotomy is repaired using wires to bring the two halves of the sternum together, and the operative wound is closed by sutures or staples.

32150-32151

The physician opens the chest cavity widely to remove a foreign body or fibrin deposit (thick insoluble protein deposit formed after the clotting of blood). Using a scalpel, the surgeon makes a long incision around the side of the chest between two of the ribs. The incision is carried through all of the tissue layers into the chest cavity. Rib spreaders are inserted into the wound and the ribs are spread apart exposing the lung. Alternately, the chest cavity can be opened and the operation performed through a vertical incision in the center of the chest through the sternum. The skin incision is carried down to the sternum bone and a saw is used to split the sternum. With the sternum split in half, the chest is entered by spreading the sternum apart with a set of rib spreaders. Space is made in the chest by packing the uninvolved lung away from the operative field using large moist gauze sponges. The foreign body or fibrin deposit is located and removed by sharp and blunt dissection. When the procedure is complete, the instruments and gauze sponges are removed. A chest tube(s) may be used to provide drainage for the chest cavity. If applicable, the sternotomy is repaired using wires to bring the two halves of the sternum together, and the operative wound is closed by sutures or staples. Report 32150 for removal of an intrapleural foreign body or fibrin deposits and 32151 for removal of an intrapulmonary foreign body.

32160

The physician opens the chest cavity widely to perform manual cardiac massage in the case of cardiac arrest. Using a scalpel, the surgeon makes a long incision around the side of the chest between two of the ribs. The incision is carried through all of the tissue layers into the chest cavity. Rib spreaders are inserted into the wound and the ribs are spread apart exposing the lung. Alternately, the chest cavity can be opened and the operation performed through a vertical incision in the center of the chest through the sternum. The skin incision is carried down to the sternum bone and a saw is used to split the sternum. With the sternum split in half, the chest is entered by spreading the sternum apart with a set of rib spreaders. Space is made in the chest by packing the uninvolved lung away from the operative field using large moist gauze sponges. The heart is exposed and squeezed rhythmically to mimic cardiac contractions, thus pumping blood through the body. The heart may be directly contra-shocked to produce spontaneous heartbeats. When the procedure is complete, the instruments and gauze sponges are removed. A chest tube(s) may be used to provide drainage for the chest cavity. If applicable, the sternotomy is repaired using wires to bring the two halves of the sternum together, and the operative wound is closed by sutures or staples.

32200

The physician treats an abscess or cyst in the lung by draining the pus or fluid directly through the chest wall. Using a scalpel, the skin between two ribs is incised and the tissues separated to expose the inside of the chest cavity. The lung is cut with scissors or a scalpel down to the abscess or the cyst. The abscess or cyst is opened and the fluid is allowed to drain through the wound created in the lung and the chest wall. A rubber drainage tube may be left in place to maintain or facilitate drainage. The incision is not sutured closed. The outside incision is dressed with bulky gauze dressing to absorb the drainage.

32215

The physician treats repeat pneumothorax by producing adhesions between the surface of the lung and the inside surface of the chest cavity. To create the adhesions, a chemical solution is injected into the chest cavity and allowed to circulate over the surface of the lung and the inside surface of the chest cavity. The physician injects the solution by passing a tube into the chest cavity. The physician passes a trocar over the top of a rib and punctures through the chest tissues between the ribs and enters the pleural cavity. With the end of the trocar in the chest cavity, the physician advances the plastic tube into the chest cavity. The sharp instrument is removed leaving one end of the plastic catheter in place within the chest cavity. A syringe is attached to the outside end of the catheter and fluid is injected into the chest cavity. The fluid selected is designed to cause the formation of adhesive scar tissue between the surface of the lung and the inside surface of the chest cavity. Once the lung adheres to the chest wall it can no longer collapse and allow the formation of a pneumothorax.

32220-32225

The physician removes a constricting membrane or layer of tissue from the surface of the lung (decortication) in order to permit the lung to fully expand. The physician opens the chest cavity widely. Using a scalpel, the surgeon makes a long incision around the side of the chest between two of the ribs. The incision is carried through all the tissue layers into the chest cavity. Rib spreaders are inserted into the wound and the ribs are spread apart exposing the lung. The constricting membrane is stripped off the surface of the lung. In 32225, only a portion of the lung surface is removed. The chest wall incision is sutured closed in layers. A chest tube(s) may be used to provide drainage for the chest cavity. Alternately, the chest cavity can be opened by a vertical incision in the front of the chest through the sternum. The skin incision is carried down to the sternum bone and a saw is used to split the sternum. With the sternum split in half, the chest is entered by spreading the sternum apart with a set of rib spreaders. When the procedure is complete, the wound is closed by using wires to bring the two halves of the sternum together and the skin is closed by suturing.

32310

The physician removes the membranous tissue lining the inside surface of the chest cavity (the parietal pleura). The physician opens the chest cavity widely to gain access to the inside surface of the chest. Using a scalpel, the surgeon makes a long incision around the side of the chest between two of the ribs. The incision is carried through all the tissue layers into the chest cavity. Rib spreaders are inserted into the wound and the ribs are spread apart exposing the lung. The parietal pleura is stripped from the inside surface of the chest. The chest wall incision is sutured closed in layers. A chest tube(s) may be used to provide drainage for the chest cavity. Alternately, the chest cavity can be opened and the operation performed through a vertical incision in the center of the chest through the sternum. The skin incision is carried down to the sternum bone and a saw is used to split the sternum. With the sternum split in half, the chest is entered by spreading the sternum apart with a set of rib spreaders. When the procedure is complete, the wound is closed by using wires to bring the two halves of the sternum together and the skin is closed over the sternum by suturing.

32320

The physician removes a constricting membrane or layer of tissue from a portion of the surface of the lung (decortication) in order to permit the lung to fully expand and also removes the membranous tissue lining the inside surface of the chest cavity (the parietal pleura). The physician opens the chest cavity widely. Using a scalpel, the surgeon makes a long incision around the side of the chest between two of the ribs. The incision is carried through all the tissue layers into the chest cavity. Rib spreaders are inserted into the wound and the ribs are spread apart exposing the lung. The constricting membrane is stripped off the surface of the lung. The parietal pleura is stripped from the inside surface of the chest. The chest wall incision is sutured closed in layers. A chest tube(s) may be used to provide drainage for the chest cavity. Alternately, the chest cavity can be opened and the operation performed through a vertical incision in the center of the chest through the sternum. The skin incision is carried down to the sternum bone and a saw is used to split the sternum. With the sternum split in half, the chest is entered by spreading the sternum apart with a set of rib spreaders. When the procedure is complete, the wound is closed by using wires to bring the two halves of the sternum together and the skin is closed over the sternum by suturing.

32400

The physician obtains a sample of the lining of the lung and/or the lining of the inside of the chest cavity by needle biopsy. Using a pleural biopsy needle, the physician passes the needle over the top of a rib, punctures through the chest tissues between two ribs, enters the pleural cavity and slightly punctures the surface of the lung. With the end of the needle in the chest cavity, the physician withdraws a piece of tissue. The needle is withdrawn and the puncture site covered with a bandage. The procedure is often done under radiological guidance to assure more precise placement of the needle.

32408

The physician obtains a sample of the lung or the mediastinum (the tissues in the center of the chest between the two lung cavities) by puncturing through the space between two of the ribs with a needle. The procedure is often done under radiological guidance, which is included in this code when performed, to assure more precise placement of the needle. Using a core biopsy needle, the physician passes the needle over the top of a rib, punctures through the chest tissues, enters the pleural cavity, and punctures the area of concern in the lung or the mediastinum. With the end of the needle in the chest cavity, the physician withdraws a piece of tissue. The needle is withdrawn and the puncture site covered with a bandage.

32440

The physician removes one lung in its entirety. The physician opens the chest cavity widely to gain access to the lung to be removed. Using a scalpel, the surgeon makes a long incision around the side of the chest between two of the ribs. The incision is carried through all of the tissue layers into the chest cavity. Rib spreaders are inserted into the wound and the ribs are spread apart exposing the lung, heart, and other structures. Alternately, the chest cavity can be opened and the operation performed through a vertical incision in the center of the chest through the sternum. The skin incision is carried down to the sternum bone and a saw is used to split the sternum. With the sternum split in half, the chest is entered by spreading the sternum apart with a set of rib spreaders. The root of the lung is found by pushing aside the deflated lung with a gloved hand and large moist gauze sponges. Within the root of the lung, the blood vessels and bronchial tubes are clamped, tied off, and cut. The lung is removed through the wide chest incision. The instruments and gauze sponges are removed. A chest tube(s) may be used to provide drainage for the chest cavity. When the procedure is complete, if applicable, the sternotomy is repaired using wires to bring the two halves of the sternum together, and the operative wound is closed by sutures or staples.

32442

The physician removes one lung in its entirety. The physician opens the chest cavity widely to gain access to the lung to be removed. Using a scalpel, the surgeon makes a long incision around the side of the chest between two of the ribs. The incision is carried through all of the tissue layers into the chest cavity. Rib spreaders are inserted into the wound and the ribs are spread apart exposing the lung, heart, and other structures. Alternately, the chest cavity can be opened and the operation performed through a vertical incision in the center of the chest through the sternum. The skin incision is carried down to the sternum bone and a saw is used to split the sternum. With the sternum split in half, the chest is entered by spreading the sternum apart with a set of rib spreaders. The root of the lung is found by pushing aside the deflated lung with a gloved hand and large moist gauze sponges. Within the root of the lung, the blood vessels and bronchial tubes are clamped, tied off, and cut. The lung and a segment of the trachea are removed through the wide chest incision. The trachea is sutured to the main bronchial tube of the remaining lung in the other half of the chest. The instruments and gauze sponges are removed. A chest tube(s) may be used to provide drainage for the chest cavity. When the procedure is complete, if applicable, the sternotomy is repaired using wires to bring the two halves of the sternum together, and the operative wound is closed by sutures or staples.

32445
The physician removes one lung in its entirety and the pleural membranes covering the lung and the inside surface of the chest cavity (the parietal pleura). The physician opens the chest cavity widely to gain access to the lung to be removed. Using a scalpel, the surgeon makes a long incision around the side of the chest between two of the ribs. The incision is carried through all of the tissue layers down to the membrane lining the chest cavity. Rib spreaders are inserted into the wound and the ribs are spread apart, taking care to preserve the integrity of the chest lining. Holding a gauze sponge, the surgeon strips away the lining inside the chest all the way around to the root of the lung. This creates a sac of the parietal pleura that contains the lung. Within the root of the lung, the blood vessels and bronchial tubes are clamped, tied off, and cut. The lung and the pleural tissues of the inside of the chest wall are removed through the wide chest incision. After the removal of the instruments and gauze sponges, the chest incision is sutured closed in layers. A chest tube(s) may be used to provide drainage for the chest cavity.

32480-32482
The physician opens the chest cavity widely to gain access to the lung to be removed. Using a scalpel, the surgeon makes a long incision around the side of the chest between two of the ribs. The incision is carried through all of the tissue layers into the chest cavity. Rib spreaders are inserted into the wound and the ribs are spread apart exposing the lung. Alternately, the chest cavity can be opened and the operation performed through a vertical incision in the center of the chest through the sternum. The skin incision is carried down to the sternum bone and a saw is used to split the sternum. With the sternum split in half, the chest is entered by spreading the sternum apart with a set of rib spreaders. The lobe(s) to be removed is identified and isolated in the operative field by pushing aside the deflated lung with a gloved hand and large moist gauze sponges. Within the lobe(s) of the lung, the main blood vessels and bronchial tubes are clamped, tied off, and cut. The lobe(s) is removed through the wide chest incision. The instruments and gauze sponges are removed. A chest tube(s) may be used to provide drainage for the chest cavity. When the procedure is complete, if applicable, the sternotomy is repaired using wires to bring the two halves of the sternum together, and the operative wound is closed by sutures or staples. Report 32480 when one lobe is removed and 32482 when two lobes are removed.

32484
The physician removes a segment of a lobe of one lung. The physician opens the chest cavity widely to gain access to the lung to be removed. Using a scalpel, the surgeon makes a long incision around the side of the chest between two of the ribs. The incision is carried through all of the tissue layers into the chest cavity. Rib spreaders are inserted into the wound and the ribs are spread apart exposing the lung. Alternately, the chest cavity can be opened and the operation performed through a vertical incision in the center of the chest through the sternum. The skin incision is carried down to the sternum bone and a saw is used to split the sternum. With the sternum split in half, the chest is entered by spreading the sternum apart with a set of rib spreaders. The segment to be removed is identified and isolated in the operative field by pushing aside the deflated lung with a gloved hand and large moist gauze sponges. Within the segment of the lung, the main blood vessels and bronchial tubes are clamped, tied off, and cut. The segment is removed through the wide chest incision. The instruments and gauze sponges are removed. A chest tube(s) may be used to provide drainage for the chest cavity. When the procedure is complete, if applicable, the sternotomy is repaired using wires to bring the two halves of the sternum together, and the operative wound is closed by sutures or staples.

32486
The physician removes a portion (lobectomy, bilobectomy, or segmentectomy) of one lung and repairs a bronchial tube that has been partially resected. The physician opens the chest cavity widely to gain access to the lung to be removed. Using a scalpel, the surgeon makes a long incision around the side of the chest between two of the ribs. The incision is carried through all of the tissue layers into the chest cavity. Rib spreaders are inserted into the wound and the ribs are spread apart exposing the lung. Alternately, the chest cavity can be opened and the operation performed through a vertical incision in the center of the chest through the sternum. The skin incision is carried down to the sternum bone and a saw is used to split the sternum. With the sternum split in half, the chest is entered by spreading the sternum apart with a set of rib spreaders. The portion of lung to be removed is identified and isolated in the operative field by pushing aside the deflated lung with a gloved hand and large moist gauze sponges. Within the lung, main blood vessels and bronchial tubes are clamped, tied off, and cut. The resected part of the lung is removed through the wide chest incision. The segment of diseased or damaged bronchial tube is removed. The healthy end of the smaller bronchial tube in the remaining lobe is sutured to the main bronchial tube in the root of the lung. The instruments and gauze sponges are removed. A chest tube(s) may be used to provide drainage for the chest cavity. When the procedure is complete, if applicable, the sternotomy is repaired using wires to bring the two halves of the sternum together, and the operative wound is closed by sutures or staples.

32488
The physician removes the remaining portion(s) of a lung from a prior partial lung removal. The physician opens the chest cavity widely to gain access to the lung to be removed. Using a scalpel, the surgeon makes a long incision around the side of the chest between two of the ribs. The incision is carried through all of the tissue layers into the chest cavity. Rib spreaders are inserted into the wound and the ribs are

spread apart exposing the lung. Alternately, the chest cavity can be opened and the operation performed through a vertical incision in the center of the chest through the sternum. The skin incision is carried down to the sternum bone and a saw is used to split the sternum. With the sternum split in half, the chest is entered by spreading the sternum apart with a set of rib spreaders. The remaining portion of lung is isolated in the operative field by pushing aside the deflated lung with a gloved hand and large moist gauze sponges. Within the root of the lung, the blood vessels and bronchial tubes are clamped, tied off, and cut. The lung is removed through the wide chest incision. The instruments and gauze sponges are removed. A chest tube(s) may be used to provide drainage for the chest cavity. When the procedure is complete, if applicable, the sternotomy is repaired using wires to bring the two halves of the sternum together, and the operative wound is closed by sutures or staples.

32491

The physician removes part of an emphysematous lung. Using a scalpel, the surgeon makes a long incision around the side of the chest between two of the ribs. The incision is carried through all of the tissue layers into the chest cavity. Rib spreaders are inserted into the wound and the ribs are spread apart exposing the lung. Alternately, the chest cavity can be opened and the operation performed through a vertical incision in the center of the chest through the sternum. The skin incision is carried down to the sternum bone and a saw is used to split the sternum. With the sternum split in half, the chest is entered by spreading the sternum apart with a set of rib spreaders. Space is made in the chest by packing the uninvolved lung away from the operative field using large moist gauze sponges. In order to perform the procedure, the pleural surface may require an operative procedure such as pneumonolysis (separation of the surface of the lung that has become adherent to the inside surface of the chest cavity). The lung tissue to be removed is identified and isolated in the operative field by pushing aside the deflated lung with a gloved hand and large moist gauze sponges. The lung tissue may be further isolated using a row of staples. The emphysematous lung tissue is removed by sharp and blunt dissection and often by folding and suturing of the tissues (plication). When the procedure is complete, the instruments and gauze sponges are removed. A chest tube(s) may be used to provide drainage for the chest cavity. If applicable, the sternotomy is repaired using wires to bring the two halves of the sternum together, and the operative wound is closed by sutures or staples.

32501

During lobectomy or segmentectomy, the physician repairs part of a bronchus. After removing the lobes or lobe segments (see codes 32480, 32482, 32484 for procedure description), the segment of diseased or damaged bronchial tube is repaired and sutured to the main bronchial tube in the root of the lung. The remaining instruments and gauze sponges are removed from the chest cavity. The chest incision is sutured closed in layers (sternal wires are used if the chest was entered through a midline sternal incision). A chest tube(s) may be used to provide drainage for the chest cavity. List this code separately in addition to the primary procedure.

32503-32504

The physician removes a tumor from the apex of the lung, such as a Pancoast tumor, as well as a portion of the chest wall. The patient may be intubated with a double lumen endotracheal tube to verify correct positioning and to evaluate endobronchial disease. The chest cavity is entered using an anterior or posterior incision. The posterior incision is made along the outline of the scapula, entering the pleural space at the third or fourth intercostal space. In some cases, an anterior transcervical approach is used. The necessary extended en bloc resection of the chest wall includes posterior portions of the first three ribs, part of the upper thoracic vertebrae (including the transverse process), the intercostal nerves, the lower trunk of the brachial plexus, the stellate ganglion, a section of the dorsal sympathetic ganglion, and the portion of the involved lung. For tumors that are situated peripherally, the apical segment of the upper lobe of the lung is separated from the remaining superior lobe. The apex of the lung is left attached to the chest wall. The first through third, fourth, or fifth ribs are sectioned anteriorly. The subclavian artery is sharply dissected from the surrounding structures. A subperiosteal dissection is performed around the first rib, which is transected, and the subclavian vessels are mobilized superiorly. If preoperative magnetic resonance imaging demonstrated vessel involvement, an initial anterior approach is performed to dissect or graft the vessels. The ribs are disarticulated and the tumor, along with the involved chest wall, is gradually mobilized. Next, the segmental vessels are identified, doubly ligated, and transected. The parietal pleura are bluntly dissected along the anterior border of the spinal column. The tumor and the involved chest wall that has remained attached to the inferior trunk of the brachial plexus is excised, using caution to spare the T1 nerve root as it crosses beneath the angle of the first rib to join the C8 nerve root. If a tumor has invaded the vertebral bodies, the subclavian artery, or the C8 to T1 nerve routes, a multidisciplinary approach may be necessary. At the completion of the procedure, two large chest tubes are placed: one at the apex of the chest to drain any residual air and the other to drain fluids. Report 32504 when chest wall reconstruction is performed.

32505-32507

The physician removes a wedge-shaped portion(s) of a lobe(s) on one or both lungs. The physician opens the chest cavity widely to gain access to the lung to be removed. Using a scalpel, the surgeon makes a long incision around the side of the chest between two of the ribs. The incision is carried through all of the tissue layers into the chest cavity. Rib spreaders are inserted into the wound and the ribs are spread apart exposing the lung. Alternately, the chest cavity can be opened and the operation performed through a vertical incision in the center of the chest through the sternum. The skin incision is carried down to the sternum bone and a saw is used to split the sternum. With the sternum split in half, the chest is entered by spreading the sternum apart with a set of rib spreaders. The area to be removed is identified and isolated in the operative field by pushing aside the deflated lung with a gloved hand and large moist gauze sponges. The healthy portions of the lung surrounding the area(s) to be removed are clamped and the unhealthy portion is removed by cutting the lung tissue isolated by the clamps. Sutures or surgical clips are used to repair the cut portion of the remaining lung tissue. The instruments and gauze sponges are removed. A chest tube(s) may be used to provide drainage for the chest cavity. When the procedure is complete, if applicable, the sternotomy is repaired using wires to bring the two halves of the sternum together and the operative wound is closed by sutures or staples. Report 32505 for the initial therapeutic wedge resection and 32506 for each additional wedge resection on the same side. Report 32507 when the wedge resection is followed by a lung resection.

32540

The physician removes an empyema (an abscess in the chest cavity between the lung and the chest wall) in its entirety, including the pleural membranes surrounding the abscess. The physician opens the chest cavity to gain access to the abscess. Using a scalpel, the surgeon makes an incision around the side of the chest between two of the ribs. The incision is carried through all the tissue layers down to the membrane lining the chest cavity. Rib spreaders are inserted into the wound and the ribs are spread apart exposing the tissues, taking care to preserve the integrity of the chest lining. Holding a gauze sponge, the surgeon strips away the lining adherent to the chest wall and the abscess and carries this all the way around the abscess. This creates a sac that contains the abscess. The intact mass is shelled out through the chest incision. After the removal of the instruments and gauze sponges, the chest incision is sutured closed in layers leaving a drainage tube or the wound is partially closed to allow drainage.

32550

The physician inserts a tunneled, indwelling pleural catheter to aid quality of life and long-term management of malignant effusion. The catheter allows drainage on an outpatient or home basis and consists of flexible rubber tubing with a safety drainage valve to provide access to the pleural cavity and prevent air and fluid entering. A polyester cuff secures the catheter in place and helps prevent infection. Using separately reportable imaging guidance, the physician inserts the catheter percutaneously through a small incision in the anterior axillary area. The pleural catheter is threaded over a guidewire to access the pleural cavity, tunneled under the skin along the chest wall, and brought out that side in the lower chest. After placement, the patient may drain pleural fluid at home periodically into vacuum bottles by connecting the matching drainage line access tip to the valve.

32551

The physician removes fluid and/or air from the chest cavity by puncturing through the space between the ribs. To enter the chest cavity, the physician passes a trocar over the top of a rib, punctures through the chest tissues between the ribs, and enters the pleural cavity. Separately reportable imaging guidance may be used. With the end of the trocar in the chest cavity, the physician advances the plastic tube into the chest cavity. The sharp trocar is removed leaving one end of the plastic catheter in place within the chest cavity. A large syringe is attached to the outside end of the catheter and the fluid (blood or pus) is removed from the chest cavity by pulling back on the plunger of the syringe. The outside end of the tube may be connected to a drainage system, such as a water seal, to prevent air from being sucked into the chest cavity and to allow continuous or intermittent removal of air or fluid.

32552

The physician removes a previously placed, indwelling tunneled pleural catheter with cuff. Following administration of local anesthesia along the subcutaneous catheter tunnel, blunt dissection is used to release the cuff and the catheter is meticulously withdrawn. Conscious sedation may be required.

32553

The physician places one or more interstitial devices such as gold seeds (fiducial markers) for radiation therapy guidance or a dosimeter to gauge the amount of radiation received. Implanted percutaneously in and/or around an intrathoracic soft tissue tumor, these act as radiographic landmarks to define the position of the target lesion. Under CT or other image guidance, the physician injects a small capsule or seed into the intrathoracic tissue using a needle injection device. Allowing for precision in targeting radiation and/or for measuring the radiation doses received, an injected fiducial marker is visible by ultrasound and fluoroscopy and permits accurate triangulation of the tissue to be treated. An injected capsule dosimeter relays radiation dose information so that the clinical team can monitor for any deviation between the radiation plan and the actual radiation received.

32554-32555

The physician removes fluid and/or air from the chest cavity by puncturing through the space between the ribs with a hollow needle (cannula) and entering the chest cavity. The fluid (blood or pus) is removed from the chest cavity by pulling back on the plunger of the syringe attached to the cannula. Report 32554 if the procedure is performed without imaging guidance. Report 32555 when imaging guidance is used during the procedure.

32556-32557

The physician removes fluid and/or air from the chest cavity. The patient is positioned dependent upon the location of the fluid (blood or pus) on preprocedural imaging. The chest cavity is accessed by puncturing through the space between the ribs with a needle. Once the fluid is accessed via the needle(s), a guidewire is inserted to the most distal point of the fluid in the pleural cavity. A catheter (i.e., pigtail catheter) is inserted the length of the guidewire and the chest cavity is drained. In some instances, the catheter is connected to a water seal system. Report 32556 if the procedure is performed without imaging guidance. Report 32557 when imaging guidance is used during the procedure.

32560

The physician instills an agent for pleurodesis, such as talc for recurrent or persistent pneumothorax, into the chest cavity via a chest tube or catheter by puncturing through the space between the ribs. The physician passes a trocar over the top of a rib, punctures through the chest tissues, and enters the pleural cavity. With the end of the trocar, the physician advances the plastic tube into the chest cavity within the pleural space, specifically between the layers of the visceral and parietal pleura. The sharp instrument is removed leaving one end of the plastic catheter in place. A syringe is attached to the outside end of the catheter and the agent is injected into the pleural space. The agent selected is designed to eradicate the pleural space preventing reoccurrence of pleural effusion.

32561-32562

The physician instills a fibrinolytic agent (one that breaks up fibrinous adhesions) into the chest cavity via a chest tube or catheter by puncturing through the space between the ribs. To enter the chest cavity, the physician passes a trocar over the top of a rib, punctures through the chest tissues, and enters the pleural cavity. With the end of the trocar in the chest cavity, the physician advances the plastic tube into the chest cavity. The sharp instrument is removed, leaving one end of the plastic catheter in place within the chest cavity. A syringe is attached to the outside end of the catheter and a fibrinolytic agent, such as a saline mixture with Streptokinase or urokinase, is injected into the chest cavity. The agent selected is designed to break up multiloculated pleural effusions and facilitate adequate drainage. Report 32561 for the first day of instillation and 32562 for each subsequent day.

32601

The physician examines the inside of the chest cavity through a rigid or flexible fiberoptic endoscope. The procedure can be done under local or general anesthesia. The surgeon makes a small incision between two ribs and by blunt dissection and the use of a trocar enters the thoracic cavity. The endoscope is passed through the trocar and into the chest cavity. The lung is usually partially collapsed by instilling air into the chest through the trocar, or if general anesthesia is used, the lung may be collapsed through a double lumen endotracheal tube inserted through the mouth into the trachea. The contents of the chest cavity are examined by direct visualization and/or the use of a video camera. Still photographs may be taken as part of the procedure. At the conclusion of the procedure, the endoscope and the trocar are removed. A chest tube for drainage and re-expansion of the lung is usually inserted through the wound used for the thoracoscopy.

32604

The physician examines the pericardial sac using a rigid or flexible fiberoptic endoscope. The procedure can be done under local or general anesthesia. The physician makes a small incision between two ribs and by blunt dissection and the use of a trocar enters the thoracic cavity. The endoscope is passed through the trocar and into the chest cavity. The lung is usually partially collapsed by instilling air into the chest through the trocar or, if general anesthesia is used, the lung may be collapsed through a double lumen endotracheal tube inserted through the mouth into the trachea. The endoscope is advanced to and into the pericardial sac as the physician views the structures and the anatomy of the area through the scope. The contents of the pericardial sac are examined by direct visualization and/or the use of a video camera. Still photographs may be taken as part of the procedure. The pericardial tissue selected for biopsy is identified and the biopsy is taken using a device inserted through the endoscope. At the conclusion of the procedure, the endoscope and the trocar are withdrawn. A chest tube for drainage and re-expansion of the lung is usually inserted through the wound used for the thoracoscopy.

32606

The physician examines the inside of the mediastinal space through a rigid or flexible fiberoptic endoscope. The procedure can be done under local or general anesthesia. The physician makes a small incision between two ribs and by blunt dissection and the use of a trocar enters the thoracic cavity. The endoscope is passed through the trocar and into the chest cavity. The lung is usually partially collapsed by instilling air into the chest through the trocar or, if general anesthesia is used, the lung may be collapsed through a special double lumen endotracheal tube inserted through the mouth into the trachea. As the physician views the structures and the anatomy of the area through the endoscope, the endoscope is advanced into the mediastinum (area inside the center of the chest cavity between the lungs). The contents of the mediastinal space are examined by direct visualization and/or by the use of a video camera. Still photographs may be taken as part of the procedure. The tissue selected for biopsy is identified and a biopsy taken using a device inserted through the endoscope. At the conclusion of the procedure, the endoscope and the trocar are withdrawn. A chest tube for drainage and re-expansion of the lung is usually inserted through the wound used for the thoracoscopy.

32607
The physician biopsies lung infiltrates through a rigid or flexible fiberoptic endoscope. This procedure can be done under local or general anesthesia. The surgeon makes a small incision between two ribs and by blunt dissection and the use of a trocar enters the thoracic cavity. The endoscope is passed through the trocar and into the chest cavity. One lung is usually partially collapsed by instilling air into the chest through the trocar or, if general anesthesia is used, the lung may be collapsed through a double lumen endotracheal tube inserted through the mouth into the trachea. The contents of the chest cavity are examined by direct visualization and/or the use of a video camera. Still photographs may be taken as part of the procedure. The lung infiltrates selected for biopsy are identified and the biopsy is taken using a device inserted through the endoscope. At the conclusion of the procedure, the endoscope and the trocar are removed. A chest tube for drainage and re-expansion of the lung is usually inserted through the wound used for the thoracoscopy.

32608
The physician biopsies a lung nodule or mass through a rigid or flexible fiberoptic endoscope. This procedure can be done under local or general anesthesia. The surgeon makes a small incision between two ribs and by blunt dissection and the use of a trocar enters the thoracic cavity. The endoscope is passed through the trocar and into the chest cavity. One lung is usually partially collapsed by instilling air into the chest through the trocar or, if general anesthesia is used, the lung may be collapsed through a double lumen endotracheal tube inserted through the mouth into the trachea. The contents of the chest cavity are examined by direct visualization and/or the use of a video camera. Still photographs may be taken as part of the procedure. The lung nodule(s) or mass(es) selected for biopsy is identified and the biopsy is taken using a device inserted through the endoscope. At the conclusion of the procedure, the endoscope and the trocar are removed. A chest tube for drainage and re-expansion of the lung is usually inserted through the wound used for the thoracoscopy.

32609
The physician biopsies the pleura through a rigid or flexible fiberoptic endoscope. This procedure can be done under local or general anesthesia. The surgeon makes a small incision between two ribs and by blunt dissection and the use of a trocar enters the thoracic cavity. The endoscope is passed through the trocar and into the chest cavity. One lung is usually partially collapsed by instilling air into the chest through the trocar or, if general anesthesia is used, the lung may be collapsed through a double lumen endotracheal tube inserted through the mouth into the trachea. The contents of the chest cavity are examined by direct visualization and/or the use of a video camera. Still photographs may be taken as part of the procedure. The area of the pleura selected for biopsy is identified and the biopsy is taken using a device inserted through the endoscope. At the conclusion of the procedure, the endoscope and the trocar are removed. A chest tube for drainage and re-expansion of the lung is usually inserted through the wound used for the thoracoscopy.

32650
The physician examines the inside of the chest cavity through a rigid or flexible fiberoptic endoscope and induces adhesion of the surface of the lung to the inside surface of the chest cavity. The procedure can be done under local or general anesthesia. The physician makes a small incision between two ribs and by blunt dissection and the use of a trocar enters the thoracic cavity. The endoscope is passed through the trocar and into the chest cavity. The lung is usually partially collapsed by instilling air into the chest through the trocar or, if general anesthesia is used, the lung may be collapsed through a double lumen endotracheal tube inserted through the mouth into the trachea. The contents of the chest cavity are examined by direct visualization and/or by the use of a video camera. Still photographs may be taken as part of the procedure. A second trocar and instruments may be inserted into the chest cavity through a second wound in the chest. Adhesion may be induced in one of two ways: by abrading the surfaces of the lung and the inside of the chest cavity or by the instillation of chemicals into the chest cavity that bath the surfaces of the lung and the inside of the chest cavity. Most commonly, a chemical solution is instilled into the chest through the endoscope or second puncture site. At the conclusion of the procedure, the endoscope and the trocar are removed. A chest tube for drainage and re-expansion of the lung is usually inserted through the wound used for the thoracoscopy.

32651-32652
The physician examines the inside of the chest cavity through a rigid or flexible fiberoptic endoscope and removes a portion of the tissue covering the surface of the lung. The procedure can be done under local or general anesthesia. The physician makes a small incision between two ribs and by blunt dissection and the use of a trocar enters the thoracic cavity. The endoscope is passed through the trocar and into the chest cavity. The lung is usually partially collapsed by instilling air into the chest through the trocar or, if general anesthesia is used, the lung may be collapsed through a double lumen endotracheal tube inserted through the mouth into the trachea. The contents of the chest cavity are examined by direct visualization and/or by the use of a video camera. Still photographs may be taken as part of the procedure. A second and/ or third trocar and instruments may be inserted into the chest cavity through a second and/or third wound in the chest. Under direct visualization through the endoscope, the physician strips away the membranous tissues covering a portion of the lung (or all of the lung ins 32652) using instruments inserted into the chest through the secondary sites. Code 32652 includes intrapleural pneumonolysis in which the physician divides the tissues attaching the lung to the wall of the

chest cavity. At the conclusion of the procedure, the endoscope and the trocar are removed. A chest tube for drainage and re-expansion of the lung is usually inserted through the wound used for the thoracoscopy.

32653

The physician examines the inside of the chest cavity through a rigid or flexible fiberoptic endoscope and removes a foreign body or a fibrin deposit (the thick tissue much like remains of a blood clot). The procedure can be done under local or general anesthesia. The surgeon makes a small incision between two ribs and by blunt dissection and the use of a trocar enters the thoracic cavity. The endoscope is passed through the trocar and into the chest cavity. The lung is usually partially collapsed by instilling air into the chest through the trocar or, if general anesthesia is used, the lung may be collapsed through a double lumen endotracheal tube inserted through the mouth into the trachea. The contents of the chest cavity are examined by direct visualization and/or by the use of a video camera. Still photographs may be taken as part of the procedure. A second and/or third trocar and instruments may be inserted into the chest cavity through a second and/or third wound in the chest. The foreign body or fibrin deposit is located and removed using instruments through the scope or the secondary sites. At the conclusion of the procedure, the endoscope and the trocar are removed. A chest tube for drainage and re-expansion of the lung is usually inserted through the wound used for the thoracoscopy.

32654

The physician examines the inside of the chest cavity through a rigid or flexible fiberoptic endoscope and controls bleeding from a wound to the chest. The procedure can be done under local or general anesthesia. The physician makes a small incision between two ribs and by blunt dissection and the use of a trocar enters the thoracic cavity. The endoscope is passed through the trocar and into the chest cavity. The lung is usually partially collapsed by instilling air into the chest through the trocar or, if general anesthesia is used, the lung may be collapsed through a double lumen endotracheal tube inserted through the mouth into the trachea. The contents of the chest cavity are examined by direct visualization and/or by the use of a video camera. Still photographs may be taken as part of the procedure. A second and/or third trocar and instruments may be inserted into the chest cavity through a second and/or third wound in the chest. Under direct visualization through the endoscope, the physician manipulates the instruments inserted through the secondary sites and localizes the site of the bleeding. The hemorrhage is controlled by clipping or cauterizing the damaged blood vessel. At the conclusion of the procedure, the endoscope and the trocar(s) are removed. A chest tube for drainage and re-expansion of the lung is usually inserted through the wound used for the thoracoscopy.

32655

The physician examines the inside of the chest cavity through a rigid or flexible fiberoptic endoscope and removes one or more lung bullae (large nonfunctional air sacs). The physician makes a small incision between two ribs and by blunt dissection and the use of a trocar enters the thoracic cavity. The endoscope is passed through the trocar and into the chest cavity. The lung is usually partially collapsed by instilling air into the chest through the trocar or the lung may be collapsed through a double lumen endotracheal tube inserted through the mouth into the trachea. The contents of the chest cavity are examined by direct visualization and/or by the use of a video camera. Still photographs may be taken as part of the procedure. A second and/or third trocar and instruments may be inserted into the chest cavity through a second and/or third wound in the chest. Under direct visualization through the endoscope, the physician manipulates the instruments inserted through the secondary sites and localizes the bullae. The bulla(e) is removed by sharp and blunt dissection of the tissues, which often requires folding and suturing of the tissues (plication). In order to perform the procedure, the pleural surface may require an operative procedure such as pneumonolysis (separation of the surface of the lung that has become adherent to the inside surface of the chest cavity). At the conclusion of the procedure, the endoscope and the trocar(s) are removed. A chest tube for drainage and re-expansion of the lung is usually inserted through the wound used for the thoracoscopy.

32656

The physician examines the inside of the chest cavity through a rigid or flexible fiberoptic endoscope and removes the inside lining of the chest cavity (the parietal pleura). The physician makes a small incision between two ribs and by blunt dissection and the use of a trocar enters the thoracic cavity. The endoscope is passed through the trocar and into the chest cavity. The lung is usually partially collapsed by instilling air into the chest through the trocar or the lung may be collapsed through a double lumen endotracheal tube inserted through the mouth into the trachea. The contents of the chest cavity are examined by direct visualization and/or by the use of a video camera. Still photographs may be taken as part of the procedure. A second and/or third trocar and instruments may be inserted into the chest cavity through a second and/or third wound in the chest. Under direct visualization through the endoscope the physician manipulates the instruments inserted through the secondary sites and strips away the parietal pleura from the inside surface of the chest. At the conclusion of the procedure, the endoscope and the trocar(s) are removed. A chest tube for drainage and re-expansion of the lung is usually inserted through the wound used for the thoracoscopy.

32658

The physician examines the inside of the pericardial sac through a rigid or flexible fiberoptic endoscope and removes a blood clot or foreign body. The procedure can be done under local or general anesthesia. The physician makes a small incision between two ribs and by blunt dissection and the use of a trocar enters the thoracic cavity. The endoscope is passed through the trocar and into the chest cavity. The lung is usually partially collapsed by instilling air into the chest through the trocar or, if general anesthesia is used, the lung may be collapsed through a double lumen endotracheal tube inserted through the mouth into the trachea. The endoscope is advanced to and into the pericardial sac as the physician views the structures and the anatomy of the area through the scope. The contents of the pericardial sac are examined by direct visualization and/or by the use of a video camera. Still photographs may be taken as part of the procedure. The clot and/or foreign body is identified and removed using a device through the endoscope or using a second instrument introduced into the area through a second insertion site in the chest. At the conclusion of the procedure, the endoscope and the trocar are withdrawn. A chest tube for drainage and re-expansion of the lung is usually inserted through the wound used for the thoracoscopy.

32659
The physician operates on the pericardial sac (the sac surrounding the heart) through a rigid or flexible fiberoptic endoscope and creates a hole in the pericardial sac for drainage. The procedure can be done under local or general anesthesia. The physician makes a small incision between two ribs and by blunt dissection and the use of a trocar enters the thoracic cavity. The endoscope is passed through the trocar and into the chest cavity. The lung is usually partially collapsed by instilling air into the chest through the trocar or, if general anesthesia is used, the lung may be collapsed through a double lumen endotracheal tube inserted through the mouth into the trachea. The endoscope is advanced to and into the pericardial sac as the physician views the structures and the anatomy of the area through the scope. The contents of the pericardial sac are examined by direct visualization and/or by the use of a video camera. Still photographs may be taken as part of the procedure. Using an instrument introduced through the endoscope or through a second wound in the chest, the physician creates an opening in the pericardial sac to allow constant drainage from the sac. The drainage opening is made by the creation of a window (a flap) in the pericardium or by resecting (cutting away) a portion of the pericardium. At the conclusion of the procedure, the endoscope and the trocar are withdrawn. A chest tube for drainage and re-expansion of the lung is usually inserted through the wound used for the thoracoscopy.

32661
The physician examines the inside of the pericardial sac through a rigid or flexible fiberoptic endoscope and removes a cyst, tumor, or mass lesion inside the pericardial sac. The procedure can be performed under local or general anesthesia. The physician makes a small incision between two ribs and by blunt dissection and the use of a trocar enters the thoracic cavity. The endoscope is passed through the trocar and into the chest cavity. The lung is usually partially collapsed by instilling air into the chest through the trocar or, if general anesthesia is used, the lung may be collapsed through a double lumen endotracheal tube inserted through the mouth into the trachea. The endoscope is advanced to and into the pericardial sac as the physician views the structures and the anatomy of the area through the scope. The contents of the pericardial sac are examined by direct visualization and/or by the use of a video camera. Still photographs may be taken as part of the procedure. The cyst, tumor, or mass is identified and removed using instruments guided through the endoscope or by using instruments introduced into the area through a second and/or third insertion site in the chest. At the conclusion of the procedure, the endoscope and the trocar are withdrawn. A chest tube for drainage and re-expansion of the lung is usually inserted through the wound initially created for the horoscope insertion.

32662
The physician removes a cyst, tumor, or mass from the mediastinum through a rigid or flexible fiberoptic endoscope. The procedure can be done under local or general anesthesia. The physician makes a small incision between two ribs and by blunt dissection and the use of a trocar enters the thoracic cavity. The endoscope is passed through the trocar and into the chest cavity. The lung is usually partially collapsed by instilling air into the chest through the trocar or, if general anesthesia is used, the lung may be collapsed through a double lumen endotracheal tube inserted through the mouth into the trachea. As the physician views the structures and the anatomy of the area through the endoscope, the endoscope is advanced to and into the mediastinum (area inside the center of the chest cavity between the lungs). The contents of the mediastinal space are examined by direct visualization and/or by the use of a video camera. Still photographs may be taken as part of the procedure. The cyst, tumor, or mass is identified and removed using instruments guided through the endoscope or by using instruments introduced into the area through a second and/or third insertion site in the chest. At the conclusion of the procedure, the endoscope and the trocar are withdrawn. A chest tube for drainage and re-expansion of the lung is usually inserted through the wound used for the thoracoscopy.

32663
The physician removes an entire lobe of one lung through a rigid or flexible fiberoptic endoscope. The physician makes a small incision between two ribs and by blunt dissection and the use of a trocar enters the thoracic cavity. The endoscope is passed through the trocar and into the chest cavity. The lung is usually partially collapsed by instilling air into the chest through the trocar or the lung may be collapsed through a double lumen endotracheal tube inserted through the mouth into the trachea. The contents of

the chest cavity are examined by direct visualization and/or by the use of a video camera. Still photographs may be taken as part of the procedure. Additional instruments may be inserted into the chest cavity through a second and/or third wound in the chest. Under direct visualization through the endoscope, the physician manipulates the instruments inserted through the secondary sites and clamps the blood vessels and bronchial tubes going to the lobe of the lung to be removed. With the clamps in place, the lobe is removed by dividing the vessel and bronchial tubes isolated by the clamps. Any cut portions of the remaining lung tissue are repaired by suturing or clipping with surgical clips. At the conclusion of the procedure, the endoscope and the trocar(s) are removed. A chest tube for drainage and re-expansion of the lung is usually inserted through the wound used for the thoracoscopy.

32664

The physician performs a sympathectomy inside of the chest cavity through a rigid or flexible fiberoptic endoscope. The procedure can be done under local or general anesthesia. The physician makes a small incision between two ribs and by blunt dissection and the use of a trocar enters the thoracic cavity. The endoscope is passed through the trocar and into the chest cavity. The lung is usually partially collapsed by instilling air into the chest through the trocar or, if general anesthesia is used, the lung may be collapsed through a double lumen endotracheal tube inserted through the mouth into the trachea. The contents of the chest cavity are examined by direct visualization and/or by the use of a video camera. Still photographs may be taken as part of the procedure. A second and/or third trocar and instruments may be inserted into the chest cavity through a second and/or third wound in the chest. Under direct visualization through the endoscope, the physician manipulates the instruments inserted through the secondary sites and localizes and isolates a portion of the sympathetic nerves as they course deeply through the chest. The sympathectomy is accomplished by clipping and/or cutting the nerves. At the conclusion of the procedure, the endoscope and the trocar(s) are removed. A chest tube for drainage and re-expansion of the lung is usually inserted through the wound used for the thoracoscopy.

32665

The physician repairs a diseased and malfunctioning esophagus by operating through a series of several ports through the chest wall, guided under direct visualization through an endoscope introduced into the chest cavity. The physician makes a small incision between two ribs and by blunt dissection and the use of a trocar enters the thoracic cavity. The endoscope is passed through the trocar and into the chest cavity. The lung is usually partially collapsed by instilling air into the chest through the trocar or the lung may be collapsed through a double lumen endotracheal tube inserted through the mouth into the trachea. The contents of the chest cavity are examined by direct visualization and/or by the use of a video camera. Still photographs may be taken as part of the procedure. Several other trocars and instruments are inserted into the chest cavity through a series of similar puncture wounds placed at various locations in the chest. A second fiberoptic endoscope is passed through the mouth and guided into the esophagus just above the stomach to assist in the procedure. Under direct visualization through the chest endoscope, the physician manipulates the instruments inserted through the secondary chest sites and operates on the esophagus just above its junction with the stomach. The esophagus is presented to the physician by flexing the tip of the scope inside the esophagus. The outer longitudinal muscle of the esophagus is identified, and cut in a longitudinal fashion and the incision is carried down through the circular muscle layer of the esophagus. The length of the incision is carried onto the surface of the stomach about one centimeter. The depth of the incision in the esophageal wall is down to but not through the mucosal tissues lining the inside of the esophagus. Care is taken not to enter the inside of the esophagus. The incision relaxes the esophagus just above the stomach and allows food to more easily enter the stomach in those patients who have difficulty swallowing due to disease in this area of the esophagus. At the conclusion of the procedure, the endoscope and the trocar(s) are removed. A chest tube for drainage and re-expansion of the lung is usually inserted through the wound used for the thoracoscopy.

32666-32667

The physician performs a wedge resection of a lung mass or nodule through a rigid or flexible fiberoptic endoscope. The physician makes a small incision between two ribs and by blunt dissection and the use of a trocar enters the thoracic cavity. The endoscope is passed through the trocar and into the chest cavity. The lung is usually partially collapsed by instilling air into the chest through the trocar or the lung may be collapsed through a double lumen endotracheal tube inserted through the mouth into the trachea. The contents of the chest cavity are examined by direct visualization and/or by the use of a video camera. Still photographs may be taken as part of the procedure. Additional instruments may be inserted into the chest cavity through a second and/or third wound in the chest. Under direct visualization through the endoscope, the physician manipulates the instruments inserted through the secondary sites and clamps the blood vessels and bronchial tubes going to the sections of lung to be removed. With the clamps in place, the tissue is removed. Any cut portions of the lung tissue are repaired by suturing or clipping with surgical clips. At the conclusion of the procedure, the endoscope and the trocar(s) are removed. A chest tube for drainage and re-expansion of the lung is usually inserted through the wound used for the thoracoscopy. Report 32666 for the initial therapeutic wedge resection and 32667 for each additional resection on the same side.

32668
The physician performs a wedge resection followed by a lung resection through a rigid or flexible fiberoptic endoscope. The physician makes a small incision between two ribs and by blunt dissection and the use of a trocar enters the thoracic cavity. The endoscope is passed through the trocar and into the chest cavity. The lung is usually partially collapsed by instilling air into the chest through the trocar or the lung may be collapsed through a double lumen endotracheal tube inserted through the mouth into the trachea. The contents of the chest cavity are examined by direct visualization and/or by the use of a video camera. Still photographs may be taken as part of the procedure. Additional instruments may be inserted into the chest cavity through a second and/or third wound in the chest. Under direct visualization through the endoscope, the physician manipulates the instruments inserted through the secondary sites and clamps the blood vessels and bronchial tubes going to the sections of lung to be removed. With the clamps in place, the tissue is removed. Any cut portions of the lung tissue are repaired by suturing or clipping with surgical clips. At the conclusion of the procedure, the endoscope and the trocar(s) are removed. A chest tube for drainage and re-expansion of the lung is usually inserted through the wound used for the thoracoscopy.

32669-32671
The physician removes a segment of the lung or an entire lung through a rigid or flexible fiberoptic endoscope. The physician makes a small incision between two ribs and by blunt dissection and the use of a trocar enters the thoracic cavity. The endoscope is passed through the trocar and into the chest cavity. The lung is usually partially collapsed by instilling air into the chest through the trocar or the lung may be collapsed through a double lumen endotracheal tube inserted through the mouth into the trachea. The contents of the chest cavity are examined by direct visualization and/or by the use of a video camera. Still photographs may be taken as part of the procedure. Additional instruments may be inserted into the chest cavity through a second and/or third wound in the chest. Under direct visualization through the endoscope, the physician manipulates the instruments inserted through the secondary sites and clamps the blood vessels and bronchial tubes going to the sections of lung to be removed. With the clamps in place, the tissue is removed. Any cut portions of the lung tissue are repaired by suturing or clipping with surgical clips. At the conclusion of the procedure, the endoscope and the trocar(s) are removed. A chest tube for drainage and re-expansion of the lung is usually inserted through the wound used for the thoracoscopy. Report 32669 when the physician removes a single lung segment, 32670 when the physician removes two lobes of a lung, and 32671 when an entire lung is removed.

32672
The physician removes part of an emphysematous lung. A small incision is made between two ribs and by blunt dissection and the use of a trocar the thoracic cavity is entered. The endoscope is passed through the trocar and into the chest cavity. The lung is usually partially collapsed by instilling air into the chest through the trocar or the lung may be collapsed through a double lumen endotracheal tube inserted through the mouth into the trachea. The contents of the chest cavity are examined by direct visualization and/or by the use of a video camera. Still photographs may be taken as part of the procedure. Additional instruments may be inserted into the chest cavity through a second and/or third wound in the chest. Under direct visualization through the endoscope, the physician manipulates the instruments inserted through the secondary sites and clamps the blood vessels and bronchial tubes going to the section(s) of lung to be removed. With the clamps in place, the emphysematous lung tissue is removed by sharp and blunt dissection and often by folding and suturing of the tissues (plication). Any cut portions of the lung tissue are repaired by suturing or clipping with surgical clips. At the conclusion of the procedure, the endoscope and the trocar(s) are removed. A chest tube for drainage and re-expansion of the lung is usually inserted through the wound used for the thoracoscopy.

32673
The physician removes one or both lobes of the thymus gland via thoracoscopic approach. A small incision is made between two ribs and by blunt dissection and the use of a trocar the thoracic cavity is entered. The endoscope is passed through the trocar and into the chest cavity. Additional instruments may be inserted into the chest cavity through a second and/or third wound in the chest. Under direct visualization through the endoscope, the physician manipulates the instruments inserted through the secondary sites and the superior lobe of the thymus is separated from the inferior aspect of the thyroid. The blood supply to the thymus is divided and the thymus is dissected free from the pericardium and removed. A chest tube for drainage is usually inserted through the wound used for the thoracoscopy.

32674
A regional and mediastinal lymphadenectomy is performed via a thoracoscopic approach. A small incision is made between two ribs and by blunt dissection and the use of a trocar the thoracic cavity is entered. The endoscope is passed through the trocar and into the chest cavity. Additional instruments may be inserted into the chest cavity through a second and/or third wound in the chest. Under direct visualization through the endoscope, the physician manipulates the instruments inserted through the secondary sites and removes the lymph nodes near the lungs, around the heart, and behind the trachea. The area is irrigated, and the operative incision is closed with sutures. A chest tube for drainage is usually

inserted through the wound used for the thoracoscopy.

32701
In stereotactic radiosurgery (SRS) and stereotactic body radiation therapy (SBRT), the skill of a surgeon and a radiation oncologist is usually required. SRS/SBRT uses a single or up to five fractionated doses of high potent biological radiation directly to a malignant tumor. Due to the high doses of radiation used, the tumor is precisely localized using four dimensional imaging and, occasionally, separately reportable fiducial markers are placed to ensure proper placement of the radiation delivery. Code 32701 reports the surgeon's determination of the location of the thoracic tumor margins and any involvement of adjacent tissues and organs using the images previously obtained for the entire course of treatment.

32800
The physician repairs a hernia of the chest wall that allows the bulging of the lung through a defect in the chest wall. The physician makes an incision through the skin overlying the defect and carries the incision down to the inside lining of the chest cavity. The defect is repaired by the folding and suturing of tissues or the rotation of muscle and/or thick fibrous tissue flaps over the area and suturing of the flap over the defect. Alternately, the defect can be covered by a synthetic mesh material which is sutured in place. The incision is closed in layers of sutures.

32810
The physician treats a draining empyema (accumulation of pus in the chest cavity) by resecting a rib, irrigating the empyema space with an antibiotic solution intermittently over an extended period of time, and closing of the empyema space in six to eight weeks. This code reports the closure portion only.

32815
The physician repairs a major bronchial fistula (an abnormal passageway between the remaining end of a bronchial tube and the chest that occurs sometimes after the removal of a lung or portion of a lung). The physician enters the chest cavity through a vertical incision made in the middle of the front of the chest. The incision is carried down to the sternum which is split in order to enter the chest cavity at the root of the lung near the center of the chest. The fistula exposure often requires the resection of one or two of the upper ribs. The end of the bronchial tube is located and the stump of the bronchial tube is reamputated and the inside lining of the bronchial tube is treated with silver nitrate to destroy the mucus forming cells lining the bronchus. The stump is sutured or stapled. The chest defect created is repaired and the sternum closed using wire sutures and the skin closed in layers of sutures. A chest tube may be inserted into the chest cavity for drainage.

32820
The physician repairs and reconstructs the chest wall following a major disfiguring injury to the chest; this reconstruction may be performed immediately, months, or years following the traumatic event. The purpose of the repair is to restore structure and coverage of the chest wall, as well as fill any vacant spaces within the chest to prevent infection. The chest wall consists of three layers: the soft tissue layer, including the skin, subcutaneous tissue, and muscle; the skeletal layer, consisting of the ribs, cartilage, and sometimes the sternum; and the pleural space (parietal cavity). During the procedure, the parietal cavity is checked for air leaks and repaired if necessary. Any empty pleural space may be filled with muscle flap, omentum, or prosthetic material. Bone grafts, muscle, or omental flaps or methyl methacrylate reinforced mesh is used to reconstruct the ribs and/or sternum damaged in the trauma. Repair of the soft tissue layer using skin flaps is included in the reconstruction. Skin autograft or substitutes required to close the defect may be reported separately.

32850
The physician performs a donor pneumonectomy(ies) for transplant from a cadaver donor. In cases where the donor has been declared brain dead, adequate functioning of the heart, lungs, and circulatory system are maintained prior to removal of the organ. During surgical removal of the lung(s), the donor may be placed on a cardiopulmonary bypass machine to maintain perfusion to the organs. The physician makes a long, mid-line vertical incision through all the layers of the skin down to the sternum bone. The sternum is split and the chest cavity entered. Each lung is removed in one block by dividing the trachea and the major arteries and veins that carry blood to and from the heart. The lung(s) is preserved for transplantation into the recipient. The organ(s) remains under refrigeration, specially packed in a sealable container with some preserving solution and kept on ice in a suitable carrier.

32851-32852
The physician performs a single lung transplantation of the recipient patient. A long, mid-line vertical incision is made through all the layers of the skin down to the sternum bone. The sternum is split, and the chest cavity entered. In 32851, the patient's oxygenation and circulation are maintained by the patient's own heart and other lung during the procedure, while in 32852, the patient is placed on a cardiopulmonary bypass machine to maintain circulation to the organs. The patient's original lung is deflated and the root of the lung isolated and the major arteries and veins that carry blood to and from the heart are identified and divided. The main bronchial tube to that lung is severed and the lung removed. The donor lung is placed in the chest cavity and its bronchial tube and arteries and veins sutured to the patients where the former lung was attached. Circulation and functioning of the donor lung are assured and the chest is closed. The sternum is closed using wire sutures and the skin closed in layers of sutures. A chest tube(s) is inserted into the chest cavity for drainage.

32853-32854
The physician performs a double lung transplantation of the recipient patient, either in a bilateral sequential fashion or performed en bloc. A long, midline vertical incision is made through all the layers of the skin down to the sternum bone. The sternum is split, and the chest cavity entered. The patient's original lungs are deflated, the root of the lung isolated, and the major arteries and veins that carry blood to and from the heart are identified and divided. The tracheal tube to the lungs is severed and the lungs are removed. The donor lungs are placed in the chest cavity as a single unit or one at a time. The tracheal tube and arteries and veins are sutured to the site where the former lungs were attached. Circulation and functioning of the donor lungs are assured and the chest is closed. The sternum is closed using wire sutures and the skin closed in layers. Chest tubes are inserted into the chest cavities for drainage. The transplantation procedure in 32853 is accomplished without cardiopulmonary bypass, while in 32854 the patient is placed on a cardiopulmonary bypass machine to maintain circulation to the organs.

32855-32856
The physician performs a standard backbench preparation of one or both lungs following procurement from a cadaver donor. Backbench or back table preparation refers to procedures performed on the donor organs following procurement to prepare the donor organs for transplant. Both lungs are removed or the heart and lungs are removed en bloc. If the heart and lungs are removed en bloc, back table separation of the heart and lungs is performed. The lungs are inspected following procurement to identify any injury or abnormality not noted prior to procurement. The physician prepares the lungs by dissecting free any residual soft tissue. Attention is focused on the pulmonary venous/atrial cuff, pulmonary artery, and bronchus. The pulmonary venous/atrial cuff is inspected and any residual tissue removed. The pulmonary artery, which was divided at its bifurcation, is inspected and any residual tissue removed. The aorta, which was divided distal to the innominate artery, is inspected and residual tissue removed. When all residual soft tissue has been removed and the vessels prepared, the lung(s) is ready for transplant. Report 32855 for backbench preparation of one lung (unilateral). Report 32856 for backbench preparation of both lungs (bilateral).

32900
The physician resects a rib(s) without entering the chest cavity. The surgeon make an incision in the skin overlying the rib to be removed and carries that incision through the tissues down to the rib. The tissues are dissected away from the rib taking care not to puncture through the pleural membrane on the inside surface of the rib. This avoids the egress of air into the chest cavity. With the tissue removed from the surface of the rib, the rib is cut at two places and the intervening section removed. The resulting defect may be covered by the use of muscle flaps grafted to the area. The remaining tissues and skin are closed by suturing in layers.

32905
The physician performs a thoracoplasty which is the removal of the skeletal support of a portion of the chest to treat chronic thoracic empyema (accumulation of pus in the chest cavity) when there is insufficient lung tissue to fill the chest space. The procedure is carried out primarily on the upper chest. An incision is made through the skin down to the ribs. The Schede operation consists of the extensive unroofing of an empyema space by resecting the overlying ribs and portions of membrane lining the chest cavity (parietal pleural peel). The muscles in the area are partially closed over gauze packing and the skin partially closed by suturing in layers. As the packing is withdrawn in stages a few days later, it is hoped that freshly granulation tissue fills in the space formerly occupied by the empyema. The original Schede type operation is rarely performed but several modifications are currently done.

32906
The physician closes a bronchopleural fistula and performs a thoracoplasty which is the removal of the skeletal support of a portion of the chest to treat chronic thoracic empyema (accumulation of pus in the chest cavity) when there is insufficient lung tissue to fill the chest space. The procedure is carried out primarily on the upper chest. An incision is made through the skin down to the ribs. The Schede operation consists of the extensive unroofing of an empyema space by resecting the overlying ribs and portions of membrane lining the chest cavity (parietal pleural peel). The bronchopleural fistula (an abnormal passageway between the remaining end of a bronchial tube that occurs sometimes after the removal of a lung or portion of a lung) is identified and resected, then closed by suturing. Closure of the fistula sometimes requires muscle flap grafts taken from outside the chest cavity. After the repair of the fistula, the muscles in the area are partially closed over gauze packing and the skin partially closed by suturing in layers. As the packing is withdrawn in stages a few days later, it is hoped that freshly granulation tissue fills in the space formerly occupied by the empyema. The original Schede type operation is rarely performed but several modifications are currently done.

32940
The physician opens the chest cavity and separates the surface of the lung, which has become adherent to the inside surface of the chest cavity. Using a scalpel, the surgeon makes an incision around the side of the chest between two of the ribs. The incision is carried through all the tissue layers down to the tissue lining the chest cavity. Rib spreaders are inserted into the wound and the ribs are spread apart exposing the membrane lining the chest cavity (the parietal pleura). The surgeon separates the tissue between the periosteal membrane adherent to the inside surface of the lung and the parietal pleural membrane. This allows the movement of the lung within the chest cavity. The area

Respiratory

or space created is packed or filled and the incision is closed in layers of sutures.

32960

The physician partially collapses a lung by injecting air into the chest cavity by puncturing through the space between the ribs. Using a needle attached to a syringe the physician passes the needle over the top of a rib and punctures through the chest tissues and enters the pleural cavity. With the end of the needle in the chest cavity, the physician injects air into the chest cavity to create a partial collapse of one lung, most commonly used to treat tuberculosis. A small plastic tube may be passed through the chest and left in place for repeated injections of air.

32997

The physician performs total lavage on one lung. The physician views the airway using a fiberoptic or rigid bronchoscopy. Under appropriate anesthesia, the bronchoscope is introduced through the nasal or oral cavity and advanced to the lungs. Saline is introduced through the bronchoscope, and the lung tissue is washed or bathed. The saline is removed by suction and the solution containing the cells that have been obtained in the procedure may be sent to pathology to diagnose certain diseases, such as cancer. This procedure may also be performed to treat specific diseases or injuries.

32998 [32994]

In 32998, the physician uses the heat created from high-frequency radiowaves to destroy one or more tumors in the lung, pleura, or chest wall. A small incision is made in the skin of the chest and the lesion is accessed by inserting an ablation probe connected to a radiofrequency generator between the ribs. Under imaging guidance, the ablation probe is advanced into the lesion of the lung, pleura, or chest wall. Treatment with the heat probe usually takes several minutes and may include repositioning the probe within the lesion so that overlapping ablations treat the entire tumor. The incision is closed with sutures. This process may be repeated for multiple lesions within the same lung. Report 32994 when the procedure is performed using cryoablation. Imaging guidance is included in these procedures, when performed.

Cardiovascular

33016

The physician drains fluid from the pericardial space. The physician may perform this procedure using anatomic landmarks or under fluoroscopic or echocardiographic (ultrasound) guidance, which is not separately reportable. The physician places a long needle below the sternum and directs it into the pericardial space. When pericardial fluid is aspirated, the physician may advance a guidewire through the needle into the pericardial space and exchange the needle over the guidewire for a drainage catheter. The physician removes as much pericardial fluid as is required, removes the needle or catheter, and dresses the wound.

33017-33018

The physician drains fluid from the pericardial space. The physician may perform these procedures using anatomic landmarks or under fluoroscopic or echocardiographic (ultrasound) guidance, which is included in these codes and not reported separately. The physician places a long needle percutaneously below the sternum and directs it into the pericardial space. When pericardial fluid flows back through the needle, the physician passes a guidewire through the needle into the pericardial space. The physician exchanges the needle over the wire for an indwelling drainage catheter. The physician attaches the catheter to a drainage bag, sutures the indwelling catheter into place on the chest wall, and dresses the wound. Report 33017 when the procedure is performed on ages 6 years and older without a congenital cardiac anomaly. Report 33018 when the procedure is performed on newborns to 5 years of age with a congenital cardiac anomaly, such as dextrocardia, heterotaxy, mesocardia, or a single ventricle anomaly, or for any age within the first 90-day postop period following surgical repair of a congenital cardiac anomaly.

33019

The physician drains fluid from the pericardial space. The physician performs this procedure under CT guidance, which is included in this code and not reported separately. The physician places a long needle percutaneously below the sternum and directs it into the pericardial space. When pericardial fluid flows back through the needle, the physician passes a guidewire through the needle into the pericardial space. The physician exchanges the needle over the wire for an indwelling drainage catheter. The physician attaches the catheter to a drainage bag, sutures the indwelling catheter into place on the chest wall, and dresses the wound.

33020

The physician removes a clot or foreign body from the pericardial space. The physician performs a midline sternotomy, incising skin, fascia, and the sternum. The pericardium is incised and the clot or foreign body is removed. The pericardium is repaired loosely, leaving gaps for blood and fluid to drain into the pleural space. The sternum is reanastomosed with sternal wires and the skin is sutured in layers. In a less invasive approach for smaller clots or foreign matter, a needle is inserted through the skin under the sternum until it reaches the pericardial sac guided by fluoroscopy or echocardiography. A catheter is inserted to retrieve foreign matter or a catheter with a balloon attachment may also be used. The inflation of the balloon creates an opening within the desired location. The balloon catheter is removed and replaced with another catheter used to retrieve the foreign matter or clot.

33025

The physician gains access to the pericardium in one of three ways: an incision into the subxiphoid space, the chest wall (thoracotomy), or thoracoscopically. The physician may make an incision in the pericardium or use electrocautery to open the pericardium large enough to allow drainage of pericardial fluid into the pleural space. This may require the use of a clamp or forceps to retract the surrounding tissues; however, if the pericardium is distended, a needle aspiration may be utilized under thoracoscopic guidance. The physician closes the sternal or chest wall incision and dresses the wound. The physician may leave chest tubes and/or a mediastinal drainage tube in place following the procedure.

33030-33031
The physician gains access to the pericardium through an incision through the sternum (median sternotomy). The physician cuts away most or all of the pericardial tissue while the heart is still beating (without cardiopulmonary bypass), taking care to leave the phrenic nerves intact. The physician closes the sternal or chest wall incision and dresses the wound. The physician may leave chest tubes and/or a mediastinal drainage tube in place following the procedure. Report 33031 if the procedure is performed with cardiopulmonary bypass.

33050
The physician gains access to the pericardium through an incision through the sternum (median sternotomy) or the chest wall (lateral thoracotomy). If cardiopulmonary bypass is performed, the physician places cardiopulmonary bypass catheters (usually through incisions in the right atrial appendage and aorta or femoral artery). The physician stops the heart by infusing cardioplegia solution into the coronary circulation. The physician cuts away the pericardial cyst or tumor. The physician takes the patient off cardiopulmonary bypass, if used, closes the surgical incisions, and dresses the sternal or chest wall wound. The physician may leave chest tubes and/or a mediastinal drainage tube in place following the procedure.

33120
Cardiopulmonary bypass is employed. Venous tubes are placed in both caval veins. The part of the heart that is opened depends on where the tumor is located. Every effort is made to avoid making an incision in any ventricular wall. After the heart is opened, the tumor is resected with a margin of normal heart tissue. Any problems created by this resection (damage to heart valves, holes in the walls between heart chambers or the outside of the heart, injury to coronary arteries) are repaired. All holes in the heart are closed. Cardiopulmonary bypass is stopped when heart function returns.

33130
Cardiopulmonary bypass is only required if a significant portion of the heart or major vessel must be removed with the tumor to get a margin of normal tissue around the tumor. The tumor and surrounding normal tissue are removed. Defects created in the heart, coronary arteries or major vessels are repaired.

33140-33141
The physician performs transmyocardial laser revascularization to restore the flow of blood and oxygen to the heart. Varying approaches may be employed. The procedure is frequently performed on the beating heart, although cardiopulmonary bypass may be initiated. In the beating heart: Using a scalpel the physician makes a 10 centimeters to 15 centimeters incision on the left side of the chest between the ribs and exposes the surface of the heart. The area of ischemia (in still vital tissue) is identified. A laser is inserted through the chest opening and is fired (between heartbeats) through the filled left ventricle. Between 10 channels to 40 channels (small holes) are created to encourage new capillary growth in the area. As the channels are created pressure is applied to each to help close the openings. When the procedure is completed the laser is removed and the wound is closed with layered sutures. If cardiopulmonary bypass was initiated it is discontinued, the patient is rewarmed, and the heartbeat is restored. Report 33140 if the transmyocardial laser revascularization is performed alone. Report 33141 when it is performed at the time of another open cardiac procedure.

33202
The physician places one or more electrical leads on the outside of the heart (epicardial electrodes) by open chest incision. The incision can be in the middle of the chest (midline sternotomy), a vertical incision just below the ribcage (subxiphoid), or between the ribs on the left side of the body (thoracotomy). The chest cavity is opened. After the heart is exposed, electrodes are affixed to the appropriate areas of the heart muscle. The electrodes are tested and then tunneled under the coastal margin to the upper abdomen to a pulse generator or to the infraclavicular area if the generator is in that area. The physician closes the incision with layered sutures.

33203
The physician places electrical leads on the outside of the heart (epicardial electrodes) using an endoscopic approach. Three trocars are placed in the left anterior chest wall and the left lung is collapsed. A small incision is made in the chest (thoracostomy) and a 12 mm trocar is placed. The thoracoscope (endoscope) is inserted. Two additional trocars are placed under thoracoscopic visualization in the inframammary anterolateral region. Under thoracoscopic guidance, the pericardium is grasped and incised. The lateral trocar is removed and the incision enlarged to allow passage of the epicardial electrode placement device and the electrodes through the intercostal space. The electrodes are placed intrapericardially. The pericardium is approximated with a single stitch to hold the electrodes in place. The electrodes are tested and then tunneled under the costal margin to the upper abdomen to a pulse generator or over the ribs to the infraclavicular area if the generator is in that area. The thoracoscope is removed and a thoracostomy tube is placed at this site. The lung is expanded and the incisions closed with layered sutures.

33206-33211

The physician inserts or replaces a permanent pacemaker with transvenous electrodes. Under appropriate anesthesia, the physician gains access to the central caval veins typically via a percutaneous approach through the subclavian vein or employing a cut-down technique to the cephalic vein. Less commonly, the axillary, internal jugular, or femoral vein may be used. The chosen vein is penetrated with a large needle and a wire is passed through it. A fluoroscope is used to guide the wire into the right atrium. A pocket for the pacemaker generator is created and the wire is tested. The wire is connected to the generator and the generator is closed in its pocket. Report 33206 if the guide and pacemaker wires are placed in the right atrium only; 33207 if the guide and pacemaker wires are placed in the right ventricle only; 33208 if the elements of 33206 and 33207 are combined; and 33210 or 33211 if the pacemaker generator is not implanted but temporarily placed outside of the body and a transvenous single chamber cardiac electrode or pacemaker catheter (33210) or transvenous dual chamber (33211) electrode(s) is inserted or replaced.

33212-33214 [33221]

A single or dual chamber pacemaker pulse generator is inserted or replaced and connected to previously placed, existing leads. If this is an initial insertion, a pocket for the pacemaker generator is created subcutaneously in the subclavicular region or underneath the abdominal muscles just below the ribcage. The generator is inserted into the pocket. The pocket is closed. Report 33212 if a single chamber (atrial or ventricular) pacemaker pulse generator is inserted, 33213 if a dual chamber (atrial and ventricular) pacemaker pulse generator is inserted, or 33221 for the insertion of the generator with multiple existing leads. In 33214, a single chamber system is converted to a dual chamber system. The existing pacemaker generator pocket is opened and the single chamber generator removed. The dual chamber generator is placed into the existing pocket. The existing pacer wire is tested and connected to the generator. A second lead is placed and tested. The pocket is closed.

33215

A previously placed transvenous right atrial or right ventricular electrode is repositioned. This is done when the system does not function due to improper placement of the electrode wire itself. The generator is removed and the wire is tested to ensure that the wire is not defective, but simply in the wrong place. It is reattached to the generator in its new position and tested again.

33216-33217

The physician inserts a single transvenous electrode in 33216 and two transvenous electrodes in 33217 when there is a malfunction or complication with the electrode wire of a permanent pacemaker or implantable defibrillator. The generator is removed and the wire is tested. When the wire is found defective, another transvenous electrode is inserted. Access to the central caval veins is obtained through the subclavian vein or jugular vein. The vein is penetrated with a large needle and a wire is passed through it. Fluoroscopy is used to guide the wire into position. The wire is connected to the generator and the wound is closed. Various head and body positions are tested again to ensure adequate pacing.

33218-33220

A previously placed transvenous electrode is repaired. The permanent pacemaker or implantable defibrillator pocket is opened and the generator is removed. The electrode wire is tested. Repairs are performed on the electrode. The wire is tested again and reconnected to the generator. The generator is placed back in its pocket and the pocket is closed. Report 33218 if a single electrode is repaired and 33220 if two electrodes are repaired.

33222-33223

The physician relocates a pacemaker or defibrillator pocket due to infection, erosion, or complications from the original generator placement. The pocket is opened and the generator is removed. A new pocket is formed in the subcutaneous tissue within the reach of the already present electrodes. The electrodes are brought through a new subcutaneous tunnel into the new pocket. The old pocket is closed. The existing or new generator is placed in the new pocket and the electrodes are connected. The pocket is closed. Report 33222 when a permanent pacemaker pocket is relocated and 33223 when an implantable defibrillator pocket is relocated.

33224

If biventricular pacing is required, an additional electrode is placed in the left ventricle. With the pacemaker or implantable defibrillator already in place, the physician gains access transvenously through the subclavian or jugular vein. This procedure is done under local anesthesia. A fluoroscope may be used for guidance and a pacing electrode is inserted in the left ventricular chamber of the heart, usually in the coronary sinus tributary. The electrode is connected to the pulse generator and the pocket is closed. The generator pocket may be revised and/or the existing generator removed, inserted, or replaced. In rare cases, when transvenous approach cannot be used, the device is implanted in the pocket underneath the skin in the lower abdomen (epicardial approach). Implantation using this approach is done under general anesthesia.

33225

If biventricular pacing is required, an additional electrode is placed in the left ventricle. During insertion of an implantable defibrillator or pacemaker pulse generator, the physician gains access transvenously through the subclavian or jugular vein. This procedure is done under local anesthesia. A fluoroscope may be used for guidance and a pacing electrode is inserted in the left ventricular chamber of the heart, usually in the coronary sinus tributary. The generator is upgraded to a dual chamber system. The electrode is connected to the pulse generator and the pocket is closed. In rare cases, when transvenous approach cannot be used, the device is implanted in the pocket underneath the skin in the lower abdomen (epicardial approach). Implantation using this approach is done under general anesthesia.

33226

The physician gains access transvenously through the subclavian or jugular vein. A fluoroscope may be used for guidance and the pacing electrode that is already in place in the ventricular chamber of the heart, usually in the coronary sinus tributary, is repositioned. The generator pocket may be revised and/or the existing generator removed, inserted, or replaced. The electrode is connected to the generator and the pocket is closed.

33233

In 33233, only the permanent pacemaker pulse generator is removed. The pacemaker generator pocket is opened. The generator is disconnected from the wire(s) and removed. The wire(s) is left in place in the pocket and the pocket is closed.

[33227, 33228, 33229]

A permanent pacemaker pulse generator is removed and replaced. The pacemaker generator pocket is opened. The existing generator is disconnected from the wire(s) and removed. The wire(s) is left in place in the pocket and a new permanent pacemaker pulse generator is inserted. The existing pacer wire(s) is tested and connected to the generator. The pocket is closed. Report 33227 for removal and replacement of a single lead system generator, 33228 for a dual lead system generator, and 33229 for a multiple lead system generator.

33234-33235

In 33234 and 33235, only the transvenous electrode(s) are removed. In 33234, the generator pocket is opened and the wire is disconnected from the generator. The wire is dissected from the scar tissue that has formed around it. Once the wire is completely freed, it is twisted in a direction opposite to that used for insertion (counterclockwise). The wire is withdrawn. Bleeding from the tracts leading to the vein is controlled with sutures. A new wire may be placed, but is reported separately. Report 33235 for a dual lead system (removal of two wires).

33236-33237

Code 33236 reports the removal of a single lead epicardial pacemaker system and electrodes. The old pacemaker pocket is opened and the generator is removed. The old wires are cut and the incision is closed. The old chest incision is opened. The wires are pulled into the chest and they are followed onto the heart surface. The electrodes are detached from the heart. The chest incision is closed. Report 33237 if a dual lead epicardial system is being removed.

33238

The physician removes a transvenous electrode(s) by thoracotomy. Prior to this procedure, the pacemaker pocket was opened, the generator removed, and the wires cut. The right chest is opened and the superior caval vein is dissected out. Tourniquets are placed around the vein above and below the planned site of opening. The tourniquets are tightened and a hole is made in the caval vein. The cut ends of the wires are pulled out through the hole in the caval vein. The ends of the wires that are still in the heart are twisted counterclockwise until they are free and are withdrawn through the caval vein. The hole in the caval vein is closed and the tourniquets released. The chest is closed.

33240 [33230, 33231]

This operation is done only when defibrillator electrodes are already in place. The previous pocket is opened or a new pocket is created for the implantable defibrillator pulse generator. The defibrillator pulse generators are implanted subcutaneously usually in an infraclavicular or abdominal pocket with the assistance of fluoroscopy. The electrodes are tested. The electrodes are connected to the defibrillator pulse generator and it is placed in the pocket. The pocket is closed with sutures, adhesive strips, or special glue. Report 33240 when there is an existing single lead (electrode); 33230 when there are existing dual leads (electrodes); and 33231 when there are existing multiple leads (electrodes).

33241

The physician removes only the implantable defibrillator pulse generator. The pulse generator may be removed due to a complication or malfunction. The subcutaneous generator pocket is opened and the generator is removed. The electrodes are detached from the generator and the electrodes are placed in the pocket. The pocket is closed.

[33262, 33263, 33264]

An implantable defibrillator pulse generator is removed and replaced. The pulse generator may be removed due to a complication or malfunction. The generator pocket is opened. The existing generator is disconnected from the wire(s) and removed. The wire(s) is left in place in the pocket and a new pulse generator is inserted. The existing wire(s) is tested and connected to the new generator. The pocket is closed. Report 33262 for removal and replacement of a single lead system generator; 33263 for a dual lead system generator; and 33264 for a multiple lead system generator.

33243

Single or dual chamber implantable defibrillator electrodes are removed. Electrodes may be removed due to a complication or malfunction. The generator pocket is opened and the electrode wires are disconnected. The old chest incision is opened and the electrodes are dissected out and removed. The chest incision is closed.

33244
Electrodes only are removed by transvenous extraction, which is currently the most common technique for removing electrodes since most implantable defibrillator electrodes are now placed transvenously. Electrodes may be removed due to a complication or malfunction. The generator pocket is opened and the wire is disconnected from the generator. The wire is dissected from the scar tissue that has formed around it. Once the wire is completely freed, it is twisted in a direction opposite to that used for insertion (counterclockwise). The wire is withdrawn. Bleeding from the tracts leading to the vein is controlled with sutures. A new wire may be placed, but it is reported separately.

33249
The physician inserts or replaces a permanent implantable defibrillator system, including the pulse generator with transvenous electrode placement. Transvenous placement is currently the most common technique for placing implantable defibrillator electrodes. An implantable defibrillator is a device designed to administer an electric shock to control cardiac arrhythmias and restore a normal heartbeat. Local anesthesia is administered. An incision is made in the infraclavicular area. The subcutaneous tissue is opened and a pocket is created for the pulse generator. The electrode catheter is advanced through the superior vena cava into the heart and placed in the appropriate site in the right ventricle (single chamber system) or in the right ventricle and atrium (dual chamber system). Multiple leads may be required for both single and dual chamber systems. Once all leads are placed, they are tested and connected to the pulse generator that is placed in the previously prepared pocket. All incisions are closed. All radiological supervision and guidance is included.

[33270, 33271]
In 33270, the physician performs initial insertion or replacement of a permanent subcutaneous implantable defibrillator (S-ICD) system, including the pulse generator and lead. The pulse generator is placed in a subcutaneous pocket on the left side of the chest next to the ribs. Two small incisions are made above the sternum and the lead wire is threaded through and sutured into place. The lead is connected to the pulse generator. The physician records cardiac electrical signals from the leads and paces the heart through the leads to determine pacing threshold. The physician uses the S-ICD pulse generator to pace the heart into an arrhythmia, such as ventricular tachycardia or fibrillation. The S-ICD detects and terminates the arrhythmia using pacing or by shocking the heart through the lead. The physician may reprogram the treatment parameters to optimize the device function to best treat the patient's arrhythmia. The incisions are closed. Report 33271 for insertion of the lead only.

[33272]
The physician performs a procedure to remove the subcutaneous implantable defibrillator lead only. The lead may be removed due to a complication or malfunction. An incision is made in the area above the sternum where the lead is located. The lead is disconnected from the pulse generator, pulled through, and removed. The incision is repaired.

[33273]
A previously placed implanted subcutaneous defibrillator lead (electrode) is repositioned. This procedure is performed when the system does not function due to improper placement of the lead. An incision is made over the previous subcutaneous pocket on the left side of the chest next to the ribs. The lead is disconnected from the pulse generator. The generator is removed and the lead is tested for proper function. It is then reattached to the generator in the new position and retested. The incision is closed.

[33274, 33275]
The physician performs transcatheter insertion, replacement, or removal of a ventricular permanent leadless pacemaker. This pacemaker is a single-chamber unit without leads that is placed into the right ventricle. The size varies based on manufacturer, but is approximately 7 mm x 26 mm and weighs 2 grams. The less invasive and shorter implantation procedure of a leadless pacemaker reduces recovery time and eliminates complications related to the transvenous leads and the subcutaneous pulse generator used in traditional pacemaker implantation, specifically infections. The battery typically lasts seven to 15 years, and the pacing, amplitude, and impedance are all relative to the traditional pacemaker. The femoral vein is entered and the device is fed into the right ventricle using a special catheter. Once attached, a continued connection allows for measurements to be taken and to determine positioning. All imaging and device evaluations are included in the procedures and should not be reported separately. For insertion or replacement of the pacemaker, report 33274; for removal of the pacemaker, report 33275.

[33276, 33277]
The physician treats central sleep apnea with insertion of a phrenic nerve stimulator system, which consists of a pulse generator much like a pacemaker, a stimulation electrode, and, when appropriate, a sensing electrode. Respiration sensing is accomplished by the electrodes determining the patient's position at rest/activity to allow for programming of applicable delivery times. This unit assists stable breathing by preventing episodes of apnea followed by rapid breathing. With the patient under appropriate anesthesia (typically conscious sedation), the physician creates a subcutaneous or submuscular pocket in the pectoral region of the chest and inserts the implantable pulse generator (IPG). Using standard transvenous implantation techniques, venous access is obtained through the axillary, cephalic, or subclavian vein;

access wires are then advanced into the inferior vena cava. The stimulating lead is inserted and placed in the left pericardiophrenic vein or the right brachiocephalic vein. The sensing electrode, if deemed necessary, is inserted into the azygos vein (on the back of the thorax, which flows into the superior vena cava). The electrodes are connected to the generator and tested prior to pocket closure. Report 33276 for insertion of the pulse generator and one or more stimulating leads; this includes the initial analysis with diagnostic mode activation if performed and all imaging guidance and vessel catheterization. In addition, report 33277 for insertion of the transvenous sensing lead if applicable.

[33278, 33279, 33280]

The phrenic nerve stimulator system for treatment of central sleep apnea consists of a pulse generator much like a pacemaker, a stimulation electrode, and a sensing electrode. Respiration sensing is accomplished by the electrodes determining the patient's position at rest/activity to allow for programming of applicable delivery times. This unit assists stable breathing by preventing episodes of apnea followed by rapid breathing. In 33279, the physician removes one or more transvenous stimulation or sensing leads. The generator pocket is opened, and the generator disconnected from the appropriate lead (electrode). The lead is dissected from any scar tissue that has formed around it and withdrawn, bleeding is controlled, and the pocket is closed with sutures. In 33280, only the pulse generator is removed. The physician opens the generator pocket. The generator is disconnected from the electrodes and removed. The electrodes remain within the pocket and the pocket is closed. In 33278, the entire system, consisting of the pulse generator and the leads, is removed. These codes include interrogation and programming if performed and all imaging guidance and vessel catheterization.

[33281]

One or more previously placed phrenic nerve stimulation and/or sensing transvenous leads are repositioned. This may be done when the system does not function due to improper placement of the electrode itself. The generator is removed, and the electrode is tested to ensure that it is not defective, but simply in the wrong place. It is reattached to the generator in its new position and tested again. This code includes all imaging guidance and vessel catheterization necessary to complete the procedure.

[33287, 33288]

The physician removes and replaces an existing phrenic nerve stimulator pulse generator in 33287. The generator pocket is opened. The existing generator is disconnected from any attached electrodes (leads) and removed. The leads are left in place in the pocket and a new pulse generator is inserted. The existing leads are tested and connected to the generator and the pocket is closed. In 33288, the physician removes and replaces one or more transvenous stimulation or sensing leads. The generator pocket is opened, and the generator disconnected from the appropriate lead. The lead is dissected from any scar tissue that has formed around it and extracted. A replacement lead is advanced into the targeted location, connected to the pulse generator, and tested. These codes include interrogation and programming if performed and all imaging guidance and vessel catheterization.

33250

The heart is exposed through the sternum. A mapping grid of electrodes is placed over the surface of the beating heart. The location of the arrhythmia source is determined. The source is destroyed using electrical current, freezing, or cutting. Any bleeding is controlled with sutures. The chest is closed.

33251

Cardiopulmonary bypass is required. The heart is exposed through the sternum. A mapping grid of electrodes is placed over the surface of the beating heart. The right atrium is opened and a long cut is made around the tricuspid valve until the cut on the outside of the heart is seen. Any other focuses of the arrhythmia are destroyed with electrical current or freezing. The right atrium is closed. Cardiopulmonary bypass is discontinued when heart function returns. Typically this open approach is reserved for patients requiring surgery for additional conditions. This procedure is being replaced by ablation performed via a catheter that is threaded through the femoral vein into the area of the heart requiring treatment.

33254-33256

The physician performs operative ablation and reconstruction of the atria to treat atrial fibrillation. Atrial fibrillation is rapid, randomized muscle contraction of the atrial myocardium causing an irregular, rapid heart rate. In a maze procedure, the physician seeks to permanently interrupt aberrant electrical conduction within the atria to restore normal sinus rhythm. The physician performs a midline sternotomy, incising the skin, fascia, muscles, and sternum. The pericardium is incised. For a limited operative ablation and reconstruction (33254), also referred to as a modified maze procedure, an incision is made into the left or right atrium. A combination of surgical incision and/or energy sources such as heat, microwave, laser, ultrasound, or cryoprobe is used to create lesions that will heal into scars that disrupt conduction. In 33255 and 33256, an extensive operative ablation and reconstruction is performed. In an extensive procedure, the right and/or left atrial tissue and/or atrial septum is treated as described in 33254, and additional operative ablation involving the atrioventricular annulus is performed. In any of these procedures, the left atrial appendage may be excised or isolated. In 33256, lines are placed for cardiopulmonary bypass. When cardiopulmonary bypass is achieved, an extensive ablation and reconstruction procedure is performed. The atrial incision lines are reanastomosed. The pericardium is repaired loosely, leaving gaps for blood and fluid to drain into the pleural space. The sternum is reanastomosed with sternal wires and the skin is sutured in layers.

33257-33259
Concurrently with other cardiac procedures, the physician performs operative tissue ablation and reconstruction of the atria to treat atrial fibrillation. Atrial fibrillation is rapid, randomized muscle contraction of the atrial myocardium causing an irregular, rapid heart rate. In this procedure, the physician seeks to permanently interrupt aberrant electrical conduction within the atria to restore normal sinus rhythm. The physician performs a midline sternotomy, incising the skin, fascia, muscles, and sternum. The pericardium is incised. For a limited operative tissue ablation and reconstruction of atria (33257), also referred to as a modified maze procedure, an incision is made into the left or right atrium. A combination of surgical incision and/or energy sources, such as heat, microwave, laser, ultrasound, or cryoprobe, is used to create lesions that will heal into scars that disrupt conduction. In 33258 and 33259, an extensive operative tissue ablation and reconstruction of the atria is performed. In these extensive procedures, the right and/or left atrial tissue and/or atrial septum is treated as described in 33257, and additional operative ablation involving the atrioventricular annulus is performed. In any of these procedures, the left atrial appendage may be excised or isolated. In 33259, lines are placed for cardiopulmonary bypass. When cardiopulmonary bypass is achieved, an extensive tissue ablation and atria reconstruction procedure is performed. The atrial incision lines are reanastomosed. The pericardium is repaired loosely, leaving gaps for blood and fluid to drain into the pleural space. The sternum is reanastomosed with sternal wires and the skin is sutured in layers.

33261
Following initiation of cardiopulmonary bypass, the physician exposes the heart through the sternum. A mapping grid of electrodes is placed over the surface of the beating heart. The location of the arrhythmia source is determined. The source is destroyed using electrical current, freezing or cutting, though not in the tricuspid valve. Any bleeding is controlled with sutures. The chest is closed.

[33267, 33268]
The physician excludes the left atrial appendage (LAA) from systemic circulation using an open approach via sternotomy or thoracotomy. Exclusion may be performed by any method (i.e., clip, excision, ligation, oversewing, plication, or stapling). In patients with atrial fibrillation, abnormal electrical impulses prevent the heart from effectively pumping the blood from the atria into the ventricles. Blood collects in the LAA, where clots can form and travel outside the heart to the brain, resulting in stroke. The LAA is the most common site of thrombosis in those with atrial fibrillation. In 33267, the LAA exclusion is the primary procedure. In 33268, the exclusion is performed during the same operative episode as another open cardiac procedure.

[33269]
The physician excludes the left atrial appendage (LAA) from systemic circulation using a thoracoscopic approach. Exclusion may be performed by any method (i.e., clip, excision, ligation, oversewing, plication, or stapling). In patients with atrial fibrillation, abnormal electrical impulses prevent the heart from effectively pumping the blood from the atria into the ventricles. Blood collects in the LAA, where clots can form and travel outside the heart to the brain, resulting in stroke. The LAA is the most common site of thrombosis in those with atrial fibrillation. One method utilizes a proprietary clip device. With the patient in a supine position and under appropriate anesthesia, three thoracoscopic ports are placed and access to the left side of the chest is obtained. Pericardial blood vessels are cauterized, and the pericardium is opened to expose the LAA. Using a sizing tool inserted through a lower port, the LAA is measured and the appropriate clip size is selected. The device holding the clip is inserted through the port, manipulated over the LAA, positioned onto the base of the LAA and closed, using echocardiographic guidance to assure complete closure. The clip may be opened and repositioned until adequate closure is obtained. The clip is then released, instruments are removed, and port sites are closed.

33265-33266
The physician performs endoscopic operative ablation and reconstruction of the atria to treat atrial fibrillation. Atrial fibrillation is rapid, randomized muscle contraction of the atrial myocardium causing an irregular, rapid heart rate. In a maze procedure, the physician seeks to permanently interrupt aberrant electrical conduction within the atria to restore normal sinus rhythm. Through multiple endoscopic incisions in the chest, the physician accesses and visualizes the outer (epicardial) surface of the heart. For a limited or modified maze procedure performed endoscopically (33265), the pulmonary veins or other anatomically defined triggers are isolated in the left or right atrium and a heat, microwave, laser, ultrasound, or cryoprobe is used to create lesions from the outside of the left atrium that will heal into scars that disrupt conduction. In 33266, the right and/or left atrial tissue and/or atrial septum is treated as described in 33265, and additional operative ablation involving the atrioventricular annulus is performed. In either of these procedures, the left atrial appendage may be excised or isolated. Once sufficient interruption of electrical conduction has been accomplished, the endoscope is removed and access incisions are sutured in layers.

33285-33286
The physician implants or removes an electronic device that is capable of recording heartrates and rhythms for over one year (subcutaneous cardiac rhythm monitor, cardiac event recorder, implantable loop recorder or ILR). In 33285, the physician uses a scalpel to make a small parasternal incision and dissects down to the level of subcutaneous tissue located over the left pectoral or mammary area. The monitor is implanted

into the subcutaneous tissue. Electrodes that sense heart activity are located on the surface of the monitor, making it unnecessary to place transvenous leads. The device continuously and automatically monitors the heart's electrical activity when sensing the patient's rapid, irregular, or slow heartrate or can also be prompted by the patient in the course of experiencing symptoms. Programming of the device is included in this service. In 33286, the physician removes the monitor when sufficient information regarding the heart's activities has been obtained or when the batteries run out by incising down to the level of the recorder and removing it. In either surgery, the incision is closed with sutures. This type of recorder is capable of storing many separate events. When appropriate, a "programmer" is used by the physician to retrieve the information that can be displayed, stored, or printed.

33289

The physician places a pulmonary pressure monitoring system. A proprietary device comprised of a battery-free sensor is placed directly in a distal portion of the pulmonary artery of a patient with heart failure to permit ongoing monitoring and measurement of the patient's heartrate, as well as systolic, diastolic, and mean pressures. The system is placed via a corresponding catheter. Pulmonary arterial pressure (PAP) readings transmitted from the sensor to a wireless electronic unit are subsequently transmitted to an online portal that can be accessed by the patient's treating health care provider. Through accurate monitoring of patients diagnosed with heart failure (HF) for exacerbations, it is possible to minimize the need for additional hospitalizations and the associated complications and allow for early pharmacological intervention. Deployment and calibration of the sensor, as well as any associated catheterizations, angiography, and radiological supervision and interpretation, are included in this service, when performed.

33300-33305

The physician gains access to the heart using an incision through the sternum (median sternotomy) or the left anterior chest wall (thoracotomy). A pericardial window may be created if the diagnosis of penetrating cardiac trauma is not confirmed. Once penetrating trauma has been confirmed, the pericardial sac is incised and clotted blood and fluid removed. The entire heart is inspected and wound site(s) identified. Small lacerations are repaired with sutures and reinforced with Teflon felt pledges to anchor the sutures. Lacerations to small coronary vessels are ligated. Lacerations to larger coronary vessels are repaired. Large myocardial wounds may require synthetic grafting to cover the wound. The surgical incision is closed. Chest tubes and/or a mediastinal drainage tube may be left in place following the procedure. Report 33300 when the procedure is performed without cardiopulmonary bypass; report 33305 when cardiopulmonary bypass is required.

33310-33315

The physician exposes the heart via the sternum. The foreign body is located by feeling the heart. If possible, the object is removed from the surface of the heart. If necessary, a hole is made in one of the ventricles or atria to remove the object or thrombus lodged there. The holes are closed with sutures and small reinforcing patches of Teflon felt. Report 33310 if cardiopulmonary bypass is not initiated; report 33315 if cardiopulmonary bypass is initiated.

33320-33322

The physician gains access to the mediastinum through an incision through the sternum (median sternotomy) or the chest wall (lateral thoracotomy). The physician repairs the aorta or great vessels while the heart is still beating. The physician closes the surgical incisions and dresses the sternal or chest wall wound. The physician may leave chest tubes and/or a mediastinal drainage tube in place following the procedure. Report 33321 if performed with a shunt bypass; report 33322 if performed with a cardiopulmonary bypass.

33330

The physician gains access to the mediastinum through an incision through the sternum (median sternotomy) or the chest wall (lateral thoracotomy). The physician sews in the aortic or great vessel graft while the heart is still beating. The physician closes the surgical incisions and dresses the sternal or chest wall wound. The physician may leave chest tubes and/or a mediastinal drainage tube in place following the procedure.

33335

The physician gains access to the mediastinum through an incision through the sternum (median sternotomy) or the chest wall (lateral thoracotomy). The physician places cardiopulmonary bypass catheters usually through incisions in the right atrial appendage and aorta or femoral artery. The physician stops the heart by infusing cardioplegia solution into the coronary circulation. The physician sews in the aortic or great vessel graft while the heart is still. The physician takes the patient off cardiopulmonary bypass, closes the surgical incisions and dresses the sternal or chest wall wound. The physician may leave chest tubes and/or a mediastinal drainage tube in place following the procedure.

33340

A left atrial appendage is closed or occluded using an endocardial implant delivered via catheter. The physician places an introducer sheath in a vein (typically, the femoral vein) using percutaneous puncture. The physician places a lumen catheter through the introducer sheath into the femoral vein and advances it, under fluoroscopic guidance, to the right atrium. The physician exchanges this catheter over a wire for a transseptal puncture needle, dilator, and sheath. The physician advances the transseptal puncture apparatus to the right atrium and punctures the intra-atrial septum (in some cases, the physician may use a patent foramen ovale if present rather than performing a septal puncture). The physician advances the needle, dilator, and transseptal sheath into the left atrium. The occlusive device is positioned over the left atrial appendage and deployed blocking the opening completely. The physician removes the catheters and sheaths from the femoral vessels. Pressure is placed on the wound for 20 to 30 minutes to stem bleeding. This code includes fluoroscopy, transseptal puncture, catheter placement, left atrial and left atrial appendage angiography, and radiological supervision and interpretation.

33361-33362

Transcatheter aortic valve replacement or implantation (TAVR/TAVI) is performed on patients with symptomatic aortic stenosis that are high risk or not eligible for traditional open chest surgery. A guidewire is placed in the femoral artery in the groin and manipulated into the left ventricle. A catheter is inserted following the guidewire to the aortic valve. A balloon is inflated to compress the native valve. A bioprosthetic valve attached to an expandable stent is deployed over the compressed native valve. The catheter and guidewire are removed. Report 33361 if the catheter access is percutaneous and 33362 when access to the femoral artery is open.

33363-33364

Transcatheter aortic valve replacement or implantation (TAVR/TAVI) is performed on patients with symptomatic aortic stenosis that are high risk or not eligible for traditional open chest surgery. A guidewire is placed in a peripheral or other artery and manipulated into the left ventricle. A catheter is inserted following the guidewire to the aortic valve. A balloon is inflated to compress the native valve. A porcine valve attached to an expandable stent is deployed over the compressed native valve. The catheter and guidewire are removed. Report 33363 if the catheter access is via an open axillary artery approach and 33364 when access is via an open iliac artery approach.

33365

Transcatheter aortic valve replacement or implantation (TAVR/TAVI) is performed on patients with symptomatic aortic stenosis that are high risk or not eligible for traditional open chest surgery. A median sternotomy or mediastinotomy is performed for direct access to the aorta. The aorta is incised and a guidewire is inserted and manipulated into the left ventricle. A catheter is inserted following the guidewire to the aortic valve. A balloon is inflated to compress the native valve. A porcine valve attached to an expandable stent is deployed over the compressed native valve. The catheter and guidewire are removed.

33366

Transcatheter aortic valve replacement or implantation (TAVR/TAVI) is performed on patients with symptomatic aortic stenosis that are high risk or not eligible for traditional open chest surgery. A small incision is made between ribs (usually the fifth or sixth intercostal space) on the lower left side of the patient's chest to achieve direct access to the heart. The pericardium is incised and opened near the left ventricular apex. A guidewire is advanced through the opening into the left ventricle, through the septum, and into the right ventricle. A catheter is inserted following the guidewire to the aortic valve. A balloon is inflated to compress the native valve. A porcine valve attached to an expandable stent is deployed over the compressed native valve. The catheter and guidewire are removed and the pericardium is closed using sutures. A chest tube may be placed. The wound is closed in layers.

33367-33368

The patient's blood is pumped to a bypass machine, oxygenated, and returned to the patient during a transcatheter aortic valve replacement or implantation (TAVR/TAVI). Its purpose is to provide mechanical support for the heart and lungs during the procedure. In 33367, the access for the intake and output of the patient's blood is via percutaneous cannulations of a peripheral artery and vein, typically the femoral vessels. Report 33368 for open peripheral arterial and venous cannulation.

33369

The patient's blood is pumped to a bypass machine, oxygenated, and returned to the patient during a transcatheter aortic valve replacement or implantation (TAVR/TAVI). Its purpose is to provide mechanical support for the heart and lungs during the procedure. Access for the intake and output of the patient's blood is via cannulations of a central artery (i.e., aorta, pulmonary artery) and vein.

33370

A cerebral embolic protection device (CEPD) is a mesh filter designed to collect debris released during transcatheter aortic valve replacement (TAVR) procedures. These devices are intended to reduce the risk of stroke by preventing embolic material from entering the carotid arteries and reaching the cerebral vasculature. A variety of CEPDs exist in various pore sizes, differing in chemical composition and deployment location. They are designed to capture materials such as arterial valve tissue, calcification, foreign matter, and thrombus. This code includes the percutaneous transcatheter placement and subsequent removal, arterial access, catheterization, imaging, and radiological supervision and interpretation.

33390-33391

The physician initiates cardiopulmonary bypass. The aorta is clamped from above the heart and a cold preserving solution is pumped through the heart. The aorta is opened near the valve. The spaces where the heart valve leaflets meet have been fused by inflammation and scarring in diseases requiring this operation. Blunt dilators are passed through the hole and across the aortic valve. Progressively larger dilators are inserted until the valve is wide open. The dilators break the scar tissues that are cut in an open aortic valvoplasty. After the valve is fully dilated, the purse string is tied off. In the simple procedure (33390), cutting into the aortic valve leaflets, debridement utilizing scalpel blades and/or forceps to remove calcium deposits or tumors, and/or simple commissural resuspension may be performed. Commissurotomy requires the physician to stretch or cut the aortic valve due to rigid or fused leaflets. In the complex procedure (33391), extensive repairs to the leaflets may be necessary and/or annuloplasty may also be performed. Annuloplasty requires the physician to attach fibrous tissue to the base of the valve or utilize an implantable ring that prevents blood from accumulating within the left atrium, essentially resizing the valve opening. This procedure assists in maintaining the shape and flexibility of the annulus. The aorta is closed and the clamp is removed. Cardiopulmonary bypass is discontinued when heart function returns.

33404
Cardiopulmonary bypass is required. Access to the heart may be achieved by median sternotomy or left thoracotomy. A hole is made in the tip of the left ventricle and another is made in the aorta above the coronary arteries. The conduit is oriented so that the valve in it will only let blood flow out of the heart, but not back in. One end of the conduit is sewn to the hole in the tip of the heart. The other end is sewn to the hole in the aorta. Air is removed from the heart and from the conduit. Cardiopulmonary bypass is discontinued when heart function returns.

33405
Cardiopulmonary bypass is initiated. A clamp is placed on the aorta well above the heart. A cold preserving solution is pumped into the coronary arteries to stop the heart. The aorta is opened just above the aortic valve. The valve leaflets are cut out and the annulus of the valve (ring of tissue where the valve leaflets normally attach to the aorta) is cleaned of calcium. The valve annulus size is measured and an appropriate artificial valve is selected. The artificial valve is sewn to the valve annulus. The aorta is closed and the clamp is taken off. Cardiopulmonary bypass is discontinued when heart function returns.

33406
Cardiopulmonary bypass is initiated. A clamp is placed on the aorta well above the heart. A cold preserving solution is pumped into the coronary arteries to stop the heart. The aorta is opened just above the aortic valve. The valve leaflets are cut out and the annulus of the valve (ring of tissue where the valve leaflets normally attach to the aorta) is cleaned of calcium. At this point an allograft is selected. The tissue valve is trimmed so that it can be sewn to the valve annulus. The aorta above the graft valve is trimmed so that the valve cusps can be suspended when the graft is in place. By doing so, the coronary arteries are not obstructed by the graft. The new valve is sewn in place. The valve annulus size is measured and an appropriate artificial valve is selected. The artificial valve is sewn to the valve annulus. The aorta is closed and the clamp is taken off. Cardiopulmonary bypass is discontinued when heart function returns.

33410
Cardiopulmonary bypass is initiated. A clamp is placed on the aorta and above the heart. A cold preserving solution is pumped into the coronary arteries to stop the heart. The aorta is opened just above the aortic valve. The valve leaflets are cut out and the annulus of the valve (ring of tissue where the valve leaflets normally attach to the aorta) is cleaned of calcium. The valve annulus size is measured and an appropriate stentless tissue valve is selected (the stentless valve is unique because unlike other valves it has no rigid external frame or sewing ring) and sutured directly into the aortic wall. The aorta is closed and the clamp is taken off. Cardiopulmonary bypass is discontinued when heart function returns. The wound is closed with layered sutures.

[33440]
Aortoventriculoplasty with pulmonary autograft (Ross-Konno procedure) is a treatment option geared toward younger patients diagnosed with left ventricular outflow tract obstructions who typically require aortic valve replacement reoperation. Cardiopulmonary bypass is initiated. The physician opens the patient using a median sternotomy approach and cold preserving solution is pumped into the coronary arteries to stop the heart. After aortic cross-clamping, the aorta and pulmonary artery are extensively excised and mobilized. Removal of the aortic valve and sinuses of Valsalva are performed. A pulmonary autograft is excised with a muscular tongue of the right ventricular front wall. A Konno technique incision is made in the interventricular septum beginning where the left and right coronary leaflets abut and toward the ventricular septal defect (VSD), if present, resecting the outflow septum. The incision length is based on the morphology of the obstruction and is made as far as needed in order to provide full relief of the left ventricular outflow tract obstruction (LVOTO). The pulmonary autograft is placed into aortic position using great care to precisely position the right ventricular front tongue and avoid injury to the left coronary artery, the pulmonary artery valves, and septal perforator of the left coronary artery. The right and left coronary buttons are implanted back into the autograft avoiding rotation, tension, or kinking. Anastomosis with the ascending aorta is made. Right ventricular (RV) and pulmonary artery (PA) connections are restored via the use of a homograft or bovine jugular vein conduit. Running sutures, including sutures at the base of the root and may include a thin strip of pericardium for reinforcement, are used. An echocardiogram should be performed once the patient has been weaned from bypass.

33411
Cardiopulmonary bypass is initiated. A clamp is placed on the aorta well above the heart. A cold preserving solution is pumped into the coronary arteries to stop the heart. The aorta is opened just above the aortic valve. The valve leaflets (cusps) are cut out and the

annulus of the valve (ring of tissue where the valve leaflets normally attach to the aorta) is cleaned of calcium. At this point, a homograft or a xenograft is selected. The tissue valve is trimmed so that it can be sewn to the valve annulus. The aorta above the graft valve is trimmed so that the valve cusps can be suspended when the graft is in place and so the coronary arteries are not obstructed by the graft. When the valve is sized, it must be greater than or equal to 19 mm on a normal sized adult. If a smaller valve is inserted, the heart will slowly fail. Aortic annulus enlargement may be performed utilizing the noncoronary sinus, located just below the aortic valve (Nick's technique). Incision is carried downward posteriorly through the noncoronary aortic sinus across the aortic ring to the origin of the mitral valve. Dacron or other appropriate material is sutured to the fibrous origin of the mitral ring with mattress sutures, which are continued along the anterior and posterior margins of the aortic incision. The valve is sutured to the aortic ring and tied into position. Alternately, the aortic annular enlargement may be performed using the Manougian technique (through the commissure between the left coronary leaflet and the noncoronary leaflet). The aorta is cut longitudinally toward the heart and through the commissure (connecting point where two valve leaflets meet on the aortic wall) between the noncoronary leaflet (no coronary is near this leaflet) and the left coronary leaflet (leaflet near the left coronary artery) and across the valve annulus for a variable distance. The cut may need to extend onto the roof of the left atrium and onto the anterior leaflet of the mitral valve. The end of the cut is determined by the point at which the aortic root accommodates at least a 19 mm valve. The anterior mitral leaflet, left atrial roof, and the aorta are repaired with patches. The new valve is sewn in place. The aorta is closed and the clamp is taken off. Cardiopulmonary bypass is discontinued when heart function returns.

33412

The physician replaces the aortic valve with transventricular aortic annulus enlargement, also referred to as the Konno procedure. Cardiopulmonary bypass is initiated. A clamp is placed on the aorta well above the heart. A cold preserving solution is pumped into the coronary arteries to stop the heart. The aorta is opened just above the aortic valve. The valve leaflets are cut out and the annulus of the valve (ring of tissue where the valve leaflets normally attach to the aorta) is cleaned of calcium. At this point a homograft or a xenograft is selected. The tissue valve is trimmed so that it can be sewn to the valve annulus. The aorta above the graft valve is trimmed so that the valve cusps can be suspended when the graft is in place and so the coronary arteries are not obstructed by the graft. When the valve is sized, it must be greater than or equal to 19 mm on a normal sized adult. If a smaller valve is inserted, the heart will slowly fail. The aorta is incised longitudinally toward a point just to the left of the right coronary artery. The cut is carried across the annulus and for a variable distance onto the right ventricular infundibulum. A triangular patch of pericardium or Dacron (e.g., a gusset) is used to close the incision in the right ventricle and aorta and to enlarge the aortic annulus. The new valve is sewn in place. The aorta is closed and the clamp is taken off. Cardiopulmonary bypass is discontinued when heart function returns.

33413

Cardiopulmonary bypass is initiated. The aorta and pulmonary artery are separated and the main pulmonary trunk is completely cleaned off. After the heart is stopped, the pulmonary trunk is detached from the branching point of the left and right pulmonary arteries. It is taken off the heart with a small lip of heart muscle. Care is taken when the muscle of interventricular septum is cut. It is possible to damage a large branch of the left anterior descending coronary artery when this muscle is cut. The aorta is opened above the valve. The coronary arteries are detached from the aorta with a surrounding "button" of aortic wall. Next, the aortic valve and its annulus are removed from the heart. A length of the ascending aorta is also removed. The pulmonary artery is sewn to the heart in the aortic position. The commissures and cusps of the pulmonary valve are lined up to be in the same positions as their aortic counterparts were before the aortic valve was removed. The open end of the pulmonary artery is sewn to the ascending aorta. The coronary arteries are re-implanted on the pulmonary artery in positions similar to their positions on the aorta. The pulmonary valve and artery from an organ donor are sewn into the pulmonary position.

33414

The physician enlarges the left ventricular outflow track by patch due to obstruction. The physician performs a midline sternotomy, incising the skin, fascia, muscles, and sternum. The pericardium is incised and lines are placed for cardiopulmonary bypass. Dissection of the aorta is performed within the aorta, right ventricle, and pulmonary artery reaching the aortic annulus. An incision is made in the aorta and the right ventricular outflow tract is opened through the septum. The cusps of the aortic valve are removed. Reconstruction of the left ventricular outflow tract is achieved using a patch of Dacron cut into a diamond shape and the septum is closed to the area of patch placement. The aortic annulus is measured with replacement of aortic valve. An additional patch is attached to broaden the right ventricular outflow tract connecting it to the left ventricular outflow tract patch. The aortic valve prosthesis is connected to the outflow tract patches. The right ventricular outflow tract patch is attached to the right ventriculotomy. The pericardium is repaired loosely, leaving gaps for blood and fluid to drain into the pleural space. The sternum is reanastomosed with sternal wires and the skin is sutured in layers.

33415-33416

Cardiopulmonary bypass is initiated. The aorta is opened and the left ventricular outflow tract is assessed below the valve. There is usually a clearly definable ring or shelf below the valve. This is taken off with a tool designed for the purpose. Usually, the left ventricular septal muscle is thickened. A trough of muscle tissue is cut out of the left ventricular septal muscle. The aorta is closed. Cardiopulmonary bypass is discontinued when heart function returns. Report 33416 if there is no ring of subvalvular tissue to remove.

33417
Aortoplasty for supravalvular stenosis is performed with a median sternotomy to gain access. Cardiopulmonary bypass is required. A piece of pericardium or Dacron is prepared. The aorta is clamped beyond the area of narrowing. The heart is stopped with a cold preserving solution. An incision is made into the narrowest point of the ascending aorta and three additional incisions are made that extend into the sinuses of Valsalva. Using patches of pericardium, the sinuses are enlarged. A patch from the noncoronary sinus is extended into the ascending aorta in order to assure symmetrical enlargement. The clamp is released. Cardiopulmonary bypass is discontinued when heart function returns.

33418-33419
A mitral valve is repaired percutaneously. The procedure is performed under general anesthesia. The physician makes an incision over a lower extremity vessel, usually the femoral vein. A catheter with a specially designed prosthesis or stent is maneuvered through the vessels to the heart under fluoroscopic imaging guidance. Depending on the approach and the device being used, the catheter may be threaded through the inferior vena cava to the right atrium where a septal puncture to access the left atrium and mitral valve is created. Once the device is positioned above the diseased valve, it is secured into place with precautions taken to ensure proper positioning and anchoring. The physician removes the catheter and the surgical wound is closed. Report 33418 for insertion of the initial device and 33419 for any additional devices used during the same operative session.

33420
The chest is opened by median sternotomy or left thoracotomy. The pericardium is opened. An incision is made within the left atrial appendage where a Tubbs dilator (or gloved physician's finger) is introduced into the left ventricle by way of the apex and opened in the valve. Calcium deposits may be removed from the annulus and leaflets with a bone nibbler. Upon completion of valvotomy, the dilator (or finger) is removed and the incisions are sutured closed.

33422
The skin and muscle are incised from the sternum to the xiphoid process. The sternum is split and a retractor is utilized to open the chest. An incision is made in the pericardium and cardiopulmonary bypass is initiated. The left atrium is opened from the right side. The mitral valve is exposed. The scar tissue between the lateral ends of the valve leaflets is divided sharply. Cardiopulmonary bypass is discontinued when heart function returns. The pericardium and left atrium are closed. Chest tubes may be inserted to allow drainage.

33425-33427
This operation is done to improve the ability of the mitral valve to close completely when the ventricle contracts. It is done in patients whose mitral valve has lost the ability to close normally. In almost all cases, this is the result of a mitral valve prolapse in which the mitral leaflets and the cords that tether them on the ventricle have become elongated. Cardiopulmonary bypass is initiated. The left atrium is opened and the mitral valve is exposed. Redundant leaflet tissue is excised and defects in the valve leaflets are closed with sutures. The cords are also shortened with sutures. Valve closure is assessed after the repair. The left atrium is closed and cardiopulmonary bypass is discontinued when heart function returns. Report 33426 if the mitral valve diameter is enlarged requiring placement of a prosthetic ring. Report 33427 if a more extensive repair, including transfer of cords from the posterior leaflet to the anterior leaflet, is performed. A prosthetic ring may be required with extensive reconstruction.

33430
The physician performs a sternotomy to gain access to the heart. Cardiopulmonary bypass is initiated. The mitral valve may be accessed by opening the right atrium followed by opening the atrial septum or the left atrium directly, exposing the mitral valve. All leaflet tissue and its attached cords are cut out. Sutures are placed in the mitral annulus. The annulus is sized and an appropriate artificial valve is selected (a totally mechanical valve or a valve with plastic supports and tissue leaflets). The sutures are passed through the sewing ring of the annulus and the sutures are tied down so the sewing ring is adherent to the annulus. The atrial septum (or left atrium) may be sutured closed or left to heal on its own. Cardiopulmonary bypass is discontinued when heart function returns. The sternotomy is closed with wires and the skin is sutured closed.

33460
Cardiopulmonary bypass is initiated. The right atrium is opened and the tricuspid valve is exposed. The valve tissue and its cords are completely excised. The right atrium is closed. Cardiopulmonary bypass is discontinued when heart function returns.

33463-33464
In 33463, cardiopulmonary bypass is initiated with venous uptake tubes in both of the caval veins. The right atrium is opened. Valvuloplasty of the tricuspid valve almost always requires nothing more than reducing the diameter of the tricuspid valve. To accomplish this, a double purse string of sutures is placed around the circumference of the valve and tightened to reduce the valve diameter. The right atrium is closed. Report 33464 if a stiff ring is used to reduce the valve's diameter rather than purse strings.

33465

The physician incises the sternum with a cut of about 7 to 9 inches to expose the heart. A minimally invasive procedure could entail a sternal incision of 2 to 4 inches or an incision between the ribs. Cardiopulmonary bypass is initiated with venous uptake tubes in both caval veins. The right atrium is opened and clamps are placed on the aorta. Typically, the tricuspid valve leaflets are left intact; however, when excessive thickening is present, several incisions into the leaflets may be necessary allowing for the best possible fit of the prosthetic. A valve of an appropriate diameter is selected (usually it is a tissue/plastic valve, although a metal valve can also be used). Sutures are placed around the circumference of the tricuspid valve annulus. They are brought through the sewing ring of the valve. The valve is seated so that the sewing ring is resting on the annulus. The sutures are tied tightly. The right atrium is closed. Cardiopulmonary bypass is discontinued when heart function returns.

33468

In this anomaly, the tricuspid valve annulus is displaced onto the right ventricle, the right ventricle becomes atrophied and the valve leaflets become tethered to the wall of the ventricle. Cardiopulmonary bypass is initiated with venous uptake tubes in both caval veins. The right atrium is opened. The valve is detached from the ventricular wall around its circumference. The edge of the cut valve is sewn circumferentially around the lone port by the true junction of the right atrium and right ventricle. The right atrium is closed. Cardiopulmonary bypass is discontinued when heart function returns.

33474

The surgeon creates an incision into the pulmonary valve in order to enlarge the opening to the pulmonary artery, allowing blood to flow more easily into the artery. The heart is exposed through the sternum and the patient is placed on cardiopulmonary bypass. Tourniquets are placed around the superior and inferior caval veins and tightened. An opening is created in the pulmonary artery to allow access to the pulmonary valve. The pulmonary valve in incised. The opening in the pulmonary artery is closed and the tourniquets are released. Cardiopulmonary bypass is discontinued, the sternum is closed with wires or sutures, and the soft tissues are closed with sutures.

33475

Cardiopulmonary bypass is initiated with venous uptake tubes in both caval veins. The pulmonary artery is opened and the pulmonary valve leaflets are cut out. Stitches are placed around the circumference of the pulmonary annulus and the valve is sized. An appropriate artificial valve is selected. The stitches are passed through the sewing ring of the valve. The sewing ring is seated against the valve annulus and the stitches are tied. The hole in the pulmonary artery is closed. Cardiopulmonary bypass is discontinued when heart function returns.

33476, 33478

Cardiopulmonary bypass is initiated. The right ventricular infundibular muscle is opened and the obstructing muscle bands are cut out. The valve may also need to be opened. If so, the valve is cut open. The hole in the right ventricle is closed with a patch of pericardium. Cardiopulmonary bypass is discontinued when heart function returns. Report 33478 if the operation is performed with a gusset, with or without commissurotomy or infundibular resection.

33477

Percutaneous placement of a prosthetic pulmonary valve is used primarily to treat patients with stenosis or regurgitation of a previously repaired right ventricular outflow tract (RVOT). The patient is prepped with general anesthesia in addition to endotracheal intubation. The provider inserts a needle through the skin and into an underlying vein, usually a lower extremity vein, although jugular access is also utilized. Angiography and hemodynamic studies are performed and a guidewire is threaded through the needle and advanced into the pulmonary artery. A balloon is inflated in the RVOT conduit to evaluate for coronary compression and an aortogram is performed to visualize the coronary arteries. Pre-stenting is commonly performed with a covered bare metal stent to decrease the risk of fractured stents and more than one stent may be required. The needle is removed and a catheter carrying the prosthetic valve is inserted. The prosthesis is positioned over the diseased pulmonary valve and a balloon is inflated, deploying the prosthetic valve in place. Angiography and hemodynamic evaluations are repeated. The catheter is removed and pressure is applied to stop bleeding at the access site. A single suture may provide hemostasis at the venous access.

33496

This procedure is typically performed to repair an artificial prosthetic valve that is malfunctioning due to leakage around the valve sewing ring or the valve is impeded by blood clot or growth of surrounding tissue (pannus) into the functioning part of the valve. The physician exposes the heart through the sternum. Cardiopulmonary bypass is initiated. The prosthetic valve is exposed and the valve is repaired. Cardiopulmonary bypass is discontinued when heart function returns. The sternum is closed with wires or sutures and the soft tissues are closed with sutures.

33500-33501

The physician repairs a coronary arteriovenous or arteriocardiac chamber fistula. In one technique, a catheter is used to advance a balloon or microcoils for embolization of the artery closest to the site of fistula termination. Open repair may be performed to ligate a complicated fistula or when other cardiac procedures are necessary. Report 33500 when cardiopulmonary bypass is used; 33501 without cardiopulmonary bypass.

33502
The physician ligates an anomalous coronary artery arising from the pulmonary artery. Ligation of the anomalous coronary artery has a poor prognosis and may be performed as a temporary measure prior to creation of a double coronary artery system during a subsequent surgical intervention. The anomalous coronary artery is exposed at the site of origin in the pulmonary artery. A suture is placed around the artery and it is ligated.

33503-33504
The physician repairs an anomalous coronary artery arising from the pulmonary artery using a graft. The anomalous coronary artery is identified and detached. The subsequent hole in the pulmonary artery is sutured closed. An opening is made in the side of the aorta and the free end of the coronary artery is anastomosed to the aorta. Report 33504 if cardiopulmonary bypass is required. This procedure will most always require the cardiopulmonary bypass.

33505
The physician repairs an anomalous coronary artery arising from the pulmonary artery by construction of an intrapulmonary artery tunnel. Cardiopulmonary bypass is required. This operation is done in cases where the anomalous coronary artery is located far from the aorta on the left lateral side of the pulmonary artery. Openings are made in the aorta and the pulmonary artery at the level of the anomalous coronary artery where the vessels touch each other. The two open areas are sewn together to create a direct aortopulmonary opening. A flap of pulmonary artery wall is created with the anomalous coronary artery at one end. The flap is fashioned into a tunnel with the flap as one side of the tunnel, the back wall of the pulmonary artery as the other side of the tunnel, the hole between the aorta and pulmonary artery as one end, and the anomalous coronary artery as the other end. In this way, blood from the aorta is diverted into the anomalous coronary artery. The hole in the pulmonary artery is closed. Cardiopulmonary bypass is discontinued when heart function returns. This procedure is less common today; surgeons typically repair the defect by direct transfer of the anomalous coronary artery from the pulmonary artery.

33506
The physician repairs an anomalous coronary artery arising from the pulmonary artery by translocation from the pulmonary artery to the aorta. The anomalous coronary artery arising from the pulmonary artery is detached. The subsequent hole in the pulmonary artery is patched with autologous pericardium. An opening is created in the side of the aorta and the coronary artery is anastomosed into the opening. Cardiopulmonary bypass is almost always required for this operation.

33507
The physician repairs an anomalous coronary artery by unroofing or translocation. Common anomalies repaired using this technique include anomalous right coronary artery arising from the left coronary sinus, anomalous left coronary artery arising from the right coronary sinus, and anomalous coronary artery arising from a single ostia. Cardiopulmonary bypass is almost always required. The physician detaches the posterior commissure of the aortic valve. Unroofing of the intramural segment of the coronary artery is accomplished by excision of a triangular portion of the internal aortic wall. The coronary arteries are excised as a single disc and divided into two cuffs. An arterial switch is performed. The posterior commissure of the aortic valve is resuspended to a pericardial patch used to reconstruct the pulmonary artery sinus.

33508
A surgical vascular endoscopy is performed, including video-assisted harvesting of a vein for a coronary artery bypass. The physician makes a portal incision above the saphenous vein. The endoscope is inserted into the incision and visualization occurs on a video monitor. CO2 gas is insufflated through the endoscope and dissection is made to the vein. A cannula is inserted and a portion of the vein to be removed is released from the surrounding structures. The vein is tied off or cauterized above and below the portion of the vein to be removed. The vein is removed through the harvesting cannula. The endoscope is removed and the incision is closed with sutures and Steri-strips. The portion of the vein removed is prepared for use in cardiac bypass surgery.

33509
Using an endoscopic approach, the physician harvests a segment of an artery from an upper extremity (arm) to use for a planned bypass procedure on a coronary artery. A 3-cm longitudinal incision is made just proximal to the wrist crease on the forearm over the radial artery. The physician separates the fascia and identifies the radial artery and its venae comitantes; these are dissected as one pedicle to avoid radial artery trauma. The endoscope is advanced directly over the radial artery, and the port trocar inserted and inflated to form a seal. Following CO2 insufflation and the establishment of a flow rate to create a tunnel, the physician performs anterior, posterior, and lateral dissection of the artery using the conical dissection tip of the endoscope. The tip is then removed, and the endoscope is placed into a proprietary vessel-harvesting cannula. Using direct energy force, the physician releases the fascia from the distal to the proximal forearm. Radial artery branches are captured between the jaws of the cannula and the artery pedicle divided and ligated. The physician makes a stab incision near the elbow, clamps the radial artery pedicle, and brings it through the stab incision. The radial artery is transected and the stump ligated. The pedicle is retrieved from the original incision at the wrist. The portion of the radial artery removed is prepared for use in a bypass procedure by flushing with papaverine and clipping the branches.

33510-33516
Cardiopulmonary bypass is initiated with a single, two-stage venous uptake tube. Saphenous vein is

Cardiovascular

harvested from either leg. Vein may also be taken from the arm, the back of the leg, or from a cadaver. A clamp is placed on the aorta above the heart. Cold preserving solution is pumped through the coronary arteries to stop the heart. A point is chosen on the diseased coronary (arteries) beyond the area of disease and a longitudinal incision is cut in it. The proximal part (the part nearest the thigh) of the vein is trimmed to the same length as the cut in the coronary artery and is cleaned off. The end of the vein is sewn to the side of the coronary artery. A 3 mm to 6 mm hole is punched in the ascending aorta and the other end of the vein graft is sewn to this hole. The clamp on the aorta is released. Cardiopulmonary bypass is discontinued when heart function returns. Report 33511 if two coronary venous grafts are needed; report 33512 if three are needed; report 33513 if four are performed; report 33514 if five are performed; report 33516 if six or more are performed.

33517-33523

The physician initiates cardiopulmonary bypass with a single, two-stage venous uptake tube. The physician harvests saphenous vein from the legs. Other vein grafts may be obtained from the arms, backs of the legs, or cadavers (organ donors.) These sources are inferior to the saphenous vein. Arterial grafts may be obtained from the internal mammary artery (along the lateral side of the breastbone), the gastroepiploic artery (from the abdomen), the inferior epigastric artery (from the abdominal wall), or the radial artery (from the nondominant hand). The most commonly used vessel is the internal mammary artery. It is left connected at one end to the subclavian artery from which it arises. Report 33517 for a single vein graft, 33518 if two venous grafts are performed, 33519 if three venous grafts are performed, 33521 if four venous grafts are performed, 33522 if five venous grafts are performed, and 33523 if six or more venous grafts are performed.

33530

For descriptions of the actual therapeutic procedure to be performed, please see the description of that procedure. The breast bone must be split again. Because the heart is invariably tightly adherent to the underside of the sternum in a redo operation, a vibrating saw is used to cut through it. After the sternum is cut, its halves are gently retracted while the tissues that have adhered to its undersurface are carefully cut down. Once the sternum can be opened, the heart is exposed by cutting any chest tissues that have adhered to it since the last operation. It is usually necessary to initiate cardiopulmonary bypass before the heart is completely cleaned off.

33533-33536

Cardiopulmonary bypass is initiated with a single, two-stage venous uptake tube. Arterial grafts may be obtained from the internal mammary artery (along the lateral side of the breast bone), the gastroepiploic artery (from the abdomen), the inferior epigastric artery (from the abdominal wall), or the radial artery (from the non-dominant hand). The most commonly used vessel is the internal mammary artery. It is left connected at one end to the arm artery from which it arises. Report 33534 if two arterial grafts are placed; report 33535 if three are placed; report 33536 if four or more are placed.

33542

This operation is almost always done in conjunction with coronary artery bypass grafting. Prior to placing the bypass grafts, the aneurysm is opened and any clot is removed from the ventricle. The aneurysm is opened widely and damaged tissue is removed from the ventricular wall. The ventricle is repaired by suturing the walls of the ventricle back together directly or with a patch of Gortex, Dacron, or other appropriate material sewn into the defect. All stitches are placed in healthy (not aneurysm) heart tissue and care is taken to avoid the coronary arteries.

33545

This operation is always done in conjunction with coronary artery bypass grafting. The heart muscle involved in the infarction extends from the septum onto the surface of the heart. The heart is opened through this dead muscle and all dead muscle on the surface of the heart is cut out as is all the dead muscle in the septum. The septum is reconstructed by sewing in a patch of Gortex, for example, or Dacron. The surface of the heart is closed directly with sutures or with a patch sewn over the hole.

33548

The physician performs a surgical ventricular restoration (SVR) procedure to treat congestive heart failure subsequent to a myocardial infarction that has caused scarring or aneurysm of the left ventricle resulting in an enlarged rounded heart. SVR restores the heart to a more normal size and shape thereby improving function. Cardiopulmonary bypass is initiated. The ventricle is collapsed. A small incision is made in the bottom of the left ventricle through the scar tissue. The heart is opened and the area between the scar and the good heart muscle is identified. Using a plastic model of the heart selected based on the body surface area of the patient, the physician reshapes the heart. Rather than closing the defect, the physician sutures a patch over the defect to restore the normal spherical shape of the heart.

33572

This operation is done when a coronary artery is so full of disease along its length that a good site for sewing on the bypass graft cannot be found. Coronary artery bypass grafts are almost always done along with the endarterectomy. The coronary artery to be cleaned out is opened along its length for a distance greater than that usually opened for a bypass alone. The plaque within the artery is separated from the outer layer of the arterial wall with a tool designed for the purpose. The plaque is removed from as much of the artery as is possible. A bypass graft is usually sewn to part of the hole left in the coronary. The rest of the hole is closed directly with suture or a patch of opened vein graft is laid over the open artery and sewn to the coronary artery wall to close the hole.

33600-33602
Cardiopulmonary bypass is initiated. The appropriate heart chamber (right atrium for the tricuspid valve; left atrium for the mitral valve) is opened and the valve is assessed. The hole in the leaflet is cleaned of any infection. If it can be closed directly without distorting the valve significantly, suture alone is used. If the hole is large, it is closed with a patch made of pericardium. The open heart chamber is closed and cardiopulmonary bypass is discontinued when heart function returns. Report 33602 if the pulmonary artery or aorta are opened to gain access to the valve.

33606
The heart is exposed by dividing the breast bone longitudinally. Mechanical, extra corporeal circulation is established and the heart is stopped (cardiopulmonary bypass). The pulmonary artery is cut just before it divides into right and left branches. The pulmonary artery end is connected to the side of the ascending aorta. A piece of Dacron graft is used to construct this connection. This allows the single ventricle to pump blood to the body.

33608
Mechanical, extracorporeal circulation is established and the heart is stopped (cardiopulmonary bypass). A hole is made in the pulmonary artery and is enlarged to cross any areas of narrowing. A cadaver ascending aorta is trimmed to the right length. A tube of artery or Dacron is sewn to the valve end of the cadaver aorta. The cadaver artery is connected to the hole in the pulmonary artery. The tube of aorta or Dacron is sewn to the hole in the ventricle to close the hole and allow blood to flow through the new valved tube that now connects the ventricle to the pulmonary artery.

33610
The heart is exposed by dividing the breast bone longitudinally. Mechanical, extra corporeal circulation is established and the heart is stopped (cardiopulmonary bypass). The heart is opened and the hole in the wall between the two ventricles is enlarged so that blood will flow freely across it. A baffle is placed to direct blood that flows across the enlarged ventricular septal defect out the aorta.

33611-33612
Cardiopulmonary bypass is initiated. A hole is made in the right ventricle free wall. This exposes the hole between the right and left ventricles. A patch of pericardium or Dacron is sewn in place to block the hole and directs blood ejected from the left ventricle (i.e., blood coming from the lungs) out the aorta. If the pulmonary artery is of adequate size, blood will flow from the right ventricle to the lungs. If it is inadequate or if the valve does not open, a conduit containing a valve (natural or artificial) is sewn to the hole in the right ventricle free wall. The far end of the conduit is attached to the pulmonary artery. This will allow blood to be pumped from the right ventricle to the lungs. Report 33612 if the obstructing muscles bundles in the outflow part of the right ventricle are excised when the heart is open.

33615
The right pulmonary artery (or left in situs inverses) is exposed from the main pulmonary trunk to the hilum of the lung. The superior vena cava is detached from the right atrium. The atrial hole is closed. A hole is made in the top part of the pulmonary artery and the cut end of the superior vena cava is connected to the hole in the pulmonary artery. Pulmonary blood flow comes directly from the venous system and bypasses the heart. Later the process is completed by performing a Fontan operation. This procedure may also be referred to as a simple Fontan or Bidirectional Glenn Shunt (BDG).

33617
This operation is usually considered to be the second stage of a Glenn repair. Cardiopulmonary bypass with or without circulatory arrest is required. In this operation, blood flow is directed from the inferior caval vein, through a tunnel created inside the right atrium to the pulmonary artery. All systemic venous return is diverted away from the heart and directly into the pulmonary circulation. The right atrium is widely opened. A large patch of pericardium or Dacron is used for one wall of the tunnel. The lateral wall of the right atrium forms the other half of the tunnel. The tunnel leads from the inferior caval vein, where it joins the right atrium, to the undersurface of the pulmonary artery. The mouth of the tunnel is connected to a hole on the undersurface of the pulmonary artery. Previously, or at the same time, the superior caval vein will already have been directly connected to the upper surface of the pulmonary artery.

33619
Cardiopulmonary bypass and circulatory arrest are required. The small aorta is opened on the inner surface of its arch up to the point where the aortic diameter becomes normal. The pulmonary artery is removed and its connection to the branched pulmonary artery is closed with a patch. A large, rectangular patch of pericardium is used to enlarge the small aorta. The pulmonary valve becomes the systemic arterial valve of the heart and is encircled by the large patch that becomes shaped like a tube as it is sewn along either side of the small ascending aorta and arch that have been opened longitudinally. The coronary arteries are small and still originate in the root of the abnormal aorta.

33620
The cardiovascular surgeon performs bilateral pulmonary artery banding (bPAB) using a hybrid stage 1 approach, which does not require open heart surgery or circulatory arrest. Hybrid procedures utilize the services of both a cardiovascular surgeon and an interventional cardiologist. This procedure is typically performed on high-risk neonates with hypoplastic left heart syndrome or related congenital anomalies for short-term palliation as part of a staged approach to

more definitive surgical repair. Following a median sternotomy, the pulmonary arteries are banded individually in order to restrict some of the pulmonary blood flow. In a separately reportable procedure, the interventional cardiologist may place a stent in the ductus arteriosus under fluoroscopic guidance. Incisions are closed.

33621

The interventional cardiologist performs a transthoracic insertion of a catheter for stent placement using a hybrid stage 1 approach, which does not require open heart surgery or circulatory arrest. Hybrid procedures utilize the services of both an interventional cardiologist and a cardiovascular surgeon. This procedure is typically performed on high-risk neonates with hypoplastic left heart syndrome or related congenital anomalies for short-term palliation as part of a staged approach to more definitive surgical repair. Because pulmonary arteries in a newborn are difficult to access for catheter interventions, access is obtained by direct puncture of the right ventricular outflow tract, typically in the same operative episode as another, separately reportable procedure performed by the cardiovascular surgeon (i.e., pulmonary artery banding, which requires sternotomy). Upon completion of the separately reportable stent placement, the catheter is removed and the incisions are closed.

33622

While a "hybrid procedure" is one that combines both surgical and transcatheter interventional approaches, a "hybrid approach" may be any of a group of staged procedures that follow (not all procedures classified as hybrid approach are true hybrid procedures). The hybrid approach stage 2 reported by 33622 is part of a planned staged approach that typically follows a hybrid procedure; it is not a hybrid procedure in and of itself. The physician performs a hybrid stage 2 reconstruction of a congenital cardiac abnormality, such as left heart hypoplasia or a single ventricle. The physician gains access to the mediastinum through a sternal incision (median sternotomy).
Cardiopulmonary bypass and circulatory arrest are required. For palliation of a single ventricle with aortic outflow obstruction and aortic arch hypoplasia, the physician performs a Norwood procedure. After the bypass pump is turned off, the small aorta is opened on the inner surface of its arch up to the point where the aortic diameter becomes "normal." The physician removes the pulmonary artery bands (placed during a previous surgery). The pulmonary artery is removed and its connection to the branched pulmonary artery is closed with a patch. A large, rectangular patch of pericardium is used to enlarge the small aorta. The pulmonary valve becomes the systemic arterial valve of the heart and is encircled by the large patch that becomes shaped like a tube as it is sewn along either side of the small ascending aorta and arch that have been opened longitudinally. The coronary arteries are small and still originate in the root of the abnormal aorta. The physician creates a cavopulmonary anastomosis. The left superior vena cava is dissected free. The left superior vena cava is divided and anastomosed in end-to-side fashion to the left pulmonary artery. The physician closes the cardiac incisions, takes the patient off cardiopulmonary bypass, closes the remaining surgical incisions, and dresses the sternal or chest wall wound. The physician may leave chest tubes and/or a mediastinal drainage tube in place following the procedure.

33641

Cardiopulmonary bypass is necessary. Two venous tubes are placed for the bypass machine—one draining the superior caval vein and the one draining the inferior caval vein. The right atrium is isolated by the putting tourniquets around the superior vena cava and inferior vena cava and their corresponding tubes. The right atrium is opened and the size and location of the arterial septal defect are assessed. If it is small enough or if the atrial septal tissue is sufficiently redundant, the defect is closed primarily with suture. If not, a patch of pericardium or Dacron is sewn to the edge of the defect to close it.

33645

The right atrium is opened and the size and location of the congenital sinus venosus defect is assessed. If it is small enough or if the atrial septal tissue is sufficiently redundant, the defect is closed primarily with suture. If not, a patch of pericardium or Dacron is sewn to the edge of the defect to close it. Care is taken to place the patch so that all pulmonary veins remain patent and there is no obstruction of the superior vena cava, right ventricle, or pulmonary veins by the patch.

33647

Cardiopulmonary bypass is established with the venous uptake tubes in the superior and inferior caval veins. A hole in the right atrium or, if needed, a hole in one of the ventricles is made. The hole in the ventricle is made in the area of scar (if the ventricular septal defect is due to ischemia) or in the anterior part of the right ventricle (if the ventricular septal defect is congenital). All dead heart muscles are cut out (in ischemic ventricular septal defect) and the ventricular septal defect is closed with a patch of Dacron or pericardium. The hole in the atrium or ventricle is closed. Cardiopulmonary bypass is discontinued when heart function is restored.

33660

Cardiopulmonary bypass is established using venous uptake tubes in both the superior and inferior caval veins. The right atrium is opened. A radially oriented cleft or division in the anterior leaflet of the mitral valve is closed with interrupted sutures. Care is taken to assure that the valve closes properly after it is repaired. There is a line of denser valve tissue marking the anatomic line between the two AV valves. The ventricular septal defect is obliterated by sewing this line to the top of the septal muscle. The arterial septal defect is closed with a patch of Dacron or pericardium. The right atrium is closed and cardiopulmonary bypass is discontinued after heart function is restored.

33665
Cardiopulmonary bypass is established with the venous uptake tubes in both the superior and inferior caval veins. A hole in the right atrium or, if needed, a hole in one of the ventricles is made. The hole in the ventricle is made in the area of scar tissue (if the ventricular septal defect is due to ischemia) or in the anterior part of the right ventricle (if the ventricular septal defect is congenital). The AV valve anatomy can be highly variable, ranging from normal mitral and tricuspid anatomy with a subvalvular ventricular septal defect to grossly abnormal AV valve leaflet with two separate valves present separated by a line of tissue. The AV valves are repaired. Repair is all that is done if valvular competence can be restored to the left AV valve. If not, the valve is replaced with a mechanical valve on a tissue valve.

33670
Cardiopulmonary bypass is established using venous uptake tubes in the superior and inferior caval veins. The right atrium is opened. A radially oriented cleft or division in the anterior leaflet of the mitral value is closed with the interrupted sutures. Care is taken to assure that the valve closes properly after it is repaired. There is a raphe or line of denser value tissue marking the anatomic line between the two AV valves. The ventricular septal defect is obliterated by sewing this line to the top of the septal muscle. The atrial septal defect is closed with a patch of Dacron or pericardium. The competency of the single AV valve is assessed as is the imaginary line where the plane extending upward from the ventricular septal defect intersects the AV valve. The AV valve leaflets are divided along this line. The ventricular septal defect patch is placed. The valve leaflets are resuspended by sewing them to the ventricular septal defect patch. The competency of the valves is assessed. The atrial septal defect is closed with a patch sewn to the top of the ventricular septal defect patch or an extension of the ventricular septal defect patch is used to close the atrial septal defect (single patch technique). The hole in the right atrium is closed. Cardiopulmonary bypass is discontinued when cardiac function has returned.

33675
The physician repairs multiple defects in the tissue separating the right and left ventricles of the heart in an open heart procedure. Cardiopulmonary bypass is established with tubes in both the caval veins. The ventricular septal defects can almost always be accessed and repaired through an incision in the right atrium. Each ventricular septal defect is usually repaired with a patch of Dacron or pericardium, but may be closed using only sutures. The septal defects may be repaired with a pair of patches, one in each ventricle. After the ventricular septal defects are repaired, the access incision in the right atrium is closed with sutures. Cardiopulmonary bypass is discontinued when heart function returns. The chest incision is repaired.

33676
The physician repairs multiple defects in the tissue separating the right and left ventricles of the heart, and surgically releases fused leaflets within the pulmonary valve or resects the anterosuperior portion of the right ventricle (infundibulum). The heart is accessed through a midline sternal incision. Cardiopulmonary bypass is established with tubes in both the caval veins. The septal and ventricular defects can almost always be accessed and repaired through an incision in the right atrium, and the pulmonary valve is usually accessed through an incision in the pulmonary artery. Each ventricular septal defect is usually repaired with a patch of Dacron or pericardium, but may be closed using only sutures. The septal defects alternately may be repaired with a pair of patches, applied on each side of the septum. Fused pulmonary valve leaflets are incised and any abnormal tethering of the leaflets to the arterial wall is released. For infundibular resection, obstructions within the right ventricle are excised and the ventricle repaired. After repairs are complete, the access incision in the right atrium is closed with sutures. Cardiopulmonary bypass is discontinued when heart function returns. The chest incision is repaired.

33677
The physician repairs multiple defects in the tissue separating the right and left ventricles of the heart, removes a previously placed band from the pulmonary artery, and may place a gusset. The heart is accessed through a midline sternal incision. The physician gains access to the mediastinum through an incision through the sternum (median sternotomy). The physician places cardiopulmonary bypass catheters through incisions in the low inferior vena cava, the superior vena cava, and aorta or femoral artery. The physician stops the heart by infusing cardioplegia solution into the coronary circulation. The septal defects can almost always be accessed and repaired through an incision in the right atrium, and the pulmonary valve is usually accessed through an incision in the pulmonary artery. Each ventricular septal defect is usually repaired with a patch of Dacron or pericardium, but may be closed using only sutures. The septal defects alternately may be repaired with a pair of patches applied on each side of the septum. The physician removes the pulmonary artery band (placed during a previous surgery) and dilates the pulmonary artery to normal size. A triangular patch (gusset) may be sutured into the incised pulmonary artery to enlarge its circumference. The physician closes the cardiac incisions, takes the patient off cardiopulmonary bypass, closes the remaining surgical incisions, and dresses the sternal or chest wall wound. The physician may leave chest tubes and/or a mediastinal drainage tube in place following the procedure.

33681
The physician repairs a solitary defect in the tissue separating the right and left ventricles of the heart in an open heart procedure. Cardiopulmonary bypass is

established with tubes in both the caval veins. The ventricular septal defect can almost always be accessed and repaired through an incision in the right atrium, except in the case of a supracristal ventricular septal defect, in which the ventricle is higher in the outflow part of the right ventricle. This type of ventricular septal defect is most often accessed and repaired through an incision in the pulmonary artery. All types of ventricular septal defects can be accessed and repaired through an incision in the muscle of the right ventricle, but this causes more damage and is avoided if possible. The ventricular septal defect is usually repaired with a patch of Dacron or pericardium, but may be closed using only sutures. After the ventricular septal defect is closed, the hole that has been created in the right atrium, right ventricle, or pulmonary artery is closed. The chest incision is repaired. Cardiopulmonary bypass is discontinued when heart function returns.

33684

The physician repairs a solitary defect in the tissue separating the right and left ventricles of the heart in an open heart procedure in conjunction with a pulmonary valvotomy or infundibular resection. Cardiopulmonary bypass is established with venous uptake tubes in both the caval veins. Prior to surgery, it is established by echocardiography, cardiac catheterization, or both that the diameter of the tricuspid valve is large enough to permit a normal cardiac output. If not, the operation is combined with a modified Blalock-Taussig shunt. The right ventricle or pulmonary artery is opened. Through either opening, the infundibular muscle blocking blood flow to the pulmonary artery can be cut out and cuts can be made in the pulmonary valve to reduce the restriction to blood flow that it presents. A singular ventricular septal defect is closed through either of these incisions, if possible. If it is not possible to close the ventricular septal defect with the exposure thus provided, the right atrium is opened and the ventricular septal defect closed. A patch is almost always used. All holes in the heart are closed. Cardiopulmonary bypass is discontinued when heart function is restored.

33688

The physician repairs a solitary defect in the tissue separating the right and left ventricles of the heart in an open heart procedure in conjunction with removal of a previously placed pulmonary artery (PA) band. The patient is prepared for cardiopulmonary bypass, but it is not established yet. The previously placed pulmonary artery band is dissected out and removed. Stenosis at the site of the pulmonary artery band is assessed before and after band removal with a pressure transducer connected to a needle probe that measures any pressure drop across the area of narrowing. Cardiopulmonary bypass is then established and the ventricular septal defect is repaired. If pulmonary artery pressures proximal to the band site remain high after band removal and ventricular septal defect closure or if the surgeon feels the residual stenosis is too tight, cardiopulmonary bypass is restarted. The surgeon then removes the stenosed segment of pulmonary artery followed by a primary repair or the surgeon makes an incision in the pulmonary artery across the area of narrowing and closes the defect with a patch graft. Heart function is restored and cardiopulmonary bypass is discontinued.

33690

Cardiopulmonary bypass is not required. The pulmonary artery is exposed through a median sternotomy or left thoracotomy. A band of heavy Dacron suture or tape is place around the base of the pulmonary artery. Once the PA pressure distal to the band is less than half of the systemic pressure and the patients arterial saturation is greater than 70 percent, the band is tight enough, but not too tight. The incision is closed.

33692

In this defect, there are four cardiac anomalies: narrowing of the pulmonary valve annulus and/or the right ventricular infundibulum that restricts normal pulmonary blood flow, a ventricular septal defect, hypertrophy of the right ventricle, and an overriding aorta. Repair of this defect assumes that the pulmonary valve and right ventricular outflow tract are of adequate size to permit normal pulmonary blood flow. Cardiopulmonary bypass is required. The surgical approach relies on the anatomical location of the VSD, by way of atrial incision or ventriculotomy. The ventricular septal defect is closed with a patch of Dacron allowing normal blood flow from the left ventricle to the aorta. The physician enlarges the pulmonary artery from the right ventricle in order to increase blood flow to the lungs allowing the proper amount of oxygen distribution to the body. Upon completion of the repair, the pericardium is closed and drainage tubes are placed.

33694

In this defect, there are four cardiac anomalies: narrowing of the pulmonary valve annulus and/or the right ventricular infundibulum that restricts normal pulmonary blood flow, a ventricular septal defect, hypertrophy of the right ventricle, and an overriding aorta. Surgical approach may be by right arteriotomy or right ventriculotomy based on the extent of obstruction within the right ventricular outflow tract. Cardiopulmonary bypass is required. Resection of the infundibular muscle is performed first. The ventricular septal defect is sutured closed. A longitudinal incision is made in the pulmonary artery and carried proximally across the pulmonary valve annulus and onto the muscles of the right ventricular outflow tract. The defect is closed with a patch placed across the pulmonary valve annulus. Cardiopulmonary bypass is discontinued when heart function returns.

33697

The physician completely repairs tetralogy of Fallot with pulmonary atresia, including construction of a conduit from the right ventricle to the pulmonary artery and closure of the ventricular septal defect.

Cardiopulmonary bypass is required. A hole is made in the right ventricle and any muscular obstruction in the outflow tract of the right ventricle is removed. The pulmonary artery or its branches are opened longitudinally until normal-sized vessels are encountered. The ventricular septal defect is closed. An aortic graft from a donor is trimmed to form a patch over the opened pulmonary artery. Any excess artery from the donor graft or a patch of pericardium or Dacron is sewn to the graft below the valve to use as a secondary patch for closing the hole in the right ventricle. The graft valve becomes the new pulmonary valve. After the patches and graft are sewn in place and heart function returns, cardiopulmonary bypass is stopped.

33702-33710

The physician repairs a sinus of Valsalva fistula. Cardiopulmonary bypass is required. After the heart is stopped, the aorta is opened and the fistula is identified. It is closed with a patch of pericardium. Any aorta valve incompetence is repaired by shortening the redundant valve leaflet diameter with stitches that reef in its free edge. The hole in the aorta is closed. Report 33710 if the sinus of Valsalva fistula is closed through the right atrium or through an incision in the aorta.

33720

Cardiopulmonary bypass is required. The aorta is opened after the heart has stopped. Thrombus (clot) in the aneurysm is removed. The neck of the aneurysm is closed with stitches. The aortic valve is usually incompetent. If the aortic annulus is sufficiently dilated by the aneurysm the aortic valve may need to be replaced with a mechanical aortic valve, a biomechanical valve or a tissue valve from an organ donor. After the valve is repaired or replaced, the aorta is closed. Cardiopulmonary bypass is discontinued after heart function returns.

33724

The physician repairs an isolated partial anomalous venous return (scimitar syndrome) using one of two open techniques. Scimitar syndrome describes a congenital condition in which an aberrant vessel connects the pulmonary vein in the right lung to the inferior vena cava. It can be diagnosed in infancy through adulthood, and symptoms occurring in infancy suggest a more severe form of the disease. Scimitar syndrome is so named because the aberrant vein casts a shadow shaped like a curved Turkish sword, a scimitar, upon x-ray. A midline sternotomy is performed. In one technique, a long pericardial patch graft is used to divert the anomalous pulmonary venous drainage from the inferior vena cava into the left atrium. In the second technique, the anomalous pulmonary vein is divided off the inferior vena cava and reimplanted into the posterior wall of the right atrium. A short pericardial baffle is used to divert flow to the left atrium through an atrial septal defect. Grafts may be required to enlarge remaining vessels. In some cases, a separately reported right pneumonectomy is performed.

33726

The physician gains access to the heart through a midline sternotomy. The physician places cardiopulmonary bypass catheters usually through incisions in the right atrial appendage and aorta or femoral artery. The physician stops the heart by infusing cardioplegia solution into the coronary circulation. Either atria may be incised for exploration to locate and better visualize the defect. The blocked pulmonary vein is opened along its length. The inner layer of the artery is removed. The outer layer of the artery is closed with suture directly or with a patch of pericardium, saphenous vein, or Dacron.

33730

The physician performs a complete repair of total anomalous pulmonary venous return (TAPVR), a rare congenital defect in which all four pulmonary veins do not connect normally to the left atrium, but rather drain to the right atrium by way of an abnormal connection. Via a midline sternotomy, the physician exposes the heart. Cardiopulmonary bypass is initiated. The abnormal veins are rerouted to the left atrium, most often by connecting them directly to the back wall of the atrium. Any abnormal routes for pulmonary venous drainage are tied off, and any existing atrial septal defect is closed. The heart is restarted, cardiopulmonary bypass is discontinued, and the sternotomy is closed.

33732

This lesion is frequently considered to be related to TAPVR, but it is distinctly different. In this anomaly, there is a wall subdividing the left atrium between the pulmonary veins and the mitral valve. This restricts blood flow to the left ventricle and therefore to the rest of the body. Cardiopulmonary bypass is readied. The left atrium is opened and the membrane is cut out. The left atrium is closed. Cardiopulmonary bypass is discontinued when heart function returns.

33735

This procedure is of historical interest only. The procedure requires access by lateral thoracotomy. An incision is made in the pericardium with the right pulmonary artery and pulmonary veins tied off. A clamp is utilized at the anterior position of the right atrium and the posterior position of the left atrium. Incisions are made within the right atrium and right pulmonary vein. The atrial septum is removed and incisions are closed. The clamps are removed and ligatures previously placed in the pulmonary veins and right pulmonary artery are released. Alternatively, a purse string may be placed in the right atrial appendage and the appendage is opened in the middle of the purse string. A finger or a dilating tool is passed through the hole in the atrium and the wall between the right and left atria is torn open. The dilating instrument is removed and the purse string is tied to stop the bleeding. The thoracotomy is closed in standard fashion.

33736
This procedure is largely of historical interest. In most pediatric cardiac surgery centers, it has been supplanted by balloon dilation of a naturally occurring hole in the wall between the atrial chambers. No incision is needed for balloon dilation. Operative septostomy/septectomy requires cardiopulmonary bypass with venous uptake tubes in both caval veins. The right atrium is opened and the thin part of the wall between the right and left atria is cut out or opened widely. The goal is to allow free mixing of the blood from the right and left atria. Cardiopulmonary bypass is discontinued when heart function returns.

33741
The physician performs a transcatheter atrial septostomy (TAS) by various methods to treat specific congenital cardiac anomalies, typically in infants ≤ 4 kg. Various congenital heart defects, particularly those involving transposition of the great vessels, require surgical creation or enlargement of an opening in the interatrial septum (wall) that separates the upper right and left chambers of the heart. In one method, the physician makes a small incision in the arm or leg. Two catheters are placed: a central venous catheter and a second catheter threaded up to the heart. When the foramen ovale has not closed, a deflated balloon (Rashkind-type) is passed through the foramen ovale, inflated, and pulled through the atrial septum, enlarging the opening and improving oxygenation of the blood. When the septum is intact, the deflated balloon is passed from the right atrium through the septum to the left atrium, inflated, and withdrawn, creating an interatrial septal defect and improving oxygenation of the blood. The catheters are removed. Pressure is placed over the incision for 20 to 30 minutes to stem bleeding and the patient is observed for a period afterward. The Park septostomy, or blade method, is an alternative to the Rashkind procedure, and is typically performed on infants older than 1 month of age. The physician makes a small incision in the femoral vein and places a transseptal sheath using standard methods, advancing the sheath to the superior vena cava under fluoroscopic or echocardiographic guidance. Using a transseptal needle to cross the atrial septum, the left atrium is entered. The physician introduces a guidewire into the left atrium and removes the transseptal catheter while leaving the wire in place. A septostomy catheter is advanced over the wire into the left atrium. This catheter has a retracted blade, which the physician extends. The physician pulls the blade slowly across the atrial septum from the left into the right atrium, under fluoroscopic or echocardiographic guidance; several passes with the blade catheter may be made in this fashion. The purpose of this procedure is to increase blood flow across the atrial septum in children with certain forms of cyanotic congenital heart disease. The physician removes the septostomy catheter and venous sheath. Pressure is placed over the incision for 20 to 30 minutes to stem bleeding. The patient is observed for a period afterward. This code includes the percutaneous access, placement of one or more access sheaths, advancement of the transcatheter delivery system, all imaging guidance that is performed, and the creation of effective intracardiac atrial blood flow.

33745-33746
The physician treats various congenital cardiac anomalies by placing one or more intracardiac stents to create a shunt that allows for more effective intracardiac blood flow. Under imaging guidance, the physician uses a transcatheter approach to place one or more stents in the same location in 33745. Included in the procedure is intracardiac stent placement, balloon angioplasty of the target zone before or after stent placement, and, when performed, all ultrasound guidance for vascular access, fluoroscopic guidance for the intervention, and complete diagnostic right and left heart catheterization. Report 33746 if additional, different intracardiac locations are treated with stents during the same session.

33750
In its unmodified form, this operation involves dividing the left subclavian artery, tying off the end of the artery going to the arm, and creating a connection between the end of this artery coming from the heart and the side of the pulmonary artery. The difficulty with this operation is making the connection to the pulmonary artery exactly the right size to supply adequate, but not excessive blood flow to the lungs. Instead, a modified version of the operation is usually performed. The artery to the arm is not divided. Instead, one end of a 3 mm to 5 mm diameter tube of Gortex is sewn to the side of the artery to the arm and the other end is sewn to the side of the pulmonary artery. The size of the tube determines the amount of blood flow to the lungs. Cardiopulmonary bypass is not required. The ductus arteriosus (a connection between the aorta and pulmonary artery that has been supplying blood to the lungs, but usually closes at birth) is tied off.

33755
This procedure is largely of historic interest. This procedure requires cardiopulmonary bypass. It is designed to allow adequate blood flow to the lungs. After cardiopulmonary bypass is initiated, the aorta is occluded above the heart. A hole may be cut in the aorta with the shunt closed from within by sutures. A more common method utilizes the pulmonary artery detached from the aorta and consequently reattached to the defect of the ascending aorta by sutures. The remaining defect in the pulmonary artery may be closed with sutures, but typically is patched with pericardium or pulmonary homograft. It is difficult to accurately control the diameter of the resulting connection and the resulting flow of blood into the lungs. Cardiopulmonary bypass is discontinued when heart function returns.

33762
This procedure is performed through the left side of the chest. Cardiopulmonary bypass is not required. The pulmonary artery is dissected from its original position

to the branches and the aorta is visualized. Occlusion of the pulmonary artery is conducted and incisions are made into both arteries. One end of a 3 mm to 5 mm diameter tube made of polytetrafluoroethylene (PTFE) (e.g., Gortex) is sewn to the side of the descending aorta and the other end is sewn to the pulmonary artery. The ductus arteriosus (a connection between the aorta and pulmonary artery that has been supplying blood to the lungs, but usually closes at birth) is tied off.

33764

The operation is done through an incision in the middle of the breast bone or through an incision in the left chest. Cardiopulmonary bypass is usually not required. One end of a 3 mm to 5 mm diameter tube made of Gortex is sewn to the side of the ascending aorta and the other end is sewn to some part of the pulmonary artery. The ductus arteriosus (a connection between the aorta and pulmonary artery that has been supplying blood to the lungs, but usually closes at birth) is tied off.

33766

This operation is performed when there is an irreparable obstruction to blood flow through the right side of the heart. It is usually done as a prelude to a bidirectional or bilateral Glenn procedure, which is usually a prelude to a Fontan procedure. Cardiopulmonary bypass is usually required. The right (or the persistent left) superior caval vein is occluded and its connection with the heart is divided. The heart end of the superior caval vein is closed. The free end of the superior caval vein is sewn to the side of the corresponding pulmonary artery. It is assumed that the corresponding pulmonary artery is isolated from the opposite lung congenitally or surgically. The goal is to permit blood to flow directly from the superior caval vein to the lungs, thereby bypassing the right side of the heart.

33767

For this procedure, it is assumed that all the pulmonary arteries from both lungs communicate freely. Cardiopulmonary bypass is required. Circulatory arrest and deep cooling of the body are usually employed. The main pulmonary artery is often tied off. The superior caval vein is detached from its connection to the right atrium. The hole left in the right atrium is closed with sutures. The free end of the superior caval vein is sewn to a hole in the side of the pulmonary artery. In this way, blood can flow to the lungs without passing through the right side of the heart. This operation is usually done as a prelude to a Fontan procedure.

33768

A cavopulmonary anastomosis of an anomalous left superior vena cava is performed in conjunction with separately reportable repair of other cardiac anomalies (e.g., bidirectional Glenn procedure, modified Fontan procedure, outflow tract augmentation). Cavopulmonary anastomosis is required when a left superior vena cava is present. The left superior vena cava is dissected free. The left superior vena cava is divided and anastomosed in end-to-side fashion to the left pulmonary artery.

33770

The physician gains access to the mediastinum through the sternum (median sternotomy). Cardiopulmonary bypass catheters are usually placed through an incision in the right atrial appendage and aorta or femoral artery and the heart is stopped by infusion of cardioplegia solution into the coronary circulation. A large Dacron patch is applied to direct oxygenated blood from the left ventricle through the large ventricular septal defect into the aortic valve and ascending aorta. The physician ligates the proximal main pulmonary artery or oversews the pulmonic valve. A fabric conduit or human cadaveric homograft is placed to direct unoxygenated blood from the right ventricle to the branch pulmonary arteries. The physician may place a bioprosthetic valve in the pulmonary outflow conduit if the pulmonary vascular resistance is elevated. The cardiac incisions are closed, the patient is removed from cardiopulmonary bypass, and the remaining surgical incisions are closed. Chest tubes and/or a mediastinal drainage tube may be inserted for drainage following the procedure.

33771

The physician gains access to the mediastinum through the sternum (median sternotomy). Cardiopulmonary bypass catheters are usually placed through incision in the right atrial appendage and aorta or femoral artery and the heart is stopped by infusion of cardioplegia solution into the coronary circulation. The physician enlarges the ventricular septal defect anteriorly to avoid damage to the conduction bundles. A large Dacron patch is applied to direct oxygenated blood from the left ventricle through the large ventricular septal defect into the aortic valve and ascending aorta. The physician ligates the proximal main pulmonary artery or oversews the pulmonic valve. A fabric conduit is placed to direct right ventricular flow to the pulmonary artery. The physician may place a bioprosthetic valve in the pulmonary outflow conduit if the pulmonary vascular resistance is elevated. The cardiac incisions are closed, the patient is removed from cardiopulmonary bypass, and the remaining surgical incisions are closed. Chest tubes and/or a mediastinal drainage tube may be inserted for drainage following the procedure.

33774

The physician gains access to the mediastinum through an incision through the sternum (median sternotomy). Cardiopulmonary bypass catheters are placed through incisions in the low inferior vena cava, the superior vena cava, and aorta or femoral artery and the heart is stopped by infusion of cardioplegia solution into the coronary circulation. The physician excises the interatrial septum and sews baffle material (pericardium or Dacron) to direct blood from the pulmonary veins to the right ventricle and the systemic venous drainage to the left ventricle. The pulmonary venous chamber may be enlarged with a woven

Dacron or pericardial patch. The cardiac incisions are closed and the patient is taken off cardiopulmonary bypass. The remaining surgical incisions are closed and the sternal and chest wounds are dressed. Chest tubes and/or mediastinal drainage tubes may be inserted for drainage following the procedure.

33775

The physician gains access to the mediastinum through an incision through the sternum (median sternotomy). Cardiopulmonary bypass catheters are placed through incisions in the low inferior vena cava, the superior vena cava, and aorta or femoral artery and the heart is stopped by infusion of cardioplegia solution into the coronary circulation. The physician removes the pulmonary artery band (placed during a previous surgery) and dilates the pulmonary artery to normal size. If this is not possible, the pulmonary band and the constricted area of pulmonary artery are removed, and a woven Dacron patch is applied over the hole. The physician excises the interatrial septum and sews baffle material (pericardium or Dacron) to direct blood from the pulmonary veins to the right ventricle and the systemic venous drainage to the left ventricle. The pulmonary venous chamber may be enlarged with a woven Dacron or pericardial patch. The cardiac incisions are closed and the patient is taken off cardiopulmonary bypass. The remaining surgical incisions are closed and the sternal or chest wall wounds are dressed. Chest tubes and/or mediastinal drainage tubes may be inserted for drainage following the procedure.

33776

The physician gains access to the mediastinum through an incision through the sternum (median sternotomy). Cardiopulmonary bypass catheters are placed through incisions in the low inferior vena cava, the superior vena cava, and aorta or femoral artery and the heart is stopped by infusion of cardioplegia solution into the coronary circulation. The ventricular septal defect is closed, usually with a Dacron patch, and the interatrial septum is excised. The physician sews baffle material (pericardium or Dacron) to direct blood from the pulmonary veins to the right ventricle and the systemic venous drainage to the left ventricle. The pulmonary venous chamber may be enlarged with a woven Dacron or pericardial patch. The cardiac incisions are closed and the patient is taken off cardiopulmonary bypass. The remaining surgical incisions are closed and sternal or chest wall wounds are dressed. Chest tubes and/or mediastinal drainage tubes may be inserted for drainage following the procedure.

33777

The physician gains access to the mediastinum through an incision through the sternum (median sternotomy). Cardiopulmonary bypass catheters are placed through incisions in the low inferior vena cava, the superior vena cava, and aorta or femoral artery and the heart is stopped by infusion of cardioplegia solution into the coronary circulation. The physician makes an incision in the right ventricular outflow tract, resects the fibrous muscular tissue causing the subpulmonic obstruction, and sews the ventriculotomy closed. The interatrial septum is excised and baffle material (pericardium or Dacron) is sewn in to direct blood from the pulmonary veins to the right ventricle and the systemic venous drainage to the left ventricle. The pulmonary venous chamber may be enlarged with a woven Dacron or pericardial patch. The cardiac incisions are closed and the patient is taken off cardiopulmonary bypass. The remaining surgical incisions are closed and the sternal or chest wall wounds are dressed. Chest tubes and/or mediastinal drainage tubes may be inserted for drainage following the procedure.

33778

The physician performs an arterial switch (or Jatene type procedure) for transposition of the great arteries, aortic pulmonary artery reconstruction. Access to the mediastinum is performed through an incision of the sternum (median sternotomy). Cardiopulmonary bypass catheters are placed through incisions in the low inferior vena cava, the superior vena cava, and aorta or femoral artery and the heart is stopped by infusion of cardioplegia solution into the coronary circulation. The physician removes the coronary ostia from the aortic root and sews them into the root of the pulmonary trunk. The pulmonary trunk and aortic root are each transected and interchanged to direct blood from the pulmonary veins through the left ventricle to the aorta, and the systemic venous drainage to the pulmonary trunk via the right ventricle. The cardiac incisions are closed and the patient is taken off cardiopulmonary bypass. The remaining surgical incisions are closed and the sternal or chest wall wounds are dressed. Chest tubes and/or mediastinal drainage tubes may be left in place following the procedure.

33779

The physician gains access to the mediastinum through an incision of the sternum (median sternotomy). Cardiopulmonary bypass catheters are placed through incisions in the low inferior vena cava, the superior vena cava, and the aorta or femoral artery and the heart is stopped by infusion of cardioplegia solution into the coronary circulation. The physician removes the pulmonary artery band placed during a previous surgery and dilates the pulmonary artery to normal size. If this is not possible, the pulmonary band and constricted area of pulmonary artery are removed and a woven Dacron patch is applied over the hole. The physician removes the coronary ostia from the aortic root and sews into the root of the pulmonary trunk. The pulmonary trunk and aortic root are each transected and interchanged to direct blood from the pulmonary veins through the left ventricle to the aorta, and the systemic venous drainage to the pulmonary trunk via the right ventricle. The cardiac incisions are closed and the patient is taken off cardiopulmonary bypass. The remaining surgical incisions are closed and the sternal or chest wall wounds are dressed. Chest tubes and/or mediastinal drainage tubes may be inserted following the procedure.

33780
The physician gains access to the mediastinum through an incision of the sternum (median sternotomy). Cardiopulmonary bypass catheters are placed through incisions in the low inferior vena cava, the superior vena cava, and the aorta or femoral artery and the heart is stopped by infusion of cardioplegia solution into the coronary circulation. The physician removes the coronary ostia from the aortic root and sews into the root of the pulmonary trunk. The pulmonary trunk and aortic root are each transected and interchanged to direct blood from the pulmonary veins through the left ventricle to the aorta, and the systemic venous drainage to the pulmonary trunk via the right ventricle. The ventricular septal defect is closed, usually with a Dacron patch. The cardiac incisions are closed and the patient is taken off cardiopulmonary bypass. The remaining surgical incisions are closed and the sternal or chest wall wounds are dressed. Chest tubes and/or mediastinal drainage tubes may be inserted following the procedure.

33781
The physician gains access to the mediastinum through an incision in the sternum (median sternotomy). Cardiopulmonary bypass catheters are placed through incisions in the low inferior vena cava, the superior vena cava, and the aorta or femoral artery and the heart is stopped by infusion of cardioplegia solution into the coronary circulation. The physician removes the coronary ostia from the aortic root and sews them into the root of the pulmonary trunk. The pulmonary trunk and aortic root are each transected and interchanged to direct blood from the pulmonary veins through the left ventricle to the aorta, and the systemic venous drainage to the pulmonary trunk via the right ventricle. An incision is made in the right ventricular outflow tract, resection of the fibrous muscular tissue causing the subpulmonic obstruction is performed, and the ventriculotomy is closed. Cardiac incisions are closed and the patient is taken off cardiopulmonary bypass. The remaining surgical incisions are closed and the sternal or chest wall wounds are dressed. Chest tubes and/or mediastinal drainage tubes may be inserted following the procedure.

33782-33783
The physician repairs anomalies of ventriculoarterial connection, ventricular septal defect (VSD), and pulmonary outflow tract obstruction (stenosis) in the Nikaidoh procedure. A median sternotomy incision is made and cardiopulmonary bypass is initiated. The physician may harvest a piece of pericardium to be used in the reconstruction of the right ventricular outflow tract, and mobilizes the branch pulmonary arteries. The physician harvests the aortic root from the right ventricle, with coronary arteries attached. The outlet septum is divided and the physician excises the pulmonary valve. The left ventricular outflow tract is reconstructed with the posteriorly translocated aortic root and the VSD patch. Using the pericardial patch, the physician reconstructs the right ventricular outflow tract. Report 33782 if no reimplantation of the coronary ostium is performed and 33783 if the physician reimplants one or both coronary ostia.

33786
Total repair, truncus arteriosus (Rastelli type operation) is performed by access to the mediastinum through an incision in the sternum (median sternotomy). Cardiopulmonary bypass catheters are placed usually through incisions in the right atrial appendage and the aorta or femoral artery. The heart is stopped by infusion of cardioplegia solution into the coronary circulation. A large Dacron patch is placed to direct oxygenated blood from the left ventricle through the large ventricular septal defect into the aortic valve and ascending aorta. The proximal main pulmonary artery is ligated or the pulmonic valve is oversewn. A fabric conduit or a human cadaveric homograft is placed to direct unoxygenated blood from the right ventricle to the branch pulmonary arteries after removing them from their origin(s) at the truncal vessel. A pericardial patch is sewn in place to close the defect(s) in the truncal vessel. A bioprosthetic valve may be placed in the pulmonary outflow conduit if the pulmonary vascular resistance is elevated. The cardiac incisions are closed and the patient is taken off cardiopulmonary bypass. The remaining surgical incisions are closed and the sternal or chest wall wounds are dressed. Chest tubes and/or mediastinal drainage tubes may be placed following the procedure.

33788
Reimplantation of an anomalous pulmonary artery is performed with access to the mediastinum through an incision in the sternum (median sternotomy). Cardiopulmonary bypass catheters are placed usually through incisions in the right atrial appendage and aorta or femoral artery and the heart is stopped by infusion of cardioplegia solution into the coronary circulation. The physician identifies the coronary artery anomaly and reattaches the unperfused pulmonary artery to the pulmonic outflow tract, directly or using a Dacron graft, and ligates the patent ductus arteriosus, if present. The cardiac incisions are closed and the patient is taken off cardiopulmonary bypass. The remaining surgical incisions are closed and the sternal or chest wall wounds are dressed. Chest tubes and/or mediastinal drainage tubes may be inserted following the procedure.

33800
Aortopexy for tracheal decompression is performed to open the tracheal lumen thereby preventing collapse. A right lateral thoracotomy or, sometimes, a midline sternotomy is performed to identify the ascending aorta. The thymus is isolated with partial removal performed to allow the ascending aorta to be mobilized and pulled forward. The physician sutures the adventitia of the ascending aorta and base of the innominate artery to the periosteum of the posterior aspect of the sternum or anterior rib. A similar

operation may be performed on the descending aorta, depending upon the site of tracheomalacia. The thoracotomy or sternotomy is closed, leaving chest or mediastinal tubes in place.

33802-33803
The physician gains access to the mediastinum through an incision through the left chest (posterolateral thoracotomy). The physician identifies the two aortic arches and occludes the smaller left arch with vascular clamps. The physician divides the arch and oversews and possibly ligates the divided ends. The physician dissects away the stumps of the divided left arch and frees them from their mediastinal attachments. The physician attaches traction sutures to the ligated stumps and to the endothoracic fascia anteriorly and posteriorly to minimize obstruction to the esophagus and trachea. The physician closes the remaining surgical incisions and dresses the chest wall wound. The physician may leave a chest tube and/or a mediastinal drainage tube in place following the procedure. Report 33803 if the procedure includes reanastomosis.

33814
The physician performs obliteration of an aortopulmonary septal defect. Access is gained to the mediastinum through an incision through the sternum (median sternotomy). Cardiopulmonary bypass catheters are placed through incisions in the low inferior vena cava, the superior vena cava, and high aorta or femoral artery, and the heart is stopped by infusing cardioplegia solution into the coronary circulation. The physician cross-clamps the aorta and places sump suction in the left atrium to obtain a bloodless surgical field. The aortopulmonary septal defect is exposed by cutting through the ascending aorta or main pulmonary artery. The physician closes the defect with a Dacron fabric patch, closes the aortic or pulmonary arterial incision, closes the remaining surgical incisions, and dresses the sternal wound. The physician may leave chest tubes and/or a mediastinal drainage tube in place following the procedure.

33820
The physician repairs patent ductus arteriosus (PDA) by ligation with access to the mediastinum through an incision of the posterolateral left chest wall (posterolateral thoracotomy). Dissection is performed through the posterior chest wall musculature to expose the superior mediastinum with continued dissection of the tissues surrounding the ductus. Several heavy ligatures are passed around the ductus followed by ligation. The surgical incisions are closed and the chest wall wound is dressed. Chest tubes and/or mediastinal drainage tubes may be inserted following the procedure.

33822-33824
The physician gains access to the mediastinum through an incision through the posterolateral left chest wall (posterolateral thoracotomy). The physician dissects through the posterior chest wall musculature to expose the superior mediastinum. The physician dissects away the tissues surrounding the ductus and passes several heavy ligatures around the ductus and ties it off (ligation) at each end. The physician occludes the ductus with vascular clamps and divides the ductus with scissors. The physician closes the aortic end with suture, then closes the pulmonary stump. The physician removes the vascular clamps, sutures the pleura closed, closes the remaining surgical incisions and dresses the chest wall wound. The physician may leave chest tubes and/or a mediastinal drainage tube in place following the procedure. Report 33824 if the patient is 18 years and older.

33840-33845
The physician gains access to the mediastinum through an incision through the posterolateral left chest wall (posterolateral thoracotomy). The physician dissects through the posterior chest wall musculature to expose the superior mediastinum, clamping and ligating large collateral vessels as they are encountered. The physician dissects away the tissues surrounding the aorta. The physician clamps the aorta on either side of the coarctation and ties off and divides the ligamentum arteriosum (or patent ductus arteriosus, if present). The physician excises the stricture sutures the two ends of the aorta to each other. The physician closes the mediastinal pleura and chest and dresses the chest wall wound. The physician may leave chest tubes and/or a mediastinal drainage tube in place following the procedure. Report 33845 if a graft is placed.

33851
The physician gains access to the mediastinum through an incision in the posterolateral left chest wall (posterolateral thoracotomy). Dissection through the posterior chest wall musculature to expose the superior mediastinum is performed with clamping and ligating of large collateral vessels as they are encountered. The tissues surrounding the aorta are dissected away and clamps are placed on the aorta at either side of the coarctation and tied off with division of the ligamentum arteriosum (or patent ductus arteriosus, if present). The aorta is opened with a longitudinal incision that extends along the subclavian artery above and for a distance distally. Any extra tissue at the stricture site is excised. The physician sews in the left subclavian artery or a Dacron patch graft to attach and enlarge the aorta at the longitudinal incision. The mediastinal pleura and chest wounds are closed and dressing is applied to the chest wall wound. Chest tubes and/or a mediastinal drainage tube may be placed following the procedure.

33852-33853
The physician surgically attaches the ascending and descending parts of the aorta, where normal connection is too small or interrupted entirely. Access to the mediastinum is achieved through an incision in the sternum (midline sternotomy). The aorta and left carotid artery are clamped to allow completion of the end-to-side attachment of a Dacron mesh graft to the ascending aorta. The physician cross-clamps the graft and releases the proximal clamp and the left carotid

artery clamp. End-to-side attachment is performed to secure the distal graft to the descending aorta. The mediastinal pleura and chest are closed with dressing applied to the chest wall wound. Chest tubes and/or a mediastinal drainage tube may be placed following the procedure. Report 33853 when cardiopulmonary bypass is utilized.

33858-33859

In 33858, the surgeon places an ascending aortic graft for aortic dissection and in 33859, for aortic disease other than dissection, such as aneurysm. Following induction of general anesthesia, a median sternotomy is performed. The physician places appropriate arterial and venous cannulation and initiates cardiopulmonary bypass. Following cross-clamp of the distal ascending aorta at the base of the innominate artery, the physician opens the proximal ascending aorta. The affected section of the ascending aorta is removed, the inside and outside of the aortic wall is lined with strips of felt for reinforcement, and a piece of synthetic graft material such as Dacron or PTFE is put in place of the missing piece of the aorta. The patient's aortic valve is preserved, although valve suspension may be performed. The physician closes the sternal incision and dresses the wound. If the patient's ascending aortic disease process includes the aortic arch and requires an aortic hemiarch graft, it is reported separately.

33863-33866

In 33863, the surgeon places an ascending aortic graft. The aorta is the largest artery in the body, extending from the heart through the chest and down into the abdomen. Cardiopulmonary bypass is required. Deep cooling of the body and circulatory arrest are often required, especially if the transverse arch of the aorta must be replaced. After circulatory arrest or if a cross-clamp can be placed on the aorta before its first branch, the aneurysm (an abnormally widened or weakened section of an artery) is opened. The hole in the aneurysm is lengthened along the aorta until the end of the aneurysm is reached. The aorta is divided at this point. A double layer of felt strips is placed circumferentially around the inner and outer circumference of the normal aorta with the aortic wall sandwiched in between. A Dacron tube graft is sewn to this end of the aorta and its felt layers. The aortic root is also replaced using a valved conduit and coronary reconstruction (e.g., Bentall procedure). In 33864, following induction of general anesthesia, the surgeon accesses the operative field via median sternotomy. Cardiopulmonary bypass is initiated. The coronary ostia are identified, detached from the aorta using dissecting scissors, and mobilized. After exposing the aneurysm site and clamping the artery above and below the aneurysm, the physician makes an incision into the aneurysm and removes any plaque deposits or clotted blood. The arterial section that is affected by the aneurysm is replaced with a synthetic graft. One end of the graft is attached to the arterial wall just above the beginning point of the aneurysm, while the other continues down through the artery to a point below the end of the aneurysm. The proximal coronary arteries are implanted into the aortic vascular graft. The physician performs a valve-sparing aortic root remodeling in which the dilated aortic root is replaced with a Dacron tube (graft) and the native aortic valve is integrated within the graft. The patient is taken off cardiopulmonary bypass and incisions are repaired. This procedure may be referred to as a David or Yacoub procedure in the operative note. When the patient's ascending aortic disease process includes the aortic arch requiring an aortic hemiarch graft, 33866 may be reported in addition to one of the procedures described above. This code describes three distinct elements: complete circulatory arrest or isolated cerebral retro- or antegrade perfusion, transverse arch incision performed under a single or multiple arch vessel(s) such as the left common carotid or innominate, and extending the ascending aortic graft beneath the aortic arch using a slanted or sloped (beveled) anastomosis. All three elements must be performed in order to use this code.

33871

The physician performs a transverse aortic arch graft in which the entire aortic arch is replaced. This operation requires cardiopulmonary bypass, profound hypothermia, total circulatory arrest, and isolated cerebral perfusion. The patient's body temperature is lowered to 18 to 21 degrees centigrade and the bypass pump is stopped. The aneurysm is opened along its length and a patch of aortic wall containing the openings of the arteries to the head and arms is cut out. Each of these vessels will have been surrounded by tourniquets that were tightened before the bypass pump was stopped. The hole in the aneurysm is lengthened along the aorta until the end of the aneurysm is reached. The aorta is divided at this point. A double layer of felt strips is placed circumferentially around the inner and outer circumference of the normal aorta with the aortic wall sandwiched between. A Dacron tube graft is sewn to this end of the aorta and its felt layers. The aortic root where the aorta emerges from the heart is assessed. This area is where the aortic valve is located. If the valve closes normally, the aortic root size is reduced using stitches that also sew a double layer of felt to the aorta as previously described. Arch vessels are reimplanted individually or using an island pedicle. The physician closes the sternal incision and dresses the wound.

33875-33877

A segment of the intrathoracic descending aorta is replaced with a tube of Dacron. This is done through an incision in the left chest cavity. The great concern in performing this operation is possible damage to the spinal cord. Preserving the spinal cord can be accomplished using a cardiopulmonary bypass circuit from above the aneurysm to below it, using deep cooling of the body and stopping the bypass machine, using perfusion of one or more spinal artery branches with blood pumped through it or using the "clamp and go" method in which no effort, except a speedy operation, is used to preserve the spinal cord. No matter what spinal cord preservation method is chosen, clamps are placed across the aorta above and below the aneurysm. The aneurysm is cut out and the ends of any small branches are closed with sutures. One end of a Dacron tube graft is sewn to the end of the aorta above the aneurysm and the other end of the graft is sewn to the aorta below the aneurysm. The clamps on the aorta are released. Report 33877 if aorta is exposed through the left chest.

33880-33881
The physician repairs the descending thoracic aorta by placing an endoprosthesis from within the artery. Endovascular repair may be performed for an aneurysm, pseudoaneurysm, dissection, penetrating ulcer, intramural hematoma, or traumatic disruption. The defect in the descending thoracic aorta is identified using aortography. The endoprosthesis, contained inside a holding device, is introduced into the artery under fluoroscopy and positioned at the target zone area of repair. Extension prostheses may be required to the level of the celiac artery origin. When the endoprosthesis is in position, it is deployed within the artery at the target site in the descending thoracic aorta, covering the origin of the left subclavian artery in 33880. A balloon angioplasty may be necessary to achieve proper positioning and functioning of the endoprosthesis. The placement position is confirmed, the catheter is removed, and the arteriotomy site is closed. Report 33880 when the repair covers the left subclavian artery origin and 33881 when the repair does not cover the left subclavian artery origin.

33883-33884
A leak, called an endoleak, may occur at the proximal fixation sites of a grafted descending thoracic aorta defect through the body of the graft or from patent arteries within the defect and may require endovascular repair. A proximal extension prosthesis is placed endovascularly to repair an endoleak in a grafted descending thoracic aortic aneurysm, pseudoaneurysm, dissection, penetrating ulcer, intramural hematoma, or traumatic disruption. The target site is identified by aortography and the proper extension prosthesis is selected. Under fluoroscopy, the extension prosthesis, contained inside a long plastic holding capsule, is threaded through the arteries to the site of the leak. Once the extension prosthesis is in place, the holding capsule is removed. The extension prosthesis, activated by heat, expands like a spring and becomes anchored to the artery wall at the site of the endoleak. If full expansion of the prosthesis does not occur automatically, a balloon catheter is threaded to the graft site and inflated within the endovascular prosthesis until full expansion is achieved. The placement position is confirmed, the catheter is removed, and the arteriotomy site is closed. Report 33883 for an initial proximal extension and 33884 for each additional proximal extension.

33886
A leak, called an endoleak, may occur at the distal fixation sites of a previously grafted descending thoracic aorta defect through the body of the graft or from patent arteries within the defect and may require endovascular repair. One or more distal extension prosthesis modules are placed endovascularly to the level of the celiac artery to repair an endoleak in a previously grafted descending thoracic aortic aneurysm, pseudoaneurysm, dissection, penetrating ulcer, intramural hematoma, or traumatic disruption. The target site is identified by aortography and the proper extension prosthesis is selected. Under fluoroscopy, the extension prosthesis, contained inside a long plastic holding capsule, is threaded through the arteries to the site of the leak. Once the extension prosthesis is in place, the holding capsule is removed. The extension prosthesis, activated by heat, expands like a spring and becomes anchored to the artery wall at the site of the endoleak. If full expansion of the prosthesis does not occur automatically, a balloon catheter is threaded to the graft site and inflated within the endovascular prosthesis until full expansion is achieved. The placement position is confirmed, the catheter is removed, and the arteriotomy site is closed. This code is reported only once regardless of the number of extension modules deployed.

33889
The physician performs a unilateral open subclavian to carotid artery transposition in conjunction with endovascular repair of the descending aorta. The physician performs a 2 to 3 cm supraclavicular incision to gain access to the carotid and subclavian arteries. The clavicular section of the sternocleidomastoid muscle is partially divided exposing the phrenic nerve, which is identified and avoided. The physician clears the adventitia of the chosen translocation site in the wall of the common carotid artery. The section of artery where the aneurysm occurs is isolated and dissected from adjacent structures. Vessel clamps are affixed above and below the defect. The repair is accomplished by excising the segment containing the aneurysm. The vessel ends are sutured in an end-to-end fashion. Next, the subclavian artery is transposed and anastomosed to the common carotid artery in an end-to-side fashion. Vessel clamps are removed and the incision is closed with layered sutures.

33891
The physician performs a transcervical retropharyngeal carotid-to-carotid bypass graft with other than vein in conjunction with endovascular repair of the descending thoracic aorta. Through incisions in the neck, the physician isolates and dissects the common carotid arteries, separating them from adjacent critical structures. The physician creates a bypass around a section of carotid artery that is damaged or blocked using a synthetic graft and one of two methods of repair. After vessel clamps have been affixed above and below the damaged area, the ends of the synthetic graft are sutured into the side of the carotid arterial wall (end-to-side). In the second method, the carotid artery may be cut above the damaged area and sutured to one end of a synthetic graft, which is sutured to the side of the carotid artery

on the opposite side of the neck (end-to-end). In either case, the blocked or damaged section of artery is not removed. When the clamps are removed, the synthetic graft forms a new path through which blood can easily bypass the blocked or damaged area. After the graft procedure is complete, the skin incisions are repaired with layered sutures.

33894-33895

The physician places an endovascular stent to repair a narrowing (coarctation) of the ascending, descending, or transverse thoracic or abdominal aorta. The aorta, the largest artery in the body, moves oxygen enriched blood from the heart to the rest of the body. Coarctation of the aorta (CoA), which is usually present at birth, forces the heart to work harder to pump blood through the aorta. Following anesthesia, the physician gains arterial access, typically via the femoral artery. A second arterial access via the brachial or radial artery may also be required for antegrade catheterization of the aortic coarctation. IV heparin is administered, and a multipurpose catheter is advanced into the descending aorta, followed by a soft-tipped glide wire through the CoA site. The catheter is replaced over the wire by a pigtail or multitrack catheter and peak pressure gradient (PPG) is obtained. Angiography is obtained and measurements are made at various points of the aorta to determine the most appropriate stent and balloon size. The soft-tipped wire is exchanged for a stiffer exchange wire, which is secured in the ascending aorta or right subclavian artery. The physician advances a long sheath from the femoral artery site and places it across the CoA segment for stent deployment. The stent is hand-crimped on the balloon catheter and the stent/balloon assembly is advanced through the sheath over the stiff wire and positioned across the CoA site. The physician withdraws the sheath enough to uncover the stent/balloon and confirms the correct position, repositioning the stent, if necessary, prior to inflation. Balloons are deflated and the balloon catheter removed over the wire while the sheath is maintained in position. Following stent deployment, another PPG across the CoA is obtained, and a final angiogram is performed to evaluate the final result and to assure there are no complications such as aortic wall injury. Report 33894 if the procedure is performed across major aortic side branches; report 33895 if no major side branches are crossed.

33897

The physician performs percutaneous transluminal angioplasty (PTA) of a native or recurrent coarctation of the aorta (CoA). Cardiac catheterization and selective angiography are first performed to confirm the clinical diagnosis, exclude other defects, and evaluate the suitability for balloon angioplasty. The aorta, the largest artery in the body, moves oxygen enriched blood from the heart to the rest of the body. Coarctation, which is usually present at birth, forces the heart to work harder to pump blood through the aorta. Following appropriate sedation, the physician gains access percutaneously via the femoral artery, introduces the catheter, and positions it across the aortic coarctation. A guidewire is passed through the catheter into the ascending aorta, where the tip is positioned. The physician then positions a balloon angioplasty catheter across the coarctation and inflates it with diluted contrast material while monitoring the pressure of inflation. The balloon is inflated for five second intervals; typically, a total of two to four inflations are performed approximately five minutes apart. Aortography is performed, as well as pressure gradient measurements across the CoA. Heartrate, systemic pressure, and cardiac index are recorded before and approximately 15 minutes following balloon dilation to confirm that the change in pressure gradient is dilation-related and not merely a change in patient status.

33900-33904

The physician performs revascularization of the pulmonary artery by percutaneous stent placement. This procedure may be used for patients with pulmonary artery stenosis, which is a narrowing of the pulmonary artery, the large blood vessel that connects the heart's right ventricle to the lungs. With the patient under appropriate anesthesia, an introducer sheath is placed into a vein (typically the femoral vein) using a percutaneous puncture and advanced to the target location. A catheter with a balloon and stent attached is inserted and threaded with a guidewire into the vessel. The wire is removed. The catheter is fed through the vascular system to the stenotic segment of the pulmonary artery. Position of the balloon and stent is confirmed angiographically. The provider employs balloon dilation as necessary to reach optimal stent diameter within the region of stenosis. Several inflations may be performed along the narrowed area. The catheter is slowly withdrawn after deflation. Pressure is applied to the puncture site to stop the bleeding after the catheter is removed. Report 33900 for an initial unilateral stent placement on a patient with normal native connections (those in which the blood flow follows the expected course through the great vessels and heart chambers); report 33901 for bilateral placement. Report 33902 for unilateral stent placement on a patient with abnormal connections (those in which alternative blood flow connections exist, as in patients with aberrant cardiac anatomy); report 33903 for bilateral placement. Report 33904 for stent placement in each additional vessel or separate lesion, whether the connections are normal or abnormal.

33910-33915

This operation is only done for patients who are in extremis following a pulmonary artery embolism (i.e., a blood clot originating in one of the large veins in the leg breaks loose and travels into the heart via the caval vein where it obstructs blood flow to the lungs). Survival is low. If cardiopulmonary bypass is used, the physician opens the right atrium widely. If cardiopulmonary bypass is not used, the right atrium is opened through a hole in the middle of a purse string. The clot is "milked" out of the pulmonary artery into the right atrium and out the hole. Report 33910 if cardiopulmonary bypass is required and the right atrium is opened widely. Report 33910 if cardiopulmonary bypass is initiated. Report 33915 if cardiopulmonary bypass is not initiated.

33916

A pulmonary endarterectomy is performed to treat patients diagnosed with chronic thromboembolic pulmonary hypertension. Cardiopulmonary bypass and hypothermia are required in order to perform this procedure. Only the main and branch pulmonary arteries can be treated. Via a median sternotomy, the pulmonary arteries are opened along their lengths. If present, any thrombotic or embolic material is extracted. The inner layer of each artery is removed. Once the endarterectomies are complete, the arteries are closed with suture directly or with a patch of pericardium, saphenous vein, or Dacron. Homeostasis is achieved and the chest is closed in layers using standard techniques.

33917

The physician reconstructs the pulmonary artery to correct any outflow tract obstruction caused by stenosis. Cardiopulmonary bypass is required. Via a median sternotomy, the stenotic pulmonary artery is opened longitudinally until healthy artery is encountered. The diseased vessel is removed. A patch is trimmed to reconstruct the defect in the artery or grafting may be performed if the defect is too complex or large for a patch. After the patch or graft is placed, homeostasis is achieved and the chest is closed in layers using standard techniques.

33920

Cardiopulmonary bypass is required. A hole is made in the right ventricle and any muscular obstruction in the outflow tract of the right ventricle is removed. The pulmonary artery or its branches are opened longitudinally until normal-sized vessels are encountered. The ventricular septal defect is closed. An aortic graft from an organ donor is trimmed to form a patch over the opened pulmonary artery. Any excess artery from the donor graft or a patch of pericardium or Dacron is sewn to the graft below the valve to use as a secondary patch for closing the hole in the right ventricle. The graft valve becomes the new pulmonary valve. After the patches and graft are sewn in place, cardiopulmonary bypass is stopped when heart function returns.

33922

Cardiopulmonary bypass is required. After it is started, cuts are made all the way across the pulmonary artery just above and just below the part of the artery containing the disease. The pulmonary artery is closed directly or is closed using a piece of the pulmonary artery or a piece of the aorta from an organ donor that is placed as an interposition graft.

33924

During a separately reportable congenital heart procedure, the physician ligates and takes down a previously formed systemic-to-pulmonary artery shunt. The shunt is ligated and the systemic arteries are returned to their correct anatomic position.

33925-33926

The physician repairs pulmonary artery arborization anomalies (i.e., stenosis of unbranched and intrapulmonary arteries) by unifocalization, a surgical technique in which the various sources of pulmonary blood supply can be perfused from a single source. In patients with pulmonary atresia or with a ventricular septal defect (VSD), the pulmonary blood supply often comes from multiple sources, particularly major aortopulmonary collateral arteries (MAPCA), which often arise from the aorta and its direct branches. Unifocalization, which may be performed as a single operation or as a staged procedure, interrupts the extracardiac sources of pulmonary arterial blood flow; restores segmental, lobar, and pulmonary arterial confluence; replaces missing central pulmonary arterial branches; and creates a central, accessible source of pulmonary arterial blood flow. The physician accesses the mediastinum through an extended median sternotomy or a bilateral transsternal thoracotomy. The major aortopulmonary collateral arteries are identified, mobilized, and dissected, using a variety of techniques, from the upper descending aorta, the aortic arch, brachiocephalic vessels, or coronary arteries, and anastomosed to the native pulmonary artery. Ligation of the collateral arteries at their origin is performed to achieve controlled perfusion. As each artery is ligated, desaturation is assessed by pulse oximetry. If desaturation approaches a compromising level, the surgeon may proceed with cardiopulmonary bypass at this point. Report 33925 when the procedure is performed without cardiopulmonary bypass and 33926 when it is performed with cardiopulmonary bypass.

33927-33929

In 33927, the physician implants a total replacement heart system, or artificial heart, as a temporary measure until transplantation or to prolong life for patients not eligible for transplant. One artificial heart system, described here, is a self-contained, electrohydraulic action heart, charged from a battery source through the skin. Once attached, the natural atria pump blood into the artificial ventricles of the replacement heart and the hydraulic pump moves the blood into circulation. The patient is prepared for open heart surgery, and an extended median sternotomy is made. A subcutaneous/submuscular pocket is created in the patient's abdominal area for the internal battery and the heart's pumping controller unit, and these internal components are placed between muscle layers. A separate incision is made over the chest wall for placement of the internal transcutaneous energy transmission coil, which is sutured into an appropriate position where the external coil may lie flat over it without much interposing tissue. Cardiopulmonary bypass is initiated, the aorta is cross-clamped, and cardiectomy is undertaken to remove the native ventricles and transect the great vessels. Outflow grafts are anastomosed to the pulmonary artery and the aorta. The artificial ventricles are anastomosed to the native atrial cuffs and all air is removed from the system. The aortic cross-clamp is released and cardiopulmonary bypass weaned onto the artificial heart support. The internal components are connected to the artificial heart and energy is transferred through the transcutaneous coils, where external battery packs transmit power across the skin to keep the internal battery charged. In 33928, the physician removes and replaces a total replacement heart system or artificial heart. The thoracic unit is the pump that consists of the artificial ventricles, which are attached to the natural atria, containing their corresponding valves, and the motor-driven hydraulic pumping system, or the pneumatic air pressure valves, depending on the system. Removal and replacement of this component requires open chest access in a procedure following the same kind of steps for implantation (see 33927). Internal components include the implanted rechargeable battery, which is continually charged by external battery packs, the internal transcutaneous coil for receiving the battery charge across the skin, or the control unit, which monitors and controls the pumping speed of the artificial heart. These components are removed and replaced back in their prepared subcutaneous/submuscular pockets and tunneled back to their connection with the thoracic unit. Report 33929 for removal of a total replacement heart system or artificial heart for heart transplantation.

33930

The physician performs a donor cardiectomy-pneumonectomy by removing the heart and lung from a donor cadaver for transplantation. This is usually performed when other organs such as the liver, kidneys, intestines, or pancreas are also acquired from the organ donor. The chest cavity is accessed and cold preserving solutions are infused into the aorta and pulmonary arteries. After enough solution has been given, the heart and lungs are removed by transection, en bloc. This includes the aorta well above the heart, the right atrium, the atrial septum, and the left atrium, completely and as close to the patient's spine (or as posteriorly) as possible. The heart/lung block is preserved for transplantation into the recipient. The organ remains under refrigeration, specially packed in a sealable container with some preserving solution and kept on ice in a suitable carrier.

33933

The physician performs a standard backbench preparation of the heart and lungs following procurement from a cadaver donor. Backbench or back table preparation refers to procedures performed on the donor organs following procurement to prepare the donor organs for transplant. The heart and lungs are removed en bloc. The heart and lungs are inspected following procurement to identify any injury or abnormality not noted prior to procurement. The physician prepares the heart and lungs by dissecting free any residual soft tissue. Attention is focused on the aorta, superior vena cava, inferior vena cava, and the trachea. The aorta, which was divided at the aortic arch, is inspected and residual tissue removed. The superior vena cava is inspected and residual tissue removed. The inferior vena cava is inspected to assure adequate length has been preserved. Any residual tissue is removed from the inferior vena cava. The trachea, which was divided as far above the carina as possible, is inspected and residual tissue removed. When all residual soft tissue has been removed and the vessels prepared, the heart and lungs are ready for transplant.

33935

The patient is placed on cardiopulmonary bypass and the heart and lungs are removed. The donor's organs are placed by sewing the left atrium of the donor to the left atrium of the recipient's first, and then sewing together the atrial septums and the right atrium. The donor aorta is trimmed to an appropriate length and sewn to the ascending aorta of the recipient. Immunosuppressive drugs may be given to the patient before, during, and after surgery. Cardiopulmonary bypass is discontinued when function returns to the donor heart.

33940

The physician performs a donor cardiectomy by removing the heart from a donor cadaver for transplantation. This is usually performed when other organs such as the liver, kidneys, intestines, or pancreas are also acquired from the organ donor. The chest cavity is accessed and cold preserving solutions are infused into the aorta. After enough solution has been given, the heart is removed by transection, en bloc. This includes the aorta well above the heart, the right atrium, the atrial septum, and the left atrium, completely and as close to the patient's spine (or as posteriorly) as possible. The heart is preserved for transplantation into the recipient. The organ remains under refrigeration, specially packed in a sealable container with some preserving solution and kept on ice in a suitable carrier to maintain hypothermia.

33944

The physician performs a standard backbench preparation of the heart following procurement from a cadaver donor. Backbench or back table preparation refers to procedures performed on the donor organs following procurement to prepare the donor organs for transplant. The heart is removed or the heart and lungs are removed en bloc. If the heart and lungs are removed en bloc, back table separation of the heart and lungs is performed. The heart is inspected following procurement to identify any injury or abnormality not noted prior to procurement. The physician prepares the heart by dissecting free any residual soft tissue. Attention is focused on the aorta, superior vena cava, inferior vena cava, and the left atrium. The aorta, which was divided at the aortic arch, is inspected and residual tissue removed. The superior vena cava is inspected and residual tissue removed. The inferior vena cava is inspected to assure adequate length has been preserved. Any residual tissue is removed. The left atrium is inspected and residual

Cardiovascular

tissue removed. When all residual soft tissue has been removed and the vessels prepared, the heart is ready for transplant.

33945

The patient is placed on cardiopulmonary bypass. Cardiac transplantation may be performed by one of two techniques: total orthotopic heart replacement or heterotopic implantation. A total orthotopic heart replacement involves excising the ventricles, atrial appendages, and most of the coronary sinus from the donor heart. The recipient heart is then opened. The atria, aorta, and pulmonary artery of the recipient heart are anastomosed to the donor heart. The sinoatrial nodes of both the donor and recipient heart are left intact. In a heterotopic implantation, the donor's organs are placed by sewing the left atrium of the donor heart to the left atrium of the recipient, and then sewing together the atrial septum and the right atrium. The donor aorta is trimmed to an appropriate length and sewn to the ascending aorta of the recipient. Immunosuppressive drugs may be given to the patient before, during, and after the operation. Cardiopulmonary bypass is discontinued when the donor heart begins functioning in the recipient.

33946-33947

The physician initiates veno-venous or veno-arterial extracorporeal membrane oxygenation (ECMO)/ extracorporeal life support (ECLS). In ECMO/ECLS, the patient's blood is pumped to a machine, oxygenated, and returned to the patient, similar to a cardiopulmonary bypass but modified for prolonged use (days to weeks) at the bedside. Its purpose is to provide mechanical support for the heart and lungs in order to allow time for recovery. Report 33946 for initiation of veno-venous ECMO/ECLS, which exchanges blood between large veins through a single double-lumen cannula. Report 33947 for initiation of veno-arterial ECMO/ECLS, which exchanges oxygen poor blood from a central vein or right atrium with oxygen rich blood pumped back into the patient within the arterial circulation through two cannulae: one into a vein and the other into an artery.

33948-33949

The physician performs daily management of extracorporeal membrane oxygenation (ECMO)/ extracorporeal life support (ECLS). In ECMO/ECLS, the patient's blood is pumped to a machine, oxygenated, and returned to the patient, similar to a cardiopulmonary bypass but modified for prolonged use (days to weeks) at the bedside. Its purpose is to provide mechanical support for the heart and lungs in order to allow time for recovery. Patients receiving ECMO/ECLS require daily management to monitor for infections of the skin along cannulas and to identify any evidence of clotting in the legs or any deposits visualized within the pump. Report 33948 for daily management of veno-venous ECMO/ECLS, which exchanges blood between large veins through a single double-lumen cannula. Report 33949 for daily management of veno-arterial ECMO/ECLS, which exchanges oxygen poor blood from a central vein or right atrium with oxygen rich blood pumped back into the patient within the arterial circulation through two cannulae: one into a vein and the other into an artery.

33951-33952

The physician inserts a peripheral cannula for extracorporeal membrane oxygenation (ECMO)/ extracorporeal life support (ECLS) percutaneously. When veno-arterial ECMO/ECLS is performed, a cannula is typically placed in the inferior vena cava or right atrium allowing for drainage. This cannula is introduced at the internal jugular or femoral vein. The blood is pumped back into the patient through a cannula placed within the femoral artery. When veno-venous ECMO/ECLS is performed, two or more cannulae are used within the large veins (jugular, femoral, or both) to assist with draining and oxygenated blood flow. A relatively new dual-chamber cannula is being utilized in some facilities for improved drainage, to reduce the risk of complications, and to improve the ability to move the patient. Report 33951 for peripheral insertion of a cannula performed percutaneously on patients from birth through age 5 and 33952 for patients age 6 years and older. Fluoroscopic guidance is included in these procedures when performed.

33953-33954

The physician inserts a peripheral cannula for extracorporeal membrane oxygenation (ECMO)/ extracorporeal life support (ECLS) using an open approach. When veno-arterial ECMO/ECLS is performed, a cannula is typically placed in the inferior vena cava or right atrium allowing for drainage. This cannula is introduced at the internal jugular or femoral vein. The blood is pumped back into the patient through a cannula placed within the femoral artery. When veno-venous ECMO/ECLS is performed, two or more cannulae are used within the large veins (jugular, femoral, or both) to assist with draining and oxygenated blood flow. A relatively new dual-chamber cannula is being utilized in some facilities for improved drainage, to reduce the risk of complications, and to improve the ability to move the patient. Report 33953 for peripheral insertion of a cannula using an open approach on patients from birth through age 5 and 33954 for patients age 6 years and older.

33955-33956

The physician inserts central cannulae for extracorporeal membrane oxygenation (ECMO)/ extracorporeal life support (ECLS) via sternotomy or thoracotomy. A cannula is placed in the inferior vena cava or right atrium allowing for drainage. This cannula is introduced at the internal jugular or femoral vein accomplished by sternotomy or thoracotomy. The blood is pumped back into the patient through a cannula surgically placed within the ascending aorta, referred to as central ECMO/ECLS. This form of introduction is typically utilized following cardiopulmonary bypass since the location of cannulae placement would be the same as location during surgery. When veno-venous ECMO/ECLS is performed, two or more cannulae are used within the large veins (jugular, femoral, or both) to assist with draining and oxygenated blood flow. A relatively new dual-chamber cannula is being utilized in some facilities for improved drainage, to reduce the risk of complications, and to improve the ability to move the patient. Report 33955 for centrally inserted cannulae by sternotomy or thoracotomy performed on patients from birth through age 5 and 33956 for patients age 6 years and older.

33957-33958

The physician repositions a peripheral cannula used for extracorporeal membrane oxygenation (ECMO)/ extracorporeal life support (ECLS) percutaneously. Repositioning of the cannula may be necessary in the event of technical and/or vascular complications, such as blood flow obstruction, movement of the cannula from the original position, and/or bleeding issues resulting from the use of heparin during ECMO/ECLS. Oftentimes this requires a pull back of the cannula until it is back in an optimal position; however, in some cases, repositioning may require another procedure to achieve an appropriate position based on the specific location of the cannula and the complication. Report 33957 for percutaneous repositioning performed on a peripheral vessel for patients from birth through age 5 and 33958 for patients age 6 years and older. These codes include fluoroscopic guidance when performed.

33959 [33962]

The physician repositions a peripheral cannula used for extracorporeal membrane oxygenation (ECMO)/ extracorporeal life support (ECLS) via an open approach. Repositioning of the cannula may be necessary in the event of technical and/or vascular complications, such as blood flow obstruction, movement of the cannula from the original position, and/or bleeding issues resulting from the use of heparin during ECMO/ECLS. Oftentimes this requires a pull back of the cannula until it is back in an optimal position; however, in some cases, repositioning may require another procedure to achieve an appropriate position based on the specific location of the cannula and the complication. Report 33959 if the reposition is performed by open approach on a peripheral vessel for patients from birth through age 5 and 33962 for patients age 6 years and older. These codes include fluoroscopic guidance when performed.

[33963, 33964]

The physician repositions a central cannula used for extracorporeal membrane oxygenation (ECMO)/ extracorporeal life support (ECLS) via a sternotomy or thoracotomy. Repositioning of the cannula may be necessary in the event of technical and/or vascular complications, such as blood flow obstruction, movement of the cannula from the original position, and/or bleeding issues resulting from the use of heparin during ECMO/ECLS. Oftentimes this requires a pull back of the cannula until it is back in an optimal position; however, in some cases, repositioning may require another procedure to achieve an appropriate position based on the specific location of the cannula and the complication. Report 33963 for reposition of a central cannula by sternotomy or thoracotomy performed on patients from birth through age 5 and 33964 for patients age 6 years and older. These codes include fluoroscopic guidance when performed.

[33965, 33966]

When extracorporeal membrane oxygenation (ECMO)/ extracorporeal life support (ECLS) therapy is complete, the physician removes the cannula. Cannulae introduced percutaneously are simply pulled out like any other percutaneous placed catheter. Pressure is applied to the site for a limited time to stop bleeding. Report 33965 for removal of a peripheral percutaneous cannula for patients from birth through age 5 and 33966 for patients age 6 and older.

[33969, 33984]

When extracorporeal membrane oxygenation (ECMO)/ extracorporeal life support (ECLS) therapy is complete, the physician removes the cannula. Cannulae placed via an open procedure require surgical intervention, sometimes performed bedside. The vessels cannulated are repaired and the skin is closed with stitches. Some patients require continued ventilation upon discontinuation of ECMO/ECLS therapy. Report 33969 for removal of a peripheral cannula performed by open approach for patients from birth through age 5 and 33984 for patients age 6 and older.

[33985, 33986]

When extracorporeal membrane oxygenation (ECMO)/ extracorporeal life support (ECLS) therapy is complete, the physician removes the cannula. Cannulae placed via sternotomy or thoracotomy requires surgical intervention. The vessels cannulated are repaired and the skin is closed with stitches. Some patients require continued ventilation upon discontinuation of ECMO therapy. Report 33985 for removal of a central cannula performed by sternotomy or thoracotomy for patients from birth through age 5 and 33986 for patients age 6 and older.

[33987]

The physician inserts a cannula(e) to provide prolonged extracorporeal circulation for cardiopulmonary insufficiency. The artery is exposed to create a graft that will broaden the vessel upwards (similar to a chimney) from the main artery being utilized. The graft is placed next to the artery often allowing for improved blood flow to smaller branches. Creating this type of graft requires special attention to the length needed to effectively use this technique. This cannula carries blood that is low in oxygen and high in carbon dioxide into the extracorporeal membrane oxygenation (ECMO) circuit. In veno-venous ECMO, if a double lumen cannula was inserted, blood that has passed through the membrane oxygenator that is now high in oxygen and low in carbon dioxide (oxygenated blood) is rewarmed to body temperature and returned via the same cannula. If a single lumen cannula is used, a second cannula is inserted into a second vein (venovenous ECMO) or a main artery (venoarterial ECMO), usually the femoral but in children the carotid may be used.

This second cannula passes from the ECMO circuit carrying oxygenated, rewarmed blood back to the vein or artery.

[33988, 33989]

The physician inserts a cannula(e) to provide extracorporeal membrane oxygenation (ECMO) or extracorporeal life support services (ECLS). A small incision is made to access the vessel. A single or double lumen cannula is inserted and passed into the inferior vena cava or right atrium. This cannula carries blood that is low in oxygen and high in carbon dioxide into the ECMO circuit. If a single lumen cannula is used, a second cannula is inserted into a main artery (venoarterial ECMO), usually the femoral but in children the carotid may be used. This second cannula passes from the ECMO circuit carrying oxygenated, rewarmed blood back to the vein or artery. This process reduces the amount of work the cardiac muscle must provide and if recovery is anticipated, ventricle expansion should be minimal and is often achieved by placing a catheter (to vent) in the left ventricle for draining. ECMO with ventricular decompression can be attained by insertion of a vent catheter directly into the left ventricle. Through an open incision into the thorax, the vent cannula is most commonly inserted into the pulmonary artery and positioned in the left ventricle. Report 33988 for insertion of the left heart vent and 33989 for removal of the left heart vent.

33967

An intra-aortic balloon catheter, usually with a 40 cc volume capacity, is inserted into the femoral artery and advanced under fluoroscopy to the distal portion of the aortic arch. After correct placement of the intra-aortic balloon assist device (IAB) in the descending aorta with its tip at the distal aortic arch, the balloon is connected to a drive console. The console consists of a pressurized gas reservoir, a monitor for ECG and pressure wave recording, adjustments for inflation/deflation timing, triggering selection switches, and battery back-up power sources. Helium or carbon dioxide is used for inflation. Inflation and deflation are synchronized to the patient's cardiac cycle. Inflation at the onset of diastole results in proximal and distal displacement of blood volume in the aorta. Deflation occurs just prior to the onset of systole. Once the patient's cardiac performance improves, weaning from the intra-aortic balloon catheter pump (IABP) begins by gradually decreasing the balloon augmentation ratio under control of hemodynamic stability.

33968

The physician removes an intra-aortic balloon assist device (IABP). In a previous separately reportable procedure an IABP was inserted. When the patient is stabilized they are weaned off of the IAPB. The pump is turned off and the IABP catheter with the attached balloon is withdrawn from the femoral artery. Pressure is placed over the wound in the groin for a specified period of time. A light dressing is applied. The patient may be placed at bed rest and observed for several hours to avoid problems that could arise from bleeding or a hematoma at the puncture site.

33970

This operation is done to help support the function of the left ventricle of the heart. The left or right femoral artery is exposed in the groin. After the vessel is occluded above and below the proposed insertion site, the artery is opened transversely. In some cases, the end of a small tube of Gortex may be sewn to the side of the artery. The tip of the balloon catheter is inserted into the artery (or Gortex tube). The clamp occluding the artery upstream is released and the balloon catheter is advanced through the femoral artery and into the aorta above the level of the kidney arteries, but not beyond the left arm artery. It is connected to a pump and the pump is turned on. The pump inflates and deflates the balloon during each heartbeat cycle.

33971

The previously placed balloon pump is withdrawn and the artery is occluded above and below the hole. If a Gortex sleeve has been used, it is simply tied off and no other repair is needed. If the balloon was directly introduced into the artery, the hole is sewn shut. If sewing the hole shut narrows the artery significantly, the hole can be patched with a piece of saphenous vein or Dacron. If the arterial diameter has been damaged, the segment of artery containing the hole can be removed and the artery replaced with an interposition graft of saphenous vein or Dacron tube.

33973

The procedure is performed when the femoral arteries cannot be readily exposed in the operating room because of patient positioning; the arteries are occluded by atherosclerosis or trauma; or there will be a need to reopen the patient's chest soon. A balloon placed in this fashion must be removed in the operating room and the chest must be reopened. A purse string is placed in the aorta. A hole is made in the aorta in the middle of the purse string. The balloon is inserted through this hole until it lies beyond the left arm artery but above the kidney arteries. The purse string is tightened with a tourniquet. The chest incision is not closed. The balloon is driven by a pump outside the patient.

33974

The physician removes an ascending aortic intra-aortic balloon assist device during performance of a primary procedure. If the sternum is open, the physician removes the aortic balloon while tightening purse-string sutures around the hole. When hemostasis is assured, the pericardium is repaired loosely with or without graft, leaving gaps for blood and fluid to drain into the pleural space. The sternum is reanastomosed with sternal wires and the skin is sutured in layers. If the sternum is closed, a Dacron-tube graft (reported separately) is used as a vehicle for balloon removal. As the balloon is removed, the Dacron-tube graft tightens around the aortic incision to create aortic hemostasis.

33975-33976

Cardiopulmonary bypass is required. For right ventricular failure, a pump uptake tube is placed in the right ventricular apex. A pump delivery tube is placed in the pulmonary artery. The pump is turned on and the patient is weaned off cardiopulmonary bypass. For left ventricular failure, the pump uptake tube is placed in one of the pulmonary veins or in the left ventricle apex. The arterial delivery tube is placed in the aorta. The pump is turned on and the patient is removed from cardiopulmonary bypass. The implanted pump is placed in a pocket formed in the upper abdominal wall, but outside the abdominal cavity. Tubes for the pump drive are brought out through separate incisions in the skin. The pump is started and the patient is weaned off cardiopulmonary bypass. The device is removed when the patient's ventricle recovers, a total artificial heart is placed or the patient undergoes heart transplantation. Report 33976 if biventricular support is needed.

33977-33978

Cardiopulmonary bypass is required. The pump is stopped. All the tubes are removed and any holes in the heart or vessels are closed. The device is removed from the patient's body. Cardiopulmonary bypass is discontinued when the patient's heart function returns. An intra-aortic balloon pump is often required to allow discontinuation of bypass. All wounds are closed. Report 33978 if biventricular support is needed.

33979-33980

The physician makes a midline incision extending from the sternal notch to the umbilicus. Sternotomy is performed prior to creation of the pocket. The preperitoneal fat is dissected from the undersurface of the rectus sheath using low-power cautery. Superiorly the dissection is carried to the undersurface of the diaphragm until the apex of the heart can be palpated just lateral to the inferior phrenic artery and vein and carried well back into the retroperitoneum. The preperitoneal space is opened to allow room for the device outflow valve and graft conduit. The muscular attachment of the right hemidiaphragm to the medial edge of the sternum is divided to allow room for the graft. A small incision is made and a tunneling device is passed subcutaneously inferiorly around the umbilicus, and into the pocket through the rectus sheath at its most inferior aspect. The tunneler is screwed onto the end of the drive line, which is pulled back through the tunnel to the skin. The drive line is not attached to the skin. Cardiopulmonary bypass is instituted using standard aortic and dual stage venous cannulae. The apex of the left ventricle is elevated. The physician cores out a piece of ventricle and places the apical cuff sutures. An apical vent is passed into the left ventricle. Pledgeted 2-0 Ethibond sutures are placed circumferentially partial thickness into the myocardium and passed through the sewing ring of the apical cuff. Once the apical cuff is secure, a cruciate incision in the diaphragm opposite the ventricular apex is made just lateral to the inferior phrenic vessels, and the inflow cannula is brought into the chest. The inflow cannula is inserted through the apical cuff until the sintered titanium surface is within the cuff. The Dacron tie of the inflow cuff is secured and an additional plastic band and Dacron tie are used to reinforce the connection and flatten out the silicone cuff. Blood is allowed to passively fill the device and exit via the outflow valve. A partial occluding clamp is placed on the right lateral aspect of the ascending aorta and a longitudinal aortotomy is performed. The periaortic adventitia is left in place and a strip of pericardium is incorporated into the anastomosis. The apex and heel of the anastomosis are reinforced with interrupted 4-0 Prolene pledgeted horizontal mattress stitches. Inotropic support is started before separating from bypass and activating the LVAD. The device is switched to automatic mode after the cessation of cardiopulmonary bypass. Transesophageal echocardiography is used to ensure adequate ventricular decompression and a bubble study is performed to rule out a patent foramen ovale. A thermodilution cardiac output is performed and compared to the output from the LVAD. In the presence of severe coagulopathy, the chest may need to be packed open. The device is removed (33980) when the patient's ventricle recovers, an artificial heart is placed, or the patient undergoes heart transplantation.

33981

The physician replaces the blood pump component of an extracorporeal ventricular assist device (VAD). The previously implanted pump, which was placed in a pocket formed in the upper abdominal wall (but outside the abdominal cavity), is removed. Pump replacement includes removal of the existing pump, insertion of a new pump, connection, de-airing, and new pump initiation. Report 33981 for one or more pumps; this code reports pump replacement of single or biventricular VAD systems.

33982-33983

The physician replaces the blood pump component of an implantable, intracorporeal, single ventricle VAD (ventricular assist device). This may be accomplished without cardiopulmonary bypass (33982) or with cardiopulmonary bypass (33983). Pump replacement includes removal of the existing pump, insertion of a new pump, connection, de-airing, and new pump initiation.

33990-33991 [33995]

The physician performs a percutaneous insertion of a ventricular assist device (VAD) into the left, right, or both ventricles (lower chambers) of the heart. This mechanical pump assists in pushing blood from the ventricles. The procedure may be temporary for some until the heart regains the ability to pump blood on its own again (bridge to recovery), for patients awaiting heart transplant (bridge to transplant), or permanent in those who are ineligible for heart transplantation due to age or medical conditions (destination therapy). A percutaneous right ventricular assist device (RVAD) is reported with 33995. One approach described by this

Cardiovascular

code involves placing two venous cannulas (typically two femoral venous cannulas or one femoral and one internal jugular venous cannula). One is positioned in the right atrium and another in the pulmonary artery. An extracorporeal centrifugal pump is used, with the inflow from the right atrial cannula and the outflow to the pulmonary artery. A left ventricular assist device (LVAD) bypasses the left ventricle during the blood oxygenation cycle, making the ventricle work less during the systolic phase. In percutaneous placement of an LVAD, a catheter is inserted in the patient's femoral vein and maneuvered to the left atrium. A centrifugal assist device is placed outside the body, usually on the patient's thigh. The catheter is attached to the device. Oxygenated blood is pumped from the left atrium to the device and distributed to one or both femoral arteries via catheter. Report 33990 when the LVAD is inserted with a single arterial access. Report 33991 if the septum is punctured for left atrial access and the procedure includes both arterial and venous access. These codes include radiological supervision and interpretation.

33992

A left ventricular assist device (LVAD) bypasses the left ventricle during the blood oxygenation cycle making the ventricle work less during the systolic phase. The device is removed when the patient's ventricle recovers, an artificial heart is placed, or the patient undergoes heart transplantation. The arterial or arterial and venous cannulas are removed, and the external centrifugal assist device is discontinued and removed. This code can only be reported for the removal of an LVAD during a different operative encounter than the insertion, and is only used for a percutaneous LVAD, not an implantable LVAD.

[33997]

A right ventricular assist device (RVAD) assists the right ventricle in pumping blood to the pulmonary artery and is typically only used for short-term, right ventricular support following left ventricular assist device (LVAD) surgery or other heart surgery. The device is removed when the patient's right ventricle recovers sufficiently. The venous cannula is removed, and the external centrifugal assist device is discontinued and removed. This code can only be reported for the removal of an RVAD during a different operative encounter than the insertion, and is only used for a percutaneous RVAD, not an implantable RVAD.

33993

A left ventricular assist device (LVAD) is the most common type of VAD, helping the left ventricle pump blood to the aorta. A right ventricular assist device (RVAD) assists the right ventricle in pumping blood to the pulmonary artery and is typically used only for short-term, right ventricular support following LVAD surgery or other cardiac surgery. Report 33993 when the components of a percutaneously placed LVAD or RVAD need to be repositioned at any time other than during the surgical encounter for insertion. This code includes imaging guidance.

34001

To remove a blood clot in the carotid, subclavian, or innominate artery, the physician makes an incision in the skin of the neck usually in front of the sternocleidomastoid muscle over the site of the clot or immediately above it. The artery is isolated and dissected from critical structures. The artery may be clamped above and below the clot and incised. The physician removes the blood clot and sutures the artery. The clamps are removed. If a catheter is required, it is threaded past the clot and a small balloon at its tip is inflated. The catheter is withdrawn, capturing and retrieving the clot. The physician may make several passes to remove the entire clot. The blood vessel is repaired with sutures and the skin incision is repaired with layered closure.

34051

The physician exposes the innominate or subclavian artery by making an incision in the anterior chest (midline sternotomy or lateral thoracotomy). The physician identifies the embolus or thrombus and occludes the artery proximal to the clot. The physician makes a small incision in the artery proximal to the clot and withdraws it using ring forceps, or by passing a Fogarty balloon catheter beyond the clot, inflating and withdrawing the balloon. The physician establishes proof of patency by injecting contrast in the artery under fluoroscope. The physician sutures the arteriotomy closed, removes the vascular clamp or tie, and closes the chest wall. The physician may leave chest tubes and/or a mediastinal drainage tube in place following the procedure.

34101

To remove a blood clot in the axillary, brachial, innominate, or subclavian artery, the physician makes an incision in the skin of the arm at the site of the blood clot or above it. The artery is isolated and dissected from critical structures. The artery may be clamped above and below the clot, and incised. The physician removes the blood clot and repairs the artery. The clamps are removed. If a catheter is required, it is threaded past the clot and a small balloon at its tip is inflated. The catheter is withdrawn, capturing and retrieving the clot. The physician may make several passes to remove all of the clot. The blood vessel is repaired with sutures and the skin incision is repaired with a layered closure.

34111

To remove a blood clot in the radial or ulnar artery, the physician makes an incision in the skin of the arm, over the site of the clot or immediately above it. The artery is isolated and dissected from adjacent critical structures. The artery may be clamped above and below the clot, and incised. The physician removes the blood clot and repairs the artery. The clamps are removed. If a catheter is required, it is threaded past the clot and a small balloon at its tip is inflated. The catheter is withdrawn, capturing and retrieving the clot. The physician may make several passes to remove all of the clot. The blood vessel is repaired with sutures and the skin incision is repaired with a layered closure.

34151
To remove a blood clot in the renal, celiac, mesentery, or aortoiliac artery, the physician makes an incision in the skin of the abdomen over the site of the clot or immediately above or below it. The artery is isolated and dissected from adjacent critical structures. The artery may be clamped above and below the clot and incised. The physician removes the blood clot. The clamps are removed. If a catheter is required, it is threaded past the clot and a small balloon at its tip is inflated. The catheter is withdrawn, capturing and retrieving the clot. The physician may make several passes to remove the entire clot. The blood vessel is repaired with sutures and the skin incision is repaired with a layered closure.

34201
To remove a blood clot in the femoropopliteal or aortoiliac artery, the physician makes an incision in the skin of the leg over the femoral artery. The artery is isolated and dissected from adjacent critical structures. The artery may be clamped above and below the clot and incised. The physician removes the blood clot and repairs the vessel. The clamps are removed. If a catheter is required, it is threaded past the clot and a small balloon at its tip is inflated. The catheter is withdrawn, capturing and retrieving the clot. The physician may make several passes to remove all of the clot. The blood vessel is repaired with sutures and the skin incision is repaired with a layered closure.

34203
To remove a blood clot in the popliteal-tibio-peroneal artery, the physician makes an incision in the skin of the leg over the femoral or popliteal artery. The artery is isolated and dissected from adjacent critical structures. The artery may be clamped above and below the clot and incised. The physician removes the blood clot. The clamps are removed. If a catheter is required, it is threaded past the clot and a small balloon at its tip is inflated. The catheter is withdrawn, capturing and retrieving the clot. The physician may make several passes to remove all of the clot. The blood vessel is repaired with sutures and the skin incision is repaired with a layered closure.

34401
The physician exposes the vena cava or iliac vein by making an abdominal incision. The physician identifies the thrombus by venogram and may perform a contralateral femoral venogram to rule out inferior vena caval involvement. The physician makes an incision in the vena cava or iliac vein. The physician withdraws the clot by passing a Fogarty balloon catheter beyond the clot, inflating and withdrawing the balloon. The physician may attempt to reduce the risk of pulmonary embolism by increasing intrathoracic pressure in a ventilated patient. The physician may establish proof of patency by repeat venography. The physician sutures the venotomy closed and closes the wound.

34421
To remove a blood clot in the vena cava, iliac, or femoropopliteal vein, the physician makes an incision in the skin of the upper leg over the site of the clot or immediately above or below it. The vein is isolated and dissected from adjacent critical structures. The vein may be clamped above and below the clot and incised. The physician removes the blood clot. The clamps are removed. If a catheter is required, it is threaded past the clot and a small balloon at its tip is inflated. The catheter is withdrawn, capturing and retrieving the clot. The physician may make several passes to remove all of the clot. The blood vessel is repaired with sutures and the skin incision is repaired with a layered closure.

34451
The physician exposes the vena cava, iliac, or femoropopliteal veins by making abdominal and leg incisions. The physician identifies the thrombus by venogram and may perform a contralateral femoral venogram to rule out inferior vena caval involvement. An incision is made over the site of the clot or immediately above or below it. The vein is isolated and dissected from adjacent critical structures. The vein may be clamped above and below the clot and incised. The physician removes the blood clot. The clamps are removed. The physician may cut down and introduce a Fogarty catheter via the popliteal vein, advancing the catheter toward the femoral vein while extruding thrombus through the femoral venotomy. The physician withdraws the clot by passing a Fogarty balloon catheter beyond the clot, inflating, and withdrawing the balloon. The physician may establish proof of patency by repeat venography. The physician sutures the venotomy closed and closes the wound.

34471
To remove a blood clot in the subclavian vein, the physician makes an incision in the skin of the neck over the site of the clot or immediately above or below it. The vein is isolated and dissected from adjacent critical structures. The vein may be clamped above and below the clot and incised. The physician removes the blood clot. The clamps are removed. If a catheter is required, it is threaded past the clot and a small balloon at its tip is inflated. The catheter is withdrawn, capturing and retrieving the clot. The physician may make several passes to remove the entire clot. The blood vessel is repaired with sutures and the skin incision is repaired with layered closure.

34490
To remove a blood clot in the axillary and subclavian vein, the physician makes an incision in the skin of the arm over the site of the clot or immediately above or below it. The vein is isolated and dissected from adjacent critical structures. The vein may be clamped above and below the clot and incised. The physician removes the blood clot. The clamps are removed. If a catheter is required, it is threaded past the clot and a small balloon at its tip is inflated. The catheter is withdrawn, capturing and retrieving the clot. The physician may make several passes to remove the

entire clot. The blood vessel is repaired with sutures and the skin incision is repaired with layered closure.

34501
The physician makes an incision in the skin overlying the site of the incompetent valve. The femoral vein is isolated and dissected from adjacent critical structures. The physician affixes vessel clamps above and below the malfunctioning valve. The physician opens the vein and repairs the valve leaflets by suture plication (tacking the excess valve material). The vein is repaired with sutures. The clamps are removed and the skin incision is repaired with a layered closure.

34502
The physician exposes the inferior vena cava by making an incision in the anterior abdomen. Clamps are placed on the vena cava proximally and any defects are sutured closed. Abnormal vena caval tissue may be replaced or bypassed with synthetic graft material. An injection of intravenous contrast may be administered under fluoroscopy to demonstrate appropriate flow. The clamps are removed and the abdominal wall incision is closed. A surgical drain may be left in place at the conclusion of the procedure.

34510
The physician makes an incision in the skin overlying the site of the malfunctioning valve. The vein is isolated and dissected from adjacent critical structures. The physician affixes vessel clamps above and below the vein and excises the section of vein containing the malfunctioning valve. A section of harvested vein containing functional valves is sutured end-to-end to the vein. The clamps are removed and the skin incision is repaired with a layered closure.

34520
The physician makes an incision in the skin overlying the site of the incompetent valve. The incompetent vein is isolated and dissected from adjacent critical structures. The physician affixes vessel clamps above and below the vein. The divided section of incompetent vein is connected to a nearby vein with functioning valves, placing competent valves above the incompetent vein. Both the vein and the skin incision are closed with sutures.

34530
The physician makes an incision in the skin overlying the site of the greater saphenous vein just below the knee. The vein is isolated and dissected from adjacent critical structures. The physician affixes vessel clamps above and below the incision site. The dissected section of saphenous vein is connected to the popliteal vein in an end-to-side anastomosis. The other end of the saphenous vein is closed with sutures. Once the saphenous vein and the popliteal vein are connected, the clamps are removed and the skin incision is repaired with layered closure.

34701-34702
The physician introduces, positions, and deploys an endograft to treat abdominal aortic conditions, with or without rupture, such as an aneurysm, pseudoaneurysm, dissection, penetrating ulcer, or traumatic disruption located in the infrarenal abdominal aorta that may or may not extend into the iliac arteries. A covered stent may be referred to using terms such as endovascular graft, endoprosthesis, endograft, or stent graft. The infrarenal aortic endograft may be an aortic tube device, a bifurcated unibody device, a modular bifurcated docking system with docking limbs, or an aorto-uni-iliac device. The abdominal aortic treatment zone is defined as the infrarenal aorta. This procedure requires a vascular surgeon and a radiologist. In 34701, an incision is made over the femoral artery, which is normally used for access, and a guidewire is threaded into the blood vessel. A catheter with a stent-transporting tip is advanced over the guidewire into the vessel. The catheter carries the aortic tube prosthesis, approximately 6 inches long and contained inside a holding capsule, through the arterial tree to the site of the aortic infrarenal aneurysm. Once the stent is in proper position, the holding capsule is removed and the stent is deployed, expanding like a spring to anchor itself to normal walls of the aorta above and below the aneurysm. The device serves as a substitute channel for blood flow. If full expansion of the prosthesis does not occur, or leaks are present, a balloon catheter is threaded to the graft site and inflated within the prosthesis until full expansion is achieved and leaking is stopped. The catheter/guidewire is removed and the arteriotomy site is closed. The aneurysm, excluded from the blood flow, typically shrinks over time. The treatment zone for endograft procedures is defined by those vessels that contain an endograft (main body, docking limbs, and/or extensions) deployed during that operative session. Report 34702 when endovascular repair is performed on a ruptured aneurysm in the aorta. Rupture is defined as clinical and/or radiographic evidence of acute hemorrhage. A chronic, contained rupture is considered a pseudoaneurysm and its endovascular treatment is reported with 34701. Nonselective catheterization is included in these codes. Balloon angioplasty and/or stenting at the sealing zone of an endograft is an integral part of the procedure. Fluoroscopic guidance and radiological supervision and interpretation in conjunction with endograft repair is not reported separately, and includes all intraprocedural imaging (e.g., angiography, rotational CT) of the aorta and its branches prior to deployment of the endovascular device, fluoroscopic guidance, and roadmapping used in the delivery of the endovascular components, and intraprocedural and completion angiography (e.g., confirm position, detect endoleak, evaluate runoff) performed at the time of the endovascular infrarenal aorta repair.

34703-34706
The physician introduces, positions, and deploys an endograft to treat abdominal aortic conditions, with or without rupture, such as an aneurysm, pseudoaneurysm, dissection, penetrating ulcer, or traumatic disruption located in the infrarenal abdominal aorta that may or may not extend into the

iliac arteries. A covered stent may be referred to as an endovascular graft, endoprosthesis, endograft, or stent graft. The infrarenal aortic endograft may be an aortic tube device, a bifurcated unibody device, a modular bifurcated docking system with docking limbs, or an aorto-uni-iliac device. In 34703 and 34704, the abdominal aortic treatment zone is typically defined as the infrarenal aorta and ipsilateral common iliac artery. In 34705 and 34706, the abdominal aortic treatment zone is typically defined as the infrarenal aorta and both common iliac arteries. These procedures require a vascular surgeon and a radiologist. In 34703, under general anesthesia, a small incision is made in the groin over one femoral artery or both femoral arteries through which the endovascular devices are inserted. If contralateral femoral access is necessary, a percutaneous sheath may be placed. An aorta-uni-iliac prosthetic graft device contained inside a plastic holding capsule is threaded through the arteries to the site of the infrarenal aneurysm. The endograft is deployed by slowly removing the holding capsule away from the endograft, with continual monitoring of exact positioning. Once the prosthesis is in place, the holding capsule is removed. Balloon angioplasty is performed at the ends of the prosthesis to expand and seat the graft. Stents are deployed within the body of the endograft to maintain expansion forces. The aorta-uni-iliac prosthetic endograft is supported along its length by a series of metal rings sutured to the graft and is held in place by the radial force applied by the rings to the patient's aorta. Once in place, the arteriotomy site is closed. Report 34705 for simultaneous bilateral iliac artery aneurysm repairs with aorto-bi-iliac endograft. Report 34704 and 34706 when endovascular repair is performed on a ruptured aneurysm in the aorta or iliac arteries. Rupture is defined as clinical and/or radiographic evidence of acute hemorrhage. A chronic, contained rupture is considered a pseudoaneurysm and its endovascular treatment is reported with 34703 and 34705. Nonselective catheterization is included in 34703, 34704, 34705, and 34706. Balloon angioplasty and/or stenting at the sealing zone of an endograft is an integral part of the procedure. Fluoroscopic guidance and radiological supervision and interpretation in conjunction with endograft repair is not separately reported, and includes all intraprocedural imaging (e.g., angiography, rotational CT) of the aorta and its branches prior to deployment of the endovascular device, fluoroscopic guidance and roadmapping used in the delivery of the endovascular components, and intraprocedural and completion angiography (e.g., confirm position, detect endoleak, evaluate runoff) performed at the time of the endovascular infrarenal aorta and/or iliac repair.

34707-34708

The physician introduces, positions, and deploys an ilio-iliac endograft for treatment of isolated arterial pathology (with or without rupture), such as an aneurysm, pseudoaneurysm, dissection, arteriovenous malformation, or trauma involving the iliac artery. The treatment zone is defined as the portion of the iliac artery (e.g., common, internal, external iliac arteries) involved. The procedure requires a vascular surgeon and a radiologist. The patient receives medication (Heparin) to help prevent blood clots prior to the procedure. In 34707, under general anesthesia, the physician makes a small incision near the patient's hip bone area to enter the iliac artery. A proprietary device is used, which is comprised of two main components: a trunk component and a contralateral leg component. The endoprosthesis, contained inside a holding device, is introduced into the artery under fluoroscopy and positioned at the target zone area of repair by threading guidewires and catheters. Nonselective catheterization is included. Report 34708 when endovascular repair is performed on a ruptured aneurysm in the iliac artery. Rupture is defined as clinical and/or radiographic evidence of acute hemorrhage. A chronic, contained rupture is considered a pseudoaneurysm, and its endovascular treatment is reported with 34707. Balloon angioplasty and/or stenting at the treatment zone of an endograft is an integral part of the procedure. Fluoroscopic guidance and radiological supervision and interpretation, in conjunction with endograft repair, are not reported separately. Included are all intraprocedural imaging (e.g., angiography, rotational CT) of the iliac artery prior to deployment of the endovascular device, fluoroscopic guidance and roadmapping used in the delivery of the endovascular components, and intraprocedural and completion angiography (e.g., confirm position, detect endoleak, evaluate runoff) performed at the time of the endovascular iliac repair.

[34717]

At the time of aorto-iliac artery endograft placement, the physician repairs a unilateral iliac artery rupture, aneurysm, pseudoaneurysm, arteriovenous (AV) malformation, dissection, penetrating ulcer, or traumatic disruption by placing an iliac branched endograft. The endograft, contained inside a holding device, is introduced into the artery under fluoroscopy and positioned at the target zone area of repair. This may require open access exposure of the artery or may be accomplished by threading guidewires and catheters through to the site. Once the endoprosthesis is in place, it is deployed within the artery at the targeted site. The position of the endoprosthesis is confirmed, any endoleaks are identified, and the status of runoff vessels is evaluated for any related stenosis, dissection, thrombosis, or embolism. All selective ipsilateral catheterization(s) necessary for device placement, device selection and preprocedural sizing, endograft extension(s), angioplasty or stenting within the treatment zone, as well as radiological supervision and interpretation are included in this procedure. Report 34717, once per side, in addition to the code for the primary procedure.

34709

The physician places an extension prosthesis distal to the common iliac artery or proximal to the renal artery for endovascular repair of an infrarenal abdominal aortic or iliac aneurysm, pseudoaneurysm, dissection or penetrating ulcer that terminates in the internal iliac, external iliac, or common femoral arteries or in the abdominal aorta proximal to the renal arteries. Using separately reportable aortography, the target site is identified. The proper extension prosthesis is selected. Under separately reportable fluoroscopy, the extension prosthesis, contained inside a long plastic holding capsule, is threaded through the arteries to the leak site. Once the extension prosthesis is in place, the holding capsule is removed. The extension prosthesis, activated by heat, expands like a spring and becomes anchored to the artery wall at the site of the endoleak. If full expansion of the prosthesis does not occur automatically, a balloon catheter is threaded to the graft site and inflated within the endovascular prosthesis until full expansion is achieved. The catheter is removed and the arteriotomy site is closed. Report 34709 once per vessel treated.

[34718]

The physician repairs a unilateral iliac artery aneurysm, pseudoaneurysm, arteriovenous (AV) malformation, dissection, or penetrating ulcer by placing an iliac branched endograft. The endograft, contained inside a holding device, is introduced into the artery under fluoroscopy and positioned at the target zone area of repair. This may require open access exposure of the artery or may be accomplished by threading guidewires and catheters through to the site. Once the endoprosthesis is in place, it is deployed within the artery at the targeted site. The position of the endoprosthesis is confirmed, any endoleaks are identified, and the status of runoff vessels is evaluated for any related stenosis, dissection, thrombosis, or embolism. All selective ipsilateral catheterization(s) necessary for device placement, device selection and preprocedural sizing, endograft extension(s), angioplasty or stenting within the treatment zone, as well as radiological supervision and interpretation is included in this procedure. Placement of an aorto-iliac artery endograft is not performed during this session.

34710-34711

The physician performs delayed endovascular placement of a distal or proximal extension prosthesis to repair an infrarenal abdominal aortic or iliac aneurysm, pseudoaneurysm, dissection, endoleak, or endograft migration. A leak may occur at fixation sites of a grafted aneurysm through the body of the graft or from patent arteries within the aneurysm sac and may require endovascular reparation. Using separately reportable aortography, the target site is identified. The proper extension prosthesis is selected. Under separately reportable fluoroscopy, the extension prosthesis, contained inside a long plastic holding capsule, is threaded through the arteries to the leak site. Once the extension prosthesis is in place, the holding capsule is removed. The extension prosthesis, activated by heat, expands like a spring and becomes anchored to the artery wall at the site of the endoleak. If full expansion of the prosthesis does not occur automatically, a balloon catheter is threaded to the graft site and inflated within the endovascular prosthesis until full expansion is achieved. The catheter is removed and the arteriotomy site is closed. These procedures include all nonselective catheterizations, sizing, and device selection prior to the procedure; radiological supervision and interpretation; and treatment zone angioplasty or stenting, when performed. These codes may only be reported once per vessel treated (e.g., multiple endograft extensions placed in a single vessel may only be reported once). Report 34710 for placement of an extension prosthesis in the initial vessel and 34711 for placement of an extension prosthesis in each additional vessel.

34712

The physician performs transcatheter delivery of accessory-enhanced fixation devices, such as an anchor, screw, or tack, to the endograft. Commonly referred to as a bioprosthesis, this procedure is used for patients with abdominal aortic and/or iliac artery conditions, such as an aneurysm with complex anatomies, or for patients who are experiencing an endoleak. Proprietary devices ensure a safe and effective treatment solution for these types of repairs. They enhance durability to the level of a surgical anastomosis and address concerns for future complications. They are used to improve fixation and sealing of an endovascular graft, either in primary cases or to fix endoleaks and stent migration. The devices lock the endograft to the abdominal aorta and/or iliac artery to secure the patient's future and maximize outcomes in challenging patients. The fixation devices quickly identify, aim, and activate a sealing mechanism to close up endoleaks. Endoanchors are used to repair an endovascular graft in cases where the original graft has moved away from the implant site and developed endoleaks. In such cases, augmented fixation and/or sealing is required to regain or maintain effective aneurysm exclusion. These devices can be placed during the initial endoprosthesis placement procedure or for a subsequent repair procedure. Percutaneous access using a sheath smaller than 12 French is included in 34712 and is not reported separately. Radiologic supervision and interpretation are included in this procedure.

34713-34714 [34812]

The femoral artery may be accessed percutaneously or by open incision. For percutaneous access the femoral artery is identified using ultrasound guidance and the guide catheter is percutaneously inserted with subsequent insertion of a large arterial sheath (i.e., 12 French or larger). Closure may involve the use of an arterial closure device (ACD). Several types of ACDs may be used for closure including a small balloon that ensures sealant coverage of the arteriotomy, four needles that anchor and close suture material upon removal, or a collagen sponge with polymer that forms a self-tightening suture seal. Alternately, the femoral artery may be examined via an open technique. With the patient in the supine position, the physician exposes the femoral artery through an incision in the groin area revealing the femoral artery on one side while underlying subcutaneous layers and muscles incised to reach the artery are placed out of the way as hemostasis is achieved in preparation for delivery of the endograft, endovascular prosthesis, or creation of a conduit. Closure may be by direct suture. Report 34713 for percutaneous access and closure of a femoral arteriotomy for delivery of an endovascular prosthesis. Ultrasound guidance is included. Report 34812 for open femoral artery exposure with delivery of an endovascular prosthesis and repair and closure of the femoral artery. Report 34714 for open femoral artery exposure with endovascular device delivery or establishment of cardiopulmonary bypass that requires creation of a prosthetic conduit utilizing a femoral artery.

[34820]

The physician makes an abdominal or retroperitoneal incision to expose the iliac artery on one side to facilitate the delivery of an endovascular prosthesis or to perform temporary iliac artery occlusion during a procedure for endovascular therapy. The patient is placed supine and the buttocks are elevated. An incision is made parallel with and just above the inguinal ligament. The incision is in the middle third of a proximally curved line extending from the anterior superior iliac spine to the pubic symphysis. Hemostasis of vessels is achieved and the aponeuroses of the external and internal oblique and the transversus muscles are incised parallel to the inguinal ligament. The structures are reflected upward and medially, the transversalis fascia is opened, and the retroperitoneal space is entered. The iliac artery is exposed in preparation for delivering an endovascular prosthesis and its sheath is opened with tape placed about it. If the artery has been exposed for the purpose of placing a temporary occlusion device, the clamp is placed.

[34833, 34834]

In 34833, a conduit is created for the delivery of an endovascular prosthesis or for the establishment of cardiopulmonary bypass via transabdominal or retroperitoneal incision. A skin incision is made parallel with and just above the inguinal ligament. The skin is incised and the retroperitoneal space is entered to access the iliac artery. Bowels, blood vessels, and other soft tissue are mobilized from the area to give clear access to the iliac artery. With adequate exposure, loops are passed around the vessel proximally and distally. Anticoagulation is achieved and vascular clamps are applied. An arteriotomy is made for creation of the conduit, which is formed by placing a tubular piece of bypass graft material that has been fashioned into the right size onto the iliac artery and suturing it together. The conduit is clamped and the vascular clamps are removed from the iliac artery. Additional sutures are placed as needed. Through the newly created conduit, endovascular repair by deployment of a prosthesis may be undertaken. After the repair is complete, the conduit may be closed in one of two ways. The open end of the conduit may be sewn to the distal external iliac artery, and thereby left in place as a channel for external iliac bypass graft, or it may be cut close to the iliac artery and simply oversewn with sutures. This code reports the creation of the conduit, not the endovascular repair. In 34834, open brachial artery exposure is done for delivery of an endovascular prosthesis. An incision is made in the skin of the upper arm and nerves, blood vessels, and other soft tissues are mobilized from the area to give clear access to the brachial artery. With adequate exposure, loops are passed around the vessel proximally and distally. Anticoagulation is achieved and vascular clamps are alternately applied and removed as needed for introduction of guidewires, sheaths, and catheters through the brachial artery for accomplishing deployment of an aortic or iliac endovascular prosthesis. After the endovascular repair is complete, the opening remaining in the brachial artery is closed with fine sutures after irrigation and trimming of the edges has been done. Hemostasis is achieved and the wound is irrigated and closed. This code reports the open brachial artery exposure, not the endovascular repair.

34715-34716

The physician exposes the axillary or subclavian artery for delivery of an endovascular prosthesis and performs closure of the artery with an arterial closure device (ACD). In one method, an ACD is inserted through the existing procedural sheath. A small balloon is inflated within the artery and pulled back to the arterial wall, serving as an anchor to ensure proper placement, and is inflated. The balloon is deflated and removed through the tract, leaving behind only the expanded sealant, which seals the arteriotomy. In an alternate method, an ACD utilizes four needles (two sutures) directed outward from within the arterial lumen. It is advanced over a guidewire until blood return indicates proper placement. When the physician pulls the device handle, the needles are deployed and pulled through the arterial wall. The needles remain contained within the device shaft and are removed by pulling them up through the device shaft, leaving behind the suture ends, which are then tied and the device is removed. Yet another method uses an ACD composed of collagen sponge and polymer anchor joined together with a self-tightening suture that seals and sandwiches the arteriotomy for a more complete closure. The device stops the flow of blood mechanically, which is supported by the platelet-inducing properties of the collagen. Report 34715 for delivery of an endovascular prosthesis by axillary or subclavian exposure through an infraclavicular or supraclavicular or sternotomy incision during endovascular aneurysm repair. The patient is placed in supine position and open incision is made. Hemostasis of vessels is achieved. The underlying subcutaneous layers and muscles are incised to reach the artery and reflected out of the way. The axillary or subclavian artery is exposed in preparation for delivery of the endovascular prosthesis and its sheath is opened with tape placed about it. Report 34716 for endovascular device delivery or establishment of cardiopulmonary bypass that requires creation of a prosthetic conduit utilizing axillary or subclavian artery exposure through an infraclavicular or supraclavicular or sternotomy incision during endovascular aneurysm repair or cardiac procedures requiring cardiopulmonary bypass.

34808

Endovascular placement of an iliac artery occlusion device is performed during separately reportable repair of an abdominal aortic aneurysm and/or endovascular graft procedure. As part of the repair, the iliac artery is occluded. Under separately reportable fluoroscopy, an iliac artery occlusion device is threaded through the arteries and placed distal to the aneurysm. When the aneurysmal repair is complete, the endovascular occlusion device may be left in the artery. Catheters and devices used for access and to deploy the occlusion device are removed and any bleeding controlled.

34813

During separately reportable endovascular repair of an aortic aneurysm, a diseased or damaged femoral artery is repaired by placing a prosthetic femoral-femoral graft. Through incisions in the skin of the upper thighs, the physician isolates and dissects a section of the affected femoral artery. Once vessel clamps have been affixed above and below the area of damaged vessel to be anastomosed, the femoral artery is cut above and below the diseased or damaged area and the new distal and proximal ends are sutured to the ends of the prosthetic graft, which now replaces the section of diseased or damaged artery. When the clamps are removed, the blood flows unobstructed through the femoral artery. After the graft is complete, the skin incisions are repaired with layered closures.

34830-34832

An attempted endovascular repair of an aortic aneurysm originating below the renal arteries (infrarenal) fails, necessitating open repair of the aneurysm as well as repair of any trauma associated with the endovascular attempt. An incision is made in the abdomen from just below the diaphragm to the umbilicus. The aorta is exposed, the aneurysm identified, and the aorta and other arteries inspected for injury resulting from the failed endovascular procedure. Repair of the aneurysm is accomplished by temporarily clamping the aorta both above and below the aneurysm. It is usually possible to place the upper clamp just below the origins of the renal arteries so that the kidneys continue to receive blood flow throughout the operation. Blood flow to the legs is interrupted while the aorta is clamped. The aneurysm is opened lengthwise and any thrombi (blood clots) removed. The aneurysm wall is not removed. The aorta is cut above and below the aneurysm and a prosthetic graft made of synthetic material is sutured in place between the two ends. The aneurysm wall is wrapped around the synthetic graft. The clamps are removed allowing blood to flow through the graft and into the vessels of the lower extremities. The surgical wound is closed. Repair using a tube prosthesis is reported with 34830; repair with an aorto-bi-iliac prosthesis is reported with 34831; and repair with an aorto-bifemoral prosthesis is reported with 34832.

34839

The physician spends at least 90 minutes planning for the placement of a fenestrated visceral aortic endograft, which requires detailed preparation prior to implantation. The planning includes review of radiological imaging enhanced by computer software to assist in the production of the device. Before placement, the physician needs to determine the size parameters of the graft that will conform to the branches of the aorta. These dimensions allow the physician to cut holes (fenestrations) in the device at each visceral artery orifice to allow side branch perfusion of these vessels. Precise planning has to allow for adequate blood flow upon completion of placement. The physician must document at least 90 minutes of planning in the medical record.

34841-34844

Endovascular repair of an abdominal aortic aneurysm, pseudoaneurysm, or dissection, using a prosthesis, and involving visceral branches (superior mesenteric, celiac, and/or renal artery) requires the skills of a vascular surgeon and a radiologist. A small incision is made in the groin over both femoral arteries. Under fluoroscopic guidance, the physician inserts an aortic component through one femoral artery. These are contained inside a plastic holding capsule that is threaded through the arteries to the site of the aneurysm. The physician places the necessary extension prostheses and cuts fenestrations (holes) at each visceral artery orifice to allow side branch perfusion of these vessels. Next, catheters are used to place overlapping stents at each fenestration and vessel orifice to secure the junction. Once the graft components and stents are in place, the holding capsule and catheters are removed and the arteriotomy site is closed. Report 34841 when one visceral artery is included, 34842 for two, 34843 for three, and 34844 for four or more arteries.

34845-34848

Endovascular repair of an abdominal aortic aneurysm, pseudoaneurysm, or dissection, using a prosthesis, and involving visceral branches (superior mesenteric, celiac, and/or renal artery) requires the skills of a vascular surgeon and a radiologist. A small incision is made in the groin over both femoral arteries through which the endovascular devices are inserted. Under fluoroscopic guidance, the physician inserts the aortic component and one iliac limb through one femoral artery. These are contained inside a plastic holding capsule that is threaded through the arteries to the site of the aneurysm. Next, the physician inserts the opposite iliac limb by contralateral femoral artery access. The physician mates the aortic and iliac limb inserted into the first femoral artery to the opposite iliac limb inserted by contralateral femoral artery access. Since this repair extends above the visceral vessels, a visceral extension prosthesis is required. The physician places the extension prosthesis and cuts fenestrations (holes) at each visceral artery orifice to allow side branch perfusion of these vessels. Catheters are used to place overlapping stents at each fenestration and vessel orifice to secure the junction. Once the graft components and stents are in place, the holding capsule and catheters are removed and the arteriotomy site is closed. Report 34845 when one visceral artery is included, 34846 for two, 34847 for three, and 34848 for four or more arteries.

35001-35002
The physician makes an incision in the neck in front of the sternocleidomastoid muscle. The section of the carotid or subclavian artery (35001) or the ruptured section (35002) is isolated and dissected from adjacent critical structures. Vessel clamps are affixed above and below the defect. The repair may be accomplished by removing the segment of artery containing the aneurysm and suturing the exposed ends of the vessel in an end-to-end fashion or the aneurysm may be bypassed with a venous or synthetic graft. If a large section is removed, a harvested or synthetic graft is inserted into the defect, or a patch may be sutured into place to open the diameter of the vessel. The skin incision is repaired with a layered closure.

35005
The physician makes an incision in the skin overlying the neck. The enlarged or blocked section of the vertebral artery is isolated and dissected from muscles and adjacent critical structures. A portion of a cervical vertebra may be removed to access the defect. Vessel clamps are affixed above and below the defect, which may be repaired or removed. The repair may be accomplished by removing the segment of artery containing the aneurysm and suturing the exposed ends of the vessel in an end-to-end fashion or the aneurysm may be bypassed with a venous or synthetic graft. If a large section is removed, a harvested or synthetic graft is inserted into the defect. Instead of a complete graft, a patch may be sutured into place to open the diameter of the vessel. Once the vessel is repaired, the clamps are removed. The skin incision is repaired with a layered closure.

35011-35013
The physician makes an incision in the skin of the arm or axilla. The enlarged or blocked section of the axillary or brachial artery (35011) or the ruptured section (35013) is isolated and dissected from adjacent critical structures. Vessel clamps are affixed above and below the defect, which may be repaired or removed. The repair may be accomplished by removing the segment of artery containing the aneurysm and suturing the exposed ends of the vessel in an end-to-end fashion or the aneurysm may be bypassed with a venous or synthetic graft. If a large section is removed, a harvested or synthetic graft is inserted into the defect. Instead of a complete graft, a patch may be sutured into place to open the diameter of the vessel. Once the vessel is repaired, the clamps are removed. The skin incision is repaired with a layered closure.

35021
The physician exposes the innominate or subclavian artery by median sternotomy or lateral thoracotomy. The physician anticoagulates the patient with heparin, clamps the aortic arch widely around the origin of the innominate artery, and clamps the right common carotid and right subclavian arteries. The physician excises the aneurysmal tissue. The physician may use a woven Dacron patch graft or harvested vein to repair the aneurysmal artery. The physician unclamps the aorta, as well as the right common carotid and right subclavian arteries. The physician closes the sternotomy or thoracotomy, leaving a chest tube in place.

35022
The physician exposes the innominate or subclavian artery by median sternotomy or lateral thoracotomy. The physician clamps the aortic arch widely around the origin of the innominate artery, and clamps the right common carotid and right subclavian arteries. The physician excises the ruptured aneurysmal tissue. The physician may use a woven Dacron patch graft or harvested vein to repair the aneurysmal artery. The physician unclamps the aorta, as well as the right common carotid and right subclavian arteries. The physician closes the sternotomy or thoracotomy, leaving a chest tube in place.

35045
The physician makes an incision in the skin overlying the arm. The enlarged or blocked section of the radial or ulnar artery is isolated and dissected from adjacent critical structures. Vessel clamps are affixed above and below the defect, which may be repaired or removed. The repair may be accomplished by removing the segment of artery containing the aneurysm and suturing the exposed ends of the vessel in an end-to-end fashion or the aneurysm may be bypassed with a venous or synthetic graft. If a large section is removed, a harvested or synthetic graft is inserted into the defect. Instead of a complete graft, a patch may be sutured into place to open the diameter of the vessel. Once the vessel is repaired, the clamps are removed. The skin incision is repaired with a layered closure.

35081
The physician exposes the abdominal aorta using a transperitoneal approach, placing a long incision in the mid abdomen. The physician retracts the transverse colon and small bowel to allow dissection and exposure of the aorta. The physician places an umbilical tape or rubber catheter around the aorta proximal to the aneurysm. The physician exposes the iliac arteries and achieves control of blood flow with umbilical tape or rubber catheters. The physician anticoagulates the patient and cross-clamps the iliac arteries and proximal aorta. The physician opens and clears the aneurysm, controls collateral bleeding from the lumbar arteries with suture, and sutures a Y-shaped knitted Dacron graft to the proximal aorta. The physician sutures the distal ends of the graft to the iliac arteries. The physician may anastomose the

inferior mesenteric arteries and any aberrant or accessory renal arteries to the Dacron graft. The physician sutures the remaining aneurysmal shell around the graft and closes the retroperitoneum. The physician closes the abdominal wound, leaving drains in place.

35082

The physician quickly exposes the abdominal aorta using a transperitoneal approach, placing a long incision in the midabdomen, and retracts the transverse colon and small bowel to allow dissection and exposure of the aorta. Bleeding control is achieved by pushing the liver aside and compressing the aorta manually against the spine. The aorta is cross-clamped proximal to the dissection. The physician exposes the iliac arteries and achieves control of blood flow with umbilical tape or rubber catheters. If bleeding is controlled, the patient receives anticoagulation while the iliac arteries and proximal aorta are cross-clamped. The physician opens and clears the aneurysm, controls collateral bleeding from the lumbar arteries with suture, and sutures a Y-shaped knitted Dacron graft to the proximal aorta. The distal ends of the graft are sutured to the iliac arteries with the remaining aneurysmal shell around the graft. The retroperitoneum and abdominal wounds are closed, leaving drains in place.

35091

The physician exposes the abdominal aorta using a transperitoneal approach, placing a long incision in the midabdomen. The physician retracts the transverse colon and small bowel to allow dissection and exposure of the aorta. The physician places an umbilical tape or rubber catheter around the aorta proximal to the aneurysm. The physician exposes the iliac arteries and achieves control of blood flow with umbilical tape or rubber catheters. The physician anticoagulates the patient and cross-clamps the iliac arteries and proximal aorta. The physician opens and clears the aneurysm, controls collateral bleeding from the lumbar arteries with suture, and sutures a Y-shaped knitted Dacron graft to the proximal aorta. The physician sutures the distal ends of the graft to the iliac arteries. The physician will anastomose the inferior mesenteric arteries and any aberrant or accessory renal arteries to the Dacron graft, when applicable. The physician sutures the remaining aneurysmal shell around the graft and closes the retroperitoneum. The physician closes the abdominal wound, leaving drains in place.

35092

The physician quickly exposes the abdominal aorta using a transperitoneal approach, placing a long incision in the midabdomen and retracting the transverse colon and small bowel to allow dissection and exposure of the aorta. Control of bleeding is achieved by pushing the liver aside and compressing the aorta manually against the spine. The aorta is cross-clamped proximal to the dissection and the iliac arteries are exposed. Control of blood flow is done with umbilical tape or rubber catheters. If bleeding is controlled, the iliac arteries and proximal aorta are cross-clamped. The physician opens and clears the aneurysm, controls collateral bleeding from the lumbar arteries with suture, then sutures a Y-shaped knitted Dacron graft to the proximal aorta. The distal ends of the graft are sutured to the iliac arteries. The physician may anastomose the celiac, inferior mesenteric, and/or renal arteries to the Dacron graft. The remaining aneurysmal shell is sutured around the graft. The retroperitoneum and abdominal wounds are closed, leaving drains in place.

35102

The physician exposes the abdominal aorta using a transperitoneal approach, placing a long incision in the midabdomen, and retracting the transverse colon and small bowel to allow dissection and exposure of the aorta. Umbilical tape or a rubber catheter is placed around the aorta proximal to the aneurysm. The iliac arteries are exposed and control of blood flow is achieved with umbilical tape or rubber catheters. The physician anticoagulates the patient and cross-clamps the iliac arteries and proximal aorta. The physician opens and clears the aneurysm, controls collateral bleeding from the lumbar arteries with suture, then sutures a Y-shaped knitted Dacron graft to the proximal aorta. The distal ends of the graft are sutured to the iliac arteries. The physician may anastomose grafts from other involved iliac vessels (common, hypogastric, external) to the Dacron graft. The remaining aneurysmal shell is sutured around the graft. The retroperitoneal and abdominal wounds are closed, leaving drains in place.

35103

The physician quickly exposes the abdominal aorta using a transperitoneal approach, placing a long incision in the midabdomen. The transverse colon and small bowel are retracted to allow dissection and exposure of the aorta. The physician quickly achieves control of bleeding by pushing the liver aside and compressing the aorta manually against the spine. The aorta is cross-clamped proximal to the dissection and the iliac arteries are exposed. Control of blood flow is achieved with umbilical tape or rubber catheters. Anticoagulation is provided (if bleeding is controlled) and the iliac arteries and proximal aorta are cross-clamped. The physician opens and clears the aneurysm, controls collateral bleeding from the lumbar arteries with suture, and sutures a Y-shaped knitted Dacron graft to the proximal aorta. The distal ends of the graft are sutured to the iliac arteries. The physician may anastomose grafts from other involved iliac vessels (common, hypogastric, external) to the Dacron graft. The remaining aneurysmal shell is sutured around the graft. The retroperitoneal and abdominal wounds are closed, leaving drains in place.

35111

The physician exposes the splenic artery using an abdominal incision. If the aneurysm involves the proximal or distal (hilar) splenic artery, the physician may repair the aneurysm using harvested venous material or synthetic graft material or may simply tie off the diseased artery and vein. If the aneurysm involves the middle splenic artery, which is surrounded by pancreatic tissue, the surgeon may tie off the artery to avoid dissection of the pancreas. The abdominal wound is closed, leaving drains in place.

35112
The physician quickly exposes the splenic artery using an abdominal incision and gains control of bleeding by clamping the proximal splenic artery. If the aneurysm involves the proximal or distal (hilar) splenic artery, the physician may repair the aneurysm using harvested venous material or synthetic graft material or may simply tie off the diseased artery and vein. If the aneurysm involves the middle splenic artery, which is surrounded by pancreatic tissue, the artery may be tied off to avoid dissection of the pancreas. The abdominal wound is closed, leaving drains in place.

35121
The physician exposes the involved hepatic, celiac, renal, or mesenteric artery using an abdominal incision, retracting and dissecting past large and small bowel. If the aneurysm involves an artery whose vascular distribution has adequate collaterals (the common hepatic artery, for example), the physician may simply tie off the diseased artery. Otherwise, the physician repairs the aneurysm, often using harvested vein graft, harvested internal iliac artery graft, or synthetic graft material. The physician closes the abdominal wound, leaving drains in place.

35122
The physician quickly exposes the involved hepatic, celiac, renal, or mesenteric artery using an abdominal incision, retracting and dissecting past large and small bowel. Bleeding is controlled by clamping or compressing the involved artery proximal to the rupture. If the aneurysm involves an artery whose vascular distribution has adequate collaterals (e.g., the common hepatic artery), the physician may simply tie off the diseased artery. Otherwise, the aneurysm is repaired, often using harvested vein graft, harvested internal iliac artery graft, or synthetic graft material. The abdominal wound is closed, leaving drains in place.

35131
The physician exposes the involved iliac arterial branches (common, hypogastric, external) using a low abdominal incision. The aneurysm is repaired by clamping off the affected artery proximally and distally and replacing the affected arterial segment with harvested venous material or synthetic graft material such as Dacron mesh. Arterial patency is confirmed with a Doppler probe or by angiography. The abdominal wound is closed, leaving drains in place.

35132
The physician quickly exposes the involved iliac arterial branches (common, hypogastric, external) using a low abdominal incision. Bleeding is controlled by clamping or compressing the proximal segment of the affected artery. The ruptured aneurysm is repaired by clamping off the affected artery proximally and distally and replacing the affected arterial segment with harvested venous material or synthetic graft material such as Dacron mesh. The arterial patency is confirmed with a Doppler probe or by angiography. The abdominal wound is closed, leaving drains in place.

35141-35142
The physician makes an incision in the skin of the leg. The enlarged or blocked section of the femoral artery (35141) or ruptured section (35142) is isolated and dissected from adjacent critical structures. Vessel clamps are affixed above and below the defect, which may be repaired or removed. The repair may be accomplished by removing the segment of artery containing the aneurysm and suturing the exposed ends of the vessel in an end-to-end fashion or the aneurysm may be bypassed with a venous or synthetic graft. If a large section is removed, a harvested or synthetic graft is inserted into the defect. Instead of a complete graft, a patch may be sutured into place to open the diameter of the vessel. Once the vessel is repaired, the clamps are removed. The skin incision is repaired with a layered closure.

35151-35152
The physician makes an incision in the skin over the leg. The enlarged or blocked section of the popliteal artery (35151) or the ruptured section (35152) is isolated and dissected from adjacent critical structures. Vessel clamps are affixed above and below the defect, which may be repaired or removed. The repair may be accomplished by removing the segment of artery containing the aneurysm and suturing the exposed ends of the vessel in an end-to-end fashion or the aneurysm may be bypassed with a venous or synthetic graft. If a large section is removed, a harvested or synthetic graft is inserted into the defect. Instead of a complete graft, a patch may be sutured into place to open the diameter of the vessel. Once the vessel is repaired, the clamps are removed. The skin incision is repaired with a layered closure.

35180
The physician makes an incision in the skin of the head or neck over the site of the unnatural opening, a congenital fistula that exists between an artery and vein. The fistula is isolated and dissected from adjacent critical structures, and vessel clamps are applied to the vein and the artery. The walls of the artery and vein creating the fistula are each sutured closed. A graft or patch graft may be required to complete the repair. The fistula is tied off, or it may be excised. Once the fistula has been eliminated, the clamps are removed and the skin incision is repaired with a layered closure.

35182
The congenital arteriovenous fistula is exposed by choosing an incision appropriate to the fistula site. The physician examines the fistulous connection and repairs it by ligation (tying it off) or may repair the fistula by clamping the connection from both sides, dividing the connection with scissors, and closing each side with suture. A synthetic graft material or vein

material harvested from the patient may be sewn in to enlarge the arterial or venous lumen. The vessel patency is confirmed with a Doppler probe or angiography prior to closing the wound. The physician may leave surgical drains in place.

35184
The physician makes an incision in the skin of an extremity over the site of the unnatural opening, a congenital fistula that exists between an artery and vein. The fistula is isolated and dissected from adjacent critical structures, and vessel clamps are applied to the vein and the artery. The walls of the artery and vein creating the fistula are each sutured closed. A graft or patch graft may be required to complete the repair. The fistula is tied off or excised. Once the fistula has been eliminated, the clamps are removed and the skin incision is repaired with layered closure.

35188-35189
The physician makes an incision in the skin of the head or neck over the site of the unnatural opening, a fistula, created through trauma. The fistula connects an artery to a vein. The fistula is isolated and dissected from adjacent critical structures, and vessel clamps are applied to the vein and the artery. The walls of the artery and vein creating the fistula are each repaired and closed. A graft or patch graft may be required to complete the repair. The fistula is tied off or excised. Once the fistula has been eliminated, the clamps are removed and the skin incision is repaired with a layered closure. Report 35189 if either fistula is in the thorax or abdomen.

35190
The physician makes an incision in the skin of an extremity at the site of the unnatural opening, a fistula, created through trauma. It connects an artery to a vein. The fistula is isolated and dissected from adjacent critical structures, and vessel clamps are applied to the vein and the artery. The walls of the artery and vein creating the fistula are each repaired and closed. A graft or patch graft may be required to complete the repair. The fistula is tied off or excised. Once the fistula has been eliminated, the clamps are removed and the skin incision is repaired with a layered closure.

35201
The physician makes an incision in the skin of the neck over the site of an injured blood vessel. The vessel is isolated and dissected from adjacent critical structures, and vessel clamps are applied. The edges of the injured vessel may be trimmed to ease repair. A patch graft may be sutured over the defect or the hole in the vessel may be repaired with sutures. The clamps are removed and the skin incision is repaired with a layered closure.

35206
The physician makes an incision in the skin of an upper extremity over the site of an injured blood vessel. The vessel is isolated and dissected from adjacent critical structures, and vessel clamps are applied. The edges of the injured vessel may be trimmed to ease repair. A patch graft may be sutured over the defect or the hole in the vessel may be repaired with sutures. The clamps are removed and the skin incision is repaired with a layered closure.

35207
The physician makes an incision in the skin of the hand or finger over the site of an injured blood vessel. The vessel is isolated and dissected from adjacent critical structures, and vessel clamps are applied. The edges of the injured vessel may be trimmed to ease repair. A patch graft may be sutured over the defect or the hole in the vessel may be repaired with sutures. The clamps are removed and the skin incision is repaired with a layered closure.

35211
The abnormal blood vessel (arterial or venous) is exposed by choosing a thoracic incision appropriate to the involved vessel. This procedure is performed with cardiopulmonary bypass, in which the heart is stopped by infusing cardioplegia solution into the coronary circulation via bypass catheters inserted through incisions in the low inferior vena cava, the superior vena cava, and high aorta or femoral artery. The physician exposes the abnormal blood vessel (arterial or venous) by choosing a thoracic incision appropriate to the involved vessel. The abnormal vessel is examined and repaired by ligation (tying it off) or may be repaired by clamping it proximally and distally to the defect, and suturing the defect closed. The physician may repair the vessel by sewing in synthetic graft material or vein material harvested from the patient in order to enlarge the lumen of the repaired vessel (patch graft). Vessel patency is confirmed with a Doppler probe or angiography prior to taking the patient off cardiopulmonary bypass and closing the wound. The physician leaves chest tubes and, possibly, mediastinal drains in place.

35216
The physician exposes the abnormal blood vessel (arterial or venous) by choosing a thoracic incision appropriate to the involved vessel. The abnormal vessel is examined and repaired by ligation (tying it off) or may be repaired by clamping it proximally and distally to the defect, and suturing the defect closed. The physician may repair the vessel by sewing in synthetic graft material or vein material harvested from the patient in order to enlarge the lumen of the repaired vessel (patch graft). Vessel patency is confirmed with a Doppler probe or angiography prior to closing the wound. The physician leaves chest tubes and, possibly, mediastinal drains in place.

35221
The physician exposes the abnormal blood vessel (arterial or venous) by choosing an abdominal incision appropriate to the involved vessel. The abnormal vessel is examined and repaired by ligation (tying it off) or may be repaired by clamping it proximally and distally to the defect. The defect is sutured closed. A patch graft may be sutured over any remaining defect. Vessel patency is confirmed with a Doppler probe or

angiography prior to closing the wound, leaving surgical drains in place.

35226
The physician makes an incision in the skin of a lower extremity over the site of an injured blood vessel. The vessel is isolated and dissected from adjacent critical structures, and vessel clamps are applied. The edges of the injured vessel may be trimmed to ease repair. A patch graft may be sutured over the defect or the hole in the vessel may be repaired with sutures. The clamps are removed and the skin incision is repaired with a layered closure.

35231
The physician makes an incision in the skin in the neck over the site of an injured blood vessel. The vessel is isolated and dissected from adjacent critical structures, and vessel clamps are applied. The defect is too extensive to repair directly, so the physician removes a short length of vein. The physician repairs the injured vessel with a length of vein harvested from another site in the body or with cadaver vein. The vein is sutured end-to-end to the vessel, replacing the excised portion, or is used as a patch to repair a large hole in the side of the vessel. A patch graft may be sutured over any remaining the defect. The clamps are removed and the skin incision is repaired with a layered closure.

35236
The physician makes an incision in the skin of an upper extremity over the site of an injured blood vessel. The vessel is isolated and dissected from adjacent critical structures, and vessel clamps are applied. The defect is too extensive to repair directly, so the physician removes a short length of vein. The physician repairs the injured vessel with a length of vein harvested from another site in the body or with cadaver vein. The vein is sutured end-to-end to the vessel, replacing the excised portion, or is used as a patch to repair a large hole in the side of the vessel. A patch graft may be sutured over any remaining defect. The clamps are removed and the skin incision is repaired with a layered closure.

35241
The physician exposes the abnormal blood vessel (arterial or venous) by choosing a thoracic incision appropriate to the involved vessel. This procedure is performed with cardiopulmonary bypass, in which the heart is stopped by infusing cardioplegia solution into the coronary circulation via bypass catheters inserted through incisions in the low inferior vena cava, the superior vena cava, and high aorta or femoral artery. The physician exposes the abnormal blood vessel (arterial or venous) by choosing a thoracic incision appropriate to the involved vessel. The physician examines the abnormal vessel and repairs it by clamping proximally and distally to the defect, and sewing in venous graft material harvested from the patient (patch graft). The physician confirms vessel patency with Doppler probe or angiography prior to taking the patient off cardiopulmonary bypass and closing the wound. The physician leaves chest and, possibly, mediastinal drains in place.

35246
The physician exposes the abnormal blood vessel (arterial or venous) by choosing a thoracic incision appropriate to the involved vessel. The physician examines the abnormal vessel and repairs it by clamping proximally and distally to the defect, and sewing in venous graft material harvested from the patient (patch graft). The physician confirms vessel patency with Doppler probe or angiography prior to closing the wound. The physician leaves chest tubes and, possibly, mediastinal drains in place.

35251
The physician exposes the abnormal blood vessel (arterial or venous) by choosing an abdominal incision appropriate to the involved vessel. The physician examines the abnormal vessel and repairs it by clamping proximally and distally to the defect, and sewing in vein material harvested from the patient (patch graft). The physician confirms vessel patency with Doppler probe or angiography prior to closing the wound. The physician leaves surgical drains in place.

35256
The physician makes an incision in the skin of a lower extremity over the site of an injured blood vessel. The vessel is isolated and dissected from adjacent critical structures, and vessel clamps are applied. The physician repairs the injured vessel by sewing in vein material harvested from the patient (patch graft). The clamps are removed and the skin incision is repaired with a layered closure.

35261
The physician makes an incision in the skin of the neck over the site of an injured blood vessel. The vessel is isolated and dissected from adjacent critical structures and vessel clamps are applied. If the defect is too extensive to repair directly, the physician repairs the injured vessel with a length of synthetic graft material (patch graft). The clamps are removed and the skin incision is repaired with layered closure.

35266
The physician makes an incision in the skin of an upper extremity over the site of an injured blood vessel. The vessel is isolated and dissected from adjacent critical structures and vessel clamps are applied. If the defect is too extensive to repair directly, the physician repairs the injured vessel with a length of synthetic graft material (patch graft). The clamps are removed and the skin incision is repaired with layered closure.

35271
The physician exposes the abnormal blood vessel (arterial or venous) by choosing a thoracic incision appropriate to the involved vessel. This procedure is performed with cardiopulmonary bypass, in which the heart is stopped by infusing cardioplegia solution into the coronary circulation via bypass catheters inserted through incisions in the low inferior vena cava, the superior vena cava, and high aorta or femoral artery.

The physician examines the abnormal vessel and repairs it by clamping proximally and distally to the defect, and sewing in synthetic graft material in order to cover the defect. The physician confirms vessel patency with Doppler probe or angiography prior to closing the wound. The physician leaves chest and, possibly, mediastinal drains in place.

35276

The physician exposes the abnormal blood vessel (arterial or venous) by choosing a thoracic incision appropriate to the involved vessel. The physician examines the abnormal vessel and repairs it by clamping proximally and distally to the defect, and sewing in synthetic graft material in order to correct the defect. The physician confirms vessel patency with Doppler probe or angiography prior to closing the wound. The physician leaves chest and, possibly, mediastinal drains in place.

35281

The physician exposes the abnormal blood vessel (arterial or venous) by choosing an abdominal incision appropriate to the involved vessel. The physician examines the abnormal vessel and repairs it by clamping proximally and distally to the defect, and sewing in synthetic graft material in order to correct the defect. The physician confirms vessel patency with Doppler probe or angiography prior to closing the wound. The physician leaves surgical drains in place.

35286

The physician makes an incision in the skin of a lower extremity over the site of an injured blood vessel. The vessel is isolated and dissected from adjacent critical structures and vessel clamps are applied. If the defect is too extensive to repair directly, the physician repairs the injured vessel with a length of synthetic graft material. The clamps are removed and the skin incision is repaired with layered closure.

35301

The physician makes an incision in the skin of the neck over the site of plaque or abnormal lining of the carotid, vertebral, or subclavian artery. The vessel is isolated and dissected from adjacent critical structures and vessel clamps are applied. A temporary vascular shunt may be placed, bypassing the area and allowing blood supply to continue uninterrupted during the procedure. The vessel is incised. Using a blunt, spatula-like tool, the plaque and the vessel lining are separated from the artery and removed. The edge of the normal artery lining may be sutured to the artery wall to prevent separation when blood flow resumes. After the plaque and lining are removed, a patch graft may be applied and sutured to the vessel. This enlarges the diameter of the artery. The vessel clamps are removed and the skin incision is repaired with layered closure.

35302-35304

The physician makes an incision in the skin of the leg over the site of a blood clot, plaque, or abnormal lining of the superficial femoral (35302), popliteal (35303), or tibioperoneal trunk (35304) arteries. The vessels are isolated and dissected from adjacent critical structures and vessel clamps are applied. The vessels are incised. Using a blunt, spatula-like tool, the plaque and the vessel lining are separated from the arteries and removed. The edge of the normal artery linings may be sutured to the artery walls to prevent separation when blood flow resumes. After the plaque and lining are removed, a patch graft may be applied and sutured to the vessels. This enlarges the diameter of the arteries. The vessel clamps are removed and the skin incision is repaired with layered closure.

35305

A thromboendarterectomy is performed on an initial tibial or peroneal artery. The physician makes an incision in the skin over the site of plaque or abnormal lining of a tibial or peroneal artery. The vessel is isolated and dissected from adjacent critical structures and vessel clamps are applied. The vessel is incised. Using a blunt, spatula-like tool, the plaque and the vessel lining are separated from the artery and removed. The edge of the normal artery lining may be sutured to the artery wall to prevent separation when blood flow resumes. After the plaque and lining are removed, a patch graft may be applied and sutured to the vessel. This enlarges the diameter of the artery. The vessel clamps are removed and the skin incision is repaired with layered closure.

35306

An additional thromboendarterectomy is performed on a tibial or peroneal artery. The physician makes an incision in the skin over the site of plaque or abnormal lining of an additional tibial or peroneal artery during a surgical session in which one tibial or peroneal artery has already been treated. The additional vessel is isolated and dissected from adjacent critical structures and vessel clamps are applied. The vessel is incised. Using a blunt, spatula-like tool, the plaque and the vessel lining are separated from the artery and removed. The edge of the normal artery lining may be sutured to the artery wall to prevent separation when blood flow resumes. After the plaque and lining are removed, a patch graft may be applied and sutured to the vessel. This enlarges the diameter of the artery. The vessel clamps are removed and the skin incision is repaired with layered closure.

35311

The physician exposes the innominate or subclavian artery by median sternotomy or lateral thoracotomy. The physician clamps the aortic arch widely around the origin of the diseased artery and clamps the distal end of the diseased artery. After making a longitudinal incision in the diseased artery, the physician uses a spatula to remove the atherosclerotic material. The physician may tack (suture) down the inner layer of the artery with a few 6-0 sutures before closing the artery with suture. A patch graft may be used to enlarge the arterial lumen. The physician unclamps the aorta, as well as the distal arterial clamp, and closes the sternotomy or thoracotomy, leaving a chest tube in place.

35321

The physician makes an incision in the skin of the axilla or arm over the site of a blood clot, plaque, or abnormal lining of the axillary or brachial artery. The vessel is isolated and dissected from adjacent critical structures and vessel clamps are applied. The vessel is incised. Using a blunt, spatula-like tool, the plaque and the vessel lining are separated from the artery and removed. The edge of the normal artery lining may be sutured to the artery wall to prevent separation when blood flow resumes. After the plaque and lining are removed, a patch graft may be applied and sutured to the vessel. This enlarges the diameter of the artery. The vessel clamps are removed and the skin incision is repaired with layered closure.

35331

The physician exposes the abdominal aorta using a transperitoneal approach, placing a long incision in the midabdomen. The transverse colon and small bowel are retracted to allow dissection and exposure of the aorta. The iliac arteries are exposed and control of blood flow is achieved with umbilical tape or rubber catheters placed proximal to the diseased area. The physician anticoagulates the patient and cross-clamps the iliac arteries and proximal aorta. A longitudinal incision down the affected portion of abdominal aorta is performed and a spatula is used to remove the atherosclerotic material. The inner layer of the aorta may be tacked down with small sutures. A patch graft may be applied and sutured to the vessel. The physician sutures the aorta closed and closes the retroperitoneum and abdominal wound, leaving drains in place.

35341

The physician exposes the involved mesenteric, celiac, or renal artery using an abdominal incision, retracting and dissecting past large and small bowel. The aorta is clamped to isolate the involved vessel with a longitudinal incision placed down the affected vessel, and a spatula is used to remove the atherosclerotic material. If there is significant stenosis at the arterial takeoff, the aorta may be opened and the atherosclerotic material removed from within the aorta before suturing the aorta and diseased artery closed. A patch graft may be applied and sutured to the vessel An arteriography may be performed or a Doppler probe may be used to establish patency of the vessel, before closing the abdominal wound, leaving drains in place.

35351

The physician exposes the involved iliac artery using an abdominal incision, retracting and dissecting past large and small bowel. The aorta is clamped to isolate the involved vessel, with a longitudinal incision down the affected vessel, and a spatula is used to remove the atherosclerotic material. If there is significant stenosis at the arterial takeoff, the aorta may be opened and the atherosclerotic material removed before suturing the aorta and diseased artery closed. A patch graft may be applied and sutured to the vessel. The physician may perform arteriography or use a Doppler probe to establish patency of the vessel before closing the abdominal wound, leaving drains in place.

35355

The physician exposes the involved iliac artery using abdominal and femoral incisions, retracting and dissecting past large and small bowel. The femoral artery is exposed via a femoral incision. The aorta is clamped to isolate the involved vessel, a longitudinal incision is performed down the involved vessel, and a spatula is used to remove the atherosclerotic material. If there is significant stenosis at the arterial takeoff, the physician may open the aorta and remove the atherosclerotic material from within the aorta before suturing the aorta and diseased artery closed. A patch graft may be applied and sutured to the vessel. An arteriography may be performed or a Doppler probe may be used to establish patency of the vessel before closing the abdominal and femoral wounds, leaving drains in place.

35361

The physician exposes the involved iliac artery using an abdominal incision, retracting and dissecting past large and small bowel. The proximal aorta is clamped above the diseased area, a longitudinal incision is performed down the distal aorta and affected iliac artery, and a spatula is utilized to remove the atherosclerotic material before suturing the aorta and iliac artery closed. A patch graft may be applied and sutured to the vessel. Arteriography or use of a Doppler probe may be necessary to establish patency of the vessel before closing the abdominal wound, leaving drains in place.

35363

The physician exposes the involved abdominal aorta and iliac artery using an abdominal incision, retracting and dissecting past large and small bowel. The involved femoral artery is exposed via a femoral incision and dissection. The proximal aorta is clamped above the diseased area, a longitudinal incision is performed down the distal aorta and affected iliac artery, and a spatula is used to remove the atherosclerotic material before suturing the aorta and iliac artery closed. A longitudinal incision is performed down the femoral artery and a spatula is used to remove any atherosclerotic material before sewing the femoral artery closed. A patch graft may be applied and sutured to the vessel. An arteriography or Doppler imaging may be performed to establish patency of the vessel. The physician closes the femoral and abdominal wounds, leaving drains in place.

35371-35372

The physician makes an incision in the skin over the leg at the site of a blood clot, plaque, or abnormal lining of the common femoral artery (35371) or the deep (profunda) femoral artery (35372). The vessel is isolated and dissected from adjacent critical structures and vessel clamps are applied. The vessel is incised. Using a blunt, spatula-like tool, the plaque and the vessel lining are separated from the artery and removed. The edge of the normal artery lining may be sutured to the artery wall to prevent separation when blood flow resumes. After the plaque and lining are removed, a patch graft may be applied and sutured to the vessel. This enlarges the diameter of the artery. The vessel clamps are removed and the skin incision is repaired with layered closure.

35390

The physician makes an incision in the skin of the neck over the site of plaque or abnormal lining of the carotid, vertebral, or subclavian artery. The vessel is isolated and dissected from adjacent critical structures, and vessel clamps are applied. A temporary vascular shunt may be placed, bypassing the area and allowing blood supply to continue uninterrupted during the procedure. The vessel is incised. Using a blunt, spatula-like tool, the plaque and the vessel lining are separated from the artery and removed. The edge of the normal artery lining may be sutured to the artery wall to prevent separation when blood flow resumes. After the plaque and lining are removed, a patch graft may be applied and sutured to the vessel. This enlarges the diameter of the artery. The vessel clamps are removed and the skin incision is repaired with layered closure.

35400

The purpose of this procedure is to use an endoscope to look inside a blood vessel. The physician places an introducer sheath in the vessel to be examined, using percutaneous puncture or a cutdown technique. The physician places an angioscopy catheter through the introducer sheath into the vessel to be examined. The physician advances the angioscope through the vessel, clearing the view with injections of saline. Once the inside of the vessel has been examined, the angioscope and sheath are withdrawn. Vessel hemostasis is achieved using sutures or manual pressure.

35500

The physician harvests a vein from an upper extremity (arm) to use for a planned bypass procedure on a lower extremity vessel (leg) or coronary artery. An incision is made over the site on the arm. Tissue is dissected to the vein. The portion of the vein to be removed is released from the surrounding structures, and is tied off above and below the portion of vein to be removed. The vein is removed. The wound is closed with layered sutures. The portion of vein removed is prepared for use in a separately reportable bypass graft procedure of a leg vessel or coronary artery.

35501

The physician bypasses a blocked segment of common carotid artery to a segment of internal carotid artery on the same side of the neck. Through an incision in the skin of the neck in front of the sternocleidomastoid muscle, the physician isolates and dissects the common carotid artery, separating it from adjacent structures. After vessel clamps are affixed above and below the defect, the physician creates a bypass around the defective section of common carotid artery. The common carotid artery may be cut through below the damaged area and sutured to one end of the harvest vein (end-to-end), which is then sutured to the internal carotid artery beyond the affected area. As an alternative, the ends of the harvested vein are sutured into the side of the common carotid arterial wall and to the side of the internal carotid arterial wall (end-to-side). Either method results in a bypass of the damaged area. When the clamps are removed, the section of vein graft forms a new path through which blood can easily bypass the blocked area. The defective common carotid artery is not removed. After the graft is complete, the skin incision is repaired with layered closure.

35506

The physician bypasses a segment of blocked common carotid or subclavian artery. Through an incision in the skin at the side of the neck, the physician isolates and dissects the subclavian and common carotid arteries, separating them from adjacent critical structures. In this procedure, a blocked common carotid arterial flow may be bypassed to the subclavian artery, or a blocked subclavian arterial flow may be bypassed to the common carotid artery. To create a bypass around a section of artery that is damaged or blocked, the physician uses a harvested vein and one of two methods of repair. After vessel clamps have been affixed above and below the damaged area, the graft is sewn to the side of the two arteries (end-to-side) or cut ends may be sewn (end-to-end). The graft is attached above the portion of blocked artery. The blocked portion of artery is not removed. When the clamps are removed in either case, the section of vein graft forms a new path through which blood can easily bypass the blocked area. After the graft is complete, the skin incision is repaired with layered closure.

35508

Through an incision in the skin of the neck, the physician isolates and dissects the vertebral and carotid arteries, separating them from adjacent critical structures. The physician creates a bypass around a section of vertebral artery that is damaged or blocked, using a harvested vein and one of two methods of repair. After vessel clamps have been affixed above and below the damaged area, the graft is sewn to the side of the carotid artery and sewn to the side of the vertebral artery beyond the affected area (end-to-side) or sewn over the cut end of the vertebral artery after dividing it beyond the affected area (end-to-end). The damaged or blocked section of the vertebral artery is not removed. When the clamps are removed, the section of vein graft forms a new path through which blood can easily bypass the blocked area. After the graft is complete, the skin incision is repaired with a layered closure.

35509

The physician performs a vein bypass graft from one carotid to the contralateral carotid. Through incisions in the skin of the neck, the physician isolates and dissects the carotid arteries, separating them from adjacent critical structures. The physician creates a bypass around a section of carotid artery that is damaged or blocked, using a harvested vein and one of two methods of repair. After vessel clamps have been affixed above and below the damaged area, the ends of the vein graft are sutured into the side of the carotid arterial wall (end-to-side). In the second method, the carotid artery may be cut through above the damaged area and sutured to one end of a harvested vein, which is sutured to the side of the carotid artery on the opposite side of the neck (end-to-end). In either case, the blocked or damaged section of artery is not removed. When the clamps are removed, the section of vein graft forms a new path through which blood can easily bypass the blocked or damaged area. After the graft is complete, the skin incisions are repaired with layered closures.

35510

Through an incision in the skin at the side of the neck, the physician dissects down to the common carotid artery, separating soft tissue and adjacent critical structures. Soft tissue must be cleared for several centimeters. Dissection through the skin and soft tissue at the distal anastomosis site of this bypass graft is also done over the brachial artery in the arm. Next, a tunnel is made from the carotid through the axilla and down the arm to the brachial artery site. To create a bypass graft around the section of brachial artery that is damaged or blocked, the physician uses a harvested vein, usually the greater saphenous. After vascular clamps have been affixed above and below the anastomosis area on the carotid artery, the proximal arteriotomy is carried out and the harvested vein is sutured to the carotid artery. When this is completed and checked for hemorrhaging, the arterial clamps are removed. The vein graft is tunneled through the prepared space to the brachial artery and the distal arteriotomy and anastomosis are carried out in the same manner. The clamps are removed, additional sutures may be placed for complete hemostasis, and the patency of the graft is checked. The incisions are closed and the appropriate pulses are checked again before dressings are applied.

35511

Through incisions in the skin at the base of the neck, the physician isolates and dissects the subclavian arteries, separating them from adjacent critical structures. The physician creates a bypass around a section of subclavian artery that is damaged or blocked, using a harvested vein and one of two methods of repair after vessel clamps have been affixed above and below the defect. In the first method of repair the ends of the vein graft are sutured into the sides of the walls of the two subclavian arteries, resulting in a bypass of the damaged area. In the second method, the subclavian artery may be cut through beyond the damaged area and sutured to one end of a harvested vein, which is sutured to the subclavian artery on the opposite side of the neck. In either case, the blocked or damaged portion of the artery is not removed. When the clamps are removed, the section of vein graft forms a new path through which blood can easily bypass the blocked area. After the graft is complete, the skin incisions are repaired with a layered closure.

35512

Through an incision in the skin at the base of the neck, the physician dissects down to the subclavian artery just above the clavicle, separating soft tissue and adjacent critical structures. Soft tissue must be cleared for several centimeters. Dissection through the skin and soft tissue at the distal anastomosis site for this bypass graft is also done over the brachial artery in the arm. Next, a tunnel is made from the subclavian, under the clavicle, through the axilla, and down the arm to the brachial artery site. To create a bypass graft around the section of brachial artery that is damaged or blocked, the physician uses a harvested vein, usually the greater saphenous. After vascular clamps have been affixed above and below the anastomosis area on the subclavian artery, the proximal arteriotomy is carried out and the harvested vein is sutured to the subclavian artery. When this is completed and checked for hemorrhaging, the arterial clamps are removed. The vein graft is tunneled through the prepared space to the brachial artery and the distal arteriotomy and anastomosis are carried out in the same manner. The clamps are removed, additional sutures may be placed for complete hemostasis, and the patency of the graft is checked. The incisions are closed and the appropriate pulses are checked again before dressings are applied.

35515

Through an incision in the skin of the neck, the physician isolates and dissects the vertebral and subclavian arteries, separating them from adjacent critical structures. The physician creates a bypass around a section of vertebral artery that is damaged or blocked, using a harvested vein and one of two methods of repair. Once vessel clamps are affixed above and below the defect, the ends of the harvested vein are sutured into the sides of the subclavian and vertebral arterial walls resulting in a bypass of the damaged area (end-to-side). In the second method, the vertebral artery can be cut through above the damaged area and sutured to one end of a harvested vein (end-to-end). The remaining end is sutured to the subclavian artery. In either case, the blocked or damaged vertebral artery is not removed. When the clamps are removed, the section of vein graft forms a new path through which blood can easily bypass the blocked area. After the graft is complete, the skin incision is repaired with a layered closure.

35516

Through an incision in the skin at the base of the neck and axilla, the physician isolates and dissects the subclavian and axillary arteries, separating them from adjacent critical structures. The physician creates a bypass around a section of subclavian artery that is damaged or blocked, using a harvested vein and one of two methods of repair. Once vessel clamps have been affixed above and below the defect, the ends of the harvested vein are sutured into the sides of the subclavian and axillary arterial walls resulting in a bypass of the damaged area (end-to-side). In the second method, the subclavian artery may be cut through before the damaged area and sutured to one end of a harvested vein, which is sutured to the axillary artery (end-to-end). The blocked or damaged portion of the subclavian artery is not removed. When the clamps are removed, the section of vein graft forms a new path through which blood can easily bypass the blocked area. After the graft is complete, the skin incisions are repaired with a layered closure.

35518

The physician makes an incision in the skin of both axillae. The physician creates a bypass around the section of axillary artery that is damaged or blocked, using a harvested vein and one of two methods of repair. Once vessel clamps have been affixed above and below the defect, the ends of the harvested vein are sutured into the sides of the two axillary arterial walls, resulting in a bypass of the damaged area. In the second method, the axillary artery may be cut through beyond the damaged area and sutured to one end of a harvested vein, which is passed across the front of the chest under the skin and sutured to the side of the contralateral axillary artery. The blocked or damaged portion of the axillary artery is not removed. When the clamps are removed, the section of vein graft forms a new path through which blood can easily bypass the blocked area. After the graft is complete, the skin incisions are repaired with layered closures.

35521

The physician makes incisions in the skin of the axilla and upper thigh. The axillary and femoral arteries are isolated and dissected from adjacent critical structures. The physician creates a bypass around the section of damaged or blocked artery using a harvested vein and one of two methods of repair. Once vessel clamps have been affixed above and below the areas of anastomosis, the harvested vein is sutured to an incision in the side of the axillary artery and passed through a subcutaneous tunnel on the side of the body and to the upper thigh. The harvested vein is sutured to the femoral artery (common, deep, or superficial) in an end-to-side or end-to-end fashion. The blocked or damaged portion of artery is not removed. When the clamps are removed, the section of vein graft forms a new path through which blood can easily bypass the blocked area. After the graft is complete, the skin incisions are repaired with layered closures.

35522

Through an incision in the skin of the chest wall, the physician dissects down to the axillary artery just below the clavicle, separating soft tissue and adjacent critical structures. Soft tissue must be cleared for several centimeters. Dissection through the skin and soft tissue at the distal anastomosis site for this bypass graft is also done over the brachial artery in the arm near the elbow. Next, a tunnel is made from the exposed axillary, through the axilla and down the arm to the brachial artery site. To create a bypass graft around the section of brachial artery that is damaged or blocked, the physician uses a harvested vein, usually the greater saphenous. After vascular clamps have been affixed above and below the anastomosis area on the axillary artery, the proximal arteriotomy is carried out and the harvested vein is sutured to the axillary artery. When this is completed and checked for hemorrhaging, the arterial clamps are removed. The vein graft is tunneled through the prepared space to the brachial artery and the distal arteriotomy and anastomosis are carried out in the same manner. The clamps are removed, additional sutures may be placed for complete hemostasis, and the patency of the graft is checked. The incisions are closed and the appropriate pulses are checked again before dressings are applied.

35523

The physician performs a brachial-ulnar or brachioradial bypass graft. Through an incision in the skin of the upper arm, the physician dissects down to the brachial artery at a site above the diseased or damaged portion of the artery. Soft tissue and adjacent critical structures are separated. Soft tissue must be cleared for several centimeters. Dissection through the skin and soft tissue at the distal anastomosis site for this bypass graft is also done over the radial or ulnar artery. A tunnel is made from the exposed proximal brachial site down the arm to the radial or ulnar artery site. To create a bypass graft around the section of the artery that is damaged or blocked, the physician uses a harvested vein, usually the greater saphenous. After vascular clamps have been affixed above and below the proximal anastomosis area on the brachial artery, arteriotomy is carried out and the harvested vein is sutured to the artery. When this is completed and checked for hemorrhaging, the arterial clamps are removed. The vein graft is tunneled through the prepared space to the distal site on the radial or ulnar artery and arteriotomy and anastomosis are carried out again in the same manner. The clamps are removed, additional sutures may be placed for complete hemostasis, and the patency of the graft is checked. The incisions are closed and the appropriate pulses are checked again before dressings are applied.

35525

Through an incision in the skin of the upper arm, the physician dissects down to the brachial artery at a site above the diseased or damaged portion of the artery, usually in the mid to distal part, and separates soft tissue and adjacent critical structures. Soft tissue must be cleared for several centimeters. Dissection through the skin and soft tissue at the distal anastomosis site for this bypass graft is also done over the distal brachial artery in the arm, most often below the elbow. Next, a tunnel is made from the exposed proximal brachial site, down the arm to the distal brachial artery site. To create a bypass graft around the section of the artery that is damaged or blocked, the physician uses a harvested vein, usually the greater saphenous. After vascular clamps have been affixed above and below the proximal anastomosis area on the brachial artery, arteriotomy is carried out and the harvested vein is sutured to the brachial artery. When this is completed and checked for hemorrhaging, the arterial clamps are removed. The vein graft is tunneled through the prepared space to the distal site on the brachial artery and arteriotomy and anastomosis are carried out again in the same manner. The clamps are removed, additional sutures may be placed for complete hemostasis, and the patency of the graft is checked. The incisions are closed and the appropriate pulses are checked again before dressings are applied.

35526

The physician exposes the aorta by median sternotomy and exposes the aortocarotid, aortoinnominate, or aortosubclavian artery extending this incision in the appropriate direction. The physician clamps the middle part of the right anterolateral aspect of the anterior ascending aorta with a J clamp. The physician makes a 2 cm to 3 cm longitudinal incision in the clamped portion of the aorta and sews the venous graft to the aortic incision. The physician clamps the vein and releases the aortic clamp to assess the anastomosis for leaks. The physician clamps the distal end of the diseased artery. The physician makes a longitudinal incision in the diseased artery, distal to the blockage, and sews the venous graft to the arterial incision. The physician may also use harvested vein to enlarge the arterial lumen (patch graft). The physician removes the clamp from the vein graft. The physician may perform arteriography or use a Doppler probe to establish patency of the graft. The physician closes the sternotomy or thoracotomy, leaving a chest tube in place.

35531

The physician exposes the involved aortomesenteric or aortoceliac artery using an upper midline abdominal incision, retracting and dissecting past large and small bowel. The physician exposes the distal thoracic aorta, administers heparin for anticoagulation, and clamps the aorta both proximal and distal to the celiac axis origin. The physician cuts out an elliptical disk of aortic wall from the anterior surface of the aorta. The physician exposes the involved vessel (aortomesenteric or aortoceliac artery) and divides it proximal to the occlusion, closing off the proximal stump with suture. The physician sews a venous graft from the clamped aorta to the nondiseased distal artery. The physician may use harvested vein to enlarge the arterial lumen (patch graft). The physician may perform arteriography or use a Doppler probe to establish patency of the graft. The physician closes the abdominal wound, leaving drains in place.

35533

Through incisions in the skin of the axilla and both upper thighs, the physician creates a bypass using a harvested vein around the section of diseased or damaged artery. Once vessel clamps have been affixed above and below the area of anastomosis, the harvested vein is sutured to the side of the axillary artery and passed through a subcutaneous tunnel to the upper thigh, where it is sutured end-to-end or end-to-side to the femoral artery. A second harvested vein is sutured end-to-side to the femoral artery or to the vein graft descending from the axilla where it joins the femoral artery, and is passed through another subcutaneous tunnel to the opposite thigh, where it is sutured end-to-end or end-to-side to the femoral artery. When the clamps are removed, the two grafted vein limbs form a new path through which blood can easily bypass the blocked area. The section of the blocked or damaged vessel is not removed. After the graft is complete, the incisions are repaired with layered closures.

35535

The physician performs hepatorenal bypass graft. With the patient placed supine, a right subcostal (beneath the ribs) incision is made and extended through the subcutaneous tissue, fat, and muscle. The abdominal cavity is entered, the stomach is retracted, and the lesser omentum is entered. The physician locates the common hepatic, proper hepatic, and gastroduodenal arteries. These are dissected and encircled with Silastic vessel loops. After the physician mobilizes the right renal vein, the right renal artery is exposed, dissected, and encircled with Silastic vessel loops. The physician harvests a greater saphenous vein segment and forms a proximal end-to-end anastomosis to the common hepatic artery. Distal anastomosis is then performed with the renal artery in either a side-to-side or end-to-end fashion. Bleeding is controlled and Doppler or duplex is performed to verify revascularization. After the graft is complete, the incisions are repaired with layered closure.

35536

The physician performs a bilateral subcostal incision from the right midrectus position extending into the left flank, and dissects past bowel and pancreas to expose the splenic vein. The physician exposes the splenic artery by careful dissection. The physician exposes the left renal artery by dissecting through the posterior parietal peritoneum, partially clamps it, and excises an ellipse of renal artery at its upper border. The physician performs end-to-side anastomosis of vein graft material from the splenic artery to the renal artery. The physician removes the clamps and assesses the anastomotic sites for leaks. The physician may perform Doppler studies or arteriography to establish patency of the graft. The physician closes the abdominal wound, leaving drains in place.

35537-35538

The physician exposes the involved abdominal aorta and iliac arteries using an abdominal incision, retracting and dissecting past large and small bowel. The physician partially clamps the aorta above the diseased area and places a longitudinal incision down the clamped portion of the aorta. The physician sews in a (two) venous graft(s), clamps the graft(s), and removes the aortic clamp to assess the anastomosis(es) for leaks. The physician clamps the iliac artery(ies) distal to the stenosis and incises and attaches the distal venous graft to the iliac artery(ies). The physician may also use harvested vein to enlarge the aortic or arterial lumen (patch graft). The physician may perform arteriography or use a Doppler probe to establish patency of the graft. The physician closes the abdominal wound, leaving drains in place. A bypass graft to a single iliac artery is performed in 35537; both iliac arteries are bypassed in 35538.

35539-35540
The physician makes an incision in the skin of the abdomen over a section of damaged or blocked lower aorta. The artery is isolated and dissected. Through a separate skin incision in the upper thigh, the femoral artery is isolated and dissected from adjacent critical structures. The physician creates a bypass around the damaged or blocked lower aorta using a harvested vein. Once vessel clamps have been affixed above the defect, the lower aorta may be cut through or tied off with sutures above the damaged or blocked area and sutured to one end of the harvested vein in an end-to-end or side-to-side fashion. In 35539, the graft to one femoral artery is passed through a tunnel on the inside of the upper thigh and sutured to the femoral artery. In 35540, a bifemoral bypass is accomplished and a second harvested vein is placed in a similar fashion to the second side. When the clamps are removed, the two grafted vein limbs form a new path through which blood can easily bypass the blocked area. The blocked or damaged portion of artery is not removed. After the graft is complete, the skin incisions are repaired with layered closures.

35556
Through incisions in the skin of the leg overlying the femoral and popliteal arteries, the physician isolates and dissects a section of artery that is damaged or blocked. The physician creates a bypass around the superficial femoral artery, using a harvested vein and one of two methods of repair. Once vessel clamps have been affixed above and below the defect, the superficial femoral artery may be cut through above the damaged or blocked area and sutured to one end of a harvested vein. The vein is passed through a tunnel down the thigh muscles and behind the knee and sutured to the popliteal artery. In the second method, the ends of the harvested vein are sutured into the side of the femoral and popliteal arterial walls, resulting in a bypass of the damaged area. When the clamps are removed, the section of vein forms a new path through which blood can easily bypass the blocked area. The blocked or damaged portion of artery is not removed. After the graft is complete, the skin incisions are repaired with layered closures.

35558
Through incisions in the skin of the upper thighs, the physician isolates and dissects a section of the femoral arteries. The physician creates a bypass using a harvested vein. Once vessel clamps have been affixed above and below the area of anastomosis, the femoral artery may be cut through below the damaged area and sutured to one end of a harvested vein, which is sutured to the femoral artery in the opposite leg, resulting in a bypass of the damaged or blocked area. When the clamps are removed, the section of vein forms a new path through which blood can easily bypass the blocked area. The blocked or damaged portion of the artery is not removed. After the graft is complete, the skin incisions are repaired with layered closures.

35560
The physician exposes the involved abdominal aorta and renal artery using an abdominal incision, retracting and dissecting past large and small bowel. The aorta is partially clamped below the renal takeoff and a small longitudinal incision is performed down the clamped portion of the aorta. The venous graft is sutured and clamped and the aortic clamp is removed to assess the anastomosis for leaks. The renal artery is clamped distal to the stenosis and incised. The distal venous graft is attached to the distal renal artery. A harvested vein may be utilized to enlarge the renal arterial lumen (patch graft). The physician may perform arteriography or use a Doppler probe to establish patency of the graft. The abdominal wound is closed, leaving drains in place.

35563
The physician exposes the iliac arteries using an abdominal incision, retracting and dissecting past large and small bowel. The patent (nondiseased) iliac artery is partially clamped and a longitudinal incision is performed down the clamped portion of the aorta. A venous graft is attached and clamped. The iliac clamp is removed to assess the anastomosis for leaks. The diseased iliac artery is clamped distal to the stenosis and a distal incision is performed. The distal venous graft is attached to the diseased iliac artery. A harvested vein may be used to enlarge the aortic or arterial lumen (patch graft). The physician may perform arteriography or use a Doppler probe to establish patency of the graft. The abdominal wound is closed, leaving drains in place.

35565
Through incisions in the skin of the lower abdomen overlying the iliac artery and in the skin of the upper thigh overlying the femoral artery, the physician isolates and dissects a section of common iliac artery. The physician creates a bypass around the iliac artery, using a harvested vein and one of two methods of repair. Once vessel clamps have been affixed above and below the defect, the iliac artery may be cut or tied off with sutures above the damaged area and sutured to one end of a harvested vein. The graft is passed through a tunnel on the inside of the upper thigh and is sutured to the side of the femoral artery. In the second method, the end of the harvested vein is sutured to the side of the iliac artery. Either method results in a bypass of the damaged area. When the clamps are removed, the section of vein forms a new path through which blood can easily bypass the blocked area. After the graft is complete, the skin incisions are repaired with layered closures.

35566
Through incisions in the skin of the leg overlying the superficial femoral artery, the physician isolates and

dissects sections of the femoral and anterior tibial, posterior tibial, or peroneal arteries. The physician creates a bypass around the affected artery using a harvested vein. Once vessel clamps have been affixed above and below the defect, the superficial femoral artery may be cut through above the damaged area and sutured to one end of a harvested vein, which is passed through an intramuscular tunnel and sutured to the anterior tibial, posterior tibial, peroneal, or other distal vessel. In the second method, the ends of the harvested vein are sutured to the side of the femoral artery and anterior tibial, posterior tibial, peroneal, or other distal vessel wall, resulting in a bypass of the damaged area. When the clamps are removed, the section of vein forms a new path through which blood can easily bypass the blocked area. The blocked or damaged portion of artery is left in place and not removed. After the graft is complete, the skin incisions are repaired with layered closures.

35570
The physician performs tibial-tibial, peroneal-tibial, or tibioperoneal trunk-tibial bypass graft. Through incisions in the skin of the leg overlying the affected tibial, peroneal, or tibioperoneal trunk artery, the physician isolates and dissects a section of arteries from adjacent critical structures. The physician creates a bypass around the affected artery using a harvested vein and one of two methods of repair. Once vessel clamps have been affixed above and below the defect, the artery may be cut through above the damaged area and sutured to one end of a harvested vein, which is sutured to the targeted tibial artery. In the second method, the ends of the harvested vein are sutured to the side of the bypassed artery and tibial vessel wall, resulting in a bypass of the damaged area. When the clamps are removed, the section of vein forms a new path through which blood can bypass the blocked area. The blocked or damaged portion of artery is left in place and not removed. After the graft is complete, the skin incisions are repaired with layered closures.

35571
Through incisions in the skin of the leg overlying the popliteal arteries, the physician isolates and dissects a section of arteries from adjacent critical structures. The physician creates a bypass around the artery, using a harvested vein and one of two methods of repair. Once vessel clamps have been affixed above and below the defect, the popliteal artery may be cut through above the damaged area and sutured to one end of a harvested vein, which is sutured to the tibial, peroneal, or other distal artery. In the second method, the ends of the harvested vein are sutured into the side of the popliteal and the tibial or peroneal arterial wall resulting in a bypass of the damaged area. When the clamps are removed, the section of vein forms a new path through which blood can easily bypass the blocked area. After the graft is complete, the incisions are repaired with layered closures.

35572
The physician harvests one segment of the femoropopliteal vein for a vascular reconstructive procedure. The leg is prepared circumferentially to make the leg accessible and provide optimal access. A single incision or multiple incisions can be made to harvest the vein. The vein is first located through an approximately 10 cm incision and dissected. The skin is cut over the course of the vein. If multiple incisions are made, the index finger is used to continue dissection along the anterior surface of the vein, with the incisions made about 2 to 4 cm from the last incision and the physician's finger underneath, or an external vein stripper is used with incisions made where the stripper meets resistance again. Branches of the vein are ligated. Dissection can begin at the proximal or distal end. The length of vein needed is estimated based on its intended purpose and the desired length is mobilized and divided at both ends. The vein is placed in a prepared solution of blood and saline at room temperature and prepared with diluted blood placed to flush the vein. A vascular device is applied, the vein is gently distended, and uncontrolled branches are closed. The vein is returned to the solution until used.

35583
Through an incision in the skin of the leg overlying the greater saphenous vein, the physician isolates and dissects the greater saphenous vein from adjacent critical structures from the upper thigh to the level of the knee. Vessel clamps are affixed above and below the site of the anastomosis to the femoral and popliteal arteries. All side branches of the saphenous vein are tied off. The vessel's valves are destroyed. The upper end of the saphenous vein is divided and sutured into the femoral artery end-to-end or end-to-side. The lower end is divided and sutured into the popliteal artery end-to-end or end-to-side. The clamps are removed, and blood flows backward toward the feet, as if the vein were an artery. When the procedure is complete, the skin incision is repaired with a layered closure.

35585
Through an incision in the skin of the leg overlying the greater saphenous vein, the physician isolates and dissects the greater saphenous vein from adjacent critical structures. Vessel clamps are affixed above and below the site of anastomosis in the femoral artery and the distal artery. All side branches of the Saphenous are tied off. The vessel's valves are destroyed. The upper end of the saphenous vein is divided and sutured end-to-end or end-to-side in the femoral artery above the blockage. The lower end is divided and sutured end-to-end or end-to-side to the anterior tibial, posterior tibial, or peroneal artery below the blockage. The clamps are removed, and blood flows backward toward the feet, as if the vein were an artery. When the procedure is complete, the skin incision is repaired with a layered closure.

35587
Through an incision in the skin of the leg overlying the greater saphenous vein from the knee to the ankle, the physician isolates and dissects the greater saphenous vein from adjacent critical structures along its length.

Vessel clamps are affixed above and below the site of anastomosis on the popliteal and peroneal arteries. All side branches of the saphenous vein are tied off. The vessel's valves are destroyed. The upper end of the saphenous vein is divided and sutured into the popliteal-tibial artery. The lower end is divided and sutured into the peroneal artery. The clamps are removed and blood flows backward through the vein toward the feet, as if it were an artery. When the procedure is complete, the incision is repaired with layered closure.

35600

The physician harvests an artery from an upper extremity (arm) to use for a planned bypass procedure on a coronary artery using an open approach. An incision is made over the site on the arm. Tissue is dissected to the artery. The portion of the artery to be removed is released from the surrounding structures and is tied off above and below the portion of artery to be removed. The artery is removed and the wound closed with layered sutures. The portion of artery removed is prepared for use in the bypass graft.

35601

Through an incision in the skin of the neck in front of the sternocleidomastoid muscle, the physician isolates and dissects the common carotid and internal carotid arteries, separating them from adjacent critical structures. The physician creates a bypass around the section of common carotid artery that is damaged or blocked, using a synthetic vein graft and one of two methods of repair involving the internal carotid artery on the same side of the neck. After vessel clamps have been affixed above and below the damaged area, the common carotid artery may be cut through below the damaged area and sutured to one end of the synthetic vein (end-to-end), which is sutured to the internal carotid artery beyond the affected area. In the second method, the ends of the synthetic vein are sutured into the side of the common carotid arterial wall and the internal carotid arterial wall (end-to-side). Either method results in a bypass of the damaged area. When the clamps are removed, the section of synthetic graft forms a new path through which blood can easily bypass the blocked area. The damaged or blocked carotid artery is not removed. After the graft is complete, the skin incision is repaired with layered closure.

35606

Through an incision in the skin at the side of the neck, the physician isolates and dissects the subclavian and carotid arteries, separating them from adjacent critical structures. To create a bypass around a section of subclavian artery that is damaged or blocked, the physician uses a synthetic vein and one of two methods of repair. After vessel clamps have been affixed above and below the damaged area, the graft is sewn to the side of the carotid artery and sewn to the side of the subclavian artery beyond the affected area (end-to-side) or sewn to the cut end of the subclavian artery after dividing it beyond the affected area (end-to-end). The damaged or blocked portion of the subclavian artery is not removed. When the clamps are removed in either case, the section of synthetic graft vein forms a new path through which blood can easily bypass the blocked area. After the graft is complete, the skin incision is repaired with a layered closure.

35612

Through incisions in the skin at the base of the neck, the physician isolates and dissects the subclavian arteries, separating them from adjacent critical structures. The physician creates a bypass around a section of subclavian artery that is damaged or blocked, using a synthetic vein and one of two methods of repair. Once vessel clamps have been affixed above and below the defect, the ends of the synthetic vein graft are sutured into the sides of the walls of the two subclavian arteries, resulting in a bypass of the damaged area. In the second method, the subclavian artery may be cut through beyond the damaged area and sutured to one end of a synthetic vein, which is sutured to the subclavian artery on the opposite side of the neck. In either case, the blocked or damaged portion of the artery is not removed. When the clamps are removed, the section of synthetic vein graft forms a new path through which blood can easily bypass the blocked area. After the graft is complete, the skin incisions are repaired with a layered closure.

35616

Through an incision in the skin at the base of the neck and axilla, the physician isolates and dissects the subclavian and axillary arteries, separating them from adjacent critical structures. The physician creates a bypass around a section of subclavian artery that is damaged or blocked, using a synthetic vein and one of two methods of repair. Once vessel clamps have been affixed above and below the defect, the ends of the synthetic vein are sutured into the sides of the subclavian and axillary arterial walls resulting in a bypass of the damaged area (end-to-side). In the second method, the subclavian artery may be cut through before the damaged area and sutured to one end of a synthetic vein, which is sutured to the axillary artery (end-to-end). The blocked or damaged portion of the subclavian artery is not removed. When the clamps are removed, the section of synthetic vein graft forms a new path through which blood can easily bypass the blocked area. After the graft is complete, the skin incisions are repaired with a layered closure.

35621

The physician makes incisions in the skin of the axilla and upper thigh. The artery is isolated and dissected from adjacent critical structures. The physician creates a bypass around a section of artery that is damaged or blocked using a synthetic vein and one of two repair methods. Once vessel clamps have been affixed above and below the areas of anastomosis, the synthetic vein is sutured to an incision in the side of the axillary artery and passed through a subcutaneous tunnel on the side of the body and to the upper thigh. The synthetic vein is sutured to the femoral artery (common, deep, or superficial) in an end-to-side or end-to-end fashion. The blocked or damaged portion of the artery is not removed. When the clamps are removed, the section of synthetic vein graft forms a new path through which blood can easily bypass the blocked area. After the graft is complete, the skin incisions are repaired with layered closures.

35623

The physician makes incisions in the skin of the axilla and behind the knee or in the lower leg. The artery is isolated and dissected from adjacent critical structures. The physician creates a bypass around a section of artery that is damaged or blocked using a synthetic vein and one of two repair methods. Once vessel clamps have been affixed above and below the areas of anastomosis, the synthetic vein is sutured to an incision in the side of the axillary artery and passed through a subcutaneous tunnel on the side of the body and behind the knee or upper thigh. The synthetic vein is sutured to the popliteal or tibial artery in an end-to-side or end-to-end fashion. The blocked or damaged portion of the artery is not removed. When the clamps are removed, the section of synthetic vein graft forms a new path through which blood can easily bypass the blocked area. After the graft is complete, the skin incisions are repaired with layered closures.

35626

The physician exposes the aorta by median sternotomy and exposes the aortocarotid, aortoinnominate, or aortosubclavian artery, extending this incision in the appropriate direction. The physician clamps the middle part of the right anterolateral aspect of the anterior ascending aorta with a J clamp. The physician makes a 2 cm to 3 cm longitudinal incision in the clamped portion of the aorta and sews the arterial or synthetic graft to the aortic incision. The physician clamps the graft and releases the aortic clamp to assess the anastomosis for leaks. The physician clamps the distal end of the diseased artery. The physician makes a longitudinal incision in the diseased artery, distal to the blockage, and sews the graft to the arterial incision. The physician may also use graft material to enlarge the arterial lumen (patch graft). The physician removes the clamp from the graft. The physician may perform arteriography or use a Doppler probe to establish patency of the graft. The physician closes the sternotomy or thoracotomy, leaving a chest tube in place.

35631

The physician exposes the involved aortomesenteric, aortoceliac, or aortorenal artery using an upper midline abdominal incision, retracting and dissecting past large and small bowel. The distal thoracic aorta is exposed, heparin is administered for anticoagulation, and the aorta is clamped both proximal and distal to the celiac axis origin. An elliptical disk of aortic wall is cut out from the anterior surface of the aorta. The involved vessel (aortomesenteric, aortoceliac, or aortorenal artery) is exposed and divided proximal to the occlusion, closing off the proximal stump with suture. A synthetic or arterial graft is sewn from the clamped aorta to the undiseased distal artery. Graft material may be utilized to enlarge the arterial lumen (patch graft). The physician may perform arteriography or use a Doppler probe to establish patency of the graft. The abdominal wound is closed, leaving drains in place.

35632-35634

The physician performs ilio-celiac (35632), ilio-mesenteric (35633), or iliorenal (35634) bypass using a synthetic graft. Through a midline abdominal incision, the physician retracts the intestines and exposes the common iliac artery and the involved vessel (celiac, mesenteric, or renal artery). The common iliac artery is clamped proximally and distally. The physician makes an oval incision on the anterolateral aspect of the common iliac artery, temporarily releases the distal clamp, and administers heparin for anticoagulation. A synthetic graft is attached to the common iliac artery at the site of the arteriotomy and sutured in place. An end-to-end anastomosis of the synthetic graft to the disease-free portion of the celiac, mesenteric, or renal artery is created. The physician may perform arteriography or Doppler to establish patency of the graft. The physician closes the abdominal wound, leaving drains in place.

35636

The physician performs a bilateral subcostal incision from the right midrectus position extending into the left flank, and dissects past bowel and pancreas to expose the splenic artery. The splenic artery is exposed by careful dissection. The left renal artery is exposed by dissecting through the posterior parietal peritoneum and partially clamped. An ellipse of renal artery is excised at its upper border. An end-to-side anastomosis of synthetic or arterial graft material from the splenic artery to the renal artery is performed. The clamps are removed and the anastomotic sites are assessed for leaks. The physician may perform Doppler studies or arteriography to establish patency of the graft. The abdominal wound is closed, leaving drains in place.

35637-35638

The physician makes an incision in the abdominal wall and separates the muscles to expose the internal organs, which are checked for any undetected disease. The aorta and iliac arteries are located and the obstruction is isolated by clamping the vessels. An artificial graft, commonly of polyester or polytetrafluoroethylene, is made ready. Synthetic grafts are preferred in aortoiliac bypass since they more closely match the luminal dimensions of the replaced arteries. The graft is sewn into place, with one end anastomosed to the aorta and the other end to the iliac artery. The clamps are removed, blood flows freely, and the anastomotic sites are assessed for leaks. The physician may perform Doppler studies or arteriography to establish patency of the graft. The abdominal wound is closed in layers. Report 35637 for an artificial bypass graft to a single iliac artery and 35638 when both iliac arteries are bypassed.

35642
Through an incision in the skin of the neck, the physician isolates and dissects the vertebral and carotid arteries, separating them from adjacent critical structures. The physician creates a bypass around a section of vertebral artery that is damaged or blocked, using a synthetic vein and one of two methods of repair. After vessel clamps have been affixed above and below the damaged area, the synthetic graft is sewn to the side of the carotid artery and sewn to the side of the vertebral artery beyond the affected area (end-to-side) or sewn to the cut end of the vertebral artery after dividing it beyond the affected area (end-to-end). The damaged or blocked section of the vertebral artery is not removed. When the clamps are removed, the section of synthetic vein graft forms a new path through which blood can easily bypass the blocked area. After the graft is complete, the skin incision is repaired with a layered closure.

35645
Through an incision in the skin of the neck, the physician isolates and dissects the vertebral and subclavian arteries, separating them from adjacent critical structures. The physician creates a bypass around a section of vertebral artery that is damaged or blocked, using a synthetic vein and one of two methods of repair. Once vessel clamps are affixed above and below the defect, the ends of the synthetic vein are sutured into the sides of the subclavian and vertebral arterial walls resulting in a bypass of the damaged area (end-to-side). In the second method, the vertebral artery can be cut through above the damaged area and sutured to one end of a synthetic vein (end-to-end). The remaining end is sutured to the subclavian artery. In either case, the blocked or damaged vertebral artery is not removed. When the clamps are removed, the section of synthetic vein graft forms a new path through which blood can easily bypass the blocked area. After the graft is complete, the skin incision is repaired with a layered closure.

35646-35647
The physician makes an incision in the skin of the abdomen over a section of damaged or blocked lower aorta. The artery is isolated and dissected. Through a separate skin incision in the upper thigh, the femoral artery is isolated and dissected from adjacent critical structures. The physician creates a bypass around the damage or blocked lower aorta using a synthetic vein. Once vessel clamps have been affixed above the defect, the lower aorta may be cut through or tied off with sutures above the damaged or blocked area and sutured to one end of the synthetic vein in an end-to-end or side-to-side fashion. The graft to one femoral artery is passed through a tunnel on the inside of the upper thigh and sutured to the femoral artery. A second synthetic vein is placed in a similar fashion to the second side. When the clamps are removed, the two grafted synthetic vein limbs form a new path through which blood can easily bypass the blocked area. The blocked or damaged portion of artery is not removed. After the graft is complete, the skin incisions are repaired with layered closure. Report 35646 when both femoral arteries are bypassed and 35647 when a single femoral artery is bypassed.

35650
The physician makes an incision in the skin of both axillae. The physician creates a bypass around a section of artery that is damaged or blocked, using a synthetic graft and one of two repair methods. Once vessel clamps have been affixed above and below the defect, the ends of the synthetic graft are sutured into the sides of the two axillary arterial walls, resulting in a bypass of the damaged area. In the second method, the axillary artery may be cut through beyond the damaged area and sutured to one end of a synthetic graft, which is passed across the front of the chest under the skin and sutured to the side of the contralateral axillary artery. The blocked or damaged portion of the axillary artery is not removed. When the clamps are removed, the section of synthetic vein graft forms a new path through which blood can easily bypass the blocked area. After the graft is complete, the skin incisions are repaired with layered closures.

35654
Through an incision in the skin of the axilla and both upper thighs, the physician creates a bypass around a section of lower aorta that is damaged or blocked, using a synthetic graft. Once vessel clamps have been affixed above and below the defect, the synthetic graft is sutured to the side of the axillary artery and passed through a subcutaneous tunnel to the upper thigh where it is sutured end-to-end or end-to-side to the femoral artery. A second synthetic graft is sutured end-to-side to the femoral artery and passed through another subcutaneous tunnel to the opposite thigh where it is sutured end-to-end or end-to-side to the femoral artery. The section of blocked artery is not removed. When the clamps are removed, the two synthetic grafted limbs form a new path through which blood can easily bypass the blocked area. After the graft is complete, the skin incisions are repaired with layered closures.

35656
Through incisions in the skin of the leg overlying the femoral and popliteal arteries, the physician isolates and dissects a section of artery that is damaged or blocked. The physician creates a bypass around the superficial femoral artery, using a synthetic vein and one of two methods of repair. Once vessel clamps have been affixed above and below the defect, the superficial femoral artery may be cut through above the damaged or blocked area and sutured to one end of a synthetic vein, which is passed through a tunnel down the thigh muscles to behind the knee and sutured to the popliteal artery. In the second method, the ends of the synthetic vein are sutured into the side of the femoral and popliteal arterial walls, resulting in a bypass of the damaged area. When the clamps are removed, the section of synthetic vein forms a new path through which blood can easily bypass the blocked area. The blocked or damaged portion of

artery is not removed. After the graft is complete, the skin incisions are repaired with layered closures.

35661
Through incisions in the skin of the upper thighs, the physician isolates and dissects a section of the femoral arteries. The physician creates a bypass using a synthetic vein. Once vessel clamps have been affixed above and below the area of anastomosis, the femoral artery may be cut through below the damaged area and sutured to one end of a synthetic vein, which is sutured to the femoral artery in the opposite leg, resulting in a bypass of the damaged or blocked area. When the clamps are removed, the section of synthetic vein forms a new path through which blood can easily bypass the blocked area. The blocked or damaged portion of the artery is not removed. After the graft is complete, the skin incisions are repaired with layered closures.

35663
The physician exposes the iliac arteries using an abdominal incision, retracting and dissecting past large and small bowel. The patent (nondiseased) iliac artery is partially clamped and a longitudinal incision is performed down the clamped portion of the aorta. A synthetic or arterial graft is sewn in, the graft is clamped, and the iliac clamp is removed to assess patency of the anastomosis. The diseased iliac artery is clamped distal to the stenosis, a distal incision is performed, and the distal graft is attached to the diseased iliac artery. Graft material may be utilized to enlarge the aortic or arterial lumen (patch graft). The physician may perform arteriography or use a Doppler probe to establish patency of the graft. The abdominal wound is closed, leaving drains in place.

35665
Through incisions in the skin of the lower abdomen overlying the iliac artery, and in the skin of the upper thigh overlying the femoral artery, the physician isolates and dissects a section of common iliac artery. The physician creates a bypass around the iliac artery, using a synthetic vein and one of two methods of repair. Once vessel clamps have been affixed above and below the defect, the iliac artery may be cut or tied off with sutures above the damaged area and sutured to one end of a synthetic vein. The graft is passed through a tunnel on the inside of the upper thigh and is sutured to the side of the femoral artery. In the second method, the end of the synthetic vein is sutured to the side of the iliac artery. Either method results in a bypass of the damaged area. When the clamps are removed, the section of synthetic vein forms a new path through which blood can easily bypass the blocked area. After the graft is complete, the skin incisions are repaired with layered closures.

35666
Through incisions in the skin of the leg overlying the superficial femoral artery, the physician isolates and dissects sections of the femoral and anterior tibial, posterior tibial or peroneal arteries. The physician creates a bypass around the affected artery using a synthetic vein. Once vessel clamps have been affixed above and below the defect, the superficial femoral artery may be cut through above the damaged area and sutured to one end of a synthetic vein, which is passed through an intramuscular tunnel and sutured to the anterior tibial, posterior tibial, peroneal, or other distal vessel. In the second method, the ends of the synthetic vein are sutured to the side of the femoral artery and anterior tibial, posterior tibial, peroneal, or other distal vessel wall, resulting in a bypass of the damaged area. When the clamps are removed, the section of synthetic vein forms a new path through which blood can easily bypass the blocked area. The blocked or damaged portion of artery is left in place and not removed. After the graft is complete, the skin incisions are repaired with layered closures.

35671
Through incisions in the skin of the leg overlying the popliteal arteries, the physician isolates and dissects a section of artery from adjacent critical structures. The physician creates a bypass around the artery, using a synthetic vein and one of two methods of repair. Once vessel clamps have been affixed above and below the defect, the popliteal artery may be cut through above the damaged area and sutured to one end of a synthetic vein, which is sutured to the tibial, peroneal, or other distal artery. In the second method, the ends of the synthetic vein are sutured into the side of the popliteal and the tibial or peroneal arterial wall resulting in a bypass of the damaged area. When the clamps are removed, the section of synthetic vein forms a new path through which blood can easily bypass the blocked area. After the graft is complete, the incision is repaired with layered closures.

35681-35683
In 35681 the physician constructs a composite graft from donor and synthetic materials. One common composite would involve the reconfiguring of a harvested vein into a length of larger diameter graft material. The harvested vein would be split lengthwise and wrapped in a spiral and sutured around a larger diameter mandrill. This length of composite graft would be used to complete the primary procedure. In 35682 a graft is constructed using tissue acquired from two veins at separate locations in the patient's body for the transplantation. In 35683 a graft is constructed using three or more segments of vein from two or more locations in the patient's body. In all three procedures veins are harvested by making an incision over the site where the vein will be removed. Tissues are dissected down to the vein and the vein is released from surrounding tissues. The vein is tied off above and below the area of vein that is to be removed. The vein is removed. The wound is closed with layered sutures. The portion of vein(s) removed is prepared for use in a separately reportable bypass graft procedure.

35685
The physician places a vein patch or cuff at a distal arterial anastomosis site during a bypass graft, synthetic conduit procedure of the lower extremity. The physician harvests the vein to be used for the vein

patch from a previously chosen site. The vein patch is positioned and anastomosed between the distal portion of the synthetic vein graft and the native artery, end-to-end or side-to-end. The physician returns to the bypass graft surgery having performed this additional procedure.

35686
The physician creates a fistula between an artery and vein during a lower extremity bypass procedure. The physician harvests the vein to be used for creation of the fistula from a previously chosen site. The vein is anastomosed between the tibial or peroneal artery and a vein at or beyond the distal bypass anastomosis site. The physician returns to the bypass graft surgery having performed this adjuvant (additional) procedure.

35691
The physician performs a supraclavicular incision and exposes the vertebral and carotid arteries by careful dissection. The adventitia of the chosen translocation site in the posterolateral wall of the common carotid artery is cleared. The physician anticoagulates the patient with heparin and divides the vertebral artery above the stenotic area. The proximal vertebral stump is ligated with sutures and a small arteriotomy in the common carotid arterial wall with an aortic punch is performed. The vertebral artery is attached using an end-to-side anastomosis to the carotid artery. The physician may perform arteriography or use a Doppler probe to establish patency of the graft. The supraclavicular wound is closed, leaving a drain in place.

35693
The physician performs a supraclavicular incision and exposes the vertebral and subclavian arteries by careful dissection. The adventitia of the chosen translocation site in the subclavian artery lateral to the thyrocervical trunk is cleared. The physician anticoagulates the patient with heparin and divides the vertebral artery above the stenotic area. The proximal vertebral stump is ligated with sutures and a small arteriotomy is made in the subclavian artery wall with an aortic punch. The vertebral artery is attached using an end-to-side anastomosis to the subclavian artery. The physician may perform arteriography or use a Doppler probe to establish patency of the graft. The supraclavicular wound is closed, leaving a drain in place.

35694
The physician performs a supraclavicular incision and exposes the carotid and subclavian arteries by careful dissection. The adventitia of the chosen translocation site in the posterolateral wall of the common carotid artery is cleared. The physician anticoagulates the patient's blood with heparin and divides the subclavian artery distal to the stenotic area. The proximal subclavian stump is ligated with sutures and a small arteriotomy in the common carotid artery wall is performed with an aortic punch. The subclavian artery is attached using an end-to-side anastomosis to the carotid artery. The physician may perform arteriography or use a Doppler probe to establish patency of the graft. The supraclavicular wound is closed, leaving a drain in place.

35695
The physician performs a supraclavicular incision and exposes the carotid and subclavian arteries by careful dissection. The adventitia of the chosen translocation site in the subclavian artery lateral to the thyrocervical trunk is cleared. The physician anticoagulates the patient's blood with heparin and divides the carotid artery above the stenotic area. The proximal carotid stump is ligated with sutures and a small arteriotomy in the subclavian artery wall is made with an aortic punch. The carotid artery is attached using an end-to-side anastomosis to the subclavian artery. The physician may perform arteriography or use a Doppler probe to establish patency of the graft. The supraclavicular wound is closed, leaving a drain in place.

35697
A reimplantation of a visceral artery to an infrarenal aortic prosthesis, each artery, is done in addition to the primary procedure of an open aortic aneurysm repair (35081). This surgery is performed when a visceral artery, such as the inferior mesenteric, has been determined not to supply sufficient blood flow to vital organs, after repair of the aortic aneurysm. After the aortic prosthesis has been placed and blood flow is re-established through the aorta, the physician dissects soft tissue from around the origin of the visceral artery in the aorta where it exits. A small button-shaped patch of aortic tissue is removed from this site. Next, a clamp is placed on the aortic prosthesis at the intended site for reimplantation and a hole is cut the size of the button patch, which is anastomosed to the recipient hole in the prosthesis. The suturing is tested by removing the clamps and placing any additional sutures for complete hemostasis.

35700
This code is only used with other codes to identify the reoperation aspect of this procedure, which usually requires more effort when performed again. Through incisions in the skin of the leg, overlying the affected artery, the physician isolates the graft. The physician makes an incision in the proximal portion of the graft and passes a Fogarty balloon catheter through the graft to clear and straighten it. If an arteriograph indicates the graft must be replaced, the physician makes a second incision distal to the inguinal incision, releases the graft, and places vein clamps above and below the stricture. The physician replaces the graft by suturing the ends of a new graft to the side of the arteries to form a bypass of the damaged area. The clamps are removed. After the stricture is controlled or the graft is otherwise complete, the incisions are repaired with layered closures.

35701-35703
Through an incision in the skin overlying the targeted artery, the physician dissects around surrounding structures as necessary to access the artery, freeing it so it can be examined. The artery is released from any surrounding scar tissue that may be compressing it. Finding no perforations or other signs of injury, the physician repairs the skin incision with a layered closure. Report 35701 for exploration of arteries of the neck (e.g., carotid or subclavian); 35702 for those of the upper extremity (e.g., axillary, brachial, radial, or ulnar); and 35703 for those of the lower extremity (e.g., common, deep, or superficial femoral, peroneal, popliteal, or tibial).

35800
Through an incision in the neck over the affected area, the physician isolates the vessel and explores it for postoperative complications such as hemorrhage, thrombosis, or infection. The physician dissects any adjacent critical structures as necessary to access the vessel. The complication is identified and corrected. A hemorrhage is controlled by ligation or suture repair of the artery. Thrombosis requires opening of the artery and the removal of the clot. Any infection is drained, and sometimes a temporary tube is placed so the infection can continue to drain. The physician sutures the skin incision with a layered closure once the postsurgical complication has been treated.

35820
The physician reopens the original incision site and inspects the operative area for active bleeding, hematoma, thrombus, and exudate. The physician removes or debrides any observed hematoma, thrombus, and infected tissues. The physician looks for and corrects any active bleeding sites using electrocautery or ligation of bleeding vessels. The physician may leave an infected wound open, but generally closes the incision, leaving drains and chest tubes in place.

35840
The physician reopens the original incision site and inspects the operative area for active bleeding, hematoma, thrombus, and exudate. The physician removes or debrides any observed hematoma, thrombus, and infected tissues. The physician looks for and corrects any active bleeding sites using electrocautery or ligation of bleeding vessels. The physician may leave an infected wound open, but generally closes the incision, leaving drains in place.

35860
Through an incision in the extremity over the affected area, the physician isolates the vessel and explores it for postoperative complications such as hemorrhage, thrombosis, or infection. The physician dissects any adjacent critical structures as necessary to access the vessel. The complication is identified and corrected. A hemorrhage is controlled by ligation or suture repair of the artery. Thrombosis requires opening of the artery and the removal of the clot. Any infection is drained, and sometimes a temporary tube is placed so the infection can continue to drain. The physician sutures the skin incision with a layered closure once the postsurgical complication has been treated.

35870
The physician opens the abdomen under antibiotic cover and exposes the graft-enteric fistula site by careful dissection (most often aortic/Dacron anastomosis with a fistulous connection to the duodenum). The fistula is disconnected and the enteric defect is repaired using two layers of suture. The vascular prosthesis is examined and removed with an appropriate new bypass graft sewn in if there is obvious graft infection. If there is no obvious infection, the graft is repaired with local sutures. The wound is closed, leaving drains in place.

35875-35876
Through an incision in the skin overlying the arterial or venous graft, the physician isolates the site of the thrombus. The physician dissects any muscle, overlying vessel, and/or adjacent critical structures to access the graft. To excise the thrombus from the graft, the blood vessel is clamped above and below the thrombus, an incision is made into the vessel or graft and the thrombus is removed. The graft or vessel is sutured at the site of the thrombectomy and the clamps are removed. To remove the thrombus with a catheter, the physician makes an incision in the vessel above or below the graft and threads the catheter past the thrombus. A balloon or tool at the tip of the catheter is inflated or extended. The physician withdraws the catheter, repeating as necessary, to capture and retrieve all of the thrombus. The blood vessel is repaired with sutures. After either procedure, the skin incision is repaired with a layered closure. In 35876, the thrombotic graft is removed, the graft site is repaired with sutures, and, avoiding the repair site, a new graft is sutured into place on the vessel. The skin incision is repaired with a layered closure.

35879-35881
The physician revises a lower extremity arterial bypass with vein-patch angioplasty or segmental vein interposition. A previous lower-extremity arterial bypass graft requires open revision due to graft-threatening stenosis. The physician makes an incision in a lower extremity over the site of a previous arterial bypass graft. Dissection is carried down to the graft. In 35879, angioplasty of the stenosed area is performed by excising the area of stenosis and using a patch of vein to close the created wound. In 35881, a segment of vein is excised from another area. The area of stenosis is excised and the vein segment is positioned between the two ends of the graft and anastomosed in an end to end fashion. A thrombectomy is not performed. The wound is closed with layered sutures.

35883-35884
The physician performs open revision of the femoral anastomosis of a synthetic arterial bypass graft in the groin using a nonautogenous patch graft such as bovine pericardium, polyester, or expanded

polytetrafluoroethylene (ePTFE) in 35883 or an autogenous vein patch graft in 35884. This procedure is performed due to formation of an anastomotic aneurysm in the femoral artery, which occurs due to a defect in the anastomosis. The physician makes an incision in the skin of the upper thigh to isolate and dissect the anastomotic aneurysm. An arteriotomy is performed and the aneurysm is excised. A patch graft is placed and the skin incision repaired.

35901

Through an incision in the skin of the neck overlying the graft, the physician dissects around any muscle, vessels, or other structures to access the graft site. The physician dissects around the vessel, and applies vessel clamps above and below the graft. The physician excises above and below the existing infected graft. The blood vessel is repaired with sutures. A catheter may be left in place to help drain infection. The skin is loosely closed. If the excised graft is replaced with a new graft, report the appropriate revascularization code.

35903

Through an incision in the skin of the extremity overlying the graft, the physician dissects around any muscle, vessels or other structures to access the graft site. The physician dissects around the vessel, and applies vessel clamps above and below the graft. The physician excises above and below the existing infected graft. The blood vessel is repaired with sutures. A catheter may be left in place to help drain infection. The skin is loosely closed. If the excised graft is replaced with a new graft, report the appropriate revascularization code.

35905

Through an incision in the skin of the thorax overlying the graft, the physician dissects around any muscle, vessels or other structures to access the graft site. The physician dissects around the vessel, and applies vessel clamps above and below the graft. The physician excises above and below the existing infected graft. The blood vessel is repaired with sutures. A catheter may be left in place to help drain infection. The skin is loosely closed. If the excised graft is replaced with a new graft, report the appropriate revascularization code.

35907

Through an incision in the skin of the abdomen overlying the graft, the physician dissects around any muscle, vessels or other structures to access the graft site. The physician dissects around the vessel, and applies vessel clamps above and below the graft. The physician excises above and below the existing infected graft. The blood vessel is repaired with sutures. A catheter may be left in place to help drain infection. The skin is loosely closed. If the excised graft is replaced with a new graft, report the appropriate revascularization code.

36000-36005

In 36000, the provider places a needle or a catheter through a puncture in the skin and into a peripheral vein. In 36002, the physician or other qualified health care provider injects a pseudoaneurysm, which is a pulsatile hematoma with a fibrous capsule that maintains persistent communication with the adjacent vessel. The vessel wall does not heal and blood flows back and forth between the vessel and hematoma during the cardiac cycle. Under ultrasound control, the physician advances a 22-gauge needle into the lumen of the pseudoaneurysm and injects thrombin to cause thrombosis of the pseudoaneurysm. In 36005, an opaque substance is injected through the catheter for venography. Once the procedure is complete, the catheter is removed and pressure is applied to stop bleeding at the injection site.

36010

The physician punctures a distal vein (typically antecubital, internal jugular, subclavian, or femoral) with a large needle and passes a guidewire via the needle into the punctured vein. The physician removes the needle while leaving the guidewire in place, and enlarges the skin opening slightly with a blade. The physician may slide an introducer sheath over the guidewire into the venous lumen, or may slide the catheter directly into the venous lumen without using an introducer sheath. If using an introducer sheath, the physician inserts the catheter into the vein through an O-ring in the introducer sheath (this prevents blood from leaking around the catheter) into the superior or inferior vena cava. The physician may check the catheter position with fluoroscope or with an x-ray.

36011-36012

Through a puncture through the skin, the physician passes a needle into the vein and threads a guidewire through the needle into the vein. The needle is removed and the wire is passed to the desired location in the venous system. A catheter follows the wire into the selected point in the vein and the wire is removed. A first order branch from the vena cava (36011) is any initial vessel draining directly into the vena cava (e.g., renal vein or jugular vein). A second order branch of the vena cava (36012) is any vein draining into a first order branch (e.g., left adrenal, petrosal sinus). Contrast material for venography is injected into the catheter that has traveled to an area upstream of the site under investigation. Once the procedure is complete, the catheter is removed, and pressure applied to stop bleeding at the injection site.

36013

The physician punctures a distal vein (typically antecubital, internal jugular, subclavian, or femoral) with a large needle and passes a guidewire via the needle into the punctured vein. The physician removes the needle while leaving the guidewire in place, and enlarges the skin opening slightly with a blade. The physician slides an introducer sheath over the guidewire into the venous lumen. The physician inserts the catheter into the vein through an O-ring in the introducer sheath (this prevents blood from leaking around the catheter) and advances the catheter into the right heart or main pulmonary artery, using fluoroscopic guidance or while measuring pressures through the catheter lumen to ensure that the catheter tip is in the desired place. The physician may use the catheter to inject contrast material to perform venography or pulmonary arteriography.

36014
The physician punctures a distal vein (typically antecubital, internal jugular, subclavian, or femoral) with a large needle and passes a guidewire via the needle into the punctured vein. The physician removes the needle while leaving the guidewire in place, and enlarges the skin opening slightly with a blade. The physician slides an introducer sheath over the guidewire into the venous lumen. The physician inserts the catheter into the vein through an O-ring in the introducer sheath (this prevents blood from leaking around the catheter) and advances the catheter into one of the main pulmonary arteries (right or left) using fluoroscopic guidance and possibly measuring pressures through the catheter lumen to ensure that the catheter tip is in the desired place. The physician may use the catheter to inject contrast material to perform venography or pulmonary arteriography.

36015
The physician punctures a distal vein (typically antecubital, internal jugular, subclavian, or femoral) with a large needle and passes a guidewire via the needle into the punctured vein. The physician removes the needle while leaving the guidewire in place, and enlarges the skin opening slightly with a blade. The physician slides an introducer sheath over the guidewire into the venous lumen. The physician inserts the catheter into the vein through an O-ring in the introducer sheath (this prevents blood from leaking around the catheter) and advances the catheter into one of the segmental or subsegmental pulmonary arteries using fluoroscopic guidance and possibly measuring pressures through the catheter lumen to ensure that the catheter tip is in the desired place. The physician may use the catheter to inject contrast material to perform venography or pulmonary arteriography.

36100
Through the skin of the neck, the physician inserts a needle into the carotid or vertebral artery. A guidewire is threaded through the needle into the artery and the needle is removed. A catheter follows the wire into the artery. The wire is removed. Contrast material is injected through the catheter into the artery for arteriography. Once the procedure is complete, the catheter is removed and pressure is applied to the puncture site to stop bleeding.

36140
Through a puncture in the skin over an upper or lower extremity artery, the physician injects a needle into the artery and threads a guidewire through it. The needle is removed. A catheter follows the wire into the artery and the wire is removed. Contrast material for arteriography is injected into the catheter placed upstream of the site under investigation. Once the procedure is complete, the catheter is removed and pressure is applied to stop bleeding at the injection site.

36160
The physician punctures the left lumbar area, typically just above a rib, to direct a large needle into the aorta. When pulsatile red blood is obtained through the needle, indicating successful aortic puncture, the physician passes a guidewire via the needle into the punctured aorta. The physician removes the needle while leaving the guidewire in place, and enlarges the skin opening slightly with a blade. The physician slides a catheter over the guidewire into the aortic lumen and secures the catheter in place with suture.

36200
The physician punctures a distal artery (typically femoral, brachial, radial, or axillary) with a large needle and passes a guidewire via the needle into the punctured artery. The physician removes the needle while leaving the guidewire in place, and enlarges the skin opening slightly with a blade. The physician slides an introducer sheath over the guidewire into the arterial lumen. The physician inserts a catheter into the artery through an O-ring in the introducer sheath (this prevents blood from leaking around the catheter) and advances the catheter into the aorta. The physician may use the catheter to inject contrast material to perform aortography, measure aortic pressures, or to administer medication.

36215-36216
The physician passes a needle into the skin into an extremity artery, usually in the upper thigh. A guidewire is threaded through the needle into the vessel. The needle is removed. The wire is threaded into the aorta and up to the thoracic aorta where it is manipulated into a branch off the aortic arch. A catheter follows the wire into a first order thoracic or brachiocephalic artery. The wire is removed. The catheter may pass through the first order vessel into a second order thoracic or brachiocephalic artery. Contrast material for arteriography is injected into the catheter that has been guided to an area upstream of the site under investigation. In 36215, the catheter remains in a first order artery. In 36216, the catheter travels further to a second order artery. Upon completion, the catheter is removed, and pressure applied to stop bleeding at the puncture site.

36217-36218
The physician punctures the skin and underlying artery with a needle and threads a guidance wire through the needle into the artery. The needle is removed. The guidewire is manipulated into the specific artery. A catheter follows the wire into a first order thoracic or brachiocephalic artery. The catheter passes through the first order vessel into the second order thoracic or brachiocephalic artery. The catheter continues to a third order vessel. Contrast material for arteriography

is injected into the catheter that has been guided to the site under investigation. Once the procedure is complete, the catheter is removed and pressure is applied to stop bleeding at the injection site. Report 36218 for an additional second order, third order, and beyond, thoracic or brachiocephalic branch, within a vascular family.

36221

The physician punctures a distal artery (typically femoral, brachial, radial, or axillary) with a large needle and passes a guidewire via the needle into the punctured artery. The needle is removed while leaving the guidewire in place, and the skin opening is enlarged slightly with a blade. An introducer sheath is inserted over the guidewire and into the arterial lumen. A catheter is introduced into the artery through an O-ring in the introducer sheath, which prevents blood from leaking around the catheter, and advanced into the thoracic aorta. The physician injects contrast material to perform angiography of the cervicocerebral arch, the extracranial carotid, and the vertebral and/or other intracranial vessels, unilaterally or bilaterally. Upon completion, the catheter is removed and pressure is applied to stop bleeding at the access site.

36222-36223

The physician passes a needle through the skin and into an extremity artery, usually in the upper thigh. A guidewire is threaded through the needle into the vessel. The needle is removed. The wire is threaded into the aorta and up to the thoracic aorta where it is manipulated into a branch off the aortic arch. A catheter follows the wire into the common carotid or innominate artery on one side. The wire is removed. Contrast material is injected into the catheter for arteriography. Report 36222 when angiography of the ipsilateral extracranial carotid circulation is also included. In 36223, angiography of the ipsilateral extracranial and intracranial carotid circulation is performed. Angiography of the cervicocerebral arch may also be performed. Upon completion, the catheter is removed and pressure is applied to stop bleeding at the access site.

36224

The physician passes a needle through the skin and into an extremity artery, usually in the upper thigh. A guidewire is threaded through the needle into the vessel. The needle is removed. The wire is threaded into the aorta and up to the thoracic aorta where it is manipulated into a branch off the aortic arch. A catheter follows the wire into the internal carotid artery on one side. The wire is removed. Contrast material is injected into the catheter for arteriography, including the intracranial carotid circulation. Angiography of the ipsilateral extracranial carotid circulation and the cervicocerebral arch may also be performed. Upon completion, the catheter is removed and pressure is applied to stop bleeding at the access site.

36225

The physician passes a needle through the skin and into an extremity artery. A guidewire is threaded through the needle into the vessel. The needle is removed. The wire is threaded into the thoracic aorta where it is manipulated into a branch off the aortic arch. A catheter follows the wire into the subclavian or innominate artery on one side. The wire is removed. Contrast material is injected into the catheter for arteriography, including the ipsilateral vertebral circulation. Angiography of the cervicocerebral arch may also be performed. Upon completion, the catheter is removed and pressure is applied to stop bleeding at the access site.

36226

The physician passes a needle through the skin and into an extremity artery. A guidewire is threaded through the needle into the vessel. The needle is removed. The wire is threaded into the thoracic aorta where it is manipulated into a branch off the aortic arch. A catheter follows the wire into the vertebral artery on one side. The wire is removed. Contrast material is injected into the catheter for arteriography, including the ipsilateral vertebral circulation. Angiography of the cervicocerebral arch may also be performed. Upon completion, the catheter is removed and pressure is applied to stop bleeding at the access site.

36227

During selective angiography of the common carotid, internal carotid, or innominate artery, the physician also manipulates the catheter to the external carotid artery. Contrast material is injected into the catheter for arteriography, including the ipsilateral external carotid circulation.

36228

During selective angiography of the internal carotid or vertebral artery, the physician further manipulates the catheter into additional intracranial branches of the artery, such as the middle cerebral or posterior inferior cerebellar arteries. Contrast material is injected into the catheter for arteriography, including the selected vessels circulation.

36245-36246

The physician inserts a needle through the skin and into an underlying artery, usually a lower extremity artery, and threads a guidewire through the needle and into the artery. The needle is removed. The wire is threaded into the specific vessel. A catheter follows the wire into the artery branch. The wire is removed. Contrast material for arteriography is injected into the catheter that has been guided to the site under investigation. In 36245, the catheter remains in a first order artery. In 36246, the catheter travels to a second order artery. Once the procedure is complete, the catheter is removed and pressure applied to stop bleeding at the injection site.

36247-36248
The physician inserts a needle through the skin and into an underlying artery. A guidewire is threaded through the needle into the artery and the needle is removed. The guidewire is manipulated into the specific artery. A catheter follows the wire into the third order abdominal, pelvic, or lower extremity artery branch. Contrast material for arteriography is injected into the catheter that has been guided to the site under investigation. Once the procedure is complete, the catheter is removed and pressure applied at the injection site. Report 36247 for a placement in the initial third order or more selective abdominal, pelvic, or lower extremity artery branch, within a vascular family. Report 36248 for any additional second order, third order, and beyond, abdominal, pelvic, or lower extremity artery branch, within a vascular family.

36251-36252
The physician inserts a needle through the skin and into an underlying artery, usually a lower extremity artery, and threads a guidewire through the needle and into the artery. The needle is removed. The wire is threaded into the main renal artery and any accessory renal arteries, first order (branch) only. A catheter follows the wire into the arteries. The wire is removed. Contrast material for arteriography is injected into the catheter. Images are taken, the catheter is removed, and pressure applied to stop bleeding at the injection site. These codes include image postprocessing, permanent recording of images, and radiological supervision and interpretation (e.g., pressure gradient measurements and flush aortogram). Report 36251 for a unilateral procedure and 36252 for a bilateral procedure.

36253-36254
A superselective catheterization is performed on one or more of the second order (branch) or higher of the renal artery branches. Superselective catheterization is needed for extremely small vessels or vessels that have sharp angles when branching to another order. The physician inserts a needle through the skin and into an underlying artery, usually a lower extremity artery, and threads a guidewire through the needle and into the artery. The needle is removed. The wire is threaded into the targeted artery and any accessory renal arteries of the second order or higher. A super fine and small catheter follows the wire into the arteries. The wire is removed. Contrast material for arteriography is injected into the catheter. Images are taken, the catheter is removed, and pressure is applied to stop bleeding at the injection site. These codes include image postprocessing, permanent recording of images, and radiological supervision and interpretation (e.g., pressure gradient measurements and flush aortogram). Report 36253 for a unilateral procedure and 36254 for a bilateral procedure.

36260
The physician performs an upper abdominal incision and exposes the hepatic artery. The physician punctures the hepatic artery with a large needle and passes a guidewire via the needle into the punctured artery. The physician removes the needle while leaving the guidewire in place. The physician slides the infusion catheter over the guidewire into the arterial lumen. The physician secures the catheter with suture and closes the abdominal wound around the proximal end of the infusion catheter. The physician may use the catheter to administer chemotherapeutic medication.

36261
The physician performs an upper abdominal incision and exposes the hepatic artery, locating the previously implanted infusion catheter. The physician may unkink the catheter or replace it over a wire. The physician secures the catheter with suture and closes the abdominal wound around the proximal end of the infusion catheter. The physician may use the catheter to administer chemotherapeutic medication.

36262
The physician performs an upper abdominal incision and exposes the hepatic artery while dissecting free the previously implanted infusion catheter. The physician removes the catheter, and may repair the arteriotomy with suture. The physician closes the abdominal wound, and may leave a drain in place.

36400
A needle is inserted through the skin to puncture the femoral or jugular vein of a child younger than age 3. The needle is inserted into the vein and used for the withdrawal of blood for diagnostic study or for the therapeutic infusion of intravenous medication. A soft flexible catheter may be placed for prolonged therapy. Once the procedure is complete, the needle or catheter is withdrawn and pressure is applied over the puncture site to control bleeding. Use this code for venipuncture when it necessitates the skill of a physician or other qualified health care professional. Do not use this code when routine venipuncture is performed.

36405-36406
A needle is inserted through the skin to puncture a vein of a child younger than age 3. In 36405, the scalp vein is punctured and in 36406, a vein other than the femoral, jugular, or scalp vein is used. The needle is inserted into the vein and used for the withdrawal of blood or for the therapeutic infusion of intravenous medication. A soft flexible catheter may be placed for prolonged therapy. Once the procedure is complete, the needle or catheter is withdrawn and pressure is applied over the puncture site to control bleeding. Use these codes when venipuncture necessitates the skill of a physician or other qualified health care professional. Do not use these codes when routine venipuncture is performed.

36410
A needle is inserted through the skin to puncture a vein of a person 3 years of age or older. The needle is inserted into the vein and used for the withdrawal of blood for diagnostic study or for the therapeutic infusion of intravenous medication. A soft flexible catheter may be placed for prolonged therapy. Once

the procedure is complete, the needle or catheter is withdrawn and pressure is applied over the puncture site to control bleeding. Use this code when the venipuncture necessitates the skills of a physician or other qualified health care professional. Do not use this code when routine venipuncture is performed.

36415-36416
A needle is inserted into the skin over a vein to puncture the blood vessel and withdraw blood for venous collection in 36415. In 36416, a prick is made into the finger, heel, or ear and capillary blood that pools at the puncture site is collected in a pipette. In either case, the blood is used for diagnostic study and no catheter is placed.

36420-36425
The physician makes an incision in the skin directly over the vessel and dissects the area surrounding the vein. A needle is passed into the vein for the withdrawal of blood or for the infusion of intravenous medication of a patient under 12 months of age (in 36420) or over 12 months of age (in 36425). A catheter may be left behind. Once the procedure is complete, the incision is repaired with a layered closure.

36430
The physician transfuses blood or blood components to a patient. The physician establishes venous access with a needle and catheter and transfuses the blood products.

36440
The physician performs a push transfusion on a child 2 years old and under. The physician calculates the amount of blood to be transfused and slowly injects it into the patient using a needle or existing catheter.

36450-36455
The physician performs an exchange transfusion on a newborn. The physician calculates the blood volume to be transfused. A needle is placed in an artery or in an existing arterial catheter. The patient's blood is removed and replaced simultaneously to maintain blood pressure. Report 36455 if the child is other than a newborn.

36456
A partial exchange transfusion (PET) is the commonly accepted method of treating polycythemia (too many red blood cells in the blood circulation) in newborns. This condition is sometimes associated with babies who are post-term, small for gestational age (SGA) or with intrauterine growth restriction (IUGR), identical twins with twin-to-twin transfusion, babies of diabetic mothers, or babies with chromosomal abnormalities. The physician or other qualified health care professional slowly removes blood from the newborn, replacing it with fluids that assist in the dilution of the red blood cell concentration, usually normal saline (crystalloid), blood, or plasma. The amount of blood to be exchanged is based on the observed and desired hematocrit, which is usually 55 percent.

36460
The physician performs a blood transfusion to a fetus. The physician uses separately reportable ultrasound guidance to locate the umbilical vein. A needle is directed through the abdominal wall into the amniotic cavity. The umbilical vein is pierced and fetal blood is exchanged with transfused blood. The needle is withdrawn and the fetus is observed under separately reportable ultrasound.

36468
The physician inserts a tiny needle through the skin and directly into the tiny, distended veins in the arm, leg, or trunk. A sclerosant for telangiectasias (spider veins) is injected into these veins. The solution causes the walls of the veins to become inflamed, collapse, and stick together so the veins close.

36470-36471
The physician inserts a tiny needle through the skin and injects sclerosant into a single, incompetent vein, other than telangiectasias (spider veins), of the leg. The patient stands while the sclerosant injection is given. The leg is elevated and wrapped in an elastic dressing. The solution causes the walls of the veins to become inflamed, collapse, and stick together so the veins close. Report 36471 for injection of sclerosant into multiple incompetent veins, other than telangiectasias, of the same leg.

[36465, 36466]
The physician performs ultrasound guided foam sclerotherapy (UGFS) of varicose veins. UGFS is a minimally invasive and relatively safe treatment of restricted amounts of small varicose veins. In UGFS, a non-compounded foam sclerosant is injected into an extremity truncal vein (e.g., great saphenous vein, accessory saphenous vein) using ultrasound-guided compression of the junction of the central vein (saphenofemoral junction or saphenopopliteal junction) to limit the dispersion of the injectate. The physician creates a detailed outline or mapping of the veins in the lower legs to identify all vein abnormalities along with additional nearby structures to include deep veins and arteries via duplex ultrasound examination. Once completed, the patient is placed in the supine position and the leg being treated is exposed. The physician guides the needle into the vein using ultrasonic guidance and injects a non-compounded foam. Foam volumes vary from 1 mL to 16 mL per treatment. The injected vein collapses and is eventually absorbed by the body. The physician may need to repeat the injection process a number of times along the vein in order to completely target the incompetent truncal vein. Report 36465 for injection of a non-compounded foam sclerosant into a single incompetent extremity truncal vein and 36466 for multiple incompetent truncal veins of the same leg.

36473-36474
The physician uses endovenous ablation therapy to treat venous incompetence in an extremity vein. Mechanochemical endovenous ablation (MOCA) uses a rotating wire in conjunction with an infused sclerosing

agent to damage the wall of the vein. The most common site of treatment is the greater saphenous vein. The procedure includes any imaging guidance and monitoring. The leg is prepared and draped and a local anesthetic is applied to the puncture site. A needle is inserted into the access site. A guidewire is placed into the vessel using ultrasound guidance. An introducer sheath is placed over the guidewire and the guidewire is removed. A wire catheter system is introduced and the tip is advanced to the site of the venous incompetence under ultrasound guidance. The wire catheter system is connected to a handle with a motor that provides the rotation to the wire. The system is started for about 10 seconds to create vasospasm and slowly withdrawn with continuous infusion of sclerosing agent. The ablation catheter and introducer sheath are removed and pressure is applied to the puncture site. A compression stocking is applied for the immediate 24 hours and replaced daily for the following two weeks. Report 36473 for the initial vein treated and 36474 for subsequent veins treated in the same extremity via different access sites.

36475-36476

The physician uses percutaneous, radiofrequency, endovenous ablation therapy to treat venous incompetence in an extremity vein. Radiofrequency energy is used to heat and seal the vein closed. The most common site of treatment is the greater saphenous vein. The procedure includes any imaging guidance and monitoring. The leg is prepared and draped and a local anesthetic is applied to the puncture site. A needle is inserted into the access site. A guidewire is placed into the vessel using ultrasound guidance. An introducer sheath is placed over the guidewire and the guidewire is removed. The radiofrequency ablation catheter system is introduced and the tip is advanced to the site of the venous incompetence under ultrasound guidance. A local anesthetic agent is injected into the tissues surrounding the vein within its fascial sheath along the course of the vein. Ultrasonography is used to position the catheter tip at the level of the terminal valve and the catheter electrodes are deployed. The electrodes should be just distal to the valve cusps of the terminal valve. Radiofrequency energy is applied until the thermocouple temperature rises to 80° to 85°C and remains at this temperature for 10 to 15 seconds. Once this temperature is reached, the catheter tip is slowly withdrawn until it reaches the introducer sheath in the distal vein. The ablation catheter and introducer sheath are removed and pressure is applied to the puncture site. Report 36475 for the first vein treated in a single extremity and 36476 for each additional vein treated through a separate access site in the same extremity.

36478-36479

The physician uses percutaneous, laser, endovenous ablation therapy to treat venous incompetence in an extremity vein. Laser energy is used to heat the vein and seal the vein closed. The most common site of treatment is the greater saphenous vein. The procedure includes any imaging guidance and monitoring. The leg is prepared and draped and a local anesthetic is applied to the puncture site. A needle is inserted into the access site. A guidewire is placed into the vessel using ultrasound guidance. An introducer sheath is placed over the guidewire and the guidewire is removed. The laser ablation catheter system is introduced and the tip is advanced to the site of the venous incompetence under ultrasound guidance. A local anesthetic agent is injected into the tissues surrounding the vein within its fascial sheath. The anesthetic is injected along the course of the vein. Ultrasonography is used to position the catheter tip at the level of the terminal valve and laser energy is applied via a laser fiber along the length of the vein as the catheter is slowly withdrawn. When the laser catheter tip reaches the introducer sheath in the distal vein, the laser energy is terminated. The ablation catheter and introducer sheath are removed and pressure is applied at the puncture site. Report 36478 for the first vein treated in a single extremity and 36479 for each additional vein treated through a separate access site in the same extremity.

[36482, 36483]

The physician creates a detailed outline or mapping of the veins in the lower legs to identify all vein abnormalities, along with additional nearby structures to include deep veins and arteries, via duplex ultrasound examination. The patient is placed in the supine position and the leg being treated is exposed. A local anesthetic is administered. Through a small incision, the physician uses a needle to position an intravenous catheter the length of the incompetent vein. A chemical adhesive, such as cyanoacrylate, is injected through the catheter via a special type of applicator and into the vein under imaging guidance. A small amount of the chemical adhesive is injected approximately every 3 cm along the vein causing sclerosis or a hardening of the vein. To minimize dispersing of the chemical adhesive, ultrasound compression of the outflow vein is often included in these procedures. Imaging guidance and monitoring are included in these procedures. Report 36482 for the first vein treated and 36483 for subsequent veins treated in a single extremity, each through separate access sites.

36481

The physician numbs the right lateral abdominal wall with local anesthetic. The physician places a large needle through the skin into the liver, maneuvering the needle through the liver into the intrahepatic portal vein, injecting contrast under fluoroscope for localization. The physician places a wire through the needle, retrograde into the portal vein. The physician removes the wire over the needle, and advances a catheter over the wire, through the skin and liver into the portal vein. The physician secures the catheter with suture. Alternative methods include placing a catheter via the internal jugular vein or using a transsplenic approach.

36500

The physician inserts a needle through the skin and into a peripheral vein. A guidewire is threaded through the needle into the vessel. The needle is removed. The wire is manipulated into the vein draining from the organ to be sampled. The catheter follows the guidewire into the vein. Once the catheter has been placed, the guidewire is removed and the blood sample obtained. The catheter is removed and pressure is applied to the puncture site to stop the flow of blood.

36510

The physician catheterizes the umbilical vein for diagnostic or therapeutic purposes. The physician cleanses the umbilical cord stump and locates the umbilical vein. A catheter is inserted in the vein for reasons including blood sampling or administering medication.

36511-36513

Therapeutic apheresis is the removal of some specific circulating blood component, cells or plasma solute, that is directly responsible for a disease process. Cells and plasma components may also be mobilized from other tissue storage during apheresis, such as from the spleen and lymph nodes, for enhanced clearance of the undesired element. The patient is prepared much the same as giving a regular blood donation. Whole blood is drawn out of one arm and into an instrument called a separator, which uses a microprocessing technique to draw the blood, anticoagulate it, and separate the component to be removed by centrifugal spinning, filtration, or column adsorption with the help of computerized calibration. The cells to be removed are collected while the remainder of the blood is recombined and returned to the patient through a tube and needle in the other arm. Report 36511 for white blood cell isolation and removal (leukapheresis or lymphocytapheresis), 36512 for red blood cell removal, and 36513 for removal of platelets.

36514-36516

Therapeutic apheresis is the removal of specific circulating blood components, cells, or plasma solute that is directly responsible for a disease process. Cells and plasma components may also be mobilized from other tissue storage during apheresis, such as from the spleen and lymph nodes, for enhanced clearance of the undesired element. The patient is prepared much the same as giving a regular blood donation. Whole blood is drawn out of one arm and into an instrument called a separator, which uses a microprocessing technique to draw the blood, anticoagulate it, and separate the component to be removed by centrifugal spinning, filtration, or column adsorption with the help of computerized calibration. Plasmapheresis, reported with 36514, is the isolation of the plasma from the blood. Plasma exchange isolates, discards, and replaces the plasma with a substitute fluid, like albumin. Plasma exchange is nonspecific since the plasma is discarded on the basis that toxins and antibodies accumulate in the plasma. The best method requires treating a disorder by removing the offending abnormal plasma component selectively. Report 36516 for extracorporeal immunoadsorption, selective adsorption, or selective filtration, such as dextran sulfate cellulose columns, to selectively remove low-density lipoproteins with plasma reinfusion.

36522

The physician draws a patient's blood and exposes the blood to light to eliminate destructive elements. The physician establishes venous access or attaches the machine to an existing central venous catheter line. The blood is removed and cycled through the pheresis machine where it is exposed to therapeutic wavelengths of light. The conditioned blood is returned to the patient through a catheter and a needle inserted in the vein.

36555-36556

A central venous access device (CVAD) or catheter is one in which the tip terminates in the subclavian, brachiocephalic, or iliac vein; the superior or inferior vena cava; or the right atrium. A centrally inserted CVAD has an entry site in the inferior vena cava or the jugular, subclavian, or femoral vein. For insertion of a non-tunneled, centrally inserted CVAD, the site over the access vein (e.g., subclavian, jugular) is injected with local anesthesia and punctured with a needle. A guidewire is inserted. The central venous catheter is placed over the guidewire. Ultrasound guidance may be used to gain venous access and/or fluoroscopy to check the positioning of the catheter tip. The catheter is secured into position and dressed. Non-tunneled catheters are percutaneously inserted for short term (five to seven days) use; to infuse medications, fluids, blood products, and parenteral nutrition; and to take blood draws. Report 36555 for insertion for children younger than 5 years of age and 36556 for a patient 5 years of age or older.

36557-36558

A central venous access device (CVAD) or catheter is one in which the tip terminates in the subclavian, brachiocephalic, or iliac vein; the superior or inferior vena cava; or the right atrium. A centrally inserted CVAD has an entry site in the inferior vena cava or the jugular, subclavian, or femoral vein. A tunneled catheter has an entrance site at a distance from its entrance into the vascular system; they are "tunneled" through the skin and subcutaneous tissue to a great vein. For insertion of a tunneled, centrally inserted CVAD, without subcutaneous port or pump, standard preparations are made and the site over the access vein (e.g., subclavian, jugular) is injected with local anesthesia and punctured with a needle or accessed by cutdown approach. A guidewire is inserted. A subcutaneous tunnel is created using a blunt pair of forceps or sharp tunneling tools, over the clavicle from the anterior chest wall to the venotomy site, which is dilated to the right size. The catheter is passed through this tunnel over the guidewire and into the target vein. Ultrasound guidance may be used to gain venous access and/or fluoroscopy to check the positioning of the catheter tip. The catheter is secured into position and any incisions are sutured. Report 36557 for insertion for children younger than 5 years of age and 36558 for a patient 5 years of age or older.

36560-36563

For insertion of a tunneled, centrally inserted CVAD, with subcutaneous port/pump, the site over the access vein (e.g., subclavian, jugular) is injected with local anesthesia and punctured with a needle or accessed by cutdown approach. A guidewire is inserted. A subcutaneous tunnel is created using a blunt pair of forceps or sharp tunneling tools, over the clavicle, from the anterior chest wall to the venotomy site, which is dilated to the right size. The catheter is passed through this tunnel over the guidewire and into the target vein. The subcutaneous pocket for the port/pump is created with an incision through the skin overlying the second rib, a few centimeters from the midline. Blunt dissection and cautery are used to create the pocket in the chest wall and the port/pump is placed. The catheter is connected to the port/pump and checked by injection. Ultrasound guidance may be used to gain venous access and/or fluoroscopy to check the positioning of the catheter tip. The catheter and port/pump are secured into position and any incisions are sutured. Report 36560 for insertion with a port for children younger than 5 years of age and 36561 for a patient 5 years of age or older. Report 36563 for insertion with a pump.

36565

For insertion of a tunneled, centrally inserted CVAD, requiring two catheters via two separate venous access sites, without subcutaneous port/pump, the sites of access (e.g., subclavian, jugular vein) for each catheter are injected with local anesthesia and two punctures are made with a needle or cutdown approach. Guidewires are inserted. Two subcutaneous tunnels are created using a blunt pair of forceps or sharp tunneling tools, over the clavicle, from the anterior chest wall to the venotomy sites, which are dilated to the right size. The catheters are each passed through their tunnel, over the guidewires, and into their venotomy sites. Ultrasound guidance may be used to gain venous access and/or fluoroscopy to check the positioning of the catheter tip. The catheters are secured into position and any incisions are sutured.

36566

For insertion of a tunneled, centrally inserted CVAD, requiring two catheters via two separate venous access sites, with subcutaneous ports, the sites of access (e.g., subclavian, jugular vein) for each catheter are injected with local anesthesia and two punctures are made with a needle or cutdown approach. Guidewires are inserted. Two subcutaneous tunnels are created using a blunt pair of forceps or sharp tunneling tools, over the clavicle, from the anterior chest wall to the venotomy sites, which are dilated to the right size. The catheters are each passed through their tunnel over the guidewires and into their venotomy sites. Two subcutaneous pockets for the ports are created with incisions through the skin in the chest wall, a few centimeters from the midline. Blunt dissection and cautery are used to create the pockets in the chest wall and the ports are placed. The catheters are connected to their respective ports and checked by injection. Ultrasound guidance may be used to gain venous access and/or fluoroscopy to check the positioning of the catheter tip. The catheters and ports are secured into position and any incisions are sutured.

36568-36569 [36572, 36573]

A central venous access device or catheter is one in which the tip terminates in the subclavian, brachiocephalic, or iliac vein; the superior or inferior vena cava; or the right atrium. A peripherally inserted central venous catheter (PICC) has an entry site in the basilic or cephalic vein in the arm and is threaded into the superior vena cava above the right atrium. PICC lines are used for antibiotic therapy, chemotherapy, total parenteral nutrition, lab work, pain medications, blood transfusions, and hydration the same as a central line. For insertion of a (non-tunneled) peripherally inserted central venous catheter, without subcutaneous port or pump, the access vein (basilic or cephalic) is injected with local anesthesia and punctured with a needle. A guidewire is inserted. The central venous catheter is placed over the guidewire. The catheter is secured into position and dressed. Report 36568 for insertion of a PICC, without imaging, for children younger than 5 years of age; for a patient 5 years of age or older, report 36569. Report 36572 for insertion of a PICC, with imaging, for children younger than 5 years age; for a patient 5 years of age or older, report 36573.

36570-36571

A central venous access device or catheter is one in which the tip terminates in the subclavian, brachiocephalic, or iliac vein; the superior or inferior vena cava; or the right atrium. A peripherally inserted central venous catheter (PICC) has an entry site in the basilic or cephalic vein in the arm and is threaded into the superior vena cava above the right atrium. PICC lines are used for antibiotic therapy, chemotherapy, total parenteral nutrition, lab work, pain medications, blood transfusions, and hydration the same as a central line. For insertion of a peripherally inserted central venous catheter with a subcutaneous port, the site over the access vein (basilic or cephalic) is injected with local anesthesia and punctured with a needle. A guidewire is inserted. The central venous catheter is placed over the guidewire and fed through the vein in the arm into the superior vena cava. The port may be placed in the chest in a subcutaneous pocket created through an incision in the chest wall, or placed in the arm through a small incision just above or halfway between the elbow crease and the shoulder on the inside of the arm. The port is attached to the catheter and checked. Ultrasound guidance may be used to gain venous access and/or fluoroscopy to check the positioning of the catheter tip. The catheter and port are secured into position and incisions are closed and dressed. Report 36570 for insertion for children younger than 5 years of age and 36571 for a patient 5 years of age or older.

36575
This code reports repair of a central venous access device (CVAD) that has external catheters with the access ports outside the body, and no subcutaneous ports or pumps, whether centrally or peripherally inserted, tunneled or non-tunneled. The repair is done on the catheter that is placed without any replacement of components. A Hickman catheter is an example of a tunneled CVAD with an external port.

36576
The physician repairs a central venous access device (CVAD) that has an internal access port/pump in a subcutaneous pocket that is connected to the catheter, whether centrally or peripherally inserted. The repair is done on the device as it is placed within the patient, without any replacement of components, catheter, or subcutaneous port/pump.

36578
The catheter only of a central venous access device with a subcutaneous port or pump is replaced, whether centrally or peripherally inserted. Local anesthesia is given and the subcutaneous pocket over the port is incised. The catheter is disconnected. A guidewire is placed through the existing catheter, which is removed over the guidewire. A new central venous catheter of correct length is placed into position and connected to the port/pump device that has not been removed or replaced. The connection with the new catheter is checked, as well as the catheter and port secured, and the wound is dressed.

36580
A non-tunneled, centrally inserted central venous catheter, without subcutaneous port or pump, is replaced through the same venous access site. Local anesthesia is given. A guidewire is first passed through the existing central line catheter and the catheter is removed. A new central venous catheter is placed back into position over the guidewire, secured into position, and dressed.

36581
A tunneled, centrally inserted central venous catheter, without subcutaneous port or pump is replaced. Local anesthesia is given and the sutures securing the cuff of the indwelling catheter are freed from the skin. A guidewire is next placed through the existing catheter, which is removed, and a new central venous catheter is inserted into the tunneled position over the guidewire. The new catheter is secured into position and the wound is dressed.

36582-36583
A tunneled, centrally inserted central venous catheter, along with a subcutaneous port (36582) or pump (36583) device is replaced. Local anesthesia is given and the subcutaneous pocket over the port/pump device is incised. The pump/port is dissected free and tested. The catheter is disconnected and the pump/port device is removed from its pocket. A guidewire is placed over the existing catheter, which is removed, and a new central venous catheter is threaded into position over the guidewire. A new pump/port device is inserted into the subcutaneous pocket and the catheter is connected. The connection is checked with an injection. The new pump/port is secured into the pocket, incisions are closed, and the wound is dressed.

36584
A peripherally inserted central venous catheter (PICC), without subcutaneous port or pump, is replaced through the same venous access site. Local anesthesia is given and the sutures securing the cuff of the catheter with external port are freed from the skin and it is partially withdrawn. A sheath is placed over the nonfunctioning catheter and it is completely withdrawn. A guidewire is inserted into the access site through the sheath and advanced. A new catheter of correct length is placed over the guidewire and the sheath and guidewire are removed. The catheter is fastened in position and the wound is dressed. This service includes all imaging guidance and documentation, as well as the supervision and interpretation.

36585
A peripherally inserted central venous catheter (PICC), along with a subcutaneous port, is replaced through the same venous access site. Local anesthesia is given, the skin over the subcutaneous pocket is incised, and the port is dissected free. A sheath is placed over the nonfunctioning catheter and it is completely withdrawn. A guidewire is inserted into the access site through the sheath and advanced. A new catheter of correct length is placed over the guidewire and the sheath and guidewire are removed. The catheter is fastened in position and the wound is dressed.

36589-36590
In 36589, a tunneled central venous catheter without subcutaneous port or pump is removed. Local anesthesia is given and the sutures securing the cuff of the tunneled catheter's external port are freed from the skin. In 36590, a tunneled central venous access device, both catheter and subcutaneous port or pump, is removed. Local anesthesia is given and the subcutaneous pocket over the port/pump device is incised and the pump/port is dissected free. The catheter is disconnected and the pump/port device is removed from its pocket. In both cases, a guidewire is placed over the existing catheter, which is withdrawn over the guidewire, and the guidewire is removed. The incisions are closed and the wound is dressed.

36591
The physician obtains a blood specimen from a previously placed, completely implantable venous access device. Completely implanted devices are those that have access through a subcutaneous port (e.g., Port-A-Cath, Infusaport). An implantable access device requires a percutaneous noncoring needle to accomplish the blood draw. The skin is cleansed with alcohol or iodine solution. The needle is placed into the port. Heparin is withdrawn. A second needle is inserted and the blood specimen obtained. The port is flushed with heparin solution.

36592
The physician obtains a blood specimen from an established central venous or peripheral venous catheter. A central venous catheter (CVC) is one that is inserted through the skin into central veins, such as the femoral, internal jugular, or subclavian veins. Peripheral catheters include those inserted in the arm veins (basilic or cephalic), such as a PICC line, saline lock, or heparin lock. In order to clear the catheter of any material that could contaminate the sample and affect the test results, a specific volume of infusing fluid and blood must be discarded before a blood specimen is obtained; this volume varies depending on the type of catheter utilized. With a central venous catheter, a three-way stopcock is attached to the catheter's hub and two syringes attached to the stopcock. Using one syringe, the catheter is flushed with normal saline. A specific amount of blood is aspirated into the same syringe used for the saline flush and discarded. The blood sample is then withdrawn using the other syringe and placed into an appropriate tube for laboratory analysis. If using a peripheral venous catheter, a specific amount of blood is also aspirated and discarded before the blood sample is drawn.

36593
To remove a clot from an implanted vascular access device or catheter, the physician injects a thrombolytic agent (e.g., Streptokinase) into the catheter to dissolve the clot. The patient is observed for any abnormal signs of bleeding.

36595
Pericatheter obstructive material such as a fibrin sheath is removed from around a central venous device via separate venous access. Central venous catheters often fail because of the accumulation of an obstructing thrombus or fibrin sheath around the tip of the catheter. The catheter is first checked that it can aspirate and flush forward. The pericatheter material is identified by contrast material injection. Generally, a right femoral vein access is used. A guidewire followed by an angiographic catheter are advanced into the superior vena cava and exchanged for a loop snare with its catheter, which are advanced cephalad along the length of the central venous catheter beyond the ports. The loop snare is tightly closed about the central venous catheter to encircle it and slowly pulled down and off the tip of the catheter, stripping off the pericatheter obstructive material. This is repeated a few times and the catheter is rechecked for infusion and injection ability of the ports. A contrast study is done again to identify any fibrin and the process may be repeated until the fibrin sheath is completely removed.

36596
Intraluminal obstructive material, such as a thrombus or fibrin sheath, is removed from inside a central venous device through the lumen of the device. This does not require a separate access incision. The central venous catheter is first checked that it can aspirate and flush forward. The obstructing material is disrupted and removed mechanically by using an angioplasty balloon or other catheter introduced into the central venous catheter through its entry site on the skin. The catheter is checked for unimpeded, restored flow and the process may be repeated until the central venous catheter is cleared.

36597
A previously placed central venous catheter needs to be repositioned. It is possible for a catheter position to change significantly after the procedure is completed. Catheter position change and tip migration occur most often with subclavian venous access in women and obese patients, because the soft tissues of the chest wall move inferiorly with standing and often cause the catheter to get pulled back. When a catheter tip is incorrectly placed, it can increase the risks of thrombosis, fibrin sheath formation, perforation of the vein, and even arrhythmias. Fluoroscopy is used to check the positioning of the catheter tip and guide it to its correct position. Local anesthesia is given, and the sutures securing the cuff of the catheter may be freed from the skin. The catheter is partially withdrawn, and a sheath may be placed over the catheter at the existing venous access site. A guidewire is inserted through the catheter and advanced. The central venous catheter is maneuvered back into correct position and monitored with fluoroscopy to view correct placement of the tip.

36598
A previously placed central venous access device is evaluated for complications that may be interfering with its proper functioning or the ability to draw blood from the catheter. Complications may include the presence of a fibrin sheath around the end of the catheter, migration of the catheter tip, patency of the tubing, kinking, fracture, or leaks. A small amount of contrast agent is injected into the catheter and the central venous access device is examined under fluoroscopy as the flow is evaluated. Images are documented and a radiological report is prepared.

36600
The physician inserts a needle through the skin and punctures the artery to withdraw blood for testing. No catheter is left in the artery. Pressure is applied to the puncture site to stop the flow of blood.

36620-36625
The physician accesses, in most cases, the ulnar or radial artery to insert a cannula, or tube-shaped portal. In 36620, the physician inserts a needle through the skin to puncture the artery and inserts a cannula. In 36625, the physician makes an incision in the skin overlying the artery and dissects the surrounding tissue to access it. The artery is sometimes nicked with a thin-bladed scalpel before the physician inserts the cannula. This cannula acts as a portal for sampling, monitoring or transfusion. Once the procedure is complete, the cannula is removed. In an open procedure, the opening in the artery may be sutured and the incision repaired with a layered closure.

Pressure is applied to the puncture if a percutaneous approach is used.

36640

The physician accesses the artery supplying the area to be treated. To insert a cannula, or tube-shaped portal for prolonged infusion therapy, the physician makes an incision above the artery and dissects the surrounding tissue to access it. The artery is sometimes nicked with a thin-bladed scalpel before the physician inserts the catheter. The catheter may be advanced to a site immediately upstream of the site to be treated. This catheter acts as a portal for the infusion of chemotherapy drugs and will remain in place until chemotherapy is completed. The catheter is removed, the hole in the artery is repaired, and the incision is repaired with a layered closure.

36660

The physician catheterizes an umbilical artery in a newborn for diagnostic or therapeutic purposes. The physician prepares the umbilical artery and passes a catheter sheath inside the lumen for arterial access. The catheter is attached to a pressure line that maintains patency of the arterial lumen. The access is used for diagnostic or therapeutic purposes, allowing the drawing of blood for tests or instillation of medication.

36680

The physician inserts a hollow needle through the skin and through the muscle tissue to puncture the bone marrow cavity, usually in the tibia or femur, of a patient whose vessels otherwise seem inaccessible. This needle is used as a method of infusing fluids into the blood vessels in the bone marrow.

36800

The physician isolates two veins, usually in the nondominant forearm, and inserts a needle through the skin and into each vessel. A guidance wire may be threaded through the needle into each vessel. The needle is removed. An end of a single cannula is inserted into each puncture, and any guidance wire removed. The cannula remains external, and may be left in place for several days. (This hemodialysis cannula is used to remove blood from the vein, route it through the dialysis machine, then reinfuse it.)

36810

The physician isolates an artery and a vein, usually in the nondominant forearm, and inserts a needle through the skin and into each vessel. A guidewire may be threaded through the needle into each vessel. The needle is removed. An end of a single cannula is inserted into each puncture, and any guidance wire removed. The Scribner cannula remains external, and may be left in place for several days. (This hemodialysis cannula is used to remove blood from the vessel, route it through the dialysis machine, then reinfuse it.)

36815

The physician repositions an external cannula or removes it. The cannula forms a ready connection between the artery and vein or vein and vein for hemodialysis or another purpose. Closure of the insertion site is performed using sutures on the vessels or skin as necessary.

36818-36819

A vascular surgeon creates a connection between an artery and a vein for a vascular access site in patients with end stage renal disease who require hemodialysis. In 36819, the surgeon dissects down to the basilic vein on the medial side of the upper arm and mobilizes the vein. A subcutaneous tunnel on the anterior side of the arm is created, and the mobilized basilic vein is transposed to this tunnel and anastomosed to the brachial artery. Report 36818 if a similar arteriovenous connection is made in the upper arm by anastomosing the cephalic vein to the brachial artery.

36820

The physician creates a connection between an artery or vein using a forearm vein in the arm inverted end to end. The physician dissects down to the vein and artery. The subfascial plane is identified and elevated laterally to the flexor carpi radialis (FCR) and medially to the brachioradialis (BR). The plane between the BR and FCR is dissected and the perforating vessels are identified and cauterized. The pedicle is followed to the antecubital fossa. The tourniquet is released, and the vessels are further cleaned of their adventitia under loupe visualization. Using microvascular techniques, a suture for the arterial anastomosis is performed and closure is completed. Suction drains are placed in the neck. If a Doppler is to be used for postoperative assessment, a suture is placed to mark the pedicle site. A splint is fabricated and secured to the arm with an elastic bandage.

36821

Through an incision, usually in the skin over an artery in the nondominant wrist or antecubital fossa, the physician isolates a desired section of artery and neighboring vein. Vessel clamps are placed on the vein and adjacent artery. The vein is dissected free, divided, and the downstream portion of the vein is sutured to an opening created in the adjacent artery, usually in an end-to-side fashion, allowing blood to flow both down the artery and into the vein. Large branches of the vein may be tied off to cause flow down a single vein. The skin incision is repaired with a layered closure. This arteriovenous anastomosis will allow an increased blood flow through the vein, usually for hemodialysis.

36823

The physician inserts arterial and venous cannula(s) for isolated extracorporeal circulation to an extremity to provide regional perfusion chemotherapy (RPC) with or without hyperthermia. The external iliac, common femoral, or subclavian artery and vein are isolated depending on the site of the tumor. A cannula is inserted into the selected artery and vein to isolate blood flow to and from the extremity. The blood flow from the isolated extremity is connected to a perfusion pump where the blood is oxygenated. The blood may be heated to between 40°-40.5° C (104°-105° F). One or more high dose chemotherapy agents are injected and perfused over an hour or more with flow rates monitored and adjusted to minimize leakage into the systemic circulation. The combination of heat and the chemotherapy agent act to destroy the cancer cells. After completion of the perfusion procedure, the cannula(s) are removed and the artery and vein repaired.

36825-36830

The physician creates an arteriovenous fistula by other than direct anastomosis. The physician makes an incision in the skin over an artery and vein, and the vein and artery are dissected free. A vessel clamp is affixed to each. A length of harvested vein from the patient is used for an autogenous graft in 36825 and is sutured to the incised artery and vein, usually in an end-to-side fashion. The graft is passed in a superficial subcutaneous tunnel that is created bluntly and connects the arterial and venous sites. The clamps are removed, allowing the blood to flow through the graft, creating an arteriovenous fistula. The skin incision is repaired with a layered closure. Report 36830 if a nonautogenous graft, such as biological collagen or a thermoplastic graft, is used.

36831

The physician removes a blood clot from a surgically created connection between an artery and a vein (arteriovenous fistula). The procedure involves making an incision over the site of an existing fistula. The fistula is isolated and dissected free. Vessel clamps are affixed above and below the fistula. The blood clot is removed, the clamps are taken off, and the incision is repaired by layered sutures. The procedure may involve a vein acquired from the patient or the construction of a synthetic graft.

36832-36833

In 36832, the physician makes an incision at the site of an already existing artificial fistula between an artery and a vein. The fistula is dissected free. Vessel clamps are affixed above and below the fistula, which is incised. Revisions are made to the fistula at its juncture to the vein and/or artery and may require creating a new anastomosis with a graft obtained from a separate site or created with synthetic material. After the repair has been made, the fistula is sutured, the clamps removed, and the skin incision repaired with a layered closure. Report 36833 when the physician removes a blood clot at the fistula site in addition to revising the existing arteriovenous fistula.

[36836, 36837]

The physician creates an arteriovenous (AV) fistula, which is a surgically created connection between an artery and a vein, in an upper extremity using a minimally invasive, catheter-based percutaneous approach. The procedure is typically performed by a vascular specialist and is created for long-term dialysis access. Conscious sedation, regional anesthesia, or local anesthesia may be used. Code 36836 is reported for the creation of an AV fistula via a single access site for the arteriovenous puncture, along with thermal energy. In one technique, the cubital vein is accessed using a standard micropuncture needle and wire. Using ultrasound guidance, the access needle is advanced intravenously into the perforating vein and into the proximal radial artery. A guidewire is positioned through the vein into the radial artery followed by a sheath, which allows the device to be inserted into the artery. The access needle is withdrawn, and a 6-F sheath is advanced over the guidewire into the artery. The device catheter is placed through the sheath and the walls of the artery and vein are engaged. The catheter is activated, creating a fistula via a low-power direct current. The device and sheath are removed, and hemostasis is accomplished with pressure. A Doppler study may be performed to confirm fistula flow and measure brachial artery flow volume, and balloon angioplasty may be performed immediately following fistula creation to quickly increase blood flow in the fistula. In an alternate method (36837), separate access sites are employed, and the AV fistula is created using magnetic-guided arterial and venous catheters along with radiofrequency (RF) energy. Most commonly, the brachial vein is accessed using a standard micropuncture needle and wire. The guidewire is advanced intravenously, under imaging guidance, through the brachial vein into the ulnar vein, and a dilator and sheath are placed. The brachial artery is accessed, also under imaging guidance, using a standard micropuncture needle and wire. The guidewire is advanced intravenously into the ulnar artery, and a dilator and sheath are placed. A magnetic catheter is inserted into the artery and a second magnetic catheter is inserted into the vein. The magnets draw the artery and vein together. Once alignment is confirmed, an RF cutting electrode is deployed in the venous catheter, which aligns with a ceramic backstop in the arterial catheter. The electrode is energized, and a channel is created between the vein and artery. The catheters are removed, and the accessed brachial vein is embolized with a coil to force blood into the superficial veins for dialysis. All prosthetic materials are removed, and hemostasis is accomplished with pressure. A fistulogram is performed to confirm fistula flow. In either procedure, the patient must have vessels that are more than 2 mm in diameter and have less than 2 mm of separation between the artery and vein at the site of fistula creation. These codes include all fistula maturation procedures such as coil embolization or transluminal balloon angioplasty if performed, and include all vascular access, imaging guidance, and any radiologic supervision/interpretation.

36835

Through an incision in the skin overlying a large vein or artery of a child, the physician dissects the vessel that will receive a synthetic shunt. The vessel may be clamped. The vessel is nicked, and a needle threads a guidance wire into the vein or artery. The shunt follows, and the wire is removed. The physician sutures the synthetic shunt end-to-end, or end-to-side, to the vein or artery. The shunt is most often used for access in hemodialysis.

36838
A DRIL procedure, distal revascularization and interval ligation, is done to treat Steal syndrome occurring in patients with a permanent indwelling access site in the arm for hemodialysis. In Steal syndrome, the hand becomes cold and painful, due to ischemia because the hemodialysis access is taking the arm's blood supply. The DRIL procedure restores blood flow to the hand and preserves the access site. It is a two-step procedure. The surgeon first creates a bypass graft around the access site, using a harvested vein conduit, usually the greater saphenous. An incision is made in the upper arm for the proximal anastomosis, which is placed above the dialysis access site, nearer to the axilla. Soft tissue is dissected to expose the brachial artery. An incision is also made lower in the arm for the site of the distal anastomosis, which is placed below the dialysis access site, down in the forearm. A tunnel is created from one site to the other and the graft is completed using the harvested vein. This is the revascularization portion of the procedure and allows a good flow of blood around the access site. The second part of the procedure is the ligation. The brachial artery is tied off at a point between the dialysis access and the distal anastomosis site of the bypass graft. Now the arterial blood flow being pumped from the heart runs through the bypass, supplying the hand with oxygen before entering the access site. The incisions are closed and pulses are checked for good perfusion before applying dressings.

36860-36861
To remove a blood clot lodged in a previously placed cannula, the physician may inject a solution containing enzymes into the cannula to dissolve the clot (in 36860) or the physician may, after injecting a solution containing enzymes, insert a balloon catheter (in 36861) into the cannula to retrieve a clot there. The balloon is inserted and inflated beyond the clot. The catheter is slowly pulled out, capturing and retrieving the clot. Once the clot is dissolved or retrieved, the catheter is removed and the cannula is left in place.

36901-36903
The physician inserts a needle or catheter into a dialysis circuit via a puncture in the skin overlying the circuit of a dialysis patient. The catheter is guided into the circuit and vessel to an area upstream of the site under investigation, and contrast material is injected into it. Report 36901 for the initial access, including shunt access, contrast injections, and all fluoroscopic imaging deemed necessary from the arterial anastomosis and adjacent artery through the entire venous outflow (inferior and superior vena cava included). In 36902, a catheter with a balloon attached is inserted into the peripheral dialysis segment and fed into the narrowed portion where its balloon may be inflated several times in order to stretch the diameter, allowing a more normal flow of blood through the area. In 36903, a catheter with a stent-transporting tip is threaded over the guidewire into the peripheral dialysis segment and the wire is extracted. The catheter travels to the point where the vessel needs additional support. The compressed stent is passed from the catheter into the vessel, where it deploys, expanding to support the vessel walls. Once the procedure is complete, the catheter is removed and pressure is applied over the puncture site.

36904-36906
The physician treats the dialysis circuit occlusion with mechanical thrombectomy and/or thrombolysis infusion. The devices used for mechanical thrombectomy include those that fragment the thrombus with or without removal of the clot, as well as those that come into contact with the vessel wall. The dialysis circuit is cannulated to gain access and 5,000 units of heparin are administered. Angiography is performed to confirm the occluded segment. A hydrophilic wire is passed across the occlusion, followed by passing of the device over a stiff exchange length wire. The distal and proximal balloons are inflated in the segment on either side of a treatment zone containing infusion to isolate the treatment zone and to sustain the fluid concentration that is infused. One milligram of tissue plasminogen activator (TPA) is infused into the treatment zone. A thrombectomy device is run at 4,000 rpm for five minutes. After the proximal balloon is deflated, small clots are removed via the integral aspiration port to prevent embolization. Thrombolysis infusion may be performed with a catheter threaded over the wire for pharmaceutical administration directly within the thrombosis. When the procedure is complete, the instruments are removed, and pressure is applied over the puncture site to stop the bleeding. This procedure is reported with 36904 and includes imaging guidance, diagnostic angiography, catheter placement, and intraprocedural pharmacological thrombolytic injections. Report 36905 when the peripheral dialysis segment is treated with balloon angioplasty. A catheter with a balloon attached is inserted into the segment and fed into the narrowed portion, where its balloon may be inflated several times to stretch the diameter allowing a more normal flow of blood through the area. Report 36906 when the peripheral dialysis segment is treated with an intravascular stent. A catheter with a stent-transporting tip is threaded over the guidewire into the vessel and the wire is extracted. The catheter travels to the point where the vessel needs additional support. The compressed stent is passed from the catheter into the vessel, where it deploys, expanding to support the vessel walls. Once the procedure is complete, the catheter is removed, and pressure is applied over the puncture site.

36907-36908
The physician inserts a needle or catheter into a dialysis circuit via a puncture in the skin. The catheter is guided into the circuit to an area upstream of the investigation site and contrast material is injected. In 36907, a catheter with a balloon attached is inserted into the central dialysis segment and fed into the narrowed portion, where its balloon may be inflated several times in order to stretch the diameter, allowing a more normal blood flow through the area. In 36908,

a catheter with a stent-transporting tip is threaded over the guidewire into the central dialysis segment and the wire is extracted. The catheter travels to the point where the vessel needs additional support. The compressed stent is passed from the catheter out into the vessel, where it deploys, expanding to support the vessel walls. Once the procedure is complete, the catheter is removed and pressure is applied over the puncture site. All imaging and radiological supervision and interpretation is included.

36909
The physician performs embolization or occlusion of a dialysis circuit (main circuit or any accessory vein) due to complications or to assist in circuit maturity and/or patency. A needle is inserted through the skin and into a blood vessel. A guidewire is threaded through the needle into the vessel. The needle is removed. A catheter is threaded into the vessel and the wire is extracted. The catheter travels to the appropriate blood vessel and beads, coils, or another vessel-blocking device are released. The beads or other device block the vessel. The catheter is removed and pressure is applied over the puncture site to stop bleeding.

37140
The physician performs portocaval venous anastomosis. The physician places a long right thoracoabdominal incision and exposes the liver. The physician exposes the inferior vena cava and portal vein through careful dissection. The physician places a plastic sling around the portal vein and ties it closed, just proximal to its bifurcation. The physician clamps and divides the portal vein. The physician applies a partial exclusion vascular clamp to the front of the vena cava and removes a small oval of tissue from the vena cava to allow end-to-side anastomosis of portal vein to the inferior vena cava. The physician removes the clamps and checks for appropriate flow without anastomotic leakage. The physician closes the incision, leaving a chest tube in place (but no abdominal drains, as this may lead to protein loss from postoperative drainage of ascites).

37145
The physician performs an abdominal incision and exposes the left renal vein and inferior vena cava. The physician transects the left renal vein and attaches it to the portal circulation by sewing the vena caval end to the portal vein, the superior mesenteric vein, or the splenic vein. Alternatively, the physician may divide the portal vein and attach its splanchnic end to the end of the transected renal vein. The physician assesses patency of the anastomosis and may measure venous pressures before closing the abdomen.

37160
The physician performs an upper midline vertical abdominal incision and retracts the transverse colon in a cephalad direction. The physician exposes the anterior surface of the inferior vena cava and frees the posterior surface of the superior mesenteric vein after careful dissection through the root of the transverse mesocolon. The physician isolates a long segment of the superior mesenteric vein with ties and partially occludes the inferior vena cava. The physician removes an ellipse of tissue from the inferior vena cava and performs and end-to-side anastomosis of Dacron graft to the inferior vena cava. The physician occludes the superior mesenteric vein, cuts an ellipse from its anterior surface, and sews the end of the Dacron graft to the side of the superior mesenteric vein. The physician assesses patency of the anastomosis and may measure venous pressures before closing the abdomen.

37180
The physician performs a bilateral subcostal incision from the right midrectus position extending into the left flank, and dissects past bowel and pancreas to expose the splenic vein. The physician dissects the splenic vein free, ligating the splenic vein toward the left and using the central (right) end of the vein for the anastomosis. The physician exposes the left renal vein by dissecting through the posterior parietal peritoneum. The physician exposes the left renal vein, partially clamps it, and excises an ellipse of renal vein at its upper border. The physician performs and end-to-side anastomosis of the splenic vein to the renal vein, using harvested vein graft material if extension is required. The physician removes the clamps. The physician may measure superior mesenteric (portal), renal, and splenic venous pressures. The physician may perform venography to establish patency of the graft. The physician closes the abdominal wound.

37181
The physician performs a bilateral subcostal incision from the right midrectus position extending into the left flank, and dissects past bowel and pancreas to expose the splenic vein. The physician dissects the splenic vein free, ligating or clipping any vessels in continuity to the vein. The physician exposes the left renal vein by dissecting through the posterior parietal peritoneum. The physician exposes the left renal vein, partially clamps it, and excises an ellipse of renal vein at its upper border. The physician performs and end-to-side anastomosis of the splenic vein to the renal vein, using harvested vein graft material if extension is required. The physician removes the clamps and divides the coronary (right gastric) vein, left gastric vein, and gastroepiploic veins. The physician may measure superior mesenteric (portal), renal, and splenic venous pressures. The physician may perform venography to establish patency of the graft. The physician closes the abdominal wound.

37182-37183
A transvenous intrahepatic portosystemic shunt (TIPS) is inserted in 37182 and replaced in 37183. Shunts are placed percutaneously to manage the complications of portal hypertension and control variceal bleeding and ascites. Once the patient is under general anesthesia or conscious sedation, the right internal jugular vein is accessed and a catheter is placed into the right hepatic vein. Catheter placement is verified using venography.

A Colapinto needle is advanced through the catheter into the wall of the right hepatic vein to access the right portal vein. A guidewire and catheter are advanced along this route into the portal vein and venography is performed again to verify placement. A self-expanding metallic stent is deployed through the catheter and dilated to the desired diameter where it bridges the portal and hepatic veins, using an angioplastic balloon. Postplacement venography and pressure measurements confirm adequate position and flow through the TIPS. The balloon, catheter, and other endoscopic tools are removed and pressure is applied to the insertion site, which may require suture. In 37183, the existing shunt is collapsed and removed through the catheter before a new one is inserted and dilated.

37184-37185

The physician treats an acute noncoronary, nonintracranial arterial occlusion with a combination of thrombolytic drugs and percutaneous mechanical thrombectomy. The devices used for mechanical thrombectomy include those that fragment the thrombus with or without removal of the clot, as well as those that come into contact with the wall of the vessel. For the procedure using the Trellis device, the artery is cannulated to gain access and 5,000 units of heparin are administered. Angiography is performed to confirm the occluded arteries. A hydrophilic wire is passed across the occlusion, followed by passing of the Trellis device over a stiff exchange length wire. The distal and proximal balloons are inflated in the artery on either side of a treatment zone containing infusion to isolate the treatment zone and to sustain the fluid concentration that is infused. One milligram of tissue plasminogen activator (TPA) is infused into the treatment zone. The Turbo Trellis is run at 4,000 rpm for five minutes. After the proximal balloon is deflated, small clots are removed via the integral aspiration port to prevent embolization. Fluoroscopic guidance services and injections administered during the course of the procedure are included in the service. Separately reportable procedures include other percutaneous interventions such as stent placement and diagnostic studies. Report 37184 for the first vessel and 37185 for the second and subsequent vessels in the same vascular family.

37186

The physician performs a secondary thrombectomy of a noncoronary, non-intracranial arterial occlusion. Prior to or after a percutaneous intervention is performed, such as balloon angioplasty or placement of a stent, the transcatheter removal of small sections of the thrombus or embolism is performed using suction, a snare basket, or a mechanical thrombectomy device under fluoroscopic guidance. Thrombolytic injections may also be used during the procedure.

37187-37188

The physician performs a percutaneous transluminal mechanical venous thrombectomy. A catheter sheath is inserted through a small incision in the vein, most commonly a groin incision in the femoral vein or an incision below the knee in the popliteal vein. Contrast is injected through the sheath and a separately reportable venography is performed to visualize the area of the vein being treated. Fluoroscopic guidance may be used. A guidewire is inserted through the sheath and advanced past the clot. A catheter is passed over the wire to the blocked area. A device at the tip of the catheter, a mechanical tool or a high-velocity liquid jet, is used to break the clot. A thrombolytic agent may be injected. When the procedure is completed, all instruments are removed and a compression bandage is applied. Report 37187 for the initial treatment. Report 37188 for repeat treatment on a subsequent day during the course of thrombolytic therapy.

37191-37193

An inferior vena cava (IVC) filter is placed most commonly for refractory deep vein thrombosis and pulmonary embolism or when anticoagulation is contraindicated. In 37191, the physician places a needle in the femoral (or internal jugular) vein, advances a guidewire through the needle, removes the needle over the wire, and advances an introducer sheath over the wire into the femoral vein. The physician advances the filter through the introducer sheath into the inferior vena cava under fluoroscopic guidance. The physician removes the introducer sheath and compresses the femoral vein manually until hemostasis is achieved. Report 37192 for the repositioning of an already placed filter utilizing an endovascular approach and associated radiologic guidance when applicable. In 37193, the physician utilizes the same approach to remove the filter.

37195

The physician remedies a stroke-causing blood clot obstructing blood flow to the brain. The physician infuses a thrombolytic ("clot-busting") drug through an intravenous catheter to help dissolve the clot and restore normal blood flow to the brain.

37197

The physician places a needle into a blood vessel. A guidewire is threaded through the needle into the vessel and the needle is removed. A catheter is threaded into the vessel and the wire is extracted. The catheter, equipped with a grasping instrument, travels to the site of the foreign body typically using imaging guidance. The instrument grasps the foreign body, typically a fractured catheter, and retrieves it. The catheter is removed and pressure is applied over the puncture site to stop the bleeding.

37200

A needle is inserted through the skin and into a blood vessel, and a guidewire is threaded through the needle into the vessel. The needle is removed. A catheter is threaded into the vessel, and the wire extracted. The catheter equipped with a biopsy instrument travels to the area to be sampled. The instrument extracts for biopsy tissue affixed to the vessel wall. Pressure is applied over the puncture site to stop bleeding after the catheter is removed. This procedure may also be performed through a skin incision with direct exposure of the access vessel.

37211-37214

Transcatheter thrombolysis infusion is most commonly used to treat symptomatic inferior vena cava thrombosis that is responding poorly to the routine anticoagulation regimen or symptomatic iliofemoral or femoropopliteal deep vein thrombosis (DVT) in patients with a low risk of bleeding. A diagnostic arteriography or venography is performed to pinpoint the extent of the thrombosis. The physician places a needle into the blood vessel. A guidewire is threaded through the needle to the site of the clot using fluoroscopic guidance and the needle is removed. An infusion catheter is threaded to the site and the wire is extracted. A thrombolytic pharmaceutical is administered directly to the thrombosis. During the infusion, the patient is on bed rest with frequent monitoring. Once the thrombosis has dissipated satisfactorily, the infusion is stopped and the catheter removed. Pressure is applied over the puncture site to stop the bleeding. Report 37211 for the first day of arterial transcatheter therapy; 37212 for the first day of venous transcatheter therapy; 37213 for each subsequent day of arterial or venous therapy, including follow-up catheter contrast injection, position change, or exchange, if applicable; and 37214 for the last day the thrombolysis is administered, including removal of the catheter and closure of the access site. These codes are not for use when thrombolysis is performed on coronary or intracranial arteries.

37215-37216

The physician places an intravascular stent via open or percutaneous approach through a catheter into the cervical carotid artery. The open procedure is carried out by making an incision exposing the cervical carotid artery and creating an arteriotomy. In the percutaneous approach, a needle is inserted through the skin into the access blood vessel, usually the brachial or femoral artery. A guidewire is threaded through the needle into the cervical carotid artery and the needle is removed. Long sheaths or guiding catheters are advanced into the stenosed cervical carotid artery. A filter protection device may be inserted distal to the stenosis to capture emboli. After filter opening, predilation of the stenosis with angioplasty balloons may be performed. A catheter with a stent-transporting tip is threaded over the guidewire into the vessel and the wire is extracted. The catheter travels to the point where the vessel needs additional support. The compressed stent is passed from the catheter out into the vessel, where it deploys, expanding to support the vessel walls. The catheter is removed and pressure is applied over the puncture site. Report 37215 when stenting is performed with a filter protection device (distal embolic protection) and 37216 when stenting is performed without a filter protection device. The procedures include radiologic supervision and interpretation, as well as angioplasty, when performed.

37217

Placing stents into the intrathoracic common carotid artery or innominate artery via a catheter is a less invasive alternative to open endarterectomy. The procedure is carried out by making an incision exposing the cervical carotid artery and creating an arteriotomy. A catheter is inserted through the artery and threaded to the target. A stent delivery system, which may also include an embolic capturing device, is loaded into a delivery pod and advanced to the blocked or narrowed artery through the catheter. The embolic protection device is deployed first, distal to the lesion so that any emboli are collected as the blood passes through the device. The stent is advanced out of the pod until it expands to open the narrowing. The instruments are removed. The artery and overlying tissues are closed. The procedure includes radiologic supervision and interpretation, as well as angioplasty, when performed.

37218

The physician places an intravascular stent via open or percutaneous antegrade approach through a catheter into the intrathoracic common carotid artery or innominate artery. A catheter is inserted through the artery and threaded to the target. A stent delivery system, which may also include an embolic capturing device, is loaded into a delivery pod and advanced to the blocked or narrowed artery through the catheter. The embolic protection device is deployed first, distal to the lesion, so that any emboli are collected as the blood passes through the device. The stent is advanced out of the pod until it expands to open the narrowing. The instruments are removed. The artery and overlying tissues are closed. The procedure includes radiologic supervision and interpretation, as well as angioplasty, when performed.

37220-37223

The physician treats an iliac artery occlusion or stenosis by endovascular revascularization (restoration of blood supply) in 37220. Access is gained using a small open incision or a percutaneous sheath. Typically, a femoral approach under local anesthesia is used. After sheath placement, intra-arterial heparin is administered. Using a retrograde approach and under angiographic guidance, the occlusion is crossed using a catheter and guidewire. The balloon catheter is inflated in order to dilate the vessel to a larger diameter. Report 37220 for revascularization of the initial vessel and 37222 for each additional vessel on the same side (ipsilateral). Report 37221 if stent placement follows; angioplasty within the same vessel is included in this code. Following dilation and stent deployment, an angiogram is performed to assure appropriate placement and to evaluate the final result. Report 37223 for each additional ipsilateral vessel into which a stent is placed.

37224-37227

The physician treats occlusive disease of a unilateral femoral or popliteal artery by endovascular revascularization (restoration of blood supply) using angioplasty in 37224. Access is gained using a femoral cutdown incision or a percutaneous sheath. Under local anesthesia, the physician accesses the femoral artery. After sheath or needle placement, intra-arterial heparin may be administered. A guidewire is inserted into the artery, followed by a catheter with an attached balloon. The catheter is advanced through the arterial system and into the narrowed portion of the targeted artery. There, the balloon is inflated in order to dilate the vessel to a larger diameter; several inflations may be necessary to achieve maximal results. The physician withdraws the deflated catheter and applies pressure to the puncture site to staunch the bleeding or closes the arteriotomy with suture. In 37225, the physician also performs atherectomy. The physician slides a guidewire through the atherectomy catheter or device, and inserts the guidewire/atherectomy catheter combination through the introducer sheath. The atherectomy device is fluoroscopically positioned at the site of the stenosis. The physician activates the device to remove the stenotic tissue and rechecks the diameter of the lesion by angiography. Several passes with the atherectomy device may be required. The physician removes the atherectomy catheter, guidewire, and introducer sheath. In 37226, the physician places one or more transluminal stents percutaneously using a guidewire or by incision. A catheter with a stent-transporting tip is threaded into the vessel. The catheter travels to the point where the vessel needs additional support, and the compressed stent is passed from the catheter into the vessel, where it deploys and expands to support the vessel walls. The catheter is removed. Pressure is applied over the percutaneous puncture site or, if performed via open approach, the vessel may be repaired and the skin incision closed by sutures. Angioplasty within the same vessel is included in 37226. Report 37227 if the physician performs both stent placement and atherectomy.

37228-37231

The physician treats occlusive disease of a unilateral tibial or peroneal artery by endovascular revascularization (restoration of blood supply) using angioplasty in 37228. Access is gained using a femoral cutdown incision or a percutaneous sheath. Under local anesthesia, the physician accesses the femoral artery. After sheath or needle placement, intra-arterial heparin may be administered. A guidewire is inserted into the artery, followed by a catheter with an attached balloon. The catheter is advanced through the arterial system and into the narrowed portion of the targeted artery. There, the balloon is inflated in order to dilate the vessel to a larger diameter; several inflations may be necessary to achieve maximal results. The physician withdraws the deflated catheter and applies pressure to the puncture site to staunch the bleeding or closes the arteriotomy with suture. In 37229, the physician also performs atherectomy. The physician slides a guidewire through the atherectomy catheter or device, and inserts the guidewire/atherectomy catheter combination through the introducer sheath. The atherectomy device is fluoroscopically positioned at the site of the stenosis. The physician activates the device to remove the stenotic tissue and then rechecks the diameter of the lesion by angiography. Several passes with the atherectomy device may be required. The physician removes the atherectomy catheter, guidewire, and introducer sheath. In 37230, the physician places one or more transluminal stents percutaneously using a guidewire or by incision. A catheter with a stent-transporting tip is threaded into the vessel. The catheter travels to the point where the vessel needs additional support, and the compressed stent is passed from the catheter into the vessel, where it deploys and expands to support the vessel walls. The catheter is removed. Pressure is applied over the percutaneous puncture site or, if performed via open approach, the vessel may be repaired and the skin incision closed by sutures. Angioplasty within the same vessel is included in 37230. Report 37231 if the physician performs both stent placement and atherectomy.

37232-37235

The physician treats occlusive disease of unilateral tibial or peroneal arteries by endovascular revascularization (restoration of blood supply) using angioplasty. Access is gained using a femoral cutdown incision or a percutaneous sheath. Under local anesthesia, the physician accesses the femoral artery. After sheath or needle placement, intra-arterial heparin may be administered. A guidewire is inserted into the artery, followed by a catheter with an attached balloon. The catheter is advanced through the arterial system and into the narrowed portion of the targeted artery. The balloon is inflated in order to dilate the vessel to a larger diameter; several inflations may be necessary to achieve maximal results. The physician withdraws the deflated catheter and applies pressure to the puncture site to staunch the bleeding or closes the arteriotomy with suture. Use 37232 in conjunction with applicable codes in range 37228–37231 to report each additional vessel. In some cases, the physician also performs atherectomy. The physician slides a guidewire through the atherectomy catheter or device, and inserts the guidewire/atherectomy catheter combination through the introducer sheath. The atherectomy device is fluoroscopically positioned at the site of the stenosis. The physician activates the device to remove the stenotic tissue and rechecks the diameter of the lesion by angiography. Several passes with the atherectomy device may be required. The physician removes the atherectomy catheter, guidewire, and introducer sheath. Use 37233 in conjunction with 37229–37231 to report each additional vessel. In other cases, the physician places one or more transluminal stents percutaneously using a guidewire or by incision. A catheter with a stent-transporting tip is threaded into the vessel. The catheter travels to the point where the vessel needs additional support, and the compressed stent is passed from the catheter into the vessel, where it deploys and expands to support the vessel walls. The catheter is removed. Pressure is applied over the percutaneous puncture site or, if performed via open approach, the vessel may be repaired and the skin incision closed by sutures. Angioplasty within the same vessel is included in the codes for this procedure. Use 37234 in conjunction with 37230 or 37231 to report each additional vessel. If the physician performs both stent placement and atherectomy on more than one vessel, use 37235 in conjunction with 37231.

[37246, 37247]

Transluminal balloon angioplasty is performed by open or percutaneous approach (except lower limb arterial occlusion, intracranial, coronary, pulmonary, or dialysis circuit). In an open procedure, the physician makes an incision in the skin overlying the vessel. The vessel is dissected from adjacent critical structures, and vessel clamps are applied. The physician may nick the vessel to create an opening into which a catheter with a balloon attached is inserted into the vessel and threaded. The catheter is fed into the narrowed portion of the vessel, where its balloon is inflated in the narrowed area. The blood vessel is stretched to a larger diameter, allowing a more normal outflow of blood through the area. Several inflations may be performed along the narrowed area. The catheter is slowly withdrawn after deflation. Occasionally, the opening in the vessel is repaired with sutures. In a percutaneous approach, the physician isolates the vessel and inserts a large needle through the skin and into the vessel. A guidewire is threaded through the needle into the vessel. The needle is removed. A catheter with a balloon attached follows the wire into the vessel. The wire is removed. The catheter is fed through the vascular system and into the narrowed portion of the affected vessel and the balloon is inflated. The blood vessel is stretched to a larger diameter, allowing a more normal outflow of blood through the area. Several inflations may be performed along the narrowed area. The catheter is slowly withdrawn after deflation. Pressure is applied to the puncture site to stop the bleeding after the catheter is removed. These codes include all radiological imaging within the same artery. Report 37246 for the initial artery treated and 37247 for each additional artery.

[37248, 37249]

Transluminal balloon angioplasty is performed by open or percutaneous approach (except dialysis circuit). In an open procedure, the physician makes an incision in the skin overlying the vessel. The vessel is dissected from adjacent critical structures and vessel clamps are applied. The physician may nick the vessel to create an opening into which a catheter with a balloon attached is inserted into the vessel and threaded. The catheter is fed into the narrowed portion of the vessel, where its balloon is inflated in the narrowed area. The blood vessel is stretched to a larger diameter, allowing a more normal outflow of blood through the area. Several inflations may be performed along the narrowed area. The catheter is slowly withdrawn after deflation. Occasionally, the opening in the vessel is repaired with sutures. In a percutaneous approach, the physician isolates the vessel and inserts a large needle through the skin and into the vessel. A guidewire is threaded through the needle into the vessel. The needle is removed. A catheter with a balloon attached follows the wire into the vessel. The wire is removed. The catheter is fed through the vascular system and into the narrowed portion of the affected vessel and the balloon is inflated. The blood vessel is stretched to a larger diameter, allowing a more normal outflow of blood through the area. Several inflations may be performed along the narrowed area. The catheter is slowly withdrawn after deflation. Pressure is applied to the puncture site to stop the bleeding after the catheter is removed. These codes include all radiological imaging within the same vein. Report 37248 for the initial vein treated and 37249 for each additional vein.

37236-37237

The physician places one or more intravascular stents through a catheter into an artery other than a coronary, cervical or intrathoracic carotid, extracranial vertebral, iliac, intracranial, or lower extremity artery. The procedure may be performed via a percutaneous or an open approach. In the percutaneous approach, a guidewire is threaded through the needle into the blood vessel and the needle is removed. In the open approach, the physician makes an incision in the skin overlying the vessel to be catheterized. The vessel is dissected and nicked with a small blade. After the approach, a catheter with a stent-transporting tip is threaded over the guidewire into the vessel and the wire is extracted. The catheter travels to the point where the vessel needs additional support. The compressed stent is passed from the catheter out into the vessel, where it deploys, expanding to support the vessel walls. The catheter is removed and pressure is applied over the puncture site or layered closure is performed. Report 37236 for stents placed in the initial artery and 37237 for each additional artery where a stent is placed. These procedures include radiologic supervision and interpretation, as well as angioplasty, when performed.

37238-37239

The physician places one or more intravascular stents through a catheter into a vein. The procedure may be performed via a percutaneous or an open approach. In the percutaneous approach, a guidewire is threaded through the needle into the blood vessel and the needle is removed. In the open approach, the physician makes an incision in the skin overlying the vessel to be catheterized. The vessel is dissected and nicked with a small blade. After the approach, a catheter with a stent-transporting tip is threaded over the guidewire into the vessel and the wire is extracted. The catheter travels to the point where the vessel needs additional support. The compressed stent is passed from the catheter out into the vessel, where it deploys, expanding to support the vessel walls. The catheter is removed and pressure is applied over the puncture site or layered closure is performed. Report 37238 for stents placed in the initial vein and 37239 for each additional vein where a stent is placed.

37241-37242
Embolization or occlusion of a blood vessel is performed. A needle is inserted through the skin and into a blood vessel. A guidewire is threaded through the needle into the vessel. The needle is removed. A catheter is threaded into the vessel and the wire is extracted. The catheter travels to the appropriate blood vessel and beads, coils, or another vessel-blocking device are released. The beads or other device block the vessel. The catheter is removed and pressure is applied over the puncture site to stop bleeding. Report 37241 for occlusion of a vein for any condition other than hemorrhage. Report 37242 when the occlusion is of an artery to treat a condition other than hemorrhage or tumor.

37243
Embolization or occlusion of an artery is performed to treat tumors or organ infarction/ischemia. A needle is inserted through the skin and into the artery. A guidewire is threaded through the needle and the needle is removed. A catheter is threaded into the vessel over the guidewire and the wire is extracted. The catheter travels to the appropriate site and beads, coils, or another vessel-blocking device are released. The beads or other device block the artery that supplies the tumor or that portion of the organ with blood. The catheter is removed and pressure is applied over the puncture site to stop bleeding.

37244
Embolization or occlusion of a blood vessel is performed to treat hemorrhage. A needle is inserted through the skin and into a blood vessel. A guidewire is threaded through the needle and the needle is removed. A catheter is threaded into the vessel over the guidewire and the wire is extracted. The catheter travels to the appropriate site and beads, coils, or another vessel-blocking device are released. The beads or other device block the vessel. The catheter is removed and pressure is applied over the puncture site to stop the bleeding.

37252-37253
Intravascular ultrasound may be used during diagnostic evaluation of the noncoronary artery or vein. It may also be used before and after a therapeutic intervention upon a noncoronary artery or vein to assess patency and integrity of the vessel. A needle is inserted through the skin and into a blood vessel. A guidewire is threaded through the needle into a noncoronary blood vessel. The needle is removed. An intravascular ultrasound catheter is placed over the guidewire. The ultrasound catheter is used to obtain images from inside the vessel to assess area and extent of disease prior to interventional therapy, as well as adequacy of therapy after interventional therapy. Report 37252 for the initial noncoronary vessel. In 37253, the physician advances the ultrasound catheter into additional noncoronary vessels to assess patency and structure. The catheter and guidewire are removed and pressure is applied over the puncture site to stop bleeding. These codes include radiological supervision and interpretation.

37500
Subfascial endoscopic perforator surgery (SEPS) is performed as a minimally invasive way to treat patients with chronic venous insufficiency (CVI) of the lower extremities. Incompetent calf perforator veins are ligated in this procedure. Perforator veins are an irregular group of veins growing as tributaries of the greater saphenous vein, which connect between it and other veins in the lower leg. They are considered incompetent when the direction of blood flow within the perforator vein changes upon applying distal pressure. SEP is carried out under regional or general anesthesia. A rollover tourniquet technique is used to exsanguinate the leg and a single stab incision is made over the medial aspect of the calf through which the operating telescope is inserted. The subfascial plane is created with blunt dissection and maintained open by insufflating with carbon dioxide gas at low pressure. The perforators are identified and ligated, or transected, with a 5 mm ultrasonic scalpel. Patients may be given elastic stockings to wear for the next two weeks.

37565
Through an incision in the skin at side of neck in front of the sternocleidomastoid muscle, the physician isolates and dissects the internal jugular vein, separating it from critical structures. Using a vascular clip or ligature, the blood flow is reduced and the vein is ligated. Once the vein has been tied off, the skin incision is repaired with a layered closure.

37600
Through an incision in the skin at the side of neck in front of the sternocleidomastoid muscle, the physician isolates and dissects the external carotid artery, separating it from critical structures. Using a vascular clip or ligature, the blood flow is reduced and the artery is ligated. Once the artery has been tied off, the skin incision is repaired with a layered closure.

37605-37606
Through an incision in the skin at the side of neck, the physician isolates and dissects the internal or common carotid artery, separating it from critical structures. After vessel clamps have been affixed above and below the injured or affected artery, the physician sutures the artery to permanently stop the flow of blood through it (37605). The physician may apply a gradual occluding clamp (37606) to assess the effect of a ligation prior to complete occlusion (37605). Once the artery has been ligated or the occluding clamp has been placed, the vessel clamp is removed and the skin incision is repaired with a layered closure.

37607
The physician exposes a surgically created arteriovenous fistula by careful dissection. The physician isolates the fistula with ties or clamps. The physician may tie the arteriovenous fistula off completely (ligation) with suture, or the physician may

partially obstruct (banding) the lumen of the fistula with a broader band in order to reduce flow. The physician closes the skin incision.

37609
Through an incision in the skin in front of the ear, the physician isolates and dissects the temporal artery, separating it from critical structures. Using a vascular clip or ligature, the artery is ligated or tissue samples are taken for biopsy. Once the artery has been tied off, the skin incision is repaired with a layered closure.

37615
Through an incision in the skin in the side of neck, usually in front of the sternocleidomastoid muscle, the physician isolates and dissects the ruptured or otherwise traumatized vessel, separating it from critical structures. Using a vascular clip or ligature, the vessel is ligated with sutures. Once the vessel has been tied off, the skin incision is repaired with a layered closure.

37616
The physician performs an incision of the chest wall (thoracotomy or median sternotomy) to best expose the involved artery. The physician identifies the injured artery and quickly clamps it to reduce blood loss. The physician ties off the artery completely (ligation), proximal and distal to the site of injury. The physician closes the chest, leaving chest tubes in place.

37617
The physician performs an abdominal incision to best expose the involved artery. The physician identifies the injured artery and quickly clamps it to reduce blood loss. The physician ties off the artery completely (ligation), proximal and distal to the site of injury. The physician closes the abdomen, leaving drains in place.

37618
Through an incision the skin of an extremity, usually over the damaged or traumatized vessel, the physician isolates and dissects the vessel, separating it from critical structures. Using a vascular clip or ligature, the vessel is ligated with sutures or vascular clips. Once the vessel has been tied off, the skin incision is repaired with a layered closure.

37619
The physician performs an upper midline abdominal incision and dissects to expose the inferior vena cava. The physician interrupts vena caval flow by tying the cava off with suture or clipping it. The physician closes the abdomen, leaving drains in place.

37650
Through a small incision in the skin of the upper leg overlying the femoral vein, the physician isolates and dissects the femoral vein from other critical structures. After affixing vessel clamps, the physician ligates the vein or inserts a catheter into the femoral vein. A guidewire may be inserted prior to the catheter, then removed. Through the catheter, the physician places an occluding device (one that blocks blood flow) in the vein. The catheter is removed and the skin incision is repaired with a layered closure.

37660
The physician performs a lower midline abdominal incision and dissects to expose the common iliac vein. The physician interrupts common iliac venous flow by tying the common iliac vein off with suture. The physician closes the abdomen, leaving drains in place.

37700
Through multiple small incisions in the skin of the upper thigh and along the femoral vein or its branches lower in the thigh, the physician isolates and separates the saphenous vein at the point it joins the femoral vein or at several points farther down the leg. The physician affixes vessel clamps and ligates sections of the saphenous vein along the leg as necessary. Once the ligations are completed, each skin incision is repaired with a layered closure.

37718-37722
The physician makes a skin incision in the upper thigh or upper leg exposing the short saphenous vein (37718) or the long saphenous veins (37722). Additional skin incisions are made at the knee and the ankle and along the leg as necessary. A long wire is threaded through the length of the vein and brought out at the ankle. The vein is tied to the end of the wire and the wire is pulled out along with the vein. Once the vein has been removed, the skin incisions are repaired with layered closures. The leg is wrapped with an elastic pressure dressing postoperatively.

37735
The physician makes a skin incision in the upper thigh and the upper leg exposing the long and short saphenous veins. Additional skin incisions are made at the ankle and along the leg as necessary. A long wire is passed through the length of the vein and brought out at the ankle. Each vein is tied to the end of the wire and the vein is pulled out along with the wire. The physician uses a scalpel to remove the skin ulcer from the leg. The ulcer site is covered with a piece of skin that has been shaved from another part of the patient's body. Veins that connect superficial veins with deep veins may be tied off. The tough, fibrous envelope containing the muscle of the leg is split and removed at points where the superficial and deep veins connect. The skin incisions are repaired with layered closures. The leg is wrapped with an elastic pressure dressing postoperatively.

37760-37761
The physician performs a radical (Linton type) subfascial ligation (tying) of the perforator veins in 37760 and an open subfascial perforator vein ligation in 37761. Through incisions along the course of the saphenous vein, the veins connecting the deep and superficial veins of the leg are isolated. They are ligated, isolating the two systems along the course of the leg. The incisions may be sutured or covered with skin grafts taken from another part of the patient's body. Code 37760 includes skin grafts, when

performed, and code 37761 includes the use of ultrasonic guidance, when performed. Both codes report a procedure involving one leg.

37765-37766

Stab phlebectomy for varicose veins is an ambulatory procedure that permits removal of nearly any incompetent vein below the saphenofemoral and saphenopopliteal junction. The varicose veins are identified with an indelible marking pen while the patient is standing. The patient is placed supine for further marking. Diluted lidocaine is injected into the tissues in large volumes until the perivenous tissues are engorged and distended with the anesthetic. Regional nerve blocks may be used for extensive areas. Tiny stab incisions are made with a scalpel or 18-gauge needle. The varicose vein is dissected with the phlebectomy hook. The vein is undermined along its course, all fibroadipose attachments to the vein are freed, and the vein is grasped with the hook and removed with mosquito forceps. Hemostasis is achieved by applying local compression to the veins already removed. The varicose vein is progressively extracted from one stab incision to the next. No skin closure is needed. Bandages are applied. Large pads are placed along the site of vein removal and covered with an inelastic bandage, followed by a second bandage of highly elastic material. Report 37765 when 10 to 20 stab incisions are made and 37766 when more than 20 are reported.

37780

The physician makes an incision in the skin overlying the short saphenous vein at its junction with the saphenopopliteal vein at the knee. The vessels are dissected and ties are placed around the short saphenous vein which is divided between the ties. Once the ties are in place and the vein has been divided, the skin incision is repaired with a layered closure.

37785

The physician ligates, divides, and/or excises varicose vein cluster(s) in one leg. The physician makes small incisions in the skin over localized areas of superficial varicose veins along the leg. These veins are isolated and dissected free of neighboring tissue, tied with sutures and divided, or stripped out bluntly. Pressure is applied over the site to stop bleeding. All incisions are repaired with a layered closure. The legs are wrapped in an elastic pressure dressing postoperatively.

37788-37790

Through an incision in the skin near the base of the penis, the physician isolates the penile artery and separates it from critical structures. In 37788, a neighboring artery in the groin or lower abdomen is also isolated and dissected and a vessel clamp applied. The end of the neighboring artery is sewn into the penile artery in an end-to-side fashion, or a piece of harvested vein may be used to connect the two arteries to establish an adequate blood flow to the penis. The clamps are removed and incision is repaired with a layered closure. In 37790, through an inguinoscrotal incision, lateral to the root of the penis, and along the spermatic cord, the physician exposes the suspensory ligaments and detaches them from the pubic bone, The physician incises the superficial layer of Buck's fascia, exposing and suture-ligating each leaking vein. A segment of deep dorsal vein is dissected, ligated at both ends, and resected. The physician reattaches the suspensory ligaments and when the procedure is complete, closes the skin incision with a layered closure.

Hemic/Lymphatic

38100-38102

The physician makes a midline incision and dissects tissue around the spleen. The short stomach vessels are doubly ligated and cut. The splenic recess is dissected and the splenic artery and vein are divided and cut individually. The physician removes the spleen. A drain may be placed and the wound is irrigated. The incision is closed with sutures or staples and a dry dressing is applied. Report 38101 if performing a partial splenectomy; report 38102 if performing a total splenectomy in conjunction with another procedure.

38115

The physician makes an upper midline incision and dissects around the spleen until it is exposed. Lacerations are sutured. The damaged segment of the spleen is resected and removed and the edges are sutured. The wound is irrigated and the incision is closed using sutures or staples and a dry dressing.

38120

The physician performs a laparoscopic splenectomy. The patient is placed in a right lateral decubitus position, left arm over the head. With the patient under anesthesia, the physician makes a small incision in the abdominal wall and inserts a trocar just below or above the umbilicus. The physician insufflates the abdominal cavity and places the laparoscope through the umbilical incision. Dissection is carried down to the level of the spleen with care taken to identify the tail of the pancreas. Electrocautery is used to divide ligaments and the spleen is mobilized. Short gastric vessels may be transected to gain additional exposure. The splenic vessels are transected and the spleen is excised and hemostasis is ensured. The freed spleen is isolated and a surgical "retrieval bag" is inserted through a trocar into the abdomen. The spleen is placed into the bag, the bag is closed, and the neck of the bag is brought through the abdominal wall. The spleen is morcellized (unless pathological purposes require an intact specimen) within the bag and the bag containing the spleen is removed. The abdomen is evaluated for accessory spleens and hemostasis. The laparoscope and trocars are removed and the incisions are closed with sutures.

38200

The physician makes an incision in the left lower axilla. An 18 or 20 gauge sheath catheter is inserted into the middle of the soft sponge-like tissue of the spleen. The splenic vein is visualized and the catheter is placed. Around 2 cc to 3 cc of dye are injected per second totaling 15 cc to 20 cc of radiopaque dye. X-rays are taken every second for 12 seconds. The catheter is removed and the incision is covered with a dressing.

[38225, 38226, 38227, 38228]

Chimeric antigen receptor (CAR)-T cell therapy is a type of immunotherapy used to treat cancer, particularly blood cancers such as leukemia. The therapy involves the use of genetically modified T cells; T-cells are a lymphocyte (type of white cell) produced by the thymus gland and are essential to healthy functioning of the immune system. The T-cells are collected from the patient by a process that involves extracting the patient's blood from the body. Plasma, platelets, and/or white blood cells are subsequently filtered out from the extracted blood and the rest of the blood is transfused back into the patient. This process is referred to as apheresis. The filtered cells are transported to a facility for processing where DNA is inserted into the cells, prompting them to produce chimeric antigen receptors (CARs) that transform the cells into CAR-T cells that can identify and destroy cancer cells. The CARs make a protein that gives the T cells the ability to identify an antigen on a cancerous cell. Once the CAR-T cells are created, they are grown in a lab to make more. Once enough cells have been created, they are cryopreserved (frozen) until the patient is ready for treatment. Prior to beginning immunotherapy, the patient may undergo a short course of chemotherapy to eradicate lymphocytes and T cells. The CAR-T cells are infused back into the patient's bloodstream where they increase in number and begin to identify and attack cells containing the antigen that identifies the cell as being malignant. The CAR-T cells stay in the body for months after the treatment, resulting in longer remission periods for patients. The codes describe the different steps required in the process. Report 38225 for collection of the blood-derived T lymphocytes; 38226 for the preparation of the T lymphocytes for transportation; 38227 for the receiving and preparation for the administration step of the process; and 38228 for the administration of the genetically engineered CAR-T cells. Collection and handling services and administration services should only be reported once per day no matter how many cells are collected or units administered.

38204

This code is used to report the management involved in carrying out a donor search to locate a suitably matched donor for a transplant patient and to physically acquire the hematopoietic progenitor cells for the recipient's transplant.

38205-38206

Hematopoietic progenitor cells, or stem cells, harvested for transplantation are used to regenerate bone marrow and immune systems destroyed by chemotherapy and/or radiation therapy. These progenitor cells are not only acquired from bone marrow, but are also found in peripheral blood, collected by apheresis. For stem cell harvesting from peripheral blood by apheresis, the donor is often given a hematopoietic growth factor to mobilize progenitor cells into the blood stream. The patient is prepared much the same as giving a regular blood donation. Whole blood is drawn out of one arm and into an instrument called a cell separator. A column in the separator sorts out the desired cells from the other cells with the help of computerized calibration. The stem cells are collected while the remainder of the blood is returned to the donor through a tube and needle in the other arm. More than one collection session may be required to acquire the amount needed for transplanting. Blood-derived progenitor cells may also be harvested from placental and umbilical cord blood after delivery for transplantation to the neonate later in life or to others. Report 38205 when the cells are collected from a donor for transplantation to another person and 38206 when the cells are harvested from the patient. Report the appropriate code for each collection done.

38207

Progenitor cells (stem cells) harvested from umbilical cord and placental blood after delivery are cryopreserved and kept for transplantation to the neonate later in life or to other recipients. Peripheral blood progenitor cells can also be frozen with ease as well as marrow. The cells are preserved in a cryoprotectant solution generally containing dimethyl sulfoxide (DMSO), hydroxyethyl starch (HES), and a plasma protein such as human serum albumin. Salt solutions are used to dilute DMSO or adjust the cell concentration before freezing. The solution with the suspended cells is cooled at 1-3 degrees Celsius per minute and stored at -80 C or colder. The concentration of cells being frozen, the source and amount of plasma protein used, and the cooling technique used may vary. The cryopreserved cells are stored in bags or vials constructed of cryogenic-tolerant plastic and kept in most laboratories below -120 C in electrical freezers or nitrogen in the vapor or liquid phase. The ultra-low storage temperature is based on the possible progressive growth of ice crystals at warmer temperatures. Storage may be done at warmer temperatures up to -80 C for short-term storage for use within a few weeks or months of harvest, in conjunction with cryoprotectant solution.

38208

A previously frozen harvest of hematopoietic progenitor stem cells is thawed, without washing. A 37 C water bath filled with water is used to thaw the cells rapidly in order to melt the intracellular ice crystals quickly and stop the melting and refreezing of larger crystals. Because small ice crystals store more free surface energy than larger ice crystals, when they are released by thawing, they move to a lower energy state by fusing and forming larger ice crystals. To conquer this phenomenon, the volume and temperature of the thawing liquid must be adequate without allowing the cells to reach a temperature above 37 C where they will suffer heat damage. Cells are removed from the warm bath right when the last of the ice thaws and are infused or processed further immediately. This code is reported for each donor's cells that are thawed.

38209

Previously prepared hematopoietic progenitor cells (HPC) are thawed and washed to remove most of the dimethyl sulfoxide (DMSO) used in the cryoprotectant solution for initial freezing and to decrease the amount of cellular debris and hemoglobin in the infusate, which leads to clumping and trapping of the progenitor cells. A 37-degree Celsius water bath filled with water is used to thaw the cells rapidly in order to melt the intracellular ice crystals quickly and stop the melting and refreezing of larger crystals. Because small ice crystals store more free surface energy than larger ice crystals, when they are released by thawing, they move to a lower energy state by fusing and forming larger ice crystals. To conquer this phenomenon, the volume and temperature of the thawing liquid must be adequate without allowing the cells to reach a temperature above 37 C where they will suffer heat damage. The thawed solution is diluted slowly at room temperature with five to 10 volumes of a selected diluent, usually buffered saline with a macromolecular substance such as sorbitol or Dextran 40 added. This is especially true in thawing umbilical cord blood to retain all possible HPCs. Thawed cord blood is diluted with a buffer of Dextran 40 and albumin then centrifuged and resuspended in the same protein-containing medium. This dilution washing method improves post-thaw viability of the cells and helps to prevent osmotic shock by bringing the cells down from their hyperosmolar state in the post-thaw solution. This code is reported for each donor's cells that are thawed.

38210

Specific cell depletion of a harvested preparation of hematopoietic progenitor cells (HPC) is sometimes needed to decrease the volume of the component or to remove certain cell populations for a particular transplant indication. T-cells within the HPC infusate are removed to help reduce the incidence and severity of chronic and acute graft vs. host disease in the recipient of cells from an allogeneic donor. More than one depletion technique may be employed, including physical and antibody-based methods such as elutriation, in which heavier constituents are made to settle out of a solution and separated from lighter elements; agglutination, in which antigen-bearing cells are made to clump together in a solution in the presence of specific antibodies (agglutinins); or complement-mediated killing. CD34+ cell enrichment technique have been recently developed in which T cells are nonspecifically separated along with other CD34- (antigen-negative) cells from the positive population. This is achieved by identifying the CD34 glycoprotein marker found on hematopoietic stem and progenitor cells and separating them from all the other negative cell population, which will include T-cells. The CD34+ cell enrichment technique can be successfully done after thawing, using the same techniques as prefreeze separation.

38211

Specific cell depletion of a harvested preparation of hematopoietic progenitor cells (HPC) is sometimes needed to decrease the volume of the component or to remove certain cell populations for a particular transplant indication. Tumor cells must be removed from autogenous harvests so the patient is not reinfused with more of his or her own cancer cells. For the removal of greater numbers of tumor cells from the harvest, combination purging techniques of cell enrichment and depletion may be employed. The recently developed CD34+ cell enrichment technique in which tumor cells are nonspecifically separated along with other CD34- (antigen-negative) cells from the positive population is employed first. The CD34 glycoprotein marker found on hematopoietic stem and progenitor cells is identified, separating them from all of the other negative cell population, which will include tumor cells. This is followed by a depletion technique for additional removal such as elutriation, in which heavier constituents are made to settle out of a solution and separated from lighter elements; centrifugation over gradients; or incubation with chemotherapeutic agents. Cell enrichment alone probably purges a number of cells about the same as a depletion technique alone, although reducing the number of tumor cells below assay detection.

38212-38213

Specific cell depletion of a harvested preparation of hematopoietic progenitor cells (HPC) is sometimes needed to decrease the volume of the component or to remove certain cell populations for a particular transplant indication. The removal of red blood cells is especially important for ABO-incompatible allogeneic donor transplantation and in cryopreserved harvests, particularly marrow. Mature blood cells do not survive the freezing process. Red cells become lysed stroma with free hemoglobin released into the solution when thawed. Damaged granulocytes and platelets also create cellular debris that further contribute to clumping in the infusate. Large quantities of mature blood cells requires freezing in large volumes which puts the patient at toxicity risk due to the corresponding large quantities of cryoprotectant used. Red cells in 38212 and platelets in 38213 are removed by centrifugation in blood transfer packs, cell washers, or apheresis devices. Peripheral blood-derived HPCs already collected by apheresis contain minimal amounts of blood cells and normally do not require this extra processing. Marrow collections, however, are processed before cryofreezing for removal of red blood cells, commonly with apheresis devices.

38214-38215

Excessive volume or cell content of harvested component can be a risk to the recipient and can complicate further processing techniques. Plasma removal is commonly done to deplete the volume of infusion given to a small patient and to reduce the isoagglutinins for allogeneic transplants for a red cell incompatible donor. Plasma volume depletion also reduces the amount of cryoprotectant used in freezing as well as the fat cell quantity in marrow harvests to alleviate respiratory difficulties. Plasma can be removed by centrifugation. Report 38214 if volume is reduced by depleting or removing the plasma. Report 38215 if the concentration of mononuclear cells or buffy coat layer of white blood cells (the leukocytes or granulocytes) within the blood plasma is reduced. This is also done with centrifugation, often by apheresis devices to enrich the mononuclear cell fraction, reducing granulocytes and reducing the storage volume with increased stem cell.

38220-38222

In 38220, diagnostic bone marrow aspiration is performed with bone marrow samples usually taken from the pelvic bone or sternum. The skin over the bone is cleaned with an antiseptic solution. A local anesthetic is injected and the physician inserts a needle beneath the skin and rotates it until the needle penetrates the cortex. At least 2.5 cc of marrow is aspirated out of the bone by a syringe attached to the needle. If more marrow is needed, the needle is repositioned slightly, a new syringe is attached, and a second sample is taken. In 38221, diagnostic bone marrow biopsies are performed. The skin over the bone is cleaned with an antiseptic solution. A local anesthetic is injected and the needle is inserted, rotated to the right, rotated to the left, withdrawn, and reinserted at a different angle. This procedure is repeated until a small chip is separated from the bone marrow. The needle is again removed, and a piece of fine wire threaded through its tip transfers the specimen onto gauze. Samples contain bone marrow of which the structure has not been disturbed or destroyed. The bone must be decalcified overnight before it can be properly stained and examined. In both procedures, samples are transferred from the syringes to slides and sent to a laboratory for analysis. Report 38222 when both bone marrow biopsies and aspirations are performed.

38230-38232

The physician removes bone marrow for later transplantation. The physician places a large bore needle into the marrow cavity of the sternum, iliac crest, or ribs. The bone marrow is aspirated with a large syringe and placed in a container. The puncture wound is covered with a dressing. Report 38230 if the bone marrow is extracted from a donor other than the patient receiving the transplant. Report 38232 if the bone marrow is extracted from the patient receiving the transplant.

38240-38241

Hematopoietic cells obtained from bone marrow, peripheral blood apheresis, and/or umbilical cord blood are implanted. The recipient's immune system is suppressed using radiation or chemotherapy. The harvested cells are injected into the recipient by intravenous drip therapy in a sterile environment. Report 38240 if the transplanted cells came from a donor other than the patient and 38241 if the transplant material is autologous and came from the patient.

[38243]

A boost of hematopoietic progenitor cell (HPC) is given to treat a relapse or posttransplant cytopenia(s).The hematopoietic cells are obtained from the original donor. The harvested cells are injected into the recipient by intravenous drip therapy in a sterile environment. The infusion may occur days, months, or years after the initial hematopoietic cell transplant.

38242

An allogeneic lymphocyte infusion is used to treat relapse, infection, or posttransplant lymphoproliferative syndrome. Harvested lymphocytes from a donor other than the patient are infused into the patient by intravenous drip therapy in a sterile environment. The infusion may occur days, months, or years after the initial hematopoietic cell transplant.

38300-38305

The physician performs this procedure to drain inflamed lymph nodes. The physician makes an incision over the affected lymph node and the abscess or infection is drained. The wound is irrigated and closed with sutures or Steri-strips. Report 38305 if the procedure is extensive.

38308

This procedure is performed to correct lymphangiomas, which are primarily found in the neck. The physician makes an incision over the site of the tumor. The tissue, muscles, nerves, and blood vessels are dissected away from the tumor. The tumor is removed. The incision is closed with sutures, wound drains are placed, and a dressing is applied.

38380-38382

The thoracic duct is sutured or ligated. The thoracic duct is a tubular structure, approximately 2 to 3 mm in diameter, that originates in the cisterna chyli, which lies above the second lumbar vertebral body. It ascends on the right, anterior to the vertebral bodies, entering the chest through the aortic hiatus. At the fourth or fifth thoracic vertebra, it crosses to the left and empties into the left jugulosubclavian venous junction. Tears or injury can occur in any segment (cervical, thoracic, abdominal) and the approach is dependent on the site of the leak. An incision is made in the left neck, right or left chest, or abdomen. The involved compartment is drained of all effluent and the leak identified. The duct is ligated a few centimeters below the leak and also a few centimeters above it. Dry gauze is placed at the site of the leak to ensure that the ligation has completely sealed the leak. When it has been determined that the leak is completely sealed, the gauze is removed and glue or other sealant is applied to the area. If the leak is repaired by thoracotomy, chest tubes are placed. Incisions are closed. Report 38380 for a cervical approach; 38381 for a thoracic approach; or 38382 for an abdominal approach.

38500-38531
The physician performs a biopsy on or removes one or more superficial lymph nodes in 38500. The physician makes a small incision through the skin overlying the lymph node. The tissue is dissected to the node. A small piece of the node and surrounding tissue are removed, or the entire node may be removed. The incision is repaired with a layered closure. Report 38505 if a needle is used, other than fine needle aspiration, for superficial lymph nodes such as those in the axillary, cervical, or inguinal regions. Report 38510 if deep cervical nodes are biopsied or removed and 38520 if the scalene fat pad is also excised. Report 38525 if the biopsy or excision involves the deep axillary nodes and 38530 for the internal mammary nodes. For biopsy or excision of the inguinofemoral (groin) nodes, report 38531. Removal of deep nodes may necessitate the placement of a subcutaneous drain, as well as a layered closure.

38542
The physician makes an incision over one of three jugular groups and retracts tissue. The nodes are isolated and excised. The incision is closed by sutures.

38550-38555
The physician removes a cystic hygroma, also called a lymphangioma, from the neck or axilla. A cystic hygroma is a congenital anomaly typically found in the neck or axilla, sometimes extending into the head or chest. Cystic hygromas may be diagnosed during fetal ultrasound or evident at birth. The majority are evident by age 2. Rarely, they are diagnosed into adulthood. Because cystic hygromas can be very large and can extend into multiple areas of the head, neck, and chest, the location and size of the incision will vary. A surgical incision is made in the area of the cyst. If the hygroma does not involve deeper neurovascular structures, the physician dissects away the surrounding tissue and exposes the sac. The sac is excised. The incision is closed and a dry, sterile dressing applied. A larger cystic hygroma may not have a defined capsule and may wrap around blood vessels, nerves, and muscles. In that case, the surgeon dissects the tissue around these vital structures before removing the cystic hygroma. Cystic hygromas may be removed in part or in full depending on whether excision would compromise nerves or blood vessels. If the entire cystic hygroma cannot be excised, the surgeon may cauterize the part remaining. Report 38550 for excision of a cystic hygroma without deep neurovascular dissection; report 38555 when deep neurovascular dissection is required.

38562-38564
The physician makes a midline abdominal incision just below the navel. The surrounding tissue, nerves, and blood vessels are dissected away, and the pelvic and/or para-aortic lymph nodes are visualized. The nodes are removed. The wound is closed with sutures or staples. Report 38564 if retroperitoneal lymphadenectomy is performed.

38570-38573
The physician performs a surgical laparoscopy. A trocar is placed at the umbilicus into the abdominal or retroperitoneal space to insufflate the abdominal, peritoneal, or retroperitoneal space. The laparoscope is placed through the umbilical trocar and additional trocars are placed into the peritoneal or retroperitoneal space. In 38570, retroperitoneal lymph node sampling is also performed. The lymph nodes are identified, dissected free of surrounding structures, and sampled for further separately reported analysis. In 38571, a bilateral pelvic lymphadenectomy is performed. The iliac vessels are identified and the lymph nodes are dissected from the surrounding structures and removed. When dissection is continued to the aorta for periaortic lymph node sampling, report 38572. In 38573, the services from 38571 and 38572 are performed, as well as peritoneal washing and biopsies, an omentectomy (removal of the membrane containing fat, lymph, and blood vessels that acts as a protective layer extending from the stomach to the transverse colon), and diaphragmatic washings. Diaphragmatic and other serosal biopsies are included in the procedure, when performed. When each procedure is complete, the trocars are removed and the incisions are closed.

38700
The physician makes a curved incision beginning below the ear curving down to the top of the hyoid bone and continuing toward the chin. The tissues are dissected and the targeted structures are exposed. The submental and submandibular lymph nodes are removed along with the submandibular gland and surrounding tissues. The incision is sutured with drain if necessary.

38720
The physician makes a large curved incision starting at the ear, going down the neck, and continuing to the chin. Incision may also be made starting at the original incision and continuing down the neck. The skin flaps are folded back and held in place with retractors. The tissue, lymph tissue, blood vessels, nerves, and muscles targeted for removal are dissected away and removed. The incision is closed with sutures.

38724
The physician performs a cervical lymphadenectomy to preserve the spinal accessory nerve, jugular vein, and the sternocleidomastoid muscles. The physician makes a large curved incision starting at the ear, going down the neck, and continuing to the chin. Other incisions may be made down the neck from the original incision. Skin and tissue are retracted and the physician removes the lymph nodes. The incision is closed with sutures, including wound drains connected to suction. A tracheotomy may be performed.

38740-38745
The physician makes a diagonal incision across the lower axilla, exposing the axillary vein. The fatty tissue, lymph nodes, and vessels beneath the vein are

dissected free. A drain is placed and connected to suction. The tissue and skin is closed with sutures. Report 38745 if a complete procedure is performed.

38746
The physician performs a regional and mediastinal lymphadenectomy via an open approach. Using a scalpel, the surgeon makes a long incision around the side of the chest between two of the ribs. The incision is carried through all of the tissue layers into the chest cavity. Rib spreaders are inserted into the wound and the ribs are spread apart exposing the lung, the heart, and other structures. Alternately, the chest cavity can be opened and the operation performed through a vertical incision in the center of the chest through the sternum. The skin incision is carried down to the sternum bone and a saw is used to split the sternum. With the sternum split in half, the chest is entered by spreading the sternum apart with a set of rib spreaders. Lymph nodes near the lungs, around the heart, and behind the trachea are removed. The area is irrigated and the retractors are removed. If applicable, the sternotomy is repaired using wires to bring the two halves of the sternum together, and the operative wound is closed by sutures or staples.

38747
The physician makes a midline abdominal incision. The abdominal contents are exposed, allowing the physician to locate the lymph nodes. Each lymph node grouping, with or without para-aortic and vena caval nodes, is dissected away from the surrounding tissue, nerves, and blood vessels, and removed. The incision is closed with sutures or staples.

38760-38765
The physician makes an incision across the groin area. The surrounding tissue, nerves, and blood vessels are dissected away, and the inguinal and femoral lymph nodes are visualized. The nodes are removed by group. The wound is closed with sutures or staples. Report 38765 if performing pelvic lymphadenectomy concurrently.

38770
The physician makes a low abdominal vertical incision. The surrounding tissue, nerves, and blood vessels are dissected away, and the pelvic lymph nodes are visualized. The nodes are removed by group. The wound is closed with sutures or staples.

38780
The physician makes a large midline abdominal incision. The surrounding tissue, nerves, and blood vessels are dissected away, and the lymph nodes are visualized. The nodes are removed by group. Some surrounding tissues may also be removed. The wound is closed with sutures or staples.

38790
Vital blue dye is injected into the subcutaneous tissues for outlining of skin lymphatics. As soon as the lymphatic vessels are visualized by their blue color, the radiologist makes a small longitudinal incision over the area. Exposure of the lymph vessel is accomplished, the vessel is made taut, and it is cannulated with a 27 or 30 gauge needle with a fine catheter attached. A small amount of dye is injected to ensure correct placement, and the needle is advanced 2 to 3 mm into the vessel. The needle and catheter are secured. Dye is injected with a 10 cc syringe. X-rays are made and repeated 24 hours later. The physician removes the needle and closes the incision with sutures.

38792
The physician injects radioactive material into the patient to identify the first lymph node to receive lymphatic drainage from a tumor (sentinel lymph node). This procedure is most commonly performed for breast cancer and melanoma. A radioactive tracer (radiotracer), such as radioactive technetium sulfur colloid, is injected around the tumor or, in cases of breast cancer, in periareolar or subareolar areas. Time is allowed for the tracer to flow to the sentinel lymph node. X-rays are taken and repeated 24 hours later.

38794
Exposure of the lymph vessel is accomplished, the vessel is made taut, and it is cannulated with a 27 or 30 gauge needle with a find catheter attached. The needle and catheter are secured. Medication is injected. The physician removes the needle and closes the incision with sutures.

38900
Intraoperative mapping may be utilized during lymph node biopsy procedures. During the procedure, a nonradioactive dye such as methylene blue is injected into the area of focus. Following the path of the dye with the aid of fluorescence imaging, the first lymph node to receive lymphatic drainage from a tumor (sentinel lymph node) is identified and a separately reportable biopsy follows.

Mediastinum and Diaphragm

39000-39010
The physician makes an incision low in the front of the neck, pulling back the sternomastoid muscles and the cranial vessels to the side and drawing the trachea and thyroid to the center. The space behind the esophagus is exposed. The foreign body is removed, biopsy of any abnormal mass performed, and Penrose drains are placed. The incision is closed with sutures or staples. Report 39010 if using a transthoracic approach.

39200
The physician makes an incision from in front of the axilla just below the nipple line. The incision extends below the tip of the shoulder blade and ascends to halfway between the spinal column and the shoulder blade. The physician exposes the rib cage, retracting muscles. A rib spreader is used to ease access to the thoracic cavity. The cyst is located and removed. The rib spreader is removed, and the wound is closed with sutures or staples.

39220
The physician makes an incision from in front of the axilla just below the nipple line. The incision extends below the tip of the shoulder blade and ascends to halfway between the spinal column and the shoulder blade. The physician exposes the rib cage by cutting through the muscles. The chest cavity is entered between the ribs by using a rib spreader. The tumor is located and dissected from the surrounding tissue. The wound is closed using sutures or staples.

39401-39402
The physician performs a mediastinoscopy. The physician makes a small incision in the notch above the sternum. The mediastinoscope is inserted and explorations are carried out between the trachea and the major vessels. The mediastinal lymph nodes, thymus, and thyroid are visualized and a biopsy(ies) may be performed through the mediastinoscope during the procedure. The scope is removed and the incision is closed with sutures or Steri-strips. Report 39401 for biopsy of a mediastinal mass. Report 39402 for a biopsy of the lymph nodes.

39501
The physician makes an abdominal or chest incision and exposes a tear in the diaphragm. The tear is repaired with nonabsorbable sutures. Occasionally the tear may be so extensive that an artificial patch is used to repair defects or reinforce sutures. The incision is closed with sutures or staples, and a dressing is applied.

39503
The physician makes an incision across the abdomen. The herniated stomach is returned to its appropriate position in the abdomen, and the hernia sac is cut away and removed. The enlarged opening in the diaphragm through which the esophagus passes is narrowed by placing sutures in the two pillars connecting the spinal column and diaphragm. Reforming the stomach, cutting the vagus nerve or altering the size of the stomach-intestinal opening may be performed as well. Drains are placed, and the wound is sutured closed.

39540-39541
A massive injury in the diaphragm is repaired, allowing organs to protrude into the chest cavity. The physician makes an incision into the chest or abdomen. The abdominal contents are drawn back into the abdomen, and the hole in the diaphragm is exposed. The opening is closed with sutures or by insertion of a patch. The tear is repaired with nonabsorbable sutures. The incision is closed with sutures or staples. Report 39541 if the hernia is chronic.

39545
The physician makes an incision across the chest or abdomen. The abdominal contents are drawn back into the abdomen, and the diaphragm is exposed. The connective tissue is used to stitch folds or tucks into the diaphragm to restore it to its original position. The incision is closed with sutures or staples.

39560
Usually performed for tumors that have invaded the diaphragm, the surgeon removes part of the large muscle separating the chest and abdominal cavities. The patient is taken to the operating room and the chest is surgically opened using a midline incision. Occasionally, the xiphoid process is divided or removed to gain access. Retractors are placed to provide an optimal view of the subphrenic space. Using electrocautery, any affected tissue from the diaphragm is dissected and removed. The liver may be mobilized to provide better access to the surgical site. Once the tissue is removed, the diaphragm is repaired using internal sutures. Hemostasis is confirmed and the operative wound is closed in layers.

39561
Usually performed for tumors that have invaded the diaphragm, the surgeon removes part of the large muscle separating the chest and abdominal cavities. The patient is taken to the operating room and the chest is surgically opened using a midline incision. Occasionally, the xiphoid process is divided or removed to gain access. Retractors are placed to provide an optimal view of the subphrenic space. Using electrocautery, any affected tissue from the diaphragm is dissected and removed. The liver may be mobilized to provide better access to the surgical site. Once the tissue is removed, the diaphragm is repaired using a muscle flap or synthetic material to correct the remaining large surgical defect. Hemostasis is confirmed and the operative wound is closed in layers.

Digestive

40490
The physician performs a biopsy of a lesion on the lip. An incision is made in the lip and a portion of the lesion together with some normal tissue is removed. The surgical wound is closed directly.

40500
The physician removes the diseased vermilion border of the lip. The mucosa from the skin to the labial mucosa is separated from the underlying muscle and removed. The remaining labial mucosa is advanced and sutured to the skin, covering the exposed muscle and forming a new vermilion.

40510
The physician removes a portion of the lip using a transverse wedge technique. Incisions are made perpendicularly through the skin and mucosa and a wedge of the lip with surrounding tissue is removed. The physician extends the incisions below the surgical wound and advances the tissue flaps. The incisions are sutured primarily.

40520
The physician removes a portion of the lip using a "V" incision technique. A "V" cut is made around the portion of lip to be removed and the lip and surrounding tissue are removed. The surgical wound is closed primarily.

40525
The physician removes a full thickness portion of the lip with local flap reconstruction. A "V" incision may be made around the lesion and through the full thickness of the lip. The lesion and surrounding tissues are removed. A local skin flap is incised and advanced to the site of the surgical wound and sutured into place with layered closure.

40527
The physician removes a full thickness portion of the lip with a cross lip flap reconstruction. A "V" incision may be made around the lesion and through the full thickness of the lip. The lesion and surrounding tissues are removed. A skin flap from the upper lip is incised and cross advanced to the surgical site of the lower lip. The flap is sutured with layered closure.

40530
The physician performs a lip resection of more than one fourth without reconstruction. An incision may be made through the midline of the lip and extended over the portion of the lip to be removed. The tumor and surrounding tissues are removed. The oral cavity is closed primarily, and the lip and surrounding structures are closed with layered sutures.

40650
The physician repairs a full thickness laceration of the lip. The tissues of the vermilion are closed with layered sutures.

40652-40654
The physician repairs a laceration extending through the full thickness of the lip. In 40652, a laceration or surgically created wound of up to one-half the vertical height of the lip is closed with layered sutures and in 40654, a wound of more than one-half the vertical height of the lip is repaired.

40700
The physician surgically corrects a partial or complete unilateral developmental cleft lip/nasal deformity. A cleft lip may range in appearance as a "notch" in the upper lip to a complete separation running into the nose. The cleft margins are incised on either side from the mouth toward the nostril and through the full-thickness layers of mucosa, muscle, and skin. The vermilion border of the cleft lip is turned downward to restore the normal shape of the lip and the muscle and skin are brought together to close the cleft separation and preserve muscle function. The nasal deformity often caused by the cleft lip may be repaired. The physician closes the prepared margins in layers from the intraoral mucosa through the muscle with final closure of the skin.

40701
The physician surgically corrects a bilateral developmental cleft lip/nasal deformity in one operation. A cleft lip may range in appearance as a "notch" in the upper lip to a complete separation running into the nose. The cleft margins are incised on either side from the mouth toward the nostril and through the full-thickness layers of mucosa, muscle, and skin on both sides of the face. The vermilion border of the cleft lip is turned downward to restore the normal shape of the lip and the muscle and skin are brought together to close the cleft separations on each side and preserve muscle function. The nasal deformity often caused by the cleft lip may be repaired. The physician closes the prepared margins in layers from the intraoral mucosa through the muscle with final closure of the skin.

40702
The physician performs one stage of two surgeries to correct a bilateral cleft lip/nasal deformity. This may be necessary because of the severity or the vascular compromise of the deformity. Typically, the cleft lip is repaired first and nasal deformities are repaired in a second surgical session. A cleft lip may range in appearance as a "notch" in the upper lip to a complete separation running into the nose. The cleft margins are incised on either side from the mouth toward the nostril and through the full-thickness layers of mucosa, muscle, and skin on both sides of the face. The vermilion border of the cleft lip is turned downward to restore the normal shape of the lip and the muscle and skin are brought together to close the cleft separations on each side and preserve muscle function. The prepared margins are closed in layers from the intraoral mucosa through the muscle with final closure of the skin. The second surgery is performed after adequate healing of the first surgical site.

40720
The physician performs a secondary cleft lip/nasal deformity repair after unfavorable results from a first surgical correction. This failure may be due to scar contracture (permanent shortening), wound dehiscence (splitting), or infection. The cleft margins are recreated to define clean edges for the defect through full-thickness layers of mucosa, muscle, and skin. The prepared margins are again closed in layers from the intraoral mucosa through muscle with final closure of the skin.

40761
The physician performs a complicated cleft lip/nasal deformity repair using pedicle flaps from the lower lip. This is necessary because of inadequate quantity or quality of upper lip soft tissue. A cleft lip may range in appearance as a "notch" in the upper lip to a complete separation running into the nose. The cleft margins are incised on either side from the mouth toward the nostril and through the full-thickness layers of mucosa, muscle, and skin. The vermilion border of the cleft lip is turned downward to restore the normal shape of the lip and the muscle and skin are brought together to close the cleft separation and preserve muscle function. A pedicle flap is designed from the lower lip based on blood supply. The flap is created with a full-thickness incision and rotated on its pedicle to the desired location. The flap is sutured in layers to the recipient tissue location. The prepared cleft margins are closed in layers from the intraoral mucosa through muscle with final closure of the skin.

40800-40801
The physician drains an abscess, a cyst, or a hematoma within the vestibule of the mouth. The vestibule consists of the mucosal and submucosal tissue of the lips and cheeks within the oral cavity, not including the dentoalveolar structures. The physician makes an incision in the tissue overlying the abscess, cyst, or hematoma. Tissues are dissected and the fluid is drained. Complicated drainage for larger lesions or drainage requiring multiple incisions is done in 40801. The physician may place a drain to facilitate healing. If a drain is placed, it is later removed.

40804-40805
The physician removes a foreign body embedded in the vestibule of the mouth. The vestibule consists of the mucosal and submucosal tissue of the lips and cheeks within the oral cavity, not including the dentoalveolar structures. The physician may simply grasp the object with an instrument and remove it or incisions may be made to free the object and remove it. Complicated removal of a large foreign body or one that is difficult to access is done in 40805. Closure of the wound may be needed.

40806
The physician performs a frenotomy by incising the labial frenum. The labial frenum is a connecting fold of mucous membrane that joins the lip to the gums at the inside midcenter. This procedure is often performed to release tension on the frenum and surrounding tissues. The frenum is simply incised and not removed.

40808
The physician performs a biopsy on a lesion in the vestibule of the mouth. The vestibule consists of the mucosal and submucosal tissue of the lips and cheeks within the oral cavity, not including the dentoalveolar structures. The physician makes an incision in the area of the vestibule to be biopsied and removes a portion of the lesion and some surrounding tissue. The incision is closed simply.

40810-40812
The physician removes a lesion in the vestibule of the mouth. The vestibule consists of the mucosal and submucosal tissue of the lips and cheeks within the oral cavity, not including the dentoalveolar structures. The physician makes an incision around the lesion and through submucosal tissue, removing the lesion. No repair of the wound is done in 40810. Simple repair of the wound is done in 40812, such as a sutured closure.

40814
The physician removes a lesion in the vestibule of the mouth with complex repair. The vestibule consists of the mucosal and submucosal tissue of the lips and cheeks within the oral cavity, not including the dentoalveolar structures. An incision is made around the lesion and through submucosal tissue, removing the lesion. Complex repair of the surgical wound left after excision of the lesion is required. This may include advancement of tissue flaps, rearrangement of tissue, or complex suturing techniques.

40816
The physician removes a lesion in the vestibule of the mouth. The vestibule consists of the mucosal and submucosal tissue of the lips and cheeks within the oral cavity, not including the dentoalveolar structures. An incision is made around the lesion and through the submucosal tissue, removing the lesion, along with the excision of underlying muscle as well. Complex repair of the surgical wound is required after excision of the lesion. This may include advancement of tissue flaps, rearrangement of tissue, or complex suturing techniques.

40818
The physician harvests mucosa from the vestibule to be used as a graft elsewhere in the mouth. The vestibule consists of the mucosal and submucosal tissue of the lips and cheeks within the oral cavity, not including the dentoalveolar structures. A retractor is used to hold the mucosa to be grafted. The physician uses a scalpel to make an incision through the mucosa, usually in an elliptical shape. The physician grasps the mucosa with an instrument and the scalpel is used to cut just beneath the mucosa, freeing it from the underlying tissues. Any remaining fat or muscle attached to the mucosa is removed and the donor tissue is ready for grafting to another part of the mouth. The surgical wound is closed directly.

40819
The physician removes the labial or buccal frenum. The buccal frenum is a band of mucosal membrane that connects the alveolar (dental) ridge to the cheek and separates the lip vestibule from the cheek vestibule. The labial frenum is a connecting fold of mucous membrane that joins the lip to the gums at the inside midcenter. Incisions are made around the frenum and through the mucosa and submucosa. The underlying muscle is removed as well. The excision may extend to the interincisal papilla. The mucosa is closed simply, or the physician may rearrange the tissue as in a Z-plasty technique.

40820
The physician destroys a lesion or a scar in the vestibule of the mouth without excising it. Destruction may be accomplished by using a laser or electrocautery to burn the lesion, cryotherapy to freeze the lesion, or chemicals to destroy the lesion.

40830-40831
The physician sutures a laceration of the vestibule of the mouth measuring 2.5 cm or less in length. The physician performs a simple closure without submucosal sutures or tissue rearrangement in 40830. Extensive tissue damage or crushing, requiring complex closure, such as retention sutures, or the closure of a laceration more than 2.5 cm is done in 40831.

40840-40844
The surgeon performs a vestibuloplasty and deepens the vestibule of the mouth by any series of surgical procedures for the purpose of increasing the height of

the alveolar ridge, allowing a complete denture to be worn. The vestibule refers to the mucosal and submucosal tissue of the inner lips and cheeks, the part of the oral cavity outside of the dentoalveolar structures. This procedure may be performed in several ways. The surgeon may rearrange the patient's own tissue or the submucosal tissue may be dissected and freed from the bone. The mucosa is moved deeper into the vestibule. Soft tissues may also be grafted into the mouth. An anterior procedure is performed in 40840; a one-sided procedure is done on the posterior portion of the mouth in 40842; and a posterior procedure is done on both sides of the mouth in 40843. Report 40844 when this procedure is done over the arch of the mouth.

40845
The surgeon performs a vestibuloplasty and deepens the vestibule of the mouth by any series of surgical procedures for the purpose of increasing the height of the alveolar ridge, allowing a complete denture to be worn. The vestibule refers to the mucosal and submucosal tissue of the inner lips and cheeks, the part of the oral cavity outside of the dentoalveolar structures. This procedure is performed for complex cases, such as those in which the physician must lower muscle attachments to provide enough space for deepening the vestibule. Soft tissue grafting from other areas of the body into the mouth is often required. Hypertrophied and hyperplastic tissue may need to be trimmed and soft tissue revised by dissecting it from the alveolar ridge and rearranging its attachment.

41000-41009
The physician makes a small intraoral incision through the mucosa of the tongue or floor of the mouth overlying an abscess, cyst, or hematoma and drains the fluid. The incision and drainage site of the cyst, hematoma, or abscess is on the tongue (lingual) in 41000. In 41005, the lesion is located superficially under the tongue (sublingual) and in 41006, the sublingual lesion is deep to the supramylohyoid muscle. The physician dissects through the anterior floor of the mouth into the supramylohyoid muscle to drain an abscess in the submental space in 41007. In 41008, the physician incises through the mucosa of the floor of the mouth to the supramylohyoid muscle and carries the dissection deeper into the tissue to reach the submandibular space. In 41009, the physician dissects down through the mucosa in the posterior floor of the mouth and into the masticator space, containing the ramus, the posterior part of the mandible, and the masticator muscles to drain the abscess.

41010
The physician makes an incision in the lingual frenum, freeing the tongue and allowing greater range of motion. The lingual frenum is the connecting fold or membrane under the tongue that attaches it to the floor of the mouth. Sutures may be placed. The frenum is simply incised and not removed.

41015-41018
The physician drains an abscess, a cyst, or a hematoma from the floor of the mouth by making an extraoral incision in the skin below the inferior border of the mandible and dissecting through the tissue to reach the affected space. In 41015, the physician dissects through the supramylohyoid muscle and submental space into the sublingual space below the tongue to drain the abscess. In 41016, dissection is taken to the supramylohyoid muscle to drain an abscess in the submental space. In 41017, the physician makes an incision under the angle of the mandible, or between the angle and the chin, and below the inferior border of the mandible. Dissection is limited to the submandibular space. In 41018, an incision is made just below the angle of the ramus of the mandible, the posterior part of the mandible, and into the masticator space containing the masticator muscles to drain the abscess, cyst, or hematoma. A drain may be placed to facilitate healing, which is later removed.

41019
The physician places needles, catheters, or other devices into the head and/or neck region for subsequent interstitial radioelement application. The route of insertion may be under the skin (percutaneous), through the mouth (transoral), or through the nose (transnasal). The radioactive isotopes that are introduced subsequently, such as iridium-192, are contained within tiny seeds that are left in place to deliver radiation over a period of time. They do not cause any harm after becoming inert. This method provides radiation to the prescribed body area while minimizing exposure to normal tissue.

41100-41105
The physician performs an excisional biopsy on a lesion in the anterior two-thirds of the tongue in 41100 or the posterior one-third of the tongue in 41105. The physician makes an incision around the lesion, usually in an elliptical shape, which typically includes the diseased tissue and part normal tissue. Incisions are carried beneath the tissue sample and the specimen is removed. The surgical wound is usually sutured simply.

41108
The physician performs an excisional biopsy on a lesion of the floor of the mouth. An incision is made around the lesion, usually in an elliptical shape, which typically includes the diseased tissue and part normal tissue. Incisions are carried beneath the tissue sample and the specimen is removed. The surgical wound is usually sutured simply.

41110
The physician removes a lesion in any area of the tongue. Incisions are made in an elliptical shape completely around and under the lesion. The lesion is excised. Due to the small size of the lesion, no suturing or closure of the surgical wound is necessary.

41112-41113
The physician removes a lesion in the anterior two-thirds of the tongue in 41112 or the posterior

one-third in 41113. Incisions are made in the tissue completely around and under the lesion, typically in an elliptical shape, and the lesion is excised. The surgical wound is sutured closed.

41114
The physician removes a lesion in any area of the tongue with a local flap for closure. Incisions are made in the tissue completely around and under the lesion, usually in an elliptical shape, and the lesion is excised. A flap of mucosa from another part of the tongue is incised, moved, and sutured to repair the surgical wound. The donor site is closed with sutures.

41115
The physician removes a tight or short lingual frenum to free the tongue and allow greater range of motion. The lingual frenum is the connecting fold or membrane under the tongue that attaches it to the floor of the mouth. The physician makes incisions in the frenum both near the tongue and near the mandible, which ultimately connect as they move posteriorly. The frenum is excised. The surgical wound may be sutured.

41116
The physician excises a lesion from the floor of the mouth. The physician makes incisions in the tissue completely around and under the lesion, usually in an elliptical shape, and the lesion is excised with some surrounding normal tissue as well. The surgical wound is typically sutured simply.

41120-41130
The physician removes less than one half of the tongue in 41120 or one half of the diseased, often malignant, tongue in 41130. The physician makes incisions around the portion of the tongue to be removed and extends the incisions through the thickness of the tongue. Scalpels, scissors, electrocautery, or lasers may be used. The diseased portion is removed. After obtaining good hemostasis (controlled bleeding), the tongue is sutured closed to repair the surgical wound. Tissue grafting to close the wound is rarely needed.

41135
The physician removes a part of the diseased, and often malignant, tongue and performs a unilateral radical neck dissection. The physician makes incisions in the tissue around the portion of the tongue to be removed and extends the incisions through the thickness of the tongue. Scalpels, scissors, electrocautery, or lasers may be used. The diseased portion is removed. After obtaining good hemostasis (controlled bleeding), the tongue is sutured to repair the surgical wound. Tissue grafting to close the wound is rarely needed. Radical neck dissection is also done to remove lymph nodes, muscles, blood vessels, and other tissue from one side of the neck.

41140-41145
The physician removes the entire tongue, with or without a tracheostomy. The physician makes incisions through the thickness of the tongue. Scalpels, scissors, electrocautery, or lasers may be used. The tongue is removed. A tracheostomy may be performed. An incision is made in the front of the neck below the larynx. The physician dissects the tissues down to the trachea. An incision is made through the tracheal wall and an artificial airway is inserted, which extends out of the neck. The patient breathes through this airway. No radical neck dissection is performed in 41140. Report 41145 if a unilateral radical neck dissection is also performed to remove lymph nodes, muscles, blood vessels, and other tissues from one side of the neck.

41150-41155
The physician removes part or all of the diseased or cancerous tongue and resects the mandible and the tissue of the floor of the mouth. The physician uses incisions both extraorally in the skin and intraorally through the mucosa. The physician removes the tongue by making incisions through the thickness of the tongue. Scalpels, scissors, electrocautery, or lasers may be used. The affected tissue of the mouth floor is removed with a scalpel and the diseased portion of the mandible is also accessed and resected. After removal of the diseased section, continuity of the mandible is reestablished. This is done with metal plates initially and bone grafting at a later time, or with immediate bone grafting. Skin or mucosal grafting may also be needed. The skin and mucosal incisions are repaired with layered sutures. No neck dissection is performed in 41150. Report 41155 if in addition, a radical neck dissection is performed and lymph nodes, muscles, blood vessels, and other tissue are removed from one side of the neck. Report 41153 if a glossectomy with resection of the floor of the mouth is done and lymph nodes and other soft tissue are removed from between the floor of the mouth and the hyoid bone for a suprahyoid neck dissection, without mandible resection.

41250-41251
The physician sutures a laceration measuring 2.5 cm or less of the mouth floor and/or anterior two-thirds of the tongue in 41250 or a laceration in the posterior one-third of the tongue in 41251. This is done simply without tissue rearrangement.

41252
The physician sutures a laceration of the mouth floor or portion of the tongue measuring 2.6 cm or more or requiring complex closure techniques. These may include tissue rearrangement, extensive submucosal suturing, debridement of grossly contaminated lacerations, or repair of through-and-through lacerations.

41510
The physician makes an incision in the commissure (corner) of the mouth. The tongue is sutured to the lip in the area previously incised to enlarge the mouth. The tongue is later sectioned from the mouth in a second surgical session.

41512
Moderate to severe obstructive sleep apnea (OSA) is often associated with collapse of the pharyngeal airway on multiple levels, including tongue base obstruction. The physician treats OSA with a tongue base suspension suture. A titanium screw is initially placed in the inner mandibular cortex. A permanent suture is placed through the posterior tongue base and secured anteriorly around the screw. This procedure is intended to support the pharynx and lessen collapse, partially reducing the respiratory severity of OSA.

41520
The physician performs a lingual or labial frenoplasty and surgically alters the frenum by rearranging the tissue, usually with a Z-plasty technique. The lingual frenum is the connecting fold or membrane under the tongue that attaches it to the floor of the mouth, and the labial frenum connects the upper lip to the gums. An incision in the shape of a "Z" is made through the frenum and the tissues are reapproximated in a different position, freeing the constriction, and sutured.

41530
Using radiofrequency, the physician ablates submucosal tissues with temperatures in the 60°C to 90°C range. The physician may perform the submucosal radiofrequency tissue volume reduction (RFTVR) of tongue base on one or more sites. RFTVR uses low levels of radiofrequency energy to create targeted coagulative submucosal lesions. When these necrotic lesions in the soft tissue heal, scar formation and retraction of tissue occur, thus producing an overall reduction in tissue volume. Code 41530 is reported per session.

41800
The physician drains an abscess, cyst, or hematoma from dentoalveolar structures. The physician may make gingival incisions to provide drainage. An artificial drain may be placed and removed at a later time. On occasion, drainage may be obtained by probing the gingival sulcus.

41805
The physician removes a foreign body embedded in the soft tissue of the dental alveolus (gingival or alveolar mucosa). The physician may simply grasp the object with an instrument and remove it. If the object is further embedded, incisions may be made in the mucosa near the object to remove it. Sutures may be necessary.

41806
The physician removes a foreign body embedded in the bone of dentoalveolar structures. The physician may simply grasp the object with an instrument and remove it. If the object is further embedded, mucosal incisions may be made to reach the foreign body in the bone, which is removed, possibly with drills or osteotomes as necessary. The incision is sutured simply.

41820
The physician excises or trims hypertrophic (overgrown) gingiva to normal contours. The physician excises the overgrown gingiva using a scalpel, electrocautery, or a laser. Periodontal dressing or packing is often placed. Use this code for each quadrant of the mouth where gingivectomy is performed.

41821
The physician removes a small piece of gingiva from the back or top of a tooth. A scalpel, a laser, or electrocautery is used to excise the tissue and establish normal gingival contours around the tooth. A periodontal dressing may be applied.

41822
The physician excises fibrous soft tissue overlying the tuberosities of dentoalveolar structures, reducing the size of the tuberosity. The physician makes wedged or elliptically shaped incisions through the soft tissue of the tuberosity. The tissue is removed and the surgical wound is sutured directly.

41823
The physician removes the osseous tissue from the tuberosities of dentoalveolar structures, producing more favorable bone contours. The physician makes an incision through the mucosa of the tuberosity and exposes the underlying bone. Drills, osteotomes, or files are used to remove and contour the bone. The tissue is sutured directly over the bone. Some soft tissue may be excised prior to closure for adaptation over the newly contoured bone.

41825-41826
The physician removes a lesion or tumor of the dentoalveolar structures. If the lesion is within the mucosa, the physician makes incisions around the lesion and dissects it away from adjacent structures. If the lesion is within the bone, the mucosa is incised and the underlying bone exposed. The lesion is removed from the bone and the incision closed with layered sutures. No repair is done in 41825 and simple repair of the surgical wound is done in 41826.

41827
The physician removes a lesion or tumor of the dentoalveolar structures. If the lesion is within the mucosa, the physician makes incisions around the lesion and dissects it away from adjacent structures. If the lesion is within the bone, the mucosa is incised and the underlying bone exposed. The lesion is removed from the bone. The resultant surgical wound is closed with complex repair techniques, such as tissue rearrangement with flaps, tissue grafting, or complex suturing.

41828
The physician excises hyperplastic or excessive mucosa from the alveolus. Incisions are made in the hyperplastic tissue, separating it from the normal mucosa. The excessive tissue is removed. The resultant defect may be directly sutured or left to heal without suturing. With large amounts of excess tissue, more

than one surgical session may be required to eliminate all of the tissue. Use this code for each specified quadrant excised.

41830
The physician removes a portion of the alveolus. Incisions are made through the mucosa to expose the alveolar bone. Curettes, drills, or osteotomes are used to remove the diseased alveolar bone or sequestrum. The mucosa may be sutured directly over the surgical wound, or it may be packed and allowed to heal secondarily.

41850
The physician destroys a lesion of the dentoalveolar structures without excision. The physician may use different techniques of lesion destruction. Electrocautery may be used to burn the lesion, cryotherapy to freeze the lesion, or chemical injections to destroy the lesion. A laser which produces high-intensity light may be used to destroy the lesion. No suturing is required and the resultant surgical wound is left to heal secondarily.

41870
The physician takes mucosa from one area of the mouth and grafts it around the teeth to repair areas of gingival recession. The physician uses a scalpel to remove a small piece of mucosa, usually from the hard palate. After preparing the recipient site, the physician sutures the graft in the area of gingival recession.

41872
The physician alters the contours of the gums by performing gingivoplasty. Areas of gingiva may be excised or incisions may be made through the gingiva to create a gingival flap. The flap may be sutured in a different position, trimmed, or both. Any incisions made are closed with sutures.

41874
The physician alters the contours of the alveolus by selectively performing alveoloplasty to remove sharp areas or undercuts of alveolar bone. The physician makes incisions in the mucosa overlying the alveolus, exposing the alveolar bone. Drills, osteotomes, or files are used to contour the bone. The mucosa is sutured in place over the contoured bone.

42000
The physician drains an abscess of the palate or uvula. The abscess is opened with a surgical instrument and the fluid is drained. The wound is allowed to heal without closure.

42100
The physician performs a biopsy on a lesion of the palate or uvula. An incision is made in the tissue, usually in an elliptical shape and typically including part diseased and part normal tissue. Incisions are made beneath the tissue and the specimen is removed. The surgical wound is closed with sutures.

42104-42107
The physician removes a lesion of the palate or uvula. Incisions are made completely around and under a lesion, typically in an elliptical shape, removing the lesion. Due to the small size of the lesion, no suturing or closure of the surgical wound is necessary in 42104. Removal of larger lesions requires simple closure in 42106 or local flap closure in 42107.

42120
The physician resects the palate or area of a lesion. The physician excises the lesion and any adjacent tissue where the lesion may have spread. The surgical wound is repaired by intermediate or complex closure, adjacent tissue transfer, or graft.

42140
The physician removes the uvula with a full-thickness incision. Electrocautery may be used to control hemorrhage. Sutures may be used to close the mucosa in a single layer.

42145
The physician removes elongated and excessive tissues of the uvula, soft palate, and pharynx. Incisions are made in the soft palate mucosa and a wedge of mucosa is excised. Excessive submucosal tissue is removed and the uvula is partially excised. The midline at the uvula is sutured first. The physician closes the remaining mucosa in a single layer, reapproximating the soft palate and thus increasing the diameter of the oropharynx.

42160
The physician destroys a lesion of the palate or uvula. Destruction may be accomplished by using a laser or electrocautery to burn the lesion, cryotherapy to freeze the lesion, or chemicals to destroy the lesion.

42180-42182
The physician repairs a laceration of the palate measuring 2 cm or less in length in 42180 and more than 2 cm or complex in 42182. The physician sutures the wound in a simple closure without submucosal sutures or tissue rearrangement for 42180. The physician sutures a laceration greater than 2 cm or one that requires complex closure, such as tissue rearrangement, submucosal sutures, or extensive cleaning due to tissue damage or crushing in 42182.

42200
The physician repairs the developmental cleft opening of the palate. The cleft size and location will dictate the type of repair to be performed. The physician closes the opening between the oral and nasal cavities with a partition of soft tissue. Typically, incisions are made in the palatal mucosa adjacent to the alveolar (tooth-bearing) bone. The mucosa is elevated and loosened from the bony palate. The margins of the cleft are incised and dissected to develop mucosal and muscular layers. These incised midline margins are closed in layers, thus closing the communication between the oral and nasal cavities.

42205
The physician repairs the developmental cleft opening of the palate which extends through the alveolar ridge (tooth-bearing region) of the maxilla. The cleft size and

location will dictate the type of repair performed. The physician closes the opening between the oral and nasal cavities with a partition of soft tissue. Closure of the alveolar ridge will benefit development of both the maxilla and the teeth. Typically, incisions are made in the palatal mucosa adjacent to the alveolar bone. The mucosa is elevated and loosened from the bony palate. The midline margins of the cleft are incised and dissected to develop mucosal and muscular layers. The physician closes the midline margins in layers.

42210
The physician repairs the developmental cleft opening of the palate and reconstructs the alveolar ridge (tooth-bearing region) of the maxilla. The cleft size and location will dictate the type of repair performed. The physician closes the opening between the oral and nasal cavities with a partition of soft tissue. Bony reconstruction of the alveolar ridge can stabilize maxillary segments, benefit development of the teeth, and aid dental rehabilitation of chewing functions. Typically, incisions are made in the palatal mucosa adjacent to the alveolar bone. The mucosa is elevated and loosened from the bony palate. The midline margins of the cleft mucosa and gingiva are incised and dissected to develop mucosal and muscular layers. Through a separate incision, the physician harvests bone from the hip or skull and closes the surgically created wound. The bone is placed in the alveolar cleft, reestablishing normal contours of the maxilla. The physician closes all midline incisions in layers and gingival incisions in a single layer.

42215
The physician revises previous repairs of the cleft palate. Wound dehiscence (splitting), infection, or scarring after initial surgeries could cause oral/nasal recommunication, developmental growth restrictions, or velopharyngeal incompetence. The defect will dictate the repair to be performed. Typically, incisions are made in the palatal mucosa adjacent to the alveolar (tooth-bearing) bone. The mucosa is elevated and loosened from the bony palate. The previous midline incisions are excised and dissected to develop mucosal and muscular layers. The physician resutures all midline incisions in layers and gingival incisions are closed in a single layer.

42220
The physician revises the previous cleft palate incisions to lengthen the soft palate. Wound dehiscence (splitting), infection, or scarring after initial surgeries could cause developmental growth restrictions or velopharyngeal incompetence. The defect will dictate the repair performed. Typically, the soft palate lengthening is accomplished with the use of mucosal advancement flaps. Incisions are made in the palatal mucosa adjacent to the alveolar (tooth-bearing) bone. The mucosa is elevated and loosened from the bony palate. The pedicle flaps utilizing posterior palatine blood supply are developed and sutured to increase the anterior-posterior length of the soft palate. The physician sutures all remaining midline incisions in layers.

42225
The physician revises previous cleft palate incisions with pharyngeal flap techniques. Through the soft palate, a midline incision is made to expose the posterior pharyngeal wall. The physician incises a flap from the posterior pharyngeal wall through the mucosa, submucosa, and muscle. This flap is sutured to the soft palate. Revision of previous surgical incisions may be necessary. All remaining midline incisions are sutured in layers.

42226
The physician uses both advancement flaps and pharyngeal flaps to lengthen the soft palate. Typically, the soft palate lengthening is accomplished with the use of mucosal advancement flaps. Correction of velopharyngeal incompetence is accomplished by pharyngeal flap techniques. A midline incision through the soft palate is made to expose the posterior pharyngeal wall. The physician incises a flap from the posterior pharyngeal wall through mucosa, submucosa, and muscle. This flap is sutured to the soft palate. Advancement flaps utilizing posterior palatine blood vessels are used to lengthen the soft palate by suturing techniques that increase the anterior-posterior length of the soft palate. All remaining midline incisions are sutured in layers.

42227
The physician uses mucosal island flaps to lengthen the soft palate. Incisions are made in the palatal mucosa adjacent to the alveolar (tooth-bearing) bone. The mucosa is elevated and loosened from the bony palate. Advancement flaps utilizing posterior palatine blood vessels are used to lengthen the soft palate by suturing techniques that increase the anterior-posterior length of the soft palate. All remaining incisions are sutured in layers.

42235
The physician repairs the hard palate by closing the communication between the oral and nasal cavities. A combination of mucosal and mucoperiosteal flaps are used to repair the defect. The margins of the defect are incised and dissected to develop mucosal, muscular, and mucoperiosteal layers. The mucoperiosteum of the vomer (nasal septum) is elevated and sutured to the mucoperiosteum of the hard palate. This closes the communication between the oral and nasal cavities. Incisions are made in the palatal mucosa adjacent to the alveolar (tooth-bearing) bone. The mucosa is elevated and loosened from the bony palate. The palatal mucosa is closed in layers.

42260
The physician repairs a fistula communication from the nasal or sinus regions to the nasolabial region of the midface. The repair is dependent on the size of the fistula tract. For small defects, an excision of the epithelized tract is made from source to skin surface. This wound is sutured in layers. In larger defects, a nasolabial flap may be necessary after excision of the fistula. A nasolabial flap is designed, incised, and

rotated to the defect region. The flap is sutured over the defect in layers.

42280
The physician takes impressions of the maxilla. A palatal prosthesis is customized from the cast model of the impression.

42281
The physician inserts a palatal prosthesis prepared by an outside laboratory. The prosthesis is retained by pins and augments the palate.

42300-42305
The physician drains an abscess of the parotid gland. An incision is made intraorally through the tissue overlying the gland. The physician dissects through the tissue overlying the abscess. The abscess is opened with a surgical instrument and the fluid is drained. Report 42305 if the excision is complicated.

42310
The physician drains an abscess of the submaxillary (submandibular) or sublingual gland. An incision is made intraorally through the tissue overlying the gland. The physician dissects through the tissue overlying the abscess. The abscess is opened with a surgical instrument and the fluid is drained.

42320
The physician drains an abscess of the submaxillary (submandibular) salivary gland. An incision is made extraorally through the skin overlying the gland. The physician dissects through the tissue overlying the abscess. The abscess is opened with a surgical instrument and the fluid is drained. A drain may be placed.

42330
The physician makes an incision in the submandibular, sublingual, or parotid ducts to remove a sialolith (a stone). An incision is made intraorally in the mucosa overlying the duct and tissue is dissected to reach the duct. The physician removes the stone in a simple sialolithotomy. The incision is usually not closed.

42335
The physician makes an incision in the submandibular duct to remove a complicated sialolith (a stone). An incision is made intraorally in the mucosa overlying the duct and tissue is dissected to reach the duct. A large stone and portion of surrounding tissue must be removed. The incision is usually not closed.

42340
The physician makes an incision in the parotid gland to remove a sialolith (a stone). An incision is made extraorally in the skin overlying the gland and dissected to reach the stone or the intraoral mucosa overlying the duct is incised. Tissue is dissected to the gland. The physician removes the stone. The incision is closed with layered sutures.

42400-42405
The physician performs a needle biopsy in 42400 or an incisional biopsy in 42405 of a salivary gland. For a needle biopsy, a needle is inserted through the skin overlying the salivary gland. The physician takes a tissue sample from the gland and withdraws the needle. For an incisional biopsy, an incision is made in the skin overlying the salivary gland. Tissues are dissected to the gland. An incision is made in the tissue of the gland and a small piece of the gland is removed. The surgical wound is sutured.

42408
The physician removes a sublingual salivary cyst. An incision is made intraorally in the floor of the mouth overlying the cyst. The physician removes the cyst.

42409
The physician incises and removes the mucosa overlying a cyst on the floor of the mouth. The roof of the cyst is removed and the remaining sides of the cyst wall are sutured to the mucosa, creating a pouch. The saliva drains through the pouch. The pouch shrinks in size to a small opening in the floor of the mouth. Saliva from the sublingual gland flows through this opening.

42410-42426
The physician excises a portion or all of the parotid gland with or without facial nerve preservation and unilateral neck dissection. The physician makes a preauricular incision with a curved cervical extension to the midpoint of the mandible. The anterior and posterior skin flaps are retracted and the tissues are retracted to expose the parotid gland, leaving the fascia over the gland intact. In 42410, the main trunk of the facial nerve is visualized and the lateral (superficial) lobe of the parotid gland is freed and excised. In 42415, the facial nerve is identified and the lateral lobe is lifted off the branches of the nerve using dissection. A nerve stimulator may be used to test nerve integrity. In 42420, the facial nerve is identified and the lateral lobe is lifted off the branches of the nerve using dissection. A nerve stimulator is used to test nerve integrity. The nerve is retracted so the deep parotid gland can be removed without damaging the facial nerve. The nerve stimulator is used often to ensure nerve integrity. In 42425, the physician removes the gland without capsule disruption, sacrificing the facial nerve. In 42426, the physician removes the gland without capsule disruption, sacrificing the facial nerve. The incision is extended inferiorly to dissect the unilateral neck for lymph node excision.

42440
The physician removes a diseased, infected, blocked, or injured submandibular gland. The physician makes an incision in the skin of the neck below the inferior border of the mandible and near the angle of the mandible. The underlying tissues are dissected to the submandibular gland. The gland is exposed, freed from the surrounding tissue, and removed. The incision is closed with sutures.

42450
The physician removes a diseased, infected, blocked, or injured sublingual gland. The physician makes an intraoral incision in the mucosa overlying the gland.

Tissues are dissected down to the gland. The gland is exposed, freed from surrounding tissue, and removed. The incision is closed with sutures.

42500-42505
The physician repairs a salivary duct by inserting a hollow plastic or silicone tube into the duct. The tube is threaded through the duct. The duct is allowed to heal and may be sutured around the tube. In 42505, repair of the duct is complex and may be delayed. The tube is later removed and patency is restored.

42507
The physician makes an intraoral incision overlying the parotid duct. The path of the duct is diverted into a new position and sutured to the mucosa so that the opening of the duct is in a different location. To bypass a blockage, the duct may be cut behind the blockage and repositioned so that saliva can flow freely into the mouth. This procedure is performed on both parotid ducts.

42509
The physician makes an intraoral incision overlying the parotid duct. The path of the duct is diverted into a new position and sutured to the mucosa so that the opening of the duct is in a different location. To bypass a blockage, the duct may be cut behind the blockage and repositioned so that saliva can flow freely into the mouth. This procedure is performed on both parotid ducts. The physician also removes both submandibular glands. The physician makes an incision in the skin of the neck below the inferior border of the mandible. The underlying tissues are dissected to the submandibular gland. The gland is exposed, freed from the surrounding tissue, and removed. The incision is closed with sutures. The mucosal incisions are closed directly.

42510
The physician makes an intraoral incision overlying the parotid duct. The path of the duct is diverted into a new position and sutured to the mucosa so that the opening of the duct is in a different location. To bypass a blockage, the duct may be cut behind the blockage and repositioned so that saliva can flow freely into the mouth. This procedure is performed on both parotid ducts. The physician ligates both submandibular ducts. An incision may be made over the duct. Suture material is tied around the ducts to stop the flow of saliva. The mucosal incisions are closed directly.

42550
The physician inserts a small catheter into the duct of a salivary gland. A radiopaque dye (a dye which projects white on x-rays) is injected into the duct. The duct is filled with the dye back to and including the gland, if possible. A separately reported x-ray is taken. The x-ray shows the duct and gland filled with the dye, demonstrating the structure, blockages or disease affecting the structure.

42600
The physician closes a salivary fistula. The physician makes an incision around the fistula and excises the fistula down to the level of the duct. After excision of the fistula, the incision is closed directly.

42650
The physician inserts a probe into the salivary duct to dilate a narrowed section. The physician repeats the procedure with progressively larger probes until the desired amount of dilation is achieved.

42660
The physician introduces a catheter and dilates or expands the salivary duct. A radiopaque dye may be injected into the duct to outline the structure of the duct and any disease process. The catheter is removed.

42665
The physician makes an intraoral incision overlying a salivary duct and dissects to the layer of the duct. The duct is ligated (tied) and the incision is closed.

42700
The physician drains an abscess near or on a tonsil. The patient is given a topical anesthetic or placed under general anesthesia. Using an intraoral approach with a mouth gag, the physician incises the mucus membrane of the abscess. The abscess cavity is opened with angulated closed forceps or hemostat. The wound is irrigated and left open.

42720
The physician drains an abscess located on or near the pharynx. Retropharyngeal indicates the abscess is located on the back of the pharynx; parapharyngeal indicates the abscess is near the pharynx. The patient is given a topical anesthetic or placed under general anesthesia. Through an intraoral approach, the physician locates the abscess using a diagnostic needle puncture and aspiration at the point of maximal fluctuation on the pharynx. The physician incises the mucous membrane to open the abscess. The pus is evacuated using suction and sponging.

42725
The physician drains an abscess located on or near the pharynx. The patient is placed under general anesthesia. The physician makes an incision beneath the angle of the jaw and carries out a blunt dissection to locate and isolate the abscess. The physician incises the mucous membrane of the abscess. The pus is evacuated and a gauze or rubber drain may be inserted into the abscess cavity. The incision is repaired in sutured layers.

42800
The physician obtains a biopsy of the oropharynx. After the airway is secured with an endotracheal tube, a mouth gag is placed. The physician obtains a tissue sample through an incisional or snare technique. Bleeding is controlled through electrocautery. The wound is not closed.

42804-42806
The physician obtains a biopsy of the oropharynx or hypopharynx. After the airway is secured with an endotracheal tube, a mouth gag is placed. The physician obtains a tissue sample through an incisional

or snare technique. Bleeding is controlled through electrocautery; the wound is not closed. In 42804, tissue with a visible in the nasopharynx is biopsied. In 42806, tissue in the nasopharynx is biopsied to survey for an unknown primary lesion. If the lesion is deep in the nasopharynx, an operating laryngoscope is used to visualize the area.

42808

The physician removes or destroys a lesion of the pharynx. The physician uses an intraoral approach to excise or destroy the lesion. Destruction may be accomplished using a laser, cryosurgery, or electrocoagulation to cause the tissue to coagulate. Methods of excision may include avulsion or curettage.

42809

The physician removes a foreign body from the pharynx. The physician uses an intraoral approach with the aid of a tongue blade to visualize the foreign body. The foreign body is grasped with forceps and removed.

42810

The physician removes a branchial cleft cyst or vestige that is confined to the skin and subcutaneous tissues of the neck. A branchial cleft is an abnormal embryological remnant that resembles gills. The physician makes a horizontal neck incision just below the jaw line to access and remove the cyst or vestige. The incision is repaired in sutured layers.

42815

The physician removes a branchial cleft cyst or vestige that has extended beyond the skin and subcutaneous tissue. A branchial cleft is an abnormal embryological remnant that resembles gills. The physician makes one or two horizontal neck incisions just below the jaw line. The cyst or vestige is dissected from the surrounding muscle and fascia. If a fistula is present, a surrounding elliptical skin excision is performed. Any ducts of the cyst are dissected and traced to a pharyngeal communication. The cyst, vestige, and ducts are removed. A tissue drain is placed and the wound is sutured in layers.

42820-42821

The physician removes the tonsils and adenoids. The physician accesses the tonsils and adenoids in an intraoral approach. First, the physician removes the tonsils by grasping the tonsil with a tonsil clamp and dissecting the capsule of the tonsil. The tonsil is removed. Bleeding vessels are clamped and tied. Bleeding may also be controlled using silver nitrate and gauze packing. Using a mirror or nasopharyngoscope for visualization, the physician uses an adenotome or a curette and basket punch to excise the adenoids. Alternate surgical techniques for a tonsillectomy and adenoidectomy include electrocautery, laser surgery, and cryogenic surgery. Report 42820 if the patient is under 12 years. For patients 12 years or older, report 42821.

42825-42826

The physician removes the tonsils. The tonsillectomy can be the first the patient has undergone, or a secondary procedure to remove tonsil regrowth since the primary procedure. The physician accesses the tonsils in an intraoral approach. First, the physician removes the tonsils by grasping the tonsil with a tonsil clamp and dissecting the capsule of the tonsil. The tonsil is removed. Bleeding vessels are clamped and tied. Bleeding may also be controlled using silver nitrate and gauze packing. Alternate surgical techniques for a tonsillectomy include electrocautery, laser surgery, and cryogenic surgery. Report 42825 if the patient is under 12 years. For patients 12 years or older, report 42826.

42830-42836

The physician removes the adenoids. Using an intraoral approach and a mirror or nasopharyngoscope for visualization, the physician uses an adenotome or a curette and basket punch to excise the adenoids. Alternate surgical techniques for an adenoidectomy include electrocautery, laser surgery, and cryogenic surgery. For adenoidectomy performed as a primary procedure (the initial removal of the adenoid), report 42830 for patients under 12 years; report 42831 for patients 12 years and older. When performed as a secondary procedure (secondary procedure to remove adenoid tissue that has grown back since an initial adenoidectomy), report 42835 if the patient is under 12 years; report 42836 for patients 12 years and older.

42842-42845

The physician removes the tonsils, tonsillar pillars, and/or the retromolar trigone, along with any affected area of the maxilla or mandible involved in the tumor. First, the physician performs a tracheostomy. The involved tissue is resected. In addition to the above areas, radical resection may include a hemiglossectomy or a total glossectomy, as well as a full neck dissection. In 42842, the wound is so extensive that it is packed open and grafted at a later session. In 42844, the wound is less extensive and can be closed primarily with sutured layers. In 42845, a flap is rotated from the chest. If the wound included a resection of the mandible or maxilla, a fibular bone graft or a metal plate may be used to reconstruct the jaw.

42860

The physician removes portions of the tonsils not excised during primary resection or that have developed polyps. The physician cauterizes and/or snares the affected tissue. No closure is required.

42870

The physician removes or destroys the lingual tonsils. Because the abscessed tonsils may restrict the airway passage, the physician is present during intubation in case an emergency airway is needed. The physician uses an endotracheal tube or an operating laryngoscope with jet ventilation to ventilate the patient. Using an intraoral approach, the physician uses a laser to destroy the lingual tonsils.

42890

The physician removes the affected portion of the pharyngeal wall. The physician makes a vertical incision in the neck and retracts the strap muscles. The affected area of the pharynx is excised and the pharyngeal walls are reapproximated and closed with sutures. The incision is sutured in layers. Occasionally, the area removed includes part of the thyroid ala, hyoid bone, and wall of the pyriform fossa. Procedures include: anterior transhyoid pharyngotomy, lateral pharyngotomy, and median labiomandibular glossotomy. Reconstructive surgery is required for closure.

42892
The physician removes the affected portion of the pharyngeal wall or pyriform sinus. The physician makes a vertical incision and retracts the strap muscles. The mucosa of the upper pyriform sinus and the affected portion of the pharynx are excised. The lateral and posterior pharyngeal walls are reapproximated and closed with sutures. The incision is sutured in layers.

42894
The physician removes the affected portion of the pharyngeal wall or pyriform sinus. The physician makes a vertical incision and retracts the strap muscles. The mucosa of the upper pyriform sinus and the affected portion of the pharynx are excised. Myocutaneous or fasciocutaneous flap reconstruction of the pharyngeal area may be achieved using the pectoralis major muscle and its overlying skin. The flap is rotated and inserted through a previously created tunnel between the clavicle and overlying skin and sutured into place to reconstruct the pharynx. Alternately, free muscle, skin, or fascial flap closure with microvascular anastomosis may be performed. The flaps used in reconstruction are separately reportable. The incisions are sutured in layers.

42900
The physician locates and sutures a wound or injury to the pharynx. The physician uses an intraoral or transhyoid approach, depending on the location and extent of the wound. For an intraoral approach, the physician uses a mirror for visualization. For a transhyoid approach, the physician makes a horizontal incision directly below the jaw line. The physician sutures the wound. If a transhyoid approach is used, the incision is sutured in layers.

42950
A variety of techniques may be used for pharyngeal reconstruction including skin grafts, tongue flaps, regional cutaneous flaps and microvascular free-tissue transfer. Skin grafts are commonly harvested from the forehead, deltopectoral, nape of the neck, and pectoralis major. Reconstruction is performed when direct wound closure or reapproximation is not possible.

42953
The physician repairs a tear at the pharyngeal esophageal junction. After the airway is secured, the physician makes a horizontal neck incision and retracts superficial tissues to expose the pharyngeal esophageal junction. The defect is identified, irrigated to reduce infection, and sutured in layers.

42955
The physician creates an opening to the pharynx for long term feeding. The physician makes a horizontal incision below the jaw line to create a communication between the pharyngeal lumen and the exterior of the patient's neck. The incision is sutured to create an opening for placement of a feeding tube.

42960-42962
The physician controls bleeding of the oropharynx. Primary hemorrhaging occurs within 24 hours after surgery; secondary hemorrhaging occurs 24 hours to two weeks after tonsillectomy. In 42960 and 42961, hemorrhaging is controlled using methods such as clot evacuation and applying pressure with sponges, electrocautery, or application of vasoconstrictor solutions such as tannic acid, silver nitrate, and epinephrine. Cellulose sponges that expand when placed in the tonsillar cavity may be used. Report 42961 when extensive bleeding requires hospitalization. In 42962, surgery is required to control hemorrhaging. Surgical intervention methods include suture ligation of bleeding vessels. In cases of profuse bleeding, emergency ligation of the external carotid artery may be performed. The tonsillar pillars may be approximated with sutures to control post-tonsillectomy bleeding.

42970-42972
The physician controls bleeding of the nasopharynx. Primary hemorrhaging occurs within 24 hours after surgery; secondary hemorrhaging occurs 24 hours to two weeks after adenoidectomy. In 42970 and 42971 hemorrhaging is controlled using methods such as clot evacuation and application of vasoconstrictor solutions such as tannic acid, silver nitrate, and epinephrine; electrocautery; and posterior or anterior nasal packing. Report 42971 when extensive bleeding requires hospitalization. In 42972, surgery is required to control hemorrhaging. Surgical intervention methods include ligation of ethmoidal arteries using silver clips and/or electrocautery. The physician may use a nasal or intraoral approach for secondary surgery.

42975
The physician performs a diagnostic drug-induced sleep endoscopy (DISE) to evaluate the airway of a patient with obstructive sleep apnea (OSA). Also known as sleep nasoendoscopy (SNE), this procedure is typically performed in conjunction with an anesthesiologist. The patient is administered a sedative infusion, often propofol. The dose is carefully titrated in order to cause obstructive apnea but avoiding central apnea. The physician passes a fiberoptic nasopharyngoscope into the nasal cavity and performs a full examination to rule out any airway obstructions. The scope is advanced into the nasopharynx. The physician pauses at this point until the patient begins snoring, at which point the examination continues of the nasopharynx,

velopharynx, and hypopharynx. The physician notes the degree of collapse using a standardized grading scale. Obstruction at the level of the palate (palate, tonsils, and lateral pharyngeal wall) and at the level of the hypopharynx (base of tongue, epiglottis, and lateral pharyngeal wall) is noted. The physician may advance the mandible 5 to 10 mm forward so that the action of a mandibular advancement device or a genioglossal advancement is reproduced. Insertion of a nasal trumpet or oral airway, or performance of a jaw thrust maneuver may also be a component of the evaluation.

43020

The physician makes an incision in the esophagus to remove a foreign body from it. The physician makes a horizontal or oblique incision in the lateral neck and into the esophagus, using forceps to grasp and extract the foreign body. The incision is closed with sutured layers.

43030

The physician incises the cricopharyngeal muscle, also known as the upper esophageal sphincter (UES). The physician makes a lateral neck incision to expose the UES, and a second lateral incision through the UES. The incision is repaired with sutured layers.

43045

The physician makes an incision in the esophagus to remove a foreign body. For a thoracic approach, the physician incises and dissects the left posterior chest wall to access the esophagus. The physician incises the esophagus and uses forceps to grasp and remove the foreign body. The esophageal incision is closed with sutures. The left posterior chest wall is closed with sutured layers.

43100

The physician removes a lesion in the esophagus. The physician makes a horizontal or oblique incision of the lateral neck. Next, the physician makes an incision in the esophagus and excises the lesion. The remaining esophageal borders are sutured together. The incision is sutured in layers.

43101

The physician removes a lesion in the esophagus. For a thoracic approach, the physician incises and dissects the left posterior chest wall to access the esophagus. For an abdominal approach, the physician makes an upper midline abdominal incision to access the esophagus transhiatally. The physician excises the lesion. The remaining esophageal borders are sutured together. The incision is closed with sutured layers.

43107

The physician removes most or all of the esophagus and attaches the stomach to the pharynx or cervical esophagus. The physician gains access to the esophagus through two incisions: an oblique cervical incision and a horizontal upper midline abdominal incision. The physician divides the esophagus at the cervical level (for an esophagogastrostomy) or at its origin at the pharynx (for a pharyngogastrostomy). The esophagus is removed through the abdominal incision and divided from the stomach. The stomach is pulled through the posterior mediastinum and anastomosed to the pharynx or the remaining cervical esophagus. If the stomach is used as the esophageal conduit, a pyloroplasty may be performed to open the pyloric sphincter. The incisions are repaired in sutured layers.

43108

The physician removes most or all of the esophagus and uses a bowel or colon graft for reconstruction. The physician gains access to the esophagus through two incisions: an oblique cervical incision and a horizontal upper midline abdominal incision. The physician divides the esophagus at the cervical level (for an esophagogastrostomy) or at its origin at the pharynx (for a pharyngogastrostomy). The esophagus is removed through the abdominal incision and divided from the stomach. A portion of the colon or small bowel is excised and freed of attachments, taking care to preserve its major vascular supply. Gastrointestinal continuity is reestablished by securing the distal and proximal bowel margins. Finally, the excised portion of the colon or bowel is attached to the pharynx or cervical esophagus and the stomach. This anastomosis creates a usable esophagus. If the stomach is used as the esophageal conduit, a pyloroplasty may be performed to open the pyloric sphincter. The incisions are repaired in sutured layers.

43112

The esophagus is removed through abdominal, chest, and neck incisions and replaced with stomach. The physician makes a midline abdominal incision. The stomach is dissected free of surrounding structures and the esophagus is mobilized as it passes through the diaphragm to the stomach. The physician makes an incision in the right chest between the ribs and exposes the esophagus. The esophagus is mobilized under direct vision in the chest from the diaphragm to the neck. A longitudinal incision is made in the left or right neck and the esophagus is identified and mobilized in the neck. The esophagus is divided at its junction with the stomach and in the neck and the esophagus is removed. The stomach is pulled through the middle of the chest into the neck and the stomach is connected to the stump of the esophagus in the neck. The incisions are closed. This procedure is also referred to as the McKeown procedure or the tri-incisional esophagectomy.

43113

The physician removes the esophagus through abdominal, chest and neck incisions and replaces the esophagus with colon or small bowel. The physician makes a midline abdominal incision. The stomach is dissected free of surrounding structures and the esophagus is mobilized as it passes through the diaphragm to the stomach. The physician makes an incision in the right chest between the ribs and exposes the esophagus. The esophagus is mobilized under direct vision in the chest from the diaphragm to the neck. The esophagus is divided at its junction with the stomach and in the neck and the esophagus is removed. The physician selects an appropriate segment of colon or small bowel. The bowel is divided proximal and distal to this segment and the bowel ends are reapproximated. The selected segment of colon or small bowel is pulled through the middle section of the chest and connected to the stump of the esophagus in the neck and to the stomach in the abdomen. The incisions are closed.

43116

The physician removes the affected portion of the esophagus and replaces it with a graft from the large or small intestine. The physician gains access to the esophagus through an oblique cervical incision. The physician resects the affected portion of the cervical esophagus. Next, the physician obtains a graft from the large or small intestine. To do this, the physician makes a midline abdominal incision and frees a portion of the large or small intestine of muscular and vascular attachments. The intestine is resected and interposed to reestablish gastrointestinal continuity in the cervical esophagus. Microsurgical techniques are used to create a new blood supply for the graft. The distal and proximal portions of the remaining intestine are reconnected (anastomosis).

43117

The physician removes the distal esophagus and possibly the proximal stomach through abdominal and chest incisions and replaces the esophagus with the remaining stomach. The physician makes a midline abdominal incision. The stomach is dissected free of surrounding structures and the esophagus is mobilized as it passes through the diaphragm to the stomach. The esophagus is divided at its connection to the stomach or the stomach may be divided near its middle portion. Next, a right chest incision is made between the ribs to expose the esophagus. The distal esophagus is mobilized under direct vision and divided above its diseased segment. The distal esophagus and attached proximal stomach are then removed. The remaining stomach is pulled into the chest and connected to the stump of the proximal esophagus. Drains are placed into the chest near the new anastomosis and the incisions are closed.

43118

The physician removes the distal esophagus and possibly proximal stomach through abdominal and chest incisions and replaces the esophagus with colon or small bowel. The physician makes a midline abdominal incision. The stomach is dissected free of surrounding structures and the esophagus is mobilized as it passes through the diaphragm to the stomach. The esophagus is divided at its connection to the stomach or the stomach may be divided near its middle portion. An appropriate segment of colon or small bowel is selected and the bowel is divided proximal and distal to this segment and the bowel ends re- approximated. One end of the selected bowel segment is connected to the remaining stomach and the other end is placed through the diaphragm into the chest. A right chest incision is made between the ribs to expose the esophagus. The distal esophagus is mobilized under direct vision and divided above its diseased segment. The distal esophagus and attached proximal stomach are removed. The remaining end of the segment of colon or small bowel that has been attached to the stomach is pulled into the chest and connected to the stump of the proximal esophagus. Drains are placed into the chest near the new anastomosis and the incisions are closed.

43121

The physician removes the affected part of the esophagus and proximal stomach and reattaches the remaining stomach to the esophageal stump. The physician accesses the esophagus through a right posterolateral thoracotomy; no abdominal incision is made. The physician resects the affected portion of the distal esophagus and sometimes a portion of the proximal stomach. The resected area is removed. The stomach or gastric remnant is pulled into the thorax and sutured to the esophageal stump. If the stomach is used as the esophageal conduit, a pyloroplasty may be performed to open the pyloric sphincter. The incision is sutured in layers.

43122

The physician removes the distal esophagus and possibly proximal stomach through a combined abdominal and chest incision and replaces the esophagus with the remaining stomach. The physician makes a midline abdominal incision. The stomach is dissected free of surrounding structures and the esophagus is mobilized as it passes through the diaphragm to the stomach. The esophagus is divided proximally above the diseased area and distally at its junction with the stomach or the middle portion of the stomach may be divided. The distal esophagus and attached proximal stomach are removed. The remaining stomach is connected to the stump of the esophagus. The incision is closed.

43123

The physician removes the distal esophagus and possibly the proximal stomach through a combined abdominal and chest incision and replaces the esophagus with colon or small bowel. The physician makes a midline abdominal incision that may extend onto the chest between the ribs. The stomach is dissected free of surrounding structures and the esophagus is mobilized as it passes through the diaphragm to the stomach. The esophagus is divided proximally above the diseased area and distally at its junction with the stomach or the middle portion of the stomach may be divided. The distal esophagus and attached stomach are removed. An appropriate segment of colon or small bowel is selected. The bowel is divided proximal and distal to the segment and the bowel ends are re- approximated. The selected segment of bowel is connected proximally to the remaining esophageal stump and distally to the remaining stomach. The incision is closed.

43124

The physician removes the esophagus with no attempt to reconstruct the esophagus. The physician first creates a permanent tracheoplasty. The physician accesses the esophagus through an oblique cervical incision, a thoracotomy, and/or a midline abdominal incision and resects the affected portion of the esophagus. The esophageal stump is sutured to the cervical incision, creating a connection from the exterior of the neck to the esophageal lumen to provide drainage of saliva and mucus. The incisions are closed with sutured layers.

43130-43135

The physician removes a diverticulum from the hypopharynx or esophagus. A diverticulum is a pouch that occurs normally or because of a defect in the muscular membrane. In 43130 (cervical approach), the physician makes a lateral incision in the neck. In 43135 (thoracic approach), the physician incises and dissects the left posterior chest wall. The physician may dissect or incise the cricopharyngeus muscle to expose the diverticulum. If a myotomy is necessary, the physician makes a vertical incision through the cricopharyngeus muscle. The physician clamps the diverticulum and closes using sutures or staples. The incision is closed with sutured layers.

43180

The physician examines the esophagus via a rigid esophagoscope inserted through the patient's mouth and into the esophagus under general anesthesia. The physician removes a diverticulum from the hypopharynx or esophagus. A diverticulum is a pouch that occurs normally or because of a defect in the muscular membrane of the upper esophagus. The physician may dissect or incise the cricopharyngeus muscle to expose the diverticulum. Cricopharyngeal myotomy is accomplished by making a vertical incision through the cricopharyngeus muscle. The physician clamps the diverticulum and closes using sutures or staples. The incision is closed with sutured layers.

43191-43193

The physician views the esophagus via a rigid esophagoscope inserted through the patient's mouth and into the esophagus under general anesthesia. In 43191, a collection of cells may be taken by brushing or washing and/or aspirating the esophageal lining for specimens. In 43192, the physician injects any substance into a specific area through the scope. In 43193, biopsy forceps are used to obtain samples of the esophageal mucosa.

43194

The physician locates and removes a foreign body(s) from the esophagus via a rigid esophagoscope passed through the patient's mouth and into the esophagus. The foreign body is located. It may be suctioned or grasped with forceps and retracted through the scope. An alternative technique is to pass a balloon beyond the foreign body. The balloon is inflated and withdrawn, capturing the foreign body.

43195-43196

The physician stretches esophageal tissue via a rigid esophagoscope passed through the patient's mouth and into the esophagus. A narrowing in the esophagus is expanded. In 43195, a balloon is advanced through the scope. After entering the obstructed region, the balloon is briefly inflated several times to achieve a satisfactory opening. In 43196, a guidewire is placed through the scope and the scope is removed. A dilator is passed over the guidewire. This process may be repeated several times using progressively larger dilators until the esophagus is opened satisfactorily.

43197-43198

Transnasal flexible esophagoscopy is the safer, less-expensive, and more accurate technique as compared to conventional esophagoscopy. The physician examines the esophagus via a flexible esophagoscope inserted through one of the patient's nasal passages into the oropharynx and down into the esophagus. In 43197, a collection of specimen cells may be obtained by brushing or washing and/or aspirating the esophageal lining. In 43198, biopsy forceps are used to obtain samples of the esophageal mucosa.

43200-43202

The physician views the esophagus via a flexible esophagoscope inserted through the patient's mouth and into the esophagus. In 43200, cells are collected for specimen by brushing or washing and/or aspirating the esophageal lining. In 43201, the physician injects any substance into a specific area through the scope while viewing the esophagus. In 43202, biopsy forceps are used to obtain samples of the esophageal mucosa.

43204-43205

The physician passes a flexible esophagoscope through the patient's mouth and into the esophagus to identify and treat varices. Varices are dilated, enlarged, tortuous veins. In 43204, the physician passes a sclerotherapy needle through the scope and injects the varices with an agent that causes fibrosis (scarring). Over time, this results in obliteration of the varices. In 43205, the physician uses a suction tip to lift the varix and places a rubber band around the base of the varix.

43206

The physician views the esophagus via a flexible esophagoscope inserted through the patient's mouth and into the esophagus. Any abnormalities of the mucosal lining of the esophagus can be seen using an endomicroscope that is attached to the esophagoscope. The endomicroscope uses laser light to magnify the cells of the mucosa in order to identify the histopathology in real time.

43215

The physician passes a flexible esophagoscope through the patient's mouth and into the esophagus to locate and remove a foreign body(s). It may be suctioned or grasped with forceps and retracted through the scope. An alternative technique is to pass a balloon beyond the foreign body. When the balloon is inflated and withdrawn, the foreign body(s) is captured.

Digestive

43216-43217
The physician uses an esophagoscope to remove tumors, polyps, or lesions from the esophagus. A flexible esophagoscope is passed through the patient's mouth and into the esophagus to locate the lesion. In 43216, the base of the lesion is electrocoagulated and severed using biopsy forceps. In 43217, a snare loop is placed around the base of the lesion and closed (the tissue is electrocoagulated and severed as the loop is closed). The severed tissue is withdrawn through the scope.

[43211]
The physician performs an endoscopic mucosal resection (EMR) to remove abnormal tissues from the esophagus. A flexible esophagoscope is passed through the patient's mouth and into the esophagus to locate the lesion in the inner lining of the esophagus. Saline or other solution is injected into the submucosa around the lesion to raise it from the surrounding deep muscle layer. Once the lesion is raised, it is removed using a snare, banding, or ligation and sent for pathology. The esophagoscope is removed.

[43212]
A flexible esophagoscope is passed through the patient's mouth and the esophagus is examined. A guidewire is placed through the scope and the stent is advanced over the guidewire. The position of the stent is confirmed and the scope is withdrawn. This procedure usually follows dilation for an obstruction.

43220 [43214]
The physician passes a flexible esophagoscope through the patient's mouth and into the esophagus. A balloon is advanced through the scope to dilate the esophagus. After entering the obstructed region, the balloon is briefly inflated several times to stretch the esophageal tissue. Report 43220 when the balloon is dilated to a diameter of less than 30 mm and 43214 when the balloon is dilated to 30 mm or more.

[43213]
The physician stretches esophageal tissue in patients where routine esophageal dilation is not feasible. The physician passes a flexible esophagoscope through a patient's gastrostomy or jejunostomy. The scope is passed to the area of the stricture. A second flexible esophagoscope is inserted through the patient's mouth to the stricture. A guidewire is passed from either esophagoscope through the stricture. A balloon or dilators are passed over the guidewire through the scope. After entering the obstructed region, the balloon is briefly inflated several times or progressively larger dilators are passed in succession. Once the diameter of the stricture is acceptable, instruments are removed, the area is examined for perforation, and the scope is removed.

43226
The physician passes a flexible esophagoscope through the patient's mouth and into the esophagus. A guidewire is placed through the scope. The scope is removed and a dilator is passed over the guidewire. This process is repeated several times using progressively larger dilators to stretch the esophageal tissue.

43227
The physician passes a flexible esophagoscope through the patient's mouth and into the esophagus to identify the source of bleeding. Several endoscopic methods may be used to control bleeding, including the use of laser therapy, electrocoagulation, rubber band ligation, and the injection of the bleeding vessel with sclerosants, ethanol, or adrenaline.

43229
The physician removes tumors, polyps, or lesions from the esophagus by inserting a flexible esophagoscope through the patient's mouth and into the esophagus to locate the lesion. Laser therapy, electrocoagulation, or injection of toxic agents may be used to destroy the lesion.

43231
The physician passes a flexible esophagoscope through the patient's mouth and into the esophagus to perform an endoscopic ultrasound examination. The esophagus is examined and the area of interest is identified. The esophagoscope is removed and replaced with an echoendoscope or an ultrasound probe is passed through the already placed esophagoscope. The echoendoscope or ultrasound probe is fitted with a water-filled balloon near the tip; the tip contains a transducer that picks up the ultrasound frequency and relays it to a processor, outside of the body. The water-filled tip is positioned in the esophagus, against the esophageal wall next to the area of interest. The area is scanned and an ultrasound image is projected through the processor to a monitor in real-time. When the ultrasound examination is complete, the echoendoscope or esophagoscope and ultrasound probe are removed.

43232
The physician views the esophagus and performs a transendoscopic ultrasound-guided intramural or transmural fine needle aspiration/biopsy. A flexible esophagoscope is passed through the patient's mouth and into the esophagus where the esophagus is examined and the area of interest is identified. The esophagoscope may be removed. A radial scanning echoendoscope is inserted and ultrasound scanning performed or an ultrasound probe is passed through the already placed esophagoscope. The site for a fine needle aspiration biopsy is determined. If a radial scanning echoendoscope is used it is removed and replaced with a curvilinear array echoendoscope. The echoendoscope or ultrasound probe is fitted with a water-filled balloon near the tip; the tip contains a transducer that picks up the ultrasound frequency and relays it to a processor outside of the body. The water-filled tip is positioned in the esophagus, against the esophageal wall next to the predetermined fine needle aspiration (FNA) biopsy site. The area is scanned and an ultrasound image is projected through

the processor to a monitor in real-time. The FNA needle is passed through the scope to the biopsy site and the needle is inserted through the wall of the esophagus to the lesion or other structure, such as a lymph node, and a biopsy is taken. When the FNA is complete, the echoendoscope or esophagoscope and ultrasound probe is removed.

43235-43236
The physician examines the upper gastrointestinal tract for diagnostic purposes. The physician passes an endoscope through the patient's mouth into the esophagus. The esophagus, stomach, duodenum, and sometimes the jejunum are viewed to determine if bleeding, tumors, erosions, ulcers, or other abnormalities are present. In 43235, specimens may be obtained by brushing or washing the esophageal lining with saline, followed by aspiration. Report 43236 if the physician injects any substance into the submucosa through the scope while viewing the upper gastrointestinal tract.

43237-43238
The physician performs an esophagogastroduodenoscopy (EGD) with a concomitant ultrasound examination for diagnostic purposes. The patient is prepped for an upper gastrointestinal exam and the scope is advanced through the mouth into the stomach and duodenum or jejunum. An examination is carried out to determine if any bleeding, tumors, erosions, ulcers, or other abnormalities are present. Report 43237 when the endoscope exam is followed by insertion of an echoendoscope for an ultrasound exam limited to the esophagus, stomach, duodenum, and adjacent structures. Report 43238 when the echoendoscope is inserted following the EGD examination and an ultrasound and transmural fine needle aspiration biopsy is performed. Using real-time ultrasonic imaging guidance, the physician inserts a 22-gauge needle through the scope to the biopsy site and tissue is removed. Several passes may be made for an adequate specimen before the scope is removed.

43239
The physician examines the upper gastrointestinal tract for diagnostic purposes. The physician passes an endoscope through the patient's mouth into the esophagus. The esophagus, stomach, duodenum, and sometimes the jejunum are viewed to determine if bleeding, tumors, erosions, ulcers, or other abnormalities are present. Single or multiple tissue samples from the upper gastrointestinal tract are obtained for biopsy specimens using biopsy forceps through the endoscope.

43240
The physician examines the upper gastrointestinal tract and performs transmural drainage of a pseudocyst. The physician passes an endoscope through the patient's mouth into the esophagus. The esophagus, stomach, duodenum, and sometimes the jejunum are examined. The site for drainage of the pseudocyst is identified. A needle is passed through the scope to the site and the needle is inserted through the small intestinal wall into the pancreatic pseudocyst. The pseudocyst is drained and the endoscope is removed.

43241
The physician examines the upper gastrointestinal tract and places a tube or catheter. The physician passes an endoscope through the patient's mouth into the esophagus. The esophagus, stomach, duodenum, and sometimes the jejunum are viewed. The physician places a tube or catheter through the endoscope. The endoscope is removed.

43242
The physician examines the upper gastrointestinal tract and performs transendoscopic ultrasound-guided intramural or transmural fine needle aspiration/biopsy. The physician passes an endoscope through the patient's mouth into the esophagus. The esophagus, stomach, duodenum, and sometimes the jejunum are viewed. The endoscope may be removed. A radial scanning echoendoscope is inserted and ultrasound scanning is performed to examine the esophagus, stomach, and the duodenum and/or jejunum; or an ultrasound probe is passed through the already placed endoscope. The site for a fine needle aspiration biopsy is determined. If a radial scanning echoendoscope is used, it is removed and replaced with a curvilinear array echoendoscope. The echoendoscope or ultrasound probe is fitted with a water-filled balloon near the tip; the tip contains a transducer that picks up the ultrasound frequency and relays it to a processor outside of the body. The water-filled tip is positioned in the esophagus, stomach, or small intestine against the tissue wall next to the predetermined fine needle aspiration (FNA) biopsy site. The area is scanned and an ultrasound image is projected through the processor to a monitor in real-time. The needle is passed through the scope to the biopsy site and a biopsy is taken of the tissue or the needle is inserted through the wall of the esophagus, stomach, or small intestine and into a lesion or other structure, such as a lymph node. The area is biopsied. When the FNA/biopsy is complete, the instruments are removed.

43243-43244
The physician examines the upper gastrointestinal tract to identify and treat esophageal and/or gastric varices. Varices are dilated, enlarged, tortuous veins. The physician passes an endoscope through the patient's mouth into the esophagus. The esophagus, stomach, duodenum and sometimes the jejunum are viewed. The physician identifies the varices. In 43243, the physician passes a sclerotherapy needle through the scope, and injects the varices with an agent that causes fibrosis (scarring). The result is obliteration of the varices. In 43244, the physician uses a suction tip to lift the varix. The physician places a rubber band around the base of the varix.

43245
The physician uses an endoscope to examine the upper gastrointestinal tract to locate an obstruction. The physician passes an endoscope through the patient's mouth into the esophagus. The esophagus, stomach, duodenum, and sometimes the jejunum are viewed. The gastric or duodenal stricture is located. The physician dilates it using various methods, such as a balloon or bogie. If balloon dilation is performed, the balloon is inflated briefly several times to enlarge the stricture. When the dilation is complete, the balloon and endoscope are removed.

43246
The physician uses an endoscope to examine the upper gastrointestinal tract to guide placement of a gastrostomy tube. The physician passes an endoscope through the patient's mouth into the esophagus. The esophagus, stomach, duodenum, and sometimes the jejunum are viewed. The endoscope is used to guide the placement of a percutaneous gastrostomy tube. The tube is inserted through an incision of the abdomen. When in place, the tube connects the gastric lumen with the exterior abdominal wall.

43247
The physician uses a flexible endoscope to examine the upper gastrointestinal tract to locate and remove a foreign body(s). The physician passes a flexible endoscope through the patient's mouth, down the esophagus, through the stomach, and into the duodenum; sometimes the jejunum is also examined. The foreign body(s) is located. It may be suctioned or grasped with forceps and retracted through the endoscope.

[43290, 43291]
In a minimally invasive endoscopic surgery, the physician inserts an intragastric bariatric balloon into an obese patient (43290). The endoscope is advanced into the esophagus, stomach, and duodenum with notation of any abnormalities. The deflated gastric balloon is then inserted through the esophagus and into the stomach. Once the balloon is in an appropriate position, the central wire from the balloon is removed. A syringe is used to fill the balloon with a sterile saline solution. At the physician's discretion, the balloon may be filled with 50 mL at a time and up to 500 mL, dependent on the balloon type. The catheter is removed, with the balloon remaining within the stomach cavity. Endoscope may be utilized to ensure the balloon is not too snug within the stomach or wedged with the potential to cause an outlet obstruction in the stomach. At the conclusion of the procedure, the endoscope is withdrawn. Light sedation, local, or general anesthesia may be utilized. In 43291, the physician removes one or more intragastric bariatric balloons. The endoscope is advanced into the esophagus, stomach, and duodenum with notation of any abnormalities. The balloon in the stomach cavity is then punctured, aspirated, or connected to suction to remove the saline or gas. The balloon is deflated, grasped with forceps, and removed through the mouth. The physician may utilize a lubricating material such as mineral oil to ease the removal of the balloon through the esophagus.

43248
The physician uses an endoscope to examine and dilate a portion of the upper gastrointestinal tract. The physician passes an endoscope through the patient's mouth into the esophagus. The esophagus, stomach, duodenum, and sometimes the jejunum are viewed. A guidewire is placed through the endoscope and the scope is removed. A dilator is passed into the esophagus over the guidewire. This may be repeated several times using progressively larger dilators.

43249 [43233]
The physician visualizes the esophagus, stomach, and proximal small bowel with an endoscope and dilates an esophageal stricture. The physician inserts the endoscope through the mouth into the esophagus. The endoscope is advanced under direct vision through the esophagus into the stomach. The stomach is visualized and the endoscope is advanced into and through the duodenum and into the proximal jejunum if possible. The endoscope is withdrawn. If an esophageal stricture is present, a balloon on a catheter is advanced through the endoscope and through the stricture. The balloon is inflated to correct volume, pressure, and duration according to the package insert. The endoscope is removed. Report 43249 if the balloon is dilated less than 30 mm and 43233 if the balloon is dilated 30 mm or more.

43250-43251
The physician uses a flexible endoscope to examine the upper gastrointestinal tract and locate and remove tumors, polyps, or other lesions. The physician passes a flexible endoscope through the patient's mouth, down the esophagus, through the stomach, and into the duodenum; sometimes the jejunum is also examined to locate the lesion. Report 43250 when the base of the lesion is electrocoagulated and severed using biopsy forceps. Report 43251 when a snare loop is placed around the base of the lesion and closed (the tissue is electrocoagulated and severed as the loop is closed). The severed tissue is withdrawn through the endoscope. The endoscope is removed.

43252
The physician examines the upper gastrointestinal tract for diagnostic purposes. The physician passes an endoscope through the patient's mouth into the esophagus. The esophagus, stomach, duodenum, and sometimes the jejunum are viewed to determine if bleeding, tumors, erosions, ulcers, or other abnormalities are present. The physician views any abnormality of the mucosal lining using an endomicroscope that is attached to the esophagoscope. The endomicroscope uses laser light to magnify the cells of the mucosa in order to identify the histopathology in real time.

43253
The physician examines the upper gastrointestinal tract and performs transendoscopic ultrasound-guided transmural injection. The physician passes an endoscope through the patient's mouth into the esophagus. The esophagus, stomach, duodenum, and sometimes the jejunum are viewed. The endoscope may be removed. A radial scanning echoendoscope is inserted and ultrasound scanning is performed to examine the esophagus, stomach, and the duodenum and/or jejunum or an ultrasound probe is passed through the already placed endoscope. The site for injection is determined. If a radial scanning echoendoscope is used, it is removed and replaced with a curvilinear array echoendoscope. The echoendoscope or ultrasound probe is fitted with a water-filled balloon near the tip; the tip contains a transducer that picks up the ultrasound frequency and relays it to a processor outside of the body. The water-filled tip is positioned in the esophagus, stomach, or small intestine against the tissue wall next to the injection site. The area is scanned and an ultrasound image is projected through the processor to a monitor in real-time. The needle is passed through the scope to the site and the injection of a diagnostic or therapeutic substance or fiducial marker is performed through the wall of the esophagus, stomach, or small intestine and into a lesion or other structure, such as a lymph node. When the injection is complete, the instruments are removed.

43254
The physician performs an endoscopic mucosal resection (EMR) to remove abnormal tissues from the upper gastrointestinal system. The physician passes an endoscope through the patient's mouth into the esophagus. The esophagus, stomach, duodenum, and sometimes the jejunum are viewed and the lesion in the inner lining of the upper gastrointestinal system is located. Saline or another solution is injected into the submucosa around the lesion to raise it from the surrounding deep muscle layer. Once the lesion is raised, it is removed using a snare, banding, or ligation and sent for pathology. The endoscope is removed.

43255
The physician uses an endoscope to access and control bleeding of the upper gastrointestinal tract. The physician passes an endoscope through the patient's mouth and into the esophagus. The esophagus, stomach, duodenum, and sometimes the jejunum are viewed. Control of bleeding may be achieved using several endoscopic methods including laser therapy, electrocoagulation, rubber band ligation, and injection of the bleeding vessel with sclerosants, ethanol, or adrenaline. The endoscope is removed.

[43266]
The physician uses an endoscope to examine the upper gastrointestinal tract and performs a stent placement. The physician passes an endoscope through the patient's mouth into the esophagus. The esophagus, stomach, duodenum, and sometimes the jejunum are viewed. The endoscope is placed at the site of an obstruction or stricture, the necessary stent length is determined, and predilation of the obstruction or stenosis may be performed. The stent (endoprosthesis) is introduced into the site of the obstruction. Using a commercial delivery system, a plastic covering over the stent is removed and the stent self-deploys, shoring-up the walls at a specific site in the esophagus or proximal small intestine. When necessary, a balloon catheter is placed into the stent and gently inflated to more fully deploy the stent. The delivery system and endoscope are removed.

43257
The physician uses thermal energy to the muscle of the lower esophageal sphincter and/or gastric cardia to treat gastroesophageal reflux disease. The physician performs an esophagogastroduodenoscopy (EGD) with a concomitant ultrasound examination for diagnostic purposes. The patient is prepped for an upper gastrointestinal exam and the scope is advanced through the mouth into the stomach and duodenum or jejunum. An examination is carried out to determine if any bleeding, tumors, erosions, ulcers, or other abnormalities are present. Radiofrequency energy is applied through the scope equipment to apply heat to the muscle of the lower esophageal sphincter and/or the gastric cardia to treat gastroesophageal reflux disease (GERD). The heat is applied by electrodes placed in the esophageal tissue at multiple points above and below the squamocolumnar junction. Thermal lesions are created at the gastroesophageal junction that is thought to ablate the nerve pathways responsible for relaxing the sphincter and allowing reflux to occur. The thermal lesions are also thought to produce a "tightened" effect due to collagen contraction.

[43270]
The physician uses an endoscope to locate and remove tumors, polyps, or lesions from the upper gastrointestinal tract. The physician passes an endoscope through the patient's mouth into the esophagus. The esophagus, stomach, duodenum, and sometimes the jejunum are viewed to locate the lesion. The lesion is destroyed using laser therapy, electrocoagulation, or injection of toxic agents. The endoscope is removed.

43259
The physician uses an endoscope to examine the upper gastrointestinal tract and performs an endoscopic ultrasound examination of the esophagus, stomach, and the duodenum and/or jejunum. The physician passes an endoscope through the patient's mouth into the esophagus. The esophagus, stomach, duodenum, and sometimes the jejunum, are viewed. The endoscope may be removed and a radial scanning echoendoscope inserted or an ultrasound probe is passed through the already placed endoscope and an ultrasound examination is performed, including the esophagus, stomach, and the duodenum and/or jejunum. The echoendoscope or ultrasound probe is fitted with a water-filled balloon near the tip, which

contains a transducer that picks up the ultrasound frequency and relays it to a processor outside of the body, where the internal images can be viewed on screen. When the ultrasound scanning is completed, the instruments are removed.

[43210]
Esophagoscopy with esophagogastric fundoplasty involves an incisionless fundoplication technique; plication is the process of suturing one tissue to another, in this case part of the stomach around the esophagus. Fundoplication allows restoration of natural gastric and esophageal positioning resulting in the elimination of reflux and providing relief of gastroesophageal reflux disease (GERD) associated symptoms. By performing this procedure, the physician is able to treat the root cause of GERD by repairing an anatomic defect at the gastroesophageal valve. One procedure uses a proprietary device with a flexible video endoscope that provides visualization throughout the procedure. Another proprietary system combines a surgical stapler, ultrasonic sights to permit proper positioning, and a miniature video camera into a single device inserted through the patient's mouth to the gastrointestinal tract to perform esophagogastric fundoplication. The fundus of the stomach is wrapped around the lower end of the esophagus and secured. At the end of the procedure, the endoscope is removed.

Digestive

43260-43261
The physician performs an endoscopic retrograde cholangiopancreatography (ERCP) for diagnostic purposes. The physician passes the endoscope through the patient's oropharynx, esophagus, stomach, and into the small intestine. The ampulla of Vater is cannulated and filled with contrast. The common bile duct and the whole biliary tract, including the gallbladder, are visualized. Diagnostic brushing and washing may be performed in 43260. Report 43261 if a biopsy is performed.

43262
The physician performs an endoscopic retrograde cholangiopancreatography (ERCP) with a sphincter/ papillotomy. The physician passes the endoscope through the patient's oropharynx, esophagus, stomach, and into the small intestine. The ampulla of Vater is cannulated and filled with contrast. The common bile duct and the whole biliary tract, including the gallbladder, are visualized. The sphincter is cannulated using a sphincterotome. The sphincter is divided using electrocautery to control bleeding.

43263
The physician performs an endoscopic retrograde cholangiopancreatography (ERCP) with sphincter of Oddi manometry for diagnostic purposes. The physician passes the endoscope through the patient's oropharynx, esophagus, stomach, and into the small intestine. The ampulla of Vater is cannulated and filled with contrast. The common bile duct and the whole biliary tract, including the gallbladder, are visualized. A catheter is inserted into the bile duct and pancreatic ducts and connected to an external monitor to allow real time reading of the pressure of the muscle that controls the flow from the ducts to the duodenum.

43264-43265
The physician performs an endoscopic retrograde cholangiopancreatography (ERCP) to destroy or remove calculi or debris. The physician passes the endoscope through the patient's oropharynx, esophagus, stomach, and into the small intestine. The ampulla of Vater is cannulated and filled with contrast. The common bile duct and the whole biliary tract, including the gallbladder, are visualized. Report 43264 if stones or debris are removed from biliary and/or pancreatic ducts. Report 43265 if stones are destroyed using any method and any remaining debris removed.

[43274]
The physician performs an endoscopic retrograde cholangiopancreatography (ERCP) to insert a stent. The physician passes the endoscope through the patient's oropharynx, esophagus, stomach, and into the small intestine. The ampulla of Vater is cannulated and filled with contrast. The common bile duct and the whole biliary tract, including the gallbladder, are visualized. A sphincterotomy may be performed. A guidewire is threaded into the biliary or pancreatic duct. The stent is advanced over the guidewire and expanded in place. Balloon dilation may be performed to achieve desired outcome. The guidewire and surgical instruments are removed.

[43275]
The physician performs an endoscopic retrograde cholangiopancreatography (ERCP) to remove a biliary stent or other foreign body. The physician passes the endoscope through the patient's oropharynx, esophagus, stomach, and into the small intestine. The ampulla of Vater is cannulated and filled with contrast. The common bile duct and the whole biliary tract, including the gallbladder, are visualized. A sphincterotomy may be performed. The previously placed stent or foreign body is located and removed using any method, including basket and snare techniques.

[43276]
The physician performs an endoscopic retrograde cholangiopancreatography (ERCP) to exchange a biliary stent. The physician passes the endoscope through the patient's oropharynx, esophagus, stomach, and into the small intestine. The ampulla of Vater is cannulated and filled with contrast. The common bile duct and the whole biliary tract, including the gallbladder, are visualized. A sphincterotomy may be performed. The previously placed stent is located and removed using any method, including basket and snare techniques. A guidewire is threaded into the biliary or pancreatic duct. A new stent is advanced over the guidewire and expanded in place. Balloon dilation may be performed to achieve desired outcome. The guidewire and surgical instruments are removed.

[43277]
The physician performs an endoscopic retrograde cholangiopancreatography (ERCP) to dilate a biliary duct or the ampulla of Vater. The physician passes the endoscope through the patient's oropharynx, esophagus, stomach, and into the small intestine. The ampulla is cannulated and filled with contrast. The common bile duct and the whole biliary tract, including the gallbladder, are visualized. A stricture or obstruction is visualized. A sphincterotomy may be performed to reach the area to be treated with the balloon dilator. Once the balloon is in place, it is expanded multiple times until the desired outcome is achieved. The endoscope and all surgical instruments are removed. Report 43277 for each biliary duct and ampulla dilated.

[43278]
The physician performs an endoscopic retrograde cholangiopancreatography (ERCP) to perform destruction of a tumor, polyp, or other lesion of the biliary system. The physician passes the endoscope through the patient's oropharynx, esophagus, stomach, and into the small intestine. The ampulla is cannulated and filled with contrast. The common bile duct and the whole biliary tract, including the gallbladder, are visualized to locate the lesion. The lesion is destroyed using laser therapy, electrocoagulation, or injection of toxic agents. The endoscope is removed.

43273
At the same time as an endoscopic retrograde cholangiopancreatography (ERCP) with or without additional therapeutic or diagnostic procedures, the physician performs endoscopic cannulation of papilla with direct visualization of the pancreatic and/or common bile duct(s). A catheter or papillotome is inserted through the channel of the ERCP scope. With or without the use of a guidewire, the pancreatic and/ or common bile duct are located and visually inspected.

43279
The physician performs laparoscopic esophagomyotomy (Heller myotomy), often for treatment of achalasia. Achalasia (a motility disorder of the esophagus) is caused by degeneration of the nerves in the esophageal wall and results in an absence of the typical wave-like motion of the esophagus and lack of relaxation of the lower esophagus. The physician makes several small incisions in the abdominal wall through which a video camera and laparoscopic instruments are inserted. An incision of the esophageal muscle is made using specialized laparoscopic instruments. To prevent reflux, a part of the upper stomach is then wrapped around the lower portion of the esophagus. Laparoscopic instruments are removed, and the small incisions are sutured. A swallowing study is typically obtained prior to discharge.

43280
The physician performs an esophagogastric fundoplasty using a laparoscope. With the patient under anesthesia, the physician places a trocar at the umbilicus into the abdomen and insufflates the abdominal cavity. The physician places a laparoscope through the umbilical incision and additional trocars are placed into the peritoneal space. Additional instruments are introduced through the trocars. The physician identifies the fundus and the esophagus and resects them. The fundus is wrapped around the lower end of the esophagus, which is rejoined to the stomach with sutures. The trocars are removed and the incisions are closed with sutures.

43281-43282
The physician repairs a paraesophageal hernia using a laparoscope and may also perform a fundoplasty when indicated. With the patient under anesthesia and in a supine position, the physician places laparoscopic ports in the upper abdomen, through which the appropriate surgical instruments are inserted. With the left lateral segment of the liver retracted, the hiatus is exposed. The physician reduces the herniated stomach into the abdomen and dissects the hernia sac and gastroesophageal fat pad using a combination of sharp and blunt dissection. If a fundoplasty is indicated, the physician identifies the fundus and the esophagus and resects them. The fundus is wrapped around the lower end of the esophagus, which is rejoined to the stomach with sutures. The instruments and trocars are removed and the incisions are closed with sutures. Report 43281 for a procedure performed without the implantation of mesh and 43282 for one requiring mesh implantation.

43283
The physician performs a laparoscopic esophageal lengthening in order to extend a short esophagus prior to a separately reportable fundoplasty. This procedure is facilitated through a thoracoabdominal incision. With the patient under anesthesia, the physician places a trocar at the umbilicus into the abdomen and insufflates the abdominal cavity. The physician places a laparoscope through the umbilical incision and mobilizes the esophagus at the arch of the aorta. In the event that additional length is necessary, a gastric tube may be manipulated by separating the stomach with clamps and fixation of the proximal stomach that runs parallel with the lesser gastric curvature. A shortened esophagus may be due to damage caused by gastroesophageal reflux disease (GERD) thereby making fundoplasty difficult due to decreased tension necessary to reposition the GE junction. The trocars are removed and the incisions are closed with sutures.

43284-43285
Esophageal sphincter augmentation is a procedure used to treat gastroesophageal reflux disease (GERD), which is the result of a malfunction in the lower esophageal sphincter (LES) that allows acidic stomach contents to enter the esophagus. Symptoms of GERD include heartburn, regurgitation, difficulty swallowing,

and gas. When untreated, acid from GERD can cause damage to the lining of the esophagus, including the formation of strictures, and increase the patient's risk for esophageal cancer. One laparoscopic procedure involves the use of a proprietary magnetic sphincter augmentation device (MSAD) that is comprised of magnetic titanium beads connected on a stainless steel cable. The MSAD encircles the LES to strengthen the barrier while the magnetic attraction is calibrated in such a way as to provide sufficient augmentation to keep the weak LES closed to reflux, ensuring restoration of the body's natural barrier, yet opened when needed to permit swallowing of solids and liquids to pass through to the stomach or with increased gastric pressure from belching or vomiting. In 43284, with the patient under general anesthesia, the physician places the device around the esophagus, just above the stomach, via a laparoscopic approach. Implantation of the device uses a minimal dissection technique with slight adjustment to the anatomy at the gastroesophageal (GE) junction, but does not alter the anatomy of the stomach. Report 43285 for removal of the esophageal sphincter augmentation device.

43286-43288

In laparoscopic or thoracoscopic esophagectomy, the physician partially or totally removes the esophagus, the upper stomach, and surrounding lymph nodes in patients diagnosed with esophageal cancer and/or Barrett's esophagus. In Barrett's esophagus, a complication resulting from chronic gastroesophageal reflux (GERD), the normal tissue lining the esophagus transforms into the tissue lining the intestine, which can develop into esophageal precancer or cancer. Laparoscopic/thoracoscopic esophagectomy is also used to treat patients who have damaged their esophagus by ingesting a caustic or burning substance or for patients with achalasia. In 43286, the physician removes all or most of the esophagus and attaches the stomach to the pharynx or cervical esophagus utilizing a combination of laparoscopic and open approaches. The physician gains access to the esophagus through an oblique cervical incision. Using a laparoscopic approach, the physician mobilizes portions of the esophagus and the proximal stomach. The esophagus is divided at the cervical level (for an esophagogastrostomy) or at its origin at the pharynx (for a pharyngogastrostomy). The esophagus is removed through the laparoscopic abdominal access site and is divided from the stomach. The stomach is anastomosed to the pharynx or the remaining cervical esophagus via the open cervical incision. The laparoscopic instruments are removed and all incisions are repaired in sutured layers. In 43287, the physician removes the distal two-thirds of the esophagus utilizing a combination of laparoscopic and thoracoscopic approaches. Also referred to as a laparoscopic/thoracoscopic Ivor Lewis esophagectomy, this procedure involves laparoscopic access to mobilize portions of the lower esophagus and stomach, to resect a portion of the proximal stomach and celiac axis lymph nodes, and to create a gastric tube. Following removal of the abdominal trocars and closure of the trocar sites by layered suture, the patient is repositioned and the physician places appropriate trocars for separate thoracoscopic access to the chest. Via upper thoracoscopic technique, the physician mobilizes the middle and upper mediastinal esophagus. The esophagus is divided above the level of the azygos vein and the proximal esophageal margin is submitted for frozen-section pathological confirmation that no tumor remains. The distal esophagus and previously formed gastric conduit are brought into the chest. The thoracoscopic port is enlarged, the specimen is removed, and the gastric margin is evaluated by frozen-section pathology to confirm that it is tumor-free. The physician creates a side-to-side esophagogastric anastomosis. Chest tubes and drains are placed, trocars are removed, and trocar sites repaired with layered sutures. In 43288, the physician removes all or most of the esophagus utilizing a combination of laparoscopic, thoracoscopic, and open cervical approaches. The physician gains access to the esophagus through an oblique cervical incision. The esophagus is divided at the cervical level (for an esophagogastrostomy) or at its origin at the pharynx (for a pharyngogastrostomy). Using a laparoscopic approach, the physician mobilizes the stomach and performs a proximal gastrectomy. Utilizing a separate thoracoscopic approach, the physician mobilizes the upper, middle, and lower mediastinal esophagus and performs the appropriate resection. Anastomosis is performed via the open cervical incision. Laparoscopic pyloric drainage is included in all three techniques, when performed.

43300-43305

The physician repairs a defect in the esophagus using plastic repair or reconstruction. The physician makes a lateral neck incision to access the esophagus. The defect is identified and repaired. In 43305, the physician also transects the tracheoesophageal fistula. The physician closes the tracheal opening and repairs the esophagus. The incision is sutured in layers.

43310-43312

The physician repairs a defect in the esophagus using plastic repair or reconstruction. The physician makes a thoracic incision to access the esophagus. In 43310, the defect is identified and repaired. In 43312, the physician also transects the tracheoesophageal fistula. The physician closes the tracheal opening and repairs the esophagus. The incision is sutured in layers.

43313-43314

There are multiple types of material and methods that may be used to repair the esophagus, including autologous grafts, nonautologous grafts, patches, and gastric tubes. In the case of an autologous graft, the graft or patch may be harvested from the patient's intestine or colon depending on the anatomy and vasculature. The patient is positioned for a right posterolateral incision at the sixth rib region. A muscle-sparing incision is made and an extrapleural approach is used to gain access to the esophageal anomaly. The anomalous part of the esophagus is opened longitudinally with significant margins above and below the affected area. The graft, patch, or tube is placed over the defect and sutured into place. Report 43314 when a transesophageal fistula is also present and repaired.

43320
The physician performs a plastic repair of the lower esophagus where it joins the upper area (cardia) of the stomach. The physician may also transect the vagus nerve and/or enlarge the pylorus, the distal portion of the stomach. The physician accesses the esophagus through an upper abdominal or lateral thoracic incision. The diseased portion of the esophagus is resected. An anastomosis between the esophageal stump and the cardiac portion of the stomach is created. If the lesion is secondary to acid reflux, a vagotomy may be performed. The anterior and posterior trunks of the vagus nerve are transected to decrease acid production. If the gastric outlet area is decreased, a pyloroplasty may be performed to enlarge the pylorus. The incision is repaired in sutured layers.

43325
The physician pulls up part of the gastric fundus to cover the affected distal esophagus. A bougie (dilating instrument) is placed in the distal esophagus to maintain the esophageal opening. The physician accesses the esophagus and stomach through a transverse abdominal incision. The physician picks up the stomach 1 cm below the gastroesophageal (GE) junction and attaches it 1 cm above the GE junction. This fundic patch is sutured to the esophagus. Next, a Nissen fundoplication is performed by wrapping the rest of the fundus around the esophagus and suturing it into place. The incision is sutured in layers.

43327-43328
The physician performs a partial or complete fundoplasty by an incision in the abdominal wall (43327) or an incision through the chest cavity (43328). Through this incision, the fundus of the stomach is wrapped around the lower 4 cm of the esophagus and sutured into position. This allows the sphincter at the distal end of the esophagus to pass through a small area within the stomach muscle, creating a new valve that prevents reflux.

43330-43331
The esophagus is repaired using a fundic flap. The physician accesses the esophagus through an upper abdominal or a thoracic incision. For an abdominal approach, report 43330. For a thoracic approach, report 43331. The physician makes an incision into the muscular layers of the distal esophagus and cardia of the stomach (myotomy), leaving a gastric fundic flap. The flap is pulled along the esophagus, and sutured onto the margins of the myotomy. Repair of a hiatal hernia is performed by restoring the herniated portion of the stomach back to the abdomen, then narrowing the hiatal opening of the diaphragm by suturing the left and right crura together. All incisions are sutured in layers.

43332-43333
The physician repairs a non-neonatal paraesophageal hiatal hernia via open approach in 43332. A paraesophageal hernia occurs when a portion of the stomach passes through the hiatus and rests in the chest next to the esophagus. The physician makes an incision into the abdomen, pulls the stomach back down into the correct position, and sutures it to the rectus sheath. The diaphragm is often secured with sutures and the hiatus is sutured along the gastroesophageal junction. Fundoplication is performed to prevent the stomach from moving out of position again. Report 43333 when mesh is sutured to the abdominal wall over the defect during the repair.

43334-43335
The physician repairs a non-neonatal paraesophageal hiatal hernia via thoracotomy approach in 43334. A paraesophageal hernia occurs when a portion of the stomach passes through the hiatus and rests in the chest next to the esophagus. The physician makes the incision into the chest wall. The physician pulls the stomach back down into the abdomen and sutures it to the rectus sheath. The diaphragm is often secured with sutures and the hiatus is sutured along the gastroesophageal junction. Fundoplication is performed to prevent the stomach from moving out of position again. Report 43335 when mesh is sutured to the abdominal wall over the defect.

43336-43337
The physician repairs a non-neonatal paraesophageal hiatal hernia via thoracoabdominal incision in 43336. A paraesophageal hernia occurs when a portion of the stomach passes through the hiatus and rests in the chest next to the esophagus. The physician makes the incision into the chest wall and abdomen. The physician pulls the stomach back down into the abdomen and sutures it to the rectus sheath. The diaphragm is often secured with sutures and the hiatus is sutured along the gastroesophageal junction. Fundoplication is performed to prevent the stomach from moving out of position again. Report 43337 when mesh is sutured to the abdominal wall over the defect.

43338
In conjunction with a separately reportable fundoplasty procedure, the physician performs an esophageal lengthening procedure (also called a wedge gastroplasty) in order to extend a short esophagus. A bougie (dilating instrument) is passed through the esophagus into the stomach so that the bougie spans the gastroesophageal junction. The stomach is divided along the bougie with a gastric stapler, forming a gastric tube that effectively lengthens the esophagus.

43340-43341
The physician removes the affected esophagus and stomach, using the remaining stomach and jejunum to restore gastrointestinal continuity. The physician accesses the esophagus and stomach through an upper abdominal or a thoracic incision. For an abdominal approach, report 43340. For a thoracic

approach, report 43341. The physician resects the affected part of the esophagus. The stomach is advanced through the hiatus and sutured to the esophageal remnant. The antral portion of the stomach is excised, and the proximal jejunum is sutured to the gastric remnant. The distal end of the duodenum is anastomosed to the jejunum; the proximal end of the duodenum is sutured closed to form a blind pouch. The incision is sutured in layers.

43351-43352
The physician connects the esophagus to the exterior of the body, creating a fistula for drainage. In 43351, the physician uses a lateral thoracotomy to access the esophagus. In 43352, access is gained through a cervical incision. The physician makes an incision in the esophagus or the esophageal stump. The proximal limb of the esophagus is exteriorized and sutured into place, creating a connection from the exterior of the body to the esophageal lumen for mucus drainage. The incision is sutured in layers.

43360-43361
The physician repairs the esophagus and other gastronomic structures for a number of reasons. The physician uses a thoracoabdominal approach as a continuous incision or separate thoracic and abdominal incisions. The stomach is mobilized and repositioned in the chest in the original esophageal bed and sutured to the esophageal stump. The incision and esophageal stoma are closed. A jejunostomy tube is left in place. Report 43361 if performed with colon interposition or small bowel reconstruction, including bowel mobilization, preparation, and/or anastomosis.

43400
The physician accesses the esophagus through a midline abdominal or thoracic incision, and makes a longitudinal incision in the esophagus. The physician locates the varices (tortuous, dilated veins) and ligates them with sutures. The esophagotomy is closed with sutures. The incision is sutured in layers.

43405
The physician ligates or staples the esophagus to promote healing of a preexisting esophageal perforation. The physician makes a midline upper abdominal incision and retracts the soft tissues to expose the gastroesophageal junction. the physician staples or ligates the junction of the stomach and esophagus. A gastrostomy is created for feeding. The distal end of the esophagus may be exteriorized as a mucus fistula. The incision is sutured in layers.

43410-43415
The physician sutures a wound or injury to the esophagus. The physician accesses the esophagus through a lateral neck, midline abdominal, or thoracic incision. For a cervical approach, report 43410. For a thoracic or transabdominal approach, report 43415. The physician exposes the affected segment of the esophagus, which is repaired by suturing. The incision is sutured in layers.

43420-43425
The physician closes an opening in the esophagus and returns it to its natural position. The physician accesses the defect through an oblique cervical incision along the border of the sternocleidomastoid muscle, a midline abdominal incision, or a thoracic incision. For a cervical approach, report 43420. For a thoracic or transabdominal approach, report 43425. The physician closes the opening with sutures and repositions the esophagus to its normal anatomical position. The incision is sutured in layers.

43450
The physician dilates the esophagus using an unguided dilator. The physician passes a dilator into the patient's throat down into the esophagus until the end of the dilator passes the stricture. A stricture is a decrease in the esophagus opening as a result of cicatricial (scar) contraction or a deposit of abnormal tissue. The dilator is withdrawn after it passes the stricture. This may be repeated several times to dilate the esophagus to an acceptable size.

43453
The physician dilates the esophagus by passing dilators over a guidewire. The physician uses a fluoroscope to place a guidewire into the patient's throat, down the esophagus, and into the stomach. A series of dilators are passed over the guidewire and withdrawn. The process is repeated until the esophagus is dilated to an acceptable size.

43460
The physician inserts a multilumen tube into the esophagus through which a balloon is passed for the tamponade of bleeding esophageal varices. The balloon is inflated to exert pressure on the varices to stop bleeding. The balloon is left inflated so coagulation can occur before the physician proceeds with definitive treatment.

43496
The physician makes an abdominal incision to gain access to the omentum. The greater omentum is reflected to reveal the underlying small intestine. The jejunum is identified and removed. The remaining jejunum is reattached and the omentum is replaced. The free section of jejunum is transferred to another site with anastomosis of its vessels to another structure. Most commonly, the free transfer of a short segment of jejunum occurs between the pharynx and esophagus with microvascular anastomosis of jejunal vessels to the external carotid artery branches and the jugular vein. Portions of the pharynx and/or esophagus have already been resected with removal of cervical esophageal and hypopharyngeal carcinoma. Operative sites are sutured closed.

43497
The physician performs a transoral lower esophageal myotomy, also known as a peroral endoscopic myotomy or POEM. This procedure is often performed for the treatment of achalasia or spastic esophageal disorders (such as nutcracker esophagus or diffuse

esophageal spasm) that have not responded to medical therapy. Prior to the procedure, an IV is inserted into a vein through which anesthesia, fluids, and antibiotics are administered. An arterial line is inserted for pressure monitoring during the procedure. The physician inserts an endoscope through the mouth and into the esophagus, observing the images on a monitor. The first incision is made into the internal lining of the esophagus, through which the endoscope is inserted. The muscle is exposed within the wall of the esophagus; the physician makes an incision (myotomy) in the inner muscle layer near the lower esophageal sphincter. Upon completion of the procedure, the physician repairs the esophageal incision using standard endoscopic clips. The patient is typically admitted for postoperative monitoring and administration of antibiotics.

43500-43510

The physician performs a gastrostomy and explores gastric area, removes a foreign body or corrects a mucosal defect. The physician makes a midline epigastric incision and retracts the skin and underlying tissues laterally. The stomach is incised and explored. In 43500, a foreign body is removed. In 43501, a bleeding ulcer is identified and bleeding is controlled with electrocautery or ligation of vessels, and the mucosa is drawn over the ulcer and sutured. In 43502, an esophagogastric laceration is identified and bleeding is controlled with electrocautery or ligation of vessels, and the mucosa is drawn over the defect and sutured. In 43510, the physician introduces dilators into the esophagus from the stomach to increase the diameter of the esophagus. When dilation is complete, a stent is placed and secured with sutures to maintain to patency. After exploration or repair, the stomach is sutured in layers, the soft tissues are returned to anatomical position, and the incision is sutured in layers.

43520

The physician incises the pyloric muscle. The physician makes a small subcostal incision over the pyloric olive. The peritoneum is incised, the tissues are retracted, and the pylorus is identified. The serosa is incised and the tension of the pyloric muscle is released with longitudinal incisions. The peritoneum is sutured closed and the operative site is sutured in layers.

43605

The physician obtains a biopsy of the stomach via open approach (laparotomy). The physician makes a midline abdominal incision. The peritoneum is incised and tissues are retracted to identify the anterior surface of the stomach. An incision is made in the stomach and the physician explores the mucosa to obtain biopsies. Once biopsies are acquired, the stomach incision is closed with sutures or staples. The peritoneum is sutured closed and the abdominal incision is closed using layered sutures.

43610

The physician performs a local excision of an ulcer or a benign tumor of the stomach. The physician makes a midline abdominal incision. Next, the stomach is dissected free of surrounding structures and the area of the tumor identified. The tumor is excised with a normal margin of stomach around the tumor. The defect created in the stomach is closed with sutures or a stapling device. The incision is closed.

43611

The physician performs a local excision of a malignant tumor of the stomach. The physician makes a midline abdominal incision. Next, the stomach is dissected free of surrounding structures and the area of the tumor identified. The tumor is excised with a normal margin of stomach around the tumor. The defect created in the stomach is closed with sutures or a stapling device. The incision is closed.

43620-43621

The physician removes the stomach and approximates a limb of small bowel to the esophagus by performing an esophagoenterostomy in 43620 or a Roux-en-Y esophagojejunostomy in 43621. The physician makes a midline abdominal incision. The stomach is dissected free of surrounding structures and its blood supply is divided. The stomach is divided at the gastroesophageal junction and at the gastroduodenal junction and removed. In 43620, the remaining duodenal end of the intestine is simply mobilized to the end of the esophagus and connected. In 43621, a measured limb of Roux, or limb of small intestine, is created by dividing the upper jejunum. The distal part of the now divided upper jejunum, the limb in continuity with the ileum, is brought up and anastomosed to the esophagus. The proximal end of the divided jejunum, the segment containing the duodenum, must be connected back into the limb of small bowel farther down from the esophageal anastomosis. This maintains continuity for the duodenal section, which was sealed upon removal of the stomach, but which is also receiving bile from the liver and gallbladder as well as pancreatic juice.

43622

The physician removes the stomach and forms a pouch of small bowel and approximates this to the esophagus. The physician makes a midline abdominal incision. Next, the stomach is dissected free of surrounding structures and its blood supply divided. The stomach is divided at the gastroesophageal junction and the gastroduodenal junction removed. The proximal jejunum is divided and the distal end of bowel is folded upon itself and approximated in such a way to form a pouch. The pouch is connected to the esophagus. The divided proximal jejunum is connected to the limb of small bowel distal to the esophageal anastomosis to restore intestinal continuity. The incisions are closed.

43631

The physician removes the distal stomach and approximates the proximal stomach to the duodenum. The physician makes a midline abdominal incision. The distal stomach (antrum) is dissected free from surrounding structures and the blood supply to the antrum is divided. Next, the gastroduodenal junction is divided and the stomach is divided in its middle portion removing the antrum. An anastomosis is made between the proximal stomach and the duodenum with staples or sutures. The incision is closed.

43632
The physician removes the distal stomach and approximates the proximal stomach to the jejunum. The physician makes a midline abdominal incision. The distal stomach (antrum) is dissected free from surrounding structures and the blood supply to the antrum is divided. Next, the gastroduodenal junction is divided and the stomach is divided in its middle portion removing the antrum. An anastomosis is made between the proximal stomach and the jejunum with staples or sutures. The incision is closed.

43633
The physician removes the distal stomach (antrum) and performs an anastomosis between the proximal stomach and a Roux-en-Y limb of jejunum. The physician makes a midline abdominal incision. Next, the distal stomach is dissected free of surrounding structures and the blood supply to the antrum is divided. The gastroduodenal junction and the middle portion of the stomach are divided and the antrum is removed. The vagus nerves, as they pass from the esophagus onto the stomach, are usually divided. The proximal jejunum is divided and the distal limb of jejunum is connected to the proximal stomach. The proximal jejunum is connected to the limb of jejunum distal to the gastrojejunostomy to restore intestinal continuity. The incisions are closed.

43634
The physician removes the distal stomach (antrum) and performs an anastomosis between the stomach and a pouch formed of jejunum. The physician makes a midline abdominal incision. The distal stomach is dissected free of surrounding structures and the blood supply to the antrum is divided. The gastroduodenal junction and the middle portion of the stomach are divided and the antrum is removed. The vagus nerves, as they pass from the esophagus onto the stomach, are usually divided. The proximal jejunum is divided and the distal end is folded upon itself and approximated in such a way to form a pouch. The pouch is connected to the proximal stomach and the proximal end of the divided jejunum is connected to the jejunal limb distal to the pouch anastomosis to establish intestinal continuity. The incision is closed.

43635
The physician performs this with a separately reportable partial distal gastrectomy and repairs the stomach and severs vagus nerves. The physician uses a midline abdominal approach. The distal stomach (antrum) is dissected free and the blood supply to the antrum divided. The distal stomach is removed and the proximal stomach is sutured to the duodenum. Truncal vagotomy is performed by severing both right and left vagus nerves just below the diaphragm.

43640-43641
The physician severs the vagus nerves and widens the pyloric canal, with or without making an incision in the stomach. The physician uses a midline upper abdominal incision to expose the muscular band surrounding the distal opening of the stomach. A longitudinal incision is made in the pylorus. The incision is closed with a single full thickness suture layer. The two branches of the vagus nerve are exposed and a truncal vagotomy is performed by severing both right and left vagus nerves. A gastrostomy may be created by inserting a tube from the stomach to the external surface of the abdominal wall. Report 43641 if performed with a parietal cell procedure.

43644
The physician performs a laparoscopic gastric bypass for morbid obesity by partitioning the stomach and performing a small bowel division with anastomosis to the proximal stomach (Roux-en-Y gastroenterostomy). This bypasses the majority of the stomach. The physician places a trocar though an incision above the umbilicus and insufflates the abdominal cavity. The laparoscope and additional trocars are placed through small portal incisions. The stomach is mobilized and the proximal stomach is divided with a stapling device along the lesser curvature, leaving only a small proximal pouch in continuity with the esophagus. A short limb of the proximal small bowel (150 cm or less) is divided and the distal end of the short intestinal limb is brought up and anastomosed to the proximal gastric pouch. The other end of the divided bowel is connected back into the small bowel distal to the short limb's gastric anastomosis to restore intestinal continuity. The instruments are removed.

43645
The physician performs a laparoscopic gastric bypass with small intestine reconstruction to limit absorption. This procedure is done to combine gastric restriction of intake with limited intestinal absorption. In one method used, the physician places a trocar though an incision above the umbilicus and insufflates the abdominal cavity. The laparoscope and additional trocars are placed through small portal incisions. The stomach is mobilized and the distal half is resected along a line from the lesser to greater curvature, leaving a "pouch" of stomach, which is connected directly to the final, distal section of small intestine. The bypassed duodenum, jejunum, and upper part of the divided ileum—the segment in connection with the gallbladder and pancreas, or the biliopancreatic loop—is anastomosed back to the common distal segment of the small intestine. This leaves a short common channel where food coming through the shortened alimentary tract combines with digestive juices from the much longer biliary tract before entering the colon. The instruments are removed.

43647-43648
The physician performs a laparoscopic placement of gastric neurostimulator electrodes. The physician

makes an incision and places a trocar at the umbilicus to insufflate the abdomen. The laparoscope is placed through the umbilical port and additional trocars are placed into the abdominal cavity. The antrum of the stomach is identified and the physician secures two electrodes into the muscle of the pyloric antrum. The electrodes are connected to a neurostimulator that has been secured in a subcutaneous pocket in the abdomen in a separately reportable procedure. The physician removes the laparoscope and tools from the abdomen, which is deflated and repaired with sutures. Report 43647 if electrodes are placed or if existing electrodes are removed and replaced with new ones. Report 43648 for the revision or removal of the electrodes.

43651

The physician performs laparoscopic truncal vagotomy. The physician places a trocar through an incision above the umbilicus and insufflates the abdominal cavity. The laparoscope is placed through the supraumbilical port and additional trocars are placed into the abdominal cavity. The fascial anterior to the esophagus is incised and the distal esophagus is mobilized. The anterior and posterior vagal nerve trunks are identified and divided. The physician removes a small segment of each nerve. The trocars are removed and the incisions are closed.

43652

The physician performs laparoscopic selective or highly selective vagotomy. The physician places a trocar though an incision above the umbilicus and insufflates the abdominal cavity. The laparoscope is placed through the supraumbilical port and additional trocars are placed into the abdominal cavity. The distal esophagus is mobilized and the anterior and posterior vagal nerve trunks are identified. The main nerve trunks are followed down onto the stomach and the branches from the nerves to the proximal half of the stomach are divided. The trocars are removed and the incisions are closed.

43653

Using a laparoscope, the physician constructs a temporary or permanent gastrostomy for feeding. With the patient under anesthesia, the physician places a trocar at the umbilicus into the abdomen and insufflates the abdominal cavity. The physician places a laparoscope through the umbilical incision. An additional trocar is inserted through the abdominal wall into the intra-abdominal cavity at a previously determined site where the gastrostomy will reside. The gastrostomy tube is pulled through the trocar from outside the abdomen into the intra-abdominal cavity. The physician identifies the stomach and introduces instruments to open the organ and create a viable receptacle for the tube. The tip of the gastrostomy tube is inserted into the stomach, and the tube is clamped off on the outside of the body and sutured into place on the stomach. Additional sutures are placed in the abdominal wall to hold the gastrostomy tube in place and to secure the tube. The trocars are removed and the incisions are closed with staples or sutures.

43752

The physician places a naso- or orogastric tube. The patient is placed in an upright position. The physician checks the nostrils for obstruction and selects the nostril for tube insertion. The physician may swab the nostril and spray the oropharynx with medication to numb the nasal passage and suppress the gag reflex. Next, the physician lubricates the tube, elevates the tip of the nose, and introduces the nasogastric tube into the nostril. The tube is advanced and the position of the tube is checked using fluoroscopy to ensure it is aligned to enter the oropharynx. As the patient swallows, the physician advances the tube through the pharynx, esophagus, and into the stomach. Air is injected into the tube (at the nose) while the physician listens with a stethoscope positioned at the stomach for the air to come out of the tube. Gastric contents are aspirated. These precautions are performed to ensure the tube is positioned in the stomach. The nasogastric tube is taped to the nostril. If the tube is fitted with a balloon (at the end of the tube in the stomach), it is inflated to hold the tube in place. This code includes the fluoroscopic guidance, image documentation, and report.

43753-43754

The physician performs therapeutic intubation and aspiration of the stomach (43753), often for indications such as poisoning or gastrointestinal hemorrhage. A gastric lavage (stomach pump) may also be performed. The physician inserts a Levin tube or other gastric lavage tube through the nose or mouth. The tube passes through the esophagus into the stomach. The stomach contents are removed by suction. The inside of the stomach may be rinsed with a salt water (saline) solution. If the intubation and aspiration are performed for diagnostic purposes (such as acid analysis) of a single specimen, report 43754.

43755

Multiple specimens are collected via gastric stimulation (gastric secretory study). The physician inserts a tube through the patient's nose or mouth and down into the stomach. Gastric contents are suctioned out for collection. Insulin, or another gastric secretion stimulant such as histamine, pentagastrin, calcium, or secretin, is given to the patient. Blood glucose is monitored while continued collection of gastric contents is done. Following sample collection, gastric contents undergo volume, pH, acid concentration, and volume measurements.

43756-43757

The physician performs diagnostic intubation and aspiration of the first portion of the small intestine (duodenum) using image guidance. A tube is inserted orally or nasally and positioned in the duodenum. In one method, the physician advances a double-lumen introducer tube containing an inflatable balloon through the esophagus. Upon reaching the stomach, the introducer tube is turned so that the balloon is positioned toward the greater curvature. As the physician inflates the balloon, it expands and conforms to the shape of the stomach. Once inflated, the distal end of the introducer tube abuts the pylorus. The physician inserts a duodenal catheter through the introducer tube into the duodenum. Following appropriate placement, the balloon is deflated and the introducer tube is removed, leaving the distal tip of the duodenal catheter within the duodenum. Report 43756 if the aspiration procedure is performed for a single specimen, such as an afferent loop culture or bile study for crystals. Report 43757 if multiple fractional specimens are collected and pancreatic or gallbladder stimulation occurs. Separately reportable chemical analysis procedures may follow. These codes include the administration of any drugs, although the drugs themselves are separately reportable.

43761

The physician repositions a nasogastric or orogastric feeding tube through the duodenum for enteric nutrition. Under separately reportable fluoroscopic guidance, the physician passes the feeding tube through the stomach into the distal duodenum.

43762-43763

In 43762, the physician replaces a gastrostomy tube via percutaneous approach that does not require revision (simple) of the gastrostomy tract. If the old gastrostomy tube has been placed endoscopically, the physician must remove it by snaring and pulling it out through the mouth. A new tube is placed percutaneously through the abdominal wall via the existing tract. In 43763, the replacement requires revision (complex). A small incision is made through the skin and fascia. A large bore needle with suture attached is passed through the incision into the lumen of the stomach. The needle is snared and the needle and suture are removed via the mouth. The gastrostomy tube is connected to the suture and passed through the mouth into the stomach and out the abdominal wall. The gastrostomy tube is sutured to the skin. No imaging or endoscopic guidance is utilized in either procedure.

43770

The physician performs a laparoscopic gastric restrictive procedure in which an adjustable gastric restrictive device, such as a gastric band with subcutaneous port components, is inserted. This is a gastric restrictive procedure for treatment of morbid obesity that does not permanently alter the gastrointestinal tract. The physician places a trocar though an incision, generally above the umbilicus, and insufflates the abdominal cavity. The laparoscope and additional trocars are placed through small portal incisions. The silicone gastric band is introduced into the peritoneal cavity via a trocar and is placed and secured around the upper stomach to form a smaller stomach pouch with a narrowed outlet. A small port, or reservoir, is placed under the skin at the time of surgery and connected to the silicone band by tubing to facilitate postoperative adjustments of the outlet size by the addition or removal of saline via the port. The instruments are removed and the incisions are closed.

43771

The physician performs laparoscopic revision of an adjustable gastric restrictive device. This revision is most often performed for slippage of the device or for dilation of the gastric pouch. The physician places a trocar though an incision, generally above the umbilicus, and insufflates the abdominal cavity. The laparoscope and additional trocars are placed through small portal incisions. Saline is removed from the gastric restrictive device and the device is repositioned around the upper stomach. Saline is slowly reintroduced through the existing port to secure the device position. Once the device is in place, the instruments are removed and the incisions are closed. This code reports revision of the device component only.

43772-43773

The physician performs laparoscopic removal of an adjustable gastric restrictive device component. The physician places a trocar though an incision, generally above the umbilicus, and insufflates the abdominal cavity. The laparoscope and additional trocars are placed through small portal incisions. Saline is removed from the gastric restrictive device and the component is removed. Once the device component has been removed, the instruments are withdrawn and the incisions are closed. Report 43772 for removal of an adjustable gastric restrictive device component only. Report 43773 for removal and replacement of an adjustable gastric restrictive device component only.

43774

The physician performs laparoscopic removal of an adjustable gastric restrictive device and subcutaneous port components. The physician places a trocar though an incision, generally above the umbilicus, and insufflates the abdominal cavity. The laparoscope and additional trocars are placed through small portal incisions. Saline is removed from the gastric device and the device is removed. Once the device has been removed, the subcutaneous port components are removed. The instruments are withdrawn and the incisions are closed.

43775

The physician performs a laparoscopic sleeve gastrectomy (LSG), a gastric restrictive procedure for the treatment of morbid obesity. Following appropriate anesthesia, the physician begins the longitudinal gastrectomy by placing a trocar though an incision, generally above the umbilicus, and insufflating the abdominal cavity. The laparoscope and additional trocars are placed through small portal incisions. The physician divides the greater curvature of the stomach from the left crus of the diaphragm to a point distal to the pylorus. The short gastric vessels are coagulated and gastric staplers are used. A gastric tube (sleeve) is formed and the remaining 80 percent of the stomach is excised. The instruments are removed and the incisions are closed.

43800
The physician repairs the pylorus. The physician makes an upper abdominal incision through skin, fascia, and muscles to expose the pylorus, a muscular band surrounding the distal opening of the stomach. A longitudinal incision is made in the pylorus. The incision is closed with a single full thickness suture layer.

43810
The physician performs a gastroduodenostomy. The physician uses an upper midline epigastric incision through fascia and muscle. The distal end of the greater curvature of the stomach is removed. The duodenum is mobilized and connected to the greater curvature. The anastomosis is closed with interrupted stitches and the abdominal incision is closed.

43820-43825
The physician performs a gastrojejunostomy to create a direct passage between the stomach and jejunum. The physician makes an upper abdominal incision to expose the stomach and small intestine. The distal portion of the stomach is incised and the jejunum is anastomosed to the gastric stump. The duodenal stump is closed. The vagal nerves are preserved. Report 43825 if a vagotomy is also performed.

43830-43831
The physician constructs a temporary or permanent gastrostomy for instillation of nutrients. After making a midline incision in the upper abdomen, the physician chooses a gastrostomy site on the middle anterior surface of the stomach. Stay sutures are placed and a small stab wound is made between purse string sutures. A gastrostomy tube is inserted and the purse string sutures are tied. The gastrostomy tube is withdrawn through a stab wound in the abdominal wall and stay sutures are placed in the posterior fascia. The abdominal incision is closed. Report 43831 if performed to facilitate feeding a neonate.

43832
The physician constructs a permanent gastrostomy for instillation of nutrients. After a small midline upper abdominal incision, the physician creates a flap with its base at the greater curvature of the stomach. The flap is converted into a tube by closure of the stomach incision. The tube is brought through the skin surface via a stab wound or tunnel. The end of the tube is everted slightly and sutured to the skin. The abdominal incision is closed with sutures.

43840
The physician repairs an ulcer, wound, or injury to the stomach or duodenum. The ulcer or wound is exposed by the physician via a midline upper abdominal incision or a transverse supraumbilical incision through skin, fascia, and muscle. The perforation is sutured closed and the peritoneal cavity is irrigated and suctioned to remove contamination. The abdominal fascia and peritoneum are closed in one layer. The skin and subcutaneous layers are closed.

43842-43843
The physician alters the stomach's size to help stem morbid obesity. The physician exposes the lesser curvature of the stomach via a midline abdominal incision through skin, fascia, and muscles. In 43842, double row of staples is placed in the upper portion of the stomach to create a small stoma. A small strip of mesh or a Silastic ring is wrapped around the stoma and stapled to itself. Report 43843 if the technique used is other than the vertical-banded gastroplasty, and allows for staples restricting other parts of the stomach.

43845
A partial gastrectomy with pylorus-preserving duodenoileostomy and ileoileostomy is done to combine gastric restriction with limited intestinal absorption for weight loss. This procedure is called a biliopancreatic diversion with duodenal switch. The stomach is resected along the greater curvature, leaving the pyloric valve intact with the remaining stomach that maintains its functionality. A portion of the duodenum is also left within the food track to preserve the pylorus/duodenum pathway. The duodenum is divided near the pyloric valve. The small intestine is also divided. The distal end of the small intestine in continuity with the large intestine is brought up and anastomosed to the short duodenal segment on the stomach. The other end of the small intestine—the duodenal segment in connection with the gallbladder and pancreas, or the biliopancreatic loop—is attached to the newly anastomosed other limb further down near the large intestine. This forms a 75 to 100 cm "common loop" where the contents of both these segments channel together before dumping into the large intestine.

43846
The physician performs a gastric bypass for morbid obesity by partitioning the stomach and performing a small bowel division and anastomosis to the proximal stomach (Roux-en-Y gastrojejunostomy). This bypasses the majority of the stomach. The physician makes a midline abdominal incision. The stomach is mobilized and the proximal stomach is divided with a stapling device along the lesser curvature, leaving only a small proximal pouch in continuity with the esophagus. A short limb of the proximal small bowel (150 cm or less) is divided and the distal end of the short intestinal limb is brought up and anastomosed to the proximal gastric pouch. The other end of the divided bowel is connected back into the small bowel distal to the short limb's gastric anastomosis to restore intestinal continuity. The incision is closed.

43847
The physician partitions the stomach and performs a small intestine anastomosis to the proximal stomach (Roux-en-Y gastrojejunostomy) in order to bypass the majority of the stomach. The physician makes a midline abdominal incision. Next, the stomach is mobilized and the proximal stomach is divided with a stapling device leaving only a small proximal pouch in

Digestive

continuity with the esophagus. The small intestine is reconstructed so that it is partially bypassed to limit the amount of area available for absorption of nutrients. The incision is closed.

43848

The physician uses an open technique to revise a failed gastric restrictive procedure for morbid obesity. Indications for revision include stomal stenosis, stomal dilation, non-emptying gastric pouch, gastroesophageal reflux, staple dehiscence, intragastric foreign body, gastric fistula, gastroesophageal fistula, failure to maintain weight loss, breakdown of staple continuity, and restored gastric continuity. This code is not used to report revision of an adjustable gastric restrictive device. Revision techniques vary depending on the technique used in initial gastric restrictive procedure (i.e., gastroplasty, partial gastrectomy, gastric bypass) and the nature of the gastric restrictive failure. Types of revision include gastroplasty, conversion of a gastroplasty to a gastric bypass, and revision of a gastric bypass. The physician makes a midline abdominal incision. Next, the stomach and previous anastomoses are dissected free of surrounding structures. This can involve painstaking lysis of adhesions between the liver, stomach, distal esophagus, colon, and/or spleen. The physician performs the required revision. If a gastroplasty is performed, a double row of staples is placed in the upper portion of the stomach to create a small stoma. A small strip of mesh or a Silastic ring is wrapped around the stoma and stapled to itself. A partial gastrectomy involves resecting the stomach along the greater curvature and leaving the pyloric valve intact with the remaining stomach to maintain functionality. If a gastric bypass is performed, the stomach is partitioned, the small bowel divided, and the small bowel is reanastomosed to the proximal stomach.

43860-43865

The physician revises an anastomoses between the stomach and the jejunum. The physician exposes the stomach and small intestine via a midline upper abdominal incision through skin, muscles, and fascia. About 8 cm to 10 cm of the jejunum limb is divided, reversed and connected to the distal end of the stomach. The short reversed segment is connected to the jejunum and the remnant of jejunum and duodenum are anastomosed to the long segment of jejunum. A partial gastrectomy or intestine resection may be performed. The abdominal incision is closed. Report 43865 if a vagotomy is performed in conjunction with this procedure.

43870

The physician closes a gastrostomy no longer needed. The physician enters through a previous gastrostomy. The stomach is dissected free of the abdominal wall. The stomach gastrostomy site is closed with sutures. The abdominal incision is closed with layered sutures.

43880

The physician closes a gastrocolic fistula. The physician exposes stomach and colon via a midline abdominal incision through skin, fascia, and muscle. The bowel is mobilized and the fistula is located. The stomach and intestinal tissue involving the fistula is resected en bloc with a margin of healthy adjacent tissue. The surgical defects of the stomach and intestine are repaired, the method depending on the extent of the defect. The abdominal incision is closed in layers.

43881-43882

The physician performs placement of gastric neurostimulator electrodes in an open procedure. Through a laparotomy, the physician enters the abdominal cavity. The antrum of the stomach is identified and the physician secures two electrodes to the muscle of the pyloric antrum. The electrodes are connected to a neurostimulator that has been secured in a subcutaneous pocket in the abdomen in a separately reportable procedure. The physician closes the laparotomy with layered sutures. Report 43881 if electrodes are placed or if existing electrodes are removed and replaced with new ones. Report 43882 for the revision or removal of the electrodes.

43886

The physician performs an open revision of the subcutaneous port component used in a gastric restrictive procedure for the treatment of morbid obesity. The subcutaneous port is the access point for infusing saline into the gastric band to adjust the band for optimal performance. The physician makes an incision through the old scar near the original port. Dissection is carried down to the port. The sutures adhering the port to the fascia may be removed so that necessary repairs and revisions can be made. The port is secured to the fascia with sutures. The incision is closed with sutures.

43887-43888

The physician performs an open removal or a removal and replacement of the subcutaneous port component used in a gastric restrictive procedure for the treatment of morbid obesity. The subcutaneous port is the access point for infusing saline into the gastric band to adjust the band for optimal performance. The physician makes an incision through the old scar near the original port. Dissection is carried down to the port and the sutures adhering the port to the fascia are removed. The physician severs the tubing connected to the port. In 43887, the subcutaneous port is removed. In 43888, the original subcutaneous port is removed and replaced with a new port to which the tubing is reattached. The replacement port is secured to the fascia with sutures. The incision is closed with sutures.

44005

The physician frees intestinal adhesions. The physician enters the abdomen through a midline abdominal incision. The bowel is freed from its attachments to itself, the abdominal wall and/or other abdominal organs. The abdominal incision is closed.

44010
The physician opens the duodenum, explores the segment, collects tissue samples for biopsy, or removes a foreign body. The physician exposes the proximal duodenum via a midline upper abdominal incision through skin, fascia, and muscles. The duodenum is incised in a longitudinal fashion and the area of concern is exposed. The physician may choose during exploration to excise tissues, biopsy, or remove foreign bodies. The duodenum is closed with transverse interrupted sutures. The abdominal incision is closed.

44015
The physician places a tube in the jejunum for feeding during a separately reportable operation. The physician makes an abdominal incision. A section of proximal jejunum is selected and a tube is placed in the jejunum and brought out through the abdominal wall. This segment of jejunum is securely tacked to the inside of the abdominal wall. The incision is closed.

44020
The physician makes an incision in the small intestine (enterotomy) for biopsy, exploration or foreign body removal. The physician makes an abdominal incision. Next, the selected segment of small intestine is mobilized and incised to expose the area of interest. A biopsy is taken or a foreign body is removed. The enterotomy is closed with staples or sutures. The abdominal incision is closed.

44021
The physician places a tube in the small bowel for decompression. The physician makes an abdominal incision. Next, the small bowel is dissected free of surrounding structures. The proximal small bowel is incised (enterotomy) and a tube is threaded through the small bowel. The proximal end of the tube is brought out through the abdominal wall. The bowel is tacked to the inside of the abdominal wall where the tube goes through. The abdominal incision is closed.

44025
The physician makes an incision in the colon (colotomy) through which the colon is explored for biopsy or foreign body removal. The physician makes an abdominal incision. Next, the selected segment of colon is mobilized and a colotomy is made in the area of interest. The colon is explored and biopsy performed or foreign body removed. The colotomy is closed with staples or sutures. The abdominal incision is closed.

44050
The physician reduces a volvulus, intussusception, or internal hernia. After appropriate anesthesia is administered, a midline abdominal incision is made. The abdomen is explored to identify the location of the bowel abnormality. The twisted segment of bowel (volvulus), telescoped segment (intussusception), or internal hernia is manually reduced. Release or lysis of adhesions is performed if necessary. The bowel is inspected to ensure viability. The incision is closed in layers by suturing.

44055
The physician corrects a malrotation of the bowel. Malrotation is a congenital condition in which sections of the intestine are not in the proper position in the abdomen. After appropriate anesthesia is administered, a midline abdominal incision is made. The abdomen is explored to identify the extent of the malrotation and identify any segments of twisted bowel (midgut volvulus). Peritoneal fibrous bands over the duodenum, also known as Ladd's bands, are divided until the duodenum lies in a straight line. The small bowel is placed in the right side of the abdomen, while the large bowel is placed on the left. The appendix may also be removed. If a midgut volvulus is present, it is manually reduced by twisting the bowel in the opposite direction. The bowel is inspected to ensure viability. The incision is closed in layers by suturing.

44100
The physician performs a peroral biopsy of the small intestine with a capsule. The physician places a biopsy capsule attached to a tube through the mouth and directs it into the small intestine usually with fluoroscopy. The capsule blade is fired by placing suction on the tube and a biopsy obtained. The tube and capsule are withdrawn.

44110
The physician removes one or more lesions in the small or large intestine through an incision in the colon (colotomy) or small intestine (enterotomy) without bowel resection. The physician makes an abdominal incision. Next, the segment of small intestine or colon containing the lesions is mobilized. An incision is made in the small intestine or colon and the lesions are removed. The enterotomy or colotomy is closed with staples or sutures. The abdominal incision is closed.

44111
The physician removes one or more lesions in the small or large intestine through multiple incisions in the colon (colotomy) or small intestine (enterotomy) without bowel resection. The physician makes an abdominal incision. Next, the segments of small intestine or colon containing lesions are mobilized. Incisions are made in the small intestine or colon and the lesions are removed. The enterotomies or colotomies are closed with staples or sutures. The abdominal incision is closed.

44120
The physician resects a segment of small intestine and performs an anastomosis between the remaining bowel ends. The physician makes an abdominal incision. Next, the selected segment of small bowel is isolated and divided proximally and distally to the remaining bowel and removed. The remaining bowel ends are reapproximated using staples or sutures. The incision is closed.

44121
The physician resects one or more segments of small intestine and performs an anastomosis between the

remaining intestinal ends. The physician makes an abdominal incision. Next, the selected segments of small intestine are isolated and divided proximally and distally to the remaining intestine and removed. The remaining intestinal ends are reapproximated using staples or sutures. The incision is closed.

44125
The physician resects a segment of small bowel and brings the proximal end of bowel through the abdominal wall onto the skin as a stoma. The physician makes an abdominal incision. Next, the selected segment of small bowel is isolated and divided proximally and distally to the remaining bowel and removed. The proximal end of the remaining small bowel is brought through a separate incision in the abdominal wall onto the skin as a stoma. The initial incision is closed.

44126-44128
The physician resects a segment of small intestine and may perform tapering to fit the area of anastomosis. The physician makes an abdominal incision. The selected segment of small intestine is isolated and divided proximally and distally to the remaining bowel and removed. An end-to-end anastomosis of the proximal rectum to the distal anal canal is performed. The remaining bowel ends are reapproximated using staples or sutures. The incision is closed. Report 44126 for a single resection and anastomosis. Report 44127 when tapering (gradually narrowing toward one end) of the bowel is performed with the resection and anastomosis. Report 44128 for each additional resection and anastomosis beyond the first one.

44130
The physician performs a small bowel anastomosis and may bring one end of small bowel through the abdominal wall onto the skin as a stoma. The physician makes an abdominal incision. A segment of small bowel may be resected. Next, a small bowel anastomosis is performed with staples or sutures. An end or loop of small bowel may be brought through a separate incision in the abdominal wall onto the skin as a stoma. The initial incision is closed.

44132-44133
The physician performs an open donor enterectomy from a cadaver donor in 44132 and an open partial enterectomy from a living donor in 44133. With the cadaver or living donor supine on the operating room table, the physician performs a midline abdominal incision. Tissue is incised and muscles are separated down to the level of the small intestine. In 44132, the small intestine can be mobilized and excised from the cadaver, as needed. In 44133, only a portion of the small intestine can be excised from the living donor and the bowel ends are anastomosed to restore continuity. Any bleeding is controlled, the area is irrigated, and the incision is closed with layered sutures. The acquired intestine is preserved for transplantation into the recipient, who may be hundreds of miles away. The organ remains under refrigeration, specially packed in a sealable container with some preserving solution and kept on ice in a suitable carrier.

44135-44136
The physician performs an intestinal allotransplantation. The patient is placed supine on the operating room table. After adequate preparation, the physician performs a midline abdominal incision, tissue is incised, and muscles are separated down to the level of the small intestine. The area of small intestine to be transplanted is located. An incision is made through the intestine, the area is examined, and the free intestinal edges are debrided or excised in order to accept the intestinal transplant. The previously excised small intestinal allograft, from a cadaver (44135) or partially excised small intestinal allograft, from a living donor (44136) are removed from the maintenance solution, and irrigated. The allograft is sized and is anastomosed first to one free end of the patient's small intestine and then the opposite end of the patient's small intestine. Any bleeding is controlled, the area is irrigated, and the small bowel is anatomically positioned in the abdominal cavity. The wound is closed with layered sutures over a drain. A dressing is applied.

44137
The physician removes a previously transplanted intestinal allograft due to complications such as infection or rejection. The physician makes an abdominal incision. The intestinal allograft is isolated and resected at sites distal and proximal to the anastomosis sites of the previously placed intestinal graft. The distal and proximal ends of the remaining intestine are reapproximated using staples or sutures. The incision is closed.

44139
The physician mobilizes the splenic flexure in conjunction with a partial colon resection. The physician makes an abdominal incision. The attachments between the splenic flexure of the colon and the lateral abdominal wall and spleen are dissected free and taken down to mobilize the colon. This is done to mobilize adequate length of colon in conjunction with a partial colon resection. At the completion of the procedure the abdominal incision is closed.

44140
The physician resects a segment of colon and performs an anastomosis between the remaining ends of colon. The physician makes an abdominal incision. Next, the selected segment of colon is isolated and divided proximally and distally to the remaining colon and removed. The remaining ends of colon are reapproximated with staples or sutures. The incision is closed.

44141
The physician resects a segment of colon and brings the proximal end of colon through the abdominal wall onto the skin as a colostomy. The physician makes an abdominal incision. Next, the selected segment of

colon is isolated and divided proximally and distally to the remaining colon and removed. The proximal end of colon is brought through a separate incision on the abdominal wall and onto the skin as a colostomy. Alternately, the remaining bowel ends may be reapproximated and a loop of colon proximal to the anastomosis brought through a separate incision on the abdominal wall onto the skin as a loop colostomy. The initial incision is closed.

44143

The physician resects a segment of colon and brings the proximal end of colon through the abdominal wall onto the skin as a colostomy. The physician makes an abdominal incision. Next, the selected segment of colon is isolated and divided proximally and distally to the remaining colon and removed. The proximal end of colon is brought through a separate incision on the abdominal wall onto the skin as a colostomy. The distal end of colon is closed with staples or sutures and left in the abdomen. The initial incision is closed.

44144

The physician resects a segment of colon. The proximal and distal ends of colon are brought through the abdominal wall onto the skin as a colostomy and mucus fistula. The physician makes an abdominal incision. Next, the selected segment of colon is isolated and divided proximally and distally to the remaining colon and removed. The proximal end of colon or terminal ileum and the distal end of colon are brought through separate incisions on the abdominal wall onto the skin as an ileostomy or colostomy and mucus fistula. The initial abdominal incision is closed.

44145

The physician resects a segment of distal colon or rectum and performs a low colorectal anastomosis in the pelvis. The physician makes an abdominal incision. Next, the distal colon and rectum are mobilized and the selected segment divided proximally and distally to the remaining colon. An anastomosis is created between the proximal colon and remaining rectum in the pelvis with staples or sutures. The incision is closed.

44146

The physician resects a segment of distal colon or rectum and performs a low colorectal anastomosis in the pelvis and creates a proximal colostomy. The physician makes an abdominal incision. Next, the distal colon and rectum are mobilized and the selected segment of diseased colon and/or rectal tissue is removed. The new ends are brought together and an anastomosis is done between the colon and the rectum low in the pelvis with staples or sutures (coloproctostomy). A loop of colon above the newly sutured anastomosis is brought out through a separate incision in the abdominal wall and fixed there so the colon will empty through this artificial opening in the skin as a colostomy, usually temporary, to divert the fecal stream while the anastomosis heals. The initial incision is closed.

44147

The physician removes a segment of colon through a combined abdominal and transanal approach and reapproximates the remaining ends of the colon. The physician makes an abdominal incision. The distal colon and rectum are mobilized also by using a transanal approach. The segment of the colon to be eliminated is divided at the appropriate distal and proximal points and the remaining ends are anastomosed. The abdominal and transanal incisions are closed.

44150

The physician removes the entire colon and performs an ileostomy or an anastomosis between the ileum and rectum. The physician makes an abdominal incision. Next, the colon is mobilized and the colorectal junction and terminal ileum is divided. The colon is removed. The terminal ileum is approximated to the rectum or brought out through a separate incision on the abdominal wall onto the skin as an ileostomy. The initial incision is closed.

44151

The physician removes the entire colon and creates a reservoir of distal ileum (Kock pouch). The reservoir is brought out through the abdominal wall as a continent stoma. The physician makes an abdominal incision. Next, the colon is mobilized. The colorectal junction and terminal ileum is divided and the colon removed. The distal ileum is folded upon itself and approximated to form a pouch and valve. The distal end of the pouch is brought through a separate incision on the abdominal wall onto the skin as a continent ileostomy. The initial incision is closed.

44155

The physician removes the entire colon and rectum and brings the terminal ileum out through the abdominal wall onto the skin as an ileostomy. The physician makes an abdominal incision. Next, the colon and rectum are mobilized, the proximal rectum and distal ileum are divided, and the colon and proximal rectum are removed. The distal rectum is mobilized and removed through a perineal approach. The terminal ileum is brought out through a separate incision on the abdominal wall onto the skin as an ileostomy. The abdominal and perineal incisions are closed.

44156

The physician removes the entire colon and rectum and creates a pouch from the terminal ileum (Kock pouch) that is brought out through the abdominal wall as a continent ileostomy. The physician makes an abdominal incision. Next, the colon and rectum are mobilized, the proximal rectum and distal ileum are divided, and the colon and proximal rectum are removed. The distal rectum is mobilized and removed through a perineal approach. The terminal ileum is folded upon itself and approximated to form a pouch with a valve. The end of the pouch is brought out through a separate abdominal incision onto the skin as a continent ileostomy. The abdominal and perineal incisions are closed.

44157-44158

The physician removes the entire colon and rectum, strips the mucosa from the distal rectum, and performs an anastomosis between the terminal ileum and anus. The physician makes an abdominal incision. Next, the colon and rectum are mobilized. The mucosa of the distal rectum is stripped from a perineal approach. In 44157, the terminal ileum and rectum are divided and the colon is removed. The terminal ileum is pulled through the remaining muscular cuff of the rectum and approximated to the anus with sutures. A loop of ileum may be brought out through the abdominal wall onto the skin as an ileostomy proximal to the anastomosis. In 44158, the terminal ileum is folded upon itself and approximated in order to form a pouch. The pouch is pulled through the remaining muscular tube of the rectum and approximated to the anus with sutures. A loop of ileum may be brought out through a separate incision on the abdominal wall onto the skin as an ileostomy proximal to the anastomosis.

44160

The physician makes an abdominal incision and removes a segment of the colon and terminal ileum and performs an anastomosis between the remaining ileum and colon. The physician makes an abdominal incision. Next, the selected segment of colon and terminal ileum are isolated and divided proximal and distal to the remaining bowel and removed. An anastomosis is created between the distal ileum and remaining colon with staples or sutures. The incision is closed.

44180

The physician performs laparoscopic enterolysis to free intestinal adhesions. With the patient under anesthesia, the physician places a trocar at the umbilicus into the abdominal or retroperitoneal space and insufflates the abdominal cavity. The physician places a laparoscope through the umbilical incision and additional trocars are placed into the abdomen. Intestinal adhesions are identified and instruments are passed through to dissect and remove the adhesions. The trocars are removed and the incisions are closed with sutures.

44186

The physician constructs a jejunostomy using a laparoscope. With the patient under anesthesia, the physician makes small incisions into the abdomen, places one trocar at the umbilicus into the abdomen, and insufflates the abdominal cavity. The physician places a laparoscope through one of the incisions with additional instruments introduced through the trocars. The tube is placed into the jejunostomy with the other end sutured to the skin at the exit point. The trocars are removed and the incisions are closed with sutures.

44187

The physician constructs a non-tube ileostomy or jejunostomy using a laparoscope. With the patient under general anesthesia, the physician places a trocar at the umbilicus into the abdomen and insufflates the abdominal cavity. The physician places a laparoscope through the umbilical incision. Additional trocars are placed through which the specialized surgical instruments are inserted. Next, the selected segment of jejunum or ileum is isolated. A loop or end of the selected segment of bowel is located and grasped. The skin and fat are excised, the fascia is opened, and the loop is exteriorized through a previously defined ileostomy or jejunostomy site. The laparoscope is removed, the ports are closed with incisions, and the stoma is matured.

44188

The physician constructs a colostomy or skin level cecostomy using a laparoscope. With the patient under general anesthesia, the physician places a trocar at the umbilicus into the abdomen and insufflates the abdominal cavity. The physician places a laparoscope through the umbilical incision. Additional trocars are placed, through which the specialized surgical instruments are inserted. The selected segment of colon or cecum is isolated. The physician brings a loop, end of colon, or cecum onto the skin as a stoma (colostomy or cecostomy) through a small incision in the abdominal wall. The laparoscope is removed, the ports are closed with incisions, and the stoma is matured.

44202-44203

The physician performs a laparoscopic single resection and anastomosis of the small intestine. With the patient under general anesthesia, a urinary catheter is inserted and the patient is placed in a supine or Trendelenburg position on the operating table. Carbon dioxide gas is used to insufflate the abdomen through a laparoscopic port placed through the umbilicus. The laparoscope is positioned in the abdominal cavity and a diagnostic laparoscopy is performed. The remaining laparoscopic ports are placed under direct vision. The transverse colon is located and maintained in upward traction. The ligament of Treitz is identified and the small intestine is run. The targeted section of small intestine is marked and suspended with traction sutures through the mesentery. The peritoneum overlying the mesentery is scored and the segment of small intestine marked for resection is devascularized. The bowel is divided proximal and distal to the segment with a stapler. The segment is brought out through an enlarged trocar site. The divided bowel ends are anastomosed with staples and inspected. The mesentery is closed with interrupted sutures. The trocars and laparoscope are removed and the incisions are closed with sutures. Report 44203 for each additional small intestine resection and anastomosis beyond the first.

44204-44205

With the patient under general anesthesia, a urinary catheter is inserted and the patient is placed supine or in a Trendelenburg position on the operating table. Carbon dioxide gas is used to insufflate the abdomen through a laparoscopic port placed through the umbilicus. The laparoscope is positioned in the abdominal cavity and a diagnostic laparoscopy is performed. The remaining laparoscopic ports are placed under direct vision. The physician incises peritoneum along both sides to mobilize the colon. The greater omentum and colon are separated by incision to mobilize the hepatic and splenic flexures. The colon is mobilized centrally onto its mesentery and the mesenteric vessels are divided intracorporeally using titanium clips. The colon is divided with an endoscopic stapler and the specimen is removed through an enlarged trocar site. If the procedure is being performed for malignancy, a wound protector is used. In 44204, the divided bowel ends are anastomosed and inspected. In 44205, for the ileocolostomy with removal of terminal ileum, the selected segment of colon and terminal ileum are isolated and divided proximal and distal to the remaining bowel and removed. An anastomosis is created between the distal ileum and remaining colon. The abdomen is deflated and the laparoscope and trocar incisions are closed.

44206-44207

The physician performs a laparoscopic partial colectomy with end colostomy and closure of the distal segment (Hartmann type) in 44206 and with anastomosis and coloproctostomy in 44207. With the patient under general anesthesia, a urinary catheter is inserted and the patient is positioned supine. Carbon dioxide gas is used to insufflate the abdomen through a laparoscopic port placed through the umbilicus. A 10 to 12 mm cannula is used to facilitate insertion of the laparoscope into the abdominal cavity. Cannulae are inserted in the right middle quadrant, the suprapubic area, and in the left middle quadrant to allow instrument access to the surgical site. The laparoscope is placed through the left cannula for mobilization of the colon. The physician dissects along the peritoneum to mobilize the colon. Once mobilized, the laparoscope is placed in the suprapubic cannula and the omentum is dissected using electrocautery and vascular clips. A 4 to 6 cm transverse incision is made at the appropriate cannula site depending on the portion of the resection. The colon is exteriorized and the distal segment is resected. In 44206, the new proximal end of the colon is brought through an opening made in the abdominal wall and anastomosed so as to exit onto the skin for a colostomy and the remaining distal end is closed off. In 44207, after the distal segment of diseased colon and/or rectal tissue is resected, the new ends are brought together and an anastomosis is done between the colon and the rectum low in the pelvis with staples or sutures (coloproctostomy). The abdominal cavity is inspected through the laparoscope for hemostasis and irrigated. The instruments are removed and the remaining abdominal wounds are closed.

44208

The physician performs a laparoscopic partial colectomy with anastomosis and coloproctostomy, with a colostomy. With the patient under general anesthesia, a urinary catheter is inserted and the patient is positioned supine. Carbon dioxide gas is used to insufflate the abdomen through a laparoscopic port placed through the umbilicus. A 10 12 mm cannula is used to facilitate insertion of the laparoscope into the abdominal cavity. Cannulae are inserted in the right middle quadrant, the suprapubic area, and in the left middle quadrant to allow instrument access to the surgical site. The laparoscope is placed through the left cannula for mobilization of the colon. The physician dissects along the peritoneum to mobilize the colon. Once mobilized, the laparoscope is placed in the suprapubic cannula and the omentum is dissected using electrocautery and vascular clips. A 4 to 6 cm transverse incision is made at the appropriate cannula site depending on the portion of the resection. The distal segment of diseased colon and/or rectal tissue is resected and the new ends are brought together and an anastomosis is done between the colon and the rectum low in the pelvis with staples or sutures (coloproctostomy). A loop of colon above the newly sutured anastomosis is brought out through a separate incision in the abdominal wall and fixed there so the colon will empty through this artificial opening in the skin as a colostomy, usually temporary, to divert the fecal stream while the anastomosis heals.

44210

The physician performs a laparoscopic total colectomy with ileostomy or ileoproctostomy. With the patient under general anesthesia, a urinary catheter is inserted and the patient is positioned supine. Carbon dioxide gas is used to insufflate the abdomen through a laparoscopic port placed through the umbilicus. A 10 to 12 mm cannula is used to facilitate insertion of the laparoscope into the abdominal cavity. Cannulae are inserted in the right middle quadrant, the suprapubic area, and in the left middle quadrant to allow instrument access to the surgical site. The laparoscope is placed through the left cannula for mobilization of the colon. The physician dissects along the peritoneum to mobilize the colon. Once mobilized, the laparoscope is placed in the suprapubic cannula and the omentum is dissected using electrocautery and vascular clips. A 4 to 6 cm transverse incision is made at the appropriate cannula site depending on the portion of the resection. After the colon has been mobilized, the colorectal junction and the terminal ileum are divided. The whole colon is removed. The terminal ileum is approximated to the rectum and the ends anastomosed together or it is brought out through a separate incision on the abdominal wall and sutured as an ileostomy artificial opening onto the skin.

44211

The physician performs a laparoscopic total colectomy with proctectomy with ileoanal anastomosis and creation of an ileal reservoir, with loop ileostomy, with or without rectal mucosectomy. With the patient under general anesthesia, a urinary catheter is inserted and the patient is positioned supine. Carbon dioxide gas is used to insufflate the abdomen through a laparoscopic port placed through the umbilicus. A 10 to 12 mm cannula is used to facilitate insertion of the laparoscope into the abdominal cavity. Cannulae are inserted in the right middle quadrant, the suprapubic area, and in the left middle quadrant to allow instrument access to the surgical site. The laparoscope is placed through the left cannula for mobilization of the colon. The physician dissects along the peritoneum to mobilize the colon. Once mobilized, the laparoscope is placed in the suprapubic cannula and the omentum is dissected using electrocautery and vascular clips. A 4 to 6 cm transverse incision is made at the appropriate cannula site depending on the portion of the resection. After the colon and rectum have been mobilized, they are removed. The mucosa of the remaining distal rectum may be stripped. The terminal ileum is folded upon itself and approximated in order to form a pouch and the terminal ileum is pulled through the remaining muscular tube of the rectum and approximated to the anus with sutures. A loop of ileum above the newly sutured ileoanal anastomosis is brought out through a separate incision in the abdominal wall and fixed there so the ileum will empty through this artificial opening in the skin as an ileostomy, usually temporary, to divert the fecal stream while the anastomosis heals.

44212

The physician performs a laparoscopic total colectomy with proctectomy, with ileostomy. With the patient under general anesthesia, a urinary catheter is inserted and the patient is positioned supine. Carbon dioxide gas is used to insufflate the abdomen through a laparoscopic port placed through the umbilicus. A 10 to 12 mm cannula is used to facilitate insertion of the laparoscope into the abdominal cavity. Cannulae are inserted in the right middle quadrant, the suprapubic area, and in the left middle quadrant to allow instrument access to the surgical site. The laparoscope is placed through the left cannula for mobilization of the colon. The physician dissects along the peritoneum to mobilize the colon. Once mobilized, the laparoscope is placed in the suprapubic cannula and the omentum is dissected using electrocautery and vascular clips. A 4 to 6 cm transverse incision is made at the appropriate cannula site depending on the portion of the resection. After the colon and rectum have been mobilized, they are removed. The terminal ileum is brought out through a separate incision on the abdominal wall and sutured as an ileostomy artificial opening onto the skin.

44213

The physician mobilizes the splenic flexure via a laparoscopic approach in conjunction with a separately reportable partial colon resection. With the patient under general anesthesia, a urinary catheter is inserted and the patient is placed supine or in a Trendelenburg position on the operating table. A 15-mmHg carbon dioxide pneumoperitoneum is established with a laparoscopic port placed through the umbilicus using a direct open technique. The laparoscope is positioned in the abdominal cavity and a diagnostic laparoscopy is performed. The remaining laparoscopic ports are placed under direct vision. The attachments between the splenic flexure of the colon and the lateral abdominal wall and spleen are dissected free and taken down in order to mobilize an adequate length of colon in conjunction with a partial colon resection. At the completion of the procedure, the abdomen is deflated and the laparoscope and trocar incisions are closed.

44227

The physician takes down (closes) a previously created enterostomy (stoma) of the large or small intestine using a laparoscope. With the patient under general anesthesia, the physician places a trocar at the umbilicus into the abdomen and insufflates the abdominal cavity. The physician places a laparoscope through the umbilical incision. Additional trocars are placed, through which the specialized surgical instruments are inserted. The stoma is mobilized and taken down from the abdominal wall. The stoma is resected and the bowel ends are reapproximated with staples or sutures. The laparoscope is removed, the ports are closed with incisions, and the stoma is matured.

44300

The physician places a tube in the small bowel for feeding or into the cecum for decompression via an open approach. The physician makes an abdominal incision. Next, a segment of proximal small bowel or the cecum is isolated. A tube is placed into the small bowel or cecum and brought out through the abdominal wall. The incision is closed.

44310

The physician brings a loop or end of jejunum or ileum through the abdominal wall onto the skin as a stoma. The physician makes an abdominal incision. Next, the selected segment of jejunum or ileum is isolated. A loop or end of the selected segment of bowel is secured through a separate incision on the abdominal wall onto the skin as a stoma. The initial incision is closed. This stoma is created for purposes other than enteral feeding.

44312

The physician revises an ileostomy through an incision around the stoma with release of scar tissue. The physician makes and incision around the ileostomy site. Next, the stoma is dissected free of the surrounding abdominal wall and constricting scar tissue is released. The stoma is reapproximated to the skin or the distal end of the stoma may be transected. Additional ileum may be pulled through the abdominal wall and approximated to the skin as a revised ileostomy.

44314

The physician revises an ileostomy by forming a new stoma site. The physician makes an abdominal incision. Next, the previous ileostomy is completely taken down. The distal ileum is brought through a new incision on the abdominal wall onto the skin as an ileostomy at a new site. The initial incision and former stoma site are closed.

44316
The physician forms a reservoir of distal ileum (Kock pouch) and brings it through the abdominal wall onto the skin as a continent ileostomy. The physician makes an abdominal incision. Next, the distal ileum is folded upon itself and approximated in such a way to form a pouch with a valve. The end of the pouch is brought through a separate incision on the abdominal wall onto the skin as a continent ileostomy. The initial incision is closed.

44320
The physician performs a colostomy or skin level cecostomy. An abdominal incision is made and the peritoneum is entered, followed by a thorough exploratory exam of abdominal organs and tissues, including lysis of any adhesions. The small bowel is mobilized and isolated out of the way. The distal bowel is measured for the appropriate length for pouch creation. A proximal point from the distal end is separated from its blood supply to be made into a pouch nipple valve. The pouch is fashioned into the right configuration and secured in place. The nipple valve component is intussuscepted and secured in place. The pouch end of colon (or cecum) is brought out through a separate incision on the abdominal wall onto the skin as a stoma (cecostomy or colostomy) and secured in place with a pouch nipple to mucocutaneous tissue anastomosis. The abdomen is irrigated, a final inspection is made, and a closed-system suction drain may be placed. The abdominal wall skin is closed and dressed and a pouch intubation catheter is placed into the nipple valve and pouch.

44322
The physician performs multiple biopsies of the colon wall and brings a loop of colon or cecum through the abdominal wall onto the skin as a stoma. The physician makes an abdominal incision. Next, multiple biopsies are obtained along the length of the colon wall. A loop of colon or cecum is brought through a separate incision on the abdominal wall onto the skin as a stoma (colostomy or cecostomy). The initial incision is closed.

44340
The physician revises a colostomy through an incision around the stoma site with release of scar tissue. The physician makes an incision around the stoma site. Next, the stoma is dissected free of the surrounding abdominal wall and constricting scar tissue is released. The stoma is reapproximated to the skin or the distal stoma is transected and additional colon pulled through the abdominal wall and approximated to the skin as a revised colostomy.

44345
The physician revises a colostomy by forming a new stoma site. The physician makes an abdominal incision. Next, the previous colostomy is completely taken down. The distal end of colon is brought through a separate incision on the abdominal wall onto the skin at a new site as a revised colostomy The initial incision and previous stoma site are closed.

44346
The physician performs a colostomy revision and repairs a paracolostomy hernia. The physician makes an abdominal incision. Next, the previous colostomy site is taken down. The hernia at the former colostomy site is repaired. The end of colon is brought through a separate incision on the abdominal wall at a new site and onto the skin as a revised colostomy. The initial incision and previous stoma site are closed.

44360
The physician performs endoscopy of the proximal small bowel and may obtain brushings or washings. The physician places an endoscope through the mouth and advances it into the small intestine beyond the second portion of the duodenum, but not including the ileum. An abdominal incision may be made to mobilize the small bowel and assist in running the bowel over the endoscope. The lumen of the small bowel is examined and brushings or washings may be obtained of suspicious areas. The endoscope is withdrawn at the completion of the procedure. If an incision was made, it is closed.

44361
The physician performs endoscopy of the proximal small bowel and obtains biopsies. The physician places an endoscope through the mouth and advances it into the small intestine. An abdominal incision may be made to mobilize the small bowel and assist in running the bowel over the endoscope. The lumen of the small bowel is examined and biopsies are obtained of suspicious areas. The endoscope is withdrawn at the completion of the procedure. If an incision was made, it is closed.

44363
The physician performs endoscopy of the proximal small bowel and removes a foreign body(s). The physician places an endoscope through the mouth and advances it into the small intestine beyond the second portion of the duodenum, but not including the ileum. An abdominal incision may be made to mobilize the small bowel and assist in running the bowel over the endoscope. The bowel lumen is examined and the foreign body(s) located. A snare or forceps is advanced through the endoscope and the foreign body(s) grasped and removed. The endoscope is withdrawn at the completion of the procedure. If an incision was made, it is closed.

44364
The physician performs endoscopy of the proximal small bowel and removes a tumor or polyp by snare technique. The physician places an endoscope through the mouth and advances it into the small intestine. An abdominal incision may be made to mobilize the small bowel and assist in running the bowel over the endoscope. The bowel lumen is examined and the

polyp or tumor is located and removed with a snare placed through the endoscope. The endoscope is withdrawn at the completion of the procedure. If an incision was made it is closed.

44365
The physician performs endoscopy of the proximal small bowel and removes a tumor or polyp with hot biopsy forceps or cautery. The physician places an endoscope through the mouth and advances it into the small intestine. An abdominal incision may be made to mobilize the small bowel and assist in running the bowel over the endoscope. The bowel lumen is examined and the polyp or tumor is located and removed with hot biopsy forceps or cautery placed through the endoscope. The endoscope is withdrawn at the completion of the procedure. If an incision was made, it is closed.

44366
The physician performs endoscopy of the proximal small bowel and controls an area of bleeding. The physician places an endoscope through the mouth and advances it into the small intestine. An abdominal incision may be made to mobilize the small bowel and assist in running the bowel over the endoscope. The bowel lumen is examined and the area of bleeding is identified and controlled. The endoscope is withdrawn at the completion of the procedure. If an incision was made, it is closed.

44369
The physician performs endoscopy of the proximal small bowel and ablates a tumor or polyp or other lesion. The physician places an endoscope through the mouth and advances it into the small intestine. An abdominal incision may be made to mobilize the small bowel and assist in running the bowel over the endoscope. The bowel lumen is examined and the tumor, polyp, or other lesion is identified and ablated. The endoscope is withdrawn at the completion of the procedure. If an incision was made it is closed.

44370
The physician uses an endoscope to examine the proximal small intestine and performs a transendoscopic placement of a stent in the small intestine. The physician places an endoscope through the mouth and advances it into the small intestine. The lumen of the entire small intestine is visualized. The endoscope is placed at the site of an obstruction or stricture, the necessary stent length is determined and predilation of the obstruction or stenosis may be performed. The stent (endoprosthesis) is introduced into the site of the obstruction. Using a commercial delivery system, a plastic covering over the stent is removed and the stent self-deploys, shoring-up the walls at a specific site in the small intestine beyond the second portion of duodenum, not including the ileum. When necessary, a balloon catheter is placed into the stent and gently inflated to more fully deploy the stent. The delivery system and endoscope are removed.

44372
The physician performs endoscopy of the proximal small bowel and places a percutaneous jejunostomy tube. The physician places an endoscope into the mouth and advances it into the small intestine. The bowel lumen is visualized and transilluminated through the abdominal skin. A needle is placed through the skin into the lumen of the jejunum under visualization of the endoscope. A wire is threaded through the needle into the bowel lumen. The needle is removed. A jejunostomy tube is placed over the wire, through the skin, into the jejunum, and secured into place. The endoscope is withdrawn.

44373
The physician performs endoscopy of the proximal small bowel and converts a percutaneous gastrostomy tube to a percutaneous jejunostomy tube. The physician places an endoscope into the mouth and advances it into the stomach. A jejunostomy tube is advanced through the previously placed gastrostomy tube. The jejunostomy tube is grasped with a snare or forceps placed through the endoscope and advanced with the endoscope into the proximal jejunum. The endoscope is withdrawn.

44376
The physician performs endoscopy of the small bowel and may obtain brushings or washings. The physician places the endoscope into the mouth and advances it into the small intestine. An abdominal incision may be made to mobilize the small bowel and assist in running the bowel over the endoscope. The lumen of the small bowel is visualized and brushings or washings may be obtained. The endoscope is withdrawn at the completion of the procedure. If an incision was made, it is closed.

44377
The physician performs endoscopy of the entire small bowel and performs biopsies. The physician places the endoscope into the mouth and advances it into the small intestine. An abdominal incision may be made to mobilize the small bowel and assist in running the bowel over the endoscope. The lumen of the small bowel is visualized and biopsies are performed. The endoscope is withdrawn at the completion of the procedure. If an incision was made, it is closed.

44378
The physician performs endoscopy of the small intestine, which may include the ileum, and controls an area of bleeding. The physician places the endoscope into the mouth and advances it into the small intestine. The lumen of the small intestine is visualized and any area of bleeding is controlled using various methods, such as cautery, injection, or laser. In some cases, a separately reportable abdominal incision is made to mobilize the small intestine and assist in running the intestine over the endoscope. The endoscope is withdrawn at the completion of the procedure.

44379
The physician uses an endoscope to examine the small intestine and performs transendoscopic placement of a stent in the small intestine. The physician performs endoscopy of the small bowel and places a transendoscopic stent. The physician places an endoscope into the mouth and advances it into the small intestine. The lumen of the small intestine is visualized. The endoscope is placed at the site of an obstruction or stricture and the necessary stent length is determined. The stent (endoprosthesis) is introduced into the site of the obstruction. Using a commercial delivery system, a plastic covering over the stent is removed and the stent self-deploys, shoring-up the walls at a specific site in the small intestine beyond the second portion of the duodenum, including the ileum. When necessary, a balloon catheter is placed into the stent and gently inflated to more fully deploy the stent. The delivery system and endoscope are removed.

44380
An ileostomy is an artificial opening (called a stoma) created in the abdomen. The physician performs endoscopy through ileostomy and may obtain brushings or washings. The physician places the endoscope into the ileostomy and advances the endoscope into the small intestine. The lumen of the ileum, the last part of the small intestine, is visualized and brushings or washings may be obtained. The endoscope is withdrawn at the completion of the procedure.

44382
The physician performs endoscopy through an ileostomy and obtains material for biopsies. The physician places the endoscope into the ileostomy and advances the endoscope into the small intestine. The small bowel lumen is visualized and biopsies are obtained. The endoscope is withdrawn at the completion of the procedure.

[44381]
An ileostomy is an artificial opening (called a stoma) created in the abdomen. The physician performs endoscopy through ileostomy and dilates strictures by balloon catheter. The physician places the endoscope into the ileostomy and advances the endoscope into the small intestine. The lumen of the ileum, the last part of the small intestine, is visualized. Areas of stenosis are identified and a balloon catheter is passed to the point of constriction and a little beyond. The balloon is inflated to the appropriate diameter and gradually withdrawn through the stenosed area, stretching the walls of the bowel at the strictured area. The endoscope is withdrawn at the completion of the procedure.

44384
The physician uses an endoscope through an ileostomy to view the ileum and places an endoscopic stent. The physician places the endoscope into the ileostomy and advances the endoscope into the small intestine. The lumen of the ileum is visualized. The endoscope is placed at the site of an obstruction or stricture and the necessary stent length is determined. The stent (endoprosthesis) is introduced into the site of the obstruction. Using a commercial delivery system, a plastic covering over the stent is removed and the stent self-deploys, shoring-up the walls at a specific site in the ileum. When necessary, a balloon catheter is placed into the stent and gently inflated to more fully deploy the stent. The delivery system and endoscope are removed. This code includes dilation before and after stent placement, as well as guidewire passage when performed.

44385
The physician performs endoscopic evaluation of an intestinal pouch and may obtain brushings or washings. The physician places the endoscope into the pouch, through the anus or abdominal wall stoma. The lumen of the pouch is visualized and brushings or washings may be obtained. The endoscope is withdrawn at the completion of the procedure.

44386
The physician performs endoscopic evaluation of an intestinal pouch and obtains biopsies. The physician places the endoscope into the pouch, through the anus or abdominal wall stoma. The lumen of the pouch is visualized and biopsies are obtained. The endoscope is withdrawn at the completion of the procedure.

44388
The physician performs colonoscopy through an abdominal wall colostomy and may obtain brushings or washings. The physician places the endoscope into the colostomy and advances the endoscope into the colon. The lumen of the colon is visualized and brushings or washings may be obtained. The endoscope is withdrawn at the completion of the procedure.

44389
The physician performs colonoscopy through an abdominal wall colostomy and obtains biopsies. The physician places the endoscope into the colostomy and advances the endoscope into the colon. The lumen of the colon is visualized and biopsies are obtained. The endoscope is withdrawn at the completion of the procedure.

44390
The physician performs colonoscopy through an abdominal wall colostomy and removes a foreign body(s). The physician places the endoscope into the colostomy and advances the endoscope into the colon. The lumen of the colon is visualized. The foreign body(s) is isolated and grasped with a snare or forceps (placed through the endoscope) and removed. The endoscope is withdrawn at the completion of the procedure.

44391
The physician performs colonoscopy through an abdominal wall colostomy and controls an area of bleeding. The physician places the endoscope into the colostomy and advances the endoscope into the colon. The lumen of the colon is visualized and the area of

bleeding is identified and controlled. The endoscope is withdrawn at the completion of the procedure.

44392
The physician performs colonoscopy through an abdominal wall colostomy and removes a tumor, polyp, or other lesion with hot biopsy forceps. The physician places the endoscope into the colostomy and advances the endoscope into the colon. The lumen of the colon is visualized and the tumor, polyp, or lesion is identified and removed with hot biopsy forceps. The endoscope is withdrawn at the completion of the procedure.

[44401]
The physician performs colonoscopy through an abdominal wall colostomy and performs ablation of a tumor, polyp, or other lesion. The physician places the endoscope into the colostomy and advances the endoscope into the colon. The lumen of the colon is visualized and the tumor, polyp, or other lesion is identified and ablated. The endoscope is withdrawn at the completion of the procedure. This code includes dilation before and after the procedure, as well as guidewire passage when performed.

44394
The physician performs colonoscopy through an abdominal wall colostomy and removes a tumor, polyp or other lesion with a snare. The physician places the endoscope into the colostomy and advances the endoscope into the colon. The lumen of the colon is visualized and the tumor, polyp or other lesion is identified and removed with a snare placed through the endoscope. The endoscope is withdrawn at the completion of the procedure.

44402
The physician uses a colonoscope to examine the colon through an abdominal wall colostomy and places an endoscopic stent. The physician places the endoscope into the colostomy and advances the endoscope into the colon. The lumen of the colon is visualized. The endoscope is placed at the site of an obstruction or stricture and the necessary stent length is determined. The stent (endoprosthesis) is introduced into the site of the obstruction. Using a commercial delivery system, a plastic covering over the stent is removed and the stent self-deploys, shoring-up the walls at a specific site in the large intestine. When necessary, a balloon catheter is placed into the stent and gently inflated to more fully deploy the stent. The delivery system and colonoscope are removed. This code includes dilation before and after stent placement, as well as guidewire passage when performed.

44403
The physician uses a colonoscope to examine the colon through an abdominal wall colostomy. The physician places the endoscope into the colostomy and advances into the colon. The lumen of the colon is visualized with an instrument containing a camera and light. The scope is directed to the affected area. A special needle is used to administer fluid under the polyp to elevate the polyp allowing for the removal from the bowel lining. Removal may be done by snare, cutting out, or suction and typically includes cautery of the attached blood vessels. The tissue is sent to pathology for analysis and the scope is withdrawn at the completion of the procedure.

44404
The physician uses a colonoscope to examine the colon through an abdominal wall colostomy and injects a substance into the submucosa, directed at specific areas through the scope while viewing the colon. The physician places the endoscope into the colostomy and advances into the colon. The lumen of the colon is visualized. Submucosal saline injections, for instance, may be done before polypectomy using snare and electrocautery to greatly enhance the effectiveness of resection for large sessile colorectal polyps. The scope is withdrawn at the completion of the procedure.

44405
The physician uses a colonoscope to examine the colon through an abdominal wall colostomy and dilates strictures by balloon catheter. The physician places the endoscope into the colostomy and advances into the colon. The lumen of the colon is visualized. Areas of stenosis are identified and a balloon catheter is passed to the point of constriction and a little beyond. The balloon is inflated to the appropriate diameter and gradually withdrawn through the stenosed area, stretching the walls of the strictured area. The scope is withdrawn at the completion of the procedure.

44406-44407
In 44406, the physician uses a flexible colonoscope to examine the colon and perform an endoscopic ultrasound (EUS) examination. Ultrasound and endoscopic imaging techniques are combined in this diagnostic modality. An endoscope equipped with an ultrasound transducer at the tip is inserted into the colon through an abdominal wall colostomy. The lumen of the colon is visualized and the probe tip is guided next to the area of concern. Sound waves are sent out from the transducer and reflect back to a receiving unit at varying speeds as they pass through different densities of tissue. The waves are converted to electrical pulses displayed as a picture on screen. Using ultrasound from within the endoscope instead of transcutaneously shortens the distance between the source and the target lesion and produces greater clarity from high frequency, high-resolution sound waves that have a short penetration distance. EUS is currently the most accurate method of staging cancer within the gastrointestinal tract. In 44407, the physician uses a colonoscope to examine the colon and perform a transendoscopic ultrasound guided intramural or transmural fine needle aspiration (FNA)/biopsy(s). An endoscope equipped with an ultrasound transducer at the tip is inserted into the colon through an abdominal wall colostomy. The lumen of the colon is visualized and the probe tip is guided next to the area of concern. Sound waves are sent out from the transducer and reflect back to a receiving unit at varying speeds as they pass through different densities

of tissue. The waves are converted to electrical pulses displayed as a picture on screen. An FNA needle is passed through the scope to the site of the lesion, lymph node, or tumor and a fine needle aspiration/biopsy(s) is taken of the abnormal tissue or fluid within the colon wall or through the intestinal wall. These codes are used for examination of the colon, cecum, and surrounding structures only.

44408
The physician uses a colonoscope to examine the colon through an abdominal wall colostomy to decompress a pathologic distention, such as a volvulus or megacolon. The physician places the endoscope into the colostomy and advances into the colon. The lumen of the colon is visualized. The scope is advanced into the area of distention decompressing it as the scope passes through the lumen. The scope is withdrawn at the completion of the procedure. This procedure includes placement of a decompression tube when utilized.

44500
A long, Miller-Abbott style gastrointestinal tube with a mercury-filled balloon at the bottom is introduced, usually nasally, and used to clear gastrointestinal strictures. The patient is seated lower than the person performing the procedure and the dilator is placed in the posterior pharynx. The patient swallows and the tube and balloon are carried into the small intestine. The balloon is inflated and withdrawn until resistance is encountered. The balloon is partially deflated, withdrawn a little more, and re-inflated. This process is repeated several times to achieve dilation of the stricture. This procedure may be done without fluoroscopy or with fluoroscopy by instilling a diluted contrast into the balloon.

44602
The physician performs suture closure of a single small bowel perforation. The physician makes an abdominal incision. Next, the abdomen is explored and the small bowel perforation is identified and repaired with sutures. The incision is closed.

44603
The physician performs suture closure of multiple small bowel perforations. The physician makes an abdominal incision. Next, the abdomen is explored and the small bowel perforations are identified and repaired with sutures. The incision is closed.

44604
The physician performs suture closure of a colon perforation. The physician makes an abdominal incision. Next, the abdomen is explored and the colon perforation is identified and repaired with sutures. The incision is closed.

44605
The physician performs suture closure of a colon perforation and forms a colostomy proximal to the repair. The physician makes an abdominal incision. Next, the abdomen is explored and the colon perforation identified and repaired with sutures. A loop or end of colon proximal to the repair is brought out through a separate incision on the abdominal wall onto the skin as a colostomy. The initial incision is closed.

44615
The physician performs an abdominal incision to gain access to the site of an intestinal narrowing (stricture). Once identified, the intestinal stricture is incised (enterotomy) in a longitudinal manner. The physician may find it necessary or prudent to dilate the stenotic intestine to complete proper repair. The intestine is repaired or sutured. The two divided portions of the incised intestine may be reapproximated after one segment is drawn into the other (invagination) end to end (enterorrhaphy). The abdominal incision is sutured or stapled closed.

44620
The physician takes down and closes an enterostomy (stoma) of the small intestine or colon. The physician makes an incision around the stoma or a separate abdominal incision may be made. Next, the stoma is mobilized and taken down from the abdominal wall and the stoma is closed. The abdominal incisions are closed.

44625
The physician takes down an enterostomy (stoma) of small intestine or colon, with resection and anastomosis other than colorectal. The stoma is resected and an anastomosis between the bowel ends is completed. The physician makes an incision around the stoma or a separate abdominal incision may be made. Next, the stoma is mobilized and taken down from the abdominal wall. The stoma is resected and the bowel ends are reapproximated with staples or sutures. The abdominal incisions are closed. Report 44625 if with resection and anastomosis other than colorectal.

44626
A surgeon closes a previously-existing enterostomy, or a surgically created opening, in the large or small intestine. This code includes both resection of the intestine and a colorectal anastomosis, or a reconnection of the colon and rectum.

44640
The physician takes down and closes an intestinal cutaneous fistula. The physician makes an abdominal incision. Next, the bowel is mobilized and the fistula is identified and taken down from the abdominal wall and skin. The segment of bowel containing the fistula is resected and the bowel ends reapproximated with staples or sutures. The abdominal wall incisions are closed.

44650
The physician closes a connection (fistula) between loops of small bowel or between the small bowel and colon. The physician makes an abdominal incision. Next, the enteroenteric or enterocolic fistula is identified and divided. The ends of the fistula may be closed with sutures or the segments of bowel involved

with the fistula may be resected and the bowel ends reapproximated in order to completely remove the involved areas. The incision is closed.

44660
The physician closes a connection between the small bowel and bladder (enterovesical fistula). The physician makes an abdominal incision. Next, the enterovesical fistula is identified and divided. The ends of the fistula are closed with sutures. The incision is closed.

44661
The physician closes a connection between the small or large intestine and bladder (enterovesical fistula) by resecting a portion of the intestine or bladder. The physician makes an abdominal incision. Next, the enterovesical fistula is identified and divided. The connection of the fistula to the bladder is resected and the bladder is closed with sutures. The segment of intestine containing the fistula is resected and the ends are reapproximated. The incision is closed.

44680
The physician folds the intestine upon itself and attaches the edges with sutures for anchoring purposes. The physician makes an abdominal incision. Next, the bowel is folded upon itself and the edges are plicated with sutures without making an anastomosis to anchor the bowel in place. The incision is closed.

44700
Prior to implementing radiation therapy, the physician uses mesh, other prosthesis, or native tissue (bladder or omentum) to lift and fix the small intestine away from the site of radiation therapy. An abdominal incision is made. If mesh or other prosthetic material is used, it is sutured into place. If native tissue is used, a sling is fashioned and sutured into place. The incision sutured closed.

44701
The patient's colon is flushed during a surgical procedure. A Foley catheter is inserted into the cecum through which the irrigation is performed. A noncrushing bowel clamp is placed across the terminal ilium to prevent the lavage fluid from flowing into the small intestine. An intravenous infusion set is connected to the catheter and a clear, corrugated scavenger tube is inserted in the distal bowel and secured in place. A closed irrigation system is created by securing a large bag to the free end of the tube, draped over the patient to the side. The colon is lavaged with warm, isotonic saline solution for 15 to 30 minutes until the flow through the tube is seen to be clear.

44705
Fecal microbiota transplantation (FMT) is the process of instilling fecal matter from a donor to a patient to treat a *Clostridium difficile* (*C. diff*) infection, most commonly. The donor stool is thinned using a normal saline solution and filtered for use in a nasogastric tube or an enema application. This code includes the screening protocol of the donor specimen for *C. diff* and other enteric bacterial pathogens and any ova or parasites.

44715
The physician performs a standard backbench preparation of an intestine allograft requiring mobilizing and fashioning of the superior mesenteric artery and vein. Backbench or back table preparation refers to procedures performed on the intestine allograft to prepare the allograft for transplant. Removal of the small intestine graft requires careful dissection of the superior mesenteric artery (SMA) and superior mesenteric vein (SMV). Backbench or back table preparation of the SMA or SMV is required when the pedicles are too short. When a cadaver donor is used, the SMA and/or SMV are lengthened using free vascular grafts from the iliac or carotid arteries and veins that were procured from the cadaver. The physician performs the grafting procedure prior to transplantation of the intestine allograft.

44720
The physician performs a backbench reconstruction of an intestine allograft requiring venous anastomosis. Backbench or back table preparation refers to procedures performed on the intestine allograft to prepare the allograft for transplant. The physician procures venous grafts from the iliac or carotid veins of the cadaver. The physician applies the venous grafts to one of more venous sites on the intestine. Report 44720 for each venous anastomosis.

44721
The physician performs a backbench reconstruction of an intestine allograft requiring arterial anastomosis. Backbench or back table preparation refers to procedures performed on the intestine allograft to prepare the allograft for transplant. The physician procures arterial grafts from the iliac or carotid arteries of the cadaver. The physician applies the arterial grafts to one of more arterial sites on the intestine. Report 44721 for each arterial anastomosis.

44800
The physician excises a Meckel's diverticulum or an omphalomesenteric duct. The physician makes an abdominal incision. Next, the Meckel's diverticulum in the terminal ileum or the omphalomesenteric duct connecting the terminal ileum to the umbilicus is identified. The Meckel's diverticulum or omphalomesenteric duct is excised and the defect in the ileum is closed with sutures or staples or the segment of ileum may be excised and reapproximated. The incision is closed.

44820
The physician excises a lesion in the mesentery. The physician makes an abdominal incision. Next, the lesion in the mesentery is identified. The lesion is removed by shelling it out of the mesentery, resecting a portion of the mesentery with the lesion, or resecting a segment of bowel and mesentery to include the lesion with reapproximation of the bowel. The incision is closed.

44850
The physician repairs a defect in the mesentery with sutures. The physician makes an abdominal incision. Next, the mesenteric defect is identified and closed with sutures. The incision is closed.

44900
The physician drains an appendiceal abscess. The physician makes an abdominal incision. Next, the abscess near the appendix is identified and incised and drained. A drain may be left in the abscess cavity. The abdominal wall incision is closed and the skin incision may be left open to heal secondarily.

44950
The physician removes the appendix through an abdominal incision. The appendix is identified and mobilized, its blood supply is divided, and the appendix is transected and removed. The incision is closed.

44955
The physician removes the appendix during a major procedure for which an incision has been made. The physician identifies and mobilizes the appendix. The blood supply to the appendix is divided and the appendix is transected and removed. The incision is closed.

44960
The physician removes a perforated appendix. The physician makes an abdominal incision. The appendix is identified and mobilized, its blood supply is divided, and the appendix is transected and removed. The abscess cavity is debrided and irrigated. The incision is closed.

44970
The physician performs a laparoscopic appendectomy. The physician places a trocar at the umbilicus and insufflates the abdomen. The laparoscope is placed through the umbilical port and additional trocars are placed into the abdominal cavity. The appendix is identified, dissected from surrounding structures and its blood supply divided. The appendix is transected with staples or suture and removed. The trocars are removed and the incisions are closed.

45000
The physician drains a pelvic abscess through the rectum. The physician identifies the area of abscess through the rectum by palpation or preoperative localizing studies. Next, a transanal incision is made through the rectum into the abscess cavity and the abscess is irrigated and drained. The incision is left open to drain.

45005
The physician drains a submucosal rectal abscess. The physician identifies the area of abscess in the rectum. Next, a transanal incision is made through the rectal lining into the abscess cavity and the abscess is drained. The incision is left open to drain.

45020
The physician drains an abscess above the pelvic floor or behind the rectum through the rectum. The physician identifies the area of abscess by palpation or preoperative localizing studies. Next, a transanal incision is made through the rectum into the abscess cavity and the abscess is drained. The incision is left open to drain.

45100
The physician performs a biopsy of the rectal wall using a transanal approach. The physician performs an incisional biopsy or a suction biopsy of the low rectal wall. The biopsy may be closed with sutures.

45108
The physician removes a muscle tumor or a section of muscle from the anorectum. The physician identifies the anorectal muscle tumor or area of interest. A transanal incision is made through the rectal wall and the tumor or identified area of muscle is excised. The incision is closed by approximating the muscle edges and closing the incision in the rectal lining.

45110
The physician removes the entire rectum and anus and forms a colostomy. The physician makes an abdominal incision. The proximal rectum is mobilized within the abdomen to the level of the sphincter muscles and the colon is divided above the pelvic brim. An incision is made around the anus from a perineal approach and the anus and distal rectum are dissected free of surrounding structures and the anus and rectum are removed. The proximal end of colon is brought out through a separate incision on the abdominal wall as a colostomy. The abdominal and perineal incisions are closed.

45111
The physician removes the proximal rectum using an open transabdominal approach. The physician makes an abdominal incision. The distal colon and rectum are mobilized and divided proximal and distal to the segment of interest and that portion of the rectum is removed. The distal end of the colon is approximated to the remaining rectum or may be closed with sutures or staples. The abdominal incision is closed.

45112
The physician removes the rectum and performs an anastomosis between the colon and the anus. The physician makes an abdominal incision. The distal colon and rectum are mobilized within the abdomen to the level of the sphincter muscles. The colon is divided above the pelvic brim and the rectum at the level of the sphincter muscles and removed. The mucosa may be stripped from the remaining distal rectum from a perineal approach. The distal colon is pulled through the sphincter complex and approximated to the anus with sutures. The incision is closed.

45113
The physician removes the proximal rectum, strips the mucosa from the distal rectum and performs an

anastomosis between an ileal pouch and the anus. The physician makes an abdominal incision. The distal colon and rectum are mobilized within the abdomen to the level of the sphincter muscles. The colon is divided above the pelvic brim and the rectum is divided above the sphincter muscles and removed. The mucosa of the distal rectum is stripped from a perineal approach. The distal ileum is folded upon itself and approximated in order to form a reservoir. The ileal pouch is pulled through the remaining muscular cuff of distal rectum and sutured to the anus. A loop ileostomy may be formed proximal to the anastomosis. The incision is closed.

45114
The physician removes a portion of the rectum through combined abdominal and transsacral approaches. The physician makes an abdominal incision. The proximal rectum and distal colon are mobilized and the colon is divided above the pelvic brim. An incision is made posteriorly at the junction of the sacrum and coccyx. The coccyx is excised. Dissection is continued posteriorly to further mobilize the rectum. The rectum is divided distally and the excised segment is removed. The distal end of colon is approximated to the remaining rectal stump with sutures or staples. The incisions are closed.

45116
The physician removes a portion of the rectum through a transsacral approach. The physician makes a posterior incision at the junction of the sacrum and coccyx. The coccyx is excised. Dissection is continued posteriorly and the rectum and distal colon are mobilized. The rectum is transected proximally and distally and a portion of the rectum is removed. The distal end of colon is approximated to the remaining rectal stump with sutures or staples. The incision is closed.

45119
The physician surgically removes the rectum. The physician makes an abdominal incision, and the distal part of the diseased colon and rectum are mobilized down to the level of the anal sphincter muscles. The rectum is incised at the level of the sphincter muscles while the colon is incised above the pelvic brim where it is disease free. The diseased colon and rectum are removed. The free end of the distal colon is brought through the sphincter complex and approximated with the anus to form a colo-anal anastomosis. The distal colon is folded and sutured in such a way as to create a colonic reservoir pouch. The physician may elect to bring a loop or end of the colon through a separate abdominal incision to create a stoma (enterostomy). The incisions are sutured closed.

45120
The physician removes or bypasses the diseased rectal segment and performs an anastomosis of the colon and anus. The physician makes an abdominal incision. The rectum and distal colon are mobilized and the colon is divided just proximal to the diseased rectal segment. The rectal segment may be removed and the distal colon pulled through the sphincter complex and approximated to the anus with sutures from a perineal approach. Alternatively, the distal colon may be pulled down and approximated to the anus with sutures, bypassing the diseased rectal segment with a combined longitudinal anastomosis between the colon and the diseased rectal segment. The incision is closed.

45121
The physician removes the rectum and part or all of the colon, and performs an anastomosis of the remaining colon or ileum and anus. The physician makes an abdominal incision. Multiple biopsies are taken of the colon wall to determine the level of disease. The involved rectum and colon are mobilized and removed. The remaining segment of colon or ileum is pulled through the sphincter complex and approximated to the anus with sutures from a perineal approach. Alternatively, the colon or ileum may be pulled down and approximated to the anus with sutures, bypassing a small remaining rectal segment with a combined longitudinal anastomosis to the rectal segment. The incision is closed.

45123
The physician removes a portion of the rectum through a perineal approach. The physician makes an incision around the anus. Dissection is continued around the anus to mobilize the anus and distal rectum. The anus and distal rectum are removed. A proximal colostomy may be formed. The incision is closed.

45126
The physician removes pelvic organs, with or without a colostomy, due to cancer of the colon and rectum. The physician makes an abdominal incision. The distal colon and rectum are mobilized and divided proximal and distal to the segment of interest. The pelvic organs are dissected free of surrounding structures and removed. The colon and rectum may be reapproximated or the proximal end of the colon may be brought out through a separate incision on the abdominal wall as a colostomy and the remaining rectum closed with staples or sutures. The initial incision is closed. In males the procedure may include removal of the prostate and bladder. In a female, the procedure may include removal of the bladder and also the uterus, cervix, fallopian tubes, and/or ovaries depending upon the extent of the disease.

45130
The physician removes a rectal prolapse through a perineal approach. The physician prolapses the rectum and colon through the anus. A circular incision is made through the distal rectum at the anorectal junction. The mesentery and blood supply to the prolapsed rectum is divided and the segment is telescoped out through the anus. The proximal rectum or colon is divided and the prolapsed segment is removed. The proximal end of rectum or colon is approximated to the anus with sutures or staples.

45135

The physician removes a rectal prolapse through a combined abdominal and perineal approach. The physician makes an abdominal incision. The proximal colon and rectum are mobilized. The rectum and colon are prolapsed through the anus. A circular incision is made through the distal rectum at the anorectal junction from a perineal approach. The mesentery and blood supply to the prolapsed rectum is divided and the segment is telescoped out through the anus. The proximal rectum or colon is divided and the prolapsed segment is removed. The proximal end of rectum or colon is approximated the anus with sutures or staples. The incision is closed.

45136

The physician excises an ileoanal reservoir and creates an ileostomy. The physician makes an abdominal incision. Dissection is carried down to the site of the ileoanal reservoir. The reservoir is excised at the level where the ileum was previously anastomosed to the anus. The anus is closed. The loose end of the ileum may be trimmed. A disk of skin is excised from the abdominal wall and the terminal ileum is brought out through the split rectus muscle and the opening in the abdomen to form a stoma on the abdominal wall. An anastomosis is performed via the transanal approach and the full thickness of the ileum is sutured to the anal canal. Interrupted sutures complete the ileostomy construction.

45150

The physician performs division of a rectal stricture. The physician makes longitudinal incisions in the scar tissue in one or more places circumferentially around the strictured area of the rectal mucosa. A dilatation of the strictured area may be performed. In addition, the internal anal sphincter may be incised as part of the procedure.

45160

The physician removes a rectal tumor through a transsacral or transcoccygeal approach. The physician makes an incision at the junction of the sacrum and coccyx. The coccyx is excised and dissection is continued posteriorly to mobilize the rectum. The tumor is identified, an incision is made in the rectum (proctotomy), and the tumor is excised. The rectum is closed with sutures or staples. The initial incision is closed.

45171-45172

The physician removes a rectal tumor through a transanal approach. The physician explores the anal canal and exposes the tumor. Report 45171 for a partial thickness excision (one that excludes the muscularis propria) and 45172 for a full thickness excision (including the muscularis propria). The defect in the rectum is closed with sutures.

45190

The physician performs destruction of a rectal tumor from a transanal approach. The physician explores the anal canal and exposes the tumor. The tumor is ablated by electrosurgery, laser, freezing (cryosurgery), or some other method.

45300

The physician performs rigid proctosigmoidoscopy and may obtain brushings or washings. The physician inserts the rigid proctosigmoidoscope into the anus and advances the scope. The sigmoid colon and rectal lumen are visualized and brushings or washings may be obtained. The proctosigmoidoscope is removed at the completion of the procedure.

45303

The physician performs rigid proctosigmoidoscopy and performs dilation of a rectal stricture. The physician inserts the rigid proctosigmoidoscope into the anus and advances the scope. The sigmoid colon and rectal lumen are visualized. The stricture is identified and dilated with a balloon or other device. The proctosigmoidoscope is removed at the completion of the procedure.

45305

The physician performs rigid proctosigmoidoscopy and obtains biopsies. The physician inserts the rigid proctosigmoidoscope into the anus and advances the scope. The sigmoid colon and rectal lumen are visualized and biopsies are obtained of suspicious areas. The proctosigmoidoscope is removed at the completion of the procedure.

45307

The physician performs rigid proctosigmoidoscopy and removes a foreign body. The physician inserts the rigid proctosigmoidoscope into the anus and advances the scope. The sigmoid colon and rectal lumen are visualized and the foreign body is identified. The foreign body is removed by a snare or forceps inserted through the scope. The proctosigmoidoscope is removed at the completion of the procedure.

45308

The physician performs rigid proctosigmoidoscopy and removes a tumor, polyp, or other lesion. The physician inserts the rigid proctosigmoidoscope into the anus and advances the scope. The sigmoid colon and rectal lumen are visualized and the tumor, polyp or other lesion is identified and removed by hot biopsy forceps or cautery. The proctosigmoidoscope is removed at the completion of the procedure.

45309

The physician performs rigid proctosigmoidoscopy and removes a tumor, polyp, or other lesion. The physician inserts the rigid proctosigmoidoscope into the anus and advances the scope. The sigmoid colon and rectal lumen are visualized and the tumor, polyp or other lesion is identified and removed by snare technique. The proctosigmoidoscope is removed at the completion of the procedure.

45315

The physician performs rigid proctosigmoidoscopy and removes multiple tumors, polyps, or other lesions. The physician inserts the rigid proctosigmoidoscope into the anus and advances the scope. The sigmoid colon and rectal lumen are visualized and the tumors, polyps, or other lesions are identified and removed by hot biopsy forceps cautery or snare technique. The proctosigmoidoscope is removed at the completion of the procedure.

45317
The physician performs rigid proctosigmoidoscopy and controls an area of bleeding. The physician inserts the rigid proctosigmoidoscope into the anus and advances the scope. The sigmoid colon and rectal lumen are visualized and the area of bleeding is identified and controlled. A variety of methods can be used to control bleeding, including injection, bipolar cautery, unipolar cautery, laser, heater probe, stapler, or plasma coagulator. The proctosigmoidoscope is removed at the completion of the procedure.

45320
The physician performs rigid proctosigmoidoscopy and ablation of a tumor polyp or other lesion. The physician inserts the proctosigmoidoscope into the anus and advances the scope. The lumen of the sigmoid colon and rectum is visualized and the tumor, polyp or other lesion is identified and ablation performed. The proctosigmoidoscope is removed at the completion of the procedure.

45321
The physician performs rigid proctosigmoidoscopy and decompresses a sigmoid volvulus. The physician inserts the proctosigmoidoscope into the anus and advances the scope. The lumen of the sigmoid colon and rectum is visualized. The proctosigmoidoscope is advanced into the volvulus, decompressing the volvulus as it passes through the bowel lumen. The proctosigmoidoscope is removed at the completion of the procedure.

45327
The physician uses a rigid proctosigmoidoscopy to examine the rectum and sigmoid colon and places a transendoscopic stent. The physician inserts the rigid proctosigmoidoscope into the anus and advances the scope. The sigmoid colon and rectal lumen are visualized. The endoscope is placed at the site of an obstruction or stricture and the necessary stent length is determined. The stent (endoprosthesis) is introduced into the site of the obstruction. Using a commercial delivery system, a plastic covering over the stent is removed and the stent self-deploys, shoring up the walls at a specific site in the sigmoid colon. When necessary, a balloon catheter is placed into the stent and gently inflated to more fully deploy the stent. The delivery system and endoscope are removed.

45330
The physician performs flexible sigmoidoscopy and may obtain brushings or washings. The physician inserts the sigmoidoscope into the anus and advances the scope through the rectum and into the sigmoid colon. The lumen of the sigmoid colon and rectum are visualized and brushings or washings may be obtained. The sigmoidoscope is withdrawn at the completion of the procedure.

45331
The physician performs flexible sigmoidoscopy and obtains biopsies. The physician inserts the sigmoidoscope into the anus and advances the scope into the sigmoid colon. The lumen of the sigmoid colon and rectum are visualized and biopsies are obtained with forceps placed through the scope. The sigmoidoscope is withdrawn at the completion of the procedure.

45332
The physician performs flexible sigmoidoscopy and removes a foreign body(s). The physician inserts the sigmoidoscope into the anus and advances the scope through the rectum and into the sigmoid colon. The lumen of the sigmoid colon and rectum are visualized. The foreign body(s) is identified and removed with a snare or forceps placed through the sigmoidoscope. The sigmoidoscope is withdrawn at the completion of the procedure.

45333
The physician performs flexible sigmoidoscopy and removes a tumor, polyp, or other lesion. The physician inserts the sigmoidoscope into the anus and advances the scope through the rectum and into the sigmoid colon. The lumen of the sigmoid colon and rectum are visualized and the tumor, polyp, or other lesion is identified and removed with hot biopsy forceps. The sigmoidoscope is withdrawn at the completion of the procedure.

45334
The physician performs flexible sigmoidoscopy and controls an area of bleeding. The physician inserts the sigmoidoscope into the anus and advances the scope through the rectum and into the sigmoid colon. The lumen of the sigmoid colon and rectum are visualized and the area of bleeding is controlled. A variety of methods can be used to control bleeding, including medication application and cauterization. The sigmoidoscope is withdrawn at the completion of the procedure.

45335
The physician performs flexible sigmoidoscopy and injects a substance into the submucosa, directed at specific areas through the scope while viewing the colon. The physician inserts the sigmoidoscope into the anus and advances the scope into the sigmoid colon. The lumen of the sigmoid colon and rectum are visualized. Submucosal saline injections, for instance, may be done before polypectomy using snare and electrocautery to greatly enhance the effectiveness of resection for large sessile colorectal polyps.

45337
The physician performs flexible sigmoidoscopy with decompression of a pathological distention, such as a volvulus or megacolon. The physician inserts the sigmoidoscope into the anus and advances the scope through the rectum and into the sigmoid colon. The

lumen of the sigmoid colon and rectum are visualized. The sigmoidoscope is advanced into the area of distention decompressing it as the scope passes through the bowel lumen. The sigmoidoscope is withdrawn at the completion of the procedure. This procedure includes placement of a decompression tube when utilized.

45338 [45346]

The physician performs flexible sigmoidoscopy and removes tumors, polyps, or other lesions. The physician inserts the sigmoidoscope into the anus and advances the scope through the rectum and into the sigmoid colon. The lumen of the sigmoid colon and rectum are visualized. The tumor, polyp, or other lesions are identified and removed by snare technique in 45338 or by ablation in 45346. The sigmoidoscope is withdrawn at the completion of the procedure. Code 45346 includes dilation before and after with utilization of a guidewire, if employed.

45340

The physician performs flexible sigmoidoscopy and dilates strictures by balloon catheter. The physician inserts the sigmoidoscope into the anus and advances the scope through the rectum and into the sigmoid colon. The lumen of the sigmoid colon and rectum are visualized. Areas of stenosis are identified and a balloon catheter is passed to the point of constriction and a little beyond. The balloon is inflated to the appropriate diameter and gradually withdrawn through the stenosed area, stretching the walls of the bowel at the strictured area. The scope is withdrawn at the completion of the procedure.

45341

The physician uses a flexible sigmoidoscopy to examine the rectum and sigmoid colon and performs an endoscopic ultrasound examination. The physician inserts the sigmoidoscopy into the anus and advances the scope into the sigmoid colon. The lumen of the sigmoid colon and rectum are visualized. The sigmoidoscope is removed and replaced with an echoendoscope or an ultrasound probe is passed through the already placed sigmoidoscope. The echoendoscope or ultrasound probe is fitted with a water-filled balloon near the tip; the tip contains a transducer that picks-up the ultrasound frequency and relays it to a processor, outside of the body. The water-filled tip is positioned in the sigmoid colon, against the colon wall next to the area of interest. The area is scanned and an ultrasound image is projected through the processor to a monitor in real-time. When the ultrasound examination is complete the echoendoscope, or esophagoscope and ultrasound probes are removed.

45342

The physician uses a flexible sigmoidoscopy to examine the rectum and sigmoid colon and performs a transendoscopic ultrasound guided intramural or transmural fine needle aspiration/biopsy. The physician inserts the sigmoidoscopy into the anus and advances the scope into the sigmoid colon. The lumen of the sigmoid colon and rectum are visualized. The sigmoidoscope may be removed. A radial scanning echoendoscope is inserted and ultrasound scanning is performed, or an ultrasound probe is passed through the already placed endoscope. The site for a fine needle aspiration biopsy is determined. If a radial scanning echoendoscope is used it is removed and is replaced with a curvilinear array echoendoscope. The echoendoscope or ultrasound probe is fitted with a water-filled balloon near the tip; the tip contains a transducer that picks-up the ultrasound frequency and relays it to a processor, outside of the body. The water-filled tip is positioned in the sigmoid colon against the colon wall next to the predetermined fine needle aspiration (FNA) biopsy site. The area is scanned and an ultrasound image is projected through the processor to a monitor in real-time. A FNA needle is passed through the scope to the biopsy site and a biopsy is taken of the tissue or the needle is inserted through the wall of the tissue into the lesion, or other structure, such as a lymph node. The area is biopsied. When the FNA is complete the echoendoscope or sigmoidoscope and ultrasound probes are removed.

45347

The physician performs flexible sigmoidoscopy to examine the rectum and sigmoid colon and places an endoscopic stent. The physician inserts the sigmoidoscope into the anus and advances the scope through the rectum and into the sigmoid colon. The lumen of the sigmoid colon and rectum are visualized. The endoscope is placed at the site of an obstruction or stricture and the necessary stent length is determined. The stent (endoprosthesis) is introduced into the site of the obstruction. Using a commercial delivery system, a plastic covering over the stent is removed and the stent self-deploys, shoring-up the walls at a specific site in the sigmoid colon. When necessary, a balloon catheter is placed into the stent and gently inflated to more fully deploy the stent. The delivery system and endoscope are removed. This code includes dilation before and after the procedure and utilization of a guidewire, if employed.

45349

The physician inserts the sigmoidoscope into the anus and advances the scope through the rectum and into the sigmoid colon. The lumen of the sigmoid colon and rectum are visualized. The scope is directed to the affected area. A special needle is used to administer fluid under the polyp, elevating the polyp and allowing its removal from the bowel lining. Removal may be done by snare, cutting out, or suction and typically includes cautery of the attached blood vessels. The tissue is sent to pathology for analysis and the scope is withdrawn at the completion of the procedure.

45350

The physician uses a flexible sigmoidoscope to examine the rectum and sigmoid colon and perform band ligation for hemorrhoids. The physician inserts the sigmoidoscope into the anus and advances the scope through the rectum and into the sigmoid colon. The lumen of the sigmoid colon and rectum are visualized. The scope is directed to the affected area. The physician identifies the hemorrhoid. The hemorrhoid is ligated at its base with a rubber band. The hemorrhoid tissue is allowed to slough over time.

45378
The physician performs flexible colonoscopy and may obtain brushings or washings. The physician inserts the colonoscope into the anus and advances the scope through the colon to the cecum. The lumen of the colon and rectum are visualized. Brushings or washings may be obtained. The colonoscope is withdrawn at the completion of the procedure.

45379
The physician performs flexible colonoscopy and removes a foreign body(s). The physician inserts the colonoscope into the anus and advances the scope through the colon to the cecum. The lumen of the colon and rectum are visualized. The foreign body(s) is identified and removed by forceps or snare placed through the colonoscope. The colonoscope is withdrawn at the completion of the procedure.

45380
The physician performs flexible colonoscopy and obtains tissue samples. The physician inserts the colonoscope into the anus and advances the scope through the colon to the cecum. The lumen of the colon and rectum are visualized and biopsies are obtained. The colonoscope is withdrawn at the completion of the procedure.

45381
The physician performs flexible colonoscopy and injects a substance into the submucosa, directed at specific areas through the scope, while viewing the colon. The physician inserts the colonoscope into the anus and advances the scope through the colon to the cecum. The lumen of the colon is visualized. Submucosal saline injections, for instance, may be done before polypectomy using snare and electrocautery to greatly enhance the effectiveness of resection for large sessile colorectal polyps.

45382
The physician performs flexible colonoscopy and controls an area of bleeding. The physician inserts the colonoscope into the anus and advances the scope through the colon to the cecum. The lumen of the colon and rectum are visualized and the area of bleeding is identified and controlled. A variety of methods can be used to control the bleeding, including medication application, laser, heat, or electric probe. The colonoscope is withdrawn at the completion of the procedure.

[45388]
The physician performs flexible colonoscopy and ablation of a tumor, polyp, or other lesion. The physician inserts the colonoscope into the anus and advances the scope through the colon to the cecum. The lumen of the colon and rectum are visualized. The tumor, polyp, or other lesions are identified and ablated by laser or other method. The colonoscope is withdrawn at the completion of the procedure. This code reports dilation before and after the procedure and utilization of a guidewire, if employed.

45384
The physician performs flexible colonoscopy and removes a tumor, polyp, or other lesion. The physician inserts the colonoscope into the anus and advances the scope through the colon to the cecum. The lumen of the colon and rectum are visualized. The tumor, polyp, or other lesions are identified and removed by hot biopsy forceps. The colonoscope is withdrawn at the completion of the procedure.

45385
The physician performs flexible colonoscopy and removes a tumor, polyp, or other lesion. The physician inserts the colonoscope into the anus and advances the scope through the colon to the cecum. The lumen of the colon and rectum are visualized. The tumor, polyp, or other lesions are identified and removed by snare technique. The colonoscope is withdrawn at the completion of the procedure.

45386
The physician performs flexible colonoscopy and dilates strictures by balloon catheter. The physician inserts the colonoscope into the anus and advances the scope through the colon to the cecum. The lumen of the colon is visualized. Areas of stenosis are identified and a balloon catheter is passed to the point of constriction and a little beyond. The balloon is inflated to the appropriate diameter and gradually withdrawn through the stenosed area, stretching the walls of the bowel at the strictured area. The scope is withdrawn at the completion of the procedure.

45389
The physician uses a colonoscope to examine the colon and place an endoscopic stent. The physician inserts the flexible endoscope into the anus and advances the scope through the colon to the cecum. The lumen of the colon is visualized. The endoscope is placed at the site of an obstruction or stricture and the necessary stent length is determined. If the area is partially occluded or obstructed, a balloon-tipped catheter is inserted through the scope and the balloon is inflated to dilate the area before stent placement. The stent (endoprosthesis) is introduced to the site of the lesion by a stent-carrying catheter inserted through the scope. The plastic covering over the stent is removed and the stent self-deploys, shoring-up the walls at the target site in the colon. When necessary, a balloon catheter is placed into the stent and gently inflated to more fully deploy the stent. The delivery system and endoscope are removed at the completion of the procedure. This code reports dilation before and after the procedure and utilization of a guidewire, if employed.

45391
The physician uses a flexible colonoscope to examine the colon and perform an endoscopic ultrasound (EUS) examination. Ultrasound and endoscopic imaging

techniques are combined in this diagnostic modality. A flexible fiberoptic endoscope equipped with an ultrasound transducer at the tip is inserted into the anus and the scope is advanced through the colon to the cecum. The lumen of the colon is visualized and the probe tip is guided next to the area of concern. Sound waves are sent out from the transducer and reflect back to a receiving unit at varying speeds as they pass through different densities of tissue. The waves are converted to electrical pulses displayed as a picture on screen. Using ultrasound from within the endoscope instead of transcutaneously shortens the distance between the source and the target lesion and produces greater clarity from high frequency, high-resolution sound waves that have a short penetration distance. EUS is currently the most accurate method of staging cancer within the gastrointestinal tract.

45392

The physician uses a flexible colonoscope to examine the colon and perform a transendoscopic, ultrasound-guided intramural or transmural fine needle aspiration (FNA)/biopsy(s). A flexible fiberoptic endoscope equipped with an ultrasound transducer at the tip is inserted into the anus and the scope is advanced through the colon to the cecum. The lumen of the colon is visualized and the probe tip is guided to the area of concern. Sound waves are sent out from the transducer and reflect back to a receiving unit at varying speeds as they pass through different densities of tissue. The waves are converted to electrical pulses displayed as a picture on screen. An FNA needle is passed through the scope to the site of the lesion, lymph node, or tumor and a fine needle aspiration/ biopsy(s) is taken of the abnormal tissue or fluid within the colon wall or through the intestinal wall. The instruments are removed.

[45390]

The physician uses a flexible colonoscope to examine the colon. The physician inserts the colonoscope into the anus and advances the scope through the colon to the cecum. The lumen of the colon and rectum are visualized with an instrument containing a camera and light. The scope is directed to the affected area. A special needle is used to administer fluid under the polyp to elevate the polyp allowing for the removal from the bowel lining. Removal may be done by snare, cutting out, or suction and typically includes cautery of the attached blood vessels. The tissue is sent to pathology for analysis and the scope is withdrawn at the completion of the procedure.

45393

The physician uses a flexible colonoscope to examine the colon and decompress a pathologic distention such as a volvulus or megacolon. The physician inserts the scope into the anus and advances the scope into the colon. The lumen of the colon and rectum are visualized. The scope is advanced into the area of distention decompressing it as the scope passes through the lumen. The scope is withdrawn at the completion of the procedure. This procedure includes placement of a decompression tube when utilized.

[45398]

The physician uses a flexible colonoscope to examine the rectum and colon and perform band ligation for hemorrhoids. The physician inserts the scope into the anus and advances the scope into the colon. The lumen of the colon and rectum are visualized. The scope is directed to the affected area. The physician identifies the hemorrhoid. The hemorrhoid is ligated at its base with a rubber band. The hemorrhoid tissue is allowed to slough over time.

45395-45397

With the patient under general anesthesia, the physician places a trocar at the umbilicus into the abdomen and insufflates the abdominal cavity. The physician places a laparoscope through the umbilical incision and additional trocars are placed, through which the surgical instruments are inserted. The physician mobilizes the sigmoid colon, tractions it upward, and incises the right pelvic peritoneum. Dissection and ligation are carried out on the inferior mesenteric artery and inferior mesenteric vein. The dissection is carried into the retrorectal space by using cautery scissors. The peritoneum is incised on both sides of the rectum and also anteriorly at the pouch of Douglas, and the mesorectum is mobilized off the sacrum. The physician frees the rectum from the posterior vaginal wall or the prostate and seminal vesicles. After the rectum is totally mobilized, a loop of sigmoid colon is brought through the small incision in a lower quadrant port, where it may be transected outside the body. The distal part is sutured shut and returned to the cavity and the stoma is matured. The specimen is removed en bloc during the perineal phase of the resection performed in a conventional fashion. The laparoscopic instruments are removed and the incisions are sutured. In 45397, the free end of the distal colon is brought through the sphincter complex and approximated with the anus to form a colo-anal anastomosis. The distal colon is folded and sutured in such a way as to create a colonic reservoir pouch. The physician may elect to bring a loop or end of the colon through a separate abdominal incision to create a stoma (diverting enterostomy).

45400-45402

The physician performs a laparoscopic proctopexy (or rectopexy) for correction of rectal prolapse. With the patient under general anesthesia, the physician places trocars into the abdomen and insufflates the abdominal cavity. Using a laparoscope, the physician completely mobilizes the rectum down to the pelvic floor and attaches the rectum to the sacrum using polypropylene mesh. The mesh is initially stapled to the sacral hollow and sutured on both sides of the rectum. The trocars are removed and the incisions are closed with sutures. In 45402, a laparoscopic sigmoid resection is performed in conjunction with the proctopexy. Using a laparoscope, the physician mobilizes the sigmoid colon and rectum. The redundant segment of sigmoid colon and rectum are excised and an anastomosis is created between the remaining bowel ends with sutures or staples. Following laparoscopic proctopexy as described above, the trocars are removed and the incision closed with sutures.

45500
The physician performs proctoplasty for an area of stenosis. The physician makes a longitudinal incision through the scar tissue at the anorectal junction or may completely excise the scar tissue to an area of normal mucosa. The surrounding perianal skin is undermined and mobilized in one of several possible fashions as a flap. The flap is approximated to the normal mucosa at the edges of the incised or excised scar, thus closing the wound.

45505
The physician performs proctoplasty for an area of prolapse of rectal mucosa (ectropion). The physician makes a circular incision just proximal to the prolapsing mucosa and mobilizes the redundant mucosa. An incision is made out onto the perianal skin to form a flap of skin on the right and left sides of the anus adjacent to the mobilized mucosa. The mucosa is excised and the flaps of skin are advanced into the anal canal. The mucosal edges are reapproximated in their normal anatomic position with sutures. The skin incisions are closed completing the procedure.

45520
The physician performs sclerotherapy for rectal prolapse. The physician identifies the anorectal ring. Sclerosing solution is injected into the submucosa of the rectum circumferentially just above the anorectal ring.

45540
The physician approximates the rectum to the sacrum (proctopexy) for rectal prolapse. The physician makes an abdominal incision. The rectum is completely mobilized from the sacrum and placed in upward tension to remove any redundancy. The rectum is reapproximated to the sacrum with sutures or a mesh may be wrapped around the rectum and attached to the sacrum. The incision is closed.

45541
Through a perineal approach, the physician approximates the rectum to the sacrum (proctopexy) for rectal prolapse. The physician makes a transverse incision between the anus and coccyx. Dissection is continued through the levator muscles to mobilize the rectum from the sacrum. The rectum is placed on upward tension to remove the redundancy and approximated to the sacrum with sutures or with a mesh wrapped around the rectum and secured to the sacrum. The incision is closed.

45550
The physician approximates the rectum to the sacrum and performs a sigmoid colon resection. The physician makes an abdominal incision. The sigmoid colon and rectum are mobilized. The redundant segment of sigmoid colon and rectum is excised and an anastomosis is created between the remaining bowel ends with sutures or staples. The rectum is approximated to the sacrum with sutures. The incision is closed.

45560
The physician repairs a rectocele, a herniation of the rectum against the vaginal wall. The physician makes an incision in the mucosa of the posterior vaginal wall over the rectocele. The rectocele is dissected free of surrounding structures and the levator muscles are identified. The rectum is plicated to surrounding fascia with multiple sutures and the levator muscles are reapproximated. The vaginal mucosa is excised and the incision is closed.

45562
The physician explores, repairs, and drains a rectal injury. The physician makes an abdominal incision. The rectal injury is explored and repaired with sutures if possible. An incision is made between the coccyx and anus and drains are placed in the presacral space. The abdominal incision is closed.

45563
The physician explores, repairs, and drains a rectal injury and performs a proximal colostomy. The physician makes an abdominal incision. The rectal injury is explored and repaired with sutures. A loop or end of sigmoid colon is brought through a separate incision on the abdominal wall as a colostomy. An incision is made between the sacrum and anus and drains are placed in the presacral space. The abdominal incision is closed.

45800
The physician closes a connection between the rectum and the bladder (rectovesical fistula). The physician makes an abdominal incision. The sigmoid colon and rectum are mobilized and the connection between the rectum and bladder is identified and divided. The fistulous openings in the rectum and bladder are debrided and closed with sutures.

45805
The physician closes a connection between the rectum and bladder (rectovesical fistula) and performs a proximal colostomy. The physician makes an abdominal incision. The sigmoid colon and rectum are mobilized and the connection between the rectum and bladder is identified and divided. The fistulous openings in the rectum and bladder are debrided and closed. The involved segment of colon or rectum may be excised. A loop or end of sigmoid colon proximal to the involved area is brought out through a separate incision on the abdominal wall as a colostomy. The abdominal incision is closed.

45820
The physician closes a rectourethral fistula. The physician makes an abdominal incision. The rectum is dissected from the prostate and the fistula is identified and divided. The fistulous opening in the rectum is closed with sutures and the opening in the urethra may be closed or left open. A pedicle of omentum is

usually mobilized and placed between the areas of repair. The incision is closed. As an alternate method an incision may be made between the anus and urethra from a perineal approach and dissection continued between the rectum and urethra. The fistula is identified and divided and the openings in the rectum and urethra are closed. The incision is closed.

45825
The physician closes a rectourethral fistula and forms a proximal colostomy. The physician makes an abdominal incision. The rectum is dissected from the prostate and the fistula is identified and divided. The fistulous opening in the rectum is closed with sutures and the opening in the urethra may be closed or left open. A pedicle of omentum is usually mobilized and placed between the areas of repair. A loop or end of proximal colon is brought through a separate incision on the abdominal wall as a colostomy. The initial incision is closed.

45900
The physician reduces a rectal prolapse (procidentia) to a patient under general anesthesia. The physician performs a manual reduction of an incarcerated rectal prolapse by pushing the prolapsed segment into the anus under the relaxation of anesthesia.

45905
The physician dilates the anal sphincter under anesthesia. The physician performs dilation of the anal sphincter digitally or with a dilating instrument under the relaxation of anesthesia.

45910
The physician dilates a rectal stricture under anesthesia. The physician performs dilation of a rectal stricture digitally or with a dilating instrument under the relaxation of anesthesia.

45915
The physician removes a foreign body or fecal impaction under anesthesia. The physician performs removal of a foreign body or fecal impaction manually or with an instrument under the relaxation of anesthesia.

45990
The physician performs a diagnostic anorectal exam. The patient is placed under general, spinal or epidural anesthesia. The physician examines the external perineal area. A pelvic examination is performed when appropriate. A digital rectal exam is performed. An anoscope is inserted into the rectum. The anal canal and distal rectum are visualized. The anoscope is removed and a rigid proctosigmoidoscope is inserted into the anus and advanced. The sigmoid colon and rectal lumen are visualized. The proctosigmoidoscope is removed.

46020
The physician makes an incision in the anal opening. A suture is passed and the seton is securely tied using a rubber band, or similar technique. A nylon suture is threaded around the sphincter and tied loosely. An elastic band is secured to the suture and a safety pin is attached. The pin is taped to the patient's thigh and the patient is instructed to adjust the amount of pull to produce minimal discomfort until the seton cuts through.

46030
The physician removes an anal seton or other marker. The physician identifies the seton stitch or other marker at the anal verge. The seton is divided and removed. The external anal sphincter at the level of the seton may be divided.

46040
The physician drains an perirectal or ischiorectal abscess. The physician identifies the location of the abscess. The perianal skin over the abscess is incised and the abscess cavity is opened and drained. The incision is packed open for continued drainage.

46045
The physician drains a perirectal abscess in the intramural, intramuscular, or submucosal position. The physician identifies the location of the abscess in relation to the sphincter muscles. The perianal skin or rectal mucosa over the abscess is incised. Dissection is carried through muscle if necessary and the abscess cavity is opened and drained. The incision is packed open for continued drainage.

46050
The physician drains a superficial perianal abscess. The physician identifies the location of the abscess. The perianal skin over the abscess is incised and the abscess cavity is opened and drained. The incision is packed open for continued drainage.

46060
The physician drains an ischiorectal or intramural perirectal abscess with fistulectomy or fistulotomy and may place a seton. The physician identifies the location of the abscess and the internal and external openings of the anal fistula in relation to the sphincter muscles. An incision is made in the perianal skin over the abscess and the abscess cavity is opened and drained. The mucosa, skin, and internal sphincter muscle overlying the fistula is incised and the fistula is completely unroofed or may be excised. If the fistula goes beneath the external sphincter muscle a stitch (seton) may be placed through the fistula tract to allow drainage and preserve continence. The incision is left open to drain and the abscess cavity is packed open for continued drainage.

46070
The physician incises a congenital anal septum. The physician identifies the anal opening and septum in the infant. The septum is sharply incised.

46080
The physician divides the anal sphincter. The patient is placed in jackknife or lithotomy position. The physician performs digital and instrumental dilation of the anus with exposure of the patient's anal canal. A small incision is made between the muscle layers of the anus

and internal muscle is divided without opening the lining of the anus.

46083
The physician performs incision of a thrombosed external hemorrhoid. The physician identifies the thrombosed external hemorrhoid. An incision is made in the skin over the hemorrhoid and the thrombus is removed. The incision is left open for continued drainage.

46200
The physician excises a fissure (fissurectomy) and may perform a sphincterotomy. The physician identifies the anal fissure and the internal sphincter muscle by palpation. An incision is made around the fissure, dissecting it free of underlying sphincter muscle, and the fissure is excised. The internal sphincter muscle may be incised, usually in a lateral position away from the fissure. The incision is usually left open to allow drainage.

46221
The physician performs hemorrhoidectomy by tying off (ligating) an internal hemorrhoid. The physician identifies the internal hemorrhoid. The hemorrhoid is ligated at its base with a rubber band. The hemorrhoid tissue is allowed to slough over time.

[46945, 46946]
The physician performs ligation (tying off) of internal hemorrhoids using methods other than rubber bands. The physician explores the anal canal and identifies the hemorrhoid column(s). Report 46945 for ligation of a single hemorrhoid column or group and 46946 for ligation of two or more columns or groups. Imaging guidance is not utilized.

[46948]
The physician performs transanal dearterialization of two or more hemorrhoid groups or columns as an alternative to excisional hemorrhoidectomy or stapled hemorrhoidopexy. With the patient under general anesthesia or IV sedation with infiltration of a local anesthetic, the physician identifies the arteries supplying blood to the hemorrhoids utilizing a proctoscope coupled with a Doppler transducer. In order to interrupt the blood supply to the hemorrhoid, each selected artery is tied off (ligated) using a 2-0 absorbable suture. Mucopexy, or lifting and suturing of prolapsed mucosal membranes, may also be performed in cases of redundant prolapse.

[46220]
The physician performs excision of a single external anal papilla or skin tag. The physician identifies the anal skin tag or papilla, which is usually associated with the external edge of a fissure or fistula. An incision is made around the skin tag or papilla and the lesion is dissected from the underlying sphincter muscle and removed. The incision is closed with sutures or may be left partially open to drain.

46230
The physician performs an excision of multiple external anal papillae or tags. Papillae are often associated with the external edge of an anal fissure or fistula. Once the physician has identified the external tags or papillae, incisions are made around the lesions. The lesions are dissected from the underlying sphincter muscle and removed. The incisions are closed with sutures or may be left partially open to drain.

[46320]
The physician performs an excision of an external hemorrhoid that has become clotted with blood (thrombosed). Following appropriate anesthesia, the physician exposes the thrombosed external hemorrhoid. The hemorrhoid is completely excised with a scalpel. The site of the excision may be closed or left open to allow continued drainage.

46250
The physician performs an excision of external hemorrhoids. The physician identifies the external hemorrhoids. Incisions are made around the hemorrhoids and the lesions are dissected from the underlying sphincter muscle and removed. The incisions are closed with sutures.

46255
The physician performs excision of a single column or group of internal and external hemorrhoids. The physician explores the anal canal and identifies the hemorrhoid column. An incision is made in the rectal mucosa around the hemorrhoids and the lesions are dissected from the underlying sphincter muscles and removed. The incisions are closed with sutures.

46257
The physician performs excision of a single column or group of internal and external hemorrhoids and an associated fissure. The physician explores the anal canal and identifies the hemorrhoid column and the fissure. An incision is made in the rectal mucosa around the hemorrhoids and the lesions are dissected from the underlying sphincter muscles and removed. An incision is made around the fissure and the fissure is dissected from the underlying sphincter muscles and excised. The incisions are closed with sutures.

46258
The physician performs excision of a single column or group of internal and external hemorrhoids with associated fistulectomy and possible fissurectomy. The physician explores the anal canal and identifies the hemorrhoid column and the fistula. If the fistula is in the same plane as the hemorrhoid, a single incision is made in the mucosa around the lesions and the lesions are dissected from the underlying sphincter muscles and removed. If the lesions are in different planes, separate incisions are used to excise the lesions. If a fissure is present, it may be excised in a similar manner. The incisions are closed with sutures.

46260
The physician performs excision of two or more columns or groups of internal and external hemorrhoids. The physician explores the anal canal and identifies the hemorrhoid columns. Incisions are made in the rectal mucosa around the hemorrhoid columns. The lesions are dissected from the underlying sphincter muscles and removed. The incisions are closed with sutures.

46261
The physician performs excision of two or more columns or groups of internal and external hemorrhoids and an associated fissure. The physician explores the anal canal and identifies the hemorrhoid columns and the fissure. Incisions are made in the rectal mucosa around the hemorrhoid columns and around the fissure. The lesions are dissected from the underlying sphincter muscles and removed. The incisions are closed with sutures.

46262
The physician performs excision of two or more columns or groups of internal and external hemorrhoids with an associated fistulectomy and possible fissurectomy. The physician explores the anal canal and identifies the hemorrhoid columns and the fistula. Incisions are made in the rectal mucosa around the hemorrhoid columns and around the fistula. The lesions are dissected from the underlying sphincter muscles and removed. If a fissure is present, it may be excised in a similar manner. The incisions are closed with sutures.

46270
The physician excises or incises a subcutaneous anal fistula. The physician explores the anal canal and identifies the location of the fistula in relation to the sphincter muscles. The skin and subcutaneous tissue overlying the fistula is excised or incised to open the fistula tract. The incision is usually left open to allow continued drainage.

46275
The physician excises or incises an intersphincteric anal fistula. The physician explores the anal canal and identifies the location of the fistula in relation to the sphincter muscles. The skin, subcutaneous tissue, and internal sphincter muscle overlying the fistula are excised or incised to open the fistula tract. If the external sphincter is involved, a portion of the external sphincter may also be safely incised. The incision is usually left open to allow continued drainage.

46280
The physician excises or incises a transsphincteric, suprasphincteric, extrasphincteric, or multiple anal fistula. The physician explores the anal canal and identifies the location of the fistula in relation to the sphincter muscles. The tissue overlying the fistula or fistulas is excised or incised to open the fistula tract. If the external sphincter or the puborectal muscular sling is involved, only a portion of the muscle is incised to open the fistula. A permanent suture is placed through the remainder of the fistula tract (seton) in order to allow drainage and preserve continence. The incisions are usually left open to allow continued drainage. This code includes the seton placement, when performed.

46285
The physician performs a second stage excision or incision of an anal fistula. The physician explores the anal canal and identifies the location of the fistula in relation to the sphincter muscles. Usually the fistula tract has been partially opened and a seton may be in place. The remainder of the fistula tract is excised or incised and a seton if present is removed. The incision is usually left open to allow continued drainage.

46288
The physician excises an anal fistula and closes the defect with a rectal advancement flap. The physician explores the anal canal and identifies the location of the fistula in relation to the sphincter muscles. The fistula tract is excised. An incision is made onto the perianal skin and a wedge of skin and subcutaneous tissue is mobilized and advanced into the defect created by the excision of the fistula. The incisions are closed with sutures.

46500
The physician performs sclerotherapy of internal hemorrhoids. The physician explores the anal canal and identifies the hemorrhoid columns. Sclerosing solution is injected into the submucosa of the rectal wall under the hemorrhoid columns.

46505
The physician utilizes chemodenervation (the use of chemical agents, including neurotoxins) to provide selective weakening of certain muscles or muscle groups by causing a neuromuscular blockade. Chemodenervation works by introducing a substance used to block the transfer of chemicals at the presynaptic membrane. Botulinum toxin type A (BTX-A) is the most common substance used. To treat chronic anal fissures, the physician injects BTX-A into the internal anal sphincter. This permits chemical denervation of the anal sphincter and promotes healing of the fissure.

46600-46601
In 46600, the physician performs anoscopy and may obtain brushings or washings. The physician inserts the anoscope into the anus and advances the scope. The anal canal and distal rectal mucosa are visualized and brushings or washings may be obtained. In 46601, the physician performs a diagnostic examination of the anal canal using high resolution anoscopy (HRA), frequently indicated for patients with abnormal anal cytology. The physician examines the anal canal using a thin round tube (anoscope) and a high resolution magnifying instrument (colposcope). A mild acidic liquid may be applied to the anal canal to facilitate evaluation of any abnormal or dysplastic tissue as it causes abnormal tissue to turn white. Code 46601 includes specimens obtained by brushing or washing,

when performed. The anoscope is withdrawn at the completion of the procedure.

46604
The physician performs anoscopy and performs anal dilation. The physician inserts the anoscope into the anus and advances the scope. The anal canal and distal rectal mucosa are visualized. Dilation of the anal sphincter or a distal stricture is performed with the anoscope, digitally, or by some other instrument. The anoscope is withdrawn at the completion of the procedure.

46606-46607
In 46606, the physician performs anoscopy and obtains tissue samples by biopsy. The physician inserts the anoscope into the anus and advances the scope. The anal canal and distal rectal mucosa are visualized and tissue samples are obtained. The anoscope is withdrawn at the completion of the procedure. In 46607, the examination is performed using high resolution anoscopy (HRA), frequently indicated for patients with abnormal anal cytology. The physician examines the anal canal using a thin round tube (anoscope) and a high resolution magnifying instrument (colposcope). A mild acidic liquid may be applied to the anal canal to facilitate evaluation of any abnormal or dysplastic tissue as it causes abnormal tissue to turn white. The anoscope is withdrawn at the completion of the procedure. Both codes include biopsy.

46608
The physician performs anoscopy and removes a foreign body. The physician inserts the anoscope into the anus and advances the scope. The anal canal and distal rectal mucosa are visualized. The foreign body is identified and removed with a snare or forceps placed through the anoscope. The anoscope is withdrawn at the completion of the procedure.

46610
The physician performs anoscopy and removes a single tumor, polyp, or other lesion. The physician inserts the anoscope into the anus and advances the scope. The anal canal and distal rectal mucosa are visualized. The tumor, polyp, or other lesion is identified and removed by hot biopsy forceps or cautery. The anoscope is withdrawn at the completion of the procedure.

46611
The physician performs anoscopy and removes a single tumor, polyp, or other lesion. The physician inserts the anoscope into the anus and advances the scope. The anal canal and distal rectal mucosa are visualized. The tumor, polyp, or other lesion is identified and removed by snare technique. The anoscope is withdrawn at the completion of the procedure.

46612
The physician performs anoscopy and removes multiple tumors, polyps, or other lesions. The physician inserts the anoscope into the anus and advances the scope. The tumors, polyps or other lesions are identified and removed by hot biopsy forceps, cautery, or snare technique. The anoscope is removed at the completion of the procedure.

46614
The physician performs anoscopy and controls an area of bleeding. The physician inserts the anoscope into the anus and advances the scope. The anal canal and distal rectal mucosa are visualized. The area of bleeding is identified and controlled. The anoscope is withdrawn at the completion of the procedure.

46615
The physician performs anoscopy and performs ablation of a tumor, polyp, or other lesions. The physician inserts the anoscope into the anus and advances the scope. The anal canal and distal rectal mucosa are visualized. The tumor, polyp, or other lesions are identified and ablation of the lesions is performed. The anoscope is withdrawn at the completion of the procedure.

46700
The physician performs anoplasty for an anal stricture in an adult. The physician explores the anal canal and identifies the stricture. An incision is made in the scar of the stricture and a portion of the stricture is excised. Incisions are extended onto the perianal skin and subcutaneous tissue and skin flaps are mobilized and advanced into the defects created by the scar excision. The flaps are sutured to the surrounding skin and anoderm thus closing the defect.

46705
The physician performs anoplasty for an anal stricture in an infant. The physician explores the anal canal and identifies the stricture. An incision is made in the scar of the stricture and a portion of the stricture is excised. Incisions are extended onto the perianal skin and subcutaneous tissue and skin flaps are mobilized and advanced into the defects created by the scar excision. The flaps are sutured to the surrounding skin and anoderm thus closing the defect.

46706-46707
The physician repairs an anal fistula using fibrin glue (46706). Fibrin glue is made with human fibrinogen pooled from the plasma of long-term donors under control methods that avoid passing infection to the recipient. The glue is composed of two components, usually applied through double lumen catheters to guide the component injections separately to the tissue and must be applied at a temperature of 37 C. The fistula is localized and cannulated and then prepped for the glue. The margins and canal of the fistula are de-epithelialized with electrocoagulation and/or roughening the fistulous canal with a brush. Some bleeding actually improves the adhesion of the fibrin clot. The gluing is done so as to completely fill the defect and around the borders of the fistula, sealing it with a clot. Fibrin glue only works on tissue capable of local regeneration for wound healing since the glue does not actually function as a seal or a plug, but provides the substrate for fibroblasts to move in. After about four weeks, the glued surface is replaced

by scar tissue and the fibrin glue totally decomposes. Mechanical stress must be avoided while this stage is developing. In 46707, the physician treats an anorectal fistula or artificial communication from the anus or rectum to the skin with a porcine small intestine submucosa (SIS) plug. The patient is in a prone position. Using a sterile probe, the physician identifies the primary fistula opening by advancing the probe through the secondary fistula opening. The fistula is irrigated. The fistula plug is introduced through the internal (primary) fistula opening and threaded into the fistula until the internal opening is occluded. The plug is trimmed flush with the mucosal wall of the anus or colon and also trimmed flush at the secondary site. Each end of the plug is secured with resorbable sutures.

46710-46712

The physician repairs an ileoanal pouch fistula or sinus by pouch advancement using a transperineal or combined transperineal and transabdominal approach. An ileoanal pouch is created as a place for the storage of stool in patients that have had their large intestines removed due to disease. The pouch is connected to the anus, allowing the patient to have a bowel movement into the anus rather than needing a colostomy bag. If a drainage tract (fistula or sinus) erodes from an ileoanal pouch to the perineal area or into the vagina, it can be repaired by dissecting the tract from its external origin, the skin of the perineum or the lining of the vagina, to its source at the ileoanal pouch, and closing the tissues. In 46710, the tract is dissected (removed) and closed starting in the perineal area. In 46712, the tract is dissected (removed) using an approach that combines dissection starting in the perineal area moving toward the pouch along with an incision in the lower abdominal wall that allows access to the ileoanal pouch internally. In both cases, any damage done to the pouch is repaired (pouch advancement).

46715

The physician performs an incision to open a low imperforate anus ("cutback" procedure). The physician exposes the perineum and identifies the fistulous opening to the imperforate anus. An incision is made through the fistula into the anus onto the skin thus opening the anus. The anus is usually dilated with Hegar dilators. The incision is usually left open to heal.

46716

The physician transposes an ectopic anal orifice. The imperforate anus has usually been previously incised and opened. The physician makes an incision around the anus. Dissection is continued circumferentially around the distal rectum. Next, a cruciate incision is made over the usual site of the anus and an opening is created through the subcutaneous tissue and what remains of the external sphincter. The rectum is tunneled down through the new orifice and sutured to the new location. The incision at the previous anal site is closed.

46730

The physician repairs a high imperforate anus through a perineal or sacroperineal approach. The physician makes an incision at the usual site of the anus. Dissection is continued through the external sphincter. The puborectalis muscle is identified and dissection is carried through the muscle to identify and mobilize the rectal stump. The rectal stump is pulled through the sphincter complex, opened, and sutured to the sphincter and skin creating an anal opening. Alternately, a posterior midline sacral incision may be made initially. Dissection is carried superiorly, the puborectalis muscle is identified and a tract is formed through the puborectalis sling to the new anal opening. A perineal incision is made and the rectal stump mobilized and pulled through the sphincter complex onto the skin as described above.

46735

The physician repairs an imperforate anus by combined transabdominal and sacroperineal approaches. The physician makes a posterior midline incision on the sacrum and removes the coccyx. The puborectalis muscle is identified and a tract is made through the puborectalis sling to the future anal site. Next, the physician makes an abdominal incision and mobilizes the distal colon and rectum. The rectum is divided and the mucosa is striped from the distal rectum. An incision is made in the bottom of the rectal muscle pouch and the proximal rectum or colon is pulled through the muscular floor and puborectalis sling to the new anal site. A skin incision is made at the new anal site and the end of the colon is sutured to the sphincter muscles and skin creating a new anus. The incisions are closed.

46740

The physician repairs a high imperforate anus with a urethral or vaginal fistula through a perineal or sacroperineal approach. The physician makes an incision at the usual site of the anus. Dissection is continued through the external sphincter. The puborectalis muscle is identified and dissection is carried through the muscle to identify and mobilize the rectal stump. The urethral or vaginal fistula is identified, divided, and closed with sutures. The rectal stump is pulled through the sphincter complex, opened and sutured to the sphincter muscles and skin creating a new anal orifice. A posterior midline sacral incision may be made initially. Dissection is carried superiorly, the puborectalis muscle is identified and a tract is formed through the puborectalis sling to the new anal opening. A perineal incision is made at the site of the new anal opening. The rectal stump is mobilized, the fistula identified and divided, and the rectum pulled through the sphincter complex onto the skin as described above.

46742

The physician repairs an imperforate anus with a urethral or vaginal fistula by combined transabdominal and sacroperineal approaches. The physician makes a posterior midline incision on the sacrum and removes the coccyx. The puborectalis muscle is identified and a tract is developed through the puborectalis sling to the future anal site. Next, the physician makes an abdominal incision and mobilizes the distal colon and rectum. The rectum is divided, the mucosa is stripped from the distal rectum and the urethral or vaginal fistula is identified and closed with sutures. An incision is made in the bottom of the rectal muscle pouch and the proximal rectum or colon is pulled through the muscular floor and puborectalis sling to the new anal site. A skin incision is made at the new anal site end of the colon is sutured to the sphincter muscles and skin creating a new anus. The incisions are closed.

46744
The physician repairs a cloacal anomaly. The patient is placed in a lithotomy position. The physician makes a small incision in the perineum. The bladder, urethra, and vagina are dissected free of each other. A new rectum is formed by interposing muscle posterior to the rectum. The incision is closed with sutures.

46746
The physician repairs a cloacal anomaly. The physician makes a small incision, using a combined abdominal and sacroperineal approach. The bladder, urethra, and vagina are dissected free of each other. A new rectum is formed by interposing muscle posterior to the rectum. The incision is closed.

46748
The physician corrects a congenital anomaly of the cloaca. A cloacal anomaly usually involves a single opening on the anterior perineum for the urethra, vagina, and rectum. The physician enters the pelvic cavity through an incision in the lower abdomen and makes a second incision in the perineum from the clitoris to the anal area. The surgeon creates separate openings and divides membranes for the urethra, vagina, and rectum by using intestinal grafts, pedicle flaps, and free skin grafts.

46750
The physician performs anal sphincteroplasty for prolapse or incontinence in an adult. The physician makes a transverse incision anterior to the anus. Dissection is carried through subcutaneous tissues to expose the anal canal. The external anal sphincter muscle is dissected from the internal sphincter in the anterior plane and divided in the midline. The ends of the external sphincter are wrapped around the anal canal in an overlapping fashion and approximated with sutures. The incision is closed.

46751
The physician performs anal sphincteroplasty for prolapse or incontinence in a child. The physician makes a transverse incision anterior to the anus. Dissection is carried through the subcutaneous tissues to expose the anal canal. The external anal sphincter muscle is dissected from the internal sphincter and divided in the midline. The ends of the external sphincter are wrapped around the anal canal in an overlapping fashion and approximated with sutures. The incision is closed.

46753
The physician places a wire, suture, or muscular graft around the anus for rectal prolapse or incontinence (Thiersch procedure). The physician makes incisions on opposite sides of the anus in the lateral perianal subcutaneous tissue. A wire, suture or muscular graft mobilized from the thigh is wrapped around the anus in the subcutaneous space and secured in place. The incisions are closed.

46754
The physician removes a wire or suture that has been placed around the anal canal for rectal prolapse or incontinence. The physician makes incisions in the lateral perianal subcutaneous tissue. The wire or suture that is encircling the anus is identified, divided and removed. The incisions are closed.

46760
The physician performs an anal sphincteroplasty with a muscular graft for incontinence in an adult. The physician makes a transverse incision anterior to the anus. Dissection is carried through subcutaneous tissue to expose the anal canal and the remaining external sphincter muscle is dissected from the internal sphincter. A muscle from the thigh is mobilized and tunneled to the perineum. The muscle is wrapped around the anal canal and approximated with sutures. The incisions are closed.

46761
The physician performs sphincteroplasty with levator muscle imbrication for incontinence in an adult (Park repair). The physician makes a transverse incision anterior to the anus. Dissection is carried through the subcutaneous tissue to expose the anal canal. The external sphincter muscle is dissected from the internal sphincter and dissection is continued between the sphincters to expose the puborectalis muscle (levator). The edges of the puborectalis muscle are imbricated around the anal canal with sutures. The external sphincter muscle is imbricated around the anal canal with sutures. The incision is closed.

[46947]
The physician performs a stapled hemorrhoidopexy for prolapsing internal hemorrhoids. After having fleet enemas or oral preparation for cleansing the colon, the patient is sedated and given local or spinal anesthesia. A circular anal dilator is inserted that reduces the prolapsed anal tissue. The center obturator piece is removed and the prolapsed mucosa falls into the dilator lumen. An anoscope is inserted through the dilator that pushes the mucosa back against the rectal wall for 270 degrees of rotation. The other tissue protrudes through a window in the scope through which a purse string suture is made, containing only mucous membrane. The anoscope is rotated until a purse-string suture is completed around the anal circumference. A circular stapler is positioned proximal to the suture. The ends are tied externally. With

traction on the purse string suture, the prolapsed mucosa is brought into the casing of the circular stapler, which is fired to release two staggered rows of staples while a circular knife removes a column of redundant mucosa from the upper anal canal. The staple line is examined and instruments are removed.

46900-46916

The physician performs destruction of anal lesions with chemicals in 46900. The physician exposes the perianal skin and identifies the lesions. The lesions are painted with destructive chemicals. In 46910, the physician performs destruction of anal lesions with electrodesiccation. The physician exposes the perianal skin and identifies the lesions. The lesions are destroyed with cautery. In 46916, the physician performs destruction of anal lesions with cryosurgery. The physician exposes the perianal skin and identifies the lesions. The lesions are frozen and destroyed, usually with liquid nitrogen.

46917-46922

The physician performs destruction of anal lesions with laser therapy in 46917. The physician exposes the perianal skin and identifies the lesions. The lesions are destroyed by laser ablation or laser excision. In 46922, the physician performs destruction of anal lesions by excision. The physician exposes the perianal skin and identifies the lesions. The lesions are surgically excised. The incisions are closed.

46924

The physician performs destruction of extensive anal lesions. The physician exposes the perianal skin and identifies the lesions. An extensive destruction of the lesions is performed by various methods, such as laser surgery, electrosurgery, cryosurgery, or chemosurgery.

46930

The physician destroys internal hemorrhoids using various forms of thermal energy. The physician explores the anal canal and identifies the hemorrhoid columns. The hemorrhoids may be destroyed by clamping and cauterization, by employing high-frequency radio waves (radiofrequency), or by infrared or laser coagulation, which causes the hemorrhoidal tissue to harden, deteriorate, and form scar tissue as the area heals. The hemorrhoidal remnants may be removed.

46940-46942

The physician performs an initial (46940) or subsequent (46942) curettage or cautery of an anal fissure with dilation of the anal sphincter. The physician exposes the perianal area and identifies the fissure. The fissure is debrided with curettage or cautery. The anal sphincter is manually dilated.

47000-47001

The physician takes tissue from the liver for examination. In 47000, the physician uses separately reportable ultrasound guidance to place a hollow bore needle between the ribs on the patient's right side. The liver biopsy is sent for pathology for separately reportable activity. Report 47001 when a liver biopsy is performed incidental to another major procedure.

47010

The physician incises the liver to drain an abscess or a cyst, sometimes taking one or two stages. The physician exposes the liver via an upper midline incision. The cyst is incised and suctioned with care to not contaminate the abdomen with purulent matter. Cultures and pathology are sent in a separately reported activity. The incision is closed.

47015

The physician performs aspiration or injection of liver parasitic cysts or abscesses. The physician makes an abdominal incision. The liver is mobilized and the parasitic cysts or abscesses are identified. The remaining abdominal contents are packed off with sponges for protection. The cysts are aspirated with a needle and syringe or unroofed and aspirated and may be injected with a hypertonic solution. The abdominal incision is closed.

47100

The physician takes a wedge-shaped section of liver tissue for biopsy. The physician exposes the abdomen via an upper abdominal incision through skin, fascia, and muscle. Interrupted mattress sutures are placed on the edge of the liver lobe. A pie-shaped wedge of the liver is resected and sent for pathology in a separately reportable activity. Electrocautery is used to obtain hemostasis of the liver edge. The abdominal incision is closed with layered sutures.

47120-47130

The physician removes a section of liver, or lobectomy. The physician exposes the liver via an upper midline incision through skin, fascia, and muscle. The fibrous connections of the liver to the diaphragm are divided and the portal structures are controlled. The portal and hepatic vessels associated with the affected lobe are divided. The portal structures are clamped. The liver parenchyma is divided by pressure or coagulation hemostasis. The portal clamp is removed and hemostasis is assured before the abdomen is closed with sutures. Report 47120 if a partial lobectomy is performed; report 47122 if a trisegmentectomy is performed; report 47125 if a total left lobectomy is performed; and report 47130 if a total right lobectomy is performed.

47133

The physician performs a donor hepatectomy by removing the liver from a cadaver donor for transplantation into another recipient. The physician accesses the liver, which is mobilized from its attachments. The blood supply and bile ducts to the liver are dissected free and isolated. The liver is removed with its attached blood vessels and bile ducts and perfused with a cold preservation solution and removed from the operative field. The liver is preserved for transplantation into the recipient. The organ remains under refrigeration, specially packed in a sealable container with some preserving solution and kept on ice in a suitable carrier.

47135

The physician performs partial or whole liver transplantation to the normal anatomic position of the liver in a patient of any age. The physician makes an abdominal incision. The diseased liver tissue is removed, hemostasis is achieved, and the liver bed is dried and prepared for the donor tissue. The donor liver is placed in the prepared liver bed. Anastomoses are created between the donor hepatic vessels and the appropriate recipient vessels. The donor bile duct is approximated to the recipient bile duct or to a limb of small bowel for drainage. Drains are placed and the abdominal incision is closed.

47140

Surgeons remove the left lateral portion only (segments II and III) of the liver from a living donor, who is oftentimes a parent of compatible blood type donating to an infant or young child. Bilateral subcostal incisions are made to the xiphoid and the peritoneum is entered. The liver is exposed and mobilized. The left hepatic vein is exposed, adhesions are removed, and the porta hepatis is encircled with a drain. The left hepatic artery is dissected free and looped. The gastrohepatic ligament is transected and any aberrant left hepatic arteries within it are dissected to the left gastric artery. The left lateral segment of the liver is now reflected forward and ligaments are dissected away. The left portal vein is dissected and encircled. The left bile duct is identified and the left hepatic duct is transected, along with any multiple bile ducts within the liver, while preserving blood supply to the main bile duct. Ultrasound is used to locate the left and middle hepatic veins and the left hepatic vein is dissected and encircled. The liver's resection lines are marked with cautery. Vessels and bile ducts within this area are sutured and divided. The liver is resected and hemostasis maintained with a laser coagulator. Clamps are applied to the left hepatic artery, hepatic vein, and portal vein. The left lateral segment is removed and perfused with preservative solution for transplant. The clamped vessels and the left bile duct are sutured. The liver is checked for complete hemostasis and any bile leaks before closing. The tissue is preserved for transplantation into the recipient. The organ remains under refrigeration, packed in a sealable container with some preserving solution and kept on ice in a suitable carrier.

47141

Surgeons remove the whole left lobe (segments II, III, and IV) of the liver from a living donor, who is oftentimes a parent of compatible blood type donating to an infant or young child. Bilateral subcostal incisions are made to the xiphoid and the peritoneum is entered. The liver is exposed and mobilized. The left hepatic vein is exposed, adhesions are removed, and the porta hepatis is encircled with a drain. The left hepatic artery is dissected free and looped. The gastrohepatic ligament is transected and any aberrant left hepatic arteries within it are dissected to the left gastric artery. The left lateral segment of the liver is now reflected forward and ligaments are dissected away. The left portal vein is dissected and encircled. The left bile duct is identified. A cholecystectomy and cholangiogram are performed with catheter insertion into the cystic duct. The left hepatic duct is transected, along with any multiple bile ducts within the liver, while preserving blood supply to the main bile duct. Ultrasound is used to locate the left and middle hepatic veins, which are dissected and encircled. The liver's resection lines are marked with cautery. Vessels and bile ducts within this area are sutured and divided. The liver is resected and hemostasis is maintained with a laser coagulator. Clamps are applied to the left hepatic artery, hepatic vein, and portal vein. The total left lobe of the liver is removed and perfused with preservative solution for transplant. The clamped vessels and the left bile duct are sutured. The liver is checked for complete hemostasis and any bile leaks before closing. A final cholangiogram is performed, the catheter is removed, and the cystic duct is sutured. The tissue is preserved for transplantation into the recipient. The organ remains under refrigeration, packed in a sealable container with some preserving solution and kept on ice in a suitable carrier.

47142

Surgeons remove the whole right lobe (segments V, VI, VII, and VIII) of the liver from a living donor, who is oftentimes a parent of compatible blood type donating to an infant or young child. Bilateral subcostal incisions are made to the xiphoid and the peritoneum is entered. The liver is exposed and mobilized. Ligaments on the right are divided and dissection is continued to the inferior vena cava. Adhesions are removed and the porta hepatis is encircled with a drain. The right hepatic artery is dissected free and looped. A cholecystectomy and cholangiogram are performed with catheter insertion into the cystic duct. The right portal vein is dissected and encircled. The right bile ducts are identified. The right hepatic duct is transected within the liver parenchyma, along with any multiple bile ducts, while preserving blood supply to the main bile duct. The caudate lobe must be mobilized from the inferior vena cava. All accessory hepatic veins are ligated and ultrasound is used to locate the right and middle hepatic veins. The right hepatic vein is dissected and encircled. The liver's resection lines are marked with cautery. Vessels and bile ducts within this area are sutured and divided, maintaining the veins from segments V and VIII, and the liver is resected. Hemostasis is maintained with a laser coagulator. Clamps are applied to the right hepatic artery, hepatic vein, and portal vein. The right lobe of the liver is removed and perfused with preservative solution for transplant. The clamped vessels and the right bile duct are sutured. The liver is checked for complete hemostasis and any bile leaks before closing. A final cholangiogram is performed, the catheter is removed, and the cystic duct is sutured. The tissue is preserved for transplantation into the recipient. The organ remains under refrigeration, packed in a sealable container with some preserving solution and kept on ice in a suitable carrier.

47143

The physician performs a standard backbench preparation of cadaver donor whole liver graft without trisegment or lobe split prior to allotransplantation. Backbench or back table preparation refers to procedures performed on the donor organ following procurement to prepare the donor organ for transplant. After removal from the body, the liver is flushed with a preserving solution and packed. The superfluous tissues that accompany the liver when it is removed en bloc are removed. If the gallbladder has been removed with the liver, it is dissected free. Next, any necessary vascular reconstruction procedures are performed with the arteries being the most common sites of reconstruction. The goal of the physician is to provide a single common inflow vessel of sufficient length so that only one anastomosis is required in the recipient. Arterial grafting is performed using previously procured iliac artery grafts as required to accomplish this goal. Other vessels, including the vena cava and portal vein, are prepared and grafting performed as needed. All vessels and grafts are tested for patency and integrity by flushing with preservation solution. Next, the common bile duct is inspected and residual tissue removed. Following liver preparation, the internal iliac arteries and veins are prepared for use as arterial and venous grafts in the recipient. When all residual tissue has been removed, vascular grafting performed as needed, and the common bile duct prepared, the liver is ready for transplant.

47144

The physician performs a standard backbench preparation of cadaver donor whole liver graft with trisegment split of whole liver graft into two partial liver grafts prior to allotransplantation. Backbench or back table preparation refers to procedures performed on the donor organ following procurement to prepare the donor organ for transplant. After removal from the body, the liver is flushed with a preserving solution and packed. The superfluous tissues that accompany the liver when it is removed en bloc are removed. If the gallbladder has been removed with the liver, it is dissected free. In split liver transplants, the liver can be split prior to procurement (in situ) or during the back table preparation (ex situ). If an ex situ split is required, it is performed at this time. A trisegment split involves dividing the liver through the falciform ligament to create a small left lateral segment graft for a child and a large extended right lobe graft for an adult. Next, any necessary vascular reconstruction procedures are performed, with the arteries being the most common sites of reconstruction. The goal of the physician is to construct a single common inflow vessel of sufficient length in the donor liver segments so that only one anastomosis is required in the recipient. Arterial grafting is performed using previously procured iliac artery grafts as required to accomplish this goal. Other vessels, including the vena cava and portal vein, are prepared and venous grafting performed as needed. All vessels and grafts are tested for patency and integrity by flushing with preservation solution. Next, the common bile duct is inspected and residual tissue removed. Following liver preparation, the internal iliac arteries and veins are prepared for use as arterial and venous grafts in the recipient. When all residual tissue has been removed, vascular grafting performed as needed, and the common bile duct prepared, the liver segments are ready for transplant.

47145

The physician performs a standard backbench preparation of cadaver donor whole liver graft with lobe split of whole liver graft into two partial liver grafts prior to allotransplantation. Backbench or back table preparation refers to procedures performed on the donor organ following procurement to prepare the donor organ for transplant. After removal from the body, the liver is flushed with a preserving solution and packed. The superfluous tissues that accompany the liver when it is removed en bloc are removed. If the gallbladder has been removed with the liver, it is dissected free. In split liver transplants, the liver can be split prior to procurement (in situ) or during the back table preparation (ex situ). If an ex situ split is required, it is performed at this time. A lobe split involves dividing the liver through the main portal fissure and gallbladder bed to create right and left lobe grafts. Next, any necessary vascular reconstruction procedures are performed, with the arteries being the most common sites of reconstruction. The goal of the physician is to construct a single common inflow vessel of sufficient length in the two donor liver lobes so that only one anastomosis is required in the recipient. Arterial grafting is performed using previously procured iliac artery grafts as required to accomplish this goal. Other vessels, including the vena cava and portal vein, are prepared and venous grafting performed as needed. All vessels and grafts are tested for patency and integrity by flushing with preservation solution. Next, the common bile duct is inspected and residual tissue removed. Following liver preparation, the internal iliac arteries and veins are prepared for use as arterial and venous grafts in the recipient. When all residual tissue has been removed, vascular grafting performed as needed, and the common bile duct prepared, the two liver lobes are ready for transplant.

47146

The physician performs venous anastomosis during a backbench reconstruction of cadaver or living donor liver graft prior to allotransplantation. Previously procured iliac vein grafts from the liver donor are anastomosed to the veins of the donor liver as required. Multiple grafts may be required depending on anatomical variations found in the liver donor. Code 47146 is reported for each venous graft performed.

47147

The physician performs arterial anastomosis during a backbench reconstruction of cadaver or living donor liver graft prior to allotransplantation. Previously procured iliac artery grafts from the liver donor are anastomosed to the arteries of the donor liver as required. Multiple grafts may be required depending on anatomical variations found in the liver donor. Code 47147 is reported for each artery graft performed.

47300

The physician creates a pouch with the lining of a cyst on the liver. The physician exposes the liver via an upper midline abdominal incision through skin, fascia, and muscles. The cyst is incised and suctioned with care not to contaminate the abdomen. Electrocautery is used to resect the cyst wall to allow open drainage into the abdomen. The abdominal incision is closed with sutures.

47350-47362

The physician sutures a liver wound to control the bleeding or repair damage. In 47350, the physician exposes the liver via an upper midline abdominal incision. The abdomen is packed to control bleeding. The patient is stabilized hemodynamically. The liver is systematically exposed with pressure on bleeding points. The liver tissue is divided to expose the points of bleeding and the bleeding is controlled by ligation of bleeding vessels. The abdominal incision is closed. Report 47360 if the procedure requires a complex suture of liver wound or injury, with or without hepatic artery ligation; report 47361 if procedure requires an exploration of a hepatic wound, extensive debridement, coagulation and/or suture, with or without packing of the liver; and report 47362 if the procedure is a re-exploration of hepatic wound for removal of packing.

47370-47371

The physician places a laparoscope via a small periumbilical port or through a small incision in the right upper quadrant, and an additional port is placed in the right upper quadrant under direct vision. Adhesions are lysed and ligamentous attachments divided to mobilize the liver. The physician examines all the parietal and visceral peritoneal surfaces, the lesser sac, the omentum, and the viscera. The gastrohepatic omentum is opened for inspection of the caudate lobe, followed by sequential laparoscopic ultrasonographic examination of all eight liver segments using an ultrasonic probe. Radiofrequency ablation is performed using a 15-gauge needle with a retractable curved electrode placed percutaneously into the abdomen at the place overlying the area of interest under direct vision. The needle is directed into the center of the lesion under real-time ultrasound guidance, tines are deployed, and alternating current is delivered to ablate the tumor. Upon completion of ablation, the probe tract is cauterized and the needle withdrawn. In microwave ablation, which is also part of the radiofrequency spectrum, microwaves are delivered from the needle to create a small region of heat that destroys the targeted cells. Report 47371 if ablation is accomplished using a cool-tipped multiple probe electrode.

47380

The physician performs radiofrequency ablation of a liver tumor via an open laparotomy. Grounding pads are placed on the patient's legs. The physician performs a midline laparotomy. Dissection is carried down to the liver. Under direct visualization, a needle-electrode, with an insulated shaft and an uninsulated distal tip, is inserted into the tumor. Each treatment session has about 10 to 15 minutes of active ablation. The energy at the needle tip causes ionic agitation and frictional heat in the surrounding tissue, which, when hot enough, leads to cell death and coagulative necrosis. This results in a 3 to 5.5 cm sphere of dead tissue per treatment session. In large tumors, the physician may create more than one sphere next to each other to try to turn the tumor edges in three dimensions. A small margin of normal tissue next to the tumor is also burned, as a precaution to destroy all tumor cells. The tumor cells are not removed, but are gradually replaced by fibrosis and scar tissue. One method uses a needle-within-a-needle electrode system with an inner needle that expands once placed into the tumor.

47381

The physician performs cryosurgical ablation of a liver tumor. The physician performs a laparotomy. Dissection is carrier down to the liver. Cryosurgical probes are inserted into the liver tumor. The cryosurgical probes rapidly freeze (liquid nitrogen at -196°C or nitrous oxide at -89.5°C) the area being treated, the liver tissue is slowly thawed, and repeated cycles of freezing and thawing are immediately performed. Cryogen may also be applied directly into or on to the tumor by probe, direct application, spraying, or by pouring. The incision is closed with layered sutures.

47382-47383

Intravenous sedation is administered and grounding pads are placed on the patient's legs. A needle-electrode, with an insulated shaft and an uninsulated distal tip, is inserted through the skin and directly into the tumor. Ultrasound, CT scan, or MRI guide the needles to the correct spot and monitor treatment. Each treatment session has about 10 to 15 minutes of active ablation. Report 47382 when the energy at the needle tip causes ionic agitation and frictional heat in the surrounding tissue, which, when hot enough, leads to cell death and coagulative necrosis. This results in a 3 to 5.5 cm sphere of dead tissue per treatment session. In large tumors, the physician may create more than one sphere next to each other to try to turn the tumor edges in three dimensions. A small margin of normal tissue next to the tumor is also burned, as a precaution to destroy all tumor cells. The tumor cells are not removed, but are gradually replaced by fibrosis and scar tissue. One method uses a needle-within-a-needle electrode system with an inner needle that expands once placed into the tumor. Report 47383 when the physician performs cryosurgical ablation of a liver tumor. Cryosurgical probes are inserted into the liver tumor.

The cryosurgical probes rapidly freeze the area being treated (liquid nitrogen at -196°C or nitrous oxide at -89.5°C), the liver tissue is slowly thawed, and repeated cycles of freezing and thawing are immediately performed. Cryogen may also be applied directly into or onto the tumor by probe, direct application, spraying, or pouring.

47400

The physician makes a midline abdominal incision. The physician makes an incision into the hepatic duct and surgically creates an artificial opening. The physician performs exploration, drainage, or removal of calculus from the hepatic duct. The hepatic duct is closed primarily or around a tube for continued drainage. If a drainage tube is placed, a separate incision is made in the abdominal wall through which the drainage tube is positioned. The abdominal incisions are closed.

47420-47425

The physician explores the common bile duct, removing calculus, draining purulent matter, and/or constructing a new duct. The physician exposes the common bile duct within the portal triad through a subcostal or upper midline incision. The common bile duct is incised, explored, and drained. The common bile duct is closed with interrupted sutures primarily or around a drainage tube (choledochostomy). If placed, the drainage tube is brought out through the skin at a site separate from the incision. The abdominal incision is closed. Report 47425 if this procedure performed with transduodenal sphincterotomy or sphincteroplasty.

47460

The physician performs a transduodenal sphincterotomy or sphincteroplasty and may repair the duodenal sphincter or remove a stone, as needed. The physician exposes the second portion of the duodenum via a subcostal or upper midline incision through skin, fascia, and muscle. The duodenum is opened using a longitudinal incision. The ampulla of Vater is identified and an incision is made in the ampulla at the two o'clock position. The common bile duct mucosa may be reapproximated to the duodenal mucosa and the duodenum transversely closed with interrupted sutures. Stones may be removed. The abdominal incision is closed.

47480

The physician performs an open cholecystotomy or cholecystostomy with exploration, drainage, or removal of calculus. The physician exposes the gallbladder through a subcostal or upper midline incision. The gallbladder is incised, explored, and may be drained. Calculi may be removed. The gallbladder is closed with interrupted sutures primarily or around a drainage tube. If placed, the drainage tube is brought out through the skin at a site separate from the incision. The abdominal incision is closed.

47490

The physician inserts a tube into the gallbladder to allow drainage through the skin. The physician uses ultrasound guidance to place a subcostal drainage tube into the gallbladder. The physician places a needle between the ribs into the gallbladder. The needle position is checked by aspiration. A guidewire is passed through the needle. A catheter is passed over the wire into the biliary tree. The wire is removed and the tube is left in place. This code reports the complete procedure and includes placement of the catheter under image guidance, a cholecystogram if performed, and radiological supervision and interpretation.

47531-47532

A radiographic medium is injected into the common bile duct, gallbladder, and/or liver for diagnostic purposes. The physician inserts a needle between the ribs into the lumen of the common bile duct and checks positioning by aspiration. Radiographic dye is injected. The needle is removed. This procedure includes imaging guidance and all radiological supervision and interpretation. Report 47531 when the service is performed through an existing access, such as a T-tube. Report 47532 when the service is performed via a new access.

47533-47537

In 47533, the physician introduces a catheter into the liver to drain fluid using ultrasound and/or fluoroscopy to guide the process. The puncture site on the right side of the body is incised, the needle inserted between the ribs, advanced into the liver, and into the bile duct. Contrast medium is injected to visualize the intrahepatic bile ducts. A guidewire is inserted and advanced to the point of obstruction through an optimal duct permitting access and drainage. A catheter is threaded over the guidewire and dilators may be used to enlarge the opening and the tract from the skin to the bile duct. The drainage catheter is inserted and positioned above the point of the obstruction and secured to the skin. All of the bile drains out of the body through the catheter and into a collection bag. Occasionally, the use of two separate catheters is necessary to drain the right and left biliary duct systems. In 47534, the physician introduces a catheter into the liver to drain fluid internally and externally, usually on patients with inoperable bile duct obstruction. The procedure is the same as in the external procedure except that a drainage catheter is inserted and positioned so that openings for drainage are above and below the obstruction and secured in place. This allows bile to flow to an external drainage system as well as into the duodenum (internal). Report 47535 for a percutaneous conversion from an external biliary drainage catheter to internal-external. Report 47536 for a percutaneous exchange, such as external, internal-external, or conversion of internal-external to external only. Report 47537 for the removal of a biliary drainage catheter. Codes 47533-47537 include diagnostic cholangiography (when performed), imaging guidance (fluoroscopy), as well as all associated radiological supervision and interpretation.

47538-47540

The physician inserts a thin needle through the skin and into the liver and injects contrast material for

Digestive

x-rays in order to diagnose and treat obstructions impacting the flow of bile from the liver to the gastrointestinal (GI) tract. Once the stricture or obstruction is identified, the physician places an introducer sheath into the biliary system. Under ultrasonic or fluoroscopic guidance, a stent delivery system is placed within a narrow section of the bile duct in order to keep the duct patent. Stents may be comprised of metallic mesh or plastic tubing. A balloon-tipped catheter may be required to achieve adequate expansion of the narrow duct. The stent may be a self-expandable stent, which means it opens by itself once deployed, or balloon expandable, meaning a balloon is required in order to open the stent. When a balloon expandable stent is used, the stent is generally placed over a balloon tipped catheter because once the balloon is expanded the catheter pushes the stent into place against the duct wall. Once the balloon tipped catheter is deflated and removed, the stent stays in place and functions similarly to a scaffold for the duct. A hilar malignancy may create an obstruction within both hepatic ducts and require the use of a bilateral stent. Report 47538 when this procedure is performed via an existing access site; 47539 when performed via a new access site without placement of separate biliary drainage catheters; and 47540 when performed via a new access site with placement of separate biliary drainage catheters (external or internal-external). The use of imaging, diagnostic cholangiography, balloon dilation, and/or the exchange or removal of catheters, as well as all supervision and interpretation, is included in these procedures, when performed.

47541

Placement of access through the biliary tree and into the small bowel is performed to assist in an endoscopic biliary procedure, such as rendezvous. The physician inserts a needle through the skin and liver moving it into the bile duct for a biliary drainage procedure. For stent placement, a drainage tube is typically placed prior to stent insertion. If this fails to resolve the obstruction, the physician inserts a guidewire and the tube is removed. A sheath is placed over the guidewire and a stent delivery system is placed within the narrow section. Tissue samples and stone removal may be performed via this access. This code includes all imaging guidance. Report this code if the access is new.

47542

Percutaneous balloon dilation of a biliary duct or repair of the ampulla is most often required to widen a stricture or remove stones. The repair is done due to damage caused by the stricture, stone, or by the dilation itself. The provider inserts a needle through the skin and into the biliary duct and the needle is advanced through the stricture, allowing for insertion of a balloon catheter. A guidewire is inserted over the needle into the biliary duct and the needle is removed. The balloon is placed over the guidewire. Under imaging guidance, the balloon is filled with saline in order to stretch the vessel. The size of inflation and continuity depend on the patient's diagnosis and dispensation. Once the procedure is complete, the instruments are removed and simple closure of the access site is performed.

47543

Endoluminal surgery, such as a biopsy, is performed in a hollow organ (biliary tree, stomach, etc.) using common surgical techniques. Because of the nature of these procedures, they must be performed under endoscopic control and, ideally, performed via natural orifices. The physician performs a percutaneous, endoluminal biopsy of the biliary tree by brush or forceps catheters or needle using real-time imaging (ultrasound, fluoroscopy), and the specimen is deposited on a glass slide. Smears are made from the biopsy specimen, which may be used for immediate analysis (e.g., Diff-Quik) or fixed in ethanol for immunohistochemical stains. If possible, the use of an on-site cytopathologist or cytotechnologist ensures an immediate interpretation of the sample. The use of ultrasound is particularly helpful to identify small lesions that may move during respiration. Fluoroscopy is often used in conjunction with percutaneous transhepatic biliary drainage (PTBD) as a means to access the biliary tract for the purposes of conducting endoluminal biopsy.

47544

The physician removes a stone from the biliary duct after previous surgery. The common bile duct is approached by placing a scope into the tract through a previously placed drainage tube (T-tube). Manipulating basket or snare tools through the scope, the physician removes the stone(s). This code reports only the radiological supervision and interpretation required in performing this procedure.

47550

The physician performs a biliary endoscopy during the same surgical session as other biliary procedures. The physician advances an endoscope through the previously made abdominal incision. With the endoscope the physician is able to directly visualize portions of the biliary tract, which may be filled with contrast medium for identifying the common bile duct, biliary tree and gall bladder (including areas of abnormality, stricture, or obstruction) under separately reportable fluoroscopy.

47552-47553

The physician makes a small incision in the abdominal wall. The physician advances an endoscope through an opening in the abdominal wall or through a T-tube inserted through the abdominal wall into the common bile duct. With the endoscope, the physician is able to directly visualize portions of the biliary tract, which may be filled with contrast medium for identifying the common bile duct, biliary tree, and gallbladder (including areas of abnormality, stricture, or obstruction) under separately reportable fluoroscopy. In 47552, the physician may collect specimens by brushing and/or washing. In 47553, the physician advances biopsy forceps along the tract or T-tube to obtain single or multiple biopsies under direct endoscopic visualization or with the use of fluoroscopy. The endoscope is removed. The T-tube is withdrawn and the defect in the common bile duct is sutured closed. The tract, peritoneum, and abdominal wall are closed with layered sutures.

47554

The physician makes a small incision in the abdomen. The physician advances an endoscope through an opening in the abdominal wall or through a T-tube inserted through the abdominal wall into the common bile duct. With the endoscope, the physician is able to directly visualize portions of the biliary tract, which may be filled with contrast medium for identifying the common bile duct, biliary tree, and gallbladder (including areas of abnormality, stricture, or obstruction) under separately reportable fluoroscopy. Calculi are identified and removed. The endoscope is removed. The T-tube is withdrawn and the defect in the common bile duct is sutured closed. The tract, peritoneum, and abdominal wall are closed using a layered technique.

47555-47556

The physician makes a small incision in the abdomen. The physician advances an endoscope through an opening in the abdominal wall or through a T-tube inserted through the abdominal wall into the common bile duct. With the endoscope, the physician is able to directly visualize portions of the biliary tract, which may be filled with contrast medium for identifying the common bile duct, biliary tree, and gallbladder (including areas of abnormality, stricture, or obstruction) under fluoroscopy. The physician advances a balloon-tipped catheter through the tract or T-tube so that it is above the site of the duct stricture, inflates the balloon, and draws it back through the site of stricture to achieve dilation. This procedure may be repeated until optimal dilation is obtained. The endoscope is removed and the tract, peritoneum, and abdominal wall are approximated. The T-tube is withdrawn and the common bile duct is sutured closed. The abdomen is sutured closed. In 47556, the physician places a stent to prevent future stricture before the endoscope is withdrawn.

47562-47564

The physician removes the gallbladder through a laparoscope. The physician makes a 1.0-centimeter infraumbilical incision through which a trocar is inserted. Pneumoperitoneum is achieved by insufflating the abdominal cavity with carbon dioxide. A fiberoptic laparoscope fitted with a camera and light source is inserted through the trocar. Other incisions are made on the right side of the abdomen and in the subxiphoid area to allow other instruments or an additional light source to be passed into the abdomen. The tip of the gallbladder is mobilized and placed in traction. The Hartmann's pouch (junction of the cystic duct and gallbladder neck) is identified. Tissue is dissected free from around the area for exposure of Calot's triangle (formed by the cystic artery, and cystic and common bile ducts). Clips are applied to the proximal area of the cystic duct and artery (close to the gallbladder) and the cystic duct and artery are cut. In 47563, a contrast study is also obtained through the cystic duct. In 47564, a contrast study of the bile ducts is usually obtained through the cystic duct. The common bile duct may be explored with a small choledochoscope through the cystic duct or a separate incision may be made in the common bile duct. The common duct is visualized with a choledochoscope and stones may be extracted from the duct with a variety of instruments. If an incision was made in the common bile duct, this is usually closed with sutures over a T-tube that is brought out through the abdominal wall. The cystic duct and artery are divided. The gallbladder is removed through the trocar site. A drain is usually placed below the liver and brought out through the abdominal wall. The trocars are removed and the incisions are closed.

47570

Through the laparoscope the physician performs an anastomosis between the gallbladder and small bowel (cholecystoenterostomy). The physician places a trocar at the umbilicus and insufflates the abdominal cavity. The laparoscope is placed through the umbilical port and additional trocars are placed into the abdominal cavity. The gallbladder and a proximal loop of small bowel are identified and mobilized. An anastomosis is created between the gallbladder and loop or limb of proximal small bowel with staples or sutures. The trocars are removed and the incisions are closed.

47600-47605

The physician removes the gallbladder by open incision. The patient is placed in the supine position and general anesthesia is administered. The physician makes a 6-inch incision into the abdomen on the right side. There are two approaches for open cholecystectomy: retrograde and antegrade, with the more common being retrograde, and discussed here. Incision into the anterior rectus sheath is performed following the length of incision with division of the muscles. An incision is then made into the posterior rectus sheath and peritoneum to open the abdomen. A retractor may be placed to allow adequate inspection of the liver and gallbladder. Inspection and palpation of the liver and gallbladder are performed. A clamp is used to grab and lift the dome of the gallbladder. If adhesions are present between the gallbladder and colon or duodenum, they are lysed by sharp dissection or use of electrocautery. The retrograde technique removes the gallbladder starting at the top and working down from the fundus toward the porta hepatis. The visceral peritoneum is cut at 1 cm from the liver and the clamp holds the fundus of the gallbladder at which time, the physician continues the incision along the gallbladder running parallel to the liver. Once the gallbladder is mobilized from the liver bed, dissection within Calot's triangle is performed and division of the cystic duct and artery are performed with ligation (suture, staple, and clip). At this point, the small veins may be present requiring division and/or ligation in order to completely remove the gallbladder.

The incision is closed with layered sutures. The entire procedure can take up to two hours and inpatient hospitalization of two to three days with full recovery at about four to six weeks. Report 47605 if this is performed with a cholangiography.

47610-47620
The physician removes the gallbladder and explores the common duct. The physician exposes the liver and gallbladder via a right subcostal incision. The cystic duct and cystic artery are ligated and the gallbladder removed using electrocautery. The common bile duct is exposed in the portal triad, incised, and the stones removed. The common bile duct is closed and the abdominal incision is closed with sutures. Report 47612 if this procedure is performed with choledochoenterostomy, establishment of communication between the intestine and the common bile duct; report 47620 if this procedure is performed with transduodenal sphincterotomy or sphincteroplasty, with or without cholangiography.

47700
The physician explores a congenital atresia of the bile ducts without making a repair, with or without liver biopsy, with or without cholangiography. The physician uses an upper midline abdominal incision to expose the liver, gall bladder, and bile ducts. Inspection and evaluation of the gallbladder, common bile ducts, and duodenum is carried out to determine the status of the bile ducts. A tissue sample may be removed. Cholangiography may be performed. A biliary drainage tube may be placed.

47701
The physician performs a portoenterostomy, a procedure in which the jejunum is connected to the bile ducts and other portal structures of the liver and gallbladder. The physician exposes the liver and gallbladder via an upper midline or subcostal incision. The bile ducts are connected to the small bowel for drainage by anastomosing a Roux-en-Y hook of jejunum to the divided extravascular portal structures. The abdominal incision is closed.

47711
The physician performs excision of an extrahepatic bile duct tumor and reconstructs bile duct drainage. The physician makes an abdominal incision and explores the abdomen. The bile duct is dissected from surrounding structures and the tumor is identified and mobilized. The tumor is excised with a margin of normal bile duct tissue proximal and distal to the tumor. An anastomosis is usually created between the proximal end of the bile duct and a loop of small bowel to allow biliary drainage. The distal end of the bile duct is oversewn. The incision is closed.

47712
The physician performs excision of an intrahepatic bile duct tumor and reconstructs bile duct drainage. The physician makes an abdominal incision and explores the abdomen. The distal bile duct is isolated. The tumor is identified and dissection is continued proximally along the bile duct into the parenchyma of the liver beyond the tumor onto the left and right hepatic ducts. The tumor is excised with a normal margin of bile duct or hepatic duct proximal and distal to the tumor. An anastomosis is created between the proximal bile duct or left and right hepatic ducts and a limb of small bowel to allow biliary drainage. The distal end of the bile duct is oversewn. The incision is closed.

47715
The physician excises a cyst in the common bile duct. The physician exposes the liver and gallbladder via an upper midline or subcostal incision made through skin, fascia, and muscle. The cyst is exposed and excised and the defect of the biliary system is repaired. The abdominal incision is closed with layered sutures.

47720-47741
The physician performs a cholecystoenterostomy, in which a communication is made between the gallbladder and an artificial anus or fistula in the abdominal wall. The physician exposes the liver and gallbladder via an upper midline or subcostal incision. The cyst is opened and connected to the small intestine for drainage. The abdominal incision is closed. Report 47721 if this procedure is performed with gastroenterostomy; report 47740 if this procedure is performed with Roux-en-Y; and report 47741 if this procedure is performed with Roux-en-Y with gastroenterostomy.

47760
The physician performs an anastomosis between an extrahepatic biliary duct and the small bowel. The physician makes an abdominal incision and explores the abdomen. The extrahepatic biliary duct is divided and anastomosis is formed between an extrahepatic biliary duct and the small bowel with sutures or staples (end-to-side). The incision is closed in layers.

47765
The physician performs an anastomosis between an intrahepatic biliary duct and the small bowel. The physician makes an abdominal incision and explores the abdomen. The intrahepatic biliary duct is divided and anastomosis is formed between an intrahepatic biliary duct and the small bowel with sutures or staples (end-to-side). The incision is closed in layers.

47780
The physician performs an anastomosis between a limb of small bowel (Roux-en-Y) and the gallbladder and stomach. The physician makes an abdominal incision and explores the abdomen. The proximal small bowel is divided and anastomoses are formed between the distal limb of jejunum and the gallbladder and the stomach with sutures or staples. The proximal end of bowel is approximated to the limb of jejunum distal to the gallbladder and stomach anastomoses. This procedure is usually performed for a mass obstructing the bile duct and stomach. The incision is closed.

47785
The physician performs an anastomosis between a limb of small bowel (Roux-en-Y) and the intrahepatic biliary ducts. The physician makes an abdominal incision. The bile duct is isolated and dissection is carried proximally along the duct into the liver parenchyma exposing the intrahepatic biliary ducts. The bile duct is divided or excised. The proximal small bowel is divided and an anastomosis is created between the distal limb of jejunum and the intrahepatic biliary ducts with sutures. The distal bile duct is oversewn. The proximal end of bowel is approximated to the limb of jejunum distal to the bile duct anastomosis. The incision is closed.

47800
The physician reconstructs the biliary ducts through anastomosis. The physician exposes the liver and gallbladder via an upper midline or subcostal incision made via skin, fascia, and muscle. The abnormal biliary tree is excised and the resected ends are reconnected. The incision is closed with layered sutures.

47801
The physician inserts a stent into the bile duct. The physician makes a small incision overlying the bile duct. Using an endoscope or percutaneous choledochostomy tube, a catheter and stent are placed to bridge a narrowing in the common bile duct. The scope or tube is removed and the incision closed.

47900
The physician performs suture closure of a biliary duct injury. The physician makes an abdominal incision. The bile duct is dissected from surrounding structures and the injury of the duct is identified. The duct injury is closed with sutures. A drain is usually placed and brought out through the abdominal wall. The incision is closed.

48000
The physician places peripancreatic drains for acute pancreatitis. The physician makes an upper transverse abdominal incision. The transverse colon and small intestines are retracted to reveal the underlying pancreas. Necrotic pancreatic tissue may be resected. Drains are placed circumferentially around the pancreas, sutured secure, and anchored through the abdominal wall. The upper transverse abdominal incision is closed with sutures.

48001
The physician places peripancreatic drains for pancreatitis and performs cholecystostomy, gastrostomy and jejunostomy. The physician makes an abdominal incision. The pancreas is exposed, necrotic pancreatic tissue may be debrided, and drains are placed around the pancreas. The gallbladder is identified and a tube is sutured into the gallbladder and brought out through the abdominal wall. An incision is made in the anterior gastric wall and a tube is sutured into the stomach and brought out through the anterior abdominal wall. An incision is made in a proximal segment of jejunum and a tube is sutured into the jejunum and brought out through the anterior abdominal wall. The abdominal incision is closed.

48020
The physician removes a stone from the pancreas. The physician exposes the pancreas via an upper midline incision through skin, fascia, and muscle. The pancreatic duct is opened and calculus removed. The pancreatic duct is connected directly to the small bowel for drainage. The abdominal incision is closed.

48100
The physician obtains a biopsy of the pancreas. The physician makes a midline epigastric incision and retracts the skin and underlying tissues laterally. The physician approaches the pancreas through the lesser sac of the omental bursa. The pancreas is palpated, the lesion is identified, and a biopsy is obtained by various methods, such as fine needle aspiration or needle core or wedge biopsy. Bleeding is controlled and the lesser sac is closed. Tissues are reapproximated to the anatomical position and the incision is sutured in layers.

48102
The physician removes tissue from the pancreas. The physician passes the biopsy needle through the skin of the upper abdomen under separately reportable computerized tomography guidance. The pancreatic lesion is removed and the specimen is sent for pathology for examination (reported separately).

48105
The physician performs resection and debridement of the pancreas for necrotizing pancreatitis. The physician makes an abdominal incision. The pancreas is exposed and necrotic areas of the pancreas and peripancreatic tissue are debrided. Drains are usually placed around the pancreas. The incision is closed.

48120
The physician excises a lesion of the pancreas. The physician makes a midline epigastric incision and retracts the skin and underlying tissues laterally. The physician approaches the pancreas through the lesser sac of the omental bursa or the through the transverse mesocolon. The pancreas is palpated, the lesion is identified and excised. Bleeding is controlled, and the lesser sac is closed. Tissues are reapproximated to anatomical position, and the incision is sutured in layers.

48140-48145
The physician removes the distal portion of the pancreas, with or without removing the spleen and jejunum. The physician makes a midline epigastric incision and retracts the skin and underlying tissues laterally. The physician approaches the pancreas through the lesser sac of the omental bursa or the through the transverse mesocolon. The pancreas is identified and freed from attachments. If the blood supply to the distal pancreas also supplies the spleen, the spleen is sacrificed in the resection. The pancreas is transected, and the distal portion is removed, with or without the spleen. In 48140, the pancreatic duct is not

obstructed, permitting free drainage of pancreatic enzymes. In 48145, the duct flow is obstructed and a jejunal loop is brought up to create a fistula for enzyme flow to the digestive tract. Bleeding is controlled, and the lesser sac is closed. Tissues are reapproximated to anatomical position, and the incision is sutured in layers.

48146
The physician performs a near-total pancreatectomy. The physician makes an abdominal incision. The pancreas is exposed and the body and tail of the pancreas are mobilized. The pancreas is transected at the junction of the head and body of the pancreas over the superior mesenteric vessels. The distal pancreas is removed. Frequently the spleen is removed with the distal pancreas. The end of the proximal pancreas is closed with staples or sutures. Drains are usually placed in the pancreatic bed. The incision is closed.

48148
The physician excises the ampulla of Vater, a saccular dilation of liver and/or pancreas. The physician exposes the duodenum and pancreas via an upper midline abdominal incision. The duodenum is opened with a longitudinal incision. The ampulla of Vater is exposed and the abnormality is excised. The common bile duct and duodenal mucosa are re-approximated as needed. The duodenum is closed with transverse interrupted sutures. The abdominal incision is closed.

48150
The physician performs excision of the proximal pancreas, duodenum, distal bile duct and distal stomach with reconstruction (Whipple procedure) but with pancreatojejunostomy. The physician makes an abdominal incision and explores the abdomen. The duodenum, proximal pancreas, and bile duct are mobilized. The distal bile duct, distal stomach, and distal duodenum are divided. The pancreas is transected at the junction of the head and body and the pancreatic head, duodenum, distal stomach, and distal bile duct are removed en bloc. The anatomy is reconstructed by performing sequential anastomoses between the proximal jejunum and the distal bile duct and distal stomach. The edge of the remaining distal pancreas is closed with sutures or staples. The incision is closed.

48152
The physician performs excision of the proximal pancreas, duodenum, distal bile duct and distal stomach with reconstruction (Whipple procedure) but without pancreatojejunostomy. The physician makes an abdominal incision and explores the abdomen. The duodenum, proximal pancreas, and bile duct are mobilized. The distal bile duct, distal stomach, and distal duodenum are divided. The pancreas is transected at the junction of the head and body and the pancreatic head, duodenum, distal stomach, and distal bile duct are removed en bloc. The anatomy is reconstructed by performing sequential anastomoses between the proximal jejunum and the distal bile duct and distal stomach. The edge of the remaining distal pancreas is closed with sutures or staples. The incision is closed.

48153
The physician performs excision of the proximal pancreas, duodenum, and distal bile duct with reconstruction (pylorus preserving Whipple procedure). The physician makes an abdominal incision and explores the abdomen. The duodenum, proximal pancreas, and bile duct are mobilized. The distal bile duct and distal duodenum are divided. The proximal duodenum is divided just distal to the pylorus. The pancreas is transected at the junction of the head and body and the proximal pancreas, duodenum and distal bile duct are removed en bloc. The anatomy is reconstructed by performing sequential anastomoses between the proximal jejunum and the remaining pancreatic tail, distal bile duct and pylorus. The incision is closed.

48154
The physician performs excision of the proximal pancreas, duodenum and distal bile duct with reconstruction but without pancreatojejunostomy. The physician makes an abdominal incision and explores the abdomen. The duodenum, proximal pancreas and bile duct are mobilized. The distal bile duct and distal duodenum are divided. The proximal duodenum is divided just distal to the pylorus. The pancreas is transected at the junction of the head and body and the proximal pancreas, duodenum, and distal bile duct are removed en block. The anatomy is reconstructed by performing sequential anastomoses between the proximal jejunum and the distal bile duct and the pylorus. The edge of the remaining distal pancreas is closed with sutures or staples and no anastomosis is performed to the pancreas. The incision is closed.

48155-48160
The physician removes all or part of the pancreas. The physician makes a midline epigastric incision and retracts the skin and underlying tissues laterally. The physician approaches the pancreas through the lesser sac of the omental bursa or the through the transverse mesocolon. The pancreas is identified and freed from attachments. In 48155, the pancreas is removed. In 48160, all or part of the pancreas is removed and pancreatic islet cells are transplanted into the abdominal tissue. Blood vessels are ligated and the affected pancreas is removed. Bleeding is controlled, and the lesser sac is closed. Tissues are reapproximated to anatomical position, and the incision is sutured in layers.

48400
The physician performs a contrast study of the pancreatic duct. The physician makes an abdominal incision. The pancreas is exposed and may be mobilized by dissecting it from its retroperitoneal attachments. A separately reported pancreatogram may be obtained by injecting contrast into the common bile duct thus filling the pancreatic duct in a retrograde fashion and a radiograph obtained. Alternately, the duodenum may be opened and the

pancreatic duct injected directly, or the tail of the pancreas may be transected and the pancreatic duct injected directly with contrast and a radiograph obtained. The duodenum is closed or the pancreatic tail is sutured closed. The incision is closed.

48500

The physician marsupializes a pancreatic cyst. The physician approaches the pancreas through a midline abdominal incision and retracts the skin and underlying tissues laterally. The physician approaches the pancreas through the lesser sac of the omental bursa or the through the transverse mesocolon. The cyst is located, and the anterior cyst wall is incised. The cut edges of the cyst are sutured to the skin edges establishing a pouch of what was formally an enclosed cyst. The remainder of the operative site is sutured in layers.

48510

The physician externally drains a pancreatic cyst. The physician approaches the pancreas through a midline abdominal incision. The physician locates the cyst through an incision and approaches the pancreas through the lesser sac of the omental bursa or the through the transverse mesocolon. Once the drain is placed, the adjacent tissues are returned to anatomic position and the operative site is sutured in layers.

48520

The physician creates an internal anastomosis of a pancreatic cyst to a portion of the gastrointestinal tract. The physician approaches the pancreas through a midline abdominal incision and retracts the skin and underlying tissues laterally. The physician approaches the pancreas through the lesser sac of the omental bursa or the through the transverse mesocolon. The cyst is located. The physician approximates the stomach wall or a loop of duodenum or jejunum and incises it. The anterior cyst wall is incised and the cyst edges are approximated with the cut edges of the gastrointestinal tract and sutured. The cyst is decompressed through the drainage tract. The surrounding tissues are returned to anatomic position and the operative site is sutured in layers.

48540

The physician creates a Roux-en-Y anastomosis to drain enzymes from the pancreatic duct. The physician approaches the pancreas through a midline abdominal incision and retracts the skin and underlying tissues laterally. The physician approaches the pancreas through the lesser sac of the omental bursa or the through the transverse mesocolon. The physician divides a loop of small intestine (usually the jejunum) and implants the distal end into the stomach or duodenum. The proximal end is anastomosed distal to the first anastomosis to prevent reflux. The pancreatic duct is fistulized to the proximal end to create a drain to the gastrointestinal tract for pancreatic enzymes. The surrounding tissues are returned to anatomic position and the operative site is sutured in layers.

48545

The physician repairs a pancreatic injury (pancreatorrhaphy). The physician makes an abdominal incision and the abdomen is explored. The pancreas is exposed and the pancreatic injury is identified and repaired with sutures. A peripancreatic drain is usually placed. The incision is closed.

48547

The physician performs duodenal exclusion and gastrojejunostomy for a pancreatic injury. The physician makes an abdominal incision and explores the abdomen. The pancreas is exposed and an injury in the duodenum or pancreas may be closed with sutures. An incision is made in the stomach (gastrotomy). The natural opening from the stomach to the duodenum is closed with sutures or staples. A limb of proximal small bowel is brought up to the stomach and an anastomosis is performed (gastrojejunostomy) at the site of the gastrotomy. The abdominal incision is closed.

48548

The physician creates a pancreaticojejunostomy to drain pancreatic enzymes through a side-to-side anastomosis. The physician makes a midline epigastric incision and retracts the skin and underlying tissues laterally. The physician approaches the pancreas through the lesser sac of the omental bursa or through the transverse mesocolon. A jejunal loop is brought up to create a fistula for enzyme flow to the digestive tract. Bleeding is controlled and the lesser sac is closed. Tissues are reapproximated to the anatomical position and the incision is sutured in layers.

48550

The physician performs a donor pancreatectomy by removing the pancreas with or without a segment of the duodenum from an organ donor. The physician makes an abdominal incision to access the pancreas and duodenum, which are mobilized and dissected free from their retroperitoneal attachments. The segments of mesenteric and splenic arteries and portal vein supplying the pancreas and duodenum are divided. The pancreas is removed en bloc with its vascular supply. Usually a segment of duodenum is also removed en bloc with the pancreas. The donor tissue is preserved for transplantation into the recipient, who may be hundreds of miles away. The organ remains under refrigeration, packed in a sealable container with some preserving solution and kept on ice in a suitable carrier.

48551

The physician performs a standard backbench preparation of a cadaver donor pancreas. Backbench or back table preparation refers to procedures performed on the donor organ following procurement to prepare the donor organ for transplant. In a separately reportable procedure, the physician removes the pancreas in conjunction with the thoracic organs, liver, and spleen from a cadaver donor. One pair of donor iliac arteries and vein are also procured for use in back table reconstruction procedures. Backbench procedures on the pancreas are accomplished at very cold temperatures to prevent the organ from deteriorating. Considerable back table preparation is required to prepare the pancreas for the transplant procedure. First, the pancreas is separated from the thoracic organs and liver. The spleen is removed by tying the individual vessels with 2-0 silk ligatures. The surrounding soft tissues are dissected from the pancreas allograft. The duodenal segment of bowel attached to the head of the pancreas is mobilized and shortened to allow for transplantation. The bile duct is ligated. Since the pancreas receives blood flow from two arteries, the superior mesenteric artery and the splenic artery, the arteries must be combined into one to allow anastomosis of the blood vessels in the transplant recipient. The physician performs a bypass graft from the previously procured iliac artery. The bypass graft consists of Y-graft arterial anastomoses of the internal iliac artery to the splenic artery and the external iliac artery to the superior mesenteric artery.

48552
The physician performs a backbench venous reconstruction of a cadaver donor pancreas allograft. Backbench or back table refers to procedures performed on the donor organ following procurement to prepare the donor organ for transplant. Backbench procedures on the pancreas are accomplished at very cold temperatures to prevent the organ from deteriorating. The physician dissects the portal vein. Venous anastomosis of the portal vein is required when there is not sufficient length or when there are anatomic variations in the donor organ. Previously procured iliac vein segments are fashioned and anastomosed as required to provide for systemic and portal drainage. More than one anastomosis may be required to accomplish this. Code 48552 is reported for each anastomosis.

48554
The physician performs pancreas transplantation. The physician makes an abdominal incision. The iliac arteries and veins in the pelvis are exposed and isolated. An anastomosis is usually performed between the artery and vein supplying the pancreas to the iliac artery and vein on one side of the pelvis. An additional anastomosis is usually performed between the attached duodenal segment and the bladder. The incision is closed.

48556
The physician removes a transplanted pancreas graft. The physician makes an abdominal incision. The pancreatic graft is mobilized. The vascular supply to the pancreatic graft is isolated, ligated and divided. The anastomosis between the duodenum and bladder is taken down and the defect in the bladder is closed with sutures. The incision is closed.

49000
To explore the intra-abdominal organs and structures, the physician makes a large incision extending from just above the pubic hairline to the rib cage. The abdominal cavity is opened for a systematic examination of all organs. The physician may take tissue samples of any or all intra-abdominal organs for diagnosis. The incision is closed with sutures.

49002
The physician reopens the incision of a recent laparotomy before the incision has fully healed to control bleeding, remove packing, or drain a postoperative infection.

49010
The physician explores the retroperitoneum and may obtain sample tissue for separately reportable diagnostic testing. The physician may approach the retroperitoneum through a flank or an abdominal incision. The surface of the retroperitoneum is inspected and any area of interest of the retroperitoneum may be opened and the retroperitoneum explored. Tissues may be sampled. The incision is closed.

49013-49014
In 49013, the physician performs local exploration and preperitoneal pelvic packing (PPP) for hemorrhage associated with pelvic trauma. This type of hemorrhage is often from venous or bony sources and not amenable to correction by angioembolization, which is effective in controlling hemorrhages from arterial sources. The physician makes a 6 to 8 cm vertical midline incision from the pubic symphysis extending upwards, through skin and subcutaneous tissue to fascia. The fascia is incised in the midline and the preperitoneal space is entered. The physician retracts the bladder to permit the placement of surgical laparotomy pads. Because of lack of visibility due to the amount of hemorrhage in the pelvic space, rapid packing is necessary. The first laparotomy pad is pressed down onto the sacrum using a blunt instrument, followed by six to nine pads to complete the packing and tamponade. If a laparotomy is necessary, a separate incision may be made that extends from the xiphoid to just below the umbilicus in order to keep abdominal and pelvic spaces separate for adequate tamponade to be achieved. Utilizing a running suture at the fascial level, the physician closes the pelvic packing incision. In 49014, the physician performs re-exploration of the pelvic wound. The previously placed preperitoneal pelvic packing is removed and, if the physician deems it necessary, the wound is repacked.

49020
The physician makes an open abdominal or flank incision (laparotomy) to gain access to the peritoneal cavity. The peritoneum is explored and the abscess or isolated area of peritoneal inflammation is identified. The abscess is incised and drained and inflamed peritoneal tissue may be excised. The abscess and surrounding peritoneal cavity may be irrigated. A drain may be placed whereby a separate abdominal incision is made and the drain is drawn through it and sutured in place. The physician may completely reapproximate the abdominal incision or leave a portion of the incision open to allow for further drainage. Specimens

taken during the procedure are typically sent to microbiology for identification and to determine antibiotic suitability. If a drain is placed, it is removed at a later date.

49040

The physician drains a subdiaphragmatic or subphrenic abscess. The physician makes an abdominal incision and the abdomen is explored. The abscess beneath the diaphragm is identified and the abscess cavity is opened and drained. Irrigation of the cavity is usually performed. A drain is usually placed into the abscess cavity and brought out through the abdominal wall. The incision is closed. The superficial portion of the incision may be packed open to allow drainage.

49060

The physician drains a retroperitoneal abscess. The physician makes an abdominal or flank incision. The abscess is identified and the retroperitoneal space is entered. The abscess cavity is opened and drained. Irrigation of the cavity is usually performed. A drain is usually placed in the abscess cavity and brought out through the abdominal wall. The incision is closed. The superficial portion of the incision may be packed open to allow drainage.

49062

The physician drains a lymphocele to the peritoneal cavity. The physician creates an opening in a lymphatic swelling or cavity (lymphocele) located outside the abdominopelvic walls to drain the material contained within to a cavity of the peritoneum. Irrigation of the lymphocele is performed. The incision is sutured closed. For radiological supervision and interpretation, see 75989.

49082-49083

The physician inserts a needle or catheter into the abdominal cavity and withdraws and drains fluid for diagnostic or therapeutic purposes. The needle or catheter is removed at the completion of the procedure. Report 49082 if imaging guidance is not used and 49083 if imaging guidance is used.

49084

Peritoneal lavage is usually performed to determine the presence and/or extent of internal bleeding within the peritoneum. The physician makes a small incision to insert a catheter into the abdominal cavity. Fluids are infused into the cavity and subsequently aspirated for diagnostic testing. The catheter is removed at the completion of the procedure and the incision is closed.

49180

Using radiological supervision, the physician locates the mass within or immediately outside the peritoneal lining of the abdominal cavity. A biopsy needle is passed into the mass, a tissue sample is removed, and the needle is withdrawn. This may be repeated several times. No incision is necessary.

49185

Sclerotherapy is the therapeutic use of sclerosing agents (e.g., ethanol, povidone-iodine, tetracycline, doxycycline, bleomycin, talc, or fibrin glue) to systematically destroy undesired fluid collections such as cysts, lymphoceles, or seromas. This procedure is usually performed with the patient under moderate conscious sedation and involves a minimally invasive, percutaneous approach; depending on the size of the cyst or lymphocele, treatment may involve catheter drainage by gravity for approximately one day with subsequent administration of a sclerosing agent, such as ethanol, into the fluid collection under fluoroscopic guidance. For larger fluid collections, a catheter is placed using ultrasound or fluoroscopy and ethanol is administered via the catheter daily until the fluid collection has been reduced. The process involves percutaneous placement of a catheter over a guidewire into the area of fluid collection where the catheter is left in place and the sclerosing agent(s) is administered via the catheter as the patient remains in the supine position. The patient may be asked to change positions after the sclerosing agent has been injected in order to allow the entire area where the fluid collection is located to have contact with the sclerosing agent. Drainage of the sclerosing agent may take between 15 minutes and one hour depending on the agent used. Occasionally, depending on the size of the fluid collection, two catheters may be used. Aspirated fluid from the lymphocele, seroma, or cyst is sent for histopathology. The catheter is removed.

49186-49190

The physician removes or destroys intra-abdominal primary or secondary tumors or cysts. An incision is made in the abdomen over the location of the growth. Prior to removal, the tumor and/or cyst is measured, not including margins. If only a portion of the growth will be excised or destroyed, only that portion is measured. The growths are removed or destroyed using various techniques such as laser ablation, debulking, electric cautery, or scalpel excision. The incision is closed with sutures. Report 49186 when the sum of the maximum length of tumors or cysts is 5 cm or less; 49187 for a sum of 5.1 to 10 cm; 49188 for 10.1 to 20 cm; 49189 for 20.1 to 30 cm; and 49190 for greater than 30 cm.

49215

The physician performs resection of a presacral or sacrococcygeal tumor. The physician makes an abdominal incision and explores the abdomen. The tumor is identified and the rectum is mobilized from the sacrum to expose the tumor. The tumor is dissected free of surrounding structures and removed. Alternately, the tumor may be approached posteriorly through an incision between the sacrum and coccyx. The coccyx is removed, the rectum is mobilized from the sacrum and the tumor is dissected from surrounding structures and removed. A portion of the sacrum may be excised en bloc with the tumor. The incision is closed.

Digestive

49250
The physician performs excision of the umbilicus. The physician makes an incision around the umbilicus and dissects the umbilicus from surrounding subcutaneous tissue. The umbilical arteries and vein, the urachal remnant, and the omphalomesenteric remnant identified and divided. The umbilicus is removed. The fascial defect is closed and the umbilicus is reconstructed with small skin flaps.

49255
The physician performs resection of the omentum or epiploectomy. The physician makes an abdominal incision and the abdomen is explored. The omentum is mobilized from the stomach and colon, divided from its blood supply and removed. One or more epiploica of the colon may be removed. The incision is closed.

49320
The physician makes a 1.0-centimeter incision in the umbilicus through which the abdomen is inflated and a fiberoptic laparoscope is inserted. Other incisions are also made through which trocars can be passed into the abdominal cavity to deliver instruments, a video camera, and when needed an additional light source. The physician manipulates the tools so that the pelvic organs, peritoneum, abdomen, and omentum can be viewed through the laparoscope and/or video monitor. Biopsy from any or all of the areas observed are obtained by brushing the surface and collecting the cells or by washing (bathing) the area with a saline solution, and suctioning out the cell rich solution. When the procedure is complete, the laparoscope, instruments, and light source are removed and the incisions are closed with sutures. If biopsy of pelvic organs is performed, the physician may also insert an instrument through the vagina to grasp the cervix and pass another instrument through the cervix, into the uterus to manipulate the uterus.

49321
The physician makes a 1.0 centimeter incision in the umbilicus through which the abdomen is inflated and a fiberoptic laparoscope is inserted. Other incisions are also made through which trocars can be passed into the abdominal cavity to deliver instruments, a video camera, and, when needed, an additional light source. The physician manipulates the tools so that the pelvic organs, peritoneum, abdomen, and omentum can be viewed through the laparoscope and/or video monitor. Biopsy from any or all of the areas observed are obtained by grasping a sample with a biopsy forceps that is capable of "biting off" small pieces of tissue. When the procedure is complete, the laparoscope, instruments, and light source are removed and the incisions are closed with sutures. If a biopsy of female pelvic organs is performed, the physician may also insert an instrument through the vagina to grasp the cervix and pass another instrument through the cervix and into the uterus to manipulate the uterus.

49322
The physician makes a 1.0-centimeter incision in the umbilicus through which the abdomen is inflated and a fiberoptic laparoscope is inserted. A second incision is made directly below the umbilicus, just above the pubic hairline, through which a trocar can be passed into the abdominal cavity to deliver instruments. The physician manipulates the tools to view the pelvic organs through the laparoscope. An additional incision may be needed for a second light source. Once the biopsy site is viewed through the laparoscope, a 5.0-centimeter incision is made just above the site. Through this incision, the physician uses an aspirating probe to aspirate a cavity or cyst or to collect fluid for culture. The instruments are removed and the incisions are sutured.

49323
The physician drains a lymphocele to the peritoneal cavity. With the patient under anesthesia, the physician places a trocar at the umbilicus into the abdominal or retroperitoneal space and insufflates the abdominal cavity. The physician places a laparoscope through the umbilical incision and additional trocars are placed into the abdomen. The lymphocele is identified and instruments are passed through to open and drain the lymphocele. The trocars are removed and the incisions are closed with sutures.

49324-49325
A permanent intraperitoneal catheter is inserted laparoscopically using a tunneling technique. The physician makes a 1 cm incision in the umbilicus through which the abdomen is inflated and a fiberoptic laparoscope is inserted. Other incisions are also made through which trocars can be passed into the abdominal cavity to deliver additional instruments. The physician manipulates the tools so that the pelvic organs, peritoneum, abdomen, and omentum can be viewed through the laparoscope and/or video monitor. Using various tunneling techniques, the physician inserts the intraperitoneal catheter, positioning the tip inside the peritoneal cavity. A separately reportable subcutaneous extension of the catheter with a remote chest exit site may also be performed. If the physician is revising an intraperitoneal catheter, the catheter is inspected and freed of occlusion or blockage. When either procedure is complete, the laparoscope and other instruments are removed and the incisions are closed with sutures. Report 49324 for the tunneled insertion of an intraperitoneal cannula or catheter and 49325 for its revision.

49326
Omentum is a strong and highly vascularized serous membrane in the abdomen. The physician makes a 1 cm incision in the umbilicus through which the abdomen is inflated and a fiberoptic laparoscope is inserted. Other incisions are also made through which trocars can be passed into the abdominal cavity to deliver instruments, a video camera, and, when needed, an additional light source. The physician manipulates the tools so the pelvic organs, peritoneum, abdomen, and omentum can be viewed through the laparoscope and/or video monitor. The physician isolates the omentum at the stomach and intestine and may cut, suture, or plicate omental tissue

to achieve the desired effect. When the procedure is complete, the laparoscope, instruments, and light source are removed and the incisions are closed with sutures.

49327
The physician makes a 1 cm incision in the umbilicus through which the abdomen is inflated and a fiberoptic laparoscope is inserted. Other incisions are also made through which trocars can be passed into the abdominal cavity to deliver instruments, a video camera, and, when needed, an additional light source. The physician manipulates the tools so that the pelvic organs, peritoneum, abdomen, and omentum can be viewed through the laparoscope and/or video monitor. In conjunction with other laparoscopic abdominal, pelvic, or retroperitoneal procedures that are performed concurrently, and using image guidance if necessary, the physician places one or more interstitial devices such as gold seeds (fiducial markers) for radiation therapy guidance or a dosimeter to gauge the amount of radiation received into the targeted soft tissue tumor. Allowing for precision in targeting radiation and/or for measuring the radiation doses received, a fiducial marker is visible by ultrasound and fluoroscopy and permits accurate triangulation of the tissue to be treated. A capsule dosimeter relays radiation dose information so that the clinical team can monitor for any deviation between the radiation plan and the actual radiation received. When the procedure is complete, the laparoscope, instruments, and light source are removed and the incisions are closed with sutures.

49400
The physician injects air contrast into the peritoneal cavity. The physician inserts a needle or catheter into the peritoneal cavity and injects air as a diagnostic procedure. An x-ray is usually obtained to define the pattern of air in the abdomen. The needle or catheter is removed at the completion of the procedure.

49402
The physician removes a foreign body from the abdominal cavity. The physician makes an abdominal incision and explores the abdominal cavity. The foreign body is identified and removed. The incision is closed.

49405
A fluid collection in the visceral organs (kidney, liver, spleen, lung, mediastinum, etc.), such as a hematoma, seroma, abscess, lymphocele, or cyst, is drained using a catheter. The area over the affected organ is cleansed and local anesthesia is administered. Imaging is performed to assist in the insertion of a needle or guidewire into the fluid collection. Small tissue samples may be collected from the site for pathological examination. A catheter is inserted to drain and collect the fluid for analysis. The catheter is removed. More imaging may be performed to ensure hemostasis. A bandage is applied. In some cases, the catheter may be attached to a bag to allow for further drainage over the course of days.

49406
A fluid collection in the peritoneum or retroperitoneum, such as a hematoma, a seroma, an abscess, a lymphocele, or a cyst, is drained using a catheter. The area over the affected site is cleansed and local anesthesia is administered. Imaging is performed to assist in the insertion of a needle or guidewire into the fluid collection. Small tissue samples may be collected from the site for pathological examination. A catheter is inserted to drain and collect the fluid for analysis and is then removed. More imaging may be performed to ensure hemostasis. A bandage is applied. In some cases, the catheter may be attached to a bag to allow for further drainage over the course of days.

49407
A fluid collection in the peritoneum or retroperitoneum, such as a hematoma, a seroma, an abscess, a lymphocele, or a cyst, is drained via a vaginal or rectal approach. An intracavitary probe is used to create access through the rectal or vaginal wall. Imaging is performed to assist in the insertion of a needle or guidewire into the fluid collection. Small tissue samples may be collected from the site for pathological examination. A catheter is inserted to drain and collect the fluid for analysis and is then removed. In some cases, the catheter may be attached to a bag to allow for further drainage over the course of days.

49411
The physician places one or more interstitial devices such as gold seeds (fiducial markers) for radiation therapy guidance or a dosimeter to gauge the amount of radiation received. Implanted percutaneously in and/or around an intra-abdominal, intra-pelvic (excluding prostate), and/or retroperitoneal soft tissue tumor, these act as radiographic landmarks to define the position of the target lesion. Under CT or other image guidance, the physician injects a small capsule or seed into the targeted tissue using a needle injection device. Allowing for precision in targeting radiation and/or for measuring the radiation doses received, an injected fiducial marker is visible by ultrasound and fluoroscopy and permits accurate triangulation of the tissue to be treated. An injected capsule dosimeter relays radiation dose information so that the clinical team can monitor for any deviation between the radiation plan and the actual radiation received.

49412
The physician places one or more interstitial devices such as gold seeds (fiducial markers) for radiation therapy guidance or a dosimeter to gauge the amount of radiation received into a targeted intra-abdominal, intrapelvic, or retroperitoneal soft tissue tumor. Implanted in conjunction with an open abdominal, pelvic, or retroperitoneal procedure performed concurrently, these act as radiographic landmarks to define the position of the target lesion. Using image guidance if necessary, the physician places a small capsule or seed into the targeted tissue. Allowing for

precision in targeting radiation and/or for measuring the radiation doses received, a fiducial marker is visible by ultrasound and fluoroscopy and permits accurate triangulation of the tissue to be treated. A capsule dosimeter relays radiation dose information so that the clinical team can monitor for any deviation between the radiation plan and the actual radiation received. When the procedures are complete, the incisions are closed with sutures.

49418
The physician places a tunneled intraperitoneal catheter for drainage, dialysis, or chemotherapy instillation using a percutaneous approach. The physician makes a small abdominal incision, opens the peritoneum (the double-layered sac covering the internal organs and lining the abdominopelvic walls), and inserts the catheter into the cavity. The proximal end of the catheter is tunneled subcutaneously away from the initial incision and brought out through the skin. The incision is closed. Alternately, the physician may percutaneously insert the catheter over a wire placed through a needle inserted into the peritoneal cavity. This code reports the complete procedure and includes placement of the catheter under imaging guidance, contrast injection if performed, and radiological supervision and interpretation.

49419
The physician inserts a tunneled intraperitoneal catheter with subcutaneous reservoir (port) for continuous drug infusion of substances such as insulin, morphine, or chemotherapeutic agents. In the case of a totally implantable, intraperitoneal insulin delivery system, the pump reservoir is inserted under general or local anesthesia into a surgically prepared pocket in the subcutaneous fat of the lower or mid-left abdomen. The infusion line catheter from the pump is placed inside the peritoneal cavity using a tunneling technique with the tip free moving.

49421
The physician places a tunneled intraperitoneal catheter for dialysis using an open technique. The physician makes a small abdominal incision, opens the peritoneum (the double-layered sac covering the internal organs and lining the abdominopelvic walls), and inserts the catheter into the cavity. The proximal end of the catheter is tunneled subcutaneously away from the initial incision and brought out through the skin. The incision is closed. A separately reportable subcutaneous extension of the intraperitoneal catheter with a remote chest exit site may also be performed at this time.

49422
The physician removes a tunneled intraperitoneal catheter. The physician makes an incision over the insertion site of the catheter. The catheter is dissected free of surrounding scar tissue, transected, and removed from the peritoneal insertion site and skin exit site. The incision at the insertion site of the catheter is closed. The skin exit site is left open to allow drainage.

49423
The physician exchanges a previously placed drainage catheter. The physician locates the drainage catheter and removes sutures that may be holding it in place. The drainage catheter is removed. With the use of fluoroscopy, the physician places a new drainage catheter and may elect to use a catheter guidewire to assist in this maneuver. Once placed and found to be patent, the new drainage catheter may be sutured in place. For radiological supervision and interpretation, see 75984.

49424
The physician injects a radio-contrast dye through a previously placed catheter to determine the existence, nature, or size of an abscess or cyst. Once the radio-contrast dye is placed, the operative site is examined under direct fluoroscopy or with radiographic studies. The contrast dye may be aspirated and/or irrigated from the cyst or abscess. For radiological supervision and interpretation, see 76080.

49425
The physician places a peritoneal-venous shunt. The physician makes a small lateral upper abdominal incision. Dissection is carried through the abdominal wall layers, the peritoneum is entered and the peritoneal end of the catheter is inserted into the peritoneal cavity and sutured into place. A subcutaneous tunnel is created from the abdominal incision up to the neck and the catheter is pulled through the tunnel into the neck. A counter incision is made in the neck over the internal jugular vein and the venous end of the catheter is inserted into the jugular vein. The incisions are closed.

49426
The physician performs revision of a peritoneal-venous shunt. The physician may remove the shunt by incisions over the venous and peritoneal insertion sites with a subcutaneous tunnel is created from the abdominal incision up to the neck and the catheter is pulled through the tunnel into the neck. A counter incision is made in the neck over the internal jugular vein and the venous end of the catheter is inserted into the jugular vein. Alternately, the physician may make an incision over the dysfunctional end of the shunt and replace that portion of the shunt and insert it back into the peritoneal cavity or jugular vein. The incisions are closed.

49427
The physician injects contrast material through the skin into the reservoir of a peritoneo-venous shunt. Radiography is used to visualize the flow of contrast through the shunt into the peritoneal and venous ends for evaluation.

49428
The physician performs ligation of a previously placed peritoneo-venous shunt. The physician makes an incision over the path of the shunt. The shunt tubing under the incision is isolated and ligated with sutures. The incision is closed.

49429

The physician performs removal of a peritoneal venous shunt. An incision is made over the abdominal insertion site of the shunt. The shunt is dissected from surrounding scar tissue and removed from the abdominal cavity. The fascia and peritoneum of the abdominal insertion site is closed. Usually the venous end of the catheter can be removed by placing traction on the shunt through the abdominal incision and pulling it through the subcutaneous tunnel. If necessary a second incision is made over the venous insertion site and the catheter removed from the jugular vein. The incisions are closed.

49435

A permanent, subcutaneous intraperitoneal catheter is lengthened with an extension and brought to the surface of the skin during the primary procedure in which a catheter/cannula is established. In the primary procedure, the physician makes a small abdominal incision, opens the peritoneum, and establishes the cannula. In 49435, the physician fits an extension to the cannula and tunnels subcutaneously to accommodate the extension. The physician makes a separate incision in the chest as an exit site for the extension. The extension is brought out through the skin and may be attached to the drug delivery system. The operative incision is closed.

49436

A previously implanted, permanent subcutaneous intraperitoneal catheter is brought to the surface of the skin. The physician makes a small abdominal incision, opens the peritoneum, and locates the end of the existing intraperitoneal cannula. An extension may be fitted to the existing cannula. The physician makes a separate incision as an exit site for the cannula. The cannula is brought out through the skin and may be attached to the drug delivery system. The operative incision is closed.

49440

The physician inserts a gastrostomy tube via percutaneous (under the skin) approach using fluoroscopic guidance. Percutaneous image-guided gastrostomy or enterostomy procedures may be indicated for patients who have an impaired swallowing mechanism, mechanical obstruction of the upper GI tract due to malignancy, or those with aberrant upper GI anatomy. Following administration of any necessary sedation, nasogastric or orogastric intubation is performed under fluoroscopic guidance and the stomach is insufflated. The skin and subcutaneous tissues overlying the stomach are anesthetized with lidocaine. Using a subcostal (below the ribs) approach and fluoroscopic guidance, the physician inserts a 7 cm, 18-gauge needle in the area of the horizontal portion of the greater curvature. A guidewire is then passed through the needle and the needle is withdrawn. A dilator is introduced over the wire and the tract is dilated. The physician places a self-retaining loop catheter into the stomach and injects a small amount of contrast material in order to confirm placement. A loop-locking suture is tied and nasogastric or orogastric tubes are removed. Antiseptic ointment and sterile dressings are applied. This code includes image documentation and report.

49441

The physician inserts a duodenostomy or jejunostomy tube via percutaneous (under the skin) approach using fluoroscopic guidance. Percutaneous image-guided gastrostomy or enterostomy procedures may be indicated for patients who have an impaired swallowing mechanism, mechanical obstruction of the upper GI tract due to malignancy, or those with aberrant upper GI anatomy. Particularly in patients who have undergone gastrectomy or gastric pull-up, the jejunum or duodenum is often a viable site for percutaneous feeding tube placement. Following administration of any necessary sedation and contrast materials, the physician identifies a suitable site for puncture of the duodenum or jejunum and a needle is inserted percutaneously. When the contrast material can be aspirated from the needle, a guidewire is inserted under fluoroscopic guidance. The tract is dilated and an appropriate catheter is inserted and secured to the skin with a stoma device. Nasogastric or orogastric tubes are removed. Antiseptic ointment and sterile dressings are applied. This code includes image documentation and report.

49442

The physician inserts a cecostomy or other colonic tube via percutaneous (under the skin) approach using fluoroscopic guidance. Following identification of the gallbladder, liver, and urinary bladder by ultrasound, the physician inserts a silicone catheter into the rectum and a retention balloon is filled with air. The abdomen is prepared and draped in sterile fashion and appropriate anesthesia is administered. The colon is inflated with air via the rectal catheter and the physician assesses the position of the cecum to determine the appropriate tract site. The physician makes a small incision in the skin and inserts a puncture needle through the skin and soft tissues. Under fluoroscopic guidance, the needle is advanced into the cecum and contrast is injected to confirm the needle's position. Still using fluoroscopic guidance, a guidewire is advanced through the needle and positions the retention sutures. The physician removes the needle and clamps the sutures. A dilator is introduced over the wire, followed by an appropriately sized catheter. The catheter is locked and the physician confirms placement with contrast. The locked portion of the catheter is pulled against the cecum's anterior wall, where the retention sutures are anchored. Antiseptic ointment and sterile dressings are applied. This code includes image documentation and report.

49446

The physician converts a gastrostomy tube to a gastrojejunostomy tube via percutaneous (under the skin) approach using fluoroscopic guidance. Following administration of any necessary sedation and contrast materials, the physician advances a jejunostomy tube through the previously placed gastrostomy tube into

Digestive

the proximal jejunum. This code includes contrast injections, image documentation, and report.

49450

The physician replaces an existing gastrostomy, cecostomy, or other colonic tube via percutaneous (under the skin) approach using fluoroscopic guidance and contrast monitoring. The existing tube is removed and the replacement is placed percutaneously via the existing tract. Contrast injection allows for correct positioning to be visualized with fluoroscopic images displayed on a screen. In order for this code to be reported, the new tube must be placed via the existing percutaneous access site. This procedure includes contrast injection, image documentation, and report.

49451

The physician replaces an existing duodenostomy or jejunostomy tube via percutaneous (under the skin) approach using fluoroscopic guidance and contrast monitoring. The existing tube is removed and the replacement is placed percutaneously through the abdominal wall via the existing tract. Contrast injection allows for correct positioning to be visualized with fluoroscopic images displayed on a screen. In order for this code to be reported, the new tube must be placed via the existing percutaneous access site. This procedure includes contrast injection, image documentation, and report.

49452

The physician replaces an existing gastrojejunostomy tube via percutaneous (under the skin) approach using fluoroscopic guidance and contrast monitoring. The existing tube is removed and the replacement is placed percutaneously through the abdominal wall via the existing tract. Contrast injection allows for correct positioning to be visualized with fluoroscopic images displayed on a screen. In order for this code to be reported, the new tube must be placed via the existing percutaneous access site. This procedure includes contrast injection, image documentation, and report.

49460

The physician mechanically removes obstructive material from an existing tube (gastrostomy, duodenostomy, jejunostomy, gastrojejunostomy, or cecostomy) by any method. Fluoroscopic guidance and contrast imaging may be utilized. This procedure includes image documentation and report.

49465

The physician injects contrast via a percutaneous approach for the radiological evaluation of existing tubes (gastrostomy, duodenostomy, jejunostomy, gastrojejunostomy, or cecostomy). Image documentation and report are included in this procedure.

49491-49492

The physician repairs an initial, reducible, inguinal hernia in a preterm infant (less than 37 weeks gestation at birth), performed up to 50 weeks postconceptual age, with or without hydrocelectomy. The physician dissects in the preperitoneal plane to present the hernia ring. The physician applies manual pressure to the inguinal region from outside while trying to dissect the hernia sac to reduce the hernia. If that fails, which can occur when there is a discrepancy in size of the hernia compared to its contents, the physician enlarges the hernia ring by an electrocautery incision in a ventral direction. The incision is made in a ventromedial direction for medial hernias and a ventrolateral direction for lateral hernias. The hernia is reduced using pleural insufflation of carbon dioxide. If a hydrocele is present, it is incised and drained. The hernia defect is repaired by suture and reinforced by staples or mesh. Report 49492 if, in the case of an incarcerated or strangulated hernia, the physician empties the contents of the hernia sac, places the contents in the lower abdomen, and repairs the hernia defect by suture.

49495-49496

The physician repairs an initial, reducible, inguinal hernia in a full-term infant under age 6 months, or a preterm infant over 50 weeks postconceptual age and under 6 months at the time of surgery, with or without hydrocelectomy. The physician dissects in the preperitoneal plane to present the hernia ring. The physician applies manual pressure to the inguinal region from outside while trying to dissect the hernia sac to reduce the hernia. If that fails, which can occur when there is a discrepancy in size of the hernia compared to its contents, the physician enlarges the hernia ring by an electrocautery incision in a ventral direction. The incision is made in a ventromedial direction for medial hernias and a ventrolateral direction for lateral hernias. The hernia is reduced using pleural insufflation of carbon dioxide. If a hydrocele is present, it is incised and drained. The hernia defect is repaired by suture and reinforced by staples or mesh. Report 49496 if, in the case of an incarcerated or strangulated hernia, the physician empties the contents of the hernia sac, places the contents in the lower abdomen, and repairs the hernia defect by suture.

49500

The physician repairs an inguinal hernia in a child between six months and 5 years of age. The physician makes a groin incision. The hernia sac is identified and dissected free of surrounding structures. The hernia sac is ligated and resected. If a hydrocele is present it is incised and drained. The groin incision is closed.

49501

The physician repairs an incarcerated inguinal hernia in a child between six months and 5 years of age. The physician makes a groin incision. The hernia sac is identified and dissected free of surrounding structures. The hernia sac is opened and the contents of the sac are examined. If the hernia contents are viable the hernia is reduced and the sac ligated and resected. If a hydrocele is present it is incised and drained. The groin incision is closed.

49505
The physician repairs an inguinal hernia in a patient age 5 or over. The physician makes a groin incision. The hernia sac is identified and dissected free from surrounding structures. The hernia sac is ligated and resected. The groin incision is closed.

49507
The physician repairs an incarcerated inguinal hernia in a patient over the age of 5 years. The physician makes a groin incision. The hernia sac is identified and dissected free from surrounding structures. The hernia sac is opened and the contents of the sac are examined. If the contents of the hernia are viable the hernia is reduced and the hernia sac is ligated and resected. The groin incision is closed.

49520
The physician repairs a recurrent inguinal hernia. The physician makes a groin incision. Dissection is continued through scar tissue and the spermatic cord and the hernia sac are identified and dissected from surrounding structures. The hernia sac may be ligated and resected. The incision is closed.

49521
The physician repairs an incarcerated recurrent inguinal hernia. The physician makes a groin incision. Dissection is continued through scar tissue and the spermatic cord and hernia sac is identified and dissected from surrounding structures. The hernia sac is opened and the contents of the sac are examined. If the contents of the hernia are viable the hernia is reduced and the hernia sac may be ligated and resected. The incision is closed.

49525
The physician repairs a sliding inguinal hernia. The physician makes a groin incision. The hernia sac is identified and dissected from surrounding structures. The hernia sac is opened and the abdominal viscera attached to the sac are dissected away from the sac if possible. The hernia contents are reduced and the hernia sac is closed and a portion of the sac may be resected. The incision is closed.

49540
The physician repairs a lumbar hernia. The physician makes an incision posteriorly over the hernia. The hernia sac is identified and dissected from surrounding structures to expose the fascial defect. The hernia is reduced and the hernia sac may be resected. The fascial defect is closed with sutures. The incision is closed.

49550
The physician repairs a femoral hernia. The physician makes a femoral or groin incision. The hernia sac is identified and dissected from surrounding structures. The femoral defect is closed with a prosthetic patch or sutures by plicating the fascia and muscles to cover the defect. The incision is closed.

49553
The physician repairs an incarcerated femoral hernia. The physician makes a groin or femoral incision. The hernia sac is identified and dissected from surrounding structures. The hernia sac is opened and the contents of the sac are examined. If the contents of the hernia are viable the hernia is reduced and the hernia sac is closed and may be resected. The femoral defect is closed with sutures by plicating the fascia and muscles to cover the defect. The incision is closed.

49555
The physician repairs a recurrent femoral hernia. The physician makes a groin or femoral incision. Dissection is continued through scar tissue and the hernia sac is identified and dissected from surrounding structures. The hernia sac is reduced and may be resected. The femoral defect is closed with sutures by plicating the fascia and muscles to cover the defect. The incision is closed.

49557
The physician repairs an incarcerated recurrent femoral hernia. The physician makes a groin or femoral incision. Dissection is continued through scar tissue and the hernia sac is identified and dissected from surrounding structures. The hernia sac is opened and the contents of the sac are examined. If the hernia contents are viable the hernia is reduced and the hernia sac is closed and may be resected. The femoral defect is closed with sutures by plicating fascia and muscle to cover the defect. The incision is closed.

49591-49596
The physician performs an initial repair of a reducible, incarcerated, or strangulated anterior abdominal hernia (epigastric, incisional, ventral, umbilical, or spigelian) using an open, laparoscopic, or robotic approach. If utilizing a laparoscopic approach, the physician places a trocar at the umbilicus and insufflates the abdominal or retroperitoneal cavity. The laparoscope is placed through the umbilical port and additional trocars are placed into the peritoneal or retroperitoneal space. The hernia sac is identified and reduced into the abdominal cavity. A sheet of mesh is often placed into the abdominal or retroperitoneal cavity and stapled into place on the pubis and abdominal wall covering the hernial defect. The trocars are removed, and the incisions are closed. Robotic assistance may also be utilized. This technique likewise employs a laparoscope, but the surgeon is positioned at a console in the surgical suite and manipulates the surgical instruments from the console. If performed via open approach, the physician makes an incision over the hernia and dissection is continued through scar tissue. The hernia sac is identified and dissected from surrounding structures. The fascial defect is identified circumferentially. The hernia is reduced, and the hernia sac may be resected. The hernia defect is closed with sutures and the incision is closed. If incarcerated or strangulated, the hernia sac is opened, and the contents of the hernia sac are examined. If the contents of the hernia sac are viable, the hernia is

reduced and the hernia sac may be resected. The hernia defect is closed with sutures and the incision is closed. These codes include the insertion of mesh, when performed. Report 49591 for repair of a reducible hernia that is less than 3 cm and 49592 if the hernia is incarcerated or strangulated. Report 49593 for a reducible hernia that is 3 to 10 cm and 49594 if incarcerated or strangulated. Report 49595 for a reducible hernia greater than 10 cm and 49596 if incarcerated or strangulated.

[49613, 49614, 49615, 49616, 49617, 49618]
The physician performs repair of a recurrent reducible, incarcerated, or strangulated anterior abdominal hernia (epigastric, incisional, ventral, umbilical, or spigelian) using an open, laparoscopic, or robotic approach. If utilizing a laparoscopic approach, the physician places a trocar at the umbilicus and insufflates the abdominal or retroperitoneal cavity. The laparoscope is placed through the umbilical port and additional trocars are placed into the peritoneal or retroperitoneal space. The hernia sac is identified and reduced into the abdominal cavity. A sheet of mesh is often placed into the abdominal or retroperitoneal cavity and stapled into place on the pubis and abdominal wall covering the hernial defect. The trocars are removed, and the incisions are closed. Robotic assistance may also be utilized. This technique likewise employs a laparoscope, but the surgeon is positioned at a console in the surgical suite and manipulates the surgical instruments from the console. If performed via open approach, the physician makes an incision over the hernia. Dissection is continued through scar tissue and the hernia sac is identified and dissected from surrounding structures. The fascial defect is identified circumferentially. The hernia is reduced, and the sac may be resected. The hernia defect is closed with sutures and the incision is closed. If incarcerated or strangulated, the hernia sac is opened, and the contents of the hernia sac are examined. If the contents of the hernia sac are viable, the hernia is reduced, and the hernia sac is closed and may be resected. The hernia defect is closed with sutures and the incision is closed. These codes include the insertion of mesh, when performed. Report 49613 for repair of a recurrent reducible hernia that is less than 3 cm and 49614 if the hernia is incarcerated or strangulated. Report 49615 for a reducible hernia that is 3 to 10 cm and 49616 if incarcerated or strangulated. Report 49617 for a reducible hernia greater than 10 cm and 49618 if incarcerated or strangulated.

[49621, 49622]
The physician performs repair of a reducible, incarcerated, or strangulated parastomal hernia, either initial or recurrent, using an open, laparoscopic, or robotic approach. If utilizing a laparoscopic approach, the physician places a trocar at the umbilicus and insufflates the abdominal or retroperitoneal cavity. The laparoscope is placed through the umbilical port and additional trocars are placed into the peritoneal or retroperitoneal space. Dissection is continued through scar tissue and the hernia is identified and reduced. The fascia is reapproximated. The defect is repaired with sutures, mesh, or by relocating the stoma to another site on the abdominal wall. The sac may be resected. The trocars are removed, and the incisions are closed. Robotic assistance may also be utilized. This technique likewise employs a laparoscope, but the surgeon is positioned at a console in the surgical suite and manipulates the surgical instruments from the console. In one open approach method, the physician performs a laparotomy, reduces the hernia, resects the sac, and reduces the stoma trephine to an appropriate size. The opening to the ostomy is covered with prosthetic mesh placed intraperitoneally and then sutured to the fascia. All codes include the insertion of mesh, when performed. Report 49621 for repair of a reducible parastomal hernia; report 49622 if incarcerated or strangulated.

[49623]
At the time of an initial or recurrent parastomal or anterior abdominal hernia repair employing an open, laparoscopic, or robotic approach, the physician performs total or near total removal of a previously placed, noninfected prosthetic material or mesh. In the open approach, the skin is incised and the tissue dissected, exposing the prosthetic material. Debridement of the tissue adjacent to or incorporated in the mesh may be performed with instruments or irrigation.

49600
The physician repairs a small omphalocele. The physician identifies the omphalocele and dissects the peritoneal sac from the umbilicus and the abdominal wall defect. The peritoneal sac is reduced and the abdominal wall defect is closed with sutures. The umbilicus is reconstructed and the skin is loosely closed.

49605
The physician repairs a large omphalocele or gastroschisis. The peritoneal sac of the omphalocele is dissected from the umbilicus and surrounding structures and reduced or the herniated contents of the gastroschisis are reduced into the abdominal cavity if possible. The abdominal wall defect is identified. If possible the abdominal wall defect is closed with sutures and the umbilicus is reconstructed. If the defect is too large or if the herniated contents cannot be reduced a prosthetic material is used to create a patch or silo that is sutured over the defect to close the defect and accommodate the herniated contents.

49606
The physician removes a previously placed prosthesis and closes an omphalocele or gastroschisis. The physician removes the previously placed prosthetic material covering the abdominal wall defect. The herniated contents are reduced and the edges of the defect are identified. The abdominal wall defect is closed with sutures. The umbilicus is reconstructed with skin flaps if possible. The remainder of the skin incision is usually left open to allow drainage.

49610

The physician performs the first stage of an omphalocele repair (Gross type operation). The physician identifies the omphalocele. Skin flaps are widely mobilized around the omphalocele and the skin flaps are closed over the intact omphalocele with sutures. The abdominal wall defect is not addressed.

49611

The physician performs the second stage of an omphalocele repair (Gross type operation). The physician makes an incision in the previously closed skin over the omphalocele. Skin flaps are mobilized off the omphalocele and the peritoneal sac of the omphalocele is dissected from the abdominal wall defect. The abdominal wall defect is closed with sutures. The skin flaps are closed over the repair thus closing the incision.

49650-49651

The physician performs laparoscopic repair of an initial (49650) or recurrent (49651) inguinal hernia. The physician places a trocar at the umbilicus and insufflates the abdominal or retroperitoneal cavity. The laparoscope is placed through the umbilical port and additional trocars are placed into the peritoneal or retroperitoneal space. The hernia sac is identified and reduced into the abdominal cavity. A sheet of mesh is placed into the abdominal or retroperitoneal cavity and stapled into place on the pubis and abdominal wall covering the hernial defect. The trocars are removed, and the incisions are closed.

49900

The physician performs a secondary closure of the abdominal wall for dehiscence or evisceration. The physician completely opens the former incision and removes the remaining sutures. Necrotic fascia is debrided to viable tissue. Any eviscerated abdominal contents are reduced into the abdominal cavity. The abdominal wall is closed with sutures.

49904-49906

The physician mobilizes an omental flap for reconstruction of a defect. The surgical recipient site of the flap is prepared. An upper abdominal transverse or midline incision is made. A laparotomy and manual exploration of the abdominal cavity is done first and the omentum and transverse colon are delivered from the cavity. The omentum is dissected from the transverse colon from left to right and small vessels are ligated. When completely separated from the transverse colon, the omentum is dissected from the stomach with careful clamping, division, and ligation of vessels. The omentum is fully mobilized and pedicled on the right or left gastroepiploic vessel, depending on the purpose. More incisions and tunneling may be necessary to bring the flap into its new location to fill a defect. The flap may be used as a pedicled transposition flap or a free microvascular transfer flap. Report 49904 when the flap is transpositioned to repair an extra-abdominal defect, such as chest wounds after radiation and mastectomy or lower extremity trauma wounds. Report 49905 when the omental flap is repositioned to repair a defect intra-abdominally. Report 49906 when the omentum is used as a free vascularized transfer flap to repair defects such as hemifacial atrophy. Microvascular anastomosis is performed to maintain blood flow to the omental flap. The abdominal incision is closed. If a separate split-thickness skin graft is required for omental coverage, it is done immediately and applied directly over the omentum and a dressing is applied.

Urinary

50010

The physician examines the kidney and renal pelvis. To access the kidney, the physician makes an incision in the skin of the flank, cuts the muscles, fat, and fibrous membranes (fascia) overlying the kidney, and sometimes removes a portion of the eleventh or twelfth rib. The physician clears away the fatty tissue surrounding the kidney, explores the area, and performs a layered closure.

50020

The physician drains an infection (abscess) on the kidney or on the surrounding renal tissue in an open procedure. To access the renal or perirenal abscess, the physician makes a small incision in the skin of the flank, cuts the muscles, fat, and fibrous membranes (fascia) overlying the kidney, and sometimes removes a portion of the eleventh or twelfth rib. After exploring the abscess cavity, the physician irrigates the site, inserts multiple drain tubes through separate stab wounds, and sutures the drain tube ends to the skin. The physician packs the wound with gauze and sutures the fascia and muscles. The skin and subcutaneous tissue are usually left open to prevent formation of a secondary body wall abscess. The drainage catheters are later removed.

50040

The physician creates an opening from the kidney to the exterior of the body by making an incision in the kidney. To access the kidney, the physician makes an incision in the skin of the flank, cuts the muscles, fat, and fibrous membranes (fascia) overlying the kidney, and sometimes removes a portion of the eleventh or twelfth rib. Using an incision to open the renal pelvis (pyelotomy), the physician passes a curved clamp into the renal pelvis, a middle or lower minor calyx, and the cortex of the kidney. The physician inserts a catheter tip through the same path as the clamp, and passes the tube through a stab incision in the skin of the flank. After suturing the incisions, the physician inserts a drain tube, bringing it out through a separate stab incision, and performs a layered closure.

50045

The physician makes a small incision in the kidney to explore the interior of the kidney. To access the kidney, the physician makes an incision in the skin of the flank, cuts the muscles, fat, and fibrous membranes (fascia) overlying the kidney, and sometimes removes a portion of the eleventh or twelfth rib. The physician makes an incision in the kidney (nephrotomy) and sometimes places fine traction sutures at the edges of the incision. After exploration, the physician sutures the incision, inserts a drain tube, bringing it out through a separate stab incision, and performs a layered closure.

50060-50070
The physician removes a kidney stone (calculus) by making an incision in the kidney. To access the calculus, the physician makes an incision in the skin of the flank, cuts the muscles, fat, and fibrous membranes (fascia) overlying the kidney, and sometimes removes a portion of the eleventh or twelfth rib. The physician isolates the calculus and removes it through an incision. After examining the kidney for other defects, the physician sutures the incision, inserts a drain tube, bringing it out through a separate stab incision, and performs a layered closure. Simple removal of the calculus by nephrotomy is reported with 50060. Report 50065 when a previous surgery on the kidney complicates the procedure. Report 50070 if the procedure is complicated because of a congenital kidney abnormality, wherein the physician usually repairs any calyces that are obstructed or abnormally narrowed.

50075
The physician removes a stone that fills the calyces and renal pelvis (staghorn calculus) by making incisions in the kidney and renal pelvis. To access the staghorn calculus, the physician makes an incision in the skin of the flank, cuts the muscles, fat, and fibrous membranes (fascia) overlying the kidney, and sometimes removes a portion of the twelfth rib. After isolating the staghorn calculus, the physician makes an incision in the renal pelvis (pyelotomy) and may make an incision in the kidney (nephrotomy). The physician removes the staghorn calculus, irrigates the area, and examines the kidney for other defects. After closing the incisions, the physician inserts a drain tube and performs a layered closure.

50080-50081
The physician creates a percutaneous passageway to remove kidney stones (nephrolithotomy) or renal pelvic stones (pyelolithotomy). The physician makes a small incision in the skin of the back, inserts a large needle, and radiologically guides it toward the kidney or renal pelvis. After passing a guidewire through the needle, the physician dilates the passageway by inserting and removing tubes with increasingly larger diameters. The physician inserts an endoscope over the guidewire and passes an instrument through the endoscope to crush (lithotripsy) or extract calculi. A ureteral stent may be passed from the pelvis into the bladder. The physician removes the guidewire and allows the passageway to seal on its own or inserts a nephrotomy or pyelostomy tube before removing the guidewire. Report 50080 for simple stones (up to 2 cm) that are nonbranching and/or exist in a single location in the kidney or renal pelvis. Report 50081 for complex stones greater than 2 cm, such as those that block more than one branch of the collecting system, stones in the ureter, or stones in multiple locations. These codes include imaging guidance, antegrade stent placement, and antegrade ureteroscopy (direct visualization of ureteral strictures when strictures are dilated via catheter), when performed. Note that these codes may be reported only once per side.

50100
The physician corrects an obstruction by cutting across or repositioning renal vessels that deviate from proper anatomical placement. To access the kidney, the physician makes an incision in the skin of the flank, cuts the muscles, fat, and fibrous membranes (fascia) overlying the kidney, and sometimes removes a portion of the twelfth rib. After repositioning the aberrant vessels to a more functional anatomic placement, the physician performs a layered closure.

50120
The physician makes an incision in the renal pelvis to explore the calyces and renal pelvis. To access the kidney, the physician makes an incision in the skin of the flank, cuts the muscles, fat, and fibrous membranes (fascia) overlying the kidney, and sometimes removes a portion of the eleventh or twelfth rib. The physician makes an incision in the renal pelvis (pyelotomy). The physician may place fine traction sutures at the edges of the pyelotomy while exploring the calyces and renal pelvis. After closing the pyelotomy, the physician inserts a drain tube, bringing it out through a separate stab incision, and performs a layered closure.

50125
The physician makes an incision in the renal pelvis to insert a pyelostomy tube for drainage. To access the kidney, the physician makes an incision in the skin of the flank, cuts the muscles, fat, and fibrous membranes (fascia) overlying the kidney, and sometimes removes a portion of the eleventh or twelfth rib. After exposing the renal pelvis, the physician makes an incision in the renal pelvis (pyelotomy). The physician inserts the tip of a catheter into the renal pelvis and passes the tube out through a stab incision in the skin of the flank. The physician performs a layered closure.

50130
The physician removes stones (calculi) or an insoluble mass (coagulum) from the renal pelvis by making an incision into the renal pelvis. To access the kidney, the physician makes an incision in the skin of the flank, cuts the muscles, fat, and fibrous membranes (fascia) overlying the kidney, and sometimes removes a portion of the eleventh or twelfth rib. The physician makes an incision in the renal pelvis (pyelotomy) to isolate and remove the calculus. The physician irrigates the area and examines the renal pelvis for other defects. The physician inserts a drain tube, bringing it out through a separate stab incision, and performs a layered closure.

50200
The physician extracts a plug of biopsy tissue from the kidney by inserting a needle or trocar in the skin of the

back. Using radiologic or ultrasonic guidance, the physician advances the instrument into the suspect tissue of the kidney. With the instrument's cutting sheath, the physician traps a specimen of renal tissue and removes the instrument. After repeating the process several times, the physician applies pressure to the puncture wound.

50205

The physician excises a specimen of biopsy tissue from the kidney through an incision. To access the kidney, the physician makes an incision in the skin of the flank and cuts the muscles, fat, and fibrous membranes (fascia) overlying the kidney. After excising a specimen of the diseased or damaged renal tissue, the physician sutures the incision and performs a layered closure.

50220-50225

The physician removes the kidney and upper portion of the ureter. To access the kidney and ureter, the physician usually makes an incision in the skin of the flank, cuts the muscles, fat, and fibrous membranes (fascia) overlying the kidney, and sometimes removes a portion of the eleventh or twelfth rib. After mobilizing the kidney and ureter, the physician clamps, ligates, and severs the upper ureter and major renal blood vessels (renal pedicle). The physician removes the kidney and upper ureter, but does not remove the adrenal gland, surrounding fatty tissue, or Gerota's fascia. After controlling bleeding, the physician irrigates the site with normal saline and places a drain tube, bringing it out through a separate stab incision in the skin. The physician removes the clamps and performs a layered closure. Report 50225 when a previous surgery on the kidney and/or ureter complicates the procedure.

50230

The physician removes the kidney, surrounding fat, Gerota's fascia, adrenal gland, periaortic lymph nodes, and upper ureter. To access the kidney and upper ureter, the physician usually makes an incision in the skin of the chest (transthoracic approach) or flank. After mobilizing the kidney and ureter, the physician clamps, ligates, and severs the upper ureter and major renal blood vessels (renal pedicle). The physician removes the kidney, upper ureter, neural and vascular structures at the apex of the renal pelvis, surrounding fat, Gerota's fascia, adrenal gland, and involved renal lymph nodes. The physician irrigates the site, places a drain tube, removes the clamps, and performs a layered closure. In a transthoracic approach, the lung is re-expanded and the chest tube left in.

50234

The physician removes the kidney, ureter, and small cuff of the bladder through one excision. To access the kidney and ureter, the physician usually makes an incision in the skin of the flank, cuts the muscles, fat, and fibrous membranes (fascia) overlying the kidney, and sometimes removes a portion of the eleventh or twelfth rib. After mobilizing the kidney, ureter, and bladder, the physician clamps, ligates, and severs the ureter, major renal blood vessels (renal pedicle), and a small cuff of the bladder. The physician pulls the kidney, ureter, and bladder cuff upward through the flank incision. The physician does not remove the adrenal gland, surrounding fatty tissue, or Gerota's fascia. After controlling bleeding, the physician irrigates the site with normal saline and places a drain tube, bringing it out through a separate stab incision in the skin. The physician sutures and catheterizes the bladder, removes the clamps, and performs a layered closure.

50236

The physician removes the kidney, ureter, and small cuff of the bladder through two incisions. To access the kidney and upper ureter, the physician usually makes an incision in the skin of the flank, cuts the muscles, fat, and fibrous membranes (fascia) overlying the kidney, and sometimes removes a portion of the eleventh or twelfth rib. After mobilizing the kidney and ureter, the physician isolates, clamps, ligates, and severs the upper ureter and major renal blood vessels (renal pedicle) and removes the kidney. The physician does not remove the adrenal gland, surrounding fatty tissue, or Gerota's fascia. After controlling bleeding, the physician irrigates the site with normal saline and places a drain tube, bringing it out through a separate stab incision in the skin. To access the lower ureter and bladder, the physician makes an incision in the skin of the abdomen. After mobilizing the bladder, the physician removes the lower ureter and a small cuff of the bladder. The physician sutures and catheterizes the bladder. After placing a drain tube behind the bladder, the physician removes the clamps and performs a layered closure.

50240

The physician removes a portion of the kidney. To access the kidney and ureter, the physician usually makes an incision in the skin of the flank, cuts the muscles, fat, and fibrous membranes (fascia) overlying the kidney, and sometimes removes a portion of the eleventh or twelfth rib. After mobilizing the kidney and the major renal blood vessels (renal pedicle), the physician clamps the renal vessels, and sometimes induces hypothermia of the kidney with iced saline slush. The physician excises a wedge containing the diseased or damaged kidney tissue. After clamping and ligating the exposed arteries and veins, the physician inserts a drain tube, bringing it out through a separate stab incision in the skin, removes the clamps, and performs a layered closure.

50250

The physician performs cryosurgical ablation of one or more renal mass lesions. The physician performs a laparotomy. Dissection is carried down to the kidney. Intraoperative ultrasound guidance and monitoring may be used to identify the lesion and monitor progress of the procedure. Cryosurgical probes are inserted into the kidney lesion. The cryosurgical probe delivers cryogen, a coolant, at subfreezing temperatures to freeze the lesion. The renal tissue is slowly thawed. A minimum of two cycles of freezing and thawing are performed. This is repeated for each lesion. When all lesions have been treated, the incision is closed with layered sutures.

50280-50290
The physician excises a cyst on the kidney or in the surrounding renal tissue. To access the kidney, the physician makes an incision in the skin of the flank, cuts the muscles, fat, and fibrous membranes (fascia) overlying the kidney, and sometimes removes a portion of the twelfth rib. After clearing away the fatty tissue surrounding the kidney, the physician excises the cyst from the renal surface. The physician destroys tiny vessels bordering the cyst with high-frequency electric current (fulguration) to minimize the need for sutures. If the cyst requires a deep excision, the physician usually sutures the renal tissue. The physician inserts a drain tube, bringing it out through a separate stab incision in the skin, and performs a layered closure. 50280 reports excision of a cyst (or cysts) on the kidney; 50290 reports excision of a cyst (or cysts) in the tissue surrounding the kidney.

50300
The physician performs a donor nephrectomy by removing the kidney and upper ureter from a cadaver for transplantation. To access the kidney and upper ureter, the physician usually makes a midline incision in the skin from the xiphoid process to the symphysis pubis. After cutting the muscles, fat, and fibrous membranes (fascia) overlying the kidney, the physician uses clamps, ties, suture ligatures, and electrocoagulation to control bleeding. Before clamping the major renal blood vessels (renal pedicle), the physician administers heparin sodium to prevent intravascular clotting. The physician dissects and removes the kidney, renal vessels, and ureter, usually removing sections of the inferior vena cava and aorta with both kidneys. The donor kidney is preserved for transplantation into the recipient. The organ remains under refrigeration, packed in a sealable container with some preserving solution and kept on ice in a suitable carrier.

50320
The physician performs an open donor nephrectomy from a living donor by removing one kidney and upper ureter for transplantation. To access the kidney, the physician usually makes an incision in the skin of the flank, cuts the muscles, fat, and fibrous membranes (fascia) overlying the kidney, and sometimes removes a portion of the eleventh or twelfth rib. After mobilizing the kidney and ureter, the physician administers an anticlogging agent. The physician clamps, ligates, and severs the upper ureter and major renal blood vessels (renal pedicle), and removes the kidney and upper ureter. The physician administers medication to reverse the effects of the anticlogging agent. After controlling bleeding, the physician irrigates the site, places a drain tube, and performs a layered closure. The donor kidney is preserved for transplantation into the recipient. The organ remains under refrigeration, packed in a sealable container with some preserving solution and kept on ice in a suitable carrier.

50323
The surgeon prepares a donor kidney from a cadaver prior to transplantation. Back table prep time is about an hour. The kidney and necessary vital structures removed en bloc usually contain some of the inferior vena cava, a cuff of aorta, perinephric tissue, the adrenal gland, and muscle, as well as some damaged blood vessels. The renal vein is dissected and the gonadal and adrenal veins are isolated and separated with ligatures. The renal artery is dissected from surrounding tissue along with the aortic patch. The adrenal gland, excess perinephric fat, and other tissue attachments are removed from the graft, taking care to leave fibrofatty tissue around the ureter to ensure its blood supply. The aortic patch, renal vein, and ureter are further repaired and/or modified to fit the recipient.

50325
The physician performs a standard backbench preparation of the kidney following procurement from a living donor. Backbench or back table preparation refers to procedures performed on the donor organ following procurement to prepare the donor organ for transplant. In a separately reportable procedure, the physician removes the kidney and upper ureter from a living donor. The kidney is flushed with a cold electrolyte solution to rinse any remaining donor blood from the kidney and lower its temperature. When the kidney is procured from a living donor, only minimal backbench preparation is required because most of the dissection is performed in situ during the nephrectomy. During the backbench preparation any excess perinephric fat and other tissue attachments are removed from the graft, taking care to leave fibrofatty tissue around the ureter to ensure its blood supply. Further separation of the renal artery or arteries from the renal veins is performed. The arterial and venous separation prevents the technical inconvenience of side-by-side anastomosis in the recipient. To reduce the risk of postoperative complications, the transplant ureter is shortened as needed leaving the vascularized periureteral fat intact. When all residual soft tissue has been removed and the blood vessels and ureters prepared, the kidney is ready for transplant.

50327
The surgeon reconstructs a donor kidney from a cadaver or living donor prior to transplantation with a venous anastomosis. This procedure consists of performing venoplasties on the donor kidney to extend the renal vein before grafting. The inferior vena cava is used from a cadaver donor. When the donor organ comes from a living donor, a cuff of the inferior vena cava attached to the renal vein is used. When the donor organ comes from a cadaveric source, the external iliac vein is also routinely procured and prepared for venous grafting to extend the renal vein for the recipient. The vessels are tested for patency by flushing with a preservation solution.

50328
The surgeon performs arterial anastomosis reconstruction of a donor kidney from a cadaver or living donor prior to transplantation. The allograft is prepared with multiple renal arteries. When the donor organ comes from a cadaveric source, the aortic patch removed with the specimen is used for creating a viable renal artery graft for transplantation. Donor iliac arteries are routinely procured from cadaveric donors to be prepared and used as arterial grafting material. The segmental renal artery may also be anastomosed to the inferior epigastric artery when an aortic patch is not available, such as when the donor kidney is from a living donor. The vessels are tested for patency by flushing with a preservation solution.

50329
The physician performs a standard backbench reconstruction of the ureter following renal allograft procurement from a cadaver or living donor. Backbench or back table preparation refers to procedures performed on the donor organ following procurement to prepare the donor organ for transplant. In a separately reportable procedure, the physician removes the kidney en bloc from a cadaver donor or the kidney and upper ureter from a living donor. The kidney is flushed with a cold electrolyte solution to rinse any remaining donor blood from the kidney and lower its temperature. After preparing the kidney and blood vessels in a separately reportable procedure, the physician turns his attention to any required ureteral anastomosis. Ureteral anastomosis is generally required when anatomic variations are present in the donor organ. Anatomic variations for kidney donors include multiple ureters. When two or more ureters are present, the ureters may be separately implanted into the bladder or a side-to-side anastomosis of the ureters may be performed during the backbench preparation prior to implantation into the bladder. Code 50329 is reported when side-to-side anastomosis is performed and is reported for each anastomosis.

50340
The physician removes the kidney and the upper portion of the ureter in a patient who is to receive a kidney transplant. To access the kidney and ureter, the physician usually makes an incision in the skin of the flank, cuts the muscles, fat, and fibrous membranes (fascia) overlying the kidney, and sometimes removes a portion of the eleventh or twelfth rib. After mobilizing the kidney and ureter, the physician clamps, ligates, and severs the upper ureter and major renal blood vessels (renal pedicle). The physician removes the kidney and upper ureter, but does not remove the adrenal gland, surrounding fatty tissue, or Gerota's fascia. After controlling bleeding, the physician irrigates the site with normal saline and places a drain tube, bringing it out through a separate stab incision in the skin. The physician performs a layered closure.

50360
The physician surgically implants a human kidney and ureter from a living donor or cadaver into a transplant patient, without performing a concurrent nephrectomy on the recipient. To access the transplant site, the physician usually makes a curved, right or left lower quadrant incision in the skin. After cutting the muscles, fat, and fibrous membranes (fascia), the physician controls bleeding with clamps, ties, and electrocoagulation. The physician surgically connects the renal vein and artery of the donor kidney to the recipient's clamped and dissected internal iliac vein and hypogastric artery. After removing the clamps, the physician checks for leakage, bleeding, and insufficient blood supply. To implant the donor ureter, the physician makes an incision into the bladder and passes the ureter through the bladder. The physician sutures the ureter as well as the opening in the bladder (cystotomy). The physician performs a layered closure. The drain tube may be left in.

50365
The physician implants a donor kidney and upper ureter after removing the recipient's kidney and upper ureter. To access the recipient's kidney and ureter, the physician usually makes an incision in the skin of the flank, cuts the muscles, fat, and fibrous membranes (fascia) overlying the kidney, and sometimes removes a portion of the eleventh or twelfth rib. The physician clamps, ligates, and severs the upper ureter and major renal blood vessels (renal pedicle), and removes the kidney and upper ureter. To implant the donor kidney and upper ureter, the physician usually makes a curved lower quadrant incision in the skin. The physician surgically connects the renal vein and artery of the donor kidney to the recipient's clamped and dissected internal iliac vein and hypogastric artery. After incising the bladder, the physician passes the donor ureter through the bladder and sutures the ureter and opening in the bladder (cystotomy). The physician performs a layered closure. The drain tube may be left in.

50370
The physician removes a transplanted donor kidney from the recipient. To access the rejected kidney, the physician usually reopens the original kidney transplant incision, and cuts the muscles, fat, and fibrous membranes (fascia) overlying the kidney. After mobilizing the kidney, the physician clamps, ligates, and severs the major renal blood vessels (renal pedicle). The physician removes the rejected kidney. After controlling bleeding, the physician irrigates the site with normal saline. The physician may place a drain tube, bringing it out through a separate stab incision in the skin. After removing the clamps, the physician performs a layered closure.

50380
The physician moves the kidney from its original anatomic site and revascularizes the kidney by connecting the renal and iliac vessels to a new site. To access the transplant site, the physician usually makes

a midline transabdominal incision in the skin and cuts the muscles, fat, and fibrous membranes (fascia). After exposing the kidney, the physician clamps, ligates, and severs the renal vessels, keeping the ureter intact. The physician flushes the kidney with cold, anticoagulant electrolyte solution, and surgically connects the renal vessels to another appropriate arterial and venous site. The physician removes the clamps and checks for leakage, bleeding, and infarction. After placing a drain tube and bringing it out through a separate stab incision in the skin, the physician removes the clamps and performs a layered closure.

50382-50384

The physician percutaneously removes an internally dwelling ureteral stent through the renal pelvis in 50384. With the patient under moderate sedation, a long, thin needle is advanced into the renal calyx under imaging guidance and the position is confirmed with contrast and fluoroscopy. A guidewire is threaded over the needle into the renal pelvis, the needle is removed, and a sheath placed over the guidewire. A snare device is threaded through the sheath into position, the indwelling stent is grasped, and pulled out partially through the sheath until the proximal end is outside the ureter. A guidewire is threaded through the stent, which is guided completely out. In 50382, the physician replaces the indwelling ureteral stent after removal of the old stent. The guidewire is left in place, the length of the old stent is noted, and the replacement stent is advanced into the ureter until the distal end is in the bladder and the distal loop is deployed. Stent position is confirmed with the proximal loop in the renal pelvis. The instruments are removed.

50385-50386

Using snare or capture, the physician removes (50386) or removes and replaces (50385) an internally dwelling ureteral stent (a thin, flexible tube that is inserted into the ureter to assist in the drainage of urine from the kidney). In one method, under appropriate sedation and sonographic guidance, a rigid biopsy forceps is introduced through the urethra, advanced to the urinary bladder, and the stent is grasped and removed. These codes are appropriate only when the procedure is performed via a transurethral approach, without the use of cystoscopy. Radiological supervision and interpretation is included and should not be reported separately.

50387

The physician removes and replaces an externally accessible nephroureteral catheter under fluoroscopic guidance. A nephroureteral catheter is placed within the renal collecting system, through the renal pelvis and into the bladder; the other end remains outside the body for drainage. Contrast may be injected at the entry site to assess anatomy and positioning. The suture holding the pigtail in place is cut and a guidewire is threaded through the stent lumen until it exits the distal end. The original stent is removed over the guidewire. Diameter and length are noted for a new stent, which is threaded over the guidewire until the distal end forms within the bladder. Fluoroscopy is used to assess the proximal position of formation within the renal pelvis. After position is verified, the guidewire is removed and the suture is put in position to hold the pigtail in place. Contrast may be injected to check position and function. Final adjustments are made for patient comfort, and the catheter may be sutured to the skin, capped, or a drainage bag may be attached.

50389

The physician removes an indwelling nephrostomy tube under fluoroscopic guidance that was previously placed concurrently with an indwelling ureteral stent. Nephrostomy tube removal may be done to avoid displacement of the stent. Contrast may first be injected through the indwelling catheter tube to verify placement and functioning of the stent. The suture holding the pigtail in place is cut and a guidewire is threaded through the nephrostomy tube under fluoroscopy, making certain that the pigtail or suture do not hook the stent and that the stent remains in proper position. The nephrostomy tube is pulled out over the guidewire, stent position is checked again, and the access site is dressed.

50390

The physician inserts a needle through the skin to inject or drain fluid from the renal pelvis or a renal cyst. The physician usually inserts a long, thin needle in the skin of the back. Using radiologic guidance, the physician advances the needle toward the renal pelvis or renal cyst and injects or drains fluid.

50391

The physician instills a therapeutic agent, such as an anticarcinogenic or an antifungal, through the tube of an established opening between the skin and kidney (nephrostomy), renal pelvis (pyelostomy), or ureter (ureterostomy). This type of intracavitary topical therapy is reliably done through a tube left in place following a previous surgery. After inserting a guidewire, an endoscope or flexible delivery catheter is passed through the tube into the kidney, renal pelvis, or ureter. To better view renal and ureteric structures, the physician may flush (irrigate) or introduce by drops (instillate) a saline solution. The physician introduces the therapeutic agent to the target area. After examination, the physician removes the instruments and reinserts the nephrostomy, pyelostomy, or ureterostomy tube or allows the surgical passageway to seal on its own.

[50436, 50437]

A guide is inserted into the renal pelvis and/or ureter to enlarge the passageway between the skin and kidney. The physician makes a small incision in the skin of the back, inserts a large needle, and ultrasonographically guides it toward the kidney. After passing a guidewire through the needle and through the kidney into the renal pelvis, the physician removes the needle by passing it backward over the guidewire. The physician enlarges (dilates) the guidewire passageway by inserting and removing tubes with increasingly larger diameters. When the passageway is sufficiently dilated, the physician passes a nephrostomy tube over the guidewire, removes the guidewire, and sutures the tube to the skin. All imaging (e.g., radiologic supervision and interpretation) is included and should not be reported separately. Report 50436 when the physician enlarges an existing percutaneous nephrostomy tract and inserts a needle into the renal collecting system to allow for the introduction of large instruments to be utilized in an endoscopic urologic procedure. Report 50437 when the physician creates new access into the renal collecting system during the same operative session in an area where a pre-existing tract was not present.

50396

The physician connects an indwelling ureteral catheter or existing pyelostomy or nephrostomy tube to a manometer line to measure pressure and flow in the kidneys and ureters. The physician connects a ureteral catheter or pyelostomy or nephrostomy tube to a manometer line filled with fluid. The physician inserts a bladder catheter that may be irrigated. The physician measures intrarenal and/or extrarenal pressure. After discontinuing perfusion of fluid, the physician aspirates residual fluid from the kidney and disconnects the manometer line. The physician may remove the ureteral catheter or pyelostomy or nephrostomy tube and dress the wound.

[50430, 50431]

The physician injects a contrast agent through a tube or indwelling catheter into the renal pelvis to study the kidney and renal collecting system. The physician determines immediate allergic response to the contrast agent by injecting a small initial dose of contrast material through an existing nephrostomy tube or indwelling ureteral catheter. If no allergic response occurs, a large quantity of contrast material is injected into the renal pelvis. The contrast is visualized as it passes from the kidneys into the ureters and the urinary bladder. Imaging guidance via fluoroscopy or ultrasound is used to observe the contrast path. When an obstruction is present, it can be readily identified on imaging because the contrast is unable to progress properly through the urinary tract. The radiologist produces a representation of the kidney, renal pelvis, and/or ureter with an x-ray. Report 50431 when this test is performed through an existing access.

[50432, 50433]

The physician inserts a catheter through the skin and into the kidney for drainage of urine and/or for an injection. With the patient lying face down and the puncture site having been identified, a local anesthetic is injected. A needle with a guidewire is slowly advanced into the kidney under fluoroscopic guidance. The needle is removed when urine flows back through and, if necessary, the tract may be dilated to accommodate the catheter or nephrostomy tube, which is advanced over the needle, and the needle is removed. The catheter or nephrostomy tube is fixed in place and secured on the skin with a drainage bag attached. These codes include diagnostic nephrostogram and ureterogram, imaging guidance, and all radiological supervision and interpretation. Report 50433 for placement of a nephroureteral catheter via a new access.

[50434]

A previously placed nephrostomy catheter is converted to a nephroureteral catheter via percutaneous approach along the current nephrostomy tract. The patient is placed face down and the conversion is performed over a stiff wire. Contrast is injected through the catheter to better visualize the kidneys and ureter. The wire is advanced and the catheter is replaced over the wire and the wire removed. Imaging guidance assures proper placement and the new catheter is secured to the skin with sutures. This procedure includes diagnostic nephrostogram and/or ureterogram, imaging guidance, and all radiological supervision and interpretation.

[50435]

The provider changes a nephrostomy catheter by replacing the existing tube. Sutures holding an existing tube in place are removed. A guidewire is inserted through the tube and pulls the tube back out over the wire. A new tube is threaded over the wire until proper placement is achieved. The wire is removed and the new catheter is sutured to the skin. This procedure includes diagnostic nephrostogram and/or ureterogram, imaging guidance, and all radiological supervision and interpretation.

50400-50405

The physician uses plastic surgery to correct an obstruction or defect in the renal pelvis or ureteropelvic junction. To access the renal pelvis and ureter, the physician usually makes an incision in the skin of the flank. The physician incises, trims, and shapes the renal pelvis and ureter, using absorbable sutures or soft rubber drains for traction. The physician usually inserts a slender tube into the renal pelvis to provide support during healing. In Foley Y-pyeloplasty, the physician advances a Y-shaped flap of the renal pelvis into a vertical incision in the upper ureter. The physician may surgically fixate (nephropexy) a floating or mobile kidney, and/or establish an opening between the kidney (nephrostomy) or renal pelvis (pyelostomy) and the exterior of the body. The physician places a drain tube, bringing it out through a separate stab incision in the skin, and performs a layered closure. Report 50405 if a congenital abnormality, secondary pyeloplasty, solitary kidney, or calycoplasty complicates the procedure.

50500

The physician uses sutures to surgically fixate a wound or injury of the kidney. To access the kidney, the physician makes an incision in the skin of the flank, cuts the muscles, fat, and fibrous membranes (fascia) overlying the kidney, and sometimes removes a portion of the eleventh or twelfth rib. After using sutures to close or surgically fixate a kidney wound or injury, the physician places a drain tube, bringing it out through a separate stab incision in the skin, and performs a layered closure.

50520

The physician closes a fistula that is an abnormal opening between the skin and the kidney (nephrocutaneous) or the renal pelvis (pyelocutaneous). After excising the fistula, the physician sutures the clean percutaneous tissues together to create a smooth surface.

50525-50526

The physician closes a fistula that is an abnormal opening between the kidney and an organ of the digestive, respiratory, urogenital, or endocrine system. In 50525, the physician usually makes an incision in the abdomen, cuts the muscles, fat, and fibrous membranes (fascia) overlying the kidney to access the fistula. In 50526, the physician makes an incision in the skin of the chest, opens the chest cavity, collapses the lung, and separates the leaves of the diaphragm to expose the kidney. After excising the fistula, the physician sutures the clean tissues together to create a smooth surface. The physician places a drain tube, bringing it out through a separate stab incision in the skin, and performs a layered closure. In 50526, the physician inserts a chest tube to re-expand the lung.

50540

The physician divides an abnormal union of the kidneys to correct a horseshoe kidney. To access the horseshoe kidney, the physician usually makes an incision in the skin of the lower abdomen and cuts the muscles, fat, and fibrous membranes (fascia) overlying the kidney. After incising the union and placing two rows of sutures to control bleeding, the physician usually performs pyeloplasty or another plastic procedure on one or both sides of the divided kidney. After completion of repair, the physician may rotate the kidney to effect drainage. The physician irrigates the site with normal saline, places a drain tube, bringing it out through a separate stab incision in the skin, and performs a layered closure.

50541-50542

The physician performs a laparoscopic surgical ablation of renal cysts in 50541 or a renal mass lesion in 50542 through the abdomen or back. With the abdominal approach, an umbilical port is created by placing a trocar at the level of the umbilicus. The abdominal wall is insufflated. The laparoscope is placed through the umbilical port and additional trocars are placed into the abdominal cavity. In the back approach, the trocar is placed at the back proximate to the retroperitoneal space near to the kidney with additional ports placed nearby for appropriate access to the operative site. The physician uses the laparoscope fitted with a fiberoptic camera and/or an operating instrument. The renal cysts or lesions are visualized through the scope and are ablated by fulguration or another method that can be utilized endoscopically, such as cryotherapy or radiofrequency thermal coagulation. The instruments are removed and the abdominal or back incisions are closed by staples or sutures. Code 50542 includes intraoperative ultrasound guidance and monitoring, if performed.

50543

The physician performs a laparoscopic partial nephrectomy to treat small renal lesions or tumors. With an abdominal approach, an umbilical port is created by placing a trocar at the level of the umbilicus. The abdominal wall is insufflated. The laparoscope is placed through the umbilical port and additional trocars are placed into the abdominal cavity. In a back approach, the trocar is placed at the back proximate to the retroperitoneal space near to the kidney with additional ports placed nearby for appropriate access to the operative site. The physician uses the laparoscope fitted with a fiberoptic camera for direct vision and/or an operating instrument. Direct vision and the use of laparoscopic ultrasonography allow the physician to identify the tumors and assess the appropriate surgical margin that should be allowed. The diseased kidney tissue is removed with emphasis on hemostasis. Methods such as electrocautery, argon beam coagulator, topical agents, and microwave thermotherapy may be employed to help reduce bleeding during resection. Retrieval pouches used in endoscopic surgery allow removal of the tumor specimen without spilling. The instruments are removed and the abdominal or back incisions are closed by staples or sutures.

50544

The physician performs a laparoscopic pyeloplasty to correct an obstruction or defect in the renal pelvis or ureteropelvic junction through the abdomen or back. With the abdominal approach, an umbilical port is created by placing a trocar at the level of the umbilicus. The abdominal wall is insufflated. The laparoscope is placed through the umbilical port and additional trocars are placed into the abdominal cavity. In the back approach, the trocar is placed at the back proximate to the retroperitoneal space near to the kidney with additional ports placed nearby for appropriate access to the operative site. The physician uses the laparoscope fitted with a fiberoptic camera and/or an operating instrument. The physician incises, trims, and/or shapes the renal pelvis and ureter using absorbable sutures or soft rubber drains for traction. A tube is usually inserted to promote healing. The instruments are removed and abdominal or back incisions are closed by staples or sutures.

50545

The physician performs a radical nephrectomy, including removal of Gerota's fascia and surrounding fatty tissue, regional lymph nodes, and the adrenal gland through a laparoscope. The physician makes a 1 centimeter periumbilical incision and inserts a trocar. The abdominal cavity is insufflated with carbon dioxide. A fiberoptic laparoscope fitted with a camera and light source is inserted through the trocar. Other incisions (ports) are made in the abdomen or flank to allow other instruments or an additional light source to be passed into the abdomen or retroperitoneum. The colon is mobilized, and the laparoscope is advanced to the operative site. The ureter is transected at the ureterovesical junction. The physician clamps, ligates, and severs the renal vein and renal artery. The Gerota's fascia is dissected to expose the upper pole of the kidney. The adrenal gland is visualized. Clips are placed on the suprarenal vein and adrenal arteries (diaphragmatic [inferior phrenic], aortic, and renal) which are cut. Any lymph nodes in the surrounding area are excised and removed. The kidney, adrenal gland, renal (Gerota's) fascia, and surrounding fat are dissected free; they are bagged and removed through an enlarged port site. The instruments are removed. The incisions are closed with staples or suture.

50546
The physician removes the kidney and a portion of the ureter through a laparoscope. The physician makes a 1 cm periumbilical incision and inserts a trocar. The abdominal cavity is insufflated with carbon dioxide. A fiberoptic laparoscope fitted with a camera and light source is inserted through the trocar. Other incisions (ports) are made in the abdomen or flank to allow other instruments or an additional light source to be passed into the abdomen or retroperitoneum. The colon is mobilized and the laparoscope is advanced to the operative site. The physician mobilizes the kidney and clamps, ligates, and severs part of the ureter and major renal blood vessels (renal pedicle). The kidney and upper ureter are bagged and brought through one of the port sites (e.g., periumbilical) that has been slightly enlarged. The instruments are removed, and the small abdominal or flank incisions are closed with staples or suture.

50547
The physician performs a donor nephrectomy from a living donor by removing the kidney and upper portion of the ureter laparoscopically through the abdomen or back. With the abdominal approach, an umbilical port is created by placing a trocar at the level of the umbilicus. The abdominal wall is insufflated. The laparoscope is placed through the umbilical port and additional trocars are placed into the abdominal cavity. In the back approach, the trocar is placed at the back proximate to the retroperitoneal space near the kidney with additional ports placed nearby for appropriate access to the operative site. The physician uses the laparoscope fitted with a fiberoptic camera and/or operating instruments to explore the area. After mobilization of the kidney and ureter, an anti-clotting agent is administered. The physician clamps, ligates, and severs the upper ureter and major renal blood vessels (renal pedicle), and removes the kidney and upper ureter. The physician administers medication to reverse the effects of the anti-clotting agent. The small abdominal or back incisions are closed by staple or suture in the usual fashion. The donor kidney is preserved for transplantation into the recipient. The organ remains under refrigeration, packed in a sealable container with some preserving solution and kept on ice in a suitable carrier.

50548
The physician removes the kidney and all of the ureter through a laparoscope. The physician makes a 1.0-centimeter periumbilical incision and inserts a trocar. The abdominal cavity is insufflated with carbon dioxide. A fiberoptic laparoscope fitted with a camera and light source is inserted through the trocar. Other incisions (ports) are made in the abdomen or flank to allow other instruments or an additional light source to be passed into the abdomen or retroperitoneum. The colon is mobilized and the laparoscope is advanced to the operative site. The physician mobilizes the kidney and clamps, ligates, and severs the all of the ureter at the ureterovesical junction and major renal blood vessels (renal pedicle). The kidney and ureter are bagged and brought through one of the port sites (e.g., periumbilical) that has been slightly enlarged. The instruments are removed, and the small abdominal or flank incisions are closed with staple or suture.

50551
The physician examines the kidney and ureter with an endoscope passed through an established opening between the skin and kidney (nephrostomy) or renal pelvis (pyelostomy). After inserting a guidewire, the physician removes the nephrostomy or pyelostomy tube and passes the endoscope through the opening into the kidney or renal pelvis. To better view renal and ureteric structures, the physician may flush (irrigate) or introduce by drops (instillate) a saline solution. The physician may introduce contrast medium for radiologic study of the renal pelvis and ureter (ureteropyelogram). After examination, the physician removes the endoscope and guidewire and reinserts the nephrostomy tube or allows the surgical passageway to seal on its own.

50553
The physician examines the kidney and ureter with an endoscope passed through an established opening between the skin and kidney (nephrostomy) or renal pelvis (pyelostomy), and inserts a catheter into the ureter. After inserting a guidewire, the physician removes the nephrostomy or pyelostomy tube and passes the endoscope through the opening into the kidney or renal pelvis. To better view renal and ureteric structures, the physician may flush (irrigate) or introduce by drops (instillate) a saline solution. The physician may introduce contrast medium for radiologic study of the renal pelvis and ureter (ureteropyelogram). After examination, the physician passes a thin tube through the endoscope into the ureter. The physician may insert a balloon catheter to dilate a ureteral constriction. The physician reinserts the nephrostomy tube or allows the passageway to seal on its own.

50555
The physician examines the kidney and ureter with an endoscope passed through an established opening between the skin and kidney (nephrostomy) or renal pelvis (pyelostomy), and biopsies renal tissue. After

inserting a guidewire, the physician removes the nephrostomy or pyelostomy tube and passes the endoscope through the opening into the kidney or renal pelvis. To better view renal and ureteric structures, the physician may flush (irrigate) or introduce by drops (instillate) a saline solution. The physician may introduce contrast medium for radiologic study of the renal pelvis and ureter (ureteropyelogram). After examination, the physician passes a cutting instrument through the endoscope into the suspect renal tissue and takes a biopsy specimen. The physician removes the endoscope and reinserts the nephrostomy or pyelostomy tube or allows the passageway to seal on its own.

50557

The physician examines the kidney and ureter with an endoscope passed through an established opening between the skin and kidney (nephrostomy) or renal pelvis (pyelostomy), and removes renal lesions by electric current (fulguration) or incision. After inserting a guidewire, the physician removes the nephrostomy or pyelostomy tube and passes the endoscope through the opening into the kidney or renal pelvis. To better view renal and ureteric structures, the physician may flush (irrigate) or introduce by drops (instillate) a saline solution. The physician may introduce contrast medium for radiologic study of the renal pelvis and ureter (ureteropyelogram). After examination, the physician passes through the endoscope an instrument that destroys lesions with electric current or incises lesions. The physician may insert a cutting instrument to biopsy renal tissue. The physician removes the endoscope and reinserts the nephrostomy/pyelostomy tube or allows the passageway to seal on its own.

50561

The physician examines the kidney and ureter with an endoscope passed through an established opening between the skin and kidney (nephrostomy) or renal pelvis (pyelostomy), and removes a foreign body or calculus. After inserting a guidewire, the physician removes the nephrostomy or pyelostomy tube and passes the endoscope through the opening into the kidney or renal pelvis. To better view renal and ureteric structures, the physician may flush (irrigate) or introduce by drops (instillate) a saline solution. The physician may introduce contrast medium for radiologic study of the renal pelvis and ureter (ureteropyelogram). After examination, the physician passes an instrument through the endoscope to remove a foreign body or calculus. The physician removes the endoscope and reinserts the nephrostomy tube or allows the surgical passageway to seal on its own.

50562

The physician examines the kidney and ureter with an endoscope passed through an established opening between the skin and kidney (nephrostomy) or renal pelvis (pyelostomy). After inserting a guidewire, the physician removes the nephrostomy or pyelostomy tube and passes the endoscope through the opening into the kidney or renal pelvis. To better view renal and ureteric structures, the physician may flush (irrigate) or introduce by drops (instillate) a saline solution. The physician may introduce contrast medium for radiologic study of the renal pelvis and ureter (ureteropyelogram). After examination, the physician passes an instrument through the endoscope to resect a tumor. The tumor may be removed by cold-cup biopsy forceps with the bulk of the tumor being grasped and removed in piecemeal fashion until the base is reached. Alternately, a cutting loop may be used to remove the tumor to the base, or the tumor may be ablated with YAG laser. After the tumor resection, the physician removes the endoscope and other instruments and reinserts the nephrostomy tube or allows the surgical passageway to seal on its own.

50570

The physician examines the kidney and ureter with an endoscope passed through an incision in the kidney (nephrotomy) or renal pelvis (pyelotomy). After accessing the renal and ureteric structures with an incision in the skin of the flank, the physician incises the kidney or renal pelvis and guides the endoscope through the incision. To better view renal and ureteric structures, the physician may flush (irrigate) or introduce by drops (instillate) a saline solution. The physician may introduce contrast medium for radiologic study of the renal pelvis and ureter (ureteropyelogram). After examination, the physician sutures the incision, inserts a drain tube, and performs a layered closure.

50572

The physician examines the kidney and ureter with an endoscope passed through an incision in the kidney (nephrotomy) or renal pelvis (pyelotomy), and inserts a catheter into the ureter. After accessing the renal and ureteric structures with an incision in the skin of the flank, the physician incises the kidney or renal pelvis and guides the endoscope through the incision. To better view renal and ureteric structures, the physician may flush (irrigate) or introduce by drops (instillate) a saline solution. The physician may introduce contrast medium for radiologic study of the renal pelvis and ureter (ureteropyelogram). After examination, the physician passes a thin tube through the endoscope into the ureter, and may insert a balloon catheter to dilate a ureteral constriction. The physician sutures the incisions, inserts a drain tube, and performs a layered closure.

50574

The physician examines the kidney and ureter with an endoscope passed through an incision in the kidney (nephrotomy) or renal pelvis (pyelotomy), and biopsies renal tissue. After accessing the renal and ureteric structures with an incision in the skin of the flank, the physician incises the kidney or renal pelvis and guides the endoscope through the incision. To better view renal and ureteric structures, the physician may flush (irrigate) or introduce by drops (instillate) a saline solution. The physician may introduce contrast medium for radiologic study of the renal pelvis and ureter (ureteropyelogram). After examination, the physician passes a cutting instrument through the endoscope into the suspect renal tissue and takes a biopsy specimen. The physician removes the endoscope, sutures the incision, inserts a drain tube, and performs a layered closure.

50575
The physician examines the kidney and ureter with an endoscope passed through an incision in the kidney (nephrotomy) or renal pelvis (pyelotomy), and dilates ureter and ureteropelvic junction. After accessing the renal and ureteric structures with an incision in the skin of the flank, the physician incises the kidney or renal pelvis and guides the endoscope through the incision. To better view renal and ureteric structures, the physician may flush (irrigate) or introduce by drops (instillate) a saline solution. The physician may introduce contrast medium for radiologic study of the renal pelvis and ureter (ureteropyelogram). For endopyelotomy, the physician places endoscope through the ureter and/or the pelvis, incises the pelvis, enlarges the ureteropelvic junction, and sutures the junction as in a Y-V pyeloplasty. The physician inserts the stent through the renal pelvis into the junction, sutures the incisions, inserts a drain tube, and performs a layered closure.

50576
The physician examines the kidney and ureter with an endoscope passed through an incision in the kidney (nephrotomy) or renal pelvis (pyelotomy), and removes renal lesions by electric current (fulguration) or incision. After accessing the renal and ureteric structures with an incision in the skin of the flank, the physician incises the kidney or renal pelvis and guides the endoscope through the incision. To better view renal and ureteric structures, the physician may flush (irrigate) or introduce by drops (instillate) a saline solution. The physician may introduce contrast medium for radiologic study of the renal pelvis and ureter (ureteropyelogram). After examination, the physician passes through the endoscope an instrument that destroys lesions by electric current or incision The physician may insert instrument to biopsy renal tissue. The physician removes the scope, sutures the incision, inserts a drain tube, and performs a layered closure.

50580
The physician examines the kidney and ureter with an endoscope passed through an incision in the kidney (nephrotomy) or renal pelvis (pyelotomy), and removes a foreign body or calculus. After accessing the renal and ureteric structures with an incision in the skin of the flank, the physician incises the kidney or renal pelvis and guides the endoscope through the incision. To better view renal and ureteric structures, the physician may flush (irrigate) or introduce by drops (instillate) a saline solution. The physician may introduce contrast medium for radiologic study of the renal pelvis and ureter (ureteropyelogram). After examination, the physician passes instruments through the endoscope to remove a foreign body or calculus, and may pass a stent through the ureter into the bladder. The physician sutures the incision, inserts a drain tube, and performs a layered closure.

50590
The physician pulverizes a kidney stone (renal calculus) by directing shock waves through a liquid medium. Two different methods are currently available to accomplish this procedure. The physician first uses radiological guidance to determine the location and size of the renal calculus. In the first method, the patient is immersed in a liquid medium (degassed, deionized water) with shock waves directed through the liquid to the kidney stone. In the second method, the one most often used, the patient is placed on a treatment table. A series of shock waves are directed through a water-cushion, or bellow that is placed against the patient's body at the location of the kidney stone. Each shock wave is directed to the stone for only a fraction of a second, and the procedure generally takes from 30 to 50 minutes. The treatment table is equipped with video x-ray so the physician can view the pulverization process. Over several days or weeks, the tiny stone fragments pass harmlessly though the patient's urinary system and are discharged during urination.

50592
The physician performs percutaneous radiofrequency ablation of one or more renal tumors. Using computerized tomography (CT), magnetic resonance imaging (MRI), or ultrasound guidance, the site for the electrode placement is identified. With the patient under moderate sedation, a small incision is made and an internally cooled radiofrequency needle electrode is introduced and placed into the renal tumor. Placement of the tip is confirmed with image guidance. Alternating current is applied as needed until correct core heat is reached in the electrode. The tumor tissue is heated to a specified temperature with monitoring done before and after each treatment, depending on the ablation device used, until sufficient time results in permanent cell damage and tumor necrosis. Overlapping tumor tissue is ablated in the same manner until all margins are satisfactory. Hemostasis is maintained after the electrode needle is withdrawn, the site is cleaned, and dressings are applied. The ablated tissue remains in place and is absorbed over time and replaced with scar tissue.

50593
The physician uses percutaneously placed cryotherapy probes to destroy tumors of the kidney. The patient is positioned for best exposure of the affected kidney. Separately reportable images are obtained using ultrasound, CT, or MRI to localize the tumor and determine the site for cryoprobe placement. After planning the skin entry site, the cryoprobe is placed in the lesion and the tip confirmed in position. Cycles of freezing and thawing are monitored to ensure encapsulation of the tumor tissue and a sufficient margin within the ice ball created by the cryotherapy. After the second active thaw cycle, the cryoprobes are removed if the ice ball is judged to cover the tumor

tissue. If freezing was insufficient, the probes may be removed and repositioned or additional probes may be added and freezing is continued until the tumor and margin receive two complete cycles. The instruments are removed, the incision site closed, and dressings are applied.

50600
The physician makes an incision in the ureter (ureterotomy) for examination of the ureter or insertion of a drainage catheter (ureterostomy tube) between the ureter and skin. To access the ureter, the physician makes an incision in the skin of the flank, and cuts the muscles, fat, and fibrous membranes (fascia) overlying the ureter. The physician makes an incision in the ureter and sometimes places fine traction sutures at the edges of the incision. The physician examines the interior of the ureter or, if the incision is for drainage, the physician inserts a catheter tip into the ureter and passes the tube through a stab incision in the skin of the flank. The physician sutures the incision and performs a layered closure.

50605
The physician makes an incision in the ureter (ureterotomy) to insert a catheter (stent) in the ureter. To access the ureter, the physician makes an incision in the skin of the flank, and cuts the muscles, fat, and fibrous membranes (fascia) overlying the ureter. The physician makes an incision in the ureter and sometimes places fine traction sutures at the edges of the incision. The physician inserts a slender rod or catheter into the ureter, sutures the incision, and performs a layered closure.

50606
A nonendoscopic endoluminal biopsy of the ureter and/or renal pelvis is accomplished by incision into the skin overlying the target area. The patient is anesthetized and the incision is made. The target area is visualized by imaging guidance. A guidewire is inserted into the biopsy site followed by a sheath over the wire. A forceps device is inserted along the wire until it reaches the biopsy site and the sheath is withdrawn exposing the forceps. With the wings of the forceps open, the device is inserted into the target area where the wings are closed trapping the tissue sample. The device is pulled back with the biopsy sample intact. Another method uses a brush biopsy to retrieve the sample. The brush may be inserted through a scope until it reaches the target area. Biopsy is obtained with rubbing of the brush within the lumen. Upon removal, the sample is retrieved from the brush for examination. The guidewire is removed and any other instruments used in the primary procedure are also removed. The incision site is closed with sutures. This code includes procurement of biopsy sample, imaging guidance, and radiological supervision and interpretation. The biopsy may be performed via transrenal access, existing renal/ureteral access, transurethral access, an ileal conduit, or ureterostomy. This code reports the biopsy only; the procedure performed for access to the biopsy site is reported separately.

50610-50630
The physician makes an incision in the ureter (ureterotomy) to remove a stone (calculus) from the ureter. To access the ureter, the physician makes an incision in the skin and cuts the muscles, fat, and fibrous membranes (fascia) overlying the ureter. For the upper or middle third of the ureter, the physician usually makes an incision in the skin of the flank; to access the lower third of the ureter, the physician usually makes a curved lower quadrant incision. The physician isolates the calculus and removes it through an incision in the ureter. After examining the ureter for other defects, the physician sutures the incision and performs a layered closure, inserting a drain tube through a stab incision in the skin. Report 50610 for calculus removal from the upper third of the ureter; 50620 for calculus removal from the middle third; and 50630 for calculus removal from the lower third.

50650
The physician removes the ureter and a small cuff of the bladder. To access the ureter, the physician usually makes a curved lower quadrant incision in the skin of the abdomen, and cuts the muscles, fat, and fibrous membranes (fascia) overlying the ureter. The physician mobilizes the bladder, dissects a small cuff of the bladder, and ligates and dissects the ureter. After removing the bladder cuff and lower ureter, the physician sutures and catheterizes the bladder. The physician places a drain tube behind the bladder and performs a layered closure.

50660
The physician removes a ureter that deviates from proper anatomical placement. To access the ureter, the physician makes an incision in the skin of the abdomen, perineum, and/or vagina. The physician cuts the muscles, fat, and fibrous membranes (fascia) overlying the ureter. After mobilizing the bladder and ureter, the physician ligates, dissects, and removes the ureter. The physician places a drain tube at the site of the incision and performs a layered closure.

50684
The physician injects a contrast agent through an opening between the skin and the ureter (ureterostomy) or via an indwelling catheter into the ureter and renal pelvis to study the renal collecting system. To determine immediate allergic response to the contrast agent, the physician injects a dose of contrast material through the ureterostomy or indwelling catheter into the ureter and renal pelvis, and takes an x-ray.

50686
The physician connects an indwelling ureteral catheter or existing ureterostomy to a manometer line to measure pressure and flow in the kidneys and ureters. The physician connects a ureteral catheter or ureterostomy to a manometer line filled with fluid. The physician inserts a bladder catheter that may be irrigated. The physician measures intrarenal and/or extra renal pressure. After discontinuing perfusion of fluid, the physician aspirates residual fluid from the

kidney and disconnects the manometer line. The physician may remove the ureteral catheter or ureterostomy tube (if applicable) and dress the wound.

50688
The physician changes an ureterostomy tube or an externally accessible ureteral stent via an ileal conduit. To remove the existing tube, the physician takes out the sutures securing the tube to the skin. The physician inserts a guidewire through the tube and passes the tube back over the guidewire. The physician passes a new tube over the guidewire, removes the guidewire, and sutures the tube to the skin. To change an externally accessible ureteral stent via an ileal conduit, a guidewire is inserted through the ileal conduit. An ileal conduit is an isolated loop of ileum to which the ureter has been anastomosed at one end with the opposite end exiting through the skin and attached to an ostomy bag. The existing stent is retrieved and a new stent is placed. The guidewire is removed.

50690
The physician injects a contrast agent through an existing ileal stoma into the renal pelvis or ureters to study the ileal conduit (where the ureters have been diverted into the ilium) or percutaneously or intravenously via a catheter to study the renal collecting system. To determine immediate allergic response to the contrast agent, the physician injects a small, initial dose of contrast material. If an allergic response is not evident, a larger amount of radiopaque dye is injected into the ureter and renal pelvis, and radiographic pictures are obtained for a ureteropyelogram or study of the ileal conduit diversion.

50693-50695
The physician inserts a catheter or stent percutaneously through the renal pelvis into the ureter for drainage of urine and/or an injection. With the patient face down, and the puncture site having been identified, a local anesthetic is injected. The physician inserts a long, thin needle with a removable probe in the skin of the back. The physician advances the needle toward the renal pelvis and into the ureter. When urine flows back through the needle, the physician advances a catheter over the needle and the needle is removed. An internal stent resides in the ureter and an external stent has one end that remains outside of the body. These codes report diagnostic nephrostogram and/or ureterogram, imaging guidance, and radiological supervision and interpretation. Report 50693 when this procedure is performed through an existing nephrostomy tract; 50694 when performed via a new access without a separate nephrostomy catheter; and 50695 when performed via a new access with a separate nephrostomy catheter.

50700
The physician uses plastic surgery to correct an obstruction or defect in the ureter. To access the ureter, the physician makes an incision in the skin and cuts the muscles, fat, and fibrous membranes (fascia) overlying the ureter. For the upper or middle third of the ureter, the physician usually makes an incision in the skin of the flank; to access the lower third of the ureter, the physician usually makes a curved lower quadrant incision. The physician inserts a catheter into the ureter to the point of obstruction. The balloon is inflated, sometimes using repeated inflation with increasing diameter of the catheter. The physician incises, trims, and shapes the ureter, using absorbable sutures or soft rubber drains for traction. The physician may insert a slender tube into the ureter to provide support during healing. The physician places a drain tube, bringing it out through a separate stab incision in the skin, and performs a layered closure.

50705
Ureteral embolization or occlusion performed non-endoscopically requires the patient to be under anesthesia. Typically a nephrostomy tube is introduced into both kidneys prior to embolization, being replaced with a sheath during the procedure. A nephrostogram may be performed. A catheter is positioned into the distal ureter with groups of coils in various sizes. These coils are used for the occlusion and it may take four to 12 coils to accomplish the end result. Gelatin sponges may also be placed within the coil groups to speed up the lumen occlusion. A nephrostogram may be performed again to verify success of the procedure at the coil positions. The sheath is replaced with a catheter allowing for drainage and may be replaced every eight weeks. This procedure may be performed via transrenal access, existing renal/ureteral access, transurethral access, an ileal conduit, or ureterostomy. It includes the embolization or dilation, imaging guidance, and radiological supervision and interpretation. The service performed for gaining access may be reported separately.

50706
The physician treats a ureteral stricture by balloon dilation by making an incision into the skin overlying the target area. The patient is anesthetized and the incision is made. The target area is visualized by imaging guidance. A guidewire is inserted through the strictured area. A catheter containing the balloon is threaded over the wire to the stricture and the wire is removed. Balloon catheter sizes are determined based on normal ureter diameter as measured by radiological images. The balloon is inflated until stricture is minimalized; the process may be repeated until the desired result is achieved. Contrast may be injected to determine adequate flow through the ureter. The instruments are removed and the incision site is sutured closed. This procedure may be performed via transrenal access, existing renal/ureteral access, transurethral access, an ileal conduit, or ureterostomy. It includes the embolization or dilation, imaging guidance, and radiological supervision and interpretation. The service performed for gaining access may be reported separately.

50715

The physician surgically frees the ureter from localized inflammatory disease of retroperitoneal fibrous tissue. To access the ureter, the physician makes a midline incision in the skin of the abdomen and cuts the muscles, fat, and fibrous membranes (fascia) overlying the ureter. The physician incises surrounding fibrotic tissue to free the ureter, and may use sutures to reposition the ureter away from obstructive fibrous tissue. The physician places a drain tube, bringing it out through a separate stab incision in the skin, and performs a layered closure.

50722

The physician surgically frees the ureter from ureteral obstruction caused by aberrant ovarian veins (ovarian vein syndrome). To access the ureter, the physician makes an incision in the skin above the pubic hairline, and cuts the muscles, fat, and fibrous membranes (fascia) overlying the ureter. The physician incises surrounding adhesions to free the ureter from the obstructing ovarian veins. The physician places a drain tube, bringing it out through a separate stab incision in the skin, and performs a layered closure.

50725

The physician divides and reconnects a ureter aberrantly positioned behind the vena cava. To access the ureter, the physician makes a midline incision in the skin of the abdomen, and cuts the muscles, fat, and fibrous membranes (fascia) overlying the ureter. The physician dissects the ureter on both sides of the vena cava, leaving the ureteric segment behind the vena cava in place. The physician connects (anastomosis) the distal end of the ureter to the upper ureter by fashioning a long, elliptical flap from the renal pelvis. The physician may alternatively dissect and connect the two ends of the vena cava, positioning the ureter in front. To provide support during healing, the physician may insert a slender tube into the renal pelvis. After wrapping the anastomosis with perinephric fat, the physician inserts a drain tube and performs a layered closure.

50727-50728

The physician revises any surgical opening (anastomosis) between the skin and ureter, bladder, or colon segment. The physician removes the sutures securing the anastomosis to the skin and revises the anastomosis. The physician may make a midline incision in the skin of the abdomen to access the urinary tract. In 50728, the physician repairs a defect in surrounding fibrous membranes (fascia), and/or a rupture (hernia) in ureteral tissues.

50740

The physician surgically connects the upper ureter and renal pelvis to allow for urinary drainage. To access the renal pelvis and ureter, the physician makes an incision in the skin of the flank, cuts the muscles, fat, and fibrous membranes (fascia) overlying the kidney, and sometimes removes a portion of the eleventh or twelfth rib. The physician ligates the renal pelvis and ureter at the point of blockage. After excising the obstructing part of the ureter or pelvis, the physician surgically connects (anastomosis) the two structures, bypassing the obstructing point. To provide support during healing, the physician may insert a slender tube into the renal pelvis. After wrapping the anastomosis with perinephric fat, the physician inserts a drain tube and performs a layered closure.

50750

The physician connects the upper ureter and a renal calyx to allow for urinary drainage. To access the renal calyces and ureter, the physician makes an incision in the skin of the flank, cuts the muscles, fat, and fibrous membranes (fascia) overlying the kidney, and sometimes removes a portion of the eleventh or twelfth rib. The physician ligates the appropriate renal arteries and performs a partial nephrectomy by removing a part of the kidney. The physician partially mobilizes the calyx and ureter, and places a nephrostomy tube and stent. After surgically joining (anastomosing) the calyx and ureter, the physician closes the renal pelvis and wraps the anastomosis with perinephric fat. The physician inserts a drain tube and performs a layered closure.

50760

The physician divides and reconnects the ureter to bypass a defect or obstruction. To access the ureter, the physician makes an incision in the skin of the abdomen and cuts the muscles, fat, and fibrous membranes (fascia) overlying the ureter. For the upper or middle third of the ureter, the physician usually makes an incision in the skin of the flank; to access the lower third of the ureter, the physician usually makes a curved lower quadrant incision. The physician ligates and dissects the ureter at the point of blockage, and surgically rejoins (anastomosis) the two ends, bypassing the obstructing point. To provide support during healing, the physician may insert a slender tube into the ureter. The physician inserts a drain tube and performs a layered closure.

50770

The physician divides and connects a diseased or obstructed ureter to the other ureter. To access the ureters, the physician usually makes a midline incision in the skin of the abdomen, and cuts the muscles, fat, and fibrous membranes (fascia) overlying the ureters. The physician ligates and dissects the ureter at the point of disease or blockage, and surgically attaches (anastomosis) the end of the usable ureteric portion to the other ureter. To provide support during healing, the physician may insert a slender tube into the ureter. The physician inserts a drain tube and performs a layered closure.

50780-50785

The physician connects the lower ureter and bladder to allow for urinary drainage. The physician usually makes an incision in the skin of the abdomen. After dissecting the ureter at the point of disease or obstruction, the physician brings the ureter through a stab incision in the bladder and sutures the ureter to the bladder. To provide support during healing, the physician may insert a catheter into the ureter. The physician inserts a drain tube and performs a layered single ureter to the bladder (50780). Report 50782 if the physician attaches a duplicated ureter to the bladder. Report 50783 if the anastomosis requires extensive ureter reconstruction. Report 50785 if the anastomosis requires suturing the bladder and psoas, or by fashioning a long, elliptical flap from the bladder.

50800

The physician connects the ureter to a segment of intestine to divert urine flow. To access the ureter and intestine, the physician makes an incision in the skin of the abdomen and cuts the corresponding muscles, fat, and fibrous membranes (fascia). The physician dissects the ureter, makes small incisions in the intestine segment, and surgically connects (anastomosis) the ureter to the intestine. To provide support during healing, the physician may insert a slender tube into the ureter. The physician inserts a drain tube and performs a layered closure.

50810

The physician connects the ureters to a segment of sigmoid colon to create a bladder with an opening to the skin. To access the ureters and sigmoid colon, the physician makes a midline incision in the skin of the abdomen and cuts the corresponding muscles, fat, and fibrous membranes (fascia). After dissecting an isolated segment of sigmoid colon, the physician reconnects (anastomosis) the divided colon to restore bowel continuity. The sigmoid section is closed by sutures on one end. The physician dissects each ureter, makes small incisions in the sigmoid segment, and surgically connects each ureter to the sigmoid segment. To provide support during healing, the physician may insert a slender tube into each ureter. The physician fashions a bladder by closing the proximal end of the sigmoid segment, and brings the distal end through an incision in the skin of the abdomen to establish an opening (colostomy) for intermittent emptying of urine. The physician inserts a drain tube and performs a layered closure.

50815-50820

The physician connects the ureters to a segment of intestine to divert urine flow through an opening in the skin. To access the ureters and intestine, the physician makes a midline incision in the skin of the abdomen and cuts the corresponding muscles, fat, and fibrous membranes (fascia). After dissecting an isolated segment of intestine, the physician reconnects (anastomosis) the divided intestine to restore bowel continuity. The colon segment is closed by sutures on one end. The physician dissects each ureter, makes small incisions in the intestine segment, and surgically connects each ureter to the colon segment. To provide support during healing, the physician may insert a slender tube into each ureter. The physician closes the proximal end of the intestine segment and brings the distal end through an incision in the skin of the abdomen to establish an opening (stoma) for direct emptying of urine. The physician inserts a drain tube and performs a layered closure. Report 50820 if the physician dissects a segment of ileal colon to divert urine flow.

50825

The physician connects the ureter(s) to loops of intestine fashioned into a reservoir with a valve opening. To access the intestine and ureters, the physician makes a midline incision in the skin of the abdomen and cuts the corresponding muscles, fat, and fibrous membranes (fascia). After dissecting an isolated segment of intestine, the physician reconnects (anastomosis) the divided intestine to restore bowel continuity. After shaping the intestine segment into a pouch, the physician dissects each ureter, makes small incisions in the intestine segment, and surgically connects each ureter to the intestine segment. To provide support during healing, the physician inserts a slender tube into each ureter, and closes the pouch. The physician brings part of the pouch out through an abdominal wall opening, or anastomosis the pouch to the male urethra. The physician inserts a drain tube and performs a layered closure.

50830

The physician restores continuity of a ureter through which urine flow was previously diverted. To access the ureter, the physician usually reopens the original ureteral diversion incision and cuts the corresponding muscles, fat, and fibrous membranes (fascia). The physician reverses the diversion by removing sutures connecting the ureter and colon, colon segment, and/or skin. The physician closes the opening in the skin used for the diversionary anastomosis. To restore ureteral continuity, the physician reconnects the upper and lower ureter segments or connects the ureter to the other ureter (ureteroureterostomy), or reimplants the ureter into the bladder (ureteroneocystostomy). To provide support during healing, the physician inserts a slender tube into the ureter. The physician inserts a drain tube and performs a layered closure.

50840

The physician replaces part or all of the ureter with a segment of intestine. To access the ureters and intestine, the physician makes a midline incision in the skin of the abdomen and cuts the corresponding muscles, fat, and fibrous membranes (fascia). After dissecting an isolated segment of intestine, the physician reconnects (anastomosis) the divided intestine to restore bowel continuity. The physician dissects and removes the diseased or defective ureteral segment, replacing it with the intestine segment. To provide support during healing, the physician may insert a slender tube into the ureter. The physician inserts a drain tube and performs a layered closure.

50845

The physician connects a segment of cecum colon (vermiform appendix) to the bladder to directly divert urine flow through an opening in the skin (cutaneous appendico-vesicostomy). To access the bladder and cecum colon, the physician makes a midline incision in the skin of the abdomen and cuts the corresponding muscles, fat, and fibrous membranes (fascia). After dissecting vermiform appendix, the physician sutures the colon to restore bowel continuity. The physician makes an incision in the bladder and surgically connects the proximal end of the vermiform appendix to the bladder. The physician brings the distal end of vermiform appendix through an incision in the skin of the abdomen to establish an opening (stoma) for direct emptying of urine. The physician inserts a drain tube and performs a layered closure.

50860
The physician connects the ureter to the skin for urinary drainage. To access the ureter, the physician makes a midline incision in the skin of the abdomen and cuts the corresponding muscles, fat, and fibrous membranes (fascia). The physician ligates the distal ureter and brings the proximal end to the skin. The physician splits the end of the ureter and sutures it to the skin with a double Z-plasty to prevent the ureter from narrowing. To provide support during healing, the physician may insert a slender tube into the ureter. The physician inserts a drain tube and performs a layered closure.

50900
The physician sutures a wound or defect in the ureter. To access the ureter, the physician makes an incision in the skin and cuts the muscles, fat, and fibrous membranes (fascia) overlying the ureter. For the upper or middle third of the ureter, the physician usually makes an incision in the skin of the flank; to access the lower third of the ureter, the physician usually makes a curved lower quadrant incision. The physician uses sutures to close or surgically fixate a ureteral wound or defect. To provide support during healing, the physician may insert a slender tube into the ureter. The physician inserts a drain tube and performs a layered closure.

Urinary

50920
The physician closes an abnormal opening (fistula) between the skin and the ureter (ureterocutaneous). After excising the fistula, the physician sutures the clean percutaneous tissues together to create a smooth surface.

50930
The physician closes an abnormal opening (fistula) between the ureter and an organ of the digestive, respiratory, urogenital, or endocrine system. To access the ureter, the physician makes a midline incision in the skin of the abdomen and cuts the corresponding muscles, fat, and fibrous membranes (fascia). After excising the fistula, the physician sutures the clean tissues together to create a smooth surface. The physician places a drain tube, bringing it out through a separate stab incision in the skin, and performs a layered closure.

50940
The physician removes a thread, wire, or constricting band (ligature) placed on the ureter during a previous operative session. To access the ureter, the physician usually reopens the incision used for the previous operative session. After removing the ligature(s) from the ureter, the physician places a drain tube, bringing it out through a separate stab incision in the skin, and performs a layered closure.

50945
The physician performs a laparoscopic surgical removal of a stone (calculus) lodged in the ureter (ureterolithotomy). In an abdominal approach, the physician creates an umbilical port by placing a trocar at the level of the umbilicus. The abdominal wall is insufflated. The laparoscope is placed through the umbilical port and additional trocars are placed into the abdominal cavity. In the back (flank) approach, the trocar is placed at the back proximate to the retroperitoneal space near the kidney with additional ports placed nearby for appropriate access to the operative site. The physician uses the laparoscope fitted with a fiberoptic camera and/or an operating instrument to isolate the calculus and remove it through an incision in the ureter. The ureter is surgically closed. The small abdominal or back (flank) incisions are closed with staples or sutures.

50947-50948
The physician repositions the ureter on the bladder (due to an obstruction of the ureterovesical junction), using a laparoscopic approach. A stent may be placed with a cystoscope. In both procedures the physician makes a 1 centimeter periumbilical incision and inserts a trocar. The abdominal cavity is insufflated with carbon dioxide. A fiberoptic laparoscope fitted with a camera and light source is inserted through the trocar. Other incisions (ports) are made in the abdomen to allow other instruments or an additional light source to be passed into the abdomen. The physician manipulates the tools so the ureter and bladder can be observed through the laparoscope. The physician transects the ureter above the point of obstruction, brings the ureter through a stab incision in the bladder, and sutures the ureter to the new site on the bladder. In 50947, the physician inserts a cystoscope and places a stent in the repositioned ureter to provide support of the ureter. In 50948, the ureter is repositioned without cystoscopy or stent placement. The instruments are removed. The incisions are closed with staples or suture.

50951
The physician examines renal and ureteral structures with an endoscope passed through an established opening between the skin and ureter (ureterostomy). The physician inserts a guidewire, removes the ureterostomy tube, and passes the endoscope into the kidney or renal pelvis. The physician may flush (irrigate) or introduce by drops (instillate) a saline solution to better view the renal and ureteral structures, and/or may introduce contrast medium for radiologic study of the renal pelvis and ureter (ureteropyelogram). The physician removes the endoscope and guidewire and reinserts the ureterostomy tube or allows the passageway to seal on its own.

50953

The physician examines renal and ureteral structures with an endoscope passed through an established opening between the skin and ureter (ureterostomy), and inserts a catheter into the ureter. The physician inserts a guidewire, removes the ureterostomy tube, and passes the endoscope into the kidney or renal pelvis. The physician may flush (irrigate) or introduce by drops (instillate) a saline solution to better view the renal and ureteral structures, and/or may introduce contrast medium for radiologic study of the renal pelvis and ureter (ureteropyelogram). The physician passes a thin tube through the endoscope into the ureter, and may insert a balloon catheter to dilate a ureteral constriction. The physician removes the endoscope and guidewire and reinserts the ureterostomy tube or allows the passageway to seal on its own.

50955

The physician examines renal and ureteral structures with an endoscope passed through an established opening between the skin and ureter (ureterostomy), and biopsies renal and/or ureteral tissue. The physician inserts a guidewire, removes the ureterostomy tube, and passes the endoscope into the kidney or renal pelvis. The physician may flush (irrigate) or introduce by drops (instillate) a saline solution to better view the renal and ureteral structures, and/or may introduce contrast medium for radiologic study of the renal pelvis and ureter (ureteropyelogram). The physician passes a cutting instrument through the endoscope into the suspect tissue and takes a biopsy specimen. The physician removes the endoscope and guidewire and reinserts the ureterostomy tube or allows the passageway to seal on its own.

50957

The physician examines renal and ureteral structures with an endoscope passed through an established opening between the skin and ureter (ureterostomy), and removes lesions by electric current (fulguration) or incision. The physician inserts a guidewire, removes the ureterostomy tube, and passes the endoscope into the kidney or renal pelvis. The physician may flush (irrigate) or introduce by drops (instillate) a saline solution to better view the renal and ureteral structures, and/or may introduce contrast medium for radiologic study of the renal pelvis and ureter (ureteropyelogram). The physician passes through the endoscope an instrument that destroys lesions by electric current or incision. The physician may insert an instrument to biopsy renal tissue. The physician removes the endoscope and guidewire and reinserts the ureterostomy tube or allows the passageway to seal on its own.

50961

The physician examines renal and ureteral structures with an endoscope passed through an established opening between the skin and ureter (ureterostomy), and removes a foreign body or calculus. The physician inserts a guidewire, removes the ureterostomy tube, and passes the endoscope into the kidney or renal pelvis. The physician may flush (irrigate) or introduce by drops (instillate) a saline solution to better view the renal and ureteral structures, and/or may introduce contrast medium for radiologic study of the renal pelvis and ureter (ureteropyelogram). The physician passes an instrument through the endoscope to remove a foreign body or calculus. The physician removes the endoscope and guidewire and reinserts the ureterostomy tube or allows the passageway to seal on its own.

50970

The physician examines renal and ureteral structures with an endoscope passed through an incision in the ureter (ureterotomy). After accessing the ureter with an incision in the skin of the flank, the physician incises the ureter and guides the endoscope through the incision. The physician may flush (irrigate) or introduce by drops (instillate) a solution to better view the renal and ureteral structures, and/or may introduce contrast medium for radiologic study of the renal pelvis and ureter (ureteropyelogram). After examination, the physician sutures the incision, inserts a drain tube, and performs a layered closure.

50972

The physician examines renal and ureteral structures with an endoscope passed through an incision in the ureter (ureterotomy), and inserts a catheter into the ureter. After accessing the ureter with an incision in the skin of the flank, the physician incises the ureter and guides the endoscope through the incision. The physician may flush (irrigate) or introduce by drops (instillate) a solution to better view the renal and ureteral structures, and/or may introduce contrast medium for radiologic study of the renal pelvis and ureter (ureteropyelogram). To catheterize the ureter, the physician passes a thin tube through the endoscope into the ureter. The physician may insert a balloon catheter to dilate a ureteral constriction. The physician sutures the incision, inserts a drain tube, and performs a layered closure.

50974

The physician examines renal and ureteral structures with an endoscope passed through an incision in the ureter (ureterotomy), and biopsies ureteral and/or renal tissue. After accessing the ureter with an incision in the skin of the flank, the physician incises the ureter and guides the endoscope through the incision. The physician may flush (irrigate) or introduce by drops (instillate) a solution to better view the renal and ureteral structures, and/or may introduce contrast medium for radiologic study of the renal pelvis and ureter (ureteropyelogram). The physician passes a cutting instrument through the endoscope into the suspect tissue and take a biopsy specimen. The physician removes the endoscope, sutures the incision, inserts a drain tube, and performs a layered closure.

50976

The physician examines renal and ureteral structures with an endoscope passed through an incision in the ureter (ureterotomy), and removes renal or ureteral lesions by electric current (fulguration) or incision. After accessing the ureter with an incision in the skin of the flank, the physician incises the ureter and guides the endoscope through the incision. The physician may flush (irrigate) or introduce by drops (instillate) a solution to better view the renal and ureteral structures, and/or may introduce contrast medium for radiologic study of the renal pelvis and ureter (ureteropyelogram). The physician passes through the endoscope an instrument that destroys lesions with electric sparks or incises lesions. The physician may insert an instrument to biopsy renal tissue. The physician removes the endoscope, sutures the incision, inserts a drain tube, and performs a layered closure.

50980
The physician examines renal and ureteral structures with an endoscope passed through an incision in the ureter (ureterotomy), and removes a foreign body or stone (calculus). After accessing the ureter with an incision in the skin of the flank, the physician incises the ureter and guides the endoscope through the incision. The physician may flush (irrigate) or introduce by drops (instillate) a solution to better view the renal and ureteral structures, and/or may introduce contrast medium for radiologic study of the renal pelvis and ureter (ureteropyelogram). The physician passes an instrument through the endoscope to remove a foreign body or calculus, and may pass a stent through the ureter into the bladder. The physician removes the endoscope, sutures the incision, inserts a drain tube, and performs a layered closure.

51020
The physician makes an incision (cystotomy) or creates an opening (cystostomy) into the bladder to destroy abnormal tissue. To access the bladder, an incision is made in the skin of the lower abdomen and the corresponding muscles, fat, fibrous membranes (fascia), and bladder wall are incised. The physician uses electric current (fulguration) or inserts radioactive material to destroy a lesion on the bladder (usually with the aid of a radiation oncologist). The bladder wall and lower abdomen is sutured closed. If a cystostomy is made, the cystostomy tube is sutured in place and the bladder and abdominal wall are closed.

51040
The physician creates an opening into the bladder (cystostomy) through an incision in the bladder (cystotomy). To access the bladder, the physician makes an incision in the skin of the lower abdomen and cuts the corresponding muscles, fat, and fibrous membranes (fascia). The physician makes a small incision and inserts a catheter (cystostomy tube) into the bladder, passing the tube through a stab incision in the skin of the abdomen. The physician may insert a drain tube for the cystostomy. If only a cystotomy is performed the wound can be repaired with a layered closure using absorbable sutures.

51045
The physician makes an incision in the bladder to insert a catheter or slender tube (stent) into the ureter. To access the bladder and ureters, the physician makes a midline incision in the skin of the abdomen and cuts the corresponding muscles, fat, and fibrous membranes (fascia). The physician incises the bladder (cystotomy) and inserts a stent or catheter in the ureter. Insertion of a ureteral catheter requires that the physician bring the tube end out through the urethra or bladder incision. The physician inserts a drain tube and performs a layered closure.

51050
The physician makes an incision in the bladder to remove a calculus. To access the bladder, the physician makes an incision in the skin of the lower abdomen and cuts the corresponding muscles, fat, and fibrous membranes (fascia). The physician performs a cystotomy, isolates the calculus, and removes it. The bladder neck is not excised. After examining the bladder for other defects, the physician sutures the incision and performs a layered closure using absorbable sutures, inserting a drain tube through a stab incision in the skin.

51060
The physician makes an incision in the bladder to remove a calculus in the ureter. To access the bladder and ureters, the physician makes a midline incision in the skin of the abdomen and cuts the corresponding muscles, fat, and fibrous membranes (fascia). The physician isolates the calculus and removes it through incisions in the bladder (cystotomy) and ureter (ureterotomy). After examining the ureter for other defects, the physician inserts a ureteral catheter and sutures the incisions. The physician inserts a drain tube and performs a layered closure.

51065
The physician makes an incision in the bladder and inserts an instrument in the ureter to remove or destroy the calculus. To access the bladder and ureters, the physician makes a midline incision in the skin of the abdomen and cuts the corresponding muscles, fat, and fibrous membranes (fascia). After isolating the calculus, the physician makes an incision in the bladder (cystotomy). The physician inserts an instrument (e.g., a stone basket) through the bladder incision into the ureter to remove or destroy a ureteral calculus. After examining the ureter for other defects, the physician inserts a ureteral catheter and sutures the incision. The physician inserts a drain tube and performs a layered closure.

51080
The physician drains an infection (abscess) near the bladder. To access the bladder, the physician makes an incision in the skin of the lower abdomen and cuts the corresponding muscles, fat, and fibrous membranes (fascia). After exploring the abscess cavity, the physician irrigates the site, inserts multiple drain tubes through separate stab wounds, and sutures the drain

tube ends to the skin. The physician inserts a urethral catheter and performs a layered closure.

51100-51102
In 51100, the physician inserts a needle through the skin into the bladder to withdraw urine. In 51101, the physician inserts a trocar or intracatheter through the skin into the bladder. In 51102, a suprapubic catheter is placed into the bladder. This procedure may also be performed after the abdomen has been surgically incised.

51500
The physician removes a cyst or dilated urachus (the remnant of bladder development that attaches from bladder to umbilicus). To access the urachus, the physician makes an incision in the skin of the lower abdomen through the umbilicus, and cuts the corresponding muscles, fat, and fibrous membranes (fascia). After isolating the urachus with a clamp, the physician excises the urachal cyst or sinus and a small cuff of the bladder. The physician sutures the bladder and removes the urachal tissue, leaving the navel intact. The physician may also repair a rupture (hernia) of tissue in the umbilicus. After inserting a drain tube and urethral catheter, the physician performs a layered closure.

51520
The physician removes part or all of the bladder neck. The physician makes an incision in the skin of the lower abdomen and cuts the corresponding muscles, fat, and fibrous membranes (fascia). Through this incision, the physician accesses the bladder neck and removes diseased or enlarged bladder neck tissue. The bladder is sutured and the abdominal wall is closed.

51525
The physician removes a diverticulum, a herniated defect of the bladder. To access the diverticulum, the physician makes an incision in the skin of the lower abdomen and cuts the corresponding muscles, fat, and fibrous membranes (fascia). The physician makes an incision in the bladder and may insert a ureteral stent if the diverticulum is close to the ureter. After dissecting the diverticulum from surrounding tissues and arteries, the physician excises the defective tissue and closes the remaining musculature and mucosa with absorbable sutures. This process may be repeated in other diverticula. The incision is repaired with a layered closure.

51530
The physician makes an incision in the bladder to remove a tumor of the bladder. To access the bladder, the physician makes an incision in the skin of the lower abdomen and cuts the corresponding muscles, fat, and fibrous membranes (fascia). The bladder is incised (cystotomy). After removing the tumor and surrounding diseased vesical tissue, the physician inserts a drain tube and performs a layered closure.

51535
The physician makes an incision in the bladder to remove or repair a saccular dilation of the ureteral end (ureterocele) that protrudes into the bladder. To access the bladder and ureters, the physician makes a midline incision in the skin of the abdomen and cuts the corresponding muscles, fat, and fibrous membranes (fascia). The physician incises the bladder (cystotomy) and excises or fulgurates the ureterocele. After examining the ureter for other defects, the physician sutures the bladder incision and inserts a ureteral catheter. The physician inserts a drain tube and performs a layered closure.

51550-51555
The physician removes a portion of diseased or damaged bladder tissue. To access the bladder, the physician makes an incision in the skin above the pubic bone and cuts the corresponding muscles, fat, and fibrous membranes (fascia). The physician mobilizes the bladder and the major vesical blood vessels, and incises the bladder wall to access the diseased or damaged bladder tissue. After removing the tissue, the physician inserts catheters into the bladder and urethra and sutures the bladder tissues. The physician performs a layered closure and inserts a drain tube, bringing it out through a separate stab incision in the skin. Report 51550 if the cystectomy presents few complications; report 51555 if the procedure is complicated because of prior administration of radiation, a previous surgery, or difficult access to the diseased or damaged bladder tissue.

51565
The physician removes diseased or damaged bladder tissue close to the ureteral orifice, and reimplants ureter(s) into the bladder (ureteroneocystostomy). To access the bladder and ureters, the physician makes a midline incision in the skin of the abdomen and cuts the corresponding muscles, fat, and fibrous membranes (fascia). The physician mobilizes the bladder, ureter(s), and the major vesical blood vessels, and may incise the bladder wall to access the diseased or damaged bladder tissue. The physician removes the diseased or damaged bladder tissue, requiring removal of the ureteral orifice and/or ureteral division. The physician brings the cut end of the ureter through a stab wound in the bladder and sutures the ureter to the bladder. To provide support during healing, the physician inserts a ureteral catheter, bringing the tube end out through the urethra or bladder incision. The physician inserts a drain tube and performs a layered closure.

51570-51575
The physician removes the bladder (cystectomy). To access the bladder, the physician makes an incision in the skin of the lower abdomen and cuts the corresponding muscles, fat, and fibrous membranes (fascia). Report 51570 if the physician dissects and ties (ligates) the hypogastric and vesical vessels, and severs the bladder from the urethra, rectum, surrounding peritoneum, vas deferens, and prostate (if applicable). After removing the bladder and controlling bleeding, the physician inserts drain tubes and performs a layered closure. If the physician bilaterally removes the pelvic lymph nodes, report 51575.

51580

The physician removes the bladder (cystectomy) and connects the ureters to the skin or sigmoid colon. To access the bladder and ureters, the physician makes a midline incision in the skin of the abdomen and cuts the corresponding muscles, fat, and fibrous membranes (fascia). The physician dissects and ligates the hypogastric and vesical vessels, and severs the bladder from the ureters and urethra. Blunt dissection from adherent rectum, surrounding peritoneum, and vas deferens and prostate may be needed. After controlling bleeding, the physician diverts urine by implanting the ureters to the skin (ureterocutaneous transplant), or connecting (anastomosing) the ureters to the sigmoid colon (ureterosigmoidostomy). To provide support during healing, the physician inserts a slender tube into each ureter. After completing the urinary diversion procedure, the physician inserts drain tubes and performs a layered closure.

51585

The physician removes the bladder (cystectomy) and pelvic lymph nodes, and connects the ureters to the skin or sigmoid colon. To access the bladder and ureters, the physician makes a midline incision in the skin of the abdomen and cuts the corresponding muscles, fat, and fibrous membranes (fascia). The physician dissects and ligates the hypogastric and vesical vessels, and severs the bladder from the ureters and urethra. Blunt dissection from adherent rectum, surrounding peritoneum, and vas deferens and prostate may be needed. The physician also removes external iliac, hypogastric, and obturator lymph nodes. After controlling bleeding, the physician diverts urine by implanting the ureters to the skin (ureterocutaneous transplant), or connecting the ureters to the sigmoid colon (ureterosigmoidostomy). The physician also inserts a slender tube into each ureter for support. After completing the urinary diversion procedure, the physician inserts drain tubes and performs a layered closure.

Urinary

51590

The physician removes the bladder (cystectomy) and diverts urine by connecting the ureters to a ureteroileal conduit or sigmoid bladder with an opening into the skin. To access the bladder and ureters, the physician makes a midline incision in the skin of the abdomen and cuts the corresponding muscles, fat, and fibrous membranes (fascia). The physician dissects and ligates the hypogastric and vesical vessels, and severs the bladder from the ureters and urethra. Blunt dissection from adherent rectum, surrounding peritoneum, and vas deferens and prostate may be needed. After controlling bleeding, the physician diverts urine by connecting the ureters to a segment of ileal or sigmoid colon fashioned into a conduit or bladder, respectively, with an opening into the skin. To provide support during healing, the physician inserts a slender tube into each ureter. After completing the urinary diversion procedure, the physician inserts drain tubes and performs a layered closure.

51595

The physician removes the bladder (cystectomy) and pelvic lymph nodes, and diverts urine by connecting the ureters to a ureteroileal conduit or sigmoid bladder with an opening into the skin. To access the bladder and ureters, the physician makes a midline incision in the skin of the abdomen and cuts the corresponding muscles, fat, and fibrous membranes (fascia). The physician dissects and ligates the hypogastric and vesical vessels, and severs the bladder from the ureters and urethra. Blunt dissection from adherent rectum, surrounding peritoneum, and vas deferens and prostate may be needed. The physician also removes external iliac, hypogastric, and obturator lymph nodes. After controlling bleeding, the physician diverts urine by connecting the ureters to a segment of ileal or sigmoid colon fashioned into a conduit or bladder, with an opening into the skin. The physician inserts a slender tube into each ureter. After completing the urinary diversion procedure, the physician inserts drain tubes and performs a layered closure.

51596

The physician removes the bladder (cystectomy) and diverts urine by any method, using any bowel segment to create a new bladder. To access the bladder and ureters, the physician makes a midline incision in the skin of the abdomen and cuts the corresponding muscles, fat, and fibrous membranes (fascia). The physician dissects and ligates the hypogastric and vesical vessels, and severs the bladder from the urethra. Blunt dissection from adherent rectum, surrounding peritoneum, and vas deferens and prostate may be needed. After controlling bleeding, the physician diverts urine by connecting the ureters to a segment of large or small bowel fashioned into a bladder with an opening into the skin. To provide support during healing, the physician inserts a slender tube into each ureter. After completing the urinary diversion procedure, the physician inserts drain tubes and performs a layered closure.

51597

The physician removes the bladder, lower ureters, lymph nodes, urethra, prostate (if applicable), colon, and rectum, due to a vesical, prostatic, or urethral malignancy. To access the bladder and ureters, the physician makes a midline incision in the skin of the abdomen and cuts the corresponding muscles, fat, and fibrous membranes (fascia). The physician dissects and ligates the hypogastric and vesical vessels, and severs the bladder, urethra, lower ureters, lymph nodes, and prostate (if applicable) from surrounding structures. The physician removes the bladder and diverts urine flow by transplanting the ureters to the skin or colon. The vagina and uterus (if applicable) and/or rectum and part of the colon may be removed and an artificial abdominal opening in the skin surface created for waste (colostomy). After completing the urinary diversion procedure, the physician inserts drain tubes and performs a layered closure.

51600-51610

The physician injects a radiocontrast agent through a catheter inserted in the bladder to study the lower urinary tract. Using radiologic instruments, the physician produces an image of the bladder with x-rays (cystogram). Filling, voiding, and post-voiding x-rays are obtained. The catheter is partially or completely withdrawn and the urethra is studied by x-ray. Report 51605 if the physician inserts a chain in the bladder or through the urethra as part of the injection procedure for contrast x-rays of the bladder and urethra (chain urethrocystogram). Report 51610 if contrast material is injected through a urethral catheter or catheter-tipped syringe for x-rays of the urethra and bladder (retrograde urethrocystogram).

51700

The physician irrigates the bladder with saline solution that is flushed, injected, or introduced by drops (instillation) through a catheter. The physician initially places the catheter into the bladder and irrigates by hand until the bladder is free of clots or debris. A three-way Foley catheter may be inserted for continuous bladder irrigation.

51701-51703

The patient is catheterized with a non-indwelling bladder catheter (e.g., for residual urine) in 51701; simple catheterization with a temporary indwelling bladder catheter (Foley) is performed in 51702. The area is properly cleaned and sterilized. A water-soluble lubricant may be injected into the urethra before catheterization begins. The distal part of the catheter is coated with lubricant. In males, the penis is held perpendicular to the body and pulled up gently and the catheter is steadily inserted about 8 inches until urine is noted. In females, the catheter is gently inserted until urine is noted. With an indwelling catheter, insertion continues into the bladder until the retention balloon can be inflated. The catheter is gently pulled until the retention balloon is snuggled against the neck of the bladder. The catheter is secured to the abdomen or thigh and the drainage bag is secured below bladder level. Report 51703 if a change in anatomy, such as enlarging of the prostate or a fractured catheter or balloon, complicate the catheterization process.

51705-51710

A cystostomy tube, also referred to as a suprapubic catheter, is inserted into the bladder through a small hole in the abdomen for patients with urinary incontinence or retention. The catheter must be changed every four to six weeks by a health care provider or the patient. The old catheter is slowly extracted after the area is cleansed and a balloon is deflated within the syringe. The new catheter is inserted and positioned in the same location. Once urine flows through the catheter, the balloon is inflated with saline or sterile water and the new catheter is attached to the collection bag. Report 51710 if complications such as infection, inflammation, hemorrhage, constriction, or dilation occur.

51715

The physician injects natural proteins or synthetic material into the urethra and bladder neck, helping to prevent urinary incontinence. Before the injection, an endoscope is placed through the urethra into the bladder. Using local anesthesia, the physician makes one to three injections into the transurethral submucous. The injections are made through the endoscope into the affected area. The procedure can also be performed through the lower abdomen.

51720

The physician introduces by drops (instillation) an anticarcinogenic agent into the bladder to treat a cancer. Prior to the instillation of the agent, a standard lavage is usually performed. The anticarcinogenic agent is introduced through a catheter and held in the bladder for a specified amount of time. This procedure may be used in conjunction with a cystostomy or with procedures such as cystectomy for the removal of a tumor.

51721

The physician inserts an ablation transducer into the urethra to deliver thermal energy for prostate tissue ablation. A catheter is placed through the urethra into the bladder, followed by a guidewire. The ultrasound applicator is advanced over the guidewire and into the prostatic urethra. An endorectal cooling device may be inserted into the rectum to protect the rectal tissue during treatment.

51725-51729

A cystometrogram (a graphic record of urinary bladder pressure at different volumes) is used to distinguish bladder outlet obstruction from other voiding dysfunctions. For a simple cystometrogram (51725), the physician inserts a pressure catheter into the bladder and connects it to a manometer line filled with fluid to measure pressure and flow in the lower urinary tract. For a complex cystometrogram (51726), the physician typically uses a transurethral catheter to fill the bladder with water or gas while simultaneously obtaining rectal pressure. As the bladder is being filled, intravesical pressure is measured by a microtip transducer or fluid-filled catheter attached to the transducer. Code 51727 reports a complex cystometrogram performed in conjunction with a study for measuring urethral pressure. In one technique, the bladder is filled with fluid and the catheter withdrawn into the urethra while bladder sensations and volume are recorded. Urethral pressure changes are recorded as the patient follows specific instructions (Valsalva maneuver, cough). For voiding pressure studies performed in conjunction with a complex cystometrogram (51728), a transducer is placed into the bladder and the bladder is filled with fluid. The patient is instructed to attempt to void upon the feeling of bladder fullness, and recordings are taken of bladder sensation and volume at specific times. Report 51729 if complex cystometrogram is combined with both voiding pressure studies and urethral pressure profile studies.

[51797]
The physician conducts an intra-abdominal voiding pressure study. In one method, the physician places a rectal catheter simultaneously with a urethral catheter in order to determine how much the patient strains while attempting to void. This measures both the amount of pressure generated and the subsequent urine flow.

51736-51741
For simple uroflowmetry (51736), the physician assesses the rate of emptying the bladder by stopwatch, recording the volume of urine per time. For complex uroflowmetry, (51741), the physician assesses the rate of emptying of the bladder by electronic equipment, recording the volume of urine per time.

51784
The physician places a pad in the anal or urethral sphincter and measures the electrical activity with the bladder filled and during emptying.

51785
The physician places a pad or needle in the anal or urethral sphincter and measures the electrical activity with the bladder filled and during emptying.

51792
The physician electrically stimulates the head of the penis. The physician measures the delay time for travel of stimulation through the pelvic nerves to the pudendal nerve.

51798
Residual urine and/or bladder capacity is measured by ultrasound after the patient has voided. A portable ultrasound scanner is used for this purpose. Operation of the scanner is done simply by directing the scanning head over the suprapubic area while the patient is lying down in the supine position. The software built in to the scanner calculates the post-void residual urine volume immediately and also does calculations for the bladder capacity based on the individual's bladder shape and not on fixed geometric formulas.

51800
The physician uses plastic surgery to correct an obstruction or defect in the bladder or vesical neck and urethra. The bladder is distended using a Foley catheter. To access the bladder, the physician makes an incision in the skin of the lower abdomen and cuts the corresponding muscles, fat, and fibrous membranes (fascia). The physician incises, trims, and shapes the bladder or vesical neck and urethra, using absorbable sutures or soft rubber drains for traction. The physician may insert a catheter through the urethra to provide support during healing. In anterior Y-plasty, the physician makes a Y-shaped flap of the bladder extending the vertical incision into the vesical neck. The vertical part of this incision is pulled up into the V-shaped incision, which becomes a straight line when sutured. The physician may remove a portion of the vesical neck. The physician places a drain tube, bringing it out through a separate stab incision in the skin, and performs a layered closure.

51820
The physician uses plastic surgery to correct a defect in the bladder and urethra, and reimplants one or both ureters into the bladder (ureteroneocystostomy). To access the bladder, urethra, and ureters, the physician makes a midline incision in the skin of the abdomen and cuts the corresponding muscles, fat, and fibrous membranes (fascia). The physician incises, trims, and shapes the bladder and urethra, using absorbable sutures or soft rubber drains for traction. The physician brings the cut end of one or both ureters through a stab wound in the bladder and sutures the ureter(s) to the bladder. To provide support during healing, the physician inserts a ureteral catheter, bringing the tube end out through the urethra or bladder incision. The physician inserts a drain tube and performs a layered closure.

51840-51841
The physician performs a vesicourethropexy or urethropexy in the Marshall-Marchetti-Krantz or Burch style. The physician makes a small horizontal incision in the abdomen above the symphysis pubis, which is the midline junction of the pubic bones at the front. The bladder is suspended by placing several sutures through the tissue surrounding the urethra and into the vaginal wall. The sutures are pulled tight so that the tissues are tacked to the symphysis pubis and the urethra is moved forward. The incision is closed by suturing. 51841 is used when the procedure is performed for the second time or if some other factor increases the time or level of complexity.

51845
The physician surgically suspends the bladder neck by suturing surrounding tissue to the fibrous membranes (fascia) of the abdomen in a female patient. After inserting a catheter through the urethra to visualize the bladder neck, the physician makes an incision in the vagina, extending it upward toward the base of the bladder. On both sides of the vesical neck, the physician passes a needle through a small incision in the skin above the pubic bone down through the vaginal incision. The physician threads the needle in the vagina and pulls the needle back through the suprapubic incision. Dacron tubing may be threaded onto the sutures to provide extra periurethral support. The physician repeats this process, using an endoscope to ensure proper placement of the suspending sutures. After placing sutures on both sides of the bladder neck, the physician uses moderate upward traction to tighten the bladder neck. The physician inserts a drain tube, bringing it out through a stab incision in the skin, and performs a layered closure.

51860-51865
The physician sutures a wound, injury, or rupture in the bladder. To access the bladder, urethra, and ureters, the physician makes an incision in the skin of the abdomen and cuts the corresponding muscles, fat, and fibrous membranes (fascia). To provide support during healing, the physician may insert a catheter through the urethra. The physician inserts a drain tube and

performs a layered closure. Constant irrigation is provided to help prevent infection. Report 51865 if the procedure is complicated by a previous surgery, congenital defect, or other reason.

51880
The physician closes an artificial opening into the bladder (cystostomy). To access the cystostomy, the physician uses the original incision creating the cystostomy or makes an incision in the skin of the lower abdomen. After removing the sutures securing the cystostomy tube to the skin and bladder, the physician removes the cystostomy tube and sutures the bladder musculature to repair the opening. The physician places a drain tube, bringing it out through a separate stab incision in the skin, and performs a layered closure of the abdominal cystostomy incision.

51900
The physician closes a vesicovaginal fistula, which is an abnormal passage between the bladder and the vagina. This procedure is done through the abdomen. The fistula and surrounding scar tissue of the vaginal wall are usually excised. The physician makes an incision in the skin, muscle, and fascia of the abdomen. The bladder wall is opened and the bladder explored. The fistula is excised along with the surrounding tissue. The resulting defect is closed with sutures in multiple layers. In some cases, a pedicle graft of tissue may be sutured between the bladder and the vagina. A urethral or suprapubic catheter is left in the bladder to prevent distension of the bladder and tension to the sutured areas.

51920-51925
The physician excises an abnormal opening between the uterus and the bladder, then sutures the clean tissues together closing the resulting defect and creating a smooth surface. In 51920, the procedure is done through the bladder with a small abdominal incision or during a laparotomy. In 51925, the physician completes the fistula closure and also removes the uterus through a small horizontal incision just above the pubic hairline. To remove the uterus, the supporting pedicles containing the tubes, ligaments, and arteries are clamped and cut free. The uterus and cervix are removed along with a narrow rim or cuff of vaginal lining. The vaginal defect may be left open for drainage. The abdominal incision is closed by suturing.

51940
The physician repairs a congenital defect in the front of the bladder wall, which is associated with lack of closure of the pubic bone at the symphysis pubis. The physician makes an incision around the exposed bladder and around the urethra to develop thick skin flaps. The physician brings the skin flaps together in the midline to close the roof of the urethra and allow the bladder and prostatic urethra to drop back beneath the bony pelvis (male patients), or lengthen the urethra (female patients). To invert the bladder and establish a functional vesical neck, the physician dissects the edge of the bladder from the rectus muscle, and divides the fibromuscular bar that unites the pubic bone to the bladder base. To support the urethra and bladder neck, the physician brings the muscles of the urogenital diaphragm toward the midline. The physician places drain tubes and performs a layered closure.

51960
The physician reconstructs or enlarges a bladder with a segment of intestine. To access the intestine and bladder, the physician makes a transverse or longitudinal incision on the lower abdomen and cuts the corresponding muscles, fat, and fibrous membranes (fascia). After dissecting an isolated segment of colonic intestine, the physician reconnects (anastomosis) the ileum end-to-end to the ascending colon, restoring continuity to the bowel. The dissected segment of colon is opened and the distal ends are sutured. An incision is made at the bladder dome, a portion of the top of the bladder is removed in preparation, and the colonic segment is sutured to the bladder. After controlling bleeding, the physician inserts a catheter and closes the abdomen in layers over the catheter for support.

51980
The physician connects the bladder to the skin (cutaneous vesicostomy) for direct urinary drainage. The Blocksom technique is usually performed on newborns. To access the bladder, the physician makes a suprapubic incision in the abdomen and cuts the corresponding muscles, fat, and fibrous membranes (fascia). After securing the bladder dome to the rectus fascia, the physician incises the bladder to create an opening that is sutured to a small incision in the skin. To support the opening during healing, the physician inserts a catheter or stent into the bladder. The physician inserts a drain tube and performs a layered closure. In adults, the Lapides technique passes a flap of bladder beneath the skin to replace a retracted section of abdominal skin. The abdominal skin is passed below the abdominal surface and sutured to the opening in the bladder, making a long-term tubular passage for urine. A catheter is placed through the stoma for two or three days.

51990
The physician treats stress incontinence in the male or female patient. The physician makes a 1 cm incision just below the umbilicus through which a fiberoptic laparoscope is inserted. A second incision is made on the left or right side of the abdomen and a second instrument is passed into the abdomen. The physician then manipulates the tools so that the pelvic organs can be observed through the laparoscope. The bladder is suspended by placing several sutures through the tissue surrounding the urethra and into support structures. The sutures are pulled tight so that the urethra is elevated and moved forward. The instruments are removed and incisions are closed with sutures.

51992
The physician inserts an instrument through the cervix into the uterus to manipulate the uterus. Next, the

physician makes a 1 cm incision just below the umbilicus through which a fiberoptic laparoscope is inserted. A second incision is made and a second instrument is passed into the abdomen. The physician manipulates the tools so that the pelvic organs can be observed through the laparoscope. The physician places a sling under the junction of the urethra and bladder. The physician places a catheter in the bladder, makes an incision in the anterior wall of the vagina, and folds and tacks the tissues around the urethra. A sling is formed out of synthetic material or from fascia harvested from the sheath of the rectus abdominis muscle. The loop end of the sling is sutured around the junction of the urethra. An incision is made in the lower abdomen and the ends of the sling are grasped with a clamp and pulled into the incision and sutured to the rectus abdominis sheath. The instruments are removed and incisions are closed with sutures.

52000

The physician examines the urethra, bladder, and ureteric openings into the bladder with a cystourethroscope passed through the urethra and bladder. No other procedure is performed at this time. After examination, the physician removes the cystourethroscope.

52001

Using a rigid or flexible cystoscope, the physician removes clots and examines the urethra, bladder, and ureteric openings into the bladder. The cystoscope is introduced into the meatus and the urethra is inspected before proceeding to the bladder. When the bladder is entered, the urine is evacuated using a syringe; the cystoscope is advanced further through the bladder and deflected upward. Following cystoscopic examination, and localization of the area of interest, the physician inserts a suction and irrigation probe with laser guide to evacuate multiple obstructing clots and to automatically remove any tissue from the operative site. The operative site is irrigated. Following completion of the procedure, the instrument is removed.

52005-52007

The physician passes the cystourethroscope through the urethra into the bladder. After insertion of a catheter into the ureter, the physician may flush (irrigate) or introduce by drops (instillate) a saline solution to better view structures, and/or may introduce contrast medium for radiologic study of the renal pelvis and ureter (ureteropyelogram, retrograde pyelogram). The physician removes the cystourethroscope. If a brush biopsy of the ureter or renal pelvis is also performed, report 52007.

52010

The physician examines the urinary collecting system with a cystourethroscope passed through the urethra and bladder, and inserts a catheter into the ejaculatory duct. The physician may flush (irrigate) or introduce by drops (instillate) a saline solution to better view structures, and may introduce contrast medium for radiologic study of ejaculatory duct (duct radiography). The physician removes the cystourethroscope.

52204

The physician examines the urinary collecting system with a cystourethroscope passed through the urethra and bladder, and extracts biopsy tissue from the bladder or urethra. To do so, the physician passes a cutting instrument through the endoscope to the suspect tissue and traps a specimen of tissue. Multiple samples may be collected. The physician removes the instrument and cystourethroscope.

52214

The physician examines the urinary collecting system with a cystourethroscope passed through the urethra and bladder, and destroys tissue of the trigone, bladder neck prostatic fossa, urethra, or periurethral glands. The physician passes through the endoscope an instrument that uses electric current to destroy lesions on the urethra, periurethral glands, bladder neck, depression below the prostate surface (prostatic fossa), and triangular area at the base of the bladder (trigone). The physician may employ endoscopic use of liquid nitrogen or carbon dioxide (cryosurgery) or lasers to destroy lesions. The physician removes the instruments and cystourethroscope.

52224

The physician examines the urinary collecting system with a cystourethroscope passed through the urethra and bladder, and uses electric current (fulguration) to destroy lesions smaller than 0.5 cm. The physician may also employ endoscopic use of liquid nitrogen or carbon dioxide (cryosurgery) or lasers to destroy lesions. The physician may insert an instrument to extract biopsy tissue from the bladder. The physician removes the instruments and cystourethroscope.

52234-52240

The physician examines the urinary collecting system with a cystourethroscope passed through the urethra and bladder, and removes tumors of the bladder by electric current (fulguration) or excision. The physician passes an instrument through the endoscope to destroy or remove tumors of the bladder by electric current (fulguration) or excision. The physician may also use liquid nitrogen or carbon dioxide (cryosurgery) or lasers to destroy lesions. The physician removes the instruments and cystourethroscope. For small tumor(s) that are 0.5 up to 2 cm in size, report 52234. For medium bladder tumor(s) that are 2 to 5 cm in size, report 52235. For large tumor(s) that are larger than 5 cm, report 52240.

52250

The physician examines the urinary collecting system with a cystourethroscope passed through the urethra and bladder, and inserts a radioactive substance. To release a radioactive substance, the physician passes an instrument through the endoscope. The physician may insert instruments through the endoscope to remove lesions or extract biopsy tissue from the bladder. The physician removes the instruments and cystourethroscope.

52260-52265
The physician examines the urinary collecting system with a cystourethroscope passed through the urethra and bladder and dilates the bladder with a balloon to relieve chronic inflammation of the bladder (interstitial cystitis). The physician removes the instrument and cystourethroscope. If general or spinal anesthesia is administered to the patient, use 52260. If the procedure is performed using local anesthesia, use 52265.

52270-52276
The physician examines the urinary collecting system with a cystourethroscope passed through the urethra and bladder. With a cutting instrument introduced through the cystourethroscope, the physician incises the inside of the urethral constriction. The physician removes the instrument and cystourethroscope. For incision of a female urethra, report 52270; for a male urethra, report 52275. If the physician incises the scar tissue or stricture within the urethra to open the lumen diameter while maintaining direct vision of the urethral lumen in either sex, report 52276.

52277
The physician examines the urinary collecting system with a cystourethroscope passed through the urethra and bladder, and makes an incision (sphincterotomy) in the musculature of the urethral closure (urethral sphincter). The physician passes a cutting instrument through the cystourethroscope for resection of the external sphincter. After the sphincterectomy, the physician removes the instrument and cystourethroscope.

52281
The physician examines the urinary collecting system with a cystourethroscope passed through the urethra and bladder. The physician inserts progressively larger urethral sounds, French Bougies, or filiforms and followers to dilate or calibrate a urethral stricture or stenosis. Alternatively, a balloon dilator may be used. The physician may pass a cutting instrument through the cystourethroscope to make an incision (meatotomy) in the opening of the urethra or inject radiocontrast for radiologic study of the bladder. After dilation, the physician removes any instrument(s) and the cystourethroscope.

52282
The physician places a permanent urethral stent via cystourethroscopy. Following appropriate anesthesia, the cystourethroscope is advanced through the urethra and bladder. A guidewire is placed through the scope and across the urethral stricture. A visual internal urethrotomy, which is reported separately, may be performed. A preloaded stent delivery device is passed through the stricture and the permanent stent is deployed. After confirming the position of the stent, the delivery system and scope are withdrawn.

52283
The physician treats a stricture with steroids. The physician examines the urinary collecting system with a cystourethroscope passed through the urethra and bladder, injecting material into a stricture. The physician passes an instrument through the cystourethroscope to inject the steroid into the urethral stricture. The physician removes the instrument and cystourethroscope.

52284
The physician examines the urinary collecting system with a cystourethroscope passed through the urethra and bladder of a male patient. A drug-coated balloon attached to the end of a urethral catheter dilates the urethral lumen, creating microfissures in the targeted tissue. The balloon's outer surface is coated with a therapeutic drug (paclitaxel), that is delivered directly to the stricture/stenosis site. The microfissures allow a pathway for the drug's absorption, which may help maintain the stricture expansion and preserve improved urinary flow. The device is removed after five minutes of inflation and the remaining drug lasts in the urothelium for up to 28 days. Fluoroscopy, when performed, is included in this code.

52285
The physician passes a cystourethroscope through the urethra and bladder to treat female urethral syndrome. The physician may pass instruments through the cystourethroscope to incise the opening of the urethra (urethral meatotomy), dilate the urethra, incise the inside the urethra, treat septal fibrosis of the urethra and vagina, incise the bladder neck, or destroy polyps of the urethra in the bladder neck or trigone with electric current (fulguration). The physician removes the instruments and cystourethroscope.

52287
Botulinum toxin A (BTX-A) injections are used to treat an overactive bladder (OAB). The physician examines the urinary collecting system with a cystourethroscope passed through the urethra and bladder. Injections are made into multiple sites of the bladder wall. All instruments and the cystourethroscope are removed.

52290
The physician examines the urinary collecting system with a cystourethroscope passed through the urethra and bladder, and makes an incision in the opening of the ureter(s) into the bladder (ureteral meatotomy). The physician passes the cystourethroscope through the urethra into the bladder, and inserts a cutting instrument through the cystourethroscope to incise the opening of one or both ureters into the bladder. The physician removes the instrument and cystourethroscope.

52300
The physician corrects an orthotopic (normally positioned) intravesical ureterocele(s). A ureterocele is a saccular dilation generally associated with single ureters. An orthotopic ureterocele is less common than an ectopic ureterocele, see 52301. The physician

passes the cystourethroscope through the urethra into the bladder, and examines the urinary collecting system. An instrument is inserted through the cystourethroscope which allows the physician the excise the ureterocele or destroy the ureterocele with electric current (fulguration). The physician removes the instrument and the cystourethroscope. The physician usually performs this procedure with local anesthesia. When an open procedure is necessary it is chosen on the basis of the anatomical location of the ureteral meatus, the position of the ureterocele, and the impairment of renal function.

52301
An ectopic (abnormally positioned) ureterocele is a saccular dilation generally located, in part, at the bladder neck or in the urethra. This type of ureterocele most often involves the upper pole of duplicated ureters. An ectopic ureterocele is four times more common than an intravesical, or orthotopic, ureterocele (52300), and in females the ectopic ureterocele may prolapse through the urethra. The physician passes the cystourethroscope through the urethra into the bladder, and examines the urinary collecting system. An instrument is inserted through the cystourethroscope which allows the physician to excise the ureterocele with electric current (fulguration). The physician removes the instrument and the cystourethroscope.

52305
The physician corrects a diverticulum in the bladder. The physician examines the urinary collecting system with a cystourethroscope passed through the urethra and bladder, and removes a saccular opening of the bladder (diverticulum) by excision or fulguration. The physician removes the instrument and cystourethroscope.

52310-52315
The physician examines the urinary collecting system with a cystourethroscope passed through the urethra and bladder, and removes a foreign body, calculus, or ureteral stent from the urethra or bladder. The physician passes the cystourethroscope through the urethra into the bladder, and inserts an instrument through the cystourethroscope to extract a foreign body, calculus, or ureteral stent from the urethra or bladder. The physician removes the instrument and cystourethroscope. Report 52315 if the procedure is complicated due to previous surgery or the size or condition of the foreign body, calculus, or ureteral stent.

52317-52318
The physician uses ultrasound to smash a calculus. The physician examines the urinary collecting system with a cystourethroscope passed through the urethra and bladder to remove a foreign body. The physician inserts an instrument that generates shock waves through the cystourethroscope. The physician crushes the calculus in the bladder (litholapaxy) and washes out the fragments through a catheter. Post-shockwave fragments too large to be easily suctioned may require manual crushing. For a calculus smaller than 2.5 cm, report 52317. For a calculus larger than 2.5 cm, report 52318.

52320-52330
The physician examines the urinary collecting system with a cystourethroscope passed through the urethra and bladder, and removes, fragments, or manipulates a calculus in the ureter. The physician passes the cystourethroscope through the urethra into the bladder, and inserts an instrument through the cystourethroscope to extract, fragment, or manipulate a calculus in the ureter. The physician inserts a ureteral catheter and removes the cystourethroscope. Report 52320 if the physician uses a stone basket or other instrument to remove the calculus. Report 52325 if the physician uses ultrasound or electrohydraulics to fragment the calculus. Report 52327 if the physician uses a subureteric injection of implant material. Report 52330 if the physician uses an instrument to manipulate, not remove, the calculus.

52332
The physician examines the urinary collecting system with a cystourethroscope passed through the urethra and bladder, and inserts an indwelling catheter (stent) in the ureter. The physician passes the cystourethroscope through the urethra into the bladder, and inserts an instrument through the cystourethroscope to insert an indwelling stent in the ureter. The stent provides support of the ureter. The physician removes the instrument and cystourethroscope.

52334
The physician examines the urinary collecting system, and creates an opening through the kidney to the exterior of the body (nephrostomy) by inserting a guidewire through a cystourethroscope. After examining the urinary collecting system through a cystourethroscope inserted through the urethra into the bladder, the physician inserts a catheter through the cystourethroscope into the ureter. The physician passes a guidewire through the ureteral catheter into the kidney and through a small incision in the skin of the flank. The physician removes the cystourethroscope and enlarges (dilates) the percutaneous opening by passing tubes with increasingly larger diameters through the skin incision over the guidewire to the kidney. The physician passes a nephrostomy tube over the guide, removes the guide, and sutures the tube to the skin. The physician usually withdraws the ureteral catheter at the end of the procedure.

52341-52343
The physician treats a ureteral stricture by balloon dilation, laser, electrocautery, or incision through a cystourethroscope. Under direct vision, the physician passes a flexible or rigid cystourethroscope through the urethra into the bladder. A balloon catheter is placed into the ureteral stricture, and the balloon is gently inflated. After approximately five minutes, the balloon is deflated and removed. In laser treatment of

a ureteral stricture, probes, in combination with laser fibers, are used to apply laser energy to the stricture. In electrocautery, heat is applied to eliminate the stricture. The ureteral stricture may be incised alone or in combination with balloon dilation, laser, or electrocautery to open the blocked ureter. Report 52341 when a ureteral stricture is treated, 52342 when a ureteropelvic junction stricture is treated, or 52343 when an intra-renal stricture is treated.

52344-52346

The physician treats a ureteral stricture by balloon dilation, laser, electrocautery, or incision through a cystourethroscope and ureteroscope. Under direct vision, the physician passes a flexible or rigid cystourethroscope through the urethra into the bladder and a ureteroscope into the ureter and examines the urinary collecting system. In balloon dilation, a balloon catheter is placed into the ureteral stricture, and the balloon is gently inflated. After approximately five minutes, the balloon is deflated and removed. In laser treatment of a ureteral stricture, probes, in combination with laser fibers, are used to apply laser energy to the stricture. In electrocautery, heat is applied to eliminate the stricture. Alternately, the ureteral stricture may be incised alone or in combination with balloon dilation, laser, or electrocautery to open the blocked ureter. Report 52344 when a ureteral stricture is treated, 52345 when a ureteropelvic junction stricture is treated, or 52346 when an intra-renal stricture is treated.

52351

The physician examines the urinary collecting system for diagnostic purposes with endoscopes passed through the urethra into the bladder (cystourethroscope), ureter (ureteroscope), and renal pelvis (pyeloscope). After examination, the physician removes the endoscopes.

52352-52353

The physician examines the urinary collecting system with endoscopes passed through the urethra into the bladder (cystourethroscope), ureter (ureteroscope), and/or renal pelvis (pyeloscope), and removes or manipulates a stone (calculus). To extract or manipulate a calculus, the physician passes the appropriate surgical instruments through an endoscope to perform the procedure. A ureteral catheter is inserted and the endoscope and instruments are removed. Report 52352 if the physician passes a stone basket through an endoscope to extract or manipulate a calculus. Report 52353 if the physician uses an ultrasonic, electrohydraulic, or laser technique to fragment the calculus.

[52356]

The physician examines the urinary collecting system with endoscopes passed through the urethra into the bladder (cystourethroscope), ureter (ureteroscope), and/or renal pelvis (pyeloscope) and removes or manipulates a stone (calculus). To extract or manipulate a calculus, the physician passes the appropriate surgical instruments through an endoscope to fragment the calculus. An ultrasonic, electrohydraulic, or laser technique is used. A ureteral stent is inserted, and the endoscope and instruments are removed.

52354

The physician examines the urinary collecting system with endoscopes passed through the urethra into the bladder (cystourethroscope), ureter (ureteroscope), and renal pelvis (pyeloscope), and takes a biopsy and/or uses electric current (fulguration) to destroy a ureteral or renal pelvic lesion. The physician may take a biopsy of suspect tissue and/or destroy a lesion with electric current. The physician removes required instruments and endoscopes.

52355

The physician examines the urinary collecting system with endoscopes passed through the urethra into the bladder (cystourethroscope), ureter (ureteroscope), and renal pelvis (pyeloscope), and excises a ureteral or renal pelvic tumor. The physician inserts a cutting instrument through the endoscope and excises the tumor. After flushing the area with saline solution, the physician may insert a ureteral stent. The physician removes the cutting instrument and endoscopes.

52400

The physician examines the urinary collecting system with a cystourethroscope passed through the urethra and bladder, and incises, excises, or uses electric current (fulguration) to correct defects of the bladder neck or the back of the urethra.

52402

Through the urethra, the physician performs a transurethral resection or a transurethral incision of the ejaculatory ducts (TUIED). The cystourethroscope is introduced into the meatus and the urethra is inspected. Instruments are inserted through the cystourethroscope to the region of the ejaculatory ducts. The seminal vesicles are compressed and the ejaculatory ducts are incised with a hook electrode or resected in one "bite" with a loop electrode. The seminal vesicles are again compressed. The area is observed through the scope and the instruments and cystourethroscope are removed.

52441-52442

The physician passes the cystourethroscope through the urethra into the bladder to evaluate the urethra and the bladder and ensure that no obstructions are present in the median lobe of the prostate. After assessment, the physician identifies the exact location in the lateral lobes where the permanent adjustable transprostatic implant will be deployed. The implant is assembled, tailored, and inserted via the use of an implant delivery device. Once inserted, the implant draws back and constricts the obstructing prostatic lobes while expanding the urethral lumen. The physician removes the delivery device and sheath and the lateral prostatic lobes remain retracted. The number of implants is determined by the physician and based on the individual patient's anatomy, prostate size, and shape of the prostatic lobes. Cystourethroscopy may be repeated to allow the physician to evaluate the final results and ensure the urethral lumen remains open without complications. An obstruction of the urethral lumen may require the insertion of multiple implants. Report 52441 for insertion of a single implant for the treatment of lower urinary tract symptoms (LUTS) associated with benign prostatic hyperplasia (BPH). Report 52442 for each additional implant inserted.

52450
Through a cystourethroscope, the physician incises the capsule of the prostate gland and into but not through the true prostate to create a larger passage for urine. A small transurethral tissue sample from the prostate is often collected at the same time. The bladder is catheterized for the immediate postoperative period.

52500
The physician relieves an obstruction of the outlet of the bladder. After the scope is passed through the urethra, instruments are inserted through the cystourethroscope to the target region. The physician excises the tissue responsible for the obstruction of urine flow.

52601
After preliminary cystourethroscopy, the physician passes the resectoscope under direct vision up the urethra to the region of the prostate. Meatotomy, cutting to enlarge the opening of the urethra, and/or dilatation of the urethra may be necessary to allow the passage of the resectoscope. The prostate gland is removed in a systematic fashion by using a series of small cuts into the glandular tissue with an electrocautery knife. The resected tissue is removed and the area is kept clear by irrigation through the resectoscope. Bleeding is controlled by fulguration. A catheter is passed into the bladder and left in place for the postoperative period.

52630
The physician inserts an endoscope through the urethra to remove residual or regrowth obstructive tissue from a previous surgical procedure. After preliminary cystourethroscopy, the physician passes the resectoscope into the urethra to the prostate. Meatotomy, cutting to enlarge the external opening of the urethra, and dilatation of the urethra may be necessary to allow the passage of the resectoscope. The physician removes residual tissue of the prostate gland through a series of small cuts. The resected tissue is removed, and the area is kept clear by irrigation through the resectoscope. Bleeding is controlled by fulguration. A catheter is passed into the bladder and left in place.

52640
Contracture of the bladder neck outlet usually results from scarring after a transurethral resection of the prostate gland. After preliminary cystourethroscopy, the physician passes the resectoscope under direct vision up the urethra to the region of the bladder neck contracture. Meatotomy, cutting to enlarge the opening of the urethra, and dilation of the urethra may be necessary to allow the passage of the resectoscope. The scar tissue is incised at one to three sites or resected, using a cutting electrocautery knife. The operative site is inspected for bleeding, which is controlled by fulguration. A catheter is passed into the bladder at the end of the procedure and left in place for the postoperative period.

52647-52649
The physician uses a laser to coagulate, vaporize, or enucleate the prostate through an endoscope or resectoscope inserted through the urethra. These procedures are typically performed to remove or destroy obstructive tissue in patients with benign hypertrophy of the prostate (BHP). Dilation of the urethra may be necessary to permit scope insertion. The entire prostate is treated; to accomplish this, vasectomy, meatotomy, cystourethroscopy, and internal urethrotomy may be necessary. Report 52647 if prostatic tissue is coagulated. This procedure may also be referred to as visual laser ablation of the prostate (VLAP) and utilizes a transurethral approach with a resectoscope, YAG continuous wave laser, and dilation of the urethra. A laser is inserted through the resectoscope and the physician directs the laser onto the prostate, without allowing the laser to touch the prostate tissue. In this procedure, the effects of the laser procedure cannot be visualized during the operative session. The prostate will shrink and slough tissue over a period of weeks. Transurethral vapor resection of the prostate (TUVRP), also known as electrovaporization of the prostate, is reported with 52648. The physician passes a contact or noncontact laser fiber through a resectoscope. High laser energy is delivered to the obstructive tissue in timed bursts; the hypertrophied tissue is vaporized, and a resected cavity is created. Unlike the noncontact laser coagulation procedure, the effects of the procedure can be visualized during the operative session. Enucleation, reported with 52649, entails the use of a holmium laser inserted via a resectoscope. The obstructive tissue is divided and removed in small pieces (morcellation) with an evacuator. Once the laser treatment is complete, a urinary catheter is inserted. All procedures include control of any postoperative bleeding.

52700
The physician inserts an endoscope through the urethra to drain an abscess on or near the prostate. The physician passes a cystourethroscope through the penile urethra to the region of the prostate and identifies the area of the abscess. A needle is passed into the abscess and purulent matter is removed by aspiration. The cystourethroscope is removed.

53000-53010
The physician makes an external incision in the urethra or creates an opening between the urethra and the skin. The physician passes a sound into the urethra until it meets the obstructing stricture. A longitudinal incision is made directly over the sound. After the

stricture is identified, the urethra is incised the length of the stricture so defects may be removed. The sound is removed and a catheter is passed through the urethra into the area of the incision and guided past it into the bladder. The urethra is repaired over the catheter, using sutures. Occasionally, the urethra is not repaired by suturing but is simply allowed to grow epithelial cells (epithelialize) around the catheter. In 53010, the physician meets the stricture in the perineal part of the urethra.

53020-53025

The physician makes an incision in the opening of the urethra (urethral meatus) using a small pointed knife and a meatotomy clamp. The meatus is opened on the ventral surface and the meatus may be dilated. Sutures may be required on the mucosa of the meatus. The physician often uses a hemostat to separate the tissue in the urethra prior to making his incision. Report 53020 if the patient is older than one year, or 53025 if the patient is younger than 1 year.

53040-53060

The physician drains an abscess in the urethra resulting from a urethral infection or traumatic injury. The physician makes an incision through the skin, subcutaneous tissue, and overlying layers of muscle, fat, and tissue (fascia) over the site of the abscess. By blunt or sharp dissection, the incision is carried into the abscess. Several drains are inserted and the incision is closed in layers. Report 53040 for drainage of a deep periurethral abscess. For an abscess or cyst in Skene's or paraurethral glands in the female, report 53060.

53080-53085

The physician drains urine that has passed out of the urethra (extravasation) into the perineal tissue. The physician makes an incision through the skin over the site. The incision is carried to the extravasation for drainage. Following drainage, the incision is closed with sutures. Report 53080 for uncomplicated extravasation and 53085 for complicated extravasation.

53200

Using an open approach, the physician excises a specimen of tissue from the urethra for biopsy. At the site to be analyzed, a portion of the suspect tissue is excised by blunt or sharp dissection. The incision is closed in layers.

53210-53220

The physician removes the urethra and creates an opening between the bladder and skin for drainage of urine. The physician makes a slightly curved, suprapubic (Cherney) incision down to the ureter and bladder. The bladder is opened and the urethral orifice is circumcised and usually tied off with sutures. Tumors of the urethra are removed by partial or complete urethrectomy or by electric current (fulguration). If the bladder has been opened, it is closed in two layers or more. Report 53210 for females; use 53215 for male-specific procedure. Report 53220 for removal of malignant tumor from the urethra.

53230-53235

The physician removes a urethral diverticulum. In a female patient, a longitudinal incision is made in the anterior vaginal wall and the urethral diverticulum is separated from the vaginal wall by a combination of blunt and sharp dissection. The urethra may be opened back to the orifice of the diverticulum in order to facilitate identification. A balloon catheter may be inserted and inflated. Once the diverticulum has been excised, the urethra is closed over a catheter and the vaginal wall is repaired with a layered closure. In a male patient, a cystourethroscope is inserted into the urethra and the diverticulum is excised through a transurethral incision. The physician may inject fluid or pass a balloon catheter into the diverticulum to allow it to be easily found and dissected. The diverticulum is isolated down to the neck and transected. The physician closes the urethra, leaving a catheter in the urethra. Report 53230 if performed on a female and 53235 if performed on a male.

53240

The physician repairs a urethral diverticulum by creating a pouch (marsupialization). In a female patient, a longitudinal incision is made in the anterior vaginal wall of the female and the borders of the urethral diverticulum are raised and sutured to create a pouch. The interior of the sac separates and gradually closes by granulation. The urethra is closed over a catheter and the vaginal wall is repaired with a layered closure. In a male patient, a cystourethroscope is inserted into the urethra and the diverticulum treated in the same manner, but through the perineum.

53250

The physician excises a bulbourethral gland. A bulbourethral gland is located on each side of the prostate gland near the external sphincter and is connected to the urethra with a one-inch duct. The gland secretes what becomes part of the seminal fluid. The physician completes this procedure through transurethral or segmental resection with end-to-end sutures (anastomosis).

53260-53275

The physician removes urethral polyps or caruncles in either sex, or in a female, removes Skene's glands or treats urethral prolapse. In a female, the physician separates the urethra from the vaginal wall. The urethra is incised. A circular excision is made around the lesion and the targeted tissue is resected. The urethra and vaginal mucosa are reattached in layers. In a male, the physician uses a transurethral approach to similarly excise the defect. Report 53260 if removing distal urethral polyps; 53265 if removing a urethral caruncle; 53270 if removing the Skene's glands; or 53275 if treating urethral prolapse.

53400-53405

The physician reconstructs the urethra in two stages. In the first stage (53400), the area of the stricture is identified by a catheter and urethrography and its location is marked with ink or dye. The incision is made over the stricture area and targeted tissue is removed.

Otherwise, the stricture is opened widely and the normal skin of the male or female is sutured to the edge of the mucosa on each side. In those areas in which mucosa had to be removed, the skin is sutured edge-to-edge. Six to eight weeks are required for complete healing of this stage. In the second stage (53405), the physician makes parallel incisions around the defect and continues around the urethral opening both proximally and distally. The lateral skin edges are closed over an indwelling catheter to create a new urethra. The corpora and muscles are closed, respectively, becoming the new urethra structure.

53410
The physician reconstructs the urethra of a male patient. The area of the urethral stricture is identified by catheterization. The physician cuts over the stricture area through the skin, fascia, corpus, and urethra. When the stricture is so severe that the urethral lumen cannot be identified, the physician removes the area involved. Otherwise, the stricture is opened widely and the normal skin is sutured to the edge of the mucosa on each side. In those areas in which the mucosa had to be removed, the skin is sutured edge-to-edge.

53415
The physician repairs the urethra. The stricture of the male perineal urethra is opened through a midline perineal or transpubic incision extending from the base of the scrotum to the anal margins. The physician makes an incision into the normal urethra distal to the stricture and opens the stricture on its ventral surface. From here a wide-based skin flap is developed by a U-shaped incision in the scrotum and advanced until it can be approximated to the posterior angle of the perineal incision without tension. The ends of the proximal and distal urethra are connected (anastomosis) to the extremities of the scrotal incision and anchored to the midline of the urethral bed to provide a stable urethral roof. When the urethra stricture has been opened but not excised, the edges of the longitudinal incision in the scrotal flap are sutured to the edges of the urethral wall. The outer edges of the flap are sutured to the edges of the original perineal skin incision.

53420-53425
Urethroplasties are performed to open a stricture, repair trauma, or correct a prolapse. In the first stage, the physician identifies the injured area using a catheter or a urethrograph. The incision is made over the injury and carried through the skin, fat, and other tissues (fascia). If a urethral prolapse is involved, other incisions may be involved. The problem is repaired or excised and layered sutures are made to provide adequate support. A catheter is placed and left for at least six to 12 days. In the second stage, to close the urethra, the physician cuts around the urethral defect, using skin from the scrotal flap to make a urethra. The right size urethra must be constructed to allow a catheter and prevent obstructions. The physician pulls the loose skin around the urethra and closes the incisions. The first stage is 53420; report 53425 for the second stage.

53430
The physician uses perineal or vaginal tissue to reconstruct the female urethra. With the patient in the lithotomy position and a catheter in the urethra, the physician cuts an inverted U-shaped flap above the urethral meatus and extending on the anterior vaginal wall. This flap is undermined with sharp dissection and spreading of the scissors around the upper portion of the urethral meatus, leaving a strip attached. The flap is sutured into a tube shape, reconstructing the distal urethra. The vaginal wall on each side is brought together in several layers to cover the new urethra. Small submucosal vessels are cauterized and a drain may be placed for one to two days.

53431
In the Tenago, Leadbetter procedure, the physician elongates the urethra by using bladder musculature. Continence is achieved due to contraction of the bladder musculature. The physician exposes the bladder through a suprapubic incision. The bladder is opened and the bladder neck incision is made 2 cm lateral to the urethra on each side. The musculature is drawn together in a tube and attached to the urethra. The urethral canal is closed in a two-layer technique. For the Tenago procedure, they are moved laterally.

53440-53442
The physician produces a mechanical obstruction in the urethra or at the bladder neck to put pressure on the muscles, which will prevent leakage but still allows the patient to force urine. A small midline scrotal or penile incision is made to introduce a sling composed of fascia or synthetic material. The sling is placed across the muscles surrounding the urethra and anchored. Three screws on each side of the pelvic bone secure the sling. Tension of the sling is adjusted to obtain a stress pressure optimal for the patient. With the procedure completed, the incision is closed with layered sutures. Report 53442 when the physician removes the previously placed sling or accesses the site again for revision of the sling.

53444
A urethral retention catheter is placed in the bladder and a midline lower abdominal incision is made to gain access to the space of Retzius. The bladder neck and urethra are exposed and the plane between the bladder neck and urethra is dissected and the urethrovaginal septum is dissected at the midline attachment at the distance required for accommodating the tandem cuff. Having freed the bladder neck, the physician measures its circumference and the tandem cuff is placed in position around the bladder neck and the tubing brought to the suprapubic area.

53445
The physician implants an artificial sphincter to stem urinary incontinence. In male patients, for whom the incontinence is caused by anything other than prostatic surgery, the prosthesis is inserted through a subpubic incision. For those patients who have undergone previous prostate surgery, the most

common approach is perineal with the cuff typically placed around the urethra. In female patients, the sphincter is inserted through a suprapubic incision. The space of Retzius (between the bladder and the pubis) is opened and the bladder neck is cut free, making space for the device. The bladder neck circumference is measured and a cuff of slightly larger size is chosen and sutured around the bladder neck. A space is created below the skin low in the scrotum, and the control pump passed into this position from the subpubic incision. The pressure balloon is placed in a pocket behind the rectus muscle on the same side as the control pump. The physician injects fluid into the pressure balloon. In females, the plane between the bladder neck and vagina is dissected to provide access for reservoir placement. The pump is placed in the scrotum for male patients and in the labia or inner thigh for female patients.

53446
In female patients, the physician makes a midline lower abdominal incision to gain access to the space of Retzius. The artificial urinary sphincter is exposed and the plane between the bladder neck and vagina is dissected. The device is removed and the opening is closed using suture for the rectus fascia. The subcutaneous tissues are closed and staples are used for skin closure. In male patients, the urethral bulb is exposed and the bulbospongiosus muscles are left intact over the urethra. The strap of the prosthesis is grasped under the crus and the muscle and the procedure is repeated distally to grasp the second lateral strap. The same maneuvers are repeated on the opposite site. The proximal straps are untied, as are the lateral straps. The incision is closed and a Foley catheter remains for several days.

53447
The physician removes and replaces an artificial sphincter (including pump, reservoir, and cuff) used to stem urinary incontinence. In male patients for whom the incontinence is caused by anything other than prostatic surgery, the prosthesis is accessed through a subpubic incision. In female patients, the sphincter is accessed through a suprapubic incision. The sphincter and pump are examined, removed, and replaced. The bladder neck circumference is measured and a cuff of slightly larger size is chosen and positioned around the bladder neck. A space is created below the skin low in the scrotum and the control pump passed into this position from the subpubic incision. The pressure balloon is placed in a pocket behind the rectus muscle on the same side as the control pump. The physician injects fluid into the pressure balloon and the connections are permanently established. In females, the plane between the bladder neck and vagina is dissected.

53448
In females, the vagina is prepared preoperatively and a urethral retention catheter is placed in the bladder. The patient is administered general anesthesia and placed supine. The physician makes a midline lower abdominal incision to gain access to the space of Retzius. The artificial urinary sphincter is exposed and the plane between the bladder neck and vagina is dissected. The device is removed. The area is irrigated with antibiotics and the physician debrides the infected tissue. Antibiotics are again used to flush the area. The tubing of the balloon of the replacement device is brought into the suprapubic area through a separate stab incision laterally in the rectus fascia. The control pump is passed through the suprapubic area through a subcutaneous track into the subcutaneous tissue of the ipsilateral labium. The device is emptied of fluid and a Hypaque solution is injected into the pressure balloon, using a 14-gauge blunt needle. The device components are connected, the pressure balloon is aspirated until empty, and the Hypaque solution is re-injected. Connections are completed between the control pump and cuff and reinforced by suture. The device is activated. The opening is closed using suture for the rectus fascia. The subcutaneous tissues are closed and staples are used for skin closure. In males, the patient is placed under general anesthesia in the lithotomy position. The urethral bulb is exposed and the bulbospongiosus muscles are left intact over the urethra. The strap of the prosthesis is grasped under the crus and the muscle and the procedure is repeated distally to grasp the second lateral strap. The same maneuvers are repeated on the opposite site. The proximal straps are untied, as are the lateral straps. The area is irrigated by antibiotic, and the infected tissue is debrided. The area is again flushed by antibiotic and the physician inserts the replacement pump using the same steps in the procedure for placement of the artificial sphincter described. The incision is closed and a Foley catheter is left indwelling for several days.

53449
The physician repairs an inability of an inflatable sphincter device to stem incontinence. In male patients the prosthesis is accessed through a subpubic incision. In female patients, the sphincter is accessed through a suprapubic incision. The space of Retzius (between the bladder and the pubis) is opened and the device is located. The physician checks the cuff and sutures around the bladder neck. The physician locates reservoir and checks for any malfunctions or abnormalities. The pressure balloon, usually located in a pocket behind the rectus muscle on the same side as the control pump, is evaluated for patency and function. Any necessary repairs are completed. The physician closes the incisions. The reservoir is filled and all connections are made. Several test inflations and deflations are performed during closure. The physician places a catheter in the bladder for about one day.

53450
The physician performs this surgery to open or reconstruct the urethra, improving voiding or allowing insertion of an instrument. The meatus, which may be congenitally small or narrowed as the result of infection, is opened and a mucosal flap is advanced and sutured to the glans.

53451-53454

These procedures describe minimally invasive, long-term, and adjustable continence therapy for stress urinary incontinence (SUI) utilizing a proprietary balloon device. Indications often include post-prostatectomy incontinence in males and intrinsic sphincter deficiency or a previously failed surgery in females. Following appropriate anesthesia (general, spinal, or local), the patient is placed in a lithotomy position that enables access to the perineum. A cystourethroscopy is performed, leaving the cystoscope sheath in place during the procedure for visualization and palpation of the ureter. Via transverse perineal incisions and under fluoroscopic guidance, implantation instruments are advanced to the area of the bladder neck and the tissue is dilated to create a space for the balloon device. The balloon is inserted to the level of the bladder neck (or at the apex of the prostatic remnant in TURP patients) under fluoroscopic guidance and inflated using a needle to inject an isotonic filling solution into the port. The procedure is repeated on the contralateral side. Titanium ports are placed under the skin of the scrotum in males and under the skin of the labia majora in females. Incisions are closed with resorbable sutures and a dressing is applied. The fluid-filled balloons provide support and pressure to stop urine leakages during sneezing, coughing, exercising, or other physical exertion. Once implanted, the clinician can adjust the device at any time as required to meet the patient's needs. Report 53451 for bilateral insertion placement and 53452 for unilateral insertion. For removal, the physician locates the balloon's port by palpation. Following administration of a local anesthetic, he makes a small incision over the port, through the subcutaneous tissue, and removes any fluid from the balloon using a syringe and needle. Once the fluid is removed, the physician places gentle traction on the port and tubing, removes the balloon, and closes the skin and subcutaneous tissues with sutures. Report 53453 for each balloon removed. Report 53454 for balloon fluid volume adjustments. Following localization of the port by palpation, the physician anesthetizes the perineum. After filling a syringe with isotonic fluid, the physician inserts the needle percutaneously to puncture the port's septum and adds 0.5 to 1.0 cc of fluid to the balloon. This is repeated on the other side.

53460

The physician widens the meatus to enhance voiding. The physician makes an incision on the ventral surface of the penis and skin is freed from the shaft. Fibrous tissue is removed. An erection is artificially induced to confirm all fibrous tissue has been removed.

53500

Transvaginal, secondary, open urethrolysis is performed in cases when voiding is obstructed due to excessive periurethral scarring caused by previous surgical repair of stress incontinence, procedures such as bladder neck suspension. Urethrolysis involves cutting obstructive adhesions or bands of fibrous tissue that have grown to fix the urethra to the pubic bone. An incision is made through the vagina. The adhering fibrous bands and periurethral scar tissue are visualized and dissected. Lysis and removal continues until the urethra is mobilized away from the surrounding fibrous tissue. Some correction to vaginal abnormalities may be accomplished before closure of the incision. Postsurgical cystourethroscopy is included in this procedure to examine the urethra following urethrolysis.

53502-53515

The physician repairs a urethral wound or injury, including the skin and even more traumatic wounds requiring more than a layered closure. Examples include debridement of cuts (lacerations) or tears (avulsion). Suturing of the urethra is done in layers to prevent later complications and fistula formations. The tissue can be constructed around a catheter. Report 53502 if the patient is female; 53505 if the patient is male; 53510 if the wound in either sex is perineal; or 53515 if repair involves the prostate.

53520

The physician closes a urethrostomy or urethrocutaneous fistula. An elliptical incision is made around the opening of the urocutaneous fistula and carried deeper into the supporting tissue toward the urethra. The entire tract is freed and excised unless it involves other important structures, such as the external sphincters. When the tract cannot be completely removed, the remaining part is cut. The defect of the urethra is closed in layers over a catheter.

53600-53605

When the physician examines the male patient, a soft rubbery urethral catheter is passed and the stricture is noted. If a stricture is found, a dilator is used. Report 53600 for the first visit and 53601 for subsequent visits. Report 53605 if spinal anesthesia is administered.

53620-53621

The physician uses fine tools to dilate the male urethra. A filiform (a small silk-like instrument with woven spiral tips, to which followers made of a similar material can be attached by a screw-like mechanism) is used when a stricture cannot be passed. With a filiform as a guide, the follower is passed through the urethra. Increasing sizes of followers are introduced, dilating the stricture. The filiform is manipulated up a lubricated urethra to the stricture. The physician attaches a follower to the filiform and the stricture is widened. Report 53621 if it is a subsequent procedure.

53660-53665

The physician uses dilators of increasing size to widen the female urethra. A suppository or instillation of a saline solution may be used. Report 53660 for initial dilation, and 53661 for subsequent dilation. Use 53665 if general or spinal anesthesia is administered for dilation of female urethral stricture.

53850

The physician performs transurethral destruction of prostate tissue by microwave thermotherapy. The physician inserts an endoscope in the penile urethra, prior to endoscope placement the urethra may need to be dilated to allow instrument passage. After the endoscope is passed, a microwave thermotherapy stylet is inserted in the urethra and the diseased prostate is treated with electromagnetic radiation. The treated prostate is examined for evidence of bleeding which may be controlled with electrocoagulation. The endoscope and instruments are removed. A urinary catheter is inserted into the bladder and left in place postoperatively.

53852

The physician performs transurethral destruction of prostate tissue by radiofrequency thermotherapy. The physician inserts an endoscope in the penile urethra, prior to endoscope placement. The urethra may be dilated to allow instrument passage. After the endoscope is placed, a radiofrequency thermotherapy stylet is inserted in the urethra and the diseased prostate is treated with thermal energy vapor. The treated prostate is examined for evidence of bleeding, which may be controlled with electrocoagulation. The endoscope and instruments are removed. A urinary catheter is inserted into the bladder and left in place postoperatively.

53854

The physician performs transurethral destruction of prostate tissue by radiofrequency generated water vapor thermotherapy. The physician inserts an endoscope in the penile urethra. The urethra may be dilated to allow instrument passage. After the endoscope is placed, a radiofrequency generated water vapor thermotherapy stylet is inserted in the urethra and the diseased prostate is treated with steam. The treated prostate is examined for evidence of bleeding, which may be controlled with electrocoagulation. The endoscope and instruments are removed. A urinary catheter is inserted into the bladder and left in place postoperatively.

53855

A physician inserts a temporary urethral stent in a patient with prostatic urethral obstruction to improve voiding function. The stent system consists of a proximal balloon to prevent distal displacement, a urine port situated above the balloon, and the stent. Topical anesthesia is administered and the physician inserts the probe to locate the external sphincter. Once the external sphincter is located, a measurement is taken and the proper size stent selected. The stent device is mounted on a single-use insertion tool and standard catheter insertion technique is used to insert it. The proximal tip, balloon, and urine port are positioned in the bladder and the balloon is inflated with 5 cc of water. The insertion device is removed. A distal anchor mechanism is secured by sutures. A retrieval suture that extends to the meatus and deflates the balloon when pulled is also secured. The stent is typically left in place for up to 30 days.

53860

The physician uses radiofrequency energy to treat female stress urinary incontinence, the involuntary loss of urine from the urethra due to increased intra-abdominal pressure. Using a small transurethral probe, the physician applies low temperature radiofrequency energy to targeted submucosal areas of the bladder neck and urethra. This results in minute structural alterations to the collagen that, upon healing, makes the tissues firmer and increases the resistance to involuntary leakage.

53865-53866

In 53865, the physician examines the urinary collecting system with a cystourethroscope passed through the urethra and bladder and inserts a temporary device for ischemic remodeling of the bladder neck and prostate to treat urinary tract symptoms due to benign prostatic hyperplasia (BPH). The folded device is advanced through a cystoscope sheath and deployed into the bladder. After rotating the anchoring leaflet into a six o'clock position, the device is retracted into the prostatic urethra using a guidewire. Proper positioning is confirmed, and the physician removes the instruments and cystourethroscope. In 53866, the temporary device is removed five to seven days after insertion. During this time, the device struts have expanded into the bladder neck and prostatic tissue to create longitudinal channels through ischemic pressure, resulting in necrosis that remodels the bladder neck and prostate. To remove the device, a retrieval suture is threaded through a silicone catheter. The catheter is advanced to the end of the device. The physician pulls on the retrieval suture, causing the device to collapse into the catheter. The device and catheter are removed.

Male/Female

54000-54001

The prepuce is the fold of penile skin commonly called the foreskin. The physician makes a cut or slit in the prepuce to relieve a constriction that prevents the retraction of the foreskin back over the head of the penis. A segment of foreskin on the dorsal or the side of the penis is crushed with forceps. Using scissors, the physician makes a cut through the crushed tissue and sutures the divided skin to control bleeding. The prepuce of a newborn is slit in 54000, while 54001 reports the slitting of the prepuce of any male other than a newborn.

54015

The physician drains a deep abscess or hematoma (pocket of blood) by incising penile tissue. After instilling a local anesthesia, the physician makes an incision through the skin and deeper tissues into the abscessed cavity. The urethra and the main arteries and nerves are avoided. Often a drain is left in place to assure adequate drainage.

54050-54055
The physician treats skin lesions of the penis by local application of a chemical (54050) or local electrodesiccation (54055) to kill the diseased tissue or organism. Using a cotton-tipped applicator soaked in the chemical or an electrodesiccator, the physician applies the treatment to the specific lesions only, taking care to avoid touching normal skin with the chemical or the electrodesiccator. Using either method, no tissue is removed and no closure is required.

54056-54057
The physician treats skin lesions of the penis by local application of liquid nitrogen or the use of a cryothermal instrument (54056) or by laser beam (54057) to kill the diseased tissue or the organism. Using a cotton-tipped applicator dipped in liquid nitrogen (-78 degrees Celsius), the physician freezes or burns with the laser only the specific lesions. No tissue is removed and no closure is required.

54060
The physician excises selected large lesions of the penis not removable by other methods. After adequate local anesthesia has been administered, the physician cuts out an elliptical piece of skin that includes the lesion and a rim of normal tissue. With a forceps or hemostat clamp, the physician grasps and elongates the involved skin containing the lesion, causing the tissue to tent. Using a scalpel or scissors, an ellipse of tissue containing the lesion is excised. The resulting defect is closed with sutures.

54065
The physician destroys extensive lesions of the penis using one or more of several methods. Extensive destruction generally means the procedure took more time or was more difficult than usual due to such factors as the size and number of lesions involved. The methods used by the physician include local application of a chemical, freezing, electrodesiccation, laser vaporization to kill the diseased tissue, or excision. Local anesthesia may be used for these procedures. The physician applies the method only to the specific lesions.

54100
The physician removes a portion of a skin lesion on the penis by punch biopsy or by excising a small portion of the lesion with scalpel or scissors. The resulting defect may require simple repair with sutures.

54105
The physician removes a portion of a penile mass by deep punch biopsy or by making an incision in the penis and dissecting tissues to the deep mass and excising a portion of the lesion. The incision may be repaired with layered sutures.

54110-54112
Peyronie's disease is an induration and severe curvature of the erect penis due to fibrosis of the cavernous sheaths. The physician corrects Peyronie's disease by excising abnormal fibrous tissue on the dorsal aspect of the penis. After an incision is made around the penis, the physician retracts the skin to expose the abnormal tissue on the underlying normal spongy tissue. Avoiding critical nerves and blood vessels, with the penis erect, the defective tissue is excised. The skin is closed by suturing. Report 54111 if a graft measuring 5 cm or less in length is required; report 54112 if a graft greater than 5 cm is required.

54115
The physician removes a foreign body from deep within the shaft of the penis by making an incision and dissecting the tissues. The foreign body, usually a penile implant, is localized and removed. The resulting defect is closed with layered sutures.

54120
The physician removes a portion of the penis due to disease or mutilating injury. The distal penis is enclosed in a rubber glove and a tourniquet is applied at the base of the penis. An incision is made completely around the penile shaft. The various structures of the penis are isolated and divided with care to leave enough of the urethra to form an opening for the passage of urine. The remaining tissues and skin are closed with layered sutures.

54125
The physician removes the penis due to disease or mutilating injury. The distal penis is enclosed in a rubber glove. An incision is made from above the penis and carried around the base of the penile shaft and down through the midline of the scrotum. The various structures of the penis are isolated and divided with care to leave enough of the urethra for drainage. The urethra is brought through the perineum below the scrotum and an opening is created for the passage of urine. The remaining tissue and skin are closed in layered sutures with drains placed in the scrotum and a catheter in the bladder.

54130
The physician removes the entire penis and surrounding lymph nodes to treat invasive cancer. The distal penis is enclosed in a rubber glove. An incision is made from above the base of the penis and carried around the base of the penile shaft and down through the midline of the scrotum. The various structures of the penis are isolated and divided with care to leave enough of the urethra for drainage. The urethra is brought through the perineum below the scrotum and an opening is created for the passage of urine. The remaining tissues and skin are closed in layered sutures with drains placed in the scrotum and a catheter in the bladder. The physician also removes the lymph nodes in the groin areas. An incision is made from the pubic bone to the lateral pelvic bone exposing the area for dissection. The fatty tissues bearing the lymph nodes are removed. The defect is covered by rotating one of the thigh muscles over the area and suturing it in place. The subcutaneous tissues and the skin are closed in layered sutures over drains placed in the region.

54135
The physician removes the entire penis and surrounding lymph nodes to treat invasive cancer. The distal penis is enclosed in a rubber glove. An incision is made from above the base of the penis and carried around the base of the penile shaft and down through the midline of the scrotum. The various structures of the penis are isolated and divided leaving enough of the urethra for drainage. The urethra is brought through the perineum below the scrotum and an opening is created for the passage of urine. The remaining tissues and skin are closed in layered sutures with drains placed in the scrotum and a catheter in the bladder. The physician also removes the lymph nodes in the groin areas. An incision is made from the pubic bone to the lateral pelvic bone exposing the area for dissection. The fatty tissues bearing the lymph nodes are removed. The defect is covered by rotating one of the thigh muscles over the area and suturing it in place. The subcutaneous tissues and the skin are closed in layered sutures over drains placed in the region. A lower midline abdominal incision is made and the pelvic cavity is entered and the lymph nodes deep in the pelvis are removed. The abdominal incision is also closed in layers of sutures.

54150
After the administration of a local anesthetic by injection(s), the physician removes the foreskin of the penis by clamping the foreskin in a plastic device and trimming the excess protruding skin. A segment of foreskin on the dorsal or the side of the penis is crushed with forceps. A cut is made through the crushed tissue with scissors, and the divided foreskin is fitted in a plastic bell-shaped clamp. The clamp crushes a ring of the foreskin and holds the skin edges together while the excess skin is trimmed from the top of the device. The clamp is left in place and simply falls off when healing has finished days later.

54160-54161
The physician removes the foreskin of the penis in a baby up to 28 days of age (54160) or in a male older than 28 days (54161) by excision of the skin. A segment of foreskin on the dorsal or the side of the penis is crushed with forceps. A cut is made through the crushed tissue with scissors, and the divided foreskin is pulled down over the head of the penis while the excess skin is trimmed from around the head of the penis. Bleeding is controlled by chemical cautery or suture ligatures. The skin edges created are sutured together with absorbable suture material.

54162
The physician releases post-circumcision penile adhesions by lysis or excision. Penile adhesions occur when the skin of the penile shaft adheres to the glans of the penis. Untreated adhesions may become thicker, forming skin bridges in which the penile shaft skin adheres to the coronal margin. Using appropriate anesthesia, the physician retracts the foreskin and cleanses the glans of debris and smegma. Adhesions are freed and the skin bridge, if present, is incised and divided. Closure of the separated skin bridge is performed in appropriate fashion to avoid any postoperative curvature (chordee) with erection. The physician excises any remaining foreskin and bleeders are coagulated. Ointment, a nonadherent dressing, and gauze is applied.

54163
A repeat circumcision may be performed if there is circumferential scarring of excessive residual skin or incomplete removal of the preputial skin during the initial circumcision. First, the skin at the base of the penis is cleansed with alcohol and allowed to dry. The physician uses an index finger to palpate the lateral side of the penis to determine the position of the root of the penis. With a tuberculin syringe and needle, the anesthetic is injected parallel to the root of the penis. While the penis is stabilized by gentle downward or ventral traction, the needle is inserted at the base of the penis and inserted beneath the skin surface. The anesthetic is injected and the needle withdrawn. An incision is made around the base of the foreskin, the foreskin is pulled back, and it is cut away from the penis. Stitches are usually used to close the skin edges.

54164
The physician performs an incision of the membrane that attaches the foreskin to the glans and shaft of the penis (frenulum). A dorsal penile nerve block is administered with a needle directed through the fascia of the symphysis pubis and into the frenum space where the anesthetic is deposited to block the dorsal nerves of the penis. A longitudinal incision is made ventrally though the outer layer of the prepuce. After retracting the prepuce, the physician extends the incision along the inner layer. Bleeding is controlled with an electrocoagulator. The resultant wound is closed.

54200-54205
Peyronie's disease is an induration and severe curvature of the erect penis due to fibrosis of the cavernous sheaths. The physician injects medication into the abnormal fibrous tissue of the penis to correct painful curvature of the penis caused by Peyronie's disease. In 54200, no incision is made. The medication is injected into the dorsal area of the penis through the skin. In 54205, the physician makes an incision in the dorsum of the penis and identifies the abnormal fibrous tissue. An injection is made directly into the abnormal fibrous tissue under direct visualization through the incision.

54220
The corpora cavernosa are the spongy bodies of the penis, the dual columns of erectile tissue that form the back and sides of the penis. In priapism, this spongy tissue is in a state of persistent erection. The physician treats priapism by irrigating the corpora cavernosa. After adequate local anesthesia, the physician passes a large bore needle into the body of the penis and aspirates a quantity of blood and irrigates the space with 20 ml to 30 ml of saline solution. This may be accompanied by injecting medication into the same

region, repeating it several times to get the abnormal erection to resolve.

54230

The corpora cavernosa are the spongy bodies of the penis, the dual columns of erectile tissue that form the back and sides of the penis. The physician injects medication into the penis for x-ray studies to evaluate erectile dysfunction. After placing a constricting rubber band around the penis, the physician passes a needle into the body of the penis and aspirates a small quantity of blood. X-ray contrast medication is injected directly into the body of the penis. The constricting band is removed and x-rays are taken to demonstrate the function and integrity of the corpora cavernosa and the blood flow of the penis.

54231

Corpora cavernosa is the spongy tissue of the penis. The physician injects vasoactive drugs into the corpora cavernosa for studies to evaluate erectile dysfunction. A rubber band is placed around the base of the penis and the intracavernous pressure is measured using instrumentation. The physician evaluates the penis for leakage between the diastolic and the systolic pressures. A swift rate of decay between the two indicates arterial and/or venous insufficiency of the penis. After the test, the band is removed and the instrumentation removed.

54235

Corpora cavernosa is the spongy tissue of the penis. The physician injects medication into the penis to treat erectile dysfunction. After placing a constricting rubber band around the penis, the physician passes a needle into the body of the penis and aspirates a small quantity of blood. The selected medication is injected directly into the body of the penis. This produces an erection in most patients that may last from minutes to hours.

54240

A plethysmograph is an instrument that measures variations in the volume of an organ and in the amount of blood in it or passing through it. The physician measures the physiological potential of the penis to attain and maintain an erection using plethysmography. The volume change of the penis is measured in response to external stimuli.

54250

The physician monitors nighttime erections in impotent patients during rapid eye movement sleep. Testing can be performed in a sleep center or in the patient's home. During the test, the patient's penis is wired to a strain gauge monitor and recordings are made of the strength and duration of any erections occurring while the patient sleeps.

54300

The physician corrects and repairs chordee, which is the abnormal curvature of the penis. To assist in planning the surgery, an artificial erection may be produced by placing a band around the base of the penis and injecting saline into the body of the penis. The area of deformity is determined and by using a combination of incisions and excisions of abnormal fibrous tissue and sometimes normal tissue, the defect is corrected. Care is taken to dissect around nerves and blood vessels. Sometimes the urethra is dissected free of its position and retracted temporarily away from the operative site. The separate tissues of the penis are closed in layers with absorbable suture material. An artificial erection may again be produced to test and demonstrate the adequacy of the repair.

54304

The physician corrects and repairs chordee, which is the abnormal curvature of the penis. The physician also prepares the penis for correction of hypospadias, an abnormal opening of the urethra on the underside of the penis or on the perineum. To assist in planning the surgery, an artificial erection may be produced by placing a band around the base of the penis and injecting saline into the body of the penis. The area of deformity is determined and the defect is corrected using a combination of incisions and excisions of the prepuce (foreskin). Care is taken to dissect around the nerves and blood vessels. Often the foreskin is used in a free graft or a flap graft to cover the ventral skin defects created to correct the chordee. The separate tissues of the penis are closed in layers with absorbable suture material. An artificial erection may again be produced to test and demonstrate the adequacy of the repair. The urethral opening is left on the ventral shaft of the penis for repair during a later stage.

54308-54312

The physician completes the repair of chordee (abnormal curvature of the penis) and hypospadias (an abnormal opening of the urethra on the underside of the penis or on the perineum) by creating a urethral opening in the end of the penis. The urethra is dissected free of the surrounding tissues to mobilize it. A distal urethra, less than 3 cm in 54308 or greater than 3 cm in 54312, is formed from the prepuce (foreskin) and an opening is created at or near the tip of the head of the penis. Urine may be diverted by the use of a catheter in the bladder. The skin is closed with sutures.

54316

The physician completes the repair of chordee (abnormal curvature of the penis) and hypospadias (abnormal opening of the urethra on the underside of the penis or on the perineum) by creating a urethral opening in the end of the penis. The urethra is mobilized by dissecting it free from the surrounding tissues. A distal urethra is formed from skin obtained from a site other than the genitalia and sutured to the existing urethra and to an opening created at or near the tip of the head of the penis. Urine may be diverted using a catheter in the bladder. The skin and tissues are closed with fine absorbable sutures.

54318

The physician completes the repair of chordee (abnormal curvature of the penis) and hypospadias (an abnormal opening of the urethra on the underside of the penis or on the perineum) by separating the temporary attachments sutured between the penis and scrotum during a previous stage of the repair. Urine may be diverted using a catheter in the bladder. The skin is closed with fine sutures.

54322

The physician corrects and repairs a chordee, which is an abnormal curvature of the penis. The physician also prepares the penis for correction of hypospadias, an abnormal opening of the urethra on the underside of the penis or on the perineum. The physician corrects hypospadias in the distal penis at the base of the head of the penis in a one-stage procedure. An incision is made around the shaft of the penis next to the glans (head) and the skin is dissected from the penile shaft taking care to avoid injury to the urethra. An erection is artificially produced to evaluate any chordee before and after the correction. Any chordee present is corrected by excising the responsible fibrous band. A second incision is made in the groove on the underside of the glans. Skin in the area is pulled up to the glans and fashioned into an opening by suturing in the head of the penis. A circumcision, or excision of some foreskin, may be performed. The original incision around the penis is closed by suturing.

54324

In a one-stage procedure, the physician corrects hypospadias, which is an abnormal opening of the urethra on the underside of the penis, in the distal or end portion of the penile shaft. An incision is made from the head of the penis around the urethral opening. An erection is artificially produced to evaluate the chordee before and after the correction. Any chordee present is corrected by excising the responsible fibrous band. A flap is created from the skin below the urethral opening and flipped up and over the opening of the urethra and sutured together forming a tube extension of the urethra. The foreskin is divided and sutured over the defect left by the flap on the ventral surface of the penis. A circumcision is usually the result of the procedure.

54326

In a one-stage procedure, the physician corrects hypospadias, which is an abnormal opening of the urethra on the underside of the penis, in the distal or end portion of the penile shaft. An incision is made on the ventral surface of the penis and around the urethral opening. An erection is artificially produced to evaluate any chordee before and after the correction. Any chordee present is corrected by excising the responsible fibrous band. The urethra is dissected free of the shaft to mobilize it. A flap of skin is created from the foreskin and sutured together to form a tube to be used as a segment of urethra. The foreskin is further divided and sutured over the defect left by the flap on the ventral surface of the penis. Foreskin excision (circumcision) may be part of this procedure.

54328

Hypospadias is an abnormal opening of the urethra on the underside of the penis or on the perineum. The physician corrects hypospadias in the distal or end portion of the penile shaft in a one-stage procedure. An incision is made on the ventral surface of the penis and around the urethral opening. An erection is artificially produced to evaluate the chordee before and after the correction. Any chordee present is corrected by excising the responsible fibrous band. The urethra is dissected free of the shaft to mobilize it. An island flap of skin is created from the foreskin and sutured together to form a tube to be used as a segment of urethra. This formed urethral tube flap is sutured in place between the urethral opening in the shaft of the penis and an opening created in the head of the penis. The foreskin is further divided and sutured over the defect left by the flap on the ventral surface of the penis. Foreskin removal (circumcision) may be part of this procedure.

54332

Hypospadias is an abnormal opening of the urethra on the underside of the penis or on the perineum. The physician corrects hypospadias in the base portion of the penis in a one-stage procedure. An incision is made on the ventral surface of the penis and around the urethral opening. An erection is artificially produced to evaluate the chordee before and after the correction. Chordee is corrected by excising the responsible fibrous band. Considerable dissection is required to mobilize the urethra. An island flap of skin is created from the foreskin and sutured together to form a tube to be used as a segment of urethra. This formed urethral tube flap is sutured in place between the urethral opening at the base of the shaft of the penis and an opening created in the head of the penis. The foreskin and skin overlying the shaft are further divided and dissected free and sutured over the defect left by the flap on the ventral surface of the penis. A circumcision is usually the result of the procedure.

54336

Hypospadias is an abnormal opening of the urethra on the underside of the penis or on the perineum. The physician corrects hypospadias in the perineal portion of the penis in a one-stage procedure. An incision is made on the ventral surface of the penis and around the urethral opening. An erection is artificially produced to evaluate the chordee before and after the correction. Any chordee present is corrected by excising the responsible fibrous band. Considerable dissection is required to mobilize the urethra in preparation for repair of the hypospadias. An island flap of skin is created from the foreskin and sutured together to form a tube to be used as a segment of urethra. This formed urethral tube flap is sutured in place between the urethral opening at the base of the scrotum in the perineum and an opening created in the head of the penis. The foreskin and skin overlying the shaft are further divided and dissected free and sutured over the defect left by the flap and dissections on the ventral surface of the penis. Circumcision is usually the result of the procedure.

54340-54348

Hypospadias is an abnormal opening of the urethra on the underside of the penis or on the perineum. The physician repairs a fistula, stricture, and/or diverticula resulting from a former hypospadias repair. The fistula (abnormal passage) or diverticula (pouch or sac) is identified and excised, often using microsurgical techniques. A stricture (narrowing) is corrected by dilating the area with dilating catheters or by incision and suture closure. Report 54340 for a simple repair. Report 54344 if the urethral defect is repaired by closure with a free patch graft or flap graft. The skin defect is closed by simple suturing or using a flap skin graft. Report 54348 if the defect in the urethra is repaired by closure with a free patch graft or a flap graft that requires extensive dissection, mobilization of tissues, and the creation of complicated grafts such as a tube graft. The skin defect is closed by simple suturing or by use of a flap skin graft. Urine may be diverted through a catheter left in the bladder. The catheter can be passed through the urethra or placed directly in the bladder through the lower abdominal wall just above the pubic bone.

54352

Hypospadias is an abnormal opening of the urethra on the underside of the penis or on the perineum. The physician repairs severe, disabling complications from former hypospadias repairs, sometimes documented as hypospadias cripple. Often using microsurgical techniques and considerable excision of scarred and damaged tissues, the deformities and malfunctions of the urethra and penis are corrected. Two or three stages may be necessary to complete this complicated task. A new urethral segment is created with a free patch graft, a flap graft, or using a tube graft. Extensive dissection and mobilization of tissues are generally required to complete the process. Skin defects are closed using flap or free skin grafts. Any strictures (narrowing of hollow structures) are corrected by dilating the area with dilating catheters or by incision and suture repair. Urine may be diverted through a catheter left in the bladder. The catheter can be passed through the urethra or placed in the bladder through an incision in the lower abdominal wall just above the pubic bone.

54360

The physician corrects an abnormal curvature of the penis using a series of excisions of tissue on the side of the penis. To assist in planning the surgery, an erection may be artificially produced by placing a band around the base of the penis and injecting saline into the body of the penis. The area of deformity is determined and using a combination of incisions and excisions of tissue, the defect is corrected. An incision is made in the skin of the penis just proximal to the glans (head of the penis) and the skin is pulled to the base of the penis, exposing the underlying tissues. Further dissection is done to expose the thick connective tissue on one side of the shaft. A series of parallel excisions are made and the resulting defects are closed by suturing. The separate tissues and the skin of the penis are closed in a layered fashion with absorbable suture material. An erection may again be induced to test the adequacy of the repair.

54380

The physician corrects epispadias, which is the congenital absence of the upper wall of the urethra. The urethra has its opening anywhere on the top surface of the penis. A closed urethra is created by reapproximating the tissues, and by using skin grafts, tube grafts, free tissue grafts, or a combination of techniques depending on the extent of the defect.

54385

The physician corrects epispadias and associated urinary incontinence in one or more stages. Epispadias with incontinence is the congenital absence of the upper wall of the urethra and the lack of function of the muscles that control the bladder neck. Through an incision in the lower abdomen, the surgeon reconstructs the bladder neck and reimplants the ureters from the kidneys away from the bladder neck outlet. A closed urethra is created by reapproximating the tissues and by using skin grafts, tube grafts, free tissue grafts, or a combination of techniques depending on the extent of the defect.

54390

The physician corrects epispadias and exstrophy of the bladder in stages. Epispadias is the congenital absence of the upper wall of the urethra. Bladder exstrophy is the turning inside out of the bladder so that the bladder is open directly to the outside and as such, urine does not collect in the bladder but simply drains without any control to the outside onto the lower abdomen. The first stage is to close the bladder through incisions in the lower abdomen. The surgeon frees the bladder from the abdominal wall and proceeds to close the bladder and reimplant the ureters from the kidneys away from the bladder neck outlet. In the second stage, a closed urethra is created by reapproximating the tissues and by using skin grafts, tube grafts, free tissue grafts, or a combination of techniques depending on the extent of the defect. In the following stages, the physician reconstructs the bladder neck to provide urinary control and, if necessary, does additional surgery on the penis and urethra.

54400-54401

The physician inserts a semi-rigid penile prosthesis in 54400, which is a hinged or malleable device, or a self-contained inflatable penile prosthesis in 54401, which is a one piece, paired hydraulic device that allows fluid to be pumped from one portion of the device to another. A transverse incision is made just above the penis over the pubic bone. With care to avoid important nerves and blood vessels, dissection is carried down to the erectile tissues at the base of the penis. Incisions are made in the thick fibrous membranes surrounding the two main erectile tissues to allow the insertion of dilators to create space for the prostheses. The paired prosthetic devices are inserted one at a time into the two erectile tissue compartments down the length of the penis. The incisions and tissues are closed by suturing. The operation can also be done in similar fashion using an incision just below the scrotum in the perineum to enter the erectile tissue or in the upper scrotum at the base of the penis.

54405
The physician inserts an inflatable penile prosthesis made of three components-the reservoir, the pump, and two inflatable cylinders. A transverse incision is made at the base of the penis in the upper scrotum. With care to avoid the urethra and important nerves and blood vessels, dissection is carried down to the erectile tissues at the base of the penis. The thick fibrous membranes surrounding the two main erectile tissues are incised and dilators are inserted to create space for the prostheses. Two prosthetic devices are inserted into the two erectile tissue compartments down the length of the penis. A pouch is made in one side of the scrotum, and the pump mechanism and tubing are inserted into the space created. Using an index finger, the surgeon creates a tunnel from the pump to the space behind the pubic bone. The reservoir is placed behind the pubic bone with tubing running from it through the tunnel to the pump in the scrotum. The incisions and tissues are closed by suturing. The operation can also be done in similar fashion using an incision just below the scrotum in the perineum to enter the erectile tissue and in the area above the pubic bone to gain access to place the reservoir.

54406
The patient is taken to the operating room, placed in a supine or lithotomy position, and the physician makes an incision using the same penoscrotal or infrapubic approach as the original procedure to remove the multi-component, inflatable penile prosthesis. The physician makes an incision into the corpus cavernosum and the prosthesis is withdrawn. The corporotomy is closed by suture. The subcutaneous tissue is closed by suture and a dressing is applied to the incision. The bladder is emptied with a catheter. An indwelling urethral catheter, if used, is removed on the first postoperative day.

54408
Under general anesthesia, the patient is placed in a supine or lithotomy position and the physician makes an incision using the same penoscrotal or infrapubic approach as the original procedure to repair the previously placed multi-component, inflatable penile prosthesis. The physician makes an incision into the corpus cavernosum to inspect the previously placed prosthesis. Repairs are made. The corporotomy is closed by suture. The subcutaneous tissue is closed by suture and a dressing is applied to the incision. The bladder is emptied with a catheter. An indwelling urethral catheter, if used, is removed on the first postoperative day.

54410
Under general anesthesia, the patient is placed in a supine or lithotomy position and the physician makes an incision using the same penoscrotal or infrapubic approach as the original procedure to remove the previously placed multi-component, inflatable penile prosthesis and to insert a replacement during the same operative session. The physician makes an incision into the corpus cavernosum and the prosthesis is withdrawn. The replacement prosthesis is brought through the glans and the deflated cylinder is drawn into the distal corporal body for insertion into the crus of the penis. The corporotomy is closed and the cylinders are inflated and deflated several times to check the flow of the fluid to and from the cylinders. The reservoir is brought through the external inguinal ring and the bladder is emptied by catheter. The existing subfascial pocket in used to place the reservoir, as well as the pump/activator mechanism, which is placed in the existing scrotal pocket. Sutures are placed to prevent upward migration, the tubing is filled with fluid, and the physician makes the connections between the tubing of the pump and reservoir and the tubing of the pump and cylinders. Before the wound is closed, the prosthesis is cycled to check proper functioning. The corporotomy is closed by suture. The subcutaneous tissue is closed by suture and a dressing is applied to the incision. The bladder is emptied with a catheter. An indwelling urethral catheter, if used, is removed on the first postoperative day.

54411
The physician removes and replaces a multi-component inflatable penile prosthesis and irrigates and debrides infected tissue. The patient is taken to the operating room and placed under general anesthesia. The physician makes an incision using the same penoscrotal or infrapubic approach as the original procedure. The physician makes an incision into the corpus cavernosum and the prosthesis is withdrawn. Any infected tissue is debrided and irrigated with an antibiotic solution. The replacement prosthesis is brought through the glans and the deflated cylinder is drawn into the distal corporal body for insertion into the crus of the penis. The corporotomy is closed and the cylinders are inflated and deflated several times to check the flow of the fluid to and from the cylinders. The reservoir is brought through the external inguinal ring and the bladder is emptied by catheter. The existing subfascial pocket is used to place the reservoir, as well as the pump/activator mechanism, which is placed in the existing scrotal pocket. Any infected tissue is debrided and irrigated with an antibiotic solution. Sutures are placed to prevent upward migration, the tubing is filled with fluid, and the physician makes the connections between the tubing of the pump and reservoir and the tubing of the pump and cylinders. Before the wound is closed, the prosthesis is cycled to check proper functioning. The corporotomy is closed by suture. The subcutaneous tissue is closed by suture and a dressing is applied to the incision. The bladder is emptied with a catheter. An indwelling urethral catheter, if used, is removed on the first postoperative day.

54415
The physician makes an incision using the same approach (i.e., penoscrotal or distal penile) as the original procedure to remove the non-inflatable or self-contained inflatable penile prosthesis in a patient who is under general anesthesia. An incision is made into the corpus cavernosum, the corporal tissue is dissected, and the prosthesis is removed from the corporal body. The wound is irrigated with antibiotics, and the corporotomy is closed by suture. The subcutaneous tissue is closed by suture and a dressing is applied to the incision. The bladder is emptied with a catheter.

54416
Under general anesthesia, the patient is placed in a supine or lithotomy position and the physician makes an incision using the same approach (i.e., penoscrotal or distal penile) as the original procedure to remove the non-inflatable (semi-rigid)or self-contained inflatable penile prosthesis and to insert a replacement prosthesis. An incision is made into the corpus cavernosum, the corporal tissue is dissected, and the prosthesis is removed from the corporal body. The wound is irrigated with antibiotics and the replacement prosthesis is advanced to the mid-glans and introduced into the corporal space. Once implanted, the wound is again irrigated with antibiotics, and the corporotomy is closed by suture. The subcutaneous tissue is closed by suture and a dressing is applied to the incision. The bladder is emptied with a catheter. An indwelling urethral catheter, if used, is removed on the first postoperative day.

54417
The physician removes and replaces a non-inflatable (semi-rigid) or inflatable (self-contained) penile prosthesis, and irrigates and debrides infected tissue. The physician makes an incision using the same intrapubic, penoscrotal, or distal penile approach as the original procedure to remove the prosthesis and to insert a replacement non-inflatable or inflatable penile prosthesis at the same operative session. Using corporal incisions, the physician is able to remove the prosthesis. A colposcopy may be performed to ensure all fibrous elements are excised, and a replacement prosthesis is implanted. Any infected tissue is debrided and irrigated with an antibiotic solution. The corporotomy is closed by suture. The subcutaneous tissue is closed by suture and a dressing is applied to the incision. The bladder is emptied with a catheter. An indwelling urethral catheter, if used, is removed on the first postoperative day.

54420
The physician treats priapism, an abnormally sustained erection, by creating a shunt for the diversion of blood from the penis to the femoral vein. An incision is made in the groin area of the thigh and the saphenous vein is cut and dissected free of its attachments creating a mobile segment about 10 cm long. A second incision is made at the base of the penis and the saphenous vein is tunneled through the subcutaneous tissues to the base of the penis. A 1 cm in diameter piece of the thick fibrous tissue of the corpus cavernosum (erectile tissue) is excised and the free end of the saphenous vein is sutured to the defect. The erection resolves as blood flows from the penis to the femoral vein through this saphenous vein segment. The incisions are closed by suturing. The procedure is sometimes repeated on the opposite side.

54430
The physician treats priapism, an abnormally sustained erection, by creating a shunt for the diversion of blood from one region of the penis to an adjacent region. With a catheter in the urethra into the bladder, an incision is made in the side of the penis. Dissection is carried to the thick fibrous tissues surrounding one of the corpus cavernosum (erectile tissue) and to the corpus spongiosum, which is the erectile tissue around the urethra. Oval discs of the fibrous tissue are excised from the adjacent surfaces of these two structures. The excisional defects are sutured together creating a shunt (passageway) for the flow of blood from the engorged corpus cavernosum to the corpus spongiosum thus relieving the erection. The tissues and the skin are sutured closed. The procedure is sometimes repeated on the opposite side.

54435
The physician treats priapism, an abnormally sustained erection, by creating a shunt for the diversion of blood from the one region of the penis to an adjacent region. With adequate local anesthesia, the head of the penis is punctured with a biopsy needle and advanced into the tip of the corpus cavernosum (erectile tissue). A portion of tissue from the head of the penis to the corpus cavernosum is removed as if taking a biopsy. This creates a passageway for blood trapped in the cavernosum to escape through the circulation to the head of the penis. The procedure is repeated to the opposite corpus cavernosum. The two puncture sites in the head of the penis are closed by suturing.

54437
Repair of traumatic corporeal tears vary depending on the surgeon and/or location of the tear. Typically the tears are transverse, near midline and the urethra. A tourniquet is placed at the base of the penis to restrict blood flow, leaving the operative field as clear as possible for visualization and exploration. A midline perineal incision is made to reveal the corporeal body. A Gittes test may be performed to aid in locating the tear. The injection of saline and erection simulation can flush out possible blood clots hiding the leak. The tear is repaired with sutures. The incision is closed in layers. Some surgeons may place a catheter overnight while other surgeons only utilize this when the trauma is very close to the urethra. Postoperative treatment can range from antibiotics to compression dressings to erection inhibitors.

54440
The physician repairs an injury of the penis using one or more of plastic surgery techniques. The repair may

require skin grafts, tissue grafts, urethral repair, extensive debridement, microsurgical repairs, or any combination.

54450
The physician treats adhesions between the uncircumcised foreskin and the head of the penis that prevent the retraction of the foreskin. Adhesions are broken by stretching the foreskin back over the head of the penis onto the shaft or by inserting a clamp between the foreskin and the head of the penis and spreading the jaws of the clamp.

54500
The physician obtains a sample of testicular tissue by needle biopsy. While the testis is held firmly with the scrotal skin stretched tightly over the testis and the epididymis positioned away from the biopsy site, a biopsy needle is inserted into the testis at the area of concern. The needle biopsy sheath is advanced over the needle and twisted to shear off the enclosed sample and withdrawn with the sample enclosed. The scrotal wound may be closed by suturing.

54505
The physician obtains a sample of testicular tissue by direct incisional biopsy. The procedure is done under local or regional anesthesia. While the testis is held firmly with the scrotal skin stretched tightly over the testis and the epididymis positioned away from the biopsy site, a small incision is made through the skin of the scrotum. The underlying tissues are incised and dissected to expose the testis. The testis is stabilized by two sutures and an ellipse of tissue is removed between the two sutures. The incisions are closed by suturing.

54512
The physician excises an extraparenchymal lesion of the testis. The physician makes an inguinal incision, incising the skin and subcutaneous fat. The testicle is delivered through the incision, the tunica vaginalis is opened, and the lesion is excised. The incision is closed with suture.

54520
An incision is made in one side of the scrotum and the tissues are separated to expose the spermatic cord. The spermatic cord is opened and the individual bundles making up the cord are cross-clamped, cut, and secured with nonabsorbable suture material. The testis is removed through the scrotal incision. If the patient so chooses, and if no contraindications are present, a prosthetic testis is inserted into the scrotum before the wound is closed in layers by suturing. An alternative method uses an incision in the groin. The testis is pulled through the incision after cutting and tying the cord in a fashion similar to the scrotal approach.

54522
The physician performs a partial excision of one testis or both testes. The surgeon makes a longitudinal incision midline in the scrotum to expose the testis. The tunica vaginalis is incised, and the testicular vessels and vas deferens are identified, clamped separately, and divided. The cords are ligated at a level slightly above the area of infection, abscess, neoplasm, or trauma and the spermatic cord is isolated for manipulation of the testicle. The testis is delivered to the wound and dissected below the ligated cords. The wound is closed by suture and a pressure dressing and scrotal supporter are applied.

54530
The physician performs a radical orchiectomy by removing en bloc the contents of half of the scrotum. An incision is made in the inguinal area from the pubic bone toward the lateral pelvic bone. The incision made deep into the tissues and the spermatic cord is dissected free and cross-clamped. The testis and all its associated structures are pushed up from the scrotum into the incision and removed. Packing is placed in the empty scrotum. When the spermatic cord is opened and the individual bundles making up the cord are cross-clamped, cut, and secured with nonabsorbable suture material, care is taken to avoid important nerves and vessels in the area. The packing is removed and bleeding controlled. A prosthetic testis may be placed in the scrotum before the incision is closed in layers by suturing. This procedure results in complete removal of the testis.

54535
The physician performs a radical orchiectomy by removing en bloc the entire contents of half of the scrotum and also explores the inside of the abdomen for evidence of tumor spread. An incision is made in the inguinal area from the pubic bone toward the lateral pelvic bone. The incision made deep into the tissues and the spermatic cord is dissected free and cross-clamped. The testis and all its associated structures are pushed up from the scrotum and delivered into the incision and removed. Packing is placed in the empty scrotum. Care is taken to avoid important nerves and vessels in the area, when the spermatic cord is opened and the individual bundles making up the cord are cross-clamped, cut and secured with nonabsorbable suture material. This results in complete removal of the testis. The packing is removed and bleeding controlled. A prosthetic testis may be placed in the scrotum before the incision is closed in layers by suturing. A midline incision is made from the upper to the lower abdomen and the abdominal cavity is entered. The back wall of the abdomen is exposed and the lymph nodes are checked for spread of tumor. Some may be removed and/or biopsied and the abdominal wound is closed in layers by suturing.

54550
The physician searches for a testis that failed to descend into the scrotum during development. An incision is made in the scrotum or the inguinal area from the pubic bone to the upper lateral pelvic area in the skin fold made by the thigh and the lower abdomen. The tissues are separated by dissection to find the testis in the area. No other procedure is performed. The incision is closed in layers by suturing.

54560
The physician searches the abdominal cavity for a testis that failed to descend into the scrotum during development. An incision is made in the inguinal area from the pubic bone to the upper lateral pelvic area in the skin fold made by the thigh and the lower abdomen. The tissues are separated by dissection and the incision is extended into the abdominal cavity. No other procedure is performed at this time. The incision is closed in layers by suturing.

54600
The physician treats a torsion of the testis, which is a twisting of the testis upon itself so that its blood supply is compromised. The physician makes an incision in the scrotum and exposes the twisted testis. The testis and spermatic cord is untwisted to restore blood flow to the organ. If the testis is viable, the surgeon anchors the testis to the inside wall of the scrotum with three or more sutures. The incision is closed in layers by suturing. Because the problem that allowed the testis to twist may affect the other testis (contralateral testis), a second procedure is commonly performed to anchor it in similar fashion.

54620
The physician makes an incision in the scrotum and exposes the testis on side opposite to the one that had previously been twisted. The surgeon anchors the testis to the inside wall of the scrotum with three or more sutures to prevent the twisting of the cord and the testis. The incision is closed in layers by suturing.

54640
Orchiopexy is the surgical fixation of an undescended testicle into the scrotum. An incision is made in the scrotum or the inguinal area from the pubic bone to the upper lateral pelvic area in the skin crease made by the thigh and the lower abdomen. The physician searches for a testis that failed to descend into the scrotum during development. The tissues are separated by dissection to find the testis in the inguinal canal area. The spermatic cord is mobilized to allow positioning of the testis in the scrotum. In the scrotum, a small pouch is created for the testis and the testis is sutured in place to prevent retraction back into the inguinal canal. The incision is closed in layers by suturing.

54650
Orchiopexy is the surgical fixation of an undescended testicle into the scrotum. An incision is made in the inguinal area from the pubic bone to the upper lateral pelvic area in the skin fold made by the thigh and the lower abdomen. The physician searches the abdominal cavity for a testis that failed to descend in to the scrotum during development. The tissues are separated by dissection and the incision is extended into the abdominal cavity to find the testis in the abdominal area. The tissues are separated by dissection to find the testis in the area. At this point several surgical options are available. The one chosen will depend on the mobility of the testis and how far it can be brought down through the inguinal canal and into the scrotum. The procedure may take two stages approximately six to 12 months apart. Eventually, the spermatic cord is mobilized sufficiently to allow positioning of the testis in the scrotum. In the scrotum a small pouch is created for the testis where the testis is sutured in place to prevent retraction back in to the inguinal canal or into the abdominal cavity. The incision is closed in layers by suturing.

54660
For cosmetic reasons, the physician places an artificial testis in the scrotum of a patient. After adequate local anesthesia, an incision is made in the inguinal area and the empty scrotal sac is dilated by passing a dissecting finger or a moist gauze sponge through the inguinal canal into the scrotum. A prosthetic testis is inserted into the scrotal sac and the neck of the scrotum is closed by suturing. The inguinal incision is closed in layers by suturing.

54670
The physician repairs injury (laceration or traumatic rupture) to the testis that occurs as a result of a blunt or penetrating injury. Often a laceration is present in the scrotum and the testis is explored and repaired through the open wound. Otherwise, an incision is made in the scrotum to expose the testis. Any devitalized testicular tissue is removed by sharp dissection and the thick tough fibrous tissue encasing the testis is closed by suturing. The scrotum is closed in layers by suturing. Often a rubber drain is placed to prevent the accumulation of fluid and blood in the scrotum.

54680
The physician transplants the testis(es) under the skin of the thigh to preserve function and viability following massive injury or surgical loss of the scrotal skin. The thigh is chosen because the temperature just under the skin is approximately the same as in the scrotum, a condition to normal testicular function. Incisions are made in the skin of the thigh adjacent to the scrotum and the testis is sutured in place with attention to preserving blood flow to the organ. The thigh incisions are closed in layers over a rubber drain brought out through the skin. In four to six weeks scrotal reconstruction is begun.

54690
The physician removes one or both testicles, which may be undescended, injured or diseased using a laparoscope. The physician places a trocar at the umbilicus into the abdominal or retroperitoneal space and insufflates the abdominal cavity. The physician places a laparoscope through the umbilical incision and additional trocars are placed into the abdomen. The testis and all its associated structures are pushed up from the scrotum or freed from their undescended intra-abdominal location and removed through the abdominal or retroperitoneal space via the trocar port. Packing may be placed in the empty scrotum. Care is taken to avoid important nerves and vessels in the area. A prosthetic testis may be placed in the scrotum before the incision is closed in layers by suturing. The

trocars are removed and the incisions are closed with sutures.

54692

The physician performs an orchiopexy (surgical fixation of an undescended testicle into the scrotum) with the assistance of a fiberoptic laparoscope. A paraumbilical port is created by placing a trocar at the level of the umbilicus. The abdominal wall is insufflated. The laparoscope is placed through the umbilical port and additional trocars are placed into the abdominal cavity. The physician uses the laparoscope fitted with a fiberoptic camera and/or an operating instrument to search the abdominal cavity for the undescended testis. The physician may have several surgical options depending on the mobility of the testis and how far it can be brought down through the inguinal canal and into the scrotum. The procedure may take two stages approximately three to 12 months apart. The spermatic cord is mobilized sufficiently to allow positioning of the testis in the scrotum, which often occurs during the first and perhaps only operative session. A small pouch is created for the testis where the testis is sutured in place to prevent retraction back into the inguinal canal or into the abdominal cavity. The small abdominal incisions are closed by staple or suture in the usual fashion.

54700

The physician drains a collection of blood or an abscess within the scrotum. If the testis is the target of the drainage, it is held firmly with the scrotal skin stretched tightly over the testis and the epididymis positioned away from the site. A small incision is made through the skin of the scrotum. The underlying tissues are incised and dissected to expose the testis and the site to be drained. The testis may be stabilized by two sutures as an incision is made into the abscess or hematoma and fluid is expressed. Packing or a rubber drain may be placed to promote drainage. The incisions are usually not closed by suturing. Similar procedures are followed if the target is the epididymis or the scrotal space.

54800

The physician obtains a sample of epididymal tissues by needle biopsy. While the testis is held firmly with the scrotal skin stretched tightly over the testis and the epididymis positioned just under the taut skin, a biopsy needle is inserted into the area of concern in the epididymis. The needle biopsy sheath is advanced over the needle and twisted to shear off the enclosed sample and withdrawn containing the sample. The scrotal wound may be closed by suturing.

54830

The physician removes a local lesion of the epididymis by direct incision. The procedure is done under local or regional anesthesia. While the testis is held firmly with the scrotal skin stretched tightly over the testis and the epididymis positioned just under the taut skin, a small incision is made through the skin of the scrotum. The underlying tissues are incised and dissected to expose the epididymis and the area of concern. The epididymis may be stabilized by two sutures placed on each side of the lesion and an ellipse of tissue is removed from the epididymis containing the lesion between the two sutures. The stabilizing sutures are tied across the excision site to close it. The scrotal incision is closed by suturing.

54840

The physician removes a spermatocele, which is a small cyst, filled with fluid and spermatozoa, between the body of the testis and the epididymis. After adequate local anesthesia, an incision is made in the scrotum and the testis with its attached epididymis is brought out of the wound. The cyst is dissected free of the testis and excised. The involved area of the epididymis is sutured to the underlying testis and the scrotal wound is closed by suturing. Alternately the epididymis may be dissected free of all of its attachments to the testis. The blood vessels involved are tied and cut and/or cauterized to control bleeding. The freed epididymis is thus removed, a rubber drain is placed in the scrotum and the incision is closed by suturing.

54860-54861

The physician removes the epididymis. After adequate local anesthesia, an incision is made in the scrotum and the testis, with its attached epididymis, is brought out of the wound. The epididymis is dissected free of all of its attachments to the testis. The blood vessels involved are tied and cut and/or cauterized to control bleeding. The freed epididymis is thus removed, a rubber drain is left in the scrotum, and the incision is closed by suturing. The epididymectomy is performed on one side in 54860 or both sides in 54861.

54865

The physician explores the epididymis by making an incision in the scrotum. The procedure is done under local or regional anesthesia. While the testis is held firmly with the scrotal skin stretched tightly over the testis and the epididymis positioned just under the taught skin, a small incision is made through the skin of the scrotum. The underlying tissues are incised and dissected to expose the epididymis. The epididymis may be biopsied by placing two sutures on each side of the area of concern and an ellipse of tissue is removed from the epididymis containing the lesion between the two sutures. The stabilizing sutures are tied across the excision site to close it. The scrotal incision is closed by suturing. Alternatively, a biopsy may be done by needle puncture under direct vision.

54900-54901

The physician treats obstruction of the flow of spermatozoa from the epididymis to vas deferens, the tube that carries the semen. After adequate anesthesia, an incision is made in the scrotum and the testis with its attached epididymis and the vas deferens is brought out of the wound. The vas deferens is transected and the selected area of the epididymis is opened and the appropriate tubule in the area is brought out of the surrounding tissues and transected. The cut ends of these two tubes are sutured together and the vas deferens is sutured to the epididymis. A rubber drain is often placed in the scrotum and the incision is closed by suturing. In 54900, the procedure is performed on one side; in 54901, the procedure is bilateral.

55000
A hydrocele is a sac of fluid in the tunica vaginalis or along the spermatic cord. The physician treats a hydrocele by aspirating the fluid. After injecting a small area with local anesthetic, the physician inserts a needle on an aspirating syringe into the fluid filled hydrocele sac and withdraws the fluid into the syringe. After the aspiration and with the needle still in place, the sac may be injected with sclerosing medication to prevent accumulation of new fluid by stimulating scarring and hardening of the empty sac.

55040-55041
A hydrocele is a sac of fluid in the tunica vaginalis or along the spermatic cord. The physician treats a hydrocele by removing it. After injecting an area with local anesthetic and using aseptic techniques, the physician makes an incision in the scrotum or in the inguinal area. Care is taken to keep the hydrocele intact while it is dissected free of its attachments to the testis and other structures. The sac is opened, drained and partially excised leaving a remnant of tissue. The remaining tissue is swung back behind the epididymis and the spermatic cord and closed by suturing the edges together. The testis is anchored to the inside of the scrotum with three sutures to prevent later torsion or twisting of the testis. A rubber drain may be left in the scrotum and the incision closed in layers by suturing. The hydrocele is on one side in 55040. In 55041, each side is treated for hydrocele.

55060
The physician treats a hydrocele by removing the abnormal fluid filled sac in the scrotum or in the inguinal canal. After injecting an area with local anesthetic and using aseptic techniques, the physician makes an incision in the scrotum or in the inguinal area. Care is taken to keep the hydrocele intact while it is dissected free of its attachments to the testis and other structures. The sac is opened high along its front surface and the testis is pushed up through the sac and out through the incision. This inverts the hydrocele sac which is tacked by suturing to the spermatic cord structures behind the testis. The testis is returned to the scrotum and is anchored to the inside of the scrotum with three sutures to prevent later torsion or twisting of the testis. A rubber drain may be left in the scrotum and the incision closed in layers by suturing.

55100
After adequate local anesthesia, the physician makes an incision directly into the abscess of the scrotal wall. Pus is expressed and a drain or medicated gauze packing placed in the abscess cavity.

55110
The physician makes an incision in the scrotum for the purpose of direct visual inspection of the contents of the scrotum. This may involve one or both sides of the scrotum and may be done through one or two incisions and require incisions through the various layers of tissues to expose the testis and other structures. A drain may be left in the scrotum and the incisions closed in successive layers of sutures.

55120
The physician makes an incision in the scrotum for the purpose of foreign body removal. This may involve one or both sides of the scrotum and may be done through one or two incisions and may require incisions through the various layers of tissues to expose and locate the object. The foreign body is identified and isolated and removed with care to avoid damaging tissues in the scrotum. A drain may be placed in the scrotum and the incisions closed in successive layers of sutures.

55150
The physician removes excessive or diseased scrotal skin by excision. The extent of the procedure is dependent upon the disease process and the degree of involvement. The physician makes incisions in the scrotal skin, taking care to avoid injury to the underlying scrotal contents. In the simple case, the excess skin is removed and the defects closed in layers by suturing. In the more involved cases the testes and spermatic cords must be mobilized and removed from the scrotum and swung out of the way by making incisions in the inguinal areas. The affected scrotal skin is excised and the testes and cord structures returned to their anatomic positions. If not enough scrotal skin remains, flaps of skin are raised from the adjacent thighs and rotated to cover the testes. These grafts or flaps are separately reported. Rubber drains may be left in the scrotum and the operative site closed in layers by suturing.

55175-55180
The physician repairs defects and developmental abnormalities of the scrotum by wound revisions or the creation and suturing of simple scrotal skin flaps in 55175. In 55180, the reconstruction is more complex and the physician uses free skin grafts, mesh grafts, and/or the extensive use of rotational pedicle grafts from adjacent skin. These flaps or grafts are separately reported.

55200
The physician enters the vas deferens (the tube that carries spermatozoa from the testis) for purpose of obtaining a sample of semen or testing the patency of the tubes. Under local anesthesia, an incision is made in the upper outer scrotum overlying the spermatic cord. The tissues are dissected to expose the vas deferens. The tube is entered by puncturing with a small needle and fluid samples removed or solution injected to check for blockages. An alternate method involves the tube being cut open with a scalpel. A blunt needle is placed in the tube under direct vision and fluid samples removed or the tube checked for patency. If an incision is made in the tube, the tube must be repaired using microsurgical techniques before the scrotal incisions are closed in layers by suturing.

55250

The physician grasps the upper scrotum near the inguinal area and holds the spermatic cord between the thumb and the index finger. The skin overlying the immobilized cord is injected with local anesthetic and an incision is made through the scrotal wall to expose the tubular structures. Another incision is made to expose the vas deferens (spermatic tube) and the tissues dissected to free it from the adjacent vessels and supporting tissues. The isolated vas deferens is cut in two places and the intervening section of tube is removed. The cut ends of the vas deferens are cauterized and tied with suture material. The incisions are closed in layers by suturing. The procedure is usually repeated on the opposite side.

55300

The physician enters the vas deferens (the tube that carries spermatozoa from the testis) for purpose of testing the patency of the spermatozoa collecting system. An incision is made in the upper outer scrotum overlying the spermatic cord and the tissues dissected to expose the vas deferens.

55400

The physician treats a blockage in the vas deferens, the tube that carries semen. After anesthesia, an incision is made in the scrotum. The testis with its attached epididymis and the vas deferens are brought out of the wound. Dye injection studies and semen sampling is often done during the operation to determine the site of the blockage and to accurately choose the segment of tube for excision. The vas deferens is transected in two places, one on each side of the blocked area and the abnormal segment removed. The created cut ends are sutured together in one or two layers with care to align accurately the lumens of the tubes. The testis and associated structures are returned to the scrotum. A rubber drain is often placed in the scrotum and the incisions closed by suturing.

55500

A hydrocele is an abnormal fluid-filled sac. The physician treats a hydrocele of the spermatic cord by removing from the spermatic cord above the testis in the scrotum or in the inguinal canal. After injecting the area with local anesthetic, the physician makes an incision in the scrotum or in the inguinal area. The hydrocele is kept intact while it is freed of its attachments to the spermatic cord. The sac is opened, drained, and excised all the way to the internal inguinal ring in the upper groin area. The remaining tissues are repaired and closed by suturing. The testis is anchored to the inside of the scrotum with three sutures to prevent later torsion or twisting of the testis. A rubber drain may be placed in the scrotum and the incision closed in layers by suturing.

55520

The physician removes a lesion of the spermatic cord by dissection and excision. After injecting the area with local anesthetic, the physician makes an incision in the scrotum or in the inguinal area and dissects the tissues to expose the lesion. Care is taken to keep the lesion intact while it is dissected free of its attachments to the spermatic cord. This may involve mobilization of the testis. The lesion is removed by cutting all of its attachments. The tissues damaged during the dissection are repaired and closed by suturing. If the testis has been mobilized, it is anchored to the inside of the scrotum with three sutures to prevent later torsion or twisting. A drain may be placed in the scrotum and the incision is closed in layers by suturing.

55530

A varicocele is an abnormal dilation of the veins of the spermatic cord in the scrotum. The physician ligates the spermatic veins and/or excises a varicocele. An incision is made in the pubic area on the affected side and carried down to the spermatic cord as passes through the inguinal canal. The cord is brought up into the incision and the structures of the cord are dissected, the veins identified, and ligated with suture material. Alternately, an incision is made in the scrotum and the dilated veins ligated separately may be removed. The incision is closed in layers by suturing.

55535

The physician ligates the spermatic veins and/or excises a varicocele which is an abnormal dilation of the veins of the spermatic cord in the scrotum. An incision is made in lateral lower abdomen just medial to the bony prominence of the pelvic bone on the affected side and carried down through the abdominal musculature to the spermatic vein and artery. The vein is identified and ligated (tied off) with suture material. The abdominal incision is closed in layers by suturing.

55540

The physician repairs an inguinal hernia and ligates the spermatic veins or excises a varicocele (an abnormal dilation of the veins of the spermatic cord in the scrotum). An incision is made in the pubic area on the affected side to expose the spermatic cord as it passes through the inguinal canal. The cord is brought into the incision, the structures of the cord are dissected, and the veins identified and ligated. The hernia is repaired through the same incision by folding and suturing of tissues to strengthen the abdominal wall and correct the weakness responsible for the hernia. Alternately, an incision is made in the scrotum and the dilated veins ligated separately and may be removed (excision) and a second incision made for hernia repair. All incisions are closed in layers by suturing.

55550

The physician ligates (ties or binds with suture) the spermatic veins and/or excises a varicocele which is an abnormal dilation of the veins of the spermatic cord in the scrotum. An umbilical port is created by placing a trocar at the level of the umbilicus. The abdominal wall is insufflated. The laparoscope is placed through the umbilical port and additional trocars are placed into the abdominal or pelvic cavity. The physician uses the laparoscope fitted with a fiberoptic camera and/or an operating instrument to explore and surgically ligate the spermatic veins to repair or remove the varicocele. The structures of the cord are dissected, the veins identified, and ligated with suture. The abdomen is deflated, the trocars removed, and the incisions are closed with sutures.

55600-55605

The physician incises or punctures one of the seminal vesicles, paired glands that lie behind the urinary bladder and produce fluid that is mixed with the semen produced in the testis. The seminal vesicle is approached through an incision in the lower abdomen or an incision in the perineum (area between the base of the scrotum and the anus). In the abdominal method, the physician retracts the bladder forward toward the pubic bone to expose the back of the bladder where the seminal vesicles are positioned, or the surgeon cuts through the front and back walls to gain access to the gland. The operative wounds are closed in layers by suturing. If the procedure does not require extensive dissection, report 55600; if extensive, report 55605.

55650

The physician removes one of the seminal vesicles, paired glands that lie behind the urinary bladder and produce a fluid that is mixed with semen from the testis. Through an incision in the lower abdomen or an incision in the perineum (area between the base of the scrotum and the anus) the seminal vesicle is approached. If the abdominal method is used the surgeon retracts the bladder forward toward the pubic bone to expose the back of the bladder where the seminal vesicles are positioned or the surgeon cuts through the front and back walls to gain access to the glands. The surgeon dissects the gland free of its attachments and clips it at its joint with the ejaculatory duct and removes it. The operative wounds are closed in layers by suturing.

55680

The physician excises a Mullerian duct cyst, a remnant of the prenatal development of the seminal vesicle. The seminal vesicles are paired glands that lie behind the urinary bladder and produce a fluid that is mixed with the semen from the testis. Through an incision in the lower abdomen or an incision in the perineum (area between the base of the scrotum and the anus) the seminal vesicle is approached. If the abdominal method is used, the surgeon retracts the bladder forward toward the pubic bone to expose the back of the bladder where the seminal vesicles are positioned or the surgeon cuts through the front and back walls to gain access to the glands. The surgeon dissects the cyst free of its attachments and clips it at the attachment to the seminal vesicle and removes it. The operative wounds are closed in layers by suturing.

55700

The physician obtains tissue from the prostate by needle or punch biopsy by any approach. In the most common technique, local anesthesia is administered, and the needle or punch cannula is passed into the rectum by guidance with the index finger and punctured through the rectal mucosa. Separately reportable imaging guidance such as ultrasound, CT, MRI, or fluoroscopy may be used to advance to the biopsy location. The specimen (core) is obtained, and the needle or punch cannula is withdrawn. This is repeated multiple times to ensure adequate sampling. Typically, biopsies are obtained from each area of the prostate for a total of six to 12 cores. Pressure is applied over the puncture site to control bleeding.

55705

The physician obtains tissue from the prostate for analysis by direct incisional sampling. The prostate is usually approached in one of three ways: through skin of the perineum (the area between the base of the scrotum and the anus), through the rectal mucosa, or by advancing a biopsy instrument through the urethra. In any case, an incision is made and the tissues dissected to expose the prostate. The area of concern is identified and an excision is performed to remove tissue for analysis. Bleeding is controlled and the dissected tissues and skin incision are closed in layers by suturing.

55706

In a facility setting, the physician obtains stereotactic template-guided saturation sampling biopsies using a transperineal approach. This method allows for systematic sampling of the entire prostate gland. General anesthesia is administered, and the patient is placed in the lithotomy position. A stereotactic template is placed over the perineum using ultrasound guidance. A needle is repeatedly advanced transperineally through the template into the prostate at 5 mm intervals until 35 to 60 specimens are obtained. Pressure is applied over the puncture sites to control bleeding.

55720-55725

The physician performs a simple prostatotomy (cutting or puncturing the prostate) through one of two usual approaches. An aspirating needle is passed into the abscessed area of the prostate by puncturing through skin of the perineum (the area between the base of the scrotum and the anus), or by advancing the needle into the rectum by guidance with the index finger and puncturing through the rectal mucosa. The needle is inserted into the abscess in the prostate guided by an index finger or by ultrasound and the contents of the abscess removed by aspiration. The needle is withdrawn and the puncture site bandaged. Report 55720 for simple drainage, or 55725 if the procedure is complicated by excessive bleeding, infection, or other problem.

55801

The physician performs a prostatectomy (removal of the prostate gland) through an incision made in the perineum. The caliber (internal diameter) of the urethra is measured and if it is not adequate, the opening of the urethra is enlarged (meatotomy) and the diameter of the penile urethra is enlarged with an instrument (internal urethrotomy). A curved instrument (tractor) is advanced into the urethra to the prostate to help identify the structures and aid in the dissection. Through the perineal incision and with manipulation of the tractor, the tissues are dissected to expose the prostate. The curved tractor instrument in the urethra is replaced with a straight tractor. A portion of the prostate or the entire gland is removed with care to preserve the seminal vesicles. The operation is "subtotal" because the seminal vesicles remain intact. The bladder outlet is revised and the vas deferens is ligated and may be partially removed (vasectomy). Bleeding is controlled by ligation or cautery. A Foley catheter is placed in the bladder. A rubber drain may be placed in the site of the operative wound and brought out through a separate stab wound. The dissected tissues and the skin incision are closed in layers by suturing.

55810-55812

The physician performs a radical prostatectomy through an incision made in the skin between the base of the scrotum and the anus. If the internal diameter of the urethra is not adequate, the opening of the urethra is enlarged (meatotomy) and the diameter of the penile urethra is enlarged with an instrument (internal urethrotomy). A curved instrument (Lowery Tractor) is advanced into the urethra to the prostate to aid in the dissection. Through the perineal incision and with manipulation of the tractor, the tissues are dissected to expose the prostate. The curved tractor instrument in the urethra is replaced with a straight tractor. The entire gland is removed along with the seminal vesicles and the vas deferens. The bladder outlet is revised and bleeding controlled by ligation or cautery. In 55812, local lymph nodes are also removed for analysis. A Foley catheter is placed and left in the bladder. A rubber drain may be placed in the site of the operative wound and brought out through a separate stab wound. The dissected tissues and the skin incision are closed in layers by suturing.

55815

The physician removes the prostate gland through an incision made in the perineum and also a pelvic lymphadenectomy through a separate lower abdominal incision. A midline abdominal incision is made from the upper to the lower abdomen and the back wall of the abdomen is exposed. All lymph nodes along back wall of the pelvic and abdominal cavities are removed. The abdominal wound is closed in layers by suturing. In preparation for removal of the prostate, the caliber (internal diameter) of the urethra is measured and if it is not adequate the opening of the urethra is enlarged (meatotomy) and the diameter of the penile urethra is enlarged with an instrument (internal urethrotomy). A curved instrument (Lowery Tractor) is advanced into the urethra to aid in the dissection. Through the perineal incision and with manipulation of the tractor, the tissues are dissected to expose the prostate. The curved tractor instrument in the urethra is replaced with a straight tractor. The gland is removed along with the seminal vesicles and the vas deferens. The bladder outlet is revised and bleeding controlled by ligation or cautery. A Foley catheter is placed and left in the bladder. A rubber drain may be placed in the site of the operative wound and brought out through a separate stab wound. The dissected tissues and the skin incision are closed in layers by suturing.

55821

The physician removes the prostate gland through an incision made in the lower abdomen just above the pubic area. In preparation for removal of the prostate, the caliber (internal diameter) of the urethra is measured and if it is not adequate the opening of the urethra is enlarged (meatotomy) and the diameter of the penile urethra is enlarged with an instrument (internal urethrotomy) and a catheter is passed into the urethra into the bladder. Through the lower abdominal incision the urinary bladder is exposed and opened by an incision in the region just above the bladder neck. During the dissection to expose the bladder a vasectomy may be performed. The bladder mucosa over the prostate is removed by excision to expose the prostate. The gland is removed by "shelling it out" by blunt dissection with the surgeon's index finger. The bladder outlet and the bladder wall are revised and bleeding controlled by packing with rolls of gauze, by ligation or cautery of bleeding vessels. A second catheter is placed and left in the bladder through the incision in the lower abdomen. A rubber drain is placed in the space between the pubic bone and the bladder and brought out through a separate stab wound. The dissected tissues and the skin incision are closed in layers by suturing.

55831

The physician removes the prostate gland through an incision made in the lower abdomen just above the pubic area. In preparation for removal of the prostate, the caliber (internal diameter) of the urethra is measured and if it is not adequate the opening of the urethra is enlarged (meatotomy) and the diameter of the penile urethra is enlarged with an instrument (internal urethrotomy) and a catheter is passed into the urethra into the bladder. Through the lower abdominal incision the urinary bladder is exposed and opened by an incision in the region just above the bladder neck. During the dissection to expose the bladder a vasectomy may be performed. The bladder mucosa over the prostate is removed by excision to expose the prostate. The gland is removed by "shelling it out" by blunt dissection with the surgeon's index finger. The bladder outlet and the bladder wall are revised and bleeding controlled by packing with rolls of gauze, by ligation or cautery of bleeding vessels. A second catheter is placed and left in the bladder through the incision in the lower abdomen. A rubber drain is placed between the pubic bone and the bladder and brought out through a separate stab wound. The dissected tissues and the skin incision are closed in layers by suturing.

55840

The physician performs a radical prostatectomy (removal of the prostate gland) through an incision made in the lower abdomen just above the pubic area. In preparation for removal of the prostate, a catheter is passed into the urethra into the bladder. Through a lower abdominal incision, with or without care to spare the nerves in the area, the urinary bladder is exposed and displaced backwards to enter the space behind the pubic bone and expose the area of the prostate. The gland with the capsule intact and the seminal vesicles and the portions of the vas deferens in the area are removed by freeing the prostate by blunt dissection and by transecting the urethra and cutting through the bladder outlet. The urinary catheter is brought into the operative site and used to create traction for the dissection. A second catheter is placed in the bladder after the first one is removed along with the prostate. The transected urethra is repaired by suturing to the newly created bladder outlet. A rubber drain is placed in the space between the pubic bone and the bladder and brought out through a separate stab wound. The dissected tissues and the skin incision are closed in layers by suturing.

55842

The physician performs a radical prostatectomy and a pelvic lymph node biopsy through a midline abdominal incision (this may be done in two stages within seven to 10 days). A midline incision is made from the upper to the lower abdomen and the abdominal cavity is entered. The back wall of the abdomen is exposed and the lymph nodes are checked for spread of tumor. Some may be removed and/or biopsied. Through the abdominal incision, with or without sparing the nerves in the area, the urinary bladder is exposed and displaced backwards to enter the space behind the pubic bone and expose the area of the prostate. The gland with the capsule intact, the seminal vesicles, and portions of the vas deferens in the area are removed by freeing the prostate by blunt dissection and by transecting the urethra and cutting through the bladder outlet. The urinary catheter is brought into the operative site and used to create traction for the dissection. A second catheter is placed in the bladder after the first one is removed along with the prostate. The transected urethra is repaired by suturing it to the newly created bladder outlet. A rubber drain is placed between the pubic bone and the bladder and brought out through a separate stab wound.

55845

The physician performs a radical prostatectomy and a pelvic lymph node biopsy through a midline abdominal incision (this may be done in two stages within seven to 10 days). A midline incision is made from the upper to the lower abdomen and the abdominal cavity is entered. The back wall of the abdomen is exposed and all of the lymph nodes along the back wall of the pelvic and abdominal cavities are removed. In preparation for removal of the prostate, a catheter is passed into the urethra and into the bladder. Through the abdominal incision, with or without care to spare the nerves in the area, the urinary bladder is exposed and displaced backwards to enter the space behind the pubic bone and expose the area of the prostate. The gland with the capsule intact, the seminal vesicles, and the portions of the vas deferens in the area are removed by freeing the prostate by blunt dissection and by transecting the urethra and cutting through the bladder outlet. The urinary catheter is brought into the operative site and used to create traction for the dissection. A second catheter is placed in the bladder after the first one is removed along with the prostate. The dissected tissues and the skin incision are closed in layers by suturing.

55860

Through an incision made in the lower abdomen just above the pubic area, the physician inserts radioactive materials in the prostate. In preparation for the radiation treatment, a catheter is passed into the urethra into the bladder and a sheath is inserted into the rectum. Through the lower abdominal incision the urinary bladder is exposed and displaced backwards to enter the space behind the pubic bone and expose the prostate gland. With a finger in the rectum to guide the placement, the physician passes a hollow needle into the prostate through the abdominal incision. The needle is positioned in the prostate tumor and radioactive seeds are introduced into the needle and implanted in the prostate using an applicator. The needle is withdrawn a few millimeters and another seed is placed. This is repeated several times through multiple needle insertions. A rubber drain(s) is placed in the space between the pubic bone and the bladder and brought out through the incision wound. The dissected tissues and the skin incision are closed in layers by suturing. Alternatively, other approaches may be used in a similar fashion.

55862

Through an incision made in the abdomen, the physician inserts radioactive materials in the prostate and examines the pelvic and abdominal lymph nodes. A midline incision is made from the upper to the lower abdomen and the abdominal cavity is entered. The back wall of the abdomen is exposed and the lymph nodes are checked for spread of tumor. Some may be removed and/or biopsied. In preparation for the radiation treatment, a catheter is passed into the urethra into the bladder and a sheath is inserted into the rectum. Through the lower abdominal incision the urinary bladder is exposed and displaced backwards to enter the space behind the pubic bone and expose the prostate gland. With a finger in the rectum to guide the placement, the physician passes a hollow needle into the prostate through the abdominal incision. The needle is positioned in the prostate tumor and radioactive seeds are introduced into the needle and implanted in the prostate using an applicator. The needle is withdrawn a few millimeters and another seed is placed. This is repeated several times through multiple needle insertions. A rubber drain(s) is placed between the pubic bone and the bladder and brought out through the incision wound. The dissected tissues and the skin incision are closed in layers by suturing. Alternatively, other approaches may be used in a similar fashion.

55865

Through an incision made in the abdomen, the physician inserts radioactive materials in the prostate and examines the pelvic and abdominal lymph nodes. A midline incision is made from the upper to the lower abdomen and the abdominal cavity is entered. The back wall of the abdomen is exposed and all the lymph nodes along back wall of the pelvic and abdominal cavities are removed. In preparation for the radiation treatment, a catheter is passed into the urethra into the bladder and a sheath is inserted into the rectum. Through the lower abdominal incision the urinary bladder is exposed and displaced backwards to enter the space behind the pubic bone and expose the prostate gland. With a finger in the rectum to guide the placement, the physician passes a hollow needle into the prostate through the abdominal incision. The needle is positioned in the prostate tumor and radioactive seeds are introduced into the needle and implanted in the prostate using an applicator. The needle is withdrawn a few millimeters and another seed is placed. This is repeated several times through multiple needle insertions. A rubber drain(s) is placed between the pubic bone and the bladder and brought out through the incision wound. The dissected tissues and the skin incision are closed in layers by suturing. Alternatively, other approaches may be used in a similar fashion.

55866

The physician performs a laparoscopic radical prostatectomy, sometimes using robotic assistance. This cannot be done on a patient with prior open prostate surgery. The patient is positioned for laparoscopic surgery with the legs in low lithotomy position for rectal access. Five trocars are placed and the cavity is insufflated with gas. The vas deferens is divided, the seminal vesicles are mobilized, and the prostate is dissected off the rectum. The space of Retzius is developed by dividing the urachus medial to the umbilical ligaments. The endopelvic fascia is incised on both sides and the prostatic levator muscle attachments are bluntly removed. A suture is passed between the urethra and dorsal venous complex and tied. A second suture is passed through the anterior prostate. The bladder neck is opened anteriorly, the posterior margin is separated from the prostate, and the underlying seminal vesicles are exposed. The two prostatic pedicles are divided close to the prostate with the involved seminal vesicle retracted. The back surface of the prostate on each side is dissected from the neurovascular bundles until the prostate remains attached only at the apex. Between the two previously placed sutures, the dorsal vein is divided, the urethra is exposed, and the catheter is removed. The urethra is completely divided. The surgeon places a finger in the rectum for guidance and divides the muscles and remaining attachments to free the prostate completely. The vesicourethral anastomosis is done next with polyglycolic acid suture in running or interrupted simple sutures. A Foley catheter is placed and the anastomosis of the bladder to the urethra is tested. A suction drain is placed through a trocar site and the prostate is removed through a small port site incision.

55867

The physician performs a laparoscopic simple (subtotal) prostatectomy, in which a portion of the prostate is removed. The prostate is composed of an external capsule and internal glandular tissue that is further divided into sections, or lobes. As men age, the prostate often enlarges (hyperplasia) and the internal tissue bulges out into benign adenomas, which may inhibit urinary flow. Simple prostatectomies can be done to remove this excess tissue. In one method, the patient is positioned for laparoscopic surgery with the legs in low lithotomy position for rectal access (for digital manipulation of the prostate as needed). The caliber (internal diameter) of the urethra is measured and if it is not adequate, the opening of the urethra is enlarged (meatotomy) and the diameter of the penile urethra is enlarged with an instrument (internal urethrotomy). Four to six trocars are used to establish the pneumoperitoneum and provide access to the surgical field. The vas deferens is divided and the seminal vesicles are mobilized. Once the physician accesses the extraperitoneal space, the bladder is filled with saline and incised open with a sharp instrument. The physician takes note of the ureteric orifice locations on the bladder wall to protect the area from surgical involvement. To enhance the visual field of the prostate from inside the bladder, the physician sutures portions of the bladder walls to the abdominal wall and retroperitoneum. Attention is turned to the prostate, where the provider makes circumferential incisions to separate the inner prostatic tissue (adenoma) from the outer capsule. Robotic assistance and sutures may be used for traction to assist dissection of the adenoma from the capsule. The urethra is transected during the procedure to completely free prostatic tissue. Once satisfactory dissection of the prostatic adenoma is complete, the tissue is removed from the body through a small port site incision. Bleeding prostatic arteries are sutured. To reconstruct the dissected urethra and bladder neck, the physician sutures together mucosa from the edge of the bladder and urethra to create a mucosal bridge between the urethra and bladder neck. The prostatic capsule is sutured closed, followed by suturing of the bladder wall in multiple layers. The bladder is filled to test for leakage and subsequently drained. A surgical drain may be left in place postoperatively for drainage. Port site incisions are stitched closed. This code includes meatotomy, internal urethrotomy, urethral calibration/dilation, vasectomy, and control of postoperative bleeding.

55870

The physician uses an electrovibratory device that stimulates ejaculation. The electrostimulator probe is placed in the rectum and positioned adjacent to the prostate gland and a current of electricity is passed into the region of the prostate, seminal vesicles and the vas deferens. The stimulation excites the nerves of the area, causing ejaculation. The semen is collected and used for artificial insemination.

55873

The physician performs cryosurgical ablation of the prostate with ultrasonic guidance and monitoring. The physician places a suprapubic catheter into the bladder through a stab incision just above the pubic hairline. Next, the physician inserts a warming catheter through the urethra and into the bladder. The scrotum is elevated out of the operative field using a gauze sling. An ultrasound probe is inserted into the rectum to monitor the freezing process, and to view in real-time the probe placement during the procedure. Under ultrasonic guidance, the surgeon inserts from three to eight needles into the perineum and advances the needles into the prostate. Into each needle the surgeon advances a guidewire used to facilitate instrumentation. The skin is incised and a dilator is inserted over each guidewire to dilate the channels. Saline is injected to aid visibility of the ultrasound, the guidewire is removed, and a cryoprobe (3 mm diameter) is inserted through each dilator for direct contact with the prostate tissue. The cryoprobes, which deliver super-cooled liquid nitrogen or argon gas (both inert materials) to the prostate, are turned on at -70°C. Up to five cryoprobes can be running simultaneously at any one time. The five cryoprobes are turned on, taking the temperature down to -190°C, while the warming catheter guards against freezing the ureter. If the prostate thaws, the probes may be repositioned, and a second freeze may be performed. Once the prostate gland is completely frozen (resembling an ice ball) and all of the visible prostate tissue is destroyed, the surgeon removes the probes and applies pressure to the perineum to prevent hematoma formation. The punctures are sutured shut and the urethral warming catheter is removed.

55874

Transperineal placement of biodegradable material is a procedure that works to position the front area (anterior) of the rectal wall away from the prostate when the patient is undergoing radiotherapy for treatment of prostate cancer and subsequently limits the radiation exposure to the anterior rectum. One proprietary system is made up of materials that break down naturally by the action of biological agents and is placed inside the patient through a needle. Imaging guidance is included in this service, when performed. The system retains its position throughout the duration of the patient's radiotherapy treatments and, because the system is biodegradable, is absorbed by the patient's body over time. This code is reported for single or multiple injections.

55875

Transperineal placement of needles or catheters into the prostate gland for interstitial radioelement application is a form of brachytherapy. Brachytherapy is the application of radioactive isotopes for internal radiation. Radioactive material is encapsulated for interstitial implantation into the prostate tissue. Using separately reportable ultrasound or fluoroscopic guidance, the physician inserts the encapsulated radioactive seeds directly into the prostate tissue transperineally, using appropriate applicators (thin catheter tubes or needles). A previous transrectal ultrasound has been done on the volume of the prostate to map out the precise locations of the radioactive seeds. The radioactive isotopes, such as Iodine-125 or Palladium-103, contained within the tiny seeds are left in place and deliver their dose of radiation over a period of months. They do not cause any harm after they have become inert. This method provides radiation to the prescribed body area while minimizing exposure to normal tissue.

55876

The physician places one or more interstitial devices for radiation therapy guidance into the prostate via needle, using various approaches. In one method, the patient is placed in the lithotomy position. Under guidance from a transrectal ultrasound wand, the physician injects a small capsule into the tissue of the prostate using a percutaneous needle injection device. The capsule allows for precision in targeting radiation and/or for measuring the radiation doses received. An injected capsule fiducial marker is visible by ultrasound and fluoroscopy, allowing for an accurate triangulation of the tissue to be treated. An injected capsule dosimeter relays radiation dose information so that the clinical team can monitor for any deviation between the radiation plan and the actual radiation received by the patient. The inserted capsule may act as a fiducial marker, dosimeter, or, in many cases, will serve in both roles. This code reports the needle insertion of one or more of these devices into the patient's prostate during a single surgical session.

55880

The physician destroys malignant prostate tissue using high intensity focused ultrasound (HIFU) ablation. With the patient typically under general or spinal anesthesia, the physician inserts an ultrasound probe into the patient's rectum. The probe is surrounded by a cooling balloon that protects the rectal mucosa from the high temperature. The ultrasound transducers are positioned at the level of the prostate. The probe provides ultrasound images of the prostate and then delivers timed bursts of heat to create coagulation necrosis in a targeted area. HIFU treatment may be repeated if necessary.

55881-55882

The physician inserts an ablation transducer into the urethra to deliver thermal energy for prostate tissue ablation. A catheter is placed through the urethra into the bladder, followed by a guidewire. The ultrasound applicator is advanced over the guidewire and into the prostatic urethra. An endorectal cooling device may be inserted into the rectum to protect the rectal tissue during treatment. Magnetic resonance imaging (MRI) is obtained for visualization to allow the physician to draw boundary lines for the intended treatment areas. Individually activated transducer elements in the ultrasound applicator emit energy to target the affected prostate tissue. Ultrasound energy is used to

Male/Female

heat and destroy prostate tissue with the heat beginning inside the urethra and spreading out to the edges of the prostate as the applicator rotates within the urethra. Treatment may address the whole prostate or specific portions as determined by the physician. Real-time MRI thermometry images are used during the procedure to show temperature changes in the prostate tissue and surrounding structures. This allows the physician to monitor the tissue heating, make adjustments as necessary, and confirm successful ablation. Report 55881 for ablation of the prostate tissue using thermal ultrasound, including MRI imaging guidance and monitoring, when the transducer is placed by a different physician. Report 55882 when the insertion of the transducer and ablation of the prostate tissue are performed by the same physician.

55920

The physician places needles or catheters into the pelvic organs and/or genitalia, excluding the prostate, for subsequent interstitial radioelement application. The radioactive isotopes that are introduced subsequently, such as iodine-125 or palladium-103, are contained within tiny seeds that are left in place to deliver radiation over a period of months. They do not cause any harm after becoming inert. This method provides radiation to the prescribed body area while minimizing exposure to normal tissue.

55970

In a series of staged procedures, the physician removes portions of the male genitalia and forms female external genitals. The penis is dissected and portions are removed with care to preserve vital nerves and vessels in order to fashion a clitoris-like structure. The urethral opening is moved to a position similar to that of a normal female. A vagina is made by dissecting and opening the perineum. This opening is lined using pedicle or split thickness grafts. Labia are created out of skin from the scrotum and adjacent tissue. A stent or obturator is usually left in place in the newly created vagina for three weeks or longer.

55980

In a series of staged procedures, the physician forms a penis and scrotum using pedicle flap grafts and free skin grafts. Portions of the clitoris are used as well as the adjacent skin. Prostheses are often placed in the penis in order to have a sexually functional organ. Prosthetic testicles are fixed in the scrotum. The vagina is closed or removed.

56405

The vulva includes the labia majora, labia minora, mons pubis, bulb of the vestibule, vestibule of the vagina, greater and lesser vestibular glands, and vaginal orifice. The perineum is the area between the vulva and the anus. The physician makes an incision into the abscess at its softest point and drains the purulent contents. The cavity of the abscess is flushed and often packed with medicated gauze to facilitate drainage.

56420

The physician incises and drains a Bartholin's gland abscess. Bartholin's gland is at the end of the bulb of the vestibule of the vagina and is connected by a duct to the mucosa at the opening of the vagina. The physician makes an incision just inside the opening of the vagina through the mucosal surface into the cavity of the abscess to flush and drain it. A small wick or catheter may be left in the cavity to facilitate drainage.

56440

The physician treats a Bartholin's gland cyst with marsupialization. Bartholin's gland is at the end of the bulb of the vestibule of the vagina and is connected by a duct to the mucosa at the opening of the vagina. The physician makes an elliptical excision over the center of the Bartholin's gland cyst and drains it. The lining of the cyst is everted and approximated to the vaginal mucosa with sutures creating a pouch. Marsupialization prevents recurrent cysts and infections.

56441

The labia majora and minora are the greater and lesser folds of skin on the pudendum on either side of the vagina. The physician separates the labia majora from the labia minora, which are fused by fibrous bands of scar tissue. Using a blunt instrument, probe, scissors, and/or clamp, the labia are separated by breaking or cutting the fibrous tissue. The procedure is accomplished using general or local anesthesia.

56442

The physician performs a hymenotomy. A hymen is a membrane that partially or wholly occludes the vaginal opening. Following local injection of an anesthetic, the physician incises the hymenal membrane with a stellate (star-shaped) incision. This procedure is sometimes preceded by aspiration of the intact membrane with a needle and syringe.

56501-56515

The vulva includes the labia majora, labia minora, mons pubis, bulb of the vestibule, vestibule of the vagina, greater and lesser vestibular glands, and vaginal orifice. After examination of the lower genital tract and perianal area, the physician destroys one or more lesions of the vulva by any method including laser surgery, electrosurgery, chemosurgery, or cryosurgery. Report 56501 for simple lesion destruction and 56515 for complicated destruction of extensive vulvar lesions.

56605-56606

The vulva includes the labia majora, labia minora, mons pubis, bulb of the vestibule, vestibule of the vagina, greater and lesser vestibular glands, and vaginal orifice. The perineum is the area between the vulva and the anus. The physician removes a sample of tissue from the vulva or perineum. After injecting a local anesthetic around the suspect tissue, the physician obtains a sample using a skin punch or sharp scalpel. A clip or suture can be used to control bleeding if pressure is not successful. Use 56605 for the biopsy of one lesion and 56606 for each additional lesion.

56620-56625
The physician removes part or all of the vulva to treat premalignant or malignant lesions. A simple complete vulvectomy includes removal of all of the labia majora, labia minora, and clitoris, while a simple, partial vulvectomy may include removal of part or all of the labia majora and labia minora on one side and the clitoris. The physician examines the lower genital tract and the perianal skin through a colposcope. In 56620, a wide semi-elliptical incision that contains the diseased area is made. In 56625, two wide elliptical incisions encompassing the vulvar area are made. One elliptical incision extends from well above the clitoris around both labia majora to a point just in front of the anus. The second elliptical incision starts at a point between the clitoris and the opening of the urethra and is carried around both sides of the opening of the vagina. The underlying subcutaneous fatty tissue is removed along with the large portion of excised skin. Vessels are clamped and tied off with sutures or are electrocoagulated to control bleeding. The considerable defect is usually closed in layers using separately reportable plastic techniques. Vaginal gauze packing may be placed in the vagina.

56630
The physician removes part of the vulva to treat malignancy. A partial radical vulvectomy includes partial or complete removal of a large, deep segment of skin from the following structures: abdomen and groin, labia majora, labia minora, clitoris, mons veneris, and terminal portions of the urethra, vagina, and other vulvar organs. The clitoris may or may not be included in the partial vulvectomy. Through incisions in the lower abdomen, thighs, and vulvar area, the physician removes skin, subcutaneous fatty tissue, and deeper tissue. Also included in the en bloc removal of tissue are portions of the saphenous veins and ligaments and the target lesion. The resulting large and disfiguring defect is usually closed using separately reported plastic surgical techniques, which may include pedicle flaps or free skin grafts. Subcutaneous rubber drains may be left in the surgical site, and vaginal gauze packing may be placed in the vagina.

56631-56632
The physician removes part of the vulva to treat malignancy. A partial radical vulvectomy includes the partial or complete removal of a large, deep segment of skin and tissue from the abdomen and groin, labia majora and minora, clitoris, mons veneris, and terminal portions of the urethra, vagina, and other vulvar organs. Through incisions in the lower abdomen, thighs, and vulvar area, the physician removes skin, subcutaneous fatty tissue, and deeper tissue. The physician also removes superficial and deep inguinal lymph nodes and adjacent femoral lymph nodes on one side in 56631 and on both sides in 56632. Also included in the en bloc removal of tissue are portions of the saphenous veins and ligaments and the target lesion. The resulting large and disfiguring defect is usually closed in layers using plastic surgical techniques, which may include pedicle flaps or free skin grafts. Subcutaneous rubber drains may be left in the surgical site, and vaginal gauze packing may be placed in the vagina.

56633
The physician removes the vulva to treat malignancy. A complete radical vulvectomy includes the removal of a large, deep segment of skin and tissue from the following structures: abdomen and groin, labia majora, labia minora, clitoris, mons veneris, and terminal portions of the urethra, vagina, and other vulvar organs. Deep tissue from more than 80 percent of the vulva is excised. Through incisions in the lower abdomen, thighs, and vulvar area, the physician removes skin, subcutaneous fatty tissue, and deeper tissues. Also included in the en bloc removal of tissue are portions of the saphenous veins and ligaments and the target lesion. The resulting large and disfiguring defect is usually closed in layers using separately reported plastic surgical techniques, which may include pedicle flaps or free skin grafts. Subcutaneous rubber drains may be used, and vaginal gauze packing may be placed in the vagina.

56634-56637
The physician removes the vulva to treat malignancy. A complete radical vulvectomy includes the removal of a large, deep segment of skin and tissue from the lower abdomen and groin, labia majora and minora, clitoris, mons veneris, and terminal portions of the urethra, vagina, and other vulvar organs. Deep tissue from more than 80 percent of the vulva is removed. Through incisions in the lower abdomen, thighs, and vulvar area, the physician removes skin, subcutaneous fatty tissue, and deeper tissues. The physician also removes the inguinal and femoral lymph nodes on one side in 56634 and on both sides in 56637. Also included in the en bloc removal of tissue are portions of the saphenous veins and ligaments and the target lesion. The resulting large and disfiguring defect is usually closed in layers using plastic surgical techniques, which may include pedicle flaps or free skin grafts. Subcutaneous rubber drains may be used, and vaginal gauze packing may be placed in the vagina.

56640
The physician removes the entire vulva to treat malignancy. A complete radical vulvectomy includes the removal of a large, deep segment of skin and tissue from the following structures: lower abdomen and groin, labia majora, labia minora, clitoris, mons veneris, and terminal portions of the urethra, vagina, and other vulvar organs. Through incisions in the lower abdomen, thighs, and vulvar area, the physician removes skin, subcutaneous fatty tissue, and deeper tissue. The physician also removes the inguinal and femoral lymph nodes on both sides as well as the iliac and pelvic lymph nodes in the pelvic cavity, which is entered through an abdominal incision. Also included in the en bloc removal of tissue are portions of the saphenous veins and ligaments and the target lesion. The resulting large and disfiguring defect is usually

closed in layers using separately reported plastic surgical techniques, which may include pedicle or free skin grafts. Subcutaneous rubber drains may be used, and vaginal gauze packing may be placed in the vagina.

56700
A hymen is a membrane that partially or wholly occludes the vaginal opening. Following local injection of an anesthetic, the physician excises a portion of the hymenal membrane. Using a scalpel or scissors, the physician removes the membrane at its junction with the opening of the vagina. The cut margins of the vaginal mucosa are sutured with fine, absorbable material.

56740
The physician removes a cystic Bartholin's gland, which lies at the tail end of the bulb of the vestibular opening just inside of the vagina. The physician makes an incision through the vaginal mucosa. The cyst is isolated through the vaginal incision by dissecting the deeper fatty tissues and excised. The remaining cavity and skin are closed in layers using absorbable material.

56800
The physician repairs and restores the anatomy of the opening of the vagina by excising scar tissue and strengthening the supporting tissues using tissue flaps and suturing techniques. This procedure varies greatly from patient to patient, depending on the defect to be corrected.

56805
The physician reduces the size of an enlarged clitoris, which has been masculinized by the production of male hormones from an abnormal adrenal gland. A portion of the body of the clitoris is resected with care to ensure preservation of vital nerves and blood vessels to the glans of the clitoris. The incisions are closed using plastic surgical techniques.

56810
With upward traction on the vagina, the physician makes an incision from the lower vaginal opening to a point just in front of the anus. The underlying weakened tissues are dissected and repaired and tightened by suturing. This restores strength to the pelvic floor, closes tissue defects, and improves function of the perineal muscles.

56820-56821
The physician performs a colposcopy of the vulva, the external genitalia region of the female that includes the labia, clitoris, mons pubis, vaginal vestibule, bulb and glands, and the vaginal orifice. The patient is placed in the lithotomy position and the vulva is inspected through the colposcope, a binocular microscope used for direct visualization of the vagina and cervix. The bright light of the colposcope is directed so as to inspect the vulva and perianal area for any lesions or ulceration. In 56821, a biopsy is taken of any vulvar tissue in question under direct vision. The number and size of the biopsy will depend on the lesions. Pressure is applied and hemostasis of the biopsy site is achieved.

57000
Colpotomy is an incision in the wall of the vagina, usually to access a recess between the rectum and uterus formed by a fold in the peritoneum (cul-de-sac). Through a speculum inserted in the vagina, the physician grasps the posterior lip of the cervix with a toothed instrument called a tenaculum. The cervix is lifted, exposing the posterior vaginal pouch. An incision is made through the back wall of the vagina into the posterior pelvic cavity. Through this opening, the pelvic cavity can be explored using instruments. After exploration, the physician closes the incision with absorbable sutures.

57010
Colpotomy is an incision in the wall of the vagina, usually to access a recess between the rectum and uterus formed by a fold in the peritoneum (cul de sac). Through a speculum inserted in the vagina, the physician grasps the posterior lip of the cervix with a toothed instrument called a tenaculum. The cervix is lifted, exposing the posterior vaginal pouch. An incision is made through the back wall of the vagina into the posterior pelvic cavity. Through this opening, the pelvic cavity can be explored. The abscess in the cavity is located, entered, and drained through the vaginal incision. Rubber drains are often inserted and left in place for several days. The physician closes the incision with absorbable sutures.

57020
Colpocentesis is the aspiration of fluid in the peritoneum through the wall of the vagina. Through a speculum inserted in the vagina, the physician grasps the posterior lip of the cervix with a toothed instrument called a tenaculum. The cervix is lifted, exposing the posterior vaginal pouch and deep back wall of the vagina. A long needle attached to a syringe is inserted through the exposed vaginal wall and the posterior pelvic cavity is entered. Fluid is aspirated through the needle into the syringe.

57022-57023
The physician incises and drains a vaginal hematoma in an obstetrical or postpartum patient. The patient is placed in a dorsolithotomy position. The physician inserts a speculum into the vagina. The hematoma is visualized, and incised. Blood and clot are drained from the hematoma. Electrocautery or suture is used to control bleeding. When needed, a Hemovac drain is placed. The vagina is irrigated, and the area of hematoma is sponged with dressings. When hemostasis is achieved, the speculum is removed. Report 57022 when the procedure is performed on an obstetrical patient and 57023 when the procedure is performed on a nonobstetrical patient. Hemovac drains may be placed if the hematoma bed is still oozing.

57061-57065
Using a colposcope, a binocular microscope used for direct visualization of the vagina and cervix, the physician identifies lesion(s) in and/or around the vagina. The physician destroys the abnormal tissue by chemosurgery, electrosurgery, laser surgery, or cryotherapy. Use 57061 if the lesions are few in number, small, or simple. Use 57065 if the lesions are numerous, large, or difficult.

57100-57105
The physician takes a sample of vaginal mucosa for examination. After injecting a local anesthetic into the suspect area, the physician obtains a sample with a skin punch or sharp scalpel. In 57100, the biopsy is simple and no sutures are required. In 57105, sutures are required as the excision site is extensive and bleeding may need to be controlled.

57106-57109
The physician excises part of the vagina. This is sometimes preceded by injection of medication to constrict blood vessels to control bleeding. The vagina is everted and sizeable sections are removed by sharp and blunt dissection. In 57107, the physician removes surrounding diseased and/or damaged tissue. In 57109, the physician removes surrounding diseased and/or damaged tissue, in addition to removing the pelvic lymph nodes, and performing biopsy of the lymph nodes of the aorta to check for the extent of disease. Remaining vaginal and/or support tissue is inverted and sutured in place to obliterate some or all of the space formerly occupied by the vagina. The perineum is closed over the former vaginal opening.

57110-57111
The physician performs a complete removal of the vaginal wall in 57110. This is sometimes proceeded by injection of medication to constrict blood vessels to control bleeding. The vagina is everted. An incision circumscribes the hymen, and the vagina is marked into four quadrants. Each quadrant of vaginal wall is removed by sharp and blunt dissection. In 57111, the physician also removes surrounding diseased and/or damaged tissue. The remaining support tissues are inverted and sutured in place obliterating the space formerly occupied by the vagina. The perineum is closed over the former vaginal opening.

57120
The physician grasps the deepest portion of the vaginal vault and everts the vagina. Two large flaps of vaginal wall are removed from opposite sides of the prolapsed vagina. The vaginal walls are sutured to one another and this structure is inverted back inside the body. The former vaginal opening is closed with sutures obliterating the vagina and preventing uterine prolapse.

57130
The physician excises a vaginal septum, an anomaly that separates the vagina into two portions. The septum can be longitudinal, creating two vaginal canals, or transverse, blocking the vagina and preventing menstrual flow. For a small, thin septum, the procedure is often done by injecting a local anesthetic in the tissues around the septum and making an incision through the narrowest portion of the septum. The divided tissue is tied off with suture material and the tissue is excised. For a thicker and more extensive septum, the procedure may be done under general anesthesia. The tissue is excised, and the resulting vaginal lining defects are closed. The vagina is packed with medicated gauze or a support device.

57135
Through a speculum inserted in the vagina, the physician uses a forceps or hemostat clamp to grasp and elongate the vaginal tissue containing the cyst or tumor, causing the mucosa to tent. With a scalpel or scissors, the physician excises an ellipse of tissue containing the lesion. The defect is closed with absorbable sutures.

57150
The physician passes a catheter or similar tube high into the vaginal canal and flushes the canal with medicated solution from a large syringe. The physician also paints infected areas with medication using a cotton-tipped applicator or similar device.

57155
The physician places a brachytherapy applicator (also called a tandem and ovoids) prior to the first brachytherapy treatment for cervical cancer. Under appropriate anesthesia, a hollow plastic sleeve that has been custom fitted to the uterine cavity is inserted into the uterus through the cervical opening and sutured into place onto the cervix. This sleeve remains in the uterus for the duration of the brachytherapy treatments, keeping the cervix open to allow for comfortable positioning of the tandem (a hollow metal tube that is inserted into the sleeve). Two ovoids, containing small radiation shields that reduce radiation doses to the bladder and rectum, are then positioned on either side of the cervix. Separately reportable brachytherapy follows, after which the tandem and ovoids are removed.

57156
A non-radioactive applicator or cylinder is placed into the uterine cavity and vagina in preparation for clinical brachytherapy. Under appropriate anesthesia, the physician inserts the applicator/cylinder and secures it into position, often using radiological guidance. The applicator is subsequently loaded with the radiation sources, often using a remote system in which the applicators are connected to an "afterloader" machine via a series of guide tubes. Remote afterloading systems provide radiation exposure protection to health care professionals by delivering radiation sources along the guide tubes into the prespecified positions within the applicator without staff presence in the treatment room. Separately reportable vaginal brachytherapy is then administered using low-dose rate (LDR) or high-dose rate (HDR) radiotherapy. Code 57156 reports insertion of the afterloading apparatus only.

57160
The physician fits a pessary to a patient, provides instructions for its use, and inserts it into the vagina. A pessary is a prosthesis that comes in different shapes and styles and is used to support the uterus, cervical stump, or hernias of the pelvic floor. The pessary selection and fitting will depend on the patient's symptoms and anatomy.

57170
The physician fits a diaphragm or cervical cap and provides instructions for use. A diaphragm is a device that acts as a mechanical barrier between the vagina and the cervical canal. Cervical caps are larger, cup-like diaphragms pressed up against the cervix to form a snug seal. Either device can be used to prevent pregnancy.

57180
The physician pushes gauze packing into the vagina to put pressure on bleeding that is not related to childbirth or pregnancy. The packing may be coated with a chemical to make the blood clot and stop hemorrhaging.

57200-57210
The physician inserts a speculum into the vagina and identifies the extent of the vaginal laceration or wound that is not related to childbirth or pregnancy. Usually a local anesthetic is used; however, some instances may require general anesthesia. The wound is closed with absorbable sutures. In 57210, after the speculum is removed, the perineal laceration is closed in layers with sutures.

57220
The physician accesses the urethral sphincter from the vagina. With a catheter in the urethra, the physician dissects the midline vaginal wall separating it from the bladder and the proximal urethra. Sutures are placed at the junction of the bladder and urethra on each side of the urethra. This supports the area. Excess vaginal tissue is excised and the vaginal wall is closed.

57230
The physician repairs a urethrocele, which is a sagging or prolapse of the urethra through its opening or a bulging of the posterior wall of the urethra against the vaginal canal. The prolapsed urethral tissue is excised from the meatus in a circular manner. The cut edges of urethral mucosa and vaginal mucosa are sutured.

57240
The physician repairs a cystocele, which is a herniation of the bladder through its support tissues and against the anterior vaginal wall causing it to bulge downward. The physician may also repair a urethrocele, which is a prolapse of the urethra. An incision is made from the apex of the vagina to within 1 cm of the urethral meatus. Plication sutures are placed along the urethral course from the meatus to the bladder neck. A suture is placed through the pubourethral ligament to the posterior symphysis pubis on each side of the urethra. The sutures are tied (ligated) and the posterior urethra is pulled upward to a retropubic position. If a cystocele is repaired, mattress sutures are placed in the mobilized paravesical tissue. The vaginal mucosa is closed. Cystourethroscopy is included when performed with this procedure.

57250
The physician repairs a rectocele by colporrhaphy. A rectocele is a protrusion of part of the rectum through its supporting tissues against the vagina causing a bulging in the vagina. Colporrhaphy involves a plastic repair of the vagina and the fibrous tissue separating the vagina and rectum. The physician makes a posterior midline incision that includes the perineum and posterior vaginal wall. In order to strengthen the area, the rectovaginal fascia is plicated by folding and tacking, and it is closed with layered sutures. The physician may also perform a perineorrhaphy, which is a plastic repair of the perineum, including midline approximation of the levator and perineal muscles. Excess fascia in the posterior vaginal wall is excised. The incisions are closed with sutures.

57260-57265
The physician repairs a cystocele and rectocele by colporrhaphy. Colporrhaphy involves a plastic repair of the vagina and the fibrous tissue separating the bladder, vagina, and rectum. A cystocele is a herniation of the bladder through its support tissues causing the anterior vaginal wall to bulge downward. A rectocele is a protrusion of part of the rectum through its support tissues causing the posterior vaginal wall to bulge. Using a combined vaginal approach and a posterior midline incision that includes the perineum and posterior vaginal wall, the physician dissects the tissues between the bladder, urethra, vagina, and rectum. The specific tissue weaknesses are repaired and strengthened using tissue transfer techniques and layered and plication suturing. In 57260, the physician may also repair a urethrocele, which is a prolapse of the urethra, and perform a perineorrhaphy, which is plastic repair of the perineum, including midline approximation of the levator and perineal muscles. In 57265, the physician performs all of the same services and also repairs an enterocele, which is a herniation of the bowel contents of the rectouterine pouch that protrudes into the septum of tissue between the bladder and vagina or between the vagina and rectum. Through the vagina, the enterocele sac is incised and ligated and the uterosacral ligaments and endopelvic fascia anterior to the rectum are approximated. In both procedures, incisions are closed with sutures. Cystourethroscopy is included when performed with these procedures.

57267
The physician inserts mesh or other prosthetic support material to repair a pelvic floor defect using a vaginal approach. Pelvic floor defects resulting in prolapse of the pelvic viscera occur when the pelvic fascia weakens or is damaged. The physician selects the appropriate type of prosthetic support material. Some mesh supports, such as horseshoe shaped mesh, are purchased preformed in the desired configuration. Other types of mesh supports, such as tension free

tapes, are cut and fashioned by the physician during surgery into the required shapes and sizes. The mesh is inserted through the vagina and placed at the site requiring support. The exact placement of the mesh is determined by the type of pelvic floor defect being repaired. For example, horseshoe mesh is placed between the pubis and sacrum to close the area between the pelvic viscera and the inferior pelvic hiatus. Report 57267 in addition to the primary procedure for each site requiring insertion of mesh or other prosthesis, such as an anterior repair for cystocele or a posterior repair for a rectocele.

57268-57270

The physician repairs an enterocele, which is a herniation of the bowel contents of the rectouterine pouch that protrudes into the septum of tissue between the bladder and vagina or between the vagina and rectum. Through the vaginal approach in 57268, the physician incises and ligates the enterocele sac and approximates the uterosacral ligaments and endopelvic fascia anterior to the rectum. In 57270, the approach is made through an incision in the lower abdominal wall. A vaginal hysterectomy, anterior (cystocele) and posterior (rectocele) colporrhaphy, and perineorrhaphy may also be performed to augment the support.

57280

Through a lower abdominal incision, the physician attaches the vault of the vagina to the prominent point of the sacrum. This is accomplished by suturing surgical fabric or a strip of abdominal wall fascia to the tissue in front of the internal sacral wall inside the pelvic cavity forming a bridge. The apex of the vagina is firmly sutured to this bridge. This stabilizes the vaginal vault and prevents prolapse of the vagina. The abdominal incision is closed with sutures.

57282

Colpopexy is performed by transvaginal, extraperitoneal approach to restore the apex or vault of the vagina to its anatomic position in cases of prolapse. Extraperitoneal transvaginal approach is used to perform a sacrospinous ligament fixation or iliococcygeus fascial suspension. Sacrospinous ligament fixation is performed using an anterior transvaginal approach through the paravaginal space or a posterior transvaginal approach by perforation of the rectal pillar. A pair of sutures are placed approximately 1 to 2 cm apart in the sacrospinous ligaments. After placing the sutures in the sacrospinous ligaments, the apex of the vagina is identified and the sutures in the sacrospinous ligaments are incorporated into the apex of the vagina allowing for maximal suspension of the vaginal vault. Iliococcygeus fascial suspension is performed by extraperitoneal transvaginal approach. The rectum is first retracted medially. The iliococcygeus muscle is located lateral to the rectum and anterior to the ischial spine. A single suture is placed in both sides of the apex of the vaginal vault to provide bilateral fixation of the vault to the iliococcygeus fascia.

57283

Colpopexy is performed by transvaginal, intraperitoneal approach to restore the apex or vault of the vagina to its anatomic position in cases of prolapse. Intraperitoneal technique is used to perform a uterosacral ligament suspension or a levator myorrhaphy, which are performed using a posterior transvaginal approach. Uterosacral ligament suspension is performed by first locating the uterosacral ligament remnant with the use of Allis clamps posterior and medial to the ischial spine. Prior to placement of sutures in the ligaments, the ureters are located by palpation. Two to three nonabsorbable sutures are placed in each ligament and tied together. The ligaments are placated and brought together in the midline. Sutures are placed in the apical portion of the anterior and posterior vaginal walls to secure and anchor the vaginal walls to the plicated uterosacral ligaments. Levator myorrhaphy uses the levator musculature to repair the vaginal vault prolapse. The levator musculature is brought together and a high levator shelf created. The shelf is created by tagging and tying together the levator muscles at a site slightly above the junction of the levator and rectum. The vaginal vault is anchored to the shelf.

57284-57285

The physician repairs a paravaginal defect, in which there is loss of the lateral vaginal attachment to the pelvic sidewall, by dissecting the tissues between the vagina and the bladder and urethra. The specific tissue weaknesses are found, repaired, and strengthened using tissue transfer techniques and plication suturing. The paravaginal repair may be performed alone or in conjunction with cystocele repair, in which a herniation of the bladder through its support tissues into the anterior vaginal wall causes it to bulge downward. These procedures help restore the normal anatomic relationships of the urethra, bladder, and vagina. Report 57284 if access is achieved via laparotomy (open abdominal approach) and 57285 if a vaginal approach is utilized.

57287

The physician removes or revises a fascial or synthetic sling previously placed to correct urinary stress incontinence. To remove a sling, the physician makes a small abdominal skin incision to the level of the rectus fascia and releases the arm of the sling from the rectus abdominis. The physician releases the sling's attachment to the junction of the urethra via canals or tunnels formed by an instrument or a finger placed through a vertical or flap incision in the vaginal wall. In revision of a sling the physician may remove and partially or completely replace the sling using fascia or a synthetic graft through an abdominal and vaginal approach. The sling may be revised by increasing the tension on the sling using suture at one or both of the attachment sites at the junction of the urethra and/or to the rectus abdominis muscle. At the end of the procedure the area is irrigated, and hemostasis is achieved. The abdominal and/or vaginal incisions are closed with layered sutures.

57288

Through vaginal and abdominal incisions, the physician places a sling under the junction of the urethra and bladder. The physician places a catheter in the bladder, makes an incision in the anterior wall of the vagina, and folds and tacks the tissues around the urethra. A sling is formed out of synthetic material or from fascia harvested from the sheath of the rectus abdominis muscle. The loop end of the sling is sutured around the junction of the urethra. An incision is made in the lower abdomen and the ends of the sling are grasped with a clamp and pulled into the incision and sutured to the rectus abdominis sheath. The abdominal and vaginal incisions are closed in layers by suturing.

57289

The physician makes an inverted U-shaped incision in the area between the vagina and the urethra. By blunt and sharp dissection, the physician creates an opening in the space on each side of the urethra as it passes into the bladder. Using a continuous suture for each side, the physician stitches the fascial tissues along the urethra to the urethrovesical junction. The physician makes an incision in the abdomen above the pubis and, doing each side in turn, drives a Pereyra ligature carrier through the tissues just lateral to the midline and takes it down to the sutured tissue. The sutures are threaded into the instrument and brought back through the abdominal incision. The urethrovesical junction is elevated by pulling on the sutures and fixing them around the rectus abdominis muscle. In addition, the physician performs an anterior colporrhaphy using a vaginal approach, which corrects a cystocele and repairs the tissues between the vagina, bladder, and urethra.

57291-57292

For construction of an artificial vagina without graft, the physician develops a vagina by a program of perineal pressure using progressively longer and wider firm obturators. Pressure is applied to the soft area between the urethra and rectum with an obturator. Over several months of consistent, daily use by the patient, a sexually functional vagina can be created. In 57292, the physician creates or enlarges the vagina using one or more skin grafts. Through a midline episiotomy incision, the physician creates a space between the urethra and rectum. Using split thickness or full thickness skin grafts, the space is lined and the vagina created. An obturator or mold is inserted into the vagina and a catheter is passed into the bladder and left for several days. The full thickness skin donor sites are closed using plastic surgical techniques. The split thickness sites are dressed with medicated gauze.

57295

The physician revises or removes a previously placed prosthetic vaginal graft via a vaginal approach. The patient is placed in the lithotomy position and a speculum is inserted. The physician visualizes the vagina. The apex of the vagina is accessed with deep retractors. Dissection is carried out to reach the affected graft material. Depending upon the type of complication (i.e., stricture or infection), the vaginal graft may be completely or partially excised to remove eroding mesh or revisions may be made in the graft and surrounding tissue. The vaginal epithelial layers and pelvic fascia are rearranged or reapproximated and closed. Vaginal packing is put in place.

57296

The physician revises or removes a previously placed prosthetic vaginal graft using an open abdominal approach in conjunction with a vaginal approach. A laparotomy incision is made and the physician dissects into the pelvis. The vagina is elevated with tools or with the physician's hand. The graft is located, the peritoneum is opened over it, and the graft is dissected free and removed. Depending upon the type of complication (i.e., stricture or infection), the vaginal graft may be completely or partially excised to remove eroding mesh or revisions may be made in the graft and surrounding tissue. Endopelvic fascia is reapproximated and the vaginal epithelial layers and pelvic fascia are rearranged or reapproximated and closed. The abdominal incision is repaired in layers. Vaginal packing is put in place.

57300

The physician closes a rectovaginal fistula, which is an abnormal passage between the rectum and the vagina. The physician also repairs the perineum, fascia, and muscle-supporting structures between the rectum and vagina. The scar tissue and tract between the rectum and vagina are excised and the clean edges sutured together. Often a flap of tissue is transplanted between the vagina and the rectum and the area is closed in layers. The rectal wall opening is closed by inverting the mucosa into the rectal canal. The vaginal wall opening is closed by inverting the mucosal layer into the vaginal wall. Sometimes the vaginal side is left open for drainage.

57305

Through a lower abdominal incision, the physician closes a rectovaginal fistula, which is an abnormal passage between the rectum and the vagina. The physician also repairs the perineum, fascia, and muscle-supporting structures between the rectum and vagina. The scar tissue and tract between the rectum and vagina are excised and the clean edges sutured together. Often a flap of tissue is transplanted between the vagina and the rectum and the area is closed in layers. The rectal wall opening is closed by inverting the mucosa into the rectal canal. The vaginal wall opening is closed by inverting the mucosal layer into the vaginal wall. Sometimes the vaginal side is left open for drainage. The abdominal incision is closed with sutures.

57307-57308

Through a lower abdominal incision, the physician closes a rectovaginal fistula, which is an abnormal passage between the rectum and vagina. The physician also repairs the perineum, fascia, and muscle-supporting structures between the rectum and vagina. The scar tissue and tract between the rectum and vagina are excised and the clean edges sutured together. Often a flap of tissue is transplanted between the vagina and rectum and the area is closed in layers. The rectal wall opening created during the excision is closed by inverting the mucosa into the rectal canal. The vaginal wall opening is closed by inverting the mucosal layer into the vaginal canal. The vaginal side may be left open for drainage. In 57307, a transverse colostomy is done to divert the flow of feces and to allow healing of the rectal colon repair. The abdominal incision is closed with sutures. Report 57308 if the physician takes a transperineal approach, reconstructing the perineal body, with or without a levator plication.

57310-57311
The physician closes a urethrovaginal fistula, which is an abnormal passage between the urethra and vagina. With a catheter in the urethra, the fistula tract is excised and the defect in the urethra is sutured closed. A pad of fatty tissue is sutured between the repaired urethral defect and the vaginal defect in 57310. In 57311, a pad of fatty tissue and a strip of the bulbocavernosus muscle are brought through a tunnel created between the vagina and one labium. The fat and muscle flap are sutured between the repaired urethral defect and the vaginal defect. In either case, the involved area in the vagina is excised and the defect is sutured closed. The catheter is left in place for several days to allow healing of the urethra.

57320
The physician closes a vesicovaginal fistula, which is an abnormal passage between the bladder and the vagina. This procedure is done through the vagina with catheters via the urethra into both ureters. The fistula and surrounding scar tissue of the vaginal wall are usually excised. Using a vaginal approach, the bladder wall is opened and the bladder explored. The fistula is excised along with the surrounding tissue. The resulting defect is closed with sutures in layers, starting with the bladder wall and ending with the vaginal mucosa. In some cases, a pedicle graft of tissue may be sutured between the bladder and the vagina. A urethral or suprapubic catheter is left in the bladder to prevent distension of the bladder and tension to the sutured areas.

57330
The physician closes a vesicovaginal fistula, which is an abnormal passage between the bladder and the vagina. The procedure is performed through the vagina and lower abdomen, with catheters through the urethra into both ureters. The physician opens the bladder wall through the lower abdominal incision and excises the fistula. The resulting defect is closed with sutures in layers, starting with the bladder wall and ending with the abdominal wall. Through the vagina, the physician excises the fistula and surrounding scar tissue of the vaginal wall. In some cases, a pedicle graft of tissue may be sutured between the bladder and the vagina. A urethral or suprapubic catheter is left in the bladder to prevent distension of the bladder and tension to the sutured areas.

57335
The physician uses various plastic surgical techniques to correct a small, underdeveloped vagina due to the overproduction of male hormones. The physician constructs a larger and more functional vagina using carefully placed incisions and skin grafts.

57400
The physician enlarges the vagina by using a set of progressively longer and wider vaginal obturator dilators. The physician inserts the vaginal dilators sequentially from smaller to larger with firm and gentle pressure while the patient is under anesthesia (other than local).

57410
Prior to the examination, the patient is placed under anesthesia, other than local, for a bimanual examination of the pelvic organs. The physician places two fingers inside the vagina to palpate the cervix, uterus, and ovaries while using the other hand to gently palpate the top of the uterus with pressure on the abdomen noting the organs' size, shape, and/or any abnormality.

57415
Using a vaginal speculum, the physician removes a foreign body lodged in the vagina. During the procedure, the patient is under anesthesia (other than local) because of the patient's inability to tolerate the procedure while fully alert or awake, as in the case of a young child or due to the type or size of the object being removed.

57420-57421
The physician performs a colposcopy of the vagina and the cervix, if present. The patient is placed in the lithotomy position and a speculum is inserted into the vagina. The vagina is inspected through the colposcope, a binocular microscope providing direct, magnified visualization of the vagina and cervix. The physician examines the tissue for discharge, inflammation, ulceration, and lesions. The cervix is exposed, cleansed, and inspected for any ulceration or lesions. Acetic acid may be applied to help enhance visualization of the columnar villi and any lesions. In 57421, the area is examined and questionable tissue is removed from the vagina and/or cervix under direct visualization. The number and size of the biopsy(ies) is variable; multiple biopsies may be taken. Pressure is applied with a cotton swab as silver nitrate or other solution is applied with another applicator directly onto the biopsy site(s) for hemostasis. The instruments are removed.

57423
The physician performs laparoscopic repair of a paravaginal defect, in which there is loss of the lateral vaginal attachment to the pelvic sidewall. Through small stab incisions in the abdomen, a fiberoptic laparoscope and trocars are inserted into the abdominal/pelvic space and the abdomen is

insufflated. The bladder may be filled with sterile water to allow the surgeon to identify the superior border of the bladder's edge and then drained to prevent injury after the space of Retzius has been entered and the pubic ramus visualized. Following identification of the defect, the surgeon inserts the nondominant hand into the vagina in order to elevate the anterior vaginal wall and pubocervical fascia to their normal positions. Nonabsorbable sutures with attached needles are introduced through the laparoscopy port and grasped using a laparoscopic needle driver. A series of four to six sutures are placed and tied sequentially along the defects from the ischial spine toward the urethra. The procedure is repeated on the opposite side if a bilateral defect is present. The paravaginal defect repair may be performed alone or in conjunction with cystocele repair, in which a herniation of the bladder through its support tissues into the anterior vaginal wall causes it to bulge downward. These procedures help restore the normal anatomic relationships of the urethra, bladder, and vagina. At completion of the procedure, laparoscopic tools are removed, excess gas expelled, and fascial defects and skin edges are sutured.

57425

The physician performs a laparoscopic colpopexy and suspends or reattaches the apex of the vagina to the uterosacral ligaments to correct a uterovaginal prolapse and restore the vaginal apex to its normal anatomic position, often post-hysterectomy. Through small stab incisions in the abdomen, a fiberoptic laparoscope and trocars are inserted into the abdominal/pelvic space. The bowel is mobilized or moved aside to provide a better view and easier access to the uterosacral ligaments. A vaginal probe is placed for manipulation and to help ensure the cul-de-sac is properly closed. The peritoneum is incised over the vaginal apex. After the vaginal vault is elevated into its normal position, and the cul-de-sac is obliterated, if necessary, a suture is placed through the base of the right uterosacral ligament and through the apex of the vagina-securing it posteriorly to the top of the rectovaginal fascia and anteriorly to the pubocervical fascia (to a dermal or mesh graft, if placed) and secured. Four total sutures are used to elevate the vagina, this being done twice through each ligament and the vaginal apex on each side.

57426

The physician revises or removes a previously placed prosthetic vaginal graft via a laparoscopic approach. Through small stab incisions in the umbilicus and/or abdomen, a fiberoptic laparoscope and trocars are inserted into the peritoneal cavity. Depending upon the type of complication (e.g., mesh erosion into the bladder or persistent vaginal/pelvic pain), the vaginal graft may be completely or partially excised to remove eroding mesh or revisions may be made in the graft and surrounding tissue.

57452

The physician inserts a speculum into the vagina to fully expose and examine the cervix to identify abnormal cells. The upper/adjacent portion of the vagina is examined through a colposcope and a binocular microscope is used for direct visualization of the vagina, ectocervix, and endocervix. This procedure is usually performed when the patient has had an abnormal Pap test. The physician swabs the vaginal walls and cervix with vinegar, iodine, or another type of solution to remove mucus and highlight abnormal cells by turning them white, making them more easily identifiable for possible biopsy. The solution may cause a slight tingling or burning sensation.

57454-57456

The physician inserts a speculum into the vagina to fully expose and examine the cervix to identify abnormal cells. The upper/adjacent portion of the vagina is examined through a colposcope and a binocular microscope is used for direct visualization of the vagina, ectocervix, and endocervix. The physician swabs the vaginal walls and cervix with vinegar, iodine, or another type of solution to remove mucus and highlight abnormal cells by turning them white, making them more easily identifiable for biopsy. In 57455, the physician biopsies the cervix by inserting an instrument into the vagina and removing one or more small tissue samples. In 57456, endocervical curettage is performed by passing a small curette into the endocervical canal, the passage between the external cervical os and the uterine cavity. A specimen is obtained by scraping in the canal with the curette. In 57454, the physician performs biopsy and endocervical curettage procedures. The instrument is removed.

57460

The physician inserts a speculum into the vagina to fully expose and examine the cervix to identify abnormal cells. The upper/adjacent portion of the vagina is examined through a colposcope and a binocular microscope is used for direct visualization of the vagina, ectocervix, and endocervix. The physician swabs the vaginal walls and cervix with vinegar or another type of solution (acetic acid) to remove mucus and highlight abnormal cells by turning them white, making them more easily identifiable for possible biopsy. Sometimes a Schiller test, iodine solution used to coat the cervix, is performed. The solution may cause a slight tingling or burning sensation. Local anesthesia may be used to numb the area. A biopsy specimen of cervical tissue is removed by the loop electrode excision procedure (LEEP). LEEP uses a thin wire loop carrying an electrical cutting current that acts as a cutting instrument to remove abnormal cells. Due to the electrical current, a grounding pad is attached to the patient's leg during the procedure. The physician may apply Monsel's solution, a special type of paste that helps to seal blood vessels to prevent bleeding.

57461

The physician inserts a speculum into the vagina to fully expose and examine the cervix to identify abnormal cells. The upper/adjacent portion of the vagina is examined through a colposcope and a binocular microscope is used for direct visualization of the vagina, ectocervix, and endocervix. The physician swabs the vaginal walls and cervix with vinegar or another type of solution (acetic acid) to remove mucus and highlight abnormal cells by turning them white, making them more easily identifiable for possible biopsy. Sometimes a Schiller test, iodine solution used to coat the cervix, is performed. The solution may cause a slight tingling or burning sensation. Local anesthesia may be used to numb the area. LEEP uses a thin wire loop carrying an electrical cutting current that acts as a cutting instrument to remove abnormal cells. Due to the electrical current, a grounding pad is attached to the patient's leg during the procedure. The cutting current is set. Using the loop, the lesion and transformation zone (the boundary of the excision to assure complete removal of the dysplasia) is removed as one specimen. If the lesion is large and another pass is required, two equal specimens are removed and labeled for the axis of orientation. The same procedure is done again with a smaller loop if an endocervical excision is necessary. The physician may apply Monsel's solution, a special type of paste that helps to seal blood vessels to prevent bleeding or bleeding vessels are cauterized. The vagina is inspected for any accidental injury and the instruments are removed.

57465
The physician performs computer-aided mapping of the cervix uteri during colposcopy, which is reported separately. Colposcopy includes the application of an acetic acid solution to differentiate between normal and abnormal tissue. This reaction, known as acetowhitening, produces a perceptible variance when compared to the normal pinkish color of the surrounding epithelia found in the cervix. By measuring the reaction of the cervical epithelium using proprietary dynamic spectral imaging (DSI), identification of cervical disease may be aided by highlighting suspicious areas, providing more accurate biopsy site selection, and ensuring a more accurate diagnosis.

57500
The physician inserts a speculum into the vagina to view the cervix. A small cut is made in the cervix and biopsy forceps are used to remove a piece or multiple pieces of tissue, or to completely remove a lesion. Bleeding, usually minimal, may be stopped by electric current (fulguration).

57505
The physician inserts a speculum into the vagina to view the cervix. A small curette is used to scrape tissue from the endocervix, which is the region of the opening of the cervix into the uterine cavity.

57510-57513
The physician inserts a speculum into the vagina to view the cervix. In 57510, electric current or heat is used to destroy the outer layers of the cervix causing them to slough off. In 57511, the outer layers of the cervix are destroyed by freezing using a liquid such as carbon dioxide, freon, nitrous oxide, or nitrogen, or a low temperature instrument. The outer layers of the cervix slough off. This code can be used for a first-time or repeat procedure. In 57513, a laser is directed at the cervix to vaporize the outer cells.

57520
The physician performs a conization of the cervix, with or without fulguration, with or without dilation and curettage, with or without repair by using the cold knife or laser technique. The physician inserts a speculum into the vagina to view and fully expose the cervix. For most cases, the appropriate local anesthesia is administered as opposed to forms of premedication. Using a scalpel or laser instrument, a cone or slice of tissue, including about 1 to 2 cm of the endocervix and exocervical cells, is cut from the end of the cervix with the axis of the cone parallel to the axis of the cervix. Bleeding may be stopped by electric current. The cervix may need to be dilated and a curette used directly after conization to scrape tissue that is to be taken from further inside the cervix, approaching the distal uterus. The physician also may need to place interrupted figure-of-eight sutures to control the bleeding site if direct cautery does not achieve hemostasis. The speculum is removed.

57522
The physician performs a conization of the cervix, with or without fulguration, with or without dilation and curettage, with or without repair by using the loop electrode excision procedure (LEEP). The physician inserts a speculum into the vagina to view and fully expose the cervix. For most cases, the appropriate local anesthesia is administered as opposed to forms of premedication. The electric grounding pad is placed and safety checks are run. The cutting current is set. Using a loop that encompasses the lesion, an excision of the ectocervix is done with every effort made to remove the lesion in one specimen. If the lesion is large and another pass is required, two equal specimens are removed and labeled for the axis of orientation. The same procedure is done again with a smaller loop if an endocervical excision is necessary. The cervix may be dilated and an endocervical curettage collected. When all specimens have been collected, the bleeding vessels are cauterized, the vagina is inspected for any accidental injury, and the speculum is removed. No colposcope is used in this procedure.

57530
The physician inserts a speculum into the vagina to view the cervix and perform an amputation of the cervix. A tool is used to pull down the cervix. A scalpel is used to divide the cervix from the uterus just after it enters the vagina. The physician removes the cervix through the vagina and stops the bleeding with cautery and sutures.

57531
The physician inserts a speculum into the vagina to view the cervix and perform a radical excision of the cervix, including removal of local lymph nodes. A tool is used to pull down the cervix. A scalpel is used to divide the cervix from the uterus just after it enters the vagina. The physician removes the cervix through the

vagina, stops the bleeding with cautery, and also removes the pelvic lymph nodes bilaterally, performs a para-aortic lymph node biopsy, and may remove one or both tubes and/or ovaries.

57540-57545
The physician makes an incision horizontally just within the pubic hairline. In 57540, the physician removes the cervical stump, which is the part of the cervix left after the supracervical uterus has been removed. The incision is closed by suturing. In 57545, the physician removes the cervical stump and repairs the muscular floor of the pelvis where the cervix rests using suture plication. This involves folding the tissues on top of each other and suturing. The incision is sutured.

57550
Through an incision at the apex of the vagina, the physician removes the cervical stump, which is the part of the cervix left after the supracervical uterus has been removed. The vaginal incision is closed with sutures.

57555-57556
Through an incision in the apex of the vagina, the physician removes the cervical stump. In 57555, the physician also repairs the relaxed or herniated tissues in the front or back wall of the vagina. Through the vaginal incision, the physician dissects the tissues between the bladder, urethra, vagina, and rectum. The specific tissue weaknesses are repaired and strengthened using tissue transfer techniques and layered and plication suturing. The incisions are closed with sutures. In 57556, the physician also repairs an enterocele, which is a herniation of the bowel against the rectouterine pouch. Through the vaginal incision, the physician incises and ligates the enterocele sac and approximates the uterosacral ligaments and endopelvic fascia anterior to the rectum. The incisions are closed with sutures.

57558
The physician performs a dilation and curettage of the cervical stump. The physician inserts a speculum into the vagina to view the cervix. The physician enlarges the cervix using a dilator and scrapes tissue from the lining of the cervical stump, which is the part of the cervix left after removal of the uterus.

57700
The physician inserts a speculum into the vagina to view the cervix of a nonpregnant patient. Suture or wire is threaded around the cervix and pulled in pursestring fashion to make the opening smaller.

57720
The physician inserts a speculum into the vagina to view the cervix. The physician performs a plastic suture repair of a laceration or wound on the cervix. A plastic repair also can encompass excising scar tissue or tightening an incompetent cervix.

57800
The physician inserts a speculum into the vagina to view the cervix. A tool is used to grasp the cervix and pull it down. A dilator or series of dilators is inserted into the endocervix and passed through the cervical canal.

58100
The physician inserts a speculum into the vagina to view the cervix. A tool is used to grasp the cervix and pull it down. The physician places a curette in the endocervical canal and passes it into the uterus. The endometrial lining of the uterus is scraped on all sides to obtain tissue for diagnosis. Biopsy(ies) may also be taken from the endocervix. Cervical dilation is not required.

58110
A tool is used to grasp the cervix and pull it down. The physician places a curette in the endocervical canal and passes it into the uterus. The endometrial lining of the uterus is scraped in several places to obtain tissue for a biopsy sample. The endometrial sampling is performed in conjunction with direct visualization of the vagina and cervix and is reported in addition to the separately reportable primary colposcopy.

58120
The physician inserts a speculum into the vagina to view the cervix. A tool is used to grasp the cervix and pull it down. A dilator is inserted into the endocervix and through the cervical canal to enlarge the opening. The physician places a curette in the endocervical canal and passes it into the uterus. The endometrial lining of the uterus is scraped on all sides for diagnostic or therapeutic purposes.

58140
The physician removes one to four fibroid tumors from the wall of the uterus (intramural myomas) with a total weight of 250 gm or less and/or removes surface myomas by abdominal approach. A transverse incision is made in the abdomen, the anterior sheath of the rectus abdominis muscle is dissected, and muscles are retracted. Vasoconstrictors are injected and a tourniquet is applied to encompass the uterine mass and the adnexa to limit blood flow. A scalpel, electrocautery, and/or laser may be used to remove small surface myomas. The physician incises the uterus through the myometrium to expose the myoma, which is grasped with a clamp and dissected free from the surrounding myometrium with sharp and blunt dissection. The pedicle is isolated, clamped, and ligated and the myoma is dissected down to the pedicular blood supply. Other myomas are identified by palpating the uterine wall through the defect created by the already excised myoma. Adjacent myomas are reached and removed by tunneling further through the initial incision to avoid additional uterine trauma. The uterine wall defects are repaired by approximating the tissues to restore previous anatomy. The serosa is closed so as to minimize adhesion formation. Antiadhesion prophylaxis may be

instilled in the abdominal cavity and the wound is closed.

58145
The physician removes one to four fibroid tumors from the wall of the uterus (intramural myomas) with a total weight of 250 gm or less and/or removes surface myomas by vaginal approach. This approach is used for pedunculated myomas protruding through the cervix and for prolapsed myomas. The cervix is dilated with laminaria to facilitate exposure and a tonsil snare or other appropriate device is passed through to reach the myoma. Prolapsed myomas are usually attached to the cervical or endometrial cavity by a stalk. The tumor is removed by ligating or twisting the stalk or a tonsil snare is employed to encircle the tumor, cut it from its stalk, and remove it. The instruments are removed.

58146
The physician removes five or more fibroid tumors from the wall of the uterus and/or intramural myomas with a total weight greater than 250 gm by abdominal approach. A transverse incision is made in the abdomen (a midline incision is made for large myomas) and the anterior sheath of the rectus abdominis muscle is dissected and muscles are retracted. Vasoconstrictors are injected and a tourniquet is applied to encompass the uterine mass and the adnexa to limit blood flow. The physician incises the uterus down through the myometrium to expose the myoma, which is grasped with a clamp and dissected free from the surrounding myometrium with sharp and blunt dissection. For deep intramural myomas, the endometrial cavity may be exposed. The pedicle is isolated, clamped, and ligated and the myoma is dissected down to the pedicular blood supply. Other myomas are identified by palpating the uterine wall through the defect created by the already excised myoma. Adjacent myomas are reached and removed by tunneling further through the initial incision to avoid additional uterine trauma. The uterine wall defects are repaired by approximating the tissues to restore previous anatomy. The serosa is closed so as to minimize adhesion formation. Antiadhesion prophylaxis may be instilled in the abdominal cavity and the wound is closed.

58150
Through a horizontal incision just within the pubic hairline, the physician removes the uterus including the cervix and may elect to remove one or both of the ovaries and one or both of the fallopian tubes (salpingo-oophorectomy). The supporting pedicles containing the tubes, ligaments, and arteries are clamped and cut free. The uterus and cervix are removed along with a narrow rim or cuff of vaginal lining. The vaginal defect may be left open for drainage. The abdominal incision is closed by suturing.

58152
Through a horizontal incision just within the pubic hairline, the physician removes the uterus, including the cervix, and may elect to remove one or both of the ovaries and one or both of the fallopian tubes (salpingo-oophorectomy). The supporting pedicles containing the tubes, ligaments, and arteries are clamped and cut free. The bladder neck is suspended by placing sutures through the tissue surrounding the urethra and into the back of the symphysis pubis, which is the midline junction of the pubic bones in the front (Marshall-Marchetti-Krantz), or sutures are placed in the fascia on either side of the bladder and then through the Cooper's ligaments above. The sutures are tied, which elevates the vesical neck (the junction of the bladder and urethra), in the direction of the Cooper's ligament (Burch procedure). The sutures are pulled tight so that the tissues are tacked to the symphysis pubis and the urethra is moved forward. The abdominal incision is closed by suturing.

58180
Through a horizontal incision just within the pubic hairline, the physician removes the uterus above the cervix and may elect to remove one or both of the ovaries and one or both of the fallopian tubes (salpingo-oophorectomy). The supporting pedicles containing the tubes, ligaments, and arteries are clamped and cut free. The uterus is cut free from the cervix leaving the cervix still attached to the vagina. The abdominal incision is closed by suturing.

58200
Through a horizontal incision just within the pubic hairline, the physician removes the uterus, including the cervix and part of the vagina. The supporting pedicles containing the tubes, ligaments and arteries are clamped and cut free and the uterus, cervix, and part of the vagina are removed. A biopsy is taken of the para-aortic and pelvic lymph nodes. The physician may elect to remove one or both of the ovaries and one or both of the fallopian tubes (salpingo-oophorectomy). The abdominal incision is closed by suturing.

58210
Through a horizontal incision just within the pubic hairline, the physician removes the uterus, including the cervix and the pelvic lymph nodes on both sides and takes a biopsy of the para-aortic lymph nodes. The supporting pedicles containing the tubes, ligaments, and arteries are clamped and cut free and the uterus, cervix, all or part of the vagina, and all pelvic lymph nodes are removed. The physician may elect to remove one or both of the ovaries and one or both of the fallopian tubes (salpingo-oophorectomy). The abdominal incision is closed by suturing.

58240
Through a horizontal incision just within the pubic hairline, the physician removes all of the organs and adjacent structures of the pelvis including the cervix, uterus, and all or part of the vagina. The supporting pedicles containing the tubes, ligaments, and arteries are clamped and cut free and the uterus, cervix, and all or part of the vagina are removed. The physician may remove one or both of the ovaries and one or both of the fallopian tubes (salpingo-oophorectomy). The physician removes the bladder and diverts urine flow by transplanting the ureters to the skin or colon. The

rectum and part of the colon may be removed and an artificial abdominal opening in the skin surface created for waste (colostomy). The abdominal incision is closed by suturing.

58260

The physician performs a vaginal hysterectomy for a uterus 250 gm or less. An incision is made around the cervix through the full thickness of the vaginal membrane. The cut vaginal edge is pulled toward the lower cervix and vaginal dissection is continued with countertraction. The posterior peritoneum is opened to admit a finger examination of the pelvis. The uterosacral ligaments are clamped and possibly shortened, cut from the uterus, and secured to the vagina. The vesicovaginal space is entered. The connective tissue fusing the bladder and vagina is dissected and the bladder is separated from the cervix. The bladder pillars are clamped, cut, and ligated near their cervical attachments, as well as the cardinal ligament tissue on each side of the cervix and the left and right uterine vessels. The physician clamps, cuts, and ligates the upper cardinal and lower broad ligament complex. Traction applied to the cervix moves the uterus down until the fundus is low in the pelvis. Hemostats are applied to the angle of the uterus on each side and the uterus is removed. The peritoneum is closed with purse-string sutures that incorporate the proximal part of the uterosacral ligaments.

58262-58263

The physician performs a vaginal hysterectomy for a uterus 250 gm or less and removes the tubes and/or ovaries. An incision is made around the cervix through the full thickness of the vaginal membrane. The cut vaginal edge is pulled toward the lower cervix and vaginal dissection is continued with countertraction. The posterior peritoneum is opened to admit a finger examination of the pelvis. The uterosacral ligaments are clamped and possibly shortened, cut from the uterus, and secured to the vagina. The vesicovaginal space is entered. The connective tissue fusing the bladder and vagina is dissected and the bladder is separated from the cervix. The bladder pillars are clamped, cut, and ligated near their cervical attachments, as well as the cardinal ligament tissue on each side of the cervix and the left and right uterine vessels. The physician clamps, cuts, and ligates the upper cardinal and lower broad ligament complex. Traction applied to the cervix moves the uterus down until the fundus is low in the pelvis. Hemostats are applied to the angle of the uterus on each side and the uterus is removed. After the uterus is exteriorized, care is taken to ensure ligation of the ovarian vessels. The ovary is excised under direct vision. For removal of both tubes and ovaries, the round ligament on one side at a time is clamped and divided. A tunnel is made through the layers of the uterine broad ligament that enclose the tube and the tube and ovary are clamped together. The structure is pulled forward, the two sheets of the broad ligament are each cut, and the broad ligament is opened completely. The whole specimen is separated from its attaching ligament, which is clamped, and the tube and ovary on that side are removed. Report 58263 if an enterocele is repaired in addition to removing the tube and/or ovary. An enterocele is a hernia of the intestine protruding against the vaginal wall. The hernia sac is bluntly and sharply dissected from the surrounding connective tissue, excised and ligated, and the surrounding tissues are strengthened and sutured. The peritoneal and vaginal wall incisions of the hysterectomy procedure are closed.

58267

The physician performs a vaginal hysterectomy for a uterus 250 gm or less with colpo-urethrocystopexy, with or without endoscopic control. An incision is made around the cervix through the full thickness of the vaginal membrane. The cut vaginal edge is pulled toward the lower cervix and vaginal dissection is continued with countertraction. The posterior peritoneum is opened to admit a finger examination of the pelvis. The uterosacral ligaments are clamped and possibly shortened, cut from the uterus, and secured to the vagina. The vesicovaginal space is entered. The connective tissue fusing the bladder and vagina is dissected and the bladder is separated from the cervix. The bladder pillars are clamped, cut, and ligated near their cervical attachments, as well as the cardinal ligament tissue on each side of the cervix and the left and right uterine vessels. The physician clamps, cuts, and ligates the upper cardinal and lower broad ligament complex. Traction applied to the cervix moves the uterus down until the fundus is low in the pelvis. Hemostats are applied to the angle of the uterus on each side and the uterus is removed. Colpo-urethrocystopexy is done in cases of urinary incontinence to elevate the lower part of the bladder that connects to the urethra (bladder neck) and the urethra to a new position higher in the pelvis so the muscles of the pelvic floor can help control urination. After the uterus has been exteriorized and the bladder and urethra separated from surrounding structures, the physician lifts the vagina upward, suspends the bladder neck and urethra by placing sutures through the fibromuscular wall of the vagina lateral to the tissue surrounding the urethra, and sutures the tissue to the symphysis pubis (the midline junction of the pubic bones at the front). An endoscope may be placed to ensure no sutures pass through the lining of the bladder and to evaluate ureteral patency. The sutures are pulled tight to tack the structures to the pubic bone and provide support.

58270

The physician performs a vaginal hysterectomy, for a uterus 250 gm or less with repair of an enterocele. An incision is made around the cervix through the full thickness of the vaginal membrane. The cut vaginal edge is pulled toward the lower cervix and vaginal dissection is continued with countertraction. The posterior peritoneum is opened to admit a finger examination of the pelvis. The uterosacral ligaments are clamped and possibly shortened, cut from the uterus, and secured to the vagina. The vesicovaginal space is entered. The connective tissue fusing the bladder and vagina is dissected and the bladder is separated from the cervix. The bladder pillars are clamped, cut, and ligated near their cervical attachments as well as the cardinal ligament tissue on each side of the cervix and the left and right uterine vessels. The anterior peritoneum is opened under direct vision to avoid damaging the bladder and admit finger exploration. The physician clamps, cuts, and ligates the upper cardinal and lower broad ligament complex now that the peritoneum is open both anterior and posterior to the uterine fundus. Hemostats are applied to the angle of the uterus on each side and the uterus is removed, usually posteriorly. The physician also repairs an enterocele, a herniation of intestine that protrudes against the vaginal wall, discovered during finger exploration. The hernia sac is bluntly and sharply dissected from the surrounding connective tissue, excised and ligated, and the surrounding tissues are strengthened and sutured. The peritoneum is closed with purse-string sutures that incorporate the proximal part of the uterosacral ligaments.

58275-58280

The physician performs a vaginal hysterectomy with total or partial vaginectomy in 58275-58280 and with enterocele repair in 58280. An incision is made around the cervix through the full thickness of the vaginal membrane. The cut vaginal edge is pulled toward the lower cervix and vaginal dissection is continued with countertraction. The posterior peritoneum is opened to admit a finger examination of the pelvis. The uterosacral ligaments are clamped and possibly shortened, cut from the uterus, and secured to the vagina. The vesicovaginal space is entered. The connective tissue fusing the bladder and vagina is dissected and the bladder is separated from the cervix. The bladder pillars are clamped, cut, and ligated near their cervical attachments, as well as the cardinal ligament tissue on each side of the cervix and the left and right uterine vessels. The anterior peritoneum is opened under direct vision to avoid damaging the bladder and admit finger exploration. The physician clamps, cuts, and ligates the upper cardinal and lower broad ligament complex now that the peritoneum is open both anterior and posterior to the uterine fundus. Traction applied to the cervix moves the uterus down until the fundus is low in the pelvis. Hemostats are applied to the angle of the uterus on each side and the uterus is removed, usually posteriorly. The vagina is everted out through its opening and totally or partially removed in sections by blunt and sharp dissection. Any remaining vaginal tissue and the supporting tissues are inverted back into the resulting defect and are sutured in place with total vaginectomy obliterating the space. Report 58280 if the physician also repairs an enterocele, a herniation of intestine protruding through the vaginal wall. The hernia sac is bluntly and sharply dissected from the surrounding connective tissue, excised and ligated, and the surrounding tissues are strengthened and sutured. The peritoneum is closed with purse-string sutures that incorporate the proximal part of the uterosacral ligaments.

58285

The physician performs a radical vaginal hysterectomy. This includes the uterus, its surrounding tissues, and the pelvic lymph nodes. An incision is made around the cervix through the full thickness of the vaginal membrane. The cut vaginal edge is pulled toward the lower cervix and vaginal dissection is continued with countertraction. The posterior peritoneum is opened to admit a finger examination of the pelvis. The uterosacral ligaments are clamped and possibly shortened, cut from the uterus, and secured to the vagina. The vesicovaginal space is entered. The connective tissue fusing the bladder and vagina is dissected and the bladder is separated from the cervix. The bladder pillars are clamped, cut, and ligated near their cervical attachments, as well as the cardinal ligament tissue on each side of the cervix and the left and right uterine vessels. The anterior peritoneum is opened under direct vision to avoid damaging the bladder and admit finger exploration. The physician clamps, cuts, and ligates the upper cardinal and lower broad ligament complex now that the peritoneum is open both anterior and posterior to the uterine fundus. Traction applied to the cervix moves the uterus down until the fundus is low in the pelvis. Hemostats are applied to the angle of the uterus on each side and the uterus is removed, usually posteriorly. The physician also removes the surrounding tissues, including part or all of the vagina and the pelvic lymph nodes. Any incisions are closed by suturing.

58290

The physician performs a vaginal hysterectomy, for a uterus greater than 250 gm. An incision is made around the cervix through the full thickness of the vaginal membrane. The cut vaginal edge is pulled toward the lower cervix and vaginal dissection is continued with countertraction. The posterior peritoneum is opened to admit a finger examination of the pelvis. The uterosacral ligaments are clamped and possibly shortened, cut from the uterus, and secured to the vagina. The vesicovaginal space is entered. The connective tissue fusing the bladder and vagina is dissected and the bladder is separated from the cervix. The bladder pillars are clamped, cut, and ligated near their cervical attachments as well as the cardinal ligament tissue on each side of the cervix and the left and right uterine vessels. The anterior peritoneum is opened under direct vision to avoid damaging the bladder and admit finger exploration. The physician clamps, cuts, and ligates the upper cardinal and lower broad ligament complex now that the peritoneum is open both anterior and posterior to the uterine fundus. Traction applied to the cervix moves the uterus down until the fundus is low in the pelvis. Hemostats are applied to the angle of the uterus on each side and the uterus is removed, usually posteriorly. When the uterus is too large to permit delivery through the anterior or posterior peritoneal opening, the myometrium may be incised circumferentially parallel to the uterine cavity axis and removed or the uterus can be dissected and removed one half at a time. The peritoneum is closed with purse-string sutures that incorporate the proximal part of the uterosacral ligaments. Colporrhaphy may be performed before the vaginal wall is closed by running or interrupted sutures placed side to side longitudinally.

58291-58292
The physician performs a vaginal hysterectomy, for a uterus greater than 250 gm and removes the tubes and/or ovaries. An incision is made around the cervix through the full thickness of the vaginal membrane. The cut vaginal edge is pulled toward the lower cervix and vaginal dissection is continued with countertraction. The posterior peritoneum is opened to admit a finger examination of the pelvis. The uterosacral ligaments are clamped and possibly shortened, cut from the uterus, and secured to the vagina. The vesicovaginal space is entered. The connective tissue fusing the bladder and vagina is dissected and the bladder is separated from the cervix. The bladder pillars are clamped, cut, and ligated near their cervical attachments, as well as the cardinal ligament tissue on each side of the cervix and the left and right uterine vessels. The anterior peritoneum is opened under direct vision to avoid damaging the bladder and admit finger exploration. The physician clamps, cuts, and ligates the upper cardinal and lower broad ligament complex now that the peritoneum is open both anterior and posterior to the uterine fundus. Traction applied to the cervix moves the uterus down until the fundus is low in the pelvis. Hemostats are applied to the angle of the uterus on each side and the uterus is removed, usually posteriorly. After the uterus is exteriorized, care is taken to ensure ligation of the ovarian vessels. The ovary is excised under direct vision. For removal of both tubes and ovaries, the round ligament on one side at a time is clamped and divided. A tunnel is made through the layers of the uterine broad ligament that enclose the tube and the tube and ovary are clamped together. The structure is pulled forward, the two sheets of the broad ligament are each cut, and the broad ligament is opened completely. The whole specimen is separated from its attaching ligament, which is clamped, and the tube and ovary on that side are removed. Report 58292 if an enterocele is repaired in addition to removing the tube and/or ovary. An enterocele is a hernia of the intestine protruding against the vaginal wall. The hernia sac is bluntly and sharply dissected from the surrounding connective tissue, excised and ligated, and the surrounding tissues are strengthened and sutured. The peritoneal and vaginal wall incisions of the hysterectomy procedure are closed.

58294
The physician performs a vaginal hysterectomy, for a uterus greater than 250 gm, with repair of an enterocele. An incision is made around the cervix through the full thickness of the vaginal membrane. The cut vaginal edge is pulled toward the lower cervix and vaginal dissection is continued with countertraction. The posterior peritoneum is opened to admit a finger examination of the pelvis. The uterosacral ligaments are clamped and possibly shortened, cut from the uterus, and secured to the vagina. The vesicovaginal space is entered. The connective tissue fusing the bladder and vagina is dissected and the bladder is separated from the cervix. The bladder pillars are clamped, cut, and ligated near their cervical attachments, as well as the cardinal ligament tissue on each side of the cervix and the left and right uterine vessels. The anterior peritoneum is opened under direct vision. The physician clamps, cuts, and ligates the upper cardinal and lower broad ligament complex now that the peritoneum is open both anterior and posterior to the uterine fundus. Traction applied to the cervix moves the uterus down until the fundus is low in the pelvis. Hemostats are applied to the angle of the uterus on each side and the uterus is removed, usually posteriorly. The physician also repairs an enterocele, a herniation of intestine that protrudes against the vaginal wall, discovered during finger exploration. The hernia sac is bluntly and sharply dissected from the surrounding connective tissue, excised and ligated, and the surrounding tissues are strengthened and sutured. The peritoneum is closed with purse-string sutures that incorporate the proximal part of the uterosacral ligaments.

58300-58301
The physician inserts a speculum into the vagina to visualize the cervix. A tool is used to gently pull down the cervix; it is dilated. In 58300, an intrauterine device (IUD), any of a variety of shapes (coil, loop, T, 7), is guided into the uterus through an insertion tube placed in the cervical os. In 58301, to remove a previously placed IUD from the uterus, a device is inserted through the cervical os and used to grasp and remove the IUD.

58321-58322
In 58321, the physician performs artificial insemination by injecting semen into the endocervical canal by applying the blunt tip of a plastic syringe to the external os (opening) of the cervix. Sometimes a cervical cap is used to keep the semen in and around the cervix for eight to 16 hours. In 58322, the physician dilates the cervix and inserts a long flexible tube into the cavity of the uterus. Semen is injected into the uterus by a syringe connected to the tube.

58323
Sperm are spun in a centrifuge that removes the superficial antibodies on the sperm in order to facilitate fertilization. The sperm are first washed in a medium three times the volume of the collected semen. This mixture is spun in a centrifuge and the layer of liquid is discarded. The sperm are resuspended in a fresh medium. This method removes debris, bacteria, antibodies, and abnormal spermatozoa.

58340
A small catheter is introduced into the cervical opening and a saline solution (for saline infusion sonohysterography [SIS]) or liquid radiographic

contrast material (for hysterosalpingography) is injected into the endometrial cavity with mild pressure to force the material into the fallopian tubes. The shadow of the contrast material appears on separately reported x-ray films, permitting examination of the uterus and fallopian tubes for any abnormalities or blockages. When sonohysterography is performed, a thin catheter is inserted into the uterus and one to two teaspoons of saline solution is injected into the uterine cavity. Separately reported, fluid enhanced endovaginal ultrasound is performed with the saline solution acting as a contrast medium to view any abnormal anatomic findings in the uterus.

58345
The physician introduces a catheter into the cervix, and takes it into the uterus and through the fallopian tube. The catheter must be made of a material that will show on x-ray film so that any blockages or abnormalities in the tube can be seen. The physician may inject radiographic contrast material into the endometrial cavity with mild pressure to force the material into the tubes. The shadow of this material on separately reported x-ray film permits examination of the uterus and tubes for any abnormalities or blockages.

58346
The physician inserts radioactive Heyman capsules into the uterus to treat endometrial cancer. Radiotherapy is often the prescribed treatment for patients who are medically inoperable for endometrial carcinoma. Brachytherapy is administered via low dose radiation (LDR) or high dose radiation (HDR) technique, with the goal of achieving coverage of all uterine tissue. This is achieved with the placement of multiple Heyman capsules, inserted through the cervical os and placed in the uterus with consideration of appropriate radiation field. For low-dose treatment, Heyman capsules are used for patients with a large uterus to help expand the uterine cavity and cover the uterus. Heyman capsules also may be prescribed for patients with early-stage disease and low-grade histology, when radiation alone is the preferred therapy. Use this code once to report multiple capsules inserted during the same session.

58350
The physician injects a liquid dye or solution into the uterine cavity or directly into the fallopian tubes. This procedure is frequently performed during a separately reported surgery, open or laparoscopic, to verify patency of tubes.

58400
The physician plicates stretched uterine broad ligaments, bringing the uterus back into place. Plication shortens the ligament by folding and tacking it. The physician may elect to plicate the round and sacrouterine ligaments as well. This procedure may be done through a small abdominal incision or through an incision in the vagina.

58410
The physician plicates stretched uterine broad ligaments, bringing the uterus back into place. Plication shortens the ligament by folding and tacking it. The physician may elect to plicate the round and sacrouterine ligaments as well. A portion of the presacral sympathetic nerve is removed or destroyed to alleviate pelvic pain. The procedure may be done through a small abdominal incision or through an incision in the vagina.

58520
The physician repairs a uterus that became lacerated or ruptured by nonobstetrical means. A large incision is made in the abdomen and the uterus is repaired with layered suturing of torn, crushed, or deeply lacerated tissue. The physician debrides the wound by removing foreign material or damaged tissue. Irrigation of the wound is performed and antimicrobial solutions are used to decontaminate and cleanse the wound. The physician may trim skin margins with a scalpel or scissors to allow for proper closure. The abdominal incision is closed.

58540
Through a small incision in the lower abdomen, the physician performs a plastic repair of a malformed uterus. This often is an extensive procedure that involves removing abnormal tissues, rearranging the uterine walls, and suturing.

[58674]
Radiofrequency ablation (RFA) of uterine fibroids is performed laparoscopically. The physician makes a small incision in the umbilicus through which the abdomen is insufflated and a fiberoptic laparoscope is inserted. Other incisions are made through which trocars can be passed into the abdominal cavity to deliver instruments, a video camera, and, when needed, an additional light source. The physician manipulates the tools so that the uterus and fibroids can be viewed through the laparoscope and/or video monitor. Using ultrasound guidance, the RFA catheter is inserted through the skin into a fibroid and electrical energy is delivered to the fibroid, heating the tissue and killing the tumor cells. The procedure is repeated as needed for additional fibroids. The catheter, laparoscope, and instruments are removed and the incisions are closed.

58541-58542
The physician performs a laparoscopic hysterectomy, removing a uterus with a total weight of 250 gm or less while preserving the cervix. The patient is placed in the dorsal lithotomy position. After the insertion of a speculum in the vagina, the physician grasps the cervix with an instrument to manipulate the uterus during the surgery. A trocar is inserted periumbilically and the abdomen is insufflated with gas. Additional trocars are placed in the right and left lower quadrants. The uterus is dissected free from the bladder and surrounding tissue and its body is separated from the cervix. Coagulation is achieved with the aid of electrocautery instruments. Alternatively, some vessels may be

ligated. The uterus is morcellized and removed using endoscopic tools. In 58542, one or both ovaries and/or one or both fallopian tubes are removed in similar fashion. Once the excisions are complete, the abdominal cavity is deflated and instruments and trocars removed. The fascia and skin are closed with sutures.

58543-58544

The physician performs a laparoscopic hysterectomy, removing a uterus with a total weight of more than 250 gm while preserving the cervix. The patient is placed in the dorsal lithotomy position. After the insertion of a speculum in the vagina, the physician grasps the cervix with an instrument to manipulate the uterus during the surgery. A trocar is inserted periumbilically and the abdomen is insufflated with gas. Additional trocars are placed in the right and left lower quadrants. The uterus is dissected free from the bladder and surrounding tissue and its body is separated from the cervix. Coagulation is achieved with the aid of electrocautery instruments. Alternatively, some vessels may be ligated. The uterus is morcellized and removed using endoscopic tools. In 58544, one or both ovaries and/or one or both fallopian tubes are removed in similar fashion. Once the excisions are complete, the abdominal cavity is deflated and instruments and trocars removed. The fascia and skin are closed with sutures.

58545

The physician performs a laparoscopic myomectomy, removing one to four fibroid tumors from the wall of the uterus (intramural myomas) with a total weight of 250 gm or less and/or removes surface myomas. The patient is placed in the dorsal lithotomy position. A trocar is inserted periumbilically and the abdomen is insufflated with gas. Additional trocars are placed in the right and left lower quadrants. Electrocautery instruments and/or laser may be used to remove small surface myomas. Pedunculated myomas are removed by ligating, twisting, or snaring the stalk. The physician incises the uterus through the myometrium to expose the myoma, which is dissected free from the surrounding myometrium. The pedicle is isolated, clamped, and ligated and the myoma is dissected down to the pedicular blood supply. The adjacent myomas may be reached and removed by tunneling further through the initial incision. The uterine wall defects are sutured laparoscopically, the trocars are removed, and the wounds are closed.

58546

The physician performs a laparoscopic myomectomy, removing five or more fibroid tumors from the wall of the uterus (intramural myomas) and/or intramural myomas with a total weight greater than 250 gm. The patient is placed in the dorsal lithotomy position. A trocar is inserted periumbilically and the abdomen is insufflated with gas. Additional trocars are placed in the right and left lower quadrants. The physician incises the uterus through the myometrium to expose the myoma, which is dissected free from the surrounding myometrium. The pedicle is isolated, clamped, and ligated and the myoma is dissected to the pedicular blood supply. The adjacent myomas may be reached and removed by tunneling further through the initial incision. After resecting large intramural myomas, removing them from the abdominal cavity may require making a culdotomy incision or using morcellation techniques. A minilaparotomy may be done with laparoscopic myomectomy as myomas are brought to the abdominal wall for removal and the uterus may be closed with some layered suturing. The laparoscopic instruments are removed and the wounds are closed.

58548

The physician performs a laparoscopic hysterectomy, bilateral total pelvic lymphadenectomy, and para-aortic lymph node sampling, and may remove all or portions of the fallopian tubes and ovaries. The patient is placed in the dorsal lithotomy position. After the insertion of a speculum in the vagina, the physician grasps the cervix with an instrument to manipulate the uterus during the surgery. A trocar is inserted periumbilically and the abdomen is insufflated with gas. Additional trocars are placed in the right and left lower quadrants. The uterus is dissected free from the bladder and surrounding tissue and its body with the cervix is dissected from the vagina. Alternately, the vagina may also be excised. Coagulation is achieved with the aid of electrocautery instruments. Some vessels may be ligated. The uterus may be morcellized prior to being removed using endoscopic tools or it may be removed via the vagina. One or both ovaries and/or one or both fallopian tubes are removed in similar fashion. The physician removes the pelvic lymph nodes on both sides and takes samples or biopsies of the para-aortic lymph nodes. Once the excisions are complete, the abdominal cavity is deflated and instruments and trocars removed. The fascia and skin of the abdomen and vagina are closed with sutures.

58550-58552

The physician performs surgical laparoscopy with vaginal hysterectomy for a uterus with a total weight of 250 gm or less. The laparoscope is used to perform the initial operative portion of the hysterectomy. The patient is placed in the dorsal lithotomy position for the endoscopic portion. For the vaginal portion, the patient is positioned in stirrups. A trocar is inserted periumbilically and the abdomen is insufflated with gas. Additional trocars are placed in the right and left lower quadrants. An intra-abdominal and pelvic survey is done and any adhesions are lysed. The round ligaments are ligated and incised. Starting on the left round ligament, the vesicouterine peritoneal fold is incised and the peritoneal vessels are dissected and desiccated. The physician continues the incision across the lower uterine segment to the round ligament on the other side and dissects the bladder off the uterus and cervix. Staples are inserted through one port on the side to be stapled or a bipolar coagulation unit is inserted for electrocautery. At this point, if tubes and/ or ovaries are to be removed, the infundibulopelvic

Male/Female

ligament is now ligated lateral to the ovary. If not, the ligation is done medial to the ovary. Staple ligation or electrodesiccation of the uterine vasculature is accomplished on both sides, followed by ligation or electrodesiccation of the cardinal ligaments. An anterior colpotomy incision is made to enter the vagina and the vaginal portion of the procedure is begun. The remaining supporting structures attached to the cervix and uterus are detached and the hysterectomy proceeds through a posterior cul-de-sac incision. The uterus is removed, the vaginal incision is closed, and hemostasis is confirmed before the trocars are removed and the skin incisions are closed. Report 58550 for removal of uterus or 58552 if uterus, tubes, and/or ovaries are removed.

58553-58554
The physician performs surgical laparoscopy with vaginal hysterectomy for a uterus with a total weight of more than 250 gm. The laparoscope is used to perform the initial operative portion of the hysterectomy. The patient is placed in the dorsal lithotomy position for the endoscopic portion. For the vaginal portion, the patient is positioned in stirrups. A trocar is inserted periumbilically and the abdomen is insufflated with gas. Additional trocars are placed in the right and left lower quadrants. An intra-abdominal and pelvic survey is done and any adhesions are lysed. The round ligaments are ligated and incised. Starting on the left round ligament, the vesicouterine peritoneal fold is incised and the peritoneal vessels are dissected and desiccated. The physician continues the incision across the lower uterine segment to the round ligament on the other side and dissects the bladder off the uterus and cervix. Staples are inserted through one port on the side to be stapled or a bipolar coagulation unit is inserted for electrocautery. At this point, if tubes and/or ovaries are to be removed, the infundibulopelvic ligament is now ligated lateral to the ovary. If not, the ligation is done medial to the ovary. Staple-ligation or electrodesiccation of the uterine vasculature is accomplished on both sides, followed by ligation or electrodesiccation of the cardinal ligaments. An anterior colpotomy incision is made to enter the vagina and the vaginal portion of the procedure is begun. The remaining supporting structures attached to the cervix and uterus are detached and the hysterectomy proceeds through a posterior cul-de-sac incision. The uterus is removed, the vaginal incision is closed, and hemostasis is confirmed before the trocars are removed and the skin incisions are closed. Report 58553 for removal of uterus or 58554 if uterus, tubes, and/or ovaries are removed.

58555
The physician performs a diagnostic inspection of the uterus using a hysteroscope. The physician advances the hysteroscope through the vagina and into the cervical os to gain entry into the uterine cavity. The physician inspects the uterine cavity with the fiberoptic scope for diagnostic purposes.

58558
The physician performs a diagnostic inspection of the uterus using a hysteroscope and removes a uterine polyp, removes uterine tissue for biopsy, and may perform cervical dilation and uterine curettage (D&C). The physician advances the hysteroscope through the vagina and into the cervical os to gain entry into the uterine cavity. The physician inspects the uterine cavity with the fiberoptic scope and removes a sample of the uterine lining and/or removes a growth (polypectomy) within the uterus and may perform a cervical dilation and uterine curettage, scraping (D&C) to take a complete sampling of the uterine lining.

58559
The physician removes scar tissue (adhesions) from within the uterus using a fiberoptic hysteroscope. The physician advances the hysteroscope through the vagina and into the cervical os to gain entry into the uterine cavity. The physician inspects the uterine cavity with the fiberoptic scope and removes or divides adhesions (fibrous scar tissue) that are artificially connecting the walls of the uterus.

58560
The physician removes tissue abnormally dividing the intrauterine cavity using a fiberoptic hysteroscope. The physician advances the hysteroscope through the vagina and into the cervical os to gain entry into the uterine cavity. The physician inspects the uterine cavity with the fiberoptic scope and resects an intrauterine septum (tissue creating an abnormal partition in the uterus).

58561
The physician surgically removes a leiomyomata (uterine fibroid tumor) with the assistance of a fiberoptic hysteroscope. The physician advances the hysteroscope through the vagina and into the cervical os to gain entry into the uterine cavity. The physician inspects the uterine cavity with the fiberoptic scope and removes uterine leiomyomata with the assistance of the fiberoptic scope.

58562
The physician surgically removes an impacted foreign body with the assistance of a fiberoptic hysteroscope. The physician advances the hysteroscope through the vagina and into the cervical os to gain entry into the uterine cavity. The physician inspects the uterine cavity with the fiberoptic scope and removes an impacted foreign body from the uterine wall with the assistance of the hysteroscope.

58563
The physician surgically removes (ablates) the inner lining of the uterus with the assistance of a fiberoptic hysteroscope. The physician advances the hysteroscope through the vagina and into the cervical os to gain entry into the uterine cavity. The physician inspects the uterine cavity with the fiberoptic scope and ablates the endometrium by various methods, such as resection, electrosurgical ablation, or thermoablation.

58565
The physician performs a hysteroscopy with bilateral fallopian tube cannulation and placement of permanent implants to occlude the fallopian tubes. The physician advances the hysteroscope through the vagina and into the cervical os to gain entry into the uterine cavity. The physician inserts a catheter into each fallopian tube. The catheter delivers a small metallic implant into each fallopian tube. The presence of the obstructive implant causes scar tissue to form, completely blocking the fallopian tube as a means of birth control.

58570-58571
The physician performs a total laparoscopic hysterectomy (TLH), removing a uterus with a total weight of 250 gm or less. Following appropriate anesthesia, the patient is placed in the dorsal lithotomy position. A Foley catheter ensures that the bladder is emptied during the procedure. A trocar is inserted periumbilically and the abdomen is insufflated with gas. Ancillary trocars are also placed suprapubically. Following abdominal pelvic inspection and lysis of any adhesions present, the uterus is mobilized. The uterine ligaments are sectioned, and the uterus and cervix are dissected free from the bladder and surrounding tissues. Coagulation is achieved with the aid of electrocautery instruments. Alternately, some vessels may be ligated. The uterus and cervix are morcellized using endoscopic tools and removed through the abdominal incisions or the vagina. In 58571, one or both ovaries and/or one or both fallopian tubes are removed in similar fashion. Once the excisions are complete, the abdominal cavity is deflated and instruments and trocars are removed. The fascia and skin are closed with sutures.

58572-58573
The physician performs a total laparoscopic hysterectomy (TLH), removing a uterus with a total weight greater than 250 gm. Following appropriate anesthesia, the patient is placed in the dorsal lithotomy position. A Foley catheter ensures that the bladder is emptied during the procedure. A trocar is inserted periumbilically and the abdomen is insufflated with gas. Ancillary trocars are also placed suprapubically. Following abdominal pelvic inspection and lysis of any adhesions present, the uterus is mobilized. The uterine ligaments are sectioned, and the uterus and cervix are dissected free from the bladder and surrounding tissues. Coagulation is achieved with the aid of electrocautery instruments. Alternately, some vessels may be ligated. The uterus and cervix are morcellized using endoscopic tools and removed through the abdominal incisions or the vagina. In 58573, one or both ovaries and/or one or both fallopian tubes are removed in similar fashion. Once the excisions are complete, the abdominal cavity is deflated and instruments and trocars are removed. The fascia and skin are closed with sutures.

58575
Through small incisions made in the abdomen, the physician performs a total hysterectomy (removal the uterus and cervix) for an ovarian, fallopian, or peritoneal malignancy. After careful inspection of the abdomen and pelvis, aspiration of any pelvic ascites or peritoneal washings submitted for cytologic evaluation and tissue samples for frozen section may be performed to determine if malignant cells are still present and/or to determine if the cancer has metastasized. Tumor debulking is a procedure where a surgeon partially removes a surgically incurable malignant tumor to allow for subsequent therapies such as chemotherapy, radiation, or other adjunctive measures more effective with the goal of increasing the patient's survival rates. The physician also performs an omentectomy (removal of the membrane containing fat, lymph, and blood vessels that acts as a protective layer extending from the stomach to the transverse colon). Removal of one or both ovaries and/or fallopian tubes is included, when performed.

[58353]
The physician performs an endometrial ablation, using heat without hysteroscopic guidance. The physician inserts a soft, flexible balloon attached to a thin catheter into the vagina through the cervix and into the uterus. The balloon is inflated with fluid, which expands to fit the size and shape of the patient's uterus. The fluid in the balloon is heated to 87°C or 188°F and maintained for eight to nine minutes while the uterine lining is treated. When the treatment cycle is complete, all the fluid is withdrawn from the balloon and the balloon and catheter are removed.

[58356]
The physician performs endometrial cryoablation with any required endometrial curettage using ultrasound guidance. The physician inserts a speculum for visualization of the cervix. A numbing block is placed in the cervix. A thin cryoablation device is inserted through the cervix into the uterus. The cryoablation device freezes targeted uterine endometrial tissue. The instrument is withdrawn following completion of the procedure. Ultrasound provides visualization of probe placement and real-time monitoring of the ice ball growth. If endometrial curettage is required, the physician passes a curette into the uterus through the endocervical canal. The lining of the uterus is scraped.

58580
The physician performs transcervical uterine fibroid ablation using radiofrequency. A single system device is utilized, which is comprised of a reusable intrauterine ultrasound (IUUS) probe and a single use, disposable articulating radiofrequency handpiece, along with integrated components that may include a radiofrequency generator and an ultrasound system with custom graphical user interface. The process enables the transcervical destruction of fibroids without incisions or general anesthesia. The patient is administered anesthesia (typically regional or conscious sedation with or without paracervical

blockade). An electrode pad is placed on each front thigh area. Transvaginal ultrasound is used to identify the location and size of each fibroid. The cervix is dilated to approximately 8 mm and the handpiece is inserted transcervically into the uterus, along with a small amount of sterile water or 1.5% glycine for acoustic coupling. Once the size, angle, and location of the ablation is established, the physician advances the trocar-tipped introducer into the fibroid under intrauterine ultrasound imaging. Once properly positioned, the physician deploys the electrodes. Each fibroid receives one or more ablations at the discretion of the physician. One ablation usually destroys a 5 cm myoma. This technique permits the physician to plan exactly what will be ablated and avoid heating the serosa and other tissues outside the uterus. Any intraoperative ultrasound guidance and monitoring is included in this code.

58600
The physician ties off the fallopian tube or removes a portion of it on one side or both. The procedure may be done through the vagina or through a small incision just above the pubic hairline.

58605
The physician ties off the fallopian tube or removes a portion of it on one side or both. This procedure is done through a small incision just above the pubic hairline or vaginally during the same hospital stay as the delivery of a baby.

58611
The physician ties off the fallopian tube or removes a portion of it on one side or both. This procedure is done at the time of a cesarean section or during intra-abdominal surgery.

58615
The physician blocks one or both of the fallopian tubes with a band, clip, or Falope ring. The physician may elect to do the procedure through the vagina or through a small incision just above the pubic hairline.

58660
The physician performs a laparoscopic surgical cutting/releasing (lysis) of scar tissue (adhesions) surrounding the ovaries and/or fallopian tubes with the assistance of a fiberoptic laparoscope. The physician may first insert an instrument through the vagina to grasp the cervix and manipulate the uterus during surgery. Next, the physician makes a small incision just below the umbilicus through which a fiberoptic laparoscope is inserted. A second incision is made in the abdomen with additional instruments being placed through these incisions into the abdomen or pelvis. The physician manipulates the tools so that the pelvic organs can be observed, manipulated and lysis of adhesions can be performed. The abdomen is deflated, the trocars removed, and the incisions are closed with sutures.

58661
The physician performs a laparoscopic surgical removal of one or both ovaries and their accompanying fallopian tubes with the assistance of a fiberoptic laparoscope. The physician may first insert an instrument through the vagina to grasp the cervix and manipulate the uterus during surgery. Next, the physician makes a small incision just below the umbilicus through which a fiberoptic laparoscope is inserted. A second incision is made on the left or right side of the abdomen with additional instruments being placed through these incisions into the abdomen or pelvis. The physician manipulates the tools so that the pelvic organs can be observed, manipulated, and removal of one or both ovaries and fallopian tubes can be performed with the laparoscope. The abdomen is deflated, the trocars removed and the incisions are closed with sutures.

58662
The physician performs a laparoscopic electrical cautery destruction of an ovarian, pelvic or peritoneal lesion with the assistance of a fiberoptic laparoscope. The physician may first insert an instrument through the vagina to grasp the cervix and manipulate the uterus during surgery. Next, the physician makes a small incision just below the umbilicus through which a fiberoptic laparoscope is inserted. A second incision is made on the left or right side of the abdomen with additional instruments being placed through these incisions into the abdomen or pelvis. The physician manipulates the tools so that the pelvic organs can be observed, manipulated and operated upon with the laparoscope. Once lesions are identified with the laparoscope, a third incision is typically made adjacent to the lesion through which an electric cautery tool, knife, or laser is inserted for lesion fulguration. The abdomen is deflated, the trocars removed and the incisions are closed with sutures.

58670
The physician performs a laparoscopic electrical cautery destruction of an oviduct (the uterine tube) with or without complete cutting through the fallopian tubes (transection) with the assistance of a fiberoptic laparoscope. The physician may first insert an instrument through the vagina to grasp the cervix and manipulate the uterus during surgery. Next, the physician makes a small incision just below the umbilicus through which a fiberoptic laparoscope is inserted. A second incision is made on the left or right side of the abdomen with additional instruments being placed through these incisions into the abdomen or pelvis. The physician manipulates the tools so that the pelvic organs can be observed, manipulated and operated upon with the laparoscope. A third incision is typically made adjacent to the fallopian tubes. To fulgurate the fallopian tube the physician inserts an electric cautery tool or a laser. The physician may cut the tubes and fulgurate or burn the ends. Additionally, the physician may transect (cut through) the fallopian tubes. The abdomen is deflated, the trocars removed and the incisions are closed with sutures.

58671

The physician performs a laparoscopic occlusion of the oviduct (the uterine tube) with the assistance of a fiberoptic laparoscope. The physician may insert an instrument through the vagina to grasp the cervix and manipulate the uterus during surgery. A small incision is made just below the umbilicus through which a fiberoptic laparoscope is inserted. A second incision is made on the left or right side of the abdomen with additional instruments placed through these incisions into the abdomen or pelvis. The physician manipulates the tools so that the pelvic organs can be observed, manipulated, and operated upon with the laparoscope. A third incision is typically made adjacent to the fallopian tubes. To occlude the fallopian tubes, the physician places silicone rings or clips around the tubes through this incision. The abdomen is deflated, the trocars removed, and the incisions are closed with sutures.

58672

The physician performs a laparoscopic surgical repair of the ovarian fimbria (fingerlike processes on the distal part of the infundibulum of the uterine tube) with the assistance of a fiberoptic laparoscope. The physician may first insert an instrument through the vagina to grasp the cervix and manipulate the uterus during surgery. Next, the physician makes a small incision just below the umbilicus through which a fiberoptic laparoscope is inserted. A second incision is made on the left or right side of the abdomen with additional instruments being placed through these incisions into the abdomen or pelvis. The physician manipulates the tools so that the pelvic organs can be observed, manipulated and operated upon with the laparoscope. A third incision is typically made adjacent to the fallopian tubes. The physician performs surgical repair of the ovarian fimbria using instruments placed through the abdomen and pelvic trocars. The abdomen is deflated, the trocars removed and the incisions are closed with sutures.

58673

The physician performs a laparoscopic surgical restoration of the patency of the uterine tube damaged typically by infection, tumor or endometriosis. The physician may first insert an instrument through the vagina to grasp the cervix and manipulate the uterus during surgery. Next, the physician makes a small incision just below the umbilicus through which a fiberoptic laparoscope is inserted. A second incision is made on the left or right side of the abdomen with additional instruments being placed through these incisions into the abdomen or pelvis. The physician manipulates the tools so that the pelvic organs can be observed, manipulated and operated upon with the laparoscope. A third incision is typically made adjacent to the fallopian tubes. The physician performs surgical restoration of the fallopian tube (salpingostomy) using instruments placed through the abdomen and pelvic trocars. The abdomen is deflated, the trocars removed and the incisions are closed with sutures.

58700

Through a small incision in the lower abdomen just above the pubic hairline, the physician removes part or all of the fallopian tube on one or both sides. The incision is closed by suturing.

58720

Through a small incision in the abdomen just above the pubic hairline, the physician removes part or all of the ovary and part or all of its fallopian tube on one or both sides. The incision is closed by suturing.

58740

The physician cuts free any fibrous tissue adhering to the ovaries or tubes through a small incision just above the pubic hairline.

58750

Through a small incision just above the pubic hairline, the physician excises the closed or blocked portion of the tube and sutures the clean edges together. The procedure is generally performed microsurgically in order to do an accurate repair.

58752

Through a small incision just above the pubic hairline, the physician removes a blocked portion of the tube near its junction with the uterus and reimplants the tube into the uterus in the same place.

58760

Through a small incision just above the pubic hairline, the physician reconstructs the existing fimbriae in a partially or totally obstructed (occluded) or closed off oviduct. Fimbriae are the hairlike fringes at the end of the fallopian tubes. Depending on the nature of the blockage, the physician may separate the fimbriae by gentle dilation or by electrosurgical dissection. The procedure is generally performed microsurgically in order to do an accurate repair.

58770

Through a small incision just above the pubic hairline, the physician creates a new opening in the fallopian tube where the fimbrial end has been closed by inflammation, infection, or injury. The procedure is generally performed microsurgically in order to do an accurate repair.

58800

The physician drains a cyst or cysts on one or both ovaries through an incision in the vagina. A cyst is a sac containing fluid or semisolid material. The cyst is ruptured with a surgical instrument, electrocautery, or a laser, and the fluid is removed.

58805

Through a small incision just above the pubic hairline, the physician drains a cyst or cysts on one or both ovaries. A cyst is a sac containing fluid or semisolid material. The cyst is ruptured with a surgical instrument, electrocautery, or a laser, and the fluid is removed.

58820
The physician drains an abscess (infection) on the ovary through an incision in the vagina. The abscess is drained, cleaned out, and irrigated with antibiotics. Temporary catheters and tubes are often left in place to help drainage.

58822
Through a small abdominal incision just above the pubic hairline, the physician drains an abscess (infection) on the ovary. The abscess is drained, cleaned out, and irrigated with antibiotics. Temporary catheters and tubes are often left in place to help drainage.

58825
The ovaries are placed behind the uterus and sutured in place prior to radiation therapy of the pelvis. The uterus acts as a shield protecting the ovaries from the radiation. The procedure is done through a small abdominal incision just above the pubic hairline.

58900
The physician takes a tissue sample from one or both ovaries for diagnosis. This procedure may be done through the vagina or abdominally through a small incision just above the pubic hairline.

58920
Through a small abdominal incision just above the pubic hairline, the physician takes a pie-shaped section or half of one or both of the ovaries to reduce the size and repairs each ovary with sutures.

58925
Through a small abdominal incision just above the pubic hairline, the physician removes a cyst or cysts on one or both of the ovaries.

58940
Through a small abdominal incision just above the top of the pubic hairline, the physician removes part or all of one or both of the ovaries.

58943
Through an abdominal incision extending from the top of the pubic hairline to the rib cage, the physician removes part or all of one or both ovaries depending on the extent of the malignancy. The physician takes a sampling of the lymph nodes surrounding the lower aorta within the pelvis and flushes the peritoneum, which is the lining of the abdominal cavity, with saline. The saline solution is suctioned from the peritoneum for separately reportable examination. Multiple tissue samples are excised. The physician also examines and takes tissue samples of the diaphragm. The physician may elect to remove one or both fallopian tubes and the omentum. The abdominal incision is closed with layered sutures.

58950
The physician performs the initial resection of an ovarian, tubal, or primary peritoneal malignancy. Through a full abdominal incision, the physician removes both tubes, both ovaries, and the omentum, which is a membrane of lymph nodes, blood vessels, and fat that forms a protective layer extending from the stomach to the transverse colon. The abdominal incision is closed with layered sutures.

58951
Through a full abdominal incision extending from just above the pubic hairline to the rib cage, the physician treats an ovarian, tubal, or peritoneal malignancy by taking out both tubes, both ovaries, and the omentum, which is a membrane of lymph nodes, blood vessels, and fat that forms a protective layer extending from the stomach to the transverse colon. The physician also removes the uterus, the pelvic lymph nodes, and a portion of the lymph nodes surrounding the lower aorta. The abdominal incision is closed with layered sutures. This code is to be used only for the initial surgical resection of the malignancy.

58952
Through a full abdominal incision extending from just above the pubic hairline to the rib cage, the physician treats an ovarian, tubal, or peritoneal malignancy by excising both tubes, both ovaries, and the omentum, which is a membrane containing fat, lymph, and blood vessels that acts as a protective layer extending from the stomach to the transverse colon. The physician also reduces the size of a tumor that has grown large enough to cause discomfort or problems. Due to the size and location, it may not be possible to remove the tumor. The abdominal incision is closed with layered sutures. This code is to be used only for the initial surgical resection of the malignancy.

58953-58954
Through a full abdominal incision extending from just above the pubic hairline to the rib cage, the physician treats an ovarian malignancy. In both procedures, the physician makes a full abdominal incision and carries dissection down to the abdominal cavity. The physician excises the fallopian tubes, both ovaries, the uterus, and the omentum, which is a membrane containing lymph, blood vessels, and fat in a protective layer that extends from the stomach to the transverse colon. The physician removes or reduces metastatic ovarian cancer implants from the abdominal cavity. In 58954, the physician also removes pelvic lymph nodes and a portion of the lymph nodes that surround the lower aorta within the pelvis. The abdominal incision is closed with layered sutures.

58956
The physician performs a bilateral salpingo-oophorectomy with total omentectomy and total abdominal hysterectomy to treat a malignancy. A full abdominal incision is made extending from just above the pubic hairline to the rib cage. Dissection is carried down to the abdominal cavity. The physician excises the fallopian tubes, ovaries, the uterus, and the omentum. The supporting pedicles containing the tubes, ligaments, and arteries are clamped and cut free. The uterus and cervix are removed along with a narrow rim or cuff of the vaginal lining. The vaginal defect is often left open for drainage. Attention is

directed to the omentum, a membrane of lymph, blood vessels, and fat that forms a protective layer that extends from the stomach to the transverse colon. The omentum is mobilized from the stomach and colon, divided from its blood supply, and removed. The physician inspects the abdominal cavity and removes any metastatic lesions. The abdominal incision is closed with layered sutures.

58958
This code reports tumor debulking in recurrent ovarian, uterine, tubal, or peritoneal malignancies. Through a full abdominal incision extending from just above the pubic hairline to the rib cage, the physician explores the abdomen, pelvis, and viscera. In addition to debulking recurrent malignancy, excision of all or portions of the omentum, which is a membrane of lymph nodes, blood vessels, and fat that forms a protective layer extending from the stomach to the transverse colon, may be performed. The physician also removes the pelvic lymph nodes and a portion of the lymph nodes surrounding the lower aorta. The physician may remove all visible tumors or only reduce their size, depending on the nature of the malignancy and the structures involved. The abdominal incision is closed with layered sutures.

58960
This procedure is the second operation to check for remaining (or a recurrence of) ovarian, tubal, or primary peritoneal malignancy. Findings are used to determine the stage of the cancer in order to plan the most appropriate treatment. Through a full abdominal incision extending from just above the pubic hairline to the rib cage, the physician may elect to remove the omentum, a membrane of lymph, blood vessels, and fat that forms a protective layer that extends from the stomach to the transverse colon. The physician may flush the lining of the abdominal cavity (peritoneum) and remove the liquid to check for cancerous cells. A tissue sample of the abdominal and pelvic peritoneum may be taken. The physician also may examine and take tissue samples of the diaphragm. The pelvic lymph nodes are removed and a portion of the lymph nodes that surrounds the lower aorta within the pelvis is removed. The abdominal incision is closed with layered sutures.

58970
The physician aspirates a mature or nearly mature egg from its follicle for in vitro fertilization. Visualization of the aspiration may be done laparoscopically or by ultrasound. The laparoscopic method uses three puncture sites in the lower abdomen: one for the laparoscope, one for the holding forceps, and one for the aspirating needle. The ultrasound guided technique involves using a transabdominal ultrasound transducer for guidance. The aspirating needle is passed through the bladder wall to the ovary or through the urethra and into the pelvic cavity. Another ultrasound method uses transvaginal ultrasound and transvaginal needle aspiration of the ovary. In all methods, the ovary and preovulatory follicle are visualized and punctured with a needle to withdraw the follicular fluid containing the egg.

58974
The physician places fertilized eggs in the uterus after the eggs have undergone 48 to 72 hours of laboratory culture. The embryos are aspirated into a small catheter. The catheter is passed through the cervical os and into the uterus. The eggs are injected into the uterus.

58976
In gamete intrafallopian transfer (GIFT), the physician mixes previously captured eggs with sperm and draws the mixture into a catheter. The catheter is passed through the cervix and uterus and into the tubes or passed through an abdominal incision and directly into the fimbrial end of the fallopian tube. The physician deposits the eggs and sperm in the tubes, permitting fertilization. In a zygote intrafallopian transfer (ZIFT), a physician draws an already fertilized egg into a catheter. The catheter is passed through the cervix and uterus and into the tube where the egg is deposited. GIFT is a one-step procedure while ZIFT is a two-step process. In ZIFT, the egg is collected and fertilized and transferred to the fallopian tube at a later time. GIFT and ZIFT can be done laparoscopically or hysteroscopically.

Maternity Care and Delivery

59000
The physician aspirates fluid from the amniotic sac for diagnostic purposes. Using separately reportable ultrasonic guidance, the physician inserts an amniocentesis needle through the abdominal wall into the interior of the pregnant uterus and directly into the amniotic sac to collect amniotic fluid for separately reportable analysis.

59001
The physician performs a therapeutic amniotic fluid reduction. Using ultrasonic guidance, the physician inserts an 18- or 20-gauge amniocentesis needle through the abdominal wall into the interior of the pregnant uterus and directly into the amniotic sac to remove excess levels of amniotic fluid (amnioreduction). Serial amniotic fluid volume reduction may be accomplished on an ongoing basis by repeating the procedure.

59012
The physician removes blood from the fetal umbilical cord for diagnostic purposes. Using separately reportable ultrasonic guidance, the physician inserts an amniocentesis needle through the abdominal wall into the cavity of the pregnant uterus and into the umbilical vessels to obtain fetal blood. This may be accomplished with a transplacental or transamniotic approach.

59015
The physician samples tissue from the placenta for diagnostic purposes. This procedure uses ultrasonic

guidance and can be done by any one of three methods. In the transcervical method, the physician inserts a catheter through the cervix and into the uterine cavity toward the placental site. A sample of the placenta (chorionic villus) is aspirated to obtain placental cells for analysis for chromosomal abnormalities. The procedure may also be performed transvaginally or transabdominally.

59020

The physician evaluates fetal response to induced contractions in the mother. The physician applies external fetal monitors to the maternal abdominal wall. Pitocin is given intravenously to the mother to cause uterine contractions. The fetal heart rate and uterine contractions are monitored and recorded for 20 minutes to determine the effect of contractions on the fetus. This procedure is usually performed during the third trimester.

59025

The physician evaluates fetal heart rate response to its own activity. The patient reports fetal movements as an external monitor records fetal heart rate changes. The procedure is noninvasive and takes 20 to 40 minutes to perform. If the fetus is not active, an acoustic device may be used to stimulate activity.

59030

The physician samples fetal scalp blood during active labor for diagnostic purposes. This test, which assesses fetal distress during labor, must be done when the cervix is dilated more than 2 cm and the fetal vertex is low in the pelvis. The physician breaks the amniotic sac in patients whose water has not broken spontaneously and inserts an amnioscope through the vagina. An incision is made in the scalp with a narrow blade that penetrates no more than 2 mm. Blood is aspirated into a tube.

59050-59051

In 59050, a consultant other than the attending physician attaches an electrode directly to the presenting fetus' scalp via the cervix. The electrocardiographic impulses are transmitted to a cardiotachometer which converts the fetal electrocardiographic pattern into recorded electronic impulses. A catheter is inserted through the dilated cervix into the amniotic sac to measure and record the intervals between contractions. The procedure is supervised during labor until delivery. The recordings are analyzed and accompanied by an interpretive written report. In 59051, the consultant initiates the monitoring, provides the analysis and interpretive report, but does not supervise the patient during labor.

59070

The physician infuses an abnormally underhydrated amniotic sac with fluid. This may be done as a prophylactic measure for the fetus or to enhance sonographic imaging. An amniocentesis needle is placed through the mother's abdomen and advanced between extremities of the fetus under separately reportable ultrasound guidance. Normal sterile saline is infused into the uterus until the fetal anatomy is adequately visualized. The needle is removed and a detailed ultrasound is carried out.

59072

Fetal umbilical cord occlusion is carried out in cases of complicated monochorionic multiple gestation pregnancies or in cases to terminate a pregnancy due to a birth defect. Ultrasound is used to locate access to the umbilical cord, avoiding the placenta. Using ultrasound guidance, small forceps are advanced into the uterus and the cord of the affected fetus is identified and grasped. The umbilical cord may be ligated, occluded, or compressed. Complete absence of flow through the cord is confirmed and the instruments are removed.

59074

Fetal fluid drainage is done in cases of pleural effusions or pulmonary cysts, and especially in fetal megavesica, a rare syndrome caused by functional obstruction of the fetal urethra. The fetus' bladder is enlarged due to the megavesica. Oligohydramnios, dilation of the lower and upper urinary tract, and hydronephrosis may also be present. Pulmonary hypoplasia can result and lead to hypoplastic abdominal musculature, urinary tract anomalies, and cryptorchidism. The fetal urinary bladder is emptied by transabdominal intrauterine vesicocentesis. Under continual ultrasound guidance, a 20 to 22 gauge needle is inserted through the mother's abdomen and advanced into the fetus' bladder. Fetal urine is aspirated and sent to the lab for analysis of urinary electrolytes and to determine renal function. The needle is removed and the patient kept for monitoring for up to another hour to check for refilling in the bladder. Similar fluid drainage is done by transabdominal intrauterine thoracocentesis for fetal pleural effusion.

59076

Fetal shunt placement is performed for pleural or vesical amniotic shunting in cases of pleural effusion, pulmonary cysts, or fetal megavesica, where the bladder is enlarged because of urethra blockage. Shunting is done to supply continuous drainage when reaccumulation of fluid is not successfully treated by isolated vesicocentesis or thoracocentesis. Fluids can be drained into the amniotic cavity through a double pigtailed catheter. The entry site on the mother's abdomen is cleaned with antiseptic solution and local anesthetic is infiltrated down to the myometrium. Under ultrasound guidance, a metal cannula with a trocar is introduced transabdominally into the amniotic cavity and inserted through the fetal chest wall in the midthoracic region, into the effusion or cyst (if megavesical fluid accumulation is the problem, the shunt is placed into the bladder). The trocar is removed and the catheter is inserted into the cannula. A short introducer rod is used to place the proximal half of the catheter into the effusion or cyst. The cannula is gradually removed into the amniotic cavity where the other half of the catheter is pushed by a longer introducer. There is now a conduit for fluid drainage into the amniotic space. Placement of the shunt is confirmed, the instruments are removed, and the patient is monitored for one to two hours. Follow-up ultrasound scans are performed at weekly intervals to check drainage and determine if the effusions reaccumulate, in which case another shunt may be inserted. The drains are immediately clamped and removed after delivery.

59100
The physician removes an embryo or hydatidiform mole through an incision in the abdominal wall and uterus. The surgery is similar to a cesarean section but the abdominal and uterine incisions are smaller. The lower abdominal wall is opened with a vertical or horizontal incision and the uterus is entered through the lower uterine segment. The physician removes the embryo or hydatidiform mole and may also remove any remaining membranes and placenta from the uterine cavity. Curettage of the uterine cavity may also be performed. The abdominal and uterine incisions are closed by suturing.

59120
The physician treats a tubal or ovarian ectopic pregnancy by removing the fallopian tube and/or ovary. Through the vagina or through an incision in the lower abdomen, the physician explores the pelvic cavity, inspects the gestation site for bleeding, and removes all products of conception, clots, and free blood. If the tube is affected, it may be excised by cutting a small wedge of the uterine wall at the junction of the fallopian tube and body of the uterus. If the ovary is affected, it may be removed. Lysis of adhesions may be indicated and the pelvis lavaged with saline solution. If an abdominal approach is used, the incision is closed with sutures.

59121
The physician treats a tubal or ovarian ectopic pregnancy by removing the embryo from the tube or ovary. Through an incision in the lower abdomen, the physician explores the pelvic cavity, inspects the gestation site for bleeding, and removes all products of conception, clots, and free blood. If the embryo is implanted in the fallopian tube, the physician may do one of the following: manually remove the embryo from the tube, make an incision to remove the embryo, or excise the section of the tube containing the embryo. If the embryo is implanted in the ovary, the physician resects the ovary to remove the embryo. Lysis of adhesions may be indicated and the pelvis lavaged with saline solution. The incision is closed with sutures.

59130
The physician removes an embryo or fetus implanted in the abdomen. The fertilized ovum may have implanted directly in the abdomen (primary) or it may have implanted after escaping from the tube through a rupture or through the fimbriated end (secondary). After making an abdominal incision, the physician surgically removes the fetus from the abdomen. The membranes are also removed and the cord is ligated near the placenta. The placenta is usually not removed unless attached to the fallopian tube, ovary, or uterine broad ligament. Abdominal lavage may also be indicated. The abdominal incision is closed with sutures. Although this procedure is rare, it can be done any time during gestation, even at or near term.

59136
The physician treats an interstitial ectopic pregnancy where the fertilized ovum has implanted in the portion of the tube that transverses the uterine wall by partially resecting the uterus. Through an incision extending from just above the pubic hairline to the rib cage, the physician resects and reconstructs the uterine wall. The physician may also remove a portion or all of the fallopian tube. Abdominal or pelvic lavage may be indicated. The abdominal incision is closed with sutures.

59140
The physician treats an ectopic pregnancy where the embryo has implanted in the cervix. If the pregnancy is less than 12 weeks gestation, the physician usually removes the embryo through the vagina. The physician ligates the hypogastric arteries or the cervical branches of the uterus to control bleeding. Curettage of the endocervix and endometrium may stop heavy bleeding. Sutures and gauze packing may also be necessary. If later than 12 weeks gestation, the physician may treat the cervical pregnancy by performing an abdominal hysterectomy. Through a horizontal incision just within the pubic hairline, the physician clamps and cuts free the supporting pedicles containing the tubes, ligaments, and arteries. The uterus is removed above the cervix, and the incision is closed by suturing.

59150
The physician treats an ectopic pregnancy by laparoscopy without salpingectomy and/or oophorectomy. The physician inserts an instrument through the vagina to grasp the cervix while passing another instrument through the cervix and into the uterus to manipulate the uterus. Next, the physician makes a 1 cm incision in the umbilicus through which the abdomen is inflated and a fiberoptic laparoscope is inserted. A second incision is made on the left or right side of the abdomen. After locating the site of the gestation, another small incision is made above the site. Instruments are passed into the abdomen through the incisions. The physician removes the ectopic pregnancy by making an incision in the tube or ovary or by segmental excision. The abdominal incisions are closed with sutures.

59151
The physician treats an ectopic pregnancy by laparoscopy with salpingectomy and/or oophorectomy. The physician inserts an instrument through the vagina to grasp the cervix while passing another instrument through the cervix and into the uterus to manipulate the uterus. Next, the physician makes a 1 cm incision in the umbilicus through which the abdomen is inflated and a fiberoptic laparoscope is

inserted. A second incision is made on the left or right side of the abdomen. After locating the site of the gestation, another small incision is made above the site. Instruments are passed into the abdomen through the incisions. The physician removes the tube and/or ovary containing the embryo and closes the abdominal incisions with sutures.

59160
The physician scrapes the endometrial lining of the uterus following childbirth. The physician passes a curette through the cervix and endocervical canal, and into the uterus. Due to the large, soft postpartum uterus that is especially susceptible to perforation, a large blunt curette, also known as a "banjo" curette, is preferable to the suction curette. The physician gently scrapes the endometrial lining of the uterus to control bleeding, treat obstetric lacerations, or remove any remaining placental tissue.

59200
The physician inserts a cervical dilator, such as a laminaria or prostaglandin, into the endocervix to chemically stimulate and dilate the cervical canal. Using a speculum, the physician views the cervix and uses a tool to grasp it and pull it down. A laminaria, which is a sterile applicator made of kelp or synthetic material, may be placed in the cervical canal where it absorbs moisture, swells, and gradually dilates the cervix prior to inducing labor. Or the physician may insert prostaglandin in the form of gel or suppositories into the cervix in order to prime it six to 12 hours before induction.

59300
A qualified health care provider, other than the provider who performed the delivery, repairs an episiotomy, vaginal tear, or laceration using sutures.

59320
The physician threads suture material or wraps banding around the cervix to close an incompetent cervix. An incompetent cervix is one that dilates during the second trimester and will eventually allow the pregnancy to fall out. After inserting a speculum into the vagina to view the cervix, heavy suture material or wire is threaded around the cervix using purse-string sutures. The sutures are pulled tight to make the opening smaller and prevent spontaneous abortion.

59325
Through a small abdominal incision just above the pubic hairline, the physician places a band around the cervix at the level of the internal os (opening) to make the cervical opening smaller and prevent spontaneous abortion from an incompetent cervix. An incompetent cervix is one that dilates during the second trimester and will eventually allow the pregnancy to fall out. The abdominal incision is closed with sutures.

59350
The physician repairs a uterus that is lacerated or ruptured during pregnancy. A large incision is made in the abdomen and the uterus is sutured in layers. The abdominal incision is closed with sutures.

59400
The physician delivers an infant and placenta through the uterus and vagina. The physician may elect to assist the delivery with the use of forceps, vacuum extraction, or rupture of membranes. The physician may also elect to do an episiotomy, which is an incision in the perineum to widen the external opening. Episiotomy and laceration repair are included as well. This procedure covers both antepartum and postpartum care. Antepartum or prenatal care includes the initial and subsequent histories, physical examinations, recording of weight, blood pressures, fetal heart tones, and routine chemical urinalysis. It includes monthly visits up to 28 weeks gestation, biweekly visits to 36 weeks gestation, and weekly visits until delivery. Postpartum care includes hospital and office visits following delivery.

59409-59410
The physician delivers an infant and placenta through the uterus and vagina. The physician may elect to assist the delivery with the use of forceps, vacuum extraction, or rupture of membranes. The physician may also elect to do an episiotomy, which is an incision in the perineum to widen the external opening. Episiotomy and laceration repair are included as well. Code 59409 represents the vaginal delivery only and does not include antepartum or postpartum care. Code 59410 covers the vaginal delivery with postpartum care, which includes hospital and office visits following delivery.

59412
The physician turns the fetus from a breech presenting position to a cephalic presenting position. External cephalic version is performed by manipulating the fetus from the outside of the abdominal wall. The physician places both hands on the patient's abdomen and locates each pole of the fetus by palpation. The fetus is shifted so that the breech or rear end of the fetus is moved upward and the head downward. The physician may elect to use tocolytic drug therapy to suppress uterine contractions during the manipulation.

59414
The physician removes a retained placenta following delivery of the fetus, usually unattended, and after separation of the placenta from its intrauterine attachment. The physician places abdominal pressure just above the symphysis to elevate the uterus into the abdomen and prevent inversion of the uterus. This also helps move the placenta downward into the vagina. The umbilical cord is very gently pulled to help guide the placenta out of the birth canal. If the placenta cannot be removed by this technique or there is brisk bleeding, manual removal of the placenta may be indicated. Manual removal requires adequate analgesia or anesthesia. It is accomplished by grasping the fundus of the uterus with a hand on the abdomen. The other hand, wearing an elbow-length glove, is passed through the vagina into the uterus to separate the placenta and remove it.

59425-59426
Antepartum or prenatal care includes the initial and subsequent histories, physical examinations, recording of weight, blood pressures, fetal heart tones, and routine chemical urinalysis. It includes monthly visits up to 28 weeks gestation, biweekly visits to 36 weeks gestation, and weekly visits until delivery. 59425 includes four to six visits. 59426 covers seven or more visits.

59430
Postpartum care includes hospital and office visits following vaginal or cesarean section delivery.

59510
The physician delivers an infant through a horizontal or vertical incision in the abdomen and uterus. Once the incisions are made, the infant is delivered and the placenta separated and removed. The uterine and abdominal incisions are closed with sutures. This procedure includes both antepartum and postpartum care. Antepartum or prenatal care includes the initial and subsequent histories, physical examinations, recording of weight, blood pressures, fetal heart tones, and routine chemical urinalysis. It includes monthly visits up to 28 weeks gestation, biweekly visits to 36 weeks gestation, and weekly visits until delivery. Postpartum care includes hospital and office visits following delivery.

59514-59515
The physician delivers an infant through a horizontal or vertical incision in the abdomen and uterus. Once the incisions are made, the infant is delivered and the placenta separated and removed. The uterine and abdominal incisions are closed with sutures. Code 59514 represents the cesarean delivery only and does not include antepartum or postpartum care. Code 59515 covers the cesarean delivery with postpartum care, which includes hospital and office visits following delivery.

59525
The physician performs a hysterectomy immediately following cesarean delivery. Through the abdominal incision, the physician clamps and cuts free the supporting pedicles containing the tubes, ligaments, and arteries. The uterus is removed and the physician may elect to remove the cervix as well. In a subtotal hysterectomy, just the uterus is removed. In a total hysterectomy, both the uterus and cervix are removed. The abdominal incision is closed with sutures.

59610
The physician delivers an infant and placenta through the vagina. The patient has previously delivered by cesarean section. The physician may elect to assist the delivery with the use of forceps, vacuum extraction, or rupture of membranes. The physician may also elect to do an episiotomy, which is an incision in the perineum to widen the external opening. Episiotomy and laceration repair are included as well. This procedure covers both antepartum and postpartum care. Antepartum or prenatal care includes the initial and subsequent histories, physical examinations, recording of weight, blood pressures, fetal heart tones, and routine chemical urinalysis. It includes monthly visits up to 28 weeks gestation, biweekly visits to 36 weeks gestation, and weekly visits until delivery (approximately 12-15 visits). Because of the previous cesarean delivery, the physician monitors the patient during labor and delivery. Postpartum care includes hospital and office visits following delivery.

59612-59614
The physician delivers an infant and placenta through the vagina. The patient has previously delivered by cesarean section. The physician may elect to assist the delivery with the use of forceps. The physician may also elect to do an episiotomy, which is an incision in the perineum to widen the external opening. Episiotomy and laceration repair are included. Because of the previous cesarean delivery, the physician monitors the patient during labor and delivery. Code 59614 includes postpartum care, hospital office visits following delivery.

59618
After first attempting a vaginal delivery, the physician delivers an infant through a horizontal or vertical incision in the abdomen and uterus. The patient has previously delivered by cesarean section. Once the incisions are made, the infant is delivered and the placenta separated and removed. The uterine and abdominal incisions are closed with layered sutures. This procedure includes both antepartum and postpartum care. Antepartum or prenatal care includes the initial and subsequent histories, physical examinations, recording of weight, blood pressures, fetal heart tones, and routine chemical urinalysis. It includes monthly visits up to 28 weeks gestation, biweekly visits to 36 weeks gestation, and weekly visits until delivery (approximately 13-15 visits). Because of the previous cesarean delivery and the attempted vaginal delivery, the physician monitors the patient during labor and delivery. Postpartum care includes hospital and office visits following delivery.

59620-59622
After first attempting a vaginal delivery, the physician delivers an infant through a horizontal or vertical incision in the abdomen and uterus. The patient has previously delivered by cesarean section. Once the incisions are made, the infant is delivered and the placenta separated and removed. The uterine and abdominal incisions are closed with layered sutures because of the previous cesarean delivery and the attempted vaginal delivery, the physician monitors the patient during labor and delivery. Only delivery is included in 59620. Postpartum care is included in 59622. Postpartum care includes hospital and office visits following delivery.

59812
The physician removes the products of conception remaining after an incomplete abortion in any trimester. To evacuate the uterus, the physician performs a dilation and suction curettage. The

physician inserts a speculum into the vagina to view the cervix. A tenaculum is used to grasp the cervix, pull it down, and exert traction. If the cervix is not sufficiently dilated, a dilator is inserted into the endocervix and through the cervical canal to enlarge the opening. The physician places a cannula in the endocervical canal and passes it into the uterus. The suction machine is activated and the uterine contents are evacuated by rotation of the cannula. After suction curettage, a sharp curette may be used to gently scrape the uterus to ensure that it is empty.

59820-59821

The physician treats a missed abortion by suction curettage in the first trimester for 59820, and in the second trimester for 59821. In missed abortion, the fetus remains in the uterus four to eight weeks following its death. Ultrasonography may be needed to determine the size of the fetus prior to the procedure. The physician inserts a speculum into the vagina to view the cervix. A tenaculum is used to grasp the cervix, pull it down, and exert traction. A dilator is inserted into the endocervix and through the cervical canal to enlarge the opening. The physician places a cannula in the endocervical canal and passes it into the uterus. The suction machine is activated and the uterine contents are evacuated by rotation of the cannula. After suction curettage, a sharp curette may be used to gently scrape the uterus to ensure that it is empty.

59830

The physician treats a septic abortion with prompt evacuation of the uterus and vigorous medical treatment of the patient. A septic abortion is one complicated by generalized fever and infection. There is also inflammation and infection of the endometrium and in the cellular tissue around the uterus. The physician treats the infection with intravenous antibiotics and blood transfusions as necessary. To evacuate the uterus, the physician inserts a speculum into the vagina to view the cervix. A tenaculum is used to grasp the cervix, pull it down, and exert traction. A dilator is inserted into the endocervix and through the cervical canal to enlarge the opening. The physician places a cannula in the endocervical canal and passes it into the uterus. The suction machine is activated and the uterine contents are evacuated by rotation of the cannula. After suction curettage, a sharp curette may be used to gently scrape the uterus to ensure that it is empty.

59840

The physician terminates a pregnancy by dilation and curettage. The physician inserts a speculum into the vagina to view the cervix. A tenaculum is used to grasp the cervix, pull it down, and exert traction. A dilator is inserted into the endocervix and through the cervical canal to enlarge the opening. The physician places a curette in the endocervical canal and passes it into the uterus. The uterine contents are removed by rotating the curette and gently scraping the uterus until all the products of conception are removed.

59841

The physician terminates a pregnancy by dilation and evacuation (D&E). Because D&E requires wider cervical dilation than curettage, the physician may dilate the cervix with a laminaria several hours to several days before the procedure. At the time of the procedure, the physician inserts a speculum into the vagina to view the cervix. A tenaculum is used to grasp the cervix, pull it down, and exert traction. The physician places a cannula in the dilated endocervical canal and passes it into the uterus. The suction machine is activated and the uterine contents are evacuated by rotation of the cannula. For pregnancies through 16 weeks, the cannula will usually evacuate the pregnancy. For later pregnancies, the cannula is used to drain amniotic fluid and to draw tissue into the lower uterus for extraction by forceps. In either case, a sharp curette may be used to gently scrape the uterus to ensure that it is empty.

59850

The physician terminates a pregnancy by inducing labor with amniocentesis and intra-amniotic injections. This method is usually used after the first trimester (13 weeks or more). The physician inserts an amniocentesis needle into the abdomen to obtain a free flow of clear amniotic fluid. A hypertonic solution is administered by gravity drip. The hypertonic solution results in fetal death and labor usually results. The fetus and placenta are delivered through the vagina.

59851

The physician begins the termination of a pregnancy by inducing labor with amniocentesis and intra-amniotic injections. This method is usually used after the first trimester (13 weeks or more). The physician inserts an amniocentesis needle into the abdomen to obtain a free flow of clear amniotic fluid. A hypertonic solution is administered by gravity drip. The hypertonic solution results in fetal death and labor usually results. Code 59851 is used when this method fails to expel all products of conception, and a dilation and curettage and/or evacuation is used to remove the remaining tissue.

59852

The physician begins the termination of a pregnancy by inducing labor with amniocentesis and intra-amniotic injections. This method is usually used after the first trimester (13 weeks or more). The physician inserts an amniocentesis needle into the abdomen to obtain a free flow of clear amniotic fluid. A hypertonic solution is administered by gravity drip. The hypertonic solution results in fetal death and labor usually results. Code 59852 is used when this method fails to expel all products of conception, and a hysterotomy, through an incision in the abdominal wall and uterus, is used to remove the remaining tissue. Following removal, the incision is closed with sutures.

59855
The physician terminates a pregnancy by inducing labor with vaginal suppositories. Before using the suppositories, a laminaria, which is an applicator made of kelp or synthetic material, may be inserted in the cervix to soften and expand the cervical canal. Once the cervix is ready, the physician inserts the vaginal suppositories and labor usually results. The fetus and placenta are delivered through the vagina.

59856
The physician begins the termination of a pregnancy by inducing labor with vaginal suppositories. Before using the suppositories, a laminaria, which is an applicator made of kelp or synthetic material, may be inserted in the cervix to soften and expand the cervical canal. Once the cervix is ready, the physician inserts the vaginal suppositories and labor usually results. 59856 is used when this method fails to expel all products of conception, and a dilation and curettage and/or evacuation is used to remove the remaining tissue.

59857
The physician begins the termination of a pregnancy by inducing labor with vaginal suppositories. Before using the suppositories, a laminaria, which is an applicator made of kelp or synthetic material, may be inserted in the cervix to soften and expand the cervical canal. Once the cervix is ready, the physician inserts the vaginal suppositories and labor usually results. 59857 is used when this method fails to expel all products of conception, and a hysterotomy, through an incision in the abdominal wall and uterus, is used to remove the remaining tissue. Following removal, the incision is closed with sutures.

59866
Selective reduction is performed to eliminate one or more fetuses of a multiple pregnancy in an attempt to increase the viability of the remaining fetuses. Fetuses are usually eliminated in this procedure until only a twin or triplet pregnancy remains. Physicians most often use ultrasound guided intracardiac injection of potassium chloride to reduce the number of fetuses, although injection of potassium chloride in any part of the fetal body accomplishes the same result. When an intracardiac injection is performed, a 22 gauge spinal needle is advanced through the abdominal and uterine walls toward a cardiac echo using high-resolution ultrasound as a guide. With the needle position in the heart, a solution of potassium chloride is injected at intervals until prolonged cardiac standstill is observed. The physician withdraws the needle and redirects it into another gestational sac, as needed. The embryo(s) or fetus(es) that have been injected shrivel and decompose, leaving the remaining fetuses in utero an increased chance of surviving to term. Any sacs that remain intact are removed during delivery of the surviving fetus(es).

59870
The physician treats a hydatidiform mole (molar pregnancy) by evacuation and curettage of the uterus. The physician inserts a speculum into the vagina to view the cervix. A tenaculum is used to grasp the cervix, pull it down, and exert traction. A dilator is inserted into the endocervix and through the cervical canal to enlarge the opening. The physician places a cannula in the endocervical canal and passes it into the uterus. The suction machine is activated and the hydatidiform mole is evacuated by rotation of the cannula. After suction curettage, a sharp curette may be used to scrape the uterus and confirm that it is empty.

59871
The physician removes a cervical cerclage, a suture that had been placed to hold the cervix closed. A cerclage is most often placed when a cervix dilates too early during pregnancy and risks a miscarriage. The physician severs the sutures and removes them. This code includes anesthesia other than local.

Endocrine

60000
The physician incises and drains an infected thyroglossal (also called thyrolingual) cyst in the neck caused by incomplete closure or persistence of the embryonic thyroglossal duct between the developing thyroid and the back of the tongue. After the physician incises the cyst and drains the infected fluid, the wound may be irrigated with normal saline and a drainage system inserted. The drainage tubes may be stitched in place. A collection unit applies gentle suction to collect fluid from the incision site.

60100
The physician removes tissue from the thyroid for examination. The physician localizes the area to be biopsied by palpation or separately reportable ultrasound. A large, hollow, bore needle is passed through skin and muscle, into the thyroid. The tissue is removed and sent for separately reportable analysis.

60200
The physician removes a cyst or adenoma from a thyroid, or transects the isthmus. The physician exposes the thyroid via a transverse cervical incision in the skin line. The platysmas are divided and the strap muscles separated in the midline. The thyroid mass is identified. Blood supply to and from the lesion is controlled and the mass is locally excised. The skin and platysmas are closed.

60210
The physician removes part of a thyroid lobe, with or without an isthmusectomy. The physician exposes the thyroid via a transverse cervical incision in the skin line. The platysmas are divided and the strap muscles separated in the midline. The superior and inferior thyroid vessels are divided in the area for resection. The thyroid parenchyma is divided and dissected with cautery dissection. The skin and platysmas are closed.

Endocrine

60212
The physician removes part of a thyroid lobe, with contralateral subtotal lobectomy, including an isthmusectomy. The physician exposes the thyroid via a transverse cervical incision in the skin line. The platysmas are divided and the strap muscles separated in the midline. The superior and inferior thyroid vessels are divided in the area for resection. The thyroid is divided and dissected with cautery dissection. The isthmus is dissected and the lobe is removed. The skin and platysmas are closed.

60220
The physician removes all of a thyroid lobe, with or without isthmusectomy. The physician exposes the thyroid via a transverse cervical incision in the skin line. The platysmas are divided and the strap muscles separated in the midline. The thyroid lobe to be excised is isolated and superior and inferior thyroid vessels serving that lobe are ligated. Parathyroid glands are preserved. The thyroid gland is divided in the midline of the isthmus over the anterior trachea. The thyroid lobe is resected. The platysmas and skin are closed.

60225
The physician removes all of a thyroid lobe with contralateral subtotal lobectomy, including isthmusectomy (removal of thyroid nodules or thyroid isthmus). The physician exposes the thyroid via a transverse cervical incision in the skin line. The platysmas are divided and the strap muscles separated in the midline. The thyroid lobe to be excised is isolated and superior and inferior thyroid vessels serving that lobe are ligated. The isthmus is severed. Parathyroid glands are preserved. The thyroid gland is divided in the midline of the isthmus over the anterior trachea. The thyroid lobe is resected. The platysmas and skin are closed.

60240
The physician removes all of the thyroid. The physician exposes the thyroid via a transverse cervical incision in the skin line. The platysmas are divided and the strap muscles separated in the midline. The thyroid gland is mobilized and the superior and inferior thyroid vessels are ligated. The parathyroid glands are preserved and the thyroid is resected free of the trachea and removed. The platysmas and skin are closed.

60252-60254
The physician removes a malignant thyroid and some lymph nodes. The physician exposes the thyroid via a transverse cervical incision in the skin line. The platysmas are divided and the strap muscles separated in the midline. The thyroid gland is mobilized and the superior and inferior thyroid vessels are ligated. The parathyroid glands are preserved and the thyroid is resected free of the trachea and removed. All enlarged lymph nodes are identified and excised. The platysmas and skin are closed. Report 60254 if a radical neck dissection is included in the procedure.

60260
The physician removes thyroid tissue remaining following a partial thyroidectomy. The physician enters through the previous incision scar. The platysmas and scar tissue are divided and the strap muscles are divided in the midline. While preserving the parathyroid glands, all the remaining scar tissue is resected. The platysmas and skin are closed.

60270-60271
The physician removes the thyroid, including the substernal thyroid gland. The physician exposes the thyroid via sternal split/transthoracic approach in 60270 or via a transverse cervical incision in the skin line in 60271. The platysmas are divided and the strap muscles separated in the midline. The thyroid gland is mobilized and the superior and inferior thyroid vessels are ligated. The parathyroid glands are preserved and the thyroid is resected free of the trachea and removed. Any substernal thyroid is bluntly dissected. Upper sternal incision may be necessary for complete excision of substernal thyroid. The platysmas and skin are closed.

60280-60281
The physician excises a thyroglossal duct cyst or sinus. The physician circumferentially incises the skin around the cyst or sinus and extends the incision along the tract to its origin. The midpart of the hyoid bone is excised. The wound is packed and allowed to heal by secondary intention. Report 60281 if thyroglossal duct cyst or sinus is recurrent.

60300
The physician aspirates or injects a thyroid cyst. The physician localizes the thyroid cyst by palpation or separately reportable ultrasound. A needle is passed through the skin into the cyst. The cyst is aspirated and tissue captured is sent for separately reportable analysis, or the cyst is injected with therapeutic or diagnostic matter.

60500
The physician removes or explores the parathyroids, glands adjacent to the thyroids. The physician exposes the thyroid via a transverse cervical incision in the skin line. The platysmas are divided and the strap muscles separated in the midline. The parathyroid glands are identified and tissue is excised for separately reportable pathological examination. The parathyroid may be removed; usually a port remains following excision. The platysmas and skin are closed.

60502
The physician re-explores the parathyroids, glands adjacent to the thyroids. The physician exposes the thyroid via the previous incision. The parathyroid glands are identified and tissue is excised for separately reportable pathological examination. The parathyroid may be removed; usually a port remains following excision. The platysmas and skin are closed.

60505
The physician removes or explores the parathyroids, glands adjacent to the thyroids with mediastinal

exploration, sternal split or transthoracic approach. The physician exposes the thyroid via a sternal split or transthoracic approach. The parathyroid glands are identified and tissue is excised for separately reportable pathological examination. The mediastinum is explored. The parathyroid may be removed; usually a port remains following excision. The platysmas and skin are closed.

60512
The physician excises and reimplants a portion of the parathyroid. The physician exposes the thyroid via a transverse cervical incision in the skin line. The platysmas is divided and the strap muscles separated in the midline. Tissue is excised for separately reportable pathological examination. All four parathyroid glands are completely removed. One half of one gland is secured to the muscle of the sternocleidomastoid or upper arm. The platysmas and skin of the neck and transplant site are closed.

60520-60522
The physician removes part or all of the thymus gland. The physician exposes the thymus via a cervical incision in the skin line in 60520. The sternum is retracted and strap muscles separated. The superior lobe of the thymus is separated from the inferior aspect of the thyroid. The blood supply to the thymus is divided and the thymus is dissected free from the pericardium and removed. The incision is closed. Report 60521 if performed with a sternal split or transthoracic approach without radical mediastinal dissection; report 60522 if performed with a sternal split or transthoracic approach, with radical mediastinal dissection.

60540-60545
The physician removes part or all of the adrenal gland with or without biopsy. The physician exposes the adrenal gland via an upper anterior midline abdominal or posterior incision. The retroperitoneal space is explored. The capsule of the kidney is incised and the adrenal capsule is opened. Blood supply to the adrenal gland is ligated and the gland is removed. The physician may remove tissue from the site for separately reportable pathological study. The physician closes the incision with sutures. Report 60545 if this procedure is performed with excision of an adjacent retroperitoneal tumor.

60600-60605
This physician removes a tumor from a small epithelioid structure (carotid body) just above the bifurcation of the carotid. The physician exposes the carotid body via an incision anterior to the sternocleidomastoid. After dissection down to the carotid sheath, the vein is retracted and the carotid bifurcation exposed. The blood supply to the tumor is ligated and the tumor resected. The incision is closed. Report 60605 if the carotid body tumor excision is performed with excision of the carotid artery.

60650
The physician performs a laparoscopic excision (removal) of the adrenal gland, or performs and laparoscopic exploration of the adrenal gland through the abdomen or back. In the abdominal approach, a trocar is placed at the level of the umbilicus and the abdomen is insufflated. The laparoscope is placed through the umbilical port and additional trocars are placed into the abdominal cavity as needed. In the back approach, the trocar is placed at the back proximal to the retroperitoneal space superior to the kidney, adjacent to the adrenal gland. The physician uses the laparoscope fitted with a fiberoptic camera and/or an operating tool to explore, biopsy, or removal of all or part of the adrenal gland. The abdomen is the deflated, the trocars are removed and the incisions are closed with sutures.

60660-60661
The physician performs percutaneous radiofrequency ablation of one or more thyroid nodules, often those associated with progressive growth that may result in compressive symptoms. Using computerized tomography (CT), magnetic resonance imaging (MRI), or ultrasound (US) guidance, the site for the electrode placement is identified. With the patient under appropriate anesthesia, a radiofrequency needle electrode is introduced percutaneously and placed into the targeted thyroid tissue. Placement of the tip is confirmed with image guidance. Alternating current is applied as needed until the correct core heat is reached in the electrode. The targeted tissue is heated to a specified temperature with monitoring done before and after each treatment, depending on the ablation device used, until sufficient time results in permanent cell damage and tumor necrosis. Hemostasis is maintained after the electrode needle is withdrawn, the site is cleaned, and dressings are applied. The ablated tissue remains in place and is absorbed over time and replaced with scar tissue. Report 60660 for the first lobe or the isthmus and 60661 for ablation of an additional lobe.

Nervous

61000-61001
The physician draws off cerebral spinal fluid through a cranial or fontanel suture in an infant in response to hydrocephalus or diagnosed meningitis. The physician places a needle through the fontanelle at the suture line until cerebral spinal fluid is obtained. The needle is withdrawn and the area is bandaged. Report 61001 for subsequent taps for cerebral spinal fluid.

61020-61026
The physician withdraws cerebral spinal fluid for study, or injects it with a therapeutic or diagnostic substance. In 61020, The physician places a ventricular catheter through a previously formed burr hole or fontanel suture and withdraws fluid for study. In 61026, the catheter is used to inject a medication or other substance for diagnosis or treatment.

Nervous

61050-61055
The physician performs a spinal puncture in the high cervical region or at the base of the skull in the cisterna magna (cerebellomedullary cistern). For lateral cervical puncture, the physician uses a paramedian approach. For cisternal punctures, the needle is placed at the base of the skull. In 61050, the physician inserts a needle through the tissues to obtain cerebrospinal fluid (CSF) from the spine or cisterna magna. In 61055, a diagnostic or therapeutic injection occurs.

61070
The physician injects or aspirates the shunt tubing or reservoir with a needle to determine function. Shunt tubing eliminates excess cerebral spinal fluid in cases of hydrocephalus. The tubing runs behind the ear, through neck tissue, and into the gut. The physician places a needle into the tube or reservoir and injects radiologic dye, or aspirates to check for effective drainage.

61105-61108
The physician uses a manually operated twist drill to create an opening in the skull. The physician incises the scalp and peels it away from the area to be drilled. The physician places the drill over the affected area of the skull and twists until the drill pierces the periosteum and the dura is exposed. Fluid may be drawn off from the subdural space or from the ventricles. In 61105, the hole is made to alleviate pressure, and is used for subsequent surgery. In 61107, the hole is used to implant a ventricular drainage catheter, a fluid pressure recording device, or other intracerebral monitoring device. In 61108, the hole is used to access and evacuate or drain a subdural hematoma.

61120
The physician uses an electric burr drill to create a ventricular puncture to inject diagnostic fluid. The physician incises the scalp and peels it away from the area to be drilled. The physician places the drill over the area to be injected, and drills until the periosteum is reached. A ventricular puncture is made. The ventricles may be injected with gas, contrast media, dye, or radioactive material for diagnostic purposes.

61140-61151
The physician uses a burr drill or trephine to create a hole in the cranium through which a brain or intracranial lesion or abscess is located. An abscess or cyst may be drained. The physician incises the scalp and peels it away from the area to be drilled. In 61140, a lesion biopsy is obtained using a forceps or curette. In 61150, a catheter is placed through the hole and into a brain abscess or cyst for drainage. Report 61151 for subsequent drainage of the abscess or cyst through the original burr hole.

61154
The physician drills a burr hole in the cranium to drain a hematoma. The hematoma is identified using separately reportable computed tomography (CT) scan. The physician incises the scalp and peels it away from the area to be drilled. The physician uses a burr drill to access the hematoma. An extradural (epidural) hematoma is located outside the dura, just under the periosteum. A subdural hematoma is located under the dura mater, which must be incised to reach the hematoma. The hematoma is decompressed and bleeding is controlled. For subdural hematomas, the dura is sutured closed. The scalp is repositioned and sutured into place.

61156-61210
The physician drills a burr hole in the cranium to aspirate a hematoma or cyst located in the brain. The hematoma or cyst is identified using a CT scan. The physician incises the scalp and peels it away from the area to be drilled. The physician drills through the cranium to the dura mater, which is incised. The brain is dissected and retracted until the hematoma or cyst is located. The hematoma or cyst is aspirated using a syringe if the fluid is to be sent to pathology. Otherwise, the fluid is irrigated and suctioned. The dura mater is sutured closed and the scalp is repositioned and sutured into place. In 61210, a ventricular catheter, reservoir, EEG electrodes, pressure recording device, or other cerebral monitoring device is placed through the burr hole following aspiration of the hematoma. These devices or monitors are used to follow intracranial pressure and cerebral function following surgery.

61215
The physician places a device for administering chemotherapy or other medication into the cerebral spinal fluid. The physician makes a skin incision at the level at which the catheter will be inserted into the reservoir. A dermal or subdermal pocket is created with blunt dissection. The reservoir is connected to the catheter and tested to ensure function. The pocket is sutured in layers.

61250-61253
The physician drills a burr hole or trephine. In 61250 the hole is made to access the supratentorial area of the brain. In 61253, the infratentorial, unilateral, or bilateral area of the brain is accessed. The physician makes an incision in the scalp over the area to be drilled, and uses a burr hole drill or a trephine to create an opening to the brain. The physician explores the area and closes the wound. No other procedures are reported at this time.

61304-61305
The physician performs an exploratory craniectomy or craniotomy. In 61304, the supratentorial area of the brain (above the tentorium of the cerebellum) is accessed. In 61305, the infratentorial (below the tentorium of the cerebellum) area of the brain is accessed. A craniectomy involves removal of skull bone. A craniotomy involves incision without bone removal. The physician incises the scalp and retracts it. The physician drills or cuts the cranium to access the area to be explored. Bone is removed and the area of the brain is explored. If performing a craniotomy, the bone is replaced. The skull pieces are screwed together and the scalp is sutured in layers.

61312-61315
The physician performs craniectomy or craniotomy to drain a hematoma. In 61312, the supratentorial hematoma is located in the epidural or subdural space. In 61313, the supratentorial hematoma is located within the brain. In 61314, the infratentorial hematoma is located in the epidural or subdural space. In 61315, the infratentorial hematoma is located within the cerebellum. The hematoma is identified using a CT scan. The physician incises the scalp and retracts it. The physician drills or cuts the cranium to access the hematoma. Bone is removed. Epidural and subdural hematomas are identified and evacuated under direct visualization. Hematomas within the brain are located using CT verified coordinates and directed dissection. After locating the hematoma, the physician evacuates it with suction and irrigates the area while monitoring for hemorrhage. The dura is sutured closed. The skull pieces are screwed together and the scalp is sutured in layers.

61316
A cranial bone graft is placed onto a part of the skull for repair following craniectomy, craniotomy, or other intracranial surgery. The donor site is already exposed for the primary procedure. The cranial bone graft harvested may be split- or full-thickness, a shaving graft, or bone dust. When a full-thickness graft is required, the dura around the edge of the graft is exposed with a burr or neurosurgical craniotomy technique. A split graft requires removing lateral bone from a contoured area, which leaves it exposed like an island, and an osteotome is correctly placed and tapped through to produce the bone graft. Shaving grafts are acquired similar to wood shaving and bone dust is produced by using a craniotome. The graft is placed to repair the defect and rigidly fixed, if necessary. Bone dust is placed and packed to fill the skull defect. Report this code in addition to the code for the primary procedure.

61320-61321
The physician performs craniectomy or craniotomy to drain an abscess. In 61320, the abscess is located in the supratentorial region. In 61321, the abscess is located infratentorial region. The abscess is identified using separately reportable CT scan. The physician incises the scalp and retracts it. The physician drills or cuts the cranium to access the abscess. Bone is removed. Epidural and subdural abscesses are identified and evacuated under direct visualization. Abscesses within the brain are located using CT verified coordinates and directed dissection. After locating the abscess, the physician evacuates it with suction and irrigates the area while monitoring for hemorrhage. The dura is sutured closed. The skull pieces are screwed together and the scalp is sutured in layers.

61322-61323
The neurosurgeon performs a decompressive craniotomy or craniectomy, with or without duraplasty, to treat intracranial hypertension usually caused by severe closed-head injury. A scalp frontotemporoparietal incision is made from the side of the head curving over the ear and extending posteriorly, continuing in a big question mark shape back to the frontal midline. When necessary, a temporal end craniectomy site is opened first and contused brain or hematoma removed for immediate decompression of hypertension before the scalp incision is finished. A bone flap is next elevated by a series of burr holes made with a trephine connected to a saw or with a high-speed drill and footplate tool for protecting the dura matter used to make cuts around the flap margin. For subdural hematoma described here (the most common result of closed-head trauma causing hypertension), a dural opening is made over the area of greatest clot size and contused brain tissue and blood clots are removed. When the brain is swollen, instead of a large dural opening, multiple slit openings are made in the dura, through which the clot is irrigated to prevent the brain tissue from herniating through the opening. In 61323, a lobectomy is done to remove severely contused frontal or temporal brain tissue. Bipolar cautery and hemostatic agents are applied to attain meticulous hemostasis, absolutely necessary for preventing recurrent hematomas. The dura is closed primarily or duraplasty may be done with a pericranial or fascia lata graft. The dura is tacked around the craniotomy margin and to the bone flap and a drain may be placed and brought out through a separate incision. The scalp is closed in layers.

61330
The physician decompresses an orbital roof fracture. The physician incises the frontal scalp area and retracts the scalp posteriorly and the forehead anteriorly. The frontal bone is cut and removed. The forebrain is retracted until the superior margins of the orbit are visualized. The roof of the orbit is decompressed after ensuring freedom of movement of extraocular eye muscles. The dura is closed, and the bone is replaced. The forehead and scalp are reanastomosed and sutured in layers.

61333
The physician explores the orbit and excises a lesion. The physician incises the frontal scalp area and retracts the scalp posteriorly and the forehead anteriorly. The frontal bone is cut and removed. The forebrain is retracted until the superior margins of the orbit are visualized. The roof of the orbit is reconstructed and freedom of movement of extraocular eye muscles is ensured. The dura is closed and the skull is replaced. The forehead and scalp are reanastomosed and sutured in layers.

61340
The physician performs a subtemporal cranial decompression for benign intracranial hypertension (pseudotumor cerebri) or slit ventricle syndrome. Slit ventricle syndrome is a complication following shunting for hydrocephalus. The physician incises and retracts the scalp over the temporal area to be decompressed. A bone flap is next elevated by a series of burr holes made with a trephine connected to a saw or with a high-speed drill and footplate tool for

protecting the dura mater used to make cuts around the bone flap margin. When intracranial access is gained, the pressure within the skull is relieved and the bone is replaced and secured to neighboring bone. The scalp is sutured in layers.

61343

The physician removes the posterior inferior occipital scalp and the posterior aspects of the cervical vertebrae to decompress the brain stem. A dural graft may be necessary. The physician makes a longitudinal incision from the occipital through the cervical spine and retracts laterally. Decompression is achieved when the inferior occiput is cut and removed and the posterior elements of the upper cervical vertebrae are removed. If a dural graft is needed to cover the resulting defect, fascia is harvested from the thigh or a cadaveric dural graft is used. The graft is positioned over the defect and sutured to the surrounding dura. The incision is sutured in layers.

61345

The physician lowers pressure in the brain caused by excess fluid. The patient is placed in a seated position or prone. The physician makes an incision in the midline extending from the posterior mid-scalp to the midcervical region. Dissection is continued to the skull. Drills and saws are used to open the occipital bone to enter the posterior fossa of the skull. The brain is decompressed by removal of blood and pathological tissue. The occipital bone is secured with sutures, wires, or plates and screws. The scalp and neck are sutured closed in layers.

61450

The physician applies or releases pressure on the sensory root of the gasserian ganglion. The gasserian ganglion supplies sensory innervation to the face via the trigeminal nerve. The physician makes a periauricular incision and retracts the scalp and raises a bone flap. The gasserian ganglion is located and decompressed or stimulated. If indicated, the nerve or a nerve branch is sectioned. The bone flap is replaced and fastened. The scalp is reanastomosed and sutured in layers.

61458-61460

The physician performs a suboccipital craniectomy to explore or release pressure from the cranial nerves or tracts in the brainstem. In 61458, the physician explores and frees affected cranial nerves from the surrounding tissue. In 61460, the physician resects one or more cranial nerves. The nerves are freed before resection. The physician incises and retracts the scalp and removes bone from the occiput. The brain is retracted to reveal the brainstem. The affected nerve tract is explored or resected. The bone is replaced and stabilized. The scalp is anastomosed and sutured in layers.

61500-61501

The physician removes a portion of the skull bone invaded by tumor or infection. In 61500, the physician removes a tumor or bony lesion. In 61501, the physician removes infected bone. The physician incises and retracts the scalp and removes bone from the affected area. A bone graft or plastic replacement may be used to reconstruct the skull. The scalp is anastomosed and sutured in layers.

61510-61516

The physician removes a supratentorial abscess or cyst. Supratentorial structures are those located above the tentorium cerebelli, the membrane that separates the cerebellum from the basal surface of the occipital and temporal lobes of the cerebrum. The physician incises and retracts the scalp and removes bone over the area of the tumor, meningioma, abscess, or cyst. The tumor, meningioma, abscess or cyst is identified and excised. The bone is replaced and stabilized. The scalp is anastomosed and sutured in layers. In 61510, the physician removes a brain tumor. In 61512, a meningioma is removed. A meningioma is a tumor of the lining of the brain. In 61514, an abscess is excised. In 61516, a cyst is excised or fenestrated. Fenestration is the surgical creation of an opening or window in the cyst to allow it to drain.

61517

A chemotherapeutic agent is implanted into a brain cavity at the time craniectomy or craniotomy is done to excise the brain tumor. The surgeon places the chemotherapeutic agent into a cavity of the brain that has already been directly accessed during surgery for excision of the tumor. This code includes cancer therapy agents other than brachytherapy radioelement ribbons or sources. This is an add-on code to be reported with the appropriate primary procedure for the brain tumor removal and cannot stand alone.

61518-61519

The physician removes an infratentorial or posterior fossa brain tumor or meningioma. Infratentorial structures are those located below the tentorium cerebelli, the membrane that separates the cerebellum from the basal surface of the occipital and temporal lobes of the cerebrum. The physician incises and retracts the scalp and removes bone from the affected area. The tumor is identified and excised. The bone is replaced and stabilized. The scalp is anastomosed and sutured in layers. In 61518, the physician removes a brain tumor other than a meningioma, cerebellopontine angle tumor, or midline tumor of skull base. In 61519, a meningioma is removed.

61520

The physician removes a brain tumor at the cerebellopontine angle. The physician makes a lateral posterior incision and removes an occipital bone flap. The cerebellum is retracted and brain stem is examined. The tumor at the cerebellopontine angle is resected. The bone is replaced and stabilized. The scalp is anastomosed and sutured in layers.

61521

The physician removes a midline brain tumor at the base of the skull. The physician uses a posterior auricular or transmastoid approach. The physician incises and retracts the scalp and removes a bone flap. The lateral cerebellum is retracted and the tumor, located near the brain stem, is identified and resected. The bone is replaced and stabilized. The scalp is anastomosed and sutured in layers.

61522-61524

The physician removes an abscess or cyst located in the infratentorium or posterior fossa. Infratentorial structures are those located below the tentorium cerebelli, the membrane that separates the cerebellum from basal surface of the occipital and temporal lobes of the cerebrum. The physician incises and retracts the scalp and removes bone over the area of the abscess or cyst. The abscess or cyst is identified and excised the bone is replaced and stabilized. The scalp is anastomosed and sutured in layers. In 61522, an abscess is excised. In 61524 the cyst is excised or fenestrated. Fenestration is the surgical creation of an opening or window in the cyst to allow it to drain.

61526-61530

The physician excises a tumor at the cerebellopontine angle. Cerebellopontine angle tumors are benign neoplasms of the 8th cranial nerve and are more often referred to as acoustic neuromas. Other terms include acoustic tumor, vestibular neurofibromatosis (NF1 or NF2), or angle tumor. Using a transmastoid approach, the physician incises the scalp and removes a bone flap. The tumor is identified and excised. The bone is replaced and stabilized. The scalp is anastomosed and sutured in layers. In 61530, a multiple approach technique is used with the tumor being accessed from both a transtemporal and a middle or posterior fossa approach.

61531

The physician implants electrodes in the subdural layer for long term seizure monitoring. The physician uses a burr drill or trephine to reach the subdural layer and implants linear strip electrodes in each hole. Subdural electrodes are placed just below the dura and do not penetrate the cerebral tissue. The scalp is sutured to close the incisions.

61533-61534

The physician implants electrodes in the subdural layer for long term seizure monitoring. A bone flap is elevated to implant a subdural electrode array along the cerebral hemispheres. The bone is replaced and stabilized. The scalp is anastomosed and sutured in layers. Report 61534 if the epileptogenic focus (the seizure center) is excised.

61535-61536

The physician removes an electrode array located in the subdural layer. The bone flap covering the electrode array is elevated and the array is removed. The bone is replaced and stabilized. The scalp is anastomosed and sutured in layers. Report 61536 if the array is removed in addition to excision of the epileptogenic focus (the seizure center).

61537

A temporal lobectomy is commonly performed for intractable epileptic seizures when the focal point of the seizures has been identified by previous exams to originate in that lobe. An access incision is made through the scalp and overlying muscle to reach the skull. Burr holes are drilled around the periphery of the bone flap area to be raised. Using a craniotome, the bone flap is freed and lifted to expose the dura, which is dissected and retracted out of the operative field. Incisions are made into the cortex and dissection is carried down deep into the cortex. The temporal horn of the lateral ventricle and the hippocampus are identified. The pia is next encountered and is incised and opened and the temporal lobe is removed, including any part of the hippocampus, amygdala, and uncus that are to be removed with the temporal lobe. Arteries are transected and coagulated, while preserving the main cerebral/choroidal arteries and the pia-arachnoid. With the temporal lobe removed, closure is begun by suturing the dura and replacing the bone flap into position. Screws or plates are placed to secure the bone flap to surrounding skull bone. The divided muscles are sutured and the galea and the scalp are closed.

61538

A temporal lobectomy with electrocorticography is commonly performed for intractable epileptic seizures when the focal point of the seizures has been identified by previous exams to originate in that lobe. An access incision is made through the scalp and overlying muscle to reach the skull. Burr holes are drilled around the periphery of the bone flap area to be raised. Using a craniotome, the bone flap is freed and lifted to expose the dura, which is dissected and retracted out of the operative field. Electrodes are prepared and placed on the brain. The electrical activity of the brain is recorded and mapped while the cortex is kept irrigated. The recording grids may be moved a few times to gain enough information about various sites. After the electrocorticography, the electrodes are removed and markers are placed. Incisions are made into the cortex and dissection is carried down deep into the cortex. The temporal horn of the lateral ventricle and the hippocampus are identified. The pia is next encountered and is incised and opened and the temporal lobe is removed, including any part of the hippocampus, amygdala, and uncus that are to be removed with the temporal lobe. Arteries are transected and coagulated, while preserving the main cerebral/choroidal arteries and the pia-arachnoid. With the temporal lobe removed, closure is done by suturing the dura and replacing the bone flap into position. Screws or plates are placed to secure the bone flap to surrounding skull bone. The divided muscles are sutured and the galea and the scalp are closed.

61539

A partial or total lobectomy with electrocorticography is done on a lobe other than the temporal lobe. This may be done for intractable epileptic seizures after the focal point of the seizures has been identified. This is typically accomplished by previous exams showing the origination site, which is often the frontal lobe. An access incision is made through the scalp and overlying muscle to reach the skull. Burr holes are drilled around the periphery of the bone flap area to be raised. Using a craniotome, the bone flap is freed and lifted to expose the dura, which is dissected and retracted out of the operative field. Electrodes are prepared and placed on the brain. The electrical activity of the brain is recorded and mapped while the cortex is kept irrigated. The recording grids may be moved a few times to gain enough information about various sites. After the electrocorticography, the electrodes are removed and markers are placed. Incisions are made into the cortex and dissection is carried down deep into the cortex. The pia is next encountered and is incised and opened to gain access to the frontal lobe. The predetermined amount of frontal lobe is removed. Arteries are transected and coagulated, while preserving the main cerebral/ choroidal arteries and the pia-arachnoid. With the frontal lobe removed, closure is done by suturing the dura and replacing the bone flap into position. Screws or plates are placed to secure the bone flap to surrounding skull bone. The divided muscles are sutured and the galea and the scalp are closed.

61540
A partial or total lobectomy is done on a lobe other than the temporal lobe. This may be done for intractable epileptic seizures after the focal point of the seizures has been identified by previous exams, often the frontal lobe. An access incision is made through the scalp and overlying muscle to reach the skull. Burr holes are drilled around the periphery of the bone flap area to be raised. Using a craniotome, the bone flap is freed and lifted to expose the dura, which is dissected and retracted out of the operative field. Incisions are made into the cortex and dissection is carried down deep into the cortex. The pia is next encountered and is incised and opened to gain access to the frontal lobe. The predetermined amount of frontal lobe is removed. Arteries are transected and coagulated, while preserving the main cerebral/ choroidal arteries and the pia-arachnoid. With the frontal lobe removed, closure is begun by suturing the dura and replacing the bone flap into position. Screws or plates are placed to secure the bone flap to surrounding skull bone. The divided muscles are sutured and the galea and the scalp are closed.

61541-61543
The physician cuts the fibers within the corpus callosum or removes all or part of a brain hemisphere. An electrode array is used to monitor brain function during surgery. In 61541, the physician transects the corpus callosum. Report 61543 if a partial or subtotal (functional) hemispherectomy is performed. The dura is sutured around the remaining brain tissue. The bone flap is replaced and stabilized. The scalp is anastomosed and sutured in layers.

61544
The physician excises or destroys the choroid plexus. The choroid plexus produces spinal fluid. The physician cuts and retracts the scalp in the affected region. A bone flap is raised and tissues are dissected to the ventricle where the affected choroid plexus is located. The choroid plexus is resected, or destroyed using electrocautery. The bone is replaced and stabilized. The scalp is anastomosed and sutured in layers.

61545
The physician excises a craniopharyngioma through a craniotomy. The physician cuts and retracts the frontal scalp and raises a bone flap. The tissues are dissected to the sella turcica, and the craniopharyngioma is resected. The bone is replaced and fastened. The scalp is anastomosed and sutured in layers.

61546
The physician uses a craniotomy to remove a pituitary tumor or resect a portion of the gland. The physician cuts and retracts the frontal scalp and raises a bone flap. The tissues are dissected to the sella turcica, and the pituitary is identified. The tumor or hypertrophic gland is resected. The bone is replaced and fastened. The scalp is anastomosed and sutured in layers.

61548
The physician uses a transnasal or transseptal approach to remove a pituitary tumor or resect a portion of the gland. The physician accesses the base of the sella turcica through the nose. The incision may be made in the mouth underneath the upper lip to avoid facial scarring (transseptal approach). A small hole is drilled in the skull base through the inferior aspect of the sella turcica. The pituitary is identified and the tumor or hypertrophic gland is resected. The hole is packed with Gelfoam, with or without bone chips. The nasal and oral mucosa are sutured closed.

61550-61552
The physician performs a craniectomy for craniosynostosis. Craniosynostosis is a premature closure of the sutures of the skull. The physician incises and retracts the scalp over the fused suture line. The bones are cut to reshape the skull into an anatomically correct position. The recreated suture line is left open and the scalp is reanastomosed and sutured in layers. Report 61550 if a single suture is reformed. Report 61552 for multiple suture lines.

61556-61557
The physician performs a craniotomy for craniosynostosis. Craniosynostosis is a premature closure of the sutures of the skull. The physician incises and retracts the scalp over the fused suture lines. Bone flaps are elevated with careful attention to maintaining blood supply to the scalp. Cuts are made in the cranium to allow the skull to change shape as the brain grows. The scalp incision is sutured in layers. Report 61556 for elevation of a frontal or parietal bone flap; 61557 for elevation of bilateral frontal bone flaps.

61558-61559

The physician performs an extensive craniectomy for craniosynostosis affecting many suture lines. Craniosynostosis is a premature closure of the sutures of the skull. In 61558, no bone grafts are used to reshape the skull. In 61559, the physician harvests bone grafts to aid in reshaping. The physician retracts most or all of the scalp to expose the skull. The cranium is removed as a single unit. The physician breaks the skull and restores correct anatomical shape. If the cranium will not supply bone necessary to provide adequate room for brain growth, bone grafts are obtained and used for skull reshaping. If the dura mater was damaged during cranium harvest, it is primarily closed, or closed with a dural graft. The reshaped cranium pieces are replaced and secured to neighboring bone. The scalp is reapproximated and sutured in layers.

61563-61564

The physician removes an intra and extracranial bone tumor. In 61563, the optic nerve is not decompressed. In 61564, the optic nerve is decompressed. The physician cuts and retracts the scalp overlying the affected bone. The affected bone is resected and removed. Grafts may be necessary for reconstruction. The bone is fastened into place and the scalp is reanastomosed and sutured in layers.

61566

Amygdalohippocampectomy (AH) is done to treat intractable mesial temporal lobe epilepsy. This surgical procedure describes AH in which excision is limited to the anterior hippocampus, amygdala, and parahippocampal gyrus and preserves the fusiform gyrus and the lateral temporal lobe. MRI is done before surgery to map the margins of the involved brain structures. The patient is prepped with a general anesthetic and placement of a lumbar drain. With the patient's head in position, the scalp is incised and the underlying temporalis muscle is dissected to expose the skull. Burr holes are drilled around the periphery of the bone flap area to be raised. Using a craniotome, the bone flap is freed and lifted to expose the dura, which is dissected and retracted out of the operative field. An operating microscope is used. A brain retractor is inserted and cerebrospinal fluid is suctioned from the ambient cistern. The uncus is elevated with the retractor and the anatomical positioning of the related structures (fusiform and parahippocampal gyri, uncus, ambient cistern, and tentorium) is examined. Landmarks for cortical incisions are identified, such as the oculomotor nerve. Cortical incisions are made and the temporal horn of the lateral ventricle is exposed, using careful suction dissection of the cortex and white matter. The horn is opened and the amygdala and hippocampus are identified. The parahippocampal gyrus is now incised, exposing the posterior aspect of the temporal horn and anterior hippocampus. The thin layer of neural tissue connecting the hippocampus and the amygdala is divided with subpial aspiration. The parahippocampal gyrus is removed subpially, the hippocampus is divided transversely, and anterior choroidal and posterior cerebral arteries are coagulated and divided. The hippocampus is completely separated from the arachnoid membrane and removed. The amygdala facing the temporal horn is excised with an ultrasonic aspirator. Closure is done by suturing the dura and replacing the bone flap into position. Screws or plates are placed to secure the bone flap to surrounding skull bone. The divided muscles are sutured and the galea and the scalp are closed.

61567

The surgeon performs a craniotomy for multiple subpial transections, with electrocorticography during surgery. This procedure is done for chronic, intractable, complex partial seizures. The multiple subpial transections are done to reach the areas in the cortex where a focal point of the seizures is identified, as in the frontal, central, or temporal region, and cut the horizontal fibers responsible for the seizure while preserving the vertical fibers responsible for motor and speech. The patient is prepped with general anesthetic and placement of a lumbar drain. With the patient's head in position, the scalp is incised and the underlying temporalis muscle is dissected to expose the skull. Burr holes are drilled around the periphery of the bone flap area to be raised. Using a craniotome, the bone flap is freed and lifted to expose the dura, which is dissected and retracted out of the operative field. Electrodes are prepared and placed on the brain. The electrical activity of the brain is recorded and mapped while the cortex is kept irrigated. The recording grids may be moved a few times to gain enough information about various sites. After the electrocorticography, the electrodes are removed and markers are placed. The cortex is pierced or incised with a curved probe at the adjacent sulcus of the gyrus identified as the focal point of the seizures. The pia is also entered and the grey matter underneath is transected in that area. The probe is removed and the same thing is repeated approximately a centimeter further along the identified gyrus for the extent of the seizure focus. Closure is done by suturing the dura and replacing the bone flap into position. Screws or plates are placed to secure the bone flap to surrounding skull bone. The divided muscles are sutured and the galea and the scalp are closed.

61570-61571

The physician removes a foreign body from the brain. The physician incises the scalp and cuts the bone or creates a bone flap as necessary to reach the foreign body. The object is identified and removed. In 61571, the brain tissue damaged by the foreign object is debrided and irrigated. The dura is sutured closed and the bone is fastened into place.

61575-61576

The physician approaches the skull base, brain stem, or upper spinal cord and obtains a biopsy, decompresses the brain stem or spinal cord, or excises a lesion. In 61575, the physician access the affected area through the patient's mouth. In 61576, the physician performs a tracheostomy and cuts through the mandible and tongue to reach an extensive defect. The physician places a gag retractor in the patient's mouth and makes a posterior pharyngeal wall incision. The mucosa is retracted to the deep muscle layers which are dissected to reach the skull base or superior spinal cord. The bone is removed to expose the area of interest. A lesion may be biopsied or excised. Decompression is accomplished by removing bone from around the structure. If incised, the dura is closed and the posterior pharyngeal wall is reapproximated and sutured in layers.

61580
In this approach procedure, the physician exposes the anterior cranial fossa using a craniofacial approach to an extradural (outside the dura) lesion or defect at the skull base. To adequately expose the lesion or defect, the physician performs a lateral rhinotomy, ethmoidectomy, and sphenoidectomy all of which are included in the approach procedure. For full exposure of the lesion, the brain may need to be retracted from the skull base.

61581
In this approach procedure, the physician exposes the anterior cranial fossa using a craniofacial approach to an extradural (outside the dura) lesion or defect at the skull base. To adequately expose the lesion or defect, the physician performs an orbital exenteration, a lateral rhinotomy, ethmoidectomy, sphenoidectomy and/or maxillectomy all of which are included in the approach procedure. For full exposure of the lesion, the brain may need to be retracted from the skull base.

61582
In this approach procedure, the physician exposes the anterior cranial fossa using a craniofacial approach to an extradural (outside the dura) lesion or defect at the skull base. To adequately expose the lesion or defect, the physician performs a unilateral or bilateral craniotomy which is included in the approach procedure. For full exposure of the lesion, the frontal lobe is elevated and retracted from the skull base. If skull base lesions extend into the bones of the face, an osteotomy of the anterior cranial fossa may be required.

61583
In this approach procedure, the physician exposes the anterior cranial fossa using a craniofacial approach to an intradural (inside the dura) lesion or defect at the skull base. To adequately expose the lesion or defect, the physician performs a unilateral or bilateral craniotomy which is included in the approach procedure. For full exposure of the lesion, the frontal lobe is elevated and retracted from the skull base. If skull base lesions extend into the bones of the face, an osteotomy of the anterior cranial fossa may be required.

61584
In this approach procedure, the physician exposes the anterior cranial fossa using an orbitocranial (transorbital) approach to an extradural (outside the dura) lesion or defect at the skull base. To adequately expose the lesion or defect, the physician performs a supraorbital ridge osteotomy which is included in the approach procedure. For full exposure of the lesion, the frontal and/or temporal lobes are elevated and retracted from the skull base.

61585
In this approach procedure, the physician exposes the anterior cranial fossa using an orbitocranial (transorbital) approach to an extradural (outside the dura) lesion or defect at the skull base. To adequately expose the lesion or defect, the physician performs a supraorbital ridge osteotomy which is included in the approach procedure. The orbital contents are completely removed. For full exposure of the lesion, the frontal and/or temporal lobes are elevated and retracted from the skull base.

61586
In this approach procedure, the physician exposes the anterior cranial fossa using a bicoronal, transzygomatic and/or LeFort I osteotomy approach to a lesion or defect at the skull base. To enter the anterior cranial fossa, the surgeon may use a bicoronal scalp incision to expose the zygoma bone. The zygoma is removed with burrs and saws to enter the anterior skull. If visualization is inadequate, the surgeon may use an intraoral approach to fracture the maxilla and enter the skull. Once the lesion is adequately exposed, a separately reportable surgical procedure is performed which may include biopsy, excision, or other treatment of the lesion. At the conclusion, of this separately reportable procedure, the surgeon responsible for the approach will replace and secure the bony structures using wires, plates or screws as needed.

61590
In this approach procedure, the physician exposes the middle cranial fossa using an infratemporal (below the temporal fossa) pre-auricular (in front of the external ear) approach to a lesion at the skull base. This is also sometimes referred to as a transparotid approach. The transparotid approach allows access to the parapharyngeal space. First, the parotid gland is mobilized. This is followed by identification and dissection of the facial nerve. Parotidectomy with facial nerve preservation is performed. If adequate exposure has not been accomplished, the muscle overlying the mandible is divided and the mandible is displaced anteriorly. This approach may be combined with a transtemporal approach to improve exposure to lesions which extend posteriorly to involve the temporal bone.

61591
In this approach, the physician exposes the middle cranial fossa using an infratemporal (below the temporal fossa), post-auricular (behind the external ear) approach. To adequately expose the lesion or defect, it may be necessary to perform a mastoidectomy, resect the sigmoid sinus and/or decompress/mobilize the contents of the auditory canal or petrous carotid artery.

61592

In this approach procedure, an orbitocranial approach to the middle cranial fossa is performed. Skin incisions are made over the zygoma, and the frontal branches of the facial nerve and infraorbital nerve are identified, tagged, and divided. Soft tissue flaps are raised from the maxilla and zygoma, and osteotomies are performed with removal of the orbitozygomaticomaxillary complex. The temporalis muscle is displaced inferiorly exposing the skull base. If intracranial access is required a subtemporal craniectomy, or frontal or temporal craniotomy is performed. Following separately reportable lesion removal, bone segments are replaced and neurorrhaphy is performed along with meticulous reconstruction and closure.

61595

In this approach code, a transtemporal approach to the posterior cranial fossa, jugular foramen, or midline skull base is used. To obtain adequate exposure of the lesion or defect, the physician performs a mastoidectomy, decompression of sigmoid sinus and/or facial nerve, with or without mobilization. The temple, anterior and posterior ear, orbits, mandible, and mastoid may be resected to reach the affected area of the posterior cranial fossa.

61596

In this approach code, a transcochlear approach is used to expose the posterior cranial fossa, jugular foramen, or midline skull base. A postauricular incision is made and the ear is reflected anteriorly. A labyrinthectomy is performed and the internal auditory canal is skeletonized. The incus is removed, the facial nerve is completely decompressed, and opened widely into the hypotympanum. The greater superficial petrosal nerve is transected and the facial nerve is completely removed from the stylomastoid foramen to the internal auditory canal and rerouted posteriorly. The fallopian canal, stapedius muscle, and the turns of the cochlea are completely exenterated, carrying the dissection forward until the internal carotid artery wall is identified.

61597

In this approach, a transcondylar approach is used to expose the posterior cranial fossa, jugular foramen, or midline skull base. This far lateral suboccipital approach is used to expose the vertebral artery and lower cranial nerve complex in the posterior fossa. A post-auricular incision is made approximately 3 cm lateral to the midline, curving back toward the mastoid eminence. The skin flap created by the incision is retracted laterally exposing the greater occipital nerve and the greater occipital artery and vein. The sternocleidomastoid is incised parallel to its attachment. The suboccipital musculature is also incised and retracted. A suboccipital craniectomy is performed. The C1-C3 vertebral bodies are resected to further expose the cerebellum and a portion of the occipital condyle is removed. The vertebral artery is identified, decompressed and mobilized.

61598

In this approach code, a transpetrosal approach is used to expose the posterior cranial fossa, jugular foramen, or midline skull base. A craniotomy is performed posterior to the sigmoid sinus. The cerebellum is retracted posteriorly, allowing access to the petrosal and sigmoid sinuses which are ligated.

61600-61601

The physician uses a separately reportable anterior cranial fossa approach to resect a neoplastic, vascular, or infectious lesion at the base of the anterior cranial fossa. The physician incises and retracts the scalp or nasal mucosa and removes a bone flap to access the anterior cranial fossa. In 61600, the extradural lesion is identified and resected. Unaffected bone is replaced and fastened to neighboring bone. Bone defects are replaced with bone grafts. In 61601, the intradural lesion is identified and resected. The dura is primarily closed, with or without a dural graft. The bone flap is replaced and fastened to neighboring bone. The scalp is reapproximated and sutured in layers.

61605-61606

The physician uses a middle cranial fossa approach to resect a neoplastic, vascular, or infectious lesion located at the base of the middle cranial fossa (infratemporal fossa, parapharyngeal space, petrous apex). The approach is reported separately. The physician makes a pre- or post-auricular incision or an orbital zygomatic incision to access the middle cranial fossa. The physician retracts the tissues and performs an osteotomy to access the lesion. In 61605, the extradural lesion is identified and resected. Unaffected bone is replaced and fastened to neighboring bone. Bone defects are replaced with bone grafts. In 61606, the intradural lesion is identified and resected. The dura is primarily closed, with or without a dural graft. The bone flap is replaced and fastened to neighboring bone. The scalp is reapproximated and sutured in layers.

61607-61608

The physician uses a middle cranial fossa approach to resect a neoplastic, vascular, or infectious lesion located at the base of the middle cranial fossa (parasellar area, cavernous sinus, clivus, or midline skull base). The approach is reported separately. The physician makes a pre- or postauricular incision or an orbital zygomatic incision to access the middle cranial fossa. The physician retracts the tissues and performs an osteotomy to access the lesion. In 61607, the extradural lesion is identified and resected. Unaffected bone is replaced and fastened to neighboring bone. Bone defects are replaced with bone grafts. In 61608, the intradural lesion is identified and resected. The dura is primarily closed, with or without a dural graft. The bone flap is replaced and fastened to neighboring bone. The scalp is reapproximated and sutured in layers.

61611

The physician transects or ligates a carotid artery in the petrous canal. The area over the petrous canal is incised. The internal carotid artery (ICA) is identified while protecting other vital structures. The ICE is ligated above and below the obstruction or aneurysm. Where possible, the ICA is reattached or a graft placed to provide continuity of the artery. No repair is performed with this procedure.

61613

The physician uses a middle cranial fossa approach to access and obliterate a carotid aneurysm, arteriovenous malformation, or carotid-cavernous fistula. The approach is reported separately. Using an orbitocranial zygomatic approach, the physician incises and retracts the skin over the zygoma. The zygoma and the base of the skull are osteotomized to reach the cavernous sinus. The aneurysm, defect, or fistula is dissected and ligated. The skull and zygoma are packed with Gelfoam or bone pieces. The skin is reanastomosed and sutured in layers.

61615-61616

The physician uses a separately reportable skull base approach to resect or excise a neoplastic, vascular, or infectious lesion in the posterior cranial fossa, jugular foramen, foramen magnum, or C1-C3 vertebral bodies. The physician incises and retracts the scalp overlying the posterior cranial fossa and uses a transtemporal, transcochlear, transcondylar, or transpetrosal approach to reach the lesion. In 61615, the extradural lesion is identified and resected. Unaffected bone is replaced and fastened to neighboring bone. Bone defects are replaced with bone grafts. In 61616, the intradural lesion is identified and resected. The dura is primarily closed, with or without a dural graft. The bone flap is replaced and fastened to neighboring bone. The scalp is reapproximated and sutured in layers.

61618-61619

The physician repairs a cerebrospinal fluid leak in the dura following a craniotomy of the skull base. The approach is dependent on the location of the dural leak. In 61618, the physician uses a dural graft obtained from fascia, tensor fascia lata, or pericranium. In 61619, a vascularized pedicle flap is rotated over the dural defect. The temporalis, frontalis, or occipitalis muscle is used. The dural leak is closed by suturing the flap to the dura. Following anastomosis, intracranial pressure may be increased to test repair success under direct visualization. The bone flap is replaced and the scalp incision is sutured in layers.

61623

Temporary balloon occlusion (TBO) controls blood flow in arteries of the neck during procedures such as intracranial or extracranial aneurysm surgery. The balloon catheter, such as a double lumen Swan-Ganz, is placed in the artery and positioned at the point where occlusion is to occur. Selective catheterization is done first. The access artery is percutaneously punctured with a needle and a guidewire is fed through the artery into the target vessel, such as the cerebral carotid. A catheter is threaded over the guidewire to the point where it is to be occluded and the guidewire is removed. The balloon is inflated under fluoroscopy and occlusion is confirmed with small amounts of contrast material injected through the catheter and checked for stasis in the contrast column. The patient is monitored for change in neurologic status. The TBO is maintained for about 20 to 30 minutes and angiographic studies may be done after occlusion to rule out postprocedure vascular injury.

61624

The physician accesses an artery of the central nervous system percutaneously to permanently occlude or embolize a vascular malformation, destroy a tumor, or achieve hemostasis for a bleeding aneurysm. The access artery is percutaneously punctured with a needle and a guidewire is fed through the artery into the target vessel of the central nervous system. A catheter is threaded over the guidewire to the point where it is to be occluded and the guidewire is removed. When the catheter is in position, the defect is occluded or embolized with materials placed through the catheter to achieve clotting. Radiographic methods are used to position the catheter and test for successful occlusion.

61626

The physician uses a percutaneous catheter to access an arterial venous malformation, tumor, or bleeding aneurysm. The defect lies outside the central nervous system, in the head or neck regions (common carotid, external carotid, vertebral and their branches). The physician places a catheter in a peripheral artery (e.g., femoral artery). Using separately reportable fluoroscopic guidance, the physician locates the lesion with the catheter. The defect is occluded or embolized with materials placed through the catheter to aid clotting.

61630

The physician performs a percutaneous balloon angioplasty of an intracranial vessel, most often as an alternative to surgical carotid endarterectomy for carotid stenosis in high-risk patients. The patient undergoes an appropriate neurological and vascular work up preoperatively. A standard percutaneous transfemoral approach is most frequently used. Light intravenous sedation is administered. Standard diagnostic carotid and cerebral angiography is performed to confirm the suspected lesion and evaluate the cerebral circulation. The patient is anticoagulated and an antiplatelet agent is given. Using the femoral approach, the balloon is introduced on the tip of an angiographic catheter passed through the circulatory tree until it reaches the stenotic lesion. Once in place, the balloon is inflated, dilating the vessel and improving blood flow to the brain.

61635

The physician places an intravascular intracranial stent most often as an alternative to surgical carotid endarterectomy for carotid stenosis in high-risk patients. A percutaneous balloon angioplasty may also be performed. The patient undergoes an appropriate neurological and vascular work up preoperatively. A standard percutaneous transfemoral approach is most frequently used. Light intravenous sedation is administered. Standard diagnostic carotid and cerebral angiography is performed to confirm the suspected lesion and evaluate the cerebral circulation. The patient is anticoagulated and an antiplatelet agent is given. Using the femoral approach, a guiding catheter is placed from the groin into the common carotid artery. A microwire is passed through the guiding catheter and crosses the stenotic lesion in the artery. In the event that the stenosis is too tight to pass a stent primarily, an angioplasty balloon is used to predilate the stenosis prior to the stent placement. The microwire is left across the dilated segment, the balloon is removed, and the stent delivery device is placed. Once positioned, the stent is deployed across the region of the stenosis. If necessary, an additional balloon can be placed inside the deployed stent for post-dilation to make sure the struts of the stent are pressed firmly against the inner surface of the wall of the vessel.

61640-61642

The physician treats intracranial vasospasm via an endovascular approach most often performed under general anesthesia. Angioplasty is performed using a percutaneous transfemoral approach, usually with a six or seven French sheath. Heparin is administered to minimize the risk of thromboembolic events. Prior to the procedure, diagnostic angiography is performed to confirm the clinical suspicion of vasospasm and to correlate the findings with the clinical symptoms, since treatment is directed only at the areas of vasospasm correlating with symptoms. The custom-designed silicone microballoon, which conforms to the shape of the vessel, is guided through the intracranial vessels, and inflated to dilate the spastic vessel. This procedure is useful in improving blood flow to ischemic cerebral tissue by treating focal, as well as diffuse, areas of spasm involving more than one vascular territory. Report 61640 for balloon dilation of the first vessel; 61641 for each additional vessel in the same vascular territory; and 61642 for vessels in different vascular territories.

61645

The physician treats an intracranial arterial occlusion by percutaneous transluminal mechanical thrombectomy and/or thrombolysis infusion. Angiography is utilized to map the blood vessels and identify the area of the clot. The skin is punctured and a needle is inserted into the blood vessel. A guidewire is inserted over the needle and the needle is removed. A catheter is fed over the guidewire into the clotted artery. The guidewire is removed. Mechanical thrombectomy uses devices inserted through the catheter within the vessel breaking down the clot and removing it with suction. For thrombolysis infusion, the physician infuses the clot-busting drug through the catheter to help dissolve the clot and restore normal blood flow to the vessel. Fluoroscopic guidance, diagnostic angiography, catheter placement, and intraprocedural injection of the thrombolytic agent utilized during the course of the procedure are included in the service.

61650-61651

A needle is inserted through the skin and into a blood vessel. A guidewire is threaded through the needle into the vessel and the needle is removed. A catheter, equipped with an infusion tip, is threaded into the vessel and the wire is extracted. The catheter travels to the intracranial vessel requiring treatment and drugs are infused. Following administration, the catheter is removed and pressure is applied over the puncture site to stop the bleeding. This procedure may also be performed through a skin incision with direct exposure of the access vessel. This therapy is used to treat non-iatrogenic central nervous system disorders. These codes include catheter placement, angiography, imaging guidance, patient monitoring, and any arteriotomy closure. Report 61650 for treatment of the initial vessel and 61651 for each additional vascular territory treated. Vascular territories are defined as the right carotid circulation, the left carotid circulation, and the vertebra-basilar circulation.

61680-61692

The physician resects an arteriovenous malformation (AVM) in the brain. This AVM is a tumor-like growth of blood vessels. After using angiography to locate the AVM, the physician performs a craniotomy in the affected area. The AVM is located and the blood vessels feeding the tumor are ligated. The tumor is resected and bleeding is controlled. The bone flap is repositioned and secured; the scalp is reanastomosed and sutured in layers. Report according to AVM location and ease of access: Report 61680 if the AVM is located in the supratentorial region and is easily accessible; 61682 if the supratentorial AVM is more difficult to access and remove; 61684 if the AVM is located in the infratentorial region and is easily accessible; 61686 if the infratentorial AVM is more difficult to access and remove; 61690 if the AVM is located in the dural layer and is easily accessible; and 61692 if the dural AVM is more difficult to access and remove.

61697

An open middle cranial fossa approach is used to locate a complex aneurysm of the internal carotid circulation. Complex aneurysms include those that are larger than 15 millimeters as well as those that contain calcifications or incorporate normal vessels at the aneurysm neck. The surgical technique used is dependent on the specific anatomic characteristics of the aneurysm. One technique involves direct treatment of the aneurysm with clipping and resection of the mass lesion. However, clipping of the aneurysm neck may not be possible if a thick, calcified wall is present. In this instance, incision of the aneurysmal sac and aneurysmorrhaphy (suturing of the aneurysm) may be necessary. When critical perforating vessels arise from the aneurysm, the patient may not be able to tolerate occlusion of the parent vessel. If this is the case, an extracranial or intracranial bypass procedure must first be performed with subsequent trapping or proximal occlusion of the vessel. In some instances, adjunctive techniques are utilized to aid in direct surgery. Techniques include cardiopulmonary bypass with cardiac arrest to allow for a slack aneurysm, which can be dissected from surrounding cerebral tissue. Another adjunctive technique is temporary occlusion of the parent vessel to allow decompression of the aneurysm. Once the aneurysm has been occluded, resected, and/or bypassed, the physician checks to make sure that the repairs are secure and that there is no bleeding. The dura is closed and the bone flap repositioned and secured. The scalp is sutured in layers.

61698

An open posterior cranial fossa approach is used to locate a complex aneurysm of the vertebrobasilar circulation. Complex aneurysms include those that are larger than 15 millimeters as well as those that contain calcifications or incorporate normal vessels at the aneurysm neck. The surgical technique used is dependent on the specific anatomic characteristics of the aneurysm. One technique involves direct treatment of the aneurysm with clipping and resection of the mass lesion. However, clipping of the aneurysm neck may not be possible if a thick, calcified wall is present. In this instance, incision of the aneurysmal sac and aneurysmorrhaphy (suturing of the aneurysm) may be necessary. When critical perforating vessels arise from the aneurysm, the patient may not be able to tolerate occlusion of the parent vessel. If this is the case, an extracranial or intracranial bypass procedure must first be performed with subsequent trapping or proximal occlusion of the vessel. In some instances, adjunctive techniques are utilized to aid in direct surgery. Techniques include cardiopulmonary bypass with cardiac arrest to allow for a slack aneurysm, which can be dissected from surrounding cerebral tissue. Another adjunctive technique is temporary occlusion of the parent vessel to allow decompression of the aneurysm. Once the aneurysm has been occluded, resected, and/or bypassed, the physician checks to make sure that the repairs are secure and that there is no bleeding. The dura is closed and the bone flap repositioned and secured. The scalp is sutured in layers.

61700

The physician resects a simple carotid aneurysm. Simple aneurysms include those that are 15 millimeters or less in size and contain no anatomical features that will complicate the surgery such as calcifications or critical perforating vessels at the aneurysm neck. After using angiography to locate the aneurysm, the physician uses a middle cranial fossa approach for access. The aneurysm is located and clipped under direct visualization. After making sure the clip is secure and there is no bleeding, the physician closes the dura. The bone flap is repositioned and secured and the scalp is sutured in layers.

61702

The physician resects a simple vertebrobasilar aneurysm. Simple aneurysms include those that are 15 millimeters or less in size and contain no anatomical features that will complicate the surgery such as calcifications or critical perforating vessels at the aneurysm neck. After using angiography to locate the aneurysm, the physician uses a posterior cranial fossa approach for access. The aneurysm is located and clipped under direct visualization. After making sure the clip is secure and there is no bleeding, the physician closes the dura. The bone flap is repositioned and secured and the scalp is sutured in layers.

61703

The physician resects an aneurysm after clamping the carotid artery to control bleeding. The physician makes a high neck incision and locates the ipsilateral carotid artery. Next, the physician performs a craniotomy to access the intracranial aneurysm. When the aneurysm is located, the carotid artery is occluded with a clamp. The physician places a clip on the aneurysm under direct visualization. Once the aneurysm has been clipped and bleeding is controlled, the carotid clamp is released. The aneurysm site is reexamined for bleeding. The physician closes the dura. The bone flap is repositioned and secured; the scalp is reanastomosed and sutured in layers. The neck incision is sutured in layers.

61705-61710

The physician clips an aneurysm, vascular malformation, or carotid-cavernous fistula. The physician makes a high neck incision and locates the ipsilateral carotid artery. Next, the physician performs a craniotomy to access the defect. In 61705, the physician performs a craniotomy to access the intracranial aneurysm, vascular malformation or carotid-cavernous fistula. Once the lesion is located, the cervical carotid is clamped and the carotid artery proximal and distal to the lesion is ligated to prevent blood flow to the lesion. The cervical carotid is unclamped while monitoring for bleeding in the craniotomy site. In 61708, the lesion is obliterated using electrothrombosis. In 61710, the physician embolizes the lesion with an intra-arterial balloon catheter or injects material to form a regional clot to obliterate the blood supply to the lesion. After the lesion has been obliterated, the dura is closed. The bone flap is repositioned and secured; the scalp is reanastomosed and sutured in layers.

61711

The physician anastomoses the arterial and extracranial-intracranial arteries. The physician performs a craniotomy in the affected area and locates the arteries to be anastomosed and dissects them from the surrounding tissue. The feeding artery is clamped and ligated and the proximal limb is sutured to the receiving artery. After verifying successful anastomosis and adequate blood flow, the dura is closed. The bone flap is repositioned and secured; the scalp is reanastomosed and sutured in layers.

61715

Magnetic resonance imaging is combined with high intensity focused ultrasound (MRgFUS) to target specific areas of the brain for thermal ablation, typically in the treatment of movement disorders and associated symptoms. The noninvasive treatment uses phased array transducers that allow the ultrasound to pass through the skull safely, allowing for an alternative treatment to open neurologic procedures. The patient's head is shaved and inspected for scars or other lesions that could potentially affect the ultrasound beam. Following administration of local anesthetic, a stereotactic frame is placed on the patient's head. Positioning of the frame is determined to encompass the center of the brain within the treatment area. After the frame is secured, a silicone membrane containing cooled, degassed water is placed over the patient's head; this membrane allows the ultrasound to pass through. The patient is placed on the MRI table and an MRgFUS helmet containing the transducer arrays is attached. Additional cooled, degassed water is added to the space between the patient's head and the helmet. The water is further cooled to a temperature of about 18 degrees Celsius. MR images are taken of the brain and target region. The surgeon views the images, evaluating the target, parameters, and treatment plan. Treatment planning software determines the parameters for focused treatment through the skull for adequate concentration on the lesion. During the treatment, the ultrasound transducer applies a focused beam (sonication) to the target area. Initially, the beam strength is weak to map temperature distribution by MRI thermometry. Beam and temperature adjustments can be made at this time for optimal results. For ablation procedures, the sonication elevates the temperature within the target area/lesion, causing a thermal coagulation result. MR images during this process provide the surgeon with quantitative and temperature images of the entire area to ensure the treatment plan is followed. This ablation is performed in increments and repeated through several interconnecting points until the entire treatment area is covered. The brain tissue temperature is monitored continuously by MR thermometry. The patient has a remote control during the entire procedure that provides them the option of discontinuing at any time. The procedure ends when the surgeon deems that all clinical and radiologic effects are acceptable.

61720-61735

The physician creates a lesion of the brain through stereotactic methods. The tissue to be lesioned is mapped by using a CT or MRI scanning technique. The physician uses the coordinates obtained from the scans to locate the area of interest. The physician incises and retracts the scalp. A burr hole is drilled. An electrocautery unit or surgical knife is directed to the area of interest. When the precise location is reached and confirmed by the coordinates, the lesion is made. In 61720, a lesion is made in the globus pallidus or in the thalamus. In 61735, a lesion is made in subcortical structures other than the globus pallidus or the thalamus. After the lesion is made, the dura is sutured and the scalp is reapproximated and sutured in layers.

61736-61737

The surgeon performs laser interstitial thermal therapy (LITT) of a brain lesion, typically using magnetic resonance imaging (MRI) guidance. Common indications for LITT include primary brain tumors, brain metastases, radiation necrosis, and epileptogenic lesions. With the patient under general anesthesia or monitored anesthesia care (MAC), the lesion is targeted using preoperative imaging. The surgeon makes a small skin incision over the entry point, creates a burr hole, and may perform a needle biopsy prior to treatment for confirmatory tissue diagnosis. A reducing cannula followed by the laser catheter containing the optical fiber is then inserted through the burr hole to the desired depth in the lesion of interest. Laser light is delivered interstitially using low power in order to heat the tissues and induce cell death. Using MRI thermometry, the lesion temperature is measured throughout the procedure. Following completion of the procedure, the catheter is removed and the skin incision is closed with absorbable sutures. The patient is observed for any adverse effects. Report 61736 for a single trajectory procedure performed for one simple lesion and 61737 for a procedure involving multiple trajectories for multiple or complex lesions.

61750-61751

The physician biopsies, aspirates, or excises an intracranial lesion stereotactically. The lesion is mapped using a CT or MRI scanning technique. The physician uses the coordinates obtained from the scans to locate the area of interest. The physician incises and retracts the scalp. A burr hole is drilled. The physician inserts a biopsy needle into the area of interest to aspirate or biopsy the tissue. If the lesion is to be destroyed the physician inserts an electrocautery unit, knife or curette into the lesion. In 61751, the physician utilizes CT or MRI scanning intraoperatively to confirm lesion location and accurate placement of surgical instruments. The physician closes the dura and reapproximates the scalp and closes it in sutured layers.

61760

The physician implants depth electrodes into the cerebrum for long-term monitoring of seizures. After the desired locations of the electrodes have been mapped by CT or MRI scanning techniques, the physician incises and retracts the scalp. The physician drills a burr hole(s) and the electrodes are placed into the desired area of the brain by following the coordinates established by the scans. The dura is sutured closed and the scalp is reapproximated and sutured in layers.

61770

The physician implants catheters or probes into a lesion of the brain for radiation therapy. After using CT or MRI scanning techniques to map the desired locations of the catheters or probes, the physician incises and retracts the scalp. The physician drills a burr hole and the catheters or probes are placed into the desired area of the brain by following the coordinates established by the scans. The dura is sutured closed and the scalp is reapproximated and sutured in layers.

61781-61783

The physician performs cranial or spinal procedures utilizing stereotactic computer-assisted navigation. These codes may only be assigned in conjunction with the primary procedure when the physician uses a computer to assist with coordinate determination established with a CT or MRI scan. Report 61781 for intradural cranial procedures; 61782 for extradural cranial procedures; and 61783 for spinal procedures.

61790-61791

The physician under stereotactic guidance percutaneously creates a neurolytic lesion in the gasserian ganglion or the medullary trigeminal tract. The area of interest is located and mapped by CT or MRI scanning techniques. The physician guides a needle into the region to be destroyed. After reaffirming position by checking the coordinates of the needle, the physician injects, or electrically destroys the tissue. In 61790, the physician destroys the gasserian ganglion. In 61791, the physician destroys the medullary trigeminal tracts.

61796-61800

Before imaging, patients undergo application of a separately reportable stereotactic head frame (61800). Using high-resolution stereotactic imaging, a precise three-dimensional location of the brain lesion is identified. The physician uses the coordinates obtained from the images to focus linear accelerator, gamma ray, or particle beam energy onto the lesion, thereby destroying or inactivating it. This is a noninvasive procedure that does not require incision of the scalp or drilling into the skull. Report 61796 (no more than once per course of treatment) for stereotactic radiosurgery on a simple cranial lesion. Simple lesions include those that are less than 3.5 cm in maximum dimension and those that do not meet the criteria for a complex lesion. Report 61797 for each additional simple cranial lesion. Report code 61798 (no more than once per course of treatment) for stereotactic radiosurgery on a complex cranial lesion. Complex lesions include those that are 3.5 cm or greater in maximum dimension; those that are within the brainstem or adjacent (5 mm or less) to the optic nerve, optic chasm, or optic tract; schwannomas; arteriovenous malformations; cavernous sinus tumors; glomus tumors; parasellar or petroclival tumors; pineal region tumors; and pituitary tumors. Code 61798 is also reported for procedures such as thalamotomy or pallidotomy that create therapeutic lesions. If multiple lesions are treated and any single lesion is complex, report 61798. Report 61799 for each additional complex cranial lesion; however, codes 61797 and 61799 may not be reported more than four times for the entire course of treatment regardless of the number of lesions treated. Codes for cranial stereotactic radiosurgery include any required computer-assisted planning, dosimetry, targeting, positioning, or blocking by the neurosurgeon.

61850

The physician uses a twist or burr drill to reach the cortex or subcortex and implant neurostimulator electrodes. The physician incises the scalp and uses a twist or burr drill to expose the cortex for neurostimulator electrode placement. The physician places an electrode through an introducer needle into the tissue to be stimulated. The electrodes are tested to verify placement and the incision is sutured in layers.

61860

The physician performs a craniectomy or craniotomy to reach the cortex and implant neurostimulator electrodes to affect the cerebrum. The cerebrum occupies the frontal portion of the cranial cavity. Its two hemispheres joined by the corpus callosum supply the majority of brain function. The physician incises the scalp and retracts it. The physician drills or cuts the cranium to expose the cortex for neurostimulator electrode placement. Bone is removed. The physician places an electrode through an introducer needle into the tissue to be stimulated, and the electrodes are tested to verify placement.

61863-61864

The surgeon performs a twist drill, burr hole, craniotomy, or craniectomy for stereotactic implantation of a deep-brain neurostimulator electrode array. This procedure is done for Parkinsonism, uncontrolled tremors, multiple sclerosis, and intractable dystonias. MRI or CT imaging (reported separately) may be done before surgery to map out the involved brain structures. Before surgery is begun, the patient has a stereotactic head frame applied and anchored to the skull. The surgery is planned with computer assistance, using the previously acquired CT or MRI images, and the target point trajectories for placing electrodes are discussed. The entry point is calculated. The patient is prepped, the head frame is assembled, and the coordinates are entered into the stereotactic system. The entry point is marked, the scalp is incised, and the skull is exposed. A twist drill or burr hole is made with a cranial drill and the dura is exposed and punctured for access. A cannula and electrode guide connected to the computer system is next inserted and the deep-brain stimulation neuroelectrode array is placed at the target point. Testing is done. Reposition and testing may be repeated several times before optimal results in tremor suppression mobility and decreased limb rigidity are observed. When the electrode array is in the best position, the guide cannula is removed. The array is fastened into position under radiographic imaging to monitor its placement. The lead has to be coiled in a pocket under the galea, which is sutured closed, followed by skin closure. Report 61864 when more than one array is placed into a target site. This also requires additional presurgical computerized trajectory planning and other entry site access through the skull to reach the additional target area.

61867-61868

The surgeon performs a twist drill, burr hole, craniotomy, or craniectomy for stereotactic implantation of a deep-brain neurostimulator electrode array with intraoperative use of microelectrode recording. This procedure is done for Parkinsonism, uncontrolled tremors, multiple sclerosis, and intractable dystonias. MRI or CT imaging (reported separately) may be done before surgery to map out the involved brain structures. Before surgery is begun, the patient has a stereotactic head frame applied and anchored to the skull. The surgery is planned with computer assistance, using the previously acquired CT or MRI images, and the target point trajectories for placing electrodes are discussed. The entry point is calculated. The patient is prepped, the head frame is assembled, and the coordinates are entered into the stereotactic system. The entry point is marked, the scalp is incised, and the skull is exposed. A twist drill or burr hole is made with a cranial drill and the dura is exposed and punctured for access. A cannula and electrode guide connected to the computer system is next inserted. The microelectrode is put into another cannula and also attached to the computer system. The cannula protecting the microelectrode is placed within the guide cannula and advanced. Microelectrode recording (MER) and stimulation is done during targeting and repositioning of the electrodes to determine the best placement. MER records the response of individual neurons and maps out the results to define the optimal target area. The microelectrode is removed from the cannula and the deep-brain stimulation neuroelectrode array is placed at the target point. Testing is carried out and the guide cannula is removed. The array is fastened into position with radiographic imaging monitoring its placement. The lead has to be coiled in a pocket under the galea, which is sutured closed, followed by skin closure. Report 61868 when more than one array is placed into a target site in the same manner. This requires additional presurgical computerized trajectory planning and other entry site access through the skull to reach the additional target area.

61880

The physician removes or revises neurostimulator electrodes. The physician incises and retracts the scalp and drills a burr hole in the cranium to locate the electrode. The electrode is removed or revised. If necessary, the electrode is replaced. The dura is closed and the scalp is reapproximated and sutured in layers.

61885-61886

The physician inserts or replaces a cranial neurostimulator pulse generator or receiver into a subcutaneous pocket. The physician selects a location site, usually the infraclavicular area, and incises the skin. Using blunt dissection, the physician creates a pocket for the generator or receiver. The unit is connected to a previously positioned single electrode array in 61885. After ensuring that the device is functioning, the generator or receiver is sutured into place within its subcutaneous pocket. In 61886, the pulse generator or receiver is inserted or replaced and connected to two or more electrode arrays. These codes include direct or inductive coupling.

61888

The physician removes or revises a pulse generator or receiver within the subcutaneous pocket. The physician incises the skin above the unit. After locating the generator or receiver, the physician removes it or makes any necessary revisions to it and closes the incision.

61889-61892

The physician inserts a skull-mounted cranial neurostimulator pulse generator or receiver for deep brain stimulation in 61889. Following appropriate anesthesia, the physician makes one or more incisions into the skin over the skull. Leads are placed against the surface of the brain and connected to a neurostimulator device that is situated within the skull. The skin and subcutaneous tissues of all incisions are closed with layered sutures and skin staples. This code includes direct or inductive coupling and connection to depth and/or cortical strip electrode arrays. Craniectomy or craniotomy are included, when performed. In 61891, the physician revises or replaces the skull-mounted cranial neurostimulator pulse generator or receiver. Incisions are made into the skin over the neurostimulator, and the device is revised or removed and replaced. After the device is reconnected to the leads, the skin and subcutaneous tissues of all incisions are closed with sutures and skin staples. This code includes connection to depth and/or cortical strip electrode arrays. In 61892, the physician removes the skull-mounted cranial neurostimulator pulse generator or receiver. Incisions are made in the skin above the neurostimulator, and dissection is performed. The neurostimulator is detached from the leads, and all components are removed. The skin and subcutaneous tissues of all incisions are closed with sutures and skin staples. This code includes cranioplasty, when performed.

62000-62010

The physician elevates a depressed skull fracture to restore anatomical position. The physician incises and retracts the scalp to expose the skull depression. In 62000, the physician drills a burr hole and pulls on the skull to elevate the bone. In 62005, there are multiple fracture lines. The bony pieces are stabilized in anatomic position. In 62010, the fracture has damaged the dura and brain. The physician removes the bony fragments and debrides the brain and dura. The dura is sutured closed and the bony fragments are approximated and stabilized in anatomic position. The scalp is reapproximated and sutured in layers.

62100

The physician repairs a dural/cerebrospinal fluid leak. The physician determines the location of the skull fracture using an MRI scan. The skin over the damaged area is incised. A bone flap is removed to access the dura which is sutured closed. The bone flap is replaced and stabilized. The scalp is reapproximated and sutured in layers.

62115-62117
The physician reduces an enlarged skull (e.g., secondary to hydrocephalus). The physician incises and retracts the scalp to expose the cranium. In 62115, the skull is cut and the bone is reshaped. In 62117, bone flaps are cut and raised. The bones are removed and reshaped; bone grafts may be used to shape the cranium. The bone is replaced and stabilized. The scalp is anastomosed and sutured in layers. Code 62117 includes bone harvest.

62120-62121
The physician corrects an encephalocele. An encephalocele is a herniation in the brain into or through a defect in the cranium. In 62120, the defect is located in the skull vault. In 62121, the defect is in the skull base. The physician incises and retracts the scalp and raises a bone flap. The bone is reshaped to increase skull size. The skull is stabilized and the scalp is reapproximated and sutured in layers.

62140-62141
The physician corrects a defect in the cranium. In 62140, the defect is less than 5 cm. In 62141, the defect is greater than 5 cm. The physician incises and retracts the scalp. The bone flaps are lifted and remodeled. A prosthesis may be used to reapproximate the bony edges. The skull is stabilized and the scalp is reapproximated and sutured in layers.

62142
The physician removes a bone flap or prosthetic plate of the skull. The physician incises the scalp above the area to be resected and retracts it. The stabilizers are removed and the bone flap lifted. The scalp is reapproximated over the dura and sutured in layers.

62143
The physician replaces a bone flap or prosthetic plate of the skull. The physician incises the scalp and retracts it to expose the dura. The bone graft or prosthetic plate is placed over dura to correct the defect. The bone or prosthetic plate is stabilized and the scalp is reapproximated and sutured in layers.

62145
The physician reshapes or reconstructs the cranium in addition to reparative brain surgery. The physician incises the scalp above the defect area. A bone flap is raised and the physician inspects the dura and the underlying brain. Any dural defects are corrected. The bone flaps are reshaped, reapproximated and stabilized. The scalp is sutured in layers.

62146-62148
The physician reshapes or reconstructs the cranium using bone grafts obtained from the patient. The physician incises the scalp above the defect area. The scalp is retracted and the defect is located. The physician incises the cranium and reshapes available skull bone. The physician obtains bone grafts from the patient. The harvested bone is reshaped to supplement the cranium. The bones are approximated and stabilized. The scalp is reanastomosed and sutured in layers. Report 62146 if the defect is 5 cm or less in size; 62147 if the defect is greater than 5 cm; and 62148 if the surgeon reaccesses the surgical site of the cranioplasty and retrieves the bone graft used whether autologous or from another source.

62160
This code reports the use of intracranial neuroendoscopic techniques when placing or replacing a ventricular catheter of a shunt or external drainage system of the brain to divert the flow and drain obstructed cerebrospinal fluid (CSF). The physician inserts the neuroendoscope into the ventricular compartment of the brain through a burr hole in the skull just big enough to allow passage of the instrument. The scope works within the fluid-filled spaces of the ventricles and gives a much better visualization of the intracranial anatomy to allow the choroid plexus to be seen at the time of shunt placement. After the choroid plexus and ventricular anatomy are identified, the neuroendoscope is removed and the ventricular catheter is placed at a specific distance in front of and above the choroid plexus. The positioning above this potentially obstructive tissue improves shunt success since catheters placed in this position using the neuroendoscope require fewer shunt revisions and there is no need for a second pass through the brain parenchyma. This is an add-on code to be listed in conjunction with the code for the primary procedure.

62161
The physician uses a neuroendoscope for intracranial dissection of adhesions, fenestration of septum pellucidum, or intraventricular cysts. A small incision is made in the scalp based on the location of the cyst and a small burr hole is made in the skull just big enough to allow passage of the instrument. From this point, the scope is inserted into the cyst within the ventricle and the wall of the cyst is fenestrated, or opened, to drain the cystic fluid into one of the natural fluid chambers of the brain where it can be absorbed naturally. This is done by the use of a laser micro contact fiber inserted through the endoscope within the ventricular cannula. In this way, cystic adhesions within the ventricles can also be dissected as well as fenestration of the septum pellucidum, the membrane separating the horns of the lateral ventricles, for cyst drainage. This code includes placement, replacement, or removal of a ventricular catheter.

62162
The physician uses a neuroendoscope for intracranial fenestration or excision of a colloid cyst. A colloid cyst is a benign tumor in the third ventricle that contains a fluid of jelly-like substance. A small incision is made in the scalp behind the hairline and a small burr hole is made in the skull just big enough to allow passage of the instrument. From this point, the scope is inserted within the third ventricle and navigated to the tumor. The wall of the tumor is coagulated with electrical current and fenestrated, or opened, with sharp

dissection. Suction catheters are used to empty the contents and the wall is excised. Any remaining tissue is destroyed with electrical current and the endoscope is removed. This code includes the placement of an external ventricular catheter for drainage.

62164

The physician uses a neuroendoscope for the intracranial excision of a brain tumor. A small incision is made in the scalp based on the location of the tumor and a small burr hole is made in the skull just big enough to allow passage of the instrument. The scope is inserted into the ventricular compartment and moved to the tumor site. Many brain tumors occur situated deep within the brain in the ventricles. The neuroendoscope works with clarity within the fluid-filled spaces of the ventricles. The tumor is easily identified because of the different tissue appearance and is resected and removed completely through the endoscope under direct vision. Using the neuroendoscope allows bleeding vessels to be seen and other important tissue within the ventricle to be avoided and eliminates the need for long scalp incisions, skull flaps, and dissection through brain tissue. This code includes the placement of an external ventricular catheter for drainage.

62165

The physician excises a pituitary tumor using neuroendoscopic techniques employed transnasally or transsphenoidally. The face and nostrils are prepped as well as the abdomen, in case a fat graft must be harvested. Vasoconstriction is achieved in the nasal mucosa and blunt dissection is used on the middle turbinate to view the uncinate process, which is removed with rongeurs. A complete ethmoidectomy is done with removal of the posterior half of the middle turbinate. A Freer elevator is used to identify the sphenoid sinus ostia behind the posterior ethmoid wall and the ostium is enlarged with pituitary rongeurs. The sphenoid anterior wall is removed for insertion of the endoscope. The sinus mucosa is removed with rongeurs and blunt dissection to expose the posterior sphenoid sinus wall and the sella floor. The pituitary fossa is entered and the sella floor is opened with an osteotome, if possible, or small, high-speed drills. The dura is coagulated with bipolar cautery and an incision is made. The tumor can now be removed with suction and angled curettes. The scope is advanced into the empty pituitary fossa as the tumor is removed to check for complete resection with the assistance of angled telescopes. Hemostasis is ensured after tumor removal. If cerebrospinal fluid is seen, the sella is packed with a fat graft harvested from the abdomen. The instruments are removed and no nasal packing is required.

62180

The physician performs a ventriculocisternostomy to form a communicating duct from the lateral ventricles to the cisterna magna to drain excess CSF into the spinal cord where it can be absorbed. The scalp is incised and retracted posterior to the ear. The physician drills a burr hole and inserts the proximal portion of the shunt toward the lateral ventricles, with or without the aid of an endoscope until CSF flows through the shunt. The distal end of the shunt is directed toward the cisterna magna until CSF flows through the shunt. The two ends are connected and tested. The dura is sutured closed and the scalp is reapproximated and sutured in layers.

62190-62192

The physician creates a shunt to form a communicating duct from the subdural or subarachnoid to the atria, jugular veins, auricular processes, pleural space, peritoneal space, or another area to drain excess CSF. The scalp is incised over the affected area. The physician drills a burr hole and inserts the proximal portion of the shunt into the subdural or subarachnoid space. The distal end of the shunt is directed and tunneled subcutaneously toward the selected drain site. The two ends are connected and tested. The dura is sutured closed and the scalp is reapproximated and sutured in layers. In an incision is required at the distal end, the incision is sutured in layers. Report 62190 if the distal end is located at the atria, jugular veins, or auricular processes. Report 62192 if it is located at the pleural space, peritoneal space, or another area.

62194

The physician irrigates or replaces a subarachnoid or subdural shunt system catheter. The physician incises and retracts the scalp over the placement origin. The dura is incised, and the catheter is irrigated to verify function. If the catheter is inoperative, it is replaced. The dura is sutured closed and the scalp is reapproximated and sutured in layers.

62200

The physician performs a ventriculocisternostomy to form a communicating duct from the third ventricle to the cisterna magna to drain excess CSF into the spinal cord where it can be absorbed. The scalp is incised and retracted posterior to the ear. The physician drills a burr hole and inserts the proximal portion of the shunt toward the third ventricle until CSF flows through the shunt. The distal end of the shunt is directed toward the cisterna magna until CSF flows through the shunt. The two ends are connected and tested. The dura is sutured closed and the scalp is reapproximated and sutured in layers.

62201

The physician performs a ventriculocisternostomy of the third ventricle (third ventriculostomy) using stereotactic, neuroendoscopic techniques. Third ventriculostomy is done in hydrocephalus cases to create a pathway for obstructed cerebrospinal fluid (CSF) by opening a communication between the third ventricle and the subarachnoid space to allow the fluid to drain internally. This method prevents the need for shunt placement in many cases. A small incision is made in the scalp and a small burr hole is made in the skull just big enough to allow passage of the endoscopic instrument. Computerized tomography (CT) guidance for stereotactic positioning is used. The neuroendoscope is inserted through the burr hole into the third ventricle. A contact laser fiber is inserted through the endoscope onto the floor of the third ventricle and the contact tip perforates the intracranial tissue at different points, avoiding arteries. The newly opened communication is verified when the circulation of CSF is unobstructed. Hemostasis is achieved, the instruments are removed, and the incision is closed.

62220-62223
The physician creates a shunt to form a communicating duct from the lateral ventricles to the atria, jugular veins, auricular processes, pleural space, peritoneal space, or another area, to drain excess CSF. The scalp is incised and retracted posterior to the ear. The physician drills a burr hole and inserts the proximal portion of the shunt toward the lateral ventricles, with or without the aid of an endoscope, until CSF flows through the shunt. The distal end of the shunt is directed and tunneled subcutaneously toward the selected drain site. The two ends are connected and tested. The dura is sutured closed and the scalp is reapproximated and sutured in layers. If an incision is required at the distal end, the incision is sutured in layers. Report 62220 if the distal end is located at the atria, jugular veins, or auricular processes. Report 62223 if it is located at the pleural space, peritoneal space, or another area. A neuroendoscope may be used to aid in placing the ventricular catheter and connecting it to the shunt system drainage site terminus, but is not an inclusive component of these codes.

62225-62230
The physician replaces or revises a previously placed, inoperative cerebrospinal fluid shunt system or component. The physician incises and retracts the scalp over the placement origin and drills a burr hole to gain access. The dura is incised, and the inoperative portion of the shunt system is located and replaced or revised. In 62225, the ventricular catheter is irrigated or replaced. In 62230, a cerebrospinal fluid shunt, obstructed valve, or distal catheter is revised or replaced. The shunt system is reconnected and tested. The dura is sutured closed; the scalp is reapproximated and sutured in layers. A neuroendoscope may be used to aid in placing the ventricular catheter and connecting it to the shunt system drainage site terminus, but is not an inclusive component of these codes.

62252
An adjustable cerebrospinal fluid (CSF) shunt is reprogrammed. Adjustable shunts have a pressure differential valve that alters resistance using a magnetic field transmitted through the skin. During a routine office visit, the valve setting is changed using an antenna whose emitted magnetic field rotates the stepper valve to the desired position. The stepper adjusts the tension of the spring, which in turn imposes resistance on the ball valve altering the flow of CSF fluid from the ventricles.

62256-62258
The physician removes a complete cerebrospinal fluid shunt system without replacement in 62256, and with replacement by a similar or other shunt in 62258. The physician incises and retracts the scalp over the placement origin. The dura is incised, and the shunt is located and removed. The dura is sutured closed; the scalp is reapproximated and sutured in layers. Report 62256 if the shunt system is only removed. Report 62258 if the shunt system is replaced during the same operation.

62263-62264
Epidural adhesions are lysed percutaneously by an injection, such as hypertonic saline or an enzyme solution, or by mechanical means. The patient is placed in the sitting or lateral decubitus position for insertion of a needle into a vertebral interspace. The site to be entered is sterilized, local anesthesia is administered, and the needle is inserted. Separately reportable contrast media with fluoroscopy may be injected to confirm proper needle placement and to identify epidural adhesions. The physician injects the adhesiolytic solution or performs mechanical adhesion destruction, such as with a catheter, to lyse epidural adhesions. The needle and/or catheter is removed and the wound is dressed. Report 62263 for multiple adhesiolysis sessions on two or more days and 62264 for multiple adhesiolysis sessions occurring only on one day.

62267
The physician removes contents within the intervertebral disc, nucleus pulposus, or paravertebral tissue with a needle for diagnostic purposes. Separately reportable computed tomography or fluoroscopic guidance verifies placement of the needle. A spinal needle is inserted, the contents of the targeted location are aspirated, and the needle is removed. The wound is dressed. If this procedure is performed under fluoroscopic guidance, injection of the contrast is an inclusive component and is not reported separately.

62268
The physician removes the contents of a cyst or syrinx with a needle. An x-ray verifies placement of the needle (separately reportable). A spinal needle is inserted once the cyst or syrinx is located. The contents of the cyst are aspirated and the needle is removed. The wound is dressed.

62269
This procedure is performed to determine the nature and extent of a suspected lesion. The patient is placed in a spinal tap position. The affected vertebrae are located and local anesthesia is administered. A biopsy needle is inserted. In some cases, blood is drawn through the needle for testing. Separately reportable imaging confirms placement, and samples are drawn from the lesion for inspection. When the procedure is completed, the needle is removed and the wound is dressed.

62270 [62328]
A diagnostic lumbar puncture, also known as a spinal tap, is performed using anatomical landmarks in 62270 and under fluoroscopic or CT guidance in 62328. The patient is placed in a spinal tap position, either lying on one side or in an upright position. The skin is sterilized and a local anesthetic may be administered. The biopsy needle is inserted and cerebrospinal fluid (CSF) is withdrawn for diagnostic testing. Upon completion of the procedure, the needle is removed and a small sterile dressing is applied to the wound.

62272 [62329]
A therapeutic spinal puncture is performed to lessen cerebrospinal fluid pressure. The patient is placed in a spinal tap position. Using anatomical landmarks (62272) or fluoroscopic or CT guidance (62329), usually the L3 and L4 vertebrae are located and local anesthesia is administered. The lumbar puncture needle is inserted. In some cases, spinal fluid is drawn through the needle as in a lumbar puncture test. In other cases, a catheter is inserted and the fluid empties into a reservoir. Pressure reading is performed with a manometer. When the procedure is completed, the needle is removed and the wound is dressed. In many cases, the patient lies prone to prevent fluid leakage.

62273
This procedure is performed following a spinal puncture to prevent spinal fluid leakage. The patient remains in a spinal tap position. The patient's blood is injected outside the dura to clot and plug the wound, preventing spinal fluid leakage. The wound is dressed and monitored.

62280-62282
This procedure is performed to destroy nerve tissue or adhesions. The patient is placed in a spinal tap position. The site is sterilized, and the needle is inserted under fluoroscopic guidance. The needle is placed at the proper level and the neurolytic substance is administered. Once the injection/infusion is completed, the needle is removed and the wound dressed. Report 62280 if the substance is administered to the subarachnoid level. Report 62281 if the needle is inserted in the epidural region of a cervical or thoracic level. Report 62282 if the needle is inserted in the epidural region of a lumbar or sacral (caudal) level.

62284
The physician injects dye into the epidural or intrathecal space for myelography and/or computed tomography (CT scan) at the lumbar spinal level, reported separately. The patient is placed in a spinal tap position. The site is sterilized, the needle is inserted and placed to the proper level, and the dye is administered. The needle is removed and the wound dressed.

62287
This decompression procedure relieves pressure on the spinal nerves by correcting a bulge in an intervertebral disc. Commonly referred to as a percutaneous discectomy, it may be accomplished by several techniques, including non-automated (manual), automated, or laser. For all techniques, the patient is placed in a spinal tap position on the left side. In a separately reportable procedure, a C-arm x-ray verifies placement of the needle in the disc. Once the disc is located, local anesthesia is injected and a small stab wound is made. A spinal needle is inserted with additional monitoring of placement and injection of anesthesia. Using a manual technique, the physician inserts one or two needles into the disc without puncturing the dura. The patient is placed on pure oxygen, and the nucleus pulposus is suctioned out until the desired decompression is accomplished. The needle is removed and the wound is dressed. The automated technique makes use of a probe that can simultaneously dissect the disc and suction it into the probe. Laser discectomy accomplishes the decompression by vaporizing the protruding disc. This code includes any epidural injections at the level being decompressed.

62290
This procedure is performed to gauge the amount of damage suffered by an intervertebral disc. The patient is placed on an image intensification table in a left lateral decubitus position with hips and knees are flexed. The injection site is determined and marked on the sterilized surface, and local anesthesia is injected. A small stab wound is made in the tissue overlying the vertebrae. The physician directs a needle at a 45 degree angle to the center line toward the spine. In a separately reported procedure, the needle is monitored radiographically. A small needle is inserted through original needle once the needle reaches the lamina. The physician pushes this needle to the disc and injects 1 ml to 2 ml of contrast medium. In separately reported procedures, radiographs are made and the procedure may be performed again on another level. The wound is dressed.

62291
This procedure is performed to gauge the amount of damage suffered by an intervertebral disc. The patient is placed on an image intensification table in a supine position with the head extended. The proper injection site is determined and marked on the sterilized surface, and local anesthesia is injected. A small stab wound is made in the tissue overlying the vertebrae. The physician directs a needle at a 35 degree angle to the sagittal plane toward the spine. In a separately reported procedure, the needle is monitored radiographically. A small needle is inserted through original needle once the needle reaches the lamina. The physician pushes this needle to the disc and injects 1 ml to 2 ml of contrast medium. In separately reported procedures, radiographs are made and the procedure may be performed again on another level. The wound is dressed.

62292
This procedure introduces a corrective chemical enzyme into a herniated disc. The patient is placed in a spinal tap position on the left side. In a separately reported procedure, an x-ray verifies location of the

Nervous

disc. Once the disc is located, local anesthesia is injected and a small stab wound is made. A spinal needle is inserted with additional monitoring of placement and injection of anesthesia. Without puncturing the dura, the physician inserts the needle into the disc. This procedure can be performed with one or two needles. A separately reportable saline acceptance test is performed to verify correct placement. Discography is performed with an opaque substance to verify location of the herniated disc. A reparative enzyme is injected. The needles are removed and the wound is dressed.

62294
This procedure is performed to locate and occlude an arteriovenous malformation (AVM) in the spinal cord. A separately reportable x-ray is used to position the patient and identify the artery to be injected. The physician directs a needle at the feeder arteries of the AVM and causes an occlusion by embolization. The needle is monitored radiographically. Once the occlusion of the AVM is completed and needle is removed, the wound is dressed.

62302-62305
In myelography, a radiographic study using fluoroscopy is performed on the spinal cord and nerve root branches when a lesion is suspected. The procedure is performed by placing a thin needle into the spinal canal into the space that contains the spinal nerves and spinal cord. The injection site is determined and marked on the sterilized surface and local anesthesia is injected. After the anesthetic is injected, the spinal needle is placed into the skin and using the fluoroscope for guidance, the needle is directed into the spinal canal. A nonionic, water-soluble, radiopaque contrast material is used to enhance visibility and is instilled through a lumbar area puncture into the subarachnoid space. The radiologist takes a series of pictures by sending an x-ray beam through the body, using fluoroscopy to view the enhanced structure on a television camera. The patient is angled from an erect position through a recumbent position with the body tilted so as to maintain feet higher than the head to help the flow of contrast into the study area. Report 62302 for myelography performed on a cervical vertebra; 62303 for a thoracic vertebra; 62304 for a lumbar vertebra; and 62305 for myelography of two or more regions performed during the same session (e.g., lumbar/thoracic, cervical/thoracic, lumbar/cervical, lumbar/thoracic/cervical). These codes include imaging supervision and interpretation.

62320-62321
The patient is placed in a sitting or lateral decubitus position for the physician to insert a needle into the vertebral interspace of the thoracic or cervical region. The site to be entered is sterilized, local anesthesia is administered, and the needle is inserted. The physician injects a solution (excluding a neurolytic substance) to provide a therapeutic or diagnostic outcome. The solution is injected into the interlaminar epidural or subarachnoid space. When the procedure is complete, the needle is removed and the wound is dressed. Report 62320 when this procedure is performed without imaging guidance and 62321 when imaging guidance is utilized.

62322-62323
The patient is placed in a sitting or lateral decubitus position for the physician to insert a needle into the vertebral interspace of the lumbar or sacral region. The site to be entered is sterilized, local anesthesia is administered, and the needle is inserted. The physician injects a solution (excluding neurolytic substance) to provide a therapeutic or diagnostic outcome. The solution is injected into the interlaminar epidural or subarachnoid space. When the procedure is complete, the needle is removed and the wound is dressed. Report 62322 when this procedure is performed without imaging guidance and 62323 when imaging guidance is utilized.

62324-62325
The patient is placed in the sitting or lateral decubitus position for the physician to insert a catheter into the vertebral interspace of the cervical or thoracic region for continuous or intermittent infusion of material. The site to be entered is sterilized, local anesthesia is administered, and the infusion catheter is inserted. The physician provides continuous infusion or intermittent bolus injection of solution to provide a therapeutic or diagnostic outcome. The solution is injected into the interlaminar epidural or subarachnoid space. When the procedure is complete, the catheter is removed and the wound is dressed. Report 62324 when this procedure is performed without imaging guidance and 62325 when imaging guidance is utilized.

62326-62327
The patient is placed in the sitting or lateral decubitus position for the physician to insert a catheter into the vertebral interspace of the lumbar or sacral region for continuous or intermittent infusion of material. The site to be entered is sterilized, local anesthesia is administered, and the infusion catheter is inserted. The physician provides continuous infusion or intermittent bolus injection of solution to provide a therapeutic or diagnostic outcome. The solution is injected into the interlaminar epidural or subarachnoid space. When the procedure is complete, the catheter is removed and the wound is dressed. Report 62326 when this procedure is performed without imaging guidance and 62327 when imaging guidance is utilized.

62350-62355
This procedure is performed to allow direct instillation of medication via the cerebrospinal fluid. If the catheter is to be implanted the patient is placed in a spinal tap position and the fascia, paravertebral muscles, and ligaments are incised and separated. The physician inserts the catheter tip into the epidural space (the space outside the dura) or through the dura placing the catheter tip into the subarachnoid space. Tissue around the catheter may be sutured to hold the catheter in place. The catheter end is tunneled to the site where an implantable reservoir or implantable infusion pump has been previously placed or where a

pump or reservoir is to be placed (subcutaneously) in a separately reportable procedure. This procedure also includes the revision of an intrathecal or epidural catheter, which may include replacing or repositioning a catheter. In 62351, the physician performs a laminectomy, making an incision and removing the lamina of the vertebra to access the dura through which the catheter is inserted. In 62355, the catheter is removed.

62360-62365
This procedure is performed to allow medication (e.g., cancer chemotherapy, pain management drugs) to be placed into a subcutaneous reservoir for intrathecal or epidural drug infusion. The physician makes a midline incision overlying the placement site. The reservoir is placed in the subcutaneous tissues and attached to a previously placed catheter. Layered sutures are used to close the incision. Report 62360 for subcutaneous reservoir implantation or replacement, 62361 for non-programmable pump implantation or replacement, 62362 for a programmable pump implantation or replacement, and 62365 for removal of the reservoir or pump.

62367-62370
The physician, physician's assistant, nurse, or physical therapist places electrodes over the site of a programmable pump and reviews performance of the generator on a computer. Report 62367 if the pump is not reprogrammed or refilled; 62368 if it is reprogrammed; 62369 if it is reprogrammed and refilled; and 62370 if it is reprogrammed, refilled, and requires a physician or other qualified health care professional's intervention.

62380
In endoscopic decompression surgery, also referred to as a laminectomy, the physician removes the bony roof covering the spinal cord and nerves in order to allow more space for the cord and nerves to move with greater ease. It can be performed from the neck (cervical) to the lower back (lumbar) of the spine. Using a very thin, two-dimensional, fiberoptic video camera, the physician can view images displayed on a monitor by the camera. The endoscope is inserted into a small incision and provides the physician with direct visualization of the spine structures and tissues and permits the passing of instruments through the scope to allow the physician to remove damaged disc material or bone spurs. Spinal decompression can be performed anywhere along the spine from the neck (cervical) to the lower back (lumbar). The physician makes a surgical incision in the back and removes the lamina, the bone that forms the backside of the spinal canal, and creates a cover over the spinal cord that provides more room for the nerves to move. Bone spurs may be removed, if present. This procedure includes laminotomy, partial facetectomy, foraminotomy discectomy, and/or excision of herniated intervertebral disc of the lumber area, when performed. The physician inserts a small guide probe under fluoroscopic guidance. Using magnified video, as well as fluoroscopic guidance, the endoscope is manipulated through the foramen and into the spinal canal. Once the guide probe has been advanced to the surgical site, a slightly larger tube is manipulated over the guide probe. Surgical instruments are advanced through the hollow center of the tube. Herniated disc fragments are removed, and the disc is reconfigured to eliminate pressure on the nerve roots. The endoscope is withdrawn. The incision is sutured or simply dressed with an adhesive bandage. Report this procedure when performed on one lumbar interspace.

63001-63011
The physician makes a posterior midline incision overlying the vertebrae. The paravertebral muscles are retracted. The physician removes the appropriate spinous process and interspinous ligament with a rongeur. The physician excises the lamina and the attached ligamentum flavum may be removed. Decompression is continued by removal of bony overgrowths or tissue until the dural sac and nerve roots are free from any compression. Free-fat grafts or Gelfoam may be placed over the exposed nerve roots. If the ligamentum flavum has not been removed or if only portions of it were removed, it may be closed over the fat graft. A drain is placed superficial to the fat graft; the fascia, subcutaneous tissue, and skin are closed in layers. Report 63003 if vertebrae are thoracic; report 63005 if vertebrae are lumbar, except in the case of spondylolisthesis; and report 63011 if vertebrae are sacral.

63012
The physician performs the laminectomy to correct spondylolisthesis, the slipping of the lumbar vertebrae forward where they join the sacral vertebrae. The physician makes a midline incision overlying the lumbar vertebrae to facilitate repair of the spondylolisthesis. The fascia are incised and the paravertebral muscles are retracted. The physician resects the spinous processes of all three vertebrae and the middle part of the loose fifth lumbar neural arch. The ligamentum flavum is freed or excised at various levels of vertebrae. The fifth lumbar nerve root is retracted. Decompression is carried out to include the facets as well as other bony or soft tissue structures that may be applying pressure to the spinal cord, nerve roots, or cauda equina. The procedure is repeated on the opposite side. The incision is closed with layered sutures.

63015-63017
The patient is face down and the physician makes a posterior midline incision overlying the vertebrae. The paravertebral muscles are retracted. A rongeur removes the appropriate spinous processes and interspinous ligaments. The physician excises the affected laminae and the attached ligamentum flavum may be removed. Decompression is continued by removal of bony overgrowths or tissue until the dural sac and nerve roots are free from compression. Free-fat grafts or Gelfoam may be placed over the exposed nerve roots. If the ligamentum flavum has not been removed or if only portions of it were removed it may be closed over the fat graft. A drain is placed superficial

to the fat graft; the fascia, subcutaneous tissue, and skin are closed in layers. Report 63015 if vertebrae are cervical; report 63016 if the laminae are thoracic; report 63017 if lumbar.

63020-63035

In one method, a midline incision is made through a posterior (back) approach overlying the vertebrae. The incision is carried down through the tissue to the paravertebral muscles, which are retracted. The ligamentum flavum, which attaches the lamina from one vertebra to the lamina of another, may be partially or completely removed. Part of the lamina is removed on one side to allow access to the spinal cord. If a disc has ruptured, fragments or the part of the disc compressing the nerves are removed. A partial removal of a facet (facetectomy) or removal of bone around the foramen (foraminotomy) may also be performed to relieve pressure on the nerve. When decompression is complete, a free-fat graft may be placed to protect the nerve root. If the ligamentum flavum was not removed, it is placed over the fat graft. Paravertebral muscles are repositioned and the tissue is closed in layers. Note that approaches represented by these codes may be open as described above or endoscopically assisted, which still requires open and direct visualization. In an endoscopically assisted approach, a small guide probe is inserted under fluoroscopic guidance. Using magnified video, as well as fluoroscopic guidance, the endoscope is manipulated through the foramen and into the spinal canal. Once the guide probe has been advanced to the surgical site, a slightly larger tube is manipulated over the guide probe. Surgical instruments are advanced through the hollow center of the tube. Herniated disc fragments are removed, and the disc is reconfigured to eliminate pressure on the nerve root(s). The endoscope is withdrawn. The incision is sutured or simply dressed with an adhesive bandage. Report 63020 if the disc is cervical; 63030 if lumbar; and 63035 for additional interspaces, cervical or lumbar.

63040-63044

Through a posterior approach, a midline incision is made overlying the vertebrae. The incision is carried through the tissue to the paravertebral muscles, which are retracted. If the ligamentum flavum (which attaches lamina from one vertebra to the lamina of another) is still present, it may be partially or completely removed. The lamina may be removed on the opposite side or more of the lamina may be removed from the previous site to allow access to the spinal cord. If ruptured intervertebral disc fragments or part of the disc continues to compress the nerve, they are removed. A partial removal of a facet or removal of bone around the foramen may also be performed if they are causing pressure on the nerve. When decompression is complete, a new or previously placed free-fat graft may be replaced over the nerve root. If the ligamentum flavum was not removed in the first surgery or in the exploration it is placed over the fat graft. Paravertebral muscles are repositioned and the tissue is closed in layers. Report 63040 if performed on a single cervical interspace; 63042 if performed on a single lumbar interspace; 63043 for each additional cervical interspace; and 63044 for each additional lumbar interspace.

63045-63048

The physician performs a unilateral or bilateral laminectomy, facetectomy, or foraminotomy of a vertebral segment with decompression of the spinal cord, cauda equina, and/or nerve roots to treat conditions such as spinal or lateral recess stenosis. The patient is face down. Magnification may be used during the procedure. The physician makes a midline incision overlying the affected vertebrae. Fascia is incised. Paravertebral muscles are retracted. The physician removes the spinous processes with rongeurs. If the stenosis is central, the physician removes the lamina out to the articular facets using a burr. If the compression is in the lateral recess, only half of the lamina is removed. A Penfield elevator peels the ligamentum flavum away from the dura. Nerve root canals are freed by additional resection of the facet, and compression is relieved by removal of any bony or tissue overgrowth around the foramen. Removal of the lamina, facets, and bony tissue or overgrowths may be performed bilaterally when indicated. The rongeur, retractor, and microscope are removed. A free-fat graft may be placed over the nerve root(s) for protection. If the ligamentum flavum was spared, it is placed over the free-fat graft. Paravertebral muscles are repositioned and the deeper tissues and skin are closed with layered sutures. Report 63046 if the procedure affects a thoracic vertebra report, 63047 if the procedure affects a lumbar vertebra, and 63048 for procedures affecting each additional vertebral segment.

[63052, 63053]

The physician performs a unilateral or bilateral laminectomy, facetectomy, or foraminotomy of the lumbar spine with decompression of the spinal cord, cauda equina, and/or nerve roots to treat conditions such as spinal or lateral recess stenosis. The procedure is performed in conjunction with posterior interbody fusion of the lumbar spine and is reported separately in addition to that procedure. Following appropriate anesthesia, the patient is positioned face down. Magnification may be used during the procedure. The physician makes a posterior midline incision overlying the affected lumbar vertebrae. Fascia is incised and paravertebral muscles are retracted. If performing a laminectomy, the physician removes the appropriate spinous processes with rongeurs. If the stenosis is central, the physician removes the lamina out to the articular facets using a burr. If the compression is in the lateral recess, only half of the lamina is removed. An elevator peels the ligamentum flavum away from the dura. Nerve root canals may be freed by additional resection of the facet, and compression may be relieved by removal of any bony or tissue overgrowth around the foramen. Removal of the lamina, facets, bony tissue, or overgrowths may be performed bilaterally when indicated. A free-fat graft may be placed over the nerve root(s) for protection. If the ligamentum flavum was spared, it may be placed over the free-fat graft. Report 63052 if the procedure is performed on a single vertebral segment; report 63053 for each additional segment.

63050-63051

Cervical laminoplasty with decompression of the spinal cord is performed to treat cases of myelopathy related to severe spinal stenosis that will not respond to conservative treatment. Intraoperative neurologic monitoring is used during the procedure. The head is immobilized. The surgeon makes an incision in the back of the neck over the target spinal area and dissects down through the soft tissues to access the spine. The spinous processes are exposed. A subperiosteal dissection is done to mobilize the muscles, taking care to preserve the ligaments. Foraminotomies may be done when foraminal stenosis or lateral disc herniation is present. A high-speed drill burr creates a gutter in the lamina on both an opening and closing side so the spinous processes may be opened like a door on a hinge. The cancellous bone and outer cortex are removed. An osteotomy is performed by lifting up on the opening side with a hook while displacing the processes to the opposite side. The laminae are opened like a door on a hinge to the side that displays the worst compression or signs of myeloradiculopathy. This opens the restriction and decompresses the previously pinched spinal cord. The hinge is held in place by small pieces of bone struts. Report 63051 when reconstruction of the posterior bony elements is performed. Fibular or tricortical iliac crest allografts are used. The prepared graft is notched and fitted into place in the "open door" position of the lamina. Titanium miniplates (or other fixation device) may be used to stabilize each level. The tissues are sutured back into place and a suction drain is placed.

63055-63057

These procedures are performed to relieve pressure on the spinal cord, equina, and nerve roots caused by a herniated disc. The physician approaches the herniated disc through the pedicle on the side of the disc's bulge. Additional exposure is made by removing the lamina and facet joint. The physician removes the disc fragments and closes the wound in layers. Report 63055 if the segment is thoracic. Report 63056 if the segment is lumbar. A far lateral herniated lumbar intervertebral disc may require an alternative approach through the facet joint (transfacet) or foramina (transforaminal). Report 63057 for each additional segment, thoracic or lumbar.

63064-63066

The physician makes an incision two inches to three inches lateral to the spine through fascia, muscles, and a section of a rib. The physician enters anterior to the transverse process and the pedicle using a Kerrington rongeur or burr. Exposure may be increased by removal of the transverse process. The spinal cord or nerve root is decompressed by removing the herniated disc. The wound is filled with saline and radiographs (separately reported) are made to assure no air is leading into the lungs. The muscles fall over a drain and the tissue is closed with layered sutures. Report 63064 if a single segment is repaired. Report 63066 for additional segments.

63075-63076

The physician performs a cervical discectomy to remove all or part of a herniated intervertebral disc. The patient is placed supine with a head halter on the jawbone (mandible). The physician makes a transverse incision overlying the intervertebral disc. The sternocleidomastoid muscle and the carotid artery are retracted. The physician excises the anterior anulus of the disc and uses pituitary forceps to remove as much disc material as possible. A spreader and microscope are used to enhance the evacuation. A drill is used to remove the transverse bar above and below. Graft material is obtained from the ilium and fashioned into a T-shape. The graft is placed into the disc space and traction is released. The muscles fall back into place and the incision is closed with layered sutures. Report 63075 if the discectomy is in a single interspace. Report 63076 for each additional cervical interspace.

63077-63078

The physician makes an incision along the rib corresponding to the second thoracic vertebra above the involved intervertebral disc, except in cases involving the top five discs. The rib is removed for access and eventually used in the graft, which is obtained through an extrapleural or transpleural approach. Vessels are tied away from the spine. The disc is removed to the posterior ligament using a microscope and nibbling instruments. The end plates are stripped of their cartilage. The physician makes a slot in one vertebral body and a hole in the other to accept the graft, which is made of several sections of rib. The physician ties the grafts together with heavy suture material and closes the tissue with layered sutures. A chest drain may be inserted. Report 63077 for a single thoracic interspace. Report 63078 for each additional thoracic interspace.

63081-63082

The patient is placed supine with traction-producing tongs. The physician makes a right transverse incision at mid-position of the planned surgical procedure, and longitudinally between the thyroid gland and the carotid sheath. The discs above and below the vertebrae are excised using a curette. Cartilaginous endplates are removed using a high-speed burr. The crushed part of the vertebral body is partially or completely removed, and the section is prepared for the graft. The anterior surfaces of the vertebrae above and below the fusion are debrided. The physician prepares a separately reportable, tricortical iliac graft and inserts it into the site, tapping it into place with an impactor. Traction is released. Bone chips are packed in and, if needed, a metal plate is screwed to the spine over the graft. The muscles fall back into place and the wound is closed with layered sutures. Report 63081 if one segment is involved and 63082 for each additional cervical segment.

Nervous

63085-63088

This procedure corrects compression on the spinal cord resulting from an anterior fracture of the vertebra. The patient is placed in a swimmer's position. The physician makes an incision through the fascia, muscles, and moves aside any organs. The discs above and below the vertebrae are excised using a curette. Cartilaginous endplates are removed using a high-speed burr. The crushed part of the vertebral body is partially or completely removed, and the section is prepared for the graft. The anterior surfaces of adjacent vertebrae are debrided. The physician prepares a tricortical iliac graft and inserts it into the site, tapping it into place with an impactor. Traction is released. Bone chips are packed in and, if needed, a metal plate is screwed to the spine over the graft. The muscles fall back into place and the wound is closed with layered sutures. Report 63085 if one thoracic segment is involved; 63086 if more than one is involved; 63087 if caudal equina, lower thoracic, or lumbar, single segment is involved; and 63088 for each additional segment.

63090-63091

The physician makes a transperitoneal or retroperitoneal approach through skin, fascia, muscles, and ligaments. The physician incises the anterior longitudinal ligament above and below the vertebral body. Using magnification, the physician removes the disc to the posterior longitudinal ligament using nipper instruments. The physician may use dowel or tricortical iliac grafts and prepares the site as appropriate using an osteotome. Usually three grafts can be inserted. They are tapped into place and surrounded with bone chips. The physician sutures the anterior longitudinal ligament. The peritoneum and abdomen are closed in the usual manner. Report 63090 for a single segment. Report 63091 for each additional segment.

63101-63103

A vertebral corpectomy with correction of spinal cord or nerve root compression is done for fractures or tumors of the vertebrae. The body of the vertebra may be partially or completely resected. The lateral extracavitary approach is done with a midline incision made in the area of the fractured segment and inferiorly curved out to the lateral plane. The paraspinous muscles are exposed, lifted off the spinous processes, and divided and lifted off the ribs. The targeted vertebral body is identified. The corresponding ribs are dissected from the intercostal muscles and the pleura and resected in one piece from the posterior curve to the costovertebral connection. The appropriate transverse process and part of the facet and pedicle are removed with a drill from the lateral aspect. The dura and the vertebral body are now exposed from the dorsolateral view. Further posterior and lateral access to the vertebral body is gained by gently retracting the nerve root and surrounding structures. The central portion of the vertebral body is removed with a drill, exposing more area, and any bone fragments or tumor masses are removed away from the spinal cord or nerve roots. Curettes and rongeurs are used to remove disc material. At this point, any necessary fusion, intervertebral reconstruction, or grafting is undertaken and reported separately. Cartilage is scraped, bone is decorticated, and an arthrodesis or reconstruction is accomplished by tapping bone graft material into the vertebral endplates. A drain is placed and closure is done in layers. Report 63101 for vertebral corpectomy by lateral extracavitary approach on a single thoracic segment, 63102 for a single lumbar segment, and 63103 for each additional thoracic or lumbar segment.

63170

This procedure is performed to alleviate peripheral pain caused by avulsion of parts of the spinal cord's white matter. The patient is face down. The physician makes a midline incision. The fascia are incised. The paravertebral muscles and ligaments are retracted. Following a laminectomy, the physician incises the dura to gain access to the spinal cord. Without disturbing the central grey matter, the physician incises the outer white matter of the spinal cord, using a laser or a radio frequency electrode to thermally coagulate the white matter. Fascia, muscles, and ligaments are allowed to fall back into place. The physician closes the incision with layered sutures.

63172-63173

This procedure is performed to alleviate the effects of a spinal cyst or syrinx. The patient is face down. The physician makes a midline incision overlying the affected vertebrae. The fascia are incised. The paravertebral muscles are retracted. Laminectomy is performed. The spinal needle is placed in the intramedullary cyst or syrinx, and the cyst or syrinx is drained to the subarachnoid space. Fascia, muscles, and ligaments are allowed to fall back into place. The incision is closed with layered sutures. Report 63172 if the drainage is to the subarachnoid space. Report 63173 if the drainage is to the peritoneal or pleural space.

63185-63190

A rhizotomy is performed on the anterior nerve roots to stop involuntary spasmodic movements associated with paraplegia or torticollis. It is also performed on the posterior nerve roots to eliminate pain in a restricted area. The patient is face down. The physician makes a midline incision overlying the affected vertebrae. The fascia are incised. The paravertebral muscles are retracted. Laminectomy is performed. The physician identifies the anterior or posterior nerve roots to be divided. Each is lifted with a nerve hook and severed. Fascia, muscles, and ligaments are allowed to fall back into place. The incision is closed with layered sutures. Report 63185 if the procedure includes one or two segments; report 63190 if the procedure includes two or more segments.

63191

This procedure is performed to alleviate chronic pain. The patient is face down. The physician makes a midline incision overlying the affected vertebrae. The fascia are incised. The paravertebral muscles are retracted. The physician removes the lamina. The physician identifies and incises the spinal accessory nerve. The lesion is removed and sutures are placed in the perineurium of the nerves. The sutures are approximated and tied. Fascia, muscles, and ligaments are allowed to fall back into place. The incision is closed with layered sutures.

63197

This procedure is performed to alleviate pain (typically refractory pain caused by cancer) by cutting the nerves of the spinal cord. The patient is face down. The physician makes a midline incision over the thoracic spine overlying the site of the planned cordotomy. The fascia is incised. The paravertebral muscles are retracted. A laminectomy is performed. The physician identifies the spinothalamic tracts in the appropriate levels. The dentate ligament is divided at the level of the cordotomy. The ligament is drawn posteriorly toward the midline to expose the anterolateral part of the cord. A cordotomy knife is introduced into the spinal cord anterior to the dentate ligament and directed toward the anterior spinal artery. The tissue in front of this artery is divided with the knife. The procedure is repeated on the other side. The incision is closed with layered sutures.

63200

This procedure is performed to correct neurological deficits in the lower extremities and sphincter dysfunctions caused by a spinal cord shortened by adhesions to the dura. The patient is face down. The physician makes a midline incision over the lumbar vertebrae. The fascia are incised. The paravertebral muscles are retracted. A laminectomy is performed. The physician may choose from a number of techniques, but generally requires a dural opening. A surgical microscope is used to dissect the adhesions and fibrous bands. The filum is identified and transected. Care is taken to avoid severing the nerves tangled with the adhesions. If no spina bifida or myelomeningocele is present, the dura is closed to make a "sac." Muscles, fascia, and ligaments are closed. The incision is closed with a layered sutures.

63250-63252

This procedure is performed for excision or purposeful occlusion of an arteriovenous malformation (AVM) of the spinal cord. The patient is face down. The physician makes an incision overlying the cervical vertebra in the area of the AVM. The fascia and paraspinal muscles are retracted and a laminectomy is performed to access the spinal cord. Microsurgical techniques are used to excise or occlude the AVM. After muscles, fascia, and ligaments are repaired, the incision is closed with layered sutures. Report 63251 if thoracic; report 63252 if thoracolumbar.

63265-63268

This procedure removes a growth in the spine. The patient is face down. The physician makes a midline incision. Fascia are incised. Paravertebral muscles are retracted. The physician removes the laminae and the spinous processes of the vertebrae to expose the outside of the dura. The extradural intraspinal lesion is excised or evacuated. The incision is closed with layered sutures. Report 63265 if the lesion is in the cervical region; report 63266 if the lesion is in the thoracic region; report 63267 if the lesion is in the lumbar region. Report 63268 if the lesion is in the sacral region.

63270-63273

This procedure removes a growth in the spine. The patient is face down. The physician makes a midline incision. The fascia are incised. The paravertebral muscles are retracted. The physician removes the laminae and the spinous processes of the vertebrae to be exposed. The dura is exposed and incised. The pia-arachnoid is incised as necessary. The lesion is removed. The incision is closed with layered sutures. Report 63270 if the lesion is located in the cervical region; report 63271 if the lesion is in the thoracic region; report 63272 if the lesion is in the lumbar region; report 63273 if the lesion is in the sacral region.

63275-63278

The patient is face down. The physician makes a midline incision. Fascia are incised. Paravertebral muscles are retracted. The physician removes the laminae and the spinous processes of the vertebrae to the dura. A biopsy is taken of the neoplasm and the neoplasm is removed. Muscles, fascia, and ligaments are repaired. The incision is closed with layered sutures. Report 63275 if the neoplasm is in the cervical area; report 63276 if it is in the thoracic area; report 63277 if it is in the lumbar area; and report 63278 if it is in the sacral area.

63280

This procedure is performed to remove a growth in the spine. The patient is face down. The physician makes a midline incision. Fascia are incised. Paravertebral muscles are retracted. The physician removes the laminae and the spinous processes of the vertebrae to be exposed. The dura is exposed and incised. The neoplasm is identified and a biopsy is taken. The neoplasm is removed. The dura is sutured with silk sutures, and the incision is closed with layered sutures.

63281

The patient is face down. The physician makes a midline incision. Fascia are incised. Paravertebral muscles are retracted. The physician removes the laminae and the spinous processes of the vertebrae to be exposed. The dura is exposed and incised. The neoplasm is identified and a biopsy is taken. The neoplasm is removed. The dura is sutured with silk sutures, and the incision is closed with layered sutures.

63282

This procedure is performed to remove a growth in the spine. The patient is face down. The physician makes a midline incision. Fascia are incised. Paravertebral muscles are retracted. The physician removes the laminae and the spinous processes of the vertebrae to be exposed. The dura is exposed and incised. The neoplasm is identified and a biopsy is taken. The neoplasm is removed. The dura is sutured with silk sutures, and the incision is closed with layered sutures.

63283
This procedure is performed to remove a growth in the spine. The patient is face down. The physician makes a midline incision. Fascia are incised. Paravertebral muscles are retracted. The physician removes the laminae and the spinous processes of the vertebrae to be exposed. The dura is exposed and incised. The neoplasm is identified and a biopsy is taken. The neoplasm is removed. The dura is sutured with silk sutures, and the incision is closed with layered sutures.

63285
This procedure is performed to remove a growth in the spine. The patient is face down. The physician makes a midline incision. Fascia are incised. Paravertebral muscles are retracted. The physician removes the laminae and the spinous processes of the vertebrae to be exposed. The dura is exposed and incised. The neoplasm is identified and a biopsy is taken. The neoplasm is removed. The dura is sutured with silk sutures, and the incision is closed with layered sutures.

63286
This procedure is performed to remove a growth in the spine. The patient is face down. The physician makes a midline incision. Fascia are incised. Paravertebral muscles are retracted. The physician removes the laminae and the spinous processes of the vertebrae to be exposed. The dura is exposed and incised. The neoplasm is identified and a biopsy is taken. The neoplasm is removed. The dura is sutured with silk sutures, and the incision is closed with layered sutures.

63287
This procedure is performed to remove a growth in the spine. The patient is face down. The physician makes a midline incision. Fascia are incised. Paravertebral muscles are retracted. The physician removes the laminae and the spinous processes of the vertebrae to be exposed. The dura is exposed and incised. The neoplasm is identified and a biopsy is taken. The neoplasm is removed. The dura is sutured with silk sutures, and the incision is closed with layered sutures.

63290
This procedure is performed to remove a growth in the spine. The patient is face down. The physician makes a midline incision. Fascia are incised. Paravertebral muscles are retracted. The physician removes the laminae and the spinous processes of the vertebrae to be exposed. The dura is exposed and incised. The neoplasm is identified and a biopsy is taken. The neoplasm is removed. The dura is sutured with silk sutures, and the incision is closed with layered sutures.

63295
The physician performs an osteoplastic reconstruction of the dorsal spine elements at the time of a separate intraspinal procedure. Osteoplastic reconstruction is performed to stabilize elements in the spine that have been damaged by benign or malignant lesions or by disease processes. Following the intraspinal procedure, the dura is closed. Dorsal spinal elements including laminae, spinous processes and supporting ligaments are replaced in anatomic position in the spine. Holes are drilled into the lateral aspect of each lamina and the dorsal spine elements are secured in place using sutures, wires, or miniplates.

63300
This procedure is performed to remove an intraspinal lesion in the extradural space of the spinal canal. The patient is placed supine with the head extended by tongs and traction. A right transverse incision or right vertical incision is made in the lateral neck. The muscles and fascia are incised and retracted. Entering between the trachea and the carotid sheath, the physician resects the vertebral body and the intraspinal lesion is excised by the physician. After repair of the muscles, fascia, and ligaments, the wound closed with layered sutures.

63301
This procedure is performed to remove a lesion from a vertebra. The patient is placed in a lateral decubitus position and the physician makes a transthoracic approach overlying the rib corresponding to the affected vertebrae. The physician removes the rib and retracts muscles, fascia, and organs to expose the spine. The tumor mass is completely excised. Following repair of the muscles, fascia, and ligaments, the wound is closed in a routine fashion over suction drains.

63302
This procedure is performed to remove a lesion of the vertebral body, which compresses the spinal cord. The patient is placed in a lateral decubitus position with supports under the buttocks and shoulder, and the muscle, fascia, ribs, and organs are incised or retracted. An incision is made in the diaphragm to purchase access to the spine. The tumor mass is completely excised. After muscles, fascia, and ligaments are repaired, the wound is closed in a routine fashion over suction drains.

63303
This procedure is performed to remove a lesion of the vertebral body, which compresses the spinal cord. The patient is placed in a lateral decubitus position with approach from the left side, and the muscle, fascia, ribs, and organs are incised or retracted. The physician makes a groove in the vertebral bodies above and below the crushed vertebra and removes the discs above and below. Tricortical iliac crest grafts are obtained, prepared, and tapped into the grooves with a Moe impactor. An AO plate is screwed to the vertebra above and below the injured level to maintain fusion. A separately reported radiograph is obtained to assure proper placement, and the wound closed with layered sutures.

63304
This procedure is performed to correct a fracture or growth of the vertebral body, which compresses the spinal cord. The patient is placed supine with the head

extended by tongs and traction. A right transverse incision or right vertical incision is made in the lateral neck. The muscles and fascia are incised and retracted. The dura may be incised. Entering between the trachea and the carotid sheath, the physician makes a groove in the vertebral bodies above and below the crushed vertebra and removes the discs above and below. Tricortical iliac crest grafts are obtained, prepared, and tapped into the grooves with a Moe impactor. Traction is removed. An AO plate is screwed to the vertebra above and below the injured level to maintain fusion. A separately reported radiograph is obtained to assure proper placement, and the wound closed with layered sutures.

63305

This procedure is performed to correct a fracture or growth of the vertebral body, which compresses the spinal cord. The patient is placed in a lateral decubitus position and the muscle, fascia, ribs, and organs are incised or retracted. The dura may be incised. The physician makes a groove in the vertebral bodies above and below the crushed vertebra and removes the discs above and below. Tricortical iliac crest grafts are obtained, prepared, and tapped into the grooves with a Moe impactor. An AO plate is screwed to the vertebra above and below the injured level to maintain fusion. A separately reported radiograph is obtained to assure proper placement, and the wound closed with layered sutures.

63306

This procedure is performed to remove a lesion of the vertebral body, which compresses the spinal cord. The patient is placed in a lateral decubitus position with supports under the buttocks and shoulder, and the muscle, fascia, ribs, and organs are incised or retracted. The dura may be incised. An incision is made in the diaphragm to purchase access to the spine. The physician makes a groove in the vertebral bodies above and below the crushed vertebra and removes the discs above and below. Tricortical iliac crest grafts are obtained, prepared, and tapped into the grooves with a Moe impactor. An AO plate is screwed to the vertebra above and below the injured level to maintain fusion. A separately reported radiograph is obtained to assure proper placement, and the wound closed with layered sutures.

63307

This procedure is performed to remove a lesion of the vertebral body, which compresses the spinal cord. The patient is placed in a lateral decubitus position with approach from the left side, and the muscle, fascia, ribs, and organs are incised or retracted. The dura may be incised. The physician makes a groove in the vertebral bodies above and below the crushed vertebra and removes the discs above and below. Tricortical iliac crest grafts are obtained, prepared, and tapped into the grooves with a Moe impactor. An AO plate is screwed to the vertebra above and below the injured level to maintain fusion. A separately reported radiograph is obtained to assure proper placement, and the wound closed with layered sutures.

63308

This procedure is performed to remove a lesion of the vertebral body, which compresses the spinal cord. The patient is placed in a lateral decubitus position with approach from the left side, and the muscle, fascia, ribs, and organs are incised or retracted. The physician makes a groove in the vertebral bodies above and below the crushed vertebra and removes the discs above and below. Tricortical iliac crest grafts are obtained, prepared, and tapped into the grooves with a Moe impactor. An AO plate is screwed to the vertebra above and below the injured level to maintain fusion. A separately reported radiograph is obtained to assure proper placement, and the wound closed with layered sutures.

63600-63610

Lesions in the spinal cord are produced to alleviate chronic pain in a particular area of the body. A common surgery involves creating a lesion in the spinothalamic tracts for pain relief. In this procedure, a stereotactic guidance system is used to enable a physician to conceptualize a position in three-dimensional space. The stereotactic frame is applied to the head with full neck flexion and fixed to the operating table with the patient in the sitting position. Following previously determined coordinates, needles are placed through the C1-C2 interspace. Electrical stimulation and other methods are applied to create a lesion that blocks the pain. The needles and the frame are removed. Wounds are dressed. Report 63610 if percutaneous stereotactic stimulation of the spinal cord is performed as a separate procedure, not followed by other surgery.

63620-63621

High-resolution stereotactic imaging identifies a precise, three-dimensional location of the spinal lesion. The physician uses the coordinates obtained from the images to focus linear accelerator, gamma ray, or particle beam energy onto the lesion, thereby destroying or inactivating it. This is a noninvasive procedure that does not require incision into the spine. Report 63620 (no more than once per course of treatment) for stereotactic radiosurgery on a single spinal lesion. Report 63621 for each additional spinal lesion; however, 63621 should not be reported more than two times for the entire course of treatment regardless of the number of lesions treated and may be reported only once per lesion. Codes for spinal stereotactic radiosurgery are reported by the surgeon and include any required computer-assisted planning, dosimetry, targeting, positioning, or blocking. These codes are assigned only when the treated tumors affect spinal neural tissue or lie alongside the dura mater.

63650

This procedure is performed to alleviate pain or control spasms. The patient is face down. A standard epidural puncture is made. A thin-walled needle is placed at the appropriate segment. A flexible wire electrode is threaded through the needle under fluoroscopic control. Intraoperative testing is carried out to assure correct electrode positioning creating maximum paresthesia in the pain region. The needle is removed and a dressing applied. A transmitter (pulse generator or receiver) is inserted in a separately reportable procedure. Stimulation may be applied as soon as four days following the procedure.

63655
This procedure is performed to alleviate pain or control spasms. The patient is face down. The physician makes a midline incision overlying the affected vertebrae. The fascia are incised. The paravertebral muscles are retracted. The lamina is removed to expose the epidural space. The physician places passive electrodes or plates or paddles in the epidural space proximate to the desired spine segment. Paravertebral muscles are reapproximated and the incision is closed with layered sutures. A transmitter (pulse generator or receiver) is inserted in a separately reportable procedure. Stimulation may be applied as soon as four days following the procedures.

63661-63662
The physician removes spinal neurostimulator electrode percutaneous arrays (63661) or spinal neurostimulator plates or paddles that were placed via laminotomy or laminectomy (63662). The patient is face down (prone). The physician makes a midline incision overlying the affected vertebrae. The fascia is incised. The paravertebral muscles are retracted. The physician removes the electrode plates or paddles in the epidural space proximate to the spine segment. Stimulation is applied. These codes include the use of fluoroscopic guidance, when performed.

63663-63664
The physician revises neurostimulator electrode percutaneous arrays or neurostimulator electrode plates or paddles that were placed via laminotomy or laminectomy. Replacement of these devices may also be performed. The patient is face down (prone). The physician makes a midline incision overlying the affected vertebrae. The fascia is incised. The paravertebral muscles are retracted. The physician revises the electrodes or plates or paddles in the epidural space proximate to the spine segment or moves them to a new vertebral segment. Stimulation is applied. These codes include fluoroscopic guidance, when performed. Report 63663 when the original electrodes were placed percutaneously. Report 63664 when the electrodes were originally placed via laminotomy or laminectomy or if a laminectomy is performed to gain access to the epidural space in the event of movement to a new segment.

63685-63688
The physician inserts or replaces a spinal neurostimulator pulse generator or receiver into a subcutaneous pocket in 63685. The physician selects a location site, usually the abdominal area, and incises the skin. Using blunt dissection, a pocket is created for the generator or receiver. In the case of a replacement, the old generator or receiver is removed from an existing pocket. A previously placed electrode array, which is separately implanted and normally positioned in a dural/epidural pocket over the spinal cord of the affected vertebral area, is tunneled under the skin to the neurostimulator pocket and connected to the unit. After ensuring that the device is functioning, the generator or receiver is sutured into place within its subcutaneous pocket. Layered sutures are used to close the incision. In 63688, the physician revises or removes the spinal neurostimulator pulse generator or receiver. A midline incision is made overlying the affected vertebrae. The fascia is incised. The paravertebral muscles are retracted. The physician detaches the connection to the electrode array. The generator or receiver is revised or removed. In the case of a revision, the electrode array is reconnected to the unit after the revision is complete. Layered sutures are used to close the incision.

63700-63702
The physician corrects a defect in which the outer coverings of the spinal cord, meninges, and (sometimes) nervous tissue bulge through a bony defect. The patient is face down, and the physician makes a midline incision and retraction through the skin, muscles, and paravertebral ligaments. The dura is incised to avoid herniated neural tissue. The physician places the neural tissue in the spinal canal. In the lumbar region, filum terminale are often identified tethering the cord and divided. The dural defect, subcutaneous tissues, and skin are closed with layered sutures. Report 63700 for meningoceles less than 5 cm diameter; report 63702 for meningoceles greater than 5 cm.

63704-63706
The physician corrects a defect in which the spinal cord, malformed nerve roots, and meninges all protrude through the defect, often directly exposed to the outside of the body. Surgery can be performed in one of many ways, though most require fusion from the thoracic region to the sacrum. The physician places the patient prone and incises the defect to the subarachnoid space. Using a microscope, the edges of the neural placode are trimmed of skin, dural remnants, and fat. The lateral edges of the placode are sutured together to form a tube. The dura is incised and closed. Skin is closed with sutures. Report 63704 if the myelomeningocele is less than 5 cm in diameter; report 63706 if the defect is more than 5 cm in diameter.

63707-63709
This procedure is performed to mend an opening in the dura, preventing a dangerous infection. The patient is face down, and the physician makes a midline incision, retracting the skin, muscles, and paravertebral ligaments. The physician removes and prepares a graft of subcutaneous fat, freeze-dried dura, fascia, or muscle. Suction is used to keep the incision free of cerebrospinal fluid. Single dural stitches are used to achieve closure. A second needle is attached to the free suture ends and the needles are passed through the graft, which is tied down over the outside

of the repaired tear to achieve watertight closure. If the dural defect is small and difficult to access, the graft can be placed inside the dura. After verifying that the repair is watertight, the physician proceeds with closure. Report 63709 if a laminectomy is required to correct a dural/cerebrospinal fluid leak or pseudomeningocele.

63710
At the end of a procedure where the dura has been incised, the physician sometimes prepares a graft of subcutaneous fat, freeze-dried dura, fascia, or muscle. Suction is used to keep the incision free of cerebral spinal fluid. Single dural stitches are used to achieve closure. A second needle is attached to the free suture ends and the needles are passed through the graft, which is tied down outside of the repaired tear to achieve watertight closure. If the dural defect is small and difficult to access, the graft can be placed inside the dura. After verifying that the repair is watertight, the physician proceeds with closure.

63740-63741
This procedure drains excess cerebral spinal fluid that may cause hydrocephalus. The patient is placed in a spinal tap position and the fascia, paravertebral muscles, and ligaments are incised and separated. The physician removes the lamina, inserting the shunt through the dura into the subarachnoid space. The shunt is passed around the flank to the peritoneal, pleural, or other space for drainage. The incisions are closed with layered sutures. Report 63740 if a laminectomy is needed to place the shunt. Report 63741 if the shunt is placed without excising the lamina.

63744
The physician makes an incision at the site of the original incision. Scar tissue, colloidal tissues, and adhesions are removed. The physician may irrigate the shunt with saline or other substances. If it is malfunctioning, the shunt is freed and replaced. A new shunt is placed in the site. Incisions are closed using layered sutures.

63746
The physician makes an incision at the site of the original incision. Scar tissue, colloidal tissues, and adhesions are removed. The shunt is freed and removed. Incisions are closed using layered sutures.

64400-64405
The physician injects one or more anesthetic agents and/or steroids near a branch of the trigeminal nerve (ophthalmic, maxillary, or mandibular) in 64400 or the greater occipital nerve in 64405. The trigeminal nerve supplies sensory and motor fibers to the face, and is usually blocked superficially. The greater occipital nerve supplies sensory fibers to the scalp; nerve blocks are often administered to provide relief from occipital neuralgia, migraines, and chronic headaches. The physician draws a local anesthetic and/or steroid into a syringe and injects it into the targeted area near the affected nerve.

64408
The physician injects one or more anesthetic agents and/or steroids near the vagus nerve. The vagus nerve supplies sensory fibers to the pharynx and glottis, and carries parasympathetic fibers to the digestive system and heart. The physician draws a local anesthetic and/or steroid into a syringe and injects it into the targeted area near the nerve.

64415-64416
The physician injects one or more anesthetic agents and/or steroids near the brachial plexus to relieve pain and inflammation in 64415. The physician draws a local anesthetic and/or steroid into a syringe and injects it into a targeted area near the brachial plexus, approached in one of several locations: interscalene, superior trunk, supraclavicular, infraclavicular, or axillary. In 64416, continuous infusion of local anesthetic and/or steroid through a catheter is done to provide a nerve block lasting longer than the block effect achieved through a single injection. An indwelling catheter is placed and positioned to provide anesthesia to the brachial plexus. An infusion pump is connected to the catheter to supply a continuous flow of infused agent at a set rate. The infusion system may be used for regional surgical anesthesia when general anesthesia is not required and for postoperative pain management. Catheter placement is included in 64416 and is not reported separately. Imaging guidance and any contrast injection, when performed, is included in both codes.

64417
The physician injects one or more anesthetic agents and/or steroids near the axillary nerve to relieve pain and inflammation to the shoulder. The physician draws a local anesthetic and/or steroid into a syringe and injects the agent into the targeted area near the axillary nerve. Imaging guidance is included, when performed.

64418
The physician injects one or more anesthetic agents and/or steroids into the targeted area near the suprascapular nerve to provide postoperative relief of pain and inflammation to the shoulder or to diagnose and treat pain caused by chronic shoulder conditions such as bursitis, degenerative disease, rotator cuff disorders, or various forms of arthritis. This nerve innervates the supraspinatus and infraspinatus muscles and also provides sensory innervation to the acromioclavicular and glenohumeral joints, the coracohumeral ligament, the subacromial bursa, and the scapula. The injection may also be used to relax the supraspinatus and infraspinatus muscles and differentiate between brachial plexus-mediated or C5- or C6-mediated pain. The physician draws a local anesthetic and/or steroid into a syringe and injects it into the targeted area near the suprascapular nerve.

64420-64421
The physician injects one or more anesthetic agents and/or steroids near the intercostal nerves, which are located underneath the ribs, to alleviate pain and

inflammation often caused by a herpes zoster infection (shingles) or a surgical incision. In 64420, a single level is injected. Report 64421 for each additional level injected.

64425

The physician injects one or more anesthetic agents and/or steroids near the ilioinguinal and iliohypogastric nerves to block the inguinal area and lower abdomen for control of pain and inflammation, often following inguinal hernia repair. These nerves provide sensory innervation to the skin of the lower abdominal wall, as well as the upper hip/thigh. The physician draws an anesthetic agent and/or steroid into a syringe and injects it in a fan-like manner medial to the hip bone toward the umbilicus.

64430-64435

In 64430, the physician injects one or more anesthetic agents and/or steroids near the pudendal nerve, which provides the majority of sensation to the perineum, rectum, urethra, and parts of the bladder and genitals. The injection may be administered for control of pain and inflammation or for diagnosis of patients with suspected pudendal neuralgia. The physician draws a local anesthetic and/or steroid into a syringe and injects it into the targeted area near the affected nerve. In 64435, the area around the cervix is injected to supply pain control during labor or surgical abortions.

64445-64446

The physician injects one or more anesthetic agents and/or steroids near the sciatic nerve to control pain and inflammation in the distal lower extremity in 64445. It may also be utilized diagnostically to determine the anatomy of pain in this area. The physician draws an anesthetic agent and/or steroid into a syringe and injects it into a targeted area near the sciatic nerve. In 64446, continuous infusion through a catheter is done to provide a nerve block lasting longer than a single injection. An indwelling catheter is placed and positioned. An infusion pump is connected to the catheter to supply a continuous flow of the infused agent at a set rate. The infusion system may be used for regional surgical anesthesia when general anesthesia is not required and for postoperative pain management. Catheter placement is included in 64446 and is not reported separately. Imaging guidance and any contrast injection, when performed, is included in both codes.

64447-64448

The physician injects one or more anesthetic agents and/or steroids near the femoral nerve to control pain and inflammation of the lower extremity in 64447. The injection may also be indicated for diagnosis and treatment of meralgia paresthetica. The physician draws an anesthetic agent and/or steroid into a syringe and injects it into a targeted area near the femoral nerve. In 64448, continuous infusion through a catheter is done to provide a nerve block lasting longer than a single injection. An indwelling catheter is placed and positioned. An infusion pump is connected to the catheter to supply a continuous flow of the infused agent at a set rate. The infusion system may be used for regional surgical anesthesia when general anesthesia is not required and for postoperative pain management. These codes include imaging guidance, when performed.

64449

The physician performs a nerve block, posterior approach, on the lumbar plexus by infusing one or more anesthetic agents and/or steroids through a catheter placed for daily management of pain and administration of anesthesia. The lumbar plexus is formed from the nerve branches in the psoas major muscle: the ilioinguinal, obturator, iliohypogastric, lateral femoral cutaneous, genitofemoral, and the femoral nerves. IV sedatives and analgesics are set up. With the patient in the right lateral decubitus position, the insertion point for the needle is marked. A local anesthetic is given. The needle is advanced toward the lumbar plexus, avoiding any transverse processes of the lumbar vertebrae until it is in proper position within the compartment of the psoas muscle, and stimulation of the plexus is seen by the contraction of certain muscles. Blood and cerebral spinal fluid is aspirated. After determining that the needle is in the correct position and that the injection will not go intravenously or intrathecally, local anesthesia is injected through the needle, and an infusion catheter is fed through the needle past the tip. Catheter placement is also checked, the catheter is secured in place, and continuous infusion is begun.

64450

The physician injects one or more anesthetic agents and/or steroids near an affected peripheral nerve or branch to control pain and inflammation or to aid in diagnosis and treatment. The physician draws an anesthetic agent and/or steroid into a syringe and injects it into the targeted area. This code is used to report nerve blocks of other nerves not specifically listed in this section.

64451

The physician injects one or more anesthetic agents and/or steroids near the nerves innervating the sacroiliac (SI) joint, including lateral branch blocks. Utilizing image guidance (computed tomography or fluoroscopy), the physician locates the target area and the insertion point for the needle is marked. The physician draws an anesthetic agent and/or steroid into a syringe and injects it into the targeted area. This procedure may be performed for control of pain and inflammation or as a diagnostic aid in determining whether the patient would benefit from radiofrequency nerve ablation in order to provide longer lasting relief of pain associated with SI joint dysfunction.

64454

Articular branches of various nerves (common peroneal, femoral, obturator, saphenous, and tibial) innervate the knee joint. These branches around the knee joint are known as genicular nerves. The physician injects one or more anesthetic agents and/or steroids near the genicular nerve branches to control pain and inflammation of the knee. The physician determines the target area using anatomic landmarks or image guidance, draws an anesthetic agent and/or steroid into a syringe, and injects it into the targeted area near the genicular nerves.

64455

The physician injects a local anesthetic agent and/or steroid into a plantar common digital nerve from the dorsal direction. This procedure is often performed to treat Morton's neuroma, a frequently occurring injury of the forefoot that affects the third web space of the toes. This code reports single or multiple injections.

64479-64484

The physician injects an anesthetic agent and/or a long-acting corticosteroid into the epidural space using a transforaminal approach. The patient, who is sedated but awake through the intervention, is placed prone on the procedure table and the injection site sterilized with iodine or chlorhexidine. A small-gauge blunt needle is inserted through the skin and into the epidural space through the bony opening of the exiting nerve root. This approach is used primarily in the treatment of herniated discs and foraminal stenosis and requires imaging guidance by fluoroscopy or CT. The injection may be performed on one or more levels. Report 64479 for a single cervical or thoracic level (including the T12-L1 level) and 64480 for each additional level. Report 64483 for a single lumbar or sacral level and 64484 for each additional level.

[64461, 64462, 64463]

The physician injects anesthetic into the paravertebral space achieving an ipsilateral nerve block. The patient is sitting or lying with knees brought up to the chest allowing for more room between the transverse processes and proper needle placement. The transverse process is usually found when the needle is inserted about 3 cm to 6 cm. Once located, the needle is pulled back to the skin level and redirected to "walk off" the transverse process. The goal is to inject at 1 cm beyond the transverse process. This procedure is typically used in patients undergoing mastectomy, cosmetic breast procedures, thoracic surgery, and/or for patients with rib fractures. Report 64461 for a single injection site; 64462 for the second and any additional injection sites; and 64463 when continuous infusion by catheter is required.

[64466, 64467, 64468, 64469]

The physician administers a thoracic fascial plane block, often to provide postoperative pain control and to minimize the need for opioids. After the targeted area on the thoracic region is prepped and draped, an ultrasound transducer is placed. Under continuous ultrasound guidance, the layers of the thoracic wall are identified, and appropriate needle location is visualized and confirmed. Following identification of pertinent anatomic structures, the physician advances the needle to the tissue plane located between the pectoralis major and minor muscles and injects a local anesthetic, either unilaterally (64466) or bilaterally (64468). Alternatively, a placement needle may be inserted deep to the erector spinae muscle, a catheter inserted through the placement needle, and the needle subsequently removed. The physician secures the catheter and places a sterile occlusive dressing. Local anesthetic is administered by continuous infusion unilaterally (64467) or bilaterally (64469) into the fascial plane.

[64473, 64474]

The physician administers a lower extremity fascial plane block, often to provide postoperative pain control and to minimize the need for opioids. After the targeted area on the lower extremity region is prepped and draped, an ultrasound transducer is placed. In one technique, the correct tissue plane for a fascia iliaca block is identified and appropriate needle location is visualized and confirmed using continuous ultrasound guidance. Following identification of the pertinent anatomic structures, the physician inserts a needle between the fascia iliaca and iliacus muscle and injects a local anesthetic in 64473. Alternatively, a placement needle may be inserted between the fascia iliaca and iliacus muscle, a catheter inserted through the placement needle, and the needle subsequently removed. The physician secures the catheter and places a sterile occlusive dressing. Local anesthetic is administered by continuous infusion unilaterally into the fascial plane; this is reported with 64474.

64486-64489

The transversus abdominis plane (TAP) block is a relatively new regional anesthesia technique with a high margin of safety and is technically simple to perform. The physician injects a local anesthetic in the space between the aponeurosis of the internal oblique and transversus abdominis muscles to anesthetize the nerves that supply the anterior abdominal wall (T6–L1) for postoperative pain control in a wide variety of abdominal procedures, including large bowel resection, open/laparoscopic appendectomy, cesarean section, total abdominal hysterectomy, laparoscopic cholecystectomy, open prostatectomy, renal transplant surgery, abdominoplasty with/without flank liposuction, iliac crest bone graft, and inguinal hernia repairs. This technique is also useful for procedures in which epidural analgesia is contraindicated (e.g., anticoagulated patients). For prolonged analgesia, continuous infusions via a catheter may also be performed. Imaging guidance, when performed, is included in these services. Report 64486 for a unilateral TAP, by injection; 64487 for a unilateral TAP, continuous infusion; 64488 for a bilateral TAP, by injection; and 64489 for a bilateral TAP, continuous infusion.

64490-64492

The physician injects a diagnostic or therapeutic agent into a cervical or thoracic paravertebral facet joint or into the nerves that innervate the joint using fluoroscopic or CT guidance. The paravertebral facet joints, also called zygapophyseal or "Z" joints, consist of the bony surfaces between the vertebrae that articulate with each other. The injection may be performed on a single level or on multiple levels. Report 64490 for a single level, 64491 for a second level, and 64492 for the third and any additional levels.

64493-64495
The physician injects a diagnostic or therapeutic agent into a lumbar or sacral paravertebral facet joint or into the nerves that innervate the joint using fluoroscopic or CT guidance. The paravertebral facet joints, also called zygapophyseal or "Z" joints, consist of the bony surfaces between the vertebrae that articulate with each other. The injection may be performed on a single level or on multiple levels. Report 64493 for a single level, 64494 for a second level, and 64495 for the third and any additional levels.

64505
The physician injects the sphenopalatine ganglion nerve with an anesthetic agent to provide anesthesia to the nasal mucosa. The anesthesia is applied by entering through the nares and injecting local anesthetic posterior to the middle turbinate.

64510
The physician performs a nerve block on the stellate ganglion, (also known as the cervicothoracic ganglion) by injecting an anesthetic agent to block sympathetically mediated pain. The stellate ganglion is located at the C7/T1 level vertebrae; its fibers distribute to the head, neck, heart, and upper limb. This block is used to provide anesthetic relief for pain in the face, neck, and upper extremity. Using fluoroscopic imaging, the physician guides the needle into correct placement in the ganglion and injects the nerve block agent .Imaging guidance may be considered an included service by CMS and other payers

64517
The physician performs a nerve block on the superior hypogastric plexus by injecting an anesthetic agent through a needle inserted in the L5/S1 interspace. The superior hypogastric plexus, also called the presacral nerve, is located in front of the upper part of the sacrum and is formed by lower lumbar nerves responsible for pain sensation in the pelvic area. This nerve block is done in such cases as severe, intractable menstrual pain and pain due to pelvic area metastases from cancer such as prostatic malignancy. The patient is placed in the prone position and prepped. A 6-inch needle is guided under radiological imaging, such as fluoroscopy (reported separately), into the ventral lateral spine and through the L5/S1 interspace. Needle position is checked by injecting contrast material and aspirating for the return of any blood, urine, or cerebral spinal fluid. With negative aspiration results and imaging verifying that the needle position is in the prevertebral space and not within a blood vessel, a ureter, or spinal nerves, local anesthetic is injected on both sides.

64520
The physician performs a nerve block on lumbar or thoracic paravertebral sympathetic nerves by injecting an anesthetic agent to block sympathetically mediated pain. The lumbar or thoracic block provides anesthetic relief for pain in the torso, pelvis, and lower extremities. Using fluoroscopic imaging, the physician guides the needle into correct placement into the paravertebral sympathetic nerve fibers and injects the nerve block agent .Imaging guidance may be considered an included service by CMS and other payers

64530
The physician injects the celiac plexus with an anesthetic to block sympathetically mediated or visceral pain. Anesthesia is provided with or without radiologic monitoring.

64553-64561
The physician places an electrode array percutaneously (through the skin) through an introducer needle into the tissue to be stimulated. Electrodes placed over sensory nerves decrease pain sensation in the distribution of the nerve. Electrodes placed over motor nerves stimulate paralyzed muscles to prevent atrophy. In 64553, the electrodes are placed over the motor or sensory points of cranial nerves. In 64555, the electrodes are placed over peripheral motor or sensory nerves, excluding sacral nerves. Report 64561 when stimulators are placed near sacral nerves (via transforaminal approach) that may require imaging guidance.

64566
The physician places an electrode percutaneously (through the skin) through an introducer needle into the targeted tissue. Posterior tibial nerve stimulation (PTNS) is often used to treat urinary frequency, incontinence, and urgency associated with such conditions as overactive bladder or interstitial cystitis. With the treatment leg elevated, the physician inserts a needle electrode into the lower inner aspect of the leg near the tibial nerve. A grounding pad in the form of a surface electrode is placed over the medial aspect of the heel bone (calcaneus) of the same leg. The electrode is then connected to an external pulse generator. An electrical pulse is delivered via the tibial nerve to the sacral plexus, which regulates bladder and pelvic floor function.

64568-64570
The physician inserts a cranial nerve neurostimulator electrode array and programmable pulse generator (e.g., for vagal nerve stimulation) in 64568. Following appropriate anesthesia, the physician makes an incision on the left side of the neck over the sternocleidomastoid muscle at the level of C5-C6 and dissects to the area between the subcutaneous fat and the platysma. The physician exposes and retracts the sternocleidomastoid muscle, omohyoid muscle, and strap muscles. Dissection continues until the vagus nerve is exposed, taking care not to damage the jugular vein, carotid artery, and laryngeal nerve. After exposing approximately 6 cm of the vagus nerve, three stimulator electrode coils are placed by wrapping each around the vagus nerve. A loop of the electrode cable

is placed near the carotid sheath and anchored to the tissue around the strap muscles. The electrode array is tested for good contact with the nerve and repositioned as necessary. The physician then selects a location site for the neurostimulator pulse generator, typically the left chest area, and creates a pocket in the subcutaneous tissue between the fat and muscle fascia. Using an electrode passer, the end of the electrode is tunneled subcutaneously to the site of the pulse generator. The distal end of the electrode cable is connected to the pulse generator and tightened, and the pulse generator is sutured into place in the pocket. The stimulator system is tested again. After ensuring appropriate functioning, the skin and subcutaneous tissues of all wounds are closed with layered sutures and skin staples. In 64569, the physician replaces or revises the electrode array. The physician incises the skin above the array and locates it. Following location, the physician replaces or revises the array and connects it to the existing pulse generator, which is accessed by sharp dissection through the old incision site. The stimulator system is checked, and the skin and subcutaneous tissues of all wounds are closed with sutures and skin staples. In 64570, the physician removes the cranial nerve neurostimulator electrode array and pulse generator. The physician incises the skin above the electrode array and performs dissection, following the old electrode cable to the vagus nerve. The cable is then cut and removed, and each of the stimulator electrode coils is removed from the vagus nerve. The physician then opens the old incision overlying the pulse generator with sharp dissection, identifies the electrode cable and pulse generator, and removes both. The skin and subcutaneous tissues of all wounds are closed with sutures and skin staples.

64575-64581

The physician implants a neurostimulator electrode array using an open approach. Using a scalpel, the physician incises the skin and dissects down to the anatomical location. The incision aides the physician in accurately placing and testing the electrode while visualizing results. After stimulating the area, the incision is closed with layered sutures. Electrodes placed over sensory nerves decrease pain sensation in the distribution of the nerve. Electrodes placed over motor nerves stimulate paralyzed muscles to prevent atrophy. In 64575, the electrodes are placed over peripheral motor or sensory nerves (excluding the sacral nerve). In 64580, the electrodes are placed at the neuromuscular junction to stimulate a specific area of muscle tissue. In 64581, the electrodes are placed at the sacral nerve for urinary control.

64582-64584

The physician implants a hypoglossal (12th cranial) nerve stimulation system to treat moderate to severe obstructive sleep apnea (OSA). One proprietary system, consisting of an implantable pulse generator (IPG), stimulation lead, sensing lead, and external components including the physician and patient programmer, detects the breathing pattern of the patient and produces mild nerve stimulation to maintain an open airway. Following appropriate anesthesia and positioning, the physician exposes the hypoglossal nerve by making a 4 cm to 6 cm incision along a natural skin crease below the edge of the mandible and retracts the submandibular gland. The hypoglossal nerve is identified and stimulated at a low setting to assure nerve function. A length of the nerve is exposed, and the physician places the stimulation lead cuff by wrapping the flaps around the hypoglossal nerve. Intraoperative test stimulation is used to confirm proper placement and the lead is repositioned as necessary. The physician anchors the stimulation lead to the tissues surrounding the hypoglossal nerve using permanent sutures. Attention is then turned to the IPG pocket. A 5 cm to 6 cm incision is made, typically below the right clavicle, and a subcutaneous pocket is created. The physician uses a tunneling tool to pass the stimulation lead to the subcutaneous pocket. To place the extrapleural respiratory sensing lead, the physician makes a 4 cm to 6 cm incision, places the sensor between the ribs, and secures it with permanent sutures. The connector end of the respiratory sensing lead is tunneled between the intercostal muscle layers to the IPG pocket using the tunneling tool and the lead is connected to the IPG and tested. The physician also connects the stimulation lead to the IPG, and then implants the pulse generator into the subcutaneous pocket. The system is tested again using the physician programmer. The implantation procedure is competed by securing the IPG with permanent sutures to the fascia and closing the surgical incisions. Report 64582 for implantation of the neurostimulator array, pulse generator, and respiratory sensor electrode/array. Report 64583 for revision or replacement of the neurostimulator array and respiratory sensor electrode/array with connection to the existing pulse generator. Report 64584 for removal of the entire system.

64585

The physician revises or removes a previously placed neurostimulator electrode array(s). The physician makes an incision overlying the electrode array. If the initial placement has not resulted in optimal pain control or motor stimulation, the electrode array may be moved to optimize results. If the neurostimulator device is no longer required, the arrays are removed. The incision is closed with layered sutures.

64590-64595

The physician inserts or replaces a peripheral, sacral, or gastric neurostimulator pulse generator or receiver into a subcutaneous pocket in 64590. Neurostimulators are used to transmit electrical impulses to nerves outside of the brain or spinal cord, such as the sacral nerve to help the bladder muscles contract and treat cases of urinary incontinence or retention, or for pain relief. Gastric neurostimulators transmit electrical impulses in the same way, to treat nausea and vomiting in patients with gastroparesis. The physician selects a location site, usually the abdominal area, and incises the skin. Using blunt dissection, the physician creates a pocket for the generator or receiver. In the case of a replacement, the old generator or receiver is removed from an existing pocket. A previously placed electrode array, which is separately implanted to stimulate the target nerve, is tunneled under the skin to the neurostimulator pocket and connected to the unit. After ensuring that the device is functioning, the generator or receiver is sutured into place within its subcutaneous pocket. In 64595, the physician revises or removes the peripheral, sacral, or gastric neurostimulator pulse generator or receiver. A midline incision is made overlying the affected area. The fascia is incised, and muscles are retracted. The physician detaches the connection to the electrode array. The generator or receiver is revised or removed. In the case of a revision, the electrode array is reconnected to the unit after the revision is complete. Layered sutures are used to close the incision.

64596-64598
In 64596, the physician inserts or replaces an electrode array with an integrated neurostimulation system percutaneously (through the skin) for stimulation of the peripheral nerve. Under local anesthesia, a small incision is made, and the electrode array is tunneled to the area of the affected nerve using fluoroscopy. Using the same incision site, a subcutaneous pocket is created. After stimulation testing is performed to confirm proper positioning, the rest of the neurostimulator device is introduced into the pocket and anchored in place. The incision is closed in layers. Report 64596 for the initial electrode array; 64597 for each additional electrode array. Imaging guidance is included, when performed. Report 64598 for revision or removal of the electrode array with integrated neurostimulator.

64600-64610
The physician destroys a portion of the trigeminal nerve using chemical, thermal, electrical, balloon compression, or nonpulsed radiofrequency techniques, which may be used independently or in combination. These procedures are often performed for medically refractory trigeminal neuralgia and are designed to block pain or motor control to the face or scalp. In one method, radiofrequency thermal rhizotomy burns the nerve fibers utilizing a specialized needle in conjunction with an electrical current. In another, chemical destruction involves injection of a neurolytic substance (e.g., alcohol, phenol, or glycerol) into the affected nerve root. In 64600, a supraorbital, infraorbital, mental, or inferior alveolar branch of the trigeminal nerve is destroyed. In 64605, the second and third division branches at the foramen ovale are destroyed. Report 64610 if the second and third division branches at the foramen ovale are destroyed under radiologic monitoring; an example is trigeminal rhizotomy with balloon compression under fluoroscopic assistance.

[64624]
Articular branches of various nerves (common peroneal, femoral, obturator, saphenous, and tibial) innervate the knee joint. These branches around the knee joint are known as genicular nerves. In one form of destruction, the physician employs radiofrequency ablation (RFA), a minimally invasive method in which a needle electrode is inserted through the skin and into the tissue to be ablated. A high frequency electrical current is applied, causing coagulation necrosis to the targeted tissue. In an alternate method, utilizing anatomic landmarks or image guidance, the physician injects a neurolytic agent, such as alcohol or phenol compounds, into a targeted area near the genicular nerve branches in order to treat chronic knee pain. Destruction of the superolateral, superomedial, and inferomedial genicular nerve branches should be achieved in order to report 64624.

[64625]
The physician employs radiofrequency ablation (RFA) to the nerves innervating the sacroiliac joint. Utilizing image guidance (computed tomography or fluoroscopy), the physician locates the target area near the sacroiliac joint. A needle electrode is inserted through the skin and into the tissue to be ablated. A high frequency electrical current is applied, causing coagulation necrosis to the targeted tissue.

[64628, 64629]
The physician performs thermal destruction of the basivertebral nerve (BVN) to treat low back pain resulting from damaged vertebral endplates (vertebrogenic pain). With the patient under appropriate anesthesia and in a prone position, the physician makes a unilateral transpedicular incision. Under imaging guidance, an introducer trocar is advanced through the pedicle and passes the posterior vertebral body wall. Once the vertebral body is penetrated, the trocar is removed from the introducer cannula and a curved cannula assembly consisting of a cannula and stylet is used to enter the vertebral body and navigate toward the BVN, which is located in the posterior half of the vertebral body (intraosseous). Once the target site is confirmed, the curved stylet is removed and a proprietary radiofrequency probe is inserted into the posterior half of the vertebral body. The probe is connected to the radiofrequency (RF) generator and energy is applied for 15 minutes to destroy the BVN. The RF probe and cannula are removed at the end of the procedure and the physician closes the skin and subcutaneous tissue with skin glue or steri-strips and applies a pressure dressing. Once ablated, these nerves no longer transmit pain signals. Report 64628 when treatment involves the first two lumbar or sacral vertebral bodies and 64629 for each additional lumbar or sacral vertebral body.

64611
The physician injects a pharmacologic compound, such as botulinum toxin or atropine, into the parotid and/or submandibular glands in order to paralyze a muscle or group of muscles, often as a treatment for sialorrhea (drooling) in patients with Parkinson's disease. The physician first evaluates gland location, size, and vascular anatomy. Using anatomic landmarks or high-resolution ultrasound, the physician

administers the injections to the glands bilaterally. Anesthesia may or may not be necessary.

64612

The physician administers a neurotoxin to paralyze dysfunctional muscle tissue innervated by the facial nerve. Chemodenervation works by introducing a substance used to block the transfer of chemicals at the presynaptic membrane. Botulinum toxin type A (BTX-A) is the substance most commonly used for chemodenervation of muscle tissue innervated by the facial nerve. The practitioner identifies the nerve(s) or muscle endplate(s) by direct surgical exposure or through the insertion of an electromyographic needle into the muscle. A small amount of BTX-A is injected into the muscle belly, inducing muscle paralysis within 24 to 48 hours. The duration of the effect can vary, but typically is three to four months. Gradually, blocked nerves form new neuromuscular junctions resulting in the return of muscle function. BTX-A is dose-dependent and reversible secondary to the regeneration process. BTX-A injections are an effective treatment for a variety of disorders of abnormal muscle tone, including muscle overactivity or spasticity. This code represents unilateral treatment.

64615

The practitioner administers a neurotoxin to paralyze dysfunctional muscle tissue, bilaterally, that is innervated by the facial, trigeminal, cervical spinal, and accessory nerves. Chemodenervation works by introducing a substance used to block the transfer of chemicals at the presynaptic membrane. Botulinum toxin type A (BTX-A), phenol (sometimes combined with botulinum toxin type A), and/or ethyl alcohol may be used. The practitioner identifies the nerve(s) or muscle endplate(s) by direct surgical exposure or through the insertion of an electromyographic needle into the muscle. A small amount of the selected agent is injected into nerve(s) or muscle endplate(s), inducing muscle paralysis. Gradually, blocked nerves form new neuromuscular junctions resulting in the return of muscle function. The duration of the effect is variable, usually one to 12 months when phenol or alcohol is used, and three to four months when BTX-A is used. BTX-A is dose-dependent and reversible secondary to the regeneration process.

64616

The physician administers a neurotoxin to paralyze dysfunctional muscle tissue of the neck. Chemodenervation works by introducing a substance used to block the transfer of chemicals at the presynaptic membrane. Botulinum toxin type A (BTX-A), phenol (sometimes combined with botulinum toxin type A), and/or ethyl alcohol may be used. The physician identifies the nerve(s) or muscle endplate(s) by direct surgical exposure or through the insertion of an electromyographic needle into the muscle. A small amount of the selected agent is injected into nerve(s) or muscle endplate(s), inducing muscle paralysis. The duration of the effect is variable, usually one to 12 months when phenol or alcohol is used and three to four months when BTX-A is used. BTX-A is dose-dependent and reversible secondary to the regeneration process. Gradually, blocked nerves form new neuromuscular junctions resulting in the return of muscle function.

64617

The physician administers a neurotoxin to paralyze the larynx. Chemodenervation works by introducing a substance used to block the transfer of chemicals at the presynaptic membrane. Botulinum toxin type A (BTX-A), phenol (sometimes combined with botulinum toxin type A), and/or ethyl alcohol may be used. The injection site is identified by the insertion of an electromyographic needle into the muscle tissue near the larynx. A small amount of the selected agent is injected into nerve(s) or muscle(s) around the larynx. The duration of the effect is variable, usually one to 12 months when phenol or alcohol is used and three to four months when BTX-A is used. BTX-A is dose-dependent and reversible secondary to the regeneration process. Gradually, blocked nerves form new neuromuscular junctions resulting in the return of muscle function.

64620

This procedure is performed to treat chronic chest pain commonly associated with pleurisy, acute herpes zoster, and post herpetic neuralgia. An intercostal nerve is destroyed using chemical, thermal, electrical, or radiofrequency techniques, which may be used independently or in combination. This procedure is designed to destroy the specific site(s) in the nerve root that produces the pain while leaving sensation intact. Generally intravenous conscious sedation is used during the initial phase of the procedure so that the patient can assist the physician in identifying the site of pain and the correct placement of the neurolytic agent, and local anesthesia is administered during the destruction phase of the procedure. Using separately reportable fluoroscopic guidance, a needle is inserted into the affected nerve root. An electrode is inserted through the needle and a mild electrical current is passed through the electrode. The current produces a tingling sensation at a site on the nerve. The electrode is manipulated until the tingling sensation is felt at the same site as the pain. Once the physician has determined that the electrode is positioned at the site responsible for the pain, a local anesthetic is administered and a neurolytic agent applied. Chemical destruction involves injection of a neurolytic substance (e.g., alcohol, phenol, glycerol) into the affected nerve root. Thermal techniques use heat. Electrical techniques use an electrical current. Radiofrequency, also referred to as radiofrequency rhizotomy, uses a solar or microwave current.

[64633, 64634]

These procedures are performed to treat chronic cervical or thoracic back pain. The affected cervical or thoracic spinal nerve is destroyed using chemical, thermal, electrical, or non-pulsed radiofrequency techniques, which may be used independently or in combination. These procedures are designed to destroy the specific site(s) in the nerve root that produces the pain while leaving sensation intact. Generally, intravenous conscious sedation is used during the initial phase of the procedure so that the patient can assist the physician in identifying the site of pain and the correct placement of the neurolytic agent; local anesthesia is administered during the destruction phase of the procedure. Using fluoroscopic guidance, a needle is inserted into the affected nerve root. An electrode is inserted through the needle and a mild electrical current is passed through the electrode. The current produces a tingling sensation at a site on the nerve. The electrode is manipulated until the tingling sensation is felt at the same site as the pain. Once the physician has determined that the electrode is positioned at the site responsible for the pain, a local anesthetic is administered and a neurolytic agent applied. Chemical destruction involves injection of a neurolytic substance (e.g., alcohol, phenol, glycerol) into the affected nerve root. Thermal techniques use heat ≥ 80 degrees Celsius. Electrical techniques use an electrical current. Non-pulsed radiofrequency, also referred to as radiofrequency rhizotomy, uses a solar or microwave current. Report 64633 for destruction of a single facet joint at the cervical or thoracic spine level and 64634 for each additional cervical or thoracic facet joint.

[64635, 64636]

These procedures are performed to treat chronic lumbar or sacral back pain. The affected lumbar or sacral spinal nerve is destroyed using chemical, thermal, electrical, or nonpulsed radiofrequency techniques, which may be used independently or in combination. These procedures are designed to destroy the specific site(s) in the nerve root that produces the pain while leaving sensation intact. Generally, intravenous conscious sedation is used during the initial phase of the procedure so that the patient can assist the physician in identifying the site of pain and the correct placement of the neurolytic agent; local anesthesia is administered during the destruction phase of the procedure. Using fluoroscopic guidance, a needle is inserted into the affected nerve root. An electrode is inserted through the needle and a mild electrical current is passed through the electrode. The current produces a tingling sensation at a site on the nerve. The electrode is manipulated until the tingling sensation is felt at the same site as the pain, after which a local anesthetic is administered and a neurolytic agent applied. Chemical destruction involves injection of a neurolytic substance (e.g., alcohol, phenol, glycerol) into the affected nerve root. Thermal techniques use heat ≥ 80 degrees Celsius. Electrical techniques use an electrical current. Nonpulsed radiofrequency, also referred to as radiofrequency rhizotomy, uses a solar or microwave current. Report 64635 for destruction of a single facet joint at the lumbar or sacral spine level and 64636 for destruction of each additional lumbar or sacral spinal joint.

64630

This procedure is performed to treat chronic pain of the external genitalia, pelvis, and anorectal region. The pudendal nerve is destroyed using chemical, thermal, electrical, or radiofrequency techniques, which may be used independently or in combination. This procedure is designed to destroy the specific site(s) in the nerve root that produces the pain while leaving sensation intact. Generally intravenous conscious sedation is used during the initial phase of the procedure so that the patient can assist the physician in identifying the site of pain and the correct placement of the neurolytic agent, and local anesthesia is administered during the destruction phase of the procedure. Using separately reportable fluoroscopic or CT guidance, a needle is inserted next to the ischial spine, contrast dye is injected, and the nerve canal anatomy is confirmed. An electrode is inserted through the needle and a mild electrical current is passed through the electrode. The current produces a tingling sensation at a site on the nerve. The electrode is manipulated until the tingling sensation is felt at the same site as the pain. Once the physician has determined that the electrode is positioned at the site responsible for the pain, a local anesthetic is administered and a neurolytic agent applied. Chemical destruction involves injection of a neurolytic substance (e.g., alcohol, phenol, glycerol) into the affected nerve root. Thermal techniques use heat. Electrical techniques use an electrical current. Radiofrequency, also referred to as radiofrequency rhizotomy, uses a solar or microwave current.

64632

This procedure is performed to treat chronic pain in the foot, most commonly used as a treatment for Morton's neuroma. The plantar nerve is destroyed using chemical, thermal, electrical, or radiofrequency techniques, which may be used independently or in combination. This procedure is designed to destroy the specific site(s) in the nerve root that produces the pain while leaving sensation intact. Generally intravenous conscious sedation is used during the initial phase of the procedure so that the patient can assist the physician in identifying the site of pain and the correct placement of the neurolytic agent, and local anesthesia is administered during the destruction phase of the procedure. Using separately reportable fluoroscopic guidance, a needle is inserted into the affected nerve root. An electrode is inserted through the needle and a mild electrical current is passed through the electrode. The current produces a tingling sensation at a site on the nerve. The electrode is manipulated until the tingling sensation is felt at the same site as the pain. Once the physician has determined that the electrode is positioned at the site responsible for the pain, a local anesthetic is administered and a neurolytic agent applied. Chemical destruction involves injection of a neurolytic substance (e.g., alcohol, phenol, glycerol) into the affected nerve root. Thermal techniques use heat. Electrical techniques use an electrical current. Radiofrequency, also referred to as radiofrequency rhizotomy, uses a solar or microwave current.

64640

This procedure is performed to treat chronic pain that originates in a peripheral nerve other than the intercostal, pudendal, plantar, or spinal nerves. The affected peripheral nerve is destroyed using chemical, thermal, electrical, or radiofrequency techniques, which may be used independently or in combination. This procedure is designed to destroy the specific site in the nerve root that produces the pain while leaving sensation intact. Generally intravenous conscious sedation is used during the initial phase of the procedure so that the patient can assist the physician in identifying the site of pain and the correct placement of the neurolytic agent, and local anesthesia is administered during the destruction phase of the procedure. A needle is inserted into the affected nerve root. An electrode is inserted through the needle and a mild electrical current is passed through the electrode. The current produces a tingling sensation at a site on the nerve. The electrode is manipulated until the tingling sensation is felt at the same site as the pain. Once the physician has determined that the electrode is positioned at the site responsible for the pain, a local anesthetic is administered and a neurolytic agent applied. Chemical destruction involves injection of a neurolytic substance (e.g., alcohol, phenol, glycerol) into the affected nerve root. Thermal techniques use heat. Electrical techniques use an electrical current. Radiofrequency, also referred to as radiofrequency rhizotomy, uses a solar or microwave current.

64642-64645

The physician administers a neurotoxin to paralyze dysfunctional muscle tissue in the extremities. Chemodenervation works by introducing a substance used to block the transfer of chemicals at the presynaptic membrane. Botulinum toxin type A (BTX-A), phenol (sometimes combined with botulinum toxin type A), and/or ethyl alcohol may be used. The physician identifies the nerve(s) or muscle endplate(s) by direct surgical exposure or through the insertion of an electromyographic needle into the muscle. A small amount of the selected agent is injected into nerve(s) or muscle endplate(s), inducing muscle paralysis. The duration of the effect is variable, usually one to 12 months when phenol or alcohol is used and three to four months when BTX-A is used. BTX-A is dose-dependent and reversible secondary to the regeneration process. Gradually, blocked nerves form new neuromuscular junctions resulting in the return of muscle function. Report 64642 when the procedure is performed on one to four muscles of a single extremity and 64643 for one to four muscles of each additional extremity. Report 64644 when five or more muscles are treated in a single extremity and 64645 for five or more muscles of each additional extremity.

64646-64647

The physician administers a neurotoxin to paralyze dysfunctional muscle tissue in the trunk, including the erector spinae, rectus abdominis, oblique, and paraspinal muscles. Chemodenervation works by introducing a substance used to block the transfer of chemicals at the presynaptic membrane. Botulinum toxin type A (BTX-A), phenol (sometimes combined with botulinum toxin type A), and/or ethyl alcohol may be used. The physician identifies the nerve(s) or muscle endplate(s) by direct surgical exposure or through the insertion of an electromyographic needle into the muscle. A small amount of the selected agent is injected into nerve(s) or muscle endplate(s), inducing muscle paralysis. The duration of the effect is variable, usually one to 12 months when phenol or alcohol is used and three to four months when BTX-A is used. BTX-A is dose-dependent and reversible secondary to the regeneration process. Gradually, blocked nerves form new neuromuscular junctions resulting in the return of muscle function. Report 64646 when one to five muscles are treated and 64647 when six or more muscles are treated.

64650-64653

The physician administers a neurotoxin to the eccrine glands to reduce hyperhidrosis (excessive sweating). The skin area to be injected is identified by applying iodine to the skin followed by a light dusting with cornstarch. The resulting chemical change caused by the patient's perspiration turns the area black. Botulinum toxin type A (BTX-A) is injected intradermally into the site with a series of injections, usually 10 to 15 injections per axilla, via a Teflon-coated 23- to 26-gauge electromyogram (EMG) needle with syringe. Since the sweat glands are between the dermis and the dermal fat tissue, the injections must be precise. BTX-A must be injected deep enough to reach the nerve endings but not so deep as to go into the fat. Report 64650 for eccrine glands of both axillae. Report 64653 for eccrine glands of other body areas.

64680

The physician destroys the celiac plexus by applying a neurolytic agent to the celiac plexus. The celiac plexus is a network of nervous tissue that mediates sympathetic pain from the abdomen. This neurolytic block is often performed for pain relief of unresectable cancer in the upper abdomen. The celiac plexus is destroyed usually by chemodenervation, injecting phenol or alcohol to paralyze the network of nervous tissue. This procedure may be performed with or without radiologic monitoring, but is normally performed under CT guidance.

64681

The physician performs a neurolysis on the superior hypogastric plexus by injecting a chemical, thermal, or electrical agent through a needle inserted in the L5/S1 interspace. The superior hypogastric plexus, also called the presacral nerve, is located in front of the upper part of the sacrum and is formed by lower lumbar nerves responsible for pain sensation in the pelvic area. Nerve destruction is done in such cases as severe, intractable menstrual pain and pain due to pelvic area metastases from cancer such as prostatic malignancy when an anesthetic nerve block does not offer sufficient relief. The patient is placed in the prone position and prepped. A 6-inch needle is guided under radiological imaging, such as fluoroscopy (reported separately), into the ventral lateral spine and through the L5/S1 interspace. Needle position is checked by injecting contrast material and aspirating for the return of any blood, urine, or cerebral spinal fluid. With negative aspiration results and imaging verifying that the needle position is in the prevertebral space and not within a blood vessel, a ureter, or spinal nerves, the neurolytic agent is injected, or delivered, to both sides.

64702-64704

In 64702, the physician releases a compressed nerve in a digit of the hand or foot. The physician makes an incision overlying the nerve. Surrounding tissues are dissected from the nerve freeing it from scar tissue or adhesions. The incision is repaired in layers. One or both of the digital nerves in a single finger or toe are decompressed. In 64704, a nerve in the hand or foot is decompressed.

64708-64714

The physician performs an open surgical decompression of a compressed major peripheral nerve in the arm or leg. The physician makes an incision in the area of nerve tension and locates the nerve. Surrounding soft tissue or scar tissue is dissected from the nerve to release pressure and the intact nerve is freed. External neurolysis or nerve transposition may also be performed to restore or repair the nerve; this is included in the codes for the decompression procedure. Report 64708 if the repair is done on a nerve of the arm or leg other than the following: sciatic nerve (64712), brachial plexus (64713), and lumbar plexus (64714).

64716

The physician frees an intact cranial nerve from scar tissue (neuroplasty) or moves an intact nerve to a new position (transposition). The physician makes an incision overlying the nerve, dissects it free of the surrounding tissue and, if necessary, moves the nerve to a new position. If the nerve is in bone and must be decompressed, freed, or moved, the overlying bone is first removed using drills and/or osteotomes.

64718

The physician decompresses a stressed ulnar nerve by freeing the nerve and the surrounding nerve tissue. The patient is given general or regional anesthesia. The physician makes an incision at the medial epicondyle and locates the nerve typically located behind the medial epicondyle. Surrounding tissues are dissected from the nerve and the nerve is freed from the underlying bed. The nerve is moved over the epicondyle to the front (anterior transposition) and stabilized with sutures in the surrounding tissue. The incision is sutured in layers. A cast or splint is set with the elbow bent at a 45-degree angle when the nerve is placed just under the skin or a 90-degree angle when the nerve is placed within the muscle of the new location. The cast remains in place for two to four weeks allowing the incision to heal at which time the patient will begin physical therapy for exercises that allow the patient to achieve full function of the elbow and help bring swelling down.

64719-64721

The physician decompresses or transposes a portion of the ulnar or median nerve to restore feeling to the hand. The physician makes a horizontal incision in the wrist at the metacarpal joints and locates the nerve. In 64719, the ulnar nerve is located and freed. In 64721, the median nerve is decompressed by freeing the nerve inside the carpal tunnel. Soft tissues are resected and the nerve is freed from the underlying bed. Care is taken to ensure tension is released and the incision is sutured in layers.

64722-64726

The physician decompresses a nerve. In 64722, the nerve is unspecified. In 64726 the nerve is located at the base of the foot and supplies sensory fibers to one of the toes. The physician makes an incision in the area of nerve tension and locates the nerve. Surrounding soft tissues are dissected from the nerve to release pressure on the nerve.

64727

The physician makes an incision over the affected nerve and locates the nerve. The physician resects the nerve sheath parallel to the fibers and releases scar tissue within the nerve.

64732-64736

The physician transects or removes a nerve that supplies motor or sensory innervation to the affected head and neck area to eliminate pain. For supraorbital nerve, report 64732, for infraorbital nerve report 64734, for the mental nerve report 64736.

64738

The physician transects or removes a nerve that supplies sensory innervation to the lower jaw and teeth. The physician makes a small osteotomy into the bone and locates the nerve. The nerve is transected to eliminate pain.

64740-64744

The physician transects or removes a nerve that supplies motor or sensory innervation to the affected head and neck area to eliminate pain. For lingual nerve, report 64740. For facial nerve (complete or any branches) report 64742. For the greater occipital nerve, report 64744. The physician incises the area at the most proximal portion of the nerve innervating the problem area. The nerve is located, and transected and the proximal portion of the nerve is buried in the surrounding tissue or bone to prevent neuroma formation.

64746

The physician transects or removes a portion of the phrenic nerve. The phrenic nerve supplies innervation to the diaphragm. The physician makes a horizontal neck incision, dissects the surrounding tissue, and locates the nerve. The nerve is transected, and the proximal portion of the nerve is buried in the surrounding tissue to prevent neuroma formation.

64755-64760
The physician transects or removes a portion of the vagus nerve. The vagus nerves supplies parasympathetic fibers to the heart and gastrointestinal tract. In 64755, the physician makes a vertical midline epigastric incision and locates specific branches of the vagus nerve responsible for acid production in the stomach. In 64760, the physician makes a vertical midline epigastric incision and locates the vagus nerve. After locating the nerve or nerve branches, the physician transects them. The incision is sutured in layers.

64763-64766
The physician transects (cuts) or avulses (pulls out) the obturator nerve. The physician makes an incision overlying the adductor muscles. The adductor muscles are separated from each other and the obturator nerve is located. The physician accesses the nerve by an extrapelvic approach in 64763 or by an intrapelvic approach in 64766. The nerve is transected or avulsed and the incision repaired in layers.

64771
The physician cuts or avulses another cranial nerve, such as branch nerves of major nerves not listed in previous codes. The physician makes an incision on the face or neck overlying the extradural portion of the other cranial nerve. The tissues are dissected and the nerve is exposed. The nerve is destroyed. The incision is sutured in layers.

64772
The physician cuts or avulses another spinal nerve, such as branch nerves of major nerves not listed in other codes. The physician incises the skin overlying the nerve from C1 to S4. The tissues are dissected and the nerve is exposed. The nerve is destroyed. The incision is sutured in layers. This procedure is also characterized as anterior or posterior interosseous neurectomy (AIN or PIN) when performed on the wrist.

64774-64778
The physician excises a neuroma of a peripheral nerve. A neuroma is a benign tumor formed secondarily by trauma to the nerve. In 64774, the physician incises the skin and locates and excises the neuroma in the subcutaneous tissue. In 64776, the physician incises the skin over the digital nerve and excises the neuroma. Report 64778 for each additional neuroma of a separate digit.

64782-64783
The physician excises a neuroma of a peripheral nerve (except digital nerve) of the hand or foot. A neuroma is a benign tumor formed secondarily by trauma to the nerve. The physician incises the affected area in a hand or foot. After locating the nerve with the symptomatic neuroma, the physician excises the tumor. The incision is sutured in layers. Report 64783 for additional neuromas of the hand or foot.

64784-64786
The physician excises a neuroma of a major peripheral nerve. A neuroma is a benign tumor formed secondarily by trauma to the nerve. In 64784, the physician incises the area over the affected major peripheral nerve except sciatic. After locating the nerve with the symptomatic neuroma, the physician excises the tumor. The incision is sutured in layers. In 64786, the physician incises the skin at the back of the upper leg or buttocks near the symptomatic neuroma and locates the tumor on the sciatic nerve. After locating the nerve with the symptomatic neuroma, the physician excises the tumor. The incision is sutured in layers.

64787
The physician implants a nerve into a bone or muscle to prevent neuroma formation after excision of a neuroma. In bony implantation, the physician drills a small hole in the bone to implant the nerve. The surrounding tissue is brought together around the nerve to secure the nerve to the bone. In muscle implantation the nerve is sutured into muscle bed. The surrounding tissue is brought together and sutured to secure the nerve in the muscle.

64788-64792
The physician excises a neurofibroma or a neurolemmoma. A neurofibroma is a tumor of peripheral nerves caused by abnormal proliferation of Schwann cells. A neurolemmoma is a tumor of a peripheral nerve sheath. To remove the tumor, the physician incises the skin over the tumor and dissects the surrounding tissue. The tumor is freed and excised from the nerve, without damaging the nerve when possible. The incision is sutured in layers. In 64788, the tumor is located on a cutaneous nerve. In 64790, the tumor lies on a major peripheral nerve. In 64792, an extensive excision is required due to size or malignancy.

64795
The physician biopsies a nerve. The physician makes an incision overlying the suspect nerve. The tissues are dissected to locate the nerve, and a biopsy specimen is obtained. The incision is sutured in layers.

64802-64804
The physician performs a cervical sympathectomy or cervical thoracic sympathectomy. The cervical sympathetic chain supplies sympathetic innervation to the head, neck, and upper extremities. The thoracic chain supplies sympathetic innervation to the chest and its contents. In 64802, the physician makes a midlateral incision of the neck and dissects the tissues to locate the sympathetic chain. In 64804, the physician makes a thoracotomy and dissects the tissues to locate the sympathetic chain along the vertebral bodies. The ganglia (nerve cell bodies which lay outside the spinal cord) are identified and resected. The incision is sutured in layers.

64809
The physician performs a sympathectomy on the thoracolumbar sympathetic nerves. The physician makes a lateral incision through the thoracic area to reach the sympathetic ganglia, which lie on the lateral

border of the vertebral column. The physician determines at which level to remove the ganglia, and dissects to the vertebral bodies. The sympathetic plexus is located and resected. The wound is sutured in layers.

64818
The physician performs a sympathectomy on the lumbar sympathetic nerves. The physician makes a lateral incision through the lumbar area to reach the sympathetic ganglia, which lie on the lateral border of the vertebral column. The physician determines at which level to remove the ganglia, and dissects to the vertebral bodies. The sympathetic plexus is located and resected. The wound is sutured in layers.

64820-64823
In 64820, the physician performs a digital sympathectomy using a microscope for visualization. The physician makes an incision along the digital artery in the medial and lateral aspects of the digit. The artery is identified and the adventitia is stripped from the blood vessel. Peripherally, the sympathetic nerves follow the arteries and lie in the adventitia layer. The incision is closed in layers. Report 64821 when the procedure is performed on the radial artery. Report 64822 when the procedure is performed on the ulnar artery. Report 64823 when the procedure is performed on the superficial palmar arch.

64831-64832
The physician repairs a digital (finger or toe) nerve. The physician locates the damaged nerve in a previously opened incision or wound of a finger or toe. The nerve is sutured to restore sensory or motor function. Report 64831 for a single nerve; report 64832 for each additional digital nerve repaired in that hand or foot, regardless of whether it is in the same digit.

64834-64840
The physician repairs a sensory or motor nerve in the hand or foot. The physician locates the damaged nerve in a previously opened incision or wound of the hand or foot. The nerve is sutured to restore sensory function. In 64834, a common sensory nerve is repaired. In 64835, the median motor thenar nerve is repaired. This nerve supplies motor innervation to the thenar eminence (proximal thumb). In 64836, the ulnar motor nerve is repaired. This nerve supplies motor innervation to the extensor muscles of the forearm and hand. Report 64837 for repair of additional nerves in the hand or foot. In 64840, the tibial nerve is repaired. The tibial nerve supplies sensory innervation to the sole of the foot. Closure or reconstruction is separately reported.

64856-64859
The physician repairs a major peripheral nerve in the arm or leg, except for the sciatic nerve. The physician locates the damaged nerve in a previously opened incision or wound of the arm or leg. The nerve is sutured to restore sensory and/or motor innervation. The nerve may be moved (transposed) to decrease tension on the nerve. Report 64856 for repair of the peripheral nerves of the arm or leg except the sciatic nerve. Report 64857 if no transposition is necessary for repair. Report 64858 for repair of the sciatic nerve. When repairing more than one nerve, report 64859 for each additional nerve. Closure or reconstruction is reported separately.

64861-64862
The physician repairs the brachial plexus nerve or the lumbar plexus nerve. The brachial plexus supplies sensory and motor innervation to the arm. The lumbar plexus supplies sensory and motor innervation to the lower back, buttocks, and legs. The physician locates the damaged nerve in a previously opened incision or wound. In 64861, the nerve damage is in the neck or axilla. In 64862, the nerve damage is in the pelvis. The nerve is sutured to restore sensory and/or motor innervation. Closure or reconstruction is separately reported.

64864-64865
The physician repairs a nerve of the face or exterior head. The physician locates the damaged nerve in a previously opened incision or wound. In 64864, the damaged nerve is located on the face or the external cranium. In 64865, the damaged nerve is located in the temple area and grafting may be required. If a nerve is grafted, the sural nerve is often the donor nerve. Graft harvest is separately reported. The nerve is sutured to restore sensory and/or motor innervation. Closure or reconstruction is separately reported.

64866-64868
The physician creates an anastomosis (connection of two nerves that are not normally connected) to restore motor innervation to the face. In 64866, the facial nerve is anastomosed with the spinal accessory nerve. The physician makes a horizontal incision in the posterior lateral neck and isolates the spinal accessory nerve. The nerve is isolated and brought forward and sutured to the facial nerve. In 64868, the physician makes a horizontal lateral neck incision and isolates the hypoglossal nerve. The nerve is brought forward and sutured to the facial nerve. The subcutaneous structures and skin are sutured in layers.

64872-64876
The physician repairs a nerve where repair was delayed because the initial wound was contaminated. The wound is explored to locate the distal portion of the nerve. In 64872, the proximal and distal nerves are sutured together to restore innervation. In 64874, the nerve was shortened during damage. To reanastomose the nerve, the distal and proximal portions of the nerve are freed from surrounding tissues, approximated, and sutured to restore innervation. Report 64876 if excessive trauma caused loss of a significant section of a major nerve. For this procedure, a portion of the parallel bone is resected in order to approximate the distal and proximal ends of the nerve.

64885-64886
The physician obtains and places a nerve graft to restore innervation to the head or neck. A typical graft

harvest is obtained from the sural nerve. To harvest the graft, the physician makes a lateral incision of the lateral malleolus of the ankle. The nerve is identified and freed. The physician cuts the nerve to obtain the length needed for the graft, elongating the incision as necessary. The proximal and distal sural nerve endings are anastomosed. The physician makes an incision over the damaged nerve and dissects the tissues to locate the nerve. The damaged area of the nerve is resected and removed. Innervation is restored by suturing the graft to the proximal and distal ends of the damaged nerve. Report 64885 if the graft is 4 cm or less in length and 64886 if the graft is greater than 4 cm.

64890-64891

The physician obtains and places a nerve graft to restore innervation to the hand or foot. In 64890, the graft is up to 4 cm long; in 64891, the graft is greater than 4 cm. A typical graft harvest is obtained from the sural nerve. To harvest the graft, the physician makes a lateral incision of the lateral malleolus of the ankle. The nerve is identified and freed. The physician cuts the nerve to obtain the length needed for the graft, elongating the incision as necessary. The proximal and distal sural nerve endings are anastomosed. The physician makes an incision over the damaged nerve and dissects the tissues to locate the nerve. The damaged area of the nerve is resected and removed. Innervation is restored by suturing the graft to the proximal and distal ends of the damaged nerve.

64892-64893

The physician obtains and places a nerve graft to restore innervation to the arm or leg. In 64892, the graft is up to 4 cm long; in 64893, the graft is greater than 4 cm. A typical graft harvest is obtained from the sural nerve. To harvest the graft, the physician makes a lateral incision of the lateral malleolus of the ankle. The nerve is identified and freed. The physician cuts the nerve to obtain the length needed for the graft, elongating the incision as necessary. The proximal and distal sural nerve endings are anastomosed. The physician makes an incision over the damaged nerve and dissects the tissues to locate the nerve. The damaged area of the nerve is resected and removed. Innervation is restored by suturing the graft to the proximal and distal ends of the damaged nerve.

64895-64896

The physician obtains and places a nerve graft to restore innervation where a cable nerve of the hand or foot is damaged. In 64895, the graft is up to 4 cm long, and in 64896, the graft is greater than 4 cm. A typical graft harvest is obtained by taking multiple sections of the sural nerve. To harvest the graft, the physician makes an incision near the lateral malleolus of the ankle. The nerve is identified and freed. The physician cuts the nerve to obtain the length needed for the graft, elongating the incision as necessary. The proximal and distal sural nerve endings are anastomosed. The physician makes an incision over the damaged nerve and dissects the tissues to locate the nerve. The damaged area of the nerve is resected and removed. Innervation is restored by suturing graft strands to multiple proximal and distal ends of the damaged nerve cable.

64897-64898

The physician obtains and places a nerve graft to restore innervation where a cable nerve of the arm or leg is damaged (e.g., sciatic nerve or lumbar plexus nerve). In 64897, the graft is less than 4 cm long, and in 64898, the graft is greater than 4 cm. A typical graft harvest is obtained by taking multiple sections of the sural nerve. To harvest the graft, the physician makes an incision near the lateral malleolus of the ankle. The nerve is identified and freed. The physician cuts the nerve to obtain the length needed for the graft, elongating the incision as necessary. The proximal and distal sural nerve endings are anastomosed. The physician makes an incision over the damaged nerve and dissects the tissues to locate the nerve. The damaged area of the nerve is resected and removed. Innervation is restored by suturing graft strands to multiple proximal and distal ends of the damaged nerve cable.

64901-64902

The physician grafts additional nerves. These codes are reported in addition to initial nerve graft codes and include graft harvest. Report 64901 for each additional single strand graft; report 64902 for each additional multiple strand graft.

64905-64907

The physician transfers a nerve pedicle from an intact nerve to a damaged nerve. A pedicle is an intact nerve used as a donor for regeneration of axons in the damaged nerve. In 64905, the first stage is completed. The physician makes an incision over the donor nerve site and locates the nerve. The nerve is freed from surrounding tissues and cut. The proximal portion of the donor nerve is transferred to the distal portion of the recipient nerve. The incision is sutured in layers. In 64907, the second stage is completed. The physician reopens the surgical incision and locates the donor and recipient nerves. The donor nerve is resected from the recipient nerve and primarily reanastomosed to its distal end. The distal end of the recipient nerve is reanastomosed to its proximal end. The nerves may be freed from surrounding tissues if necessary to complete anastomosis. The incision is sutured in layers.

64910

The physician repairs a nerve and uses a graft to restore innervation. The physician makes an incision over the damaged nerve and dissects tissues to locate the nerve. The damaged area of the nerve is resected and removed. Innervation is restored by building a bridge to each end of the resected nerve and suturing the proximal and distal ends of the bridge into place around each severed nerve end. This technique is usually limited to nerve gaps of 3 cm or less. The bridge is usually 1 cm longer than the defect so that it covers the distal and proximal ends of the resected nerve. The bridge is composed of a bioabsorbable, corrugated synthetic conduit of polyglycolic acid. Once the bridge is sutured into place, the artificial nerve conduit is infused with a solution of heparin and saline to prevent clot formation. The operative wound is repaired in layers. Over time, the nerve conduit is restored and the tube is resorbed by surrounding tissue.

64911

The physician repairs a nerve and uses a vein graft to restore innervation. The physician obtains the venous graft by making an incision over the donor site and locating the vein. The vein is freed from surrounding tissues and excised, and vessels are tied or cauterized. The incision is sutured in layers. The physician makes an incision over the damaged nerve and dissects tissues to locate the nerve. The damaged area of the nerve is resected and removed. Innervation is restored by building a bridge of vein to each end of the resected nerve and suturing the proximal and distal ends of the bridge into place around each severed nerve end. This technique is usually limited to nerve gaps of 3 cm or less. The bridge is usually 1 cm longer than the defect so that it covers the distal and proximal ends of the resected nerve. Once the bridge is sutured into place, it is infused with a solution of heparin and saline to prevent clot formation. The operative wound is repaired in layers. Over time, the nerve conduit is restored.

64912-64913

The physician repairs a peripheral nerve injury using a processed human nerve allograft to restore innervation. Peripheral nerves, unlike nerves in the central nervous system, can heal but nerve function restoration may begin to diminish over a period of time. A processed human peripheral nerve graft is donated in the same manner as other tissues and organs involving donor screening. Donated nerves are processed and sterilized to avoid risk of disease transmission from the donor to the patient and, as a result of the processing procedure, the allograft does not require a patient to take immunosuppressant drugs. An allograft offers surgeons the ability to reconnect severed nerves without the potential complications or interactions associated with using another surgical site to harvest the donor nerve. In addition, a processed human nerve allograft may minimize costs and time requirements involved when the physician must harvest a nerve from the patient. The physician makes an incision over the damaged nerve and dissects tissues to locate the nerve. The damaged area of the nerve is resected and removed. Innervation is restored by building a bridge of the decellularized and processed human nerve allograft to each end of the resected nerve and suturing the proximal and distal ends of the bridge into place around each severed nerve end. This technique is usually limited to nerve gaps of 3 cm or less. The bridge is usually 1 cm longer than the defect so that it covers the distal and proximal ends of the resected nerve. Once the bridge is sutured into place, it is infused with a solution of heparin and saline to prevent clot formation. The operative wound is repaired in layers. The allograft is designed to function with the natural structural pathways for axon regeneration and over time is absorbed into, and becomes part of, the patient's own body. Report 64912 for the first strand and 64913 for each additional strand.

Eye and Ocular Adnexa

65091-65093

The physician removes the contents of the eyeball: the vitreous, retina, choroid, lens, iris, and ciliary muscles. Retained is the tough, white outer shell (the sclera). After an ocular speculum has been inserted, the physician dissects the conjunctiva free from the sclera. An elliptical incision is made in the sclera surrounding the cornea, and the contents of the anterior chamber are removed. The physician uses a spoon to remove the contents of the posterior chamber, and scrapes the inside of the sclera with gauze on a curette. Only the scleral shell remains. The conjunctiva may be removed. A temporary (65091) or permanent (65093) implant is inserted into the scleral shell at this time. The sclera is attached to the implant, usually with sutures.

65101-65105

The physician severs the eyeball from the extraorbital muscles and optic nerve and removes it. After an ocular speculum has been inserted, the physician dissects the conjunctiva free at the corneal-scleral juncture (the limbus). The physician cuts each extraocular muscle at its juncture to the eyeball and severs the optic nerve. The eyeball, and sometimes the conjunctiva, is removed but the extraocular muscles remain attached at the back of the eye socket. A spherical implant is placed in the eye socket. This implant, if unattached to the extraocular muscles, may be temporary (65101) or permanent (65103). The extraocular muscles may be attached to the permanent implant to allow normal movement of the prosthesis (65105).

65110-65112

The physician sutures the eyelids closed. An elliptical incision is cut through the skin, subcutaneous tissue, muscle and periosteum to the bone beginning at the upper nasal orbital rim and is carried below the brow to the lateral canthus. The incision is extended from the upper nasal quadrant along the nasal and inferior orbit rim to the lateral canthus, terminating in a wide canthotomy. The periosteum is freed around the orbital rim with a periosteum elevator, beginning in the upper temporal quadrant. The trochlea is detached with a sharp dissection. In the upper temporal quadrant, the lacrimal gland is removed. The lacrimal sac is separated from its attachments and removed. The medial and lateral canthal ligaments are cut with a blunt dissection. A blunt dissection is also used to separate the periorbital to the apex, and the firm attachment of the periosteum is cut from the bone with scissors. The orbital contents are removed. Pieces of orbital bone may be excised (65112). The orbit is packed with dry gauze and pressure is applied to control bleeding.

65114
The physician splits the upper and lower eyelids at the gray line throughout their length, leaving the cilia and the skin anteriorly, and the tarsus, the orbicularis muscle, the conjunctiva, the palpebral muscle and the fascial planes posteriorly. The margins of the posterior halves of the lids are sutured together. The lateral bony wall and the temporal fossa are exposed by lateral canthotomy and dissection of the skin, continuous with both lids. The orbital septum is incised. The trochlea is detached with a sharp dissection. The lacrimal gland and lacrimal sac are removed. The medial and lateral canthal ligaments are cut with a blunt dissection. A blunt dissection is also used to separate the periorbital to the apex. The firm attachment of the periosteum is cut from the bone with scissors. The orbital contents are removed. An incision is made in the fascia at the origin of the temporalis muscle. Fascia and muscle are reflected from the temporal fossa. Adherent fascia is excised from the upper margin of the zygomatic process. The muscle is dissected beneath the process. The temporalis muscle and its fascia are taken through the opening into the orbit. After the muscle and the fascia are spread to fill the orbit, they are sutured to the periosteum.

65125
The physician modifies an ocular implant that has been created elsewhere. The modifications may include the addition of screws or other prosthetic appendages to alter the shape of the prosthesis so that it better fits the patient's eye. The physician may drill holes to accommodate the screws.

65130-65140
The physician inserts a permanent ocular prosthesis into a patient's orbit. In each case, an ocular speculum is placed in the eye, any conjunctiva is retracted, and any temporary prosthesis is removed. In a patient whose eye has been eviscerated, the implant is attached to the remaining sclera (65130). In a patient following enucleation, the implant is otherwise secured (65135). In some cases, eye muscles are attached to corresponding niches in the prosthesis to provide for more natural movement of the artificial eye following enucleation (65140).

65150-65155
The physician returns an ocular prosthesis to the patient's eye socket. After an ocular speculum is inserted, the physician places the ocular prosthesis back into an eye from which it had been previously removed. The prosthesis is attached to the sclera in an eviscerated eye, or otherwise secured in an enucleated eye (65150). In 65155, foreign material may be required to better secure the prosthesis and/or the prosthesis may be reattached to extraocular muscles. In either procedure, conjunctival tissue may be grafted over the prosthesis once it is secured.

65175
The physician removes the ocular implant from the eye socket. After placing an ocular speculum, the physician cuts and retracts any conjunctival tissue or Tenon's capsule overlying the prosthesis. Any connection between the implant and extraocular muscle or sclera is severed and the ocular implant is removed.

65205-65210
The physician picks the foreign body or mineral deposit from the conjunctiva with the side of the beveled edge of a needle (65205). A small incision may be required to remove an embedded foreign body (65210). In this case, the physician may cut a V-shaped incision to access the defect through a flap, or a straight incision may be made. The incision may penetrate the conjunctiva, but it does not penetrate the sclera. Generally, a slit lamp is used when removing any embedded foreign body. After the removal, the physician may apply a broad spectrum antibiotic and a moderate pressure patch over the closed lid for 24-48 hours.

65220-65222
The physician may remove a superficial foreign body or mineral deposit from the cornea with the side of the beveled edge of a needle (65220). An incision may be required to remove an embedded foreign body (65222). If so, the physician may cut a V-shaped incision to access the defect through a flap, or a straight incision may be made. The incision does not penetrate the cornea. Generally, a slit lamp is used with any embedded foreign body. After the removal, the physician may apply a broad spectrum antibiotic and a moderate pressure patch over the closed lid for 24-48 hours.

65235
The physician removes a foreign body, intraocular, from the anterior chamber of the eye or lens. The physician makes a small incision in the connective tissue between the cornea and the sclera (the limbus) and retrieves the foreign body through the opening with intraocular forceps or another small instrument. Generally, foreign bodies that pierce the lens are self-sealing and removal is not attempted. The incision is sutured. The physician applies an antibiotic ointment. Sometimes a pressure patch is placed on the eye for 24-48 hours.

65260
Diagnostic tests locate the foreign body before surgery is attempted. The physician will use an electromagnetic or magnetic probe to retrieve a metallic foreign body from the area behind the lens (the posterior segment). In the anterior route, the physician first dilates the patient's pupil. In a series of moves aligning the magnet to the metallic foreign body, the physician draws the foreign body to the front of the eye and around the lens into the anterior chamber. The physician makes an incision in the connective tissue between the cornea and the sclera (the limbus) and retrieves the foreign body. In the posterior route, the physician makes a small incision in the conjunctiva over the site of the foreign body. A magnet is applied and the foreign body removed. The incision from either is repaired, and an injection may

be required to reestablish proper fluid levels in the anterior and/or posterior chamber of the eye. A broad spectrum antibiotic or a pressure patch may be applied. Among the tools common to this procedure are Gruning's, Haab's, or Hirschberg's magnets.

65265
Diagnostic tests locate the foreign body before surgery is attempted. The physician will use intraocular forceps to retrieve the nonmetallic foreign body from the area behind the lens (the posterior segment). The physician makes an incision through the conjunctiva overlying the site of the foreign body. The foreign body is retrieved with intraocular forceps. Nonmetallic foreign bodies in the vitreous or retina may be removed through a pars plana approach. Either incision is repaired with a layered closure, and an injection may be required to reestablish proper fluid levels in the anterior or posterior chambers of eye. A broad spectrum antibiotic or a pressure patch may be applied.

65270-65273
An ocular speculum may be placed in the patient's eye. The physician irrigates the laceration and sutures the conjunctival wound (65270). In mobilization and rearrangement (65272), an extensive conjunctival laceration requires the creation of a flap or graft sutured over the wound, and the eyes are patched to limit their movement while the injury heals. A graft may be obtained from conjunctival tissue of the upper eyelid or from a sliding flap formed following a circumcorneal incision. Extensive repair of the eye of a child may require hospitalization to further limit eye movement (65273).

65275-65285
The physician removes any foreign body from the cornea with a hollow needle or forceps and the wound is irrigated. The nonperforating tear in the cornea (65275) is repaired with sutures. In 65280 and 65285, the perforating tear in the cornea and any tear in the sclera may be sutured. The cornea may be splinted using a soft contact lens bandage. An air or saline injection may be required to reestablish proper ocular pressure in the anterior chamber. If the laceration involves the uveal tissue (the vascular layer beneath the sclera), injured tissue may be cut out or repositioned before the uvea is sutured (65285), and the sclera and conjunctiva may each require separate closure. In any of the three procedures, topical antibiotic or a pressure patch may be applied.

65286
Tissue glue, also called medical adhesive or cyanoacrylate tissue adhesive, acts as a suture in laceration repairs of the cornea and/or sclera. If the cornea is perforated, the physician may seal the perforation with tissue adhesive after debriding the outermost layer of cornea (the epithelium) to enhance adhesion. The patient may be fitted with a soft contact lens to be worn during the healing process. Antibiotic ointment is applied. A pressure patch may be used.

65290
The physician repairs a deep laceration to the orbital complex. This laceration extends through the extraocular muscles that aid the eye in directional movement. The laceration extends through tendinous attachment of the muscles to the bony orbit and may include the deep connective tissue envelope encasing the eyeball. Each anatomic structure is identified and reapproximated with sutures. The wound is closed in layers.

65400-65410
The physician removes the corneal lesion (65400) using a blade and forceps or scleral scissors. The edges of the lesion are undermined following a superficial incision in the cornea. Sutures are not required. Antibiotic ointment and possibly a 24-hour pressure patch is applied. The lesion is superficial; the cornea is not perforated by the excision. Sometimes, only a portion of the lesion is removed for diagnostic purposes (65410).

65420-65426
A pterygium is a fleshy, wedge of the bulbar conjunctiva covering a portion of the medial cornea. The physician excises the pterygium with a blade and forceps or scleral scissors. The edges of the pterygium are undermined following a superficial incision in the clear cornea. Forceps retract the freed pterygium and it is excised as gentle pressure pulls it away from the corneal tissue and across the limbus and sclera. The physician applies sutures to the sclera and conjunctiva as needed. Often, no graft or tissue rearrangement is needed (65420). However, the physician may transpose the pterygium with normal conjunctival tissue to move it out of the field of vision in what is sometimes called McReynold's operation, or may make a circumcorneal incision and use a conjunctival flap to repair the pterygium site (65426). A topical antibiotic and a pressure patch may be applied in either procedure.

65430
In the office, the physician scrapes the surface of the corneal defect with a spatula. The scrapings will be cultured to determine a diagnosis.

65435-65436
In cases of corneal erosion or degeneration, the physician may attempt to stimulate new growth of the cornea's outermost layer by essentially "wounding" it. The physician removes the outermost layer of the cornea (epithelium) by scraping or cutting it with a spatula or curette (65435). Chemical cauterization may be applied. An alternative to cutting or scraping is the application by swab of ethylenediaminetetraacetic acid (EDTA), an acid that destroys the corneal epithelium (65436). In either case, an antibiotic ointment or pressure patch may be applied once the procedure is complete.

65450
The physician applies a freezing probe, a laser beam, or a heat probe directly to a corneal defect to destroy it.

Eye and Ocular Adnexa

Freezing is the most common method used for this procedure. The physician applies antibiotic ointment and sometimes, a pressure patch.

65600

In cases of corneal erosion or degeneration, the physician may attempt to stimulate new growth of the cornea's outermost layer by essentially "wounding" it. The physician places a speculum in the eye and uses a fine needle to create hundreds of tiny pricks in the surface of the outermost layer of the cornea (the epithelium). A topical antibiotic and patch may be applied. This procedure is sometimes called a corneal "tattoo."

65710

The physician performs an anterior lamellar corneal transplant (keratoplasty). "Lamellar" means thin layer and refers to the outermost layers of the cornea. The physician measures the patient's cornea to select the size of trephine that will be used to excise corneal tissue. The physician punches a circular hole in the outermost layers of the cornea of a donor eye, using the trephine. The physician removes the round layer of corneal tissue, threads it with sutures, and sets it aside. The trephine is used to repeat this process in the cornea of the patient, removing the defective corneal tissue. The donor cornea is of similar diameter and thickness as the removed tissue. The donor cornea is positioned with the preplaced sutures; additional sutures secure it to the cornea. The physician may use a saline or air injection into the anterior chamber during the procedure. When the procedure is completed, the speculum is removed. Antibiotic ointment and a pressure patch may be applied. This code includes preparation of the donor material.

65730-65755

Penetrating refers to the thickness of the donor cornea, indicating its full thickness. The physician measures the patient's cornea to select the size of trephine that will be used to excise corneal tissue. The physician punches a circular hole in the cornea of the donor eye using the trephine. The physician removes the disc of corneal tissue, threads it with preplaced sutures, and sets it aside. In aphakic patients, vitreous and/or aqueous humor may be withdrawn from the eye before the cornea is removed. A metal ring may be sutured to the sclera of an aphakic patient to stabilize the operative field. The defective cornea of the patient is removed with the trephine. The donor cornea is positioned with sutures; additional sutures secure it to the cornea. The physician may use a saline or air injection to restore proper intraocular pressure. Report 65730 for patients who still have a natural lens or are phakic (with lens). Report 65750 for patients who have had cataract extraction surgery or are aphakic (without lens). Report 65755 for patients who have an artificial lens or are pseudophakic (without natural lens).

65756-65757

Endothelial cells line the cornea's inner surface and constantly produce fluid to keep the cornea clear. There are a limited number of these cells, and they do not increase in number (proliferate). If they become diseased or damaged or if there are not enough cells, the cornea may become cloudy. There are several endothelial keratoplasty techniques to replace diseased corneal endothelium while maintaining the integrity of the anterior corneal surface. Deep lamellar keratoplasty (DLKP) entails complete removal of diseased corneal stromal tissue down to Descemet's membrane (the basement membrane found between the cornea's stromal and endothelial layers), with subsequent transplant of donor tissue. Later adapted due to redesigned instrumentation, the procedure was renamed deep lamellar endothelial keratoplasty (DLEK). In DLEK, the physician removes a disc of endothelial cell tissue from the patient's cornea and replaces it with a disc of endothelial cell tissue of the same size that has been removed from the donor cornea. The disc may be created with a mechanical device or with a laser microkeratome. The physician approaches from the front side of the patient's cornea and creates a lamellar incision just anterior to Descemet's membrane. After making this circular incision, the physician makes side incisions from the level of the lamellar incision back through the bottom of the cornea, creating a disc consisting only of Descemet's and endothelium. An identical disc from donor tissue is then created using the same process. The physician rolls the recipient's disc up and removes it through a tiny incision at the edge of the cornea. The donor disc is also rolled and is placed inside the eye through the same incision. The physician unfolds the disc and fits it into the site created by removal of the recipient's disc. With successive revisions, the procedure further evolved into the Descemet's stripping endothelial keratoplasty (DSEK), which involves scraping of the Descemet's membrane and endothelium from the recipient cornea rather than the lamellar dissection and excision performed in DLKP and DLEK. An alternative of DSEK is Descemet's stripping automated endothelial keratoplasty (DSAEK), which involves preparation of the donor epithelium with an automated microkeratome instead of manually. Following any of these techniques, an antibiotic ointment and a pressure patch may be applied. The physician performs an endothelial corneal transplant (keratoplasty) using a fresh or preserved graft in 65756. Preparation of the donor material is reported separately with 65757.

65760

The cornea is one of several structures in the eye that contributes to refraction. Altering the shape of the cornea therefore alters visual acuity. The physician retracts the patient's eyelids with an ocular speculum. Using a planing device, the physician removes a partial-thickness central portion of the patient's cornea, freezes it, and reshapes it on an electronic lathe. The revised cornea is positioned and secured with sutures. This is done to correct optical error. The physician may use a saline or air injection into the anterior chamber during the procedure. The speculum is removed. Antibiotic ointment and a pressure patch may be applied.

65765

The cornea is one of several structures in the eye that contributes to refraction. Altering the shape of the cornea therefore alters visual acuity. The physician retracts the patient's eyelids with an ocular speculum and measures the patient's cornea to select the size of trephine that will be used to excise corneal tissue. The physician punches a circular hole in the cornea of the donor eye using the trephine. The physician removes the disk of corneal tissue and sets it aside. An incision is made at the juncture of the cornea and the sclera (the limbus) and the patient's cornea is separated into two layers. The physician inserts the donor cornea between layers of the recipient's cornea. The resulting change in the corneal curvature alters the refractive properties of the cornea to correct the preexisting refractive error. The speculum is removed. Antibiotic ointment and a pressure patch may be applied.

65767

The cornea is one of several structures in the eye that contributes to refraction. Altering the shape of the cornea therefore alters visual acuity. The physician retracts the patient's eyelids with an ocular speculum and measures the patient's cornea to select the size of trephine that will be used to excise corneal tissue. The physician punches a circular hole in the cornea of the donor eye using the trephine. The physician removes the disk of corneal tissue and sets it aside. On a lathe, the physician shapes a lens made of two layers from a donor cornea, the stroma and Bowman's membrane. The physician sutures this donor cornea to the surface of the patient's cornea. The resulting change in the corneal curvature alters the refractive properties of the cornea to correct the preexisting refractive error. The speculum is removed. Antibiotic ointment and a pressure patch may be applied.

65770

The physician creates a new anterior chamber with a plastic optical implant that replaces a severely damaged cornea that cannot be repaired. Sometimes the corneal prosthesis is sutured to the sclera; other times, extensive damage to the eye requires the implant be sutured to the closed and incised eyelid.

65771

The cornea is one of several structures in the eye that contributes to refraction. Altering the shape of the cornea therefore alters visual acuity. The physician retracts the patient's eyelids with an ocular speculum and measures the patient's cornea. The physician places multiple nonpenetrating cuts in the cornea in a bicycle spoke on the patient's cornea to reduce myopia, or a variety of peripheral cornea tangential cuts for astigmatic correction. There are two basic surgical approaches: Russian, in which the incisions are made from the edges to the center of the cornea; and American, in which the incisions are made from the center to the periphery. The number and length of the incisions depend upon the patient's age and degree of myopia. The resulting change in the corneal curvature alters the refractive properties of the cornea to correct the preexisting refractive error. The speculum is removed. Antibiotic ointment and a pressure patch may be applied.

65772-65775

The cornea is one of several structures in the eye that contributes to refraction. Altering the shape of the cornea therefore alters visual acuity. When a previous surgery (e.g., for insertion of an intraocular lens or a corneal procedure) results in astigmatism, the physician at a later date returns the patient to the operating room to correct the problem. The physician retracts the patient's eyelids with an ocular speculum. In corneal relaxing (65772), an "X" cut is made on the cornea to repair the error. Slices along the "X" are removed and its edges are sutured. In the corneal wedge resection (65775), a wedge is cut from the cornea and the edges sutured. The resulting change in the corneal curvature alters the refractive properties of the cornea to correct the preexisting refractive error. The speculum is removed. Antibiotic ointment and a pressure patch may be applied.

65778-65779

The physician places a temporary amniotic membrane (AM) patch or bandage on the surface of the eye to promote wound healing, typically in cases of acute chemical burns, corneal scars and defects, or other ocular surface conditions. Amniotic membrane patches may also be used to cover glaucoma drainage devices to promote healing. The cryopreserved or dehydrated AM patch, prepared from placentas obtained following cesarean section births, is provided by a tissue bank. In 65778, the physician places anesthetic drops in the eye and inserts a lid speculum. Using blunt forceps or fingers, the physician grasps the plastic rim of the AM patch, lifts the lid speculum, and inserts the patch underneath. The patch conforms to the corneal surface like a contact lens, requiring no sutures. Following insertion, antibiotic drops are applied. In 65779, sutures are used to hold the device in place.

65780

Amniotic membrane transplantation for ocular surface reconstruction is done for corneal defects such as burns, scarring, thinning, ulcer, and perforation. Human amniotic membrane obtained during cesarean deliveries is used. The tissue is then prepared and preserved via cryopreservation (freezing) or dehydration for transplantation at a later date. Use of this tissue induces rapid re-epithelialization of corneal epithelium to a good surface for successful reconstruction. The eye is properly draped before incision. A lid speculum is used to keep the lids and lashes from the operative field. Using an operative microscope, any necrotic corneal epithelium is debrided. The preserved amniotic membrane tissue is trimmed to fit the defect area. The membrane must be placed with the surface of basement membrane cells facing upward and the stromal cell surface facing down. The membrane is sutured into place and the sutures are trimmed and made flush or even below the surface of the corneal epithelium. This process is repeated until all of the thinning areas or defect areas are repaired in line with the surrounding normal-thickness of corneal tissue. The instruments are removed and a topical antibiotic/steroid treated bandage contact lens is placed. This code reports reconstruction of multiple layers of the ocular surface.

65781

Limbal/conjunctival stem cell allografting for ocular surface reconstruction is done for corneal defects or damage resulting in a total loss of stem cell function. Corneal tissue relies on stem cells located in the limbal epithelium (the zone where corneal and conjunctival epithelia meet) to regenerate. The graft is taken from a cadaver or another living donor, not the patient. When harvesting grafts from a cadaver, they are taken from the corneoscleral rim, which is too deep and cannot be done when harvesting from a living donor. The central part of the cornea is excised and the remaining rim of cornea and sclera is sectioned into two halves, leaving a tiny rim of sclera around the limbus. The posterior part of each half is removed with a crescent blade and the donor tissue is placed with the epithelial layer upwards into a preparation solution until placement. The recipient eye of the patient is prepped and draped. Any adherent conjunctiva is excised along with any subconjunctival scar tissue. The conjunctiva is resected from the limbus in 360 degrees. The recipient beds are prepared by removing conjunctival tissue to expose the sclera. Abnormal corneal epithelium is dissected so as to leave a smooth surface. The eye is kept moist to await the graft transplantation. The previously removed corneoscleral pieces of limbal grafting tissue are centered over the damaged recipient eye and sutured into place with the corneal donor edges overlying the limbus of the damaged eye. A graft harvested from a living donor (see 68371) will be a conjunctival limbal graft and is placed with the limbal edge of the graft at the recipient limbus. The instruments are removed, the eye is patched, applying antibiotic and steroid cream, and a shield is placed.

65782

Limbal conjunctival autograft or autograft limbal transplantation (ALT) for ocular surface reconstruction is done for corneal defects or damage resulting in a total loss of stem cell function. Corneal tissue relies on stem cells located in the limbal epithelium (the zone where corneal and conjunctival epithelia meet) to regenerate. The graft is taken from the patient's other healthy eye to replace the lost stem cell population in the diseased eye. Both eyes are draped for surgery. The recipient eye is done first. Any adherent conjunctiva is excised along with any subconjunctival scar tissue. The conjunctiva is resected from the limbus in 360 degrees. The recipient beds are prepared by removing conjunctival tissue to expose the sclera. Abnormal corneal epithelium is dissected to leave a smooth surface. The eye is kept moist and attention is turned to the donor eye. The borders of the graft are marked to match the recipient beds. Saline solution is injected to raise the conjunctiva from the Tenon's layer. Incisions are made on the lateral borders of the graft first, undermining is done between, the posterior ridge is incised, and the graft is reflected. Dissection is carried to the conjunctival/limbal junction and anterior dissection is finished. The epitheliectomy removes tissue only at a superficial level and does not include sclera or corneal stroma. The free graft is removed and prepared in an appropriate storage medium. The posterior conjunctiva is advanced and anchored to the episclera. Topical antibiotics and steroids are instilled and the lids closed. The speculum is inserted again into the recipient eye, the graft is sutured into position, and the ends are cut at the knot and flushed with the corneal surface. The instruments are removed and the eyes are patched and protected.

65785

Intrastromal corneal ring segments are prescription corneal inserts made of ultrathin, biocompatible polymethylmethacrylate and implanted for the surgical treatment of mild myopia and corneal ectatic disease. The corneal ring is inserted between layers of the outer edge of the cornea, causing flattening of the center of the cornea to gently reshape the contour of the eye. Insertion is done under topical anesthesia and only takes about 15 minutes. The incision positions and segment placement are marked on the cornea and a radial incision is made with a diamond blade on the marked zone. Microfine nylon interrupted sutures are placed to close the initial incision.

65800

Though constantly flushed and renewed, the overall pressure of aqueous is constant in a healthy eye's anterior chamber. Too little or too much fluid can cause permanent damage. The practitioner aspirates aqueous from between the iris and the cornea (the anterior chamber) with a needle in what is typically called an "anterior chamber tap." The needle usually enters the anterior chamber through the corneal-scleral juncture (the limbus).

65810

The physician aspirates the gel-like vitreous that has pushed forward into the space between the iris and the cornea (the anterior chamber). Using a needle that enters the eye through the corneal-scleral juncture (the limbus), the prolapsed vitreous is removed. A laser might be used to destroy part of the membrane between the lens and the vitreous (the anterior hyaloid membrane). The physician may inject air to normalize eye pressure after fluid has been removed.

65815

Blood in the anterior chamber can coagulate and block the flow of aqueous. It can also cause cornea staining. The physician aspirates blood from between the iris and the cornea (the anterior chamber) with a needle that enters the eye through the corneal-scleral juncture (the limbus). In some cases, the physician may inject saline to flush the blood and make its removal easier. The physician may inject air to normalize eye pressure after fluid has been removed.

65820
To improve drainage of fluids in the eye, the physician enters the anterior chamber through an incision in the scleral-corneal juncture (the limbus) and cuts with a gonioknife. The blade passes across the anterior to the opposite limbus and a sweep is made to open the angle of the ring of meshlike tissue at the iris-scleral junction (the trabecular meshwork) of the opposite portion of the eye. De Vincentiis operation and Barkan's operation are both goniotomy procedures.

65850
To improve drainage of fluids in the eye, the physician inserts a trabeculotome into Schlemm's canal and rotates it into the anterior chamber to open the ring of meshlike tissue (the trabecular meshwork). The name (ab) externo, meaning outside the eye, refers to the surgical approach from outside the eye cutting toward the anterior chamber.

65855
The physician uses an argon laser to selectively burn the ring of mesh-like tissue at the iris-scleral junction (the trabecular meshwork) to improve the drainage of fluids in the anterior segment. The physician begins by placing a special contact on the eye to be treated. This lens allows the physician to view the angle structures of the eye and the trabecular network while using the laser. Though the trabecular network runs along the circumference of the iris, the physician burns holes in only a portion of that circumference during a treatment session. In this way, the physician can measure the effects of each treatment upon the eye's fluid, and suspend treatment once the proper intraocular fluid pressure is reached. No incision is made during this procedure.

65860
Sometimes scar tissue or adhesions bind structures within the eye, interfering with vision or with intraocular pressure. The physician uses a YAG laser to selectively sever vitreal, corneal, or ciliary strands or adhesions binding the iris to adjunct structures and interfering with vision. The physician begins by placing a special contact on the eye to be treated. This lens allows the physician to view the angle structures of the eye and the trabecular network while using the laser. The strands or adhesions are not removed; they simply fall out of the visual field.

65865
Sometimes scar tissue or adhesions bind structures within the eye, interfering with vision or with intraocular pressure. Through an incision in the corneal-scleral juncture (the limbus) the physician enters the anterior segment to sever vitreal, corneal, or ciliary strands or adhesions binding the iris to adjunct structures interfering with vision. The strands or adhesions are not removed; they simply fall out of the visual field.

65870-65875
The physician enters the anterior segment through the limbus to sever strands or adhesions binding the iris to adjunct structures interfering with vision. In the anterior synechiae (65870) the physician severs adhesions of the base of the iris to the cornea. For posterior synechiae (65875), the adhesions between the iris to the capsule of the lens or to the surface of the vitreous body are severed. Once the adhesions have been severed, the intraocular pressure may be restored with an injection of fluid or air. The incision is closed and an antibiotic and pressure patch may be applied.

65880
The physician enters the anterior segment through the limbus to sever strands or adhesions binding the cornea to the gel-like vitreous that has prolapsed into the anterior chamber. Once the adhesions have been severed, the intraocular pressure may be restored with an injection of fluid or air. The incision is closed and an antibiotic and pressure patch may be applied.

65900
Epithelial downgrowth describes the improper healing of surgical or traumatic wound to the cornea. The outer lining of the cornea (the epithelium) fails to close properly over the wound, instead growing around to the inner side of the cornea, sometimes continuing its growth to other structures of the eye. Disturbances in intraocular pressure and vision can result. The physician retracts the patient's eyelids with an ocular speculum. The physician locates and excises the extraneous epithelial tissue from where it has spread into the anterior chamber. The original wound may be trimmed and revised. Injections may be required to restore pressure in the anterior or posterior chambers. The procedure may require sutures or tissue glue, antibiotic ointment or a pressure patch.

65920
The clouding of the lens capsule (cataract) causes visual loss. To correct this problem, a bad lens is replaced with an artificial one. Sometimes complications require the removal of the artificial lens. The physician retracts the patient's eyelids with an ocular speculum. The physician cuts and retracts the conjunctiva and makes an incision at the juncture of the cornea and sclera (the limbus). The physician removes from the anterior segment the previously placed artificial lens (called an intraocular lens or IOL). It is not replaced. The limbus and the conjunctiva are closed with sutures. Antibiotic or a pressure patch may be applied.

65930
A blood clot in the anterior segment can block the flow of aqueous, thereby elevating intraocular pressure. It can also stain the cornea. Either condition can lead to permanent visual loss. The physician retracts the patient's eyelids with an ocular speculum. The physician uses a needle to aspirate a blood clot which has pooled in the anterior section between the iris and the cornea. The needle may enter the anterior segment through the cornea or through the limbus (the juncture of the cornea and sclera). Topical antibiotic or

a patch may be applied when the procedure is complete.

66020-66030

Though constantly flushed and renewed, the overall pressure of aqueous is constant in a healthy eye's anterior chamber. Too little or too much fluid can cause permanent damage. The physician administers a needle injection of air or liquid (66020) or medication (66030) to the anterior of the eye. The needle may enter the anterior segment through the cornea or through the limbus (the juncture of the cornea and sclera).

66130

The sclera, coming from the Greek word for "hard," is the tough, white, outer coat of the eye. To remove a scleral lesion, the physician cuts through the thin, transparent conjunctiva and snips the lesion with scleral scissors. The scleral and conjunctival wounds may not require sutures. The physician applies antibiotic ointment and possibly a 24-hour pressure patch.

66150-66155

To create a new pathway for fluids in the eye, the physician makes an incision in the conjunctiva near the limbus (the corneal-scleral juncture). Using a trephine to remove a circular portion of sclera and iris (66150) or by destroying a portion of the sclera and iris by burning it with a hot probe (66155), the physician creates a collection area to improve the flow of aqueous. One method of this procedure is called Elliot's operation. The physician closes the incision with sutures and may restore the intraocular pressure with an injection of water or saline. A topical antibiotic or pressure patch may be applied.

66160

To improve the flow of aqueous, the physician makes an incision in the conjunctiva near the limbus (the corneal-scleral juncture). By using a punch or scleral scissors, the physician removes a portion of sclera and iris, creating a collection area for fluids in the anterior chamber. Various methods of sclerectomy include Lindner's, LaGrange, Knapp's, Holth's and Herbert's operations. The physician closes the incision with sutures and may restore the intraocular pressure with an injection of water or saline. A topical antibiotic or pressure patch may be applied.

66170-66172

Though constantly flushed and renewed, the overall pressure of aqueous is constant in a healthy eye's anterior chamber. Too little or too much fluid can cause permanent damage. The physician places an ocular speculum in the patient's eye, and accesses the anterior chamber through an incision through the limbus (the corneal-scleral juncture). To promote better drainage of fluid, the physician removes a partial thickness portion of the ring of meshlike tissue at the iris-scleral junction (the trabecular meshwork), and a scleral trap door is left open so that aqueous may flow through the new channel into the space between the conjunctival and the sclera or cornea (bleb). The physician closes the incision with sutures and may restore the intraocular pressure with an injection of water or saline. A topical antibiotic or pressure patch may be applied. This procedure is performed in absence of previous surgery (66170) or as a repeated surgery where adhesions are reduced (66172). The adhesions may also have been caused by trauma.

66174-66175

The physician dilates the aqueous outflow canal (canaloplasty) for the treatment of glaucoma. Via scleral cutdown, the physician dilates the circular canal in the eye that drains aqueous humor from the anterior chamber into the anterior ciliary veins (Schlemm's canal) using a flexible microcatheter and viscoelastic gel in 66174; no device or stent is retained. In 66175, a device (e.g., flexible stent, suture) is attached to the distal tip of the microcatheter and positioned into the canal. At the conclusion of the procedure, the microcatheter is removed from the canal and the outer scleral flap and conjunctiva are sutured closed to seal the surgical site.

66179-66180

Aqueous drainage devices are employed to treat all forms of glaucoma, but are primarily used in patients with elevated intraocular pressure (IOP) despite aggressive medical treatment. An aqueous shunt creates an alternate path for aqueous humor to leave the anterior chamber of the eye and thus lower IOP. The physician places an ocular speculum in the patient's eye, makes an incision in the conjunctiva, places tubing into the anterior portion of the eye at the juncture of the sclera and cornea (the limbus), and sutures tubing to the sclera. This improves the aqueous flow in the anterior chamber. The tube implant connects to an equatorial reservoir plate (a bleb) sutured into place behind the pars plana between the extraocular muscles. The physician stretches conjunctival tissue over the shunt and reservoir and sutures it into place. The physician closes the incision with sutures and may restore the intraocular pressure with an injection of water or saline. A topical antibiotic or pressure patch may be applied. Report 66180 if the procedure includes a graft.

66183

The physician treats a refractory, primary, open-angle glaucoma by draining aqueous humor from the anterior chamber directly into the Schlemm's canal by shunting or stenting, lowering intraocular pressure (IOP) without the formation of a filtering bleb using an external approach. The physician inserts the implant via a superficial scleral flap through the trabeculum and into the anterior chamber. IOP is reduced by diverting the excess aqueous fluid from the anterior chamber to a subconjunctival bleb rather than to an extraocular reservoir.

66184-66185

The physician revises a previously placed aqueous shunt to extraocular equatorial plate reservoir. The physician places an ocular speculum in the patient's eye and opens the previous incision in the conjunctiva. The tubing from the anterior chamber to the reservoir is revised or replaced. The physician stretches conjunctival tissue over the shunt and reservoir and sutures it into place. The physician may restore the intraocular pressure with an injection of water or saline. A topical antibiotic or pressure patch may be applied. Report 66184 for revision without graft and 66185 for revision with graft.

66225
A staphyloma is a bulging protrusion of the vascular coating of the eyeball (uvea) into a thin, stretched portion of the sclera. To repair the staphyloma, the physician places an ocular speculum in the patient's eye and makes an incision in the conjunctiva and sclera over the site of a staphyloma. The physician excises the full-thickness staphyloma. A piece of stretched sclera may also be removed. A graft involving donor sclera tissue is used to close the surgical defect. The physician uses sutures or tissue glue in the layered repair. Antibiotic ointment and a patch may be applied.

66250
The physician reexplores an eye wound that is the site of previous surgery to revise post-operative defects. The physician uses a number of techniques, based on the wound and previous surgery. Surgery may be major or minor.

66500-66505
Though constantly flushed and renewed, the overall pressure of aqueous is constant in a healthy eye's anterior chamber. Too little or too much fluid can cause permanent damage. To enhance the flow of fluids in the anterior chamber, the physician makes an incision in the corneal-scleral juncture (the limbus). The physician slices through the iris in a side-to-side motion in an effort to increase the flow of aqueous hampered by a pupillary block (66500). No tissue is removed. In the iris bombe, where the iris balloons forward blocking aqueous outflow channels, the surgeon pierces the iris in two places (66505). The physician closes the incision with sutures and may restore intraocular pressure with an injection of water or saline. A topical antibiotic or pressure patch may be applied.

66600-66605
The physician places a contact lens on the patient's eye to direct the laser's beam. The excision of a full-thickness piece of the iris is usually accomplished with an argon laser. The physician uses the "chipping away technique" until the iris is penetrated for the excision. With cyclectomy (66605), the burn is deeper, going through the iris into the ciliary body.

66625
After placing an ocular speculum in the patient's eye, the physician makes an incision at the juncture of the cornea and sclera (the limbus). The physician removes a piece of iris, providing a direct passageway for aqueous. This causes the intraocular pressure to fall as aqueous from behind the iris can flow forward and drain from the eye. This procedure is also called basal, buttonhole, or stenopeic iridectomy. The physician may close the incision with sutures and may restore the intraocular pressure with an injection of water or saline. A topical antibiotic or pressure patch may be applied.

66630
Though constantly flushed and renewed, the overall pressure of aqueous is constant in a healthy eye's anterior chamber. Too little or too much fluid can cause permanent damage. To enhance the flow of fluids in the eye, the physician makes an incision at the juncture of the cornea and sclera (the limbus). The physician removes a wedge piece from the iris leaving what is often referred to as a keyhole pupil. This causes the intraocular pressure to fall as aqueous from behind the iris can flow forward and drain from the eye. The physician may close the incision with sutures and may restore the intraocular pressure with an injection of water or saline. A topical antibiotic or pressure patch may be applied.

66635
After placing an ocular speculum in the patient's eye, the physician makes an incision at the juncture of the cornea and sclera (the limbus). The physician trims an inner ring of iris as a means of widening an abnormally small pupil and improving vision. The physician may close the incision with sutures and may restore the intraocular pressure with an injection of water or saline. A topical antibiotic or pressure patch may be applied.

66680-66682
After placing an ocular speculum in the patient's eye, the physician makes an incision at the juncture of the cornea and sclera (the limbus) to approach and repair a trauma-caused tear of the iris from the ciliary body. The wedge shaped tear is affixed to the ciliary body with dissolving sutures, or with stitches that can be removed through an incision prepared for that retrieval. This procedure includes the later removal of the McCannel suture. The physician may close the incision with sutures and may restore the intraocular pressure with an injection of water or saline. A topical antibiotic or pressure patch may be applied. Report 66682 for a suture of the iris or ciliary body.

66683
The physician inserts a biocompatible prosthetic iris (the colored part of the pupil). Made of thin, pliable, medical-grade silicone, the prosthesis mimics the function of the natural iris and creates an artificial pupil that reduces the amount of light entering the eye. Indicated for those with congenital or traumatic aniridia (complete or partial absence of the iris), as well as iris defects due to conditions such as albinism or surgical removal due to melanoma, the device can be sized and colored for each individual patient. Repair or removal of the iris may be performed in conjunction with the insertion. In one method of implantation, a small incision is made and the rolled device is inserted under the incision into the sulcus ciliaris. Using surgical

instruments, the device is unfolded and the edges smoothed. It may be held in place by the eye's anatomical structures or, if necessary, by sutures. In another method, a proprietary injector is used to place the prosthesis into the capsular bag.

66700-66710
The ciliary body supplies the anterior chamber with aqueous humor. In cases where high intraocular pressure cannot otherwise be controlled, portions of the ciliary body are destroyed to reduce the production of aqueous humor. The physician makes an incision in the conjunctiva and through the sclera in the pars plana opposite the site of the ciliary body to be treated. The physician uses a heat probe (diathermy) or laser (cyclophotocoagulation) to burn holes in the ciliary body. The physician closes the incision with layered sutures and may restore the intraocular pressure with an anterior and/or posterior injection. A topical antibiotic or pressure patch may be applied. Report 66700 when diathermy is used and 66710 if transscleral cyclophotocoagulation is used.

66711
The ciliary body supplies the anterior chamber with aqueous humor. In cases where high intraocular pressure cannot otherwise be controlled, portions of the ciliary body are destroyed to reduce the production of aqueous humor. Endoscopic cyclophotocoagulation (ECP) is performed on the ciliary body and may be accomplished by different methods. In one method, with the pupil dilated, a limbal incision is made and any posterior synechiae are lysed. Viscoelastic material is injected under the iris to partially fill and expand the ciliary sulcus. The ECP probe is inserted under the iris. The probe allows simultaneous visualization with the photocoagulation. Approximately half the circumference of the ciliary body is treated through the first limbal incision. Another incision is made 180 degrees from the first and the other half of the ciliary body circumference is treated. The viscoelastic material is removed by irrigation and aspiration and the wounds are closed. The crystalline lens is not removed during this procedure.

66720
The ciliary body supplies the anterior chamber with aqueous humor. In cases where high intraocular pressure cannot otherwise be controlled, portions of the ciliary body are destroyed to reduce the production of aqueous humor. The physician applies a freezing probe to the sclera over the ciliary body with the purpose of destroying the ciliary process. This is especially useful in aphakic patients.

66740
The ciliary body supplies the anterior chamber with aqueous humor. In cases where high intraocular pressure cannot otherwise be controlled, portions of the ciliary body are destroyed to reduce the production of aqueous humor. The physician makes an incision in the conjunctiva and sclera in the pars plana adjacent to the portion of ciliary body to be treated. The physician passes a spatula through the incision and into the suprachoroidal space of the anterior chamber. The spatula separates the ciliary body from the scleral spur. This may result in a lowering of intraocular pressure by a decrease in aqueous humor formation from the now detached ciliary body or by increasing uveovascular scleral outflow of aqueous. The physician closes the incision with layered sutures and may restore the intraocular pressure with an anterior and/or posterior injection. A topical antibiotic or pressure patch may be applied.

66761
After applying a topical anesthetic, the physician places a special contact lens on the patient's eye. The argon or YAG laser is focused on the iris and multiple short bursts of laser light create holes in the iris. This procedure allows fluids in the eye to pass from behind the iris through the openings into the space between the iris and the cornea (the anterior chamber), lowering intraocular pressure. This code is reported once per session.

66762
The physician places a special contact lens on the eye of the patient and uses multiple bursts of light from an argon laser to create an additional hole in the iris.

66770
The physician places a special contact lens on the eye of the patient. The YAG or Argon laser is focused on the cyst or lesion and multiple short bursts of light destroy the abnormal tissue.

66820
The patient initially had extracapsular cataract surgery in which the posterior shell of the lens was not removed from the eye. But the capsule and/or the membrane adjacent to it (the anterior hyaloid) has since become opaque and must be opened in this new surgery. After placing an ocular speculum in the patient's eye, the pupil is dilated. The physician inserts a small needle, a Ziegler or Wheeler knife or special scissors into the corneal-scleral juncture (the limbus) and advances it to the edge of the capsule and through to the membrane, cutting a flap in the opaque membrane in the field of vision. The physician maneuvers the instrument around any artificial lens. No tissue is removed from the eye; the flap simply opens a window of vision. The physician may close the incision with sutures and may restore the intraocular pressure with an injection of water or saline. A topical antibiotic or pressure patch may be applied.

66821
The patient initially had extracapsular cataract surgery in which the posterior shell of the lens was not removed from the eye. But the capsule and/or the membrane adjacent to it (the anterior hyaloid) has since become opaque and must be destroyed in this new surgery. After a topical anesthetic is applied to the eye, the pupil is dilated. A number of YAG laser shots are focused to a point on the capsule, cutting it. Bursts from the YAG open a flap in the capsule, resulting in

immediate improvement in vision. Multiple sessions may be needed to create an adequate opening in the lens capsule.

66825
The physician inserts a lid speculum between the patient's eyelids and the eye is secured by a suture. The physician cuts an opening at the juncture of the cornea and sclera (limbus) to access the artificial lens. The physician adjusts the artificial lens so that the attachments (haptics) of the implant are secured. The physician may close the incision with sutures and may restore the intraocular pressure with an injection of water or saline. A topical antibiotic or pressure patch may be applied.

66830
The patient initially had extracapsular cataract surgery, in which the posterior shell of the lens was not removed from the eye. But the capsule and/or the membrane adjacent to it (the anterior hyaloid) has since become opaque and must be removed in this new surgery. The physician inserts an ocular speculum into the patient's orbit, and makes an incision at the juncture of the cornea and sclera (the limbus). A small cutting needle and suction device (an irrigating cystotome) is inserted to chip away the posterior lens capsule. In some cases, the iris must be cut or a piece of iris removed to access the lens capsule. The adjacent membrane (the anterior hyaloid) may also be removed. The physician irrigates the area during aspiration. The physician may close the incision with sutures and may restore the intraocular pressure with an injection of water or saline. A topical antibiotic or pressure patch may be applied.

66840
The physician makes an incision at the juncture of the cornea and sclera (the limbus). The anterior wall of the lens is incised. A probe attached to an irrigating/aspirating machine is inserted into the lens and the lens is destroyed and sucked away. The physician may close the incision with sutures and may restore the intraocular pressure with an injection of water or saline. A topical antibiotic or pressure patch may be applied.

66850
The physician makes an incision in the cornea or the pars plana. The anterior wall of the lens is cut out. The same type of irrigating/aspirating machine used for extracapsular surgery is used for phacofragmentation, but this time the probe is a needle that vibrates 40,000 times per second (phacofragmentation), or sound waves (phacoemulsification, ultrasound) that break up the lens. The physician uses irrigation and suction to remove the once hard nucleus, now liquefied by mechanical or sound vibrations. The physician may close the incision with sutures or may design a sutureless "self-sealing" incision. The physician may restore the intraocular pressure with an injection of water or saline. A topical antibiotic or pressure patch may be applied.

66852
To remove a cataract obstructing the view of the retina during retinal surgery, or to remove a piece of natural lens retained following cataract surgery, the physician makes an incision in the conjunctiva, sclera, and choroid of the pars plana. The physician approaches the lens capsule from behind. If the lens is being removed, the wall of the posterior lens capsule is removed and a small suction device is inserted into the lens. The lens material is sucked out. The physician irrigates the area during aspiration. If a retained portion of the lens is removed, a portion of the clear gel in the back of the eye may be removed as well (vitrectomy). The incision is closed with layered sutures. The physician may restore anterior or posterior intraocular pressure with an injection of water or saline. A topical antibiotic or pressure patch may be applied.

66920-66930
In intracapsular cataract extraction (ICCE), the lens and capsule are removed intact. The physician inserts an ocular speculum. An incision is made in the corneal-scleral juncture (the limbus). To enhance the flow of fluids in the eye, the physician may punch a hole in the iris before inserting a surgical instrument filled with coolant (cryoprobe) into the anterior chamber. The lens adheres to the cryoprobe as it freezes, and when the cryoprobe is removed, the lens comes with it (66920). The same technique is used to remove a dislocated lens (66930). The physician may close the incision with sutures and may restore intraocular pressure with an injection of water or saline. A topical antibiotic or pressure patch may be applied.

66940
In extracapsular cataract extraction (ECCE), the anterior shell and the nucleus of the lens capsule are both removed, leaving the posterior shell of the lens capsule in place. The physician inserts a lid speculum between the patient's eyelids and makes an incision in the corneal-scleral juncture (the limbus). To enhance the flow of fluids in the eye, the physician may punch a hole in the iris. Using a method other than aspiration or phacofragmentation, the physician removes the lens in parts: first the anterior lens, then the inner, hard nucleus. The clear, posterior capsule remains. The physician may close the incision with sutures and may restore the intraocular pressure with an injection of water or saline. A topical antibiotic or pressure patch may be applied.

66982 [66987, 66989]
The physician performs a complex extracapsular cataract removal with insertion of an intraocular lens prosthesis in a one-stage procedure. A local anesthetic is injected into the periorbital area. The physician makes a small horizontal incision where the cornea and sclera meet and, upon entering the eye through the incision, gently opens the front of the capsule and removes the hard center, or nucleus, of the lens. Using a microscope, the ophthalmologist suctions out the

soft lens cortex, leaving the capsule in place. The area is irrigated and aspirated and an intraocular lens (IOL), a plastic disc that replaces the natural lens, is inserted. The ophthalmologist sutures the incision and instills antibiotic ointment and applies an eye patch. A metal shield is secured over the eye with tape. Standard phacoemulsification may be performed if the lens capsule is intact and sufficient zonular support remains. In capsulorrhexis, the ophthalmologist shatters the cataract nucleus with an ultrasonic oscillating probe. After fragmentation, the phaco probe is inserted into the eye and the cataract is suctioned out through an irrigation-aspiration probe. An IOL is inserted once all the material is removed. Suture fixation is chosen if both capsular and zonular supports are insufficient and the angle is minimally damaged. In 66987, endoscopic cyclophotocoagulation (ECP) is also performed on the ciliary body and may be accomplished by different methods. In one method, with the pupil dilated, a limbal incision is made and any posterior synechiae are lysed. Viscoelastic material is injected under the iris to partially fill and expand the ciliary sulcus. The ECP probe is inserted under the iris. The probe allows simultaneous visualization with the photocoagulation. Approximately half the circumference of the ciliary body is treated through the first limbal incision. Another incision is made 180 degrees from the first and the other half of the ciliary body circumference is treated. The viscoelastic material is removed by irrigation and aspiration and the wounds are closed. In 66989, one or more anterior segment aqueous drainage devices are inserted. Aqueous drainage devices are employed to treat refractory, primary, open-angle glaucoma. These are minimally penetrating methods to drain aqueous humor from the anterior chamber into Schlemm's canal or the suprachoroidal space by shunting or stenting, lowering intraocular pressure (IOP) without the formation of a filtering bleb. Using an internal approach and no external reservoir, the physician makes a corneal incision through which one or more stents are inserted using a microdelivery system into the trabecular meshwork, the supraciliary space, or the suprachoroidal space.

66983

In intracapsular cataract extraction (ICCE), the lens and capsule are removed intact. The physician inserts an ocular speculum. An incision is made in the corneal-scleral juncture (the limbus). To enhance the flow of fluids in the eye, the physician may punch a hole in the iris before inserting a surgical instrument filled with coolant (cryoprobe) into the anterior chamber. The lens adheres to the cryoprobe as it freezes, and when the cryoprobe is removed, the lens comes with it. The physician injects a bubble of air into the anterior chamber to protect the cornea. The physician places an intraocular lens in the anterior chamber. The optic, or center, of the implant lies centered at the pupil and the haptics (securing attachments) of the implant are wedged in the anterior chamber, fixating the implant so it cannot move. The physician may close the incision with sutures and may restore the intraocular pressure with an injection of water or saline. A topical antibiotic or pressure patch may be applied.

66984 [66988, 66991]

In extracapsular cataract extraction (ECCE), the anterior shell and the nucleus of the lens capsule are removed, leaving the posterior shell of the lens capsule in place. The physician inserts a lid speculum between the patient's eyelids and makes an incision in the corneal-scleral juncture (the limbus). To enhance the flow of fluids in the eye, the physician may create a hole in the iris. Using a cutting and suction or ultrasonic device, the physician removes the lens in parts: first the anterior lens, then the inner, hard nucleus. The clear, posterior capsule remains. The physician injects a bubble of air into the anterior chamber to protect the cornea. The physician guides the intraocular implant into the eye. The haptics (securing attachments) lodge into the ciliary sulcus or the lens capsule, occupying the exact position of the original cataract. The physician may close the incision with sutures and may restore the intraocular pressure with an injection of water or saline. A topical antibiotic or pressure patch may be applied. In 66988, endoscopic cyclophotocoagulation (ECP) is also performed on the ciliary body and may be accomplished by different methods. In one method, with the pupil dilated, a limbal incision is made and any posterior synechiae are lysed. Viscoelastic material is injected under the iris to partially fill and expand the ciliary sulcus. The ECP probe is inserted under the iris. The probe allows simultaneous visualization with the photocoagulation. Approximately half the circumference of the ciliary body is treated through the first limbal incision. Another incision is made 180 degrees from the first and the other half of the ciliary body circumference is treated. The viscoelastic material is removed by irrigation and aspiration and the wounds are closed. In 66991, one or more anterior segment aqueous drainage devices are inserted. Aqueous drainage devices are employed to treat refractory, primary, open-angle glaucoma. These are minimally penetrating methods to drain aqueous humor from the anterior chamber into Schlemm's canal or the suprachoroidal space by shunting or stenting, lowering intraocular pressure (IOP) without the formation of a filtering bleb. Using an internal approach and no external reservoir, the physician makes a corneal incision through which one or more stents are inserted using a microdelivery system into the trabecular meshwork, the supraciliary space, or the suprachoroidal space.

66985

The physician inserts an ocular speculum. An incision is made in the corneal-scleral juncture (the limbus). For an anterior lens, the physician places an intraocular lens in the fluid-filled space between the iris and cornea (the anterior chamber). The optic, or center, of the implant lies just in front of the pupil and the haptics (securing attachments) of the implant are wedged between the iris and cornea, fixating the implant so it cannot move. For a posterior lens, the physician injects a bubble of air into the anterior chamber to protect the cornea. The physician guides the intraocular implant into the eye. The haptics lodge into the ciliary sulcus or the lens capsule. The physician may close the incision with sutures and may restore the intraocular pressure with an injection of water or saline. A topical antibiotic or pressure patch may be applied.

66986
Early models of intraocular lens (IOL) implants sometimes cause irritation in the patient's eye. They can also become dislocated. Here, the physician exchanges the problematic lens for a newer one. For anterior IOL, the physician replaces an intraocular lens in the fluid-filled space between the iris and cornea (the anterior chamber). The optic, or center, of the implant lies just in front of the pupil and the haptics (securing attachments) of the implant are lodged between the iris and cornea, fixating the implant so it cannot move. For posterior IOL, the physician injects a bubble of air into the anterior chamber through a syringe to protect the cornea. The physician replaces the intraocular implant in the eye. The haptics lodge into the ciliary sulcus or the lens capsule. The physician may close the incision with sutures and may restore the intraocular pressure with an injection of water or saline. A topical antibiotic or pressure patch may be applied.

66990
The ophthalmic endoscope is used for diagnostic purposes or in conjunction with another procedure. The endoscope is properly focused prior to the procedure. Once prepared, an 18- to 20-gauge endoscopic probe tip is inserted through a sclerotomy site. The physician maintains a working distance of 2 to 10 mm to allow visualization of the internal eye structures. It is commonly used when visualization is impaired by pathological changes or poor pupillary dilatation. Once the procedure is complete, the endoscope is removed and the physician may close the incision with sutures. A topical antibiotic or pressure patch maybe applied. This code is used in addition to the primary procedure.

67005-67010
The physician inserts a needle at the limbus or through the cornea (open sky technique) and passes the needle to the back of the anterior segment where a portion of displaced vitreous humor is aspirated (67005). If most or all of the vitreous is extracted, mechanical tools are used (67010). When this is done, the physician extracts the vitreous, using a mechanical cutting and suctioning process that may involve a rotoextractor or vitreous infusion suction cutter (VISC). In either case, the aspirated vitreous is usually replaced by an injection of a vitreous substitute or aqueous. Any incision is closed with sutures.

67015
The physician inserts a needle into the posterior chamber through the pars plana to aspirate vitreous. Sometimes a posterior sclerotomy is made to release the fluid. When this is done, the physician extracts the vitreous, using a mechanical cutting and suctioning process that may involve a rotoextractor or vitreous infusion suction cutter (VISC). This is often called a vitreous chamber tap in operative reports. Once completed, the incision is repaired with sutures. Intraocular pressure may be adjusted with an injection. A pressure patch may be applied.

67025
The physician inserts a syringe in the pars plana to inject a material like Healon or silicone. The injection may be required to replace vitreous that has been aspirated as part of this procedure, to restore intraocular pressure lost in another manner.

67027
The physician implants an intravitreal drug delivery system to provide consistent delivery of a drug to an area of the eye affected by disease. Implants are capable of releasing a controlled amount of a specific drug for months, avoiding drug toxicity and other problems associated with prolonged intravenous therapies. Using a scalpel, the physician makes an inferotemporal pars plana incision. Approximately 0.5 milliliter of vitreous is removed. The implant (e.g., ganciclovir or fluocinolone acetonide) in the form of a small pellet is placed through the wound, implanted into the vitreous, and sutured to the sclera. The wound is closed and intraocular pressure is restored.

67028
The physician introduces medication such as antibiotics, anticoagulants, or anti-inflammatory agents into the posterior segment via a small syringe. Local anesthetic drops are used to numb the eye prior to the procedure, followed by a solution such as povidone iodine to clean and disinfect the eye. A lid retractor or speculum is employed to avoid contamination of the needle by the lashes. Following injection, topical antibiotic drops are applied. A vision check is performed, and the patient observed for increased intraocular pressure (IOP). This medication administration does not require any sutures.

67030
The physician makes a small incision in the conjunctiva, sclera, and choroid in the pars plana. A narrow knife is inserted to cut vitreous strands that obstruct the patient's vision. The strands generally fall away from the visual field and are not retrieved. The physician repairs the pars plana incision with a layered closure and may restore the intraocular pressure with an injection of aqueous or vitreal substitute. A cataract specialist might approach the dissection through a limbal incision (at the corneal-scleral juncture), instead of through the pars plana. A topical antibiotic or pressure patch may be applied after either approach.

67031
The vitreous is the clear gel filling the posterior cavity of the eyeball. After applying a topical anesthetic and dilating the patient's pupil, the physician applies a special contact lens to the cornea of the patient. The physician uses a YAG laser to cut vitreous strands, adhesions, or opacities that obstruct the patient's vision. No tissue is removed and no incision is made. More than one treatment may be required.

67036
The physician performs a mechanical vitrectomy, utilizing a pars plana approach. The physician applies a special contact lens to the cornea to better visualize the back of the eye. Three small incisions are made in the eyeball, each about 4 mm from the juncture of the cornea and sclera. One incision is for a light cannula, one for an infusion cannula, and one for the cutting or suction instruments. The physician extracts the vitreous, using a mechanical cutting and suctioning process that may involve a rotoextractor or vitreous infusion suction cutter (VISC). This is often called a posterior sclerotomy in operative reports. The cannulas are extracted and the incisions repaired with layered closures. Injections may be required to reestablish intraocular pressure. A topical antibiotic or pressure patch may be applied.

67039-67040
The vitreous is the clear gel filling the posterior cavity of the eyeball. The physician applies a special contact lens to the cornea to better visualize the back of the eye. Three small incisions are made in the eyeball, each about 4 mm from the juncture of the cornea and sclera. (This is the pars plana approach.) One incision is for a light cannula, one for an infusion cannula and one for the laser. The physician extracts the vitreous, using a mechanical cutting and suctioning process that may involve a rotoextractor or vitreous infusion suction cutter (VISC). With focal endolaser photocoagulation (67039), the physician uses a laser to treat minor retinal disorders. If the physician performs endolaser panretinal photocoagulation (67040), a stronger laser treats larger retinal problems, like retinal detachments, diabetic retinopathy, or retinal holes. The cannulas are extracted and the incisions repaired with layered closures. Injections may be required to reestablish the intraocular pressure. A topical antibiotic or pressure patch may be applied.

67041
In macular pucker, or cellophane retinopathy, scar tissue forms a membrane across the central retina of the eye (the macula) and interferes with central vision. The vitreous is the clear gel filling the posterior cavity of the eyeball. The physician applies a special contact lens to the cornea to better visualize the back of the eye. Three small incisions are made in the eyeball, each about 4 mm from the juncture of the cornea and sclera. (This is the pars plana approach.) One incision is for a light cannula, one for an infusion cannula, and one for the cutting or suction instruments. The physician extracts the vitreous, using a mechanical cutting and suctioning process that may involve a rotoextractor or vitreous infusion suction cutter (VISC). This is often called a posterior sclerotomy in operative reports. To repair a macular pucker, the physician uses specialized microsurgical instruments to gently peel and remove the scar tissue from the surface of the retina in order to alleviate the traction and lessen the retinal surface distortion. The cannulas are extracted and the incisions repaired with layered closures. Injections may be required to reestablish intraocular pressure. A topical antibiotic or pressure patch may be applied.

67042
The vitreous is the clear gel filling the posterior cavity of the eyeball. The physician applies a special contact lens to the cornea to better visualize the back of the eye. Three small incisions are made in the eyeball, each about 4 mm from the juncture of the cornea and sclera. (This is the pars plana approach.) One incision is for a light cannula, one for an infusion cannula, and one for the cutting or suction instruments. To repair a macular hole or treat diabetic macular edema, the physician uses specialized microsurgical instruments to grasp and peel the internal limiting membrane of the retina. The cannulas are extracted and the incisions repaired with layered closures. Injections of air, gas, or silicone oil may be required to stabilize the retina. A topical antibiotic or pressure patch may be applied.

67043
The vitreous is the clear gel filling the posterior cavity of the eyeball. The physician applies a special contact lens to the cornea to better visualize the back of the eye. Three small incisions are made in the eyeball, each about 4 mm from the juncture of the cornea and sclera. (This is the pars plana approach.) One incision is for a light cannula, one for an infusion cannula, and one for the cutting or suction instruments. Using a subretinal pick or infusion cannula, the physician performs a retinotomy to access the subretinal membrane. The membrane is carefully elevated and grasped with subretinal forceps, then gently peeled and removed through the retinotomy site. Focal endolaser coagulation may also be performed to treat minor retinal disorders, or the physician may perform endolaser panretinal photocoagulation using a stronger laser to treat larger retinal problems such as retinal detachments, diabetic retinopathy, or retinal holes. Injections of air, gas, or silicone oil may be required to stabilize the retina. The cannulas are extracted and the incisions repaired with layered closures.

67101
When the retina detaches, it separates from its nourishing blood supply and falls into the posterior cavity of the eye, resulting in vision loss. The physician reattaches the retina by freezing (cryotherapy) and thus sealing the retinal tissue to the back of the eye. The physician explores the sclera and stay sutures are placed under the involved rectus muscles so the eye can be rotated to expose the area to be treated. Sometimes a rectus muscle is temporarily detached to permit adequate exposure. Cryotherapy is performed

without entering the posterior chamber. The probe is pressed against the sclera overlying the site of the retinal defect, sealing it against the choroid. If subretinal fluid must be drained, the physician makes an incision in the sclera (sclerotomy) to permit access to the middle layer of the eye's shell (the choroid), which is perforated so that fluid drains out. Any incisions are repaired with layered closures. Injections may be required to reestablish proper intraocular pressure. A topical antibiotic or pressure patch may be applied.

67105
When the retina detaches, it separates from its nourishing blood supply and falls into the posterior cavity of the eye, resulting in vision loss. Using a laser light or xenon arc that goes through a dilated pupil without an incision, the physician burns spots at the site of the retinal detachment or retinal tear to seal the retina back into place against the choroid (vascular, middle layer of the eye's shell). If subretinal fluid must be drained, the physician cuts through the conjunctiva and into the sclera (sclerotomy) to access the choroid, which is perforated so that fluid drains out. Any incisions are repaired with layered closures. Injections may be required to reestablish the intraocular pressure. A topical antibiotic or pressure patch may be applied.

67107
The physician explores the sclera to locate the site overlying a retinal detachment. Stay sutures are placed under involved rectus muscles so the eye may be exposed to the area that will be treated. The physician treats the retinal tear externally, by placing a cold or hot probe over the scleral and depressing it. The burn seals the choroid to the retina at the site of the tear. The physician cuts a groove in the sclera and mattress sutures are placed across this incision. Any subretinal fluid is drained. A silastic band is laid in the scleral bed and sutured in place. Sometimes a silicone sponge is placed under the band. Additional cryotherapy or photocoagulation may be accomplished at this time. When the tear has been adequately repaired and supported, the rectus muscle sutures are removed.

67108
When the retina detaches, it separates from its nourishing blood supply and falls into the posterior cavity of the eye, resulting in loss of vision. The physician reattaches the retina by freezing (cryotherapy), heat application (diathermy), or laser light to seal the retinal tissue to the back of the eye. Cryotherapy and diathermy are performed without entering the posterior chamber; either probe is pressed against the sclera overlying the site of the retinal defect, sealing it against the choroid. If a laser is used, the light goes through a dilated pupil without an incision to burn spots at the site of the retinal detachment or retinal tear and seals the retina back into place against the choroid (vascular, middle layer of the eye's shell). A scleral buckle may be placed by suturing a silicone band around the scleral bed and securing it. The buckle supports the healing retinal tear and holds the retina against the choroid by increasing the pressure within the eye. Expendable gas may also be injected into the eye to flatten out the retinal detachment against the choroid. The physician removes any vitreous opacity or vitreous traction. The lens may be removed if it interferes with the physician's view of the retina or if the lens is in the way of the removal of scar tissue. Any incisions may be repaired with sutures. Antibiotic ointment and a pressure patch may be applied.

67110
When the retina detaches, it separates from its nourishing blood supply and falls into the posterior cavity of the eye. Loss of vision results. The physician uses a needle to inject expandable gas into the eye to flatten the retinal tear and applies laser or cryotherapy to seal the retinal tear. The physician explores the sclera to locate the site overlying a retinal detachment. Stay sutures are placed under involved rectus muscles so the eye may be exposed to area that will be treated. Air or other gas is injected through the sclera into the posterior segment of the eye to flatten the retinal detachment against the choroid. The patient is instructed to maintain a posture that will position the bubble against the detachment. The physician treats the retinal tear externally, by placing a cold (cryotherapy) or hot (diathermy) probe over the sclera and depressing it. The burn seals the choroid to the retina at the site of the tear. This procedure is often called pneumatic retinopexy.

67113
When the retina detaches, it separates from its nourishing blood supply and falls into the posterior cavity of the eye, resulting in loss of vision. To repair a complex retinal detachment, the physician first extracts the vitreous, using a mechanical cutting and suctioning process that may involve a rotoextractor or vitreous infusion suction cutter (VISC). This is often called a posterior sclerotomy. To strip the epiretinal membrane, the physician uses a retinal cutting instrument to peel membrane or scar tissue creating tension on the retinal surface. To reattach the retina, the physician may also use freezing (cryotherapy) or laser light to seal the retinal tissue to the back of the eye. Cryotherapy is performed without entering the posterior chamber; a probe is pressed against the sclera overlying the site of the retinal defect, sealing it against the choroid. If a laser is used, the light goes through a dilated pupil without an incision to burn spots at the site of the retinal detachment or retinal tear and seals the retina back into place against the choroid (vascular, middle layer of the eye's shell). A scleral buckle may be placed by suturing a silicone band around the scleral bed and securing it. The buckle supports the healing retinal tear and holds the retina against the choroid by increasing the pressure within the eye. Expendable gas, air, or silicone oil may also be injected into the eye to flatten out the retinal detachment against the choroid. If subretinal fluid must be drained, the physician cuts through the conjunctiva and into the sclera (sclerotomy) to access

the choroid, which is perforated so that fluid drains out. The physician removes any vitreous opacity or vitreous traction. The lens may be removed if it interferes with the physician's view of the retina or if the lens is in the way of the removal of scar tissue. Any incisions may be repaired with sutures. Antibiotic ointment and a pressure patch may be applied.

67115

The physician inserts an ocular speculum. To release the tension in a previously placed scleral buckle, the physician makes an incision in the conjunctiva and sclera, adjusts the buckle, and repairs the surgical wound with sutures.

67120

The physician inserts an ocular speculum. The physician removes a previously implanted extraocular tube, reservoir, buckle, or other prosthetic device from the eye. The physician may close the incision with sutures and may restore the intraocular pressure with an injection of water or saline. A topical antibiotic or pressure patch may be applied.

67121

An incision is made in the pars plana near the site of an intraocular lens that has fallen into the posterior segment of the eye. The physician removes the extracapsular IOL from the eye. The physician closes the incision with sutures and may restore the intraocular pressure with an injection of vitreous substitute. A topical antibiotic or pressure patch may be applied.

67141-67145

When the retina detaches, it separates from its nourishing blood supply and falls into the posterior cavity of the eye. Loss of vision results. In 67141, the physician secures a degenerating retina by freezing (cryotherapy) and thus sealing the retinal tissue to the back of the eye, or by diathermy, where heat is used for the same purpose. The physician explores the sclera and stay sutures are placed under the involved rectus muscles so the eye can be rotated to expose the area to be treated. Sometimes, a rectus muscle is temporarily detached to permit adequate exposure. Cryotherapy and diathermy are performed without entering the posterior chamber; either probe is pressed against the sclera overlying the site of the retinal defect, sealing it against the choroid. In 67145, the physician treats retinal detachment with photocoagulation, often using a laser light or xenon arc that goes through a dilated pupil without an incision. The physician burns spots at the site of the retinal weakness to seal the retina into place against the choroid (vascular, middle layer of the eye's shell). No incision is made into the globe.

67208

The physician destroys a lesion of the retina by freezing (cryotherapy), or by heat (diathermy). The physician explores the sclera and stay sutures are placed under the involves rectus muscles so the eye can be rotated to expose the area to be treated. Sometimes, a rectus muscle is temporarily detached to permit adequate exposure. Cryotherapy and diathermy are performed without entering the posterior chamber; either probe is pressed against the sclera overlying the site of the retinal lesion until it is destroyed or until the session is completed. Any muscle incision is repaired and any stay sutures removed. A topical antibiotic or pressure patch may be applied.

67210

The physician destroys a lesion of the retina using a laser or xenon arc. After the patient's eye has been dilated, the physician places a special contact on the eye of the patient. Photocoagulation by laser or xenon arc is performed without entering the posterior chamber; the destructive light beam is guided through the contact and to the retinal lesion, which is destroyed in one session or in a series of sessions. A topical antibiotic or pressure patch may be applied.

67218

The physician treats a malignancy, tumor, growth, or edema by exposing it to a radioactive implant. The plaque-like implant is secured with sutures to the sclera overlying the site of a malignancy. At a future time, the physician recovers the implant. The incision is repaired. An antibiotic ointment and pressure patch may be applied.

67220

The physician destroys a localized lesion of the choroid using photocoagulation. In one or more sessions the physician directs short spots of a laser's beam at new blood vessels that have grown beneath the macula to seal leaking blood or fluid that can damage vision. Or, the physician may scatter the laser spots through the sides of the retina to reduce abnormal blood vessel growth (choroidal neovascularization) and seal the retina to the back of the eye.

67221-67225

The physician performs photodynamic therapy. This is a two-step procedure used for wet type macular degeneration to treat the abnormal blood vessels that grow under the retina. The fluid and blood present from the new blood vessel growth causes scar formation that destroys vision. Photodynamic therapy closes the abnormal blood vessels to stop or stabilize leakage and improve vision. First, the physician injects the drug Visudyne (verteporfin) intravenously into the patient's arm. This is a dye that marks the abnormal blood vessels under the retina by binding to them. A few minutes after the injection, the ophthalmologist shines a non-thermal 689-nanometer laser light into the patient's eye to activate the drug. The light reacts with the photosensitive chemical in verteporfin, and releases active oxygen molecules that cause cell death in the leaking blood vessels but not healthy ones. When the dye interacts with the light, the abnormal vessels are destroyed and closed off but the normal ones are spared. Report 67221 when photodynamic therapy is performed on one eye and 67225 when photodynamic therapy is performed on the second eye during the same session.

67227-67228
The physician destroys small vessels that are leaking blood on the retina by freezing (cryotherapy), by heat (diathermy) (67227), or treats them with photocoagulation (67228). Cryotherapy and diathermy may be performed without entering the posterior chamber; either probe is pressed against the sclera overlying the site of the retinopathy until it is destroyed. With a laser light or xenon arc aimed through a dilated pupil without an incision, the physician may burn spots at the site of diabetic retinopathy to seal vessels that have been leaking into the retina. At least 500 Xenon arc burns or 2000 burns from an argon laser are applied. This procedure is often referred to as "scattered destruction."

67229
The physician treats extensive or progressive retinopathy by freezing (cryotherapy) or by laser (photocoagulation) in a preterm infant (less than 37 weeks gestation at birth), performed from birth up to 1 year of age. Performed under topical or general anesthesia, cryotherapy may be performed without entering the posterior chamber. Under direct visualization, the physician applies a freezing probe to the avascular retina; approximately 50 applications may be required. Alternately, the physician may ablate the targeted area using a laser photocoagulation device. Multiple sessions may be required, although this code should be reported only once during a defined treatment period.

67250-67255
To repair a thin, weakened sclera, the physician places an ocular speculum in the patient's eye, and makes an incision in the conjunctiva and sclera over the site of the defect. The sclera may be cinched and overlapped for reinforcement (67250) or a patch of donor sclera may be sutured over the weakened area (67255). A piece of stretched sclera may also be removed. The physician uses sutures or tissue glue in the layered repair. Antibiotic ointment and a patch may be applied.

67311-67312
Strabismus is an imbalance in the muscles of the eyeball that control eyeball movement. Surgery can sometimes correct this imbalance. A speculum is placed in the patient's eye (no previous surgery). The physician makes incisions in the conjunctiva at the juncture of the sclera and cornea (the limbus) or in the cul-de-sac (Parks incision). Radial relaxing incisions in the conjunctiva are made and the muscle (either medial or lateral rectus) is isolated with a muscle hook. The muscle is strengthened by resection (removal of a measured segment) or weakened by recession (retroplacement of the muscle attachment). The muscles are secured with sutures. The operative wound is closed with sutures. In 67311, one horizontal muscle is treated; in 67312 two horizontal muscles in the same eye are treated.

67314-67316
Strabismus is an imbalance in the muscles of the eyeball that control eyeball movement. Surgery can sometimes correct this imbalance. A speculum is placed in the patient's eye, the physician makes incisions in the conjunctiva at the juncture of the sclera and cornea (the limbus) or in the cul-de-sac (Parks incision). Radial relaxing incisions in the conjunctiva are made and the muscle (either superior or inferior rectus) is isolated with a muscle hook. The muscle is strengthened by resection (removal of a measured segment) or weakened by recession (retroplacement of the muscle attachment). The muscles are secured with sutures. The operative wound is closed with sutures. In 67314, one vertical muscle is treated; in 67316 two vertical muscles in the same eye are treated.

67318
Strabismus is an imbalance in the muscles of the eyeball that control eyeball movement. Surgery can sometimes correct this imbalance. A speculum is placed in the patient's eye (no previous surgery). The physician makes incisions in the conjunctiva about 7 mm posterior to the juncture of the sclera and cornea (the limbus) in the superior nasal quadrant of the globe. An incision is made to expose the sclera and a muscle hook is used to engage the superior rectus muscle initially. The tendon of the superior oblique may be located about 12 mm behind the medial or nasal edge of the insertion of the superior rectus. The physician repairs, recesses, or resects the superior oblique muscle. The operative wound is closed with layered sutures.

67320
A speculum is placed in the patient's eye, the physician makes incisions in the conjunctiva at the juncture of the sclera and cornea (the limbus) to expose the muscle. The extraocular muscle or muscles to be transposed are isolated, and the physician exposes the area of sclera to which the transposed muscles are to be attached. The insertions of the transposed muscles are relocated generally adjacent to the paretic or weak muscle. They are attached to the sclera with sutures, and the surgical wound is closed with sutures. Occasionally, the transposed muscle may be split and one-half of the muscle relocated.

67331
Strabismus is an imbalance in the muscles of the eyeball that control eyeball movement. Surgery can sometimes correct this imbalance. A speculum is placed in the patient's eye, the physician makes incisions in the conjunctiva at the juncture of the sclera and cornea (the limbus) to expose the muscle. The extraocular muscle or muscles involved are isolated, and the appropriate definitive primary strabismus surgery (any of those reported with codes 67311-67318) is performed: recession or resection on horizontal or vertical muscles, or any procedure on oblique extraocular muscles. This is an add-on code used in conjunction with any strabismus surgery to denote the increased level of difficulty involved in both

the planning and performance of the chosen strabismus surgery on an eye that has had previous surgery or injury, but not involving the extraocular muscles.

67332

Strabismus is an imbalance in the muscles of the eyeball that control eyeball movement. Surgery can sometimes correct this imbalance. A speculum is placed in the eye of a patient and the physician makes incisions in the conjunctiva at the juncture of the sclera and cornea (the limbus) to expose the muscle. The extraocular muscle is isolated, and the physician performs the appropriate definitive primary strabismus surgery after freeing the muscle from surrounding fibrotic or scarred tissues. The muscle or muscles are dissected posteriorly to ensure lack of incarceration and repositioned if necessary. The surgical wound is closed with sutures. This is an add-on code used in conjunction with the appropriate strabismus surgery to denote the increased level of difficulty involved in surgery on extraocular muscles that have scarring due to previous strabismus or retinal detachment surgery, injury, or myopathy.

67334

Strabismus is an imbalance in the muscles of the eyeball that control eyeball movement. Surgery can sometimes correct this imbalance. A speculum is placed in the patient's eye, the physician makes incisions in the conjunctiva and sclera to expose the muscle. During strabismus surgery, the extraocular muscle is isolated far posterior to its insertion. The borders or edges of the muscle are sutured to the eye far back of the insertion in what is commonly called the Faden procedure. The surgical wound is closed with sutures. This is an add-on code used in conjunction with the appropriate strabismus surgery to denote that the posterior fixation suturing technique was employed on an extraocular muscle.

67335

Strabismus is an imbalance in the muscles of the eyeball that control eyeball movement. Surgery can sometimes correct this imbalance. The muscle or muscles to be placed on an adjustable suture are isolated in the usual fashion during separately reportable strabismus surgery. Instead of permanently suturing the muscle to the eyeball by tying and cutting the suture distal to the knot, the sutures are tied and brought out through the overlying conjunctiva. Tension on the muscle is adjusted later when the anesthetic is no longer affecting the position of the globe.

67340

Strabismus is an imbalance in the muscles of the eyeball that control eyeball movement. Surgery can sometimes correct this imbalance. The physician makes an extensive incision of the conjunctiva at the juncture of the cornea and the sclera (the limbus). This is called a peritomy. In the plane of the detached muscle, retractors afford increased visibility. Extensive posterior dissection may be necessary in an effort to locate the severed, lost, or detached muscle and reapproximate it to the eyeball with sutures. Once the repair is completed, the incision is repaired. This is an add-on code used in conjunction with the definitive strabismus surgery to report the exploration and/or repair required when an extraocular muscle was detached.

67343

During the performance of separately reported horizontal muscle surgery, scar tissue from a vertical muscle is excised. Or, during the performance of separately reported vertical muscle surgery, horizontal muscle scar tissue is excised. The scar tissue of the extraocular muscle is isolated, and the physician uses a scalpel to dissect the scars and fibrotic tissue from the muscle affecting the muscle itself. The surgical wound is closed with sutures.

67345

The extraocular muscle is identified through direct surgical exposure or through the insertion of an electromyographic needle into the muscle. A small quantity of botulin toxin is injected into the belly of the muscle. Onset of paralysis takes 24 to 48 hours and lasts from four to eight weeks.

67346

A speculum is placed in the patient's eye and the physician makes incisions in the conjunctiva and sclera to expose the muscle. The extraocular muscle to be tested is isolated and the physician uses a scalpel to remove a small portion of the muscle. The excision will not affect overall action of the eye muscle. The surgical wound is closed with sutures.

67400-67405

The physician accesses the orbit through a subciliary, extraperiosteal, or transconjunctival incision. In the subciliary incision, an incision is made in the upper eyelid. In the extraperiosteal incision, the approach is through an incision anterior, superior, interior, or medial to the eye allowing access to the bone beneath the periosteum. In the transconjunctival approach, the lower lid is everted and an incision is made over the infraorbital rim through the inferior cul-de-sac. In 67400, soft tissue or bone may be excised for examination, but no other tissue is removed or repaired. In 67405, fluid is drained from the orbit. In either case, the incision is closed with layered sutures.

67412-67413

The physician removes a lesion or a foreign body from the orbit through a subciliary, frontal, or transconjunctival incision. In the subciliary incision, an incision is made in the lower eyelid. In the frontal approach, an incision is made in the lid crease with a further postseptal dissection for removal of a lesion or foreign body in this portion of the orbit. In the transconjunctival approach, the lower lid is everted and an incision is made over the infraorbital rim through the inferior cul-de-sac. In 67412, the lesion is excised. In 67413, the foreign body is removed. In either case, the incision is closed with layered sutures.

67414
The physician removes bone from the orbit through a subciliary or transconjunctival incision. In the subciliary incision, an incision is made in the lower eyelid. In the transconjunctival approach, the lower lid is everted and an incision is made over the infraorbital rim through the inferior cul-de-sac. Bone is excised for decompression. The incision is closed with layered sutures.

67415
The physician performs a diagnostic percutaneous procedure using a fine gauge needle (often 25 to 30 gauge) and a syringe to sample fluid or remove clusters of cells from a lesion or tumor of the orbit. Imaging guidance such as ultrasound or computed tomography (CT) may be utilized. The needle tip is inserted into the target area of the orbit. The contents are aspirated, and the needle is carefully withdrawn along the path of insertion. Pressure is applied at the needle entry site with a cotton tipped applicator.

67420-67430
The physician makes an incision in the lateral aspect of the orbit. A C-shaped incision is made down to the periosteum overlying the lateral orbital rim. The periosteum is incised posterior to the rim itself. The temporalis muscle is moved aside and the globe is protected with pliable retractors. A vibrating saw removes the bone of the lateral orbital rim. In 67420 the lesion is excised from the orbit. In 67430, a foreign body is removed. In either case, the bone is replaced and wired into position and the operative wound is closed in layers.

67440
The physician makes an incision in the lateral aspect of the orbit. A C-shaped incision is made down to the periosteum overlying the lateral orbital rim. The periosteum is incised posterior to the rim itself. The temporalis muscle is moved aside and the globe is protected with pliable retractors. A vibrating saw is used to remove the bone from the lateral orbital rim. Fluid is excised from the orbit and the bone is replaced and wired into position. The operative wound is closed in layers.

67445
The physician makes an incision in the lateral aspect of the orbit. A C-shaped incision is made down to the periosteum overlying the lateral orbital rim. The periosteum is incised posterior to the rim itself. The temporalis muscle is moved aside and the globe is protected with pliable retractors. A vibrating saw removes the bone of the lateral orbital rim. A piece of orbital bone is removed for decompression. The bone flap is replaced and wired into position. The operative wound is closed in layers.

67450
The physician makes an incision in the lateral aspect of the orbit. A C-shaped incision is made down to the periosteum overlying the lateral orbital rim. The periosteum is incised posterior to the rim itself. The temporalis muscle is moved aside and the globe is protected with pliable retractors. A vibrating saw removes the bone of the lateral orbital rim. The physician explores the orbit and may remove tissue for examination. No other procedure is performed. The bone is replaced and wired into position. The operative wound is closed in layers.

67500-67505
The physician injects a therapeutic or anesthetic medication (67500) or alcohol (67505) into the orbit through the lower eyelid or in a transconjunctival method.

67515
A blunt or sharp-tipped needle is guided along the surface of the globe beneath the conjunctiva and between the sclera and Tenon's capsule. When the tip of the needle is in the appropriate location, medication or other substance is injected into the Tenon's capsule.

67516
The physician administers a suprachoroidal injection of a pharmacologic agent to the space between the sclera and choroid in the posterior segment of the eye. A suprachoroidal injector with an attached 900-micron or 1100-micron needle is positioned perpendicular to the sclera and manipulated into the suprachoroidal space using pressure dimpling, or localized depression, of the conjunctiva and sclera. An agent such as a corticosteroid (triamcinolone acetonide) is slowly administered into the space. After the needle is removed, pressure is applied to the injection site to avoid reflux of the medication.

67550-67560
The physician inserts a prosthesis in the eye in 67550 or revises or removes an orbital implant in 67560. An orbital implant lies outside the muscle cone and is usually secured with sutures.

67570
The physician makes an incision in the lateral or medial aspect of the fornix. In a lateral approach, a C-shaped incision is made down to the periosteum overlying the lateral orbital rim. The periosteum is incised posterior to the rim itself. The temporalis muscle is moved aside and the globe is protected with pliable retractors. The bone is removed to access the optic nerve. In a medial approach, the conjunctiva is incised and the medial rectus muscle is temporarily disinserted. Sutures are passed through the terminal portion of the medial rectus muscle and its insertion into the globe is noted. The eye is rotated laterally to gain access to the optic nerve medially. In either case, once the nerve has been identified, several small fenestrations are made. A dissection is carried down through the outer meningeal layer covering the optic nerve until the subarachnoid space is reached. An egress of cerebral spinal fluid indicates decompression of the nerve sheath. The operative wound is closed in layers.

67700
The eyelid is prepped and draped and local anesthetic is applied. A transverse incision is made to drain the

abscess in the lid. The wound is irrigated and may be closed with sutures.

67710

This procedure generally follows a previously performed tarsorrhaphy (closure of the eyelid), usually attempted to protect the cornea. The eyelid is prepped and draped, and local anesthetic is applied. The previously formed seam or union between the upper and lower lid is delineated and divided using sharp scissors.

67715

Under local anesthesia, the face and eyelids are draped and prepped. Scissors cut the lateral canthus to further divide the upper and lower lid to extend the division.

[67810]

A local anesthetic is applied and the face and eyelid are prepped and draped. A small amount of tissue is excised from the suspect portion of the eyelid, which may include the lid margin. Sutures may be required to repair the incision.

67800-67808

A chalazion is a small mass in the eyelid that results in chronic inflammation. The face and eye are prepped and draped and local anesthesia (67800, 67801, and 67805) or general anesthesia (67808) is administered. Usually, general anesthesia and hospitalization is reserved for very young or otherwise uncooperative patients. The physician applies a chalazion clamp to expose the posterior surface of the eyelid. The chalazion is incised with a blade and a curette is used to explore the lid after the incision has been drained. Any pockets of infection are drained. The lips of the wound are generally cauterized to prevent excessive bleeding. The clamp is released.

67820

Trichiasis is a condition wherein eyelashes are ingrown or misdirected in their growth so that they irritate the tissues of the eye. Using a biomicroscope, the physician plucks the offending eyelashes with forceps. The lash follicles are not treated.

67825

Trichiasis is a condition wherein eyelashes are ingrown or misdirected in their growth so that they irritate the tissues of the eye. The physician treats the area of trichiasis with local anesthetic. In cryotherapy, the freezing probe is applied to the area of trichiasis. After a period of repeated freezing and thawing, the lash follicles are usually destroyed. In electrosurgery, electrolysis directed at the follicles destroys them.

67830-67835

Trichiasis is a condition wherein eyelashes are ingrown or misdirected in their growth so that they irritate the tissues of the eye. The physician treats the area of trichiasis with a local anesthetic and preps and drapes the face and eye. The physician uses a scalpel to split the eyelid margin at the gray line (the junction of the palpebral mucosa and skin). The area of abnormal eyelash growth is excised in both 67830 and 67835. Additionally in 67835, tissue for a split-thickness graft is harvested from the buccal mucosa inside the patient's mouth. No repair is required at the graft harvest site. The graft is inlaid between the palpebral conjunctiva and the skin. In either case, sutures may be required.

67840

The physician administers a local anesthetic and the face and eyelid are draped and prepped for surgery. The eyelid lesion is outlined in a marking pen. The lesion is incised and the surgical wound is repaired with sutures if necessary.

67850

The physician administers a local anesthetic and the face and eyelid are draped and prepped for surgery. An electrocautery tool or photocoagulation is used to destroy the small eyelid lesion.

67875

The constant action of the eyelid opening and closing against the cornea can cause problems in patients with chronic corneal conditions. Temporary closure of the eyelid may provide relief for an eroded or painful cornea. The physician administers local anesthetic to the eyelids. Sutures are passed through the skin and eyelid margin at the gray line of the upper lid and corresponding portion of the lower lid. The sutures are usually tied over a bolster to prevent erosion of the suture through the lid.

67880

The constant action of the eyelid opening and closing against the cornea can cause problems in patients with chronic corneal conditions. Temporary closure of the eyelid may provide relief for an eroded or painful cornea. The physician administers a local anesthetic and preps and drapes the face and eyelids for surgery. Tissue along the mucocutaneous junction at the margins of the eyelids is excised. A suture is passed through the skin and eyelid margin at the gray line of the upper lid and corresponding portion of the lower lid. This process is repeated several times in each eye, creating a permanent marginal adhesion. The sutures are usually tied over a bolster to prevent erosion of the suture through the lid. The sutures are removed a week to 10 days later, after the lid margins have adhered.

67882

The constant action of the eyelid opening and closing against the cornea can cause problems in patients with chronic corneal conditions. Temporary closure of the eyelid may provide relief for an eroded or painful cornea. The physician administers a local anesthetic and preps and drapes the face and eyelids for surgery. Tissue along the mucocutaneous junction at the margins of the eyelids is excised. A tongue of tarsal plate is isolated from above the upper or lower lid. The tarsal plate is sutured into a corresponding area of the opposite lid. The physician passes a suture through the skin and eyelid margin at the gray line of the upper lid and corresponding portion of the lower lid. This process is repeated several times in each eye, creating a permanent marginal adhesion. The sutures are usually tied over a bolster to prevent erosion of the suture through the lid. The sutures are removed a week to 10 days later, after the lid margins have adhered.

67900

Ptosis refers to a droop or displacement resulting from paralysis. The physician makes an incision directly above the brow (supraciliary), through the mid-forehead or near the hairline (coronal). A dissection is carried down to the area of the brow. The skin is pulled superiorly and the brow approximated to its proper position above the supraorbital rim. The incision is repaired with sutures.

67901

The physician performs a repair of blepharoptosis by frontalis muscle technique using suture or other material. Blepharoptosis is a droop or displacement of the upper eyelid resulting from paralysis. The physician makes an incision directly above the brow (supraciliary). The frontalis fixation technique is a mechanical suspension that transfers the movement of the upper lid to the frontalis muscle above the eyelid. Banked fascia from a cadaver donor or other material such as Mersilene mesh may be used to create a sling to the frontalis muscle. It is sutured in place. The incision is repaired with sutures.

67902

The physician performs a repair of blepharoptosis by frontalis muscle technique using an autologous fascia to create a sling. The fascia is harvested, usually from the knee, in a separately reportable procedure. Blepharoptosis is a droop or displacement of the upper eyelid resulting from paralysis. The physician makes an incision directly above the brow (supraciliary). The frontalis fixation technique is a mechanical suspension that transfers the movement of the upper lid to the frontalis muscle above the eyelid. It is sutured in place. The physician obtains fascia from the patient's thigh and uses this fascia to create a sling to the frontalis muscle. This sling helps suspend the lid. The incisions are repaired with sutures.

67903

Blepharoptosis is a droop or displacement of the upper eyelid resulting from paralysis. The physician administers local anesthetic and the patient's face and eyelid are draped and prepped for surgery. The eyelid is everted and the physician makes an incision along the upper posterior edge of the tarsus. The levator complex, including Mueller's muscle, is isolated for a distance superiorly to correspond with the amount of ptosis to be corrected. The levator aponeurosis is advanced onto the tarsal plate internally until the eyelid margin falls at the appropriate location below the limbus. The incision is repaired.

67904

Blepharoptosis is a droop or displacement of the upper eyelid resulting from paralysis. The physician administers local anesthetic and the patient's face and eyelid are draped and prepped for surgery. An incision line is outlined along the crease of the upper eyelid. A dissection is carried down the normal insertion point of the distal point of the levator tendon. The levator tendon is isolated. The physician uses sutures to advance the levator tendon onto the tarsal plate in an adjustable fashion. If the patient is old enough to undergo the procedure under local anesthetic, the patient is placed in a sitting position and eyelid height and contour are evaluated under the effect of gravity. The amount that the levator tendon is advanced corresponds to the degree of preoperative ptosis. If the patient is not able to undergo the procedure under local anesthetic, general anesthesia is used and a predetermined amount of advancement is performed. In either case, the incision is repaired with sutures once the tendon has been secured in its new location.

67906

Blepharoptosis is a droop or displacement of the upper eyelid resulting from paralysis. The physician administers local anesthetic and the patient's face and eyelid are draped and prepped for surgery. The physician performs a repair that provides a mechanical suspension of the upper lid, transferring the movement of the upper lid to the frontalis muscle action of the eyebrow. The most common technique involves the creation of three horizontal incisions extending to the level of the tarsal plate approximately 3 mm above the upper eyelid margin in the midline, nasal, and lateral quarters. Three corresponding incisions are made just above the brow down to the periosteum of the bone. The lid is suspended in a double rhomboid configuration as the physician passes the suspending material deep in the lid tissue at the depth of the anterior surface of the levator aponeurosis through the orbital septum in front of the bone and out through the medial and lateral brow incisions. The knots are pulled up and tied to elevate the eyelid margin to the level of the superior limbus. The ends of the sutures are burned in the wound. The incisions are repaired with sutures.

67908

The physician administers local anesthetic and the patient's face and eyelid are draped and prepped for surgery. The physician everts the upper eyelid and a series of curved clamps are placed across the everted undersurface of the upper lid. All of the tissue distal to the clamps is removed or resected. This includes conjunctiva, tarsus, Muller's muscle, and the distal insertion of the levator aponeurosis. A running suture or purse string suture is used to consolidate the remaining tissues.

67909

The physician reduces overcorrection of ptosis. The physician administers a local anesthetic and the patient's face and eyelid are draped and prepped for surgery. With an incision usually at the site of the previous incision, the physician attempts to reduce a previous overcorrection of ptosis. The levator aponeurosis is cut free of or disinserted from its attachment to the levator aponeurosis, and the incision is repaired with sutures.

67911
The physician administers local anesthetic and the patient's face and eyelid are draped and prepped for surgery. The physician outlines the incision line, usually in the crease of the upper lid. The distal portion of the tendon responsible for elevating the lid (levator aponeurosis) is isolated from its attachment to the tarsal plate. The levator aponeurosis is allowed to retract itself posteriorly or autogenous graft materials are inserted between the levator aponeurosis and the tarsal plate. The patient is generally placed in a sitting position and the amount of the retraction of the levator aponeurosis is judged by the position of the eyelid while the patient is sitting on the table. Alternatively, the eyelid margin may be placed approximately 2 mm below the limbus. When the lid is positioned satisfactorily, it is affixed. The incision is closed with sutures.

67912
Lagophthalmos is a condition in which the upper eyelid is not providing complete closure to the eye, causing dryness and other complications. This code reports lagophthalmos correction using the insertion of a gold weight or other lid load into the upper eyelid for gravity-assisted closure. The surgical field is prepared around the eye and a traction suture is placed into the lid margin. An incision is made in the lid crease and dissection is carried out on the upper lid structures to expose the anterior surface of the tarsus. The weight to be used has been predetermined; it is centered over the exposed upper tarsal surface and sutured into place. After irrigation, the orbicularis oculi muscle must be closed over the inserted weight and the crease in the eyelid is restored through suturing. Antibiotics are applied and the eye is patched.

67914
An ectropion is a turning outward of the margin of the eyelid. The physician administers local anesthetic and the patient's face and eyelid are draped and prepped for surgery. The physician uses absorbable sutures to foreshorten the posterior tissues of the eyelid in an effort to redirect the rotation of the eyelid posteriorly. No incisions are required for this treatment of ectropion.

67915
An ectropion is a turning outward of the margin of the eyelid. The physician administers local anesthetic and the patient's face and eyelid are draped and prepped for surgery. Bipolar or unipolar cautery is employed to shrink the posterior tissues of the eyelid margin in an effort to rotate the lid margin posteriorly toward the globe. No incision is made.

67916
An ectropion is a turning outward of the margin of the eyelid. The physician administers local anesthetic and the patient's face and eyelid are draped and prepped for surgery. A section of tarsus and conjunctiva in the configuration of a diamond or rhomboid is taken from the posterior or back surface of the lower lid. Incisions are closed with interrupted absorbable sutures to rotate the eyelid margin posteriorly toward the globe.

67917
An ectropion is a turning outward of the margin of the eyelid. The physician administers local anesthetic and the patient's face and eyelid are draped and prepped for surgery. The physician makes an incision in the lower lid and isolates a tongue or strip of tarsus in the lateral one third of the lower lid. Nonabsorbable sutures are passed through the tarsal strip. The periosteum of tough fibrous tissue that lines the bone of the lateral orbital rim is isolated. The sutures from the tarsal strip are passed through the periosteum overlying the bone of the lateral orbital rim. The physician tightens the sutures. Eyelid margin tension and contour are evaluated and adjusted. The incision or incisions are repaired with sutures.

67921
An entropion is an inversion of the margin of the eyelid. The physician administers local anesthetic and the patient's face and eyelid are draped and prepped for surgery. The physician threads sutures through the inferior fornix or inferior cul-de-sac externally to the lash line. The sutures are placed in the medial, middle, and lateral third of the eyelid in a mattress fashion. These absorbable sutures are tied on the skin side. The sutures act to evert the eyelid margin anteriorly, correcting the malposition of the eyelid. No incision is made in this procedure.

67922
An entropion is an inversion of the margin of the eyelid. The physician administers local anesthetic and the patient's face and eyelid are draped and prepped for surgery. The physician uses bipolar or monopolar cautery to create a central tissue shrinkage to rotate the eyelid margin anteriorly. This corrects the malposition of the eyelid. No incisions are made in this procedure.

67923
An entropion is an inversion of the margin of the eyelid. The physician administers local anesthetic and the patient's face and eyelid are draped and prepped for surgery. A triangular section of tarsus is excised from the eyelid. A large chalazion clamp may be used to evert the lid and excise the triangle of tarsus, which usually measures 8 mm to 10 mm at the base. A piece of exposed orbicularis muscle is removed with the wedge. The edges of the excision site are approximated and repaired with sutures.

67924
An entropion is an inversion of the margin of the eyelid. The physician administers local anesthetic and the patient's face and eyelid are draped and prepped for surgery. The physician makes the incision along approximately 80 percent of the width of the eyelid for extensive repair. The physician uses deep sutures to sever the eyelid margin outwardly. Strips of tarsus may also be excised from the eyelid. All incisions are

repaired with sutures. This procedure is sometimes performed under general anesthesia.

67930-67935

The physician administers local anesthetic and the patient's face and eyelid is draped and prepped for surgery. The physician irrigates the wound and approximates its edges. The wound is repaired in layered sutures. In 67930, the wound is through a partial thickness of eyelid; in 67935, the wound is through the full thickness of the eyelid.

67938

The physician administers local anesthetic and the patient's face and eyelid are draped and prepped for surgery. The physician locates the foreign body through palpation. An incision is made through the anterior surface if the foreign body is principally on the anterior of the lid; the lid is everted if the foreign body is near the posterior surface. An attempt is made to conceal the incision line in the crease of the upper lid, or through a subciliary incision, when possible. The foreign body is removed and the wound is irrigated. The wound is repaired with layered sutures.

67950

The physician administers local anesthetic and the patient's face and eyelid are draped and prepped for surgery. The physician increases the lid margin by cutting the medial or lateral canthus (juncture of upper and lower eyelid). The physician rearranges the anterior tissues of the lids to prevent adherence.

67961-67966

The physician administers local anesthetic and the patient's face and eyelid are draped and prepped for surgery. A section of full-thickness eyelid is excised from the upper or lower eyelid. The section includes the defect and a margin of normal tissue. The edges of the excision site are approximated to reconstitute the eyelid contour and the wound is closed with layered sutures. Sometimes, a separately reported skin graft or pedicle flap is required to achieve proper cosmetic results. In 67961, up to one-fourth of the lid margin is removed; in 67966, more than one-fourth is removed.

67971

The patient's face and eyelid are draped and prepped for surgery. Local or general anesthesia may be administered. The patient has already undergone a separately reported excision that has created a significant eyelid defect requiring reconstruction of up to two-thirds of the eyelid. Because the defect is too large for direct closure, portions of the opposing eyelid are excised and grafted to reconstruct the eyelid. The opposite lid is everted and a horizontal incision through the tarsus and conjunctival approximately 4 mm from the eyelid margin is performed. Vertical incisions are made through the conjunctiva to match the width of the flap. The dissection is carried down through Muller's muscle toward the fornix or cul-de-sac. The advancing tarsal conjunctival flap is grafted to the opposing lid and secured with sutures. A separately reportable free, full-thickness skin graft may be applied to complete the reconstruction.

67973-67974

The patient's face and eyelid are draped and prepped for surgery. Local or general anesthesia may be administered. The patient has already undergone a separately reported excision that has created a significant eyelid defect requiring reconstruction. Because the defect is too large (e.g., total lower lid for 67973 and total upper lid for 67974), portions of the opposing eyelid are excised and grafted to reconstruct the eyelid. The opposite lid is everted and a horizontal incision through the tarsus and conjunctival approximately 4 mm from the eyelid margin is performed. Vertical incisions are made through the conjunctiva to match the width of the flap. The dissection is carried down through Muller's muscle toward the fornix or cul-de-sac. The advancing tarsal conjunctival flap is grafted to the opposing lid and secured with sutures. A separately reported free, full-thickness skin graft may be applied to complete the reconstruction.

67975

The patient's face and eyelid are draped and prepped for surgery. Local or general anesthesia may be administered. Approximately six weeks after a separately reported reconstruction of the eyelid, the tissue is divided to create an upper and lower lid. Any redundant tissue is trimmed.

68020

The patient's face and eyelid are draped and prepped for surgery. Local anesthesia is administered. A vertical or horizontal incision is made in the posterior surface of the eyelid margin. The incision does not extend to the eyelid margin itself. The contents of the cyst are drained with a cotton-tipped probe or a curette.

68040

Trachoma is a chronic inflammation of the eye causing granulations to form on conjunctival tissue. The patient's face and eyelid are draped and prepped for surgery. Local anesthesia may be administered. Under biomicroscopic guidance, the physician everts the eyelid margin and removes the conjunctival follicles with a cotton-tipped swab or a curette. No incision is required.

68100

The patient's face and eyelid are draped and prepped for surgery. Local anesthesia may be administered. A portion of the bulbar or palpebral conjunctival is excised with a curette. Sutures may be required to repair the wound.

68110-68115

The patient's face and eyelid are draped and prepped for surgery. Local anesthesia is administered. A lesion on the bulbar or palpebral conjunctival is excised with a curette. Sutures may be required to repair the wound. The lesion is up to 1 cm in size in 68110 and larger than 1 cm in 68115.

68130
The patient's face and eyelid are draped and prepped for surgery. Local anesthesia is administered and a lid speculum is inserted. A lesion on the conjunctiva and adjacent superficial sclera is excised with a curette. No sutures usually are required.

68135
The patient's face and eyelid are draped and prepped for surgery. Local anesthesia is administered and a lid speculum is inserted. A freezing probe (cryotherapy) is applied to a lesion on the conjunctiva. No repair is required.

68200
The physician applies a drop of topical anesthetic to the eye. A small gauge needle is inserted to deliver a medication such as a cortical steroid or antibiotic into the subconjunctival space.

68320
The patient's face and eyelid are draped and prepped for surgery. Local anesthesia is administered. With the aid of an operating microscope, the physician separates the conjunctival epithelial tissue from the underlying Tenon's capsule. The site to which the harvested tissue is to be grafted is prepared to accept the tissue. Its margins are freshened and the conjunctival graft is arranged and sutured into place. The tissue for graft can be a free graft or extensive rearrangement of existing tissue.

68325
The patient's face and eyelid are draped and prepped for surgery. Local anesthesia is administered. The physician separates the buccal mucous membrane that will be used for the graft from its location within the patient's mouth. The site to which the donor tissue is to be grafted is prepared to accept the tissue. Its margins are freshened and the conjunctival graft is arranged and sutured into place. The donor graft site does not usually require a repair.

68326
The patient's face and eyelid are draped and prepped for surgery. Local anesthesia is administered. With the aid of an operating microscope, the physician separates the conjunctival epithelial tissue from the underlying Tenon's capsule. The tissue for graft can be a free graft or extensive rearrangement of existing tissue. The site to which the donor tissue is to be grafted is prepared to accept the tissue. Its margins are freshened and the conjunctival graft is sutured into a foreshortened, or scarred inferior cul-de-sac or fornix. The fornix can be reformed with the use of a cul-de-sac suture fixation or with the use of a silicon stent attached to the orbital rim. The stent is used to mold the fornix and is sutured into place securely and left for up to two weeks.

68328
The patient's face and eyelid are draped and prepped for surgery. Local anesthesia is administered. The physician separates the buccal mucous membrane that will be used for the graft from its location within the patient's mouth. The donor graft site does not usually require a repair. The site to which the donor tissue is to be grafted is prepared to accept the tissue. Its margins are freshened and the conjunctival graft is sutured into a foreshortened, or scarred inferior cul-de-sac or fornix. The fornix can be reformed with the use of a cul-de-sac suture fixation or with the use of a silicon stent attached to the orbital rim. The stent is used to mold the fornix and is sutured into place securely and left for up to two weeks.

68330
A symblepharon is an adhesion between the conjunctiva on the eyeball (bulbar conjunctiva) and the conjunctiva on the inner eyelid (tarsal conjunctiva). The patient's face and eyelid are draped and prepped for surgery. Local anesthesia is administered. The physician divides the adhesions between the globe and palpebral conjunctiva and repairs the conjunctival wound with adjacent tissue transfer. Sutures are required, and a silicon stent may be placed in the eye to prevent the development of further adhesions during the healing process.

68335
A symblepharon is an adhesion between the conjunctiva on the eyeball (bulbar conjunctiva) and the conjunctiva on the inner eyelid (tarsal conjunctiva). The patient's face and eyelid are draped and prepped for surgery. Local anesthesia is administered. The physician separates the conjunctival adhesions and grafts replacement tissue over the site of the symblepharon. The tissue for graft can be a free graft of conjunctival tissue from the same or other eye, or buccal mucosa obtained from inside the patient's mouth. The site to which the donor tissue is to be grafted is prepared to accept the tissue. Its margins are freshened and the conjunctival graft is sutured in place. A silicon stent or contact lens may be placed in the eye to prevent the development of further adhesions during the healing process.

68340
A symblepharon is an adhesion between the conjunctiva on the eyeball (bulbar conjunctiva) and the conjunctiva on the inner eyelid (tarsal conjunctiva). The patient's face and eyelid are draped and prepped for surgery. Local anesthesia is administered. The physician divides the adhesions between the globe and palpebral conjunctiva. No other repair is usually needed, although a conformer or contact lens may be placed in the eye to prevent the development of further adhesions during the healing process.

68360
The patient's face and eyelid are draped and prepped for surgery. Local anesthesia is administered. The physician elevates the conjunctiva from the Tenon's capsule and a small tongue of free conjunctiva is advanced via a flap to another site where it is secured with sutures.

68362
The patient's face and eyelid are draped and prepped for surgery. Local anesthesia is administered. The physician elevates the conjunctiva from the Tenon's capsule and the conjunctiva is advanced cover the de-epithelialized cornea. The leading edge of the conjunctival flap is sutured along the medial extent of the corneal defect.

68371
A conjunctival allograft is harvested from a living donor for transplantation to another recipient to help the process of re-epithelialization in cases of corneal epithelial damage and disease when the normal population of conjunctival/limbal stem cells has been depleted. The donor eye is prepped and draped. The lid speculum is inserted to maintain the lids and lashed from the operative field. The conjunctival borders of the graft to be removed are marked with a surgical marking pen to approximate the recipient bed dimensions. Saline solution is injected subconjunctivally to raise the conjunctiva from the Tenon's layer. Incisions are made on the lateral borders of the graft first, with undermining done between those borders. The posterior ridge is incised and the graft is reflected. Dissection is carried to the conjunctival/limbal junction and anterior dissection is finished, moving into the peripheral cornea. The epitheliectomy from a living donor is kept at a superficial level like that of a keratectomy with limbal and peripheral corneal tissue, no sclera or corneal stroma. The free graft is removed and prepared in an appropriate storage medium. The wound is closed. Topical antibiotics and steroids are instilled and the lids are closed and patches applied.

68400
The lacrimal system serves to keep the conjunctiva and cornea moist through the production, distribution, and elimination of tears. The physician administers a local anesthetic along the edge of the supratemporal portion of the orbital rim over the lacrimal gland. An incision is made beneath the superior orbital rim or in the lid crease of the upper lid. The incision is extended to the lacrimal fossa where the abscess is drained. The wound is irrigated and repaired with layered sutures.

68420
The lacrimal system serves to keep the conjunctiva and cornea moist through the production, distribution, and elimination of tears. The lacrimal sac is an enlarged portion of the lacrimal duct that drains these tears. The physician administers a local anesthetic along the medical canthal tendon. A stab incision is made directly into the lacrimal sac and the pressure created by the sequestered abscess is relieved. The wound may be irrigated and repaired with layered sutures.

68440
The lacrimal system serves to keep the conjunctiva and cornea moist through the production, distribution, and elimination of tears. Tears produced by the lacrimal gland are eliminated through the lacrimal punctum, a small openings in the inner canthus. The physician administers a local anesthetic at the lacrimal punctum and uses sharp scissors to snip the lacrimal punctum, usually posteriorly. A dilating probe is introduced to ensure that enlargement of the punctum has been achieved.

68500-68505
The lacrimal system serves to keep the conjunctiva and cornea moist through the production, distribution, and elimination of tears. The tears are produced in the lacrimal gland. The physician makes an incision beneath the superior orbital rim or in the lid crease of the upper lid. The incision Is extended to the periosteum overlying the bone of the supraorbital rim. A periosteal elevator is used to isolate and dissect the lacrimal gland from its position in the lacrimal fossa. The gland is removed in total in 68500 and a part of the gland is removed in 68505. In either case, the wound is repaired with layered sutures.

68510
The lacrimal system serves to keep the conjunctiva and cornea moist through the production, distribution, and elimination of tears. The tears are produced in the lacrimal gland. The physician makes an incision beneath the superior orbital rim or in the lid crease of the upper lid. The incision is extended to lacrimal fossa. A previously determined portion of the lacrimal gland is excised for analysis. The wound is repaired with layered sutures.

68520
The lacrimal system serves to keep the conjunctiva and cornea moist through the production, distribution, and elimination of tears. The lacrimal sac is an enlarged portion of the lacrimal duct that eliminates these tears. The physician administers a local anesthetic along the medial canthal tendon. An incision is made midway between the bridge of the nose and the medial canthal tendon. The dissection is carried down to the periosteum overlying the bone of the superior lacrimal crest. A periosteal elevator is used to separate the lacrimal sac from its normal location. The sac is removed. The wound is repaired with layered sutures.

68525
The lacrimal system serves to keep the conjunctiva and cornea moist through the production, distribution, and elimination of tears. The lacrimal sac is an enlarged portion of the lacrimal duct that eliminates these tears. The physician administers a local anesthetic along the medial canthal tendon. An incision is made midway between the bridge of the nose and the medial canthal tendon. The dissection is carried down to the periosteum overlying the bone of the superior lacrimal crest. A portion of the lacrimal sac is removed. The wound is repaired with layered sutures.

68530
The lacrimal system serves to keep the conjunctiva and cornea moist through the production, distribution, and elimination of tears. Ducts distribute the tears to the eye and nose. The physician administers a local anesthetic along the medial canthal tendon. An

incision is made midway between the bridge of the nose and the medial canthal tendon. The dissection is carried down to the foreign body or lacrimal stone. It is removed and the wound is repaired with layered sutures.

68540

The lacrimal system serves to keep the conjunctiva and cornea moist through the production, distribution, and elimination of tears. The tears are produced in the lacrimal gland. The physician makes an incision beneath the superior orbital rim or in the lid crease of the upper lid. The incision is extended to the periosteum overlying the bone of the supraorbital rim or to the lacrimal fossa. The tumor is isolated and removed with a rim of normal lacrimal gland tissue. The wound is repaired with layered sutures.

68550

The lacrimal system serves to keep the conjunctiva and cornea moist through the production, distribution, and elimination of tears. The tears are produced in the lacrimal gland. The physician makes an incision beneath the superior orbital rim or in the lid crease of the upper lid. The incision is extended to the periosteum overlying the bone of the supraorbital rim or to the lacrimal fossa. The tumor has invaded the lacrimal fossa, so an osteotome is used to remove the portion of affected bone. The wound is repaired with layered sutures.

68700

The lacrimal system serves to keep the conjunctiva and cornea moist through the production, distribution, and elimination of tears. Lacrimal canaliculi are the ducts that carry the tears from the lacrimal gland where they are produced to the nose. The physician uses a probe to locate the distal and proximal ends of the canaliculi in the injured eye of patient. The ends are freshened and reattached with sutures. The wound is closed with layered sutures.

68705

The lacrimal system serves to keep the conjunctiva and cornea moist through the production, distribution, and elimination of tears. Tears produced by the lacrimal gland are released into the eye through the lacrimal punctum, a small opening in the inner canthus. The physician administers a local anesthetic at the lacrimal punctum and applies bipolar or monopolar cautery to the palpebral conjunctiva just below the level of the inferior punctum. The result is a repositioning of the punctum itself. No incisions are made and no repairs required in this procedure.

68720

The lacrimal system serves to keep the conjunctiva and cornea moist through the production and distribution of tears. The lacrimal sac is an enlarged portion of the lacrimal duct that distributes these tears. The physician administers a local anesthetic along the medial canthal tendon. A 1 cm incision is made in the skin midway between the bridge of the nose and the medial canthal tendon. The dissection is carried down to the periosteum overlying the bone of the superior lacrimal crest. The lacrimal sac is opened and a communication is established been the lacrimal sac and underlying bone and nasal mucosa. The lacrimal mucosa is exposed and a connection between the medial portion of the lacrimal sac and the nasal mucosa is created and secured with sutures. The incision is repaired with layered sutures.

68745-68750

The lacrimal system serves to keep the conjunctiva and cornea moist through the production and distribution of tears. The lacrimal sac is an enlarged portion of the lacrimal duct that distributes these tears. The physician administers a local anesthetic along the medial canthal tendon. A 1 cm incision is made in the skin midway between the bridge of the nose and the medial canthal tendon. The dissection is carried down to the periosteum overlying the bone of the superior lacrimal crest. The lateral portion of lacrimal sac is connected by a series of interrupted sutures to the nasal mucosa. A glass tube is inserted to create a connection from the lacrimal system to the nasal mucosa in 68750. The incision is repaired with layered sutures.

68760

The lacrimal system serves to keep the conjunctiva and cornea moist through the production, distribution, and elimination of tears. Tears produced by the lacrimal gland are drained from the eye through the lacrimal punctum, a small opening in the inner canthus. The physician administers a local anesthetic at the lacrimal punctum and uses a heat source such as cautery or argon laser to close the proximal portion of the canalicular and lacrimal system including the lacrimal punctum.

68761

The lacrimal system serves to keep the conjunctiva and cornea moist through the production, distribution, and elimination of tears. Tears produced by the lacrimal gland are drained from the eye through the lacrimal punctum, a small opening in the inner canthus. The physician administers a local anesthetic at the lacrimal punctum and closes the punctum by inserting a plug. The plug may be a permanent silicone plug or a temporary collagen plug.

68770

The lacrimal system serves to keep the conjunctiva and cornea moist through the production, distribution, and elimination of tears. Tears produced by the lacrimal gland are drained from the eye through the lacrimal punctum, a small opening in the inner canthus. The physician administers a local anesthetic at the lacrimal punctum and uses a probe to locate the lacrimal fistula. The fistula is dissected and its core is removed. The incision is repaired with layered sutures.

68801

The physician treats a suspected injury or blockage of the lacrimal punctum, the opening on the medial eyelids, to assist in drainage of secretions. The physician inserts a plastic probe, catheter, or large

Eye and Ocular Adnexa

suture. The physician may irrigate the punctum to evaluate the patency of lacrimal drainage system.

68810-68811
The lacrimal system keeps the conjunctiva and cornea moist through the production, distribution, and elimination of the watery lacrimal secretion, called tears. Tears produced by the lacrimal gland are drained from the eye through the lacrimal punctum, a small opening near the margin of each eyelid. The physician dilates the proximal portion of the lacrimal system and threads a probe along the canaliculus to the lacrimal sac. No incisions are made and no repairs are necessary. This is performed with the patient under local anesthetic in 68810. In 68811, less patent ducts or a less cooperative patient requires general anesthesia.

68815
The lacrimal system keeps the conjunctiva and cornea moist through the production, distribution, and elimination of the watery lacrimal secretion, called tears. Ducts distribute the tears to the eye and nose. The physician dilates the proximal portion of the lacrimal system and threads a probe along the canaliculus to the lacrimal sac. Canalicular stents are passed through the duct and placed in the distal portion of the lacrimal system. The tubes remain in place for three to six months before they are removed. No incisions are made and no repairs are necessary.

68816
The lacrimal system keeps the conjunctiva and cornea moist through the production, distribution, and elimination of the watery lacrimal secretion, called tears. Ducts distribute the tears to the eye and nose. Using topical anesthesia, the physician treats an obstructed nasolacrimal duct by dilating the puncta and canaliculi and threading a probe into the lacrimal system. The probe is removed and the balloon catheter is advanced through the superior punctum, canaliculus, lacrimal sac, and into the nasolacrimal duct down to the nasal floor. An inflation device filled with sterile water is attached to the balloon catheter and used to inflate the balloon. The balloon is deflated and the inflation procedure is repeated. The physician pulls the balloon proximally and positions it within the lacrimal sac and nasolacrimal duct junction, where the inflation procedure is again repeated. The balloon is then fully deflated and the catheter withdrawn from the lacrimal system.

68840
The lacrimal system serves to keep the conjunctiva and cornea moist through the production, distribution, and elimination of tears. Ducts distribute the tears to the eye and nose. The physician threads a probe along the canaliculi. No incisions are made and no repairs are necessary. The canaliculi may be irrigated during the procedure.

68841
Drug-eluting implants or plugs placed within the lacrimal canaliculus are used to treat inflammation, pain, or to reduce ocular pressure. The implants vary according to the drug administered and the condition being treated. The physician administers a local anesthetic at the lacrimal punctum, the punctum is dilated if needed, and the drug-eluting punctal implant is inserted. The implant is often absorbed at the end of the treatment.

68850
The lacrimal system serves to keep the conjunctiva and cornea moist through the production, distribution, and elimination of tears. A cannula is inserted into the lacrimal duct. Under radiographic guidance, radiopaque dye is introduced into the lacrimal system through the cannula. The supervision and interpretation of the radiographic results of the injection are reported separately; this code reports only the injection of the contrast medium.

Auditory

69000-69005
Through a small incision in the skin or at times into the perichondrium external ear at the site of the abscess or hematoma (collection of blood), the physician drains the contents of the abscess in a simple procedure (69000). Occasionally, a small drain tube is inserted and packing is placed to facilitate healing. A bolster with through-and-through sutures is placed to prevent accumulation of fluid. In a complicated procedure (69005), the physician also devotes more time to cleaning the abscess cavity, and a soft sponge is placed in the canal after antibiotic ear drops have been applied.

69020
The physician makes an incision in the skin and drains an abscess in the external auditory canal. Occasionally, packing is inserted to absorb the drainage and facilitate healing. Usually no further treatment is needed and no closure is required.

69090
The physician or technician uses a sharp instrument such as a sterile needle or a piercing gun to form an opening in the ear lobe. After the puncture is complete, the area is cleaned with a disinfectant and an earring is inserted to keep the opening patent. No further treatment is usually necessary.

69100
The physician uses a scalpel or punch forceps to excise a portion of a lesion on the external ear for diagnostic purposes. Unless the incision is large, a sutured closure is usually unnecessary.

69105
The physician uses a scalpel, curette, or small biopsy forceps to excise a portion of a lesion in the external auditory canal for diagnostic purposes. Ear canal packing may be required.

69110
The physician removes a full-thickness section of the external ear, often as a triangular wedge. The portion of the ear removed will vary from case to case, but

most frequently it is in the curved upper portion of the ear. A small portion of normal tissue surrounding the defect is also removed. The wound is closed with layered sutures.

69120

The physician performs a complete amputation of the external ear. This procedure is commonly performed for infection or cancer of the ear. Under appropriate anesthesia, incisions are made through the skin and cartilage, and the affected ear is detached. Portions of the skin and connective tissue may be preserved to facilitate wound repair or reconstruction. Skin grafts, flap closures, or other reconstruction procedures are reported separately.

69140

Entering through the external opening of the ear, the physician makes an incision in the skin covering the exostosis to expose the bone beneath it. The bony growth is removed with a curette or drill. The skin is replaced over the site and the canal is packed to provide hemostasis and to hold the skin in position.

69145

Through the external opening of the ear, the physician uses a knife to excise a soft tissue lesion with surrounding margin or normal tissue. Some limited drilling of the ear canal may be done. The external ear canal may be packed. If extensive skin is removed, a separate grafting procedure may be required at this time.

69150

Through a postauricular incision, the physician uses a scalpel to remove an extensive lesion in the ear canal. Depending upon whether the lesion involves bone, a section of supporting hard tissue may be excised. The tympanic membrane, parotid gland, facial nerve, and portions of the mandible and mastoid may also be removed. A separately reported graft or flap may be performed at this time, or the surgical wound may be repaired with a layered closure.

69155

Through a postauricular incision, the physician uses a scalpel to remove an extensive lesion of the ear canal. A section of supporting hard tissue may be excised as well as the tympanic membrane, parotid gland, facial nerve, and portions of the mandible and mastoid. The physician performs a neck dissection, removing the lymph nodes from that side of the neck. The jugular vein, spinal accessory nerve, or sternocleidomastoid muscle may be removed as well. The carotid artery, vagus, sympathetic, phrenic, brachial plexus, hypoglossal and lingual nerves are spared. A separately reported graft or flap may be performed at this time, or the surgical wound may be repaired with a layered closure.

69200-69205

Under direct visualization, the physician or technician removes a foreign body from the external auditory canal using delicate forceps, a cerumen spoon, or suction. In the case of a live insect, oil is dropped into the ear to immobilize it before it is removed. No anesthetic or local anesthetic is used in 69200. If a child or an adult cannot tolerate the procedure while awake, it is performed under general anesthesia in 69205. Code 69205 is also reported in cases where the foreign body is so large, an incision is made in the external meatus to enlarge the opening before the foreign body can be extracted.

69209-69210

Under direct visualization, the physician removes impacted cerumen (ear wax) using irrigation or lavage (69209), or via suction, a cerumen spoon, or delicate forceps (69210). A typical solution used for lavage is water and saline, warmed to body temperature to avoid causing dizziness, placed in the ear approximately 15 to 30 minutes prior to removal. When instrumentation is used and no infection is present, the ear canal may also be irrigated.

69220-69222

Routine mastoid cavity debridement is required every three to six months in patients who have undergone a radical or modified radical mastoidectomy. Under direct visualization, the physician uses suction, a cerumen spoon, and delicate forceps to remove skin debris and drainage from the mastoid cavity, a bony extension of the ear canal. The cavity is cleaned simply in 69220. The cavity may require more extensive cleaning, as in the case of infection or extensive debris, in 69222. Sometimes this extensive cleaning requires general anesthesia or the use of a laser to remove granulation tissue.

69300

The physician corrects a protruding ear. The physician makes an incision on the posterior auricle and raises the posterior skin off the cartilage. A new antihelical fold is created with multiple sutures through the cartilage. Some techniques employ limited cartilage cutting. A small ellipse of posterior skin is removed and the skin is closed with sutures. Packing corresponding to the anterior ear contours is placed. The size of the auricle may be reduced.

69310

The physician makes a postauricular incision and removes the thick, stenotic plug of soft tissue from the external auditory canal. Some drilling of the bony canal may be needed to enlarge the bony canal. Thin skin grafts are used to reline the canal and are held in place by packing. The posterior incision is repaired with sutures.

69320

The physician makes a postauricular incision and drills just behind and above the temporomandibular joint region. Drilling is continued until the ossicles are identified. The new bony canal is enlarged. The eardrum is reconstructed and split thickness skin grafts are used to line the new canal. A large canal opening is made by removing skin and soft tissue. The canal is packed and the incision is repaired with sutures.

69420-69421
After the application of a local anesthetic (69420) or a general anesthetic (69421) and using a microscope for guidance, the physician makes an incision in the patient's tympanic membrane. Fluid is suctioned from the middle ear space and may be reserved for analysis. The eustachian tube may be inflated. No closure is required.

69424
Assisted by microscopic visualization and using delicate forceps or hook, the physician removes from the tympanic membrane a previously placed ventilating tube with the patient under general anesthesia. No other treatment is required.

69433-69436
In a patient who has received a local or topical anesthetic (69433) or a general anesthetic (69436), the physician inserts a ventilating tube. Under direct visualization with a microscope, the physician makes a small incision in the tympanum (eardrum). Any middle ear fluid is suctioned and may be reserved for analysis. The physician inserts a ventilating tube into the opening in the tympanum. No other treatment is required.

69440
Entering through the external ear canal opening or through a postauricular incision (behind the ear) and into the ear canal, the physician performs exploratory surgery of the middle ear. The eardrum is lifted posteriorly and the middle ear is explored including testing the mobility of the ossicular chain. No major treatment is rendered at this time. The eardrum and canal skin are repositioned and the canal is packed. Any postauricular incision is sutured.

69450
Through the external ear canal opening, the physician treats a lesion or other irritation to the tympanic membrane. The physician makes an incision in the posterior canal skin and reflects the eardrum forward. Under microscopic guidance, the physician removes adhesions from the tympanic membrane (tympanolysis). When tympanolysis is complete, the eardrum and canal skin are repositioned and packing is placed in the ear canal.

69501
Through a postaural or endaural incision, the physician removes the mastoid cortex (outer bone) and drills out some of the mastoid air cells to enter the mastoid antrum. This is usually done as a drainage procedure for mastoid disease limited to the antrum region. A myringotomy with or without tube placement may be performed. A temporary drain may be placed and the incision is sutured.

69502
Through a postaural or endaural incision, the physician drills out the mastoid cavity. The mastoid sinus is exposed posteriorly. The tegmen (bony plate separating the mastoid and middle cranial fossa) is exposed superiorly. The posterior ear canal wall remains intact. The horizontal semicircular canal and part of the incus are visualized. Cholesteatoma or diseased mastoid mucosa is removed. The incision is sutured. A temporary drain may be placed, and a dressing is applied.

69505
The physician makes incisions in the ear canal to develop a posterior tympanomeatal flap that is reflected forward. Through a postaural or endaural incision, the physician drills out the mastoid cortex. The mastoid antrum is identified. Granulations and any cholesteatoma are removed. The posterior bony canal wall is taken down to the level of the facial nerve. If cholesteatoma involves the ossicles, they are removed. The posterior skin flap and eardrum are repositioned to cover the facial ridge and part of the mastoid cavity. A meatoplasty is performed. The mastoid cavity and ear canal are packed, the incision sutured, and a dressing placed.

69511
The physician makes incisions in the ear canal to develop a posterior tympanomeatal flap that is reflected forward. Through a postaural or endaural incision, the physician drills out the mastoid cells. The posterior and superior bony canal walls are taken down to the level of the facial nerve. The ossicles, except for the stapes if possible, are removed as well as the eustachian tube orifice mucosa, middle ear mucosa, granulations, and cholesteatoma. The middle ear and mastoid are exposed to the exterior through the ear canal. A large meatoplasty is performed. Packing is placed, the incision is sutured, and a dressing is applied.

69530
Through a postaural or endaural incision, the physician drills out the mastoid cavity. The mastoid sinus is exposed posteriorly. The tegmen (bony plate separating the mastoid and middle cranial fossa) is exposed superiorly. The posterior ear canal wall remains intact. The horizontal semicircular canal and part of the incus are visualized. Various cell tracts around the semicircular canals are explored to drain the petrous apex. If this is unsuccessful, the posterior and superior bony canal walls are taken down to the level of the facial nerve. The ossicles, except for the stapes if possible, are removed as well as the eustachian tube orifice mucosa, middle ear mucosa, granulations, and cholesteatoma. Cell tracts between the carotid artery and cochlea or the jugular bulb and cochlea are followed to open the petrous apex and drain any infection. A meatoplasty is performed. A temporary drain may be placed. The incision is sutured, and a dressing is applied.

69535
The physician elevates the auricle with a superior flap. If the auricle and surrounding skin is involved, a wide excision of the skin and subcutaneous tissues is performed. The sternocleidomastoid muscle is separated from the mastoid tip, exposing the internal jugular vein. The seventh nerve is sacrificed. The

zygomatic arch is divided. The middle fossa dura is exposed and elevated from the temporal bone. The head of the mandible is removed to expose the internal carotid artery. With a drill and chisel, the carotid canal is opened. The sigmoid sinus is skeletonized and a chisel is used to make the final bony cuts through the medial temporal bone. Hemostasis is obtained with cautery and packing. A parotidectomy and/or neck dissection may also be required. A separately reportable reconstructive procedure may be performed at this time. Otherwise, the incisions are repaired with a layered closure.

69540

Through the external ear canal opening, the physician removes the aural polyp with a cup forceps or an ear snare. Bleeding is controlled with packing or epinephrine on a cotton ball. Antibiotic drops may be instilled.

69550

Through the external auditory canal, the physician makes an incision in the posterior canal skin and reflects the skin flap and eardrum forward. Under microscopic visualization, the small vascular tumor is grasped with a cup forceps and gently removed. Hemostasis is obtained with packing soaked in epinephrine. Once bleeding is controlled, the middle ear is packed with absorbable material. The eardrum and skin flap are repositioned and the ear canal is packed.

69552

Through a postaural incision, the physician drills out the mastoid cavity. The mastoid sinus is exposed posteriorly. The tegmen (bony plate separating the mastoid and middle cranial fossa) is exposed superiorly. The posterior ear canal wall remains intact. An extended facial recess is sometimes needed to completely visualize the tumor. The vascular tumor is grasped and removed with cup forceps. Hemostasis is obtained using absorbable packing. Usually, the ossicles can be left undisturbed. For larger tumors, the posterior canal wall and ossicles may be removed. The incision is repaired with sutures and a dressing is applied.

69554

The surgeon makes an incision in front of the ear. The facial nerve, hypoglossal nerve, spinal accessory nerve, internal jugular vein, and carotid artery are identified in the neck. A complete mastoidectomy with extended facial recess is performed. The tip of the mastoid is removed and the jugular bulb is exposed and ligated inferiorly. The mastoid sinus is skeletonized, opened, and packed. Hemostasis is obtained with packing. If the tumor extends intracranially, a craniotomy may be necessary. A parotidectomy may also be needed if further mobilization of the facial nerve is required. The ear canal and ossicles may be removed. The incision is repair with a layered closure. Dressings are applied.

69601

Using a postaural incision, the physician revises a previously performed simple mastoidectomy with a complete mastoidectomy. The physician drills out the mastoid cavity. The mastoid sinus is exposed posteriorly. The tegmen (bony plate separating the mastoid and middle cranial fossa) is exposed superiorly. The posterior ear canal wall remains intact. The horizontal semicircular canal and part of the incus are visualized. Cholesteatoma or diseased mastoid mucosa are removed. The incision is sutured. A temporary drain may be placed and a dressing is applied.

69602

Using a postaural incision, the physician revises a previously performed simple or complete mastoidectomy with a modified radical mastoidectomy by removing all the mastoid cells, granulations, pus, and the bony partitions of the mastoid cavity. A tympanomeatal flap is developed and reflected anteriorly. The posterior and superior bony canal walls are taken down to the level of the facial nerve. If cholesteatoma is present around the ossicles, the ossicles are removed. The tympanomeatal flap is repositioned over the facial ridge and into the mastoid cavity. Some middle ear space is thus maintained. A large meatoplasty is performed. The ear canal and mastoid cavity are packed and the incision is closed with sutures.

69603

Using an endaural or postauricular incision, the physician revises a previously performed complete or modified radical mastoidectomy with a radical mastoidectomy. The posterior and superior bony canal walls are taken down to the level of the facial nerve. The ossicles, except for the stapes if possible, are removed as well as the eustachian tube orifice mucosa, middle ear mucosa, granulations, and cholesteatoma. The middle ear and mastoid are exposed to the exterior through the ear canal. A large meatoplasty is performed. Packing is placed, the incision is sutured, and a dressing is applied.

69604

Through a postauricular or endaural incision, the physician revises the site of a previous mastoidectomy. The posterior canal may be taken down. Ossicles may be removed. The physician performs a tympanoplasty in conjunction with the revision mastoidectomy. The edges of the tympanic membrane perforation are roughened ("rimming the perforation") and a fascia graft is placed under or over the tympanic membrane remnant. No ossicular reconstruction is done. Absorbable packing may be placed in the middle ear. The canal and mastoid cavity are packed, and the incision is sutured. A dressing is applied.

69610

Under microscopic visualization, the tympanic membrane is repaired. The physician may roughen the tympanic membrane perforation ("rimming the perforation") to prepare the site before closure and may apply a paper patch. In some cases, the edges of a traumatic perforation of the eardrum may need to be elevated from the middle ear with a delicate hook.

69620

Through the external ear canal, the physician visualizes the tympanic membrane and the eardrum defect. The edges of the eardrum perforation are roughened ("rimming the perforation"). Some dissolvable packing may be placed through the perforation into the middle ear space. A fat graft plug may be placed in the perforation or a piece of fascia may be placed medial to the eardrum over the dissolvable packing. A tympanomeatal flap may be raised. Any incisions are sutured and a dressing is applied.

69631

The physician makes an incision in the ear canal skin through a postauricular or transcanal approach. The edges of the tympanic membrane are roughened ("rimming the perforation"). The physician reflects the eardrum forward. The middle ear is explored, and lysis of any adhesions is performed. Any squamous debris or middle ear cholesteatoma is removed and the physician inspects and palpates the ossicles. No ossicular reconstruction is done at this time. Some drilling or curetting of the canal wall may be necessary. Some fascia from the temporalis muscle or other tissues is harvested as a graft to repair the tympanic membrane perforation. Some packing may be placed in the middle ear to support the graft. The graft may be placed under (underlay or medial graft technique) or on top of the remaining eardrum (overlay or lateral graft technique). The canal skin is repositioned and the canal is packed. Any external incisions are sutured, and a dressing is applied.

69632

The physician makes an incision in the ear canal skin through a postauricular or transcanal approach. The edges of the tympanic membrane are roughened ("rimming the perforation"). The physician reflects the eardrum forward. The middle ear is explored, and lysis of any adhesions is performed. Any squamous debris or middle ear cholesteatoma is removed and the physician inspects and palpates the ossicles. The ossicular chain can also be reconstructed by sculpting and repositioning the patient's own ossicles. The natural ossicle may be replaced with a donor cadaver ossicle, or a sculpted bone strut or piece of cartilage. Some packing may be placed in the middle ear to support the reconstructed ossicle prior to final positioning of the eardrum graft. Some drilling or curetting of the canal wall may be necessary. Some fascia from the temporalis muscle or other tissues is harvested as a graft to repair the tympanic membrane perforation. The graft may be placed under (underlay or medial graft technique) or on top of the remaining eardrum (overlay or lateral graft technique). The canal skin is repositioned and the canal is packed. Any external incisions are sutured, and a dressing is applied.

69633

The physician makes an incision in the ear canal skin through a postauricular or transcanal approach. The edges of the tympanic membrane are roughened ("rimming the perforation"). The physician reflects the eardrum forward. The middle ear is explored, and lysis of any adhesions is performed. Any squamous debris or middle ear cholesteatoma is removed and the physician inspects and palpates the ossicles. The ossicular chain is reconstructed using a synthetic reconstructive prosthesis. A partial ossicular prosthesis (PORP) is used when the stapes suprastructure is present. If the stapes suprastructure is absent, a total ossicular replacement prosthesis (TORP) is used. A piece of cartilage may be placed between the eardrum and prosthesis. Some packing may be placed in the middle ear to support the reconstructed ossicle prior to final positioning of the eardrum graft. Some drilling or curetting of the canal wall may be necessary. Some fascia from the temporalis muscle or other tissues is harvested as a graft to repair the tympanic membrane perforation. The graft may be placed under (underlay or medial graft technique) or on top of the remaining eardrum (overlay or lateral graft technique). The canal skin is repositioned and the canal is packed.

69635

Through a postauricular incision, the physician removes the mastoid cortex (outer bone) and drills out some of the mastoid air cells to enter the mastoid antrum. The edges of the tympanic membrane are roughened ("rimming the perforation"). The physician reflects the eardrum forward. The middle ear is explored, and lysis of any adhesions is performed. Any squamous debris or middle ear cholesteatoma is removed and the physician inspects and palpates the ossicles. No ossicular reconstruction is done at this time. Some drilling or curetting of the canal wall may be necessary. Some fascia from the temporalis muscle or other tissues is harvested as a graft to repair the tympanic membrane perforation. Some packing may be placed in the middle ear to support the graft. The graft may be placed under (underlay or medial graft technique) or on top of the remaining eardrum (overlay or lateral graft technique). The canal skin is repositioned and the canal is packed. Any external incisions are sutured, and a dressing is applied.

69636

Through a postauricular incision, the physician removes the mastoid cortex (outer bone) and drills out some of the mastoid air cells to enter the mastoid antrum. The edges of the tympanic membrane are roughened ("rimming the perforation"). The physician reflects the eardrum forward. The middle ear is explored, and lysis of any adhesions is performed. Any squamous debris or middle ear cholesteatoma is removed and the physician inspects and palpates the ossicles. The ossicular chain can be reconstructed by sculpting and repositioning the patient's own ossicles. The natural ossicle may also be replaced with a donor cadaver ossicle, or a sculpted bone strut or piece of cartilage. Some packing may be placed in the middle ear to support the reconstructed ossicle prior to final positioning of the eardrum graft. Some drilling or curetting of the canal wall may be necessary. Some fascia from the temporalis muscle or other tissues is harvested as a graft to repair the tympanic membrane perforation. The graft may be placed under (underlay or medial graft technique) or on top of the remaining eardrum (overlay or lateral graft technique). The canal skin is repositioned and the canal is packed. Any external incisions are sutured, and a dressing is applied.

69637

Through a postauricular incision, the physician removes the mastoid cortex (outer bone) and drills out some of the mastoid air cells to enter the mastoid antrum. The edges of the tympanic membrane are roughened ("rimming the perforation"). The physician reflects the eardrum forward. The middle ear is explored, and lysis of any adhesions is performed. Any squamous debris or middle ear cholesteatoma is removed and the physician inspects and palpates the ossicles. The ossicular chain is reconstructed using a synthetic reconstructive prosthesis. A partial ossicular prosthesis (PORP) is used when the stapes suprastructure is present. If the stapes suprastructure is absent, a total ossicular replacement prosthesis (TORP) is used. A piece of cartilage may be placed between the eardrum and prosthesis. Some packing may be placed to support the reconstructed ossicle prior to positioning of the eardrum graft. Some drilling or curetting of the canal wall may be necessary. Some fascia from the temporalis muscle or other tissues is harvested as a graft to repair the perforation. The graft may be placed under (underlay or medial graft technique) or on top of the remaining eardrum (overlay or lateral graft technique). The canal skin is repositioned and the canal is packed.

69641

The physician makes incisions in the ear canal to develop a posterior tympanomeatal flap that is reflected forward. Through a postaural or endaural incision, the physician drills out the mastoid cortex. The mastoid antrum is identified. Granulations and any cholesteatoma are removed. The posterior bony canal wall is taken down to the level of the facial nerve. The middle ear is explored, and lysis of any adhesions is performed. Any squamous debris or middle ear cholesteatoma is removed and the physician inspects and palpates the ossicles. No ossicular reconstruction is done at this time. Some fascia from the temporalis muscle or other tissues is harvested as a graft to repair the tympanic membrane perforation. Some packing may be placed in the middle ear to support the graft. The graft may be placed under (underlay or medial graft technique) or on top of the remaining eardrum (overlay or lateral graft technique). The posterior skin flap and reconstructed eardrum are repositioned to cover the facial ridge and part of the mastoid cavity. A meatoplasty is performed. The mastoid cavity and ear canal are packed, the incision sutured, and a dressing placed.

69642

The physician makes incisions in the ear canal to develop a posterior tympanomeatal flap that is reflected forward. Through a postaural or endaural incision, the physician drills out the mastoid cortex. The mastoid antrum is identified. Granulations and any cholesteatoma are removed. The posterior bony canal wall is taken down to the level of the facial nerve. The middle ear is explored, and lysis of any adhesions is performed. Any squamous debris or middle ear cholesteatoma is removed and the physician inspects and palpates the ossicles. The ossicular chain can be reconstructed by sculpting and repositioning the patient's own ossicles. The natural ossicle also may be replaced with a donor cadaver ossicle, or a sculpted bone strut or piece of cartilage. Some packing may be placed in the middle ear to support the reconstructed ossicle prior to final positioning of the eardrum graft. Some fascia from the temporalis muscle or other tissues is harvested as a graft to repair the tympanic membrane perforation. Some packing may be placed in the middle ear to support the graft. The graft may be placed under (underlay or medial graft technique) or on top of the remaining eardrum (overlay or lateral graft technique). The posterior skin flap and reconstructed eardrum are repositioned to cover the facial ridge and part of the mastoid cavity. A meatoplasty is performed. The mastoid cavity and ear canal are packed, the incision sutured, and a dressing placed.

69643

Through a postauricular incision, the physician removes the mastoid cortex (outer bone) and drills out the mastoid air cells. The edges of the tympanic membrane are roughened ("rimming the perforation"). The physician reflects the eardrum forward. The middle ear is explored, and lysis of any adhesions is performed. Any squamous debris or middle ear cholesteatoma is removed and the physician inspects and palpates the ossicles. No ossicular reconstruction is done at this time. If the posterior canal wall is taken down, it is reconstructed with cartilage, bone, or hydroxyapatite (i.e., Wehr's canal wall reconstruction). Some fascia from the temporalis muscle or other tissues is harvested as a graft to repair the tympanic membrane perforation. Some packing may be placed in the middle ear to support the graft. The graft may be placed under (underlay or medial graft technique) or on top of the remaining eardrum (overlay or lateral graft technique). The canal skin is repositioned and the canal and mastoid cavity are packed. Any external incisions are sutured, and a dressing is applied.

69644

Through a postauricular incision, the physician removes the mastoid cortex (outer bone) and drills out the mastoid air cells. The edges of the tympanic membrane are roughened ("rimming the perforation"). The physician reflects the eardrum forward. The middle ear is explored, and lysis of any adhesions is performed. Any squamous debris or middle ear cholesteatoma is removed and the physician inspects and palpates the ossicles. The ossicular chain may be reconstructed by sculpting and repositioning the patient's own ossicles. The natural ossicle also may be replaced with a donor cadaver ossicle, or a sculpted bone strut or piece of cartilage. Some packing may be placed in the middle ear to support the reconstructed ossicle prior to final positioning of the eardrum graft. If the posterior canal wall is taken down, it is reconstructed with cartilage, bone, or hydroxyapatite (i.e., Wehr's canal wall reconstruction). Some fascia from the temporalis muscle or other tissues is harvested as a graft to repair the tympanic membrane perforation. Some packing may be placed in the middle ear to support the graft. The graft may be placed under (underlay or medial graft technique) or on top of the remaining eardrum (overlay or lateral graft technique). The canal skin is repositioned and the canal and mastoid cavity are packed. Any external incisions are sutured, and a dressing is applied.

69645

Through a postauricular incision, the physician removes the mastoid cortex (outer bone) and drills out the mastoid air cells. A posterior canal skin flap and remaining eardrum are preserved and reflected forward. The middle ear is explored, and lysis of any adhesions is performed. Any squamous debris or middle ear cholesteatoma is removed and the physician inspects and palpates the ossicles. The posterior canal wall is taken down to the level of the facial nerve. The ossicles are inspected and all or part of the ossicles may be removed. The middle ear mucosa may be removed. No ossicular reconstruction is attempted. Some fascia from the temporalis muscle or other tissues is harvested as a graft to repair the tympanic membrane perforation. Some packing may be placed in the middle ear to support the graft. The graft may be placed under (underlay or medial graft technique) or on top of the remaining eardrum (overlay or lateral graft technique). A piece of Silastic may be placed in the middle ear to develop an air-containing space. The canal skin is repositioned and the canal and mastoid cavity are packed. Any external incisions are sutured, and a dressing is applied.

69646

Through a postauricular incision, the physician removes the mastoid cortex (outer bone) and drills out the mastoid air cells. A posterior canal skin flap and remaining eardrum are preserved and reflected forward. The middle ear is explored, and lysis of any adhesions is performed. Any squamous debris or middle ear cholesteatoma is removed and the physician inspects and palpates the ossicles. The posterior canal wall is taken down to the level of the facial nerve. All or part of the ossicles are removed in addition to the middle ear mucosa. Reconstruction is accomplished with the sculpting of the patient's own ossicle, or through the placement of a donor cadaver ossicle, cartilage, or bone graft, or prosthetic device. A reconstructed eardrum is positioned over the reconstructed ossicular chain. Some packing may be placed in the middle ear to support the graft. The graft may be placed under (underlay or medial graft technique) or on top of the remaining eardrum (overlay or lateral graft technique). Some fascia from the temporalis muscle or other tissues is harvested as a graft to repair the tympanic membrane perforation. Some packing may be placed in the middle ear to support the graft. The graft may be placed under (underlay or medial graft technique) or on top of the remaining eardrum (overlay or lateral graft technique). The canal skin is repositioned and the canal and mastoid cavity are packed. Any external incisions are sutured, and a dressing is applied. The canal skin is repositioned and the canal and mastoid cavity are packed. Any external incisions are sutured, and a dressing is applied.

69650

The physician makes an incision in the posterior canal skin through the external ear canal opening. Under microscopic visualization, the physician reflects the skin flap and posterior eardrum forward. A small amount of the posterior bony canal may need to be removed with a curette or drill. The incus and stapes are visualized and palpated. If the stapes is fixated it can be mobilized by applying pressure to it with delicate instruments. The canal skin and eardrum are repositioned and the ear canal is packed.

69660

The surgeon makes an incision in the posterior canal skin through the external canal opening. Occasionally, a postauricular incision may be substituted. Under microscopic guidance, the physician reflects the canal skin flap and posterior eardrum forward. Some posterior canal bone may be removed with a curette or drill. The ossicular chain is palpated. If the stapes is fixed, it is separated from the incus. The stapes can be removed (stapedectomy) or an opening can be made in the stapes footplate with a laser or drill (stapedotomy). A prosthesis is placed on the incus to replace the stapes. A piece of fascia, vein, perichondrium, or fat might be applied around or under the prosthesis. The skin and eardrum are repositioned, and the ear canal is packed.

69661

The surgeon makes an incision in the posterior canal skin through the external canal opening. Occasionally, a postauricular incision may be substituted. Under microscopic guidance, the physician reflects the canal skin flap and posterior eardrum forward. Some posterior canal bone may be removed with a curette or drill. The ossicular chain is palpated. If the stapes is fixed, it is separated from the incus. The stapes is removed (stapedectomy). The physician drills an opening in the markedly thickened footplate through which the prosthesis is inserted and attached to the incus. A piece of fascia, vein, perichondrium, or fat might be applied around or under the prosthesis. The skin and eardrum are repositioned, and the ear canal is packed.

69662

The physician revises a stapedectomy or stapedotomy. The physician makes an incision over the previous incision site in the posterior canal or through the external canal opening. Alternately a previous postauricular incision may be reincised. Under microscopic guidance, the physician reflects the canal skin flap and posterior eardrum forward. Some posterior canal bone may be removed with a curette or drill. The ossicular chain is palpated. If the stapes has become fixed since the previous surgery it is separated from the incus. The footplate may be opened with a laser or drilled out. The prosthesis may be repositioned, revised, or removed and replaced. A piece of fascia, vein, perichondrium, or fat previously placed may be removed and replaced around or under the prosthesis. The skin and eardrum are repositioned, and the ear canal is packed.

69666

The physician makes a posterior canal incision through the external ear canal opening. Sometimes, a postauricular incision is performed instead. Under microscopic guidance, the physician reflects the skin flap and posterior eardrum forward. The oval window area is inspected for fluid leak from the inner ear. The lining around the oval window is gently roughened. The area is packed with fat, fascia or muscle tissue. The eardrum and skin flap are replaced and the canal is packed. If a postauricular incision is made, it is sutured.

69667

The physician makes a posterior canal incision through the external ear canal opening. Sometimes, a postauricular incision is performed instead. Under microscopic guidance, the physician reflects the skin flap and posterior eardrum forward. The round window area is inspected for fluid leak from the inner ear. The lining around the round window is gently roughened. The area is packed with fat, fascia or muscle tissue. The eardrum and skin flap are replaced and the canal is packed. If a postauricular incision is made, it is sutured.

69670

Through a postauricular incision, the physician accesses the mastoid cavity of a previous mastoidectomy. Any remaining mastoid disease is removed. To lessen the size of a large mastoid cavity or to stop a cerebrospinal leak, the cavity is obliterated with a rotation flap of fascia or muscle and/or free fat graft and skin. The flap is sutured into place, and the incision is sutured.

69676

The physician makes an incision in the posterior canal wall skin and raises a skin flap and the eardrum forward. Jacobson's nerve is identified in the middle ear and is divided. The eardrum and canal skin are repositioned and packing is placed in the ear canal.

[69714, 69717, 69726]

The physician performs implantation, replacement, or removal of a bone-anchored (osseointegrated) hearing aid that features a percutaneous attachment to an external speech processor. Bone conduction implants transfer sound to the inner ear through direct vibration of the skull. The implant is composed of an internal prosthesis embedded into the skull, an exposed outer external abutment that is connected to the implant at the time of surgery, and an external speech processor. A percutaneous device directly attaches the speech processor to the implant that protrudes through the scalp. The internal portion of the implant (made of titanium or other material) stimulates the cochlea through direct bone conduction. The external sound processor transforms sound into vibrations, which are transferred by the implant to the skull bone and then to the cochlea. In one implantation procedure, reported by 69714, the physician makes a small break in the skin to expose the mastoid cortex, and a skin flap and periosteal flap are created. A tunnel is drilled into the skull and tapped to create a passage for the stem of the implant pedestal. The stem is placed in the tunnel adjacent to the cochlea and the abutment is attached and secured to the stem. The soft tissue surrounding the pedestal is thinned to prevent local movement and minimize the incidence of infection at the site. The implant remains in place and fuses, or osseointegrates, with the living skull bone. Report 69717 for replacement of this implant. The physician makes an incision and dissects to the pericranium. The previous implant abutment is removed and the wound inspected, after which the new placement site of the implant is identified, marked on the skull, and exposed. A hole is drilled through the cranium and the implant is installed and secured to the transcutaneous abutment. A separate incision is made in the overlying skin flap so that the percutaneous abutment can extend through the soft tissues. The wound is irrigated and closed. Report 69726 for removal of the entire osseointegrated implant. The physician makes an incision, dissects through the pericranium, and exposes the previous implant. The cranial bone surrounding the fixture in the patient's skull is drilled and the entire implant removed. The wound is inspected, irrigated, and debrided, followed by layered closure. In all scenarios, if a mastoidectomy is performed during the same operative session, it is reported separately.

[69716, 69719, 69727, 69728, 69729, 69730]

The physician performs implantation, replacement, or removal of a bone-anchored (osseointegrated) hearing aid that features a magnetic transcutaneous attachment that couples the implant and the speech processor through an intact scalp via magnet. Bone conduction implants transfer sound to the inner ear through direct vibration of the skull. The implant is composed of an internal prosthesis embedded into the skull with a magnet under the skin and an external sound and speech processor. The internal portion of the implant (made of titanium or other material) stimulates the cochlea through direct bone conduction. The external sound processor transforms sound into vibrations, which are transferred by the implant to the skull bone and then to the cochlea. In

Auditory

one implantation procedure, the physician makes an incision and dissects through the pericranium, where a subpericranial pocket for the implant coil and magnet is created. The area for the transducer is identified and marked. The physician drills the skull to create a well in the bone that will accommodate the transducer device. The entire device, including the coil, magnet, and transducer, is placed and fixed to the skull via a fixation screw. The flap overlying the magnet/coil portion of the device is trimmed to a sufficient thickness to permit transcutaneous transmission. The wound is irrigated and closed. The acoustic transmission occurs by the magnetic attachment of the external sound processor and the internally implanted device components. Since the processor adheres magnetically to the implanted device, no percutaneous abutment is necessary to connect the internal and external components. Report 69716 when the provider attaches the magnetic implant within the mastoid and/or removes less than 100 sq mm surface area of bone deep to the outer cranial cortex and 69729 if attached outside the mastoid, resulting in removal of 100 sq mm or more of surface area of bone deep to the outer cranial cortex. Report 69719 for replacement (including removal of the existing device) of an implant within the mastoid and/or involving a bony defect less than 100 sq mm surface area of bone deep to the outer cranial cortex and 69730 if the implant is outside the mastoid and involves a bony defect 100 sq mm or more of surface area of bone deep to the outer cranial cortex. Report 69727 for removal of the entire implant if within the mastoid and/or involves a bony defect less than 100 sq mm surface area of bone deep to the outer cranial cortex and 69728 if outside the mastoid involving a bony defect 100 sq mm or more of surface area of bone deep to the outer cranial cortex. In all scenarios, if a mastoidectomy is performed during the same operative session, it is reported separately.

69700

The physician makes an incision around the postauricular fistula, a skin-lined tunnel. The fistula tract is excised, and the incision site is repaired with sutures.

69705-69706

The physician performs balloon dilation of the eustachian tube (ET) via nasopharyngoscopic approach. In one method, a proprietary balloon catheter is inserted under direct endoscopic visualization and inflated in the cartilaginous portion of the eustachian tube for treatment of ET dysfunction. The tip, balloon, and rigid shaft portion of the balloon dilation system are passed into a guide catheter. The physician inserts the guide catheter through the nose to the orifice of the eustachian tube. Using an actuator designed to advance and retract the balloon catheter, the balloon is inserted into the ET by advancing the catheter. The balloon is inflated to the desired pressure by injecting sterile saline or sterile water through an inflation port. Once the desired inflation is achieved, the balloon is deflated. The balloon catheter is retracted into the guide catheter, and the system is removed from the patient. Report 69705 if the procedure is performed unilaterally and 69706 if performed bilaterally.

69710

Through a postauricular incision, the physician drills a circular depression in the outer skull cortex behind the mastoid cavity. The internal coil is seated in the circular depression and secured to the skull with titanium screws. The subcutaneous tissue over the internal coil may be thinned. The wound is irrigated and repaired with sutures. A dressing is applied.

69711

Through a postauricular incision, the physician accesses a previously implanted electromagnetic bone conduction hearing device. The device is repaired or removed. The wound is irrigated and repaired with sutures. A dressing is applied.

69720

Through a postauricular incision, the physician drills out the mastoid cavity. The sigmoid sinus is exposed posteriorly. The posterior ear canal wall remains intact. The horizontal semicircular canal and part of the incus are visualized. The vertical portion of the facial nerve is exposed. The facial recess is opened and the bone over the horizontal portion (middle ear) of the facial nerve is removed. The incus may be separated from the stapes. The incus and part of the malleus may be removed. The facial nerve sheath is incised from the stylomastoid foramen to the geniculate ganglion. The postauricular wound is sutured and a dressing is applied.

69725

Through a postauricular incision, the physician drills out the mastoid cavity. The sigmoid sinus is exposed posteriorly. The posterior ear canal wall remains intact. The horizontal semicircular canal and part of the incus are visualized. The vertical portion of the facial nerve is exposed. The facial recess is opened and the bone over the horizontal portion (middle ear) of the facial nerve is removed. Decompression continues medial to the geniculate ganglion. The incus and part of the malleus are usually removed. Sometimes, a combined transmastoid and middle fossa approach is required to access the nerve adequately, in which case, a piece of temporal bone is excised to access the middle cranial fossa.

69740

Through a postauricular incision, the physician drills out the mastoid cavity. The posterior ear canal wall remains intact. The horizontal semicircular canal and part of the incus are visualized. The vertical portion of the facial nerve is exposed. The facial recess is opened and the bone over the horizontal portion (middle ear) of the facial nerve is removed. The incus may be separated from the stapes. The incus and part of the malleus may be removed. The nerve defect is identified, and the nerve is decompressed. Cut ends of the facial nerve are sutured to each other, or grafted to a harvested nerve in an end-to-end fashion. The postauricular wound is sutured and a dressing is applied.

69745

Through a postauricular incision, the physician drills out the mastoid cavity. The posterior ear canal wall remains intact. The horizontal semicircular canal and part of the incus are visualized. The vertical portion of the facial nerve is exposed. The facial recess is opened and the bone over the horizontal portion (middle ear) of the facial nerve is removed. The incus and part of the malleus are usually removed. The nerve defect is identified, and the nerve is decompressed. Cut ends of the facial nerve are sutured to each other, or grafted to a harvested nerve in an end-to-end fashion. Sometimes, a combined transmastoid and middle fossa approach is required to access the nerve adequately, in which case, a piece of temporal bone is excised to access the middle cranial fossa.

69801

The physician administers drugs such as aminoglycosides, corticosteroids, antibiotics, or local anesthetics into the middle ear through the eardrum (tympanic membrane) to treat inner ear conditions such as Meniere's disease, tinnitus, hearing loss, and certain forms of labyrinthine dysfunction. In a transcanal approach, the physician makes a small incision into the anesthetized tympanic membrane, inserts a small catheter or needle into the middle ear, and infuses the drug.

69805-69806

Through a postauricular incision, the physician drills out the mastoid cavity. The posterior ear canal wall remains intact. The horizontal and posterior semicircular canals are visualized. Drilling is continued until the endolymphatic sac is identified. The physician uses a diamond burr and fine picks to remove the bone around the sack (decompression) in 69805. A shunt is inserted into the sac in 69806. In either case, the mastoid cavity is packed with absorbable packing and the outer incision is sutured and a pressure dressing is applied.

69905

The physician makes an incision in the posterior canal skin and reflects the skin flap and posterior eardrum forward. Under microscopic visualization through the external ear opening, the incus and stapes are removed. A right angle hook is fed through the oval window to remove the contents of the vestibule. The physician may drill a connection between the oval and round windows. The middle ear is packed with gelatin foam. The eardrum and canal skin are repositioned, and the ear canal is packed.

69910

Through a postauricular incision, the physician drills out the mastoid cavity. The posterior ear canal wall remains intact. The horizontal, posterior, and superior semicircular canals are removed along with the lining of the labyrinth. The incision is repaired with sutures and a dressing is applied.

69915

Through a postauricular incision, the physician drills out the mastoid cavity. The posterior ear canal wall remains intact. The horizontal, posterior, and superior semicircular canals are removed along with the lining of the labyrinth. The internal auditory canal is identified. The bone over the internal auditory canal is removed, exposing the dura. The dura is opened and the vestibular nerve is identified and cut. The facial nerve is preserved. The dura is closed and the mastoid cavity is packed. The incision is repaired with sutures and a dressing is applied.

69930

The physician makes a U-shaped incision, creating a skin flap well behind the mastoid, and drills a circular depression in the squamous portion of the temporal bone in which the internal coil will be housed. The mastoid air cells are removed with a drill, and a facial recess approach is used. The bony ear canal is preserved. The internal coil is secured in the depressed area of the temporal bone, and the electrode is introduced through the facial recess and the round window into the cochlea. The ground wire attached to the internal coil is introduced into the temporalis muscle. The incision is sutured.

69950

A vertical incision is made just anterior to the auricle and is extended superiorly to expose the temporalis muscle. The muscle is divided. A section of the skull (craniotomy) is removed to expose the dura over the temporal lobe of the brain. The dura is elevated off the floor of the middle fossa. The physician drills to thin the bone over the floor of the middle fossa to identify the facial nerve. The facial nerve is followed to the internal auditory canal. The canal is decompressed with the drill and the dura covering the vestibular nerves is opened. The vestibular nerves are cut while preserving the facial and cochlear nerves. A muscle graft is placed over the internal auditory canal, and the bone is replaced in the skull defect. The incision is sutured and a dressing is applied.

69955

A vertical incision is made just anterior to the auricle and is extended superiorly to expose the temporalis muscle. The muscle is divided. A section of the skull (craniotomy) is removed to expose the dura over the temporal lobe of the brain. The dura is elevated off the floor of the middle fossa. The bone over the facial nerve is removed with the drill. If there is a tumor of the facial nerve, it is resected. If the nerve has been transected because of trauma, it is repaired with sutures. A nerve graft may be needed. A transmastoid approach may also be needed if extensive decompression is required. A muscle graft is placed over the floor of the middle cranial fossa. The bone plug is replaced in the skull defect. The incision is sutured and a dressing is applied.

69960
A vertical incision is made just anterior to the auricle and is extended superiorly to expose the temporalis muscle. The muscle is divided. A section of the skull (craniotomy) is removed to expose the dura over the temporal lobe of the brain. The dura is elevated off the floor of the middle fossa. The physician identifies the internal auditory canal. A drill is used to remove bone to open the canal (decompression). A muscle graft is placed over the internal auditory canal and the bone is replaced in the skull defect. The incision is sutured and a dressing is applied.

69970
A vertical incision is made just anterior to the auricle and is extended superiorly to expose the temporalis muscle. The muscle is divided. A section of the skull (craniotomy) is removed to expose the dura over the temporal lobe of the brain. The dura is elevated off the floor of the middle fossa. The physician isolates and dissects a tumor of the temporal bone. The internal auditory canal may be decompressed. A muscle graft is placed over the internal auditory canal. The bone plug is returned to the skull, the incision is sutured, and a dressing is applied.

69990
The physician uses a surgical microscope when the services are performed using the techniques of microsurgery, except when the microscopy is part of the procedure (such as in 15756). This code is reported in addition to the primary procedure.

Radiology

70010
A radiographic study using fluoroscopy is performed on the posterior fossa when a lesion is suspected, or to detect cerebrospinal fluid (CSF) leaks or normal pressure hydrocephalus (NPH). Contrast medium, usually barium sulfate, may be used to enhance visibility and is instilled in the patient through a lumbar area puncture into the subarachnoid space. The radiologist takes a series of pictures by sending an x-ray beam through the body, using fluoroscopy to view the enhanced structure on a television camera. The patient is angled from an erect position through a recumbent position with the body tilted so as to maintain feet higher than the head to help the flow of contrast into the study area.

70015
A radiographic study is performed that maps the tumor pathology of a mass within the posterior fossa. The brainstem and cerebellum are contained within the posterior fossa and the cerebellopontine angle cistern is often the location of a mass, such as a schwannoma or meningioma. Images are taken sequentially over a period of hours and days after introducing a radiotracer intrathecally by lumbar puncture. Cisternography may also be used to detect cerebrospinal fluid (CSF) leaks or normal pressure hydrocephalus (NPH).

70030
X-rays of the eyes are obtained to determine the location of a foreign body in the eye. After positioning the patient, a one- or two-view x-ray is obtained. Transparent objects such as glass may not be good candidates for x-ray visualization. The physician supervises the procedure and interprets and reports the findings.

70100-70110
The lower jaw bone is x-rayed. In 70100, three or less projections are taken for a partial view of the bone structure and in 70110, four or more projections are taken for a complete view of the bone structure.

70120
Films are taken of the mastoid processes, or lower portion of the temporal bone of the skull, which protrudes just behind the ear. Both mastoid processes are always examined for comparison purposes, and it is essential that the radiographs be exact duplicates in both positioning of the site and technical quality. Several varying views may be taken, but the key element of this procedure is that it reports less than three views per side.

70130
Films are taken of the mastoid processes, or lower portion of the temporal bone of the skull, which protrudes just behind the ear. Both mastoid processes are always examined for comparison purposes, and it is essential that the radiographs be exact duplicates in both positioning of the site and technical quality. Several varying views may be taken, but the key element of this procedure is that it reports a complete exam, or minimum of three views per side.

70134
Films are taken of the petrous portions of the skull to demonstrate internal auditory meati, or organs of hearing. Several different views may be taken, both with varying angulation of the x-ray beam, as well as varying the position of the patient's skull.

70140
X-rays of the facial bones are obtained to determine an injury, fracture, or neoplasm. After positioning the patient, less than three views of the facial bones are obtained. The physician supervises the procedure and interprets and reports the findings.

70150
X-rays of the facial bones are obtained to determine an injury, fracture, or neoplasm. After positioning the patient, a complete series of x-rays of the facial bones, with a minimum of three views, is obtained. The physician supervises the procedure and interprets and reports the findings.

70160
Films are taken of the nasal bones to include a complete exam, or minimum of three views. Typically, this exam would consist of both right and left lateral (side to side) for comparison, as well as a tangential projection in which the x-ray beam is directed from a

position above the patient's head down through the nose. This view is primarily used to demonstrate the medial or lateral (side to side) displacement of nasal fractures.

70170

Dacryocystography is the radiographic evaluation of the lacrimal system to localize the site of an obstruction. One cc of a water-soluble contrast medium is injected through the lower canaliculus and x-rays of the excretory system are obtained. The physician supervises the procedure and interprets and reports the findings.

70190

Radiological examination of the optic foramina is useful in the evaluation of trauma, tumors, or foreign bodies. After positioning the patient, the radiologist obtains x-rays of the optic foramina. The physician supervises the procedure and interprets and reports the findings.

70200

Radiological examination of the orbits is useful in the evaluation of trauma, tumors, or foreign bodies. After positioning the patient, the radiologist obtains a minimum of four x-ray views of the orbits. Standard methods include posteroanterior (PA) exposures from two different positions, lateral views, optic canal projections, and oblique views of each side for comparison. The physician supervises the procedure and interprets and reports the findings.

70210

Films are taken of the paranasal sinuses in one or two views. Although there are several sinus projections, each serving a specific purpose, many of them are used only when required to visualize a specific lesion. Typically, but not necessarily, this code calls for a side to side (lateral) view and a back to front (PA) view, depending on the specific sinus in question. The projections are routinely taken with the patient in an erect position to demonstrate presence or absence of fluid.

70220

Films are taken of the paranasal sinuses for a complete study, with a minimum of three views. There are several sinus projections used when required to visualize a specific lesion. Projections routinely taken consist of four to five standard views of the skull, which adequately demonstrate all the paranasal sinuses on most patients. Specific exams may be included to test a particular sinus (e.g., frontal sinus, maxillary sinus, and sphenoid or ethmoid sinuses). These projections are routinely taken with the patient in an erect position to demonstrate presence or absence of fluid.

70240

Films are taken of the sella turcica, the depression within the sphenoid bone that houses the pituitary gland. The patient is placed in the prone semioblique position and the x-ray beam is directed to a spot slightly anterior and superior to the external auditory meatus while the patient's head is maintained in a lateral position.

70250-70260

Films are taken of the skull bones. In 70250, three or less views are taken, and in 70260, a complete exam with a four view minimum is performed. The most common projections for routine skull series are AP axial (front to back), lateral, and PA axial (back to front). X-rays may be taken with the patient placed erect, prone, or supine and either code may include stereoradiography, which is a technique that produces three-dimensional images.

70300-70320

Films are taken of the mouth to show teeth and/or surrounding bone. In dental radiography, the film may be placed inside or outside the mouth. Code 70300 reports a single view only, 70310 reports a partial examination, and 70320 reports a complete full mouth exam.

70328-70330

The temporomandibular joint is x-rayed in two projections on one side only in 70328 and in two projections on both sides in 70330. One film is taken with the mouth open and one with the mouth closed.

70332

A radiographic contrast study is performed on the temporomandibular joint. A contrast material is injected into the joint spaces, followed by x-ray examination of the joint. This allows the physician to see the position of the structures not normally seen on conventional x-rays.

70336

Magnetic resonance imaging (MRI) is a radiation-free, noninvasive, technique to produce high quality sectional images of the inside of the body in multiple planes. MRI uses the natural magnetic properties of the hydrogen atoms in our bodies that emit radiofrequency signals when exposed to radio waves within a strong electro-magnetic field. These signals are processed and converted by the computer into high-resolution, three-dimensional, tomographic images. Patients with metallic or electronic implants or foreign bodies cannot be exposed to MRI. The patient must remain still while lying on a motorized table within the large, circular MRI tunnel. A sedative may be administered as well as contrast material for image enhancement. This code reports an exam of the temporomandibular joint(s).

70350

A lateral or frontal x-ray projection is taken to examine the skull, jaw, and related tooth positions. The machine holds the patient's head in the same position each time so that a series of cephalograms can be directly compared for growth and development over time.

70355

A panoramic radiographic study is performed on the mandibular arch and its supporting structures. A single image is produced of the mandible for diagnostic purposes. The physician evaluates trauma, third molar, and other unique disease conditions. Tooth development and anomalies may also be studied.

70360
The technologist uses x-rays to obtain soft tissue images of the patient's neck rather than bone. The radiologist obtains two views, typically front to back (AP), and side to side (lateral). This procedure is performed to visualize abnormal air patterns or suspected foreign bodies or obstructions within the throat or neck.

70370
A radiologic examination is performed to visualize the pharynx, which serves as passage for both food and air, and larynx, or the organ of voice. Films are typically taken to show soft tissues of the neck. The films are often taken while the patient inhales or makes phonetic sounds. The key element of this code is that it includes x-ray fluoroscopy and/or magnification technique in addition to the radiologic exam.

70371
A radiologic study is performed for pharyngeal and speech evaluation. Cineradiography, or video recording, is employed, as the physiologic event of speech and swallowing occur too rapidly for normal fluoroscopic viewing. High-speed frame rates are used to evaluate speech and swallowing, and later reviewed and interpreted by the radiologist.

70380
Films are taken to visualize a salivary gland for possible calculus (calcium deposit). Typically, a front to back (AP) or back to front (PA) view is taken of the side in question. The patient is asked to fill his cheek with air, if possible, to enhance detail of the x-ray, particularly for demonstration of calcific deposits. A lateral, or side to side view, as well as an intra-oral projection, may also be taken.

70390
A radiographic contrast study is performed to visualize the salivary glands and ducts, typically to demonstrate possible lesions or tumors, salivary fistulae, or to localize calcium deposits within the gland. The radiologist injects the main salivary duct with radiopaque dye (contrast), after which it flows into the duct system and is examined with x-ray fluoroscopy. The projected image is amplified and displayed on a TV monitor for the radiologist to review and interpret.

70450-70470
Computed tomography directs multiple narrow beams of x-rays around the body structure being studied and uses computer imaging to produce thin cross-sectional views of various layers (or slices) of the body. It is useful for the evaluation of trauma, tumor, and foreign bodies as CT is able to visualize soft tissue as well as bones. Patients are required to remain motionless during the study and sedation may need to be administered as well as a contrast medium for image enhancement. These codes report an exam of the head or brain. Report 70450 if no contrast is used. Report 70460 if performed with contrast and 70470 if performed first without contrast and again following the injection of contrast.

70480-70482
Computed tomography directs multiple narrow beams of x-rays around the body structure being studied and uses computer imaging to produce thin cross-sectional views of various layers (or slices) of the body. It is useful for the evaluation of trauma, tumor, and foreign bodies as CT is able to visualize soft tissue as well as bones. Patients are required to remain motionless during the study and sedation may need to be administered as well as a contrast medium for image enhancement. These codes report an exam of the orbit, sella, posterior fossa, or outer, middle, or inner ear. Report 70480 if no contrast is used. Report 70481 if performed with contrast and 70482 if performed first without contrast and again following the injection of contrast.

70486-70488
Computed tomography directs multiple narrow beams of x-rays around the body structure being studied and uses computer imaging to produce thin cross-sectional views of various layers (or slices) of the body. It is useful for the evaluation of trauma, tumor, and foreign bodies as CT is able to visualize soft tissue as well as bones. Patients are required to remain motionless during the study and sedation may need to be administered as well as a contrast medium for image enhancement. These codes report an exam of the maxillofacial area. Report 70486 if no contrast is used. Report 70487 if performed with contrast and 70488 if performed first without contrast and again following the injection of contrast.

70490-70492
Computed tomography directs multiple narrow beams of x-rays around the body structure being studied and uses computer imaging to produce thin cross-sectional views of various layers (or slices) of the body. It is useful for the evaluation of trauma, tumor, and foreign bodies as CT is able to visualize soft tissue as well as bones. Patients are required to remain motionless during the study and sedation may need to be administered as well as a contrast medium for image enhancement. These codes report an exam of the soft tissue of the neck. Report 70490 if no contrast is used. Report 70491 if performed with contrast and 70492 if performed first without contrast and again following the injection of contrast.

70496-70498
Computed tomographic angiography (CTA) is a procedure used for the imaging of vessels to detect aneurysms, blood clots, and other vascular irregularities. Contrast medium is rapidly infused intravenously, at intervals, usually with an automatic injector, and the patient is scanned with thin section axial or spiral mode x-ray beams. The images obtained are acquired with narrower collimation and reconstructed at shorter intervals than standard CT images. Three-dimensional images are generated and postprocessing reconstruction is done at a workstation

on the scanner. CTA also provides information unavailable with conventional angiography, such as vessel wall thickness (mural thrombus) and the venous anatomy of a target organ and/or associated organs within the scan range. Report 70496 for an exam of the head and 70498 for an exam of the neck. These codes report exams with contrast materials and image postprocessing. Noncontrast images, if performed, are also included in these procedures.

70540-70543

Magnetic resonance imaging (MRI) is a radiation-free, noninvasive technique to produce high-quality sectional images of the inside of the body in multiple planes. MRI uses the natural magnetic properties of the hydrogen atoms in our bodies that emit radiofrequency signals when exposed to radio waves within a strong electromagnetic field. These signals are processed and converted by the computer into high-resolution, three-dimensional, tomographic images. Patients with metallic or electronic implants or foreign bodies cannot be exposed to MRI. The patient must remain still while lying on a motorized table within the large, circular MRI tunnel. A sedative may be administered, as well as contrast material for image enhancement. These codes report an exam of the orbit, face, or neck, or any combination of these. Report 70540 if no contrast is used; 70542 if performed with contrast; and 70543 if performed first without contrast and again following the injection of contrast.

70544-70546

Magnetic resonance angiography (MRA) is magnetic resonance imaging (MRI) that specifically visualizes blood vessels and blood flow to evaluate vascular disorders within the structure being studied. Unlike CT, it does not rely on the absorption of x-ray energy. Magnetic resonance imaging uses the natural magnetic properties of the hydrogen atoms in our bodies that emit radiofrequency signals when exposed to radio waves within a strong electro-magnetic field. These signals are processed and converted by the computer into high-resolution, three-dimensional tomographic images. Patients with metallic or electronic implants or foreign bodies cannot be exposed to MRI. The patient must remain still while lying on a motorized table within the large, circular MRI tunnel. A sedative may be administered as well as contrast material for image enhancement. These codes report an exam of the head. Report 70544 if no contrast is used. Report 70545 if performed with contrast and 70546 if performed first without contrast and again following the injection of contrast.

70547-70549

Magnetic resonance angiography (MRA) is a special type of magnetic resonance imaging (MRI) that specifically visualizes blood vessels and blood flow to evaluate vascular disorders within the structure being studied. Unlike CT, it does not rely on the absorption of x-ray energy. Magnetic resonance imaging uses the natural magnetic properties of the hydrogen atoms in our bodies that emit radiofrequency signals when exposed to radio waves within a strong electro-magnetic field. These signals are processed and converted by the computer into high-resolution, three-dimensional tomographic images. Patients with metallic or electronic implants or foreign bodies cannot be exposed to MRI. The patient must remain still while lying on a motorized table within the large, circular MRI tunnel. A sedative may be administered as well as contrast material for image enhancement. These codes report and exam of the neck. Report 70547 if no contrast is used. Report 70548 if performed with contrast and 70549 if performed first without contrast and again following the injection of contrast.

70551-70553

Magnetic resonance imaging (MRI) is a radiation-free, noninvasive, technique to produce high quality sectional images of the inside of the body in multiple planes. MRI uses the natural magnetic properties of the hydrogen atoms in our bodies that emit radiofrequency signals when exposed to radio waves within a strong electro-magnetic field. These signals are processed and converted by the computer into high-resolution, three-dimensional, tomographic images. Patients with metallic or electronic implants or foreign bodies cannot be exposed to MRI. The patient must remain still while lying on a motorized table within the large, circular MRI tunnel. A sedative may be administered as well as contrast material for image enhancement. These codes report an exam of the brain, including the brain stem. Report 70551 if no contrast is used. Report 70552 if performed with contrast and 70553 if performed first without contrast and again following the injection of contrast.

70554-70555

Functional magnetic resonance imaging (fMRI) captures metabolic changes in the working brain using progressive magnetic resonance imaging (MRI). MRI is a radiation-free, noninvasive technique to produce high-quality sectional images of the inside of the body in multiple planes. MRI uses the natural magnetic properties of the hydrogen atoms in our bodies that emit radiofrequency signals when exposed to radio waves within a strong electromagnetic field. These signals are processed and converted by the computer into high-resolution, three-dimensional, tomographic images. In fMRI, the patient's head is immobilized by a brace and the patient's table is placed in the MRI machine. The clinician asks the patient to perform small tasks that can be accomplished in the confined setting of the MRI equipment. Images are recorded while the patient is at rest and a series of progressive images is taken when a task is being performed. These images are analyzed to determine the effect of the task upon brain function. Report 70554 for repetitive testing without a physician or psychologist and 70555 when the entire test is performed by a physician or psychologist.

70557-70559

Magnetic resonance imaging (MRI) is a radiation-free, noninvasive technique to produce high quality sectional images of the inside of the body in multiple planes. MRI uses the natural magnetic properties of the hydrogen atoms in our bodies that emit radiofrequency signals when exposed to radio waves within a strong electro-magnetic field. These signals are processed and converted by the computer into high-resolution, three-dimensional, tomographic images. Patients with metallic or electronic implants or foreign bodies cannot be exposed to MRI. These codes report an exam of the brain, including the brain stem and skull base, performed during an open intracranial procedure to look for residual tumor tissue or vascular malformation. Report 70557 if no contrast is used; 70558 if the MRI imaging is performed with contrast; and 70559 if during surgery, the MRI is performed first without contrast and again following the injection of contrast.

71045-71048

In 71045, a single x-ray is taken of the patient's chest. Report 71046 for two views; 71047 for three views; and 71048 for four or more views.

71100

Films are taken unilaterally of the affected side of the ribs with two views in AP (front to back) or PA (back to front) views.

71101

Films are taken unilaterally of the affected side of the ribs for a minimum of three views, including the posterior ribs.

71110

Films are taken bilaterally of the ribs for three views of the ribcage, with the patient placed supine and the x-ray directed at the thorax midpoint, above or below the xiphoid process for a bilateral view.

71111

A minimum of four films are taken bilaterally of the ribcage, including the posterior ribs, with the patient placed supine for AP and PA views and the x-ray directed at the thorax midpoint, above or below the xiphoid process for a bilateral view.

71120

Films are taken of the sternum with a minimum of two views from an anterior oblique and lateral position.

71130

Films are taken of the sternoclavicular joint or joints with a minimum of three views from posteroanterior and oblique projections.

71250-71270

Computed tomography directs multiple narrow beams of x-rays around the body structure being studied and uses computer imaging to produce thin cross-sectional views of various layers (or slices) of the body. It is useful for the evaluation of trauma, tumor, and foreign bodies as CT can visualize soft tissue as well as bones. Patients are required to remain motionless during the study and sedation may need to be administered as well as a contrast medium for image enhancement. These codes report a diagnostic exam of the thorax. Report 71250 if no contrast is used. Report 71260 if performed with contrast and 71270 if performed first without contrast and again following the injection of contrast.

71271

Lung cancer screening is performed by low-dose computed tomography (LDCT) scanning of the chest. Indicated for individuals who have a high risk of developing lung cancer but who have no signs or symptoms, the LDCT technique utilizes specialized x-ray equipment combined with state-of-the-art computer systems. Using up to 90 percent less ionizing radiation than a conventional chest CT (computed tomography) scan, LDCT produces numerous cross-sectional images of sufficient quality to detect many abnormalities. The patient reclines on a table and is required to remain motionless while the CT scanner uses a low dose of radiation to make detailed images of the lungs. No contrast material is used.

71275

Computed tomographic angiography (CTA) is a procedure used for the imaging of vessels to detect aneurysms, blood clots, and other vascular irregularities, excluding the heart. Contrast medium is rapidly infused intravenously, at intervals, usually with an automatic injector, and the patient is scanned with thin section axial or spiral mode x-ray beams. The images obtained are acquired with narrower collimation and reconstructed at shorter intervals than standard CT images. Three-dimensional images are generated and postprocessing reconstruction is done at a workstation on the scanner. CTA provides information unavailable with conventional angiography, such as vessel wall thickness (mural thrombus) and the venous anatomy of the target organ. This code reports an exam of the chest with contrast materials and image postprocessing. Noncontrast images, if performed, are also included in this procedure.

71550-71552

Magnetic resonance imaging (MRI) is a radiation-free, noninvasive, technique to produce high quality sectional images of the inside of the body in multiple planes. MRI uses the natural magnetic properties of the hydrogen atoms in our bodies that emit radiofrequency signals when exposed to radio waves within a strong electro-magnetic field. These signals are processed and converted by the computer into high-resolution, three-dimensional, tomographic images. Patients with metallic or electronic implants or foreign bodies cannot be exposed to MRI. The patient must remain still while lying on a motorized table within the large, circular MRI tunnel. A sedative may be administered as well as contrast material for image enhancement. These codes report an exam of the chest. Report 71550 if no contrast is used. Report 71551 if performed with contrast and 71552 if performed first without contrast and again following the injection of contrast.

71555

Magnetic resonance angiography (MRA) is magnetic resonance imaging (MRI) that specifically visualizes blood vessels and blood flow to evaluate vascular disorders within the structure being studied. Unlike CT, it does not rely on the absorption of x-ray energy. Magnetic resonance imaging uses the natural magnetic properties of the hydrogen atoms in our bodies that emit radiofrequency signals when exposed to radio waves within a strong electro-magnetic field. These signals are processed and converted by the computer into high-resolution, three-dimensional tomographic images. Patients with metallic or electronic implants or foreign bodies cannot be exposed to MRI. The patient must remain still while lying on a motorized table within the large, circular MRI tunnel. A sedative may be administered as well as contrast material for image enhancement. This code reports an exam of the chest.

72020

One film is taken of the spine that requires specification of the level examined.

72040-72052

A radiologic examination of the cervical spine is performed. Report 72040 for two or three views, 72050 for four or five views, and 72052 for a complete study (six or more views). The complete study includes films taken in oblique (angled) positions and in flexion and/or extension positioning.

72070-72074

A radiologic examination of the thoracic spine is performed that includes two views in 72070, three views in 72072, and a minimum of four views in 72074. These procedures do not specify that a certain view must be performed.

72080

Films are taken of the thoracolumbar junction of the spine with a minimum of two views.

72081-72084

A scoliosis series consists of images taken of the entire thoracic and lumbar spine and may include the skull, cervical, and sacral spine. Typical views including standing from front to back (AP), supine or lying down AP, and supine views with alternate right and left flexion. These images are taken to detect any curvature of the spine when scoliosis or other pathology may be present. Report 72081 for one view; 72082 for two or three views; 72083 for four or five views; and 72084 for a minimum of six views.

72100-72110

A radiologic examination of the lumbosacral spine is performed that includes two or three views in 72100, and a minimum of four views in 72110. These procedures do not specify that a certain view must be performed.

72114

Six or more films are taken of the lumbosacral spine, or lower back, for a complete radiologic study. A complete lumbar spine series typically includes x-rays taken from front to back (AP), side to side (lateral), and oblique, or angled right and left views. In addition, this code includes bending views, films taken with the patient bending to the left and right to demonstrate mobility of the intervertebral joints, and/or films taken with the patient in both flexion and extension, typically in cases of disc protrusion to localize the involved joint.

72120

Two to three films are taken of the lumbar spine, or lower back, with the patient bending to the left and right to demonstrate the mobility of the intervertebral joints and/or with the patient in both flexion and extension, typically in cases of disc protrusion to localize the involved joint.

72125-72127

The cervical spine is examined through computed tomography. Computed tomography directs multiple narrow beams of x-rays around the body structure being studied and uses computer imaging to produce thin cross-sectional views of various layers (or slices) of the body. It is useful for the evaluation of trauma, tumor, and foreign bodies as CT is able to visualize soft tissue as well as bones. Patients are required to remain motionless during the study and sedation may be necessary. For CT of the spine, contrast material may be administered intravenously (part of the procedure) or intrathecally (reported separately). Report 72125 if no contrast is used, 72126 if performed with contrast, and 72127 if performed first without contrast and again following the injection of contrast.

72128-72130

The thoracic spine is examined through computed tomography. Computed tomography directs multiple narrow beams of x-rays around the body structure being studied and uses computer imaging to produce thin cross-sectional views of various layers (or slices) of the body. It is useful for the evaluation of trauma, tumor, and foreign bodies as CT is able to visualize soft tissue as well as bones. Patients are required to remain motionless during the study and sedation may be necessary. For CT of the spine, contrast material may be administered intravenously (part of the procedure) or intrathecally (reported separately). Report 72128 if no contrast is used, 72129 if performed with contrast, and 72130 if performed first without contrast and again following the injection of contrast.

72131-72133

The lumbar spine is examined through computed tomography. Computed tomography directs multiple thin beams of x-rays at the body structure being studied and uses computer imaging to produce thin cross-sectional views of various layers (or slices) of the body. It is useful for the evaluation of trauma, tumor, and foreign bodies as CT is able to visualize soft tissue as well as bones. Patients are required to remain motionless during the study and sedation may be necessary. For CT of the spine, contrast material may be administered intravenously (part of the procedure) or intrathecally (reported separately). Report 72131 if no contrast is used, 72132 if performed with contrast, and 72133 if performed first without contrast and again following the injection of contrast.

72141-72142, 72156

Magnetic resonance imaging (MRI) is a radiation-free, noninvasive, technique to produce high quality sectional images of the inside of the body in multiple planes. MRI uses the natural magnetic properties of the hydrogen atoms in our bodies that emit radiofrequency signals when exposed to radio waves within a strong electro-magnetic field. These signals are processed and converted by the computer into high-resolution, three-dimensional, tomographic images. Patients with metallic or electronic implants or foreign bodies cannot be exposed to MRI. The patient must remain still while lying on a motorized table within the large, circular MRI tunnel. A sedative may be administered as well as contrast material for image enhancement. For cervical spinal canal and contents, report 72141 if no contrast is used; report 72142 if performed with contrast and 72156 if performed first without contrast and again following the injection of contrast.

72146-72147, 72157

Magnetic resonance imaging (MRI) is a radiation-free, noninvasive, technique to produce high quality sectional images of the inside of the body in multiple planes. MRI uses the natural magnetic properties of the hydrogen atoms in our bodies that emit radiofrequency signals when exposed to radio waves within a strong electro-magnetic field. These signals are processed and converted by the computer into high-resolution, three-dimensional, tomographic images. Patients with metallic or electronic implants or foreign bodies cannot be exposed to MRI. The patient must remain still while lying on a motorized table within the large, circular MRI tunnel. A sedative may be administered as well as contrast material for image enhancement. For thoracic spinal canal and contents, report 72146 if no contrast is used; report 72147 if performed with contrast and 72157 if performed first without contrast and again following the injection of contrast.

72148-72149, 72158

Magnetic resonance imaging (MRI) is a radiation-free, noninvasive, technique to produce high quality sectional images of the inside of the body in multiple planes. MRI uses the natural magnetic properties of the hydrogen atoms in our bodies that emit radiofrequency signals when exposed to radio waves within a strong electro-magnetic field. These signals are processed and converted by the computer into high-resolution, three-dimensional, tomographic images. Patients with metallic or electronic implants or foreign bodies cannot be exposed to MRI. The patient must remain still while lying on a motorized table within the large, circular MRI tunnel. A sedative may be administered as well as contrast material for image enhancement. For lumbar spinal canal and contents, report 72148 if no contrast is used; report 72149 if performed with contrast and 72158 if performed first without contrast and again following the injection of contrast.

72159

Magnetic resonance angiography (MRA) is magnetic resonance imaging (MRI) that specifically visualizes blood vessels and blood flow to evaluate vascular disorders within the structure being studied. Unlike CT, it does not rely on the absorption of x-ray energy. Magnetic resonance imaging uses the natural magnetic properties of the hydrogen atoms in our bodies that emit radiofrequency signals when exposed to radio waves within a strong electro-magnetic field. These signals are processed and converted by the computer into high-resolution, three-dimensional tomographic images. Patients with metallic or electronic implants or foreign bodies cannot be exposed to MRI. The patient must remain still while lying on a motorized table within the large, circular MRI tunnel. A sedative may be administered as well as contrast material for image enhancement. This code reports an exam of the spinal canal and contents.

72170

One or two views are taken of the pelvis. The most common view is from front to back (AP) with the patient lying supine with feet inverted 15 degrees to overcome the anteversion (or rotation) of the femoral necks. The pelvic girdle, femoral head, neck, trochanters, and upper femurs are also shown.

72190

A minimum of three films are taken of the pelvis, typically front to back (AP) with the patient lying supine. The patient's legs are placed in what is termed a "frogleg" lateral position, wherein the patient's feet are drawn up toward the buttocks, at which point the knees are allowed to drop down to the table with feet together. A third film may be taken with the patient lying on his or her side for a lateral view of the pelvis, as well as unilateral views of the hips, if necessary.

72191

Computed tomographic angiography (CTA) of the pelvis is performed with contrast materials and image postprocessing. CTA produces images of vessels to detect aneurysms, blood clots, and other vascular irregularities. Contrast medium is rapidly infused intravenously, at intervals, usually with an automatic injector, and the patient is scanned with thin section axial or spiral mode x-ray beams. The images are acquired with narrower collimation and reconstructed at shorter intervals than standard CT images. Three-dimensional images are generated and postprocessing reconstruction is done at a workstation on the scanner. CTA also provides information unavailable with conventional angiography, such as vessel wall thickness (mural thrombus) and the venous anatomy of a target organ and/or associated organs within the scan range. Noncontrast images, if performed, are also included in this procedure.

72192-72194
Computed tomography directs multiple narrow beams of x-rays around the body structure being studied and uses computer imaging to produce thin cross-sectional views of various layers (or slices) of the body. It is useful for the evaluation of trauma, tumor, and foreign bodies as CT is able to visualize soft tissue as well as bones. Patients are required to remain motionless during the study and sedation may need to be administered as well as a contrast medium for image enhancement. These codes report an exam of the pelvis. Report 72192 if no contrast is used. Report 72193 if performed with contrast and 72194 if performed first without contrast and again following the injection of contrast.

72195-72197
Magnetic resonance imaging (MRI) is a radiation-free, noninvasive, technique to produce high quality sectional images of the inside of the body in multiple planes. MRI uses the natural magnetic properties of the hydrogen atoms in our bodies that emit radiofrequency signals when exposed to radio waves within a strong electro-magnetic field. These signals are processed and converted by the computer into high-resolution, three-dimensional, tomographic images. Patients with metallic or electronic implants or foreign bodies cannot be exposed to MRI. The patient must remain still while lying on a motorized table within the large, circular MRI tunnel. A sedative may be administered as well as contrast material for image enhancement. These codes report an exam of the pelvis. Report 72195 if no contrast is used. Report 72196 if performed with contrast and 72197 if performed first without contrast and again following the injection of contrast.

72198
Magnetic resonance angiography (MRA) is magnetic resonance imaging (MRI) that specifically visualizes blood vessels and blood flow to evaluate vascular disorders within the structure being studied. Unlike CT, it does not rely on the absorption of x-ray energy. Magnetic resonance imaging uses the natural magnetic properties of the hydrogen atoms in our bodies that emit radiofrequency signals when exposed to radio waves within a strong electro-magnetic field. These signals are processed and converted by the computer into high-resolution, three-dimensional tomographic images. Patients with metallic or electronic implants or foreign bodies cannot be exposed to MRI. The patient must remain still while lying on a motorized table within the large, circular MRI tunnel. A sedative may be administered as well as contrast material for image enhancement. This code reports an exam of the pelvis.

72200-72202
Films are taken of the articulation between the sacrum, the triangular bone beneath the lumbar vertebrae, and the ilium, or upper portion of the hip bone. The exam may be performed in both anteroposterior and right and left posterior oblique views. Code 72200 reports one or two views and 72202 reports three or more views.

72220
Films are taken (minimum of two views) of the sacrum and the coccyx. The sacrum is a triangular bone located between the fifth lumbar vertebra and the coccyx. It is formed by five connected vertebrae and is wedged between the two innominate bones. The coccyx is the small bone at the very base of the spinal column, and is formed by the fusion of four vertebrae. The sacrum and the coccyx form the posterior (back) boundary of the pelvis. While anteroposterior (AP; front to back) and lateral (side) views are the most common views taken, this procedure is used for any two or more views reported.

72240-72270
In myelography, a radiographic study using fluoroscopy is performed on the spinal cord and nerve root branches when a lesion is suspected. A nonionic water-soluble radiopaque contrast media is used to enhance visibility and is instilled in the patient through a lumbar or cervical area puncture into the subarachnoid space. The radiologist takes a series of pictures by sending an x-ray beam through the body, using fluoroscopy to view the enhanced structure on a television camera. The patient is angled from an erect position through a recumbent position with the body tilted so as to maintain feet higher than the head to help the flow of contrast into the study area. Code 72240 reports a cervical myelogram; 72255 reports a thoracic myelogram; 72265 reports lumbosacral myelogram; and 72270 reports a myelogram of two or more regions, such as lumbar/thoracic, cervical/thoracic or lumbar/thoracic/cervical.

72285-72295
Individual intervertebral discs are imaged and examined in discography, also known as nucleography. Iodinated contrast medium is injected into the center of the disc. A series of images is taken by the radiologist and interpreted and reported. This technique is used to determine the extent of the target disc(s) disease. Report 72285 for the cervical or thoracic discs and 72295 for the lumbar discs.

73000
Films are taken of the clavicle for a complete radiologic examination. The number of films is not specified. The patient is placed supine for a front to back (AP) view and the x-ray is directed to the midpoint and perpendicular to the clavicle.

73010
Films are taken of the scapula for a complete examination. The number of films is not specified. Anteroposterior (AP) and lateral views may be taken. The patient is placed supine for a front to back (AP) view and may be erect or recumbent for a lateral view. The arm is abducted to make a 90 degree angle to the body with the elbow flexed.

73020-73030
Films are taken of the shoulder. The patient is supine with the arm extended to a 90 degree angle from the body and externally rotated while the head is turned to face opposite the affected side. Code 73020 is for reporting one view only and 73030 specifies a minimum of two views.

73040
The synovial joint of the shoulder is visualized internally through arthrography, the direct injection of air and/or contrast material into the joint for radiological examination. Local anesthesia in injected into the joint followed by the contrast material and/or air. A series of images are taken and interpreted. Fluoroscopic films and guidance for needle localization is included. Arthrography helps diagnose conditions of cartilage abnormalities, arthritis and bursitis, rotator cuff tear, and frozen joint. AP (front to back) views are taken with the affected arm rotated externally and internally and with the arm in a neutral, flexed position lying over the abdomen.

73050
A radiologic examination is made of the acromioclavicular joints bilaterally, with no specified amount of views. The patient is placed in a sitting or standing upright position with arms at the side for an anteroposterior view. The patient may also be given weights to hold in each hand for weighted distraction radiographs of each joint.

73060
Two or more films are taken of the humerus with the x-ray beam aimed midshaft. The patient is supine with the hand also supinated for an AP view and with the hand rotated internally for an oblique view.

73070-73080
A radiologic examination of the elbow joint is made. Films of the elbow may be taken in the AP position with the hand supinated, oblique positioning with the hand pronated and/or externally rotated, and in the lateral position with the wrist lateral and the elbow flexed at 90 degrees. Code 73070 reports two views and 73080 reports a complete exam with a minimum of three views.

73085
The synovial joint of the elbow is visualized internally through arthrography, the direct injection of air and/or contrast material into the joint for radiological examination. Local anesthesia in injected into the joint followed by the contrast material and/or air. A series of images are taken by the radiologist and interpreted. Fluoroscopic films and guidance for needle localization is included. Arthrography helps diagnose conditions of cartilage abnormalities, arthritis and bursitis, and frozen joint.

73090
Two films of the forearm are taken with the x-ray beam aimed at the midforearm. Films may be taken in the AP position with the hand supinated, in the true lateral position and in oblique positioning.

73092
A minimum of two films of an infant's forearm are taken with the x-ray beam aimed at the midforearm. The infant must first be immobilized to prevent movement during the film taking. Films may be taken in the AP position with the hand supinated, in the true lateral position, and in oblique position.

73100-73110
A radiologic examination of the wrist is made in posteroanterior, oblique, or lateral views. Code 73100 reports two views only and 73110 reports three or more views.

73115
The wrist is visualized internally through arthrography, the direct injection of air and/or contrast material into the joint for radiological examination. Local anesthesia in injected into the joint followed by the contrast material and/or air. A series of images are taken and interpreted. Fluoroscopic films and guidance for needle localization is included. Arthrography helps diagnose conditions of cartilage abnormalities, arthritis and bursitis, and frozen joint. The hand and wrist is placed in the posteroanterior (PA) position with the hand rotated outward and the x-ray beam aimed vertically at the wrist or with the hand and wrist in PA position with the beam aimed at the wrist from a few degrees below the elbow.

73120-73130
A radiologic exam of the hand is made with films being taken in the PA (posteroanterior), internal or external oblique, or lateral positions. Code 73120 reports two views only. Code 73130 reports three or more views.

73140
Two or more views of the fingers (first through fifth digits) are taken. The x-ray beam is aimed at the proximal interphalangeal joint for all positions, back to front, external or internal oblique, or lateral views.

73200-73202
Computed tomography directs multiple narrow beams of x-rays around the body structure being studied and uses computer imaging to produce thin cross-sectional views of various layers (or slices) of the body. It is useful for the evaluation of trauma, tumor, and foreign bodies as CT is able to visualize soft tissue as well as bones. Patients are required to remain motionless during the study and sedation may need to be administered as well as a contrast medium for image enhancement. These codes report an exam of the upper extremity. Report 73200 if no contrast is used. Report 73201 if performed with contrast and 73202 if performed first without contrast and again following the injection of contrast.

73206
Computed tomographic angiography (CTA) is a procedure used for the imaging of vessels to detect aneurysms, blood clots, and other vascular irregularities. Contrast medium is rapidly infused intravenously, at intervals, usually with an automatic injector, and the patient is scanned with thin section

axial or spiral mode x-ray beams. The images obtained are acquired with narrower collimation and reconstructed at shorter intervals than standard CT images. Three-dimensional images are generated and postprocessing reconstruction is done at a workstation on the scanner. CTA also provides information unavailable with conventional angiography, such as vessel wall thickness (mural thrombus) and the venous anatomy of a target organ and/or associated organs within the scan range. This code reports an exam of the upper extremity with contrast materials and image postprocessing. Noncontrast images, if performed, are also included in this procedure.

73218-73220

Magnetic resonance imaging (MRI) is a radiation-free, noninvasive, technique to produce high quality sectional images of the inside of the body in multiple planes. MRI uses the natural magnetic properties of the hydrogen atoms in our bodies that emit radiofrequency signals when exposed to radio waves within a strong electro-magnetic field. These signals are processed and converted by the computer into high-resolution, three-dimensional, tomographic images. Patients with metallic or electronic implants or foreign bodies cannot be exposed to MRI. The patient must remain still while lying on a motorized table within the large, circular MRI tunnel. A sedative may be administered as well as contrast material for image enhancement. For upper extremity other than joint, report 73218 if no contrast is used; 73219 if performed with contrast; and 73220 if performed first without contrast and again following the injection of contrast.

73221-73223

Magnetic resonance imaging (MRI) is a radiation-free, noninvasive, technique to produce high quality sectional images of the inside of the body in multiple planes. MRI uses the natural magnetic properties of the hydrogen atoms in our bodies that emit radiofrequency signals when exposed to radio waves within a strong electro-magnetic field. These signals are processed and converted by the computer into high-resolution, three-dimensional, tomographic images. Patients with metallic or electronic implants or foreign bodies cannot be exposed to MRI. The patient must remain still while lying on a motorized table within the large, circular MRI tunnel. A sedative may be administered as well as contrast material for image enhancement. For any joint of the upper extremity. Report 73221 if no contrast is used; 73222 if performed with contrast; and 73223 if performed first without contrast and again following the injection of contrast.

73225

Magnetic resonance angiography (MRA) is magnetic resonance imaging (MRI) that specifically visualizes blood vessels and blood flow to evaluate vascular disorders within the structure being studied. Unlike CT, it does not rely on the absorption of x-ray energy. Magnetic resonance imaging uses the natural magnetic properties of the hydrogen atoms in our bodies that emit radiofrequency signals when exposed to radio waves within a strong electro-magnetic field. These signals are processed and converted by the computer into high-resolution, three-dimensional, tomographic images. Patients with metallic or electronic implants or foreign bodies cannot be exposed to MRI. The patient must remain still while lying on a motorized table within the large, circular MRI tunnel. A sedative may be administered as well as contrast material for image enhancement. This code reports an exam of the upper extremity.

73501-73503

X-rays are taken of the right or left hip, including the pelvis, when performed. For a front to back (AP) view, the patient is placed supine with the toes on the affected side inverted. For a frogleg view, the affected hip is flexed with the knee bent. The patient is supine with the knee on the unaffected side flexed and abducted away from the side to be studied. These codes may be reported for an exam of an infant or child's pelvis and hips. The infant or child must first be immobilized to prevent movement during the imaging process. These studies may also be performed during an operative procedure. Report 73501 for one view; 73502 for two to three views; and 73503 for a minimum of four views.

73521-73523

A radiological exam is taken of the hips and pelvis. For a front to back (AP) view, the patient is placed supine with toes inverted. For a frogleg view, the knees are bent as much as possible with the soles of the feet touching each other. Report 73521 for two views; 73522 for three to four views; and 73523 for a minimum of five views.

73525

This code reports the radiological supervision and interpretation for hip arthrography. Using a fluoroscope, the physician marks the point of the femoral neck on the skin with ink. The femoral artery is palpated and marked as well to avoid inadvertent puncture. Skin traction may be applied to increase the space between the femoral head and acetabulum. The physician inserts a needle into the capsule (located by fluoroscope) and aspirates the synovial fluid for a culture check. After aspiration, a contrast agent is injected into the hip joint and the needle is removed. X-rays are taken with the hip in neutral, external, and internal rotation. A second set of x-rays may be taken following the hip movements.

73551-73552

A radiological exam is taken of the femur, or thigh bone, the longest and largest in the body. In the front to back or lateral views, the x-ray beam is aimed at the midshaft. For the AP (front to back) view, the patient is placed supine with the foot turned inward a few degrees. For a lateral view, the patient is placed laterally with the knee flexed and the affected side down. Report 73551 for one view and 73552 for a minimum of two views.

73560-73564
A radiologic examination of the knee is done. The patient is positioned for the desired view(s) of the knee and x-ray films are taken. These codes do not specify which views must be taken. Code 73560 reports one or two views only. Use 73562 to report three views and 73564 for a complete exam of the knee with a minimum of four views.

73565
An x-ray is taken of the knees bilaterally in a front to back (anteroposterior) projection while the patient is standing.

73580
The patient is placed supine (lying on the back) on an x-ray table with the knee flexed over a small pillow. The knee is cleansed with Betadine and covered with a drape. A skin anesthetic may be applied. The physician passes a 20-gauge needle into the femoropatellar space. Air and a contrast agent is injected. After the injection, the patient is asked to move the knee to produce an even coating of the joint structures. Multiple x-rays are taken of the knee. This code reports the radiological supervision and interpretation only. Use a separately reportable code for the arthrography.

73590
Two films of the lower leg bones are taken. The physician interprets and reports the findings.

73592
Two or more films are taken of an infant's right or left lower extremity. The infant or child must first be immobilized to prevent movement during the film taking. The physician interprets and reports the findings.

73600-73610
Two films are taken of the ankle in 73600 and a complete radiologic exam of the ankle is performed in 73610 with three or more films taken. The codes do not specify that a specific view must be performed. The physician interprets and reports the findings.

73615
The physician injects radiopaque fluid into the ankle for arthrography. The physician inserts a needle into the joint and aspirates if necessary. Opaque contrast solution is injected into the ankle and the needle is removed. Films are taken of the ankle. This code reports the radiological supervision and interpretation only. Use a separately reportable code for the injection.

73620-73630
Two films are taken of the foot in 73620 and a complete radiologic exam of the foot is performed in 73630 with three or more films taken. The codes do not specify that a specific view must be performed. The physician interprets and reports the findings.

73650
Two or more films are taken of the calcaneus or heel bone. The physician interprets and reports the findings.

73660
Two or more films are taken of the toes. The physician interprets and reports the findings.

73700-73702
Computed tomography (CT) directs multiple narrow beams of x-rays around the body structure being studied and uses computer imaging to produce thin cross-sectional views of various layers (or slices) of the body. CT is useful for the evaluation of trauma, tumor, and foreign bodies as CT is able to visualize soft tissue as well as bones. Patients are required to remain motionless during the study and sedation may need to be administered as well as a contrast medium for image enhancement. These codes report an exam of the lower extremity. Report 73700 if no contrast is used. Report 73701 if performed with contrast and 73702 if performed first without contrast and again following the injection of contrast.

73706
Computed tomographic angiography (CTA) is a procedure used for the imaging of vessels to detect aneurysms, blood clots, and other vascular irregularities. Contrast medium is rapidly infused intravenously, at intervals, usually with an automatic injector, and the patient is scanned with thin section axial or spiral mode x-ray beams. The images obtained are acquired with narrower collimation and reconstructed at shorter intervals than standard CT images. Three-dimensional images are generated and postprocessing reconstruction is done at a workstation on the scanner. CTA also provides information unavailable with conventional angiography such as vessel wall thickness (mural thrombus) and the venous anatomy of a target organ and/or associated organs within the scan range. This code reports an exam of the lower extremity with contrast materials and image postprocessing. Noncontrast images, if performed, are also included in this procedure.

73718-73720
Magnetic resonance imaging (MRI) is a radiation-free, noninvasive, technique to produce high quality sectional images of the inside of the body in multiple planes. MRI uses the natural magnetic properties of the hydrogen atoms in our bodies that emit radiofrequency signals when exposed to radio waves within a strong electro-magnetic field. These signals are processed and converted by the computer into high-resolution, three-dimensional, tomographic images. Patients with metallic or electronic implants or foreign bodies cannot be exposed to MRI. The patient must remain still while lying on a motorized table within the large, circular MRI tunnel. A sedative may be administered as well as contrast material for image enhancement. For lower extremity other than joint, report 73718 if no contrast is used; 73719 if performed with contrast; and 73720 if performed first without contrast and again following the injection of contrast.

73721-73723
Magnetic resonance imaging (MRI) is a radiation-free, noninvasive, technique to produce high quality

sectional images of the inside of the body in multiple planes. MRI uses the natural magnetic properties of the hydrogen atoms in our bodies that emit radiofrequency signals when exposed to radio waves within a strong electro-magnetic field. These signals are processed and converted by the computer into high-resolution, three-dimensional, tomographic images. Patients with metallic or electronic implants or foreign bodies cannot be exposed to MRI. The patient must remain still while lying on a motorized table within the large, circular MRI tunnel. A sedative may be administered as well as contrast material for image enhancement. For any joint of the lower extremity, report 73721 if no contrast is used; 73722 if performed with contrast; and 73723 if performed first without contrast and again following the injection of contrast.

73725

Magnetic resonance angiography (MRA) is magnetic resonance imaging (MRI) that specifically visualizes blood vessels and blood flow to evaluate vascular disorders within the structure being studied. Unlike CT, it does not rely on the absorption of x-ray energy. Magnetic resonance imaging uses the natural magnetic properties of the hydrogen atoms in our bodies that emit radiofrequency signals when exposed to radio waves within a strong electro-magnetic field. These signals are processed and converted by the computer into high-resolution, three-dimensional tomographic images. Patients with metallic or electronic implants or foreign bodies cannot be exposed to MRI. The patient must remain still while lying on a motorized table within the large, circular MRI tunnel. A sedative may be administered as well as contrast material for image enhancement. This code reports an exam of the lower extremity.

74018-74021

In 74018, a single x-ray is taken of the patient's abdomen. Because an abdominal x-ray usually precedes another diagnostic imaging procedure, it is not coded separately unless performed as a separately identifiable examination. Report 74019 for two views and 74021 for three or more views.

74022

Films are taken of the abdominal cavity. Two or more views are made, with the patient lying flat, standing, and/or lying on the side. This procedure includes a single view chest x-ray. Because an abdominal x-ray usually precedes another diagnostic imaging procedure, it is not coded separately unless performed as a separately identifiable examination.

74150-74170

Computed tomography directs multiple thin beams of x-rays at the body structure being studied and uses computer imaging to produce thin cross-sectional views of various layers (or slices) of the body. It is useful for the evaluation of trauma, tumor, and foreign bodies as CT is able to visualize soft tissue as well as bones. Patients are required to remain motionless during the study and sedation may need to be administered as well as a contrast medium for image enhancement. These codes report an exam of the abdomen. Report 74150 if no contrast is used. Report 74160 if performed with contrast and 74170 if performed first without contrast and again following the injection of contrast.

74174

Computed tomographic angiography (CTA) of the abdomen and pelvis is performed with contrast material and image postprocessing. CTA is a procedure used for the imaging of vessels. CTA of the abdomen and pelvis may detect aneurysms, thrombosis, and ischemia in the arteries supplying blood to the digestive system, as well as locate gastrointestinal bleeding. Contrast medium is rapidly infused at intervals, usually with an automatic injector, and the patient is scanned with thin section axial or spiral mode x-ray beams. The images obtained are acquired with narrower collimation and reconstructed at shorter intervals than standard CT images. Three-dimensional images are generated and postprocessing reconstruction is done at a workstation on the scanner. Noncontrast images, if performed, are also included in this procedure.

74175

Computed tomographic angiography (CTA) of the abdomen is performed with contrast material and image postprocessing. CTA is a procedure used for the imaging of vessels. CTA of the abdomen may detect aneurysms, thrombosis, and ischemia in the arteries supplying blood to the digestive system, as well as locate gastrointestinal bleeding. Contrast medium is rapidly infused at intervals, usually with an automatic injector, and the patient is scanned with thin section axial or spiral mode x-ray beams. The images obtained are acquired with narrower collimation and reconstructed at shorter intervals than standard CT images. Three-dimensional images are generated and postprocessing reconstruction is done at a workstation on the scanner. Noncontrast images, if performed, are also included in this procedure.

74176-74178

Computed tomography directs multiple thin beams of x-rays at the body structure being studied and uses computer imaging to produce thin, cross-sectional views of various layers (or slices) of the body. It is useful for the evaluation of trauma, tumor, and foreign bodies as CT is able to visualize soft tissue as well as bones. Patients are required to remain motionless during the study and sedation may need to be administered, as well as a contrast medium for image enhancement. These codes report an exam of the abdomen and pelvis. Report 74176 if no contrast is used; 74177 if performed with contrast; and 74178 if performed first without contrast in one or both body regions followed by the injection of contrast and further sections in one or both body regions.

74181-74183

Magnetic resonance imaging (MRI) is a radiation-free, noninvasive, technique to produce high quality sectional images of the inside of the body in multiple planes. MRI uses the natural magnetic properties of the hydrogen atoms in our bodies that emit radiofrequency signals when exposed to radio waves within a strong electro-magnetic field. These signals are processed and converted by the computer into high-resolution, three-dimensional, tomographic images. Patients with metallic or electronic implants or foreign bodies cannot be exposed to MRI. The patient must remain still while lying on a motorized table within the large, circular MRI tunnel. A sedative may be administered as well as contrast material for image enhancement. These codes report an exam of the abdomen. Report 74181 if no contrast is used; 74182 if performed with contrast; and 74183 if performed first without contrast and again following the injection of contrast.

74185
Magnetic resonance angiography (MRA) is magnetic resonance imaging (MRI) that specifically visualizes blood vessels and blood flow to evaluate vascular disorders within the structure being studied. Unlike CT, it does not rely on the absorption of x-ray energy. Magnetic resonance imaging uses the natural magnetic properties of the hydrogen atoms in our bodies that emit radiofrequency signals when exposed to radio waves within a strong electro-magnetic field. These signals are processed and converted by the computer into high-resolution, three-dimensional tomographic images. Patients with metallic or electronic implants or foreign bodies cannot be exposed to MRI. The patient must remain still while lying on a motorized table within the large, circular MRI tunnel. A sedative may be administered as well as contrast material for image enhancement. This code reports an exam of the abdomen.

74190
A radiographic exam is done on the peritoneal cavity to define the pattern of air in the cavity after injection of air or contrast. The physician inserts a needle or catheter in to the peritoneal cavity and injects air or contrast as a diagnostic procedure. X-rays are taken. The needle or catheter is removed. This code reports the radiological supervision and interpretation for a peritoneogram. Use a separately reportable code for the procedure.

74210
Films are taken of the pharynx and/or the cervical esophagus, often to evaluate the underlying cause of difficulty swallowing (dysphagia). A scout film (one obtained without the use of a contrast medium) may initially be taken of the neck to rule out any abscess, fistula, or foreign body. The patient swallows the contrast material, which consists of barium sulfate. With the patient in an upright position, one or more radiographic views are obtained, with or without delayed images.

74220-74221
Images are obtained of the esophagus, often to evaluate structural abnormalities of the esophagus and vessels. A scout film (one obtained without the use of a contrast medium) may initially be taken of the chest. The patient then swallows a single-contrast (barium sulfate) material in 74220 or a double-contrast (high-density barium and effervescent agent) material in 74221, after which one or more radiographic views are obtained, with or without delayed images. This study is commonly referred to as a "barium swallow."

74230
In this study, also known as a modified barium swallow, the patient is seated and positioned upright or in a semi-reclining position. A scout film (one obtained without the use of a contrast medium) may initially be taken of the neck to rule out any abscess, fistula, or foreign body. Foods and liquids of different quantities and textures are soaked in or mixed with barium and ingested by the patient for the study. The patient is fluoroscoped while he/she swallows the various test items, and the fluoroscopic image is recorded on videotape for later review. This procedure includes observation of the food/liquid while in the mouth and during chewing, the tongue's mobility, movement of the hyoid bone and larynx, closing of the larynx and contraction of the pharynx, the extent of the pharyngoesophageal opening, and any aspiration or penetration of the swallowed bolus into the upper airway. Muscle strength may also be measured. This examination may be performed with or without delayed images.

74235
The physician uses an esophagoscope to locate and remove a foreign body from the esophagus. The physician passes a rigid or flexible esophagoscope through the patient's mouth and into the esophagus. The foreign body is located. It may be suctioned, or grasped with forceps ad retracted through the scope. An alternative technique that may be used for objects too large to grasp is to pass a deflated balloon beyond the foreign body. The balloon is inflated and withdrawn simultaneously with the scope and the foreign body. This code reports the radiological supervision and interpretation. Use a separately reportable code for the procedure.

74240-74246
Images are taken of the upper gastrointestinal tract to help diagnose neoplasms, ulcers, obstructions, and other diseases. The upper GI tract is generally considered to be the tract from the mouth to the major papilla in the duodenum. A scout film (one obtained without the use of a contrast medium) may initially be taken of the abdomen. The patient swallows a single-contrast material (barium) in 74240. In 74246, the patient swallows a double-contrast material (high-density barium and effervescent agent), including glucagon when administered. One or more radiographic views are obtained, with or without delayed images.

74248
Following an upper GI radiologic exam, the patient may undergo an additional study, known as a small intestine or small bowel follow-through. The patient ingests a dilute liquid barium, which is a contrast

medium that enhances radiographic images. Following ingestion, the radiologist utilizes an x-ray machine to follow the barium's passage through the stomach and into the small intestine. Depending on the amount of time that it takes the barium to progress from the stomach to the large intestine (colon), the examination may last from one to four hours.

74250-74251

In 74250, a radiologic exam is performed of the small intestine. A scout film (one obtained without the use of a contrast medium) may initially be taken of the abdomen. The patient swallows a single-contrast material (barium), after which multiple serial images are obtained. In 74251, a double-contrast study is undertaken, utilizing high-density barium and air via an enteroclysis tube. For enteroclysis, the physician inserts a tube through the patient's nose and into the stomach and the small intestine. The tube is connected to a pump that sends barium through the tube for visualizing the GI tract and small bowel. X-rays are taken in a series of multiple images. Glucagon may also be administered, which relaxes smooth muscle found in the GI tract and inhibits the muscle motility, thereby making better quality images.

74261-74263

Computed tomographic (CT) colonography, also referred to as virtual colonoscopy (VC), provides detailed, cross-sectional views of the colon by use of an x-ray machine linked to a computer. The aim of screening (74263) is to detect and remove precancerous polyps in asymptomatic patients. Diagnostic CT colonography (74261, 74262) is a noninvasive technique that is being investigated for use in symptomatic patients to diagnose and stage colon cancer. The patient is prepared for CT colonoscopy with bowel cleansing. Intravenous contrast and a spasmolytic agent may be administered via a rectal tube, but neither is required. An enema tip is inserted and the colon is distended with air or CO2. Once patient preparation is complete, one of several CT techniques can be used. One of the more common techniques uses thin collimation and three-dimensional (3-D), endoluminal computerized reconstructed images. A variation of this technique is CT pneumocolon that uses thicker collimation and intravenous contrast without 3-D reconstruction. Report 74261 for diagnostic CT colonography without contrast material and 74262 for that with contrast materials (including noncontrast images when performed). Report 74263 for screening CT colonography. All codes include image postprocessing.

74270-74280

A radiological exam of the large intestine is carried out, often as an aid in the diagnosis of cancer, colitis, and other diseases of the colon. A scout film (one obtained without the use of a contrast medium) may initially be taken of the abdomen. In 74270, following administration of a barium enema to instill contrast into the colon, fluoroscopy and x-rays are used to observe the image as the contrast fills the colon. After the patient has emptied the colon, more films are taken. In 74280, glucagon may be administered through IV. Glucagon relaxes smooth muscle found in the GI tract and inhibits muscle motility, thereby making better quality of images. A double-contrast barium enema, also known as an air-contrast barium enema, is performed. High-density barium, which coats the mucosal surface of the colon, is administered via a flexible rectal catheter. Air is introduced through the catheter, which distends the colon and aids in the identification of any abnormalities as the radiographic images are taken. These examinations may be performed with or without delayed images.

74283

An enema of air or barium contrast is administered to reduce an intussusception or obstruction. An intussusception is a section of bowel that has slipped into another loop of bowel and can cause necrosis of the tissue, perforation and infection, even death. With the patient in position, the air or contrast is instilled into the colon through the anus to reduce the intussusception or clear the intraluminal obstruction.

74290

Oral cholecystography provides radiographic visualization of the gallbladder after the oral ingestion of a radiopaque, iodinated dye that comes in the form of pills. Adequate visualization of the gallbladder requires concentration of this dye within the gallbladder. On x-ray film, the biliary calculi (gallstones) are visualized as radiolucent shadows within a dye-filled gallbladder. Gallbladder polyps and tumors can also occasionally be seen as filling defects.

74300-74301

In intraoperative cholangiography, the common bile duct is directly injected with radiopaque material. The surgeon removes the gallbladder. Stones appear as radiolucent shadows. Gallstones, tumors, or strictures cause partial or total obstruction of the flow of dye into the duodenum. This code reports only the radiological supervision and interpretation. Since the surgeon performs the dye injection in an intraoperative cholangiogram, this is the only code that the radiologist can report for this procedure. 74301 is an add-on code and cannot stand-alone. This code is used in conjunction with 74300, in the event that the surgeon would request another set of plain x-ray films to be taken during the operative session.

74328-74330

The physician performs an endoscopic retrograde cholangiopancreatography (ERCP) for diagnostic or therapeutic reasons. The physician passes the endoscope through the patient's oropharynx, esophagus, stomach, and into the small intestine. A smaller subscope may be inserted through the sphincter of Oddi into the system of ducts that drain the pancreas (74329) or into the biliary ductal system that drains the gallbladder (74328), or both (74330). These codes report only the radiological supervision and interpretation required in performing this procedure to the respective extent of catheterization.

74340
A long, Miller-Abbott gastrointestinal tube with a mercury-filled balloon at the bottom is introduced, usually nasally, and used to clear gastrointestinal strictures. The patient is seated lower than the person performing the procedure and the dilator is placed in the posterior pharynx. The patient swallows and the tube and balloon are carried into the small intestine. The balloon is inflated and withdrawn until resistance is encountered. The balloon is partially deflated, withdrawn a little more, and re-inflated. This process is repeated several times to achieve dilation of the stricture. This procedure may be done without fluoroscopy or with fluoroscopy by instilling a diluted contrast into the balloon. This code includes the fluoroscopies, images, and radiological supervision and interpretation. Use a separately reportable code for the tube placement.

74355
The physician places a tube in the jejunum for feeding through an abdominal incision. A section of proximal jejunum is selected and a tube is placed in the jejunum and brought out through the abdominal wall. This segment of jejunum is securely tacked to the inside of the abdominal wall. This code reports only the radiological supervision and interpretation required in performing this procedure.

74360
The physician passes a balloon dilator into the patient's mouth and uses a fluoroscope to place the dilator at the point of constriction. The balloon is briefly inflated several times until the area of narrowing is sufficiently enlarged. It is possible to use a guide wire to place the balloon. This code reports only the radiological supervision and interpretation required in performing this procedure.

74363
The physician advances an endoscope through an incision in the abdominal wall or an existing T-tube into the common bile duct. The biliary tract may be filled with contrast medium for identifying areas of abnormality, stricture, or obstruction in the common bile duct, biliary tree, and gallbladder. The physician advances a balloon-tipped catheter through the tract or T-tube so that it is above the site of the duct stricture, inflates the balloon, and draws it back through the stricture to achieve dilation. This may be repeated until optimum dilation is achieved. The physician may place a stent to prevent future stricture. This code reports only the radiological supervision and interpretation required in performing this procedure.

74400
Radiographic imaging of the kidneys and ureters is done before and after the administration of an intravenous contrast material to identify abnormalities of the kidneys and urinary tract. Abdominal films are obtained and contrast medium is injected into a vein. Radiographs are again obtained while the contrast material is being excreted. This is also known as intravenous pyelography or IVP. This procedure may be done with or without KUB, a general abdominal x-ray, or with or without tomography, x-rays taken onto film moving opposite the beams to yield a single plane shadowless image.

74410-74415
Radiographic imaging of the kidneys and ureters is done immediately following an infused intravenous drip or a rapid bolus injection of contrast agent. A front to back film of the abdomen is taken after contrast administration. Report 74415 if done with nephrotomography, x-rays taken onto film moving opposite the beams to yield a single plane shadowless image. This can be used to check the patency of a nephrostomy tube.

74420
Radiographic imaging of the kidneys and ureters is performed following retrograde (against the normal flow) administration of a radiopaque contrast material. A catheter is passed into the bladder and on through a ureter into the kidney. The contrast material is injected through the catheter or tube. Films are taken to show the flow of contrast as it moves through the urethra and into the upper urinary tract. This may be performed with KUB, a general x-ray of the abdomen.

74425
A radiographic exam of the urinary tract is performed with injection or instillation of a contrast medium. This test is done to follow the normal flow of urine through the tract (antegrade) and may identify obstructions, abnormalities in the urinary tract, or assess function following surgery. Contrast medium is introduced percutaneously with a needle or through an existing tube, catheter, or stoma. For percutaneous needle injection, the skin is anesthetized and the needle inserted under fluoroscopic guidance into a calyx of the kidney. Contrast medium is injected and radiographs are taken. This code reports the radiological supervision and interpretation. Use a separately reportable code for the surgical procedure.

74430
A radiographic exam of the bladder with a minimum of three views is performed using contrast material to diagnose rupture, injury, or stress incontinence. A catheter is inserted into the bladder and contrast medium is instilled using mild pressure injection. The catheter is clamped after the contrast medium has filled the bladder and the bladder is fully expanded. Films are taken to observe any medium that is outside the bladder. The bladder is next drained and more films may be taken to look for other evidence of rupture following the flow of contrast outside the bladder. This code reports the radiological supervision and interpretation. Use a separately reportable code for the surgical procedure.

74440
A radiographic exam is done to determine obstruction in the epididymis, seminal vesicle duct, or vas deferens. Methylene blue is injected into the vas to test for obstruction of the ejaculatory duct. If during

cystoscopy, dye is seen, the ducts are patent and vesiculography may be obtained to further determine obstruction. The vas is approached through an incision in the scrotum. The testis is freed and the vas separated. After a catheter is threaded into the vas, saline or lactated Ringers are instilled to determine patency or blockage. Flow resistance may require more formal vasography, with water-soluble contrast media instilled through a ureteral catheter fed to the seminal vesicles through a dilated vas. Epididymography requires taking images of the coiled tube connecting the testis to the vas deferens. This code reports the radiological supervision and interpretation for epididymography, vesiculography, or vasography.

74445

Corpora cavernosography is performed to determine the area and degree of a venous leakage. The penis is anesthetized and prepped with tubing attached to a pressure transducer that is connected to an infusion pump. Needles are inserted into the cavernosa and contrast material injected at a rate that will maintain a certain pressure so the penis can remain erect while the x-rays are taken. Fluoroscopy locates the leakage, which is determined to be minimal, moderate, or diffuse. This code reports the radiological supervision and interpretation for the procedure.

74450

A radiographic exam of the urethra and bladder is performed using contrast material to diagnose strictures, obstructions and abnormalities, or as postoperative function assessments. It is most often performed on males. A balloon catheter is threaded into the urethra and the balloon is inflated. Fluoroscopy is used to aid in injecting the contrast medium through the catheter. Films are taken to show the flow of contrast as it moves retrograde (against the normal flow) through the urethra and into certain parts of the bladder. The bladder is next drained and more images may be taken of the urethra. This code reports the radiological supervision and interpretation. Use a separately reportable code for the surgical procedure.

74455

A radiographic exam of the urethra and bladder is performed using contrast material to evaluate voiding function. The patient first empties the bladder. A catheter is inserted through the urethra into the bladder and any excess fluid is drained. Contrast medium is slowly instilled until it fills the bladder while the flow is observed via fluoroscopy. Films may be taken if reflux of medium is seen backing into the ureters. Once voiding commences, the catheter is removed and the voiding function is imaged on films or video. This code reports the radiological supervision and interpretation. Use a separately reportable code for the surgical procedure.

74470

A renal cyst is studied using contrast medium by inserting a spinal needle into the affected kidney. With the patient face down, the site for the puncture is identified with separate radiographic localization of the cyst and kidney. The skin of the puncture site is anesthetized and the needle is inserted and advanced to the kidney, while being observed on a fluoroscopic video monitor. Some of the cyst's contents are removed and a small amount of contrast is injected. This is repeated with films being taken intermittently throughout the process. When the cyst is filled with the contrast medium, more images are taken with the patient in various positions. This code reports the radiological supervision and interpretation. Use a separately reportable code for the surgical procedure.

74485

The ureter(s) or urethra is dilated under fluoroscopic control. A series of dilators in increasing size are inserted into the ureter or urethra, usually over a guidewire. A balloon may also be used. The ureters may be dilated by advancing the dilators into the ureters from the bladder. For urethral dilation, a guidewire may be advanced through the urethral stricture and one or more catheters of increasing size placed over the guidewire. A balloon is inserted and inflated until the stricture is dilated. This code reports the radiological supervision and interpretation. Use a separately reportable code for the surgical procedure.

74712-74713

Magnetic resonance imaging (MRI) is a radiation-free, noninvasive technique that produces high quality sectional images of the inside of the body in multiple planes. MRI uses the natural magnetic properties of the hydrogen atoms in our bodies that emit radiofrequency signals when exposed to radiowaves within a strong electromagnetic field. These signals are processed and converted by the computer into high-resolution, three-dimensional tomographic images. Patients with metallic or electronic implants or foreign bodies cannot be exposed to MRI. The patient must remain still while lying on a motorized table within the large, circular MRI tunnel. A sedative may be administered, as well as contrast material for image enhancement. These codes report examinations performed on the fetus, including placenta and maternal pelvis, when performed. Report 74712 for a single or first gestation and 74713 for each additional gestation.

74740

In hysterosalpingography, the uterine cavity and fallopian tubes are visualized radiographically after the injection of contrast material through the cervix. Uterine tumors, intrauterine adhesions, and developmental anomalies can be seen. Tubal obstruction caused by internal scarring, tumor, or kinking can also be detected. This code reports only the radiological supervision and interpretation. The injection portion of this study is reported separately.

74742

The physician introduces a catheter into the cervix and takes it into the uterus and through the fallopian tube to diagnose any blockages or to re-establish patency. The physician may elect to inject liquid radiographic contrast material into the endometrial cavity with mild pressure to force the material into the tubes (hysterosalpingogram). The shadow of this material on x-ray film permits examination of the uterus and tubes for any abnormalities or blockages. This code reports only the radiological supervision and interpretation. The introduction of the catheter into the fallopian tube is reported separately.

74775

The perineum, which is the area between the vulva and the anus in the female, is viewed to determine the sex of the patient. It is used mainly in cases where an infant is born with ambiguous genitalia. The procedure also may be used to check for an abnormal opening (fistula) between the vagina and bladder or the vagina and rectum. When locating a fistula, the use of contrast material is included.

75557-75559

Cardiac magnetic resonance imaging (MRI) is a radiation-free, noninvasive technique that produces high quality, detailed, three-dimensional imaging of complex congenital heart defects, as well as functional cardiac analysis. MRI uses the natural magnetic properties of the hydrogen atoms in our bodies that emit radiofrequency signals when exposed to radio waves within a strong electromagnetic field. These signals are processed and converted by the computer into high-resolution images. Patients with metallic or electronic implants or foreign bodies cannot be exposed to MRI. The patient must remain still while lying on a motorized table within the large, circular MRI tunnel. A sedative may be administered. Imaging is performed by obtaining tomographic cuts from the base to the apex and/or the interior to the posterior in order to interrogate the entire heart. Function studies may include observation of the atria and/or ventricles, qualitative and quantitative assessment of ventricular function, and obtaining numerical values for ejection fraction (EF) ventricular volumes, ventricular mass, and cardiac output. Report 75557 for observation of the cardiac function and morphology without administration of a contrast agent. Report 75559 if stress imaging is included. Following dobutamine injection, which mimics the effects of exercise on the heart and induces ischemia, the physician evaluates the left ventricular wall's ability to move during physical stress.

75561-75565

Cardiac magnetic resonance imaging (MRI) is a radiation-free, noninvasive technique that produces high quality, detailed, three-dimensional imaging of complex congenital heart defects, as well as functional cardiac analysis. MRI uses the natural magnetic properties of the hydrogen atoms in our bodies that emit radiofrequency signals when exposed to radio waves within a strong electromagnetic field. These signals are processed and converted by the computer into high-resolution images. Patients with metallic or electronic implants or foreign bodies cannot be exposed to MRI. The patient must remain still while lying on a motorized table within the large, circular MRI tunnel. A sedative may be administered. Images are first obtained without contrast materials, followed by administration of contrast materials and further sequences. Imaging is performed by obtaining tomographic cuts from the base to the apex and/or the interior to the posterior in order to interrogate the entire heart. Function studies may include observation of the atria and/or ventricles, qualitative and quantitative assessment of ventricular function, and obtaining numerical values for ejection fraction (EF) ventricular volumes, ventricular mass, and cardiac output. Report 75561 for observation of cardiac function and morphology. Report 75563 if stress imaging is included. Following dobutamine injection, which mimics the effects of exercise on the heart and induces ischemia, the physician evaluates the left ventricular wall's ability to move during physical stress. If velocity flow mapping is performed, report 75565 in addition to the code for the primary procedure.

75571

Computed tomography directs multiple narrow beams of x-rays around the body structure being studied and uses computer imaging to produce thin, cross-sectional views of various layers (or slices) of the body. It is useful for the evaluation of calcium deposits on the coronary tree. Patients are required to remain motionless during the study. This code reports the CT of the heart and quantitative evaluation of calcium deposits in the coronary tree. High levels of calcium deposits in the heart triple a person's likelihood of suffering an adverse coronary event (e.g., myocardial infarct, cardiac arrest, etc.).

75572-75574

The physician performs computed tomography (CT) of the heart utilizing contrast materials to evaluate cardiac structure and morphology. CT directs multiple, thin beams of x-rays at the body and uses computer imaging to produce thin, cross-sectional views of various layers of the body. It is useful in the evaluation of soft tissue. Because patients are required to be motionless during CT, this creates issues when producing CT images of the heart, which is continually moving rhythmically. In a cardiac gating technique, the patient is undergoing CT while attached to ECG leads. CT image acquisition is triggered by the ECG, allowing for coordination of imaging with periods of movement and rest within the heart. Code 75572 includes 3D image postprocessing, assessment of cardiac function, and evaluation of venous structures, if performed. Code 75573 reports CT of a heart with congenital anomalies, also performed utilizing contrast materials to evaluate cardiac structure and morphology. This code includes 3D image postprocessing, assessment of left ventricular (LV) cardiac function, right ventricular (RV) structure and function, and evaluation of vascular structures, if performed. Report 75574 for CT of the heart utilizing contrast materials in conjunction with computerized tomographic angiography (CTA) to evaluate the heart, coronary arteries, and any bypass grafts that are present. In addition to the CT imaging of the heart as described previously, a CTA of native and anomalous coronary arteries and coronary bypass grafts is obtained. CTA is a procedure used for imaging of vessels to detect aneurysms, blood clots, and other vascular irregularities. Contrast media is rapidly infused intravenously, at intervals, usually with an automatic injector. The patient's heart is scanned with thin section axial or spiral mode x-ray beams. Three-dimensional images are generated and postprocessing reconstruction is done at a workstation on the scanner. Vessel wall thickness and the venous anatomy of the heart are evaluated. This code also includes 3D image postprocessing (including evaluation of cardiac structure and morphology, assessment of cardiac function, and evaluation of venous structures, if performed).

75580

A proprietary noninvasive fractional flow reserve (FFR) technology is used to assist a physician in evaluating the degree of coronary artery disease (CAD) that a patient has, including how a CAD blockage can affect blood flow to the heart with much greater accuracy based on combining anatomy (coronary CT angiogram) and physiology. This technology allows clinicians to personalize a patient's care plan and reduce the likelihood of needing more invasive procedures. The patient undergoes a coronary computed tomography (CT) angiogram. Data from this test is securely uploaded from the hospital's system to a cloud server. The FFR process creates a personalized, digital, three-dimensional representation of the patient's coronary arteries and employs robust algorithms to help determine and replicate coronary blood flow. The model can also determine any potential effect of blockages on coronary blood flow. Once the process is complete, the physician receives the patient's results through a secure web interface and selects the best treatment course for the patient. This artificial intelligence technology is considered augmentative, which means the machine analyzes and/or quantifies the data to produce clinically meaningful output, and a physician or other qualified health care professional provides an interpretation and report.

75600

A local anesthetic is applied over the common femoral artery. The artery is percutaneously punctured with a needle and a guidewire is fed through the artery into the thoracic aorta. A catheter is threaded over the guidewire to the point of study and the guidewire removed. Contrast medium is injected and films are taken. This code reports the radiological supervision and interpretation. Use separately reportable code for the catheterization.

75605

A local anesthetic is applied over the common femoral artery. The artery is percutaneously punctured with a needle and a guidewire is fed through the artery into the thoracic aorta. A catheter is threaded over the guidewire to the point of study and the guidewire is removed. Contrast medium is injected and films are taken by serialography, producing a series of individual x-ray films. This code reports the radiological supervision and interpretation. Use a separately reportable code for the catheterization.

75625

A local anesthetic is applied over the common femoral artery. The artery is percutaneously punctured with a needle and a guidewire is fed through the artery into the abdominal aorta. A catheter is threaded over the guidewire to the point of study and the guidewire is removed. Contrast medium is injected and films are taken by serialography, producing a series of individual x-ray films. This code reports the radiological supervision and interpretation. Use a separately reportable code for the catheterization.

75630

A local anesthetic is applied over the common femoral artery. The artery is percutaneously punctured with a needle and a guidewire is fed through the artery into the abdominal aorta. A catheter is threaded over the guidewire to the point of study and the guidewire is removed. Contrast medium is injected into the abdominal aorta and a series of continuous films are taken of the contrast flow through the aorta and its runoff into the arteries of both legs. This code reports the radiological supervision and interpretation. Use a separately reportable code for the catheterization.

75635

Computed tomographic angiography (CTA) is a procedure used for the imaging of vessels to detect aneurysms, blood clots, and other vascular irregularities. Contrast medium is rapidly and regularly infused at intervals, usually with an automatic injector, and the patient is scanned by CT for images of the abdominal aorta and both lower extremities as the contrast runs down through the iliofemoral pathway. The images obtained are acquired with narrower collimation and reconstructed at shorter intervals than standard CT images. Three-dimensional images are generated and postprocessing reconstruction is done at a workstation on the scanner. This code reports an exam of the abdominal aorta with bilateral iliofemoral lower extremity runoff with contrast materials and image postprocessing. Noncontrast images, if performed, are also included in this procedure.

75705

A local anesthetic is applied over the artery of access, usually the common femoral artery. The artery is percutaneously punctured with a needle and a guidewire is fed through the artery into the aorta. Under fluoroscopic guidance, a catheter is threaded over the guidewire to the aorta and advanced directly into a spinal artery suitable for viewing the study area. The guidewire is removed. Contrast medium is injected in the lowest level first and just above that in sequence and films are taken until the study has covered the area of interest. This code reports the radiological supervision and interpretation only. Use a separately reportable code for the catheterization.

75710
The arteries of one arm, leg, hand, or foot that are not normally seen in an x-ray are examined radiologically by injecting contrast material. A local anesthetic is applied over the area of access which could be femoral, brachial, subclavian, or axillary artery. The artery is percutaneously punctured with a needle and a guidewire is fed through the artery to the point of study. A catheter is threaded over the guidewire until it, too, reaches the point of study and the guidewire is removed. Contrast medium is injected through the catheter and a series of x-rays or fluoroscopic images taken to visualize the vessels and evaluate any abnormalities. The catheter is removed and pressure applied to the site. This code reports the radiological supervision and interpretation. Use a separately reportable code for the catheterization.

75716
The arteries of bilateral extremities such as both arms or legs, that are not normally seen in an x-ray are examined radiologically by injecting contrast material. A local anesthetic is applied over the area of access which could be femoral, brachial, subclavian, or axillary artery. The artery is percutaneously punctured with a needle and a guidewire is fed through the artery to the point of study. A catheter is threaded over the guidewire until it, too, reaches the point of study and the guidewire is removed. Contrast medium is injected through the catheter and a series of x-rays or fluoroscopic images taken to visualize the vessels and evaluate any abnormalities. The catheter is removed and pressure applied to the site. This code reports the radiological supervision and interpretation. Use a separately reportable code for the catheterization.

75726
An artery supplying the abdominal organ of concern is examined radiologically by injecting contrast material. A local anesthetic is applied over the area of access, usually the common femoral artery. The artery is percutaneously punctured with a needle and a guidewire is fed through the artery to the point of study. A catheter is threaded over the guidewire until it, too, reaches the point of study and the guidewire is removed. Contrast medium is injected through the catheter and a series of x-rays or fluoroscopic images taken to visualize the vessels and evaluate any abnormalities. If an aortogram is performed, the catheter is directed to the origin of the coronary arteries and dye is injected into them as x-rays are taken to look for plaque build-up. The catheter is removed and pressure applied to the site. This code reports the radiological supervision and interpretation. Use separately reportable code for the catheterization.

75731
The left or right adrenal gland, located on top of the upper end of each kidney is examined radiologically by injecting contrast material. A local anesthetic is applied over the common femoral artery. The artery is percutaneously punctured with a needle and a guidewire is fed through the artery, the aorta, and further into the renal artery. A catheter is threaded over the guidewire until it, too, reaches the point of study and the guidewire is removed. Contrast medium is injected through the catheter and a series of x-rays or fluoroscopic images taken to visualize the vessels and evaluate any abnormalities. The catheter is removed and pressure applied to the site. This code reports the radiological supervision and interpretation. Use separately reportable code for the catheterization.

75733
The adrenal glands located on top of the upper end of each kidney are examined radiologically by injecting contrast material. A local anesthetic is applied over the common femoral artery. The artery is percutaneously punctured with a needle and a guidewire is fed through the artery, the aorta, and further into the renal arteries. A catheter is threaded over the guidewire until it, too, reaches the point of study and the guidewire is removed. Contrast medium is injected through the catheter and a series of x-rays or fluoroscopic images taken to visualize the vessels and evaluate any abnormalities. The catheter is removed and pressure applied to the site. This code reports the radiological supervision and interpretation. Use separately reportable code for the catheterization.

75736
An angiogram is done on operative candidates for pelvic fixation to rule out retroperitoneal arterial bleeding. A local anesthetic is applied over the common femoral artery. The artery is percutaneously punctured with a needle and a guidewire is fed through the artery into the study area in the pelvic region. A catheter is threaded over the guidewire until it, too, reaches the point of study and the guidewire is removed. Contrast medium is injected through the catheter and a series of x-rays or fluoroscopic images taken to visualize the vessels and evaluate for any transected or bleeding arteries. Embolization may be dictated by angiography results to hemorrhaging for definitive stabilization treatment. The catheter is removed and pressure applied to the site. This code reports the radiological supervision and interpretation. Use separately reportable code for the catheterization.

75741
A local anesthetic is applied over the site where the catheter is to be introduced; this is most often the common femoral or internal jugular vein. The vein is percutaneously punctured and the catheter selectively manipulated through the vena cava, right atrium, and right ventricle into the left or right pulmonary artery. Contrast medium is injected and films are taken to visualize the vessels and evaluate any abnormalities. This code reports the radiological supervision and interpretation only. Use a separately reportable code for the catheterization.

75743
A local anesthetic is applied over the site where the catheter is to be introduced; this is most often the common femoral or internal jugular vein. The vein is percutaneously punctured and the catheter selectively

manipulated through the vena cava, right atrium, and right ventricle into the pulmonary arteries. Contrast medium is injected and films taken bilaterally to visualize the vessels and evaluate any abnormalities. This code reports the radiological supervision and interpretation only. Use a separately reportable code for the catheterization.

75746

A local anesthetic is applied over the site where the catheter is to be introduced; this is most often either the common femoral or internal jugular vein. The vein is percutaneously punctured and the catheter manipulated through to the main pulmonary artery or the right atrium. Contrast medium is injected and films are taken to visualize the vessels and evaluate any abnormalities such as blockages, narrowing, or aneurysms. This code reports the radiological supervision and interpretation only. Use a separately reportable code for the catheterization.

75756

A local anesthetic is applied over the site where the catheter is to be introduced; this is most often the common femoral or brachial artery. The artery is percutaneously punctured with a needle and a guidewire is fed through the artery to the internal mammary. A catheter is threaded over the guidewire to the point of study and the guidewire is removed. Contrast medium is injected and a series of x-rays performed to visualize the vessels and evaluate any abnormalities. This code reports the radiological supervision and interpretation only. Use a separately reportable code for the catheterization.

75774

This procedure reports each additional vessel studied after the basic, initial study. It involves manipulating the catheter into additional second, third, or higher order vessels within a vascular family and performing injection of contrast and taking additional films. This code is an add-on code and cannot stand alone.

75801-75803

Vital blue dye is injected into the subcutaneous tissues for outlining of skin lymphatics. As soon as the lymphatic vessels are visualized by their blue color, the physician makes a small incision to gain access. The lymph vessel is cannulated with a needle and a fine catheter is attached. A small amount of dye is injected to ensure correct placement and the needle is advanced a few millimeters into the vessel. The needle and catheter are secured and dye is injected with a syringe. X-rays are made. Code 75801 reports the radiological supervision and interpretation for lymphangiography of an extremity on one side only; 75803 reports the radiological supervision and interpretation for lymphangiography of extremities on both sides. Use a separately reportable code for the injection procedure.

75805-75807

Vital blue dye is injected into the subcutaneous tissues for outlining of skin lymphatics. As soon as the lymphatic vessels are visualized by their blue color, the physician makes a small incision to gain access. The lymph vessel is cannulated with a needle and a fine catheter is attached. A small amount of dye is injected to ensure correct placement and the needle is advanced a few millimeters into the vessel. The needle and catheter are secured and dye is injected with a syringe. X-rays are made. Code 75805 reports the radiological supervision and interpretation for lymphangiography on one side only of the pelvic/abdominal region. Code 75807 reports the radiological supervision and interpretation for lymphangiography on both sides of the pelvic/abdominal region. Use a separately reportable code for the injection procedure.

75809

The physician injects contrast material through the skin into the reservoir of a peritoneal-venous shunt or directly into shunt tubing or reservoir with a needle. Shunt tubing is a drain to eliminate excess cerebral spinal fluid in cases of hydrocephalus. The tubing of a peritoneal-venous shunt drains the accumulation of fluids in cases of ascites into a major vein. The physician places the needle and injects radiologic dye. Pictures are taken to visualize the flow of contrast and check for effective drainage. This code reports the radiological supervision and interpretation only. Use a separately reportable code for the shuntogram injection procedure.

75810

The physician makes an incision in the lower left axilla. An 18 or 20-gauge sheath catheter is inserted into the middle of the soft, sponge-like tissue of the spleen. The splenic vein is visualized and the catheter is placed. 2.0-3 cc of radiopaque dye is injected per second, totaling about 15.0-20 cc of dye. X-rays are taken every second for about 12 seconds. The catheter is removed and the incision covered with a dressing. This code reports the radiological supervision and interpretation only. Use a separately reportable code for the splenoportography injection procedure.

75820-75822

The physician performs a radiographic study on the veins of a left or right extremity, upper or lower, in 75820 and both the left and right legs or arms in 75822. This type of study is most often performed on the lower extremities as opposed to the arms and commonly involves the femoral vein, described here. A local anesthetic is applied over the site where the catheter is to be introduced. The vein is percutaneously punctured with a needle and a guidewire is fed through the vein to the point where dye will be injected. A catheter is threaded over the guidewire and the guidewire is removed. Contrast medium is injected and a series of x-rays performed to visualize the vessels and evaluate any abnormalities. In venography, contrast medium is injected into the catheter that has traveled to an area upstream of the site under investigation. These codes report the radiological supervision and interpretation only. Use a separately reportable code for the catheterization.

75825-75827

A local anesthetic is applied over a distal vein (typically antecubital, internal jugular, subclavian, or femoral) and the vein is percutaneously punctured with a needle. A guidewire is fed through the vein to the inferior vena cava in 75825 and the superior vena cava in 75827. The physician may slide an introducer sheath over the guidewire into the venous lumen before inserting a catheter. The catheter is inserted into the vein and threaded over the guidewire to the inferior (75825) or superior (75827) vena cava. The guidewire is removed. Contrast medium is injected and a series of x-rays performed to visualize and evaluate any abnormalities. In venography, contrast medium is injected into the catheter that has traveled to an area upstream of the site under investigation. These codes report the radiological supervision and interpretation only. Use a separately reportable code for the catheterization.

75831-75833

A local anesthetic is applied over the site where the catheter is to be introduced; this is most often the common femoral vein. The vein is percutaneously punctured with a needle and a guidewire is inserted and selectively fed through the vein until it reaches the desired location in the venous system. A catheter is threaded over the guidewire into the selected point in the vein and the wire is removed. Contrast medium for venography is injected through the catheter that has traveled to an area upstream of the site under investigation. X-rays are taken. Code 75831 reports the radiological supervision and interpretation only for venography of the left or right renal vein and 75833 is used for both renal veins. Use a separately reportable code for the catheterization.

75840-75842

A local anesthetic is applied over the site where the catheter is to be introduced; this is most often the common femoral vein. The vein is percutaneously punctured with a needle and a guidewire is inserted and selectively fed through the vein until it reaches the desired location in the venous system. A catheter is threaded over the guidewire into the selected point in the vein and the wire is removed. Contrast medium for venography is injected through the catheter that has traveled to an area upstream of the site under investigation. X-rays are taken. Code 75840 reports the radiological supervision and interpretation only for venography of the left or right adrenal vein and 75842 is used for both adrenal veins. Use a separately reportable code for the catheterization.

75860

A local anesthetic is applied over the site where the catheter is to be introduced and the access vein is percutaneously punctured with a needle. A guidewire is inserted and advanced through the vein until it reaches the desired location in the venous system for imaging the sinus (petrosal, inferior sagittal) or jugular vein. A catheter is threaded over the guidewire to the selected point and the wire is removed. Non-ionic diluted contrast medium is injected over approximately 30 seconds through the catheter that has traveled to an area upstream of the site under investigation. Images are acquired. This code reports the radiological supervision and interpretation only. Use a separately reportable code for the catheterization.

75870

A local anesthetic is applied over the site where the catheter is to be introduced and the access vein is percutaneously punctured with a needle. A guidewire is inserted and advanced through the dominant jugular vein until it reaches the desired location for studying the superior sagittal sinus, which is the primary venous drainage for the cranial vasculature. A catheter is threaded over the guidewire into the selected point in the vein and the wire is removed. Non-ionic diluted contrast medium is injected through the catheter that has traveled to an area upstream of the site under investigation. Images are acquired. This code reports the radiological supervision and interpretation only. Use a separately reportable code for the catheterization.

75872

In epidural venography, a needle is inserted into the epidural space of the spine while the patient is sitting in a position with the chin on the chest and the knees pulled up or positioned on the left side. A catheter is threaded over the needle until it reaches the epidural space around the spinal cord and the needle is removed. Contrast is injected into the catheter and radiographic pictures are taken. This is done on patients with a penetrating trauma to the area, or subarachnoid or parenchymal hemorrhage. This code reports the radiological supervision and interpretation only. Use a separately reportable code for the catheterization.

75880

The physician introduces a needle or catheter through a puncture site in the skin into a peripheral vein. A guidewire is inserted and selectively fed through the vein until it reaches the desired location in the venous system for imaging the orbital veins. A catheter is threaded over the guidewire into the selected point in the vein and the wire is removed. Radiopaque dye is administered into the facial or frontal veins, and x-rays are taken to visualize the orbital veins and cavernous sinuses. This code reports the radiological supervision and interpretation only. Use a separately reportable code for the catheterization.

75885

A radiographic exam of the portal vein of the liver is done by inserting a needle through the abdomen. The patient's right side is cleansed and a local anesthetic given at the puncture site. A needle is inserted into the skin just under the ribs and diaphragm and advanced to the liver under fluoroscopic guidance. The needle is aimed at the portal vein and when blood returns from the needle, a small amount of contrast is injected to confirm placement into the portal vein. When in place, a guidewire is inserted and a catheter follows. More contrast is injected, radiographs taken and intravenous, hemodynamic pressures in the portal vein are recorded. This code reports the radiological supervision and interpretation only. Use a separately reportable code for the catheterization.

75887
A radiographic exam of the portal vein of the liver is done by inserting a needle through the abdomen. The patient's right side is cleansed and a local anesthetic given at the puncture site. A needle is inserted into the skin just under the ribs and diaphragm and advanced to the liver under fluoroscopic guidance. The needle is aimed at the portal vein and when blood returns from the needle, a small amount of contrast is injected to confirm placement into the portal vein. When in place, a guidewire is inserted and a catheter follows. More contrast is injected and radiographs are taken. This code reports the radiological supervision and interpretation only. Use a separately reportable code for the catheterization.

75889-75891
A local anesthetic is applied over the common femoral vein and a guidewire is fed through until it reaches the hepatic vein. A catheter is threaded over the guidewire and the guidewire is removed. For wedged hepatic venography, the catheter is wedged into a small hepatic vein branch to approximate the portal pressure occurring in liver disease. For free hepatic venography, the catheter tip lies free in the hepatic vein. Correct positioning of the catheter is monitored by fluoroscopy. Contrast medium is injected into the vein and x-rays are taken. Report 75889 if this is done together with hemodynamic evaluation in which blood movement through the liver is monitored by indwelling catheters connected to transducers. The pressure forces within the arteries and veins are converted to electrical signals and displayed on screen. Report 75891 if hepatic venography is performed without the hemodynamic evaluation. These codes report the radiological supervision and interpretation only.

75893
Venous sampling involves withdrawing blood from a patient's vein into a vacuum tube to test the blood for excess hormones. Single or double catheters may be used for sampling. The catheter(s) is inserted in the femoral vein(s) and maneuvered to the vein in the anatomical location in which the testing is to be performed. When the catheter is correctly placed, several blood samples are withdrawn. Angiography performed in conjunction with the sampling is included in 75893. This code reports the radiological supervision and interpretation only.

75894
A blood vessel is blocked by inserting an occlusive agent under fluoroscopic monitoring to stop or restrict the blood flow. This is done to restrict blood supply to a tumor, treat vascular malformations, or control hemorrhaging. A local anesthetic is given at the puncture site and a needle is inserted into the selected vessel followed by a guidewire. The needle is removed. A catheter is inserted over the guidewire and advanced to the vessel requiring treatment. A blocking agent is injected or inserted and monitored. The effect may remain permanent or require another transcatheter embolization with time. This code reports the radiological supervision and interpretation only. Use a separately reportable code for the catheterization.

75898
Angiography is performed during or following transcatheter infusion or embolization through the existing catheter to reassess the therapy's effectiveness. A radiopaque contrast medium is injected through the catheter and by fluoroscopic images recorded of the vessel, the radiologist interprets the status of the blood vessel and the effectiveness of treatment rendered.

75901
Pericatheter obstructive material, such as a fibrin sheath, is removed from around a central venous device via separate venous access. Central venous catheters often fail because of the accumulation of an obstructing thrombus or fibrin sheath around the tip of the catheter. The catheter is first checked that it can aspirate and flush forward. The pericatheter material is identified by contrast material injection. Generally, a right femoral vein access is used. A guidewire followed by an angiographic catheter are advanced into the superior vena cava and exchanged for a loop snare with its catheter, which are advanced cephalad along the length of the central venous catheter beyond the ports. The loop snare is tightly closed about the CV catheter to encircle it and slowly pulled down and off the tip of the catheter, stripping off the pericatheter obstructive material. This is repeated a few times and the catheter is rechecked for infusion and injection ability of the ports. A contrast study is done again to identify any fibrin and the process may be repeated until the fibrin sheath is completely removed. This code reports only the radiological supervision and interpretation required for this procedure.

75902
Intraluminal obstructive material, such as a thrombus or fibrin sheath, is removed from inside a central venous device through the lumen of the device. This does not require a separate access incision. The central venous catheter is first checked that it can aspirate and flush forward. The obstructing material is disrupted and removed mechanically by using an angioplasty balloon or other catheter introduced into the central venous catheter through its entry site on the skin. The catheter is checked for unimpeded, restored flow and the process may be repeated until the CV catheter is cleared. This code reports the radiological supervision and interpretation only required for this procedure.

75956-75957
The physician repairs the descending thoracic aorta by placing an endoprosthesis from within the artery. Endovascular repair may be performed for an

aneurysm, pseudoaneurysm, dissection, penetrating ulcer, intramural hematoma, or traumatic disruption. The defect in the descending thoracic aorta is identified using aortography. The endoprosthesis, contained inside a holding device, is introduced into the artery under fluoroscopy and positioned at the target zone area of repair. Extension prostheses may be required to the level of the celiac artery origin. In 75956, when the endoprosthesis is in position, it is deployed within the artery at the target site in the descending thoracic aorta, covering the origin of the left subclavian artery. A balloon angioplasty may be necessary to achieve proper positioning and functioning of the endoprosthesis. The placement position is confirmed, the catheter is removed, and the arteriotomy site is closed. These codes report only the radiological supervision and interpretation required for this procedure. Report 75956 when the repair covers the left subclavian artery origin and 75957 when the repair does not cover the left subclavian artery origin.

75958

A leak, called an endoleak, may occur at the proximal fixation sites of a grafted descending thoracic aorta defect through the body of the graft or from patent arteries within the defect and may require endovascular reparation. A proximal extension prosthesis is placed endovascularly to repair an endoleak in a grafted descending thoracic aortic aneurysm, pseudoaneurysm, dissection, penetrating ulcer, intramural hematoma, or traumatic disruption. The target site is identified by aortography and the proper extension prosthesis is selected. Under fluoroscopy, the extension prosthesis, contained inside a long plastic holding capsule, is threaded through the arteries to the site of the leak. Once the extension prosthesis is in place, the holding capsule is removed. The extension prosthesis, activated by heat, expands like a spring and becomes anchored to the artery wall at the site of the endoleak. If full expansion of the prosthesis does not occur automatically, a balloon catheter is threaded to the graft site and inflated within the endovascular prosthesis until full expansion is achieved. The placement position is confirmed, the catheter is removed, and the arteriotomy site is closed. This code reports only the radiological supervision and interpretation required for this procedure.

75959

A leak, called an endoleak, may occur at the distal fixation sites of a previously grafted descending thoracic aorta defect through the body of the graft or from patent arteries within the defect and may require endovascular reparation. One or more distal extension prosthesis modules are placed endovascularly to the level of the celiac artery to repair an endoleak in a previously grafted descending thoracic aortic aneurysm, pseudoaneurysm, dissection, penetrating ulcer, intramural hematoma, or traumatic disruption. The target site is identified by aortography and the proper extension prosthesis is selected. Under fluoroscopy, the extension prosthesis, contained inside a long plastic holding capsule, is threaded through the arteries to the site of the leak. Once the extension prosthesis is in place, the holding capsule is removed. The extension prosthesis, activated by heat, expands like a spring and becomes anchored to the artery wall at the site of the endoleak. If full expansion of the prosthesis does not occur automatically, a balloon catheter is threaded to the graft site and inflated within the endovascular prosthesis until full expansion is achieved. The placement position is confirmed, the catheter is removed, and the arteriotomy site is closed. This code reports only the radiological supervision and interpretation required for this procedure and is reported only once regardless of the number of extension modules deployed.

75970

A biopsy specimen is obtained through a catheter. The biopsy catheter may be inserted through an already existing drainage tube or catheter, through a tract or pathway, such as the urethra during cystourethroscopy, or through the skin and into the access artery. Fluoroscopy is used to guide the catheter through its course from entry to the point of study to be biopsied. A biopsy brush, fine biopsy needle, or biting forceps may be inserted through the catheter to obtain the cells or tissue for examination. This code reports the radiological supervision and interpretation only.

75984

An existing percutaneous drainage tube or catheter (e.g., genitourinary system or abscess) is replaced with contrast monitoring. A guidewire is usually inserted into the existing catheter to guide the new one. The old catheter is removed and the replacement catheter is threaded back over the guidewire. Contrast injection allows for correct positioning to be visualized with fluoroscopic images displayed on a screen. This code reports the radiological supervision and interpretation only.

75989

Fluoroscopic, ultrasonic, or CT guidance may be used for percutaneous drainage of an abscess or to obtain a specimen and place a tube or catheter. Once the abscess is located, the skin is punctured with a needle to begin draining. A catheter may be advanced over a guidewire inserted through the needle and into the abscess cavity. The tract to the outside is dilated to facilitate placing a percutaneous drainage tube. The cavity is aspirated and the drainage tube placed at the lowest point to ensure complete drainage. The drainage tube is secured to suction drainage. This code reports the radiological supervision and interpretation only for this procedure.

[76014, 76015]

A technologist or clinical staff trained in magnetic resonance (MR) safety perform an assessment to determine if an implant or foreign body poses a health hazard for a patient scheduled to undergo a magnetic resonance imaging (MRI) diagnostic study or MR imaging guidance on a different date of service. Strong magnetic field exposure can cause injury or death during an MRI for a patient with an implant or foreign body if appropriate safety protocols are not followed. The technologist identifies the presence of any implant and associated components using appropriate sources such as the patient's previous medical records and device databases. The assessment may include a questionnaire or verbal interview to identify previous surgeries, injuries, or other circumstances that may indicate the presence of an implant or foreign body. Published professional guidance is consulted to determine appropriate safety protocols; for an implant, this may include Food and Drug Administration (FDA) approved labeling or the manufacturer's safety declaration. A written report is required to identify the results of the safety assessment with any contraindications for MRI or adjustments necessary to proceed with the MRI examination. Report 76014 for the initial 15 minutes of the assessment. Report 76015 for each additional 30 minutes; this code is used when complex, multiple, or insufficiently documented implants require a prolonged safety assessment for an implant or foreign body.

[76016]

A physician or other qualified health care professional makes a safety determination for a patient scheduled to undergo a magnetic resonance imaging (MRI) diagnostic study or MR imaging guidance on a different date of service. The risk of harm versus clinical benefit of performing the MRI is considered along with any additional safety protocols necessary when the patient has an implant and/or foreign body that could increase the risk of the examination. For example, additional preparation of the implant may be required prior to the MRI or there may be limits on the scan time, energy deposition, or anatomical regions examined due to the presence of an implant or foreign body. The physician determines the type of equipment, accessories, and expertise required to provide a safe environment for the patient. A written report is required to identify the results of the safety determination with any contraindications for MRI or adjustments necessary to proceed with the MRI examination.

[76017]

A medical physicist or magnetic resonance safety expert (MRSE) performs MR safety examination customization, planning, and performance monitoring under supervision by a physician or other qualified health care professional on the same date as magnetic resonance imaging (MRI). Strong magnetic field exposure can cause injury or death during MRI for a patient with an implant or foreign body if appropriate safety protocols are not followed. An implant that is labeled as MR conditional is only compatible with the MRI machine under certain conditions that are provided on the implant label. Acquisition of the MRI must be customized to meet these conditions. For non-conditional implants or foreign bodies, adjustments may still be required to reduce the risk of harm to the patient. After the required conditions and/or risks are identified, the appropriate number of views and imaging sequences are selected to create a safe environment for the patient. A written report is required to identify the results of the safety customization, planning, and performance monitoring with any adjustments necessary to proceed with the MRI examination.

[76018]

A technologist or staff trained in magnetic resonance safety prepares an electronic implant on the same date as a magnetic resonance imaging (MRI) examination under supervision by a physician or other qualified health care professional. For example, cardiac or neurostimulation implant devices require additional preparation. The technologist places the implant in a protective mode prior to the patient entering the MR room. The device may also require programming to maintain device integrity and additional protection measures to shield internal circuitry from electromagnetic fields. Risks to the patient including unintentional stimulation or heating while in the MR room should be minimized prior to beginning the examination. A written report is required to identify the safety measures taken in preparation of the electronic implant prior to the MRI.

[76019]

A technologist or staff trained in magnetic resonance safety positions or immobilizes an implant on the same date as a magnetic resonance imaging (MRI) examination under supervision by a physician or other qualified health care professional. The technologist determines the appropriate position for the implant that will minimize risks such as radiofrequency burns, magnetically induced charges, or translational/vibrational forces while the patient is in the MR room. A written report is required to identify the safety measures taken to position or immobilize the implant prior to the MRI.

76000

A radiologist or other qualified health care provider supplies separate fluoroscopic monitoring of the body for up to one hour for procedures that do not include fluoroscopy as an integral component. This code is reported separately to describe the professional work component entailed in providing fluoroscopic monitoring. If formal contrast x-ray studies are done and included as a part of the procedure to produce films with written interpretation and report, fluoroscopy is already included and cannot be separately reported.

76010

Children frequently ingest foreign objects that can be diagnosed by plain film radiography. A single view is taken of the gastrointestinal pathway from nose to rectum to locate a foreign body.

76080

An injection of radiopaque material is made directly into a sinus tract (a canal or passage leading to an abscess) or through a previously placed catheter, to determine the existence, nature, or size of an abscess or fistula (an abnormal tube-like passage from a normal body cavity to a free surface or to another body cavity). This code reports the radiological supervision and interpretation only.

76098
Immediately after excision or biopsy of a suspected breast lesion, the specimen is evaluated by pathology to assist in localizing and/or ensuring clear margins of the tissue removed. The information is immediately returned to the surgeon so the procedure can be completed.

76100
A radiological exam is done on a body section in a single plane by scanning an x-ray beam across the body in one direction to take pictures of the structures under study in the selected plane. The films show detailed images of the structures within the single selected plane by blurring out the images above and below. Use this code for a single plane radiological exam of a single body section other than urography.

76120-76125
Cineradiography uses high speed x-ray films to take a series of images of an organ or system in motion such as the vocal cords or heart. These images taken in exposure ranges of nanoseconds to milliseconds are like the individual frames of a motion picture. This allows the movement to be frozen and tracked very minutely to gather information about time-varying characteristics. Use 76120 when performed alone and not specifically included as part of the procedure. Use 76125 when cineradiography is performed in conjunction with a routine exam.

76140
A radiologist provides a consultation and a written report after reviewing an x-ray exam that was performed elsewhere.

76145
The FDA encourages tracking of safety metrics for radiation, such as adverse events and dose data, by advocating development of national databases and registries. Additionally, they recommend that individual facilities, in conjunction with medical physicists, determine whether radiation doses usually related to their protocols both fall below skin-injury thresholds and parallel the values that are widely reported in medical literature. This code reports medical physics dose evaluation for radiation exposure that exceeds institutional review threshold. A report is included in this code.

76376-76377
The physician provides concurrent supervision for image postprocessing of computerized tomography (CT), magnetic resonance imaging (MRI), ultrasound, or other tomographic modality with 3D manipulation of volumetric data sets and image rendering. The exact nature of the 3D manipulation is dependent upon the type of study being performed and the purpose of the diagnostic imaging. Image manipulation can include 3D image segmentation (i.e., removing skeletal structure to better visualize vascular structure followed by identifying and segmenting vessels for individual analysis and review), 3D volume and surface rendering, and 3D image restoration by deconvolution (i.e., unfolding the colon or straightening tortuous blood vessels). Work can include diagnostic imaging and surgical planning with 3D images, scientific modeling and simulation, and other work involving volumetric data. Report 76376 for 3D rendering not requiring image postprocessing on an independent workstation. Report 76377 when image postprocessing on an independent workstation is required.

76380
Computed tomography (CT) scanning directs multiple narrow beams of x-rays around the body structure(s) being studied and uses computer imaging to produce thin cross-sectional views of various layers (or slices) of the body. It is able to visualize soft tissue as well as bones. This code reports a limited or a localized follow-up study.

76390
Magnetic resonance spectroscopy (MRS) is used to determine chemical and metabolic properties of a particular region, organ, or structure within the body. MRS can be done at the same time as standard MRI, which yields cross-sectional, anatomic information about the spatial properties of a region relative to its surrounding areas; MRS however, provides rich information about the biochemical composition or metabolite concentration levels of the localized region, identifying very subtle changes. In vivo spectroscopy is a noninvasive method that relies on nuclear magnetic resonance principles: MRS requires the patient to be placed in a strong magnetic field with a radiowave transmit pulse set at a very particular frequency in order to observe the signal produced by the nuclei specific to the type of atom chosen for the study, such as hydrogen or phosphorus. The spectrum results are in the form of a frequency axis in parts per million and a signal amplitude axis. The specific nuclei within a chosen metabolite will give rise to peaks uniquely positioned along the frequency axis; the position of the peak is called the chemical shift. The signal amplitude of a peak is quantified and correlates directly to the concentration of the assigned metabolite.

76391
Magnetic resonance elastography (MRE) is used to identify hardening of tissue particularly liver tissue since liver disease often causes fibrosis or scarring, which contributes to the stiffness of tissue in people with a known diagnosis or suspected liver disease. It is also being used in the outline of tumors and other abnormalities in other areas of the body before they have progressed enough to be detected by touch, allowing for earlier diagnosis and treatment of diseases. MRE has also been used as a noninvasive biomarker to detect, evaluate, and differentiate tissue stiffness between pancreatic ductal adenocarcinoma (PDAC) and autoimmune pancreatitis (AIP) since PDAC

has greater stiffness than AIP. It can also be used as a method of assessing AIP response to steroid treatment. MRE can be done at the same time as a standard MRI and merges conventional MRI imaging with soundwaves to essentially "palpate by imaging," in a noninvasive manner, regions of the body not reachable by a clinician's hand, to create an elastogram (i.e., visual map) that demonstrates stiffness in body tissue. MRE is noninvasive and provides the ability to detect scarring much earlier than other imaging methods, is beneficial for obese patients, and can also help to anticipate risk of complications such as ascites (i.e., fluid buildup in the abdomen) in patients with liver disease. The MRE system consists of a small, circular, drum-like device placed on the patient's abdomen that generates small, exact vibrations; accompanying software analyzes the resulting MRI images and identifies areas of the liver or other body organs or sites where stiffness is indicated.

76506

Echoencephalography is done to determine ventricular size, investigate suspected fluid masses or other intracranial abnormalities, and define cerebral contents. During the test, the radiation technician guides the transducer over the area of the brain to be examined. The transducer sends an ultrasound beam through the tissue. The reflected sound waves are converted into electrical impulses and displayed on a video screen for interpretation or photographing for later interpretation. Abnormal results may indicate cerebral edema, lesions, or subdural and extradural hemorrhage. The gray (Gy) scale refers to the amount of energy absorbed by the tissue. Real-time scan is a two-dimensional scanning procedure with display of both two-dimensional structure and motion with time. A-mode is a one-dimensional measurement procedure. This code includes A-mode encephalography as a secondary component where indicated.

76510

Diagnostic ophthalmic ultrasound, also called echography, is performed to image intraocular anatomy or to differentiate orbital lesions or disease. A-scan is a one-dimensional measurement procedure using high-frequency sound waves introduced into the eye in a straight line. B-scan utilizes sound waves in a two-dimensional scanning procedure to display a two-dimensional image of the internal ocular structures. Through a transducer placed on the eye, high-frequency sound waves are sent through the eye, which reflect back to a receiver, are converted into electrical pulses, and displayed on screen. In quantitative A scan, the resulting single-dimensional image provides information about tissue structure and reflective/sound absorptive properties. B-scan can locate structures in the eye that may be obscured by cataract, hemorrhages, or opacities and provides information as to a lesion's shape, mobility, insertion, or relationship to neighboring structures. This code reports both types of scanning performed in the same patient encounter.

76511

Diagnostic ophthalmic ultrasound, also called echography, is done to image intraocular anatomy or to differentiate orbital lesions or disease. A-scan is a one-dimensional measurement procedure using high-frequency sound waves introduced into the eye in a straight line by a transducer placed on the eye. As the waves reflect off the eye tissue, they are picked up by the same transducer, converted to electrical pulses, and displayed on screen. The resulting single-dimensional image is composed of vertical spikes that vary according to the tissue density. Quantitative A-scan only is applied for this code. Quantitative A-scan provides information about a lesion's tissue structure, and reflective/sound absorptive properties.

76512

Diagnostic ophthalmic ultrasound, also called echography, is done to image intraocular anatomy or to differentiate orbital lesions or disease. B-scan utilizes sound waves in a two-dimensional scanning procedure to display a two-dimensional image of the internal ocular structures. A transducer placed on the eye sends high-frequency sound waves into the eye, which reflect back to a receiver, are converted into electrical pulses, and displayed on screen. B-scan can locate structures in the eye that may be obscured by cataract, hemorrhages, or opacities and provides information as to a lesion's shape, mobility, insertion, or relationship to neighboring structures. Diagnostic B-scan is applied for this code with or without superimposed non-quantitative A-scan. Superimposed non-quantitative A-scan may be topographical and can give more precise measurements along one parallel sound beam, and identify the borders or maximum height of the tumor.

76513

Diagnostic ophthalmic ultrasound, also called echography, is done to image intraocular anatomy or to differentiate orbital lesions or disease. Anterior eye segment ultrasound is accomplished using B-scan of 20 to 50 MHz. This high-frequency ultrasound imaging produces pictures of the eye that approach microscopic resolution (50 microns). B-scan utilizes sound waves in a two-dimensional scanning procedure to display a two-dimensional image of the internal ocular structures. A transducer sends high-frequency sound waves into the eye that reflect to a receiver, are converted into electrical pulses, and displayed on screen. In the immersion (water bath) method, the eye is maintained in direct contact with a water bath, using a special cup filled with saline solution inserted between the eyelids. The tip of the transducer is not in direct contact with the eye. This code reports a unilateral or bilateral exam.

76514

Diagnostic ophthalmic ultrasound is done to determine corneal thickness on one or both eyes by using corneal pachymetry, which is non-invasive and painless. Measuring the cornea is done by administrating a topical anesthetic into the eye and placing a plastic ultrasonic probe onto the central cornea. A pachymeter uses ultrasound to determine the thickness of the cornea in any given location. A short wave burst of sound is generated by a transmitter and sent through the eye tissue. The detector positioned close to the transmitter detects the echo. The echo reflected from near the surface reaches the detector faster than echoes reflected at lower-lying levels. The structure of the tissue, the thickness of the corneal structure at any given location, is determined on the basis of the echo's time distribution. Pachymetry is an essential measurement prior to certain surgical procedures, such as LASIK, that require removing tissue from the cornea. These measurements ascertain whether the cornea will retain enough thickness to prevent complications.

76516-76519

A-scan uses ultrasonography, or echography, to image intraocular anatomy to determine the axial length of the eye (from the cornea to the retina) for calculating the power required for an intraocular lens implant. High-frequency sound waves are introduced into the eye in a straight line by a transducer placed on the eye. As the waves reflect off the eye tissue, they are also picked up by the same transducer, converted to electrical pulses and displayed on screen. The resulting single-dimensional image is composed of vertical spikes that vary according to the tissue density. Report 76516 for ophthalmic measurements by ultrasound echography and 76519 if intraocular power lens calculation is done.

76529

B-scan utilizes sound waves in a two-dimensional scanning procedure to display a two-dimensional image of the internal ocular structures and ultrasonically locate a foreign body in the eye. A transducer placed on the eye sends high-frequency sound waves into the eye which reflect back to a receiver, are converted into electrical pulses, and displayed on screen. B-scan can also locate structures or objects in the eye that may be obscured by cataract, hemorrhages, or opacities.

76536

Diagnostic ultrasound is an imaging technique bouncing sound waves far above the level of human perception through interior body structures. The sound waves pass through different densities of tissue and reflect back to a receiving unit at varying speeds. The unit converts the waves to electrical pulses that are immediately displayed in picture form on screen. Real time scanning displays structure images and movement with time. This code reports ultrasound, real time with image documentation, for the soft tissues of the head and neck (e.g., thyroid, parathyroid).

76604

Diagnostic ultrasound is an imaging technique bouncing sound waves far above the level of human perception through interior body structures. The sound waves pass through different densities of tissue and reflect back to a receiving unit at varying speeds. The unit converts the waves to electrical pulses that are immediately displayed in picture form on screen. Real time scanning displays structure images and movement with time. This code reports ultrasound and real time for the chest, including the mediastinum.

76641-76642

Breast ultrasound is a noninvasive diagnostic imaging technique that produces images used to assess breast tissues. Ultrasound uses a transducer that sends out ultrasound waves at a frequency too high to be heard. The ultrasound transducer is placed on the skin, and the ultrasound waves move through different densities of breast tissue. The sound waves bounce off the tissues like an echo and return to the transducer. The transducer processes the reflected waves, which are then converted by a computer into an image of the breast tissues being examined. Real time scanning displays structure images and movement with time. Report 76641 for a complete ultrasound, which includes examination of all four quadrants of the breast, as well as the retroareolar region. Report 76642 for a limited ultrasound, which pays particular attention to one or more, but not all, of the elements described by 76641. Examination of the axilla is included in both codes, when performed.

76700-76705

Diagnostic ultrasound is an imaging technique bouncing sound waves far above the level of human perception through interior body structures. The sound waves pass through different densities of tissue and reflect back to a receiving unit at varying speeds. The unit converts the waves to electrical pulses that are immediately displayed in picture form on screen. Real time scanning displays structure images and movement with time. Report 76700 for ultrasound and real time of the entire abdomen and 76705 for a single quadrant or organ of the abdomen.

76706

Screening ultrasound of the abdominal aorta with real time image documentation is the imaging technique of bouncing sound waves far above the level of human perception through interior body structures. The sound waves pass through different densities of tissue and reflect back to a receiving unit at varying speeds. The unit converts the waves to electrical pulses that are immediately displayed in picture form on screen. Real time scanning gathers and displays structural images and movement with time. This procedure is used as a tool to evaluate for abdominal aortic aneurysms (AAA) by viewing how the flow of blood moves through the abdominal aorta, which shows defects within the artery typical for an AAA. The U.S. Preventive Services Task Force has suggested screening be performed on men ages 65 to 75 who are or have been smokers, as well as men age 60 and older with family history of AAA.

76770-76775

Diagnostic ultrasound is an imaging technique bouncing sound waves far above the level of human perception through interior body structures. The sound waves pass through different densities of tissue and reflect back to a receiving unit at varying speeds. The unit converts the waves to electrical pulses that are immediately displayed in picture form on screen. Real time scanning displays structure images and movement with time. Report 76770 for ultrasound and real time for a complete retroperitoneal exam that includes renal, aortic, and lymphatic structures and 76775 for a limited retroperitoneal exam.

76776

This code reports ultrasound of a transplanted kidney, with duplex Doppler studies. Diagnostic ultrasound is an imaging technique bouncing sound waves far above the level of human perception through interior body structures. The sound waves pass through different densities of tissue and reflect back to a receiving unit at varying speeds. The unit converts the waves to electrical pulses that are immediately displayed in picture form on screen. Duplex studies combine real time with Doppler, which uses the frequency shifts of the emitted waves against their echoes to measure velocity, such as for blood flow.

76800

Diagnostic ultrasound is an imaging technique bouncing sound waves far above the level of human perception through interior body structures. The sound waves pass through different densities of tissue and reflect back to a receiving unit at varying speeds. The unit converts the waves to electrical pulses that are immediately displayed in picture form on screen. Ultrasonography of the spinal canal and its contents includes imaging of the spinal cord, the vertebrae, and the intervertebral discs.

76801-76802

Diagnostic ultrasound is an imaging technique bouncing sound waves far above the level of human perception through interior body structures. The sound waves pass through different densities of tissue and reflect back to a receiving unit at varying speeds. The unit converts the waves to electrical pulses that are immediately displayed in picture form on screen. Real time scanning displays both two-dimensional structure images and movement with time. Use 76801 to report real time ultrasound, transabdominal, with image documentation on a pregnant uterus for fetal and maternal evaluation in the first trimester of a single or first gestation. This includes determining the number of fetuses and gestational sacs and taking their measurements, surveying the visible fetal and placental structure, assessing amniotic fluid volume and sac shape, and examining the maternal uterus and adnexa. Report 76802 for each additional gestation evaluation.

76805-76810

Diagnostic ultrasound is an imaging technique bouncing sound waves far above the level of human perception through interior body structures. The sound waves pass through different densities of tissue and reflect back to a receiving unit at varying speeds. The unit converts the waves to electrical pulses that are immediately displayed in picture form on screen. Real time scanning displays both two-dimensional structure images and movement with time. Use 76805 to report real time ultrasound, transabdominal, with image documentation on a pregnant uterus for fetal and maternal evaluation after the first trimester of a single or first gestation. This includes determining the number of fetuses and amniotic/chorionic sacs, taking measurements appropriate for gestational age, surveying intracranial, spinal, abdominal, and heart chamber anatomy as well as the insertion site of the umbilical cord and the location of the placenta, and assessing amniotic fluid and maternal adnexa. Report 76810 for each additional gestation evaluation.

76811-76812

Diagnostic ultrasound is an imaging technique bouncing sound waves far above the level of human perception through interior body structures. The sound waves pass through different densities of tissue and reflect back to a receiving unit at varying speeds. The unit converts the waves to electrical pulses that are immediately displayed in picture form on screen. Real time scanning displays both two-dimensional structure images and movement with time. Use 76811 to report real time ultrasound, transabdominal, with image documentation on a pregnant uterus for fetal and maternal evaluation plus detailed fetal anatomic examination of a single or first gestation. This includes determining the number of fetuses and amniotic/chorionic sacs, taking measurements appropriate for gestational age, and surveying intracranial, spinal, abdominal, and heart chamber anatomy plus a detailed evaluation of the brain and ventricles, face, heart and outflow tracts, chest, abdominal organs, and number, length, and structure of the limbs. Assessing amniotic fluid, maternal adnexa, and any other fetal anatomy is also done with a detailed evaluation of the umbilical cord and the placenta. Report 76812 for each additional gestation evaluation.

76813-76814

Fetal nuchal translucency provides a noninvasive method to screen for chromosomal abnormalities or heart defects in the first trimester. Nuchal pertains to the back of the neck. Until the lymphatic system of the fetus develops, the back of the neck is a good predictor of fetal health, because the fetus will lie on its back and edema will form in the neck if circulatory problems are present. In a fetal nuchal translucency test, ultrasound transducers on the maternal abdomen or vagina focus on the fetal neck, and the depth of tissue there is measured. The examination includes a calculation of fetal length, and the two measurements are correlated. Fetal nuchal edema does not provide a definitive diagnosis, but would warrant further testing (e.g., chorionic villus sampling). Report 76813 for fetal nuchal translucency testing of one fetus and 76814 for each additional fetus.

76815
Diagnostic ultrasound is an imaging technique bouncing sound waves far above the level of human perception through interior body structures. The sound waves pass through different densities of tissue and reflect back to a receiving unit at varying speeds. The unit converts the waves to electrical pulses that are immediately displayed in picture form on screen. Real time scanning displays both two-dimensional structure images and movement with time. Use 76815 to report real time ultrasound with image documentation on a pregnant uterus for a limited evaluation focused on the assessment of one or more of the following: fetal heartbeat, placental location, fetal position, and/or qualitative amniotic fluid volume for one or more fetuses.

76816
Diagnostic ultrasound is an imaging technique bouncing sound waves far above the level of human perception through interior body structures. The sound waves pass through different densities of tissue and reflect back to a receiving unit at varying speeds. The unit converts the waves to electrical pulses that are immediately displayed in picture form on screen. Real time scanning displays both two-dimensional structure images and movement with time. Use 76816 to report real time ultrasound, transabdominal, with image documentation on a pregnant uterus for a follow-up to reassess fetal size by measuring standard growth parameters and amniotic fluid volume, and to re-evaluate an organ system suspected or confirmed to be abnormal on a previous scan. Report 76816 per fetus evaluated.

76817
Diagnostic ultrasound is an imaging technique bouncing sound waves far above the level of human perception through interior body structures. The sound waves pass through different densities of tissue and reflect back to a receiving unit at varying speeds. The unit converts the waves to electrical pulses that are immediately displayed in picture form on screen. Real time scanning displays both two-dimensional structure images and movement with time. Use 76817 to report real time ultrasound on a pregnant uterus done transvaginally, with image documentation.

76818-76819
The health of a term or near-term fetus is assessed using ultrasound to monitor the fetus' movements, tone, and breathing, as well as to check amniotic fluid volume. The fetal heart rate is also monitored electronically in a biophysical profile. The physician conducts a non-stress test which monitors the baby's heart rate over a period of 20 minutes or more to look for accelerations with the baby's movement. Report 76819 if the fetal profile is done without non-stress testing.

76820-76821
Doppler ultrasonography, or echography, is performed for fetal surveillance to determine the velocity of blood flow through the umbilical artery (76820) or the middle cerebral artery (76821). Doppler works off the principle that when emitted sound waves reflect back off a moving object, the frequency of the reflected waves will vary in relation to the speed of the moving object. The frequency of sound waves bouncing back off moving blood cells is converted to the velocity of blood flow through the vessel and is seen on screen as a wave with peak, systole, and diastole. Velocity waveforms through the umbilical artery of a normally growing fetus are different from those of a growth-retarded fetus. The peak systolic velocity through the middle cerebral artery is inversely related to the amount of hematocrit in fetal blood. These tests determine the timing of labor induction and when fetal anemia is severe enough to require a transfusion. The ultrasound is carried out transabdominally or endovaginally.

76825-76826
Diagnostic ultrasound is an imaging technique bouncing sound waves far above the level of human perception through interior body structures. The sound waves pass through different densities of tissue and reflect back to a receiving unit at varying speeds. The unit converts the waves to electrical pulses that are immediately displayed in picture form on screen. These codes report fetal echocardiography, real time, with or without M-mode recording. Real time scanning displays both two-dimensional structure images and movement with time. M-mode is a single dimension method of recording amplitude and velocity of a moving structure producing the echoes being studied. Report 76825 for a complete evaluation of a fetal cardiovascular system and 76826 for a follow-up or repeat study.

76827-76828
Diagnostic ultrasound is an imaging technique bouncing sound waves far above the level of human perception through interior body structures. The sound waves pass through different densities of tissue and reflect back to a receiving unit at varying speeds. The unit converts the waves to electrical pulses that are immediately displayed in picture form on screen. These codes report fetal doppler echocardiography by pulsed or continuous sound wave. Fetal echocardiography is done to study the unborn baby's heart in much greater detail than is possible with a routine pregnancy ultrasound when the mother is at risk for giving birth to a baby with heart defects. Doppler echography uses the frequency shifts of the emitted waves against their echoes to measure velocity, such as for blood flow through the heart. Pulsed wave transmits and records from a single source to determine a precise site of signal origin but not high velocity. Continuous wave uses two transducers: one to continually transmit and the other to record. This scan determines high velocities. Report 76827 for a complete fetal echocardiographic evaluation and 76828 for a follow-up or repeat study.

76830
Diagnostic ultrasound is an imaging technique bouncing sound waves far above the level of human

perception through interior body structures. The sound waves pass through different densities of tissue and reflect back to a receiving unit at varying speeds. The unit converts the waves to electrical pulses that are immediately displayed in picture form on screen. This code reports transvaginal ultrasonography.

76831

Diagnostic ultrasound is an imaging technique bouncing sound waves far above the level of human perception through interior body structures. The sound waves pass through different densities of tissue and reflect back to a receiving unit at varying speeds. The unit converts the waves to electrical pulses that are immediately displayed in picture form on screen. This code reports saline infusion sonohysterography, with or without color flow Doppler. The addition of color flow Doppler monitors the behavior of a moving structure, such as flowing blood. The color image that is produced depicts the various levels of fluid concentration within a given area. In the case of saline infusion sonohysterography, a thin catheter, the size of uncooked spaghetti, is introduced into the cervical opening and into the uterus and one to two teaspoons of saline solution is injected into the uterine cavity. Fluid enhanced endovaginal ultrasound is done with the saline solution acting as a contrast medium to view any abnormal anatomic findings in the uterus that needs to be further evaluated. This code reports only the radiological supervision and interpretation.

76856-76857

Diagnostic ultrasound is an imaging technique bouncing sound waves far above the level of human perception through interior body structures. The sound waves pass through different densities of tissue and reflect back to a receiving unit at varying speeds. The unit converts the waves to electrical pulses that are immediately displayed in picture form on screen. Real time scanning displays both structure images and movement with time. Report 76856 for a complete pelvic evaluation in a patient who is not pregnant and 76857 for a limited or follow-up pelvic evaluation, for example, to monitor real time follicle development on the ovary to evaluate gonadotrophin therapy.

76870

Diagnostic ultrasound is an imaging technique bouncing sound waves far above the level of human perception through interior body structures. The sound waves pass through different densities of tissue and reflect back to a receiving unit at varying speeds. The unit converts the waves to electrical pulses that are immediately displayed in picture form on screen. This code reports ultrasonography of the scrotum and scrotal contents.

76872-76873

Diagnostic ultrasound is an imaging technique bouncing sound waves far above the level of human perception through interior body structures. The sound waves pass through different densities of tissue and reflect back to a receiving unit at varying speeds. The unit converts the waves to electrical pulses that are immediately displayed in picture form on screen. Report 76872 for transrectal ultrasound or echography for either sex; Report 76873 for a prostate volume evaluation for planning brachytherapy treatment, which involves planting tiny radioactive elements into a treatment area.

76881-76882

Diagnostic ultrasound is an imaging technique that bounces soundwaves far above the level of human perception through interior body structures. The soundwaves pass through different tissue densities and reflect back to a receiving unit at varying speeds. The unit converts the waves to electrical pulses that are immediately displayed in picture form on a screen. Real time scanning displays structure images and movement in real time. In 76881, ultrasonography of a complete joint (including joint space and other periarticular soft tissue structures) is performed. Report 76882 for a limited study of a joint or a focal evaluation of one or more nonvascular structures in an extremity other than a joint, such as a fluid collection, nerves, or a soft tissue mass. Imaging documentation is included in these services.

76883

Comprehensive ultrasonography of one or more nerves and accompanying structures in one extremity is performed throughout their entire anatomic course. Cross-sectional areas of a nerve are measured at various sites throughout the length of the limb, ratios are calculated, vascularity is checked, and echo intensity of affected muscles is evaluated. Patterns of peripheral nerve involvement are evaluated and cine loops (a series of rapidly recorded multiple images that are taken at sequential cycles of time and displayed on a monitor) are saved. Diagnostic ultrasound is an imaging technique that bounces soundwaves far above the level of human perception through interior body structures. The soundwaves pass through different tissue densities and reflect back to a receiving unit at varying speeds. The unit converts the waves to electrical pulses that are immediately displayed in picture form on a screen. Real-time cine imaging with image documentation is included. Report 76883 once per extremity.

76885-76886

Diagnostic ultrasound is an imaging technique bouncing sound waves far above the level of human perception through interior body structures. The sound waves pass through different densities of tissue and reflect back to a receiving unit at varying speeds. The unit converts the waves to electrical pulses that are immediately displayed in picture form on screen. Real time imaging displays two-dimensional structure images and movement with time. Report 76885 for dynamic ultrasonography of an infant's hips requiring physician or other qualified health care provider's manipulation involving compressing the leg at the knee and prying the hip outward as the sound wave transducer is applied to the hip area. Report 76886 for static ultrasonography of an infant's hips requiring the legs to be still while the sound wave transducer is applied to the hip area.

76932
The physician takes a biopsy of muscle tissue from within the heart guided by ultrasound. Ultrasound is an imaging technique bouncing sound waves far above the level of human perception through interior body structures. The sound waves pass through different densities of tissue and reflect back to a receiving unit, which converts the waves to electrical pulses that are immediately displayed in picture form on screen. The physician threads a biopsy catheter to the heart through a central intravenous line often inserted into the femoral vein and takes tissue samples of the heart's septum. This code reports the imaging supervision and interpretation only for this procedure.

76936
After sedation, the pseudoaneurysm or arteriovenous fistula is examined with a duplex scanner. The physician assesses the feasibility of compression repair by compressing the neck of the pseudoaneurysm. If the pseudoaneurysm can be completely ablated visually, therapeutic compression therapy is attempted. The physician applies directed pressure to ablate the pseudoaneurysm while blood flow is maintained. Continuous compression is maintained for 10-minute intervals (20-minute intervals if the patient is anticoagulated) until the pseudoaneurysm is thrombosed. If thrombosis has not occurred after four intervals, further attempts to noninvasively thrombose the aneurysm are usually abandoned. If successful ablation has occurred, the patient is kept flat in bed for 6-8 hours with a sandbag on the groin. At 24 hours, the patient is reexamined for evidence of pseudoaneurysm recurrence. At the completion of ablation, the arteries and veins are assessed for patency with the duplex scanner.

76937
This is an add-on code to report ultrasound guidance used in conjunction with procedures requiring vascular access. For example: a tunneled, centrally inserted CVAD is inserted without subcutaneous port or pump. The site over the access vein (e.g., subclavian, jugular) is injected with local anesthesia and punctured with a needle or accessed by cutdown approach. A guidewire is inserted. A subcutaneous tunnel is created using a blunt pair of forceps or sharp tunneling tools, over the clavicle from the anterior chest wall to the venotomy site, which is dilated to the right size. The catheter is passed through this tunnel over the guidewire and into the target vein. Report 76937 for the ultrasound guidance used for this procedure, including the evaluation of potential vascular access sites or the patency of selected vessels; guidance during needle entry and catheter manipulation; and verification of final catheter positioning. This code includes permanent recording and reporting.

76940
Ultrasound guidance is used during tissue ablation of a vital organ. Diagnostic ultrasound is an imaging technique bouncing sound waves far above the level of human perception through interior body structures. The sound waves pass through different densities of tissue and reflect back to a receiving unit at varying speeds. The unit converts the waves to electrical pulses that are immediately displayed in picture form on screen. Report this code when intraoperative ultrasound guidance and monitoring is done with laparoscopic or open ablation.

76941
The physician performs a blood transfusion to a fetus or inserts an amniocentesis needle through the abdominal wall into the umbilical vessels of the pregnant uterus and obtains fetal blood guided by ultrasound. Ultrasound is an imaging technique bouncing sound waves far above the level of human perception through interior body structures. The sound waves pass through different densities of tissue and reflect back to a receiving unit, which converts the waves to electrical pulses that are immediately displayed in picture form on screen. For fetal blood transfusion, the physician locates the umbilical vein. A needle is directed through the abdominal wall into the amniotic cavity. The umbilical vein is pierced and fetal blood is exchanged with transfused blood. This code reports the imaging supervision and interpretation only for this procedure.

76942
Ultrasonic guidance is used for guiding needle placement required for procedures such as breast biopsies, needle aspirations, injections, or placing localizing devices. Ultrasound is the process of bouncing sound waves far above the level of human perception through interior body structures. The sound waves pass through different densities of tissue and reflect back to a receiving unit at varying speeds. The unit converts the waves to electrical pulses that are immediately displayed in picture form on screen. Once the exact needle entry site is determined along with the depth of the lesion, the optimal route from the skin to the lesion is decided. The needle is inserted and advanced to the lesion under ultrasonic guidance. This code reports the imaging supervision and interpretation only for this procedure.

76945
The physician aspirates cells from the chorionic villus (early stage of the placenta) under ultrasonic guidance. Ultrasound is an imaging technique bouncing sound waves far above the level of human perception through interior body structures. The sound waves pass through different densities of tissue and reflect back to a receiving unit, which converts the waves to electrical pulses that are immediately displayed in picture form on screen. In the transcervical method, a catheter is inserted through the cervix and into the uterine cavity toward the chorionic villus or early placenta. Aspirated cells are obtained for abnormal chromosome analysis. The procedure may also be done transvaginally or transabdominally. The transabdominal approach can be done throughout pregnancy while the other approaches are usually

done between 9 and 12 weeks gestation. This code reports the imaging supervision and interpretation only for this procedure.

76946

The physician withdraws fluid from the amniotic sac under ultrasonic guidance. Ultrasound is an imaging technique bouncing sound waves far above the level of human perception through interior body structures. The sound waves pass through different densities of tissue and reflect back to a receiving unit, which converts the waves to electrical pulses that are immediately displayed in picture form on screen. Following preparation of the skin and administration of a local anesthetic, a small gauge needle is introduced into the amniotic sac and fluid aspirated. This code reports the imaging supervision and interpretation only for this procedure.

76948

The physician aspirates ova under ultrasonic guidance. Ultrasound is an imaging technique bouncing sound waves far above the level of human perception through interior body structures. The sound waves pass through different densities of tissue and reflect back to a receiving unit, which converts the waves to electrical pulses that are immediately displayed in picture form on screen. Following preparation of the skin and administration of a local anesthetic, a small gauge needle is introduced into the ovary and the ova are aspirated. This code reports the imaging supervision and interpretation only for this procedure.

76965

Ultrasonic guidance is used for the accurate guiding and placement of an interstitial radioactive implant into a tumor during the course of brachytherapy for malignant neoplasms, such as in the prostate. Ultrasound is an imaging technique bouncing sound waves far above the level of human perception through interior body structures. The sound waves pass through different densities of tissue and reflect back to a receiving unit, which converts the waves to electrical pulses that are immediately displayed in picture form on screen. Radioactive implants may be enclosed in various apparatus modes such as tubes, needles, wires, or seeds. Common materials used are radium, cobalt-60, cesium-137, gold-198, and iridium-192.

76975

The physician uses endoscopic ultrasound to examine the esophageal and gastric wall. Ultrasound is an imaging technique bouncing sound waves far above the level of human perception through interior body structures. The sound waves pass through different densities of tissue and reflect back to a receiving unit, which converts the waves to electrical pulses that are immediately displayed in picture form on screen. The physician passes an endoscope equipped with the ultrasound transducer through the patient's mouth into the esophagus. The esophagus, stomach, duodenum, and sometimes jejunum are viewed through ultrasonic images to determine the extent of cancerous tissue. This code reports the imaging supervision and interpretation only for this process.

76977

Bone mineral density studies are used to evaluate diseases of bone and/or the responses of bone disease to treatment. Densities are measured at the wrist, hip, spine, or calcaneus. The studies assess bone mass or density associated with such diseases as osteoporosis, osteomalacia, and renal osteodystrophy. This code reports using low level ultrasound for measuring bone density instead of ionizing radiation.

76978-76979

Contrast-enhanced ultrasound (CEUS) imaging using microbubbles as an intravascular contrast agent has shown to be extremely effective in measuring blood flow in the heart and other organs; imaging blood perfusion in organs; describing and defining lesions, particularly focal liver lesions; and evaluating therapy responses. Microbubbles are approximately the same size as a red blood cell and are made up of a gas (e.g., perfluoro gas) enclosed with a phospholipid shell and have the ability to reflect ultrasound waves, enhance the reflections of the ultrasound waves, and create a unique image. There is a variety of microbubble contrast agents that vary based on the shell and gas core composition, as well as whether they are targeted or untargeted. Currently, all FDA-approved microbubbles are considered "untargeted," meaning they are used in clinics today; "targeted" microbubbles are in preclinical development. The microbubbles are administered using a small bolus or via continuous intravenous infusion into the circulation system and remain in the bloodstream for about five minutes. The technician directs the ultrasound waves to the area being evaluated; once the microbubbles pass into the ultrasound waves, the microbubbles produce a "fingerprint-like" harmonic reverberating sound within the ultrasound field vastly different from surrounding tissue that can be detected using microbubble-specific software. The system subsequently produces a contrast-enhanced real-time image. Microbubbles as a contrast agent are better tolerated over MR and CT agents, do not have as many side-effects and, when present, the side effects are typically less severe, and are not as toxic to the kidneys. Report 76978 for the initial lesion targeted and 76979 for each additional lesion with separate injection.

76981-76983

Ultrasound elastography (USE), also known as sonoelastography, is a noninvasive imaging technique that can be used to measure and depict relative tissue stiffness (shear wave) or displacement (strain) in response to an imparted force. Although the most common clinical application for USE is for chronic liver disease, tumor identification using this imaging modality is also effective since tumors are usually stiffer, or less elastic, than the surrounding soft tissue. The ultrasound technician takes a normal image followed by an image while pushing down or compressing the organ area. This happens multiple times and the images are generated in real time by using algorithms to give a clearer picture of the motion of the tissue being imaged. Report 76981 for imaging of an organ; 76982 for the initial target lesion; and 76983 for each additional target lesion.

76984

Diagnostic epiaortic ultrasonography is used to evaluate the ascending aorta during a cardiac procedure and identify aspects of the procedure that may affect the intraoperative plan (e.g., change in bypass targets or cannulation strategy, identifying additional anomalies). It is often performed when other diagnostic modalities such as transesophageal echocardiography (TEE) or visual or manual inspection are not adequate. Ultrasound is an imaging technique that produces bouncing sound waves far above the level of human perception through interior body structures. The sound waves pass through different densities of tissue and reflect back to a receiving unit, which converts the waves to electrical pulses that are immediately displayed in picture form on a screen. A diagnostic epiaortic ultrasound examination may include the aortic arch, sinotubular junction, innominate artery origin, and the proximal, mid, and distal segments of the ascending aorta.

76987-76989

Diagnostic epicardial ultrasonography is used to evaluate cardiac structures for a patient with congenital heart disease during a cardiac procedure and identify aspects of the procedure that may affect the intraoperative plan (e.g., change in bypass targets or cannulation strategy, identifying additional anomalies). This type of cardiac ultrasound, or echocardiography, is often performed on pediatric or adult patients when a transesophageal echocardiography (TEE) is not feasible or is contraindicated. Ultrasound is an imaging technique that produces bouncing sound waves far above the level of human perception through interior body structures. The sound waves pass through different densities of tissue and reflect back to a receiving unit, which converts the waves to electrical pulses that are immediately displayed in picture form on a screen. An ultrasound probe is placed directly on the epicardial surface of the heart. The resulting two-dimensional image allows the provider to detect any residual or previously undetected cardiac defects in a patient with congenital heart disease. Report 76987 for placement and manipulation of the transducer, including obtaining images and interpretation and report; 76988 for placement and manipulation of the transducer and obtaining images only; and 76989 for interpretation and report only.

76998

Ultrasonography is used during a procedure to guide the physician in successfully accomplishing the surgery. Ultrasonic guidance may be used by the physician intraoperatively during many different types of operations on various areas of the body. Examples of intraoperative ultrasonic guidance include evaluating tissue removal in anatomical structures such as the breast, brain, abdominal organs, etc. This procedure may also be used to determine the location and depth of incisions to be made. This code is not to be used for ultrasound guidance for open or laparoscopic radiofrequency tissue ablation.

77001

This code reports the fluoroscopic guidance for placement, replacement, or removal of a central venous access device (CVAD) to be used in conjunction with the code for the procedure. For example, a tunneled, centrally inserted CVAD is inserted without subcutaneous port or pump. The site over the access vein (e.g., subclavian, jugular) is injected with local anesthesia and punctured with a needle or accessed by cutdown approach. A guidewire is inserted. A subcutaneous tunnel is created using a blunt pair of forceps or sharp tunneling tools over the clavicle from the anterior chest wall to the venotomy site, which is dilated to the right size. The catheter is passed through this tunnel over the guidewire and into the target vein. Fluoroscopy is used throughout the procedure to guide catheter placement and to check the positioning of the catheter tip. This code includes any contrast injections done through the access site or through the catheter with the necessary corresponding radiological supervision and interpretation of the venography, and the radiographic check of final catheter position.

77002

Fluoroscopic guidance produces x-ray images shown on a screen to assist in visualization of the anatomy, instrument insertion, and/or contrast. This code is specifically reported when utilized for needle biopsy or fine needle aspiration. A cutting biopsy or fine needle is inserted into the target area and the position reaffirmed by fluoroscopy. This is done for an internal mass or lesion that has been positively identified by other diagnostic imaging performed earlier.

77003

Spinal and certain paraspinal diagnostic or therapeutic nerve injection procedures (e.g., epidural or subarachnoid injections) are guided by fluoroscopy before and during catheter or needle insertion. The target structure is localized, the needle is placed and advanced, and the contrast injection is visualized under fluoroscopic monitoring.

77011

For stereotactic localization, a movable arm holding a needle is guided by computerized tomography (CT) to locate the lesion from different angles at different fixed points. The CT images tell the computer where the coordinates are to correctly align the needle.

77012

Computed tomography (CT) is used for guiding needle biopsies. CT scanning directs multiple narrow beams of x-rays around the body structure being studied and uses computer imaging to produce thin cross-sectional views of various layers (or slices) of the body. It is able to visualize soft tissue, as well as bones. Patients are required to remain motionless during the study. Once the exact needle entry site is determined, along with the depth of the lesion, the optimal route from the skin to the lesion is decided. The needle is inserted and advanced to the lesion and another CT scan image is done to confirm placement for the biopsy. This code reports the radiological supervision and interpretation only for this procedure.

77013

Computed tomographic guidance is used for the ablation of parenchymal (vital organ) tissue. The patient receives intravenous pain medication and sedation. Grounding pads are placed on the patient's thigh. A needle-electrode with an insulated shaft and a noninsulated distal tip is inserted through the skin and directly into the tissue to be ablated. Computed tomography (CT) is used to guide the needle to the correct spot and to monitor treatment. Each treatment session has about 10 to 15 minutes of active ablation. The energy at the needle tip causes ionic agitation and frictional heat in the surrounding tissue, which leads to cell death and coagulative necrosis. This results in a 3 to 5 cm sphere of dead tissue per treatment session. In large tumors, the physician may create more than one sphere next to each other to try to turn the tumor edges in three dimensions. A small margin of normal tissue next to tumors is also burned. The dead tumor cells are not removed, but are gradually replaced by fibrosis and scar tissue. This code reports the CT guidance and monitoring of the ablation procedure.

77014

Computed tomography (CT) is used in guiding the placement of radiation therapy fields. CT scanning directs multiple narrow beams of x-rays around the body structure being studied and uses computer imaging to produce thin cross-sectional views of various layers (or slices) of the body. It is able to visualize soft tissue, as well as bones. Patients are required to remain motionless during the study. Cross-sectional images of both normal and abnormal tissue structures are obtained and the treatment field area volume is determined. The normal tissues surrounding the treatment area are also defined. Acquiring this data is an important step in planning the patient's radiation treatment.

77021

Magnetic resonance imaging guidance is used for guiding needle placement required for procedures such as breast biopsies, needle aspirations, injections, or placing localizing devices. Magnetic resonance imaging (MRI) guidance offers a radiation-free, noninvasive technique that produces high-quality images. MRI uses the natural magnetic properties of the hydrogen atoms in our bodies that emit radiofrequency signals when exposed to radiowaves within a strong electromagnetic field. These signals are processed and converted by the computer into high-resolution, three-dimensional, tomographic images. Some methods for magnetic resonance needle placement include coating the needle with contrast material, placing metallic ringlets along the needle, or using a receiving coil in the tip of the needle. This code reports the radiological supervision and interpretation only for this procedure.

77022

A needle electrode with an insulated shaft and a noninsulated distal tip is inserted through the skin and directly into the tissue to be ablated. Magnetic resonance imaging (MRI) guidance is used to guide the needle to the correct spot and to monitor treatment. Each treatment session has about 10 to 15 minutes of active ablation of parenchymal (vital organ) tissue. The energy at the needle tip causes ionic agitation and frictional heat in the surrounding tissue, which leads to cell death and coagulative necrosis. This results in a 3 to 5 cm sphere of dead tissue per treatment session. In large tumors, the physician may create more than one sphere next to each other to try to turn the tumor edges in three dimensions. A small margin of normal tissue next to tumors is also burned. The dead tumor cells are not removed, but are gradually replaced by fibrosis and scar tissue. This code reports the magnetic resonance imaging guidance and monitoring of the ablation procedure.

77046-77047

Magnetic resonance imaging (MRI) is a radiation-free, noninvasive technique to produce high-quality sectional images of the inside of the body in multiple planes. MRI uses the natural magnetic properties of the hydrogen atoms in our bodies that emit radiofrequency signals when exposed to radiowaves within a strong electromagnetic field. These signals are processed and converted by the computer into high-resolution, three-dimensional, tomographic images. Patients with metallic or electronic implants or foreign bodies cannot be exposed to MRI. The patient must remain still while lying on a motorized table within the large, circular MRI tunnel and a sedative may be administered. Report 77046 for magnetic resonance imaging of one breast and 77047 for both breasts.

77048-77049

Computer-aided detection (CAD) software is used with breast magnetic resonance imaging (MRI), a radiation-free, noninvasive technique that produces high-quality sectional images of the inside of the body in multiple planes. MRI uses the natural magnetic properties of the hydrogen atoms in the body that emit radiofrequency signals when exposed to radiowaves within a strong electromagnetic field. These signals are processed and converted by the computer into high-resolution, three-dimensional, tomographic images. Patients with metallic or electronic implants or foreign bodies cannot be exposed to MRI. The patient must remain still while lying on a motorized table within the large, circular MRI tunnel. A sedative may be administered, as well as an IV injected contrast material for image enhancement. The use of a CAD system allows breast images to be converted into digital form; the software scans the images, looking for any areas of abnormality such as density, calcifications, or a mass, and alerts the radiologist who can then notify the referring physician of the need for additional evaluation. Report 77048 for magnetic resonance imaging of one breast and 77049 for both breasts.

77053-77054

The physician performs an injection procedure for mammary ductogram or galactogram. A needle and cannula are inserted into the duct of the breast. Contrast medium is introduced into the breast duct for the radiographic visualization. A dissecting microscope may be used to aid in placing the cannula. The needle and cannula are removed when the study is complete. Report 77053 for a single duct studied and 77054 for multiple ducts. These codes report the radiological supervision and interpretation only for this procedure.

77061-77063

Digital breast tomosynthesis technology (DBT) is rapidly being implemented as it provides a higher diagnostic accuracy compared to conventional mammography. It is also referred to as three-dimensional (3D) mammography, which creates a three-dimensional picture of the breast from many angles using low-dose x-rays. The breast is positioned in a similar fashion to a conventional mammogram, with slightly less compression, while a scanner rotates around the breast in an arc formation. Several images, usually between 10 and 15, are taken over approximately seven seconds. While more images are taken, DBT does not require any more radiation than conventional mammography. Once the images have been taken, computer programs produce clear and highly-focused 3D representations of the breast that the radiologist can then view as thin layers of breast tissue, similar to CT scan images. This technology allows for greater accuracy, easier identification of abnormalities, better morphological analysis of masses and architectural distortions, and a reduction in callbacks for additional testing. Report 77061 when DBT is performed on one breast and 77062 when DBT is performed on both breasts. Report 77063 for bilateral screening DBT performed in addition to a primary procedure.

77065-77066

Diagnostic mammography is a radiographic technique used to diagnose breast cysts or tumors in women with symptoms of breast disease. Mammography is done using a different type of x-ray than is used for routine exams that do not penetrate tissue as easily. The breast is compressed firmly between two planes and pictures are taken. This spreads the tissue and allows for a lower x-ray dose. When performed in conjunction with a diagnostic mammogram, computer-aided detection (CAD) utilizes the x-ray taken of the breast, scans the analog mammography film with a laser beam, and analyzes the video display for suspicious areas, most often converting it into digital data for the computer first. The patient does not need to be present for the CAD process. Report 77065 for a unilateral diagnostic mammogram including CAD, when performed and 77066 when performed on both breasts.

77067

Screening bilateral mammography is a radiographic technique used to detect breast cysts or tumors before they are palpable in women who are asymptomatic. Mammography is done using a different type of x-ray than is used for routine exams that do not penetrate tissue as easily. The breasts are compressed firmly between two planes and two views of each breast are taken. The planes spread the breast tissue and allows for a lower x-ray dose. When performed in conjunction with a screening mammogram, computer-aided detection (CAD) utilizes the x-ray taken of the breasts, scans the analog mammography film with a laser beam, and analyzes the video display for any suspicious areas, most often converting it into digital data for the computer first. The patient does not need to be present for the CAD process.

77071

Joint radiography is done under manual stress application conditions performed by the physician or other qualified health care provider to visualize characteristics of the joint that would not normally be seen on films taken in routine positioning. The provider puts on lead-lined gloves and forcibly holds the body part in the desired position to maintain stress on the joint while x-rays are taken. This code includes radiography of the contralateral joint, if indicated.

77072

Bone age studies are a way of estimating the stage of development or skeletal decline of a child based on an x-ray, usually of the nondominant hand and wrist. The x-ray is compared to the bone structure standards equal to the child's chronological age. This allows for identifying growth failure and the need for treatment before the child's bones fuse, after which additional growth is not possible. For children younger than age 3, films of multiple areas (e.g., wrist, knee, and foot) lead to greater accuracy.

77073

Bone length studies accurately measure the length of the long bones in the skeleton. Typically, four film exposures are performed during a scanogram, as it is usually called. Views of the hip, leg, knee, and ankle are usually taken. However, there is no number or type of views specified for this code.

77074

Various bones in the body are x-rayed. A limited study is reported when specific symptomatic sites are examined. This procedure is rarely performed to determine any spread of cancer, having been replaced by nuclear bone scanning, a more precise study for diagnosing metastases.

77075

A radiologic exam is performed in which the axial (head and trunk) and appendicular (extremities) skeleton is surveyed for evidence of metastatic disease. It may also be performed on children to identify current and/or old healed fractures in the case of suspected child abuse. This procedure is rarely performed for metastatic disease, having been replaced by nuclear bone scanning, a more precise study for diagnosing metastases.

77076
A radiologic exam is performed in which an infant's axial (head and trunk) and appendicular (extremities) skeleton is surveyed for evidence of current and/or old healed fractures in the case of suspected child abuse or to identify signs of lesions due to leukemic infiltrates.

77077
A radiologic exam is done in which two or more joints are surveyed. A single view only is taken of the joints being examined. The joints surveyed require specification and are not delineated in the code.

77078
A CT density study is performed to measure the patient's bone mass. Bone mineral density is evaluated as a screening test for osteoporosis, to evaluate diseases of bone, and to review the responses of bone disease to treatment. Densities can be measured at the wrist, hip, spine, or calcaneus. The studies assess bone mass or density associated with such diseases as osteoporosis, osteomalacia, and renal osteodystrophy. This particular bone density study uses computerized tomography (CT) for the imaging modality. CT directs multiple, narrow beams of x-rays around the body structure being studied and uses computer imaging to produce thin cross-sectional views of various layers (or slices) of the body.

77080-77081 [77085]
Dual-energy x-ray absorptiometry (DXA) is an enhanced form of x-ray technology that is performed to measure bone mineral density (BMD). BMD is evaluated as a screening test for osteoporosis, to evaluate diseases of bone, and to review the responses of bone disease to treatment. Densities can be measured at the wrist, radius, hip, pelvis, spine, or heel. DXA is a two-dimensional projection system that involves two x-ray beams with different levels of energy: one beam is high energy while the other is low energy, being pulsed alternately. The results are given in two scores reported as standard deviations from bone density of a person 30 years of age, which is the age of peak bone mass. Report 77080 for DXA of the hips, pelvis, or spine (axial skeleton); 77081 for DXA of peripheral bones, such as the wrist or heel bone (appendicular skeleton); and 77085 for a study conducted on the hips, pelvis, or spine (axial skeleton), including fracture assessment.

[77086]
Dual-energy x-ray absorptiometry (DXA) is an enhanced form of x-ray technology that is performed to measure bone mineral density (BMD). DXA is a two-dimensional projection system that involves two x-ray beams with different levels of energy: one beam is high energy while the other is low energy, being pulsed alternately. The results are given in two scores reported as standard deviations from bone density of a person 30 years of age, which is the age of peak bone mass. This study is specific for assessing fractures occurring in the vertebra.

77084
Magnetic resonance imaging (MRI) is a radiation-free, noninvasive technique to produce high-quality sectional images of the inside of the body in multiple planes. MRI uses the natural magnetic properties of the hydrogen atoms in our bodies that emit radiofrequency signals when exposed to radio waves within a strong electromagnetic field. The signals are transformed into images based on the differing densities of tissues. Bone marrow contains fat cells, with high water content, and nonfat cells. MRI can give information about early changes in the marrow of the bone and the medullary cavity's composition and distribution of red and yellow marrow cells to evaluate for avascular necrosis of bone. Metastatic tumors are visualized directly because of the differences in signal intensity between normal bone marrow and tumor tissue.

77089-77092
The trabecular bone score (TBS) is a diagnostic software tool that analyzes the internal structure of the lumbar spine bones. It is used in conjunction with dual-energy x-ray absorptiometry (DXA), which is an enhanced form of x-ray technology that is performed to measure bone mineral density (BMD). TBS uses standard DXA lumbar spine images to measure the structure of trabecular (cancellous) bone, providing additional information to be used in conjunction with BMD results in calculating fracture risk. Using a software program installed on a standard DXA computer, TBS provides an index of bone structure and quality without requiring additional radiation exposure or scan time. Report 77089 for TBS using DXA or other imaging data on grayscale variogram, calculation, and interpretation/report on fracture risk. Report 77090 for the technical preparation and transmission of data for an analysis to be performed elsewhere. Report 77091 for the technical calculation only. Report 77092 for the interpretation and report on fracture risk only by a qualified health care professional.

77261-77263
Treatment planning is conducted for radiation therapy. Treatment planning for oncology patients is the process of developing a complete plan for the course of radiation therapy. The best way to deliver the treatment to the malignancy while blocking the dose received by normal tissues must be determined. This requires localizing the tumor, determining its extent of malignancy and the volume to be treated, choosing the best method of treatment, the number and size of treatment ports, and calculating time and dosage among other procedures. A port is the site where the treatment beam will enter the skin and concentrate upon the malignant area(s). Simple planning, reported in 77261, consists of a single area of malignancy with a single port or opposing ports parallel to each other and basic or no blocking. Intermediate planning, reported in 77262, consists of two separate areas of

malignancy with three or more ports that converge, multiple blocks, or time or dosage considerations. Complex planning, reported in 77263, consists of three or more separate areas of malignancy with tangential ports, wedges or compensators, complex blocking, a combination of two or more modes of treatment, or rotating or other beam considerations.

77280-77290

Simulation-aided field setting is done prior to beginning the course of radiation treatment. This is done to determine the size and location of the ports to be used so that they surround the tumor. A port is the site where the treatment beam will enter the skin and concentrate upon the malignant area(s). Simulation can be done on a dedicated simulator, a radiation therapy treatment unit, an x-ray machine, or CT scanner. Simulation allows visualization and definition of the exact treatment area(s). Simple simulation, reported in 77280, is done for a single area of malignancy with a single port or opposing ports parallel to each other and basic or no blocking. Intermediate simulation, reported in 77285, is done for two separate areas of malignancy with three or more ports and multiple blocks. Complex simulation, reported in 77290, is done for three or more areas of malignancy with tangential ports and complex blocking that may require customized shielding blocks, rotation or arc therapy, brachytherapy source and hyperthermia probe verification, and use of contrast materials.

77293

Treatment of patients with certain thoracic, abdominal, and pelvic tumors present challenges posed by respiratory motion during external-beam radiation therapy. Prior to application of radiation, the motion of the tumor should be measured when respiratory motion is a concern or when the management of the movement may spare healthy tissue. Measurements are taken using ultrasound, CT, MRI, or fluoroscopy during defined respiratory conditions, including but not limited to motion-encompassing methods, respiratory-gated techniques, breath-hold techniques, forced shallow-breathing methods, and respiration-synchronized techniques. These measurements are used to adjust the radiation application area based on the motion of the tumor and healthy surrounding tissue.

[77295]

Three-dimensional (3-D) radiotherapy planning is done prior to beginning the course of radiation treatment. Using 3-D imaging and planning, the treatment team determines the type of radiation and the dosage that will provide optimal treatment while preserving healthy tissue. The physician chooses the energy level and modality of photon or electron beams to be used for each simulated port, even if only one treatment area is concerned. Once the tentative treatment fields have been determined, the dosimetry of the treatment portals can be calculated.

77300

Dosimetry is the calculation of the radiation dose to be delivered to the tumor. The physician chooses the energy level and modality of photon or electron beams to be used for each simulated port, even if only one treatment area is concerned. Once the tentative treatment fields have been determined, the dosimetry of the treatment portals can be calculated. A basic radiation dosimetry calculation is a photon calculation that includes central axis depth dose, time dose factor (TDF), nominal standard dose (NSD), gap calculation, off-axis and tissue inhomogeneity factors, as well as calculation of nonionizing radiation surface and depth dose. Dosimetry may be repeated during the course of treatment as required.

77301

Intensity modulated radiotherapy (IMRT) is capable of varying the intensity of radiation exposure in a portion of a field depending on whether tumor or critical normal structures are present in the beam pathway. The radiation therapy consists of multiple pencil thin beams or beamlets, calculated to hit tumors with high dose radiation beams and sensitive normal tissues with modulated lower intensity beams, leaving them mostly unaffected. Planning for IMRT uses powerful computer programs that calculate the optimal arrangement of beam angle configurations and dosage intensities to deliver the best treatment. If the isodose distribution for target and critical structure partial tolerance specification and dose-volume histograms are not satisfactory, the optimization is repeated with modifications to clinical parameters, until an acceptable solution is reached.

77306-77307

For the initial setting of the treatment portals, an isodose distribution of the beams is required. Usually done by computer, a teletherapy isodose plan plots the lines of the same dosage levels to be delivered within the treatment field, usually from a combination of beams converging upon the treatment field. Only one plan may be reported per any therapy course to a specific treatment field. A simple teletherapy isodose plan, reported in 77306, consists of one or two unmodified ports directed to a single area of interest. A complex teletherapy isodose plan, reported in 77307, consists of multiple treatment areas, tangential ports, blocking, the use of wedges, and rotating or special beam considerations. Both of these codes include basic dosimetry calculations.

77316-77318

Brachytherapy is the application of radioactive isotopes for internal radiation therapy that is used to treat cancer. Some radioactive material is encapsulated in metal seeds, wires, tubes, or needles for intracavitary or interstitial implantation and some are prepared in solutions for instillation or oral administration. Sealed sources are inserted by the physician in or around the tumor. Sources are intracavitary or permanent interstitial placements and ribbons are temporary interstitial placements. Brachytherapy gives greater control over localized malignancy while preserving function and reducing damage to surrounding tissue. Brachytherapy isodose plans are necessary to determine the amount of radiation that the tumor will absorb and the distribution of radiation around the sources. Report 77316 for a simple calculation made from one to four sources/ribbons or remote afterloading, one channel. Report 77317 for an intermediate calculation made from five to 10 sources/ribbons or remote afterloading, two to 12 channels. Report 77318 for a complex calculation made from more than 10 sources/ribbons or remote afterloading, more than 12 channels. These codes include basic dosimetry calculations.

77321
Special teletherapy port plans are usually done in connection with a complex level of treatment. These are electron calculations and cannot be submitted for the same field with a basic radiation dosimetry calculation, which is photon. Electron beams require attention because of their characteristics in interacting with living tissue. A special teletherapy port plan calculates the dosage level of the treatment portal for the use of electrons or heavy particles when used in a portion of or as the main mode of treatment for the field of interest.

77331
Dosimetry is the calculation of the radiation dose to be delivered to the tumor. The physician chooses the energy level and modality of photon or electron beams to be used for each simulated port, even if only one treatment area is concerned. Once the tentative treatment fields have been determined, the dosimetry of the treatment portals can be calculated. Special dosimetry uses measuring and monitoring devices when the physician deems it necessary to calculate the total amount of radiation that a patient has received at any given point. The results determine whether to uphold or alter the current treatment plan.

77332-77334
Treatment devices used in radiation oncology are customized blocks or shields to protect healthy tissue surrounding the treatment area and are made from energy-absorbing material such as cerrobend. Treatment device services contain a professional and technical component. The professional component is based upon the physician's participation in the actual design of the block. The technical component is based on each individual block requiring time and materials to be fabricated. 77332 reports a simple block; 77333 reports intermediate device services for multiple blocks; 77334 reports complex, irregular blocks, shields, compensators, wedges, molds, or casts.

77336
This code reports ongoing medical physics consultation services to benefit patients undergoing radiation therapy. It includes quality assurance of dose delivery such as verification of dose calculation data, measuring for safe and effective use of software and equipment such as simulators, linear accelerators, and block devices. It also includes assessment of treatment parameters and review of treatment documentation, reported weekly during therapy.

77338
A multi-leaf collimator (MLC) device is used in conjunction with the delivery of intensity modulated radiation therapy (IMRT). Multi-leaf collimators are devices that are composed of individual 'leaves" of a material, often tungsten, that can block a particle beam by moving independently in and out of the beam's path. Used on linear accelerators, MLCs provide conformal shaping of the radiotherapy treatment beams. Code 77338 reports the design and construction of the MLC device based upon the IMRT plan and should be reported only once per IMRT plan.

77370
A special medical radiation physics consultation requires a written analysis on the course of treatment and is done at direct request of the radiation oncologist when the complexity of the treatment plan is great. Problems analyzed may include photon and electron treatment plans and their consequences, complex dosage calculations because of interactions between multiple treatment fields, intensity modulating radiation, total body irradiation, blocking procedures, or stereotactic or brachytherapy services.

77371-77372
Stereotactic radiosurgery (SRS) is a radiation therapy technique designed to deliver a large radiation dose to discrete cranial lesion sites, while minimizing damage to healthy tissue. Indications may include neoplasms (benign or malignant) of the brain, cranial nerves, and/or meninges; arteriovenous malformations (AVMs) of the cerebral vessels; and non-neoplastic conditions such as trigeminal neuralgia, Parkinson's disease, and essential or other disabling tremor. Computers have previously mapped the exact location of the targeted cranial region. The patient's head is precisely positioned and immobilized by a headframe or frameless, image-based immobilization and localization device so that the radiation can be aimed accurately from several directions. Radiation is delivered to one or more cranial sites. Report 77371 for a single session that is multi-source Cobalt 60 based and 77372 for a single session that is linear accelerator (LINAC) based. These codes report a complete course of treatment, given in a single day, for one or more cranial lesions and are not reported for cranial SRS treatments specified as fractionated.

77373
Fractionated stereotactic body radiation therapy (SBRT) is a radiation therapy technique designed to deliver a large radiation dose to discrete tumor sites anywhere in the body, while minimizing damage to healthy tissue. Computers have previously mapped the exact location of the tumor. The body part has been immobilized with a plastic mold/cast or a headframe to keep the targeted area still so that the radiation can be aimed accurately from several directions. Report 77373 exclusively for any SRBT or stereotactic radiosurgery

(SRS) delivery specified as fractionated, including the first fraction, regardless of the anatomic location. This includes SRS treatment of a cranial lesion that requires more than a single session (but no more than five sessions), and one to five sessions for non-cranial lesions.

77401

Radiation treatment delivery involves the delivery of a beam of radioactive electromagnetic energy onto cancerous cells within the body from a treatment machine distanced from the treatment area. External radiation is often delivered by linear accelerator (also called as LINAC), which can deliver x-rays (photon radiation) or electrons (particle radiation) to a targeted area. Cobalt teletherapy units and cesium teletherapy units are also used to direct gamma rays from a distance to the targeted area. Photons can target deeper lying tumor tissue, while electrons are used for the maximum dose of radiation near the skin surface, making the method suitable to treat skin, superficial lesions, and shallow tumor volumes where underlying tissues need to be protected. Radiation treatment delivery codes are dependent upon the number and complexity of treatment areas, as well as the energy level. Use this code to report superficial and/or orthovoltage energy levels, which are kilovoltage doses and usually treat superficial skin lesions. This code is reported per day.

77402

Radiation treatment delivery involves the delivery of a beam of radioactive electromagnetic energy onto cancerous cells within the body from a treatment machine distanced from the treatment area. External radiation is often delivered by linear accelerator (also called LINAC), which can deliver x-rays (photon radiation) or electrons (particle radiation) to a targeted area. Cobalt teletherapy units and cesium teletherapy units are also used to direct gamma rays from a distance to the targeted area. Photons can target deeper lying tumor tissue, while electrons are used for the maximum dose of radiation near the skin surface, making the method suitable to treat skin, superficial lesions, and shallow tumor volumes where underlying tissues need to be protected. This code is used to report simple treatment delivery for a single treatment area, one to two ports, and two or less simple blocks.

77407

Radiation treatment delivery involves the delivery of a beam of radioactive electromagnetic energy onto cancerous cells within the body from a treatment machine distanced from the treatment area. External radiation is often delivered by linear accelerator (also called LINAC), which can deliver x-rays (photon radiation) or electrons (particle radiation) to a targeted area. Cobalt teletherapy units and cesium teletherapy units are also used to direct gamma rays from a distance to the targeted area. Photons can target deeper lying tumor tissue, while electrons are used for the maximum dose of radiation near the skin surface, making the method suitable to treat skin, superficial lesions, and shallow tumor volumes where underlying tissues need to be protected. This code is used to report intermediate treatment delivery for two distinct treatment areas, three or more ports for a single treatment area, or three or more simple blocks.

77412

Radiation treatment delivery involves the delivery of a beam of radioactive electromagnetic energy onto cancerous cells within the body from a treatment machine distanced from the treatment area. External radiation is often delivered by linear accelerator (also called LINAC), which can deliver x-rays (photon radiation) or electrons (particle radiation) to a targeted area. Cobalt teletherapy units and cesium teletherapy units are also used to direct gamma rays from a distance to the targeted area. Photons can target deeper lying tumor tissue, while electrons are used for the maximum dose of radiation near the skin surface, making the method suitable to treat skin, superficial lesions, and shallow tumor volumes where underlying tissues need to be protected. This code is used to report complex treatment delivery for three or more distinct treatment areas, custom-made blocks, tangential ports, wedges, rotating beams, and field-within-field or other compensation not meeting IMRT or electron beam treatment parameters.

77417

Therapeutic radiology port images are taken at regular intervals to verify correct positioning of all treatment portals on patients undergoing external beam radiation therapy, since discrepancies in the field placements can happen frequently and this negatively affects the treatment outcomes. The beam of the radiation treatment machine is used to make radiographic portal images. Portal images like a snapshot are taken for localization with a partial dose or recorded for the treatment for verification. Port image charges are a technical service only.

[77385, 77386]

Intensity modulated radiation therapy (IMRT) is an advanced mode of high-precision radiotherapy that enables radiation oncologists to precisely target and attack cancerous tumors with higher doses of radiation using strategically positioned beams while minimizing collateral damage to healthy cells. The radiation therapy consists of multiple, pencil thin beams or beamlets calculated to hit tumors with high-dose radiation and sensitive normal tissues with modulated, lower-intensity beams, leaving them mostly unaffected. By dividing the radiation beam into multiple slices, the intensity of the beam in any slice can be varied by computer-controlled dynamic multileaf collimation (MLC) during the radiation exposure. MLC systems consist of multiple narrow leaves that are modulated under computer control and allow custom-shaped beam apertures without fabricated blocks. During IMRT delivery, the leaves of the MLC are adjusted while the beam is on to modify the delivery of radiation across the portal. Report 77385 for simple treatment delivery and 77386 for complex treatment delivery.

[77387]

Radiation treatment delivery involves the transfer of a beam of radioactive electromagnetic energy onto cancerous cells within the body from a treatment machine distanced from the treatment area. Stereotactic body radiation therapy is a radiation therapy technique designed to deliver a large radiation dose to discrete tumor sites in the lungs, liver, brain, or elsewhere while minimizing damage to healthy tissue. Stereoscopic x-ray guidance utilizes infrared and/or camera technology to precisely localize targets in conjunction with intensity modulated radiation therapy and stereotactic radiotherapy. This code reports the guidance for localization of target volume of radiation treatment and includes intrafraction tracking, when performed.

[77424-77425]

Radiation treatment delivery involves the delivery of a beam of radioactive electromagnetic energy from a treatment machine distanced from the treatment area. Intraoperative radiation therapy (IORT) is often delivered by a miniature, mobile linear accelerator, which can deliver x-rays (photons) or electrons to a targeted area. Photons can target deeper lying tumor tissue, while electrons are used for the maximum dose of radiation near the surface, making the method suitable to treat skin, superficial lesions, and shallow tumor volumes where underlying tissues need to be protected. IORT isolates concentrated radiation to target tumors, leaving normal tissue unscathed, while a tumor is exposed during surgery. These codes represent a single radiation treatment session. Report 77424 for x-ray (photon) radiation therapy and 77425 for electron radiation therapy.

77423

External beam radiotherapy is radiation delivered from a distant source outside the body and directed at the patient's cancer site. High-energy neutron radiotherapy destroys the cells ability to divide and grow by damaging the cells through nuclear interactions, which decreases the damaged cells chances of repairing themselves. Since high-energy neutron radiotherapy works in the absence of oxygen, unlike conventional radiation therapy, it is used to treat larger tumors and is particularly effective in treating inoperable salivary gland tumors, bone cancers, and certain types of advanced malignancies of the pancreas, bladder, lung, prostate, and uterus. Due to the high potency of neutron radiation, the required dose is much less than with conventional radiotherapy, and a full course may be delivered in 10 to 12 treatments rather than the usual 30 to 40. This service includes treatment of one or more isocenters with coplanar or noncoplanar geometry with blocking and/or wedge and/or compensator(s).

77427

The physician reviews the port films. The dosimetry, dose delivery, and treatment parameters are reviewed. Treatment setup and positioning of the patient is evaluated including the assessment of immobilization devices, blocks, wedges, or other devices. The physician also provides care of infected skin, prescribes necessary medications, and manages fluid and electrolytes as well as pain management. Nutritional counseling may be provided as necessary. This radiation treatment management code is accurately reported using units of five fractions or treatment sessions. This code is reported at the completion of each five sessions with the exception of the completion of the treatment course when it may be used for three or more sessions.

77431

The physician reviews the port films. The dosimetry, dose delivery, and treatment parameters are reviewed. The treatment setup and positioning of the patient is evaluated including the assessment of immobilization devices, blocks, wedges, or other devices. The physician also provides care of infected skin, prescribes necessary medications, manages fluid and electrolytes as well as pain management. Nutritional counseling may be provided as necessary. This radiation treatment management code is used when the course of therapy consists of only one or two fractions (treatment sessions), excepting single application brachytherapy which does not require management.

77432

This service involves using multiple megavoltage treatment ports that are directed to a specific area within the brain. When a linear accelerator is used, the extremely narrow x-ray beam from the machine remains focused on the tumor volume of the cranial lesion while the movement of the machine is coordinated to distribute the beam entry points over a wider radius. Stereotactic treatment delivery requires three-dimensional simulation for accuracy. This code is for a complete course of treatment consisting of one session and reports the radiation oncology services performed as part of the stereotactic radiosurgery procedure.

77435

Stereotactic body radiation therapy (SBRT) is a radiation therapy technique designed to deliver a large radiation dose to discrete tumor sites within the body (excluding brain) while minimizing damage to healthy tissue. This code reports treatment management for a course of SBRT. Treatment management includes review of port films; review of dosimetry, dose delivery, and treatment parameters; treatment set up; positioning of the patient; assessment of immobilization devices, blocks or wedges; ongoing evaluation of the patient's response to treatment; coordination of care; and ordering and review of laboratory or other tests.

77469

The physician reviews the port films. The dosimetry, dose delivery, and treatment parameters are reviewed. Treatment setup and positioning of the patient are evaluated, including the assessment of immobilization devices, blocks, wedges, or other devices. This radiation treatment management code is accurately reported for only the intraoperative radiation management and does not include medical evaluation and management occurring outside of the operative session.

77470

This service covers the extra planning and monitoring effort involved in the use of special radiation therapy procedures, such as total or hemibody irradiation given via oral or endocavitary methods.

77520-77525

Protons are positively charged particles that are particularly beneficial in treating malignancies and other neoplastic abnormalities near sensitive structures such as the optic nerve and spinal cord. Proton beam treatment delivers higher doses of radiation to tumors than photon beams and at the same time does not exceed radiation tolerance of normal, healthy tissue next to the targeted area. Because of the physical properties of the positively-charged protons, they stop short just at the target and do not deposit a dose beyond that boundary, making proton beam treatment advantageous for deep seated and solid tumors in any body site. Report 77520 for simple proton treatment delivery to a single treatment area utilizing a single non-tangential/oblique port and custom blocking without compensation and 77522 with compensation (custom-made devices attached to the treatment unit for manipulating the radiation dose). Report 77523 for intermediate proton delivery to one or more treatment areas utilizing two or more ports or one or more tangential/oblique ports, with custom blocks and compensators; and report 77525 for complex proton treatment delivery to one or more treatment areas utilizing two or more ports per treatment area with matching or patching fields and/or multiple isocenters, with custom blocks and compensators.

77600-77620

Hyperthermia uses heat in an attempt to speed cell metabolism. This is performed to increase potential cell destruction in the treatment of a malignancy by making tumors more susceptible to the therapy. The heat can be generated by a variety of sources, including microwave, ultrasound and radio frequency conduction. Report 77600 for hyperthermia, externally generated, superficial (i.e., heating to a depth of 4 cm or less) and 77605 for deep (i.e., heating to depths greater than 4 cm). For heat generated by interstitial probes acting like small antennae or microwave radiators placed directly into the tumor area, report 77610 for 5 or fewer interstitial applicators and 77615 for more than 5 interstitial applicators. For hyperthermia generated by intracavitary probes placed into a body cavity, report 77620.

77750

The physician infuses or instills a radioactive solution to kill cancerous cells. Brachytherapy is the application of radioactive isotopes for internal radiation. Radioactive material is encapsulated for intracavitary or interstitial implantation or prepared in solutions for instillation or oral administration. For this brachytherapy procedure, the physician intravenously injects a radioactive substance (e.g., Strontium -89) in solution into a vein or the physician may instill a radioactive substance in solution into a body cavity. This type of brachytherapy may be referred to as unsealed internal radiation therapy. This code includes three months of follow-up care.

77761-77763

Brachytherapy is the application of radioactive isotopes for internal radiation. Radioactive material is encapsulated for intracavitary or interstitial implantation or prepared in solutions for instillation or oral administration. For intracavitary application, the physician inserts encapsulated radioactive elements (e.g., metal seeds, wires, tubes, or needles) into the affected body cavity using appropriate applicators, surgically inserted under ultrasound or fluoroscopic guidance. The physician may suture the applicator into or near the tumor. A radioactive isotope, usually Cesium, Iridium, or Cobalt, is placed in the applicator. The isotopes are left in place for two to three days, but may be left longer. This method provides radiation to a limited body area while minimizing exposure to normal tissue. Report 77761 for simple intracavitary application of 1 to 4 sources/ribbons; 77762 for intermediate intracavitary application of 5 to 10 sources/ribbons; and 77763 for complex intracavitary application of more than 10 sources/ribbons.

77767-77768

Brachytherapy is the application of radioactive isotopes that are placed on the tumor or target lesion. For remote afterloading high-dose rate radionuclide brachytherapy, tiny catheters are used together with a single, high-intensity radioactive material to produce the desired radiation distribution pattern around the tumor area. Extremely tiny catheters are fixed in place around the tumor and connected to the treatment machine. These catheters, or applicators, usually do not require surgical manipulation to set them in place. Once in position, the machine loads its radioactive source into each catheter, set at predetermined positions along each catheter for previously calculated dwelling times. The radioactive isotopes are left in place for a short period, usually only three to five minutes, due to the high radioactivity of the source that makes it thousands of times more powerful than normal brachytherapy sources. Report 77767 for one channel or a lesion diameter up to 2 cm and 77768 for two or more channels, multiple lesions, or a lesion diameter over 2.0 cm.

77770-77772

Brachytherapy is the application of radioactive isotopes for internal radiation. Radioactive material is encapsulated for intracavitary or interstitial implantation. For remote afterloading high-dose rate radionuclide brachytherapy, tiny catheters are used together with a single, high-intensity radioactive material to produce the desired radiation distribution pattern around the tumor area. Extremely tiny catheters are fixed in place around the tumor and connected to the treatment machine. These catheters, or applicators, usually do not require surgical manipulation to set them in place. Once in position, the machine loads its radioactive source into each catheter, set at predetermined positions along each catheter for previously calculated dwelling times. The radioactive isotopes are left in place for a short period, usually only three to five minutes, due to the high radioactivity of the source that makes it thousands of times more powerful than normal brachytherapy sources. For intracavitary application, the physician inserts encapsulated radioactive elements (e.g., metal seeds, wires, tubes, or needles) into the affected body cavity using appropriate applicators. For interstitial application, the physician inserts encapsulated radioactive elements directly into the affected tissue using appropriate applicators. The physician may suture the applicator into or near the tumor. A radioactive isotope, usually Cesium, Iridium, or Cobalt, is placed in the applicator. The isotopes are left in place for two to three days, but may be left longer. These codes include basic dosimetry when performed. Report 77770 for one channel; 77771 for two to 12 channels; and 77772 for more than 12 channels.

77778

Brachytherapy is the application of radioactive isotopes for internal radiation. Radioactive material is encapsulated for intracavitary or interstitial implantation or prepared in solutions for instillation or oral administration. For interstitial application, the physician inserts encapsulated radioactive elements (e.g., metal seeds, wires, tubes, or needles) directly into the affected tissue using appropriate applicators, surgically inserted under ultrasound or fluoroscopic guidance. The physician may suture the applicator into or near the tumor. A radioactive isotope, usually Cesium, Iridium, or Cobalt, is placed in the applicator. The isotopes are left in place for two to three days, but may be left longer. Tiny seeds of radioactive material may be inserted directly into the tumor area and left there permanently. This method provides radiation to a limited body area while minimizing exposure to normal tissue.

77789

The physician performs a surface application of a low-dose rate radionuclide source. The physician places the radioactive source sealed in a small holder against a tumor. When surface application is used for treating pterygium, radioactive seeds are placed into a soft, plastic template, which is inserted into an eye plaque that is implanted during surgery for a specified duration and removed.

77790

The use of radiation sources for therapy requires attention and preparations for proper and safe handling of the radioelement. This code reports the supervision, handling, and loading of the radiation source used for conventional brachytherapy, not depending on the number of sources or complexity of the source used. The care of instruments involved in radioelement usage is also included.

78012-78014

The structure and function of the thyroid gland is examined. The patient is given a small dose of radioactive iodine, usually in the form of a pill or liquid, and is asked to return once or twice in a four- to 24-hour period for a thyroid uptake test and/or scan. During the thyroid uptake test, a specialized probe is placed in front of the patient's thyroid and the amount of radiotracer absorbed by the thyroid is measured as an indication of the thyroid's function. This may be performed a second time in the 24-hour period for comparative purposes. Thyroid stimulation, suppression, or discharge tests may also be performed at this time. On occasion, the radioactive iodine is given intravenously during the thyroid scan, rather than by mouth 30 minutes prior to the examination. The patient is placed supine with the head tilted backwards, extending the neck. A gamma camera is used to capture images of the thyroid from different angles. Report 78012 when only the thyroid uptake is performed. Report 78013 when only the scan is performed. Report 78014 if the uptake and scan are completed.

78015-78018

An imaging scan for thyroid cancer metastases is done only after ablation of normal thyroid tissue, six to 12 months after therapy treatment. Post-thyroidectomy patients with thyroid cancer are referred for whole body and area scanning to evaluate the thyroidectomy and demonstrate the presence and location of metastatic disease. Radioactive sodium iodide is given to the patient orally. The patient is placed supine with the neck extended and the head immobilized. Images are acquired of the neck, chest, or other clinically suspect areas with a scintillation or gamma camera that detects the radiation from the tracer in the target tissue. Report 78015 for a limited study (i.e., head and neck only); report 78016 for additional studies, such as a urinary recovery test in which urine is collected at intervals for radioactivity counts; and report 78018 for a whole body imaging scan.

78020

The uptake test is a measure of thyroid function to determine how much iodine the thyroid will take up and is expressed as the percentage of the administered radioactivity present in the thyroid gland at a given time after administration. An uptake for thyroid cancer metastases is done only after ablation of normal thyroid tissue. Radioactive iodine is given to the patient orally. The neck is extended with the patient supine and the probe is placed over the gland. Since total thyroidectomy has been done to treat the cancer, and any remaining thyroid tissue would not be functioning, the radioactive iodine uptake noted to occur in the neck would be concentrated by metastatic lesions.

78070-78072

Parathyroid imaging is a diagnostic tool for localizing parathyroid adenomas and hyperplastic glands. Planar imaging uses dual radiotracer imaging and two sets of pictures. Thallium-210, which is taken up by the thyroid gland, is injected and the patient is placed supine with the neck extended and the camera centered over the neck. Sixty-second images are taken five to 20 minutes following the injection. 99m-technetium is also injected and thyroid images are taken five to 10 minutes after injection. The images are normalized to each other and the technetium images are subtracted, distinguishing normal tissue from the parathyroid tissue. A thyroid image may be obtained 16 to 24 hours after oral administration of Iodine-123 and subtracted from thallium images to yield a more optimal subtraction image due to a better thyroid-to-background ratio. To further localize abnormal parathyroid tissue, single-photon emission computed tomography (SPECT) with or without concurrent CT imaging may be performed. SPECT provides three-dimensional imaging using gamma radiation and multiple images of the parathyroid region. The computerized tomography (CT) imaging performed in conjunction with SPECT provides further anatomic information resulting in more precise localization. Report 78070 for parathyroid planar imaging with subtraction. Report 78071 when planar imaging and SPECT are performed. Report 78072 if SPECT with concurrent CT are performed with the planar imaging.

78075

Nuclear adrenal imaging is used to evaluate biochemical evidence of adrenal cortical functioning. The adrenal cortex is responsible for steroid hormone production which is dependent on the availability and movement of cholesterol. Radiolabeled cholesterol is therefore the logical choice for adrenal cortex imaging. Depending on the underlying diagnosis, additional medications to aid in imaging are given at prescribed intervals and lengths of time in preparation for the study. After patients are injected with the radiocholesterol NP-59, they return for imaging a few days later. Optimal imaging intervals have also been empirically determined for different underlying diagnoses. All patients are given a solution to block thyroid uptake and a laxative to hasten excretion of the radiocholesterol metabolites. The patient is placed in the prone position for imaging and the gamma camera is centered to detect the radioactivity in the adrenal region.

78102-78104

Radiolabeled sulphur colloid is the most commonly used radiopharmaceutical for bone marrow imaging. The radiotracer is injected into the patient and images are obtained after a two or three-hour delay for optimal evaluation. A scintillation or gamma camera takes planar images of the study area on computer screen or film by detecting the gamma radiation from the radionuclide that has traveled to the bone marrow as it "scintillates" or gives off energy in a flash of light when coming in contact with the camera's detector. The bone marrow scan provides information about the distribution of functioning bone marrow and any irregular pattern of marrow tissue expansion occurring in different clinical states such as malignancy or infection. Report 78102 for bone marrow imaging of a limited area; 78103 for multiple areas; and 78104 for whole body imaging.

78110-78111

The radiopharmaceutical volume-dilution technique is performed to determine the patient's plasma volume by using a radiolabeled protein tracer such as iodinated serum albumin. The tracer is injected intravenously into one arm and a blood sample is withdrawn from the opposite arm 15 minutes after the injection. A standard solution is prepared by diluting a known volume of the injected radiopharmaceutical with water to a known volume. The dilution factor is figured. The blood sample is centrifuged and divided into 5-ml aliquots for plasma calculation using a formula involving the dilution factor from the standard sample. Report 78110 for a single sampling and 78111 if multiple samplings are collected at 15, 25, and 35 minutes after the injection.

78120-78121

The red cell volume determination test is done by using radioactive chromium to label red blood cells (RBCs). One or two vials of blood are withdrawn from the patient, the RBCs are separated out of the sample, and mixed with the radioisotope. One sample is saved to prepare the standard sample by diluting the known volume of radiolabeled RBCs with water to a known volume. Another sample is injected back into the patient's arm and after a 15 minute delay, blood is withdrawn from the opposite arm. The red cell volume is calculated using a formula that applies the dilution factor from the standard. Report 78121 if multiple samplings are collected at 15, 25, and 35 minutes after the injection.

78122

The radiopharmaceutical volume-dilution technique is performed to determine the patient's plasma volume and red cell volume simultaneously by using a radiolabeled protein tracer such as iodinated serum albumin and autologous radiolabeled red blood cells. The procedure involves collecting blood and recording the blood counts to calculate the volumes using respective formulas that apply the dilution factor from a standard sample of each radiotracer. The radioactive protein tracer is injected intravenously into the arm as well as the radiolabeled autologous red blood cells and blood samples are withdrawn at 15, 25, and 35 minute intervals after the injection. Standard samples are prepared of each radiotracer by diluting a known volume with water until a known volume is reached. The blood samples are centrifuged and divided into 5-ml aliquots for separate red blood cell volume and plasma volume calculations which require different formulas.

78130

Normal human red blood cells (RBCs) survive in the circulation for approximately 115 days after they are released from the bone marrow. Most techniques used to estimate RBC survival require that a label be placed on the cells that can be followed while the RBCs age in the circulation. One form of red cell survival study uses radioactive chromium to tag autologous red blood cells to evaluate the rate of red blood cell destruction, or lifespan, in patients with suspected hemolytic anemia. Prior to the procedure, the RBC volume is measured. Blood is withdrawn from the patient, the red blood cells are separated, mixed with the radioisotope, and injected back into the patient. The initial blood sample is taken on the first day and repeated at intervals for the next two to three weeks or until half of the initial radioactive chromium labeled RBCs are present. Whole blood samples are withdrawn and the hematocrit levels recorded.

78140

Red blood cell (RBC) sequestration is a test using Chromium-51 labeled autologous red blood cells to determine if the liver or spleen is the major site of sequestration. An aliquot of the patient's own radiolabeled RBCs is saved for a standard measurement and another is reinjected. The patient's skin is marked over the liver and spleen for detector placement. Over the following weeks, surface counting is performed at the desired locations with a probe, or scintillation counter, and the different ratios (organ-to-standard, liver-spleen) are compared. Since extravascular RBC destruction occurs mainly in the liver and spleen, the sequestration counts of radiolabeled RBC accumulation in the liver or spleen over time indicate the organs' related roles in RBC destruction.

78185

Radiolabeled sulphur colloid is the most commonly used radiopharmaceutical for spleen imaging. The radiotracer is injected into the patient and images are obtained after a 15-20 minute delay. A scintillation or gamma camera takes planar images of the study area on computer screen or film by detecting the gamma radiation from the radionuclide that has traveled to the spleen as it "scintillates" or gives off energy in a flash of light when coming in contact with the camera's detector. The imaging is done first with a lead strip placed on the left costal margin and again after the strip is removed. If the imaging is done with a vascular flow study, radiolabeled damaged red blood cells are injected and their flow is followed in the spleen visualization. Splenic imaging is an indirect way of evaluation for liver disease since the disease will shunt the radiocolloid away from the liver.

78191

Once released from the bone marrow, platelets normally circulate in the blood for 8 to 10 days. In patients with certain types of chronic disease such as immune thrombocytopenic purpura (chronic ITP), an autoimmune disorder in which patients produce platelet autoantibodies that destroy blood platelets, the platelet survival time is shortened due to their destruction by the autoantibodies. The patient develops a low platelet count (thrombocytopenia). For the procedure, blood is withdrawn from the patient, the platelets are separated and labeled with Indium-111, and reinjected intravenously. Samples are withdrawn at intervals and the platelet levels recorded until a certain level of tagged platelets are left in circulation.

78195

Diagnostic nuclear lymphatic and lymph node imaging is a tool for studying diseases involving nodal tissue and evaluating lymphatic transport. The patient is placed in a supine position and radioactive antimony sulfide colloid is injected according to the lymph node to be visualized. For axillary and apical lymph nodes, for example, the injection is into the medial two interdigital webs of the hand and imaging is done two to four hours later. For the internal mammary lymph nodes, the injection is into the posterior rectus sheath below the rib cage and imaging is dependent upon the study. For the iliopelvic nodes, injection is into the perianal region with the patient in a knee to chest position. A scintillation or gamma camera takes planar images of the study area on computer screen or film by detecting the gamma radiation from the radiopharmaceutical in the lymphatic tissue as it "scintillates" or gives off energy when coming in contact with the camera's detector.

78201

Diagnostic nuclear medicine uses small amounts of gamma-emitting radioactive materials, or tracers, to determine the cause of the medical problem based on the function, or chemistry, of the organ or tissue. In a static test, the radionuclide travels to the intended organ. Radiolabeled sulphur colloid is the most commonly used radiopharmaceutical for liver imaging. The radioisotope is injected into a peripheral vein and extracted by the liver. A scintillation or gamma camera takes planar images of the study area on computer screen or film by detecting the gamma radiation from the radiopharmaceutical in the body tissue as it "scintillates" or gives off energy in a flash of light when coming in contact with the camera's detector, usually a sodium iodide crystal. Uniform distribution throughout the liver is normal; but an uneven distribution may indicate a tumor.

78202

Radiolabeled sulphur colloid is the most commonly used radiopharmaceutical for diagnostic nuclear imaging of the liver because it is taken up by the reticuloendothelial cells. The radioisotope is injected into a peripheral vein and extracted by the liver. For imaging done with a vascular flow test, red blood cells are labeled to image the blood flow. A scintillation or gamma camera takes images of the liver on computer screen or film by detecting the gamma radiation from the radiopharmaceutical in the tissue and the blood as it flows through the liver. This helps characterize lesions or tumors and determine vascular complications in the liver. Impaired blood flow and reticuloendothelial function can show up as patchy colloid uptake in the liver with preferential bone marrow and spleen uptake.

78215-78216
Radiolabeled sulphur colloid is the most commonly used radiopharmaceutical for diagnostic nuclear imaging of the liver. Radiolabeled heat-denatured red blood cells are used for detecting asplenia and polysplenia. The radioisotope is injected into a peripheral vein and extracted by the liver and spleen. For imaging done with a vascular flow test, red blood cells are labeled to image the blood flow through the liver and spleen. A scintillation or gamma camera takes images of the liver and spleen on computer screen or film by detecting the gamma radiation from the radiopharmaceutical in the tissue and/or the blood as it flows through the study organs. This helps characterize lesions or tumors and determine vascular complications. Report 78215 for static liver and spleen imaging without vascular flow and 78216 for liver and spleen imaging with vascular flow.

78226-78227
Nuclear imaging is performed of the hepatobiliary ductal system, including the gallbladder if present. Special radiolabeled aminoacetic acids that are rapidly cleared by hepatocytes and excreted in the bile are injected into a peripheral vein. A scintillation or gamma camera takes planar images of the ductal system on computer screen or film by detecting the gamma radiation from the radiopharmaceutical in the body tissue as it "scintillates" or gives off energy in a flash of light when coming in contact with the camera's detector. This imaging may be done with or without pharmacologic intervention to aid in visualizing the gallbladder and/or measuring its function. An oral agent is administered that concentrates in the gallbladder after being absorbed in the intestine and excreted by the liver. The resulting opacification or even nonvisualization of the gallbladder can diagnose disease such as stones, polyps, and cholesterolosis. Report 78226 for imaging of the hepatobiliary system. Report 78227 when the imaging is accompanied by pharmacological intervention and qualitative measurements when applicable.

78230-78231
Diagnostic nuclear medicine uses small amounts of gamma-emitting radioactive materials, or tracers, to determine the cause of the medical problem based on the function, or chemistry, of the organ or tissue. In a static test, the radionuclide travels to the intended organ. For salivary gland imaging, the patient is injected with a low-level radiotracer and immediately imaged with a scintillation or gamma camera that takes planar images of the salivary, or parotid, gland by detecting the gamma radiation from the radiopharmaceutical in the body tissue. Report 78231 if the imaging is done by serial imaging and another set for comparison is taken after the patient has been given lemon candy to stimulate the salivary glands.

78232
In a nuclear imaging salivary gland function study, the patient is given a radiolabeled sulfur colloid mixture under the tongue that allows the visualization of the flow of saliva from the oral cavity through to the esophagus and the stomach. A gamma camera takes planar images by detecting the gamma radiation from the radiopharmaceutical in the saliva as it moves through the body. The test usually is conducted for an hour after the administration of the radiotracer to follow the saliva pathway.

78258
Diagnostic nuclear medicine uses small amounts of gamma-emitting radioactive materials, or tracers, to determine the cause of the medical problem based on the function, or chemistry, of the organ or tissue. For esophageal motility imaging, a radioactive sulfur colloid in water is administered orally and followed by a scintillation, or gamma camera, that takes planar images by detecting the gamma radiation from the radiopharmaceutical as it gives off energy while being swallowed down the esophagus. This test is done to diagnose motility and neurodegenerative disorders, reverse peristalsis, and dysphagia.

78261
Radiolabeled pertechnetate is administered intravenously for a nuclear imaging study of gastric mucosa, especially in children. A scintillation, or gamma camera, scans a wide vision field from the xiphoid to the symphysis pubis and takes planar images by detecting the gamma radiation from the radiopharmaceutical. Gastric mucosa surfaces of the stomach will selectively collect and secrete the pertechnetate. Gastric mucosa in an ectopic site, such as Meckel's diverticulum, will accumulate the radiotracer the same as in the stomach, and allow visualization of the ectopic area as long as there is sufficient mucosa to focally concentrate the tracer.

78262
Diagnostic nuclear medicine uses small amounts of gamma-emitting radioactive materials, or tracers, to determine the cause of the medical problem based on the function, or chemistry, of the organ or tissue. For a gastroesophageal reflux study, a sulfur colloid radioisotope in liquid form such as milk is given to the patient to drink. A scintillation, or gamma camera, takes images on camera or film by detecting the gamma radiation from the radiotracer in the liquid in the stomach to visualize any gastroesophageal reflux. The test is usually done for an hour following ingestion of the material.

78264-78266
Diagnostic nuclear medicine uses small amounts of gamma-emitting radioactive materials, or tracers, to determine the cause of the medical problem based on the function, or chemistry, of the organ or tissue. For a gastric emptying study, a sulfur colloid radioisotope in liquid form, such as milk, is given to the patient to drink. A scintillation, or gamma camera, takes images on camera or film by detecting the gamma radiation from the radiopharmaceutical in the liquid as it moves through the stomach to measure the gastric emptying time. The test is usually done for an hour following

ingestion of the material. The bowel transit time measures the amount of time it takes for ingested material to travel from the mouth through the body until it is expelled from the anus. Colon transit time measures the amount of time for ingested material to travel through just the colon. Due to varying people's transit times, the usefulness of this testing method is questionable. The timeframe in which the imaging occurs varies based on the study being performed. In some cases, images are taken five days after the material is swallowed, showing how the radiopharmaceutical moves through the intestines. The patient may be instructed to swallow multiple tracers for a few days in a row with images taken over the course of several days. At any rate, the percent of tracers visualized on the images indicates if bowel transit time is normal. Report 78264 for the gastric emptying study; 78265 for a study that includes small bowel transit; and 78266 for a study that includes small bowel and colon transit, requiring multiple days.

78267-78268

Diagnostic nuclear medicine uses small amounts of gamma-emitting radioactive materials, or tracers, to determine the cause of the medical problem based on the function, or chemistry, of the organ or tissue. The urea breath test is a noninvasive method of diagnosing a *Helicobacter pylori* infection of the stomach. The patient swallows a pill or drinks a solution containing the chemical urea, labeled with the radioactive isotope C-14. The bacteria will produce an enzyme that breaks down the urea into ammonia and carbon dioxide gas, if they are present. The gas contains the tagged carbon and is quickly absorbed into the bloodstream and expelled in the breath. Breath samples are taken six, 12, and 20 minutes after swallowing the pill. Urease activity produced by the bacteria, when present, will be made manifest in the breath samples collected by the presence of exhaled tagged carbon molecules. Analysis is done using a scintillation counter in a nuclear medicine or radiology department. Report 78267 for the isotope administration and sample collection and 78268 for the breath test analysis.

78278

Diagnostic nuclear medicine uses small amounts of gamma-emitting radioactive materials, or tracers, to determine the cause of the medical problem based on the function, or chemistry, of the organ or tissue. For acute gastrointestinal blood loss imaging, a radioactive colloid is injected intravenously and images are scanned over a large field of vision including the abdomen and pelvis by a camera that detects the gamma radiation from the radioactive tracer introduced into the patient. Detection of a hemorrhage depends on the localization of radiotracer that has filtered out of the blood vessel and into the surrounding bowel lumen. Different angle images may be necessary to rule out bleeding that may be obstructed by other organs, such as the liver and spleen.

78282

A diagnostic gastrointestinal protein loss study is done through nuclear medicine to quantitate the amount of protein loss that is occurring through the GI tract. Two equal doses of chromic chloride are prepared-one for the patient and one to be used as the standard measurement. The patient is injected intravenously via a stopcock and the port of the stopcock is flushed with saline. The stools are collected for the next 4 days in containers with lids to be returned to nuclear medicine. The standard dose is dispensed into a gallon bucket filled with water. When the stool samples return, they are filled with water to the top and mixed. The counts of both the standard and stool samples are taken and compared for diagnosis.

78290

Intestine imaging done with nuclear scintigraphy involves injecting the patient with radioactive sodium pertechnetate. With the patient supine, the scintillation, or gamma camera, scans a wide field of view covering the abdominal area and takes images on camera or film by detecting the gamma radiation from the radioactive tracer introduced into the patient. Structural abnormalities, such as ectopic gastric mucosa, diverticula, or twisting of the bowel causing obstruction may be detected and localized. Gastric mucosa surfaces in an ectopic site will selectively collect and secrete the pertechnetate. Patients suspected of Meckel's diverticulum are given a medication to increase gastric uptake of the pertechnetate. When scanning for inflammatory disorders of the bowel, such as Crohn's disease and ulcerative colitis, autologous radiolabeled white blood cells, which focus on inflammation sites, are used as the radiotracer for imaging purposes.

78291

Diagnostic nuclear medicine imaging can test peritoneovenous shunt patency in patients with intractable ascites. The shunt is plastic tubing equipped with a pressure valve that is inserted to connect the peritoneal cavity to the internal jugular or subclavian vein and permit the return of ascites fluid and proteins to the venous system. Normal inspiration creates the necessary intra-abdominal versus intrathoracic pressure change that allows the pressure valve to open and drain the ascites fluid. The ascites fluid is radiolabeled and followed by imaging with a camera that detects the gamma radiation from the radiotracer introduced into the patient. If the fluid is circulating into the systemic system correctly through a patent shunt, the radiotracer will appear in the cells of the liver.

78300-78315

Various radiopharmaceutical agents are used for diagnostic nuclear imaging of bones and/or joints. Gallium, a calcium analogue, is the radiopharmaceutical of choice when scanning for an inflammatory process because it accumulates in areas of bone mineral turnover, such as fractures, and localizes to infected or inflamed areas like inflammatory arthritis. Combining gallium with radiolabeled white blood cells, which also localize at infection sites, adds more diagnostic specificity when searching for acute osteomyelitis or osteoarthropathy. Radioactive diphosphonates are used for bony metastatic disease screening. A camera scans the area of study and detects the gamma radiation from the radiotracer introduced into the patient to detect and localize the disease process. Report 78300 for bone and/or joint imaging of a limited area; 78305 for multiple areas; 78306 for a whole body scan; or 78315 for a three-phase scan.

78350-78351

Single and dual photon absorptiometry are both noninvasive techniques to measure the absorption of the mono or dichromatic photon beam by bone material. The painless study device is placed directly on the patient and uses a small amount of radionuclide to measure the bone mass absorption efficiency of the energy used. This provides a quantitative measurement of the bone mineral density of cortical bone in diseases like osteoporosis and can be used to assess an individual's response to treatment at different intervals. Report 78350 for single photon energy and 78351 for dual photon energy.

78414

Measurement of central cardiovascular hemodynamics, such as left ventricular ejection fraction, is performed noninvasively using a scintillation probe. Using chest x-rays or echocardiography, the proper location for the probe is marked on the chest wall. An intravenous bolus of radiotracer and/or exercise may be introduced. The probe is applied and the variations in left ventricular volume changes are recorded and measured.

78428

For detecting right to left cardiac shunts, radiolabeled macroaggregated albumin is used, which is trapped by the lungs and will be identified in the systemic circulation if a right to left shunt is present. For left to right shunts, the first pass technique is used. A bolus of radionuclide is injected and rapid image frames are acquired as it moves in the venous system through the chambers of the heart. Early recirculation detected would identify a left to right shunt.

78445

Nuclear imaging for non-cardiac vascular flow studies may be performed to test for arterial or venous peripheral vascular diseases or injuries, graft patency, and even catheter malfunctions. In radionuclide angiography, for example, red blood cells from the patient are tagged with radioactivity and injected intravenously. A scintillation camera positioned over the arterial area of interest detects the radioactivity in the blood and takes a series of dynamic images every 2 to 3 seconds immediately after injection, followed by static images. These are recorded on computer and/or film to be studied at different frame rates, times, and intensities. Normal flow is demonstrated as swift and unimpeded. Luminal narrowing or widening, blood flow obstructions and occlusions, and extraluminal accumulation of the radioactive cells can be visualized for diagnostic purposes.

78451-78452

For tomographic myocardial perfusion imaging, the patient receives an intravenous injection of a radionuclide, usually thallium or technetium-99m, which localizes only in nonischemic tissue. SPECT (single photon emission computed tomographic) images of the heart are taken immediately to identify areas of perfusion vs. infarction. SPECT imaging differs from planar imaging by using a single or multiple-head camera that rotates around the patient to give three-dimensional tomographic imaging of the heart displayed in thin slices. In the nonstress version of the procedure, radionuclide is injected and images are taken without stress induction. In 78451, a single study is performed at rest or stress. If the test is to be done at a stress condition, it is induced with the standard treadmill exercise test or pharmacologically with the infusion of a vasodilator. In 78452, multiple studies are done at rest and/or stress with a second injection of radionuclide given again in the redistribution and/or resting phase just prior to resting images being taken. These codes also include attenuation correction (AC), which provides a more accurate diagnostic image for diagnosing defects or infarcted areas by raising the importance of radioactivity distribution counts arising from certain areas. For instance, counts from the anterior wall may be reduced or impeded by the presence of the breast. These codes also include qualitative or quantitative wall motion, ejection fraction (EF) by first pass or gated technique, and additional quantification, when performed.

78453-78454

For planar myocardial perfusion imaging, stress is induced with the standard treadmill exercise test or pharmacologically with the infusion of a vasodilator, if the test is to be done at stress conditions. The patient receives an intravenous injection of a radionuclide, usually thallium or technetium-99m, which localizes only in nonischemic tissue. Planar images of the heart are scanned immediately with a gamma camera that detects the radiation in the heart tissue to identify areas of infarction. In the nonstress version of the procedure, radionuclide is injected and images taken without stress induction. In 78453, a single study is performed at rest or stress. In 78454, multiple procedures are done at rest and/or at stress with a second injection of radionuclide given again in the redistribution or resting phase just prior to resting images being taken. For tests performed during pharmacological or exercise-induced stress, report the appropriate stress testing code. These codes also include qualitative or quantitative wall motion, ejection fraction (EF) by first pass or gated technique, and additional quantification, when performed.

78456

Diagnostic nuclear imaging for acute venous thrombosis imaging uses radiolabeled peptides.

Peptides are short-string proteins that attach to platelets, which are essential in blood clotting, and localize at sites where clots are present or beginning to form. Images from a scintillation, or gamma camera, are taken by detecting the gamma radiation from the radiotracer in the peptides attached to the blood component and these images can identify clots as soon as 10 minutes after the injection. Usually another set of images is done after 60 to 90 minutes following the injection as the image quality tends to improve with time after the injection. If a scan showed significantly increased uptake in any region of one leg compared to the other, or more intense uptake on delayed imaging, deep venous thrombosis is suspected.

78457-78458

A diagnostic nuclear venogram is done to identify the presence and location of thrombi (blood clots) within the venous system. An intravenous injection of a radiopharmaceutical into one or both extremities, most often the legs, is first performed. This is followed by rapid sequence imaging as the radiopharmaceutical passes through the venous system. Unilateral imaging for venous thrombosis is reported with 78457; bilateral imaging is reported with 78458. Bilateral studies may be performed even when only one leg is symptomatic for deep-vein thrombus as the normal extremity if used for comparison purposes.

78459 [78429]

In 78459, the cardiac muscle is imaged using data received from positron-emitting radionuclides administered to the patient by intravenous injection. The collision of the positrons emitted by the radionuclide with the negatively-charged electrons normally present in tissue is computer-synthesized to produce an image, usually in color. This image shows the presence or absence of ischemic or fibrotic cardiac tissue and allows evaluation of metabolic functioning of cardiac tissue. A test to determine the percentage of blood that is pumped out of a filled ventricle with each heartbeat, known as the ejection fraction, may also be undertaken at this time, as well as evaluation of ventricular wall motion. In 78429, a computed tomography (CT) scan is performed concurrently with the above-described PET study utilizing a combination PET/CT camera. Data sets obtained from the CT and PET are joined electronically by the scanner's computer system and can be viewed interactively by the clinician on a workstation, combining both excellent anatomic detail and physiologic information regarding metabolic activity.

78466-78469

A radionuclide is injected intravenously that localizes in recently (under 72-hours) infarcted myocardial tissue. Multiple cardiac images are obtained between one and four hours after injection of the isotope. The location and extent of infarct can be determined by the presence of the radionuclide in the heart tissue. In 78468, first-pass technique is utilized. In first-pass technique, a bolus of Technetium-99m or other radionuclide is injected and visualized as it moves through the venous system into the right atrium, right ventricle, pulmonary artery, lungs, left atrium, left ventricle, and aorta. Several cardia cycles are generally observed. Ejection fraction measurements from both the right and left ventricle are calculated by determining the change in radioactivity over time. In 78469, SPECT images are obtained. SPECT images are tomographic reconstructions derived from a single- or multiple-head gamma camera that rotates around the patient. Tomographic imaging displays the heart in thin slices allowing better separation of myocardial and nonmyocardial structures. SPECT imaging is helpful in identifying small infarcts that are sometimes missed using planar imaging alone.

78472-78473

Radionuclide, which will adhere to the patient's red blood cells, is injected intravenously for cardiac blood pool imaging. Multiple images of the heart, synchronized with the electrocardiographic RR interval (ECG gated), are taken several minutes later, after the radionuclide has spread through the blood pool. These images are computer synthesized and data is generated to produce a video display of cardiac wall motion, calculation of left ventricular ejection fractions, and images based on computer manipulation of the data received. In 78472, the procedure is performed as a single study at rest or stress, not both; in 78473, the procedure is performed at both rest and stress. For tests performed during pharmacological or exercise-induced stress, report the appropriate stress testing code also.

78481-78483

A bolus of radionuclide is injected intravenously for cardiac blood pool imaging, first pass technique. As the radioisotope passes through the cardiac chambers, rapid sequence imaging and computer generation of data and images is done to produce a video display of cardiac wall motion, calculation of ventricular ejection fractions, and images based on computer manipulation of the data received. This technique provides information about the functional status of the heart at rest or in response to stress. In 78481, the procedure is performed as a single study at rest or stress, not both; in 78483, the procedure is performed at rest and stress. For tests performed during pharmacological or exercise-induced stress, report the appropriate stress testing code also.

78491, 78492

The cardiac muscle is imaged using data received from positron-emitting radionuclides administered to the patient by intravenous injection. The collision of the positrons emitted by the radionuclide with the negatively-charged electrons normally present in tissue is computer-synthesized to produce an image, usually in color, which shows the presence or absence of perfusion into normal or ischemic cardiac tissue. A determination of the percentage of blood that is pumped out of a filled ventricle with each heartbeat, known as the ejection fraction, may also be made at this time, as well as evaluation of ventricular wall motion. Report 78491 if the procedure is performed as a single study at rest or during exercise or pharmacologic-induced stress. Report 78492 for multiple studies at rest and during exercise or pharmacologic-induced stress.

[78430, 78431]
The cardiac muscle is imaged using data received from positron-emitting radionuclides administered to the patient by intravenous injection. The collision of the positrons emitted by the radionuclide with the negatively-charged electrons normally present in tissue is computer-synthesized to produce an image, usually in color, which shows the presence or absence of perfusion into normal or ischemic cardiac tissue. A determination of the percentage of blood that is pumped out of a filled ventricle with each heartbeat, known as the ejection fraction, may also be made at this time, as well as evaluation of ventricular wall motion. A computed tomography (CT) scan is performed concurrently with the aforementioned PET study utilizing a combination PET/CT camera. Data sets obtained from the CT and PET are joined electronically by the scanner's computer system and can be viewed interactively by the clinician on a work station, combining both excellent anatomic detail and pertinent physiologic information. Report 78430 if the procedure is performed as a single study at rest or during exercise or pharmacologic-induced stress. Report 78431 for multiple studies at rest and during exercise or pharmacologic-induced stress.

[78432, 78433]
In 78432, a myocardial viability study is undertaken using dual radiotracers such as rubidium-82 (to measure blood flow) and 18F-fluorodeoxyglucose or FDG (to measure whether heart muscle cells are alive) that are administered to the patient by intravenous injection. The collision of the positrons emitted by the radionuclide with the negatively-charged electrons normally present in tissue is computer-synthesized to produce an image, usually in color, which shows the presence or absence of ischemic or fibrotic cardiac tissue and allows evaluation of its metabolic functioning. It also reveals the presence or absence of perfusion into these tissues. A determination of the percentage of blood that is pumped out of a filled ventricle with each heartbeat, known as the ejection fraction, may also be made at this time, as well as evaluation of ventricular wall motion. The procedure is performed to assess myocardial viability. In 78433, a computed tomography (CT) scan is performed concurrently with the above-described PET study utilizing a combination PET/CT camera. Data sets obtained from the CT and PET are joined electronically by the scanner's computer system and can be viewed interactively by the clinician on a workstation, combining both excellent anatomic detail and pertinent physiologic information.

[78434]
The physician performs absolute quantitation of myocardial blood flow during rest and pharmacologic stress using positron emission tomography (PET). Absolute quantitation of myocardial blood flow (MBF) by PET is an established method and superior tool in the detection, analysis, and management of epicardial and microvascular coronary artery disease (CAD) and provides clinicians the ability to measure, in a noninvasive manner, MBF in milliliters per minute, per gram of tissue. Positron emission tomography is a radionuclide imaging technique for noninvasive quantification of MBF. The process of evaluating myocardial perfusion is a key aspect in diagnosing and determining outcomes for cases of suspected or known CAD. Resting MBF is the total amount of blood flow received by the myocardium per minute, per gram of tissue and may be impacted by a myriad of factors including, but not limited to, the patient's age, gender, blood pressure, and heart rate. Normal values for MBF at rest range from 0.6 to 1.3 mL/min/g. Stress MBF, also referred to as hyperemic blood flow, describes the highest amount of blood flow that can be provided to the heart during the topmost period of vasodilation of the heart's vascular bed. Typically, to reach this maximum vasodilation, the patient receives vasodilators or inotropic agents via IV to simulate stress as well as a cold pressor test (CPT) and mental stress tests. Stress MBF may be impacted by a number of factors including, but not limited to, caffeine, increased microvascular tone and resistance, and coronary risk factors. Report 78434 in addition to the code for the primary procedure.

78494
Radionuclide, which will adhere to the patient's red blood cells, is injected intravenously for cardiac blood pool imaging, gated equilibrium. Multiple SPECT (single photon emission computed tomography) images of the heart, synchronized with the electrocardiographic RR interval (ECG gated), are taken several minutes later, after the radionuclide has spread through the blood pool. These SPECT images are taken by a rotating single or multiple-head camera for three-dimensional views of cross-sectional slices and provide better contrast in imaging and greater accuracy than planar scans. The SPECT images are computer synthesized and data is generated to produce a video display of cardiac wall motion, calculation of ventricular ejection fractions, and images based on computer manipulation of the data received.

78496
A bolus of radionuclide is injected intravenously for cardiac blood pool imaging with right ventricular ejection fraction by first pass technique. As the radioisotope in the venous system passes through the cardiac chambers, rapid sequence imaging, synchronized with the electrocardiographic RR interval (ECG gated), is done. This first pass technique provides information for right ventricular ejection fraction calculation not possible with static gated images which do not show right ventricular count in isolation. This test for functional status of the heart is done as a single study at rest in addition to the primary procedure.

78579
Nuclear ventilation imaging of the lungs is designed to show the regional distribution of inspired air throughout the lung tissue and the uptake and clearance dynamics of the lungs. The patient is usually placed supine and breathes in a radioaerosol or gas through a tube that is attached to a nebulizer. Once the aerosol or gas is inhaled, the radioactivity stays in the area where it was deposited long enough to take images with a camera that detects the gamma radiation being given off from the aerosol or gas in the air spaces. Increased central deposition occurs in severe obstructive airway disorders. Rapid clearance from the lungs reflects interstitial lung disease, such as in smokers, where systemic absorption rises due to increased alveolar capillary permeability.

78580
Nuclear pulmonary perfusion imaging uses a venous injection of radioactive macroaggregated albumin particles that are too large to pass through the pulmonary capillary bed and accumulate there as they are strained out. A scintillation or gamma camera takes planar images on computer screen or film by detecting the gamma radiation from the radiopharmaceutical in the lungs as it "scintillates" or gives off energy in a flash of light when coming in contact with the camera's detector. Localization of the radioactive particles is proportional to the blood flow and thereby maps lung perfusion. Standard perfusion imaging usually consists of eight planar images from different projections with the posterior oblique views being most important since they image the lower lobes, the most common site for pulmonary embolism.

78582
Ventilation and perfusion imaging of the lungs is used to detect pulmonary embolisms and the percentage of total perfusion and ventilation attributable to each lung. Perfusion imaging is done after a venous injection of radioactive macroaggregated albumin is given to the patient. The albumin particles are too large to pass through the pulmonary capillary bed and accumulate there as they are strained out. This localization of particles is proportional to the blood flow and thereby maps lung perfusion. A nuclear ventilation image is obtained to complement the perfusion image. For a single breath image, a posterior view of the thorax is taken as the patient inhales radiolabeled Xenon gas in a single breath and holds it as long as possible. This image obtained from the gamma camera that detects the radioactivity from the gas in the lungs shows well-ventilated areas having uniform activity and poorly ventilated areas with decreased or absent radioactivity.

78597-78598
Ventilation and perfusion imaging of the lungs is used to detect pulmonary embolisms and the percentage of total perfusion and ventilation attributable to each lung. Ventilation imaging of the lungs shows the regional distribution of inspired air throughout the lung tissue and the uptake and clearance dynamics of the lungs by having the patient inhale a radioaerosol or gas. Perfusion imaging uses an injection of radioactive albumin, which are particles too big to pass through the pulmonary capillary bed and accumulate there, mapping blood perfusion as they are strained out. Standard perfusion imaging usually consists of eight planar images from different projections with the posterior oblique views being most important since they image the lower lobes, the most common site for pulmonary embolisms. The two types of images complement each other for diagnosis purposes. When the data for these studies are acquired on a digital computer, lung perfusion and ventilation can be quantitated for gradient comparisons and function differential calculations. Report 78597 for pulmonary perfusion testing only. Report 78598 for pulmonary perfusion and ventilation testing.

78600, 78605
Diagnostic nuclear medicine uses small amounts of gamma-emitting radioactive materials, or tracers, to determine the cause of the medical problem based on the function, or chemistry, of the organ or tissue. This is in contrast to diagnostic tests that determine disease presence based on structural appearance. In a static test, the radionuclide travels to the intended organ. The organ, tissue, or bone under study determines the type of radioactive material used and it is introduced by injection, swallowing, or inhalation. A scintillation or gamma camera takes planar images of the study area on computer screen or film by detecting the gamma radiation from the radiopharmaceutical in the body tissue as it "scintillates" or gives off energy in a flash of light when coming in contact with the camera's detector. Report less than four static views of the brain with 78600 and four or more with 78605.

78601, 78606
Diagnostic nuclear medicine uses small amounts of gamma-emitting radioactive materials, or tracers, to determine the cause of the medical problem based on the function, or chemistry, of the organ or tissue. This is in contrast to diagnostic tests that determine disease presence based on structural appearance. In a static test, the radionuclide travels to the intended organ. The organ, tissue, or bone under study determines the type of radioactive material used and it is introduced by injection, swallowing, or inhalation. A scintillation or gamma camera takes planar images of the study area on computer screen or film by detecting the gamma radiation from the radiopharmaceutical in the body tissue as it "scintillates" or gives off energy in a flash of light when coming in contact with the camera's detector. Report 78601 for less than four static views of the brain with vascular flow and 78606 for four or more views with vascular flow.

78608
Positron emission tomography (PET) produces thin slice images of the body that can be reassembled into three-dimensional representations by detecting positron-emitting radionuclides from a radiopharmaceutical introduced into the body. These radionuclides must be produced in a cyclotron or

generator that can bombard chemicals with neutrons to produce unstable, short-lived radioisotopes, such as carbon-11, nitrogen-13, and oxygen-15. These can be readily incorporated into common and important, biological body compounds for administration. Data from the imaging yields metabolic or biochemical function information depending on the type of molecule tagged. In PET imaging of the brain with metabolic evaluation, the radionuclide in injected intravenously and carried to the brain where the scanner detects the radioactivity as the compound accumulates in different regions of the brain. By using specifically tagged compounds, information on glucose, oxygen, or drug metabolism in the brain is obtained.

78609
Positron emission tomography (PET) produces thin slice images of the body that can be reassembled into three-dimensional representations by detecting positron-emitting radionuclides from a radiopharmaceutical introduced into the body. These radionuclides must be produced in a cyclotron or generator that can bombard chemicals with neutrons to produce unstable, short-lived radioisotopes, such as carbon-11, nitrogen-13, and oxygen-15. These can be readily incorporated into common and important, biological body compounds for administration. Data from the imaging yields metabolic or biochemical function information depending on the type of molecule tagged. In PET imaging of the brain with perfusion evaluation, the radionuclide in injected intravenously and carried to the brain where the scanner detects the radioactivity as the tracer accumulates in different areas of the brain proportional to the rate of delivery of blood to that volume of brain tissue.

78610
Diagnostic nuclear medicine uses small amounts of gamma-emitting radioactive materials, or tracers, to determine the cause of the medical problem based on the function, or chemistry, of the organ or tissue. In a vascular flow test, the radionuclide labels red blood cells and therefore goes wherever the blood flows. The radionuclide is administered to the patient and a scintillation or gamma camera takes time-delayed, dynamic images of the study area on computer screen or film by detecting the gamma radiation from the radiopharmaceutical in the blood as it flows through the study area. This helps characterize lesions or tumors and determine vascular complications in an organ. Use this code for a vascular flow study only of the brain.

78630
Diagnostic nuclear medicine uses small amounts of gamma-emitting radioactive materials, or tracers, to determine the cause of the medical problem based on the function, or chemistry, of the organ or tissue. Cisternography is done to determine if there is any abnormal cerebral spinal fluid flow occurring in or around the brain. A lumbar puncture is necessary to inject the radiotracer into the lower spinal canal region. A scintillation or gamma camera takes planar images of the study area on computer screen or film by detecting the gamma radiation from the radiopharmaceutical in the body tissue as it "scintillates" or gives off energy when coming in contact with the camera's detector. Cisternography is a multiple-day procedure requiring 6-hour, 24-hour, and 48-hour scan sessions.

78635
Diagnostic nuclear ventriculography is done to measure ventricular size in the brain, especially for patients with hydrocephalus who have shunts to drain abnormal accumulations of cerebrospinal fluid (CSF) in the brain due to ventricular obstruction of the normal cerebrospinal fluid pathways. A lumbar puncture may be necessary to inject the radiotracer into the lower spinal canal region or it may be injected into a reservoir or valve of the shunt. A scintillation or gamma camera takes images of the study area on computer screen or film by detecting the gamma radiation from the injected radiopharmaceutical.

78645
A shunt is a tube placed in the interior ventricles of the brain that drains fluid by a pressure controlled valve away from the brain to another part of the body, usually the abdominal cavity, where it is reabsorbed. In order to detect any malfunction and assess the shunt's patency in a noninvasive manner, a radiotracer is injected into a reservoir or valve of the shunt. A scintillation or gamma camera takes images of the head, chest, and abdomen by detecting the radiation from the injected radiopharmaceutical to determine the movement of the tracer from the shunt in the brain to the peritoneal cavity.

78650
Diagnostic nuclear medicine uses small amounts of gamma-emitting radioactive materials, or tracers, to determine the cause of the medical problem based on the function, or chemistry, of the organ or tissue. Intracranial trauma, surgery, infection, malformation, or disease such as hydrocephalus or neoplasms can cause cerebrospinal fluid (CSF) to leak into and drain from nasal or oral cavities. A lumbar puncture may be necessary to inject the radiotracer into the lower spinal canal region. A scintillation or gamma camera takes images of the study area on computer screen or film by detecting the gamma radiation from the radiopharmaceutical to detect fluid levels in sinuses that suggest leakage and determine the leakage location.

78660
Dacryocystography is the radiographic evaluation of the lacrimal system to localize the site of an obstruction. In diagnostic nuclear medicine, a drop of a radiotracer is instilled in the eye and subsequent imaging by a scintillation or gamma camera is performed to follow the passage of the radioactivity and the rate at which it disappears into the lacrimal system to assess if there is a stone or other blockage that interferes with normal tearing function.

78700
Diagnostic nuclear medicine uses small amounts of gamma-emitting radioactive materials, or tracers, to determine a structural cause of the medical problem in the kidney. For kidney imaging, a radionuclide such as 99mTc-DMSA is chosen because it will travel to the kidney and remain in the functional tissue there. It is injected into the patient and a scintillation or gamma camera takes planar images of the kidney on computer screen or film by detecting the gamma radiation from the radiopharmaceutical in the renal tissue as it "scintillates" or gives off energy in a flash of light when coming in contact with the camera's detector. Supply and injection of the radionuclide are reported separately.

78701
For diagnostic nuclear imaging of the kidney with a vascular flow test, the radionuclide 99mTc-DTPA is commonly chosen because it will follow the blood as it flows through the kidney and also identify any obstruction in the collecting system to determine the rate at which the kidneys are filtering. It is injected into the patient and a special scintillation or gamma camera takes planar images of the study area on computer screen or film by detecting the gamma radiation from the radiopharmaceutical as it flows through the kidney.

78707-78709
For a diagnostic nuclear imaging study of kidney structure with vascular flow and function test, a radiopharmaceutical is injected that follows the blood flow through the kidneys in the normal pathway for urine production. Obstructions in the collecting system are identified, along with the rate at which the kidneys are filtering the blood, and how well the tubules and ducts are functioning. A scintillation or gamma camera scans the study area and takes images on computer screen or film by detecting the gamma radiation from the radiopharmaceutical as it flows through the kidney. If pharmacological intervention is used, a diuretic may also be injected that will increase urine flow during the exam. If the radiotracer accumulates and the kidney fails to clear it after diuretic administration, surgery may be necessary to correct the obstruction. Report 78707 for a single study without pharmacological intervention; 78708 for a single study with intervention; and 78709 for multiple studies, done with and without intervention.

78725
A non-imaging radioisotopic study of kidney function requires a radioisotope that is cleared from the body only by the glomerular filtration action of the kidneys. Measuring the glomerular filtration rate (GFR) is the best assessment of total renal function. The radioisotope is injected and blood samples are taken at two, three, and four hours for radioactive concentration counts. The filtration rate of the kidneys is proportional to the clearance rate of the radioisotope from the blood and is calculated using this information together with the distribution volume. The GFR can also be calculated by using urine collections but this method has more intrinsic complications than blood sampling.

78730-78740
In 78740, a ureteral reflux study, or radiopharmaceutical voiding cystogram, determines if the patient has vesicoureteral reflux where urine flows backwards from the bladder, through the ureters, and into the kidneys. A physician or technician inserts a Foley catheter into the urethra and advances it into the bladder. A radiopharmaceutical agent is administered through the catheter until the bladder is full. At the same time, imaging is obtained with a gamma camera to identify any reflux of urine. After the catheter is removed, the patient is asked to void, and imaging continues until the bladder is empty. Report add-on code 78730 when a urinary bladder residual study is performed in addition to the ureteral reflux study. After the patient has voided, additional imaging is obtained to measure the residual volume of urine that remains in the bladder.

78761
For testicular diagnostic nuclear imaging, 99mTc-pertechnetate is injected into a vein in the arm and travels to the testicle where it accumulates. In a vascular flow test, the radionuclide labels red blood cells and therefore goes wherever the blood flows. A scintillation or gamma camera takes images of the study area on computer screen or film by detecting the gamma radiation from the radiotracer concentrated in the testicle or the blood as it flows through the testicle. This test determines whether the blood supply to the testis is compromised. Administration and supply of the radionuclide are reported separately.

78800-78802 [78804]
Diagnostic nuclear medicine uses small amounts of gamma-emitting radioactive materials, or tracers, to determine the cause of the medical problem based on the function, or chemistry, of the organ or tissue. Monoclonal antibodies used for diagnosing certain cancers are developed from tumor-associated antigens and radiolabeled. This becomes the radiopharmaceutical used for tumor localization. Gallium, a calcium analogue, is the radiopharmaceutical of choice when scanning for an inflammatory process because it localizes to infected areas by attaching to plasma proteins found at infection sites and accumulating in areas of bone mineral turnover, such as fractures and inflammatory arthritis. Gallium is often combined with radiolabeled white blood cells, which also accumulate at infection sites but not at areas of increased bone replenishing, to augment accuracy in inflammatory localization. After administration of the specialized radiotracer, a camera, called a scintillation or gamma camera, takes planar images of the study area on computer screen or film by detecting the gamma radiation from the radiopharmaceutical focused in the body tissue. Report 78800 for localization of tumor or inflammatory process or distribution of the radiopharmaceutical within a single area in a single day imaging. Report

78801 for multiple planar (two or more areas) performed in one or more days imaging, or a single area imaging performed over two or more days. Report 78802 for scanning over the whole body done on a single day, and 78804 for whole body scanning requiring two or more days. These tests include vascular flow and blood pool imaging, when performed.

78803 [78830]

Tomographic SPECT (single photon emission computed tomography) imaging permits an in-depth evaluation of complex anatomy and can localize tumors and inflammatory processes within organs and body structures by introducing a radionuclide and detecting the distribution of gamma radiation emitted from the radiotracer introduced into the tissue being studied. Monoclonal antibodies used for diagnosing certain cancers are developed from tumor-associated antigens and radiolabeled for use as the radiopharmaceutical in tumor localization. Gallium, a calcium analogue, is the radiopharmaceutical of choice when scanning for an inflammatory process because it localizes to infected areas by attaching to plasma proteins found at infection sites and accumulating in areas of bone mineral turnover, such as fractures and inflammatory arthritis. When combined with labeled white blood cells, which also accumulate at infection sites but not at areas of increased bone replenishing, accuracy in localizing an inflammatory process is increased. Tomographic SPECT images differ from the usual planar scans of the gamma camera by rotating a single or multiple-head camera mounted on a gantry around the patient to give three-dimensional computer reconstructed views of cross-sectional slices of the body. Report 78803 for SPECT of a single area or acquisition performed in a single day. Vascular flow and blood pool imaging are included, when performed. Report 78830 for a procedure using an integrated device containing both a CT scanner and a SPECT γ-camera with a single patient table. This yields a SPECT/CT fusion, which is the combined display of image sets, providing both functional and anatomic information. This reports a SPECT/CT of a single or acquisition area performed in a single day.

[78831, 78832]

Tomographic SPECT (single photon emission computed tomography) imaging permits an in-depth evaluation of complex anatomy and can localize tumors and inflammatory processes within organs and body structures by introducing a radionuclide and detecting the distribution of gamma radiation emitted from the radiotracer introduced into the tissue being studied. Monoclonal antibodies used for diagnosing certain cancers are developed from tumor-associated antigens and radiolabeled for use as the radiopharmaceutical in tumor localization. Gallium, a calcium analogue, is the radiopharmaceutical of choice when scanning for an inflammatory process because it localizes to infected areas by attaching to plasma proteins found at infection sites and accumulating in areas of bone mineral turnover, such as fractures and inflammatory arthritis. When combined with labeled white blood cells, which also accumulate at infection sites but not at areas of increased bone replenishing, accuracy in localizing an inflammatory process is increased. Tomographic SPECT images differ from the usual planar scans of the gamma camera by rotating a single or multiple-head camera mounted on a gantry around the patient to give three-dimensional computer reconstructed views of cross-sectional slices of the body. Vascular flow and blood pool imaging are included, when performed. Report 78831 for SPECT of a minimum of two areas (such as knees and pelvis or abdomen and chest) or separate acquisitions (such as lung ventilation and perfusion) in a single day, or a single area or acquisition over two or more days. Report 78832 for a procedure using an integrated device containing both a CT scanner and a SPECT γ-camera with a single patient table. This yields a SPECT/CT fusion, which is the combined display of image sets, providing both functional and anatomic information. This reports a SPECT/CT of a minimum of two areas or separate acquisitions in a single day or a single area or acquisition over two or more days.

[78835]

Radiopharmaceutical quantification is performed. SPECT/CT is used to quantify the radiopharmaceutical uptake in the myocardium, a tumor, or other target utilizing patient-specific information obtained from the CT data in a SPECT/CT scanner.

78808

This code reports the injection procedure for radiopharmaceutical localization of structures such as a parathyroid adenoma prior to gamma probe localization.

78811-78813

Positron emission tomography (PET) produces thin slice images of the body that can be reassembled into three-dimensional representations by detecting positron-emitting radionuclides from a radiopharmaceutical introduced into the body. These radionuclides must be produced in a cyclotron or generator that can bombard chemicals with neutrons to produce unstable, short-lived radioisotopes, such as carbon-11, nitrogen-13, and oxygen-15. These can be readily incorporated into common and important, biological body compounds for administration. Data from this kind of imaging yields metabolic or biochemical function information depending on the type of molecule tagged. In PET tumor imaging, information about the tumor's glucose and oxygen utilization is obtained, which reveals the tumor's behavior compared to normal tissue or benign tumors. Report 78811 for PET imaging of a limited area such as the chest alone; 78812 for imaging from the skull base to the mid-thigh; and 78813 for imaging of the whole body.

78814-78816

Positron emission tomography (PET) produces thin slice images of the body that can be reassembled into three-dimensional representations by detecting positron-emitting radionuclides from a radiopharmaceutical introduced into the body. Computed tomography (CT) directs multiple narrow beams of x-rays around a body structure to produce thin, cross-sectional views of anatomical layers (or slices) of the body. The PET scan is highly sensitive to metabolic activity of the tumor while CT provides a detailed internal picture of the size, shape, and location of the tumor. PET, alone, has a definite limitation with respect to spatial resolution and physiological uptake of the radiopharmaceutical tracer, in some areas, can be underestimated or misinterpreted without accurate, anatomical correlations. Scanners that concurrently utilize PET with CT imaging correct for this limitation of PET, by fusing the data for precise anatomical location together with highly sensitive metabolic imaging. Report 78814 for concurrently acquired PET/CT imaging of a limited area, such as the head and neck alone; 78815 for imaging from the skull base to the mid-thigh; and 78816 for whole body scanning.

79005

Radiopharmaceutical therapy is given to the patient via oral administration. The patient swallows the radiolabeled substance prepared in a form to be given by mouth. The strategy for using radiopharmaceutical therapy is to combine radioactive, beta-particle emitters with relatively short half-lives to specific tissue-seeking molecules that can be administered to the patient. The treatment is designed to target certain types of cancers or malfunctioning tissue. An example is radioactive iodine, I-131, given to the patient orally, to treat thyroid cancers and hormone overproduction (hyperthyroidism) since iodine is specifically taken up by thyroid cells.

79101

Radiopharmaceutical therapy is given to the patient via intravenous administration. The patient is given a radiolabeled substance prepared in a form to be injected or instilled directly into a vein. The strategy for using radiopharmaceutical therapy is to combine radioactive, beta-particle emitters with relatively short half-lives to specific tissue-seeking molecules that can be administered to the patient. The treatment is designed to target certain types of cancers or malfunctioning tissue. An example is radioactive phosphorous, P-32, as sodium phosphate administered by intravenous injection. Since phosphorus-32 has a high bone marrow toxicity, it is used for treating polycythemia vera and chronic leukemia to slow the rate at which bone marrow produces cells and induce a state of remission.

79200

Radiopharmaceutical therapy is given to the patient via intracavitary administration. Intracavitary radiotherapy refers to the placement of radioactive sources within a body space or cavity, such as the bladder, esophagus, lung, vagina, or uterus, to give high doses of radiation to the cancer, while giving only low doses to the surrounding tissues. An applicator designed for placing the radioactive source within the specific body cavity is inserted and the radiotherapy is administered through the applicator.

79300

Colloids are a mixture in which one substance divided into minute, insoluble particles (called colloidal particles) is dispersed uniformly throughout a second substance, the suspension medium. Radioactive colloidal solutions that contain natural or synthetic molecules are relatively impermeable to the vascular membrane and are useful for interstitial radioactive therapy. Interstitial radiopharmaceutical therapy by radioactive colloid administration refers to the placement of this type of radioactive source directly into the affected tissue to give high doses of radiation to the cancer, while giving only low doses to the surrounding tissues. An applicator designed for placing the radioactive source within the specific body tissue is inserted and the radiotherapy is administered through the applicator. An example is inserting plastic tubes into prostate tissue and placing rapid dose radioactive colloid solutions within the tubes.

79403

Radiopharmaceutical therapy using radiolabeled monoclonal antibodies infused intravenously is given to the patient as a method of cancer treatment. Monoclonal antibodies are developed from tumor-specific associated antigens and radiolabeled to form a highly stable metal complex. This type of therapy is often called radioimmunotherapy because it combines the very specific targeting capability of a single antibody with the cancer killing power of a radioisotope. The radiolabeled monoclonal antibodies are infused intravenously where they circulate systemically, seeking out the targeted cancer cells, such as in cases of non-Hodgkin's lymphoma, in which this type of radioimmunotherapy has been found effective. This treatment may be done on an outpatient basis, but the patient is observed for immune reaction before discharge.

79440

Each episode of joint bleeding causes inflammation and swelling of the synovial membrane. If bleeding occurs often or is not treated adequately, the inflammation may become chronic and can lead to thickening of the synovial membrane and the release of substances that can destroy cartilage and bone. The administration of intra-articular radiopharmaceutical therapy is done to destroy the membrane through radiation, rather than performing a surgical procedure to remove the damaged membrane. A radioactive substance, such as phosphorus-32, is injected into the joint at a time when the patient has not been bleeding, and after a period of prophylactic therapy has already been done to reduce swelling of the membrane as much as possible.

79445

Radiopharmaceutical therapy is given to the patient via intra-arterial particulate administration. The patient is given a radiolabeled substance prepared in a form to be introduced directly into an artery. The treatment is designed to target certain types of cancers or malfunctioning tissue by blocking blood supply to the tumor while increasing the concentration of local radioactive drug therapy. An example is transcatheter selective hepatic chemoembolization using a suspension of cisplatin and particulate polyvinyl alcohol for liver metastases or carcinomas. After a catheter is selectively placed within the target hepatic artery and the distribution of arteries feeding the tumor is determined, a microcatheter is inserted and nonabsorbable polyvinyl alcohol particles are injected to obstruct blood flow to the tumor, along with an injection of intra-arterial cisplatin suspension. The intra-arterial particulate administration increases the drug concentration in the area of the hypoxic tumor.

Pathology and Laboratory

80047
A basic metabolic panel with ionized calcium includes the following tests: calcium (ionized) (82330), carbon dioxide (82374), chloride (82435), creatinine (82565), glucose (82947), potassium (84132), sodium (84295), and urea nitrogen (BUN) (84520). Blood specimen is obtained by venipuncture. See the specific codes for additional information about the listed tests.

80048
A basic metabolic panel with total calcium includes the following tests: total calcium (82310), carbon dioxide (82374), chloride (82435), creatinine (82565), glucose (82947), potassium (84132), sodium (84295), and urea nitrogen (BUN) (84520). The blood specimen is obtained by venipuncture. See the specific codes for additional information about the listed tests.

80050
A general health panel includes the following tests: albumin (82040), total bilirubin (82247), calcium (82310), carbon dioxide (bicarbonate) (82374), chloride (82435), creatinine (82565), glucose (82947), alkaline phosphatase (84075), potassium (84132), total protein (84155), sodium (84295), alanine amino transferase (ALT) (SGPT) (84460), aspartate amino transferase (AST) (SGOT) (84450), urea nitrogen (BUN) (84520), and thyroid stimulating hormone (84443). In addition, this panel includes a hemogram with automated differential (85025 or 85027 and 85004) or hemogram (85027) with manual differential (85007 or 85009). Blood specimen is obtained by venipuncture. See specific codes for additional information about the listed tests.

80051
An electrolyte panel includes the following tests: carbon dioxide (82374), chloride (82435), potassium (84132), and sodium (84295). Blood specimen is obtained by venipuncture. See specific codes for additional information about the listed tests.

80053
A comprehensive metabolic panel includes the following tests: albumin (82040), total bilirubin (82247), total calcium (82310), carbon dioxide (bicarbonate) (82374), chloride (82435), creatinine (82565), glucose (82947), alkaline phosphatase (84075), potassium (84132), total protein (84155), sodium (84295), alanine amino transferase (ALT) (SGPT) (84460), aspartate amino transferase (AST) (SGOT) (84450), and urea nitrogen (BUN) (84520). Blood specimen is obtained by venipuncture. See the specific codes for additional information about the listed tests.

80055 [80081]
An obstetric panel (80055) includes the following tests: hepatitis B surface antigen (HBsAg) (87340), rubella antibody (86762), qualitative non-treponemal antibody syphilis test (VDRL, RPR, ART) (86592), RBC antibody screen (86850), ABO blood typing (86900), and Rh (D) blood typing (86901). In addition, this panel includes an automated complete blood count (CBC) and automated differential white blood count (WBC) as described by 85025 or 85027 and 85004 OR automated CBC (85027) and appropriate manual differential WBC count (85007 or 85009). Blood specimen is obtained by venipuncture. See specific codes for additional information about the listed tests. Report 80081 when the obstetric panel also includes HIV-1 antigen(s) with HIV-1 and HIV-2 antibodies reported as a single result (87389).

80061
A lipid panel includes the following tests: total serum cholesterol (82465), high-density cholesterol (HDL cholesterol) by direct measurement (83718), and triglycerides (84478). Blood specimen is obtained by venipuncture. See specific codes for additional information about the listed tests.

80069
A renal function panel includes the following tests: albumin (82040), total calcium (82310), carbon dioxide (bicarbonate) (82374), chloride (82435), creatinine (82565), glucose (82947), inorganic phosphorus (phosphate) (84100), potassium (84132), sodium (84295), and urea nitrogen (BUN) (84520).

80074
An acute hepatitis panel includes the following tests: hepatitis A antibody (HAAb), IgM antibody (86709), hepatitis B core antibody (HbcAb), IgM antibody (86705), hepatitis B surface antigen (HbsAg) (87340), and hepatitis C antibody (86803).

80076
A hepatic function panel includes the following tests: albumin (82040), total bilirubin (82247), direct bilirubin (82248), alkaline phosphatase (84075), protein, total (84155), alanine amino transferase (ALT) (SGPT) (84460), and aspartate amino transferase (AST) (SGOT) (84450). Blood specimen is obtained by venipuncture. See the specific codes for additional information about the listed tests.

[80305, 80306]
These tests may be requested as drug screenings for all drugs and all drug classes performed by the respective

technology and process per date of service. In addition, each code encompasses all sample validations performed and may include, but is not limited to, pH, specific gravity, and nitrite. These codes describe two different process categories. Report 80305 for results obtained by direct visual reading, such as in the case of viewing urine dipsticks, urine cups, test cards, or cartridges. Report 80306 for direct visual reading of test results assisted by instrumentation. Presumptive tests may be confirmed with a definitive test that designates the drug. Specimen type varies. These codes should only be reported once per date of service no matter how many procedures or results are performed.

[80307]

This test may be requested as drug screenings for all drugs and all drug classes performed by the respective technology and process per date of service. In addition, this service encompasses all sample validations performed and may include, but is not limited to, pH, specific gravity, and nitrite. This code is reported for tests performed utilizing instrument chemistry analyzers, such as immunoassay (e.g., EIA, ELISA, EMIT, FPIA, IA, KIMS, RIA), chromatography (e.g., GC, HPLC), and mass spectrometry with or without chromatography (e.g., DART, DESI, GC-MS/MS, LC-MS, LC-MS/MS, LDTD, MALDI, TOF). Presumptive tests may be confirmed with a definitive test that designates the drug. Specimen type varies. This code should only be reported once per date of service no matter how many procedures or results are performed.

[80320, 80321, 80322]

Alcohol biomarkers are physiological signs of exposure to, or ingestion of, alcohol and may suggest the possibility of an alcohol use disorder. There are two categories of alcohol biomarkers: direct and indirect. Indirect alcohol biomarkers typically screen for specific types of liver serum elevations that may occur as the result of heavy drinking; other indirect biomarkers may include identification of changes in red blood cells that may indicate nutritional problems from alcohol use. Direct alcohol biomarkers such as the breathalyzer evaluate the blood alcohol concentration. Other direct biomarkers, also known as analytes of alcohol metabolism, include tests for EtG (ethyl glucuronide) and EtS (ethyl sulfate), which are most commonly measured in urine. These tests may register a positive result even with low level alcohol exposure and remain detectable over a several day period. Specimen may be blood (serum) or urine. Method is commonly enzymatic rate analysis (alcohol dehydrogenase). Report 80320 when testing for alcohols; 80321 when testing one or two biomarkers; and 80322 when testing three or more biomarkers.

[80323]

Alkaloids are nitrogenous substances found in plants, many of which are pharmacologically active. Common alkaloids include morphine, quinine, atropine, and strychnine. Methods may include liquid chromatography-tandem mass spectrometry (LC-MS) or high performance liquid chromatography (HPLC). This test may be used to characterize (qualitative), measure (quantitate), or characterize and measure a specific alkaloid present in a specimen. Test specimens may include random urine, whole blood, serum, or plasma.

[80324, 80325, 80326]

These tests may be requested as a qualitative, quantitative, or combination analysis of amphetamine/methamphetamine. Methods used for analysis include gas-liquid chromatography (GLC) and gas chromatometry/mass spectrometry (GC/MS). This is a definitive drug test, meaning testing methods would not be performed by enzymatic or immunoassays. Specimen type varies. Report 80324 for one to two analytes; 80325 for three to four analytes; and 80326 for five or more analytes.

[80327, 80328]

Anabolic steroids are synthetic substances related to the male hormone androgen testosterone, also referred to as anabolic-androgenic steroids (AAS) or performance enhancing drugs (PED). This test describes the ordering of definitive drug testing of one to two steroid types (e.g., DHT, or dihydroxytestosterone, a powerful androgenic hormone formed in the peripheral tissues). It is believed to be responsible for the development of most male secondary characteristics at puberty. Method is radioimmunoassay (RIA). Another type of steroid is Epiandrosterone, a steroid hormone metabolite in the androgen series that is measured for evaluation of syndromes of androgen excess such as hirsutism and polycystic ovary syndrome. It has been measured typically by methods involving extraction and chromatography, followed by detection and quantification by colorimetric or immunometric techniques. The most reliable and commonly employed specimen for detecting anabolic steroid is urine, although specimens may also include both blood and hair samples for this purpose. Measurement of this compound has largely been replaced by determination of other specific plasma androgens (e.g., testosterone) by modern, sensitive assays. For three or more steroid types, report 80328.

[80329, 80330, 80331]

Analgesics include over-the-counter (OTC) pain killers, including nonsteroidal anti-inflammatory drugs (NSAID) such as salicylates and aspirin/acetaminophen. Methods used for analysis include gas-liquid chromatography (GLC) and gas chromatometry/mass spectrometry (GC/MS). This is a definitive drug test, meaning testing methods would not be performed by enzymatic or immunoassays. Analgesic levels may be seen in overdose situations and measurement is useful in determining toxicity and potential kidney or liver damage. The expected half-life of acetaminophen is one to three hours. The expected half-life of ibuprofen is one to two hours. Serum/plasma and urine are the specimens of choice. Apart from serum/plasma and urine, other specimens, including saliva, synovial fluid, and cerebrospinal fluid (CSF), are used for monitoring acetaminophen and some NSAIDs. Report 80329 for one to two analytes; 80330 for three to five analytes; and 80331 for six or more analytes.

[80332, 80333, 80334]

Serotonergic antidepressants work by blocking the reabsorption of the neurotransmitter serotonin, a chemical that assists the brain in sending and receiving messages and in turn boosts mood. They are labeled as selective serotonin reuptake inhibitors (SSRI) because they tend to chiefly target serotonin as opposed to other neurotransmitters such as norepinephrine. Test specimens are frequently collected at the trough period, which is about 12 hours after the last dose when serum concentration is at its lowest. This approach is effective in determining a therapeutic drug level. Drug overdose may be the reason for the test as well. Definitive methods include liquid or gas chromatography with mass spectrometry, excluding immunoassays and enzymatic methods. These drugs are widely recognized as the most commonly prescribed antidepressants used to treat moderate to severe depression and are considered fairly safe with fewer side effects than other antidepressant classes. Report 80332 for one or two serotonergic antidepressants; 80333 for three to five; and 80334 for six or more.

[80335, 80336, 80337]

Tricyclic and tetracyclic antidepressants work by blocking the absorption of neurotransmitters serotonin and norepinephrine, making a greater number of these chemicals available in the brain. These chemicals assist the brain in sending and receiving messages, which in turn boosts mood. They are labeled as tricyclic or tetracyclic based on the number of rings in their chemical structure: three (tri) or four (tetra). Test specimens are frequently collected at the trough period, which is about 12 hours after the last dose when serum concentration is at its lowest. This approach is effective in determining a therapeutic drug level. Drug overdose may be the reason for the test as well. Method is typically high performance liquid chromatography (HPLC) or gas liquid chromatography (GLC). These drugs may be prescribed for disorders outside of depressive states, such as anxiety disorders or nerve-related (neuropathic) pain. While they are effective as an antidepressant, they have mostly been replaced with antidepressants that are known to have fewer side effects. Report 80335 for one or two tricyclic and other cyclical antidepressants; 80336 for three to five; and 80337 for six or more.

[80338]

Some antidepressants work by increasing the levels of neurotransmitters that are associated with depression. These chemicals assist the brain in sending and receiving messages, which in turn boosts mood. Each type or class of antidepressants affects neurotransmitters in somewhat different ways. This code describes testing of antidepressants not classified to a specific class or type. Test specimens are frequently collected at the trough period, which is about 12 hours after the last dose when serum concentration is at its lowest. This effective approach helps determine a therapeutic level of drug. Drug overdose may be the reason for the test as well. Method is typically high performance liquid chromatography (HPLC) or gas liquid chromatography (GLC). These drugs may be prescribed for disorders outside of depressive states, such as anxiety disorders or nerve-related (neuropathic) pain. While they are effective as an antidepressant, they have mostly been replaced with antidepressants that are known to have fewer side effects.

[80339, 80340, 80341]

Antiepileptic drugs (AED) are the main form of treatment for epilepsy. They work by lowering excessive electrical activity in the brain that causes seizures. There is no definitive explanation as to how AEDs do this; it is thought that each type of AED may work in a somewhat different manner. Test specimens are frequently collected at the trough period, which is about 12 hours after the last dose when serum concentration is at its lowest. Test specimens may include whole blood, serum, plasma, or saliva. These codes describe testing of unspecified antiepileptics. Methods include radioimmunoassay (RIA), gas-liquid chromatography (GLC), and enzyme high-performance liquid chromatography (HPLC). Report 80339 for one to three analytes; 80340 for four to six, and 80341 for seven or more.

[80342, 80343, 80344]

Antipsychotics are drugs that are used for treatment of some types of mental disorders, mainly schizophrenia and manic depression (bipolar disorder). They can also be used to help severe anxiety or depression. Antipsychotics work by blocking the effect of dopamine, the main neurotransmitter of brain. Test methods may include high performance liquid chromatography (HPLC), thin-layer chromatography (TLC), gas chromatography (GC), fluorometry, thin-layer chromatography (TLC), gas-liquid chromatography (GLC), or radioimmunoassay (RIA). Test specimens may include blood, serum, urine, saliva, or hair samples. These tests are performed to evaluate the amount of antipsychotic present. Report 80342 for one to three analytes; 80343 for four to six analytes; and 80344 for seven or more analytes.

[80345]

Barbiturates are a type of depressant drug that cause relaxation and sleepiness. This test may be requested as a qualitative, quantitative, or combination analysis for barbiturates. Methods used for analysis include gas-liquid chromatography (GLC) and gas chromatometry/mass spectrometry (GC/MS). Test specimens may include blood, serum, plasma, or urine. This is a definitive drug test, meaning methods of testing would not be performed by enzymatic or immunoassays.

[80346, 80347]

Benzodiazepines are a class of psychoactive drugs that are used as sedatives, hypnotics, anxiolytics, anticonvulsants and muscle relaxants. Methods used for analysis include gas chromatography (GC), gas chromatography-mass spectrometry (GC-MS), high performance liquid chromatography (HPLC), or thin layer chromatography (TLC). Test specimens may include urine, or blood. This test measures (quantitates) the amount of the drug present. Report 80346 for one to 12 analytes and 80347 for 13 or more analytes.

[80348]
This test may be requested as a qualitative, quantitative, or combination analysis of buprenorphine, which is prescribed to treat opioid dependence. The main use of this test is to monitor patients to determine if they are following dependence therapy. The specimen is urine. Methods used for analysis include gas-liquid chromatography (GLC) and gas chromatometry/mass spectrometry (GC/MS). This is a definitive drug test, meaning methods of testing would not be performed by enzymatic or immunoassays.

[80349, 80350, 80351, 80352]
These tests may be requested as qualitative, quantitative, or combination analysis of cannabinoids. Naturally occurring cannabinoids are found in the resin composition of the cannabis plant. Synthetic drugs have been constructed that follow the same courses within the brain, but work differently than the natural version. Methods used for analysis include gas-liquid chromatography (GLC) and gas chromatometry/mass spectrometry (GC/MS). The most reliable specimen for the test is urine, although specimens may also include blood, serum, saliva, and hair samples. This is a definitive drug test, meaning methods of testing would not be performed by enzymatic or immunoassays. Report 80349 when testing for natural cannabinoids; 80350 when testing for one to three synthetic cannabinoids; 80351 when testing for four to six synthetic cannabinoids; and 80352 when testing for seven or more.

[80353]
Cocaine is a refined derivative of the coca plant and is a frequently abused drug. Test specimens may include urine, blood, saliva, sweat, and hair samples. This test may be requested as a qualitative, quantitative, or combination analysis for cocaine. Methods used for analysis include gas-liquid chromatography (GLC) and gas chromatometry/mass spectrometry (GC/MS). This is a definitive drug test, meaning methods of testing would not be performed by enzymatic or immunoassays.

[80354]
This test may be requested as a qualitative, quantitative, or combination analysis of fentanyl. This drug is classified as a fast acting synthetic opiate and due to the sensation that is similar to heroin, it may be abused. It is prescribed for symptoms coinciding with chronic pain, often administered when other pain medications fail. The half-life varies depending on method of delivery. Methods used for analysis include gas-liquid chromatography (GLC) and gas chromatometry/mass spectrometry (GC/MS). This is a definitive drug test, meaning methods of testing would not be performed by enzymatic or immunoassays. Specimen is serum, plasma, or urine.

[80355]
Gabapentin is used to treat seizures, neuropathies, and a variety of neurological and psychological disorders. Methods may include liquid chromatography-tandem mass spectrometry (LC-MS) or high performance liquid chromatography (HPLC). This code is reported for specimens other than blood (e.g., urine).

[80356]
This test may be requested as a qualitative, quantitative, or combination analysis for heroin metabolite. Heroin is a manufactured opiate with a morphine base and is difficult to determine through body fluids. The half-life is just a few minutes, but in analysis, the proportion of morphine to codeine found in the specimen can assist in determining heroin versus codeine. Methods used for analysis include gas-liquid chromatography (GLC) and gas chromatometry/mass spectrometry (GC/MS). Test specimens may include urine or blood. This is a definitive drug test, meaning methods of testing would not be performed by enzymatic or immunoassays.

[80357]
This test may be requested as a qualitative, quantitative, or combination analysis for ketamine and/or norketamine. Ketamine is used for anesthesia, but is also sold/abused based on hallucinogenic properties. It has a half-life of three to four hours. Test specimens may include blood, serum, plasma, or urine. Norketamine, the breakdown product of Ketamine, is detectable in blood and urine for seven to 14 days. Methods used for analysis include gas-liquid chromatography (GLC) and gas chromatometry/mass spectrometry (GC/MS). This is a definitive drug test, meaning methods of testing would not be performed by enzymatic or immunoassays.

[80358]
Methadone is a synthetic opioid that is used clinically to relieve pain and to treat opioid and heroin addiction. This test may be requested as a qualitative, quantitative, or combination analysis for methadone. This test is used to measure toxicity and the determination of methadone in the system in cases of drug abuse. Test specimens may include blood, serum, or urine. Methods used for analysis include gas-liquid chromatography (GLC) and gas chromatometry/mass spectrometry (GC/MS). This is a definitive drug test, meaning methods of testing would not be performed by enzymatic or immunoassays.

[80359]
This test may be requested as a qualitative, quantitative, or combination analysis of amphetamine/methamphetamine. Methods used for analysis include gas-liquid chromatography (GLC) and gas chromatometry/mass spectrometry (GC/MS). This

is a definitive drug test, meaning methods of testing would not be performed by enzymatic or immunoassays. Test specimens may include blood, serum, plasma, or urine.

[80360]
This test may be requested as a qualitative, quantitative, or combination analysis for methylphenidate. This test would be ordered to monitor therapy in patients with attention deficit hyperactivity disorder (ADHD). Methods used for analysis include gas-liquid chromatography (GLC) and gas chromatometry/mass spectrometry (GC/MS). This is a definitive drug test, meaning methods of testing would not be performed by enzymatic or immunoassays. The most commonly used specimen for detecting methylphenidate is urine, although specimens may also include blood, serum, plasma, or hair samples.

[80361, 80362, 80363, 80364]
These tests may be requested as qualitative, quantitative, or combination analyses for opiates and opioids/opiate analogs. These tests measure the amount of a given opiate present and may be ordered to measure toxicity or possible drug abuse of opiates such as morphine or meperidine. These drugs are prescribed for treatment of chronic pain, but recent studies are evaluating the benefits of this type of therapy given the complex side effects and chronic conditions that can be caused by long-term use of these drugs. Methods used for analysis include gas-liquid chromatography (GLC) and gas chromatometry/mass spectrometry (GC/MS). The most reliable and commonly employed specimen for detecting opiate is urine, although specimens may also include blood, hair, saliva, sweat, or nails. This is a definitive drug test, meaning methods of testing would not be performed by enzymatic or immunoassays. Report 80361 when testing for one or more opiates; 80362 when testing for one to two opioids and/or opiate analogs; 80363 when testing for three to four opioids and/or opiate analogs; and 80364 when testing for five or more opioids and/or opiate analogs.

[80365]
Oxycodone is an opioid pain medication used to treat moderate to severe pain. This test may be requested as a qualitative, quantitative, or combination analysis of oxycodone and can detect several opiates. Methods used for analysis include gas-liquid chromatography (GLC) and gas chromatometry/mass spectrometry (GC/MS). This is a definitive drug test, meaning methods of testing would not be performed by enzymatic or immunoassays. Specimen can be blood or urine.

[83992]
This test is performed to evaluate the presence of phencyclidine (also known as PCP, or angel dust), an illegal street drug. Methodology may include immunoassay, thin-layer chromatography (TLC), gas chromatography (GC), and gas chromatography/mass spectrometry (GC/TC), which quantifies the amount of drug.

[80366]
This test may be requested as a qualitative, quantitative, or combination analysis of pregabalin. It falls within the anticonvulsant drugs and is used to reduce pain in conditions that affect the nerves (e.g., shingles, fibromyalgia) and in conjunction with other medications to treat epileptic seizures. Methods used for analysis include gas-liquid chromatography (GLC) and gas chromatometry/mass spectrometry (GC/MS). This is a definitive drug test, meaning methods of testing would not be performed by enzymatic or immunoassays. Test specimens may include serum, plasma, or urine.

[80367]
This test may be requested as a qualitative, quantitative, or combination analysis of propoxyphene. This is an opiate and was prescribed for pain relief; however, the FDA suggested removal of this drug in 2010 due to toxic effects it can have on the heart. At that time, all products containing propoxyphene were discontinued. Methods used for analysis include gas-liquid chromatography (GLC) and gas chromatometry/mass spectrometry (GC/MS).This is a definitive drug test, meaning methods of testing would not be performed by enzymatic or immunoassays. Specimen is plasma, serum, or urine.

[80368]
This test may be requested as a qualitative, quantitative, or combination analysis for sedative hypnotics, specifically non-benzodiazepines. This classification of drugs includes eszopiclone, zaleplon, and zolpidem. These drugs are typically used to treat insomnia. The effect allows the patient to fall asleep faster and promotes continued and/or extended sleep cycles. These drugs have a shorter half-life than other sedatives, reducing risk of dependence, but suggested use is for one to four weeks only. Methods used for analysis include high performance liquid chromatography (HPLC), gas chromatography (GC), gas chromatography/mass spectrometry (GC/MS), liquid chromatography mass spectrometry (LCMS), and liquid chromatography/tandem mass spectrometry (LC/MS/MS). This is a definitive drug test, meaning methods of testing would not be performed by enzymatic or immunoassays. Test specimens may include whole blood, serum, plasma, urine, or hair samples.

[80369, 80370]
These tests may be requested as a qualitative, quantitative, or combination analysis. There are several drugs classified as skeletal muscle relaxants, which may not all work the same way but are typically prescribed to reduce pain and spasms within the musculoskeletal system. The main symptoms include stiff muscles due to disorders that affect the brain or spinal cord, typically of lengthy duration, and spasms that tend to be transient in nature. Methods used for analysis include gas-liquid chromatography (GLC) and

gas chromatometry/mass spectrometry (GC/MS). This is a definitive drug test, meaning methods of testing would not be performed by enzymatic or immunoassays. Test specimens may include blood, plasma, or urine. Report 80369 when testing for one or two relaxants and 80370 when testing for three or more relaxants.

[80371]

There are a number of drugs classified as synthetic stimulants (e.g., methylenedioxypyrovalerone). These stimulants, such as bath salts, may be obtained by prescription or through illicit drug use and many consider these designer drugs. A chemical stimulant affects the central nervous system resulting in increased heart rate and altered realistic thinking. Methods used for analysis include gas-liquid chromatography (GLC) and gas chromatometry/mass spectrometry (GC/MS). This is a definitive drug test, meaning methods of testing would not be performed by enzymatic or immunoassays. Test specimens may include blood, serum, plasma, or urine.

[80372]

This test may be requested as a qualitative, quantitative, or combination analysis for tapentadol. This drug is an opioid-based analgesic prescribed for pain, most often for patients experiencing pain due to diabetic peripheral neuropathy. The half-life is about four hours. Similar to other opioid based analgesics, this drug can be highly addictive. Methods used for analysis include gas-liquid chromatography (GLC) and gas chromatometry/mass spectrometry (GC/MS). This is a definitive drug test, meaning methods of testing would not be performed by enzymatic or immunoassays. Test specimens may include blood, serum, plasma, or urine.

[80373]

This test may be requested as a qualitative, quantitative, or combination analysis for tramadol. This drug is an opioid-based analgesic prescribed for pain. The half-life is about seven hours. Similar to other opioid-based analgesics, this drug can be highly addictive. Methods used for analysis include gas-liquid chromatography (GLC) and gas chromatometry/mass spectrometry (GC/MS). This is a definitive drug test, meaning methods of testing would not be performed by enzymatic or immunoassays. Test specimens may include blood, serum, plasma, or urine.

[80374]

This test may be requested as a qualitative, quantitative, or combination analysis for stereoisomer or enantiomer, single drug class. Essentially, these are chemical compositions that have the same atoms and are connected in the same matter, but arranged in a different proportional pattern. Based on this composition, different chemical compounds can have different effects on the human body. Methods used for analysis include gas-liquid chromatography (GLC) and gas chromatometry/mass spectrometry (GC/MS). This is a definitive drug test, meaning methods of testing would not be performed by enzymatic or immunoassays.

[80375, 80376, 80377]

These tests may be requested as drug screen confirmation. They are performed when the initial drug screen is positive. Confirmatory tests must be sensitive and specific and involve a different technique than the initial screen. Methods used for analysis include gas-liquid chromatography (GLC) and gas chromatometry/mass spectrometry (GC/MS). This is a definitive drug test, meaning methods of testing would not be performed by enzymatic or immunoassays. Report 80375 for one to three analytes; 80376 for four to six analytes; and 80377 for seven or more analytes.

80143

This test determines the level of acetaminophen in the blood and is used to monitor therapeutic levels as well as to evaluate for acetaminophen toxicity. This widely used analgesic-antipyretic medication is indicated to treat arthralgia and chronic pain due to cancer, fever, headache, myalgia, and postoperative or postpartum pain, and is rapidly absorbed from the GI tract. The most common cause of toxic hepatitis in North America and Europe, acetaminophen is also one of the most common poisonings from intentional or accidental overdose. Specimen type may be whole blood, serum, or plasma; examination is quantitative.

80145

This test determines the therapeutic level of adalimumab. Adalimumab is used to treat conditions including, but not limited to, moderate to severe rheumatoid arthritis (RA), polyarticular idiopathic arthritis, psoriatic arthritis, Crohn's disease, ulcerative colitis, and chronic plaque psoriasis. Specimen type is serum. Methodology is an assessment of monoclonal antibodies to adalimumab using enzyme-linked immunosorbent assay (ELISA).

80150

Amikacin is a type of antibiotic. Test specimens are frequently collected at peak and trough periods, which is shortly after administration of amikacin and again just before the next administration when serum concentration is at its lowest. This is an effective approach to determine a therapeutic level of drug. Method is radioimmunoassay (RIA) or high performance liquid chromatography (HPLC).

80151

This test determines the level of amiodarone, an antiarrhythmic agent, in the blood. It is used to monitor amiodarone therapy and assess patient compliance and can also evaluate possible amiodarone toxicity. Amiodarone is typically used for ventricular tachyarrhythmias. Specimen type is serum or plasma; methodology is liquid chromatography/tandem mass spectrometry (LC/MS-MS).

80155

Caffeine is the most widely consumed stimulant in the world and is found in beverages, foods, and medications. This drug may cause moderate to severe symptoms and/or caffeine toxicity. Blood specimen is collected via venipuncture. Test specimens are collected randomly rather than at trough level. A quantitative analysis of caffeine in the bloodstream does not influence medical management of the patient. This test is most commonly used on neonatal patients that are not responding to caffeine therapy or have suspected toxicity of caffeine. Method is enzyme immunoassay (EIA).

80156
Carbamazepine is an enzyme inducer. Blood specimen collection is by venipuncture. CSF is obtained by spinal puncture, which is reported separately. Test specimens for total levels are frequently collected at the trough period, which is about 12 hours after the last dose when serum concentration is at its lowest. This is an effective approach to determine a therapeutic level of drug. This drug is absorbed slowly and erratically by the GI tract and a total concentration may be required, depending on the treatment underway. Methods include high performance liquid chromatography (HPLC) or gas liquid chromatography (GLC). Carbamazepine may be administered for such conditions as trigeminal neuralgia, epilepsy, and manic disorders. It is known for its anticonvulsant and pain management properties.

80157
Carbamazepine is an enzyme inducer. Specimen collection is by venipuncture. Test specimens for free drug concentrations may be collected near peak levels about two to eight hours after ingestion. Methods include high performance liquid chromatography (HPLC) or gas liquid chromatography (GLC). This drug is absorbed slowly and erratically by the gastrointestinal (GI) tract and a free plasma concentration may be assayed, depending on the type of treatment underway. Carbamazepine may be administered for such conditions as trigeminal neuralgia, epilepsy, and manic disorders. It is known for its anticonvulsant and pain management properties.

[80161]
Carbamazepine, an anticonvulsant, is indicated for certain types of seizures and is frequently used in combination with other anticonvulsants. It may also be indicated in the treatment of bipolar disorder, alcohol withdrawal, and alleviation of certain types of nerve pain. This test determines the level of its metabolite, carbamazepine-10, 11-epoxide, in the blood. Test specimens are frequently collected at the trough period, immediately prior to the next dose when serum concentration is at its lowest. This approach is effective in determining a therapeutic drug level as well as potential toxicity. Specimen type is serum or plasma; methodology is liquid chromatography/ tandem mass spectrometry (LC/MS-MS).

80158
Cyclosporine is an immunosuppressant and is often monitored. Test specimens are frequently collected at the trough period, which is typically about 12 hours after the last dose when serum concentration is at its lowest. Method is high performance liquid chromatography (HPLC) or fluorescence polarization immunoassay (FPIA).

80159
Clozapine is an atypical antipsychotic used to treat severe cases of schizophrenia in which the patient is a threat to themselves and/or others. It changes the activity of certain chemical processes in the brain. Agranulocytosis is the most common side effect and therefore white blood cell and absolute neutrophil count are required weekly for the first six months, biweekly for the second six months, and every four weeks after a year of being maintained on clozapine. Blood specimen is collected by venipuncture usually during the trough period. Methods include liquid chromatography and tandem mass spectrometry.

80162-80163
Digoxin is used principally to treat conditions surrounding congestive heart failure, such as arrhythmias, atrial fibrillation, and tachycardia. Test specimens may be drawn during peak and trough periods, which is shortly after administration and again just before the next administration when serum concentration is at its lowest. Method for total digoxin (80162) is high performance liquid chromatography (HPLC) or gas liquid chromatography (GLC) and is used to determine dosage. Free digoxin levels are useful in determining digoxin toxicity. A protein-free ultrafiltrate is prepared from the patient's serum, and the digoxin in the ultrafiltrate (free digoxin) is measured by fluorescence polarization immunoassay. Report 80162 for total serum levels and 80163 when free digoxin is assayed.

80168
Ethosuximide is an anticonvulsant medication. Test specimens may be drawn during peak and trough periods, which is shortly after administration of Zarontin and again just before the next administration when serum concentration is at its lowest. Methods include high performance liquid chromatography (HPLC), radioimmunoassay (RIA), and microbiology assay.

80169
Everolimus is most commonly used to treat kidney transplant rejection and renal cell carcinoma. Blood specimen is collected via venipuncture during the trough period. This is an effective way to determine a therapeutic level of the drug. Methods include tandem mass spectrometry or high performance liquid chromatography (HPLC).

[80167]
Felbamate is an antiepileptic drug used to treat patients with various types of partial seizures. It is also approved for Lennox-Gastaut syndrome in children ages 2 and older. This test determines the level of felbamate in the blood and is useful for dose optimization, toxicity avoidance, and monitoring changes in serum concentrations due to interactions

with drugs administered concurrently, such as barbiturates and phenytoin. Optimal time for sample collection is one hour prior to the next dose. Specimen type is serum or plasma; methodology is liquid chromatography/tandem mass spectrometry (LC/MS-MS).

[80181]
Flecainide is an antiarrhythmic drug indicated for the treatment and prophylaxis of supraventricular tachycardia (SVT) and atrial fibrillation. This test is useful for monitoring compliance, optimizing dosage, and assessing toxicity. Specimen type is serum or plasma, which should be collected at the trough period, immediately before the next scheduled dose. Test methodology is liquid chromatography/tandem mass spectrometry (LC/MS-MS).

[80171]
Gabapentin is used to treat seizures, neuropathies, and a variety of neurological and psychological disorders. Test specimens are collected immediately before the next scheduled dose. Methods may include liquid chromatography-tandem mass spectrometry (LC-MS) or high performance liquid chromatography (HPLC). Test specimens are whole blood, serum, or plasma.

80170
Gentamicin is classified as an aminoglycoside, an antibiotic. In its injectable form, the drug may be prescribed for gram-negative infections, septicemia, and other serious infections, as well as unknown causative organisms. A typical course will run seven to 10 days. Monitoring may be initiated to measure drug clearance via the kidneys. Patients with impaired renal function may accumulate the drug. Peak serum concentrations can be expected about 30 to 60 minutes following an intramuscular injection though concentrations occur just before the next dose. Dosage is highly dependent on the severity of infection. Methodology varies.

80173
This drug, also known as Haldol, is a well-established tranquilizer with antipsychotic and other properties. Blood concentrations of haloperidol do not correspond well with therapeutic dosages; therefore, assays may be performed to establish compliance or to measure the body's ability to metabolize the drug. Methods may include high performance liquid chromatography (HPLC), gas liquid chromatography (GLC), and radioimmunoassay (RIA).

[80220]
Hydroxychloroquine, an antimalarial drug used to treat or prevent malaria, is also used to treat symptoms of systemic lupus erythematosus (SLE) or acute or chronic rheumatoid arthritis. It accumulates in various organs, particularly the skin and melanin-containing retina. Mild to moderate overdose can lead to headache, vision or hearing difficulties, neuromuscular symptoms, or GI symptoms such as abdominal pain, nausea and vomiting. Therapeutic doses may result in acute hepatitis, cardiotoxicity, or retinopathy. Specimen is serum; method is liquid chromatography-tandem mass spectrometry (LC-MS/MS) for this therapeutic drug assay.

[80230]
This test is used to determine patients who have a loss of response to infliximab, which is used to treat conditions including, but not limited to, moderate to severe rheumatoid arthritis (RA), polyarticular idiopathic arthritis, psoriatic arthritis, Crohn's disease, ulcerative colitis, and chronic plaque psoriasis. Sample type is trough serum (drawn immediately before scheduled dose). The patient is advised to abstain from multivitamins and other supplements 24 hours prior to venipuncture. Methodology is liquid chromatography-tandem mass spectrometry (LC-MS/MS) testing for antibodies to infliximab.

[80189]
Itraconazole is indicated for the treatment of susceptible fungal infections, including blastomycosis and histoplasmosis, in immunocompromised and immunocompetent patients. Indications also include aspergillosis and onychomycosis of the toenail and fingernail. Routine monitoring may be recommended during the first week of therapy to ensure therapeutic levels are achieved; continued monitoring may be recommended if there is a decline or a lack of improvement in clinical presentations. This test is useful for verifying systemic absorption of orally administered itraconazole and for monitoring for drug interactions. Specimen type is serum or plasma; methodology is liquid chromatography/tandem mass spectrometry (LC/MS-MS).

[80235]
The patient is tested to determine therapeutic levels of lacosamide (also known as Vimpat®), an antiepileptic drug (AED). Specimen type is serum. When the patient is prescribed the sustained release form of the drug, blood should be drawn 12 hours after last dosage. Peak plasma concentrations occur one to four hours after oral dosing, and the elimination half-life is approximately 13 hours. Methodology is liquid chromatography-tandem mass spectrometry (LC-MS/MS).

80175
Lamotrigine is also known as Lamictal. It is used to treat and control seizures. Test specimen is blood collected via venipuncture. This is an effective approach to determine a therapeutic level. Method is enzyme immunoassay (EIA).

[80193]
This test measures the level of leflunomide, a pyrimidine synthesis inhibitor indicated for the treatment of active rheumatoid arthritis, in the blood. It is useful for optimizing therapy as well as assessment of elimination in those patients who require enhanced elimination of the drug (i.e., those who wish to become pregnant or who are experiencing toxicity). Test specimens are frequently collected at the trough period, approximately 12 hours after the last dose.

Specimen type is serum; methodology is liquid chromatography/tandem mass spectrometry (LC/MS-MS).

80177
Levetiracetam is used to treat and control seizures. Test specimen is blood collected via venipuncture. Therapeutic levels may be difficult to determine. Method is enzyme immunoassay (EIA).

[80176]
Lidocaine is widely used in its various forms, including nonprescription ointments. However, lidocaine may be injected as an intravenous bolus as a treatment for ventricular arrhythmias and for cardiac manipulation. Any of a number of testing methods may be used, including high performance liquid chromatography (HPLC), gas liquid chromatography (GLC), gas chromatography-mass spectrometry (GC-MS), and fluorescence polarization immunoassay (FPIA).

80178
Lithium is a naturally-occurring mineral and its salts may be used in the treatment of mental disorders, in particular bipolar depression. Steady state test specimens are frequently collected at the trough period, which is about 12 hours after the last dose when serum concentration is at its lowest. This is an effective approach to determine a therapeutic level of drug. Methods may include flame emission spectroscopy (FES), atomic absorption spectrophotometry (AAS), and ion-specific electrode (ISE).

[80204]
This test measures the level of methotrexate, an antineoplastic agent that inhibits DNA synthesis, in the blood. Methotrexate is used in adult rheumatoid arthritis, severe psoriasis, and certain neoplastic diseases, including malignancies characterized by rapid cell proliferation. This test is useful in verifying that a nontoxic concentration has been achieved following therapy as well as determining whether methotrexate is being cleared appropriately. Specimen type is serum or plasma; methodology is liquid chromatography/tandem mass spectrometry (LC/MS-MS) or immunoassay.

80180
Mycophenolate is an immunosuppressive given to patients to treat autoimmune diseases, such as lupus, rheumatoid arthritis, Crohn's disease, among others and is also prescribed to help manage organ transplant rejection. Test specimen is blood collected via venipuncture. This is an effective approach to determine a therapeutic level. Methods include tandem mass spectrometry or high performance liquid chromatography (HPLC).

80183
Oxcarbazepine is an anticonvulsant and mood stabilizer used to treat epilepsy, motor tics, bipolar disorder, and anxiety. Test specimen is blood collected via venipuncture. This is an effective approach to determine a therapeutic level. Methods include tandem mass spectrometry or liquid chromatography.

80184
Phenobarbital may be administered to control seizures. Test specimens are frequently collected at the trough period, which is about 12 hours after the last dose when serum concentration is at its lowest. This is an effective approach to determine a therapeutic level of drug. Methodology may include gas liquid chromatography (GLC) and high performance liquid chromatography (HPLC).

80185-80186
Phenytoin may be administered to control seizures. Steady state test specimens are frequently collected at the trough period, which is about 12 hours after the last dose when serum concentration is at its lowest. This is an effective approach to determine a therapeutic level of drug. Report 80185 for total serum levels and 80186 when free phenytoin is assayed. Methodology may include high performance liquid chromatography (HPLC), gas liquid chromatography (GLC), radioimmunoassay (RIA), and fluorescence polarization immunoassay (FPIA). Free phenytoin is assayed by ultracentrifugation. Phenytoin is a known teratogen (cause of birth defects) and lowest therapeutic levels possible are often sought.

80187
Posaconazole is an antifungal agent used as a prophylaxis for *Aspergillus* and *Candida* infections in patients who are at high risk of developing fungal infections. Sample type is serum. Methodology is liquid chromatography-tandem mass spectrometry (LC-MS/MS) testing.

80188
Primidone may be administered to control seizures. Test specimens are frequently collected at the trough period, which is about 12 hours after the last dose when serum concentration is at its lowest. This is an effective approach to determine a therapeutic level of drug. Methodology may include high performance liquid chromatography (HPLC), gas liquid chromatography (GLC), or enzyme immunoassay (EIA).

80190
Procainamide is often administered as an antiarrhythmic. Test specimens are frequently collected at the trough period, which is about 12 hours after the last dose when serum concentration is at its lowest. This is an effective approach to determine a therapeutic level of drug. Methodology may include high performance liquid chromatography (HPLC), gas liquid chromatography (GLC), and enzyme immunoassay (EIA).

80192
This procedure tests for procainamide as well as metabolites, known as NAPA (n-acetyl procainamide).

80194
Quinidine is often administered as an antiarrhythmic. Test specimens are frequently collected at the trough

period, which is about 12 hours after the last dose when serum concentration is at its lowest. This is an effective approach to determine a therapeutic level of drug. Methodology may include high performance liquid chromatography (HPLC) and gas liquid chromatography (GLC).

[80210]
Rufinamide, an antiepileptic drug, is indicated for the treatment of focal seizures in adults and adolescents and as an add-on treatment of Lennox-Gastaut-associated seizures in children ages 4 years and older. The test is useful for monitoring serum concentrations to assess patient compliance, dosage optimization, and evaluation of potential interaction with other drugs. Test specimens are frequently collected at the trough period. Specimen type is serum or plasma; methodology is liquid chromatography/ tandem mass spectrometry (LC/MS-MS).

[80179]
This test determines the amount of aspirin, an analgesic, antipyretic, anti-inflammatory drug, in the blood and is useful for assessing therapeutic level as well as potential toxicity. Optimal sampling time after dosage is two to six hours. Specimen type is serum or plasma; methodology is liquid chromatography/ tandem mass spectrometry (LC/MS-MS).

80195
This procedure tests for the level of sirolimus, a potent immunosuppressant in the blood. Sirolimus blood levels may be affected by cytochrome P450 3A4 inducers or inhibitors or by patient liver function (hepatic insufficiency). Therapeutic drug monitoring (TDM) of sirolimus concentrations are frequently performed to monitor blood concentration levels and evaluate dosage.

80197
Tacrolimus is an immunosuppressant and may be prescribed for a number of conditions, including post-transplant therapies. Blood concentration monitoring may be ordered with this drug, particularly when delivered by IV. In this event, specimen collection may be random. Methodology may include high performance liquid chromatography (HPLC).

80198
Theophylline is available in several different forms, which may affect the type of assay run. Samples may be drawn about 30 minutes after oral administration. When delivered by IV, specimen collection may be random. The drug is widely used as a bronchodilator and to relieve bronchospasms. Methodology may include high performance liquid chromatography (HPLC) or gas liquid chromatography (GLC).

80199
Tiagabine is an anticonvulsant used to treat partial seizures. Test specimen is blood collected via venipuncture. This is an effective approach to determine a therapeutic level. Methods include tandem mass spectrometry or high performance liquid chromatography (HPLC).

80200
Tobramycin has bactericidal properties and is usually injected. Specimen collection is at peak and trough. Peak will occur about one hour after an intramuscular injection and trough will occur about 12 hours after that. Method will often be by radioimmunoassay (RIA), microbiological assay, or high performance liquid chromatography (HPLC).

80201
Topiramate is a broad-spectrum, antiepileptic drug. Indications include Lennox-Gastaut syndrome (a form of childhood onset epilepsy), other various types of seizures, and migraine prophylaxis. Specimen is serum and test method is liquid chromatography-tandem mass spectrometry (LC-MS/MS).

[80164, 80165]
Valproic acid is often used to treat epilepsy and manic episodes associated with bipolar disorder. The valproic acid test is used to measure and monitor the amount of valproic acid in the blood (serum) and determine whether the drug concentration is within the therapeutic range. Test specimens are frequently collected at the trough period, which is about 12 hours after the last dose when blood (serum) concentration is at its lowest. This is an effective approach to determine the therapeutic level of drug. Method is gas liquid chromatography (GLC), gas chromatography-mass spectrometry (GC-MS), and enzyme immunoassay (EIA). Report 80164 for total and 80165 for free.

80202
Specimen collection for vancomycin assay may be drawn during the trough period. This occurs around 30 minutes prior to the next dose. It is sometimes also drawn at peak. Toxic and therapeutic dosages for vancomycin can be difficult to determine due to the way the drug is metabolized. Methods include radioimmunoassay (RIA), high performance liquid chromatography (HPLC), and microbiological assay.

[80280]
Vedolizumab is used for the treatment of patients with moderate to severe ulcerative colitis or Crohn's disease. This therapeutic drug assay is an aid to achieving desired trough serum levels of vedolizumab to determine patient response and dosing levels. Specimen type is serum. The patient is advised to avoid taking multivitamins or dietary supplements containing biotin (vitamin B7). It should also be noted that nivolumab must be discontinued at least four weeks prior to testing for vedolizumab quantitation to be accurate. Methodology is liquid chromatography.

[80285]
Voriconazole is an antifungal drug used to treat serious fungal infections, such as aspergillosis, candidemia, scedosporiosis, and fusariosis. Monitoring trough levels is often performed to determine trough levels in patients who are not responding as expected or who are taking other medications that may decrease

voriconazole levels. Specimen type is serum. Methodology is chromatography-mass spectrometry.

80203
Zonisamide is a sulfonamide anticonvulsant used to treat partial-onset seizures. Test specimen is blood collected via venipuncture. Therapeutic levels may be difficult to determine. Methods include enzyme immunoassay (EIA).

80400
This test is sometimes ordered as corticotropin-releasing factor stimulation (or CRF) test, adrenocorticotropic hormone (ACTH) infusion test, rapid ACTH test, or cosyntropin test. Method is immunoassay. A chemistry test must be performed to determine baseline serum cortisol (serum ACTH may also be ordered). Shortly thereafter, cosyntropin, an ACTH-like drug, is administered to the patient, typically by IV bolus. Blood is again drawn and assayed for a change in serum cortisol. Variations are seen in administering a 24-hour test and a three-day test. This code reports the test for adrenal insufficiency (Addison's disease), which is an ordinary reason for the test. See 82533 for serum cortisol testing specifics.

80402
This test may be ordered as an enzyme deficiency ACTH stimulation test. This code specifically cites 21-hydroxylase deficiency. The classic 21-hydroxylase deficiency is noted in ambiguous genitalia in neonates, but a later onset is also found. Cosyntropin, an ACTH-like drug, is administered to the patient, typically by IV bolus. Overproduction of the metabolite 17-hydroxyprogesterone is often associated with this condition and it is tested for as a baseline and following the ACTH stimulation injection. Cortisol levels are tested in a similar fashion in this panel.

80406
This test may be ordered as a 3B-HSD panel. The official description for the code is for 3 beta-hydroxydehydrogenase deficiency or congenital adrenal hyperplasia. The panel may often be performed on infants and small children, but adult patients are also tested. The condition involves defects in steroid synthesis. A bolus infusion of ACTH is given to the patient after baseline cortisol and 17-hydroxypregnenolone have been drawn. Cortisol and 17-hydroxypregnenolone are drawn again and the results interpreted.

80408
This panel may be ordered as a saline infusion test. Specimen is drawn from the patient while in an upright position and the product saved for baseline aldosterone and renin testing. The patient is administered saline, usually intravenously, while in a recumbent position. Specimen is again drawn for aldosterone and renin levels. In healthy individuals, aldosterone output is suppressed when the volume of blood is expanded. The test is useful in the evaluation of kidney function.

80410
This test may be ordered as human calcitonin test (HCT) or thyrocalcitonin panel. Calcitonin is a hormone secreted by the thyroid gland in response to elevated serum calcium levels. Calcitonin secretion causes the calcium to be excreted by the kidneys. A baseline calcitonin level is drawn. Stimulation of the thyroid for this panel is typically pentagastrin delivered by IV. Blood is again drawn at five and 10 minutes from stimulation. The patient should be fasting.

80412
This test may be ordered as CRH "Stim" panel. This panel allows for multiple specimens to be drawn before administration of CRH. Orders may call for blood draws from both petrous sinus veins as well as from a peripheral source. Note the high number of cortisol and ACTH tests to be run. The timing of specimen draws for cortisol and ACTH may differ somewhat. The panel is useful to differentiate Cushing's disease and certain ACTH-secreting tumors, among other disorders.

80414
This test may be ordered as a HCG "Stim" or human chorionic gonadotropin panel. Blood specimens may be drawn on two separate mornings before HCG is administered, usually by intramuscular injection. Injections may be repeated on two following days. Blood collection times may vary following HCG administration. The test is useful in diagnosis of certain cases of hypogonadotrophism as well as certain steroid deficiencies.

80415
This test may be ordered as an HCG "Stim" or human chorionic gonadotropin panel. Blood specimens may be drawn on two separate mornings before HCG is administered, usually by intramuscular injection and sometimes in several sessions. Timing of blood draws may vary, but just prior to the first administration of HCG and four hours after is common for women. Estradiol is among the more active endogenous estrogens. The panel is useful in the diagnosis of certain menstrual disorders, fertility problems, and estrogen-producing tumors.

80416-80417
These tests may be ordered as renin "Stim" panel, renin activity panel, or plasma renin activity (PRA) panel. Baseline samples may be drawn from the renal vein (80416) or peripheral vein (80417) and tested for renin. Renin is an enzyme synthesized in the kidney. A renin-stimulating agent, such as the diuretics captopril and furosemide, is administered, usually orally and usually in several stages. The patient remains upright for several hours before again testing for renin, once again, usually in stages. The panel is a useful screen and diagnostic tool for various forms of hypertension, renal artery disorders, and other disorders of the renal/circulatory system.

80418
This series of tests may also be ordered as a pituitary panel and many large facilities will have an internal code name for this panel. This is a complex panel with numerous tests. Facilities with proper capabilities can offer a rapid, combined series where stimulation agents (i.e., insulin, thyrotropin-releasing hormone, and luteinizing hormone-releasing hormone) are administered simultaneously on a single day. This panel may be used most often for a suspected pituitary tumor. See individual code listings for specifics about portions of the panel.

80420
Baseline samples are usually drawn. Dexamethasone is the suppression agent and it is usually administered orally at night. The next morning a fasting blood sample is drawn and rendered to serum. The cortisol level is measured as described in 82533. The free cortisol is a urine test as described in 82530. This panel is a 48-hour work up to differentiate diagnoses, such as Cushing's syndrome from alcoholism, obesity, and depression.

80422
Arginine is a powerful stimulator of glucagon in healthy patients and may be administered as the stimulating agent for this panel. Baseline blood work is typically performed prior to stimulating glucagon. This glucagon tolerance panel tests for insulinoma, a type of benign tumor of cells in the islets of Langerhans portion of the pancreas. Insulinoma is a prime cause of the condition known as hypoglycemia. Glucagon is a hormone secreted in the pancreas in response to hypoglycemic conditions.

80424
Arginine is a powerful stimulator of glucagon in healthy patients and may be administered as the stimulating agent for this panel. Baseline blood work is typically performed prior to stimulating glucagon. Pheochromocytoma is usually a benign tumor of the adrenal gland. Glucagon is a hormone secreted in the pancreas in response to hypoglycemic conditions. Abnormally high levels of glucagon have been linked to pheochromocytomas. The panel includes a test for fractionated catecholamines, as described by 82384. This test further differentiates a diagnosis of adrenal tumor from hypothymia and hypertension.

80426
This panel may be ordered as a GnRH "Stim." The panel tests for a variety of disorders, including pituitary disorders and premature sexual development in children. Baseline blood work is usually drawn. The gonadotropin-releasing hormone (GnRH) is typically administered by intravenous bolus. The peak response for follicle stimulating hormone (FSH) will be somewhat different than for luteinizing hormone (LH). Blood is often drawn at 30 minutes, 60 minutes, and 120 minutes.

80428
This panel may be ordered as a GH provocation test, insulin tolerance test (ITT), and as the Arginine test. Baseline blood work is typically drawn. Stimulation of growth hormone is often achieved through an intravenous infusion of arginine hydrochloride, L-dopa, or clonidine. This may be administered over about 30 minutes. Blood specimens are collected at 15 minutes, 30 minutes, and 45 minutes. These samples will be tested for HCG as specified in 83003.

80430
This panel may be ordered as a GH suppression test. Blood work is typically drawn before the test as a baseline. Glucose is the suppression agent for GH and administration may be orally. Blood is again drawn, often at 60 and 120 minutes for glucose, with one more specimen drawn for HCG.

80432
This panel may be ordered as connecting peptide insulin, insulin C-peptide, or proinsulin C-peptide. C-peptide is formed in the islets of Langerhans in the pancreas along with insulin. Both are released into the portal vein. C-peptide levels generally correlate to insulin levels and may reflect pancreatic function. Blood work is usually performed prior to the test to establish a baseline. Insulin is injected intravenously and blood is drawn at intervals for C-peptide and glucose; insulin is tested for only once.

80434
The insulin tolerance panel for ACTH insufficiency typically involves baseline blood work before testing. The insulin is administered following a fasting period, typically by an indwelling needle. The panel is specifically for adrenocorticosteroid hormone (ACTH). The cortisol test is an indirect but accurate measure of ACTH. The panel is useful to assess hypothalamic/pituitary/adrenal interaction.

80435
The insulin tolerance panel for growth hormone insufficiency typically involves baseline blood work before testing. The insulin is administered following a fasting period, typically orally. The panel is specifically for growth hormone or human growth hormone (GH or HGH). Glucose is administered, typically by IV bolus, and specimens are drawn at regular intervals following dosage. Note the number of times each component is drawn.

80436
The metyrapone panel typically involves baseline blood work before testing. The metyrapone is typically administered orally with the cortisol and 11 deoxycortisol tested for again the following morning. The test is sometimes administered outpatient and is useful in determining secondary adrenal insufficiencies, among other disorders.

80438-80439
These tests are also known as TRH test or thyrotropin releasing factor (TRF) test. The thyrotropin-releasing hormone is typically administered by IV bolus shortly

after collecting a sample to baseline for thyroid stimulating hormone. Report 80438 for a one-hour version of the test and 80439 for a two-hour version. Either test is useful in testing the anterior pituitary gland's ability to secrete TSH (normal response is for a rise in secretion following administration of TRH).

80503-80506

A clinical pathology consultation is a service performed by a physician (pathologist) in response to a written, electronic, face-to-face, or phone request from another physician/qualified health care professional who may be located at the same facility or another facility/institution. The consultation entails clinical assessment, evaluation of pathology or laboratory results or other pertinent clinical or diagnostic information such as operative/procedure notes or radiology findings that require additional medical interpretive judgment, and includes a written report. A clinical pathology consultation may also be provided by a pathologist when directed by state or federal regulation, such as Clinical Laboratory Improvement Amendments (CLIA). Code 80503 reports a consultation requiring a limited review of the patient's history and medical records. Medical decision making is straightforward; five to 20 minutes are typically spent on the date of consultation. Code 80504 reports a consultation for a moderately complex problem that requires a review of the patient's history and medical records, moderate medical decision making, and approximately 21 to 40 minutes of total time spent on the date of consultation. Code 80505 reports a consultation for a highly complex problem requiring a comprehensive review of the patient's history and medical records, a high level of medical decision making, and 41 to 60 minutes of total time spent on the date of consultation. Report 80506 for prolonged services; this code is reported in addition to the code for the primary pathology consultation and is reported once for each additional 30 minutes.

81000

This type of test may be ordered by the brand name product and the analytes tested. Although screens are considered to show the presence of an analyte (qualitative), some newer products are semi-quantitative. Many are plastic strips that contain sites impregnated with chemicals that react with urine when the strip is dipped into a specimen. The result is a color change that is compared against a standardized chart. Most strips will test for numerous analytes, as well as for pH and specific gravity. Tablets work in a similar fashion. A drop of urine is placed on the tablet and a chemical reaction causes a color change that is compared to a standard chart. Usually only a single analyte is under consideration, per tablet. Code 81000 involves a manual (nonautomated) test and includes a microscopic examination. Microscopy involves examination of the urine sediments or solids. The urine is first centrifuged in a graduated tube to concentrate the sediments. Samples (either wet or dry) are examined, usually under both high and low power, and abnormal constituents are noted. These may include a wide range of biological abnormalities, such as blood cells, casts, and bacteria, as well as chemical anomalies, such as crystals.

81001

This type of test may be ordered by the type of processor used and the analytes tested. The testing methodology is similar to the manual strips, except that the color change caused by the chemical reaction with urine is processed and read mechanically. The strip is exposed to the urine sample and is mechanically fed through a processor that reads the colors emitted by the reaction. The unit will be calibrated according to international standards and readings have a high degree of accuracy. The result may be displayed on a monitor, but is always printed or recorded in some form. Code 81001 also includes a microscopy. Microscopy involves examination of the urine sediments or solids. The urine is first centrifuged in a graduated tube to concentrate the sediments. Samples (either wet or dry) are examined, usually under both high and low power, and abnormal constituents are noted. These may include a wide range of biological abnormalities, such as blood cells, casts, and bacteria, as well as chemical anomalies, such as crystals.

81002

This type of test may be ordered by the brand name product and the analytes tested. Although usually considered screens to show the presence of an analyte (qualitative), some newer products are semi-quantitative. Many are plastic strips that contain sites impregnated with chemicals that react with urine when the strip is dipped into a specimen. The result is a color change that is compared against a standardized chart. Most strips will test for numerous analytes, as well as for pH and specific gravity. Tablets work in a similar fashion. A drop of urine is placed on the tablet and a chemical reaction causes a color change that is compared to a standard chart. Usually only a single analyte is under consideration per tablet, however. Code 81002 does not include a microscopic examination of the urine sample or its components.

81003

This type of test may be ordered by the type of processor used and the analytes tested. The testing methodology is similar to the manual strips, except that the color change caused by the chemical reaction with urine is processed and read mechanically. The strip is exposed to the urine sample and is mechanically fed through a processor that reads the colors emitted by the reaction. The unit will be calibrated according to international standards and readings have a high degree of accuracy. The result may be displayed on a monitor, but is always printed or recorded in some form. Code 81003 does not include a microscopic examination of the urine sample or its components.

81005

This test may be ordered by the type of processor used and the analytes under examination. The method will be any type of automated analyzer, usually colorimetry. The results of a semi-quantitative test indicate the presence or absence of an analyte and may be expressed as simply positive or negative. A qualitative result may be indicated as trace, 1+, 2+, etc.

81007

This type of test may be ordered by the brand name of the commercial kit used and the bacteria that the kit screens for. Human urine is normally free of bacteria. However, bacteria can easily be introduced upon voiding. In addition, specimens containing any amount of pathological bacteria can have the organisms rapidly multiply after collection. For this reason, specimens are often examined shortly after collection. Method includes any method except culture or dipstick. The test is often performed by commercial kit. The type of kit used should be specified in the report.

81015

This test may be ordered as a microscopic analysis. Human urine is normally free of bacteria. However, bacteria can easily be introduced upon voiding. In addition, specimens containing any amount of pathological bacteria can have the organisms rapidly multiply after collection. For this reason, specimens are often examined shortly after collection. The sample may first be centrifuged into a graduated tube to concentrate the sediments, or solid matter, held in suspension. The concentration of bacteria as well as cell types, crystals, and other elements seen is reported.

81020

This test may be ordered as a two-glass or three-glass test, a MacConkey-blood agar test, an MC-blood agar test, or any of the previous with a gram-positive plate. This is a culture for bacteria and will typically involve a culture plate of 5 percent sheep's blood agar and a MacConkey plate (a medium containing differentiate for lactose and nonlactose fermenters). A third plate of gram-positive media may offer further discrimination of bacteria cultured. The test is useful in determining the types and prevalence of bacteria in the urine.

81025

This test may be ordered by any of the brand name kits available. The tests typically involve a dipstick impregnated with reagents that chemically react upon contact with urine. A change in color indicates positive or negative for the presence of hormones found in the urine of women in early pregnancy.

81050

This test may be ordered as simply a volume measurement, a flow study, uroflowmetry, or urodynamic study. Timed collections are typically collected over a given period (24 hours is common). This test may be performed as a preliminary study to determine the volume of urine voided per second. A flowmeter device may be used or a simple timing of the flow into a graduated container may be employed. The test is sometimes also administered as a baseline or otherwise in conjunction with urinary tract procedures that might affect flow.

81170

Testing is performed for the translocation between the long arms of chromosomes 9 and 22 (Philadelphia chromosome). This mutation results in the hybrid gene ABL proto-oncogene 1, non-receptor tyrosine kinase (ABL). ABL encodes a fusion protein with tyrosine kinase activity, which leads to uncontrolled cell growth and has been linked to chronic myeloid leukemia (CML). This test is useful in detecting those patients who have a mutation in the ABL fusion gene, which results in a secondary resistance to imatinib, a drug used to treat CML patients, and thereby assisting providers to determine specific therapeutic treatment options. The method of testing is PCR amplification. Specimen type varies. When a specimen tests positive for the mutation, confirmation by repeat sequencing may be performed.

81171-81172

AFF2 gene analysis looks at genetic data for the occurrence of Fragile XE syndrome. In this syndrome, a segment (allele) of the AFF2 gene, located on the X chromosome, is repeated more than normal. This excess repetition makes the gene unstable, and the gene is turned off (silenced) because of the instability. The silenced gene can no longer produce AFF2 protein. The AFF2 protein binds to DNA and controls the expression and function of other genes. Absence, or low levels, of the protein causes Fragile XE syndrome. This syndrome is a form of X-linked intellectual disability that can cause aggressive behavior and/or significant language development deficits. Methodology for 81171 is PCR and/or Southern blotting. In 81172, the analysis is performed, and methyl groups are added to the DNA molecule.

[81201, 81202, 81203]

This test may be requested as APC (adenomatous polyposis coli), familial adenomatosis polyposis (FAP), or attenuated FAP analysis. Specimen is peripheral blood leukocytes. Methodology is bi-directional sequence analysis and/or multiplex ligation-dependent probe amplification (MLPA). A normal APC gene produces a protein that prevents polyps and tumors from forming. When this gene is mutated, the protein no longer is effective and polyps develop. This test screens for mutations in the APC gene that cause polyposis conditions such as FAP, colon cancer predisposition, Gardner syndrome, and Turcot syndrome. Report 81201 when the full gene sequence is analyzed. Report 81202 for the analysis of known familial variants only. Report 81203 if only the duplication/deletion variants are analyzed.

[81173, 81174, 81204]

This procedure is performed to analyze the androgen receptor gene responsible for X-linked spinal and bulbar muscular atrophy (spinobulbar muscular atrophy [SBMA] or Kennedy disease). This is an X-linked disease; males manifest this disorder and females are generally asymptomatic carriers. Specimen is blood.

Methodology is PCR-based assay, which is used to detect amplification-type mutations (CAG-repeat expansion) within the AR gene. Report 81204 for gene analysis (molecular confirmation of clinically suspected cases); 81173 for full gene sequence; and 81174 for a known familial variant.

[81200]
This test may be requested as ASPA genetic analysis, CANW, or Canavan disease mutation analysis. Specimen is whole blood. Methodology is multiplex PCR amplification. This is a blood test that screens for the missing enzyme aspartoacylase or for mutations in the gene that controls aspartoacylase. A mutation of the gene for the enzyme aspartoacylase results in Canavan disease, a common gene-linked birth disorder manifesting as cerebral degeneration during infancy. Canavan disease occurs in any ethnic group, however, it is more prevalent among Ashkenazi Jews from eastern Poland, Lithuania, and western Russia, and Saudi Arabians. Both parents must be carriers of the Canavan gene mutation, and there is a one in four (25 percent) chance with each pregnancy that the child will be affected.

81175-81176
These tests are used in the evaluation of acute myeloid leukemia (AML) at the time of diagnosis or gene mutation at the time of AML relapse. Specimen type varies but includes bone marrow, peripheral blood, and extracted DNA. Extracted DNA from the clinical specimen is fragmented and adapter ligated, and a sequence library of fragments is prepared using a custom capture hybridization method. Report 81175 when a full gene sequence (full exon) is performed. Report 81176 when a targeted gene sequence (exon 12 or hot spot) is analyzed.

81177
This test is performed to confirm the diagnosis of dentatorubral-pallidoluysian atrophy (DRPLA) for symptomatic patients or for screening patients with a family history of DRPLA and a documented expansion in the ATN1 gene in an affected family member. Specimen type varies. Methodology is A PCR-based assay to amplify across the region of the ATN1 (DRPLA) gene containing the CAG repeats.

81178-81183
These studies are used to detect CAG triplet repeat expansion in the SCA (spinocerebellar ataxia) genes responsible for symptoms including ataxia, poor coordination of hand, speech and eye movements, uncoordinated and unsteady gait. Specimen is blood. Methodology is PCR-based assay, which is used to detect amplification-type mutations (CAG-repeat expansion). Code selection is dependent upon the gene analyzed.

[81205]
This test may be ordered as BCKDHB analysis, MSUD gene analysis, or maple syrup disease analysis. Specimen is whole blood. Methodology is multiplex PCR amplification. Maple syrup urine disease is an inherited disease in which some amino acids are not processed by the body. A symptom of the disease is a distinct sweet odor of the urine of affected infants, thus the name of the disease.

[81206, 81207, 81208]
These tests may be ordered as a MBCR. Specimen is whole blood or bone marrow. Methodology is FISH (fluorescence in situ hybridization). This test is used to detect the location of an abnormality within chromosome 22 that causes the BCR gene to "break" and reattach to the ABL (chromosome 9) gene. This abnormality is called the Philadelphia or Ph chromosome. The Ph chromosome is a cause of acute and chronic myeloid leukemia and acute lymphoblastic leukemia. Report 81206 when the major breakpoint is determined; code 81207 when the minor breakpoint is determined, and 81208 when other breakpoints are determined.

[81209]
This test may be ordered as a Bloom syndrome analysis. Specimen is whole blood, chorionic villi, or amniotic fluid. Methodology is multiplex PCR amplification. Bloom syndrome causes growth problems, immune deficiencies, and places the patient at high risk for all types of cancer. It is the result of mutations of the BLM gene.

[81210]
Specimen is normal/tumor colon tissue or melanoma. Methodology is PCR-based assay. Analysis is performed to detect the presence of the V600 mutation within the BRAF (B-Raf proto-oncogene, serine/threonine kinase) gene and is used to assist in distinguishing somatic versus germline events in patients being treated for colon cancer or melanoma.

81212 [81162, 81163, 81164]
BRCA1 and BRCA2 genes are a class of genes that are known as tumor suppressors. Mutations to the BRCA1 and BRCA2 gene have been linked to hereditary breast and ovarian cancers. Specimen is blood. These tests are performed to determine what, if any, mutations have affected the BRCA1 and BRCA2 genes. Code selection is dependent on the type of mutation being tested.

81215 [81165, 81166]
BRCA1 gene is a class of genes that are known as tumor suppressors. Mutations to the BRCA1 gene have been linked to hereditary breast and ovarian cancers. Specimen is blood. These tests are performed to determine what, if any, mutations have affected the BRCA1 gene. Code selection is dependent on the type of mutation being tested.

81216-81217 [81167]
BRCA2 gene is a class of genes that are known as tumor suppressors. Mutations to the BRCA2 gene have been linked to hereditary breast and ovarian cancers. Specimen is blood. These tests are performed to determine what, if any, mutations have affected the BRCA2 gene. Code selection is dependent on the type of mutation being tested.

[81233]
This test is performed for analysis of common variants to the Bruton's tyrosine kinase (BTK) gene, which is responsible for chronic lymphocytic leukemia. Specimen type is blood. Methodology is PCR-based assay.

[81184, 81185, 81186]
These tests may also be ordered as SCA 6 DNA FORWARD, SCA 6 FORWARD, SCA Type 6 FORWARD, or Spinocerebellar Ataxia Type 6 (SCA6). The CACNA1A gene is one of a family of genes that provides instructions for making calcium channels and plays a key role in a cell's ability to generate and transmit electrical signals. Specimen type is blood. Methodology is repeat expansion detection by PCR. Code selection is dependent on the type of mutation being tested.

[81219]
Code 81219 is used to report CALR mutation analysis that is performed to distinguish between reactive thrombocytosis and/or leukocytosis and myeloproliferative neoplasm. A positive mutation status is highly suggestive of a myeloid neoplasm. This test may also be used to monitor treatment responsiveness and myeloproliferative neoplasm recurrence. Specimen types vary. Methodology is PCR amplification with analysis to detect insertions and deletions.

[81168]
This test is useful in diagnosis confirmation of mantle cell lymphoma, which can be challenging to differentiate morphologically from other B-cell malignant lymphomas. Specimen type varies; methodology is fluorescence in situ hybridization (FISH).

81218
Code 81218 is reported when testing for mutations in the CEBPA gene is performed on patients with acute myeloid leukemia (AML). Mutations within this gene predict a favorable prognosis in patients with AML. The method of testing is PCR amplification followed by DNA sequencing. Specimen type is whole blood.

81220-81221
Specimen may be blood, amniotic fluid, or chorionic villus sample. Methodology is PCR sequencing or multiplex ligation dependent probe amplification (MLPA). Testing is performed to identify the specific gene mutation when a diagnosis of cystic fibrosis has been made. Code 81220 is used to report analysis for the more common variants of the CFTR gene mutations. Report 81221 for the familial mutation(s) only, which does not rule out the presence of other mutations within the CFTR gene.

81222-81223
Specimen is whole blood. Methodology is PCR sequencing or multiplex ligation dependent probe amplification (MLPA). Mutations to the CFTR gene found on chromosome 7 are numerous and therefore there is a wide variability in clinical manifestation of cystic fibrosis. Report 81222 when analysis is performed for the identification of mutations in individuals with atypical presentations of cystic fibrosis or 81223 when full gene sequence analysis is performed. Full gene sequence analysis is usually performed when detection rates by targeted mutation analysis are low or unknown.

81224
Specimen is blood. Methodology is PCR amplification of specific regions of the CFTR gene followed by probing of the amplified regions using oligonucleotide ligation assay. The frequency of CFTR gene mutations is increased among men with congenital bilateral absence of the vas deferens (CBAVD), indicating that CBAVD is a CFTR-associated disease with incomplete penetrance. Cases of obstructive azoospermia caused by CFTR gene mutations may be considered CF cases with incomplete expression. Approximately 70 percent of men with CBAVD have at least one CF mutation. In CBAVD patients with one CF mutation, 63 percent also have the 5T variant. The most common cause of the CBAVD phenotype is a combination of one CF mutation and the 5T variant present on opposite copies (trans) of the CFTR gene.

[81267, 81268]
Specimen is blood or bone marrow. Methodology is short tandem repeat (STR). Allogenic hematopoietic stem cell transplantation (allo-HSCT) is frequently performed on patients who are at increased-risk for or have advanced hematologic malignancies and congenital or acquired aplastic anemias. In the context of the significant risk of graft failure after allo-HSCT from alternative donors and the risk of relapse in transplant recipients, precise monitoring of posttransplant hematopoietic chimerism is often necessary. Cell selection is useful in evaluating graft-versus-host disease in post-hematopoietic stem cell transplantation. Report 81267 when cell selection is not performed and 81268 once for each cell selection performed.

[81187]
This test may be ordered as CNBP DNA (DM2) or myotonic dystrophy, type 2. It is used to detect mutations to the Zinc Finger Protein 9 (ZNF9) gene in patients presenting with symptoms, including significant muscle wasting, cardiac complications, ptosis, and myotonia. Specimen type is blood. Methodology is repeat expansion detection by PCR or Southern blot.

[81265, 81266]
Short tandem repeat (STR) sequences are used as identity markers. This test is useful in fraternal and identical twin determination, donor matches, and maternal cell contamination (MCC). The potential presence of MCC in chorionic villus or amniotic fluid samples poses a serious risk for prenatal misdiagnosis. Report 81265 for the first specimen and 81266 for each additional specimen.

[81188, 81189, 81190]
These tests may also be ordered as CPI-B, CST6, cystatin B (stefin B), CYTB_HUMAN, EPM1, liver thiol proteinase inhibitor, PME, stefin B, or STFB. This gene provides instructions for making the protein cystatin B. Significant levels of cystatin B may result in a neurodegenerative disorder known as Unverricht-Lundborg disease. Code selection is dependent on the type of mutation being tested.

81225-81226 [81227]
Methodology is PCR amplification followed by DNA sequence analysis and mutation detection with hybridization probes. Specimen varies. These tests identify patients who are poor metabolizers or extensive metabolizers of drugs because of mutations to certain genes. This allows physicians to adjust drug levels, including nonconventional doses, or to select drugs that are not affected by the mutation. Report 81225 for CYP2C19, 81226 for CYP2D6, and 81227 for CYP2C9 gene analysis.

[81230, 81231]
These tests are used to aide therapeutic strategies for lipid lowering drugs that are metabolized by CYP3A4, including atorvastatin, simvastatin, and lovastatin. These tests are commonly referred to as Cytochrome P450 3A4, CYP3A, or 3A4. Specimen is blood. Methodology is polymerase chain reaction (PCR) to amplify the variant. Report 81230 when cytochrome P450 family 3 subfamily A member is 4 and 81231 when cytochrome P450 family 3 subfamily A member is 5.

81228-81229 [81349]
These codes report genome-wide analysis for constitutional chromosomal abnormalities. These tests are useful in identifying chromosomal abnormalities in patients with intellectual disabilities, developmental delay, autism, dysmorphic features, or multiple congenital anomalies, particularly those patients with normal chromosome or FISH studies. Other indications may include evaluation of fetuses with structural abnormalities discovered on fetal ultrasound or magnetic resonance imaging, or fetal tissue analysis in the evaluation of stillbirth or fetal death. Report 81228 for microarray analysis for copy number variants and 81229 when this analysis includes single nucleotide polymorphism (SNP) variants. The most common type of genetic variation occurs at the SNPs (pronounced "snips"). While most SNPs have no effect on an individual's health or normal development, some may help to predict a patient's response to certain drugs or to risk factors for developing certain diseases such as cancer, diabetes, and heart disease. Specimen may consist of blood, buccal swab, saliva, tissue, or products of conception. Methodology for 81228 and 81229 is comparative genomic hybridization (CGH) microarray analysis. In an alternate method to microarray analysis, 81349 reports low-pass sequencing analysis for copy number and loss-of-heterozygosity variants.

[81277]
Copy number variations (CNV) and loss-of-heterozygosity (LOH) variants for chromosomal abnormalities is performed to identify cancers. Specimen type is whole blood. Methodology is fluorescence in situ hybridization (FISH) using locus-specific probes targeted to the number gain or loss (CNV) and loss of heterozygosity (LOH) variants identified by the patient's chromosomal microarray testing.

[81195]
Optical genome mapping (OGM) is a technology that produces a detailed map of genomic variation by analyzing DNA molecules. By evaluating patterns generated by fluorophore tags labeled to specific sequence motifs within very long DNA molecules, this nonsequencing technology can analyze large eukaryotic genomes and their structural features at a high resolution. This code reports genome-wide analysis for hematological malignancies, which include neoplastic diseases of hematopoietic and lymphoid tissues, roughly divided into leukemias, lymphomas, myelodysplastic neoplasms, myeloproliferative neoplasms, and plasma cell neoplasms.

[81161]
This test is performed to detect abnormal alleles associated with DMD (dystrophin). Duchenne and Becker muscular dystrophy (DMD and BMD) are X-linked diseases resulting from a defect in the dystrophin gene located on Xp21. DMD is the most frequent neuromuscular disease. Specimen types vary. Multiple ligation-dependent probe amplification (MLPA) is utilized to test for the presence of large deletions and duplications within the DMD gene.

[81234, 81239]
These tests are used to detect CTG repeat expansions in the muscle protein kinase (DMPK) gene. They are performed on patients who have a range of symptoms including, but not limited to, significant muscle wasting, cardiac complications, ptosis and myotonia, infants who present with severe hypotonia, skeletal deformities, developmental delay, and intellectual disabilities. Specimen is blood. Methodology is PCR with repeat expansions. Report 81234 for evaluation to detect abnormalities and 81239 when characterization of alleles is also performed.

81232
This test is useful in identifying individuals at increased risk of toxicity when considering 5-fluorouracil (5-FU) and capecitabine chemotherapy treatment. The specimen is whole blood, saliva, or DNA. Methodology is polymerase chain reaction. Sequenced and trace files are analyzed for variations in the exons and intro/exon boundaries.

81235
Specimen is a non-small cell lung cancer (NSCLC) tumor sample. Methodology is PCR amplification and bidirectional gene sequencing. These studies are used to determine gene mutations of epidermal growth

factor receptor (EGFR). Patients that are positive for mutations of this gene generally respond well to tyrosine kinase inhibitors (TKI) treatment for the NSCLC.

81236-81237
These tests may also be ordered as enhancer of zeste homolog 2 (Drosophila), ENX-1, EZH2 HUMAN, histone-lysine N-methyltransferase EZH2, KMT6, KMT6A, or lysine N-methyltransferase 6. This gene delivers instructions for making histone methyltransferase, an enzyme. This gene analysis is used in the diagnosis and treatment of myelodysplastic and myeloproliferative neoplasms. Specimen is tumor tissue. Methodology may vary. Some test methods include fluorescence in situ hybridization (FISH), immunohistochemistry (IHC), next-generation sequencing (NGS), polymerase chain reaction (PCR), comparative genomic hybridization (CGH), karyotyping, mRNA analysis, tissue microarrays (TMAs), and southern/northern/western/eastern blot tests. Code 81237 is specific to the analysis of diffuse large B-cell lymphomas. Report 81236 for analysis of the full gene sequence and 81237 for analysis of the common variants.

81240-81241
These studies are used to determine gene mutations that directly affect coagulation. Specimen is whole blood. Methodology is direct mutation analysis. Report 81240 to detect a prothrombin mutation 20210G>A (affecting coagulation factor II). Report 81241 to detect a factor V (Leiden) mutation.

[81238]
This test is useful in diagnosing certain coagulation disorders such as hemophilia B (Christmas disease), in assessing the impact of liver disease on hemostasis, and for evaluating causes of prolonged activated partial thromboplastin time. Specimen type is plasma. Methodology is polymerase chain reaction of full gene sequence.

81242
Specimen is whole blood. Methodology is PCR-based assay using Luminex. Mutations that have been associated with Fanconi anemia have been found in several genes; however, the IVS4(+4)A->T mutation is common in the Ashkenazi Jewish population. Fanconi anemia, an aplastic anemia, causes bone marrow failure and myelodysplasia or acute myelogenous leukemia.

[81245, 81246]
This test may also be ordered as a soft FLDV. Methodology is multiplex polymerase chain reaction (PCR) assay. Test specimen is whole blood or bone marrow samples. Studies have shown the location of ITD of the FLT3 gene was restricted to exons 14 and 15. FLT3 internal tandem duplication (ITD) mutations in patients with acute myeloid leukemia (AML) portend poor prognosis in adult and pediatric patients. Report 81245 when testing for ITD variant exons 14 or 15. Report 81246 when testing for tyrosine kinase domain (TKD) variants like D835 or I836.

81243-81244
FMR1 gene analysis looks at genetic data for the occurrence and carrier status of Fragile X syndrome (FXS). In this syndrome, a portion of the FMR1 gene, located on the X chromosome, is repeated more than normal. This causes the FMR1 gene to malfunction or not work at all, producing little or no FMRP protein. FMRP protein is present in the ovaries, testes, and brain nerve synapses, playing a role in brain development and cell-to-cell communication. Absence, or low levels, of the FMRP protein causes Fragile X syndrome. This genetic syndrome affects both males and females, though females tend to have milder symptoms, which include developmental delays, learning disabilities, and behavioral challenges. Methodology for 81243 is PCR and/or Southern blotting. In 81244, the analysis is performed, and methyl groups are added to the DNA molecule.

[81284, 81285, 81286, 81289]
These tests may also be referred to as Ataxia Friedreich FORWARD, Frataxin FORWARD, FRDA FORWARD, Friedreich Ataxia TNR Analysis FORWARD, Friedreich FORWARD, or FXN FORWARD. These tests are used to diagnose or determine carrier status for Friedreich ataxia (FA), an autosomal recessive disease. Specimen is blood. Methodology is PCR or southern blot. Report 81284 when evaluating abnormal alleles, 81285 for characterization of alleles, 81286 for analysis of full gene sequence, and 81289 when analysis is made for familial variants.

[81250]
Specimen type varies. Methodology is PCR-assay. The G6PC gene family contains three members designated G6PC, G6PC2, and G6PC3. The tissue-specific expression patterns of these genes differ, and mutations in all three genes have been linked to distinct diseases in humans. This test is useful for genetic screening, as well as definitive diagnosis.

81247-81249
These tests are used to identify G6PD deficiency status, to differentiate heterozygous females with skewed X-inactivation from homozygous and compound heterozygous females, to determine the definitive diagnosis of carrier status in females, or to evaluate neonates (particularly male) with unexplained jaundice. This gene analysis can also be used to identify patients who are at risk of drug-induced acute hemolytic anemia (AHA) related to G6PD deficiency. Specimen is DNA extracted from whole blood. Methodology is polymerase chain reaction (PCR). For common variants only, report 81247. For known familial variants, report 81248. When full gene sequence is performed, report 81249.

81251
This test is for the analysis of the GBA gene (Gaucher disease). Sample can be blood, amniotic fluid, or chorionic villus. Prenatal sampling must be

accompanied by maternal blood specimen. Methodology is PCR-based assay. This test is used for prenatal diagnosis in high-risk pregnancies, for genetic screening, or as confirmation of a clinical diagnosis.

81252-81253

This test may be requested as GJB2 (gap junction protein, beta 2, 26kDa, connexin 26) or nonsyndromic hearing loss gene analysis. Specimen is whole blood. Methodology is bidirectional sequence analysis and/or PCR amplification. This test screens for a genetic mutation of GJB2, which is accountable for a high frequency of nonsyndromic autosomal recessive deafness (DFNA3). Report 81252 for the analysis of the full gene sequence. Report 81253 if only the known familial variants are analyzed.

81254

This test may be requested as GJB6 (gap junction protein, beta 6, 30kDa, connexin 30) or nonsyndromic hearing loss gene analysis. Specimen is whole blood. Methodology is bidirectional sequence analysis and/or PCR amplification. This test screens for a genetic mutation of GJB6, which is accountable for a high frequency of recessively inherited deafness (DFNB1).

[81257, 81258, 81259, 81269]

Specimen is whole blood or amniotic fluid. Prenatal screening of amniotic fluid must be accompanied by maternal blood sample. Methodology is PCR amplification followed by bidirectional sequencing. Alpha thalassemia is one of the most common inherited disorders of hemoglobin worldwide. There are two main forms of this condition: Hb Bart hydrops fetalis syndrome where there is loss of all four alpha globin genes and Hemoglobin H disease where there is loss of three alpha globin gene functions. Carrier states include the loss of two alpha globin genes (trait carrier status) and the loss of a single alpha globin gene (silent carrier status). Report 81257 for common gene deletions or variants; 81258 for known familial variants; 81259 for full gene sequencing; and 81269 for other duplication/deletion variants only.

[81361, 81362, 81363, 81364]

Hemoglobin subunit B can be used to diagnose beta thalassemia intermedia or major; to identify specific beta thalassemia mutations (i.e., unusually severe beta thalassemia trait); to evaluate abnormal hemoglobin electrophoresis identifying a rare beta globin variant, chronic hemolytic anemia of unknown etiology, or hereditary erythrocytosis; and in screening when there is a concern for a beta hemoglobin disorder based on family history prior to conception. Specimen type is whole blood. Methodology is polymerase chain reaction (PCR) then purified and sequenced in both directions using fluorescent dye-terminator chemistry. Report 81361 when common variants are analyzed, 81362 for familial variants, 81363 when duplication deletion is performed, and 81364 for full gene sequencing.

81255

This test is performed for the analysis of the HEXA gene (Tay-Sachs disease). Sample can be blood, amniotic fluid, or chorionic villus. Prenatal sampling must be accompanied by maternal blood specimen. Methodology is PCR-based assay. This test is used for prenatal diagnosis in high-risk pregnancies, for genetic screening, or as confirmation of a clinical diagnosis.

81256

Sample is whole blood. Methodology is PCR-based assay. This study is useful in establishing or confirming the clinical diagnosis of hereditary hemochromatosis. It is not recommended for general patient genetic screening; however, it is appropriate for predictive testing of patients who have a family history of hereditary hemochromatosis.

[81271, 81274]

These tests may be ordered as HD, Huntington chorea, or chorea HTT and are used for presymptomatic testing for individuals with a family history of Huntington disease and a documented expansion in the HTT gene. Specimen type varies. Methodology is PCR.

[81105, 81106, 81107, 81108, 81109, 81110, 81111, 81112]

These tests are commonly ordered to diagnose maternal immunization against fetal platelet alloantigens that may result in severe newborn thrombocytopenia or intracranial hemorrhage. Specimen is blood. Methodology is polymerase chain reaction (PCR) to amplify the variant alleles. Report 81105 for HPA-1, 81106 for HPA-2, 81107 for HPA-3, 81108 for HPA-4, 81109 for HPA-5, 81110 for HPA-6, 81111 for HPA-9w, and 81112 for HPA-15.

[81120, 81121]

These tests are useful in diagnosing grade II or III astrocytoma, oligodendroglioma, oligoastrocytoma, or secondary glioblastoma, as well as stratifying the prognosis of gliomas. Specimen type is tissue. Polymerase chain reaction is amplified specific to regions surrounding the IDH1 codon 132 and IDH2 codon 172. Samples are pyrosequenced and the pyrograms are analyzed for the presence or absence of IDH1 codon 132 (81120) or IDH2 codon 172 mutations (81121).

[81283]

This test is used to determine a patient's response to interferon lambda used for the treatment of hepatitis C. Specimen type varies. Methodology is next-generation sequencing.

[81261, 81262, 81263]

Sample may be blood, bone marrow, tissue, or spinal fluid. Immunoglobulin heavy locus (IGH@) is located on chromosome 14 and contains a gene for the heavy chains of human antibodies that recognize foreign antigens and initiate immune responses to those antigens. Each immunoglobulin contains two identical heavy changes and two identical light chains. As B-cells develop, these segments are rearranged. These tests are useful in determining if B-cell or plasma cell population is polyclonal or monoclonal. Code selection is dependent upon methodology. Report 81261 when the PCR assay method is used, 81262 when direct probe methodology is performed, and 81263 when somatic mutation analysis is performed. These tests are clinically useful for identifying neoplastic cells as having B-cell or plasma cell differentiation and in detecting immunoglobulin gene rearrangement that is similar to a previous neoplastic specimen in patients with a persistent neoplasm.

[81278]
The IGH@/BCL2 gene mutation is associated with almost 80 percent of follicular lymphomas and 20 percent of diffuse large B-cell lymphomas. Translocation analysis involves the major breakpoint region (MBR), minor cluster region (MCR), and 3' MBR sub-cluster regions of BCL2. It is also useful to monitor therapy effectiveness and to detect minimal residual disease or recurrence. Specimen type varies. Methodology is PCR and fragment analysis.

[81264]
Sample may be blood or bone marrow. Immunoglobulin kappa light chain locus (IGK@) is found on chromosome 2. Polymerase chain reaction (PCR)-based assays are commonly used to detect clonal immunoglobulin (IG) gene rearrangements during the evaluation of lymphocyte infiltrates.

81260
Sample is whole blood, amniotic fluid, or chorionic villus sampling. Prenatal testing should be accompanied by maternal whole blood sample. Methodology is PCR-based assay and fluorescent hybridization probes. This study is useful in carrier screening, prenatal diagnosis, and clinical diagnosis confirmation. Mutations in the IKBKAP gene result in the manifestations of familial dysautonomia. There are two common mutations prevalent in the Ashkenazi Jewish population: IVS20(+6)T->C and R696P, and the carrier rate is one in 31.

81270
Specimen is whole blood. Methodology is PCR assay. This test may also be ordered as a Tyrosine kinase mutation or Janus kinase 2 gene. Myeloproliferative disorders (MPD) are a large group of relatively rare, pathogenetically related diseases arising in the bone marrow. These diseases are characterized by the proliferation of one or more myeloid cell lines in the bone marrow, resulting in increased numbers of relatively mature neoplastic cells in the peripheral blood. It has been determined that the V617F mutation in the Janus Kinase 2 gene is present in patients with polycythemia vera (PV), essential thrombocythemia (ET), and myelofibrosis with myeloid metaplasia (MMM).

[81279]
The JAK2 gene provides instructions for making a protein that promotes the growth and division of cells. It is important for controlling the production of blood cells from hematopoietic stem cells. It is associated with essential thrombocythemia, polycythemia vera, as well as leukemia and other bone marrow disorders. Specimen type varies. Methodology is RT-PCR and bidirectional sequencing.

81272-81273
These codes are used to report KIT gene mutation analysis that is performed using PCR amplification with analysis to detect insertions and deletions. Specimen types vary. Code selection is dependent upon whether specific exons (8, 11, 13, 17, and 18) are being amplified (81272) or if a screening for a specific mutation (D816V) is being performed (81273). Mutations in the KIT gene have been identified in gastrointestinal stromal tumors, as well as melanoma and acute myeloid leukemia. The KIT D816V mutation has been associated with systemic mastocytosis in patients with acute myeloid leukemia.

81275-81276
Specimen is tumor tissue block. Methodology is PCR-assay. KRAS mutation is predictive of a very poor response to antiepidermal growth factor receptor (anti-EGFR) therapy in colorectal cancer. Variants in the exon 2 can form alternate protein within the KRAS gene, resulting in an amino acid exchange that has shown particular interference with some tumor medication making them less effective as potential treatment alternatives. KRAS mutations found in these exons have been known to show very little response to epidermal growth factor receptor (EGFR) therapy. Report 81275 when the test is checking exon 2 variants; report 81276 for additional variants, such as exon 3 for codon 61.

81290
Specimen is blood, amniotic fluid, or chorionic villus. Prenatal samples should include a maternal blood specimen. Methodology is PCR-based assay. This test is useful for carrier status testing in individuals of Ashkenazi Jewish ancestry, prenatal screening for at-risk pregnancies, and confirmation of clinical diagnosis of mucolipidosis IV. Mucolipidosis IV is a lysosomal storage disease that results in intellectual disabilities, hypotonia, corneal clouding, and retinal degeneration.

[81302, 81303, 81304]
Specimen is blood. Methodology is PCR-analysis. Genetic mutations in MECP2 can be associated with variable phenotypes in females, including classic Rett syndrome, variant or atypical Rett syndrome, mild intellectual disabilities, and asymptomatic carriers. Males with MECP2 mutations can present with variable phenotypes as well. These tests can be useful in the screening and diagnosis of Rett syndrome. Report 81302 for full gene sequence analysis, 81303 when analysis is for known familial gene variations, and 81304 when duplication/deletion variants are determined.

[81287]
This test is useful for determining the likelihood that glioblastoma tumor cells will be responsive to

alkylating medications and have enhanced chemosensitivity helping to determine the patient's prognosis. Glioblastoma is the most common and aggressive form of primary brain cancer associated with high mortality rates. Specimen is cryopreserved glioblastoma tumor specimen. Methodology is promoter methylation-specific polymerase chain reaction (MSP), pyrosequencing (PSQ), and methylation-specific multiplex ligation-dependent probe amplification (MS-MLPA).

[81301]

Specimen is normal and tumor tissue. Methodology is fluorescent PCR-based assay. Microsatellite instability is the reduced fidelity of the replication of repetitive DNA most commonly occurring in tumor cells. Basically, MSI analysis involves a comparison of the allelic profiles of microsatellite markers generated by amplification of DNA from normal and tumor samples. Alleles that are present in the tumor sample but not found in the corresponding normal samples indicate MSI. This test may also be ordered as an MSI analysis.

[81288, 81292, 81293, 81294]

Specimen is whole blood. A variety of techniques may be used to perform these studies. These tests are useful in the screening and diagnosis of hereditary nonpolyposis colon cancer (Lynch syndrome) by examining the MLH1 gene for mutation (mute L). About 50 percent of all cases of Lynch syndrome with an identified gene mutation are associated with mutations in the MLH1 gene. Patients with Lynch syndrome develop colon cancer at a younger age. Report 81292 when a full sequence screening is performed; 81293 when screening for known familial mutations; 81294 when screening for duplication/deletion variances; and 81288 when promoter methylation analysis is performed. Methylation can be discovered within the promoter parts of genes and this discovery implicates a disease process due to alteration in the DNA.

[81338, 81339]

The MPL gene provides instructions for making the thrombopoietin receptor protein, which promotes the growth and division of cells. MPL W515 mutations are associated with primary myelofibrosis (PMF) or essential thrombocythemia (ET). The S505 mutation is associated with familial essential thrombocythemia. Specimen type varies. Bidirectional sequencing of exon 10 is completed to detect all possible mutations at the W515 and S505 codons.

81296-81297 [81295]

Specimen is whole blood. A variety of techniques may be used to perform these studies. These tests are useful in the screening and diagnosis of hereditary non-polyposis colon cancer (Lynch syndrome) by examining the MSH2 gene for mutation (mute S). Patients with Lynch syndrome develop colon cancer at a younger age. Report 81295 when a full sequence screening is performed, 81296 when screening for known familial mutations is performed, and 81297 when screening for duplication/deletion variances is performed.

81298-81300

Specimen is whole blood. A variety of techniques may be used to perform these studies. These tests are useful in the screening and diagnosis of hereditary non-polyposis colon cancer (Lynch syndrome) by examining the MSH6 gene for mutation (mute S). Patients with Lynch syndrome develop colon cancer at a younger age. Report 81298 when a full sequence screening Is performed, 81299 when screening for known familial mutations is performed, and 81300 when screening for duplication/deletion variances is performed.

[81291]

Specimen is whole blood. Methodology is direct mutation analysis based on the amplification of fluorescent signal released by cleavage of sequence specific alleles. Several MTHFR mutations have been associated with homocystinuria. Homocystinuria presents with a wide range of clinical manifestations, including developmental delay, intellectual disabilities, and premature vascular disease.

81305

This test may be ordered as B-cell lymphoma, L265P, LPL/WM, Lymphoplasmacytic lymphoma, MYD88, or Waldenstrom Macroglobulinemia. It is used to establish the diagnosis of lymphoplasmacytic lymphoma/Waldenstrom macroglobulinemia (LPL/WM), aid in distinguishing LPL/WM low-grade B-cell lymphoma from other subtypes, or to assist in the management of LPL/WM. Specimen types vary. After extracting DNA from the specimen, the algorithm sensitive to MYD88 L265P testing by allele-specific polymerase chain reaction (PCR) is performed for the MYD88 L265P mutation.

81310

Sample is whole blood or bone marrow. Methodology is PCR-assay. This analysis examines the NPM1 gene targeting exon 12 mutations. This test is clinically significant in the prognosis of patients newly diagnosed with acute myeloid leukemia.

81311

The NRAS gene is analyzed to determine if there are mutations in the exon 2 (codons 12 and 13) and exon 3 (codon 61). Methodology is PCR amplification. Specimen types vary but are usually tissue. This testing is useful in determining patient response to cetuximab or panitumumab treatment as several studies have shown that patients with NRAS-mutated tumors are less likely to respond to these treatments.

[81191, 81192, 81193, 81194]

The NTRK1 gene provides instructions for making a protein that is necessary for the development and survival of nerve cells that transmit information about sensations such as pain, temperature, and touch. It is associated with congenital insensitivity to pain with anhidrosis (CIPA) and papillary thyroid carcinoma. The NTRK2 gene is a membrane-bound receptor that phosphorylates itself upon binding and becomes part of the MAPK pathway. Signaling through this kinase leads to cell differentiation. Gene mutations have been associated with mood disorders and obesity. The NTRK3 gene is also a membrane-bound receptor that upon binding, phosphorylates itself and becomes part of the MAPK pathway. Signaling through this kinase contributes to cell differentiation and may assist in the development of proprioceptive neurons that sense body position. Mutations in this gene have been associated with medulloblastomas, secretory breast carcinomas, and other cancers. Gene defects may also be associated with susceptibility of congenital heart defects. Fusions involving the NTRK1, NTRK2, or NTRK3 genes act as oncogenic drivers of multiple types of pediatric and adult solid tumors and can be useful in guiding treatment of individuals. There are various methodologies to test for NTRK gene fusion, including immunohistochemistry (IHC), FISH, and RNA fusion by next-generation sequencing (NGS).

[81306]

This test is used for predicting the potential for toxicity to thiopurine drugs (6-mercaptopurine, 6-thioguanine, and azathioprine). Specimen type varies. Methodology is performed using PCR to amplify the segment of DNA comprising the polymorphism. If the detection probe is an exact match to the target DNA, the 5'-nuclease polymerase damages the probe, reporter dye is released, and a fluorescent signal is detected.

[81312]

This test is used to diagnose oculopharyngeal muscular dystrophy (OPMD), a genetic disorder characterized by slowly progressing muscle disease (myopathy) affecting the muscles of the upper eyelids and the throat. Onset of OPMS usually manifests between the age of 40 and 60 years. Symptoms may include eyelid drooping (ptosis), arm and leg weakness, and difficulty swallowing (dysphagia). This condition may be distinguished by its patterns of inheritance, either the autosomal dominant and autosomal recessive types, both of which are caused by mutations in the PABPN1 gene. The specimen is blood. Methodology is repeat expansion detection by PCR.

[81307, 81308]

This test is performed for gene analysis for breast and pancreatic cancer. The PALB2 gene is called the partner and localizer of the BRCA2 gene and provides instructions to make a protein that works with the BRCA2 protein to repair damaged DNA and to stop tumor growth. Specimen type is whole blood. Both male and female patients with mutations of the PALB2 gene have an increased risk for breast cancer and pancreatic cancer. Methodology is next-generation sequencing. Report 81307 for full gene sequence analysis and 81308 when only known familial sequencing variants are analyzed.

81313

This test analyzes the prostate cancer antigen 3 (PCA3) and the kallikrein-related peptidase 3 (PSA) ratio. Target RNA molecules are isolated from urine specimens. Methodology is quantitative nucleic acid amplification testing. The PCA3 converts a prostate-specific messenger ribonucleic acid (mRNA) that can be recognized as a possible link to prostate cancer. The PCA3 score is calculated as 1,000 times the ratio of the concentration of PCA3 RNA to the concentration of PSA RNA ([PCA3 mRNA]/[PSA mRNA] x 1000). This ratio may verify the production of prostate-specific RNA, as well as specify accuracy, reliability and mRNA production.

81314

Code 81314 is reported when testing is performed for mutations in the PDGFRA gene on patients with gastrointestinal stromal tumors (GIST). Analysis of the PDGFRA gene helps to confirm GIST diagnosis and is useful to the clinician for therapeutic planning. The method of testing is PCR amplification followed by DNA sequencing to determine if there are mutations in exons 12, 14, and 18. Specimen type is tumor tissue.

[81309]

PIK3CA is a gene that provides instructions for making the p110 alpha protein, and mutation is associated with certain cancers, particularly colorectal and breast cancers, and other conditions. Specimen type is formalin-fixed paraffin-embedded (FFPE) tumor resection or biopsy samples. Methodology is real-time qualitative PCR assay.

[81320]

This test is used to determine if mutations are present to the phospholipase C gamma 2 (PLCG2) gene associated with chronic lymphocytic leukemia (CLL). The PLCG2 gene provides instructions to the phospholipase C gamma 2 protein for communication between a cell and the immune system and other cells. Particularly, this test is to perform the analysis for mutations for common variants to R665W, S707F, and L845F. Methodology and specimen types vary.

81315-81316

Specimen is whole blood or bone marrow. Methodology is PCR-assay. These tests are useful in the diagnosis of acute promyelocytic leukemia (APL), the detection of residual or recurrent APL, and in monitoring the level of promyelocytic leukemia/retinoic acid receptor alpha in patients with APL. Report 81315 for common breakpoint analysis or 81316 when a single breakpoint is analyzed.

[81324, 81325, 81326]

This test screens for mutations in the peripheral myelin protein 22 gene, which is responsible for development and maintenance of myelin in the nervous system. Specimen is whole blood. Methodology is multiplex ligation-dependent probe amplification (MLPA). Mutations of this gene, most commonly duplication, result in Charcot-Marie-Tooth syndrome type 1A. Deletion of this gene causes demyelinization, resulting in hereditary neuropathy with liability to pressure palsies. Report 81324 if only the duplication/deletion variants are analyzed. Report 81325 when the full gene sequence is analyzed. Report 81326 if only the known familial variants are analyzed.

81317-81319
Specimen varies. A variety of techniques may be used to perform these studies. These tests are useful in the screening and diagnosis of hereditary non-polyposis colon cancer (Lynch syndrome) by examining the PMS2 gene for mutation. Patients with Lynch syndrome develop colon cancer at a younger age. Report 81317 when a full sequence screening is performed, 81318 when screening for known familial mutations is performed, and 81319 when screening for duplication/deletion variances is performed.

[81343]
This test is used to repeat expansion in the SCA (spinocerebellar ataxia) gene protein phosphatase 2 regulatory subunit Bbeta (PPP2R2B) for mutation. PPP2R2B is responsible for symptoms of spinocerebellar ataxia, including poor coordination of hand, speech, and eye movements and uncoordinated and unsteady gait. Specimen is blood. Methodology is repeat expansion detection of amplification-type mutations by PCR.

81321-81323
This test may be requested as PTEN (phosphatase and tensin homolog), Cowden syndrome, or PTEN hamartoma tumor syndrome gene analysis. Specimen is whole blood or saliva. Methodology is bidirectional sequence analysis and FISH (fluorescent in situ hybridization) testing. This test screens for mutations of the PTEN gene, which causes defects in or omission of the PTEN enzyme, a tumor suppressor. A mutation of this gene results in diseases such as Cowden syndrome, which presents a high risk for benign and malignant tumors of the thyroid, breast, and endometrium, and hamartoma tumor syndrome. Report 81321 for analysis of the full gene sequence. Report 81322 if only the known familial variants are analyzed. Report 81323 when only the duplication/deletion variants are analyzed.

[81334]
Runt related transcription factor 1 (RUNX1) is useful in the diagnosis and treatment of myeloid leukemia and familial platelet disorders with associated myeloid malignancy. Specimen varies. Methodology varies and includes in situ hybridization, immunohistochemistry, next-generation sequencing, and Polymerase chain reaction (PCR) targeted on exons 3-8.

81327
This test may be referred to as methylated septin 9/SEPT9 DNA. It screens for mutations in the peripheral myelin protein 22 gene, which is responsible for development and maintenance of myelin in the nervous system. The SEPT 9 DNA analysis can determine colorectal cancer in all stages and specific locations. The specimen is plasma and method is real-time polymerase chain reaction with promoter methylation analysis. This test is not to be used as a replacement for colonoscopy due to decreased sensitivity for detecting polyps.

[81332]
Specimen is both whole blood and serum. Methodology is PCR-assay. This test is clinically useful for the diagnosis, prognosis, and genetic screening for alpha-1-antitrypsin (A1A) deficiency. A1A deficiency results in lung tissue degradation and places the patient at increased risk for early onset of panlobar emphysema.

[81347]
The SF3B1 gene encodes subunit 1 of the splicing factor 3b protein complex. The splicing encodes part of the U2 small nuclear ribonucleoproteins complex involved in DNA damage repair. It is associated with chronic lymphocytic leukemia (CLL), myelodysplastic syndrome (MDS), and MDS with ring sideroblasts (RS). Specimen varies. Methodology includes next generation (NGS)/massively parallel sequencing (MPS).

81328
The SLCO1B1 is responsible for the liver's uptake and metabolism of statins, which are used to treat high cholesterol and to predict statin-associated myopathy. The specimen is blood. Genotyping is performed using a polymerase chain reaction (PCR).

81329 [81336, 81337]
These tests are performed to determine if there are two or more SMN1 gene copies and no point mutations identified in SMN1 or SMN2. Mutations of the SMN1 or SMN2 genes are associated with spinal muscular atrophy. Specimen is blood. Methodology is Sanger sequencing with PCR. Report 81329 when carrier status is performed; 81336 for full gene sequence analysis; and 81337 when only known familial sequencing variants are analyzed.

81330
Specimen is whole blood. Methodology is PCR-assay. There are three types of Niemann-Pick disease: A, B, and C. Niemann-Pick disease type A is a lysosomal storage disease resulting from three common gene mutations (R4961, K302P, and fsP330). These mutations cause a deficiency of the enzyme acid sphingomyelinase resulting in jaundice, the progressive loss of motor skills, difficulties with feeding, enlargement of the liver and spleen, and learning disabilities. This test is useful for carrier screening. The mutation is more common in patients of the Ashkenazi Jewish heritage.

81331
This test is useful for the confirmation of Prader-Willi or Angelman syndromes. These syndromes result in global developmental delay, as well as other symptoms, and are thought to be the result of mutations to chromosome 15. Specimen is blood or amniotic fluid. Amniotic fluid must be accompanied by maternal blood. Methodology is methylation-sensitive multiple ligation-dependent probe amplification (MLPA).

[81348]
The SRSF2 gene is a component of the RNA splicing complex. It is associated with systemic mastocytosis and myeloid disorders that have a poor prognosis. Testing is used to establish diagnosis by distinguishing myeloid neoplasms from a reactive process and used to assess prognosis. Specimen includes peripheral blood or bone marrow; methodology is molecular.

[81344]
This test is performed for gene analysis to detect triplet repeat expansion in the SCA17 gene. This mutation is associated with spinocerebellar ataxia type 17 (SCA 17). Specimen type is blood. Methodology is repeat expansion detection by PCR.

[81345]
This test is performed to detect the presence of a mutation in the promoter region of the TERT gene. It may also be ordered as TERT promoter. TERT mutations in the promoter of the gene for telomerase reverse transcriptase are common mutations in cancer. Specimen type varies. Methodology is PCR-based next-generation sequencing.

81333
The TGFBI gene provides instructions for making the protein transforming growth factor beta induced and is associated with an anterior corneal dystrophy resulting in opacities of spots and lines in the central portion of the anterior cornea. This causes haziness that spars the periphery sight. There are two mutation hotspots particular at positions 124 and 555. Specimen type varies. Methodology is PCR.

[81351, 81352, 81353]
The TP53 gene provides instructions for making a protein called tumor protein p53 (or p53). The p53 protein is in the nucleus of cells throughout the body and binds directly to DNA. This protein acts as a tumor suppressor by regulating cell division and keeping cells from growing and dividing too fast. It is associated with at least 50 percent of all adult tumors with a poor prognosis. Mutations in TP53 are the cause of Li-Fraumeni syndrome. Specimen varies and may include peripheral blood, bone marrow, or FFPE solid tumor tissue. Methodology is molecular bidirectional sequencing of TP53 exons 4-9. Report 81351 for a full gene sequence; 81352 for a targeted sequence analysis; and 81353 for a known familial variant.

81335
Thiopurine S-methyltransferase (TPMT) gene analysis is useful in predicting potential toxicity to thiopurine drugs (6-mercaptopurine, 6-thioguanine, and azathioprine) for patients undergoing this drug therapy. Thiopurine drug therapy is used in patients with acute lymphoblastic leukemia, autoimmune disorders (e.g., Crohn disease, rheumatoid arthritis), and organ transplant recipients. Specimen is blood. Methodology is polymerase chain reaction (PCR)-based 5'-nuclease assay.

81340-81342
Specimen varies. Methodology can be PCR-assay (81340 [TRB] or 81342 [TRG]) or direct probe (81341). T-cell gene rearrangement is used to determine if T-cell population is polyclonal or monoclonal. This can be clinically significant in determining malignancy.

81346
Thymidylate synthetase (TYMS) gene analysis is used to determine toxicity in patients who are at increased risk of toxicity when considering 5-fluorouracil (5-FU) chemotherapy for colorectal cancer and other solid tumors. Specimen varies. The tandem repeat arrays show variation between sequences and assist in predicting patient toxicity.

[81357]
The U2AF1 gene belongs to the splicing factor SR family of genes. It encodes the small subunit that plays an important role in both constitutive and enhancer-dependent RNA splicing by directly facilitating interactions between the large subunit and proteins bound to the enhancers. It is associated with myelodysplastic syndrome and myeloid leukemia. Specimens may include bone marrow aspirate or peripheral blood; methodology includes molecular testing using next-generation sequencing (NGS) technology.

81350
This test is used to identify the UGT1A1 mutation and carrier status. Specimen is whole blood. Methodology is PCR-assay. Mutations to the UGT1A1 gene result in hyperbilirubinemia.

81355
This test may also be ordered as Coumadin genotype or warfarin genotype. Specimen is whole blood. Methodology is PCR-assay. This test is used to identify patients who are poor metabolizers or extensive metabolizers of warfarin because of mutations to the VKORC1 gene. This allows physicians to adjust drug levels, including nonconventional doses, or to select drugs that are not affected by the mutation.

81360
The ZRSR2 gene encodes for a member of the spliceosome, U2 auxiliary factor, which plays an important role in RNA splicing. Spliceosome mutations are seen in diseases such as MDS, chronic lymphocytic leukemia (CLL), AML, and chronic myelomonocytic leukemia. ZRSR2 mutations include clear loss-of-function variants that are commonly found in tumor suppressor genes. Mutations have diagnostic and prognostic relevance. Specimen type may include bone marrow and peripheral blood; methodology is molecular next generation sequencing (NGS)/ massively parallel sequencing.

81370-81371
These tests are commonly used to determine the histocompatibility between a patient and a donor to predict and prevent graft versus host disease (GVHD). Variations may also be used to detect susceptibility to certain genetic autoimmune diseases. Human

leukocyte antigens (HLA) are a group of genes found on chromosome 6. There are two types of HLA: class I and class II. Low resolution (or generic) HLA typing can be performed via serology, cellular, or molecular technique, the molecular technique being the most common. In this technique, whole blood must be obtained and DNA extracted. The genes of interest are amplified and identification of HLA type is made via detection of the DNA sequence polymorphism. High resolution typing involves identifying groups of alleles and approximating the specific HLA characteristics. Report 81370 for low resolution typing of HLA-A-, -B, -C, -DRB1/3/4/5, and -DQB1. Report 81371 for low resolution typing of HLA-A, -B, and DRB1.

81372-81374

These tests are commonly used to determine the histocompatibility between a patient and a donor to predict and prevent graft versus host disease (GVHD). Variations may also be used to detect susceptibility to certain genetic autoimmune diseases. Human leukocyte antigens (HLA) are a group of genes found on chromosome 6. There are two types of HLA: class I and class II. Low resolution (or generic) HLA typing can be performed via serology, cellular, or molecular technique, the molecular technique being the most common. In this technique, whole blood must be obtained and DNA extracted. The genes of interest are amplified and identification of HLA type is made via detection of the DNA sequence polymorphism. High resolution typing involves identifying groups of alleles and approximating the specific HLA characteristics. Report 81372 for complete low resolution HLA class I typing, including HLA-A, -B, and -C. Report 81373 for HLA low resolution typing of each individual class I loci (HLA-A, -B, or -C) when complete class I typing is not performed. Report 81374 for low resolution class I typing of each serological HLA equivalent or subtype (e.g., HLA-B*27).

81375-81377

These tests are commonly used to determine the histocompatibility between a patient and a donor to predict and prevent graft versus host disease (GVHD). Variations may also be used to detect susceptibility to certain genetic autoimmune diseases. Human leukocyte antigens (HLA) are a group of genes found on chromosome 6. There are two types of HLA: class I and class II. Low resolution (or generic) HLA typing can be performed via serology, cellular, or molecular technique, the molecular technique being the most common. In this technique, whole blood must be obtained and DNA extracted. The genes of interest are amplified and identification of HLA type is made via detection of the DNA sequence polymorphism. High resolution typing involves identifying groups of alleles and approximating the specific HLA characteristics. Report 81375 for complete low resolution HLA class II typing, including HLA-DRB1/3/4/5 and HLA-DQB1. Report 81376 for HLA low resolution typing of each individual class II loci (HLA-DRB1, -DRB3/4/5, -DQB1, -DQA1, -DPB1, or -DPA1) when complete class II typing is not performed. Report 81377 for low resolution class II typing of each serological HLA equivalent or subtype.

81378

This test is commonly used to determine the histocompatibility between a patient and a donor to predict and prevent graft versus host disease (GVHD). Variations may be used to detect susceptibility to certain genetic autoimmune diseases. Human leukocyte antigens (HLA) are a group of genes found on chromosome 6. There are two types of HLA: class I and class II. Low resolution (or generic) HLA typing can be performed via serology, cellular, or molecular technique, the molecular technique being the most common. In this technique, whole blood must be obtained and DNA extracted. The genes of interest are amplified and identification of HLA type is made via detection of the DNA sequence polymorphism. High resolution typing involves identifying alleles or allele groups by examining and determining the specific HLA characteristics. Code 81378 is reported for high resolution typing of both HLA class I and II (HLA-A, -B, -C, and -DRB1).

81379-81381

These tests are commonly used to determine the histocompatibility between a patient and a donor to predict and prevent graft versus host disease (GVHD). Variations may also be used to detect susceptibility to certain genetic autoimmune diseases. Human leukocyte antigens (HLA) are a group of genes found on chromosome 6. There are two types of HLA: class I and class II. Low resolution (or generic) HLA typing can be performed via serology, cellular, or molecular technique, the molecular technique being the most common. In this technique, whole blood must be obtained and DNA extracted. The genes of interest are amplified and identification of HLA type is made via detection of the DNA sequence polymorphism. High resolution typing involves identifying alleles or allele groups by examining and determining the specific HLA characteristics. Report 81379 for complete high resolution HLA class I typing, including HLA-A, -B, and -C. Report 81380 for HLA high resolution typing of each individual class I loci (HLA-A, -B, or -C) when complete class I typing is not performed. Report 81381 for high resolution typing of each class I allele or allele group (e.g., B*57:01P).

81382-81383

These tests are commonly used to determine the histocompatibility between a patient and a donor to predict and prevent graft versus host disease (GVHD). Variations may also be used to detect susceptibility to certain genetic autoimmune diseases. Human leukocyte antigens (HLA) are a group of genes found on chromosome 6. There are two types of HLA: class I and class II. Low resolution (or generic) HLA typing can be performed via serology, cellular, or molecular technique, the molecular technique being the most common. In this technique, whole blood must be obtained and DNA extracted. The genes of interest are amplified and identification of HLA type is made via detection of the DNA sequence polymorphism. High resolution typing involves identifying alleles or allele groups by examining and determining the specific HLA characteristics. Report 81382 for high resolution typing of an individual HLA class II locus, including HLA-DRB1, -DRB3/4/5, -DQA1, -DQB1, -DPB1, or -DPA1. Report 81383 for high resolution typing of each individual class II allele or allele group (e.g., HLA-DQB1*06:02P).

81400-81408

These tier 2 molecular pathology procedure tests are used to analyze nucleic acid for abnormalities that may indicate a variety of genetic-based disorders occurring at a low disease incidence. Portions of DNA/RNA are reviewed for variation, repetition, or mutation. Cell lysis, nucleic acid stabilization, extraction, digestion, amplification, and detection are included in the molecular pathology procedure codes. Any procedures prior to cell lysis may be reported separately. Code selection is dependent upon the gene and the specific mutation examined. Specimens may vary widely and include amniotic fluid, peripheral blood, bone marrow, and skin biopsy. The gene and type of mutation that are being analyzed are identified as molecular pathology levels one through nine; they are arranged by level of resources and provider interpretation required. For the specific gene mutation assignment, reference the code description in the CPT book.

81410-81411

This test is performed as an evaluation for hereditary conditions that fall under aortic dysfunction or dilation. It is a genomic sequencing procedure (GSP) that looks for changes in the order, number, organization, and irregular arrangements within the gene chain specific to the medical condition. Specimen is whole blood. Report 81410 for a panel that includes a minimum of nine genes, including fibrillin 1 (FBN1); transforming growth factor, beta receptor 1 (TGFBR1); transforming growth factor, beta receptor 2 (TGFBR2); collagen, type III, alpha 1 (COL3A1); myosin, heavy chain 11, smooth muscle (MYH11); actin, alpha 2, smooth muscle, aorta (ACTA2); solute carrier family 2 (facilitated glucose transporter), member 10 (SLC2A1); SMAD family member 3 (SMAD3); and myosin light chain kinase (MYLK). Report 81411 for duplication/deletion analysis to include TGFBR1, TGFBR2, MYH11, and COL3A1.

81412

This test is performed as an evaluation for the Ashkenazi Jewish associated disorders. These rare conditions tend to affect people of Eastern European descent. The evaluation is typically performed if the parent(s) is a carrier of the disease. It is a genomic sequencing procedure (GSP) that looks for changes in the order, number, organization, and irregular arrangements within the gene chain specific to the medical condition. Specimen is whole blood. Report this code for a panel that includes a minimum of nine genes, including Aspartoacylase (ASPA); Bloom Syndrome, RecQ Helicase-Like (BLM); Cystic Fibrosis Transmembrane Conductance Regulator (CFTR); Fanconi Anemia, Complementation Group C (FANCC); Glucosidase, Beta, Acid (GBA); Hexosaminidase A (Alpha Polypeptide) (HEXA); Inhibitor Of Kappa Light Polypeptide Gene Enhancer In B-Cells, Kinase Complex-Associated Protein (IKBKAP); Mucolipin 1 (MCOLN1); and Sphingomyelin Phosphodiesterase 1, Acid Lysosomal (SMPD1).

81413-81414

These tests are performed to determine factors that may play a role in idiopathic ventricular fibrillation (IVF) or sudden cardiac death due to various cardiac conditions by evaluating possible genetic markers. It is suggested that ion channel deviations may contribute to these conditions and genetic testing may assist in diagnosing family members predisposed to such conditions. It is a genomic sequencing procedure (GSP) that looks for changes in the order, number, organization, and irregular arrangements within the gene chain specific to the medical condition. Specimen is blood, saliva, or body tissue. Report 81413 for a panel that includes a minimum of 10 genes, including Ankyrin 2, Neuronal (ANK2); Calsequestrin 2 (CASQ2); Caveolin 3 (CAV3); Potassium Voltage-Gated Channel Subfamily E Regulatory Subunit 1 (KCNE1); Potassium Voltage-Gated Channel Subfamily E regulatory Subunit 2 (KCNE2); Potassium Voltage-Gated Channel Subfamily H Member 2 (KCNH2); Potassium Voltage-Gated Channel Subfamily J Member 2 (KCNJ2); Potassium Voltage-Gated Channel Subfamily Q Member 1 (KCNQ1); Ryanodine Receptor 2 (RYR2); and Sodium Voltage-Gated Channel Alpha Subunit 5 (SCN5A). Report 81414 for duplication/deletion analysis to include KCNH2 and KCNQ1.

[81418]

Genomic sequencing procedures are DNA or RNA sequence analysis methods that assay multiple genes or genetic regions concurrently that are pertinent to a clinical situation. Numerous antidepressants, atomoxetine, and various antipsychotics are metabolized by CYP2D6 and CYP2C19. Report 81418 for a drug metabolism genomic sequence analysis panel that includes testing of at least six genes, including CYP2C19, CYP2D6, and CYP2D6 duplication/deletion analysis.

[81419]

This test is performed for the analysis of genes associated with syndromic and nonsyndromic causes of epilepsy. Defined as a disorder in which a person has recurrent, unprovoked seizures, epilepsy affects approximately five to 10 per 1,000 individuals. The underlying causes of epilepsy are varied, although a substantial percentage are felt to be genetic in origin. Specimen type varies but may include whole blood, DNA, or saliva/assisted saliva. Analysis is performed by next generation sequencing (NGS).

81415-81417

Exome sequence analysis is a test for identifying disease causing DNA variants within the human genome. An exome is part of the human genome that houses inherited traits in a chain of DNA and instructs the body to create the proteins needed to operate appropriately. The exome represents less than 2 percent of the human genome, but contains about 85 percent of known disease-causing variants, making whole-exome sequencing a cost-effective alternative to whole-genome sequencing. This test may be requested when a history or exam implies a possible genetic factor is present. The patient may have previously undergone other genetic testing without results pointing to the cause. Some providers request this test initially to help facilitate a diagnosis. This test can recognize alterations to DNA that may be related to the medical issues. This newer technology allows the analysis of large quantities of genes all at once versus the current testing methods that evaluate minimal genes at a given time. Report 81415 for initial sequence analysis; 81416 for sequence analysis where a comparative exome is available from an immediate family member; and 81417 for the re-evaluation analysis when additional information becomes available or additional conditions arise.

81420

Aneuploid cell are cells with an abnormal number of chromosomes, either extra or missing, and is associated with miscarriage and congenital birth defects. The most common condition associated with aneuploidy is Down syndrome (trisomy 21). This test is considered a useful and inexpensive tool to calculate age adjusted risk for the presence of neural tube defects (NTD) and fetal aneuploidy. Indications for performing this test include a maternal age of 35 years or older, ultrasonogram findings demonstrating an increased risk of aneuploidy, personal history of a prior pregnancy with a trisomy, positive blood serum or biochemical test result for aneuploidy, and/or or parental balanced Robertsonian translocation with high risk of fetal trisomy 13 or 21. The specimen is maternal serum free DNA.

81422

This test is one of a number of noninvasive prenatal screening (NIPS) tests done to detect common genetic conditions such as trisomy 21, as well as to identify fetal genomic microdeletions such as 22q11.2 deletion for DiGeorge syndrome. However, this test does not report whether the genomic coordinates or whether the deletion is maternal or fetal. NIPS is considered more reliable than standard screening with higher detection rates, greater specificity, and higher positive predictive values but is more expensive, which prohibits it from being used universally. Method is by next-generation sequencing of cell-free DNA (cfDNA). Source is maternal blood or plasma.

[81443]

This test is performed for the genomic analysis of at least 15 genes for carrier screening of individuals with inherited conditions. Specimen type varies. Methodology is a multiplex PCR-based assay.

81425-81427

These codes represent genomic sequencing procedures (GSP) that look for changes in the order, number, organization, and irregular arrangements within the gene chain specific to the medical condition. The human genome is the set of genetic information encoded in 46 chromosomes found in the nucleus of each cell. Each genome contains all of the information needed to build and maintain that person and given the advancements in DNA studies, researchers and other personnel can now examine them. These codes are looking for abnormalities that may shed light on hereditary and/or constitutional diseases. Report 81425 for the initial genome sequence analysis (GSP); 81426 for sequence analysis of immediate family members in conjunction with the initial genome study; and 81427 for re-evaluation of a previous study due to more current information related to disorders.

81430-81431

These tests evaluate conditions that fall under hearing loss. They are genomic sequencing procedures (GSP) that look for changes in the order, number, organization, and irregular arrangements within the gene chain specific to the medical condition. Specimen is whole blood. Report 81430 for a panel that includes a minimum of 60 genes, including cadherin-23 (CDH23); clarin 1 (CLRN1); gap junction protein, beta 2, 26kDa (GJB2); G protein-coupled receptor 98 (GPR98); mitochondrially encoded 12S RNA (MTRNR1); usher syndrome type 1 gene (MY07A); gene located at the DFNB3 locus on chromosome 17p11.2 (MYO15A), protocadherin-related 15 (PCDH15), otoferlin (OTOF); solute carrier family 26 (anion exchanger), member 4 (SLC26A4); transmembrane channel-like 1 (TMC1); transmembrane protease, serine 3 (TMPRSS3); usher syndrome 1C (autosomal recessive, severe) (USH1C); usher syndrome 1G (autosomal recessive) (USH1G); usher syndrome 2A (autosomal recessive, mild) (USH2A); wolfram syndrome 1 (wolframin) (WFS1). Report 81431 for duplication/deletion analysis to include copy number analyses for STRC and DFNB1 deletions in GJB2 and GJB6 genes.

81432

Genomic sequencing and analysis is performed on at least five genes pertaining to hereditary breast cancer related disorders; interrogation for sequence variants and copy number variants is included. Genomic sequencing procedures (GSP) look for changes in the order, number, organization, and irregular arrangements within the gene chain specific to the medical condition. Specimen is whole blood. Methodology includes massively parallel sequencing (MPS) such as next-generation sequencing (NGS) or other molecular techniques such as microarray or polymerase chain reaction (PCR). These testing methods allow several genomes to be sequenced simultaneously in a single instrument.

81434

This test is performed as an evaluation for hereditary retinal disorders. It is a genomic sequencing procedure (GSP) that looks for changes in the order, number, organization, and irregular arrangements within the gene chain specific to the medical condition. Specimen is whole blood. This panel must include a minimum of 15 genes, including ATP-Binding Cassette, Sub-Family

A (ABC1), Member 4 (ABCA4); Cyclic Nucleotide Gated Channel Alpha 1 (CNGA1); Crumbs Family Member 1, Photoreceptor Morphogenesis Associated (CRB1); Eyes Shut Homolog (Drosophila)(EYS); Phosphodiesterase 6A, CGMP-Specific, Rod, Alpha (PDE6A); Phosphodiesterase 6B, CGMP-Specific, Rod, Beta (PDE6B); Pre-MRNA Processing Factor 31 (PRPF31); Peripherin 2 (Retinal Degeneration, Slow)(PRPH2); Retinol Dehydrogenase 12 (All-Trans/9-Cis/11-Cis)(RDH12); Rhodopsin (RHO); Retinitis Pigmentosa 1 (Autosomal Dominant)(RP1); Retinitis Pigmentosa 2 (X-Linked Recessive)(RP2); Retinal Pigment Epithelium-Specific Protein 65kDa (RPE65); Retinitis Pigmentosa GTPase Regulator (RPGR); and Usher Syndrome 2A (Autosomal Recessive, Mild)(USH2A).

81435
Genomic sequencing and analysis is performed on at least five genes pertaining to hereditary colon cancer related disorders; interrogation for sequence variants and copy number variants is included. Genomic sequencing procedures (GSP) look for changes in the order, number, organization, and irregular arrangements within the gene chain specific to the medical condition. Specimen is whole blood. Methodology includes massively parallel sequencing (MPS) such as next-generation sequencing (NGS) or other molecular techniques such as microarray or polymerase chain reaction (PCR). These testing methods allow several genomes to be sequenced simultaneously in a single instrument.

81437
Genomic sequencing and analysis is performed on at least five genes pertaining to neuroendocrine tumor related disorders; interrogation for sequence variants and copy number variants is included. Genomic sequencing procedures (GSP) look for changes in the order, number, organization, and irregular arrangements within the gene chain specific to the medical condition. Specimen is whole blood. Methodology includes massively parallel sequencing (MPS) such as next-generation sequencing (NGS) or other molecular techniques such as microarray or polymerase chain reaction (PCR). These testing methods allow several genomes to be sequenced simultaneously in a single instrument.

[81448]
This test evaluates for peripheral neuropathies including, but not limited to, Charcot-Marie-Tooth and spastic paraplegia. A genomic sequencing procedure (GSP) is performed to look for changes in the order, number, organization, and irregular arrangements within the gene chain specific to the medical condition. Specimen is whole blood. This panel must include a minimum of five genes associated with peripheral neuropathies, such as BSCL2, GJB1, MFN2, MPZ, REEP1, SPAST, SPG11, and SPTLC1.

81439
This test is performed to determine possible genetic factors for inherited cardiomyopathies. It is a genomic sequencing procedure (GSP) that looks for changes in the order, number, organization, and irregular arrangements within the gene chain specific to the medical condition. Specimen is whole blood. This panel includes at least five cardiomyopathy-related genes including Desmoglein 2 (DSG2); Myosin Binding Protein C, Cardiac (MYBPC3); Myosin, Heavy Chain 7, Cardiac Muscle, Beta (MYH7); Plakophilin 2 (PKP2); and Titin (TTN).

[81441]
This test is performed to determine possible genetic factors for inherited bone marrow failure syndromes (IBMFS), such as congenital amegakaryocytic thrombocytopenia, Diamond-Blackfan anemia, dyskeratosis congenita, Fanconi anemia, GATA2 deficiency syndrome, and Shwachman-Diamond syndrome. It is a genomic sequencing procedure (GSP) that looks for changes in the order, number, organization, and irregular arrangements within the gene chain specific to the medical condition. Specimen is whole blood. This panel includes sequencing of at least 30 specific genes.

81440
This panel represents comprehensive genetic testing for diagnosing mitochondrial disorders caused by mitochondrial (mtDNA) or nuclear gene mutations. They are genomic sequencing procedures (GSP) that look for changes in the order, number, organization, and irregular arrangements within the gene chain specific to the medical condition. Each genome contains all of the information needed to build and maintain that person and given the advancements in DNA studies, researchers and other personnel can now examine them. Specimen is whole blood. Mitochondrial DNA (mtDNA) is found in large quantities within each cell that can lead to the probability of mutation. The number of mutations varies depending on the tissue and can result in specific manifestations. While the typical mitochondrial genome has 13 coding genes, nuclear-encoded genes make up 99 percent of the proteins that contribute to this morphology. This test is evaluating neurologic or myopathic traits within the genome and must include the analysis of at least 100 genes, including BC1 (ubiquinol-cytochrome c reductase) synthesis-like (BCS1L); chromosome 10 open reading frame 2 (C10orf2); coenzyme Q2 4-hydroxybenzoate polyprenyltransferase (COQ2); cytochrome c oxidase assembly homolog 10 (yeast)(COX10); deoxyguanosine kinase (DGUOK); MpV17 mitochondrial inner membrane protein (MPV17); optic atrophy 1 (autosomal dominant)(OPA1); prenyl (decaprenyl) diphosphate synthase, subunit 2 (PDSS2); polymerase (NDA directed), gamma (POLG); polymerase (DNA directed), gamma 2, accessory subunit (POLG2); ribonucleotide reductase M2 HB (TP53 inducible)(RRM28); SCO1 cytochrome c oxidase assembly protein (SCO1); SCO2 cytochrome c oxidase assembly protein (SCO2); solute carrier family 25 (mitochondrial carrier; adenine nucleotide translocator), member 4 (SLC25A4); succinate-CoA

ligase, ADP-forming, beta subunit (SUCLA2); succinate-CoA ligase, alpha subunit (SUCLG1); tafazzin (TAZ); thymidine kinase 2, mitochondrial (TK2); and thymidine phosphorylase (TYMP).

81442

This test is performed as an evaluation for Noonan spectrum disorders. It is a genomic sequencing procedure (GSP) that looks for changes in the order, number, organization, and irregular arrangements within the gene chain specific to the medical condition. Preferred specimen is blood, but other specimens may be obtained by oral rinse, dried blood spot (DBS), and/or buccal swab. Report this code for a panel that includes a minimum of 12 genes, including B-Raf Proto-Oncogene, Serine/Threonine Kinase (BRAF); Cbl Porto-Oncogene, E3 Ubiquitin Protein Ligase (CBL); Harvey Rat Sarcoma Viral Oncogene Homolog (HRAS); Kirsten Rat Sarcoma Viral Oncogene Homolog (KRAS); Mitogen-Activated Protein Kinase Kinase 1 (MAP2K1); Mitogen-Activated Protein Kinase Kinase 2 (MAP2K2); Neuroblastoma RAS Viral (V-Ras) Oncogene Homolog (NRAS); Protein Tyrosine Phosphatase, Non-Receptor Type 11 (PTPN11); Raf-1 Proto-Oncogene, Serine/Threonine Kinase (RAF1); Ras-Like Without CAAX 1 (RIT1); Soc-2 Suppressor Of Clear Homolog (C. Elegans) (SHOC2); and Son Of Sevenless Homolog 1 (Drosophila) (SOS1).

81445, 81449

These codes report a genomic sequencing procedure (GSP) that looks for mutations or changes in the order, number, organization, and irregular arrangements within the gene chain specific to a solid organ neoplasm. Test specimens may include whole blood or bone marrow samples. Identification of mutations may enable more targeted diagnostic and prognostic care for the patient. Report these codes for a GSP that evaluates five to 50 genes using samples taken from a solid organ neoplasm. These codes include interrogation for sequence variants and copy number variants or rearrangements when performed. Report 81445 for DNA analysis or combined DNA/RNA analysis. Report 81449 if using RNA analysis only.

81450-81451

These codes report genomic sequencing procedures (GSP) that look for mutations or changes in the order, number, organization, and irregular arrangements within the gene chain specific to a hematolymphoid neoplasm or disorder. Hematolymphoid neoplasms are cancers of the blood, bone marrow, and lymphoid organs, such as acute lymphoblastic leukemia, chronic lymphocytic leukemia (CLL), and non-Hodgkin lymphoma (NHL). Identification of mutations may enable more targeted diagnostic and prognostic care for the patient. Report 81450 for a panel that evaluates five to 50 genes using samples taken from a hematolymphoid neoplasm or for testing for a hematolymphoid disorder with DNA analysis or combined DNA/RNA analysis. Report 81451 if using RNA analysis only. These codes include interrogation for sequence variants and copy number variants/ rearrangements, or isoform expression or mRNA expression levels when performed.

81455-81456

These codes report genomic sequencing procedures (GSP) that look for mutations or changes in the order, number, organization, and irregular arrangements within the gene chain specific to a solid organ or hematolymphoid neoplasm or disorder. Hematolymphoid neoplasms are cancers of the blood, bone marrow, and lymphoid organs, such as acute lymphoblastic leukemia, chronic lymphocytic leukemia (CLL), and non-Hodgkin lymphoma (NHL). Identification of mutations may enable more targeted diagnostic and prognostic care for the patient. Report 81455 for a panel that evaluates 51 or more genes using samples taken from a solid organ or hematolymphoid neoplasm or for testing for a hematolymphoid disorder with DNA analysis or combined DNA/RNA analysis. Report 81456 if using RNA analysis only. These codes include interrogation for sequence variants and copy number variants or rearrangements, or isoform expression or mRNA expression levels, when performed.

81457-81459

These codes report genomic sequencing procedures (GSP) that look for sequence variants within the gene chain specific to a solid organ neoplasm with analysis of tumor tissue. Report 81457 for a panel that evaluates solid organ neoplasm tissue if using DNA analysis and microsatellite instability. Report 81458 if using DNA analysis, copy number variants, and microsatellite instability. Report 81459 if using DNA analysis or combined DNA and RNA analysis; this also includes interrogation for sequence variants and copy number variants or rearrangements, microsatellite instability, and tumor mutation burden.

[81462, 81463, 81464]

These codes report a genomic sequencing procedure (GSP) of cell-free nucleic acid that looks for changes in the order, number, organization, and irregular arrangements within the gene chain specific to a solid organ neoplasm. Cell-free nucleic acid consists of fragments of DNA or RNA and is released from tumor cells into the blood and other bodily fluids. Analysis of this acid is also known as a tumor liquid biopsy. Report 81462 for a panel that evaluates cell-free nucleic acid if using DNA analysis or combined DNA and RNA analysis, copy number variants, and rearrangements. Report 81463 if using DNA analysis, copy number variants, and microsatellite instability. Report 81464 if using DNA analysis or combined DNA and RNA analysis, copy number variants, microsatellite instability, tumor mutation burden, and rearrangements.

81460

This panel represents genomic sequencing procedures (GSP) that look for changes in the order, number, organization, and irregular arrangements within the gene chain specific to the medical condition. Each genome contains all of the information needed to build and maintain that person and given the advancements in DNA studies, researchers and other personnel can now examine them. Test specimens may include whole blood or muscle tissue samples. This test is evaluating the whole mitochondrial genome for the entire mitochondrial genome with heteroplasmy detection and consists of sequencing of the mitochondrial genome. Sequencing detects known and novel point mutations associated with a number of diseases, such as Leigh syndrome, Leber hereditary optic neuropathy (LHON), myoclonic epilepsy with ragged-red fibers (MERRF), and neurogenic weakness with ataxia and retinitis pigmentosa (NARP). Mitochondrial DNA (mtDNA) is found in large quantities within each cell that can lead to the probability of mutation. The number of mutations varies depending on the tissue and can result in specific manifestations. The use of this code must include heteroplasmy detection, which is looking for the presence and ratio of mutant mtDNA within a patient previously found by less direct methods. This analysis can specify the natural expression and structure of an organism and the internal traits that are passed on among family members leading to understanding of the specific disorders presented.

81465

This panel represents genomic sequencing procedures (GSP) that look for changes in the order, number, organization, and irregular arrangements within the gene chain specific to the medical condition. Each genome contains all of the information needed to build and maintain that person and given the advancements in DNA studies, researchers and other personnel can now examine them. This test evaluates the mitochondrial genome for large deletions. If the patient's condition suggests Kearns-Sayre syndrome (KSS), the specimen is ideally muscle tissue. If the patient's condition suggests Pearson syndrome, the specimen is ideally blood. Mitochondrial DNA (mtDNA) is found in large quantities within each cell that can lead to the probability of mutation. The number of mutations varies depending on the tissue and can result in specific manifestations. This code includes heteroplasmy detection, when performed, which is looking for the presence and ratio of mutant mtDNA within a patient previously found by less direct methods. This analysis can specify the natural expression and structure of an organism and the internal traits that are passed on among family members leading to understanding of the specific disorders presented.

81470-81471

These tests evaluate conditions that fall under X-linked intellectual disability (XLID), such as syndromic and non-syndromic XLID. It is a genomic sequencing procedure (GSP) that looks for changes in the order, number, organization, and irregular arrangements within the gene chain specific to the medical condition. Specimen is whole blood. Report 81470 for a panel that includes a minimum of 60 genes, including aristaless related homeobox (ARX); alpha-thalassemia x-linked intellectual disability syndrome (ATRX); cyclin-dependent kinase-like 5 (CDKL5); FYVE, RhoGEF, and PH domain containing 1 (FGD1); fragile X messenger ribonucleoprotein 1 (FMR1); HECT, UBA, and WWE domain containing 1, E3 ubiquitin protein ligase (HUWE1); Interleukin 1 receptor accessory protein-like 1 (IL1RAPL1); lysine (K)-specific demethylase 5C (KDM5C); L1 cell adhesion molecule (L1CAM); methyl CpG binding protein 2 (MECP2); mediator complex subunit 12 (MED12); midline 1 (MID1); oculocerebrorenal syndrome of Lowe (OCRL); ribosomal protein S6 kinase, 90kDa, polypeptide 3 (RPS6KA3); and solute carrier family 16, member 2 (thyroid hormone transporter) (SLC16A2). Report 81471 for duplication/deletion analysis to include ARX, ATRX, CDKL5, FGD1, FMR1, HUWE1, IL1RAPL1, KDM5C, L1CAM, MECP2, MED12, MID1, OCRL, RPS6KA3, and SLC16A2.

81490

Autoimmune biomarker analysis by immunoassay can be a valuable tool in detecting, evaluating, and therapy monitoring for rheumatoid arthritis (RA). While the exact cause of this disease is unknown, general consensus indicates that genetics and environment can play a part in this disease. A biomarker is any criterion evaluated and measured for normal, abnormal, or therapy response within the body processes. The prevalent biomarkers shown to have risk factors for RA are found within chromosome 6 and the major histocompatibility complex (MHC) region of that chromosome. This determination accounts for about 50 percent of the genetic predisposition. There are several tests available to score multiple biomarkers contributing to RA. The multi-biomarker disease activity (MBDA) scores tests the blood using 12 biomarkers to establish a number between 0 and 100. Another method, the Disease Activity Score (DAS28), evaluates 28 joints in addition to the patient's activity tracking, and evaluation of C-reactive protein (CRP) or erythrocyte sedimentation rate (ESR). This test may allow for simpler testing methods, reducing the need for the extensive joint examination and patient interpretation. Report this code for the analysis of 12 biomarkers by immunoassay, using serum sample and prognostic algorithm to achieve a DAS.

[81595]

Gene expression profiling is the ability to examine expression of multiple genes at the same time. In doing so, it allows recognition of gene expression patterns that may be able to serve as disease markers. The most common gene expression method is gene expression array where a DNA segment representing a single gene is placed onto an area attached to a glass slide or fibrous mesh membrane. Hundreds or even thousands of DNA spots, each representing a single gene, may be placed onto a single slide or chip. Once this is done, RNA is removed from the sample, amplified and labeled with fluorescent dye, and incubated for hybridization. This process, real-time reverse transcription-polymerase chain reaction (RT-PCR), can detect and quantify the mRNA. The chip/

slide is then automatically scanned and relative levels of fluorescence, representing increased or decreased levels of RNA message for each sample compared to the control, are collected and analyzed using sophisticated statistical techniques. In most cases, the vast majority of genes (so-called "house-keeping" genes) are neither up- nor down-regulated compared to control RNA. However, when cells or tissues from one state are compared to another, a small minority (often no more than 100 to 200) of genes are found to be over- or underexpressed by magnitudes of two- to three-fold or more. These expression patterns can be displayed in a format in which the expression of each gene is provided as a rejection risk score.

81493

Gene expression profiling is the ability to examine expression of multiple genes at the same time. In doing so, it allows recognition of gene expression patterns that may be able to serve as disease markers. The most common gene expression method is gene expression array where a DNA segment representing a single gene is placed onto an area attached to a glass slide or fibrous mesh membrane. Hundreds or even thousands of DNA spots, each representing a single gene, may be placed onto a single slide or chip. Once this is done, RNA is removed from the sample, amplified and labeled with fluorescent dye, and incubated for hybridization. This process, real-time reverse transcription-polymerase chain reaction (RT-PCR), can detect and quantify the mRNA. The chip/slide is then automatically scanned and relative levels of fluorescence, representing increased or decreased levels of RNA message for each sample compared to the control, are collected and analyzed using sophisticated statistical techniques. In most cases, the vast majority of genes (so-called "house-keeping" genes) are neither up- nor down-regulated compared to control RNA. However, when cells or tissues from one state are compared to another, a small minority (often no more than 100 to 200) of genes are found to be over- or underexpressed by magnitudes of two- to three-fold or more. These expression patterns can be displayed in a format in which the expression of each gene is provided as a risk score.

81506

Multianalyte assays with algorithmic analyses (MAAA) are procedures that are typically performed by a single clinical laboratory or manufacturer. These analyses utilize results obtained from assays of various types, including molecular pathology, fluorescent in situ hybridization, and non-nucleic acid based assays. Proprietary analysis, using the results as well as other patient information, is performed by the laboratory or manufacturer and reported typically as a numeric score(s) or as a probability. Report this code for the PreDx Diabetes Risk Score analysis utilizing the results of glucose, HbA1c, insulin, hs-CRP, adoponectin, ferritin, and interleukin 2-receptor alpha analytes in the algorithm.

81507

Fetal aneuploidy is a condition in which the fetus' DNA has an abnormal number of chromosomes. Approximately 3 to 13 percent of the total cell free DNA in the mother's bloodstream belongs to the fetus and is thought to be derived from the placenta. In 81507, the mother's plasma is screened using a highly sensitive microassay known as massively parallel genomic sequencing to detect trisomy 13, 18, and 21 as early as the tenth week of pregnancy. The probability that the fetus has any of the chromosomal abnormalities being screened for is generated for each abnormality in the form of a risk score.

81508-81512

These analyses utilize results obtained from assays of various types, including molecular pathology, fluorescent in situ hybridization, and non-nucleic acid based assays. Analysis, using the results as well as other patient information, is then performed and reported typically as a numeric score(s) or as a probability. Report 81508 or 81509 for analyses utilizing proteins in the algorithm. Code 81508 represents two proteins (PAPP-A and any form of hCG). Code 81509 includes three proteins (PAPP-A, DIA, and any form of hCG). Report 81510, 81511, or 81512 when the analyses use analytes in the algorithm. Code 81510 is reported for three analytes (AFP, uE3, and any form of hCG); 81511 is reported for four analytes (AFP, uE3, any form of hCG and DIA), and 81512 is reported for five analytes (AFP, uE3, total hCG, DIA, and hyperglycosylated hCG).

81513

This molecular test is used for diagnosing bacterial vaginosis (BV), the most common cause of vaginal discharge in women of reproductive age. Utilizing vaginal fluid specimens and quantitative real-time amplification of specific bacterial RNA markers, this test uses an algorithm that reports a positive or negative result for BV.

81514

This molecular test is used to diagnose bacterial vaginosis and vaginitis by employing quantitative real-time amplification of specific DNA markers. Using amplified probe analysis, this panel evaluates various types of infectious pathogens (bacterial, fungal, and parasitic) from a single vaginal fluid specimen. The test's algorithm, which reports as a positive or negative for high likelihood of bacterial vaginosis, can also include separate detection of *Trichomonas vaginalis* and/or *Candida* species.

81515

This automated test uses vaginal fluid to assist in the diagnosis of bacterial vaginosis and vaginitis. A swab sample is taken from the vagina and placed in a transport reagent. The sample is transferred to a cartridge, which is placed into a proprietary instrument for detection of DNA markers associated with vaginosis or vaginitis, including *Atopobium vaginae*, *Atopobium* species, *Megasphaera* type 1, and Bacterial Vaginosis Associated Bacteria-2 (BVAB-2). An algorithm is used, based on the DNA markers identified, to indicate whether there is a high likelihood of bacterial vaginosis in the sample. This is reported as a positive or negative result. Methodology is real-time polymerase chain reaction (PCR) amplification. This code also includes detection of *Trichomonas vaginalis* and *Candida* species (*C. albicans*, *C. tropicalis*, *C. parapsilosis*, *C. dubliniensis*) or *Candida glabrata/Candida krusei* when results from these genera and species are reported.

[81596]

This test is used in the detection of acute hepatitis C virus (HCV) infection before the appearance of HCV antibodies in serum (i.e., <2 months from exposure) either a Hepatitis C: Testing Algorithm for Screening and Diagnosis or Chronic Hepatitis C Treatment and Monitoring Algorithm: Interferon-Free Combination Therapy. Specimen is serum. Methodology is Real-Time Reverse Transcription-Polymerase Chain Reaction (RT-PCR).

81517

Lab results are combined with patient clinical information to determine risk and prognosis of liver fibrosis, progression to cirrhosis, and risk of liver-related clinical events within five years. A risk score is generated using lab tests that detect and measure specific serum biomarkers associated with formation and degradation of extracellular matrix components in the liver. The specimen is serum. Methods include immunoassay. Presence and elevation of these biomarkers (hyaluronic acid [HA], procollagen III amino terminal peptide [PIIINP], tissue inhibitor of metalloproteinase 1 [TIMP-1]) indicate damage from liver disease. Findings from the biomarker analysis are evaluated with other patient clinical information using a prognostic algorithm to generate a risk score for predicting severity of fibrosis and liver-related clinical events.

81518-81521, 81523 [81522]

Gene expression profiling is the ability to examine expression of multiple genes at the same time. In doing so, it allows recognition of gene expression patterns that may be able to serve as tumor markers. The most common gene expression method is gene expression array where a DNA segment representing a single gene is placed onto an area attached to a glass slide or fibrous mesh membrane. In doing so, hundreds or even thousands of DNA spots, each representing a single gene, may be placed onto a single slide or chip. Once this is done, RNA is removed from the sample, amplified and labeled with fluorescent dye, and incubated for hybridization. The chip/slide is then automatically scanned and relative levels of fluorescence, representing increased or decreased levels of RNA message for each sample compared to the control, are collected and analyzed using sophisticated statistical techniques. In most cases, most of the genes (so-called "house-keeping" genes) are neither up- nor down-regulated compared to control RNA. However, when cells or tissues from one state are compared to another, a small minority (often no more than 100 to 200) of genes are found to be over- or under-expressed by magnitudes of two- to three-fold or more. These expression patterns can be displayed in a format in which the expression of each gene is provided for each tumor, usually based on color differences. Specimen type is formalin-fixed paraffin-embedded tissue. Report 81518 when algorithms are reported as a percentage risk for metastatic recurrence and includes the likelihood of benefit from extended endocrine therapy. Report 81519 for gene expression profiling of 21 genes. Report 81520 for gene expression profiling of 50 content genes and eight housekeeping genes. Report 81521 for gene expression profiling of 70 content genes and 465 housekeeping genes. Report 81522 for gene expression profiling of eight content genes and four housekeeping genes. Report 81523 for next-generation sequencing of 70 content genes and 31 housekeeping genes; the algorithm is reported as index related to risk to distant metastasis.

81525

Gene expression profiling is the ability to examine expressions of multiple genes at the same time. In doing so, it allows recognition of gene expression patterns that may be able to serve as tumor markers. The most common gene expression method is gene expression array where a DNA segment representing a single gene is placed onto an area attached to a glass slide or fibrous mesh membrane. Hundreds or even thousands of DNA spots, each representing a single gene, may be placed onto a single slide or chip. Once this is done, RNA is removed from the sample, amplified and labeled with fluorescent dye, and incubated for hybridization. The chip/slide is then automatically scanned and relative levels of fluorescence, representing increased or decreased levels of RNA message for each sample compared to the control, are collected and analyzed using sophisticated statistical techniques. In most cases, the vast majority of genes (so-called "house-keeping" genes) are neither up- nor down-regulated compared to control RNA. However, when cells or tissues from one state are compared to another, a small minority (often no more than 100 to 200) of genes are found to be over- or underexpressed by magnitudes of two- to three-fold or more. These expression patterns can be displayed in a format in which the expression of each gene is provided for each tumor, usually based on color differences. Code 81525 is reported when the gene expression profiling is performed specifically for colon tumor markers by analyzing 12 genes (seven content and five house-keeping genes).

81528

Abnormally methylated genes characterize markers used for cancer diagnosis. The methodology is a quantitative allele-specific real-time target and signal amplification (QuARTS) that combines a polymerase-based target amplification process with invasive cleavage-based signal amplification. The fluorescence signal is detected in a fashion similar to real-time PCR. The dynamic range and analytical sensitivity of multiplex QuARTS reactions with titrated plasmid DNA is measured. Specimen is stool. Results are stated as a positive or negative for colorectal cancer.

81529

Gene expression profiling (GEP) is the ability to examine expression of multiple genes at the same time. In doing so, it allows recognition of gene expression patterns that may be able to serve as tumor markers. This GEP test uses real-time reverse transcription polymerase chain reaction (rRT-PCR) to identify the risk of recurrence or metastasis in various stages of cutaneous melanoma. The test is based on the biological profile of 31 genes (28 prognostic/content genes and 3 control/housekeeping genes) within the sample tissue. Specimen is formalin-fixed paraffin-embedded tumor tissue.

81535-81536

This test or assay measures (quantifies) the likely response that a patient's gynecological tumor will have to different chemotherapy treatments, such as how sensitive or resistant the tumor may be to the therapy, aiding in the most appropriate treatment selection. The assay is designed to be used as a tool with other treatment guidelines to ensure the patient receives the ultimate standard of care in treating the tumor. The ability to test a number of different chemotherapies on the patient's cancer cells before actually administering to the patient permits the physician to determine efficacy and avoid ineffective treatments. Report 81535 for the first single drug or drug combination and 81536 for each additional single drug or drug combination.

81538

Mass spectrometry targeted protein quantification is performed to identify specific quantitative proteins used in the diagnosis and treatment of lung cancer. Specimen is analyzed for 8-protein signatures, one of which must include amyloid A, which is significantly increased in lung cancer patients. A number of different mass spectrometric platforms may be used, including triple quadrupole (triple Q), matrix assisted laser desorption/ionization time of flight tandem mass spectrometer (MALDI TOF/TOF), or an ion trap instrument using selective ion monitoring (SIM) mode. Techniques for performing the test are dependent upon the platform used. A prognostic and predictive algorithm addressing the prognosis and/or likelihood of recurrence (using statements such as good versus poor overall survival) must be included with the report.

[81500, 81503]

Multianalyte Assays with Algorithmic Analyses (MAAA) are procedures that are typically performed by a single clinical laboratory or manufacturer. These analyses utilize results obtained from assays of various types, including molecular pathology, fluorescent in situ hybridization, and non-nucleic acid based assays, to perform proprietary analysis using the results, as well as other patient information, to assess risk. This risk factor is reported typically as a numeric score(s) or as a probability. Report 81500 for the Risk of Ovarian Malignancy Algorithm analysis, also known as ROMA, which utilizes the results of CA-125 and HE4 tests in the algorithm. Report 81503 when the OVA1 analysis, utilizing CA-125, apolipoprotein A1, beta-2 microglobulin, transferrin, and pre-albumin tests in the algorithm, is performed.

81539

This biochemical assay is performed to evaluate compound binding to receptors and/or how they hinder enzyme movement specifically in relation to high-grade prostate cancer. Specimen is plasma or serum. This code reports the assay of PSA proteins and human kallikrein-2 (hK2). The assay measures the proteins and combines with patient age, results of digital rectal exam, and if previous biopsy was negative to determine algorithm that provides a score determining the patient's risk of developing prostate cancer and may assist in the decision to perform a prostate biopsy.

81541-81542

Gene expression profiling is the ability to examine expression of multiple genes at the same time. In doing so, it allows recognition of gene expression patterns that may be able to serve as tumor markers. The most common gene expression method is gene expression array where a DNA segment representing a single gene is placed onto an area attached to a glass slide or fibrous mesh membrane. In doing so, hundreds or even thousands of DNA spots, each representing a single gene, may be placed onto a single slide or chip. Once this is done, RNA is removed from the sample, amplified and labeled with fluorescent dye, and incubated for hybridization. The chip/slide is then automatically scanned and relative levels of fluorescence, representing increased or decreased levels of RNA message for each sample compared to the control, are collected and analyzed using sophisticated statistical techniques. In most cases, the vast majority of genes (so-called "house-keeping" genes) are neither up- nor down-regulated compared to control RNA. However, when cells or tissues from one state are compared to another, a small minority (often no more than 100 to 200) of genes are found to be over- or under-expressed by magnitudes of two- to three-fold or more. These expression patterns can be displayed in a format in which the expression of each gene is provided for each tumor, usually based on color differences. Report 81541 when 31 content and 15 housekeeping genes associated with prostate malignancy is performed. Report 81542 when the specimen type is formalin-fixed, paraffin-embedded prostate tissue and algorithms are reported as a percentage risk for metastatic recurrence.

81551

This test detects the probability of prostate cancer on repeat biopsy for three specific genes: GSTP1, PC, and RASSF1. Specimen type is tissue. Methodology is a modification of the real-time, methylation-specific PCR assay and includes an algorithm with an interpretation for the likelihood of early prostate cancer detection.

[81546]

Genetic alterations associated with thyroid cancer can be evaluated using gene expression profiling, or the analysis of messenger RNA (mRNA) expression levels of numerous genes at once. This test evaluates 10,196 genes using fine needle aspirate from thyroid nodules as a way of categorizing a patient's risk status for cancer. The algorithm is reported as a categorical result of benign or suspicious.

[81504]

Gene expression profiling, also known as the tissue of origin (TOO) test, is used to evaluate the site of origin in a secondary malignancy metastasized from an unknown primary and also to distinguish primary from secondary tumors. A formalin-fixed paraffin embedded (FFPE) tissue sample from the tumor is analyzed using microarray technology. The tissue's RNA expression patterns are compared to other RNA expressions of common malignancies contained in the database. The more similar the tissue, the higher the similarity score. The higher the similarity score, the more likely that type of malignancy is the tissue of origin.

[81540]

Gene expression profiling is the ability to examine expression of multiple genes at the same time. In doing so, it allows recognition of gene expression patterns that may be able to serve as tumor markers. The most common gene expression method is gene expression array where a DNA segment representing a single gene is placed onto an area attached to a glass slide or fibrous mesh membrane. Hundreds or even thousands of DNA spots, each representing a single gene, may be placed onto a single slide or chip. Once this is done, RNA is removed from the sample, amplified and labeled with fluorescent dye, and incubated for hybridization. The chip/slide is then automatically scanned and relative levels of fluorescence, representing increased or decreased levels of RNA message for each sample compared to the control, are collected and analyzed using sophisticated statistical techniques. In most cases, the vast majority of genes (so-called "house-keeping" genes) are neither up- nor down-regulated compared to control RNA. However, when cells or tissues from one state are compared to another, a small minority (often no more than 100 to 200) of genes are found to be over- or under-expressed by magnitudes of two- to three-fold or more. These expression patterns can be displayed in a format in which the expression of each gene is provided for each tumor, usually based on color differences. Code 81540 is reported when the gene expression profiling is performed for tumor markers by analyzing 92 genes (87 content and 5 house-keeping genes).

81552

Uveal melanoma is the most common primary intraocular malignancy and the leading primary intraocular disease, which can be fatal in adults. Development of metastases affects prognosis significantly. Current advances in genetics and cytogenetics have provided a significant insight in tumors with high metastatic potential and the molecular mechanisms that underlie their development. Biopsy of those lesions may prove to be important for prognostication and to allow further research into genetic mutations and potential new therapeutic targets in the future.

81554

This gene expression analysis uses RNA sequencing of 190 genes to determine the probability that a patient has idiopathic pulmonary fibrosis (IPF), a chronic interstitial lung disease whose characteristics include progressive decline in lung function and worsening dyspnea. The molecular test, using tissue obtained by transbronchial biopsies, is intended to be used in conjunction with high-resolution chest CT to differentiate IPF from other interstitial lung diseases. The algorithm provides a categorical result that is positive or negative for high probability of usual interstitial pneumonia (UIP), which is the histopathological pattern of IPF.

81558

Gene expression profiling is performed to detect kidney allograft rejection after transplantation. Using a sample of whole blood, ribonucleic acid (RNA) is extracted, and complementary DNA (cDNA) synthesis is performed. This is followed by quantitative polymerase chain reaction (qPCR) amplification and analysis of 139 genes. Certain genes may be activated and produce patterns that indicate injury or rejection of the transplanted kidney. A proprietary algorithm is used to indicate transplant excellence or the possibility of subclinical rejection. The results are reported as a binary categorization.

81560

This cell-based test is ordered to predict acute cellular rejection in pediatric patients who have undergone liver or small bowel transplantation. Rejection occurs when T-lymphocytes from the recipient directly attack and destroy cells in the transplanted liver or intestine. As opposed to biopsy, which can detect but not predict rejection, this test measures the CD154 expression on T-cytotoxic memory cells. It is a qualitative test that predicts the risk of transplant rejection as either decreased or increased. Sample is whole peripheral blood; method is flow cytometry.

82009-82010

These tests are also referred to as blood ketone analysis, serum ketone, plasma ketone, beta-hydroxybutyrate, acetone, acetoacetic acid, or blood nitroprusside reaction. Method is nitroprusside reaction (colorimetry). These tests are usually performed to screen for, detect, and monitor for diabetic ketoacidosis. This condition may also be present in starvation, alcoholism, and high-fat low-carbohydrate diets. Qualitative analysis (82009) tests for the presence of acetone or other ketone bodies while quantitative analysis (82010) measures the amount of acetone or other ketone bodies.

82013
This test is also referred to as red blood cell (RBC) acetylcholinesterase, erythrocytic cholinesterase, or true cholinesterase. Method is colorimetric or spectrophotometric rate of hydrolysis determination. This test may be performed to determine certain RBC disorders such as thalassemias, spherocytosis, and other anemias. It may also be used to determine toxicity or exposure to certain insecticides. For amniotic fluid specimen, a separately reportable amniocentesis is performed. The presence of acetylcholinesterase activity and increased alpha-fetoprotein in amniotic fluid are presumptive evidence of an open neural tube defect in the fetus.

82016-82017
These tests may be requested as qualitative acylcarnitine (carnitine esters) and quantitative acylcarnitine (carnitine esters). Acylcarnitine is a condensation product formed from carboxylic acid and carnitine. It has a variety of metabolic roles and may be an indicator of inborn errors of metabolism, chronic disease, or acute and critical illness. Methods include enzymatic, chromatography, and mass-spectrometry. Qualitative analysis (82016) tests for the presence of acylcarnitine while quantitative analysis (82017) measures the amount of acylcarnitine.

82024
This test is also referred to as adrenocorticotropic hormone (ACTH) or corticotropin. Method is radioimmunoassay. This test may be performed to determine the presence of Cushing's disease, depression, or pheochromocytoma, among other conditions.

82030
This test is also referred to as cyclic adenosine monophosphate (AMP) or cAMP. Methodology is radioimmunoassay (RIA). This test may be performed in the presence of hypercalcemia for determination of hyperparathyroidism.

82040
This test measures the concentration of albumin in serum, plasma, or whole blood. It is often used to determine nutritional status, renal disease, and other chronic diseases, particularly those involving the kidneys or liver. A blood sample is typically drawn from a vein in the hand or forearm. The skin over the vein is cleaned with an antiseptic, and a tourniquet is wrapped around the upper arm to enlarge the lower arm veins by restricting the blood flow. A thin needle is inserted into the vein, the tourniquet is removed, and blood flows from the vein through the needle and is collected into a vial or syringe. The needle is withdrawn and the puncture site covered to prevent bleeding. The blood sample is sent to the laboratory for testing.

82043-82044
Microalbuminuria is defined as albuminuria of 30 to 300 mg/24 hours and is requested to determine early increase of proteinuria, usually in diabetes and in pre-eclampsia before protein becomes evident by conventional urinalysis. Patients commonly perform specimen collection over a 24-hour period. Methods include radioimmunoassay (RIA) or enzyme-linked immunosorbent assay (ELISA). Report 82043 for quantitative microalbumin and 82044 for semi-quantitative or reagent strip microalbumin.

82045
Ischemia modified albumin (IMA) is a blood assay that measures cobalt albumin binding. In the presence of myocardial ischemia, there is decreased ability of the N-terminal region of human albumin to bind cobalt. This test may also be requested as Co(II)-albumin binding assay. Method is colorimetric assay with results recorded in absorbance units (ABSU). The test is used to detect early onset unstable angina and myocardial infarction.

[82042]
This code reports quantitative analysis for albumin on CSF or amniotic fluid. Method is colorimetry. CSF analysis requires separately reportable spinal puncture and the test is performed using nephelometry. Amniotic fluid analysis requires separately reportable ultrasound guidance and amniocentesis and is usually performed by autoanalyzer.

82075-82077
Alcohol level quantitation may be used for multiple medical or legal purposes, including the detection of alcohol intoxication or dependence and determination of appropriate therapy; testing of unconscious or comatose patients to differentiate between alcohol intoxication and conditions such as cerebral trauma, diabetic coma, or drug overdose; or monitoring of ethanol treatment for methanol intoxication. Report 82075 for an alcohol breath test. This test may be used primarily in screening for ethanol levels above the legal limit for driving. The legal limit varies from state to state with levels above 0.08-0.1 g/dL usually being defined as legally intoxicated. Report 82077 for any specimen except for breath and urine; test methods are enzymatic and immunoassay.

82085
This test may also be requested as aldolase (ALD) or fructose biphosphate aldolase. Methods may include ultraviolet, kinetic, coupled enzymatic and colorimetric. This test can be useful in the identification of a variety of degenerative diseases, myopathies, and inflammations.

82088
For serum aldosterone, blood is obtained by post-fasting venipuncture. Extreme care must be taken in preparing the patient before specimen collection and handling the specimen in order to obtain an accurate measurement. Blood specimens are usually taken early in the morning and a notation is made as to whether the patient was sitting or supine. A second test may be performed approximately four hours later. A radioimmunoassay (RIA) is typically employed for analysis of the specimen. This test is most commonly

used in the diagnosis of specific types of adrenal adenomas, or secondary aldosteronism caused by cirrhosis, congestive heart failure, nephrosis, potassium loading, toxemia of pregnancy, and other states of contraction of plasma volume. Urine aldosterone requires a 24-hour non-fasting urine specimen. The patient flushes the first urine of the day. All voided urine for the next 24 hours is collected. Method is radioimmunoassay.

82103
This test may also be requested as A1 AT, AAT, Acute Phase Proteins, or -1-Antitrypsin. Method is by radial immunodiffusion (RID), or nephelometry. This test is used to detect hereditary decreases in the production of alpha1-antitrypsin, chronic obstructive lung disease, or liver disease.

82104
This test may also be requested as A1AT phenotype, AAT phenotype, and Pi phenotype. This test is used to detect hereditary decreases in the production of alpha1-antitrypsin by specific phenotype. There are more than 75 inherited variants of AAT. Two variants, Pi ZZ and Pi SZ phenotypes, represent severe deficiencies and are associated with chronic obstructive lung disease, liver disease, and hepatoma. Method is by radial immunodiffusion (RID).

82105
This test may be abbreviated as AFP. It may also be referred to as fetal alpha globulin. While this test is most often associated with pregnancy, it is also used to diagnose a variety of other conditions. During pregnancy, the test is normally performed between the 16th and 18th week of gestation. If levels are abnormal, it may be repeated approximately one week after the first test. Analysis is normally performed by radioimmunoassay (RIA).

82106
The test may be abbreviated as AFP. The test is normally performed on pregnant women initially between the 16th and 18th week of gestation. An amniotic AFP may be performed when serum AFP (82105) results are abnormal to confirm a diagnosis. An ultrasound is performed to determine the exact location of the fetus. AFP levels are measured, generally by radioimmunoassay (RIA).

82107
This test may also be ordered as an AFP-L3. The test is a measure of the L3 form of alpha fetoprotein in a patient with chronic liver disease. The specimen is blood. Using a special fluorescent reagent, the L3 form of AFP is separated from other forms of alpha fetoprotein and tagged with a special fluorescent reagent. L3 is then measured as a percentage of total AFP. The calculations occur within an instrument developed for this test. The test is primarily used in the clinical evaluation of patient risk, as elevated levels of AFP-L3 in a patient with chronic liver disease are associated with hepatocellular carcinoma.

82108
This test may be abbreviated as Al. The test is used to monitor patients at risk for aluminum toxicity due to exposure or disease states, which cause aluminum accumulation (e.g., chronic renal failure). Blood specimen is obtained by venipuncture. A random urine sample is obtained. Method is atomic absorption spectrophotometry (AAS).

82120
This test is administered to determine the specific cause of vaginitis and may be performed following negative testing for yeasts or trichomonas. Disturbances in normal anaerobic flora are usually the etiological source. A saline wet slide is prepared and characteristic cells are identified microscopically, namely epithelial cells with bacilli clinging to the surfaces. A solution of potassium hydroxide (KOH) is added to the mount to activate amines. A characteristic odor is released when amines are present and become volatile.

82127-82128
These tests may also be referred to as a metabolic screen for amino acids. Several methods may be used including thin layer chromatography (TLC), gas chromatography (GC), and ion-exchange chromatography. These tests determine whether an amino acid is or is not present (qualitative analysis). Code 82127 tests for the presence of single amino acids while 82128 tests for the presence of multiple amino acids.

82131
This test may be requested as specific amino acid (e.g., cystine, tyrosine, methionine, propionic acid). Method is ion-exchange chromatography. This test measures (quantifies) amounts of single specified amino acids.

82135
This test may be requested as aminolevulinic acid (ALA), delta ALA or DALA. Aminolevulinic acid is a precursor of heme, produced from glycine and succinyl-CoA. This test is used to diagnose genetic disorders that allow porphyrin products, specifically aminolevulinic acid, to accumulate in the liver or red blood cells. Methodology includes spectrophotometry or ion exchange resin columns.

82136-82139
These tests may be requested as specific amino acids (e.g., cystine, tyrosine, methionine, propionic acid). Method is ion-exchange chromatography. This test measures (quantifies) amounts of multiple specified amino acids. Report 82136 for two to five amino acids. Report 82139 for six or more.

82140
This test may be requested as NH3. Elevated levels may indicate that the liver is not able to detoxify ammonia from the blood due to severe liver disease. A number of methods are used including enzymatic, resin enzymatic, and ion-selective electrode (ISE).

82143
This prenatal procedure may be requested as an amniotic fluid spectral analysis, Lily test, and amniotic fluid OD 450 spectral analysis. Amniotic fluid is collected by amniocentesis and the specimen is protected from exposure to light. A separately reported ultrasound is performed to determine the exact location of the fetus prior to the amniocentesis. Method of testing is spectrophotometry. This test measures the amount of free bilirubin in the amniotic fluid.

82150
Serum amylase is elevated in acute pancreatitis and is, therefore, a common test when abdominal pain, epigastric tenderness, nausea, and vomiting are present. There are multiple methods of testing for amylase.

82154
This test may be requested as 3-Alpha-diol G. Androstanediol glucuronide is an androgen formed in the peripheral tissues. Elevated levels are frequently seen in females with hirsutism (excessive body hair). When androstanediol glucuronide is elevated, treatment of hirsutism is directed at the peripheral tissue sites rather than at other sites that are sometimes responsible for overproduction of androgens (adrenal cortex, ovary). Method is radioimmunoassay (RIA).

82157
An androgenic steroid secreted by the testes, adrenal cortex, and ovaries. This test is used primarily to evaluate androgen production in females with hirsutism. Blood is obtained by venipuncture. Method is radioimmunoassay (RIA).

82160
Androsterone is a steroid hormone metabolite in the androgen series that is measured for evaluation of syndromes of androgen excess such as hirsutism and polycystic ovary syndrome. It has been measured typically by methods involving extraction and chromatography, followed by detection and quantification by colorimetric or immunometric techniques. Measurement of this compound has largely been replaced by determination of other specific plasma androgens (e.g., testosterone) by modern, sensitive assays.

82163
This hormone acts as a powerful vasopressor, raising blood pressure and reducing fluid loss in the kidney by restricting blood flow. It also stimulates aldosterone secretion. Blood is obtained by venipuncture. The patient must remain in a recumbent position for 30 minutes prior to obtaining the blood specimen. Angiotensin II is difficult to measure accurately and great care must be taken in both collection and storage of the specimen. Method is radioimmunoassay (RIA). Degradation products and interfering peptides must be removed from the specimen prior to RIA.

82164
This test may be requested as ACE or peptidyl-dipeptidase A. ACE converts angiotensin I to angiotensin II. Method is spectrofluorometric combined with various synthetic substrates or radioimmunoassay (RIA).

82166
This test detects the presence and level of anti-mullerian hormone (AMH) in the blood. Testing may be used in reproductive-aged women to evaluate their ovarian egg (oocyte) reserve and quality of eggs. Findings aid in fertility assessment, treatment planning, and the diagnosis of certain reproductive conditions such as polycystic ovary syndrome (PCOS). Alternatively, AMH levels can help determine menopausal status, detect granulosa cell ovarian tumors, or confirm conditions such as early or delayed puberty or intersex disorders. In males, the AMH assay results can be used to detect abnormalities in the testes and gonadal function. Specimen is serum. Method is immunoassay.

82172
This test may be requested as Apolipoprotein A, Apolipoprotein A-1, Apolipoprotein B, Apolipoprotein E, Apo-A, Apo-A1, Apo-B, or Apo-E. Apolipoproteins are the components of lipoprotein complexes found in high-density lipoprotein (HDL), low-density lipoprotein (LDL), and very low-density lipoprotein (VLDL). There are numerous variables that are designated as A, B, C, D, and E with some further subdivided (e.g., A1, A2, B48, B100, C1). Those of primary interest for laboratory testing are Apo-A1, Apo-B, and Apo-E. Multiple methods are used, including radioimmunoassay (RIA), radial immunodiffusion (RID), and enzyme-linked immunosorbent assay (ELISA).

82175
Arsenic is a toxic metallic element with exposure occurring by inhalation or ingestion. Urine is the preferred specimen for acute exposure and when the patient is symptomatic. A 24-hour urine specimen is required. Method is colorimetry, atomic absorption spectrophotometry (AAS), or neutron activation analysis (NAA). This test measures (quantifies) the amount of arsenic present.

82180
This test is used to evaluate vitamin C deficiency. It may be performed with or without vitamin C saturation. When performed as a saturation test, megadoses of vitamin C are given over a three-to-four day period. The amount of vitamin C is measured (quantified).

82190
AAS is a method for detecting the absorption of specific wavelengths of light by analyte that have been vaporized in a flame. The analysis is performed using an instrument known as an atomic absorption spectrometer. Analytes are typically pure elements, since each element has a specific absorption spectrum.

82232
This test may be requested as Beta2M. Beta2M is a small (micro) nonpolymorphic protein. CSF is obtained by spinal puncture, which is reported separately. Method is by radioimmunoassay (RIA), enzyme immunoassay (EIA), or immunoradiometric assay (IRMA).

82233-82234
This test is used to measure beta-amyloid peptides 1-40 (82233) or 1-42 (82234) in a patient with cognitive decline to assist in determining the underlying condition (e.g., Alzheimer's disease) by quantitative immunoassay. The 1-40 and 1-42 peptides are often tested together to calculate a beta-amyloid ratio, which is a surrogate marker of amyloid plaque burden. The specimen is cerebrospinal fluid.

82239-82240
This is sometimes referred to as glycocholic acid. Bile acids are steroid acids derived from cholesterol. Cholylglycine is a bile salt formed by glycine and cholic acid. Method is enzymatic or gas-liquid chromatography (GLC). Code 82239 reports total concentration of all bile acids. Code 82240 reports total concentration of cholylglycine only.

82247-82248
Bilirubin is a bile pigment formed by the breakdown of hemoglobin during both normal and abnormal erythrocyte destruction. Direct (conjugated) bilirubin is that portion of the bilirubin that has been taken up by the liver cells to form bilirubin diglucuronide. Indirect (unconjugated) bilirubin is that portion of the bilirubin that has not been taken up by the liver cells. Total bilirubin is the sum of direct and indirect bilirubin present in the specimen. Method is diazotization. Spectrophotometry may be used in neonates six weeks or younger. Report 82247 for total bilirubin. Report 82248 for direct bilirubin.

82252
Bilirubin is not normally present in feces, appearing only in cases of rapid peristaltic movement of the gut or disturbances in normal intestinal flora. Detection may be useful in evaluation of some types of diarrhea. It can be detected with the dipstick or tablet tests commonly used for urine, by testing the supernatant fluid from watery feces, or adding water to solid feces.

82261
This test may be requested as an indirect test for biotin. Biotinidase is an enzyme required for the recycling of biotin. Biotinidase deficiency is a genetic condition. Newborn screening tests may include testing for deficiency of this enzyme. Method is colorimetry or enzymatic.

82270
This test may be requested as a screening guaiac, screening stool guaiac, or by a variety of brand names. The patient is instructed to obtain three consecutive stool specimens and send the kit to a lab or physician office for performance of the test. The method is peroxidase activity. This test reports the presence (qualitative analysis) of blood in the stool, but does not quantify the amount. This code is used to report the service when performed as colorectal neoplasm screening.

82271
A specimen, other than stool, is obtained for detection of blood. The method is peroxidase activity. This test reports the presence (qualitative analysis) of blood in a specimen other than stool, but does not quantify the amount.

82272
This test may be requested as a screening guaiac or screening stool guaiac, or by a variety of brand names. The patient is instructed to obtain one to three consecutive stool specimens and send the kit to a lab or physician office for test performance. The method is peroxidase activity. This test detects the presence (qualitative analysis) of blood in the stool, but does not quantify the amount. This code is used to report the service when performed for reasons other than colorectal neoplasm screening. If more than one sample is required, each must be obtained from a separate bowel movement.

82274
Fecal sample is dispersed in a diluent with antibodies for hemoglobin antigen to form a complex of antibody and antigen. A complex of antibody and antigen is separated from the specimen and exposed to a second antibody for the hemoglobin antigen. A sample from the first complex is bound to a solid carrier, and a sample from the second antibody exposure is labeled with a detection agent to determine the presence of hemoglobin antigen in the original fecal specimen. This code requires one to three consecutive stool samples, which must be obtained from separate bowel movements, and each sample must be placed in a sterile, leakproof container with a screw-cap lid for transport to the laboratory.

82286
Bradykinin is a biologically active peptide, found in plasma and many other tissues and fluids, important in the inflammatory response. A pathogenic role for Bradykinin has been suggested in diseases ranging from asthma to hereditary angioedema, as well as other kinds of swelling disorders and allergic-type diseases. It is measured in body fluids by techniques including immunoassay, capillary electrophoresis, chromatography and mass-spectrometry.

82300
Cadmium may be abbreviated as Cd. Cadmium is a bivalent metal. This test is used to evaluate toxic levels of cadmium after industrial exposure to cadmium fumes or ingestion of cadmium. A 24-hour urine specimen is recommended and must be collected in a plastic container. The patient flushes the first urine of the day and discards it. All voided urine for the next 24 hours is collected. Method is atomic absorption spectroscopy (AAS).

82306
This test may be requested as 25-OHD3, 25(OH) Calciferol, Vitamin D 25-Hydroxy, Vitamin D3 25-OH, or Calciferol 25-Hydroxy. Specimen is serum or plasma and method is high performance liquid chromatography (HPLC), competitive protein binding (CPB), or radioimmunoassay (RIA). This code includes fractions, if performed.

[82652]
This test may be requested as 1,25 (OH) Vitamin D, 1,25-Dihydroxy Vitamin D, 1,25-Dihydroxycholecalciferal, and Vitamin D, 1,25-Dihydroxy. This is the most active form of Vitamin D. It is formed by the renal cells and is essential for calcium absorption. Specimen is serum or plasma, and method is radioimmunoassay (RIA) or column chromatography. This code includes fractions, if performed.

82308
This test may be requested as thyrocalcitonin. This test may be used to screen for specific malignant neoplasms. A fasting blood specimen should be taken. The specimen is collected in a chilled tube and the test performed within 10 minutes of collection. Serum (plasma) is separated in a refrigerated centrifuge and frozen. The test is performed by assay or radioimmunoassay (RIA).

82310
This test may be abbreviated Ca. Blood is obtained by venipuncture or heel stick. Specimen is obtained in the morning and a fasting sample is preferable. Postural changes and venous stasis may provide misleading results. Accurate diagnosis may require obtaining additional specimens on subsequent days. Method is spectrophotometry or atomic absorption spectroscopy (AAS). The test may be used to assess thyroid and parathyroid function.

82330
This test may also be referred to as free calcium. It may be abbreviated iCa, Ca++ or Ca+2. Ionized or free calcium refers to calcium that is not bound to proteins in the blood. It is the metabolically active portion of the calcium in the blood. Blood is obtained by venipuncture and collected anaerobically. Method is by ion-selective electrode (ISE). The test may be used to assess thyroid and parathyroid function.

82331
The calcium infusion test is a provocative test for evaluation of medullary thyroid carcinoma (MTC). Calcitonin levels are measured following an IV infusion of calcium solution, and sometimes calcium levels are also measured to evaluate calcium incorporation or monitor hypercalcemia.

82340
This test may be abbreviated Ca urine, Ca++ or Ca+2. A 24-hour urine specimen is generally required. The patient flushes the first urine of the day and discards it. All voided urine for the next 24 hours is collected and refrigerated. Method is spectrophotometry or atomic absorption spectrometry (AAS).

82355-82360
These tests may be requested as a stone analysis or nephrolithiasis analysis. The specimen should be rinsed to remove any tissue or blood. Chemical analysis generally includes testing for the presence of calcium, carbonate, cystine, magnesium, oxalate, phosphates and urates. The analysis may be qualitative (82355), identifying only the chemicals that are present, or it may be quantitative (82360) measuring the amounts of each of the chemicals identified.

82365
This test may be requested as a stone analysis or nephrolithiasis analysis. The specimen should be rinsed to remove any tissue or blood. The stone is analyzed for the presence of calcium, carbonate, cystine, magnesium, oxalate, phosphates, and urates. This code is specific for analysis by infrared spectroscopy, which is generally performed only by reference laboratories.

82370
This test may be requested as a stone analysis or nephrolithiasis analysis. The specimen should be rinsed to remove any tissue or blood. The stone is analyzed for the presence of calcium, carbonate, cystine, magnesium, oxalate, phosphates, and urates. This code is specific for analysis by x-ray diffraction, which is generally performed only by reference laboratories. X-ray diffraction can separately analyze the nidus (center), which often differs chemically from the cortex (external layer).

82373
This test may be ordered as a CDT or CDT percentage. Blood specimen is obtained by venipuncture. The specimen is clotted and separated. Method is nephelometry or turbidimetric immunoassay. Carbohydrate deficient transferrin is a protein formed in the liver and abnormally high elevations are linked to a prolonged period of high alcohol use. The test may be ordered to confirm diagnosis of alcoholism or to measure compliance with an abstinence program.

82374
This test may be requested as CO2, HCO3, or bicarbonate. Bicarbonate (carbon dioxide) is an indicator of electrolyte and acid-base status (alkalosis, acidosis). It is elevated in metabolic alkalosis, compensated respiratory acidosis, and hypokalemia. It is decreased in metabolic acidosis, compensated respiratory alkalosis, and in diabetic ketoacidosis. Blood specimen is normally obtained by arterial puncture, but venipuncture may also be used. Bicarbonate is usually calculated using the Henderson-Hasselbalch equation (HCO3 = Total CO2 – H2CO3). However, it can also be determined by titration.

82375-82376
These tests may be requested as carboxyhemoglobin, CO, or COHb. Carbon monoxide is a colorless, odorless,

tasteless, poisonous gas formed by burning fuels, including natural gas, wood, and gasoline. These tests are used to identify the level of carbon monoxide poisoning in individuals with known or suspected exposure to the toxic gas. Method is colorimetry, spectrophotometry, or gas-liquid chromatography (GLC). Report 82375 when testing for the amount (quantitative analysis) of carbon monoxide. Report 82376 when testing (qualifying) the presence of carbon monoxide.

82378

This test may be abbreviated as CEA. While CEA occurs normally in the gastrointestinal tract, it may be elevated for certain benign and malignant neoplasms and other diseases. CEA is used primarily to monitor patients with colorectal cancer and to a lesser extent advanced breast cancer. Method is immunofluorescence, enzyme immunoassay (EIA), and radioimmunoassay (RIA).

82379

Carnitine has a variety of metabolic roles and may be an indicator of inborn errors of metabolism, chronic disease, or acute and critical illness. Method is enzymatic. This test measures (quantifies) the amount of both total and free carnitine present.

82380

This test may also be requested as beta-carotene. Carotene is an isomeric pigment found in a number of vegetables and fruits. In the liver, carotene is converted to Vitamin A, which, in turn, is converted to retinal, the major molecule that enables vision. Method is high performance liquid chromatography (HPLC), colorimetry.

82382

Catecholamines are biogenic amines that include epinephrine, norepinephrine, and dopamine. This test is used to diagnose hypertension caused by increased levels of catecholamines secreted by specific types of tumors. A 24-hour urine specimen is preferred but shorter timed collections may also be used. The patient flushes the first urine of the day and discards it. All voided urine for the next 24 hours is collected and refrigerated. Method is fluorometry. Code 82382 reports total catecholamines and therefore does not differentiate between epinephrine, norepinephrine, and dopamine.

82383

Catecholamines are biogenic amines that include epinephrine, norepinephrine, and dopamine. This test is used to diagnose hypertension caused by increased levels of catecholamines secreted by specific types of tumors. Blood specimen is obtained by venipuncture. Preferred method is high performance liquid chromatography (HPLC), but radioimmunoassay (RIA) or radiochemical assay may also be used. Code 82383 tests for total catecholamines and does not differentiate between epinephrine, norepinephrine, and dopamine.

82384

Catecholamines are biogenic amines that include epinephrine, norepinephrine, and dopamine. This test is used to diagnose hypertension caused by increased levels of catecholamines secreted by specific types of tumors. Preferred method is high performance liquid chromatography (HPLC), but radioimmunoassay (RIA) or radiochemical assay may also be used. Code 82384 reports fractionated catecholamines and quantifies total epinephrine, norepinephrine, and dopamine separately. Most assays measure only free catecholamines, but some measure both free and conjugated types.

82387

Cathepsin D is an indicator of metastatic breast cancer. Neoplastic tissue must be dissected free of fat and normal breast tissue, sliced into small pieces, placed in a tube, and quick frozen in liquid nitrogen. The tissue is analyzed by means of enzymatic immunoassay (EIA) or immunoradiometric assay (IRMA).

82390

This test may be requested as Cp, copper oxidase, or ferroxidase. Ceruloplasmin is a copper oxidase enzyme found in plasma. Decreased levels of ceruloplasmin are found in Wilson's disease, a disorder of copper metabolism. Several methods may be used, including spectrophotometry, nephelometry, or radial immunodiffusion (RID) for blood specimens. RID is the method for urine.

82397

Chemiluminescent assay refers to a detection method, whereby a chemiluminogenic substrate is converted to a chemiluminescent (light emitting) product.

82415

This test may be requested as a chloramphenicol, Chloromycetin, or Mychel-S level. Chloramphenicol is a broad spectrum antibiotic. This test is used to monitor therapeutic and toxic levels. Several methods may be used, including high performance liquid chromatography (HPLC), gas-liquid chromatography (GLC), microbiological assay (MB), colorimetry, or enzymatic immunoassay (EIA).

82435

This test may be requested as Cl, blood. Chloride is a salt of hydrochloric acid and is important in maintaining electrolyte balance. Methods include colorimetry, coulometry, and ion-selective electrode (ISE).

82436

This test may be requested as Cl, urine. Chloride is important in maintaining proper electrolyte balance. A 24-hour urine test is preferred, but shorter timed collections and random specimens may also be used. If a timed specimen is used, the patient flushes the first urine of the day and discards it. All voided urine for the next 24 hours (or shorter time increment) is collected and refrigerated. Methods include colorimetry, coulometry, and ion-selective electrode (ISE).

82438
This test may be requested as a cystic fibrosis sweat test or Cl, sweat. Saliva is sometimes used for cystic fibrosis evaluation, but is not as reliable as sweat. Sweat is obtained from the forearm by pilocarpine iontophoresis, which is reported separately. Method is usually ion-selective electrode (ISE), but colorimetry, coulometry, Schales and Schales method, and Cotlove titration are also used.

82441
Chlorinated hydrocarbons are contained in solvents and are absorbed cutaneously and by inhalation. While they vary in toxicity, all are CNS depressants and can cause liver and kidney damage with prolonged exposure. This test is used to screen for toxic levels. Levels of one or more of the following substances are screened: carbon tetrachloride, chloroform, dichloromethane, trichloroethylene, and tetrachloroethylene. Testing methods include gas chromatography flame ionization detection (GC-FID) and gas chromatography electron capture detector (GC-ECD). Colorimetry measurement of metabolites may also be used but is nonspecific.

82465
Cholesterol level is a risk indicator for atherosclerosis and myocardial infarction. Blood specimen is obtained by venipuncture. Method is enzymatic. This test reports total cholesterol in serum or whole blood.

82480
This test may be requested as acylcholine acylhydrolase, cholinesterase II, EC, PchE, pseudocholinesterase, SChE, or S-Pseudocholine Esterase. Cholinesterase is an enzyme of the hydrolase class with serum cholinesterase being specific to choline esters. Serum cholinesterase is requested primarily for diagnosis of an inherited hypersensitivity to the certain anesthetics or when organophosphate or carbamate insecticide poisoning is suspected. Methods are colorimetry, kinetic enzyme with substrates, and fluorometry. This procedure is specific to serum cholinesterase.

82482
This test may be requested as acetylcholinesterase, cholinesterase I, erythrocytic cholinesterase, or true cholinesterase. Cholinesterase is an enzyme of the hydrolase class with RBC cholinesterase being specific to the substrate acetylcholine. RBC cholinesterase is requested when organophosphate or carbamate insecticide poisoning is suspected. Blood specimen is obtained by venipuncture. Methods include colorimetry, fluorometry, and spectrophotometry. This procedure is specific to RBC cholinesterase.

82485
The test may be called dermatan sulfate. It is a glycosaminoglycan (formerly called a mucopolysaccharide) found mostly in skin, but also in blood vessels, heart valves, tendons, and lungs. It accumulates abnormally in several of the mucopolysaccharidosis disorders and plays a role in coagulation, cardiovascular disease, carcinogenesis, infection, wound repair, and fibrosis. The specimen is a 24 hour or timed urine. Chondroitin B Sulfate has been measured using chromatographic techniques such as high performance liquid chromatography (HPLC).

82495
Chromium is an essential nutrient that is toxic in large doses. The test monitors for environmental or occupational chromium toxicity that is associated with skin respiratory and other diseases such as lung cancer. Blood, urine or hair may be tested. Methods used include atomic absorption spectrometry (AAS) and neutron activation analysis (NAA).

82507
Citrate determinations in urine are useful in evaluating nephrolithiasis. A 24-hour urine specimen is required. The patient flushes the first urine of the day and discards it. All voided urine for the next 24 hours is collected and refrigerated. Citrate may be measured using enzymatic/spectrophotometric methods or chromatography.

82523
This test may be ordered as collagen crosslink N-telopeptide or pyridinium collagen crosslinks. Pyridinium includes pyrinoline and deoxypyridinoline. Collagen cross-links are markers for bone resorption and are useful in evaluating and managing osteoporosis. A timed urine specimen is required. When testing for N-telopeptide, a two-hour specimen is usually obtained. Pyridinium, including pyrinoline and deoxypyridinoline, requires a 24-hour specimen. When a timed specimen is used, the patient flushes the first urine of the day and discards it. All voided urine for the next 24 hours (or shorter time increment) is collected and refrigerated. Method is enzyme-linked immunosorbent assay (ELISA) for N-telopeptide and high performance liquid chromatography (HPLC) for pyridinium.

82525
This test may be abbreviated as Cu. Copper is an essential trace mineral. Copper deficiency is rare, however, copper may accumulate to excessive levels in patients with Wilson's disease (a disorder of copper metabolism), primary biliary cirrhosis, and chronic extrahepatic biliary obstruction. Liver specimen is obtained by separately reportable liver biopsy. Methods include colorimetry and atomic absorption spectrometry (AAS) and specimen types vary.

82528
This test may be requested as Compound B. Corticosterone is a natural corticosteroid, similar to cortisol except that it does not possess anti-inflammatory qualities. Blood specimen is obtained by venipuncture. Method is radioimmunoassay.

82530
Cortisol is a naturally occurring glucocorticoid responsible for metabolism of glucose, protein, and fats and is important in immune system function.

Urinary free cortisol is used in initial screening for Cushing's syndrome. Amniotic fluid levels of free cortisol are useful in evaluating fetal lung maturation. To obtain an amniotic fluid specimen, an ultrasound is performed to determine the exact location of the fetus. Methods include high performance liquid chromatography (HPLC) for urine and radioimmunoassay (RIA) for amniotic fluid. This test measures free (unbound) cortisol only.

82533

Cortisol is a naturally occurring glucocorticoid responsible for metabolism of glucose, protein, and fats and is important in immune system function. To obtain an amniotic fluid specimen, an ultrasound is performed to determine the exact location of the fetus. The fluid is sent to the lab for analysis. Method is radioimmunoassay (RIA), competitive protein binding (CPB), or fluorescent assay. This test measures total cortisol (both free and bound) in various specimen types.

82540

Creatine is measured in urine or serum to evaluate certain conditions involving increased muscle tissue breakdown. It has been measured in erythrocytes as an indicator of erythrocyte survival time in the evaluation of hemolytic disorders. It can be measured by colorimetric or enzymatic/spectrophotometric methods.

82542

This code reports specific chromatography techniques combined with mass spectrometry for analyzing non-drug substances that are not specifically listed elsewhere in the chemistry section. Chromatography uses different techniques to separate and analyze the specimen components. Code 82542 reports column chromatography combined with mass spectrometry. Column chromatography uses a sorbent packed in a column. The specimen is dissolved in a solvent and poured into the column. Some of the specimen components bind to the sorbent and are retained in the column, while others escape. Subsequent washings with the same or different solvents cause more strongly bound components to escape. These components can be individually analyzed. Mass spectrometry represents one of the most powerful tools available for studying complex substances. Mass spectrometry isolates specific substances by sorting a stream of electrified particles (ions) based on their mass. This code describes screening for the presence (qualitative analysis) of, and the amount (quantitative analysis) of, non-drug analytes using a single stationary and mobile phase.

82550

This test may be requested as creatine kinase (CK) or creatine phosphokinase (CPK). Blood specimen is obtained by venipuncture. Method is enzymatic, kinetic, or spectrophotometry. This code reports total CK. Creatine kinase is an enzyme found in striated muscle and it is released following injury. Elevated CK levels are primarily associated with myocardial infarction, trauma and surgery, but CK levels may be elevated with a number of other conditions as well.

82552

This test may be requested as creatine kinase (CK) isoenzymes or creatine phosphokinase (CPK) isoenzymes. Method is electrophoresis (EP), column ion-exchange chromatography. Creatine kinase consists of three isoenzymes, each of which is composed of two units, muscle (MM), brain (BB), or muscle and brain (MB). CK1 (BB) is found primarily in the brain and smooth muscle, CK2 (MB) in cardiac muscle, and CK3 (MM) in skeletal muscle. Because elevated CK levels are indicative of injury to the cells, quantifying the levels of each isoenzyme may assist in pinpointing the injured site.

82553

This test may be requested as creatine kinase (CK) MB fraction, creatine phosphokinase (CPK) MB fraction, or CK2. Methods include immunochemical, fluorometric radial partition, microparticle enzyme immunoassay, immunoenzymetric, or chemiluminometric. Creatine kinase consists of three isoenzymes, which are each composed of two units, muscle (MM), brain (BB), or muscle and brain (MB). CK1 (BB) is found primarily in the brain and smooth muscle, CK2 (MB) in cardiac muscle, and CK3 (MM) in skeletal muscle. This code tests for the MB or CK2 fraction only.

82554

This test may be requested as CK isoforms or CPK isoforms. Blood specimen is obtained by venipuncture. Methods include electrophoresis (EP), high performance liquid chromatography (HPLC), and isoelectric focusing (IEF). Creatine kinase consists of three isoenzymes, which are each composed of two units, muscle (MM), brain (BB), or muscle and brain (MB). CK1 (BB) is found primarily in the brain and smooth muscle, CK2 (MB) in cardiac muscle, and CK3 (MM) in skeletal muscle. These isoenzymes can be further subdivided into isoforms which are designated by the isoenzyme (MM, MB, BB) followed by a number (e.g., 1, 2, 3) Examples include CK-MB1, CK-MB2.

82565

Serum creatinine is the most common laboratory test for evaluating renal function. Method is enzymatic or colorimetry.

82570

Urine creatinine levels are not normally used to evaluate disease processes except as part of a creatinine clearance test, but they are a good indicator of the adequacy of timed urine specimens. Amniotic fluid creatinine is used to evaluate fetal maturity. For amniotic fluid specimen, a separately reportable amniocentesis is performed. Method is enzymatic, Jaffe reaction, or manual.

82575

This test may be requested as urea clearance or urea nitrogen clearance. Both blood and urine specimens are required. Blood specimen is obtained by venipuncture. A 24-hour urine specimen is preferred, but timed shorter increments may also be acceptable. Method is enzymatic or Jaffe reaction, or alkaline picrate. Creatinine clearance is a calculation of urine and serum creatinine content adjusted by urine volume and body size. The test is a general indicator of glomerular filtration function of the kidneys.

82585
Fibrinogen with an abnormal physical property causing it to precipitate in the cold (4 degrees C) and dissolve again when warmed to 37 degrees C is known as cryofibrinogen. This test is performed to evaluate cold intolerance. Blood specimen is obtained by venipuncture in a prewarmed tube and must be kept warmed. Method is cold precipitation.

82595
Cryoglobulin is a serum globulin with an abnormal physical property causing it to precipitate at cold temperatures (4 degrees C) and dissolve again when warmed to 37degrees C. It is indicative of lymphoproliferative disorders, collagen vascular disease, and a variety of infections and other diseases. Blood specimen is obtained by venipuncture in a prewarmed tube and must be kept warmed. Method is cold precipitation.

82600
This test may be requested as CN, hydrocyanic acid, or potassium or sodium cyanide. Cyanide is poisonous, both as a gas (inhaled) and as a salt (ingested). It binds to cytochrome oxidase, preventing cellular respiration. Multiple methods may be used, including colorimetry, spectrophotometry, microdiffusion, gas chromatography-mass spectrometry (GC-MS), and high performance liquid chromatography (HPLC).

82607
This test may be requested as antipernicious anemia factor, true cyanocobalamin, or Vitamin B12. It is essential for red blood cell maturation and for gastrointestinal and neurologic health. Decreased levels may be indicative of certain anemias. Method is chemiluminescence, competitive protein binding (CPB) radioassay, or radioimmunoassay (RIA).

82608
This test may be requested as unsaturated Vitamin B12 binding capacity (UBBC) and Vitamin B12. It is essential for red blood cell maturation and for gastrointestinal and neurologic health. This test may be used to evaluate for certain anemias, myeloproliferative disorders, and the congenital absence of transcobalamin II or cobalophilin. Method is radioimmunoassay (RIA).

82610
Code 82610 reports the quantitative determination of Cystatin C, which is used to diagnose impaired kidney function. Serum Cystatin C is a useful indicator of glomerular filtration rate (GFR), particularly in elderly, very obese, and malnourished patients whose serum creatinine can be misleading. It is also used in renal function assessment in patients suspected of having renal disease, and for monitoring the response to treatment in those with kidney disease. The method of testing varies by laboratory.

82615
Cystine and homocystine are amino acids indicative of disease when found in the urine. Method is ion exchange chromatography or spectrophotometry.

82626
This test may be requested as unconjugated DHEA. Serum DHEA levels may be used to evaluate delayed puberty and hirsutism. Elevations may be indicative of ovarian disorders, neoplasm of the adrenal gland, Cushing's disease, or ectopic ACTH-producing neoplasm. Decreased levels in amniotic fluid may be indicative of congenital adrenal hypoplasia. For amniotic fluid specimen, a separately reportable amniocentesis is performed. Method is radioimmunoassay (RIA) or gas-liquid chromatography (GLC).

82627
This test may be requested as DHEA-S or DHEAS. Serum DHEA-S levels may be used to evaluate hirsutism. Elevations may be indicative of ovarian or adrenal disorders, neoplasm of the adrenal cortex, Cushing's disease, or ectopic ACTH-producing neoplasm. Decreased levels in amniotic fluid may be indicative of anencephaly. For amniotic fluid specimen, an amniocentesis is performed. Method is typically radioimmunoassay (RIA).

82633
This test may be requested as DOC. Deoxycorticosterone is a hormone produced in small quantities by the adrenal cortex. A normal circadian rise and fall in levels is noted. Method is radioimmunoassay (RIA). The test may be ordered during pregnancy for a variety of reasons, including preeclampsia.

82634
This test may be requested as Compound S. This test may be ordered to evaluate adrenocortical function. Do not confuse with metyrapone stimulation panel (see comments). Blood specimen is obtained by venipuncture. Methods include radioimmunoassay (RIA) and chromatography.

82638
This test may be requested as cholinesterase or pseudocholinesterase inhibition test. Dibucaine is used in this test as an inhibitor of cholinesterase to evaluate for unusual phenotypes with hypersensitivity to certain drugs. Individuals with these phenotypes experience apnea (cessation of breathing) when certain drugs are administered. Method is enzymatic.

82642
This test is used to monitor patients undergoing chemotherapy or 5 alpha-reductase inhibitor therapy. Specimen is serum. Methodology is liquid chromatography on a multiplexed LC system and analysis on a tandem mass spectrometer equipped with an electrospray ion.

82656 [82653]
Pancreatic elastase (EL-1) is a marker for exocrine pancreatic function. The test identifies pancreatic exocrine insufficiency due to conditions such as chronic pancreatitis, gallstones, cystic fibrosis, and other conditions. A random stool sample is obtained. Method is enzyme-linked immunosorbent assay (ELISA). Report 82656 for a qualitative or semi-quantitative test and 82653 for a quantitative test.

82657-82658
These codes report enzyme assays using a variety of different methods, some established and some relatively new. Code 82657 reports enzyme assay with nonradioactive substrate (substance upon which an enzyme acts), while 82658 reports enzyme assay with radioactive substrate.

82664
This code reports various electrophoretic techniques. Electrophoresis is a test method that uses an electrical field to move particles toward electrical poles. It separates ionic substances based on differences in their rates of migration toward the poles. Some types of electrophoresis include disc, gel, isoenzyme, and thin layer.

82668
This test may be requested as EPO or S-EPO. Erythropoietin is a hormone that regulates the production of erythrocytes (red blood cells). Method is radioimmunoassay (RIA) or chemiluminescent immunoassay.

82670 [82681]
Estradiol is derived from ovaries, testes, and the placenta and is the most active endogenous estrogen. The free estradiol blood test (82681) is a direct measure of free estradiol in serum and is the most commonly ordered fertility test for women with infertility problems. It is also indicated for in vitro fertilization support and to monitor estradiol levels in fertile males as well as females. Methodology is high performance liquid chromatography/tandem mass spectrometry (LC/MS) and quantitative equilibrium dialysis. Report 82670 for total estradiol.

82671
This test may be requested as fractionated estrogens. Estrogens are the female sex hormones and include estradiol, estrone, and estriol. Blood specimen is obtained by venipuncture. Method is radioimmunoassay. Fractionation involves separating total estrogen into its components.

82672
This test may be requested as total estrogen in serum or urine. Because the serum assay does not measure estriol levels, urine assay is perhaps more commonly ordered. Estrogens are the female sex hormones and include estradiol, estrone, and estriol. Method is spectroscopy or fluorometry.

82677
This test may be requested as estriol (E3). Estriol is a relatively weak estrogen, present in high concentrations during pregnancy. Low levels may be indicative of maternal complications (e.g., diabetes, preeclampsia), fetal growth retardation, or fetal anomaly (e.g., anencephaly). For amniotic fluid specimen, a separately reportable amniocentesis is performed. Method is radioimmunoassay (RIA) for serum or urine and gas-liquid chromatography (GLC) for amniotic fluid.

82679
This test may be requested as estrone (E1). Estrone is a moderately potent estrogen, derived primarily from oxidation of estradiol, but also secreted by the ovaries. For amniotic fluid specimen, a separately reportable amniocentesis is performed. Method is radioimmunoassay (RIA) for serum or urine and gas-liquid chromatography-mass spectrometry (GLC-MC) for amniotic fluid.

82693
This test may be requested as 1,2-ethanediol. Ethylene glycol is toxic substance and a component of common automotive antifreeze. The substance has a natural sweet odor and exposure is by accidental or intentional ingestion. Methods include gas chromatography-flame ionization detection (GC-FID), liquid chromatography (LC), enzymatic assay, photometry, and fluorometry.

82696
Etiocholanolone is a steroid hormone metabolite in the androgen series that is measured for evaluation of syndromes of androgen excess such as hirsutism and polycystic ovary syndrome. It has been measured typically by methods involving extraction and chromatography, followed by detection and quantification by colorimetric or immunometric techniques. Measurement of this compound has largely been replaced by determination of other specific plasma androgens (e.g., testosterone) by modern, sensitive assays.

82705
This test is used to evaluate steatorrhea, which is an abnormal amount of fat in the stool sometimes found with celiac disease and malabsorption syndromes. This is a qualitative test that assesses the presence of fat in the stool. A random stool specimen is obtained. Method is microscopic screen.

82710
This test is used to evaluate malabsorption and steatorrhea, which is an abnormal amount of fat in the stool. This test may be requested as 24-hour, 48-hour, or 72-hour stool collection for fat analysis. A 72-hour collection period is preferred. The patient is placed on a diet containing 50-150 grams of fat/day beginning at least two days prior to testing. All stool is collected in a plastic container for the designated time period. Method is gravimetry or titrimetry.

82715
Quantitative fecal fat analysis is used in the evaluation of diarrhea and malabsorption. Differentiation of the types of fat excreted can be useful in identifying the cause of steatorrhea, such as differentiating pancreatic insufficiency from other causes of malabsorption. Generally, fecal fat is differentiated as neutral fat (triglycerides) and nonesterified fat (free fatty acids), but it may be more specifically differentiated as long or short chain fatty acids, and may include cholesterol analysis. Methods used for analysis include differential extraction with gravimetric quantification, enzymatic analysis of fecal extracts, or chromatography.

82725
This test may be requested as nonesterified fatty acids (NEFA) or free fatty acids (FFA). Method is colorimetry, spectrophotometry, or enzymatic.

82726
Very long chain fatty acid levels are elevated in certain demyelinating diseases such as adrenoleukodystrophy and adrenomyeloneuropathy, and in several paroxysmal disorders including Zellweger syndrome and infantile Refsum's disease. Skin fibroblasts may be obtained by scraping. Methods include new techniques such as capillary gas chromatography, mass spectrometry, and stable isotope dilution.

82728
Serum ferritin level measures available iron stores and is a reliable indicator of normal, as well as deficient, levels. Blood specimen is obtained by venipuncture. Method is radioimmunoassay (RIA), immunoradiometric assay (IRMA), enzyme immunoassay (EIA), or enzyme linked immunosorbent assay (ELISA).

82731
Fibronectin is an adhesive glycoprotein. The presence of fetal fibronectin in cervicovaginal secretions is an indicator that a pregnant woman will soon go into labor, and it is tested for the purpose of predicting premature labor. Rapid enzyme-linked immunosorbent assay (ELISA) tests are available to perform the assay on cervical swab specimens. The test is a semi-quantitative (positive or negative) test.

82735
Fluoride is available as hydrogen fluoride and its organic salts. These salts are used in industry and as components of insecticides. Fluoride is also given as a dietary supplement in areas where it is not available in drinking water. However, fluoride is toxic in excessive quantities. This test is performed to evaluate fluoride toxicity. Method is fluoride specific electrode, ion-selective potentiometry, or gas-liquid chromatography (GLC).

82746
This test may be requested as serum folate. This test is used to detect folic acid deficiency. Folic acid is a B vitamin necessary for normal red blood cell production. It is stored in the body as folates. Folic acid deficiency results in a form of megaloblastic anemia. Method is competitive binding protein (CPB) radioimmunoassay, chemiluminescence, or microbiological assay.

82747
This test may be requested as RBC folate or red cell folate. It is used to detect folic acid deficiency. Folic acid is a B vitamin necessary for normal red blood cell production. It is stored in the body as folates. Folic acid deficiency results in a form of megaloblastic anemia. Method is radioimmunoassay (RIA), competitive binding protein (CPB) radioimmunoassay, or chemiluminescence.

82757
This test may be requested as levulose analysis. Fructose is normally present in semen, but may be absent with some congenital anomalies of the male genital tract. A semen specimen is obtained. Method is colorimetry.

82759
Galactokinase is an enzyme necessary for galactose utilization. This test evaluates galactosemia resulting from galactokinase deficiency. Method is radioisotope.

82760
Galactose levels are normally measured shortly after a galactose-rich meal or a glass of milk. Galactose is derived from dietary lactose. It appears in urine when lactose is not converted to glucose due to an inherited enzyme deficiency. This test is performed on blood or urine after ingestion of a galactose-rich meal. Multiple specimens may be required for a galactose tolerance test. Method is enzymatic.

82775-82776
These tests may be requested as UDP-G-1-P. Galactose-1-phosphate uridyl transferase is an enzyme necessary for utilization of galactose. This test is performed to identify deficiency in this enzyme. Method is radiometric or uridine diphosphoglucose (UDPG) consumption assay. Report 82775 when enzyme levels are measured (quantitated). Report 82776 when screening only for the presence (qualitative analysis) of the enzyme.

82777
This test is used to evaluate for elevated levels of galectin-3, a protein associated with a more serious form of chronic heart failure that is more likely to exacerbate than typical heart failure. The specimen is serum or ethylenediaminetetraacetic acid (EDTA) plasma. Method is enzyme-linked immunosorbent assay (ELISA).

82784
This test may be requested as immunoglobulin, IgA, IgD, IgG, or IgM. Immunoglobulins are in the group of proteins classified as antibodies. Immunoglobulins are produced in response to foreign proteins referred to antigens. IgG is the most abundant immunoglobulin. It is produced in response to secondary exposure to viral and bacterial antigens. IgA is found primarily in the respiratory, gastrointestinal, and genitourinary tracts,

as well as in tears and saliva. It is responsible for protecting the mucous membranes from viral and bacterial antigens. Congenital IgA deficiency is also associated with autoimmune disease. IgM is produced following primary exposure to an antigen and is active against rheumatoid factors, gram-negative organisms, and the ABO blood group. IgD properties are not well understood but increases with chronic infection, connective tissue disorders, and some liver disease. Serum immunoglobulins may be tested for the four types (IgA, IgD, IgG, and IgM) reported with this code. Saliva may be tested for IgA. CSF may be tested for IgA, IgD, IgG, and IgM. CSF is obtained by spinal puncture, which is reported separately. Method is dependent on specimen source and specific immunoglobulins being tested. Serum is usually analyzed using radial immunodiffusion (RID), enzyme linked immunosorbent assay (ELISA), nephelometry, or turbidimetry. Urine uses electroimmunodiffusion (EID). Saliva uses radial immunodiffusion (RID). CSF is analyzed with radioimmunoassay (RIA).

82785

This test may be requested as immunoglobulin, IgE. Immunoglobulins are in the group of proteins classified as antibodies. Immunoglobulins are produced in response to foreign proteins referred to as antigens. IgE is produced in response to allergic reactions and anaphylaxis. CSF is obtained by spinal puncture, which is reported separately. Method is radioimmunoassay (RIA). Paper radioimmunosorbent test may also be used for serum specimen only.

82787

This test may be requested as immunoglobulin subclasses or IgG subclasses. There are four IgG subclasses, which are designated as IgG1, IgG2, IgG3, and IgG4. IgG is part of the body's defense system against infection. Deficiencies of single subclasses, particularly IgG1, can significantly impair this defense. Blood specimen is obtained by venipuncture. Method is radial immunodiffusion (RID), enzyme linked immunosorbent assay (ELISA), nephelometry, or turbidimetry.

82800

This test may be requested as blood pH. Blood pH is tested to identify acidemia or alkalemia. Arterial puncture is preferred, but venipuncture may also be performed. Method is glass pH electrode or potentiometry.

82803-82805

These tests may be requested as arterial blood gases (ABGs). Blood gases are usually requested to evaluate disturbances of acid-base balance, which may be caused by respiratory or metabolic disorders. Blood specimen is obtained by arterial puncture. Code 82803 reports any combination of pH, pCO_2, pO_2, CO_2, and HCO_3, including calculated O_2 saturation. Code 82805 reports any combination of the same gases, but O_2 saturation is performed by direct measurement. Method is selective electrode, potentiometry, or spectrophotometry (O_2 saturation).

82810

This test may be requested as O_2. Oxygen saturation is the percent of the oxygen in the blood that combines with hemoglobin. Blood specimen is obtained by arterial puncture. Method is spectrophotometry.

82820

This test may be requested as oxygen, P50 or as pO_2, P50. This test is performed to measure the affinity of hemoglobin for oxygen, which allows evaluation of oxygen delivery to body tissues. Blood specimen is obtained by arterial puncture. Method is spectrophotometry or potentiometry.

82930

Gastric acid analysis is performed on stomach contents obtained via oral or nasogastric (NG) tube. The tube is inserted and the gastric contents are aspirated and discarded. Gastric juices are then collected intermittently for a specified time frame and used to measure the gastric output in both a basal and a stimulated state. Measurement of pH is included, if performed. Report this code once for each specimen obtained.

82938

Gastrin stimulation test with secretin may be performed to evaluate patients with suspected gastrinoma and Zollinger-Ellison syndrome. Blood specimen is obtained prior to secretin injection and at five-minute to 15-minute intervals over the next 30 to 60 minutes. Method is radioimmunoassay (RIA).

82941

Gastrin, produced by G cells in the antrum of the stomach, stimulates production of gastric acid. Gastrin may be measured to evaluate patients with suspected gastrinoma and Zollinger-Ellison syndrome. Method is radioimmunoassay (RIA).

82943

Glucagon is a hormone secreted by the pancreas. It stimulates the conversion of glycogen stored in the liver to glucose. Glucagon levels may be requested to evaluate suspected diabetes mellitus or glucagonoma. Method is radioimmunoassay (RIA).

82945

Glucose is the end product of carbohydrate metabolism, providing energy for living organisms. It is found in body fluids including joint fluid and CSF. Both elevated and decreased levels of glucose may be indicative of disease processes. Joint fluid specimen is obtained by separately reportable arthrocentesis. CSF specimen is obtained by separately reportable spinal puncture. Method is enzymatic.

82946

Glucagon is a hormone secreted by the pancreas. It stimulates the conversion of glycogen stored in the liver to glucose. Glucagon tolerance test may be requested to evaluate suspected diabetes mellitus or glucagonoma. A fasting glucagon level is obtained. A high carbohydrate meal or an oral dose of glucose is given. Glucagon levels are tested at 30, 60, and

120-minute intervals. Method is radioimmunoassay (RIA).

82947
This test may be requested as a fasting blood sugar (FBS). This quantitative test is used to evaluate disorders of carbohydrate metabolism. The patient has ordinarily fasted for eight hours. Method is enzymatic.

82948
This test is used to monitor disorders of carbohydrate metabolism. Blood specimen is obtained by finger stick. A drop of blood is placed on the reagent strip for a specified amount of time. When the prescribed amount of time has elapsed, the strip is blotted and the reagent strip is compared to a color chart. Method is reagent strip with visual comparison.

82950
This test may also be requested as glucose, postprandial (PP). This test is used to monitor disorders of carbohydrate metabolism. The patient consumes a high carbohydrate meal or an oral glucose solution. Blood glucose levels are checked two hours after the meal or glucose solution. A one-hour postprandial screen may be used to evaluate pregnant women for gestational diabetes mellitus. Method of testing varies.

82951-82952
These tests may be requested as GTT, oral GTT, OGTT, intravenous GTT, or IVGTT. They monitor disorders of carbohydrate metabolism. These tests are normally performed using an oral dose of glucose, but may also be performed using intravenous glucose. A blood specimen is obtained prior to glucose administration and at intervals following glucose administration. Report 82951 for up to three specimens and 82952 for each additional specimen. Testing method varies.

82955-82960
These tests may be requested as G6PD quantitative or G6PD screen. This test is used to identify genetic G6PD deficiency, which causes hemolytic anemia after ingestion of certain drugs and foods and may also cause hemolytic disease of the newborn (HDN). Blood specimen is obtained by venipuncture. Method is methemoglobin reduction (Brewer's test), modified Bishop (ultraviolet), dye reduction, or ascorbic or fluorescent spot tests. Code 82955 is used to report measurement of amount (quantitation) of G6PD in erythrocytes, while 82960 reports screening (qualitative analysis) for the presence of G6PD only.

82962
This test is used to monitor disorders of carbohydrate metabolism. This test reports blood glucose monitoring by an FDA-approved device. While the code states that it is for home use, these devices may also be used in the physician office. Blood is obtained by finger stick. Method is enzymatic, electrochemical, or spectrophotometry by small portable device designed for home glucose testing.

82963
Deficiencies of this enzyme occur in metabolic disorders, particularly Gaucher disease. The enzyme is increased following liver ischemic injury, making it favorable to monitor serum levels for this condition. Blood specimen is obtained by venipuncture. Tissue is obtained by surgical excision or biopsy, reported separately. It can be measured by enzymatic methods using spectrophotometry.

82965
This test may be abbreviated as GLD or GLDH. GLD is an enzyme found primarily in the liver, but also in erythrocytes. GLD may be requested to evaluate liver and biliary disease as well as Reye's syndrome. Blood specimen is obtained by venipuncture. Method is spectrophotometry.

82977
This test may be requested as GGT or glutamyl transpeptidase. GGT is an enzyme. This test may be used to evaluate liver disease in children or as a screening test for alcoholism. Method is radioimmunoassay (RIA).

82978
Glutathione is a red blood cell tripeptide whose synthesis is generated by two enzymes. It is normally present in blood and serves an important role in protecting red blood cells against oxidant stress produced during infections and by certain drugs. A deficiency of glutathione is commonly associated with hemolytic anemia. Literature on methodology is somewhat unclear, but cyanide-ascorbate may be among the approaches.

82979
Glutathione reductase is an enzyme. This test may be performed to evaluate riboflavin deficiency or G6PD deficiency. Method is enzymatic or spectrophotometry.

82985
This test may be requested as serum fructosamine test. It is used to assess the level of blood glucose control in the recent past. It is useful in evaluating patient compliance and the accuracy of the patient's blood glucose self-monitoring. Blood specimen is obtained by venipuncture. Method is colorimetry, nitroblue tetrazolium (NBT).

83001
This test may be requested as FSH or follitropin. FSH is a gonadotropic hormone produced by the pituitary gland. It stimulates growth and maturation of the ovarian follicle in females and promotes spermatogenesis in males. This test may be requested in an infertility work-up. Method is immunoassay.

83002
This test may be requested as LH, lutropin, or interstitial cell-stimulating hormone (ICSH). LH is a gonadotropic hormone secreted by the pituitary gland. LH required for ovulation in females and stimulates testosterone production in males. LH may

be ordered as part of an infertility work-up. Method is immunoassay.

83003

This test may be requested as GH, HGH, or somatotropin. This test may be used to evaluate pituitary gigantism or dwarfism, acromegaly, hypopituitarism, adrenocortical hyperfunction, fetal anencephaly (amniotic fluid analysis), as well as other conditions. Amniotic fluid sample is obtained by amniocentesis, which is reported separately. Method is radioimmunoassay.

83006

The growth stimulation expressed gene is a biomarker being investigated for its appearance and contribution to several medical conditions, including cardiovascular diseases. ST2 is a member of the interleukin-1 (IL-1) receptor family and is secreted by cardiac muscle cells under conditions of mechanical stress. Test specimens may include serum or plasma. Test method is quantitative enzyme immunoassay. The current studies have found that the presence of this gene could help determine death rates in patients with heart failure and has the potential of predicting the chances of encountering some form of negative cardiovascular event.

83009

The urease activity blood test is a noninvasive method of diagnosing a *Helicobacter pylori* infection of the stomach. The patient swallows a pill or drinks a solution containing the chemical urea, labeled with the nonradioactive isotope C-13. The bacteria will produce an enzyme that breaks down the urea into ammonia and carbon dioxide gas, if they are present. The gas contains the tagged carbon and is quickly absorbed into the bloodstream and later expelled in the breath. A blood sample is taken 30 minutes after ingesting the radiolabeled urea. Urease activity produced by the bacteria, when present, will be made manifest in the blood sample by the presence of tagged carbon molecules. Analysis is done by gas isotope ratio mass spectrometry.

83010

This test may be requested as Hp, HPT, hemoglobin-binding protein. Method is turbidimetry or nephelometry. This procedure measures (quantifies) the amount of haptoglobin present in serum. Haptoglobin is a plasma glycoprotein. Haptoglobin prevents loss of free hemoglobin in the blood by binding with it and removing it to the liver. This test may be indicated to evaluate anemia or other indicators of hemolysis, pregnancy induced hypertension, transfusion reactions, as well as other conditions.

83012

This test may be requested as Hp phenotype, HPT phenotype, or hemoglobin-binding protein phenotype. Haptoglobin is a plasma glycoprotein. Method is turbidimetry or nephelometry. Haptoglobin prevents loss of free hemoglobin in the blood by binding with it and removing it to the liver. There are three common phenotypes, Hp 1-1, Hp 2-1, Hp 2-2. Hp 1-1 is a monomer, while Hp 2-1 and Hp 2-2 are polymers with much greater molecular weights. This is important in evaluating nephritic syndrome because Hp 1-1 is excreted resulting in a decreased haptoglobin level, while Hp 2-1 and Hp 2-2 are retained resulting in an increase. Method is turbidimetry or nephelometry.

83013-83014

Helicobacter pylori (*H. pylori*), formerly referred to as *Campylobacter pylori,* is a gram-negative microaerophilic bacteria that causes gastritis and pyloric ulcers. Testing for *H. pylori* used to require a gastric or duodenal biopsy; however, these bacteria can now be identified using a simple breath test. The patient swallows a pill or drinks a solution containing the chemical, urea, labeled with a stable, nonradioactive isotope, C-13. The bacteria produces an enzyme that breaks down the urea into ammonia and carbon dioxide gas if they are present. The gas contains the tagged carbon and is quickly absorbed into the bloodstream and expelled in the breath. Breath samples are taken six, 12, and 20 minutes after swallowing the pill. Urease activity produced by the bacteria is detected in the breath samples collected by the presence of exhaled tagged carbon molecules. Analysis is done in a pathology laboratory using a mass spectrometer. Report 83013 for the breath test analysis and 83014 for the isotope administration and sample collection.

83015

This test may be requested as a toxic metal or poisonous metal screen. Method is atomic absorption spectrometry (AAS), colorimetry, or neutron activation analysis (NAA). This test reports qualitative analysis to detect and identify the presence of heavy metals regardless of the number of analytes.

83018

This test may be requested as a toxic metal or poisonous metal quantitation. Method is atomic absorption spectrometry (AAS), colorimetry, or neutron activation analysis (NAA). This test measures (quantifies) the amount of each single metal present and not specified elsewhere within another code descriptor. Each metal quantified is reported separately.

83020

This test may be requested as Hb electrophoresis. This test uses electrophoresis to test for several hemoglobin variants. It is used to identify the different types of hemoglobin present in the blood and measure (quantify) the amounts of each. The normal types of hemoglobin are Hb A1, Hb A2, and Hb F (fetal). When Hb F exceeds five percent of total hemoglobin after age 6 months, it may be an indicator of thalassemia. Increased amounts of Hb A2 may also indicate thalassemia. Abnormal variants, which can be identified by electrophoresis, include Hb S and Hb C. Hb S is the most common hemoglobin variant and is indicative of sickle cell anemia. Hb C is indicative of hemolytic anemia.

83021

This test may be requested as Hb chromatography. This test uses chromatography to test for several hemoglobin variants. It is used to identify the different types of hemoglobin present in the blood and measure (quantify) the amounts of each. The normal types of hemoglobin are Hb A1, Hb A2, and Hb F (fetal). When Hb F exceeds five percent of total hemoglobin after age 6 months, it may be an indicator of thalassemia. Increased amounts of Hb A2 may also indicate thalassemia. Abnormal variants, which can be identified by electrophoresis, include Hb S and Hb C. Hb S is the most common hemoglobin variant and is indicative of sickle cell anemia. Hb C is indicative of hemolytic anemia.

83026

The copper sulfate method for measuring hemoglobin is performed by placing a drop of blood into each of a series of containers containing copper sulfate solutions of varying specific gravity. If the drop sinks, the blood has greater specific gravity than the copper sulfate solution. The specific gravity of whole blood strongly correlates to the hemoglobin concentration, so the hemoglobin concentration may be accurately estimated. Specimen collection is by venipuncture.

83030

This is also known as Hb F. Hemoglobin F is the normal hemoglobin of the fetus. Most Hb F is replaced by hemoglobin A in the first days after birth. Hb F has an increased capacity to carry oxygen and is present in increased amounts in some pathologic conditions, including sickle cell anemia, aplastic anemia, and leukemia. Small amounts are produced throughout life.

83033

Hemoglobin F (Hb F) is the normal hemoglobin of the term fetus. Most Hb F is replaced by hemoglobin A in the first days after birth. Elevated levels after age 6 months may be indicative of a blood disorder. Hb F has an increased capacity to carry oxygen and the test is also useful in determining whether bleeding disorders may have occurred preterm. Method for blood specimen is electrophoresis. Method for stool specimen may be by alkali denaturation visual screening. Hemoglobin F is alkali resistant. The procedure is used to examine fresh "red" blood taken from a fresh stool sample.

83036-83037

These tests may also be known as HbA1C. A blood specimen is collected. Glycosylated hemoglobin levels reflect the average level of glucose in the blood over a three-month period. Methods may include high-performance liquid chromatography and ion exchange chromatography (83036) or FDA approved home monitoring device (83037).

83045

This test is performed after the onset of symptoms to detect the presence of the derivative methemoglobin in hemoglobin. This derivative occurs when the iron in hemoglobin is changed to different state due to certain compounds introduced into the blood stream (e.g., sulfonamides, chlorates, nitrates, nitrites, aniline). This is a qualitative test to determine the presence of methemoglobin. Method is typically co-oximetry (spectrophotometry).

83050

This test is performed after the onset of symptoms to detect and measure (quantitative) the percentage of total hemoglobin containing the derivative methemoglobin. This derivative occurs when the iron in hemoglobin is changed to a different state due to certain compounds introduced into the blood stream (e.g., sulfonamides, chlorates, nitrates, nitrites, aniline, and phenacetin). Methods may include co-oximetry (spectrophotometry).

83051

This test evaluates hemolytic anemia, especially intravascular hemolysis. Plasma hemoglobin is increased with intravascular hemolysis, ABO incompatible transfusion, traumatic hemolysis, falciparum malaria, burns, and other conditions. Increase may occur in some cases of extravascular hemolysis, delayed transfusion reaction, slight increase in sickle cell anemia, and β-thalassemia. One method of testing is spectrophotometry.

83060

This test is performed after the onset of symptoms to measure (quantitative) the percentage of total hemoglobin containing the derivative sulfhemoglobin. Method is co-oximetry (spectrophotometry). The derivative occurs when certain compounds (e.g., phenacetin or sulfonamides) bind with hemoglobin.

83065

This is also known as the unstable hemoglobin heat denaturation test. Unstable hemoglobin is a chronic fall in the stable baseline of hemoglobin. Method is by heat denaturation. This test changes the physical properties of the globin (the protein constituent of hemoglobin) and the results in the subsequent loss of its biological activity.

83068

This test screens for unstable hemoglobin (a fall in the stable baseline of hemoglobin). The stability of the hemoglobin is checked against isopropanol hemoglobin prep solubility. Falling or unstable hemoglobin levels may indicate viral or bacterial infections or, in severe cases, there may be evidence of hepatic dysfunction and renal insufficiency due to anemia. Evaluation and treatment depends on changes in the hematologic levels from baseline and symptoms, rather than absolute values that are stable.

83069

Method is spectrophotometry. It tests the presence of hemoglobin in the urine without the concurrent presence of red blood cells. Hemoglobin appears in urine only when levels in the blood are higher than the amount that can be reclaimed by the protein haptoglobin. Hemoglobin detected in the urine may indicate hemolytic anemia, or the hemolysis that can result from a transfusion reaction or other process.

83070
This test is performed to detect the presence (qualitative) of hemosiderin. Methods may include slide preparation and stain for microscopic examination. A sample from a morning collection of urine is preferable. Hemosiderin is an iron containing pigment derived from hemoglobin. The presence of hemosiderin may indicate immune hemolytic anemia secondary to drugs (e.g., penicillins, cephalosporins, levodopa, methyldopa, quinidine, and sulfonamides).

83080
The test may be performed to detect the deficiency of hexosaminidase. Specimen collection is by venipuncture; if female, patient should not be pregnant. Methods may include chromatography and automated heat inactivation/fluorometry. Levels of hexosaminidase can identify patients and carriers of Tay-Sachs disease. This genetic disorder results in degeneration of the central nervous system.

83088
This test detects the presence and measures the levels of histamine. Method may be radioimmunoassay for blood or urine. Histamine is stored in mast cells and basophils and is released from cells in the tissues upon injury, causing local inflammation. Histamine also plays a part in controlling gastric secretions, smooth muscle control, cardiac stimulation, stimulation of sensory nerve endings and alertness. Certain medications may result in an excess of histamine in the blood stream, producing sedation, weight gain, and hypotension.

83090
This test may be requested as total homocysteine (tHcy). The presence of homocysteine in urine or blood may be indicative of metabolic disorders. More recently, plasma homocysteine has been identified as a possible predictor for cardiovascular disease with risk increasing progressively with homocysteine concentration. This code reports quantitative analysis of homocysteine levels. Method is high performance liquid chromatography (HPLC), ion exchange chromatography, or spectrophotometry.

83150
This test is performed for the analysis of catecholamines or catecholamine metabolites homovanillic acid (HVA). Specimen collection is random or 24-hour urine test. Method may be high performance liquid chromatography. The test is performed to assist in diagnosing and monitoring pheochromocytoma or neuroblastoma. Catecholamines are produced by a part of the adrenal gland and metabolized to inactive substances excreted in the urine. They are also the main metabolites of neuroblastomas.

83491
This test is used to measure the cortisol metabolites (17-OCHS) for assessing adrenocortical function. Specimen collection is by 24-hour urine sample. A 24-hour test is necessary due to variations in cortisol metabolite excretion. Method is commonly Porter-Silber. Low levels of 17-OCHS indicate hyposecretion of glucocorticoids that can result in Addison's disease (primary adrenal insufficiency). Elevated levels of 17-OCHS indicate hypersecretion of glucocorticoids, especially cortisol and cortisone, which can result in a condition called Cushing's syndrome.

83497
This test may be performed to measure the levels of 5-HIAA for detecting and following the clinical course of patients with carcinoid tumors. Specimen collection is urine, collected over a 24-hour period. Method is high performance liquid chromatography. These tumors contain enteroendocrine cells that secrete stomach gastrin, a secretory hormone released upon nerve impulse. Neurohormones, such as gastrin, are metabolized by the liver and excreted in the urine. Rising levels of 5-HIAA may indicate a tumor is progressing; falling levels of 5-HIAA may indicate that a tumor is responding to antineoplastic therapy. This test measures (quantifies) the level of 5-HIAA present in the specimen.

83498
This test may also be known as 17-OHP. Methodology may involve radioimmunoassay. This test is performed to diagnose and manage certain metabolic diseases. Insufficient amounts of hydroxyprogesterone can block the synthesis of cortisol, resulting in conditions such as adrenal hyperplasia, hirsutism (excessive body and facial hair, especially in women), and infertility.

83500
This test may also be known by the abbreviation Hyp. Specimen collection is by venipuncture for serum or plasma; separately reportable lumbar puncture for CSF; or a 24-hour urine specimen. Methods may include high performance liquid chromatography, ion-exchange chromatography, and colorimetry. This test detects the presence of free hydroxyproline, due to a defect in the enzyme hydroxyproline oxidase. A defect in the enzyme carried by both parent results in hyperhydroxyprolinemia. This condition has no effect on collagen metabolism.

83505
This test is performed to detect the percentage of total hydroxyproline. Methods may include high performance liquid chromatography and colorimetry. This test may be useful in measuring response to therapy in Paget's disease.

83516-83518
Immunoassay uses highly specific antigen to antibody binding to identify specific chemical substances. This

code reports a number of immunoassay techniques for identifying analytes (chemical substances) that are not specifically identified elsewhere, excluding infectious agent antibody or infectious agent antigen. More specific methods reported with these codes include enzyme immunoassay (EIA) and fluoroimmunoassay (FIA). This test identifies (qualitative analysis) the substance or roughly measures (semi-quantitative analysis) the amount of the substance. Code 83516 reports multiple step method, while 83518 reports single step method.

83519
Immunoassay uses highly specific antigen to antibody binding to identify specific chemical substances. This code reports measurement (quantitative analysis) using radioimmunoassay (RIA) technique for identifying analytes (chemical substances) that are not specifically identified elsewhere, excluding infectious agent antibody or infectious agent antigen.

83520
Immunoassay uses highly specific antigen to antibody binding to identify specific chemical substances. This code reports measurement (quantitative analysis) using a technique other than radioimmunoassay (RIA) for identifying analytes (chemical substances) that are not specifically identified elsewhere, excluding infectious agent antibody or infectious agent antigen.

83521
This test may be requested as a free kappa/lambda ratio or an immunoglobulin free light chains test. It is used to help diagnose or monitor plasma cell disorders such as multiple myeloma and amyloidosis. Plasma cells, a type of white blood cell, make up two types of proteins known as light chains (lambda and kappa). These proteins link with other proteins (heavy chains) to form immunoglobulins. Free light chains refer to those that are not part of intact immunoglobulins and are present in the blood. If the amount is higher or lower than normal, it can indicate a plasma cell disorder. Specimen is serum; method is turbidimetry.

83525
This test measures total insulin, which includes both the protein bound and free hormone present in the blood. Method is radioimmunoassay (RIA). This test is used to evaluate hypoglycemia, which may be caused by insulin producing neoplasm or islet cell hyperplasia.

83527
This test measures free insulin. Free insulin may also be referred to as active or unbound insulin. A fasting blood specimen is obtained by venipuncture. Method is radioimmunoassay. In rare instances, the level of total insulin (protein bound and unbound) may be normal or elevated when free insulin is actually low.

[83529]
An Interleukin-6 (IL-6) test may be ordered to monitor inflammatory responses when an individual has signs or symptoms of (or has been diagnosed with) system processes, such as lupus, rheumatoid arthritis, or sepsis. It may also be used to evaluate cardiovascular disease, diabetes, or stroke. Specimen is plasma or serum; method is electrochemiluminescence immunoassay.

83528
Intrinsic factor (IF) is a glycoprotein secreted by the gastric glands and necessary for the absorption of vitamin B12. Method is guinea pig intestinal mucosal homogenate (GPIMH) or radioassay. Indications are that this test is not frequently performed.

83540
This test may be requested as Fe. Iron is an essential constituent of hemoglobin, which is present in foods and absorbed through the small bowel (duodenum and jejunum). Method is colorimetry or atomic absorption spectrophotometry. This test is often used in combination with other tests to evaluate anemia, acute leukemia, lead poisoning, acute hepatitis, and vitamin B6 deficiency. It is also used to evaluate iron poisoning caused by accidental overdose (children) or excessive use of supplements.

83550
This test may be abbreviated as TIBC. Iron is an essential constituent of hemoglobin, which is present in foods and absorbed through the small bowel (duodenum and jejunum). Method is colorimetry or atomic absorption spectrophotometry. TIBC measures the total amount of iron capable of binding to the protein transferrin. This test is often used in combination with other tests to evaluate anemia, various neoplasms, acute hepatitis and other liver disease, hemochromatosis, thalassemia, and renal disease.

83570
This test may be abbreviated as ICD or IDH. CSF is obtained by spinal puncture, which is reported separately. Method is enzymatic or colorimetry. Isocitrate dehydrogenase is an enzyme. Elevated serum or plasma levels may indicate hepatitis, malignant neoplasm metastatic to liver, or other liver disease. Elevated CSF levels may indicate acute bacterial meningitis, vascular lesions of the brain, or malignant neoplasms of the cerebrospinal system.

83582
This test may be referred to as a 17-KGS. Urine specimen collection is performed over a 24-hour period. Method is Norymberski reaction, which is the Zimmerman color reaction after treatment with a strong oxidizing agent (e.g., periodate, bismuthate). This test is used to assess for increased adrenal function as in Cushing's Syndrome, stress, and some cases of adrenogenital syndrome, or decreased adrenal function as with Addison's disease and hypopituitarism. It measures 17-ketosteroids (KS) after cortols, cortolones, pregnanetriol, and 17-OHCS are oxidized to 17-KS. 17-KS are metabolites of the androgenic sex hormones (i.e., testosterone) that are secreted from the adrenal cortex and testes.

83586
This test may be ordered as 17-KS. Urine specimen collection is performed over a 24-hour period. Method is Zimmerman reaction, which is colorimetry after extractions. This test is used to assess for adrenal androgens. The 17-ketosteroids (KS) may be elevated in Cushing's Syndrome, some adrenal and gonadal tumors, pregnancy, and female pseudohermaphrodism. The 17-KS are metabolites of the androgenic sex hormones (i.e., testosterone) secreted from the adrenal cortex and testes. This test does not detect major androgens, testosterone, and dihydrotestosterone.

83593
This test may be ordered as 17-KS fractionation. Urine specimen collection is performed over a 24-hour period. Method is column chromatography or gas-liquid chromatography (GLC). This test is for the quantitation of androsterone, etiocholanolone, and dehydroepiandrosterone (DHEA), the three major metabolites in the urine. It evaluates the presence of adrenal and gonadal abnormalities.

83605
This test is used to assess lactic blood levels to document the presence of tissue hypoxia, determine the degree of hypoxia, and monitor the effect of therapy in blood, plasma, or cerebrospinal fluid (CSF). Specimen collection is CSF from a spinal puncture or arterial or venous blood. Hand clenching and the use of a tourniquet should be avoided to prevent the build-up of potassium and lactic acid. Method is enzymatic or gas chromatography (GS). This test may be used to determine lactic acidosis when unaccountable anion gap metabolic acidosis is detected.

83615
This test may also be ordered as LD or LDH. The test is a measure of LD or LDH, which is found in many body tissues, particularly the heart, liver, red blood cells, and kidneys. Methods used are lactate to pyruvate or pyruvate to lactate. This test may be ordered for a wide variety of disorders, including renal diseases and congestive heart failure.

83625
This test may be ordered as LDH isoenzymes or LD isoenzymes. Three serial blood specimens are collected at 6-8 hour intervals to detect changes in the LD isoenzymes. Shifts in the values of five clinically significant LD fractions monitored over time create diagnostic patterns that correlate with diseases such as myocardial infarction, renal infarction and hepatic congestion. This allows for the differential diagnosis of numerous conditions. Method is by electrophoresis or immunochemical methods, including immunoprecipitation. This test may be ordered for a wide variety of reasons, and results may point to numerous diagnoses.

83630-83631
Lactoferrin in feces is a marker for intestinal inflammation in patients with abdominal pain and/or diarrhea. It aids in discrimination and monitoring progression of inflammatory bowel disease. Lactoferrin is produced by white blood cells in the intestines. A random stool sample is obtained and preserved in enteric transport media. Method is enzyme-linked immunosorbent assay (ELISA). Report 83630 for a qualitative study and 83631 for a quantitative study.

83632
This test may be called maternal serum hPL. Specimen collection is obtained by venipuncture. Method used is radioimmunoassay (RIA) or turbidimetric latex immunoassay. This test may be used to evaluate antepartum placental function and fetal health. It is also used as an indicator of intrauterine growth retardation in twin pregnancy, evaluation of placental function, and may be used to assess gestational age. Other uses are in detecting non-germ cell neoplasms.

83633
This is a diagnostic urine test to identify the presence of lactase in the small intestine. When there are high levels of lactose in the gut, lactose is absorbed and excreted in the urine. It is an indicator of lactose intolerance or intestinal disease. Method is gas chromatography. The absence of lactose implies a decrease in calcium absorption.

83655
This test may be ordered using Pb, the chemical abbreviation for lead. A whole blood test may be used to identify more recent lead exposures; the urine test is used to determine lead body burden, rather than to diagnose lead poisoning. In some instances, serum, hair samples, or bronchoalveolar lavage fluids may be tested. Specimen collection for urine is usually a 24-hour collection. Method used is source dependent, but commonly electrothermal atomic absorption spectrometry (AAS). Bronchoalveolar lavage specimens may be tested by x-ray fluorescence spectrometry.

83661
Specimen collection is by amniocentesis, but amniotic fluid may be collected vaginally after rupture of the amniotic membrane. This test determines fetal pulmonary maturation and may be an indicator for the possibility of development of respiratory distress syndrome (RDS). Method used is thin-layer chromatography (TLC) and a 1D or 2D approach may be specified.

83662
This test may also be ordered as pulmonary surfactant or the "shake test." Specimen collection is by amniocentesis. Method involves diluting amniotic fluid with ethanol and shaking the specimen. This test indicates fetal pulmonary maturation and newborn risk for respiratory distress syndrome. The test may also be useful in managing other conditions in both mother and fetus during late stages of pregnancy.

83663
Specimen collection is by amniocentesis. The amniotic fluid is analyzed by fluorescent polarization (FPOL). A fluorescent phospholipid analogue is added to amniotic fluid and its fluorescence polarization is measured using a fluorescence polarimeter. The presence of increased amounts of surfactant indicating increased lung maturity result in lower polarization levels. Therefore, polarization values decrease during gestation in conjunction with maturation of the pulmonary surfactant system. This test indicates fetal pulmonary maturation and newborn risk for respiratory distress syndrome.

83664
Specimen collection is by amniocentesis. Lamellar body density is calculated by measuring the number of surfactant containing particles per microliter of amniotic fluid. Method is automated cell count. This test indicates fetal pulmonary maturation and newborn risk for respiratory distress syndrome.

83670
This test may also be ordered as LAP or leucyl aminopeptidase. Methods are commonly colorimetry, fluorometry, and enzyme assay. The test is commonly used to measure biliary excretory function for differential diagnoses of liver and pancreatic disorders.

83690
This test may also be called triacylglycerol acylhydrolase. Method is often by turbidimetric, a specialized processor. The test is used generally to indicate pancreatic, hepatic duct, and renal disorders.

83695
This test may also be requested as Lp (a). Lipoprotein (a) is a low-density lipoprotein associated with clot formation, hardening and narrowing of the arteries. The patient is instructed to fast for 12 hours prior to this test. A blood specimen is obtained through venipuncture. Lipoprotein (a) is measured using an enzyme-linked immunosorbent assay (ELISA).

83698
This test is also ordered as a PLAC. The test measures an enzyme called lipoprotein-associated phospholipase A2. Persons at risk for heart disease or stroke may have higher levels of this enzyme. The specimen is blood serum or plasma. The PLAC test is typically a microplate-based enzyme-linked sandwich immunosorbent assay. The test is a component of clinical risk assessment for coronary artery disease and ischemic stroke associated with atherosclerosis.

83700
Lipoproteins are comprised of subclasses of lipoprotein particles. These subclasses are of different sizes, lipid and apolipoprotein composition, and function. Elevated levels of lipoproteins serve as a marker for premature coronary heart disease. The patient is fasting. Venipuncture is performed to obtain a blood sample. The test is performed using electrophoretic methods on plasma using a homogeneous gel to separate particles based on size.

83701
This test may be referred to as Type III fractionation. Type III hyperlipoproteinemia is an inherited disorder whereby both the cholesterol and triglycerides show high plasma concentrations. This particular test is usually performed following previous tests to further isolate abnormal beta-lipoproteins. The patient is told to fast. Blood is drawn by venipuncture. The test may be performed by various methods including ultracentrifugation or electrophoresis. Ultracentrifugation is more common and is considered the traditional standard for accuracy in high-density lipoproteins (HDL) subclass quantitation.

83704
This test is used to measure the subclasses of lipoprotein contained in plasma by measurement of the plasma nuclear magnetic resonance (NMR) spectrum followed by computerized reversal of the optical distortion creating a clearer image (deconvolution) of the spectral data and calculation of the subclass concentrations. Each lipoprotein particle in plasma "broadcasts" a distinctive lipid NMR signal that is graphed. The deconvolution and calculation steps are computed by using analysis software. The test is performed on plasma, acquired by venipuncture. The patient is requested to fast prior to this test.

83718
This test may be requested as HDL, HDLC, or HDL cholesterol. Lipoproteins are compounds composed of lipids bound to proteins, which are transported through the blood. High-density lipoprotein (HDL) is frequently referred to as "good cholesterol," or "friendly lipid," as it is responsible for decreasing plaque deposits in blood vessels. High levels of HDL decrease the risk of premature coronary artery disease. This code reports direct measurement only, normally performed using an enzymatic or precipitation method.

83719
This test measures VLDL, the lipoprotein that carries triglycerides in the blood. The test is useful to determine a patient's risk of arteriosclerotic occlusive disease, as well as other cholesterol-related disorders. The method used is electrophoresis and may first involve ultracentrifugation.

83721
This test may also be referred to as LDL-C. It measures the amount of low-density lipoprotein (LDL), also known as "bad cholesterol." The test is useful to determine the patient's risk of coronary heart disease (CHD), among other disorders. Method may be by precipitation procedure with results derived by the Friedewald formula.

83722
This test may be ordered as sd-LDL. It measures the heavier, small dense LDL, the lipoprotein that carries triglycerides in the blood. This test is useful in determining a patient's risk for arteriosclerotic

occlusive disease, as well as other cholesterol-related disorders. Specimen is serum. The method used is automated colorimetry.

83727

This test may also be referred to as the LH-RH test. Natural bursts of LH-RH govern the release of luteinizing hormone and follicular stimulating hormone, both essential to ovulation. The test is useful in diagnosing problems in LH-RH transport or production, as well as associated fertility problems. Methodology may entail administration of a stimulation agent with a baseline blood sample drawn before the injection and several after. Samples may be tested by immunoassay.

83735

Magnesium, abbreviated Mg, is an inorganic cation essential for many physiochemical processes. It is an enzyme activator found in body fluids and cells. Magnesium depletion is clinically associated with weakness and neuromuscular disorders including cardiac arrhythmias and seizures. IV therapy, malabsorption, dialysis, pregnancy, toxicity and conditions such as hyperparathyroidism and hyperaldosteronism deplete magnesium. Specimen types and methods of testing vary. Colorimetry or spectrophotometry are methods frequently used.

83775

This test may also be known as MDH, or MD. This enzyme is widely distributed in the system's cellular makeup and levels follow lactate dehydrogenase activity. The test is probably considered of general usefulness and indications are that it is not frequently run. Specimen collection is by venipuncture for blood; surgical excision or biopsy for tissue. Methodology may be by electrophoresis.

83785

This test is usually performed to determine manganese toxicity, exposure, or poisoning. Specimen collection may be venipuncture, 24-hour urine collection, or random or spot urine samples. Hair is sometimes analyzed as is fluid from bronchoalveolar lavage. Methods are source dependent and include neutron activation and atomic absorption spectrophotometry (AAS) with Zeeman background correction for blood and urine. Hair may be processed with acetone and nitric acid before testing with AAS as well. Fluids are likely to be x-ray fluorescence spectrum.

83789

This test identifies the presence of (qualitative), and measures the amount of (quantifies), specific analytes in protein. Specimen varies. Method is mass spectrometry (MS). The test is used for identifying the chemical makeup and structure of a substance. Tandem MS (MS/MS) is one type of MS using sequential analysis to provide structural information by establishing relationships between substances. Others include quadrupole/time-of-flight (Q/TOF) and matrix-assisted laser desorption/ionization (MALDI). This test assists in identifying the chemical makeup and structure of a substance, analyzing viruses, sequencing and analyzing peptides and proteins, and providing information on such life-threatening diseases as AIDS and various types of skin cancers as well as quantifies (measures) the amount of analyte in the specimen.

83825

This test may also be ordered as Hg. The specimen is whole blood, a 24 hour urine sample or hair cut close to the scalp. Methods are electrothermal atomic absorption, gold electrode deposition, or gas chromatography. Mercury toxicity may cause neurological defects, pneumonitis, and other problems depending on mode of entry into the body (e.g., vapor, ingestion) and which form it enters as: elemental, inorganic, and organic.

83835

The test is performed to determine metanephrine or normetanephrine concentrations. The specimen is urine collected over a 24-hour period. Method is high performance liquid chromatography (HPLC). Metanephrine or normetanephrine concentrations may be associated with neuroendocrine tumors or even associated with intense physical activity, life threatening illness and drug interferences.

83857

This test measures methemalbumin. It is representative of intravascular hemolysis. The specimen is serum or amniotic fluid. Methods may include Schumm test, ether, ammonium sulfide, EP for serum, and spectrophotometry for serum or plasma.

83861

An osmolarity test is performed for dry eye disease (DED), a condition in which the eye does not produce sufficient tears to keep the eye surface lubricated. Using a specialized collection and analysis device, microfluidic analysis is performed. Using this method, less than 50 nanoliters (nL) of tear fluid is needed and a result can be obtained in less than 30 seconds.

83864

This test may also be known as glycosaminoglycans, Keratosulfate, AMPS, and GAGS. Methods may include turbidimetry, paper spot test, and colorimetry. It may be used to detect the presence of mucopolysaccharides in solution. Mucopolysaccharides are important in the diagnosis of certain genetic metabolic disorders, such as Scheie's syndrome (also called a-L-iduronidase deficiency, Scheie type, and mucopolysaccharidosis IS).

83872

This test may also be referred to as a mucin coagulation test or joint fluid test, in addition to Rope's test. This test analyzes the hyaluronic acid in synovial fluid. Specimen collection is by arthrocentesis. Method involves adding a few drops of synovial fluid into a weak solution of acetic acid. The mixture is evaluated for clumping and change of fluid opacity. Test results may be a general guide to numerous rheumatological disorders.

83873
This test may be ordered as an MBP assay. The specimen is spinal fluid. In rare instances, serum may be tested for myelin basic protein from patients with recent head injuries. Ordinarily, the CSF sample is taken when a patient is experiencing certain symptoms characteristic of disease activity, typically multiple sclerosis. Test methods include radial immunodiffusion (RIA), electroimmunodiffusion, immunofluorometry, immunoprecipitation, or immunonephelometry. This test is typically used as an evaluation of disease activity, rather than for diagnostic purposes.

83874
Myoglobin is a principle protein of skeletal and cardiac muscle tissue. Elevated serum levels may be found in severe muscle conditions, such as polymyositis and crushing traumas to muscle and bone. This test may be used in association with other disorders as well, such as acute myocardial infarct and infections. Methods include radioimmunoassay (RIA), fluorometric immunoassay, and immunoturbidimetry for blood. Urine specimens may be processed by antigen-antibody reaction nephelometry.

83876
Myeloperoxidase (MPO) is a quantitative cardiac marker for ischemic heart disease. Plasma MPO levels help to identify patients who are at risk for myocardial infarction, particularly when used in addition to existing markers for cardiovascular disease. Code 83876 reports a myeloperoxidase enzyme immunoassay for use in identifying troponin-negative patients without EKG changes presenting with chest pain who are at higher risk, and may also be used in myeloproliferative disorders.

83880
Plasma levels of natriuretic peptides, particularly B-type, help predict left ventricular hypertrophy and systolic dysfunction, determine CHF in asymptomatic patients, and provide risk assessment after ischemic symptoms in coronary syndromes. The specimen is plasma. Radioimmunoassay (RIA) may be used.

83883
Nephelometry is a method to measure the concentration of a suspension using an instrument (nephelometer) for assessing turbidity of a solution. For example, this code can be used to measure the concentration of albumin in body fluid. Albumins make up about 60 percent of plasma proteins, and exert considerable pressure in maintaining water balance between blood and tissues. Report this nephelometry test when the analyte is not specifically cited elsewhere in this section.

83884
Neurofilament light chain (NfL) is a biomarker for neurodegenerative conditions such as Alzheimer's disease and multiple sclerosis. NfL testing by quantitative immunoassay is used for a patient with cognitive decline to determine if it is likely that the decline is due to neurodegeneration; an elevation in NfL biomarkers indicates increased likelihood. This test can also be used to monitor disease progression and treatment response over time. The specimen is plasma.

83885
This test may also be known as Nickel U or as Ni. Specimen types vary. Methods may include atomic absorption spectrophotometry and x-ray fluorescence spectrometry. Measurement of nickel is useful to determine chronic environmental exposure of manufactured products containing nickel.

83915
This test is also known as 5'-N'TASE, and 5'-NT. The specimen is serum or synovial fluid. Methods vary greatly, and may include molybdate color reaction, high performance liquid chromatography, and colorimetry. The test may be ordered to assist in identifying the cause of increased 5'-nucleotidase, a liver-related enzyme.

83916
The specimen is cerebrospinal fluid (CFS) and serum. Methods may include thin-gel agarose high-resolution electrophoresis and isoelectric focusing. This test may be used to identify diagnoses of inflammatory and autoimmune diseases of the CNS and other degenerative states.

83918
This test also may involve analyzing patterns of excretion for specific diagnosis. Urine is the preferred specimen due to concentration of the metabolites excreted by the kidney. Urine collection is typically over a 24-hour period. Methods may include gas chromatography, followed by mass spectroscopy. There are many sources for organic acids, though most come from the metabolism of amino acids, fatty acids, carbohydrates, and cholesterol, and hormones such as steroids. Abnormal patterns of organic acids in excretion may be due to genetic metabolic disorders, vitamin deficiencies, and certain drugs.

83919
This test may involve analyzing patterns of excretion for specific diagnosis. Urine is the preferred specimen due to concentration of the metabolites excreted by the kidney, but blood testing may also be performed. There are many sources for organic acids, though most come from the metabolism of amino acids, fatty acids, carbohydrates, and cholesterol, and hormones such as steroids. Abnormal patterns of organic acids in excretion may be due to genetic metabolic disorders, vitamin deficiencies, certain drugs, and identification of inborn errors of metabolism. Qualitative screening tests are typically performed by thin layer chromatography, but may involve other chemical or chromatographic techniques.

83921
This test is a quantitative test for organic acids and the preferred specimen is urine due to concentration of metabolites excreted by the kidney. Methods may include gas chromatography, followed by mass spectroscopy. The test may be performed on acutely ill

neonates, suspected cases of Reye's syndrome, or failure-to-thrive syndrome, and patients with metabolic acidosis, (associated with severe infections).

83930
This test is also known as osmolal gap and serum osmolality. The specimen is serum or plasma. Methodology may involve freezing point depression or vapor pressure techniques. The test measures the amount of molecules or ions (particles) in a solution of water or the presence of osmotically active molecules in serum. The test may be used to determine liver disease and disorders, electrolyte and water balance.

83935
This test may also be known as osmolal gap. The specimen is a random urine sample. Method may be by freezing point depression. The test may be used to determine renal disease and disorders, electrolyte and water balance. The results may be high or low urine osmolality, depending on the differential diagnosis.

83937
Osteocalcin is a test developed to measure bone formation and for monitoring therapy of preexisting bone conditions. An imbalance between the two (formation and reabsorption) may account for many of the metabolic bone diseases, such as Paget's disease and osteomalacia. The specimen is serum or plasma. Methods may include enzyme-linked immunosorbent assay (ELISA).

83945
This test is also known as oxalic acid. Urine collection is over a 24-hour period, or a first morning. The specimen may be taken as an estimate of daily output. Methods of testing may include colorimetry and high performance liquid chromatography. The test may be performed to determine patients at risk of forming oxalate calculi (stones), which are common in the urinary tract.

83950-83951
Proteins that are involved in tumor growth (oncoproteins) are coded for by a gene with a DNA sequence that causes cancer (oncogene). The human epidermal growth factor receptor 2 gene, a proto-oncogene, encodes for the HER-2/neu protein, a cell surface growth factor receptor that is expressed on the cytoplasmic membrane of some epithelial cells and regulates normal cell growth and division. Gene amplification causes overexpression of the HER-2/neu oncoprotein, which correlates to higher cell growth rates and oncogenic transformation. Immunohistochemical methods are often used to measure the overexpression of HER-2/neu protein. Code 83950 reports the evaluation of the staining pattern for intensity and the degree to which the cytoplasmic membrane is encircled with stain, indicating overexpression of the protein. Des-gamma-carboxy-prothrombin (DCP) is an oncoprotein whose levels are used to detect liver cancer at an early stage and to monitor its progression. Increased levels may also indicate the development of portal vein invasion (PVI), making it a valuable tool in the prediction of disease progression and worsening prognosis. When used in combination with AFP-L3%, DCP can help identify patients at risk of developing hepatocellular cancer. The test is by enzyme immunoassay; the sample is serum. Report DCP testing with 83951.

83970
This test may also be ordered as a PTH or parathyrin. The specimen is post-fasting serum requiring special handling. Methods may include immunochemiluminometric assay (ICMA), radioimmunoassay (RIA), and immunoradiometric assay (IRMA). Testing determines the PTH levels and may be used to differentiate between primary or secondary causes of parathyroid disorders.

83986
This test may also be called fecal pH, pleural fluid pH, or thoracentesis pH. The specimen for pleural fluid is by thoracentesis; for stool, fresh random sample; for urine, random sample; or ascitic fluid by paracentesis, etc. Methods may include a pH meter for pleural fluid; aqueous stool suspension with pH paper for stool; dipstick double indicator principal or pH meter for urine. The test may be ordered to differentiate among numerous diagnoses, depending on the sample taken and the method used.

83987
Exhaled breath condensate pH is used to ascertain the underlying cause of chronic cough and airway irritation (e.g., acid reflux disease). The patient uses a specialized breath collection/condensation device to collect breath condensate. The breath condensate is then degassed and analyzed using a special pH electrode in order to obtain accurate results.

83993
This test is used to diagnose and monitor inflammatory bowel disease (IBD). Calprotectin is a calcium-binding protein produced primarily by neutrophils. Elevated fecal calprotectin levels may be indicative of IBD or gastrointestinal (GI) tract infections, and often signal an upcoming clinical relapse in patients with inactive IBD. The test employs a quantitative enzyme immunoassay methodology to detect calprotectin in a fecal sample.

84030
This test is used to screen for phenylketonuria (PKU), a condition resulting in the inability of the body to break down the amino acid phenylalanine. Untreated PKU may lead to increased phenylalanine levels resulting in intellectual disabilities. A blood sample is placed on special paper and is usually collected within 48 to 72 hours after birth. This test may be ordered as a Guthrie, Phenylketonuria, PKU test, or phenylalanine screen. Additional testing is needed to confirm the diagnosis of PKU if this screening test is positive.

84035
This test detects the presence of phenylketone, a metabolite created in the breakdown of the amino acid

phenylamine. Methods may include gas chromatography. The amino acid is essential to developing infants and normal protein metabolism throughout life. This is a qualitative screening test for the presence of phenylketones.

84060
This is also known as phosphoric monoester phosphohydrolase and ACP. This test is often performed on individuals with diagnoses such as skeletal metastasis, myelocytic leukemia, and is useful in staging prostatic cancer rather than initial diagnosis of prostate cancer. The specimen is post-fasting serum. Methods may include radioimmunoassay (RIA), enzyme immunoassay (EIA), and spectrophotometry.

84066
This test may also be known as PAP and prostatic phosphatase. The specimen is post-fasting serum. Methods may include radioimmunoassay (RIA), enzyme monophosphate, alpha naphthylphosphate, and titrate inhibition. This test may be used to stage prostate cancer, to diagnose metastatic prostate adenocarcinoma and to monitor treatment of those diagnosed with prostatic carcinoma.

84075
This test may be requested as ALP. ALP is an enzyme. It is an indicator of liver cell damage. Amniotic fluid ALP may be screened for cystic fibrosis in mothers who have had a child affected with the disease. Methods include a number of kinetic spectrophotometry and fluorescent techniques, as well as 4-nitrylphenophosphate (4-NPP) and diethanolamine (DEA).

84078
This test may be performed to identify general liver and bone diseases. Methodology involves heat inhibition at 56 degrees Celsius.

84080
This test may also be known as ALP isoenzymes. This test may be ordered for patients with increased serum total alkaline phosphatase, or to compare total alkaline phosphatase to placental, liver, bone, and Regan isoenzymes. Methods may include electrophoresis or enzymatic.

84081
These tests together are frequently ordered as LS/PG. Testing is performed in conjunction with an L/S (lecithin/sphingomyelin) ratio for assessment of fetal maturity based on pulmonary surfactant. This test may be performed to determine fetal lung maturity and to establish the possibility of the development of respiratory distress syndrome in the fetus. The specimen is by amniocentesis, a separately reportable procedure Methods may include thin-layer chromatography (TLC) and immunologic and enzymatic assays.

84085
This test may also be known as 6-PGD. The specimen is whole blood. Methodology may involve spectrophotometry. The test may be performed to detect the presence and measure the levels of phosphogluconate, 6-, dehydrogenase, RBC, an enzyme present in the metabolic breakdown of sugars.

84087
This is also known as glucose-6-phosphate isomerase. The specimen is whole blood. Methods may include spectrophotometry and colorimetric. The test may be performed to detect the presence and measure the levels in serum of phosphohexose isomerase, an enzyme present in the breakdown of fructose.

84100
This test may be ordered as PO4. Methods may include phosphomolybdate-colorimetric and modified molybdate-enzymatic, and colorimetric. The testing may be performed to measure high or low levels of phosphorus to determine a variety of differential diagnoses. Potassium supplements increase phosphate levels. Also, phosphate levels may increase during the last trimester of pregnancy.

84105
This test is performed to identify the calcium/ phosphorus balance. High values may be associated with primary hyperparathyroidism, vitamin D deficiency, and renal tubular acidosis; low values may be due to hypoparathyroidism, pseudohypoparathyroidism, and vitamin D toxicity. The test may also be used for nephrolithiasis assessment.

84106
This test may also be known as Watson-Schwartz, PCG and Hoesch tests. The specimen is random urine which requires special handling. Methods are the Watson-Schwartz and Hoesch tests, and Ehrlich's reagent. The Hoesch test does not respond to urobilirubin. The test may be used to screen for acute intermittent porphyria and for acute attacks of abdominal and extremity pain.

84110
This test may also be known as Porphobilinogen (PBG), urine. The specimen is a 24-hour or a random urine sample, requiring special handling. Urine colored amber-red or burgundy, which darkens in light, indicates the presence of abnormally high levels. This test may be used to detect levels of porphobilinogen associated in the diagnosis of genetic or drug-induced abnormal porphyrin metabolism. Methods may involve gas chromatography, colorimetry, and spectrophotometry. This test measures (quantifies) porphobilinogen present in the specimen.

84112
This is a noninvasive test to evaluate possible rupture of membranes (ROM) in a pregnant patient. During pregnancy, large quantities of placental alpha microglobulin-1 (PAMG-1) are secreted into the amniotic fluid. If the fetal membranes are intact, a low background level of PAMG-1 is measured in cervicovaginal secretions. High levels may be indicative of ROM. A swab is inserted two to three

inches into the vagina and is withdrawn after one minute. The swab tip is placed into a vial and rinsed with solvent. A test strip is then placed into the vial with the solvent. Depending on the size of the amniotic fluid leak, results may be visible within five to 10 minutes.

84119
This test may be used to detect the presence (qualitative) of porphyria cutanea tarda (PCT). The patient typically collects a 24-hour urine Methods may include high performance liquid chromatography. Urine porphyrins are useful for evaluating photosensitivity due to abnormal metabolism of the protein used in the synthesis of the iron (heme) in hemoglobin.

84120
This test is performed for the quantitative evaluation (measurement) of porphyrias, which may include enzyme deficiencies that are necessary for heme synthesis and chemical porphyrias. Specimen is urine collected by the patient over a 24-hour period. Methods may include chromatography, fluorometry, and high performance liquid chromatography (HPLC).

84126
This test measures the levels of coproporphyrin (a nitrogen-containing substance excreted in the feces from the breakdown of bilirubin from hemoglobin decomposition) and protoporphyrin (a form of porphyrin that combines with iron and protein to form organic molecules such as hemoglobin). The specimen is feces, which may be a random or timed collection. Method is high performance liquid chromatography and fluorometry.

84132
This test may be requested as K or K+. Potassium is the major electrolyte found in intracellular fluids. Potassium influences skeletal and cardiac muscle activity. Very small fluctuations outside the normal range may cause significant health risk, including muscle weakness and cardiac arrhythmias. Blood specimen is serum, plasma, or whole blood. Methods include atomic absorption spectrometry (AAS), ion-selective electrode (ISE), and flame emission spectroscopy (FES).

84133
This test may be ordered as urine K+. The specimen is collected by the patient over a 24-hour period or is random urine sample. Methods may include flame emission photometry and ion-selective electrode (ISE). The test may be ordered to determine elevated levels for the differential diagnoses of chronic renal failure, renal tubular acidosis, and for diuretic therapy.

84134
The test may also be known as PAB, thyroxine-binding prealbumin (TBPA), thyretin, and transthyretin. The specimen may be serum, a random or a 24-hour urine specimen, or spinal fluid. A lumbar puncture, which is reported separately, is performed to obtain cerebrospinal fluid (CSF). Methods may include electrophoresis and nephelometry (serum). The test may be used as an indicator of nutrition, liver injury, chronic kidney disease, and in the diagnosis of Hodgkin's disease.

84135
This test measures pregnanediol to evaluate progesterone production by the ovaries and placenta. Methods may involve gas-liquid chromatography and radioimmunoassay. Progesterone initiates the phase in ovulation that prepares the endometrium for implantation of a fertilized ovum. The serum and urine level of the progesterone metabolite pregnanediol increases rapidly during this phase, making it a useful measure in documenting and charting ovulation.

84138
This test is also known as 17-Hydroxyprogesterone or 17-OH-Progesterone. Methods may include extraction/gas-liquid chromatography (GLC) and spectrophotometry. This test may be performed to determine differential diagnoses of adrenogenital syndrome, tumors of ovary and adrenal cortices, Stein-Leventhal syndrome, and congenital adrenal hyperplasia, among others.

84140
This test is used for detecting and measuring the levels of pregnenolone, a steroid involved in the synthesis of numerous hormones. The specimen is blood (to include cord blood) or a 24 hour timed urine collection. Method is typically radioimmunoassay.

84143
Serum or urine from a female patient may be examined using radioimmunoassay in this test for detecting and measuring the levels of 17-hydroxypregnenolone, a hormonal metabolite.

84144
This test is performed to determine corpus luteum function, confirm ovulation, and to diagnose incompetent luteal phase and insufficient progesterone production, which may be the cause of habitual abortions. The specimen is serum. Methods may include radioimmunoassay (RIA) and direct time-resolved fluorescence immunoassay.

84145
Procalcitonin (PCT) is produced in the thyroid cells of healthy individuals as a precursor for the hormone calcitonin and is not normally found in human blood. However, bacterial infections may cause many of the body's organs to produce PCT, resulting in a rapid elevation of PCT blood levels. This increase is not caused by viral infections. PCT blood levels reflect the severity of bacterial infection, making it a useful biomarker in the diagnosis of bacterial infection and sepsis. Specimen is serum or plasma; test method is by various assays.

84146
Prolactin is a hormone secreted by the anterior pituitary gland. This test may be performed for the differential diagnoses of prolactinemia, galactorrhea

(lactation disorder), pituitary adenomas, pituitary prolactinoma, and other pituitary tumors. The specimen is post-fasting serum. Methods may include immunoassay and radioimmunoassay (RIA).

84150

Method is enzyme immunoassay. Prostaglandin (PG) is a potent unsaturated fatty acid that can act against organs in exceedingly low concentrations, and in their pharmaceutical form may be used for terminating pregnancy or treating asthma. This test may also be known as PG.

84152-84154

The specimen is serum. Methods may include radioimmunoassay (RIA) and monoclonal two-site immunoradiometric assay. These tests may be performed to determine the presence of cancer of the prostate, benign prostatic hypertrophy (BPH), prostatitis, post prostatectomy to detect residual cancer, and to monitor therapy. There are several forms of PSA present in serum. PSA may be complexed with the protease inhibitor alpha-1 antichymotrypsin (PSA-ACT). Complexed PSA is the most measurable form. PSA is also found in a free form. Free PSA is not complexed to a protease inhibitor. Higher levels of free PSA are more often associated with benign conditions of the prostate than with prostate cancer. Total PSA measures both complexed and free levels to provide a total amount present in the serum. A percentage of each form is sometimes calculated to distinguish benign from malignant conditions. Code 84152 reports complexed PSA; 84153 is for total serum PSA; 84154 is for free (not complexed) PSA.

84155-84157

A total protein test may be performed to assess nutritional status. Serum, plasma, or whole blood is tested for protein in 84155. Synovial, cerebrospinal, or other fluid is obtained in 84157. A urine specimen is required for 84156. For amniotic fluid specimen (84157), a separately reportable amniocentesis is performed. Aspiration of other body fluids (CSF, bronchial fluid, exudates) may also require separately reportable procedures. The method is biuret for blood (serum) and amniotic fluid. The method is turbidimetry or nephelometry for urine and CSF. For other body fluids, the method is turbidimetry or biuret.

84160

A total protein test may be performed to assess nutritional status. This code reports any source of specimen. Collection/aspiration of other body fluids (CSF, amniotic fluid, exudates) may require separately reportable procedures. This code reports protein tested for by refractometry. The method determines the velocity of light through a refractive material (plasma).

84163

Pregnancy associated plasma protein-A (PAPP-A, PAPPA) is a large zinc binding protein that acts as an enzyme. The test is used as a marker for Down's syndrome in the fetus. It can also be used as a marker for acute coronary syndromes such as angina and acute myocardial infarction. Blood specimen is obtained by venipuncture. Testing for Down's syndrome requires a maternal blood sample. Purified human PAPP-A is used as the immunogen (antigen). Methods include enzyme linked immunosorbent assay (ELISA) and Western blot.

84165-84166

Serum protein electrophoretic fractionation and quantitation is performed primarily to evaluate for multiple myeloma or to test for hypogammaglobulinemia. The specimen is serum. Methods may be cellulose acetate and agarose electrophoresis. The value of this testing lies in the proportion of these proteins and the patterns they create on the graph, giving diagnostic clues for some diseases. Report 84165 when serum is tested and 84166 when another fluid such as urine or cerebral spinal fluid is tested.

84181-84182

Western blot is an immunoassay technique that detects and confirms certain antibody proteins in blood or other body fluid. Combining an electrophoresis process with a process that blots or transfers the separated proteins onto a membrane, the western blot is frequently utilized as a follow-up confirmatory test to assist in diagnosing a specific disease. Examples of confirmatory testing include that for HIV and Lyme disease. Report 84182 for each immunological probe that is utilized for band identification. These codes include interpretation and report.

84202-84203

This test is performed to diagnose various anemias and lead toxicity. Code 84203 is a qualitative test used as a screen to determine if protoporphyrin is present in the specimen. Code 84202 measures (quantifies) the level of protoporphyrin present. The specimen is whole blood. Methods may include hematofluorometry methods and high performance liquid chromatography.

84206

This test may be performed for the differential diagnoses of insulinoma, renal failure, factitious hypoglycemia, and diabetes mellitus. The specimen is post-fasting serum, requiring special handling. Method is radioimmunoassay.

84207

This test may also be known as PLP. Vitamin B6 is also known as pyridoxine and pyridoxal 5-phosphate. The specimen is plasma, requiring special handling. Methods may include enzyme assay, high performance liquid chromatography (HPLC) with fluorometric detection, and immunoradiometric assay. This test may be performed to identify vitamin B6 deficiency (i.e., nutritional deficiencies as a result of other diseases including chronic alcoholism).

84210
This test is also known as pyruvic acid test. The specimen is blood. Methods are usually enzymatic and colorimetry. This test measures the level of pyruvate in whole blood. The abnormal breakdown of red blood cells and subsequent release of hemoglobin characterize a congenital deficiency of pyruvate.

84220
The specimen is washed red blood cells. Method is spectrophotometric kinetic assay. This test may be performed to identify pyruvate kinase deficiency and hemolytic anemia in newborns.

84228
Quinine is used in the treatment of malaria, atrial fibrillation, and other disorders of muscular tissues. Urine is collected by a patient over a 24-hour period. Method is thin-layer chromatography.

84233
This test may be ordered to assist in identifying a breast cancer patient's ability to respond to chemotherapy and endocrine therapy. The specimen is surgical tissue. The surgical procedure is separately billable. Methods may include biochemical measurement in cytosol fractions of tumor homogenate, dextranestradiol conjugate, immunoperoxidase using tissue sections, enzyme immunoassay (EIA), and in situ hybridization.

84234
This test assists in identifying a patient's ability to respond to treatment in breast and other cancers and may be ordered as a PgR assay. The specimen is surgical tissue. Methods may include sucrose density gradient, steroid binding assay, and enzyme immunoassay.

84235
The test may be used to predict or monitor patient response to hormonal therapy. The specimen is whole blood or plasma; separately reportable biopsy or surgical excision for tumor tissue. Methods are radioimmunoassay (most commonly used technique), gas-liquid and liquid chromatography or electrophoresis.

84238
This test may be used to predict or monitor patient response to therapy, including AChR. Methods include radioimmunoassay (most commonly used technique), gas-liquid and liquid chromatography, or electrophoresis. The test is performed to determine the concentration of the target substance.

84244
This test may be ordered as plasma renin activity, or PRA. The specimen is plasma. Certain medications such as beta-blockers, may affect testing outcome. Methodology may include radioimmunoassay.

84252
This test may be used primarily to determine nutritional deficiency of this vitamin. The specimen is plasma which requires special handling or a 24-hour urine specimen. Methods may include high performance liquid chromatography (HPLC) or fluorometry.

84255
This test may also be known by the abbreviation Se. The specimen is serum or urine collected over a 24-hour period. Methods may include fluorometry and atomic absorption. The blood and the urine test may be performed simultaneously. This test may be ordered to monitor nutritional therapy and for possible toxic exposure.

84260
This test may also be called 5-HT or 5-Hydroxytryptamine. The specimen is whole blood or serum or spinal fluid. A separately reportable lumbar puncture is performed to collect cerebrospinal fluid (CSF). Methods may include fluorometry, radioimmunoassay (RIA), and gas or liquid chromatography spinal puncture to obtain specimen is reported separately, see 62270. This test may be performed to diagnose carcinoid syndrome and severe depression.

84270
The test may be used to predict or monitor patient response to hormonal therapy and to assist in certain diagnoses, including hypothyroidism and hyperthyroidism. This test may also be ordered as SHBG. The specimen is serum which requires special handling or amniotic fluid. Methods include CMA or radioimmunoassay.

84275
This test may also be known by Lipid Associated Sialic Acid or LASA. The specimen is serum. The term "sialic acids" comprises a group of natural neuraminic acid derivatives. The activity of the enzyme, neuraminidase, is also referred to as sialidase. Deficiency of the enzyme may result in the clinical disease sialidosis, a syndrome that may involve involuntary twitching of the muscular group affected and cherry-red spots on the skin. Methods include enzyme assay and spectrometry.

84285
Silica is a naturally occurring and common mineral found in sands, clays, and quartz deposits. Exposure is commonly by inhalation of dusts during rock mining and certain manufacturing. Deposition on the eyes and mucosal surfaces may also be a pathway of exposure. Most commonly, however, phagocytic cells may distribute the silica along lymph channels once the particles are inhaled and collect in lung alveoli. Long-term exposure is linked to numerous illnesses, including silicosis. Sputum induction is performed and silica is detected using light microscopy, electron microscopy, or polarized light.

84295-84302
Sodium is an electrolyte found in extracellular fluid. Blood specimen for serum, plasma, or whole blood sodium (Na) in 84295 is obtained by venipuncture. Methods include atomic absorption spectrometry

(AAS), flame emission photometry, and ion-selective electrode (ISE). The specimen for urine Na in 84300 is collected over a 24-hour period or by random urine sample. Methods may include flame emission photometry and ISE. This test is used to identify increased (hypernatremia) and decreased (hyponatremia) levels of sodium due to various conditions or disease states. Report 84302 for a sodium level test done on another source of specimen other than blood serum or urine.

84305
Somatomedin is a protein mainly produced in the liver. It is a peptide dependent on growth hormone for its actions. This test may be used to diagnose and evaluate response to therapy for a variety of growth disorders. The test may be performed to diagnose acromegaly, dwarfism, pituitary disease and disorders, nutritional deficiencies, and to monitor response to therapies. The specimen is plasma, which requires special handling. Methodology may use a process of dissociation from binding protein and chromatography, followed by radioimmunoassay (RIA).

84307
This test may be performed to measure somatostatin, a hormone found in the pancreas and in the gut. Specimen is plasma, requiring special handling. Method is usually radioimmunoassay. This hormone regulates the body's production of insulin, glucagon, gastrin, secretin, and renin. Somatostatin also may control how the body secretes insulin and glucagon.

84311
Specimen types include blood, random urine, or a 24-hour timed urine collection. Method is typically spectrophotometry, which provides a quantitative measure of the amount of a material in a solution absorbing applied light. Report this test for an analyte not elsewhere specified. Measuring the absorption of visible, ultraviolet or infrared light makes quantitative measurements of concentrations of reagents. The specimen is by the bodily fluid chosen as a sample (e.g., gastric secretions). Method is by specific gravity, which measures the concentration or the weight of a substance as compared to an equal volume of water. For laboratory testing, specific gravity shows the density of a specific material.

84315
Specific gravity is a measure of concentration. It is the weight of a substance, as compared with that of an equal volume of water. Body fluids are typically collected by needle aspiration or lavage. The method of testing is refractometer.

84375
Fructose, galactose, lactose, maltose and l-xyulose are sugars found in urine of patients with inherited metabolic disorders. Thin layer chromatography or paper chromatography is a method to separate and identify sugars in urine when a metabolic order is suspected.

84376-84379
These tests may be used for infants who are failing to thrive due to lactose, sucrose, or fructose imbalances. Methods include gas chromatography and mass spectrometry to test for sugars, mono-, di-, and oligosaccharides in body fluids.

84392
This test may be ordered to determine kidney stone risk and in the investigation of sulfur metabolism studies. Sulfates may be measured for the diagnosis of metachromatic leukodystrophy (sulfatide lipidosis), an inherited lipid metabolism that results in the accumulation of metachromatic lipids in the tissues of the central nervous system, leading to paralysis and often death in early adolescence. The specimen is a random or timed urine collection. Method is spectrophotometry.

84393-84394
Total Tau (84394) and phosphorylated Tau (84393) are biomarkers for neurodegenerative conditions such as Alzheimer's disease and Creutzfeldt-Jakob disease. Tau proteins are primarily found in central nervous system neurons but are also found in astrocytes and oligodendrocytes. Tau testing by quantitative immunoassay is used in a patient with cognitive decline to assist in determining the underlying condition; elevated Tau biomarkers indicate increased likelihood of a neurodegenerative condition. The specimen is plasma or cerebrospinal fluid.

84402-84410
These tests may be used to evaluate testosterone levels. Testosterone is an androgenic hormone responsible for, among other biological activities, secondary male characteristics in women. Increased testosterone levels in women may be linked to a variety of conditions, including hirsutism. Report 84403 for total testosterone, which includes protein bound and free testosterone. Report 84402 for testosterone as a free unbound protein. This test may be ordered to assist in diagnosis of hypogonadism, hypopituitarism, and Klinefelter's syndrome, among other disorders. The specimen is serum. Method may be by radioimmunoassay (RIA) and immunoassay (non-isotopic). Report 84410 for bioavailable testosterone. The majority of circulating testosterone is bound to sex hormone-binding globulin (SHBG) or testosterone-binding globulin. Slightly less than one-third of testosterone in the blood binds to albumin and a smaller proportion circulates as free testosterone; the free testosterone and the testosterone bound to albumin is called the bioavailable testosterone, which is all non-SHBG bound testosterone. This test is performed in cases where the patient's level of SHBG is abnormal. The specimen is serum. Method may be based on the differential precipitation of SHBG by ammonium sulfate and subsequent equilibration of the specimen and trace amounts of tritium-labeled testosterone. This test may be ordered to provide more detailed information to assist in diagnosing patients presenting

with decreased SHBG levels and other conditions such as obesity, hypothyroidism, androgen use, and a type of kidney disease called nephritic syndrome.

84425
This is also known as Vitamin B1. The specimen is whole blood. Methods are high performance liquid chromatography and thiochrome-fluorometry. Mild thiamine deficiency occurs during pregnancy, in alcoholics, the elderly and in cases of persistent vomiting and fasting. Severe thiamine deficiency, called beriberi, is characterized by peripheral neuritis or cardiac failure. The quantitation of thiamine provides the sensitivity and specificity necessary for clinical evaluation of thiamine nutritional status.

84430
This drug may also be known as Nipride, Nitroprusside, Thanite, Lithane, or KCN. The specimen is serum or plasma or random urine sample. Methods may include photometry or chromatography. The test may be ordered to evaluate thiocyanate toxicity, nitroprusside therapy and poisoning, or cigarette use.

[84433]
Thiopurine S-methyltransferase (TPMT) deficiency is a condition in which there is a significant reduction in activity of an enzyme that helps the body process drugs called thiopurines. These drugs, which include 6-thioguanine, 6-mercaptopurine, and azathioprine, suppress the body's immune system, and are often prescribed to prevent organ transplant rejection or to treat autoimmune diseases or leukemia. This enzyme activity test detects TPMT deficiency and determines the risk of developing severe side effects if treated with this class of immune-suppressing drugs. Test method is liquid chromatography/tandem mass spectrometry (LC-MS/MS); specimen is whole blood.

84431
This immunoassay is used to measure thromboxane metabolites, including thromboxane, if performed. The specimen is urine. Determination of the total level of thromboxane production is useful in identifying patients who remain at risk of a cardiovascular event despite being on aspirin therapy.

84432
This test is also known as Tg. The specimen is serum. This test is performed to determine thyroglobulin levels to identify thyroid disorders and tumors.

84436
This test may be ordered as a T4. The specimen is serum. Methods may include radioimmunoassay (RIA), enzyme-linked immunosorbent assay (ELISA), fluorescence polarization immunoassay (FPIA), and chemiluminescence assay (CIA). The test is performed to determine thyroid function as screening test; total thyroxine makes up approximately 99 percent of the thyroid hormone.

84437
This test may be ordered as a neonatal T4. The specimen is whole blood. The specimen may be taken at the same time as a PKU (Phenylalanine) test. Method is typically radioimmunoassay (RIA). The test may be performed to determine hypothyroidism in newborns (performed in all 50 states) to prevent intellectual disabilities and to monitor suppressive and replacement therapy.

84439
This test may be ordered as a FT4, free T4, FTI or FT4 index. The specimen is serum, requiring special handling. Methods may include radioimmunoassay and equilibrium dialysis for reference method. Free thyroxine is a minimal amount of the total T4 level (approximately one percent). This test is not influenced by thyroid-binding abnormalities and perhaps correlates more closely with the true hormonal status. It may be effective in the diagnosis of hyperthyroidism and hypothyroidism.

84442
Thyroxin binding globulin is a plasma protein that binds with thyroxine and transports it in the blood. Elevated levels may be associated with pregnancy and newborn states, hepatitis, and other disorders. Decreased levels may be associated with liver diseases and acromegaly, among other disorders. The specimen is serum. Methods may include chemiluminescent immunoassay, equilibrium dialysis, ultrafiltration, and solid phase enzyme immunoassay (EIA) technology.

84443
TSH is produced in the pituitary gland and stimulates the secretion of thyrotropin (T3) and thyroxine (T4); these secretory products monitor TSH. The specimen is serum, requiring special handling. Heel stick or umbilical cord sample is drawn from newborns and may be collected on a special paper. Methods may include radioimmunoassay (RIA), sandwich immunoradiometric assay (IRMA), fluorometric enzyme immunoassay with use of monoclonal antibodies, or microparticle enzyme immunoassay on IMx (MEIA). This test may be performed to determine thyroid function, to differentiate from various types of hypothyroidism (e.g., primary, and pituitary/hypothalamic), or to diagnose hyperthyroidism. The test may be ordered to evaluate therapy in patients receiving hypothyroid treatment, and to detect congenital hypothyroidism.

84445
This test may also be ordered as TSI. This serum test measures the amount of thyroid stimulating antibody, which stimulates the thyroid to produce excessive amounts of thyroid hormone. Methods may include vitro bioassay and radioimmunoassay. The test may be useful in diagnosis of Grave's disease (hyperthyroidism).

84446
This test may also be known as a-tocopherol. The specimen is serum or plasma, requiring special handling. Methods may include high performance liquid chromatography (HPLC), fluorometry after solvent extraction, and colorimetry. The test may be

performed to determine vitamin E deficiency, to evaluate patients on long-term parenteral nutrition, and to evaluate numerous disorders.

84449
Cortisol-binding globulin (Transcortin) is a type of glycoprotein. This test is performed to evaluate adrenal activity. It plays a role in fat and water metabolism. The specimen is serum. Method may include chemiluminescent. Levels of cortisol help in the diagnosis of Cushing's syndrome, and Addison's disease.

84450
This test is usually referred to as aspartate aminotransferase (AST) or as serum glutamic oxaloacetic transaminase (SGOT). AST is an enzyme found primarily in heart muscle and the liver. Serum levels are low unless there is cellular damage, at which time large amounts are released into circulation. AST levels are increased following acute myocardial infarction (MI). Liver disease may also cause elevated levels of AST. Blood specimen is serum or plasma. Method is spectrophotometry, kinetic assay, and enzymatic.

84460
This test is usually referred to as alanine aminotransferase (ALT) or as serum glutamic pyruvic transaminase (SGPT). ALT is an enzyme found primarily in liver cells and elevations may be indicative of liver disease. Blood specimen is serum or plasma. Method is spectrophotometry or enzymatic.

84466
An alternative name for this test is siderophilin. The specimen is serum. Measurement of transferrin levels in serum aids in the diagnosis of malnutrition, acute inflammation, infection, and red blood cell disorders, such as iron deficiency anemia. Methods of testing vary to include immunologic or turbidimetric assay.

84478
This test may be requested as trig. Triglycerides are blood lipids that are transported through the circulatory system by lipoproteins. Triglycerides contribute to atherosclerosis and other arterial diseases. Blood specimen is serum or plasma. Method is enzymatic or colorimetry.

84479
This test may be requested as T3 uptake and T4 uptake or THBR. The specimen is serum. Method is chemiluminescent immunoassay.

84480
This test may be ordered as a T3 (RIA) or total T3. The specimen is serum. Methods may include radioimmunoassay (RIA), immunochemiluminometric assay, and fluorometric immunoassay. Abnormal results may be diseases and disorders related to the thyroid.

84481
This test may also be known as FT3, or free T3. The specimen is serum. Method may involve equilibrium dialysis (tracer). This test may be used to identify thyroid dysfunction, such as hyperthyroidism and hypothyroidism.

84482
Reverse T3 (rT3) is an inactive form of the thyroid hormone T3, and is found in the blood of normal people. The specimen is serum. Measurement of rT3 has been suggested in differentiating euthyroid sick syndrome from true hypothyroidism, and in identifying factitious hyperthyroidism. RT3 is typically measured by radioimmunoassay.

84484
This test may also be known as troponin regulatory complex. The specimen is serum. Methods may include radioimmunoassay, enzyme-linked immunosorbent assay, and immunoenzymatic assay. This quantitative test measures the levels of troponin, found in muscle tissues. Elevated levels of troponin may be related to myocardial infarction and ischemic heart disease.

84485
This test may also be referred to as duodenal trypsinogen. Trypsin in duodenal aspirate has been measured by both radioimmunoassay and enzymatic methods. Measurement is useful in evaluation of pancreatic disease, such as primary biliary cirrhosis and cystic fibrosis, and malabsorption syndromes.

84488-84490
These tests may be called fecal tryptic activity or immunoreactive trypsin. The specimen is fresh random stool sample. Methods may be kinetic and potentiometric, and x-ray film method. Trypsin is an enzyme that acts to degrade protein and it may be referred to as proteolytic enzyme, or proteinase. This test is performed to screen for pancreatic exocrine function and malabsorption syndromes in children under the age of four. Three specimens may be taken for an accurate assessment of pancreatic function. For qualitative screening, report 84488; for quantitative measurement, see 84490.

84510
This test may also be known by the abbreviation Tyr. Measurement of tyrosine is useful in the evaluation of certain amino-acidopathies or inborn errors of metabolism, and to determine possible thyroid disorders and various other diseases Tyrosine has been measured by chromatographic techniques such as HPLC or gas chromatography combined with a variety of detection/evaluation technologies, including mass-spectrometry. Specimen types vary.

84512
This may also be known as troponin regulatory complex. The specimen is plasma. Cardiac troponins are markers for myocardial muscle damage. Qualitative tests (positive/negative results) are primarily used to rule-in or rule-out myocardial infarction. Several bedside, point-of-care type assays are available. Methods are radioimmunoassay, enzyme-linked immunosorbent assay, and immunoenzymatic assay may also be seen.

84520
This test may be requested as blood urea nitrogen (BUN). Urea is an end product of protein metabolism. BUN may be requested to evaluate dehydration or renal function. Blood specimen is serum or plasma. Method is colorimetry, enzymatic, or rate conductivity. This test measures (quantitates) the amount of urea in the blood.

84525
This test may also be ordered as a BUN. This test may provide useful information regarding carbohydrate metabolism (diabetes), kidney function, and acid-base balance. The specimen type is plasma. Method is reagent strip.

84540
This test may provide useful information regarding carbohydrate metabolism (diabetes), kidney function, and acid-base balance, in addition to dietary protein. Urea is a measure of protein breakdown in the body. Urine urea excretion can be measured to obtain a ratio between the plasma (blood) urea and the urine urea; this ratio is an indicator of kidney function. Urine collection over a 24-hour period. Methods may include enzymatic assay, colorimetry, and conductometric.

84545
This test is also known as BUN-blood urea nitrogen. The specimen is taken over a 24-hour period. Urea nitrogen is formed in the liver as an end product of protein metabolism. Increased or decreased levels of urea nitrogen can indicate renal disease, dehydration, congestive heart failure, and gastrointestinal bleeding, starvation, shock or urinary tract obstruction (by tumor or prostate gland).

84550
This test may be requested as urate. Uric acid may be ordered to evaluate gout, renal function and a number of other disorders. Blood specimen is serum or plasma. Method is enzymatic or high performance liquid chromatography (HPLC).

84560
Uric acid is also known as urate. Methods may include high performance liquid chromatography, uricase, and phosphotungstate. The test may be ordered to determine the possible occurrence of calculus formation, evaluate uric acid in gout, and to identify genetic defects and some malignancies in body fluids other than blood.

84577
This also is known as the urobilinogen 48-hour feces test. The specimen is by random stool sample. Method is colorimetry. It is used to detect the presence of the yellow substance called urobilin that develops from the chemical breakdown of urobilinogen, which is excreted in the feces.

84578
This test is used to detect the presence of urobilinogen in urine. The specimen is random urine sample. Urobilinogen determination in urine is a useful liver function test, and can be helpful in evaluating some hemolytic anemias. Urobilinogen can be detected qualitatively by a simple, visual colorimetric test or by urine dipstick. Methods may include Ehrlich's aldehyde reagent, para-dimethylaminobenzaldehyde reacts with urobilinogen with a color enhancer.

84580-84583
These tests are used to report quantitative or semi-quantitative measurement of urobilinogen present in the urine. The specimen may be performed over a two-hour period. Elevated levels of urobilinogen can be early indicators of various types of liver disorders. Methods may include Ehrlich's aldehyde reagent, Watson's method, and Urobilistix. This test identifies some cases of liver diseases and hemolytic anemias. Report 84580 for a timed quantitative measurement urobilinogen; report 84583 for a semi-quantitative measurement of urobilinogen.

84585
This test is also called 3-methoxy-4-hydroxymandelic acid test, and also as VMA. Urine collection is over a 24-hour period and requires special handling. Methods may include colorimetry, spectrophotometry, gas chromatography, and high performance liquid chromatography (HPLC). The test may be performed to evaluate hypertensive states and to diagnose certain tumors and to monitor the efficacy of treatment modalities.

84586
VIP (vasoactive intestinal peptide) is found in and released from the central nervous system. It is found in the gut and affects the cells of the immune system. The specimen is plasma. Method is radioimmunoassay. The test may be used to determine the concentration of vasoactive intestinal peptide (VIP) in serum.

84588
This test is also known as Arginine Vasopressin Hormone and Antidiuretic Hormone (ADH). The specimen is plasma. Method is radioimmunoassay. Vasopressin, secreted by the hypothalamus and stored and released by the posterior pituitary gland, increases blood pressure and the rate at which the kidneys absorb water.

84590
This vitamin is also known as retinol. The specimen is serum, and requires special handling. Methods are electrochemical, high performance liquid chromatography (HPLC), and fluorescence or UV/VIS spectroscopy. Levels of vitamin A can be increased in specific diseases and toxic states, and decreased levels are seen in other conditions, such as, nutritional deficiency.

84591
This test is used to analyze vitamin levels that are not specified elsewhere such as biotin and niacin. Methods are dependent on the specific vitamin level being analyzed and on the type of specimen, but include microbiological assay (urine biotin levels), high performance liquid chromatography (HPLC) (urine

niacin levels) solid phase (cellulose) binding assay (plasma biotin levels), chemiluminescence (serum biotin levels).

84597
This test is used to analyze vitamin K, a fat-soluble vitamin that plays an important role in blood clotting. The specimen is serum which requires special handling. Method is high-performance liquid chromatography A. A deficiency in vitamin K is characterized by the increased tendency to bleed, including internal bleeding. Such bleeding episodes may be severe in newborn infants.

84600
Volatiles, also known as volatile toxicology, include acetic oxide, acetyl oxide, ethyl ether, and ethane. Test specimens may include whole blood, serum, plasma, urine, or gastric samples (collected by gastric lavage). Method may be gas-liquid chromatography (GLC). This test is performed to determine systemic alcohol levels and possibly as surveillance for drug abuse and to evaluate methanol and isopropanol toxicity due to ingestion, inhalation, or contact.

84620
This test may also be ordered as a xylose tolerance test. The test measures the intestines' ability to absorb D-xylose, a simple sugar, as an indicator of whether nutrients are being properly absorbed. Multiple blood and/or urine specimens are collected at timed intervals after dosing with a standardized dose of D-Xylose. Samples and sampling collection times are physician specified based on patient age and other parameters.

84630
This test is also known as Serum Zn. The specimen is serum or whole blood or a 24-hour urine sample. Methods may include atomic absorption spectrometry (AAS). Zinc is a trace mineral in the body, linked to thyroid hormone function and blood clotting. The test may be performed to determine nutrient levels for patients on total parenteral nutrition (TPN) and for burn victims and critically ill patients. The test may also be ordered to evaluate possible zinc toxicity.

84681
This test may also be known as a connecting peptide insulin test or a pro-insulin c-peptide. The specimen is post-fasting serum or urine is over a 24-hour period. Methods may include radioimmunoassay (RIA). The test is primarily performed to determine hypoglycemia and to measure pancreatic beta cell secretory function. It may also be used to determine residual beta cell function in insulin-dependent diabetes, and to differentiate between insulin and non-insulin diabetics.

84702
This test may be ordered as hCG or as a serum pregnancy test. The specimen is serum. Method may be radioimmunoassay (RIA), two-site immunoradiometric assay (IRMA), two-site enzyme-linked immunosorbent assay (ELISA), and radioreceptor assay (RRA). This test is quantitative and measures the amount of hCG present, a determinate of pregnancy and certain tumors.

84703
This test is also known as a beta-subunit human chorionic gonadotropin. The specimen is serum or random urine sample. Methods may include radioimmunoassay (RIA), immunoradiometric (IRMA), and enzyme immunoassay. The test may be ordered to determine pregnancy, ectopic pregnancy, and hCG tumors, and as a screening prior to select medical care (e.g., sterilization).

84704
Free beta human chorionic gonadotropin (hCG) is a biochemical marker used in early (first trimester) screening to detect such abnormalities as Down syndrome, Trisomy 18, and neural tube defects. Maternal serum levels of free beta hCG are elevated in Down syndrome pregnancies and markedly reduced in Trisomy 18. This test is quantitative and identifies the free beta chain of human chorionic gonadotropin using an enzyme immunoassay methodology.

84830
This test is used for the qualitative detection of the luteinizing hormone (LH) in urine. The specimen is urine. Method is rapid chromatographic immunoassay. LH is always present in the blood and urine, though its levels are higher in urine during ovulation. The LH surge and actual release of the egg is considered as the most fertile time of the cycle, and the most likely time for becoming pregnant.

85002
This test may be ordered as a bleeding time or as an Ivy bleeding time. A small, superficial wound is nicked in the patient's forearm. Essentially, the amount of time it takes for the wound to stop bleeding is recorded at bedside. The Ivy bleeding time test is one standardized method. All methods are manual or point of care. A bleeding time is a rough measure of platelet (thrombocyte) function. The test is often performed on a preoperative patient.

85004
This test may be ordered as a blood count with automated differential. The specimen is whole blood. Method is automated cell counter. The blood count typically includes a measurement of normal cell constituents including white blood cells or leukocytes, red blood cells, and platelets. In addition, this test includes a differential count of the white blood cells or "diff" in which the following leukocytes are differentiated and counted automatically: neutrophils or granulocytes, lymphocytes, monocytes, eosinophils, and basophils.

85007-85008
These tests may be ordered as a manual blood smear examination, RBC smear, peripheral blood smear, or RBC morphology without differential parameters in 85008 and with manual WBC differential in 85007. The specimen is whole blood. The method is manual testing. A blood smear is prepared and microscopically

examined for the presence of normal cell constituents, including white blood cells, red blood cells, and platelets. In 85008, the white blood cell and platelet or thrombocyte counts are estimated and red cell morphology is commented on if abnormal. In 85007, a manual differential of white blood cells is included in which the following leukocytes are differentiated: neutrophils or granulocytes, lymphocytes, monocytes, eosinophils, and basophils.

85009

This test may be ordered as a buffy coat differential or as a differential WBC count, buffy coat. Specimen is whole blood. Other collection types (e.g., finger stick or heel stick) do not yield the volume of blood required for this test. Method is manual testing. The whole blood is centrifuged to concentrate the white blood cells, and a manual WBC differential is performed in which the following leukocytes are differentiated: neutrophils or granulocytes, lymphocytes, monocytes, eosinophils, and basophils. This test is usually performed when the number of WBCs or leukocytes is abnormally low and the presence of abnormal white cells (e.g., blasts or cancer cells) is suspected clinically.

85013

This test may be ordered as a microhematocrit, a spun microhematocrit, or a "spun crit." The specimen (whole blood) is by finger stick or heel stick in infants. The sample is placed in a tube and into a microcentrifuge device. The vials can be read manually against a chart for the volume of packed red cells or a digital reader in the centrifuge device. A spun microhematocrit only reports the volume of packed red cells. It is typically performed at sites where limited testing is available, the patient is a very difficult blood draw, or on infants.

85014

This test may be ordered as a hematocrit, Hmt, or Hct. The specimen is whole blood. Method is automated cell counter. The hematocrit or volume of packed red cells (VPRC) in the blood sample is calculated by multiplying the red blood cell count or RBC times the mean corpuscular volume or MCV.

85018

This test may be ordered as hemoglobin, Hgb, or hemoglobin concentration. The specimen is whole blood. Method is usually automated cell counter but a manual method is seen in labs with a limited test menu and blood bank drawing stations. Hemoglobin is an index of the oxygen-carrying capacity of the blood.

85025-85027

These tests may be ordered as a complete automated blood count (CBC). The specimen is whole blood. Method is automated cell counter. These codes include the measurement of erythrocytes (red blood cells or RBC), leukocytes (white blood cells or WBC), hemoglobin, hematocrit (volume of packed red blood cells or VPRC), platelet or thrombocyte count, and indices (mean corpuscular hemoglobin or MCH, mean corpuscular hemoglobin concentration or MCHC, mean corpuscular volume or MCV, and red cell distribution width or RDW). Code 85025 includes an automated differential of the white blood cells or "diff" in which the following leukocytes are differentiated: neutrophils or granulocytes, lymphocytes, monocytes, eosinophils, and basophils. Report 85027 if the complete CBC, or automated blood count, is done without the differential WBC count.

85032

This code reports a manual cell count done for red blood cells (erythrocytes), white blood cells (leukocytes), or platelets (thrombocytes), each. The specimen is whole blood. The method is manual examination and counting.

85041

This test may be ordered as red blood cell count or RBC. The specimen is by whole blood. Method is automated cell counter.

85044

This test may be ordered as a manual reticulocyte count or as a manual "retic." The specimen is whole blood. Method is manual. A blood smear is prepared and stained with a dye that highlights the reticulum in the immature red blood cells, or the reticulocytes. The reticulocytes reported as a percentage of total red blood cells.

85045

This test may be ordered as an automated reticulocyte count, an "auto retic," or a reticulocyte by flow cytometry. The specimen is whole blood. Method is automated cell counter or flow cytometer. Reticulocytes are immature red blood cells that still contain mitochondria and ribosomes. The reticulocytes are reported as a percentage of total red blood cells.

85046

This test may be ordered as a reticulocyte count and hemoglobin concentration, "retics" and Hgb, or as an "auto retic" and hemoglobin. The specimen is whole blood. Method is automated cell counter. The blood is stained with a dye that marks the reticulum in immature red blood cells, or reticulocytes. The reticulocytes are reported as a percentage of total red blood cells. The automated reticulocyte blood count also includes one or more cellular parameters, such as the hemoglobin content of the reticulocytes (CHr), the fraction of immature reticulocytes (IRF), the RNA content, or the volume of reticulocytes.

85048-85049

These tests may be ordered as an automated white blood cell or WBC count, white cell count, or leukocyte count for 85048 and as an automated platelet count in 85049. The specimen is whole blood. Method is automated cell counter. In 85048, the population of white blood cells, or WBCs in the blood sample, is counted by machine. Only the number of white blood cells or leukocytes is reported. In 85049, the population of platelets or thrombocytes in the blood sample is counted by machine. Only the number of platelets is reported.

85055
Reticulated platelets (RP) are the newly released, or most recently produced, platelets in circulation that contain some residual RNA in their cytoplasm. The specimen is whole blood. The measurement of reticulated platelets is used in thrombocytopenic patients to estimate the thrombocytopoietic status of bone marrow, and evaluate whether the pathophysiology is due to increased peripheral platelet destruction or decreased platelet production. RP counts are also used to monitor the state of megakaryopoiesis in patients with post-chemo or post-transplant status. The method is flow cytometry.

85060
This test may be ordered as a peripheral blood smear with interpretation by a physician, with a written report. It would usually be ordered following a hemogram with WBC differential where the technologist noted the presence of significant abnormalities and requested a pathology review. Although lacking specificity, peripheral smears also provide a quick and cost-effective screening for the presence of bacteremia. The specimen is whole blood. The method is manual. A blood smear is prepared and reviewed by a physician/pathologist, who submits a written interpretation of the findings.

85097
This test may be ordered as a bone marrow smear interpretation with or without differential cell count. The specimen is by aspiration with a syringe. The bone marrow aspirate may be collected from a variety of sites, including the posterior iliac crest (preferred) and the sternum. The method is manual. Slides or smears are prepared from the aspirate and stained. The slides are reviewed by a physician/pathologist and a written interpretation of the findings is submitted. This report may include a differential count of the white blood cells present.

85130
This test may be ordered as a chromogenic substrate assay but would more likely be ordered as a specific clotting factor assay (e.g., factor V, fibrinogen, or antithrombin III) by chromogenic analysis. The specimen is plasma. The method is usually automated coagulation instrument but may be manual.

85170
This test may be ordered as a clot retraction or a clot retraction study. The specimen whole blood. The method is manual. Clot retraction time is a measurement of blood platelet function. Normal blood begins to retract 30 to 60 minutes after collection. The test is an older method to measure platelet or thrombocyte function.

85175
This test may be ordered as a whole blood dilution clot lysis time. The specimen is whole blood. The method is manual. This is a non-specific test of fibrinolytic or clot-lysing activity. The tubes are examined at 24 and 48-hour intervals to assess degeneration of the clots. The test is rarely used today, as there are other specific assays that provide more useable information to the physician.

85210
This test may be ordered as a factor II, clotting factor II, or a prothrombin factor assay. The specimen is plasma. The method is usually automated coagulation instrument but may be manual. This factor is one of several essential to clot formation. A decreased amount of this factor may be associated with clotting impairment.

85220
This test may be ordered as a factor V, clotting factor V, or labile factor assay. It may be ordered as a proaccelerin assay or an AcG factor assay. The specimen is plasma. The method is usually automated coagulation instrument, but may be manual. This factor is one of several essential to clot formation. A decreased amount of this factor may be associated with blood clotting disorders.

85230
This test may be ordered as a factor VII assay, stable factor assay, or clotting factor VII assay. It may also be ordered as a proconvertin assay. The specimen is plasma. The method is usually automated coagulation instrument, but may be manual. This factor is one of several essential to clot formation. A decreased amount of this factor may be associated with blood clotting disorders.

85240
This test may be ordered as a factor VIII assay, AHF, or an anti-hemophilic globulin or AHG assay. The specimen is plasma. The method is automated coagulation instrument, but may be manual. This factor is one of a number of factors essential for clot formation. A decreased amount or absence may be associated with blood clotting disorders (i.e., hemophilia A). This test is essentially an assay for the presence and quantity of the AHG.

85244
This test may be ordered as factor VIII related antigen or VIIIR: Ag. The specimen is plasma. The method is automated coagulation instrument, but may be manual. The presence of Factor VIII related antigen is associated with carriers of the bleeding disorder hemophilia. The test may be useful for the detection of carriers of hemophilia A and in prenatal diagnoses.

85245
This test may be ordered as a ristocetin cofactor, VIIR:Rco, or Von Willebrand factor ristocetin cofactor. The specimen is plasma. The method is automated coagulation instrument, but may be manual. This test measures platelet aggregation in response to introduction of ristocetin into the tube. The resulting level of ristocetin cofactor may be interpreted to assess the function of the Von Willebrand Factor, which may be indicative of the presence of Von Willebrand's disease and the variant or type of the disorder.

85246
This test may be ordered as factor VIII related antigen, VIIR:Ag, Von Willebrand factor or vWF, or Von Willebrand factor antigen vWF:Ag. The specimen is plasma. The method is automated coagulation instrument, but may be manual. A deficiency or low level of Von Willebrand factor antigen is associated with Von Willebrand's disease (a bleeding disorder). A diminished VW factor antigen with reduced function of VW factor can lead to a diagnosis of a variant of Von Willebrand's known as Type I. An absence of VW factor antigen, with undetectable function of VW factor, can lead to a diagnosis of a variant of Von Willebrand's known as Type III.

85247
This test may be ordered as factor VIII assay with multimeric analysis of Von Willebrand factor, agarose gel electrophoresis of Von Willebrand factor, or vWF:Ag multimeric analysis. The specimen is plasma. The method is agarose gel electrophoresis. This test provides a differential diagnosis for variants of Von Willebrand's disease. The absence of multimeric VW factor may be indicative of a variant of Von Willebrand's known as Type II.

85250
This test may be ordered as a factor IX assay, a PTC assay, or a Christmas disease assay. The specimen is plasma. The method is automated coagulation instrument, but may be manual. This factor is one of a number of factors essential to clot formation. A decreased amount of this factor may be associated with a form of homeostasis disorder. A factor IX deficiency is the second most common clotting factor deficiency that results in a variant of hemophilia known by the suffix B or simply Christmas disease.

85260
This test may be ordered as a factor X assay or rarely as a Stuart-Prower assay. The specimen is plasma. The method is automated coagulation instrument but may be manual. This factor is one of a number of factors essential for clot formation. A decreased amount of this factor may be associated with a systemic coagulation disorder known as Factor X deficiency.

85270
This test may be ordered as a factor XI assay or as a PTA assay or antihemophilic C assay. The specimen is plasma. The method is automated coagulation instrument, but may be manual. This factor is one of a number of factors essential for clot formation. A decreased amount of this factor XI may be associated with systemic blood clotting disorder known as Hemophilia C..

85280
This test may be ordered as a factor XII assay or as a Hageman factor assay. The specimen is plasma. The method is automated coagulation instrument, but may be manual. This factor is one of a number of factors involved in clot formation. A decreased amount of this factor may be associated with blood clotting problems.

85290
This test may be ordered as a factor XIII assay or as a fibrin stabilizing factor assay. The specimen is plasma. The method is automated coagulation instrument but may be manual. This factor is one of a number of factors involved in clot formation. A decreased amount of this factor may be associated with clot dissolution and bleeding problems.

85291
This test may be ordered as a factor XIII solubility screen or a fibrin stabilizing factor solubility screen. The specimen is plasma. The method is manual. This factor is one of a number of factors involved in clot formation. A decreased amount of this factor may be associated with clot dissolution and bleeding problems. This code does not measure the amount of factor XIII antigen but is a measure of factor XIII function.

85292
This test may be ordered as a prekallikrein assay. The method is usually automated coagulation instrument but may be manual. A prekallikrein deficiency results in a prolonged clotting time but is not associated with abnormal bleeding.

85293
This test may be ordered as a high molecular weight kininogen or HMWK assay, a HMW kininogen assay, a Fitzgerald factor assay, or rarely as a Williams factor assay or a Flaujeac factor assay. The specimen is plasma. The method is automated coagulation instrument, but may be manual. A Fitzgerald or HMWK factor deficiency results in a prolonged clotting time but is not associated with abnormal bleeding.

85300
This test may be ordered as an antithrombin III activity assay, an AT-III functional assay, or as a functional antithrombin III assay. The specimen is plasma. The method is automated coagulation instrument, but may be manual. A decrease in antithrombin III function or activity is associated with thrombosis or episodes of abnormal clot formation.

85301
This test may be ordered as an antithrombin III antigen assay, an immunological antithrombin III assay, or an AT-III antigen assay. The specimen is plasma. The method is automated coagulation instrument but may be manual. Levels of antithrombin III antigen may be normal even though the antithrombin III activity is decreased, see 85300. Deficiencies of this antigen are associated with thrombosis or episodes of abnormal clot formation.

85302
This test may be ordered as a protein C antigen assay or an immunological protein C assay. The specimen is plasma. The method is enzyme immunoassay. A decrease in protein C antigen levels is associated with thrombosis or episodes of abnormal clot formation.

85303
This test may be ordered as a protein C activity assay, or as a functional protein C assay. The specimen is plasma. The method is enzyme immunoassay. A decrease in protein C activity or functional levels is associated with thrombosis or episodes of abnormal clot formation.

85305
This test may be ordered as a total protein S assay, protein S antigen assay, or immunological protein S antigen assay. The specimen is plasma. The method is enzyme immunoassay. A decrease in protein S antigen levels is associated with thrombosis or episodes of abnormal clot formation.

85306
This test may be ordered as a free protein S assay, a protein S functional assay, or a protein S activity assay. The specimen is plasma. The method is enzyme immunoassay. A decrease in protein S activity or functional levels is associated with thrombosis or episodes of abnormal clot formation.

85307
This test may be requested as activated protein C (APC) resistance test. Blood specimen is plasma. Method is clotting assay. This test is used to evaluate patients with thrombosis. APC is an important natural anticoagulant present in the blood which functions by inactivating the coagulation factors FVa and FVIIIa. The APC resistance test consists of a standard activated partial thromboplastin time (APTT) test performed both in the absence and presence of commercially available activated protein C. In the normal response, the presence of APC will prolong the clotting time due to the anticoagulant action of this protein. Failure to prolong the clotting time in the presence of APC is an abnormality resulting from resistance to this protein. The results are reported as a ratio of the APC-APTT/APTT.

85335
This test may be ordered as a factor inhibitor test or a Bethesda qualitative test. The specific factor will be ordered (i.e., factor VIII). The specimen plasma. The method is automated coagulation instrument, but may be manual. This test is used to detect the presence of inhibitors or inactivators against a coagulation factor. It is rare but not impossible to exhibit inhibitors against more than one coagulation factor. This assay may be ordered several times before the inhibitor's target factor is identified.

85337
This test may be ordered as a thrombomodulin assay. The specimen is plasma. The method is usually automated coagulation instrument but may be manual. Thrombomodulin is a protein involved in activation of the clot dissolution or lysis process.

85345
This test may be ordered as a clotting time, a whole blood clotting time, or a Lee-White clotting time. The specimen is whole blood. The method is manual. The Lee-White clotting time measures the ability of blood to clot and is performed at the patient's bedside to monitor anticoagulant therapy such as heparin, warfarin, or coumadin.

85347
This test may be ordered as an activated clotting time, an activated whole blood clotting time, or an activated Lee-White clotting time. The specimen is whole blood. The method is manual. The activated clotting time measures the ability of blood to clot and is a precursor to the activated partial thromboplastin time (85730), or PTT.

85348
This test may be ordered as a clotting time. The specimen is whole blood finger stick or, in infants, heel stick. Methods vary, as the formal description implies. Point-of-care testing often involves a hand held instrument that gives some measurement of whole blood clotting time.

85360
This test may be ordered as euglobulin lysis time, euglobulin clot lysis time, or an EGT. The specimen is plasma. The method is manual. This test is a measure of fibrinolytic or clot dissolving activity and is useful in the diagnostic workup for numerous disorders.

85362
This test may be ordered as fibrin (or fibrinogen) degradation products (FDP) or fibrin (or fibrinogen) split products (FSP). Specimen is blood or urine. The test method is latex agglutination. The degradation products of fibrinogen have characteristic biological properties, including the inhibition of clotting. This test measures the products of fibrinolytic or clot dissolving activity. FDP tests on urine are performed primarily post kidney transplant and are helpful as a predictor of rejection.

85366
This test may be ordered as a protamine paracoagulation, fibrin monomer, ethanol gelation or ethanol gel, protamine sulfate, or protamine gelation test. The specimen is blood. The degradation products of fibrinogen have characteristic biological properties, including the inhibition of clotting. This test measures the products of fibrinolytic or clot dissolving activity. The test is not in common usage.

85370
This test may be ordered as quantitative fibrin (or fibrinogen) degradation products (FDP) or quantitative FDP, quantitative fibrin (or fibrinogen) split products (FSP). The specimen is blood. The method is radioimmunoassay (RIA). The degradation products of fibrinogen have characteristic biological properties, including the inhibition of clotting. This test measures the products of fibrinolytic or clot dissolving activity. The degradation products are quantitated.

85378-85379
These tests may be ordered as D-dimer, latex agglutination, or slide D-dimer, semi-quantitative or

qualitative. The specimen is plasma. The degradation products of fibrinogen have characteristic biological properties, including the inhibition of clotting. Code 85378 is a semi-quantitative or qualitative measure of two degradation fragments known as the D-dimer. The method typically includes latex agglutination, specific antisera. Code 85379 is a quantitative measure using enzyme-linked immunosorbent assay (ELISA).

85380
The ultrasensitive test for fibrin-degradation products, specifically D-dimer, is a simple and rapid qualitative or semiquantitative in vitro whole blood agglutination assay test that relies on an antibody specific for D-dimer. A small amount of venous (non-clotted) whole blood is required. D-dimer is a specific fibrin degradation product that is produced in the body by the activation of the plasmin enzyme, which breaks down clots and fibrinogen, such as when deep venous thrombosis or pulmonary embolism is present. Elevated levels of D-dimer indicate that active fibrinolysis is occurring. Positive results are not as specific as negative results, which can rule out active fibrin breakdown and, therefore, the diagnosis of embolism accurately.

85384
This test may be ordered as, Factor I, clotting Factor I, fibrinogen, or fibrinogen activity. The specimen is plasma. The method is usually by automated coagulation instrument but may be done manually. This factor is one of a number essential to clot formation. A decreased amount of this factor may be associated bleeding disorders.

85385
This test may be ordered as Factor I, clotting Factor I, or fibrinogen antigen. The specimen is plasma. The method is usually automated coagulation instrument but may be manual. This factor is one of a number essential to clot formation. A decreased amount of this factor may be associated with bleeding disorders.

85390
This test may be ordered as a fibrinolysin screen, as a coagulopathy screen, or as a disseminated intravascular coagulopathy (DIC) screen. The specimen is blood. The method combines automated coagulation instrument, latex agglutination, and automated cell counter. This test typically screens for intravascular coagulation disorders. A pathology interpretation and report is included with the screen.

85396
A coagulation/fibrinolysis assay is done on whole blood to assess the viscoelastic properties of blood as it clots. Information about the kinetics of clot formation and growth and the strength and stability of the formed clot provides a more global assessment about hemostatic function as a whole dynamic process. The interaction between fibrinogen, platelets, and the protein coagulation process are measured in viscoelastic assays as clotting happens, and followed through to clot lysis. This is invaluable in surgical circumstances for patients who have been treated with anticoagulants, or are suspected of thromboembolic disease.

85397
This test is used to measure the functional activity of ADAMTS-13, an enzyme whose malfunction may lead to thrombotic thrombocytopenic purpura (TTP) or other thrombocytopenic conditions. It also measures the functional activity of other proteases and proteins involved in coagulation and fibrinolysis for which there are no more specific codes. Specimen is plasma and test method is enzyme-linked immunosorbent assay (ELISA) or fluorescence energy transfer (FRET). Report 85397 for each analyte tested.

85400
This test may be ordered as euglobulin lysis time, plasmin level, or plasmin activity. The specimen is plasma. The method is chromogenic substrate. Plasmin is an important agent in the dissolution of clots. Increased plasmin levels are present during fibrinolytic or clot dissolving activity.

85410
This test may be ordered as alpha-2-antiplasmin. The specimen is plasma. The method is typically radial immunodiffusion. Increased alpha-2-antiplasmin levels are present during fibrinolytic or clot dissolving activity.

85415
This test may be ordered as plasminogen activator, plasminogen activator inhibitor (PAI). The specimen is plasma. The method is chromogenic substrate or enzyme linked immunosorbent assay. Increased plasminogen activator levels are present during fibrinolytic or clot dissolving activity.

85420
This test may be ordered as plasminogen level, functional plasminogen, or plasminogen activity. The specimen is plasma. The method is chromogenic substrate. Increased plasminogen levels are present during fibrinolytic or clot dissolving activity, intrauterine death, and some metastatic cancers.

85421
This test may be ordered as plasminogen antigen level. The specimen is plasma. The method is radial immunodiffusion. Increased plasminogen antigen levels may be present during fibrinolytic or clot dissolving activity, intrauterine death, and some metastatic cancers.

85441
This test may be ordered as a Heinz body stain, or a direct Heinz body stain. Heinz bodies are anomalous intracellular erythrocytic (red blood cell) inclusions, composed of denatured hemoglobin that attach to the cell membrane. The specimen is whole blood or finger stick in adults, or heel stick in infants. The method is phase contrast microscopy or supravital stain (e.g., methyl violet, crystal violet, and brilliant cresyl blue, new methylene blue). Elevated numbers of Heinz

bodies are found following exposure to certain drugs and toxic chemicals, some enzyme deficiencies, and as a result of inherited disorders of blood hemoglobin.

85445
This test may be ordered as an induced Heinz body stain. Heinz bodies are anomalous intracellular erythrocytic (red blood cell) inclusions, composed of denatured hemoglobin that attach to the cell membrane. The specimen is whole blood or finger stick in adults, or heel stick in infants. The method is phase microscopy or supravital stain (e.g., methyl violet, crystal violet, and brilliant cresyl blue, new methylene blue). A blood sample is treated with a chemical (usually acetyl phenylhydrazine) and a blood smear is prepared and examined for the presence of Heinz bodies in the red blood cells. This test may be necessary to identify patients with certain types of unstable blood hemoglobin disorders.

85460
This test may be ordered as a Kleihauer-Betke stain or K-B stain, a Kleihauer-Betke stain for fetal hemoglobin, a Kleihauer-Betke stain for fetomaternal hemorrhage, acid-resistant fetal cells, or a differential lysis stain. The specimen is whole blood or finger stick. This test is not performed on infants. The method is semi-quantitative stain following acid elution. The blood smear is stained and examined microscopically. The number of red cells containing fetal hemoglobin or acid-resistant hemoglobin red cells are counted and reported as a percentage of the normal adult hemoglobin-containing red cells. This test is usually performed on post-partum mothers to determine if the newborn bled during delivery. The number of acid-resistant, or fetal cells, present is useful in developing postpartum treatment plans, especially with Rh-negative mothers.

85461
This test may be ordered as a fetal hemoglobin screening test, a fetal red cell rosette, a FetalDex screen, or a fetal screen. The specimen is whole blood or finger stick. This test is not appropriate for infants. The blood is treated with a chemical (anti-D) that causes fetal cells to form a rosette, or circle, of cells. This test is a screen usually performed on Rh-negative post-partum mothers to determine if the newborn bled during delivery.

85475
This test may be ordered as an acid hemolysin test, positive acidified serum test, or as a Ham test. The specimen is whole blood or finger stick in adults, or heel stick in infants. The method is manual. The patient's red blood cells are incubated with a mildly acidic solution and observed for hemolysis. Patients with paroxysmal nocturnal hemoglobinuria (PNH) have a positive acid hemolysin test.

85520
This test may be ordered as a heparin assay, a quantitative heparin analysis, or as a heparin level. The specimen is plasma. The method is chromogenic assay. This test measures the amount of heparin in a patient's blood and is usually ordered when the patient is on low-dose heparin therapy.

85525
This test may be ordered as a heparin neutralization test, a heparin-thrombin coagulation time test, or as protamine neutralization test. The specimen is plasma. The method is manual. This test is used to determine the dose of protamine needed to neutralize heparin-induced bleeding.

85530
This test may be ordered as a heparin-protamine tolerance test. Protamine is given as an antidote to heparin overdose. However, some patients develop hypersensitivity to protamine and may go into anaphylactic shock if they receive a dosage. Method is point of care testing. This test is used to assess hypersensitivity to protamine and measures the amount of protamine that can be safely administered.

85536
This test may also be ordered as a Prussian blue stain, hemosiderin stain, or red cell iron stain. The test is performed to identify abnormal iron accumulations in peripheral red blood cells. The specimen is blood stored unclotted. Method is slide preparation with Perl's Prussian blue stain and visual microscopy. The stain binds to iron in the blood cell and the test may be used to classify anemias as well as other disorders.

85540
This test may be ordered as a leukocyte alkaline phosphatase test (LAP), LAP score. The specimen is whole blood. The method is enzyme reaction with leukocyte alkaline phosphatase liberating naphthol, which is manually stained. Smears from freshly collected whole blood are prepared, stained, and examined microscopically. One hundred cells are counted and phosphatase activity scores (0 to 4+) totaled. The amount of leukocyte alkaline phosphatase present aids in the differential diagnosis of various leukemias.

85547
This test may be ordered as a red blood cell mechanical fragility test, or as a mechanical red cell fragility. The specimen is whole blood or finger stick in adults, or heel stick in infants. The method is manual. Some disorders of red blood cells cause variations in the cell membrane, which may be demonstrated by stressing the red cells.

85549
This test may be ordered as a muramidase test, a myelomonocytic lysozyme test, or as a malignant lymphoma lysozyme test. The specimen is serum, bone marrow aspirate or 24-hour urine specimen. The method is flow cytometry, gel diffusion assay, radioimmunoassay or enzymatic. The presence of this protein aids in the differential diagnosis of certain leukemias and lymphomas.

85555
This test may be ordered as an osmotic fragility test, a red blood cell fragility, an uninucleated osmotic fragility, or as a red blood cell osmotic fragility. The specimen is whole blood. The method is manual. Certain diseases cause red cells to change from their normal shape, which may increase or decrease their ability to take up water without lysing. The red cells are diluted with increasing concentrations of sodium chloride. The concentration that demonstrates hemolysis, or bursting, of the red cells, is compared to a normal patient's red cells.

85557
This test may be ordered as an incubated osmotic fragility test, an incubated red blood cell fragility, or as an incubated red blood cell osmotic fragility. The specimen is whole blood. The method is manual. Certain diseases cause red cells that have been incubated at 37 degrees for 24 hours to change from their normal shape, which may increase or decrease their ability to take up water without lysing. The red cells are diluted with increasing concentrations of sodium chloride. The concentration that demonstrates hemolysis or bursting of the red cells is compared to a normal patient's red cells.

85576
This test may be ordered as a platelet aggregation study, or as an in vitro platelet aggregation study. Specimen is plasma. The method may be platelet aggregometer. Platelet function is measured by observing the amount of platelet clumping that occurs when certain chemicals are added to a solution of platelets. The test is an in vitro enactment of the platelet aggregation that occurs naturally at the site of vascular injury. The test may be used to detect von Willebrand's disease or other inherited platelet-related disorders.

85597-85598
These are confirmatory tests for lupus anticoagulants (or other autoimmune diseases) using phospholipids derived from platelets (85597) or "hexagonal phase" phospholipids (85598). Some patients with systemic lupus develop an anticoagulant that reacts with platelet or hexagonal phase phospholipids. This test is very sensitive to this anticoagulant. The specimen is by venipuncture.

85610
This test may be ordered as a prothrombin time (PT), a prothrombin, or as simply PT. The specimen is plasma. Method is one-stage using an automated device. The prothrombin time is prolonged when deficiencies of coagulation factors II, V, VII, or X are present. More commonly, this test monitors the effectiveness of the anticoagulant drug Coumadin or warfarin, prescribed to patients who have had blood clots or myocardial infarction.

85611
This test may be ordered as a diluted prothrombin time (PT), a prothrombin 1:1, or as plasma diluted PT. The specimen is plasma. Addition or dilution with normal plasma differentiates between a clotting factor deficiency and a circulating anticoagulant. Prolonged prothrombin times due to a clotting factor deficiency will shorten to normal with the addition of normal plasma while a prolonged prothrombin time due to a circulating anticoagulant may increase with the addition of normal plasma.

85612
This test may be ordered as a Stypven time, Russell viper venom time, or as an undiluted Russell viper venom time. The specimen is plasma. Method is automated with a phospholipid being added to the test system to neutralize platelet activity. This test is used to confirm fibrinogen deficiency, deficiencies of Factors II and V, and some types of Factor X deficiency.

85613
This test may be ordered as a diluted Russell viper venom time. The specimen is plasma. Method is automated. This test is used to confirm the presence of a lupus anticoagulant.

85635
This test may be ordered as a reptilase test or, more commonly, reptilase time (RT). The specimen is plasma. Method involves adding venom of pit viper to a sample of the patient's plasma and recording the clotting time. This test is most often used to monitor the effectiveness of thrombolytic or clot-lysing drugs such as streptokinase or urokinase. It may also be used to detect the presence of coagulation disorders such as dysfibrinogenemias (non-functional or abnormal fibrinogen) and clotting disorders such as disseminated intravascular coagulation (DIC).

85651
This test may be ordered as an erythrocyte sedimentation rate (ESR), a Westergren sedimentation rate, Wintrobe sedimentation rate, or simply as a "sed rate." The specimen is whole blood. This test is a non-specific screening test for a number of diseases including anemia, disorders of protein production such as multiple myeloma, other conditions that alter the size and/or shape of red cells or erythrocytes, and to screen diseases that cause an increase or decrease in the amount of protein in the plasma. Further studies are often launched by ESR results. The method is manual. A variety of procedures have been used over time to study sedimentation rate. A common one performed manually is the Westergren tube.

85652
This test may be ordered as a Zeta sedimentation rate or as a Zeta sed rate. Specimen is whole blood. Method is centrifugation; this is an automated test. This test is a non-specific screening test for a number of diseases including anemia, disorders of protein production such as multiple myeloma, and other conditions that alter the size and/or shape of red cells or erythrocytes. This test may also be used to screen diseases that cause an increase or decrease in the amount of protein in the plasma or liquid portion of the blood.

85660
This test may be ordered as a sickle cell metabisulfite test, a sickle cell reduction test, an erythrocyte (RBC) sickling test, or as an RBC reduction sickle cell test. Specimen is whole blood. The method is manual. Whole blood is mixed with a reducing agent that causes erythrocytes that contain abnormal amounts of hemoglobin S to sickle or change their shape to an elongated 'sickle' cell. The solution is examined microscopically and the numbers of sickle cells are reported as a percentage of normal erythrocytes or RBCs.

85670
This test may be ordered as a thrombin time or as a TT. The specimen is plasma. The method is manual clotting. This test is used to measure the last stage of clotting which is the conversion of fibrinogen to fibrin following the addition of thrombin. This test is prolonged during heparin therapy, in the presence of fibrin split products, and other circulating anticoagulants, and in disorders of fibrinogen.

85675
This test may be ordered as a thrombin time titer or as a diluted thrombin time. The specimen is plasma. The method is manual clotting. This test is used to detect the presence of clotting inhibitors other than heparin. Dilutions of thrombin are used in 85675.

85705
This test may be ordered as a tissue thromboplastin inhibition test (TTI), or as a lupus anticoagulant (LA) test. Extravascular tissue requires a biopsy, which is reported separately. The method is manual clotting. This test is used when the patient has prolonged prothrombin time (85610) and/or partial thromboplastin time (85730) not due to coagulation factor deficiencies or drug therapy, such as heparin or Coumadin. Some patients with suspected or diagnosed diseases such as lupus erythematosus and AIDS may be candidates for this test.

85730
This test may be ordered as a partial thromboplastin time or PTT, or as an activated partial thromboplastin time or APTT. The specimen is plasma. The method is automated coagulation instrument. The partial thromboplastin time is prolonged when deficiencies of coagulation factors VIII, IX, XI, and XII are present. This test is used to monitor the effectiveness of the anticoagulant drug heparin, which is prescribed for patients who have had blood clots or heart attacks.

85732
This test may be ordered as a diluted partial thromboplastin time, a PTT or APTT 1:1, or as a plasma diluted PTT or APTT. The specimen is plasma. The method is automated coagulation instrument. Addition of or dilution with normal plasma differentiates between a clotting factor deficiency and a circulating anticoagulant. Prolonged partial thromboplastin times due to a clotting factor deficiency will shorten to normal with the addition of normal plasma while a prolonged PTT due to a circulating anticoagulant may increase with the addition of normal plasma.

85810
This test may be ordered as a serum viscosity test or as a viscosity. Specimen is serum. Finger stick or heel stick is not acceptable. Method is viscometer. This test measures the viscosity or thickness of serum as compared to saline. Increased viscosity may be found in disorders such as Waldenstrom macroglobulinemia.

[86041]
This test may also be called AChR antibody or myasthenia gravis (MG) binding antibody. The specimen is serum. Methods may include immunoassay, such as radioimmunoassay (RIA). The test measures the concentration of acetylcholine receptor (AChR) binding antibodies in the blood. Antibodies are proteins created by the immune system to fight foreign substances; autoantibodies can also develop and react with self-antigens, such as in MG. Binding antibodies work by binding to their specific antigen and alerting the immune system to send white blood cells to destroy the receptor and site. An increased blood concentration of AChR is associated with a higher likelihood of having MG; however, a lack of AChR does not rule out MG. AChR antibody affects the portion of nerve cell that transfers signals from nerves to muscles.

[86042]
This test measures the presence and concentration of acetylcholine receptor (AChR) blocking antibodies in the blood and is an indicator for myasthenia gravis (MG). The specimen is serum. Methods may include immunoassay. Antibodies are proteins created by the immune system to fight foreign substances; autoantibodies can also develop and react with self-antigens, such as in MG. AChR blocking antibodies work by functionally blocking nerve cell receptors so that the neurotransmitter acetylcholine is unable to bind to the nerve cell. These AChR blocking antibodies are usually seen in association with AChR binding antibodies. Therefore, the presence of AChR blocking antibodies in the blood may indicate the condition of MG. AChR antibody affects the portion of nerve cell that transfers signals from nerves to muscles.

[86043]
This test measures the presence and concentration of acetylcholine receptor (AChR) modulation antibodies in the blood and is an indicator for myasthenia gravis (MG). The specimen is serum. Methods may include immunoassay. Antibodies are proteins created by the immune system to fight foreign substances; autoantibodies can also develop and react with self-antigens, such as in MG. AChR modulation antibodies cause antigenic modulation, an internalization and degradation of antibody receptors that occurs when the antibodies crosslink receptor units. The presence of AChR modulating antibodies is associated with an increased risk of thymoma occurring with MG.

[86015]

Smooth muscle antibodies (SMA) are proteins produced by the body's immune system that attack smooth muscle tissues in the liver and other parts of the body. An actin (smooth muscle) antibody blood test (ASMA) detects these antibodies in the blood and is used primarily to diagnose various autoimmune diseases such as primary biliary cirrhosis and autoimmune hepatitis. In cases of autoimmune hepatitis, it also aids in the determination of whether the disorder is type 1 (the most common form) or type 2. Specimen is serum; method is enzyme-linked immunosorbent assay (ELISA). Report 86015 for each actin antibody tested.

86000

This test may be ordered as febrile agglutinins or febrile agglute; or separately as Brucella antibody titers, Francisella Murine typhus antibody titers, Q fever antibody titers, Rocky Mountain spotted fever titers. Method is agglutination. If positive at a screening dilution, quantitation may be performed. Serologic agglutination may be used to identify and measure an antigen/antibody response to an infectious disease.

86001

IgG is an immunoglobulin that may be a factor in some allergic reactions. Allergen IgG testing may be performed by RAST (radioallergosorbent) methodology or FETA.

86003

Method may be by agar gel diffusion, ELISA, or Western blot. Immunoglobulin E (IgE) testing may be used when skin testing is unreliable due to generalized dermatitis or severe dermatographism, or when the patient is unable to discontinue use of antihistamines. This study is reported once per each crude allergen extract.

86005

This test may be ordered as a RAST (radioallergosorbent test) or by any of the several brand name products available. Blood specimen is serum. Method is contact reagent. A disk, sponge, or card is exposed to the patient's blood. A change in color indicates the presence of antibodies, indicating an "allergic" status.

86008

Method is agar gel diffusion, ELISA, or Western blot. Immunoglobulin E (IgE) testing is used when skin testing is unreliable due to generalized dermatitis or severe dermatographism, or when the patient is unable to discontinue use of antihistamines. This code is reported once per recombinant or purified allergen component.

86021

This test may also be ordered as alloantibody identification, or alloagglutinin identification (the term "isoantibodies" is archaic). The term autoantibody may also be used. Leukocyte antibodies correlate closely to human leukocyte antigens, a complex genetic code for the immune system. The leukocyte antibody side of the equation may be referred to as alloagglutinins. This type of test is usually ordered to predict for one of several disorders: severe immune reactions from fetomaternal leukocyte incompatibility and/or neonatal incompatibilities, post-blood transfusion reactions, and poor blood component viability following transfusion. Alloantibodies arising from previous pregnancies and transfusions may be evident years after antigen exposure. Autoantibodies are usually identified with autoimmune disorders and infectious diseases. Methods may include agglutination and flow cytometry.

86022

This test may also be requested as serotonin release test. Platelets are small irregularly shaped cells, lacking a nucleus. Platelets serve a variety of functions, including providing a surface area for a variety of reactions. Autoantibodies develop in response to the body's own platelets as a result of idiopathic thrombocytopenia. Alloantibodies develop following exposure to outside antigens, often from blood transfusions. Certain drugs may also induce platelet antibodies. Blood specimen is serum, requiring special handling. Methods include indirect immunofluorescence (IIF), flow cytometry, enzyme linked immunosorbent assay (ELISA).

86023

This test may be ordered as a platelet-associated IgG. Platelets are small irregularly shaped cells, lacking a nucleus. Platelets serve a variety of functions, including providing a surface area for a variety of reactions. This test may be associated with idiopathic thrombocytopenia purpurea (ITP), a serious disorder involving low platelet counts. Method may commonly be by immunofluorescence (IF) or radial immunodiffusion (RID). IgG may also be detected by indirect assay involving interaction between patient blood product and normal platelets.

86036-86037

Antibodies are proteins created by the immune system to fight foreign substances such as bacteria and viruses. However, the antineutrophil cytoplasmic antibodies (ANCA) attack the type of white blood cells known as neutrophils by mistake, which can lead to autoimmune vasculitis. Causing inflammation and swelling of the blood vessels, the disorder is differentiated by which of the two main types of ANCA are present; each targets a specific protein inside the neutrophils. The ANCA screen identifies and differentiates the antibodies in the blood, which aids in diagnosis and treatment. Specimen type is serum; method is indirect fluorescent antibody (IFA) or enzyme-linked immunosorbent assay (ELISA). Report 86036 once for each antibody screen. If the ANCA screen is positive, a titer may be performed to determine the amount of antibody present. A serum sample is diluted in steps; each dilution is tested for the antibody's presence. The titer is the greatest dilution at which the antibody can be found. The higher the titer, the more antibody is present in the blood. Report 86037 for each antibody titer performed.

86038
This test may be ordered as antinuclear antibodies (ANA) test or, less commonly, nuclear binding antibody (NBA). The specimen is serum. Methods include indirect immunofluorescent methodology and enzyme-linked immunoassay (ELISA). This test is used to measure autoantibodies to the nucleus of human cells and may be used as a screening test for autoimmune diseases such as systemic lupus erythematosus (SLE) and the family of diseases commonly known as scleroderma.

86039
This test may be ordered as antinuclear antibodies (ANA) titer or, less commonly, nuclear binding antibody (NBA) titer. The specimen is serum. Methods include indirect immunofluorescent methodology and enzyme-linked immunoassay (ELISA). The test is used to measure autoantibodies in the nucleus of human cells and may be used as a screening test for autoimmune diseases such as systemic lupus erythematosus (SLE) and the family of diseases known as scleroderma.

86060
The test is ordered as antistreptolysin O (ASO) titer. The specimen is serum. Method is hemagglutination. The test is used for serological documentation of a group A streptococcal infection and may be used as a screening test for acute rheumatic fever, or glomerulonephritis.

86063
This test may be ordered as antistreptolysin O (ASO) screen. The specimen is serum. Methods include hemagglutination and slide agglutination. The test is used for serological documentation of a group A streptococcal infection and may be used as a screening test for acute rheumatic fever or glomerulonephritis.

[86051, 86052, 86053]
The aquaporin-4 protein (AQP4) is a normal protein found in several body systems, particularly in central nervous system tissues. Approximately 70 percent of individuals with neuromyelitis optica (NMO), an autoimmune disorder that affects the nerves of the eyes and the central nervous system, produce an antibody (an immune protein) that binds to the AQP4 protein. Although antibodies normally bind to certain foreign particles and germs, targeting them for destruction, the antibody in those with NMO attacks a normal human protein and is referred to as an autoantibody. Test may be requested as NMOFS. In 86051, the AQP4 antibody is detected using enzyme-linked immunosorbent immunoassay (ELISA); in 86052 using cell-based immunofluorescence assay (CBA), each; and in 86053 using fluorescence-activated cell sorting (also referred to as FACS or flow cytometry), each. Specimen type is serum.

86077
This physician service is an assessment of crossmatch blood work and/or evaluation of irregular antibody prior to transfusion. This type of physician review may be called for when anomalies arise in the antibody evaluation. An interpretation and written report are specifically required in the code description.

86078
This physician service is an assessment of transfusion reaction, including suspicion of transmissible disease. This type of assessment occurs following transfusion and an interpretation and written report are specifically required in the code description. Common reactions include fever and hives. Of greater concern are anaphylactic shock, graft-versus-host disease, and pulmonary edema.

86079
This physician service involves a written authorization to deviate from standard blood banking procedures. Many facilities maintain rare antigen variants well beyond recommended storage life simply to ensure availability. The code reports the authorization to transfuse this type of blood product, as well as product with incompatible Rh to the recipient. A written report is required.

86140
This test may be ordered as a C-reactive protein (CRP). The specimen is serum. The test may be performed by one of several methods, including latex agglutination and enzyme-linked immunoassay (ELISA). Elevated levels of C-reactive protein may be used as a measure for nonspecific inflammatory response. High levels of CRP may be present in bacterial infection, some tumors and various types of tissue damage, but more commonly in acute rheumatic fever and rheumatoid arthritis.

86141
C-reactive protein is released into the bloodstream when the blood vessels leading to the heart are damaged, which qualifies it is a nonspecific marker of inflammation. Measurement of C-reactive protein by high sensitivity CRP (hsCRP) assays adds to the predictive value of other markers used to assess a variety of conditions which can lead to elevated serum concentration of CRP, including inflammation, infection, and malignancy. C-reactive protein, hsCRP is also used to assess cardiovascular and peripheral vascular disease. Serum or plasma is the specimen. CRP assay involves the coating of artificially produced particles (i.e., Latex) with an antibody specific to human CRP aggregate in the presence of CRP from the patient sample of formed immune complex. The immune complex causes an increase in light scattering that is proportional to the concentration of CRP in the sample. The light scattering is quantified optically by measuring turbidity.

86146
Beta 2 glycoprotein 1 antibody actually refers to a group of autoantibodies used as serological markers for antiphospholipid syndrome (APS). APS is characterized by recurrent arterial and venous thrombosis as well as recurrent fetal loss. These autoantibodies are natural regulators of the blood coagulation cascade. Blood specimen is serum or

citrated plasma. Method is enzyme-linked immunoassay (ELISA). The test may be repeated at regular intervals.

86147
This test may also be ordered as antiphospholipid antibody or anticardiolipin antibodies (ACA). The specimen is serum. Method is enzyme-linked immunoassay (ELISA). The test may be used to classify patients with recurrent venous or arterial thrombosis, thrombocytopenia (low platelet count), recurrent fetal loss, and acquired valvular heart disease, and systemic lupus erythematosus (SLE).

[86152, 86153]
A sample of blood (or other fluid) is taken. Techniques are used to isolate certain types of cells (e.g., metastatic malignancy cells) within the sample. These cells are counted and reported. Technology today allows a single malignant cell to be identified in a vial of blood, helping determine if a more aggressive or different therapy modality should be tried. Report 86152 for the cell enumeration test. Report 86153 for the interpretation and report of the test when applicable.

86148
Testing for antiphosphatidylserine antibodies, a class of phospholipid antibodies, identifies various autoimmune disorders and antiphospholipid syndrome in patients that are negative for anticardiolipin antibodies. Antiphospholipid syndrome (APS) is an autoimmune condition that may manifest with fetal loss, thrombosis, or autoimmune thrombocytopenia. The specimen is serum. The method of testing is enzyme immunoassay.

86155
This test may be ordered as phagocytic cell function evaluation, NBT slide assay, or DCF assay. The specimen is whole blood. The method is gel agar diffusion. Live neutrophils are required for a successful test. This test may be used for screening infections, perinatal abscesses, multiple episodes of pneumonia, or delayed wound healing may be tested. Patients under treatment for malignancy or those treated with immunosuppressive antiviral therapies may also be candidates.

86156
This test may be ordered as cold agglute or thermal amplitude assay. The specimen is serum. Method is hemagglutination. The test may be used to provide an early detection of an immunoglobulin M (IgM) class antibody, which may be present in acute primary atypical pneumonia (Mycoplasma pneumoniae) and certain hemolytic anemias. Low levels of cold agglutinins have been demonstrated in malaria, peripheral vascular disease, and common respiratory diseases.

86157
This test may be ordered as cold agglute titer or thermal amplitude assay. The specimen is serum The method is hemagglutination. This test may be used to screen immunoglobulin M (IgM) class antibody, which may be present in acute primary atypical pneumonia (Mycoplasma pneumoniae) and certain hemolytic anemias. Low levels of cold agglutinins have been demonstrated in malaria, peripheral vascular disease, and common respiratory diseases.

86160
This test may be ordered as individual complement components 2-5 or Factor B. The specimen is serum. Methodology is radial immunodiffusion or nephelometry. Complement activation is a multi-component biological response function of the immune system present in inflammatory conditions; the degree of complement activation may be used to indicate the intensity of the inflammatory process. Syndromes associated with complement activation include rheumatoid arthritis, systemic lupus erythematosus (SLE), gram negative sepsis, and chronic hepatitis.

86161
This test may be ordered as an individual complement component. The specimen is serum. Methodology is radial immunodiffusion or nephelometry. Complement activation is a multi-component biological response function of the immune system present in inflammatory conditions; the degree of complement activation may be used to indicate the intensity of the inflammatory process. Syndromes associated with complement activation include rheumatoid arthritis, systemic lupus erythematosus (SLE), gram negative sepsis, and chronic hepatitis.

86162
This test may be ordered as complement CH50, total. The specimen is serum. Methodology involves an indicator system using predetermined amounts of sheep red blood cells coated with antibody and is measured by spectrophotometry. Complement activation is a multi-component biological response function of the immune system present in inflammatory conditions; the degree of complement activation may be used to indicate the intensity of the inflammatory process. Syndromes associated with complement activation include rheumatoid arthritis, systemic lupus erythematosus (SLE), gram negative sepsis, and chronic hepatitis.

86171
This test may be ordered as a complement assay. The complementary system involves enzymes and regulatory proteins synthesized in the liver. Activation of the system triggers a cascading, or sequential, response that may lead to histamine release, inflammation, and other normal activities of the immune system. Blood specimen is serum. Complement fixation is widely used test that relies on these principles. The test may be used for a wide variety of suspected illnesses, including viral infections.

86200
This test may also be known as anti-CCP or CCP antibodies. The test is used to diagnose rheumatoid

arthritis (RA) in the earliest stages. The specimen is serum and the method of testing is by enzyme linked immunosorbent assay. (ELISA).

86215
This test may be ordered as DNA antibody. This test is probably a remnant of an earlier test to detect the DNA antibody and is not in common use.

86225
This test may be ordered as anti-DNA, anti-ds-DNA, dsDNA antibody, or anti-native DNA. The specimen is serum. Methods include indirect immunofluorescent assay and enzyme-linked immunosorbent assay (ELISA). This test may be performed for patients previously diagnosed with systemic lupus erythematous (SLE). These patients may exhibit a high level of antibody against their own native double-stranded DNA, and results of the test may indicate renal involvement. This test for the double-stranded DNA. Low levels of the antibody may be found in other autoimmune disorders such as Sjogren's syndrome, mixed connective tissue disease, and progressive systemic sclerosis.

86226
This test may be ordered as ssDNA, antibody IgG, or anti-single stranded DNA. The specimen is serum. Method is enzyme-linked immunosorbent assay (ELISA). Single stranded DNA antibodies are found in 20 to 30 percent of all cases of systemic lupus erythematosus (SLE), and less specific in the diagnosis of SLE compared to double-stranded DNA antibodies. Lower levels of double-stranded DNA antibodies are associated with chronic inflammatory processes, malignancy, drug-induced lupus, or cardiolipin antibodies (cross-reaction).

86231
This test looks for specific antibodies in the blood that may indicate celiac disease, an autoimmune disease in which the immune system responds abnormally to the protein gluten. Antibodies to gluten, known as endomysial antibodies or EMA, cause the intestine to swell and may damage the small intestine if not detected. Specimen is serum; method is indirect fluorescent antibody. Report 86231 once for each immunoglobulin (Ig) class. The IgA EMA test is the most specific test for celiac disease, having a specificity of close to 100 percent.

86235
Examples of antibodies covered by this code are listed in the CPT description; however, other antibodies may also be reported with this code. This test is performed to detect antibodies associated with systemic lupus erythematosus (SLE) and mixed connective tissue disease. Anti-Sm is highly specific for SLE. Anti-RNP is found with a variety of rheumatoid diseases. The specimen is serum. The most common method of testing is flow cytometry.

86255-86256
These codes report detection of noninfectious agents using fluorescent agent antibody technique. A number of noninfectious agents are reported with codes 86255 and 86256. Some antibodies reported with these codes include: acetylcholine receptor antibody (anti-AChR); adrenal cortex antibodies; anti D. S., DNA, IFA using C. Luciliae; mitochondrial antibody, liver; smooth muscle antibody; antineutrophil antibody; endomysial antibody; parietal cell antibody; and myositis-specific auto antibody. Code 86255 is a screen and reports the presence of the antibody only. Code 86256 is a titer and reports the level of antibody present.

86258
This test looks for levels of deamidated gliadin antibodies in the blood. These are indicative of celiac disease, an autoimmune disease in which the immune system responds abnormally to the protein gluten. Most individuals with untreated celiac disease have elevated levels of these antibodies. If undiagnosed, the small intestine may be damaged and malnutrition may occur. The test may be requested as deamidated gliadin peptide antibodies, DGP, DGP-AGA, or DGP IgA and IgG. Specimen is serum; method is enzyme-linked immunosorbent assay (ELISA). Report 86258 once for each immunoglobulin (Ig) class.

86277
This test may also be ordered as somatotropin antibody, GH antibody test, or IGF (insulin-like growth factor) antibody. Portions of the pituitary gland secrete growth hormone. Serum levels normally rise and fall throughout the day. Radioimmunoassay (RIA) is the method of choice.

86280
This is a general methodology code for any test that measures the ability of soluble antigen to inhibit the agglutination of antigen-coated red blood cells by antibodies. In this test, a fixed amount of antibodies to the antigen in question is mixed with a fixed amount of red blood cells coated with the antigen (see passive hemagglutination above). Also included in the mixture are the sample to be analyzed for the presence of the antigen. If the sample contains the antigen, the soluble antigen will compete with the antigen coated on the red blood cells for binding to the antibodies, thereby inhibiting the agglutination of the red blood cells. The sample varies. This test is useful in identifying secretor status of an individual in saliva and used for antibody identification workups.

86294
This code may be requested as a single step qualitative or semi-quantitative immunoassay to identify the presence of a specific tumor antigen. The specimen is serum. Method is immunoassay.

86300
This test may also be requested as CEA carbohydrate antigen 15-3. Method is immunoassay or ICMA. Quantitative analysis for CA 15-3 is used primarily to monitor patients for recurrence of breast cancer after diagnosis and initial treatment or to evaluate response

to therapy. Elevated levels are often indicative of a recurrence or a failed treatment.

86301
This test may also be requested as carbohydrate antigen 19-9. The specimen is serum. Method is immunoassay. Quantitative analysis for CA 19-9 is used primarily as a marker for pancreatic cancer. It identifies recurrence and monitors patients. It is also used to monitor gastrointestinal, head/neck, and gynecological cancer. It may identify recurrence of stomach, colorectal, liver, gallbladder, and urothelial malignancies.

86304
This test may also be requested as cancer antigen 125. The specimen is serum. Method is immunoassay. CA 125 is found in ovarian cancers, and some endometrium and fallopian tube cancers. Testing for CA 125 is performed primarily to detect residual tumor in women who have been previously diagnosed with ovarian malignancy.

86305
The gene for human epididymis protein 4 (HE4) is among those most often identified in gene expression profiles of epithelial ovarian carcinomas and has been shown to be elevated in a high percentage of women with ovarian cancer. This test is used as an aid in monitoring disease progression or recurrence; the specimen is blood.

86308-86310
These tests may be requested as a heterophile antibody screen and/or titer. Heterophile antibodies are commonly tested to diagnose infectious mononucleosis. Blood specimen is serum or plasma. Method is agglutination. Code 86308 is a screen that identifies the presence of the antibody only; while 86309 is a titer that identifies the level of antibody present. Code 86310 reports a more specific methodology for testing heterophile titers using both beef cells and guinea pig kidneys.

86316
This test is an immunoassay for tumor antigen and may be requested by the specific antigen. Some of the more common tumor antigens include carbohydrate antigen 549 (CA 549), carbohydrate antigen 72-4 (CA 72-4, TAG 72), and carbohydrate antigen 50 (CA 50). Each of these antigens is specific for certain types of cancer. CA 549 is found in Stage IV metastatic breast cancer and is used primarily to evaluate response to therapy.

86317
This code may be requested to measure the amount of specific infectious disease antibodies in the blood that are not otherwise specified. It would normally be obtained subsequent to qualitative or semi-quantitative immunoassays (86318, 86602-86804), which identify the presence of specific antibodies but do not measure the amount of antibody present. Method is immunoassay.

86318
This code may be requested as a single step qualitative or semi-quantitative immunoassay to identify the presence of specific infectious agent antibodies. Specimen is serum. Method is immunoassay. Single step methods frequently use a reagent strip for the specific antibody.

[86328]
This code reports immunoassay antibody testing for severe acute respiratory syndrome coronavirus 2 using a single-step method such as a reagent strip. The test may be requested as single-step qualitative or semi-quantitative; infectious agent specificity may also include terminology such as SARS-CoV-2, coronavirus disease, or COVID-19. In one method, a reagent strip, pre-coated with appropriate IgM and IgG antibodies, is taken from its sealed container following collection of blood or serum from the patient. The sample is placed in the specimen well and diluent is added. Once the specimen and reagents react with the strip's test area, the specimen is read and results are interpreted and reported.

86320
This code may be abbreviated as serum IEP. Blood specimen is serum. This code is used to report a technique most often used to identify monoclonal gammopathy or lymphoproliferative processes, specifically myelomas. It combines electrophoresis and immunodiffusion. This test is qualitative only.

86325
This code may be abbreviated as IEP. A random urine specimen is obtained. CSF is obtained by separately reportable spinal puncture. This code is used to report a technique most often used to identify monoclonal gammopathy or lymphoproliferative processes, specifically myelomas. It combines electrophoresis and immunodiffusion. This test is qualitative only.

86329-86331
These tests may be abbreviated as ID. Immunodiffusion (86329) involves an antibody-antigen reaction that causes a visible precipitate to form. It is a technique used in identifying immunoglobulin. Ouchterlony gel diffusion (86331) involves evaluation of the precipitin reaction in a clear gel. Immune complex assays were once thought to be a promising diagnostic technique. However, they have generally been replaced with tests that are more specific, more standardized, and less expensive. Blood specimen is serum which requires special handling. Method is a complement binding (CP) technique.

86332
Immune complex assays were once thought to be a promising diagnostic technique. However, they have generally been replaced with tests that are more specific, more standardized, and less expensive. Blood specimen is obtained by venipuncture. Method is a complement binding (CP) technique.

86334-86335
Immunofixation electrophoresis (IFE) is a method or technique used to detect the presence of aberrant proteins, especially monoclonal proteins, and to identify when certain protein groups are being increased or decreased in blood serum or urine, particularly. This test can help diagnose and monitor the progression of diseases like multiple myeloma, monoclonal gammopathies, and kidney-damaging diseases. The specimen is serum. For urine testing, a 24-hour urine specimen is required. IFE involves high-resolution electrophoresis combined with immunoprecipitation The value in performing immunofixation electrophoresis is identifying the presence of a particular type of protein, or immunoglobulin. Report 86334 for a serum test and 86335 for another fluid, such as urine or cerebral spinal fluid.

86336
Inhibin A is a protein hormone related to pregnancy which is a screening marker of Down Syndrome. Testing for high levels of Inhibin A may be considered as a fourth hormone check that increases the accuracy of screening for Down Syndrome in addition to alpha-fetoprotein (AFP), human chorionic gonadotropin (HCG or hCG), and estriol levels. In Down Syndrome, Inhibin A and HCG protein hormone levels tend to be high while the other two tend to be low. The Inhibin A pregnancy hormone level is tested from maternal serum in the 16th to 18th week of gestation. A serum sample is from the mother and radioimmunoassay (RIA) may be used to analyze the sample.

86337
This test may be requested as insulin antibody or anti-insulin Ab. It usually includes testing for antibodies to both beef and pork insulin. Insulin dependent diabetics sometimes develop IgG antibodies to insulin, which can cause insulin resistance making larger doses of insulin necessary to achieve the same level of control. However, they may also develop IgA, IgM, IgD, and IgE antibodies. Most of these antibodies do not cause clinical problems. The specimen is serum. Method is radioimmunoassay (RIA), radiobinding assay, or enzyme linked immunosorbent assay (ELISA).

86340
This test may be requested as intrinsic factor (IF) antibody. There are two types of IF antibody. Type I, blocking antibody, is the more common of the two. It prevents binding of B12 with intrinsic factor but will not react with complex intrinsic factor. Type II antibody, binding antibody, reacts with either free of complex IF. The specimen is serum. Method is radioimmunoassay (RIA).

86341
This test detects the formation of antibodies to the pancreatic islet cell, which causes destruction of those cells and, therefore, loss of an individual's ability to produce insulin. The presence of islet cell antibodies are helpful in establishing an initial diagnosis of Type I, insulin-dependent diabetes mellitus (IDDM) and in identifying those individuals at high risk of developing IDDM. It is also useful in identifying potential transplant donors for pancreatic islet cells. The specimen is serum. Various methods are used.

86343
This test is performed to quantify the levels of histamine. The specimen is plasma. Urine is collected over a 24-hour period. Methods are fluorometric, radioenzymatic, and immunoassay. Allergic and non-allergic intolerance to drugs, insect venom, paints or cosmetics, as well as heat or cold, or stress may induce histamine release. By using the histamine release test it is possible to identify a broad spectrum of allergies.

86344
Abnormalities in leukocyte phagocytosis may be used as a screen for a variety of disorders. The specimen is whole blood. Method is flow cytometry or fluorescence microscopy. Leukocytes protect against infection and immunological disease in a process called phagocytosis. It involves ingesting and killing invading microbes inside biological compartments called phagolysosomes.

86352
The human immune system consists of two separate yet interrelated forms of immunity: humoral immunity and cell-mediated immunity (CMI). The measurement of CMI is useful in many applications, including clinical management of organ transplant recipients, management of infectious diseases such as HIV or HCV, cancer, autoimmunity, and development of drugs and vaccines. This cellular function assay detects CMI in whole blood in immunosuppressed patients by measuring their early response to immune system stimulation and detection of adenosine triphosphate (ATP), a biomarker.

86353
This test may also be requested as lymphocyte mitogen response test or phytohemagglutinin (PHA) stimulation. Lymphocytes are normally produced early in an immune response. This test is used to determine the adequacy of early immune response using nonspecific mitogens or specific antigens as transforming agents capable of inducing blastogenesis. This process involves isolation of lymphocytes in peripheral blood and culture of the isolated lymphocytes in microtiter plates for three to seven days. Prior to harvest of cultured cells, the lymphocytes are pulsed with triturated thymidine. Incorporated thymidine is measured. Control values are used to calculate a stimulation index.

86355
This test may also be referred to as a B lymphocyte assay. B cells, also known as B lymphocytes, are responsible for making antibodies. B cells develop and mature in the bone marrow. An increased B cell count may be indicative of such diseases as chronic

lymphocytic leukemia, multiple myeloma, Waldenstrom's macroglobulinemia, and DiGeorge syndrome. Decreased B cell count may indicate such conditions as acute lymphoblastic leukemia and congenital and acquired immunoglobulin deficiency disorders. The specimen is whole blood. The quantitative number of B lymphocytes is determined using flow cytometry.

86356

Using specific antibody labeling with flow cytometry measurement, this test detects the amount of specific antigens on mononuclear cells (lymphocytes, dendritic cells, monocytes, macrophages). This test distinguishes cellular disorders such as cancer and autoimmune diseases that have different antigen markers. This code is reported for each antigen.

[86366]

This test measures the presence and concentration of muscle-specific kinase (MuSK) antibody in the blood as a diagnostic indicator of myasthenia gravis (MG). The specimen is serum. Methods include radioimmunoprecipitation assay (RIPA). This test may be used when an acetylcholine receptor (AChR) antibody test is negative, but MG is still suspected. While a positive MuSK antibody test may indicate the condition of MG, a negative test does not rule out MG. MuSK antibodies occur at neuromuscular junctions where nerve endings and muscle fibers meet and interfere with signal transmission between nerves and muscles.

[86362, 86363]

The presence of myelin oligodendrocyte glycoprotein (MOG-IgG1) antibodies may be indicative of certain autoimmune spectrum disorders. This antibody test may be ordered to aid in the diagnosis of inflammatory demyelinating diseases (IDD) such as optic neuritis, transverse myelitis, neuromyelitis optica (NMO), or acute disseminated encephalomyelitis (ADEM). Report 86362 for each test performed by cell-based immunofluorescence assay (CBA); report 86363 for each test performed by flow cytometry (fluorescence-activated cell sorting or FACS). Specimen is serum.

86357

This is a blood test that provides a total count of target cells that are killed by natural killer (NK) cells. The total count of cells killed by NK cells is compared to total live cells to determine NK activity. NK cells are lymphocytes that have many functions, one of which is to produce a cytotoxic chemical called tumor necrosis factor (TNF). This is a chemical that kills malignant (cancer) cells in the body. However, in some women NK cells attack the embryo in early pregnancy causing spontaneous abortion. The specimen is whole blood. NK cells are separated from the blood and are cultured at different dilutions with target cells from an embryonic cancer cell line. These target cells have been tagged with cytoplasmic dye. Flow cytometry is used to identify the target cells that have been killed by the NK cells. Flow cytometry is used to precisely count the percentage of dead to live cells at the different dilutions.

[86364]

This test may be ordered for individuals suspected of having celiac disease (an autoimmune disease in which the immune system responds abnormally to the protein gluten) and will be positive in approximately 98 percent of those with celiac disease who are on a diet that contains gluten. It may also be ordered as a screening test for dermatitis herpetiformis (a chronic skin condition caused by a reaction to the ingestion of gluten). Other indications for this test include monitoring the adherence to gluten-free diets in patients with these diseases. The test may be requested as tTG. Specimen is serum; method is enzyme-linked immunosorbent assay (ELISA).

86359

This test may also be referred to as T-cell assay, T-cell analysis, or T-cell study. It is used to quantitate total T-cell lymphocytes without providing absolute counts of the different types of lymphocytes. Examples of different types of lymphocytes included in the total count are CD3, CD4, CD8, CD20, CD38, etc. The specimen is whole blood. Whole blood is added to fluorochrome-labeled antibodies, also referred to as monoclonal antibodies, which bind specifically to cell surface antigens on lymphocytes. This is used in conjunction with flow cytometry to obtain the total T-cell count. This test is used to type and classify different types of lymphomas and lymphocytic leukemias as well as to monitor immunodeficiency states, including HIV infections.

86360

This test may also be requested as T4/T8 ratio, CD4/CD8 ratio, T-cell assay for CD4/CD8. It is used to quantitate CD4 and CD8 specifically, and from those counts to obtain a CD4 to CD8 ratio. Whole blood is added to fluorochrome-labeled antibodies, also referred to as monoclonal antibodies, which bind specifically to cell surface antigens on lymphocytes. This is used in conjunction with flow cytometry to obtain the CD4 and CD8 cell counts. This test is used primarily in staging HIV infection and monitoring the effects of treatment. It may also be useful in diagnosing and monitoring congenital immunodeficiencies.

86361

This test may also be requested as T-cell assay for CD4. The specimen. Whole blood is added to fluorochrome-labeled antibodies, also referred to as monoclonal antibodies, which bind specifically to cell surface antigens on lymphocytes. This is used in conjunction with flow cytometry to obtain the CD4 cell count. This test is used primarily in staging HIV infection and monitoring the effects of treatment. It may also be useful in diagnosing and monitoring congenital immunodeficiencies.

86367
Many different subsets of stem cells are present in the blood and bone marrow. Some stem cell subtypes are able to differentiate into several cell types. These are called multipotent or multilineage stem cells. Multipotent stem cells have the capacity to differentiate into myeloid, lymphoid, erythroid, and megakaryocytic lineages. Other stem cell subtypes are lineage specific and differentiate only to a single cell type. While there is no test to specifically identify the multipotent stem cells, it has been discovered that high counts of progenitor cells with surface antigen CD34+ enhance engraftment in stem cell transplant recipients. This test quantifies the total number of specific stem cells subtypes in the body, such as stem cells with surface antigen CD34+ cells. Periodic blood samples are obtained to determine total amounts of circulating CD34+ cells. Flow cytometry is used to identify specific stem cell subtypes and to determine total counts of CD34+ cells. Using this test the physician can determine when the total number of circulating stem cells containing CD34+ is sufficient to begin harvesting stem cells for subsequent transplant.

86376
This test is performed to determine the presence of antithyroid microsomal antibodies. The specimen is serum. A hemagglutination test for thyroid antigens is used and, if that test is positive, it is followed by a fluorescent scan to show a decrease or absence of thyroid-stable iodine. Other methods include ELISA (enzyme linked immunosorbent assay) or particle agglutination (PA). The anti-microsomal antibody or microsomal antibody test may be used to diagnose conditions such as Hashimoto's thyroiditis and other autoimmune disorders. Hashimoto's disease is an autoimmune thyroid disorder characterized by the production of antibodies in response to thyroid antigens. Normal thyroid structures are replaced by lymphocytes and lymphoid germinal centers.

86381
A mitochondrial antibody test (M2 test) may be ordered to establish a diagnosis of primary biliary cirrhosis (PBC). A progressive disease of the liver caused by a buildup of bile, PBC can eventually lead to cirrhosis and liver failure. This test may also be performed on other mitochondrial antibodies, of which there are several (M1-M9) that are associated with various conditions; these antibodies are often used to detect specific liver cancers. Specimen type is serum; method is enzyme immunosorbent assay (EIA). Report 86381 for each mitochondrial antibody.

86382
Tissue samples may be collected by biopsy. Fluorescent dye may be used to identify the target virus directly from clinical specimens or tissue. Neutralization tests are used in various serological tests to identify antibodies to the target virus in serum (i.e., Herpes simplex virus). The identification aids in the diagnosis of diseases caused by the virus. Specimen type varies.

[86408, 86409]
Neutralizing antibodies (Nab) are responsible for defending cells against pathogens, or disease-causing organisms. Produced naturally by the body, their production can be prompted by infections and by vaccinations against infections. Code 86408 reports a SARS-CoV-2 neutralizing antibody screen. The patient's serum, diluent, and pseudovirion expressing the SARS-CoV-2 spike protein are combined with cultured cells. An incubation period follows, after which a substrate is added. This will luminesce if a viral infection is present. The signal is measured on a multi-well plate reader and the specimen compared to the control specimen. A qualitative result is generated. Code 86409 reports a SARS-CoV-2 neutralizing antibody titer. Dilutions of the patient's serum, target cells, and pseudovirion expressing the SARS-CoV-2 spike protein are incubated. Using quantitative or semi-quantitative assessment of the signal activity changes, the antibody-neutralizing activity is measured. The results are compared to the control specimen, interpreted, and reported. These tests are used to determine if antibodies present in a patient's specimen can directly block infection of cells from the COVID-19 virus.

[86413]
This antibody assay provides quantitative measurements of SARS-CoV-2 antibodies in order to examine the patient's adaptive immune response to the virus. Provision of precise measurement of the antibodies may help assess treatment effectiveness. Patient serum and diluent added to a SARS-CoV-2 spike protein receptor binding domain (RBD)-complexed solid-phase surface is incubated and washed. Antihuman-signal antibodies are then added to detect bound anti-RBD antibodies. The relative amount of the signal that is measured is directly proportionate to the specimen's anti-RBD antibody concentration. Interpretation is made using a standards-generated calibration curve. Results are reported in quantitative units.

86384
This code also may be ordered as Nitroblue Tetrazolium (NBT). The specimen is whole blood. A biochemical assay and simple laboratory equipment (microscope, incubator and centrifuge) are used to detect phagocytosis and intracellular killing of microorganisms by normal polymorphonuclear neutrophils. The test has been found to have several applications, including the detection of certain immunodeficiency disorders (i.e., AIDS), Hodgkin's disease, and chronic lymphocytic leukemia.

86386
Nuclear Matrix Protein 22 (NMP-22) is a tumor indicator for bladder cancer when found in significant quantities in a urine specimen. If a tumor is present, NMP-22, which is found within a cell's nucleus, increases 25 fold causing the NMP22 to shed into the urine.

86403-86406
These tests may be ordered as PA. The specimen is serum. There are several methods used in tandem with PA tests, such as fluorescence enzyme assay and scattered light flow cytometry. Particle agglutination (PA) tests may be performed to evaluate immune status to and diagnosis certain viruses (i.e., measles virus infection). Use 86403 to report each separate antibody screen, and 86406 to report each antibody tested according to titer.

86430
This test may be ordered as rheumatoid antibody (RA), arthritis screen, or rheumatoid factor (RF). The specimen is serum. The test is most significantly used as a qualitative measurement in evaluating patients with inflammatory polyarthritis. The presence of RF is not by itself usually considered sufficient to establish a diagnosis of rheumatoid arthritis, but as a contributing factor or a prognostic marker to a diagnosis. Testing methodology is by latex agglutination, ELISA, or nephelometry.

86431
This test may be ordered as rheumatoid antibody (RA) titer, arthritis screen, or rheumatoid factor (RF) titer. The specimen is serum. The test is most significantly used as a quantitative measurement in evaluating patients with inflammatory polyarthritis. The presence or quantity of RF is not by itself usually considered sufficient to establish a diagnosis of rheumatoid arthritis, but as a contributing factor or a prognostic marker to a diagnosis. Testing methodology is by latex agglutination, ELISA, or nephelometry.

86480-86481
Blood tests known as Interferon-Gamma Release Assays (IGRA) are used to diagnose both latent (non-active) tuberculosis (TB) infection and tuberculosis disease and may be performed instead of a skin test. The blood test can be accomplished in a single patient visit and, unlike the skin test, its results do not require subjective interpretation of a health worker. White blood cells from most individuals infected with *Mycobacterium tuberculosis* release interferon-gamma when mixed with substances that can produce an immune response (antigens) derived from *M. tuberculosis*; IGRAs measure an individual's immune reactivity. Testing is conducted by mixing fresh blood samples with antigens and controls; antigens, methods of testing, and criteria for interpretation differ. While both codes describe cell-mediated immunity (CMI) antigen response measurement, code 86480 is specific to gamma interferon, while 86481 specifies the enumeration of gamma interferon-producing T-cells in cell suspension.

86485
This test may be ordered as candida delayed hypersensitivity testing (DHT or DHR). The methods are the intradermal test and the prick test. Candida albicans is a common environmental yeast, and this testing is usually a control for immunocompetence or anergy. A standardized concentration of the yeast is introduced into the skin of the arm, usually by needle or skin prick. The test site is examined within 30 minutes and again at 24, 48, and 72-hour intervals. Evidence of a reaction is recorded.

86486
This code reports skin tests for antigens other than those for which a more specific code exists. Testing methods may consist of the intradermal test and the prick test. A standardized concentration of the antigen is introduced into the skin of the arm, usually by needle or skin prick. The test site is examined within specified time frames and evidence of a reaction is recorded.

86510
This test may be ordered as histoplasma skin test. Two testing methods are: the intradermal test and the prick test. A standardized concentration of antigen is introduced into the skin of the arm, usually be needle or skin prick. The site is examined within 30 minutes and again at 24, 48, and 72- hour intervals. Evidence of a reaction is recorded. This test has limited value diagnostically.

86580
This test may be ordered as TB skin test, TB delayed hypersensitivity testing (DHT or DHR), Tuberculin skin test, Mantoux test, or purified protein derivative test (PPD). A standardized concentration of tuberculin PPD is introduced into the skin of the arm. The method is intradermal. The test may screen individuals in high-risk circumstances, or as routine surveillance among certain populations regularly exposed (i.e., health care workers). Patients showing certain signs or symptoms are also tested. Culture extracts of tuberculin proteins in a test dosage is injected intradermally (forearm). The test site is examined at 24, 48, and 72-hour intervals for evidence of induration. Evidence of a reaction is recorded.

86581
Streptococcus pneumoniae immunoglobulin G (IgG) antibody levels are evaluated using multiplex immunoassay in a patient who has received a pure polysaccharide or protein conjugated pneumococcal vaccine. This test is performed to determine the patient's immune response to the vaccine and ensure that adequate antibody levels were produced. Various serotypes responsible for pneumococcal infections are tested. Quantitative results are reported. The specimen is serum.

86590
This test is commonly ordered as ASO. The specimen is serum. The test is useful for detection of antibody to an extracellular antigenic product of group A streptococci and commonly used to detect previous exposure to group A strep. The test may be performed by latex agglutination or enzyme-linked immunosorbent assay (ELISA).

86592
This nontreponemal (screening) antibody test is commonly ordered as RPR (rapid plasma reagin), STS

(serologic test for syphilis), VDRL (venereal disease research laboratory), or ART (automated reagin test). It may also be ordered as standard test for syphilis. The specimen is serum. The test is commonly used to provide a diagnosis (screening test) for syphilis. The method is by nontreponemal rapid plasma reagin (RPR)-particle agglutination test. More recently, it is being performed by automated methodology, such as enzyme-linked immunosorbent assay (ELISA).

86593
This nontreponemal (screening) test is commonly ordered as quantitative RPR (rapid plasma reagin), STS (serologic test for syphilis), VDRL (venereal disease research laboratory), or ART (automated reagin test). This test may also be ordered as a standard test for syphilis. The specimen is serum. It is most commonly used to provide a monitor for treatment, or to establish a diagnosis of reinfection with syphilis. The method is nontreponemal rapid plasma reagin-particle agglutination test or anticardiolipin antibodies. More recently, it is being performed by automated methodology, such as by enzyme-linked immunosorbent assay (ELISA).

86596
Voltage-gated calcium channels (VGCC) are immunologic targets for a variety of diseases, and are divided into five types (L, N, P/Q, R, and T) depending on tissues and pharmacological properties. This test detects VGCC antibodies and is used to aid in the evaluation of autoimmune diseases such as Lambert-Eaton myasthenic syndrome (LEMS), paraneoplastic as well as non-paraneoplastic cerebellar degeneration, and small cell lung cancer. Detection of these antibodies may also aid in the diagnosis of autoimmune responses in individuals with a history of cancer. Specimen is serum; method is quantitative radioimmunoassay. Report 86596 for each antibody tested.

86602
This test is commonly ordered as anti-actinomyces or actinomyces antibody titer. The specimen is serum. The test is used as a rapid serological method to diagnose for nocardial infections (infections caused by *Nocardia*, a genus of gram-positive bacteria). The methods are: complement fixation (CF), immunodiffusion, agglutination assay, and Western blot (immunoblot).

86603
This test is commonly ordered as anti-adenovirus titer or adenovirus antibody titer. The specimen is serum. The test is traditionally used as a rapid serological method to diagnose for adenovirus infections. The methods are: complement fixation (CF), immunofluorescent, and enzyme-linked immunosorbent assay (ELISA).

86606
This test is commonly ordered as anti-aspergillus titer or aspergillus antibody titer. The specimen serum. The test is used as a rapid serological method to diagnose for aspergillus infection. The methods are: complement fixation (CF), counterimmunoelectrophoresis, radioimmunoassay, immunofluorescence, enzyme-linked immunosorbent assay (ELISA), and immunodiffusion.

86609
This test is commonly ordered as a generic test for any bacterium that has not otherwise been specified. This test will usually utilize the words anti, titer, or antibody. The specimen is serum. The test is traditionally used as a rapid serological method to diagnose bacterial infections. The methods are: complement fixation (CF), immunofluorescence, and enzyme-linked immunosorbent assay (ELISA).

86611
This test may also be known as bacillary angiomatosis (BA) or bacillary peliosis (BP) antibody. IgG testing may be used to identify current or past infection whereas IgM is more specific for current infection. The specimen is serum. Methods include enzyme immunoassay (EIA) and indirect fluorescence antibody test. The *Bartonella genus* of bacteria is implicated in a variety of life-threatening infections. Exposure to the bacillus and presence of antibodies may remain asymptomatic. An opportunistic infection arising in some AIDS patients is linked to the *Bartonella genus* and is noted for vascular lesions.

86612
This test is commonly ordered as anti-Blastomyces or Blastomyces antibody titer. It may occasionally be ordered as "blasto" titer. The specimen is serum. The test is used as a rapid serological method to diagnose for Blastomyces infections. The methods are: complement fixation (CF), immunodiffusion, agglutination assay, immunofluorescence, enzyme-linked immunosorbent assay (ELISA), and Western blot (immunoblot).

86615
This test may be ordered as pertussis or whooping cough antibody. *Bordetella pertussis* is the causative agent of whooping cough. This test demonstrates antibodies, which is not a common approach to developing a clinical diagnosis due to the time required for seroconversion. However, it may be used to evaluate immunity following immunization. Blood specimen is serum. Methods include enzyme-linked immunosorbent assay (ELISA), microhemagglutination, complement fixation (CF), and toxin neutralization.

86617
This test may be ordered as a Lyme disease confirmation test. *Borrelia burgdorferi* is the causative agent of Lyme disease (the vector being a tick). Antibodies usually build up in patients several weeks or longer into an infection. This test is confirmatory, meaning previous diagnostic work has been performed. Blood specimen is serum. CSF specimen is obtained by spinal puncture that is reported separately. This test reports a second test for

confirmation by immunoblot or Western blot. It may also be used to establish a diagnosis following indeterminate ELISA results.

86618
This test may be ordered simply as a Lyme disease antibody test. *Borrelia burgdorferi* is the causative agent of Lyme disease (the vector being a tick). Antibodies usually build up in patients several weeks or longer into an infection. Blood specimen is serum. CSF specimen is obtained by spinal puncture, which is reported separately. Methods include enzyme-linked immunosorbent assay (ELISA), enzyme immunoassay (EIA), indirect fluorescent antibody (IFA), or specific IgG, IgM, and IgA by antibody capture.

86619
This test may be ordered as a relapsing fever antibody. Relapsing fever is caused by spirochetes of the genus *Borrelia,* and those infected suffer alternating fevers and chills. Ticks and body lice are the vectors to humans. Blood specimen is serum. Literature is unclear about methods and reasons to order such testing. Indications are that this test is rarely performed.

86622
Brucellosis is a rare illness caused by bacteria from the genus *Brucella*. Humans contract the disease by ingesting meat or dairy products of infected cattle, sheep, or wild game animals. Direct infection from animals to humans may also occur and is found predominantly in workers in the livestock and meat processing industries. Blood specimen is serum. Standard tube agglutination method is common. Other methods used include complement fixation (CF) and enzyme linked immunosorbent assay (ELISA). Because this disease is almost eliminated from United States and Canadian cattle and sheep populations, this test is not commonly performed.

86625
Campylobacter is a genus of bacteria, some of which are responsible for a wide variety of illnesses in humans. Enteritis is among the more common illnesses. *Campylobacter* is also implicated in Guillain-Barre syndrome, a form of peripheral neuropathy. Blood specimen is obtained by venipuncture. The literature is unclear about methods and reasons to order such testing. Most clinical cases of *Campylobacter* infection resolve themselves spontaneously or following drug therapy.

86628
Candida is a ubiquitous genus of fungi, some species of which are pathogenic to humans. The range of illnesses is quite large. This test is performed primarily to evaluate suspected systemic invasions by *Candida.* If confirmed, tests may be obtained at biweekly intervals to assess effectiveness of drug therapy. Blood specimen is serum. Methods include latex agglutination (LA), immunodiffusion (ID), crossed (2-dimensional) immunoelectrophoresis, and enzyme-linked immunosorbent assay (ELISA).

86631
This test may be ordered as *Chlamydia psittaci* or LVG titer. The specimen is serum or finger stick in adults, or heel stick in infants. Methods are complement fixation (CF), enzyme-linked immunosorbent assay (ELISA), and immunofluorescent antibody (IFA). This test may be used to determine exposure to chlamydia, though the test should not be used as a specific type. *Chlamydomonas* is a genus of algae that can cause nongonococcal urethritis, among other infections.

86632
This test may be ordered as chlamydia IgM titer. The specimen is serum or finger stick in adults, or heel stick in infants. Complement fixation (CF), enzyme-linked immunosorbent assay (ELISA), and immunofluorescent antibody (IFA) are methods commonly used to determine previous exposure to chlamydia or a current infection. *Chlamydomonas* is a genus of algae that can cause nongonococcal urethritis, among other infections.

86635
This test may be ordered as Coccidioides titer, Coccidioides antibody titer, Cocci titer or Cocci precipitins. The specimen is serum or finger stick in adults, or heel stick in infants. Methods include complement fixation (CF), enzyme-linked immunosorbent assay (ELISA), immunofluorescent antibody (IFA), immunodiffusion, and precipitin test. The test may be performed to determine current infection or assess prognosis of Coccidioides immitis, a fungus that causes coccidioidomycosis.

86638
This test may be ordered as Q fever titer, Q fever antibody titer, or C. brunetti titer. The specimen is serum. Methods are complement fixation (CF), enzyme-linked immunosorbent assay (ELISA), immunofluorescent antibody (IFA), immunodiffusion, or indirect hemagglutination (IHA). The test may be performed to determine Q fever due to Coxiella brunetti.

86641
This test may be ordered as AB cryptococcus antibody titer, or cryptococcosis. The specimen is serum. Methods are complement fixation (CF), enzyme-linked immunosorbent assay (ELISA), and immunofluorescent antibody (IFA). This test may be performed to determine exposure and prognosis of cryptococcosis, an infectious disease caused by the fungus Cryptococcus neoformans characterized by nodular lesions or abscesses in the lungs, subcutaneous tissues, joints, and the brain and meninges.

86644
This test may be ordered as CMV-IFA, CMV titers, Cytomegalic inclusion titers, or CMV IgG. The specimen is serum. Methods are complement fixation (CF), enzyme-linked immunosorbent assay (ELISA), immunofluorescent antibody (IFA), and latex agglutination. This test may be performed to determine current cytomegalovirus (CMV) infection.

CMV is any of several viruses that can cause severe disease especially in newborns by infecting the salivary glands, brain, kidneys, liver, and lungs.

86645
This test is commonly ordered as CMV IgM antibody titer, CMV IgM titer, cytomegalovirus IGM antibody titer, or CMV IgM. The specimen is serum or finger stick in adults, or heel stick in infants. Methods are complement fixation (CF), enzyme-linked immunosorbent assay (ELISA), immunofluorescent antibody (IFA), and latex agglutination. This may be performed to determine previous exposure to cytomegalovirus (CMV) or an acute CMV infection. CMV is any of several viruses that can cause severe disease especially in newborns by infecting the salivary glands, brain, kidneys, liver, and lungs.

86648
This test may be ordered as Diphtheria antibody titer, or DPT titer. The specimen is serum. Methods are complement fixation (CF), enzyme-linked immunosorbent assay (ELISA), immunofluorescent antibody (IFA), and latex agglutination. The test may be performed to determine exposure to Diphtheria, a bacterial disease that can cause inflammation to the heart and nervous system.

86651
This test may be ordered as La Crosse virus titer, California encephalitis titer, or bunyavirus titer. The specimen is serum. Methods are complement fixation (CF), or enzyme-linked immunosorbent assay (ELISA). This test may be performed to confirm the presence of the California encephalitis viral infection. There are several strains of the encephalitis virus that can cause inflammatory conditions, especially in the tissues of the brain.

86652
This test may be ordered as Eastern equine encephalitis titer. The specimen is serum. Methods are complement fixation (CF), or enzyme-linked immunosorbent assay (ELISA). This test may be performed to confirm the presence of Eastern equine encephalitis. There are several strains of the encephalitis virus that can cause inflammatory conditions, especially in the tissues of the brain.

86653
This test may be ordered as St. Louis virus titer or St. Louis encephalitis titer. The specimen is serum. Methods are complement fixation (CF), or enzyme-linked immunosorbent assay (ELISA). This test may be performed to confirm the presence of St. Louis encephalitis. There are several strains of the encephalitis virus that can cause inflammatory conditions, especially in the tissues of the brain.

86654
This test may be ordered as Western equine encephalitis titer. The specimen is serum. Methods are complement fixation (CF), or enzyme-linked immunosorbent assay (ELISA). This test may be performed to determine the presence of the Western equine encephalitis virus. There are several strains of the encephalitis virus that can cause inflammatory conditions, especially in the tissues of the brain.

86658
This test may be ordered as enterovirus antibody panel (IgG or IgM), coxsackie A titer, or poliovirus titer. The panel includes coxsackie, A and B, echovirus, and poliovirus. The specimen is serum. Methods are complement fixation (CF), viral neutralization, or enzyme-linked immunosorbent assay (ELISA). This test may be performed to determine presence of the coxsackie A virus, poliovirus, or other enteroviruses that typically occur in the gastrointestinal tract, but may also cause respiratory ailments, meningitis, and neurological disorders.

86663-86665
These tests may be ordered as EBV-EA titer, EBNA (IgG or IgM) titer, or EBV.VCA (IgG or IgM), or EB-VCA (IgG or IgM) titer. The specimen is serum. The test has been used as a serological method to detect previous exposure to EBV or acute EBV disease. Methods are complement fixation (CF) or enzyme-linked immunosorbent assay (ELISA), indirect fluorescent antibody, or immunofluorescent antibody (IFA). Code 86663 identifies an early antigen (short-lived); 86664 is reported for nuclear antigen; 86665 is used for viral capsid antigen (VCA). The VCA test may be the most effectual of the three tests for determining EB viral infection, which is the main cause of infectious mononucleosis.

86666
This test may also be ordered as *Ehrlichia* IgM or IgG. The specimen is serum. Methods include indirect fluorescent antibody (IFA) and immunofluorescent antibody (IFA). The *Ehrlichia* genus of rickettsia bacteria is implicated in a form of tick fever similar to Rocky Mountain Spotted Fever, sometimes referred to as "spotless" fever. Testing may occur during acute or convalescent phases of illness.

86668
This test is also known as Tularemia antibody titer, rabbit fever antibodies, and Francisella tularensis antibodies. The specimen is serum. Methods include complement fixation (CF), enzyme-linked immunosorbent assay (ELISA), or immunofluorescent antibody (IFA) agglutination, and hemagglutination. The test may be performed to determine the presence of the bacteria *F. tularensis*, a bacterium transmitted by insect bite that causes tularemia marked by toxemia.

86671
This code should be used to report antibody testing for fungi, which do not have a more specific genus or species code listed in this section. For example, antibody testing for sporotrichosis would be reported with this code. Blood specimen is serum. Methods are varied and may include: complement fixation (CF), immunodiffusion, latex agglutination (LA), immunofluorescence, Western blot (immunoblot),

crossed (2-dimensional) immunoelectrophoresis, and enzyme-linked immunosorbent assay (ELISA).

86674

This test may be requested as Giardia antibody or Giardia titer. Giardia lamblia is the causative protozoal organism of the intestinal disorder known as Giardia. Blood specimen is serum. Methods such as commercial kit, enzyme immunoassay (EIA), and indirect immunofluorescence may be employed.

86677

This test may be ordered as *H. pylori* antibody titer or *Campylobacter pylori* serology. The specimen is serum. Method is enzyme-linked immunosorbent assay (ELISA) or chemiluminescence. The test may be performed to determine the presence of *Helicobacter Pylori*, a common cause of intestinal disease and suspected as a cause of ulcerated stomach tissue.

86682

This code reports antibody testing for any of species of helminths not elsewhere classified in this section. Helminths are parasitic worms and many are further classified as nematodes. Helminthic infections may be intestinal or of tissues. Blood specimen is serum. Test methodologies will vary according to the suspected parasite. Methods may include enzyme immunoassay (EIA) and bentonite flocculation. Tissue parasites are easier to assay for antibodies than are those affecting the GI tract.

86684

This test may be ordered as a H. Influenza (type A or B) antibody titer. The specimen is serum. Method is complement fixation, EIA, or enzyme-linked immunosorbent assay (ELISA). This test is performed to determine the presence of H. Influenza, a common cause of chronic intestinal disease.

86687

This test is commonly ordered as HTLV-I antibody titer or Human T Cell Leukemia I Virus titer. The specimen is by venipuncture or finger stick in adults, or heel stick in infants. Methods are Western blot, radioimmunoprecipitation, and screen enzyme immunoassay. This test may be performed to determine the presence of HTLV-I virus and to screen blood and blood products used for transfusions.

86688

This test is commonly ordered as HTLV-II antibody titer or human T cell leukemia II virus titer. The specimen is serum. Methods are Western blot, radioimmunoprecipitation, and screen enzyme immunoassay. This test may be performed to determine the presence of HTLV-II virus and to screen blood and blood products used for transfusions.

86689

This test is commonly ordered as HTLV or HIV by Western blot. The specimen is serum. This test may be performed as a confirmation of a positive test for human T cell leukemia II virus or human immunodeficiency virus (HIV), often by a previous enzyme-linked immunoassay (ELISA).

86692

This test may be ordered as hepatitis D antibody, hepatitis delta antibody, or superinfection antibody. Hepatitis D occurs concurrently with hepatitis B and may lead to more severe clinical symptoms than hepatitis B alone, a condition known as superinfection. Specimen is serum. Methodology may involve enzyme immunoassay (EIA).

86694-86696

These tests may be ordered as HSV antibody titer, HSV titer, herpes simplex antibody titer, or HSV IgG/IGM. The specimen is serum or finger stick in adults, or heel stick in infants. A number of methodologies have been employed, such as complement fixation (CF), enzyme-linked immunosorbent assay (ELISA), indirect fluorescent antibody (IFA), enzyme immunoassay, and latex agglutination. This test has been used as a serologic method to detect previous or recent exposure to herpes simplex. To report non-specific type testing, see 86694; testing for type 1, see 86695; testing for type 2, see 86696.

86698

This test may be requested as histoplasma antibody. Histoplasma capsulatum is a fungus that may be infectious in humans. Incidence seems tied to certain regions. Many infections are asymptomatic or feature mild symptoms. Blood specimen is serum. Complement fixation (CF) is quantifiable and is considered one of the best methods. Immunodiffusion (ID), agar diffusion, latex agglutination (LA), radioimmunoassay (RIA), or enzyme immunoassay (EIA) may also be used.

86701

This test may be ordered as an HIV-1 serological test, an HIV-1 antibody, or by an internal code. HIV is a retrovirus and the causative agent of acquired immunodeficiency syndrome (AIDS). Specimen is serum. Numerous kits are now available that use a variety of viral proteins and serumsynthetic peptides as antigens. Methodology is enzyme immunoassay (EIA), enzyme-linked immunosorbent assay (ELISA), radioimmunoprecipitation assay (RIPA), or indirect fluorescent antibody (IFA). A negative test does not guarantee negative status and the test is often repeated several times.

86702

This test may be ordered as an HIV-2 serological antibody. This is an antibody test for HIV-2, a retrovirus closely related to simian AIDS and found initially in West African nations and Portugal, but with cases also being reported in the United States since 1987. Blood specimen is serum. Specific kits are now available that use a variety of viral proteins and synthetic peptides as antigens to test for HIV-2. Methodology is enzyme immunoassay (EIA), enzyme-linked immunosorbent assay (ELISA), radioimmunoprecipitation assay (RIPA), or indirect fluorescent antibody (IFA). A negative test does not guarantee negative status and the test is often repeated several times.

86703
This test may be ordered as a combined HIV-1 and -2 serological or a combined HIV-1 and -2 antibody. This is an antibody test that tests for both HIV-1 and HIV-2 with a single result. Both are retroviruses. HIV-1 is the causative agent of acquired immunodeficiency syndrome (AIDS), while HIV-2 is closely related to simian AIDS. Blood specimen is serum. Specific kits are now available that use a variety of viral proteins and synthetic peptides as antigens to test for both HIV-1 and HIV-2. Methodology is enzyme immunoassay (EIA), enzyme-linked immunosorbent assay (ELISA), radioimmunoprecipitation assay (RIPA), or indirect fluorescent antibody (IFA). A negative test does not guarantee negative status and the test is often repeated several times.

86704
This test may be ordered as hepatitis Bc Ab (HBcAb), total. It may also be ordered as HBcAb, anti-HBc, HBVc Ab, anti-HBVc. This test identifies Hepatitis B core total antibodies (IgG and IgM), which are markers available to identify individuals with acute, chronic, or past infection of hepatitis B. The presence of high-titered IgM specific HBcAb is always indicative of an acute infection. The presence of IgG may indicate acute or chronic infection. Blood specimen is serum. Methods include radioimmunoassay (RIA) and enzyme-linked immunosorbent assay (ELISA).

86705
This test may be ordered as hepatitis Bc Ab (HBcAb), IgM. It may also be ordered as HBcAb, anti-HBc, HBVc Ab, anti-HBVc. This test identifies Hepatitis B core IgM antibodies, the presence of which always indicates an acute infection. Blood specimen is serum. Methods include radioimmunoassay (RIA) and enzyme-linked immunosorbent assay (ELISA).

86706
This test may be requested as Hepatitis B surface antibody (HBsAb), Hepatitis Bs Ab, HBV surface antibody, or anti-HBs. The presence of HBsAb is indicative of a previous resolved infection or vaccination against hepatitis B. Blood specimen is serum. Methods include radioimmunoassay (RIA), enzyme immunoassay (EIA), immunoradiometric assay (IRMA), and immunoenzymatic assay (IEMA).

86707
This test may be ordered as hepatitis Be antibody (HBeAb) as Hepatitis Be Ab, HBVe, or anti-HBe. The presence of HBeAb usually indicates a high likelihood of a lesser infectivity and usually points to a benign outcome, although some individuals with HBeAb have chronic hepatitis. Blood specimen is serum. Methods include immunoradiometric assay (IRMA) and enzyme immunoassay (EIA).

86708
This test may be ordered as hepatitis A antibody (HAAb), HAV antibody, or anti-Hep A. The presence of HAV IgG antibody may indicate acute infection or previous resolved infection, while IgM antibody always indicates acute infectious disease. Blood specimen is serum. Methods include radioimmunoassay (RIA), enzyme immunoassay (EIA), immunoradiometric assay (IRMA), immunoenzymatic assay (IEMA), and microparticle enzyme immunoassay (MEIA).

86709
This test may be ordered as hepatitis A antibody (HAAb), HAV IgM antibody, anti-Hep A IgM, or anti-HAV IgM. The presence of IgM antibody indicates acute infectious disease. Blood specimen is serum. Methods include radioimmunoassay (RIA), enzyme immunoassay (EIA), immunoradiometric assay (IRMA), immunoenzymatic assay (IEMA), and microparticle enzyme immunoassay (MEIA).

86710
This test may be ordered as Flu A or Flu B, or Influenza A/B antibody titers. It may also be ordered as anti-Influenza A/B. The presence of IgG antibody usually indicates previous exposure, while IgM indicates a current acute infection. Blood specimen is serum. Methods vary with hemagglutination inhibition (HI) (HAI) being preferred for influenza A and complement fixation (CF) for influenza B. Other methods currently in use are immunofluorescent assay (IFA), enzyme-linked immunosorbent assay (ELISA), radial immunodiffusion (RID), and enzyme immunoassay (EIA).

86711
This test may be ordered as JCV antibody test. This test is usually performed on patients that are immunocompromised due to disease or medication to assess the risk of developing progressive multifocal leukoencephalopathy (PML). Specimen is serum. Method is enzyme-linked immunosorbent assay (ELISA).

86713
This test may be ordered as Legionella antibody titers or as anti-Legionella. Both IgG and IgM antibodies should be tested. IgA testing may also be indicated. The presence of IgG antibody usually indicates previous exposure. The demonstration of IgM or IgA antibodies may establish the diagnosis of a current acute or recent Legionella infection. Blood specimen is serum. Methods include: immunofluorescent assay (IFA) and enzyme-linked immunosorbent assay (ELISA).

86717
This test is ordered as Leishmania antibody titers or anti-Leishmania. This protozoan infection may also be referred to as kala-azar. The presence of IgG antibody usually indicates previous exposure. The demonstration of IgM or IgA antibodies may establish the diagnosis of a current acute or recent Leishmania infection. Blood specimen is serum. Preferred methods are complement fixation (CF) and enzyme-linked immunosorbent assay (ELISA). However, a number of other methods are employed including indirect

hemagglutination (IHA), immunofluorescent assay (IFA), immunoblot, and enzyme immunoassay (EIA).

86720
This test may be ordered as Leptospira antibody titers or anti-Leptospira. Blood specimen is serum. The presence of IgG antibody usually indicates previous exposure. The demonstration of IgM or IgA antibodies may establish the diagnosis of a current acute or recent Leptospira infection. Methods include complement fixation (CF); hemagglutination, immunofluorescent assay (IFA) and enzyme-linked immunosorbent assay (ELISA).

86723
This test may be ordered as Listeria antibody titers or anti-Listeria. Blood specimen is serum. The presence of IgG antibody usually indicates previous exposure. The demonstration of IgM or IgA antibodies may establish the diagnosis of an acute or recent Listeria infection. Methods include immunofluorescent assay (IFA) and enzyme-linked immunosorbent assay (ELISA).

86727
This test is ordered as LCM or LCMC antibody titers. It may also be ordered as anti-LCM. The presence of IgG antibody usually indicates previous exposure. The demonstration of IgM or IgA antibodies may establish the diagnosis of a current acute or recent LCM infection. Blood specimen is serum. A separately reportable spinal puncture is used to collect CSF. Immunofluorescent assay (IFA), direct fluorescent antibody (DFA), and enzyme-linked immunosorbent assay (ELISA) methods are among those employed in identifying antibody response to the specific LCMC. A positive direct examination by electromicroscopy or direct fluorescent microscopy is indicative of active disease.

86732
This test may be ordered as Rhizopus antibody titer, Rhizomucor antibody titer, or Cunninghamella antibody titer. These are the common species of molds that cause mucormycosis, a rare opportunistic infection usually found in patients with pre-existing conditions. Blood specimen is serum or finger stick. Literature is unclear, but immunofluorescent assay (IFA) is a common method to detect antibody responses.

86735
This test may be ordered as mumps antibody titers or anti-mumps titers. Testing may be performed to diagnose an acute infection or to evaluate immune status. The presence of IgG antibody alone usually indicates previous exposure and immunity. IgM antibodies in combination with IgG establish the diagnosis of a current acute or recent mumps infection. Blood specimen is serum. Preferred methods include enzyme immunoassay (EIA) and virus neutralization test (NT). Other methods that may be employed include hemagglutination inhibition (HAI), complement fixation (CF), indirect fluorescent antibody (IFA), and hemolysis in gel.

86738
This test is ordered as Mycoplasma antibody titers. It may also be ordered as anti-walking pneumonia, primary atypical pneumonia (PAP), pleuropneumonia-like organism (PPLO), or anti-Mycoplasma titers. The presence of IgG antibody usually indicates previous exposure to Mycoplasma. The demonstration of IgM antibodies is required to establish the diagnosis of a current acute or recent Mycoplasma infection. Blood specimen is serum. Methods include immunofluorescent assay (IFA), complement fixation (CF), and enzyme immunoassay (EIA), and IgM antibody agglutination.

86741
This test is ordered as N. meningitidis antibody titers. It may also be ordered as anti-Neisseria meningitidis. This is the causative agent of meningococcal meningitis. The presence of IgG antibody usually indicates previous exposure to N. meningitidis. The demonstration of IgM or IgA antibodies may establish the diagnosis of a current acute or recent meningitidis infection. Blood specimen is serum. CSF is obtained by spinal puncture that is reported separately. Method is enzyme-linked immunosorbent assay (ELISA).

86744
This test is ordered as Nocardia antibody titers. It may also be ordered as anti-Nocardia titers. Pathogenic species of Nocardia include N. asteroides, N. brasiliensis, N. caviae, N. farcinica, N. transvalensis, and N. nova. Nocardiosis generally occurs only in immunosuppressed individuals and presents as suppurative or cavitary pneumonia, cutaneous abscesses, or mycetoma formation on an extremity. The presence of IgG antibody usually indicates previous exposure to Nocardia. The demonstration of IgM or IgA antibodies may establish the diagnosis of a current acute or recent Nocardia infection. Blood specimen is serum. Method is enzyme-linked immunosorbent assay (ELISA) or Western blot.

86747
This test may be ordered as Parvovirus antibody titers, anti-Parvovirus titers, or Parvo B19 antibody titers. The presence of IgG antibody usually indicates previous exposure to Parvovirus B19. The demonstration of IgM antibodies may establish the diagnosis of a current acute or recent Parvovirus B19 infection. Blood specimen is serum. Enzyme-linked immunosorbent assay (ELISA), radioimmunoassay (RIA), and Western blot are among methods employed in identifying an antibody response to Parvovirus B19.

86750
This test is ordered as malaria antibody titers. This test is used primarily to screen blood donors. Specimen is whole blood. Method is indirect immunofluorescence (IIF).

86753
This test is for antibodies to any of the clinically significant simple, single-celled organisms within the subkingdom of protozoa not specified by a more

specific code in this section of CPT. For example, detection of Entamoeba histolytica antibodies would be reported 86753. The specimen is serum. Enzyme-linked immunosorbent assay (ELISA), radioimmunoassay (RIA) complement fixation, Western Blot, indirect hemagglutination (IHA) are among the methods employed in identifying an antibody response to the specific protozoa.

86756
This test is ordered as RSV antibody titers. It may also be ordered as anti-respiratory syncytial viral titers, and anti-RSV titers. The presence of IgG antibody usually indicates previous exposure to respiratory syncytial virus. The demonstration of IgM antibodies may establish the diagnosis of a current acute or recent infection. Blood specimen is serum. Enzyme-linked immunosorbent assay (ELISA), enzyme immunoassay (EIA), and complement fixation (CF) are among methodologies employed in identifying an antibody response.

86757
This test may also be ordered by the name of the suspected rickettsial pathogen (e.g., Rocky Mountain Spotted Fever, typhus). Blood specimen is serum. Methods include enzyme-linked immunoassay (ELISA) with indirect fluorescent antibody (IFA) confirmation.

86759
This test is ordered as rotavirus antibody titer. It may also be ordered as anti-rotavirus titer, Adenovirus 40-41 antibody titer, and anti-rotavirus titer. The presence of IgG antibody usually indicates previous exposure to rotavirus. The demonstration of IgM antibodies may establish the diagnosis of a recent or current rotavirus infection. Blood specimen is serum. Enzyme-linked immunosorbent assay (ELISA) and radioimmunoassays (RIA) are among methods employed in identifying antibody response to the specific to rotavirus.

86762
This test is ordered as rubella antibody titers. It may also be ordered as German measles antibody titers, and anti-rubella titers. The test is used primarily to evaluate immune status. The presence of rubella IgG and IgM antibodies may indicate previous exposure, vaccination, or current acute infection. Blood specimen is serum. Enzyme-linked immunosorbent assay (ELISA), enzyme immunoassay (EIA), and latex agglutination (LA) are among methods used in identifying antibody response, with ELISA being more common in larger, high volume laboratories.

86765
This test is ordered as rubeola antibody titers. It may also be ordered as measles antibody titers, anti-measles titers and anti-rubeola titers. This test is used primarily to evaluate immune status as clinical symptoms related to acute infection make laboratory testing unnecessary. CSF specimen is used for diagnosis of subacute sclerosing panencephalitis (SSPE). The presence of rubeola IgG antibody alone usually indicates previous exposure to rubeola. Both IgG and IgM antibodies are present with a current acute or recent rubeola infection. Blood specimen is serum. CSF specimen is reported separately. Hemagglutination inhibition test (HAI) is the preferred method of testing for immune status. Enzyme-linked immunosorbent assay (ELISA), enzyme immunoassay (EIA), complement fixation (CF), and neutralization test (NT) are other methods commonly employed in identifying an antibody response.

86768
This test is ordered as Salmonella antibody titers. It may also be ordered as anti-Salmonella titers, S. typhi antibody titers or Salmonella typhi antibody titers. The presence of Salmonella IgG antibody usually indicates previous exposure to salmonella. The demonstration of Salmonella IgM antibodies may establish the diagnosis of a recent or current salmonella infection. The specimen is serum. Enzyme-linked immunosorbent assay (ELISA) principles are most commonly employed in identifying an antibody response to the specific Salmonella. Agglutination principles may be utilized for the identification of S. typhi antibody.

86769
This code reports testing to identify the presence of antibodies to the SARS-CoV-2 virus. Infectious agent specificity may also include terminology such as severe acute respiratory syndrome coronavirus 2, coronavirus disease, or COVID-19. In one method, following dilution in buffer of the plasma or serum sample, a measured portion of the diluted sample and controls are added to a sample plate. After incubation and washing, appropriate IgG and IgM antibodies are added and incubated. It is combined with a substrate, incubated, and read immediately.

86771
This test is ordered as Shigella antibody titers. It may also be ordered as anti-Salmonella titers. The presence of Shigella IgG antibody usually indicates previous exposure to Shigella. The demonstration of Shigella IgM antibodies may establish the diagnosis of a recent or current Shigella infection. Blood specimen is serum. Enzyme-linked immunosorbent assay (ELISA) principles are most commonly employed in identifying an antibody response to the specific to Shigella. Agglutination principles may also be utilized for the identification of Shigella.

86774
This test is ordered as tetanus antibody titers. It may also be ordered as anti-tetanus titers or *Clostridium tetani* antibody titers. This test is not commonly used as a diagnostic test for acute infection. It may be used to evaluate immune status. Blood specimen is serum. Titration of tetanus antitoxin neutralization principles is the most common method. Agglutination, passive hemagglutination, or enzyme-linked immunosorbent assay (ELISA) principles may also be utilized.

86777
This test is ordered as Toxoplasma IgG antibody titers. It may also be ordered as anti-Toxoplasma IgG titers, or toxo IgG titers. The presence of Toxoplasma IgG antibody may indicate current or past infection. Blood specimen is serum. Amniotic fluid is collected by amniocentesis that is reported separately. Enzyme-linked immunosorbent assay (ELISA) or immunofluorescent assay (IFA) principles may be used for the identification of Toxoplasma antibody.

86778
This test is ordered as Toxoplasma IgM antibody titers. It may also be ordered as anti-Toxoplasma IgM titers, or toxo IgM titers. The demonstration of Toxoplasma IgM antibodies may establish the diagnosis of a recent or current infection. Blood specimen is serum amniotic fluid collected by amniocentesis that is reported separately. Enzyme-linked immunosorbent assay (ELISA) or immunofluorescent assay (IFA) principles may be used for the identification of toxoplasma IgM antibody.

86780
Treponema pallidum antibody tests are used to screen and confirm syphilis. This test may be ordered as a screening or confirmatory test for syphilis or as a screening or confirmatory test for a positive venereal disease research lab test (VDRL), rapid plasma reagent (RPR), or serologic test (STS) for syphilis. Blood specimen is serum. Fluorescent antibody (FA) or FTA principles are most commonly employed in identifying an antibody response to the specific syphilis. Agglutination or flocculation of cardiolipin principles may also be used for the identification of syphilis antibody.

86784
This test is ordered as trichinella antibody titers. It may also be ordered as trichinosis antibody titers. Trichinella antibody titers are to diagnose infestation with the parasitic roundworm Trichinella spiralis that is transmitted by eating undercooked pork or bear meat. Blood specimen is serum. Methods include bentonite flocculation test (BFT); indirect immunofluorescence (IIF), complement fixation (CF), latex agglutination (LA), enzyme immunoassay (EIA), and enzyme-linked immunosorbent assay (ELISA).

86787
This test may be requested as VZV antibody titers, chicken pox antibody titers, or herpes zoster antibody titers. This test is performed primarily to evaluate immune status. Blood specimen is serum. Methods may include enzyme immunoassay (EIA), enzyme-linked immunosorbent assay (ELISA), complement fixation, and fluorescent antibody against membrane antigen (FAMA).

86788
This code is commonly ordered as WNV IgM. Specimen is cerebrospinal fluid or blood serum. Method used is an antibody capture enzyme-linked immunosorbent assay. WNV IgM of cerebrospinal fluid is the most definitive test for WNV of the central nervous system, as antibodies may persist in the blood for more than a year following a resolved infection. WNV IgM will be positive only if a WNV infection has been active for at least eight days. West Nile virus usually causes a mild infection, but in some cases, leads to life-threatening encephalitis or meningitis.

86789
This code is commonly ordered as WNV IgG. Specimen is cerebrospinal fluid or blood serum. Method used is enzyme immunoassay, plaque reduction neutralization, or hemagglutination inhibition. WNV IgG will be positive only if a WNV infection has been active for at least three weeks. West Nile virus usually causes a mild infection, but in some cases, leads to life-threatening encephalitis or meningitis.

86790
This test is ordered as viral antibody titers not elsewhere specified. The specimen is serum The presence of viral IgG antibody usually indicates previous exposure, while viral IgM antibodies may establish the diagnosis of a recent or current infection. Methods include enzyme-linked immunosorbent assay (ELISA), indirect fluorescent antibody (IFA), and agglutination.

86793
This test is ordered as Yersinia antibody titers or by species name including Y. enterocolitica antibody and Y. pestis (bubonic plague) antibody. Blood specimen is serum. A common method used is agglutination. However, newer techniques are also used that include an immunoblot, enzyme-linked immunosorbent assay (ELISA), indirect fluorescent antibody (IFA).

86794
This code tests for antibodies to the Zika virus. Symptoms of Zika infection include fever, rash, headache, joint pain, red eyes, and/or muscle pain. Patients may be infected with the Zika virus from the bite of an infected mosquito or it can be passed from a pregnant woman to her fetus causing certain birth defects. It is recommended that asymptomatic pregnant patients be screened due to the risk of birth defects. The preferred specimen is serum; however, in some instances urine may be used. Methodology is enzyme-linked immunosorbent assay (ELISA), M antibody capture ELISA (MAC-ELISA), or polymerase chain reaction (PCR).

86800
This test is ordered as thyroglobulin antibody titers or anti-thyroglobulin. The presence of thyroglobulin antibody usually indicates presence of circulating autoantibodies in patients with endocrine disease (i.e., thyroiditis, Graves' disease). The specimen is serum. Methods may include enzyme-linked immunosorbent assay (ELISA), tanned RBC agglutination test, radiobinding assay, and immunoradiometric assay (IRMA).

86803
This test may be ordered as hepatitis C antibody titers. It may also be ordered as anti-hepatitis C titers, HCV Ab titers, and anti-HCV titers. This test is normally used for an initial hepatitis C screen. Positive or unequivocal tests are repeated using different techniques that are reported separately. Blood specimen is serum. Methods may include enzyme-linked immunosorbent assay (ELISA) or enzyme immunoassay (EIA).

86804
These tests may be ordered as hepatitis C antibody titers, anti-hepatitis C titers, HCV Ab titers, or anti-HCV titers. The specimen is serum. Recombinant immunoblot assay (RIBA) principles may be employed in identifying an antibody response to the specific hepatitis C virus. The presence of IgG antibody by RIBA is a confirmatory test.

86805-86806
These tests may also be referred to as compatibility tests or major histocompatibility complex (MHC) tests. These tests pertain primarily to matching potential donor tissues to transplant patients, but uses may also include bench research. Methodology involves mixing purified donor lymphocytes with recipient sera or known antibodies. Cytotoxic reaction (cell death) is visually monitored, usually by incubation method. Indicator dyes may be used to identify dead cells. Titration involves methodology to determine quantities. Report 86805 for testing with titration; 86806 for testing without titration.

86807-86808
These tests may be requested as PRA screen. This test is a preliminary screen to measure cytotoxicity, or cell death, when blood product is mixed. The standard method involves culturing and monitoring cytotoxicity, using marker dyes, and the corresponding buildup of antibodies, through replication and DNA. Code 86807 reports standard testing methods. Code 86808 reports a rapid method, where antibody growth and cytotoxicity are more immediately evident.

86812
This test may also be ordered as a histocompatibility antigen test, Class I (or Class III) antigen test, or according to a specific antigen (e.g., A10). This test pertains primarily to matching potential donor tissues to transplant patients. This test determines HLA compatibility of specific antigens. Method involves mixing purified donor lymphocytes with a known sera and complement. A culture is prepared and cytotoxic reaction (cell death) is monitored.

86813
This test may also be ordered as histocompatibility antigens test, Class I (or Class III) antigens test, or according to specific multiple antigens (e.g., A10-B-7). This test pertains primarily to matching potential donor tissues to transplant patients This test determines HLA compatibility of multiple antigens. Method involves mixing purified donor lymphocytes with a known sera and complement. A culture is prepared and cytotoxic reaction (cell death) is monitored.

86816
This test may also be ordered as a Class II antigen test, or simply HLA-D antigen. This test pertains primarily to matching potential donor tissues to transplant patients. The D human lymphocyte antigens (HLA) are located separately from the Class I and Class III antigens on the chromosome. Subregion names DR, DQ, and DP are described. This test determines HLA compatibility of a single Class II antigen. Method involves mixing purified donor lymphocytes with the sera and complement. A culture is prepared and cytotoxic reaction (cell death) is monitored.

86817
This test may also be ordered as a Class II antigens test, or simply HLA-D antigens. This test pertains primarily to matching potential donor tissues to transplant patients. The D human leukocyte antigens (HLA) are located separately from the Class I and Class III antigens on the chromosome. Subregion names DR, DQ, and DP are described. This test determines HLA compatibility for multiple Class II antigens. Method involves mixing purified donor lymphocytes with the sera and complement. A culture is prepared and cytotoxic reaction (cell death) is monitored.

86821
This test may also be ordered as a mixed lymphocyte culture (MLC) reaction, Class II antigen test, or simply HLA-D antigen. Donor and recipient blood samples are often collected at the same time. This test pertains primarily to matching potential donor tissues to transplant patients. The D human leukocyte antigens (HLA) are located separately from the Class I and Class III antigens on the chromosome and the MLC method is particularly good at identifying them. This test determines HLA compatibility of Class II antigens. The method is described in literature as mixing purified donor lymphocytes with the recipient's lymphocytes. A culture is prepared and the recipient's lymphocytic response is monitored. The greater the response, the greater the degree of antigen disparity.

86825-86826
This test describes non-cytotoxic crossmatches, such as flow cytometry, and identifies a subgroup of potential organ transplant recipients whose risk of graft failure or post-transplant complications may be elevated because of low levels of an antibody that is undetected by lymphocytotoxic crossmatch procedures. When used as part of a pre-transplant risk assessment, cytotoxic and flow cytometry crossmatches provide differing, but complementary, information. Using three color fluorescent tests with CD3 and CD19 monoclonals and conjugated anti-human immunoglobulin, histocompatibility crossmatching is performed to optimize allocation of organs to the most compatible donor/recipient pairs. Report 86825 for the first serum sample or dilution and 86826 for each additional sample or dilution.

86828-86829

These tests are commonly used to predict the histocompatibility between a patient and a donor to predict and prevent graft versus host disease (GVHD) or transplanted organ rejection. Human leukocyte antigens (HLA) are a group of genes found on chromosome 6. There are two types of HLA: class I and class II. The higher number of anti-HLA antibodies the higher the chance of a reaction to donor tissue. The specimen is blood. The method is enzyme-linked immunosorbent assay (ELISA) technique and the use of fluorescent beads with HLA molecules bound to their surface, which can be used in conventional flow cytometry or in conjunction with Luminex instrumentation. Report 86828 if the presence or absence of both HLA class I and II antibodies are assessed. Report 86829 when only one HLA class antibody is qualified.

86830-86831

These tests are commonly used to predict the histocompatibility between a patient and a donor to predict and prevent graft versus host disease (GVHD) or transplanted organ rejection. Human leukocyte antigens (HLA) are a group of genes found on chromosome six. There are two types of HLA: class I and class II. The higher the number of anti-HLA antibodies the higher the chance of a reaction to donor tissue. The specimen is serum. The method is enzyme-linked immunosorbent assay (ELISA) technique and the use of fluorescent beads with HLA molecules bound to their surface, which can be used in conventional flow cytometry or in conjunction with Luminex instrumentation. Report 86830 for a panel of complete HLA class I phenotypes to identify antibodies to approximately 80 antigens using a 50 or more bead array. Report 86831 for a panel of complete HLA class II phenotypes to identify antibodies to approximately 40 antigens using a 30 or more bead array.

86832-86833

These tests are commonly used to predict the histocompatibility between a patient and a donor to predict and prevent graft versus host disease (GVHD) or transplanted organ rejection. Human leukocyte antigens (HLA) are a group of genes found on chromosome six. There are two types of HLA: class I and class II. The higher the number of anti-HLA antibodies the higher the chance of a reaction to donor tissue. The specimen is blood. Antibodies to individual HLA antigens are identified using fluorescence bead-based assays. These assays utilize color-coded beads coated with cloned HLA to identify complement-binding and non-complement-binding HLA class I and II antibodies. Report 86832 to qualify HLA class I with a panel to identify antibodies to all 80+ HLA ABC antigens using a bead array of up to 98 beads. Report 86833 when HLA class II is qualified using a panel to identify antibodies to individual HLA DRB1/3/4/5, DQA1, DQB1, DPA1, and DPB1 antigens using a bead array of up to 98 beads.

86834-86835

These tests are commonly used to monitor treatment of antibody mediated transplant rejection, assess potential rejection in potential transplant patients, or test for pretransplant desensitization potential. Human leukocyte antigens (HLA) are a group of genes found on chromosome six. There are two types of HLA: class I and class II. The higher the number of anti-HLA antibodies the higher the chance of a reaction to donor tissue. The specimen is blood. The method is enzyme-linked immunosorbent assay (ELISA) technique and the use of fluorescent beads with HLA molecules bound to their surface, which can be used in conventional flow cytometry or in conjunction with Luminex instrumentation. Report 86834 if the panel is to quantify HLA class I antibodies. Report 86835 when HLA class II antibodies are quantified.

86850

This test may be ordered as an RBC antibody detection. The test is a screen for particular antibodies to red cell antigens that may present problems during a blood transfusion or childbirth. Blood specimen is whole blood. The test may be performed using tubes, microtiter plates, or gel cards. Another method is agglutination.

86860

Elution is a technique for removing antibody from antibody/antigen complex on RBCs for identification purposes. Blood specimen is whole blood. The process is usually part of a workup to aid in diagnosis of certain autoimmune disorders such as autoimmune hemolytic anemia, and for resolution of incompatible crossmatches due to unidentified antibodies, and to identify the antibody causing hemolytic disease of a newborn (HDN).

86870

This test is also known as an antibody panel. Blood specimen is whole blood. The test identifies an antibody isolated by techniques reported by 86850 and/or 86860 above. The test may be performed using tubes, microtiter plates, or gel cards. This code can be reported up to four times during the same session for differences in technique necessary for identification (i.e., regular panel, cold-panel, pre-warmed panel, and enzyme treated panel).

86880

This test is also known as a direct Coombs or sometimes as a direct antiglobulin test (DAT). Blood specimen is whole blood. The test is used to detect coating of the RBCs by antibody or complement. It is useful in diagnosis of hemolytic disease of the newborn (HDN), detection of autoimmune hemolytic anemia, investigation of transfusion reactions, and detection of red cell sensitization reactions caused by medication. Method may be by gel test, flow cytometry, or enzyme-linked immunosorbent assay (ELISA) or hemagglutination.

86885
This test is also known as an indirect Coombs, IAT, or sometimes as selective antibody screen. The indirect antiglobulin test indicates whether there is antibody in the serum, which will react to combine with antigen on the red cell. Uses for the IAT include determining if there are IgG antibodies (coating antibodies) in the patient's serum; investigating the ability to sensitize red blood cells; crossmatching, detection of Du (weak D) antigen; and investigation of transfusion reactions. The specimen is whole blood. Methodology includes agglutination, hemolysis of Type 0 test cells, flow cytometry, or enzyme-linked immunosorbent assay (ELISA). Report this code for each reagent red cell.

86886
This test is also known as an antibody titer. The test determines the strength of antibody identified through test described in 86870. The specimen is whole blood. Method is serial dilution with saline, enzyme, or low ionic strength saline followed by antiglobulin. Report this code for each antibody titer.

86890
This reports the donation of blood for one's own use. This procedure is used for patients requiring surgery who pre-deposit their own blood for use during the surgery. The procedure is most useful for patients with complex antibody production or extremely rare antibodies that make location of compatible blood difficult.

86891
This procedure may also be known as a cell-saver. This is a device used in surgeries where large blood losses are inherent to the procedure (i.e., total hip, certain heart and lung procedures, liver and spleen operations). The device aspirates spilled blood in the surgical cavity, washes it, and returns the RBCs to the patient. This reduces the need for stored blood. In postoperative patients, there may be major seepage and the patient is not physically up to additional surgery to correct the problem. The cell-saver washes the seepage and transfuses it back to the patient.

86900
This serologic test may also be known as blood group. The test determines whether a patient is O, A, B, or AB by testing for the presence or absence of these antigens on the RBC surface. This typing of blood is the oldest and most widely recognized. Blood specimen is whole blood. The classic test method is by agglutination but gel testing is common.

86901
This serologic test is known as Rh type. The test determines whether a patient is "positive" or "negative" by identifying the presence (Rh positive) or absence (Rh negative) of Rh antigens on the RBC surface. Blood specimen is whole blood. Method is enzyme-linked immunosorbent assay (ELISA), but may be performed by agglutination or gel test.

86902
This serologic test screens donated units of blood prior to a transfusion using reagent serum. The test confirms the absence of the antigen associated with the antibody identified by the antibody identification test (86870). If more than one blood unit is being tested for the same antigen, report 86902 once for each unit tested.

86904
This serologic test is used to screen for compatible blood using patient serum when there is insufficient time to identify an antibody and screen units for the associated antigen prior to transfusion. The test is also helpful when commercial antiserum to the antigen is not available.

86905
This serologic test is used to confirm the absence of antigens corresponding to antibodies identified by the antibody identification test (86870).

86906
Serologic Rh phenotyping may be required to assist in confirming the identity of an Rh antibody detected during screening, or when a family study is being undertaken for any number of reasons. Some donor centers maintain limited supplies of phenotyped blood to issue to patients who have corresponding antibodies.

86910-86911
These tests are a method to determine percentages of whether a particular male is the biological father of a particular child. These codes essentially group elements of 86900, 86901, and 86905 (MN refers to M antigen and N antigen, important in phenotyping). Code 86911 is reported when calculations using the antigen system in 86910 are indeterminate and additional systems must be analyzed. These codes also report all mathematical calculations of probability. These tests result in only a statistical probability of paternity. 86920 This test is one of the crossmatch components of tests ordered as "type and crossmatch." This step checks mainly for ABO compatibility of the unit being transfused. It may be the only step in the compatibility phase of the crossmatch when the patient has no demonstrated antibodies, or after a massive transfusion where very little of the patient's blood volume is his/her own. DNA testing is more commonly done.

86920
This test is one of the crossmatch components of tests ordered as "type and crossmatch." This step checks mainly for ABO compatibility of the unit being transfused. It may be the only step in the compatibility phase of the crossmatch when the patient has no demonstrated antibodies, or after a massive transfusion where very little of the patient's blood volume is his/her own.

86921
This test is one of the crossmatch components of tests ordered as "type and crossmatch." This test is an

intermediate step using incubation technique, in a full major compatibility test (86920, 86921, and 86922). It is a crucial step in sensitization of IgG antigens.

86922

This test is the final step in a major crossmatch. A full, major crossmatch will always be performed when antibodies are present in the patient's serum, unless more than 10 units have been given in a 24-hour period.

86923

This computer check is referred to as an electronic crossmatch, computer-assisted crossmatch, or E-XM. Some labs match donor blood for transfusions to specific patients based on patient test results previously performed and stored in the blood bank computer system. The sole purpose of the electronic crossmatch is to confirm ABO compatibility between patient and donor.

86927

Fresh frozen plasma (FFP) is frozen within six hours of donation. It maintains clotting factors in the frozen state and for this reason is used to treat certain clotting disorders, such as over-medication with Coumadin, liver diseases (i.e., parenchymal liver disease), and disseminated intravascular coagulation (DIC). It may also be used for plasma exchanges to treat diseases like thrombotic thrombocytopenic purpura (TTP), Raynaud's disease, and glomerulonephritis. This code reports only the thawing process.

86930-86932

The preparation for freezing is also known as glycerolization. Freezing allows reasonably long-term storage of pre-deposited blood. The preparation of frozen blood with thawing is also known as deglycerolization. The product is thawed and washed to remove preservative. Certain cold-insoluble proteins, such as factor VIII and fibrinogen, may be removed when the blood is close to thawing. Report 86930 for freezing, including preparation, each unit of blood. Report 86931 for thawing, each unit of blood and 86932 for freezing (including preparation) and thawing, each unit of blood.

86940-86941

These tests are used for screening (86940) or incubation (86941) of hemolysins and cold agglutinins. Cold agglutinins may mask antibodies that are not expected to be present in the blood and hemolysins are substances that lyse or dissolve red blood cells. In these tests red cells subject to incubation with and without various additives, such as glucose to determine the degree that red blood cells will lyse or clump. Irradiation is used primarily to prevent graft versus host disease (GVHD) in certain immunosuppressed patients, newborns, and patients that share the same human lymphocyte antigen (HLA) haplotype as the donor. The process inactivates the lymphocytes. Irradiation is also required when the donor is a blood relation of the recipient (GVHD).

86945

Irradiation is used primarily to prevent graft versus host disease (GVHD) in certain immunosuppressed patients, newborns, and patients that share the same human lymphocyte antigen (HLA) haplotype as the donor. The process inactivates the lymphocytes. Irradiation is also required when the donor is a blood relation of the recipient (GVHD).

86950

Granulocyte transfusion is indicated in patients on chemotherapy for leukemia or those with severe infection whose absolute granulocyte count is less than 500/cu mm.

86960

Volume reduction of blood is usually performed by an extra centrifugation step that removes plasma during processing of a blood product. Removal of excess donor plasma is indicated in patients who cannot tolerate the full volume or when ABO incompatible single donor platelets are transfused. Volume reduction may be helpful in patients with febrile transfusion reactions that persist despite leukocyte reduction.

86965

Pooling in this sense means to blend blood product from a variety of sources. Platelets and cryoprecipitate units are pooled in order to provide an adequate amount of product for the transfusion to be therapeutic. Cryoprecipitate is the fraction of blood which contains cold-insoluble proteins, such as factor VIII and fibrinogen. Cryoprecipitate is collected from frozen blood that is brought to thawing temperature.

86970

The incubation of red blood cells with certain chemical agents or drugs is performed to enhance the agglutination reaction of red blood cells during antibody identification. IgM antibodies are easily detected in saline at room temperature as IgM antibodies are able to bridge between RBC's owing to their large size, efficiently creating what is seen as agglutination. IgG antibodies are smaller and require assistance to bridge well enough to form a visual agglutination reaction

86971

The enzyme pretreatment of red blood cells is undertaken when there are multiple antibodies or one that is too weak to demonstrate without pre-treatment of the reagent RBCs. The enzyme used depends on the suspected antibody. Certain enzymes enhance particular antibodies while destroying others.

86972

In some red cell typing and antibody detection procedures it is desirable to exclude other cellular components of whole blood, such as white blood cells or platelets. Isolation of RBCs from whole blood may be accomplished by centrifugation in a density gradient.

86975
This method removes antibodies to certain drugs by using pre-treated red blood cells and the patient's serum. Serum is incubated with the treated RBCs (to attach the drug antibody) and centrifuged. The serum is removed and used in further testing.

86976
This is code is similar to 86975. There are times when the amount of antibody exceeds the amount of antigen attached to the RBCs. In these cases, the serum is diluted prior to adsorption or re-adsorption.

86977
In some instances, cell adsorption of the interfering substance will not work, and inhibitor is incubated with the patient's serum to "neutralize" the substance. The antibody to Sda is one of these substances.

86978
Incubation of the patient's cells and patient's serum together prior to testing can remove some autoimmune complexes. This can be done refrigerated for cold autoantibodies or warm for warm autoantibodies. In cases of multiple antibodies, each antibody may be absorbed out in turn by using reagent RBCs of known antigenicity.

86985
In transfusion cases where the patient is a child or where transfusion of a full unit of product will overload the circulatory system, a unit will be split into multiple smaller units.

87003
Animal inoculation with infected tissue, blood, or other specimen source is used in the diagnosis of several diseases, including rabies, Colorado tick fever, and infantile botulism. There are different specimen types for the different tests. Contact the reference lab that is performing the test for type of specimen and transport. This test is used to observe signs of illness in inoculated mice for as long as three weeks and for the dissection of mice and preparation of tissue for microscopy to confirm diagnosis when mice become ill or die.

87015
Concentration may also be referred to as thick smear preparation. The source samples are treated to concentrate the presence of suspect organisms, usually through sedimentation or flotation. There are two common methods of concentration for ova and parasite exams: formalin concentration and zinc sulfate flotation. The most common concentration methods for AFB stains or cultures are the N-acetyl-L cysteine method, cytocentrifugation, and the Zephiran-trisodium phosphate method.

87040
Samples for bacterial blood culture are drawn by venipuncture and usually consist of a set of bottles, an aerobic and an anaerobic bottle. Drawing at least two sets of cultures increases the effectiveness of the test. This code includes anaerobic culture along with aerobic, if appropriate. Presumptive identification of aerobic pathogens or microorganisms in the blood sample is by means of identifying colony morphology. The test includes gram staining and subculturing to selective media for the detection of bacterial growth. There are several automated systems that detect the presence of bacteria using colorimetric, radiometric, or spectrophotometric means. The purpose of blood culture tests is to detect the presence of aerobic and anaerobic bacteria in blood and to identify the bacteria, but not to the specific level of genus or species requiring additional testing, such as slide cultures.

87045
This test may be called a stool culture, culture for *Salmonella* and *Shigella*, or routine culture when stool or rectal swab is the specimen. The testing method includes gram staining and subculturing to selective media for the detection of bacterial growth. This test cultures specifically for the initial identification of enteric pathogens *Salmonella* and *Shigella*.

87046
This test may be requested by the name of the suspected pathogenic organism. Presumptive identification of aerobic pathogens or microorganisms in the stool sample is by means of identifying colony morphology. The test includes gram staining and subculturing to selective media for the detection of bacterial growth. There are several automated systems that detect the presence of bacteria using colorimetric, radiometric, or spectrophotometric means. The purpose of this stool culture test is to detect the presence of enteric pathogens in the form of aerobic bacteria and to identify the micro-organism(s), but not to the specific level of genus or species requiring additional testing, such as slide cultures. Report this code once for each plate prepared. Stool or rectal swab is the specimen.

87070-87071
Common names for this test are numerous and may include routine culture, aerobic culture, or, using a body or source site, may be referred to as vaginal culture, cerebral spinal fluid culture, etc. Presumptive identification of aerobic pathogens or microorganisms in the sample is by means of identifying colony morphology. The test includes gram staining and subculturing to selective media for the detection of bacterial growth. There are several automated systems that detect the presence of bacteria using colorimetric, radiometric, or spectrophotometric means. The purpose of this culture test is to detect the presence of any or multiple aerobic bacteria from a body source or site, except urine, blood, or stool samples, and to identify the micro-organism(s), but not to the specific level of genus or species requiring additional testing, such as slide cultures. The collection and transport of specimen is varied and specimen dependent. Report 87071 when the identified aerobic isolate(s) is quantified in growth numbers.

87073

The most common name for this procedure is anaerobic culture. Presumptive identification of anaerobic pathogens or microorganisms in the sample is by means of identifying colony morphology. The test includes gram staining and subculturing to selective media for the detection of bacterial growth. There are several automated systems that detect the presence of bacteria using colorimetric, radiometric, or spectrophotometric means. This culture test detects the presence of anaerobic bacteria in a body site or source, except blood, urine, or stool, and identifies the micro-organism(s), but not to the specific level of genus or species requiring additional testing, such as slide cultures. The isolate(s) identified is quantified in growth numbers. Tissues, fluids, and aspirations, except from blood, urine, or stool samples, are collected in anaerobic vials or with anaerobic transport swabs and transported immediately. Anaerobic bacteria are sensitive to oxygen and cold.

87075

The most common name for this procedure is anaerobic culture. Presumptive identification of anaerobic pathogens or microorganisms in the sample is by means of identifying colony morphology. The test includes gram staining and subculturing to selective media for the detection of bacterial growth. There are several automated systems that detect the presence of bacteria using colorimetric, radiometric, or spectrophotometric means. The purpose of this culture test is to detect the presence of any or multiple anaerobic bacteria from any body source or site, except blood, and to identify the micro-organism(s), but not to the specific level of genus or species requiring additional testing, such as slide cultures. Tissues, fluids, and aspirations, except blood samples, are collected in anaerobic vials or with anaerobic transport swabs and transported immediately. Anaerobic bacteria are sensitive to oxygen and cold.

87076-87077

This code reports definitive anaerobic (87076) or aerobic (87077) organism identification of an already-isolated anaerobic or aerobic bacterium. The pathogen has already been presumptively identified, but additional testing is required to identify the specific genus or species. The additional definitive testing methods include biochemical panels and slide cultures. Studies using chromatography, molecular probes, or specific immunological techniques may be employed for definitive testing, but are not included in this code and are reported separately.

87081-87084

These codes describe presumptive screening cultures for one or more pathogenic organisms. The methodology is by culture and the culture should be identified by type (e.g., anaerobic, aerobic) and specimen source (e.g., pleural, peritoneal, bronchial aspirates). If a specific organism is suspected, the person ordering the test typically uses common names, such as strep screen, staph screen, etc., to specify the organism for screening. Presumptive identification includes gram staining as well as up to three tests, such as a catalase, oxidase, or urease test. Screenings included in this code are nonmotile, catalase-positive, gram-positive rod bacteria. Report 87084 when an estimation of the number of organisms is also made, based on a density chart.

87086-87088

These codes report the performance of a urine bacterial culture with a calibrated inoculating device so that a colony count accurately correlates with the number of organisms in the urine. In 87088, isolation and presumptive identification of bacteria recovered from the sample is done by means of identifying colony morphology, subculturing organisms to selective media and the performance of a gram stain or other simple test to identify bacteria to the genus level. There are several automated systems that detect the presence of bacteria using colorimetric, radiometric, or spectrophotometric means. In 87086, quantified colony count numbers within the urine sample are measured.

87101

Dermatophyte culture and fungal culture are common names for this test. Fungi are divided into two broad categories, yeasts and molds. Skin, hair or nail scrapings from infected site are transferred to appropriate agar. Growth and confirmation by microscopic methods identify, or confirm, a presumptive identification of fungus isolated. Alternately, the scrapings are dropped onto dermatophyte test media (DMT) at the time of collection. The media changes color to indicate dermatophyte growth.

87102

Fungal culture, yeast culture, and mold culture are common names for this procedure. Collection is as varied as the sources and the same specimen may be used for other tests. This test is to culture and isolate fungi (yeast or mold) with presumptive identification. Presumptive identification may include fungi (yeast or mold) present or a genus name with no species (e.g., Aspergillus).

87103

Fungal blood culture and blood culture for yeast are common names for this procedure. Blood is subcultured to fungal media. This test procedure is a culture to isolate fungi (yeast or mold) with presumptive identification. Presumptive identification may include fungi (yeast or mold) present or a genus name with no species (e.g., Aspergillus).

87106

This test is commonly known as a fungal yeast identification. Yeast isolates from fungal cultures are further tested for definitive identification. This code reports testing only for yeast pathogens. Various identification procedures, including growth patterns, and macroscopic and microscopic characteristics, are employed. Examples of fungal yeast pathogens that might require definitive identification include: Histoplasma, Coccidioides and Blastomyces.

87107
This test is commonly known as a mold identification. Molds are filamentous fungi that can cause severe, life-threatening infections in immunocompromised individuals. Mold isolates from fungal cultures are further tested for definitive identification. Various identification procedures, including growth patterns, and macroscopic and microscopic characteristics, are employed. Examples of conidium-forming filamentous fungi species that might require definitive identification include: Aspergillus sp., Fusarium sp., Rhizopus arrhizus, Scedosporium apiospermum and Sporothrix schenckii.

87109
A common name for this test is Mycoplasma culture. Specimens are typically transported in viral transport media (VTM). Mycoplasma culture methods are employed. This procedure is for the isolation and identification of Mycoplasma.

87110
This test is commonly known as a Chlamydia culture. A swab of the infected site is placed in a vial of sucrose transport media containing antibiotics and glass beads. The specimen is generally kept refrigerated. The test method is by cell culture, fluorescent stain. The cell culture technique is to isolate for Chlamydia.

87116
Common names include AFB culture, TB culture, mycobacterium culture, and acid-fast culture. Collection methods are source dependent. The methodology is by culture for the isolation and presumptive identification of mycobacterium. An acid-fast smear should be done at the time the specimen is cultured. Media for isolation should include both solid and liquid types.

87118
This procedure is a definitive identification of mycobacterial organisms isolated by procedure 87116. This procedure may be performed by a reference laboratory after isolation by a primary lab. Methodology is traditional biochemical tests for identification of mycobacterium.

87140
Specific antisera are combined with a fluorescent dye and used to stain slides of organisms. Stained slides are scanned with a fluorescent microscope to look for fluorescing organisms. Typing of organisms by immunofluorescent technique is usually to determine whether an organism is of a more pathogenic strain, to determine a treatment, or for epidemiological purposes.

87143
This procedure is performed to provide more specific typing of cultured pathogenic organisms. The methodology is gas liquid chromatography (GLC) or high pressure liquid chromatography (HPLC) to analyze byproducts of rapidly growing organisms. GLC is an automated technique in which the culture specimen is dissolved in a solvent, vaporized, and transported by an inert gas through an adsorbent gas-liquid column containing detectors that analyze and graph the components of the specimen. HPLC is similar to GLC except that the liquid is forced under high pressure through a column packed with sorbent and separated by various methods including adsorption, gel filtration, ion-exchange, or partition. This procedure is performed on an isolated organism as in the definitive identification of mycobacterium.

87147
This test is used for more specifically identifying cultured specimens using an immunologic method other than immunofluorescence. For example, agglutination technique may be used to more specifically identify Salmonella usually to a group level since there are more than 2,000 serovar of Salmonella. The different species have been grouped by common antigens and are tested with polyvalent antisera and reported by group (e.g., Salmonella Group D).

87149-87150
Organisms from any type of culture are identified by nucleic acid probes. Nucleic acid (DNA or RNA) probes may be used to diagnose and monitor infectious diseases. These probes can be used to detect fungi and other organisms after they have been grown in culture. Culturing is required for many organisms because direct staining does not produce accurate results. Specificity using this culture technique is nearly 100 percent for many organisms. Report 87149 for direct probe technique and 87150 for amplified probe technique.

[87154]
This code describes the identification of pathogens in the blood using nucleic acid probes. Nucleic acid (DNA or RNA) probes may be used to diagnose and monitor infectious diseases by detecting organisms grown in a culture. The testing includes a multiplex amplified probe technique and multiplex reverse transcription, when performed. Report 87154 for each culture or isolate of six or more targets; resistance typing, when performed, is included.

87152
This test may also be known by the acronym PFGE (pulsed field gel electrophoresis), CHEF (contour-clamped homogeneous electric field), or a combination of the two. A bacterial culture and nucleic acid isolation precedes the test and cells are harvested by centrifugation and washing. The PFGE method resolves and separates very large DNA molecules for cloning and direct visualization of small chromosomes (among other genetic analysis). This emerging method provides information about macromolecular structure and function and has been used to detect in vivo chromosome breakage and degradation, the number and size of chromosomes, and to identify invasive infection in humans.

87153
This code describes the identification of organisms from any type of culture using the nucleic acid sequencing method. Isolation and identification of the genetic material of organisms known to be the infectious agent in certain diseases are helpful in determining the most precise therapy and antimicrobials for treatment of the patient. For example, identification of bacterial isolates by 16S rRNA gene sequencing identifies uncommon bacteria that cannot be identified using conventional methods. Report 87153 for each isolate. If additional studies involving molecular probes, chromatography, or immunologic techniques are performed, these should be reported separately.

87158
Any methodology that would identify a microbial organism to the species level or a type level that does not involve the use of biochemical substrates (traditional bacteriology), antigen specific fluorescent stain, gas chromatography, phage testing, or agglutination or precipitation from antigen-antibody reactions. Lectin assays and bacteriocin typing are two tests that fit in this procedure description.

87164-87166
Names commonly used include dark field for syphilis and dark field exam. Dark field microscopic exams have generally been limited to the bacteria called spirochetes. *Treponema pallidum*, the agent of syphilis; *Borrelia burgdorferi*, the agent of Lyme disease; and *Leptospira* are among the better known spirochetes. Specimens for dark field exam are typically examined within 30 minutes of collection. Certain immunological tests have rendered this method to be somewhat outdated. The term "dark field" refers to the staining method. If the lab is responsible for specimen collection, report 87164. If the lab is not responsible for collection of the specimen, report 87166.

87168
This test is performed to identify arthropods that might be vectors of disease causing organisms in man. Arthropods are small animals having a hard, jointed exoskeleton and paired legs. This group of animals includes lice and ticks. Method is visual examination (macroscopic) of the source specimen.

87169
This test is performed to identify parasites other than arthropods that might be vectors of disease causing organisms in man. Method is visual examination (macroscopic) of the source specimen.

87172
This test may be requested as pinworm examination. Clear tape is applied to the perianal area. The tape is removed and submitted to the laboratory on a clean slide. Method is microscopic examination.

87176
This test may be called grinding or homogenization of tissue. The methodology is mechanical disruption of the tissue to enhance extraction of endotoxin. It may involve the use of sterile equipment, such as scissors, mortar and pestle, or disposable grinders.

87177
Common names for this procedure are ova and parasite exam or O & P. Stool is collected in a clean, leak-proof container (when processed within one hour) or the specimen is added to formalin or fixative (both available in commercial kits). The methodology of an ova and parasite exam for stool includes a direct smear and smear of concentrated material, such as formalin concentration technique or zinc flotation method. Identification is by observing parasites with the aid of a microscope.

87181
A susceptibility study is performed to determine the effectiveness of an antimicrobial agent against microorganisms. This test is performed to assist the treating provider in determining which drug will be the most effective for treatment of an infection. The methodology is agar dilution. Varying concentrations of an antimicrobial agent are introduced into agar, a culture medium used to grow microorganisms. This introduction is performed using an instrument such as an antibiotic gradient strip. The test result is expressed as the minimum inhibitory concentration (MIC), which is the lowest concentration of the antimicrobial agent needed to inhibit growth of an organism. This code is reported once per agent.

87184
This test may also be known as a Kirby-Bauer test. A susceptibility study is performed to determine the effectiveness of an antimicrobial agent against microorganisms. This test is performed to assist the treating provider in determining which drug will be the most effective for treatment of an infection. The methodology is disk diffusion. An agar plate is a petri dish that includes agar, a culture medium used to grow microorganisms. A paper disc containing an antimicrobial compound is placed on the agar surface to measure the reaction of the agent with the microorganism. Results are expressed as susceptible, intermediate, or resistant. This code is reported once per plate.

87185
A susceptibility study is performed to determine the effectiveness of an antimicrobial agent against microorganisms. This test is performed to assist the treating provider in determining which drug will be the most effective for treatment of an infection. The methodology is enzyme detection. One example is extended-spectrum beta-lactamase (ESBL) testing. Some organisms produce enzymes that are resistant to certain antimicrobial agents. Screening for the presence of enzyme activity is performed with the introduction of different antimicrobial agents. This code is reported once per enzyme.

87186
A susceptibility study is performed to determine the effectiveness of an antimicrobial agent against

microorganisms. This test is performed to assist the treating provider in determining which drug will be the most effective for treatment of an infection. The methodology is microdilution or agar dilution. Varying concentrations of an antimicrobial agent are introduced into agar, a culture medium used to grow microorganisms. This introduction is performed using a plate with individual wells that hold predetermined concentrations of antimicrobial agents. The test result is expressed as the minimum inhibitory concentration (MIC), which is the lowest concentration of the antimicrobial agent needed to inhibit growth of an organism. This code is reported once for each multi-antimicrobial, per plate.

87187

A susceptibility study is performed to determine the effectiveness of an antimicrobial agent against microorganisms. This test is performed to assist the treating provider in determining which drug will be the most effective for treatment of an infection. The methodology is microdilution or agar dilution. Varying concentrations of an antimicrobial agent are introduced into agar, a culture medium used to grow microorganisms. This introduction is performed using a plate with individual wells that hold predetermined concentrations of antimicrobial agents. The test result is expressed as the minimum lethal concentration (MLC), which is the lowest concentration of the antimicrobial agent needed to almost completely destroy an organism. This may also be referred to as the minimum bactericidal concentration (MBC) or minimum fungicidal concentration (MFC). This add-on code is reported once for each plate in addition to the code for the primary procedure.

87188

A susceptibility study is performed to determine the effectiveness of an antimicrobial agent against microorganisms. This test is performed to assist the treating provider in determining which drug will be the most effective for treatment of an infection. The methodology is macrobroth dilution. Varying concentrations of an antimicrobial agent are introduced into agar, a culture medium used to grow microorganisms. This introduction is performed using tubes that each contain a minimum volume of 2 mL of the agent/agar mixture. The test result is expressed as the minimum inhibitory concentration (MIC), which is the lowest concentration of the antimicrobial agent needed to inhibit growth of an organism. This code is reported once for each agent.

87190

A susceptibility study is performed to determine the effectiveness of an antimicrobial agent against microorganisms. This test is performed to assist the treating provider in determining which drug will be the most effective for treatment of an infection. The methodology is agar proportion testing. Mycobacteria are introduced into agar, a culture medium used to grow microorganisms. Growth is assessed with and without an antimycobacterial drug. The test result is expressed as the proportion or percentage of resistance. The bacterium is considered resistant when the number of colonies that grow when the drug is introduced is 1 percent or more of the number of colonies that grew without the drug. This code is reported once for each agent.

87197

This procedure is called a serum cidal level, a serum bactericidal titer, or a Schlichter test. This test cannot be performed without a bacterial organism that has been previously isolated from the same patient. The killing power of the patient's serum against the isolated pathogen is measured. Blood is usually drawn and tested at peak and trough level of the antibiotic.

87205

Any smear done on a primary source (e.g., sputum, CSF, etc.) to identify bacteria, fungi, and cell types. An interpretation of findings is provided. Bacteria, fungi, WBCs, and epithelial cells may be estimated in quantity with an interpretation as to the possibility of contamination by normal flora. A gram stain may be the most commonly performed smear of this type.

87206

A fluorescent or acid-fast stain for bacteria, fungi, parasites, viruses, or cell types. These are stains usually for specific groups of organisms (e.g., mycobacterium and *Nocardia*). Identification of *Cryptosporidium* and related parasites are examples of parasites that can be identified by fluorescent or acid fast stain. An interpretation is included.

87207

This is a stain to look for inclusion bodies or parasites (e.g., malaria inside red cells). Its use to detect herpes has been outdated by amplification and immunological methods. An interpretation is included.

87209

This is a stain to look for the inclusion of trichome or iron hematoxylin indicating the presence of parasites or their eggs. An interpretation is included.

87210

This test may be requested as a KOH prep. A wet mount is prepared from a primary source to detect bacteria, fungi, or ova and parasites. Motility of organisms is visible on wet mounts and the addition of a simple stain, such as iodine, India ink, or simple dyes, may aid detection of bacteria, fungi, and parasites. An interpretation of findings is included.

87220

Potassium hydroxide (KOH) prep and calcofluor stains are the most common methods of looking for hyphal elements and/ or yeast in tissue. The KOH causes a clearing of the specimen to make fungus more visible. The preparation is enhanced for microscopic observation by adding a drop of calcofluor, a type of fluorescent dye, to the slide and reading the preparation with a fluorescent microscope.

87230

This procedure is a toxin assay for diagnosis of toxin producing organisms, such as *Clostridium difficile, E. coli*

0157, enterotoxigenic *E. coli*, and *Vibrio cholerae*. Stool is collected for testing. Filtrates of the stool are inoculated into cell cultures and observed for CPE (cytopathic effect) microscopically. Confirmation of toxin production may be done by toxin neutralization. Different cell cultures are used to test for different toxins, so organism must be specified.

87250
Embryonated egg or small animal inoculation with specimen source is used in the diagnosis of some viruses. There are different specimen types for the different viruses. Contact the reference lab that is performing the test for type of specimen and transport. There are, however, more rapid tests to diagnose most viral infections. This code includes observation for signs of illness in inoculated mice for as long as three weeks and dissection of mice and preparation of tissue for microscopy to confirm diagnosis when mice become ill or die.

87252
Cell culture is a procedure used particularly for viral detection. There is a general viral culture which can detect most viruses, but when a specific agent is suspected such as CMV, HSV, Influenzae A or B, mumps, or varicella zoster, more specific and rapid culture techniques can be used. This procedure provides presumptive identification by cytopathic effect only. Specimens may be collected by swab, washings and fluids, and blood draw.

87253
This code reports additional tissue culture studies required for specific virus identification and is reported for each isolate.

87254
This test may also be ordered as a shell vial (SV) culture, a rapid shell assay, or an immediate early antigen test. Specimen collection is by separately reportable appropriate procedure. Shell vial isolation cultures offer more immediate results (often 48-hours) than conventional cultures. The technique is particularly useful in identification of respiratory organisms. Immunofluorescence is a technique in which antibody reacts with an antigen on a fixed slide. The antibody in turn reacts with antihuman globulins for the diagnosis of infectious diseases. The fluorescence is best viewed with a laser-scanning confocal microscope.

87255
A peptide substrate specific for a viral enzyme proteolytic activity is used for detection of viral infection in primary source biological samples, such as serum and whole cells. Enzyme proteolytic activity is the splitting of protein peptide bonds with the formation of smaller polypeptides. This peptide cleavage, catalyzed by the specific enzyme, causes an increase in fluorescence, which allows determination of the specific enzymatic activity by visualizing the protease activity with a fluorescence microscope.

87260
This test may be requested as adenovirus by DFA or by immunofluorescence. It is most commonly used to diagnose serotypes that cause infantile gastroenteritis. A random stool sample is obtained. Infectious agent antigen detection by immunofluorescence includes direct and indirect fluorescent antibody technique and involves using monoclonal antibodies and immunofluorescence microscopy. Cellular material must be obtained from the site for immunofluorescence to be an effective diagnostic technique.

87265
This test may be requested as *Bordetella pertussis* or parapertussis by DFA or by immunofluorescence. *Bordetella pertussis* is the causative agent of whooping cough. Infectious agent antigen detection by immunofluorescence includes direct and indirect fluorescent antibody technique and involves using monoclonal antibodies and immunofluorescence microscopy. Cellular material must be obtained from the site for immunofluorescence to be an effective diagnostic technique.

87267
An enterovirus is detected by direct fluorescent antibody (DFA) staining technique. Molecules of a fluorescent dye are chemically linked to antibodies that are introduced into the specimen sample and bind with their specific antigen (e.g., the enterovirus) to form an antibody-antigen complex. The presence of the infectious agent microorganism is detected indirectly when the fluorescent reaction of the dye is seen under a special microscope. The enterovirus is isolated in cell culture for the test. Specimens include throat swabs, CSF, and blood samples. An enterovirus includes polio, Coxsackie, and echovirus.

87269
This procedure may be requested as Giardia by direct fluorescent antibody (DFA) stain or by immunofluorescence. The Giardia lamblia parasite causes severe diarrhea, cramps, and stomach-ache, and can lead to weight loss and dehydration. Contamination occurs in soil, food, water, or surfaces in contact with infected feces. Giardia is a very common cause of waterborne disease in humans in the United States. Infectious agent antigen detection by immunofluorescence includes direct and indirect fluorescent antibody technique and involves using monoclonal antibodies and immunofluorescence microscopy. Cellular material must be obtained from the site for immunofluorescence to be an effective diagnostic technique.

87270
This test may be requested as *Chlamydia trachomatis* or *C. trachomatis* by DFA or by immunofluorescence. *C. trachomatis* is a frequently occurring sexually transmitted disease. It may cause nonspecific urethritis or pelvic inflammatory disease (PID), although it is frequently asymptomatic in women. Another serotype also causes conjunctivitis. Infectious agent antigen

detection by immunofluorescence includes direct and indirect fluorescent antibody technique and involves using monoclonal antibodies and immunofluorescence microscopy. Cellular material must be obtained from the site for immunofluorescence to be an effective diagnostic technique.

87271
A cytomegalovirus is detected by direct fluorescent antibody (DFA) staining technique. The presence of the infectious agent microorganism is detected indirectly when the fluorescent reaction of the dye is seen under a special microscope. The cytomegalovirus is isolated in cell culture for the test. Specimens include throat swabs, CSF, and blood samples. A cytomegalovirus is any virus in the Betaherpesvirinae subfamily.

87272
This procedure may be referred to as a direct fluorescent antibody (DFA) or immunofluorescent stain for cryptosporidium. This parasite infects the gastrointestinal tract causing symptoms such as diarrhea, weight loss, fever, and abdominal pain. Infectious agent antigen detection by immunofluorescence includes direct and indirect fluorescent antibody technique and involves using monoclonal antibodies and immunofluorescence microscopy.

87273
This test may be requested as HSV 2 by DFA or HSV 2 by immunofluorescence. HSV 2 is a sexually transmitted disease with lesions occurring primarily in the genitourinary tract. Infectious agent antigen detection by immunofluorescence includes direct and indirect fluorescent antibody technique and involves using monoclonal antibodies and immunofluorescence microscopy. Cellular material must be obtained from the site for immunofluorescence to be an effective diagnostic technique.

87274
This test may be requested as HSV 1 by DFA or HSV 1 by immunofluorescence. HSV 1 is primarily responsible for oral lesions frequently referred to as fever blisters or cold sores. Infectious agent antigen detection by immunofluorescence includes direct and indirect fluorescent antibody technique and involves using monoclonal antibodies and immunofluorescence microscopy. Cellular material must be obtained from the site for immunofluorescence to be an effective diagnostic technique.

87275
This test may be requested as influenza B (less common strain) by DFA or by immunofluorescence. Infectious agent antigen detection by immunofluorescence includes direct and indirect fluorescent antibody technique and involves using monoclonal antibodies and immunofluorescence microscopy. Cellular material must be obtained from the site for immunofluorescence to be an effective diagnostic technique.

87276
This test may be requested as influenza A (most common strain) by DFA or by immunofluorescence. The causative agent is subject to wide variation in antigenic type. This is referred to as antigen shift and causes new variations of the Type A virus to appear at two to three year intervals. Infectious agent antigen detection by immunofluorescence includes direct and indirect fluorescent antibody technique and involves using monoclonal antibodies and immunofluorescence microscopy. Cellular material must be obtained from the site for immunofluorescence to be an effective diagnostic technique.

87278
This procedure may be requested as Legionella pneumophila by direct fluorescent antibody (DFA) stain or by immunofluorescence. L. pneumophila is the bacterium associated with Legionnaires' disease and Pontiac fever. Infectious agent antigen detection by immunofluorescence includes direct and indirect fluorescent antibody technique and involves nonculture (primary source) detection of infected cells using monoclonal antibodies and immunofluorescence microscopy. Cellular material must be obtained from the site for immunofluorescence to be an effective diagnostic technique. For DFA procedure it is acceptable to prepare and send two air-dried smears. This method may be a rapid diagnosis, but is not as accurate as cultured tests.

87279
This test may be requested as parainfluenza virus by DFA or by immunofluorescence. Parainfluenza is a group of viruses that cause upper respiratory infections that are often the causative agents in croup, bronchitis and bronchiolitis. Infectious agent antigen detection by immunofluorescence includes direct and indirect fluorescent antibody technique and involves using monoclonal antibodies and immunofluorescence microscopy. Cellular material must be obtained from the site for immunofluorescence to be an effective diagnostic technique.

87280
This test may be requested as DFA or immunofluorescent stain for respiratory syncytial virus (RSV). RSV causes respiratory disease that can be particularly severe in infants. Infectious agent antigen detection by immunofluorescence includes direct and indirect fluorescent antibody technique and involves using monoclonal antibodies and immunofluorescence microscopy. Cellular material must be obtained from the site for immunofluorescence to be an effective diagnostic technique.

87281
This test may be requested as pneumocystis carinii or PCP by DFA or by immunofluorescence. Pneumocystis carinii causes lung infection or pneumonia in

premature infants, cancer patients, patients being treated with immunosuppressive medications for the management of organ transplantation or cancer, and AIDS patients. Infectious agent antigen detection by immunofluorescence includes direct and indirect fluorescent antibody technique and involves using monoclonal antibodies and immunofluorescence microscopy. Cellular material must be obtained from the site for immunofluorescence to be an effective diagnostic technique.

87283

This test may be requested as rubeola stain or rubeola IFA. Rubeola, more commonly referred to as measles, is characterized by fever, coryza, cough, and conjunctivitis after which Koplik's spots appear in the mouth with pharyngitis and inflammation of the laryngeal and tracheobronchial mucosa. Infectious agent antigen detection by immunofluorescence includes direct and indirect fluorescent antibody technique and involves using monoclonal antibodies and immunofluorescence microscopy. Cellular material must be obtained from the site for immunofluorescence to be an effective diagnostic technique.

87285

The spirochete Treponema pallidum is the causative agent of syphilis. Infectious agent antigen detection by immunofluorescence includes direct and indirect fluorescent antibody technique and involves using monoclonal antibodies and immunofluorescence microscopy. Cellular material must be obtained from the site for immunofluorescence to be an effective diagnostic technique.

87290

This test may be requested as direct fluorescent stain for varicella zoster virus. This is the causative agent of chickenpox. Infectious agent antigen detection by immunofluorescence includes direct and indirect fluorescent antibody technique and involves using monoclonal antibodies and immunofluorescence microscopy. Cellular material must be obtained from the site for immunofluorescence to be an effective diagnostic technique. This test has a high specificity, but sensitivity is dependent on adequacy of the sample collected. A negative sample should be cultured.

87299

This code reports immunofluorescent technique of specific infectious agents not identified by more specific codes. Infectious agent antigen detection by immunofluorescence includes direct and indirect fluorescent antibody technique and involves using monoclonal antibodies and immunofluorescence microscopy. Cellular material must be obtained from the site for immunofluorescence to be an effective diagnostic technique.

87300

This code reports immunofluorescent technique to identify multiple strains of bacteria or other infectious organisms in a single test. Infectious agent antigen detection by immunofluorescence includes direct and indirect fluorescent antibody technique and involves using monoclonal antibodies and immunofluorescence microscopy. Cellular material must be obtained from the site for immunofluorescence to be an effective diagnostic technique.

87301

This test may be requested as adenovirus enteric types 40/41 by qualitative or semiquantitative enzyme immunoassay (EIA), enzyme-linked immunosorbent assay (ELISA), fluorescence immunoassay (FIA), or immunochemiluminometric assay (IMCA). These serotypes cause infantile gastroenteritis. A random stool sample is the specimen. This test detects if an analyte is present, as well as providing a count of the analyte in comparison to normal thresholds.

87305

This test may be requested as qualitative or semiquantitative enzyme immunoassay (EIA), enzyme-linked immunosorbent assay (ELISA), fluorescence immunoassay (FIA), or immunochemiluminometric assay (IMCA) for the detection of *Aspergillus* or *Aspergillus* galactomannan antigen. Specimen is blood serum. *Aspergillus* is a life-threatening infection in patients with immune systems compromised by leukemia, organ or bone marrow transplant, or chemotherapy.

87320

This test may be requested as *Chlamydia trachomatis* or *C. trachomatis* by qualitative or semiquantitative immunoassay techniques, such as enzyme immunoassay (EIA), enzyme-linked immunosorbent assay (ELISA), fluorescence immunoassay (FIA), or immunochemiluminometric assay (IMCA). *C. trachomatis* is a frequently occurring sexually transmitted disease. It may cause nonspecific urethritis or pelvic inflammatory disease (PID), although it is frequently asymptomatic in women. Another serotype also causes conjunctivitis. Enzyme immunoassay refers to a technique that utilizes a chemical bond between an enzyme and an antigen or antibody as a label to identify specific chemical or infectious agents. Special reagents and equipment are required for *C. trachomatis* EIA. Sensitivity of EIA is approximately 75 to 85 percent.

87324

This test may be requested as qualitative or semiquantitative enzyme immunoassay (EIA), enzyme-linked immunosorbent assay (ELISA), fluorescence immunoassay (FIA), or immunochemiluminometric assay (IMCA) for the detection of *Clostridium difficile* toxin or more simply referred to as a *C. difficile* toxin test. A random stool sample is obtained. Fresh stool should be kept refrigerated and transported in a clean, leak-proof container.

87327
This test is conducted for the detection of *Cryptococcus neoformans* by enzyme immunoassay (EIA), enzyme-linked immunosorbent assay (ELISA), fluorescence immunoassay (FIA), or immunochemiluminometric assay (IMCA). Blood is obtained by venipuncture. CSF is obtained by lumbar puncture, which is reported separately. Cryptococcosis is a life-threatening infection of the meninges in patients with compromised immune systems due to diseases such as acquired immune deficiency syndrome (AIDS). This test is most effective when performed on CSF of patients with symptoms of cryptococcal meningitis; however, serum may also contain detectable levels of antigen.

87328
This procedure is for the detection of *Cryptosporidium* by qualitative or semiquantitative enzyme immunoassay (EIA), enzyme-linked immunosorbent assay (ELISA), fluorescence immunoassay (FIA), or immunochemiluminometric assay (IMCA). This parasite infects the gastrointestinal tract causing symptoms such as diarrhea, weight loss, fever, and abdominal pain. A random stool sample is obtained. The fresh or preserved stool must be transported in a clean, leak-proof container. This test detects if an analyte is present, as well as providing a count of the analyte in comparison to normal thresholds.

87329
This procedure is for the qualitative or semiquantitative detection of *Giardia lamblia* by enzyme immunoassay (EIA), enzyme-linked immunosorbent assay (ELISA), fluorescence immunoassay (FIA), or immunochemiluminometric assay (IMCA). The *Giardia lamblia* parasite causes severe diarrhea, cramps, and stomachache, and can lead to weight loss and dehydration. Contamination occurs in soil, food, water, or surfaces in contact with infected feces. *Giardia* is a very common cause of waterborne disease in humans in the United States. The specimen is a random stool specimen.

87332
This test may be requested as cytomegalovirus (CMV) by qualitative or semiquantitative immunoassay techniques such as enzyme immunoassay (EIA), enzyme-linked immunosorbent assay (ELISA), fluorescence immunoassay (FIA), or immunochemiluminometric assay (IMCA). CMV is part of the viral family that includes herpes zoster, Epstein-Barr, and Varicella zoster infections. CMV usually causes only mild symptoms except in fetal infection or immunosuppressed patients, including AIDS and transplant patients. Blood specimen is obtained by venipuncture. Enzyme immunoassay refers to a technique that utilizes a chemical bond between an enzyme and an antigen or antibody as a label to identify specific chemical or infectious agents.

87335
This test may be requested as qualitative or semiquantitative immunoassay (EIA), enzyme-linked immunosorbent assay (ELISA), fluorescence immunoassay (FIA), or immunochemiluminometric assay (IMCA) for the detection of *Escherichia coli* (*E. coli*) 0157. *E. coli* 0157 is the causative agent of hemorrhagic colitis in food-borne epidemics. A random stool sample is obtained. Stool or rectal swabs may be transported in Carey-Blair transport media. Fresh stool can be sent in a clean, leak-proof container, but if transport time exceeds two hours, the specimen should be frozen at -70 C. This test detects if an analyte is present, as well as provides a count of the analyte in comparison to normal thresholds.

87336-87337
Code 87336 is ordered for the detection of *Entamoeba histolytica dispar* group. *E. histolytica* is an enteric protozoan that exists in trophozoite or cyst form. Code 87337 may be ordered as an *H. pylori* antibody titer, stool. Specimen collection is from a stool sample, particularly drawn from mucous in the specimen. *H. pylori* may be found along the gastric mucosa and on the mucosal cells of the GI tract, and its presence is linked to several serious disorders of the stomach. Three to six stool examinations are recommended, each permanently stained using a trichrome stained for both studies. Method is qualitative or semiquantitative, enzyme immunoassay (EIA), enzyme-linked immunosorbent assay (ELISA), fluorescence immunoassay (FIA), or immunochemiluminometric assay (IMCA).

87338
This test may be ordered as an *H. pylori* antibody titer, stool. Specimen collection is from mucous in the specimen. Method is qualitative or semiquantitative, enzyme immunoassay (EIA), enzyme-linked immunosorbent assay (ELISA), fluorescence immunoassay (FIA), or immunochemiluminometric assay (IMCA). *H. pylori* may be found along the gastric mucosa and on the mucosal cells of the GI tract, and its presence is linked to several serious disorders of the stomach.

87339
This test may be ordered as an *H. pylori* antibody titer. Method is qualitative or semiquantitative, enzyme immunoassay (EIA), enzyme-linked immunosorbent assay (ELISA), fluorescence immunoassay (FIA), or immunochemiluminometric assay (IMCA). *H. pylori* may be found along the gastric mucosa and on the mucosal cells of the GI tract and its presence is linked to several serious disorders of the stomach.

87340
This test may be requested as HBsAg by immunoassay techniques such as enzyme immunoassay (EIA), enzyme-linked immunosorbent assay (ELISA), fluorescence immunoassay (FIA), or immunochemiluminometric assay (IMCA). Hepatitis B is a retrovirus that can cause persistent infection leading to cirrhosis and hepatocellular carcinoma. HBsAg is a lipoprotein that coats the surface of the hepatitis B virus. Blood specimen is serum; method is qualitative or semiquantitative.

87341
This test may be requested as qualitative or semiquantitative HBsAg by enzyme immunoassay (EIA), enzyme-linked immunosorbent assay (ELISA), fluorescence immunoassay (FIA), or immunochemiluminometric assay (IMCA) confirmation. This assay is performed only when a specimen is repeatedly reactive for Hepatitis B surface antigen. Elevated HBsAg levels beyond six months may indicate a chronic carrier (i.e., chronic hepatitis). The HBsAg neutralization test is performed to identify false positives. False positives on a standard HBsAg test will not neutralize with anti-HBs in the confirmatory assay. Hepatitis B is a retrovirus that can cause persistent infection leading to cirrhosis and hepatocellular carcinoma. HBsAg is a lipoprotein that coats the surface of the hepatitis B virus. Blood specimen is obtained by venipuncture. Enzyme immunoassay refers to a technique that utilizes a chemical bond between an enzyme and an antigen or antibody as a label to identify specific chemical or infectious agents.

87350
This test may be requested as HBeAg by immunoassay techniques such as enzyme immunoassay (EIA), enzyme-linked immunosorbent assay (ELISA), fluorescence immunoassay (FIA), or immunochemiluminometric assay (IMCA). Hepatitis B is a retrovirus that can cause persistent infection leading to cirrhosis and hepatocellular carcinoma. HBeAg is normally tested only on individuals who are chronically HBsAg positive. Blood specimen is serum; method is qualitative or semiquantitative.

87380
This test may be requested as hepatitis delta agent (HDAg) by qualitative or semiquantitative immunoassay techniques such as enzyme immunoassay (EIA), enzyme-linked immunosorbent assay (ELISA), fluorescence immunoassay (FIA), or immunochemiluminometric assay (IMCA). Hepatitis delta agent is normally tested only on individuals who are chronically HBsAg positive or have an exacerbation of their hepatitis, as HDAg requires the presence of HBsAg to become an infectious virus. Blood specimen is serum.

87385
This test may be requested as *Histoplasma capsulatum* by qualitative or semiquantitative immunoassay techniques such as enzyme immunoassay (EIA), enzyme-linked immunosorbent assay (ELISA), fluorescence immunoassay (FIA), or immunochemiluminometric assay (IMCA). *Histoplasma capsulatum* infection results from inhalation or ingestion of spores and is common in the midwestern United States. It is usually asymptomatic, but on occasion causes acute pneumonia, disseminated reticuloendothelial hyperplasia with hepatosplenomegaly and anemia, or influenza-like symptoms with joint effusion and erythema nodosum. Reactivated infection is common in immunocompromised individuals affecting the lungs, meninges, heart, peritoneum, and adrenal glands. Blood specimen is serum.

87389
This test may be requested as human immunodeficiency virus type 1 (HIV-1) and type 2 (HIV-2) by qualitative or semiquantitative immunoassay techniques such as enzyme immunoassay (EIA), enzyme-linked immunosorbent assay (ELISA), fluorescence immunoassay (FIA), or immunochemiluminometric assay (IMCA). HIV-1 is the causative agent of acquired immunodeficiency syndrome (AIDS). HIV-2 is a retrovirus closely related to simian AIDS and was found initially in West African nations and Portugal, but cases have been reported in the United States since 1987. Blood specimen is obtained by venipuncture.

87390
This test may be requested as human immunodeficiency virus Type 1 (HIV-1) by qualitative or semiquantitative immunoassay techniques such as enzyme immunoassay (EIA), enzyme-linked immunosorbent assay (ELISA), fluorescence immunoassay (FIA), or immunochemiluminometric assay (IMCA). HIV-1 is the causative agent of acquired immunodeficiency syndrome (AIDS). Blood specimen is obtained by venipuncture. If the specific immunoassay technique is positive, it is repeated. Two out of three tests must be positive before the test is reported as positive. All positive tests are confirmed with an additional test using a different technique, usually Western blot, which is reported separately.

87391
This test may be requested as human immunodeficiency virus Type 2 (HIV-2) by qualitative or semiquantitative immunoassay techniques such as enzyme immunoassay (EIA), enzyme-linked immunosorbent assay (ELISA), fluorescence immunoassay (FIA), or immunochemiluminometric assay (IMCA). HIV-2 is a retrovirus closely related to simian AIDS and found initially in West African nations and Portugal, but with cases also being reported in the United States since 1987. Blood specimen is serum. If the test is positive, it is repeated. Two out of three tests must be positive before the test is reported as positive. All positive tests are confirmed with an additional test using a different technique, usually Western blot, which is reported separately.

87400
This test may be requested as influenza A or influenza B by immunoassay techniques such as enzyme immunoassay (EIA), enzyme-linked immunosorbent assay (ELISA), fluorescence immunoassay (FIA), or immunochemiluminometric assay (IMCA). Blood specimen is serum; method is qualitative or semiquantitative. Other specimens may be collected by procedures that are reported separately. Influenza A and B are a genus of the virus that causes the acute respiratory illness known as influenza. The designation is based on antigenic testing. Testing may occur during

the acute phase of illness and again 10 to 14 days after onset of symptoms.

87420
This test may be requested as respiratory syncytial virus (RSV) by immunoassay techniques such as enzyme immunoassay (EIA), enzyme-linked immunosorbent assay (ELISA), fluorescence immunoassay (FIA), or immunochemiluminometric assay (IMCA). RSV causes respiratory disease that can be particularly severe in infants. Blood specimen is serum; method is qualitative or semiquantitative.

87425
This test may be ordered as rotavirus. Rotavirus can cause severe infectious gastroenteritis in infants and young children. Adults may contract a milder infection. Blood specimen is serum. Method is qualitative or semiquantitative, enzyme immunoassay (EIA), enzyme-linked immunosorbent assay (ELISA), fluorescence immunoassay (FIA), or immunochemiluminometric assay (IMCA).

87426
This test may be requested as severe acute respiratory syndrome coronavirus (SARS-CoV or SARS-CoV-2 [COVID-19]) antigen detection. Methods include qualitative or semiquantitative immunoassay techniques such as enzyme immunoassay (EIA), enzyme-linked immunosorbent assay (ELISA), fluorescence immunoassay (FIA), or immunochemiluminometric assay (IMCA). Assays currently available are incapable of differentiating between SARS-CoV and SARS-CoV-2; this immunoassay detects antigenic proteins for either. A nasopharyngeal swab is collected and placed into a reagent tube, where it is swirled to release viral nucleoprotein antigen. A portion of the sample is transferred to the test cassette sample well, which is placed into the analyzer along with quality control cassettes. The result is obtained and reported to the ordering health care professional.

[87428]
This code reports a single test that measures antigens for severe acute respiratory syndrome coronavirus(es), including that which causes COVID-19, as well as influenza A and influenza B. This multiplex viral pathogen panel uses immunoassay techniques such as qualitative or semiquantitative enzyme immunoassay (EIA), enzyme-linked immunosorbent assay (ELISA), fluorescence immunoassay (FIA), or immunochemiluminometric assay (IMCA). Specimen is a nasopharyngeal swab, which is placed in a supplied reagent tube and swirled to disrupt and release the viral nucleoprotein antigens. A portion of the sample is transferred to the sample well of the test cassette and placed into the analyzer. Results are reported to the ordering health care professional.

87427
This test may be ordered as a *Shigella* Type 1 by EIA or *S. dysenteriae* test. Blood specimen is serum. Method is qualitative or semiquantitative, enzyme immunoassay (EIA), enzyme-linked immunosorbent assay (ELISA), fluorescence immunoassay (FIA), or immunochemiluminometric assay (IMCA). *Shigella* is an enteric pathogen known for its ability to produce protein toxins that cause acute gut inflammation and dysentery. Serology tests are usually conducted during the acute phase of illness.

87430
This test may be requested as *Streptococcus A* by immunoassay techniques such as qualitative or semiquantitative enzyme immunoassay (EIA), enzyme-linked immunosorbent assay (ELISA), fluorescence immunoassay (FIA), or immunochemiluminometric assay (IMCA). This test is used to determine group A *Streptococcus* (GAS) infectious antigens. GAS is a form of beta hemolytic *Streptococcus* that causes a wide variety of infections, including but not limited to pharyngitis, bronchitis, pneumonia, rheumatic fever, necrotizing fasciitis, and glomerulonephritis.

87449-87451
These codes report detection of infectious agents that are not specifically identified elsewhere. Testing is performed by qualitative or semiquantitative immunoassay techniques such as enzyme immunoassay (EIA), enzyme-linked immunosorbent assay (ELISA), fluorescence immunoassay (FIA), or immunochemiluminometric assay (IMCA). Report 87449 for each organism tested by these methods. Report 87451 for polyvalent testing for multiple organisms; report once for each polyvalent antiserum. The term polyvalent, when used in reference to microbiology, denotes an antibody molecule with multiple antigen binding sites.

87467
This test may be requested as quantitative HBsAg by immunoassay techniques such as enzyme immunoassay (EIA), enzyme-linked immunosorbent assay (ELISA), immunochemiluminometric assay (IMCA), or fluorescence immunoassay (FIA). Hepatitis B is a retrovirus that can cause persistent infection leading to cirrhosis and hepatocellular carcinoma. HBsAg is a lipoprotein that coats the surface of the hepatitis B virus. Quantitative HBsAg testing is not intended for the diagnosis of HBV infection; rather, it is intended for use in individuals with a confirmed diagnosis of Hepatitis B virus infection as determined by positive HBsAg, anti-HBs antibody, and/or anti-core antigen (anti-HBc) antibody test results. Blood specimen is serum or frozen plasma.

87468
This test is used to diagnose anaplasmosis, an infection caused by the bacterium *Anaplasma phagocytophilum*. Although predominantly transmitted to humans through the bite of an infected tick, it may also be associated with organ transplant or the transfusion of blood products. Infectious agent detection is by nucleic acid (DNA or RNA), amplified probe technique. The amplified probe technique entails detection methods in which either target, probe, or signal

amplification is used to improve the assay's sensitivity over direct probe techniques, without quantification of nucleic acid amounts.

87469
This test is used to detect *Babesia microti*, a microscopic parasite that is the primary cause of human babesiosis in the United States. Typically transmitted by the bite of certain infected ticks, these parasites infect red blood cells and may cause nonspecific flu-like symptoms such as body aches, chills, fatigue, fever, headache, and loss of appetite. Since red blood cells are infected and destroyed, babesiosis can also cause hemolytic anemia, which can lead to yellowing of the skin (jaundice) and dark urine. Detection is by nucleic acid (DNA or RNA), amplified probe technique. The amplified probe technique entails detection methods in which either target, probe, or signal amplification is used to improve the assay's sensitivity over direct probe techniques, without quantification of nucleic acid amounts.

87471
This test may be requested as *B. henselae* or *B. quintana*. These organisms are gram-negative bacilli that infect the red blood cells and epithelial cells of the lymph nodes, liver, and spleen. Blood specimen is serum. Tissue specimen requires a biopsy that is reported separately. The specimen is treated to isolate the nucleic acid (DNA, RNA) and eliminate substances that inhibit amplification. The nucleic acid is amplified using specific primers for *B. henselae* and *B. quintana* sequences.

87472
This test may be requested as *B. henselae* or *B. quintana*. These organisms are gram-negative bacilli that infect the red blood cells and epithelial cells of the lymph nodes, liver, and spleen. Blood specimen is serum. Tissue specimen requires a biopsy that is reported separately. The specimen is treated to isolate the nucleic acid (DNA, RNA). This code reports quantification only and is used primarily to assess extent of disease or disease progression.

87475
This test may be requested as DNA direct probe for Lyme disease. *Borrelia burgdorferi* is bacteria transmitted by tick bite and the causative agent of Lyme disease, acrodermatitis chronica atrophicans, and erythema chronicum migrans. Blood specimen is serum. CSF requires a spinal puncture, which is reported separately. Synovial fluid is obtained by arthrocentesis and is reported separately. A random urine specimen is obtained. DNA from spirochete *Borrelia burgdorferi* is analyzed using direct probe technique.

87476
This test may be requested as DNA amplified probe for Lyme disease. *Borrelia burgdorferi* is bacteria transmitted by tick bite and the causative agent of Lyme disease, acrodermatitis chronica atrophicans, and erythema chronicum migrans. Blood specimen is serum. CSF requires a spinal puncture, which is reported separately. Synovial fluid is obtained by arthrocentesis and is reported separately. A random urine specimen is obtained. DNA from spirochete *Borrelia burgdorferi* is analyzed using amplified probe technique. The DNA is amplified using specific primers for *Borrelia burgdorferi* sequences.

87478
This test is used to detect *Borrelia miyamotoi*, a spiral shaped tickborne bacterium. Those infected can experience body and joint pain, fatigue, fever, chills, and headache. Detection is by nucleic acid (DNA or RNA), amplified probe technique. The amplified probe technique entails detection methods in which either target, probe, or signal amplification is used to improve the assay's sensitivity over direct probe techniques, without quantification of nucleic acid amounts.

87480
This test is used to diagnose an infection by any species of *Candida*, but usually *C. albicans*. This test would normally be performed to diagnose systemic (invasive) candidiasis. Blood is serum. The specimen is treated to isolate nucleic acid (DNA, RNA). Nucleic acid is analyzed using direct probe technique.

87481
This test is used to diagnose an infection by any species of *Candida*, but usually *C. albicans*. This test would normally be performed to diagnose systemic (invasive) candidiasis. Blood is serum. The specimen is treated to isolate the nucleic acid (DNA, RNA) and eliminate substances that inhibit amplification. The nucleic acid is amplified using specific primers.

87482
This test is used to diagnose an infection by any species of *Candida*, but usually *C. albicans*. This test would normally be performed to diagnose systemic (invasive) candidiasis. Blood is serum. The specimen is treated to isolate the nucleic acid (DNA, RNA). This code reports quantification only and is used primarily to assess extent of disease or disease progression.

87483
This test is requested to determine central nervous system pathogens. The specimen is spinal fluid. Specimen retrieval achieved by spinal puncture is reported separately. The specimen is treated to isolate the nucleic acid. Nucleic acid is analyzed using multiplex amplified probe technique and includes multiplex reverse transcription when performed. This testing method has the ability to evaluate for several pathogens during the same test: multiple types/ subtypes, 12 to 25 targets.

87485
Chlamydia pneumoniae causes upper and lower respiratory tract infections and is a causative agent in many community-acquired pneumonias. Blood is serum. Sputum may be obtained by deep coughing or aerosol induced technique. The specimen is treated to

isolate nucleic acid (DNA, RNA). Nucleic acid is analyzed using direct probe technique.

87486
Chlamydia pneumoniae causes upper and lower respiratory tract infections and is a causative agent in many community-acquired pneumonias. Blood is serum. Sputum may be obtained by deep coughing or aerosol induced technique. The DNA is amplified using a technique such as polymerase chain reaction (PCR).

87487
Chlamydia pneumoniae causes upper and lower respiratory tract infections and is a causative agent in many community-acquired pneumonias. Blood is serum. Sputum may be obtained by deep coughing or aerosol induced technique. The specimen is treated to isolate the nucleic acid (DNA, RNA). This code reports quantification only and is used primarily to assess extent of disease or disease progression.

87490
This test may be requested as *Chlamydia trachomatis* or *C. trachomatis* by direct DNA probe. *C. trachomatis* is a frequently occurring sexually transmitted disease. It may cause nonspecific urethritis or pelvic inflammatory disease (PID), although it is frequently asymptomatic in women. Another serotype also causes conjunctivitis. The specimen is treated to isolate the DNA using direct probe.

87491
This test may be requested as *Chlamydia trachomatis* or *C. trachomatis* by polymerase chain reaction. *C. trachomatis* is a frequently occurring sexually transmitted disease. It may cause nonspecific urethritis or pelvic inflammatory disease (PID), although it is frequently asymptomatic in women. Another serotype also causes conjunctivitis. The DNA is amplified using a technique such as polymerase chain reaction (PCR).

87492
This test may be requested as *Chlamydia trachomatis* or *C. trachomatis* DNA quantification. *C. trachomatis* is a frequently occurring sexually transmitted disease. It may cause nonspecific urethritis or pelvic inflammatory disease (PID), although it is frequently asymptomatic in women. Another serotype also causes conjunctivitis. This code reports quantification only.

87493
This code reports infectious agent detection by nucleic acid (DNA, RNA) amplified probe for *Clostridium difficile* toxin B (tcdB). This test is used to diagnose patients whose symptoms include persistent non-bloody diarrhea, decreased appetite, abdominal discomfort, and elevated temperature following antibiotic therapy. Nucleic acid detection, also referred to as molecular pathology, is a rapidly developing diagnostic technique that is especially useful in identifying microorganisms that require tedious isolation and incubation and/or those that cannot be cultured. Another advantage of molecular methods is that they can detect infectious agents at much lower levels than required using other techniques. Amplified probe involves isolating and identifying the infectious agent DNA or RNA. This involves cell lysis and extraction of the DNA using phenol or chloroform. The nucleic acids are amplified using one of several techniques. Polymerase chain reaction (PCR) is the most frequently used amplification technique.

87495
This test may be requested as cytomegalovirus (CMV) direct DNA probe technique. CMV is part of the viral family that includes herpes zoster, Epstein-Barr, and varicella zoster infections. CMV usually causes only mild symptoms except in fetal infection or immunosuppressed patients, including AIDS and transplant patients. Blood specimen is serum. A random urine specimen is obtained. A separately reportable tissue biopsy is obtained. The specimen is treated to isolate the DNA using direct probe.

87496
This test may be requested as cytomegalovirus (CMV) by polymerase chain reaction (PCR). CMV is part of the viral family that includes herpes zoster, Epstein-Barr, and varicella zoster infections. CMV usually causes only mild symptoms except in fetal infection or immunosuppressed patients, including AIDS and transplant patients. Blood specimen is serum. A random urine specimen is obtained. A separately reportable tissue biopsy is obtained. The DNA is amplified using a technique such as polymerase chain reaction (PCR).

87497
This test may be requested as cytomegalovirus (CMV) quantification. CMV is part of the viral family that includes herpes zoster, Epstein-Barr, and varicella zoster infections. CMV usually causes only mild symptoms except in fetal infection or immunosuppressed patients, including AIDS and transplant patients. Blood specimen is serum. A random urine specimen is obtained. A separately reportable tissue biopsy is obtained. This code reports quantification only and is usually performed following amplification that is reported separately.

[87484]
This test is used to detect *Ehrlichia chaffeensis*, a bacterium that causes most reported cases of ehrlichiosis. Typically transmitted by the bite of an infected tick, the bacteria may also spread through blood transfusion and organ transplant in rare cases. Those infected will often experience chills, fever, headache, myalgia, and sometimes stomach upset. Detection is by nucleic acid (DNA or RNA), amplified probe technique. The amplified probe technique entails detection methods in which either target, probe, or signal amplification is used to improve the assay's sensitivity over direct probe techniques, without quantification of nucleic acid amounts.

87498
This test may be requested as enterovirus by polymerase chain reaction (PCR). Detection of

enterovirus nucleic acid provides a differential diagnosis of meningitis. Specimen is usually cerebrospinal fluid or throat swab. In an amplified probe technique, a small amount of DNA is manipulated using heating and cooling to reproduce the target. Because the generated DNA can also be used to replicate, the DNA is recreated exponentially. This test typically uses a real time reverse transcription polymerase (RT-RTP) chain reaction methodology in the collected clinical samples. In reverse transcription, the RNA from the organism is mapped to a single strand DNA allowing it to replicate. The test results are usually available significantly faster than viral culture results.

87500

Vancomycin is an antibiotic. The ability of certain microorganisms to withstand vancomycin treatment is called vancomycin resistance (VR). VR resistance is increasingly problematic in hospitals, nursing homes, and other health care facilities where vancomycin has been used as the drug of "last resort" to treat urinary tract, wound infections, and other serious disease processes resistant to other antibiotics. Testing organisms from clinical specimens with DNA amplified probe tests can identify vancomycin resistance genes, such as vanA and vanB genes of the Enterococcus that have a particularly high resistance to vancomycin, so other treatment options can be initiated.

87501-87503

These codes report influenza virus infectious agent detection by nucleic acid (DNA or RNA) using reverse transcription, when performed, and amplified probe technique. Nucleic acid detection, also referred to as molecular pathology, is a rapidly developing diagnostic technique that is especially useful in identifying microorganisms that require tedious isolation and incubation and/or those that cannot be cultured. Nucleic acid amplification tests are among the most sensitive and specific influenza tests. Specimen may be nasal, nasopharyngeal, or oropharyngeal swab; nasal or endotracheal aspirate; bronchoalveolar lavage (BAL); or pleural fluid. Testing for the influenza virus by amplified probe requires a molecular method referred to as reverse transcription polymerase chain reaction (RT-PCR). Report 87501 for each type or subtype and 87502 for the first two types or subtypes when testing for multiple types/subtypes. A separately reportable code (87503) is reported for each additional type or subtype beyond two.

87505-87507

These multiplexed nucleic acid tests are intended for the simultaneous qualitative detection and identification of multiple viral, parasitic, and bacterial nucleic acids in human stool specimens for the evaluation of gastrointestinal (GI) infections. These tests allow the analyst to distinguish the DNA or RNA of the pathogen by various magnification methods, including multiplex reverse transcription, when performed. The specimen is treated to isolate the nucleic acid, which is then examined. This enlarged specimen(s) can also determine the number of contagium within the sample. Quantifying the contagium at any given time can provide insight to effective therapy. Report 87505 for examination of three to five targets; 87506 for six to 11 targets; and 87507 for 12 to 25 targets.

87510

This test may also be requested as haemophilus vaginalis by direct nucleic acid probe. Gardnerella vaginalis is a gram-negative bacterium which causes an infection of the female genital tract producing a gray or yellow discharge. The specimen is treated to isolate nucleic acid (DNA, RNA). Nucleic acid is analyzed using direct probe technique.

87511

This test may also be requested as haemophilus vaginalis by amplified nucleic acid probe. Gardnerella vaginalis is a gram-negative bacterium which causes an infection of the female genital tract producing a gray or yellow discharge. The nucleic acid is amplified using specific primers for Gardnerella vaginalis sequences.

87512

This test may also be requested as haemophilus vaginalis. Gardnerella vaginalis is a gram-negative bacterium which causes an infection of the female genital tract producing a gray or yellow discharge. The specimen is treated to isolate the nucleic acid (DNA, RNA). This code reports quantification only and is used primarily to assess extent of disease or disease progression.

87513

This test is used for the detection of *Helicobacter pylori* (*H. pylori*). *H. pylori* may be found along the gastric mucosa and on the mucosal cells of the GI tract, and its presence is linked to several serious disorders of the stomach. In addition, the fecal sample is tested to determine resistance to clarithromycin by identifying the presence or absence of alterations in the 23S ribosomal ribonucleic acid (RNA) gene. Clarithromycin is an antibiotic used to treat *H. pylori*. Methodology is real-time polymerase chain reaction (PCR) amplification. The specimen is typically feces.

87516

This test may be requested as HBV DNA by polymerase chain reaction (PCR). Hepatitis B is a retrovirus that can cause persistent infection leading to cirrhosis and hepatocellular carcinoma. Molecular (DNA) tests are useful in identifying potentially infectious individuals as well as chronic progression of the disease. Blood specimen is serum. A liver biopsy is required for analysis of liver tissue and is reported separately The DNA is amplified using a technique such as polymerase chain reaction (PCR).

87517

This test may be requested as HBV DNA quantification. Hepatitis B is a retrovirus that can cause persistent infection leading to cirrhosis and hepatocellular carcinoma. Blood specimen is serum. A liver biopsy is required for analysis of liver tissue and is reported separately. Quantification is used primarily to monitor response to therapy in chronic hepatitis B. This code reports quantification only.

87520
This test may be requested as HCV RNA direct probe. Hepatitis C is also referred to as non-A non-B (NANB) hepatitis. Blood specimen is serum. A liver biopsy is required for analysis of liver tissue and is reported separately. The specimen is treated to isolate the RNA using direct probe. This test is used primarily by research facilities.

87521-87522
Hepatitis C is also referred to as non-A non-B (NANB) hepatitis. Blood specimen is plasma or serum. This test is used to detect infectious agents using the organism's DNA/RNA. In reverse transcription, the RNA from the organism is mapped to a single strand DNA allowing it to replicate. Report 87521 when the testing includes an amplified probe technique or reverse transcription polymerase chain reaction (RT-PCR) in which the reversely transcribed DNA is repeatedly duplicated (amplified) and detected using various methods. This test is used primarily by research facilities. Report 87522 if quantification of the RNA/DNA to monitor the effects of treatment is all that is performed.

87523
Hepatitis D is also referred to as delta hepatitis. It is caused by the hepatitis D virus (HDV) and only occurs in individuals who are also infected with the hepatitis B virus. Blood specimen is serum or plasma. This test is used to detect infectious agents using the organism's DNA/RNA with quantification. This test is used to confirm and quantify the presence of HDV to monitor disease progression or effects of treatment. Testing may also include reverse transcription; the RNA from the organism is mapped to a single strand DNA allowing it to replicate.

87525
This test may be requested as HGV-RNA direct probe. Blood specimen is serum. A liver biopsy is required for analysis of liver tissue and is reported separately. The specimen is treated to isolate the RNA using direct probe. This test is used primarily by research facilities. HGV is associated with acute and chronic hepatitis and active infection has been observed to persist for up to nine years. HGV is transmissible via blood transfusion and also can be acquired by exposure to blood and blood products.

87526
This test may be requested as HGV RNA amplified probe or as HCGV RNA RT-PCR. Blood specimen is serum. A liver biopsy is required for analysis of liver tissue and is reported separately. Testing for HGV by amplified probe requires a molecular method referred to as reverse transcription polymerase chain reaction (RT-PCR). This test is used primarily by research facilities. HGV is associated with acute and chronic hepatitis and active infection has been observed to persist for up to nine years. HGV is transmissible via blood transfusion and also can be acquired by exposure to blood and blood products.

87527
This test may be requested as HGV RNA quantification using molecular technique. Blood specimen is serum. A liver biopsy is required for analysis of liver tissue and is reported separately. This code reports quantification only. HGV is associated with acute and chronic hepatitis and active infection has been observed to persist for up to nine years. HGV is transmissible via blood transfusion and also can be acquired by exposure to blood and blood products.

87528
This test may be requested as HSV by direct DNA probe. Herpes simplex may be classified as HSV type 1 (HSV 1) or HSV type 2 (HSV 2). HSV 1 is primarily responsible for oral lesions frequently referred to as fever blisters or cold sores. HSV 2 is a sexually transmitted disease with lesions occurring primarily in the genitourinary tract. Lesion swab/scrapings are obtained. CSF is obtained by spinal puncture. Blood specimen is serum. The specimen is treated to isolate the DNA using direct probe. Detection and typing (HSV1, HSV2) by direct DNA probe is superior to culture methods.

87529
This test may be requested as HSV by amplified DNA probe. Herpes simplex may be classified is HSV type 1 (HSV 1) or HSV type 2 (HSV 2). HSV 1 is primarily responsible for oral lesions frequently referred to as fever blisters or cold sores. HSV 2 is a sexually transmitted disease with lesions occurring primarily in the genitourinary tract. Lesion swab/scrapings are obtained. CSF is obtained by spinal puncture. Blood specimen is serum. The DNA is amplified using a technique such as polymerase chain reaction (PCR). Detection and typing (HSV 1, HSV 2) by amplified DNA probe is superior to culture methods.

87530
This test may be requested as HSV quantification by molecular technique. Herpes simplex may be classified as HSV type 1 (HSV 1) or HSV type 2 (HSV 2). HSV 1 is primarily responsible for oral lesions frequently referred to as fever blisters or cold sores. HSV 2 is a sexually transmitted disease with lesions occurring primarily in the genitourinary tract. Lesion swab/scrapings are obtained. CSF is obtained by spinal puncture. Blood specimen is serum. This code reports quantification only.

87531
This test may be requested as HHV-6 direct DNA probe. Human herpes virus-6 is most commonly associated with roseola in children, but also causes pneumonitis, encephalitis, and hepatitis in immunosuppressed individuals. Sputum is obtained by deep coughing or by separately reportable aerosol induced technique. Respiratory fluids may also be obtained endoscopically using bronchial alveolar lavage and reported

separately. CSF is obtained by spinal puncture and reported separately. Blood specimen is serum. Liver tissue is obtained by biopsy, also reported separately. The cells are lysed and DNA is extracted. HHV-6 DNA is identified by direct probe.

87532
This test may be requested as HHV-6 amplified DNA probe. Human herpes virus-6 is most commonly associated with roseola in children, but also causes pneumonitis, encephalitis, and hepatitis in immunosuppressed individuals. Sputum is obtained by deep coughing or by separately reportable aerosol induced technique. Respiratory fluids may also be obtained endoscopically using bronchial alveolar lavage and reported separately. CSF is obtained by spinal puncture, which is reported separately. Blood specimen is serum. Liver tissue is obtained by biopsy, also reported separately. The cells are lysed and DNA is extracted. HHV-6 DNA is amplified using specific primers.

87533
This test may be requested as HHV-6 quantification using nucleic acid technique. Human herpes virus-6 is most commonly associated with roseola in children, but also causes pneumonitis, encephalitis, and hepatitis in immunosuppressed individuals. Sputum is obtained by deep coughing or by separately reportable aerosol induced technique. Respiratory fluids may also be obtained endoscopically using bronchial alveolar lavage, which is reported separately. CSF is obtained by spinal puncture and reported separately. Blood specimen is serum. Liver tissue is obtained by biopsy, also reported separately. The cells are lysed and DNA is extracted. This code reports quantification only.

87534-87535, 87537-87538
HIV is the causative agent of acquired immunodeficiency syndrome (AIDS). In 87534, the test may be requested as human immunodeficiency virus Type 1 (HIV-1) by direct nucleic acid (DNA, RNA) probe. A random urine sample is obtained. Tissue is obtained by separately reportable biopsy procedure. The specimen is treated to isolate the DNA using direct probe. In 87535, the testing includes an amplified probe technique or reverse transcription polymerase chain reaction (RT-PCR) in which the reversely transcribed DNA is repeatedly duplicated (amplified) and detected using various methods. In 87537 and 87538, the tests may be requested as human immunodeficiency virus Type 2 (HIV-2) by EIA. HIV-2 is a retrovirus closely related to simian AIDS and found initially in West African nations and Portugal, but with cases also being reported in the United States since 1987. In 87537, the specimen is treated to isolate the DNA using direct probe. In 87538, the test is used to detect infectious agents using the organism's DNA/RNA. In reverse transcription, the RNA from the organism is mapped to a single strand DNA allowing it to replicate. Report 87538 when the testing includes an amplified probe technique or reverse transcription polymerase chain reaction (RT-PCR) in which the reversely transcribed DNA is repeatedly duplicated (amplified) and detected using various methods. Blood specimen for these tests is serum. These tests are used primarily by research facilities.

87536, 87539
HIV is the causative agent of acquired immunodeficiency syndrome (AIDS). These codes may be requested as human immunodeficiency virus Type 1 (HIV-1) (87536) or human immunodeficiency virus Type 2 (HIV-2) (87539). HIV-2 is a retrovirus closely related to simian AIDS and found initially in West African nations and Portugal, but with cases also being reported in the United States since 1987. The tests are used to detect infectious agents using the organism's DNA/RNA. In reverse transcription, the RNA from the organism is mapped to a single strand DNA allowing it to replicate. Report these codes if quantification of the RNA/DNA is all that is performed to monitor the effects of treatment. Blood specimen is serum for both tests. These tests are used primarily by research facilities.

[87623, 87624, 87625, 87626]
These tests may be requested as human papillomavirus (HPV) according to low-risk types (6, 11, 42, 43, and 44) (87623), high-risk types (16, 18, 31, 33, 35, 39, 45, 51, 52, 56, 58, 59, and 68) (87624, 87626), or by specified types 16 and 18 only with type 45 included, when performed (87625). Human papillomaviruses are a genus of viruses that cause warts (benign neoplasms of skin and mucous membranes). There are at least 58 known types. HPV is commonly associated with plantar and genital warts. HPV infection of the cervix is of particular concern as it may be associated with cervical cancer. Methodology is in situ hybridization (ISH) by chromogenic or fluorescence techniques, which are based on the complementary pairing of a labeled probe to HPV antigens or nucleic acids (DNA or mRNA) within paraffin-embedded tissue biopsies or cervical smears. Report 87623 for an assay for low-risk HPV types; 87624 for a singular pooled result of high-risk types; 87625 for types 16 and 18 only, including type 45, when performed; and 87626 for detection of five or more separately reported high-risk types with high-risk pooled results.

87540
This test may also be requested as nucleic acid probe for Legionnaire's disease. The bacteria responsible for the disease, *Legionella pneumophila*, cause a fulminating pneumonia. It can also cause an influenza-like illness known as Pontiac fever. Sputum is obtained by deep coughing or by separately reportable aerosol induced technique. The specimen is treated to isolate nucleic acid using direct probe.

87541
This test may also be requested as nucleic acid probe for Legionnaire's disease. The bacteria responsible for the disease, *Legionella pneumophila*, cause a fulminating pneumonia. It can also cause an influenza-like illness known as Pontiac fever. Sputum is obtained by deep coughing or by separately

reportable aerosol induced technique. The specimen is treated to isolate nucleic acids, which are then amplified using a technique such as polymerase chain reaction (PCR).

87542
This test may also be requested as nucleic acid quantification for Legionnaire's disease. The bacteria responsible for the disease, *Legionella pneumophila*, cause a fulminating pneumonia. It can also cause an influenza-like illness known as Pontiac fever. Sputum is obtained by deep coughing or by separately reportable aerosol induced technique. This code reports quantification only.

87550
This test may be requested as Mycobacterial direct DNA probe. Blood specimen is serum. A random urine sample is obtained. Sputum is obtained by deep coughing or by separately reportable aerosol induced technique. Tissue is obtained in a separately reportable biopsy procedure. DNA is isolated directly from the specimen or following culture. The specimen is treated to isolate the Mycobacterial species. The DNA probe is hybridized and the excess probe removed. The bound probe is analyzed using chemiluminescence, color detection, or autoradiography.

87551
This test may be requested as mycobacterial amplified DNA probe or mycobacterial polymerase chain reaction (PCR). Blood specimen is serum. A random urine sample is obtained. Sputum is obtained by deep coughing or by separately reportable aerosol induced technique. Tissue is obtained in a separately reportable biopsy procedure. DNA is isolated directly from the specimen or following culture. DNA amplification is performed using PCR or transcription-based techniques. DNA amplification assay provides increased accuracy in diagnosis.

87552
This test may be requested as mycobacterial nucleic acid quantification. Blood specimen is serum. A random urine sample is obtained. Sputum is obtained by deep coughing or by separately reportable aerosol induced technique. Tissue is obtained in a separately reportable biopsy procedure. DNA is isolated directly from the specimen or following culture. The specimen is treated to isolate the mycobacterial species. This code reports quantification only.

87555
This test may be requested as tuberculosis (TB) test by direct nucleic acid probe. Tuberculosis was once diagnosed only by conventional culture techniques, which required four to six weeks for identification of mycobacteria tuberculosis. Nucleic acid probes allow for accurate identification in as little as 36-48 hours. Sputum is obtained by deep coughing or by separately reportable aerosol induced technique. The specimen is treated to isolate nucleic acid using direct probe.

87556
This test may be requested as tuberculosis (TB) test by amplified nucleic acid probe. Tuberculosis was once diagnosed only by conventional culture techniques, which required four to six weeks for identification of mycobacteria tuberculosis. Nucleic acid probes allow for accurate identification in as little as 36-48 hours. Sputum is obtained by deep coughing or by separately reportable aerosol induced technique. The specimen is treated to isolate nucleic acid using an amplified probe technique such as polymerase chain reaction (PCR). To enhance sensitivity PCR may be followed by oligonucleotide hybridization or nested PCR studies.

87557
This test may be requested as tuberculosis (TB) quantification by nucleic acid technique. Tuberculosis was once diagnosed only by conventional culture techniques, which required four to six weeks for identification of mycobacteria tuberculosis. Nucleic acid probes allow for accurate identification in as little as 36-48 hours. Sputum is obtained by deep coughing or by separately reportable aerosol induced technique. This code reports quantification only.

87560
This test may be requested as mycobacterial avium-intracellulare direct DNA probe. Blood specimen is serum. A random urine sample is obtained. Sputum is obtained by deep coughing or by separately reportable aerosol induced technique. Tissue is obtained in a separately reportable biopsy procedure. DNA is isolated directly from the specimen or following culture. The DNA probe is hybridized and the excess probe removed. The bound probe is analyzed using chemiluminescence, color detection, or autoradiography.

87561
This test may be requested as mycobacterial avium-intracellulare amplified DNA probe or mycobacterial avium-intracellulare polymerase chain reaction (PCR). Blood specimen is serum. A random urine sample is obtained. Sputum is obtained by deep coughing or by separately reportable aerosol induced technique. Tissue is obtained in a separately reportable biopsy procedure. DNA is isolated directly from the specimen or following culture. DNA amplification is performed using PCR or transcription-based techniques. DNA amplification assay provides increased accuracy in diagnosis.

87562
This test may be requested as mycobacterial avium-intracellulare nucleic acid quantification. Blood specimen is serum. A random urine sample is obtained. Sputum is obtained by deep coughing or by separately reportable aerosol induced technique. Tissue is obtained in a separately reportable biopsy procedure. DNA is isolated directly from the specimen or following culture. The specimen is treated to isolate the mycobacterial avium-intracellulare. This code reports quantification only.

[87564]
This test concurrently detects *Mycobacterium tuberculosis* complex (MTBC) and resistance to rifampin, which is one of the most effective drugs used in treating tuberculosis. One proprietary test employs nucleic acid amplification (NAA) that uses a disposable cartridge. A sputum sample is collected from a patient with suspected TB, the sputum is mixed with the reagent provided with the assay, and a cartridge containing this mixture is placed in the proprietary testing machine. All processing from this point on is fully automated. Assay results are interpreted in conjunction with clinical, radiographic, and other laboratory findings.

87563
Assays based on nucleic acid amplification tests (NAATs) are highly sensitive and specific for detecting many infectious organisms, including *Mycoplasma genitalium*. A sexually transmitted pathogen, it causes urethritis, epididymitis, and prostatitis in men and cervicitis, urethritis, and salpingitis in women. Specimen is typically vaginal or urethral swab. This code reports infectious agent detection by nucleic acid (DNA or RNA) and amplified probe technique.

87580
This test may be requested as Mycoplasma pneumoniae direct DNA probe. Mycoplasma pneumoniae is responsible for anywhere from one to eight percent of all community acquired pneumonias diagnosed each year. Sputum is obtained by deep coughing or by separately reportable aerosol induced technique. Specimen may also be obtained endoscopically using bronchial alveolar lavage, reported separately. Direct nucleic acid probe is a rapid and sensitive test for Mycoplasma pneumoniae nucleic acids, specifically rRNA, in respiratory fluids. Cells must be lysed to release the Mycoplasma pneumoniae specific rRNA.

87581
This test may be requested as Mycoplasma pneumoniae amplified DNA probe. Mycoplasma pneumoniae is responsible for anywhere from one to eight percent of all community acquired pneumonias diagnosed each year. Sputum is obtained by deep coughing or by separately reportable aerosol induced technique. Specimen may also be obtained endoscopically using bronchial alveolar lavage, reported separately. Nucleic acid probe is a rapid and sensitive test for Mycoplasma pneumoniae nucleic acids, specifically rRNA, in respiratory fluids. Cells must be lysed to release the Mycoplasma pneumoniae specific rRNA. They are amplified using polymerase chain reaction (PCR).

87582
This test may be requested as Mycoplasma pneumoniae nucleic acid quantification. Mycoplasma pneumoniae is responsible for anywhere from 1 to 8 percent of all community acquired pneumonias diagnosed each year. Sputum is obtained by deep coughing or by separately reportable aerosol induced technique. Specimen may also be obtained endoscopically using bronchial alveolar lavage, reported separately. Nucleic acid probe is a rapid and sensitive test for Mycoplasma pneumoniae nucleic acids, specifically rRNA, in respiratory fluids. Cells must be lysed to release the Mycoplasma pneumoniae specific rRNA. This code reports quantification only.

87590
This test may be requested as gonorrhea direct DNA probe, gonorrhea molecular probe assay, or DNA detection of gonorrhea. Neisseria gonorrhea is one of the most common sexually transmitted infections. Molecular (nucleic acid probe) techniques offer rapid, accurate identification of Neisseria gonorrhea. While a cervical or urethral swab is preferred, molecular techniques are sensitive enough to detect the organism in urine also. Neisseria gonorrhea can be detected by DNA, RNA, or rRNA probes.

87591
This test may be requested as gonorrhea amplified DNA probe, gonorrhea molecular probe assay, or DNA detection of gonorrhea. Neisseria gonorrhea is one of the most common sexually transmitted infections. Molecular (nucleic acid probe) techniques offer rapid, accurate identification of Neisseria gonorrhea. While a cervical or urethral swab is preferred, molecular techniques are sensitive enough to detect the organism in urine also. Neisseria gonorrhea can be detected by DNA or rRNA probes. Amplification can be performed using a number of techniques. Polymerase chain reaction (PCR) and ligase chain reaction (LCR) detect gonorrhea DNA. An assay is also available which detects gonorrhea ribosomal RNA (rRNA)

87592
This test may be requested as gonorrhea nucleic acid quantification. Neisseria gonorrhea is one of the most common sexually transmitted infections. Molecular (nucleic acid probe) techniques offer rapid, accurate identification of Neisseria gonorrhea. While a cervical or urethral swab is preferred, molecular techniques are sensitive enough to detect the organism in urine also. Neisseria gonorrhea can be detected by DNA or rRNA probes. This code reports quantification only.

87593
This code reports infectious agent detection by nucleic acid (DNA, RNA) amplified probe for orthopoxvirus (viruses that include cowpox, monkeypox, and vaccinia), and is reported for each species tested. The sample is a swab from a skin lesion. Amplified probe involves isolating and identifying the infectious agent DNA or RNA using a technique such as polymerase chain reaction (PCR).

87594
This test is used to detect *Pneumocystis jirovecii*, an opportunistic fungal pathogen. Specimen is typically fluid obtained via bronchoalveolar lavage. The amplified probe technique is utilized; this entails detection methods in which either target, probe, or signal amplification is used to improve the assay's

sensitivity over direct probe techniques, without quantification of nucleic acid amounts. The nucleic acids are amplified using one of several techniques; polymerase chain reaction (PCR) is the most frequently used. Qualitative results are reported.

87631-87633
These tests detect the RNA/DNA of multiple types of respiratory viruses during a single test. In reverse transcription, the RNA from the organism is mapped to a single strand DNA allowing it to replicate. The testing includes a multiplex amplified probe technique and multiplex reverse transcription polymerase chain reaction (RT-PCR) in which the reversely transcribed DNA is repeatedly duplicated (amplified) and detected using various methods, when performed. Specimens may include nasal, nasopharyngeal, or oropharyngeal swab; nasal or endotracheal aspirate; bronchoalveolar lavage (BAL); or pleural fluid. Report 87631 when three to five viruses are targeted; 87632 for six to 11 viruses; and 87633 for 12 to 25 viruses.

87634
This test is useful in the diagnosis of a recent respiratory syncytial virus (RSV) infection and carrier status. Specimen varies. The specimen is treated to isolate the nucleic acid (DNA, RNA) and eliminate substances that inhibit amplification. The nucleic acid is amplified using specific primers for RSV sequences.

87635-87637
This test is for the detection of SARS-CoV-2 and any pan-coronavirus types or subtypes. Specimens have been collected using one or more methods (bronchoalveolar lavage, lower respiratory tract or nasal/nasopharyngeal aspirate/wash, nasopharyngeal/oropharyngeal swab, or sputum induction), placed into appropriate containers, and transported to the laboratory. The test uses specific primers and amplified probe assay to detect DNA or RNA sequences specific for the SARS-CoV-2 virus. Infectious agent specificity may also include terminology such as severe acute respiratory syndrome coronavirus 2, coronavirus disease, or COVID-19. Report 87635 for severe acute respiratory syndrome coronavirus 2 (SARS-CoV-2) (coronavirus disease [COVID-19]), amplified probe technique; report 87636 for severe acute respiratory syndrome coronavirus 2 (SARS-CoV-2) (coronavirus disease [COVID-19]) and influenza virus types A and B, multiplex amplified probe technique; report 87637 for severe acute respiratory syndrome coronavirus 2 (SARS-CoV-2) (coronavirus disease [COVID-19]), influenza virus types A and B, and respiratory syncytial virus, multiplex amplified probe technique.

87640
This test may be requested as *Staphylococcus aureus* by amplified probe assay. Specimen is blood or other body fluid. This test uses amplified probe assay to detect DNA or RNA sequences (usually DNA) specific for *S. aureus*. The specimen is treated to isolate the DNA or RNA and eliminate substances that inhibit amplification. The *S. aureus* DNA or RNA is amplified using specific primers.

87641
This test may be requested as MRSA by amplified probe assay. Specimen is blood or other body fluid. This test uses amplified probe assay to detect DNA or RNA sequences (usually DNA) specific for methicillin-resistant *Staphylococcus aureus*. The specimen is treated to isolate the DNA or RNA and eliminate substances that inhibit amplification. The MRSA DNA or RNA is amplified using specific primers. This assay establishes the presence of both *S. aureus* and methicillin resistance. MRSA is resistant to not only methicillin, but also common antibiotics including oxacillin, penicillin, and amoxicillin.

87650
This test may be requested as *Streptococcus* A by direct nucleic acid probe. *Streptococcus* A is a form of beta hemolytic *streptococcus*, which causes pharyngitis. Untreated infection can cause rheumatic fever or glomerulonephritis. The specimen is treated to isolate the DNA using a direct probe.

87651
This test may be requested as *Streptococcus* A by amplified nucleic acid probe. *Streptococcus* A is a form of beta hemolytic *streptococcus*, which causes pharyngitis. Untreated infection can cause rheumatic fever or glomerulonephritis. The specimen is treated to isolate the DNA and eliminate substances that inhibit amplification. The *Streptococcus* A DNA is amplified using specific primers.

87652
This test may be requested as *Streptococcus* A nucleic acid quantification. *Streptococcus* A is a form of beta hemolytic *streptococcus*, which causes pharyngitis. Untreated infection can cause rheumatic fever or glomerulonephritis. This code reports quantification only.

87653
This test may be requested as GBS by direct nucleic acid probe. Group B *Streptococcus* is generally performed on pregnant women in labor or at any time during their pregnancy. The specimen is vaginal or rectal swab. The specimen is treated to isolate the DNA using an amplified probe assay to detect nucleic acid sequences specific to GBS. Results can be obtained in an hour, allowing for neonatal intervention or antibiotic treatment of the pregnant mother.

87660-87661
A microbiology test for *Trichomonas vaginalis* may be requested as *T. vaginalis* DNA probe, molecular probe assay, or DNA detection of *T. vaginalis*. *Trichomonas vaginalis* is a common cause of vaginitis and culture is limited by poor sensitivity. In 87660, a direct probe method is used to detect DNA of the organism by using DNA probes that hybridize to whole chromosomes or specific target sequences for detection. The target DNA in the sample is fixed onto a slide and denatured from double-stranded DNA to

single-stranded DNA. The target DNA is hybridized with that of the probe, reassociating into double-stranded nucleic acid. The unbound DNA is removed and the remaining DNA is counterstained and placed under fluoroscopy to visualize the hybridized probe attached to the target material. In 87661, an amplified probe technique is used to detect the organism. A small amount of DNA is manipulated using heating and cooling to reproduce the target. Because the generated DNA can also be used to replicate, the DNA is recreated exponentially.

87662

This code tests for antibodies to the Zika virus. Symptoms of Zika infection include fever, rash, headache, joint pain, red eyes, and/or muscle pain. Patients may be infected with the Zika virus from the bite of an infected mosquito or it can be passed from a pregnant woman to her fetus causing certain birth defects. It is recommended that asymptomatic pregnant patients be screened due to the risk of birth defects. The specimen is treated to isolate the nucleic acid (DNA, RNA) and eliminate substances that inhibit amplification. The nucleic acid is amplified using specific primers for Zika fever sequences.

87797

This code reports infectious agent detection by nucleic acid (DNA, RNA) direct probe for microorganisms that are not identified with a more specific code in range 87470-87652. Nucleic acid detection, also referred to as molecular pathology, is a rapidly developing diagnostic technique that is especially useful in identifying microorganisms which require tedious isolation and incubation and/or those which cannot be cultured. Another advantage of molecular methods is that they are able to detect infectious agents at much lower levels than required using other techniques. Direct probe involves isolating and identifying the infectious agent DNA or RNA. This involves cell lysis and extraction of the DNA using phenol or chloroform.

87798

This code reports infectious agent detection by nucleic acid (DNA, RNA) amplified probe for microorganisms that are not identified with a more specific code in range 87470-87652. Nucleic acid detection, also referred to as molecular pathology, is a rapidly developing diagnostic technique that is especially useful in identifying microorganisms which require tedious isolation and incubation and/or those which cannot be cultured. Another advantage of molecular methods is that they are able to detect infectious agents at much lower levels than required using other techniques. Amplified probe involves isolating and identifying the infectious agent DNA or RNA. This involves cell lysis and extraction of the DNA using phenol or chloroform. The nucleic acids are amplified using one of several techniques. Polymerase chain reaction (PCR) is the most frequently used amplification technique. Other techniques include ligase chain reaction (LCR) and the signal detection method (bDNA).

87799

This code reports infectious agent quantification using nucleic acid (DNA, RNA) technique for microorganisms that are not identified with a more specific code in range 87470-87652. Nucleic acid detection, also referred to as molecular pathology, is a rapidly developing diagnostic technique that is especially useful in identifying microorganisms which require tedious isolation and incubation and/or those which cannot be cultured. Another advantage of molecular methods is that they are able to detect infectious agents at much lower levels than required using other techniques. Quantification may be performed following direct or amplified probe. It measures the amount of the microorganism DNA/RNA present.

87800-87801

Code 87800 reports multiple infectious agent detection by nucleic acid (DNA or RNA) using direct probe technique. Nucleic acid detection, also referred to as molecular pathology, is a rapidly developing diagnostic technique that is especially useful in identifying microorganisms that require tedious isolation and incubation and/or those that cannot be cultured. Another advantage of molecular methods is that they are able to detect infectious agents at much lower levels than required using other techniques. The test is useful in that absolute specificity of hard-to-identify organisms can be attained. Report 87801 when the multiple DNA target sequences are amplified using any of several techniques, such as polymerase chain reaction (PCR), or ligase chain reaction (LCR), or signal detection (bDNA).

87802

This test may be requested as a rapid antigen test for group B strep (GBS). This code describes a visually read immunoassay for group B *Streptococcus* that is typically performed on pregnant women in labor or at any time during their pregnancy. The specimen may be vaginal or rectal swab. When referring to primary source infectious disease codes, direct optical observation is a testing platform that produces a signal, such as a colored band, on the reaction chamber that can be interpreted visually.

87803

Clostridium difficile is the major cause of antibiotic-associated diarrhea and colitis and is the cause for virtually all cases of pseudomembranous colitis (PMC). The organism is found in stools of most patients with these diseases. One gram of stool is collected and sent to the laboratory unpreserved. The fecal sample is dispersed in a diluent with antibodies for *Clostridium difficile* antigen to form a complex of antibody and antigen. A complex of antibody and antigen is separated from the specimen and exposed to a second antibody for the antigen, and a portion of the antibody. A sample from the first complex is bound to a solid carrier and a sample from the second antibody exposure is labeled with a detection agent to determine the presence of *Clostridium difficile* antigen in the original fecal specimen. Method is immunoassay with direct optical (i.e., visual) observation.

[87806]
This qualitative immunoassay point-of-care test is ordered to aid in the diagnosis of HIV infection, detecting antibodies to HIV-1 and HIV-2. Specimen may be oral fluid, plasma, or whole blood obtained by fingerstick or venipuncture. In one method, a fingerstick whole blood specimen is collected and placed into a vial of developer solution. The test device is then inserted, and the developer solution enables the specimen to flow into the device and to migrate up the test strip. If antibodies are contained in the specimen that react with the antigens on the test device membrane, a colored line will appear that can be interpreted visually and indicates the presence of antibodies to HIV-1 and/or HIV-2 in the specimen.

87804
This test may be requested as a rapid antigen test for influenza. A highly contagious, acute viral infection of the respiratory tract, influenza is caused by a single-strand RNA virus known as an influenza virus. Sample is respiratory secretion, such as nasal aspirate, a nasopharyngeal or throat swab, or sputum sample; detection is by immunoassay with direct optical (i.e., visual) observation. When referring to primary source infectious disease codes, direct optical observation is a testing platform that produces a signal, such as a colored band, on the reaction chamber that can be interpreted visually. Various tests may be utilized consisting of one sample, one analysis, and one strip. Depending on the test, the result may be non-differentiating, identifying whether the patient has influenza virus infection but not providing the specificity of influenza A or B; a positive or negative result that is specific only to influenza virus type A; or a positive or negative result that is specific only to influenza virus type B.

87807
This test may be requested as a rapid antigen test for respiratory syncytial virus (RSV). Specimen collection is typically by nasal swab, nasopharyngeal aspirate, or nasal wash. In one method, a nasal swab is dipped into a solution provided with a proprietary test kit and a measured sample from the swab solution is pipetted onto the rapid test. Results are ready in approximately 15 minutes and are interpreted as negative or positive. Detection is by immunoassay with direct optical (i.e., visual) observation. When referring to primary source infectious disease codes, direct optical observation is a testing platform that produces a signal, such as a colored band, on the reaction chamber that can be interpreted visually.

[87811]
This test may be requested as a rapid antigen test for SARS-CoV-2 or COVID-19. This immunoassay provides qualitative (positive or negative) detection of the nucleocapsid protein antigen from SARS-CoV-2; samples typically include nasopharyngeal or nasal swabs. In one method, a nasal swab specimen is collected from the patient and a specified number of drops of extraction reagent are added to the top hole of the swab well. The sample is then inserted into the test card via the bottom hole of the swab well and pushed upwards. Once the swab tip is visible through the top hole, the swab is rotated three times clockwise. The card is closed, which brings the sample into contact with the test strip. Results are interpreted visually at 15 minutes.

87808
This test may be requested as a rapid antigen test for trichomonas. Sample is vaginal swab; detection is by immunoassay with direct optical observation. When referring to primary source infectious disease codes, direct optical observation is a testing platform that produces a signal, such as a colored band, on the reaction chamber that can be interpreted visually. In one proprietary method, a swab is collected from the vaginal cavity and mixed in sample buffer to make the trichomonas proteins more soluble. The test stick is placed into the sample mixture, which migrates along the membrane surface. Within approximately 10 minutes, the results are available. Positivity is indicated by the appearance of a visible blue test line along with the red control line.

87809
This test may be requested as a rapid antigen test for adenovirus. Human adenoviruses (HAdV) are significant sources of eye and respiratory tract disease and are some of the most commonly isolated viruses. Viral conjunctivitis is often difficult to distinguish, since the presence of an upper respiratory infection (URI), conjunctival follicles, preauricular nodes, or watery discharge provides no definitive differentiation from bacterial conjunctivitis. In one method, the patient's eyelid is lowered and the inside is dabbed to saturate a sample pad of a rapid screening device. The pad is placed in a buffer solution to active; results develop in approximately 10 minutes. Detection is by immunoassay with direct optical (i.e., visual) observation. When referring to primary source infectious disease codes, direct optical observation is a testing platform that produces a signal, such as a colored band, on the readout window that can be interpreted visually.

87810
This test may be requested as a rapid antigen test for *Chlamydia trachomatis*. *C. trachomatis* is a frequently occurring sexually transmitted disease. It may cause nonspecific urethritis or pelvic inflammatory disease (PID), although it is frequently asymptomatic in women. Samples include endocervical swab and cytology brush specimens; detection is by immunoassay with direct optical observation. When referring to primary source infectious disease codes, direct optical observation is a testing platform that produces a signal, such as a colored band, on the reaction chamber that can be interpreted visually. In one proprietary method, an endocervical specimen is obtained and placed into a tube containing an extraction solution reagent. After two minutes, a

neutralization solution reagent is added. Following extraction and neutralization, a specific number of drops of the extracted sample is added to the test cassette sample well. If the extracted sample contains chlamydial antigen, a positive result is indicated by a red test line along with a blue control line.

87850

This test may be requested as a rapid antigen test for *Neisseria gonorrhea*, one of the most common sexually transmitted infections. Specimen may include urethral or endocervical swab; detection is by immunoassay with direct optical observation. When referring to primary source infectious disease codes, direct optical observation is a testing platform that produces a signal, such as a colored band, on the reaction chamber that can be interpreted visually. In one proprietary method, a swab specimen is collected from the patient's urethra. The swab is placed into an extraction tube to which a specified amount of extraction buffer has been added. The swab is rotated against the tube to express the liquid; after two minutes, another extraction buffer is added. Extraction is performed for another minute in the same way. A specified amount of extracted specimen is added to the specimen well of the test cassette. A positive result is indicated by two colored bands appearing on the membrane and may be interpreted visually in approximately 15 minutes.

87880

This test may be requested as a rapid antigen test for Strep A. *Streptococcus* A is a form of beta hemolytic *Streptococcus*, which causes pharyngitis. Untreated infection can cause rheumatic fever or glomerulonephritis. Sample is throat swab; detection is by immunoassay with direct optical observation. When referring to primary source infectious disease codes, direct optical observation is a testing platform that produces a signal, such as a colored band, on the reaction chamber that can be interpreted visually. In one test method, a throat swab specimen is collected, and antigen is extracted from the specimen with reagents. A dipstick is added to the extracted sample. If the sample contains Strep A antigen, a positive result is indicated by the appearance of a pink to red test line along with a blue control line on the dipstick.

87899

This test may be requested as a rapid antigen detection test. Samples vary; detection is by immunoassay with direct optical observation. When referring to primary source infectious disease codes, direct optical observation is a testing platform that produces a signal, such as a colored band, on the reaction chamber that can be interpreted visually. This code should be reported only when the infectious agent being tested does not have a more specific code.

87900

This test directly and quantitatively measures resistance of a patient's viral infection to drugs in order to help the physician select appropriate drugs. The test uses nucleic acid application to derive protease (PR) and reverse transcriptase (RT) sequences from a patient's plasma sample. A resistance test vector (RTV) is constructed by incorporating the patient-derived segment into a viral vector with an indicator gene, firefly luciferase, inserted within a portion of the viral envelope gene. The completion of a single round of viral replication results in the production of luciferase. Drug susceptibility is measured by comparing luciferase activity produced in the presence and absence of drugs. Susceptible viruses produce low levels of luciferase activity in the presence of PR and/or RT inhibitors, whereas viruses with reduced susceptibility to these drugs produce higher levels of luciferase.

87901-87902 [87906, 87910, 87912, 87913]

Genotype assays are useful in detecting potential or actual drug resistance in a particular virus. A genotype assay that can predict expected HIV antiviral drug resistance for most individuals is reported with 87901 (reverse transcriptase and protease regions) or 87906 (other regions; for example, integrase or fusion). Each of the procedures described by 87901 and 87906 require the analysis of eight separate sequence segments of nucleic acid. In 87910, the DNA of cytomegalovirus is isolated for and amplified by polymerase chain reaction to detect mutations that are related to antiretroviral pharmaceutical resistance. In 87902, hepatitis C virus (HCV) DNA is isolated using reverse transcription. A line probe assay (LiPA) of HCV genotypes 1 through 6 and subtypes 1a and 1b is utilized to determine the efficacy, dose, and duration or treatment with common HCV drugs. Code 87912 is reported for the isolation and analyzing of 10 hepatitis B virus (HBV) genomes that identify those at risk of HBV disease progression and to determine optimal antiviral therapy. Report 87913 for genotyping tests for the identification and differentiation of SARS-CoV-2 lineages, mutations, or variants. One such test is a next-generation sequencing (NGS) based test used on respiratory samples such as anterior nasal or nasopharyngeal swab samples.

87903-87904

Treatment of human immunodeficiency virus (HIV) requires multiple antiviral drugs administered in combination to suppress virus replication. However, over time, HIV can become resistant to one or more of these. Resistance can be recognized by identifying increases in the viral load and declines in the CD4 counts. These codes are used to report assays that help identify HIV antiviral drug resistance. Report 87903 for a phenotype assay that may be required when newer drugs are being considered for treatment of HIV, as newer drugs sometimes do not have sufficient data to predict expected outcomes based on genotype studies alone. Phenotype analysis reported by 87903 includes drug resistance tissue culture analysis of up to 10 drugs. Report 87904 for each additional drug tested.

87905

This code is used to report the enzymatic activity of an infectious agent, other than a virus, using an immunologic technique.

88000
This code reports the examination of a body after death. The body is dissected. The organs and tissues (excluding the brain and central nervous system) are systematically examined and described. This is usually done to determine the cause of death, to improve diagnosis and treatment of diseases, or to benefit family members in cases of heritable illnesses.

88005
This code reports the examination of a body after death. The body is dissected. The organs and tissues are systematically examined and described, including the brain. This is usually done to determine the cause of death, to improve diagnosis and treatment of diseases, or to benefit family members in cases of heritable illnesses.

88007
This code reports the examination of a body after death. The body is dissected. The organs and tissues are systematically examined and described, including the brain and spinal cord. This is usually done to determine the cause of death, to improve diagnosis and treatment of diseases, or to benefit family members in cases of heritable illnesses.

88012
This code reports the examination of an infant's body after death (birth through 12th month). The body is dissected. The organs and tissues are systematically examined and described, including the brain. This is usually done to determine the cause of death, to improve diagnosis and treatment of diseases, or to benefit family members in cases of heritable illnesses.

88014
This code reports the examination of a newborn's body after death (birth through 28th day), or the examination of a stillborn fetus. The body is dissected. The organs and tissues are systematically examined and described, including the brain. This is usually done to determine the cause of death, to improve diagnosis and treatment of diseases, or to benefit family members in cases of heritable illnesses.

88016
This code reports the examination of a stillborn fetus whose body tissues have become softened, as happens when there is a delay from the time of death in utero to the delivery. The body is dissected. The organs and tissues are systematically examined and described, including the brain. This is usually done to determine the cause of death, to improve diagnosis and treatment of diseases, or to benefit family members in cases of heritable illnesses.

88020
This code reports the examination of a body after death. The body is dissected. The organs and tissues are systematically examined (gross and microscopic) and described (except the brain and central nervous system). Representative samples from the organs are taken and microscopically examined and described. Laboratory tests may also be performed on tissue samples. This is usually done to determine the cause of death, to improve diagnosis and treatment of diseases, or to benefit family members in cases of heritable illnesses.

88025
This code reports the examination of a body after death. The body is dissected. The organs and tissues are systematically examined (gross and microscopic) and described (including the brain). Representative samples from the organs are taken and microscopically examined and described. Laboratory tests may also be performed on tissue samples. This is usually done to determine the cause of death, to improve diagnosis and treatment of diseases, or to benefit family members in cases of heritable illnesses.

88027
This code reports the examination of a body after death. The body is dissected. The organs and tissues are systematically examined (gross and microscopic) and described (including the brain and spinal cord). Representative samples from the organs are taken and microscopically examined and described. Laboratory tests may also be performed on tissue samples. This is usually done to determine the cause of death, to improve diagnosis and treatment of diseases, or to benefit family members in cases of heritable illnesses.

88028
This code reports the examination of an infant's body after death (birth through 12th month). The body is dissected. The organs and tissues are systematically examined (gross and microscopic) and described (including the brain). Representative samples from the organs are taken and microscopically examined and described. Laboratory tests may also be performed on tissue samples. This is usually done to determine the cause of death, to improve diagnosis and treatment of diseases, or to benefit family members in cases of heritable illnesses.

88029
This code reports the examination of a newborn's body after death (birth through 28th day), or the examination of a stillborn fetus. The body is dissected. The organs and tissues are systematically examined (gross and microscopic) and described (including the brain). Representative samples from the organs are taken and microscopically examined and described. Laboratory tests may also be performed on tissue samples. This is usually done to determine the cause of death, to improve diagnosis and treatment of diseases, or to benefit family members in cases of heritable illnesses.

88036
This code reports the examination of a body after death. The body is dissected. Certain organs and tissues within a system or region of the body are systematically examined (gross and microscopic) and described. Representative samples from the organs are taken and microscopically examined and described. Laboratory tests may also be performed on tissue

samples. This is usually done to determine the cause of death, to improve diagnosis and treatment of diseases, or to benefit family members in cases of heritable illnesses.

88037

This code reports the examination of a body after death. The body is dissected. A single organ and its related tissues are systematically examined (gross and microscopic) and described. Representative samples from the organ are taken and microscopically examined and described. Laboratory tests may also be performed on organ tissue samples. This is usually done to determine the cause of death, to improve diagnosis and treatment of diseases, or to benefit family members in cases of heritable illnesses.

88040

This code reports the examination of a body after death. The body is dissected. The organs and tissues are systematically examined (gross and microscopic) and described. Representative samples from the organs are taken and microscopically examined and described. Laboratory tests may also be performed on tissue samples. This is usually done for the purpose of gathering and preserving evidence for presentation in a court of law.

88045

A coroner is a public official, elected or appointed, who investigates the causes and circumstances of deaths from unnatural causes that occur within a specific legal jurisdiction (i.e., county). In many jurisdictions, coroners must present themselves and sign death certificates of all persons who die while not under the care of a physician. In some instances, a preliminary gross exam is performed on-site and procedural arrangements are made for a more thorough examination under laboratory conditions. As with all codes in the postmortem examination range, 88045 reports physician services. Only four states require coroners to be physicians. A medical examiner is a physician.

88104-88106

These tests have many different names, depending on the type of specimen obtained for analysis (e.g., bronchial cytology, esophageal cytology, etc.). Specimen is obtained by separately reportable washing or brushing procedure. Code 88104 reports cytopathology evaluation of smear specimens, including alcohol fixed, Papanicolaou, direct smear with 95 percent ethanol, or liquid fixative. Report 88106 for a simple filter method only.

88108

Cytopathology, concentration technique, (e.g., Saccomanno, cytocentrifugation, and cytospins) may be done on many different types of specimen samples like bronchial, cervicovaginal, and conjunctival brushings, nipple discharge, sputum, and gastrointestinal epithelial cell specimens. Cellular smear preparations (cervicovaginal, conjunctival, bronchial brushings, nipple discharge) are immediately fixated in 95 percent ethanol or pap fixative to eliminate drying. GI, urologic, and sputum samples are collected with a Saccomanno fixative added. Following preparation, the sample is centrifuged to yield a pellet at the bottom of the tube and overlying supernatant. The clear fluid supernatant is decanted completely and the pellet is used to make direct smears of the concentrated sample for cytopathology and cell counts. Cytocentrifugation, cytospins, smears and interpretations are then preformed.

88112

Selective cellular enhancement for cytopathology, such as liquid based slide preparation method, is reported when both concentration and enrichment of cytology specimens is done beyond a concentration technique alone reported with 88108 (e.g., Saccomanno, cytocentrifugation, and cytospins). Enhancement technologies allow not only for concentration of the diagnostic material, but also for removing of background debris on complicated specimens that cannot be evaluated with typical concentration techniques alone (see 88108). One liquid based slide preparation method uses a filtration system with a disposable filter, support, and means of drawing fluid where cells are caught within a large enough area to provide a high-quality, high-yield monolayer slide that has good quantity, distribution, and clarity for diagnostic purposes. When a sample is prepared using enhanced cytopathology, the slide preparation is examined and compared to previous studies. Report this for any specimen except cervical or vaginal.

88120-88121

Fluorescence in situ hybridization (FISH) DNA probe technology is a technique used to determine nucleic acid sequences within cells. Probes (short sequences of fluorescently labeled, single-strand DNA) are created. These probes match target sequences and bind to complementary strands of DNA, which aids in locating the targeted chromosomes. FISH DNA probe technology can be used to detect chromosomal abnormalities in urinary tract specimens, aiding in the initial identification of bladder cancer, as well as in bladder cancer surveillance. Analysis is done using three to five molecular probes to determine the organization, structure, form, and composition within the cells being studied, either manually in 88120 or using computer-assisted technology in 88121. These codes are reported once for each specimen.

88125

For this cytopathology code, biological samples from crime scenes are studied using techniques common to DNA testing, such as fluorescent staining. Forensic cytopathology is the application of this type of testing for legal purposes. Forensic scientists study biological evidence and samples collected at crime scenes, such as hair, blood, and sperm for DNA testing to assist in the inclusion or the exclusion of an individual in the crime.

88130
This screening test will identify the presence or lack of sex chromatin. Specimen collection is by buccal mucosa scraping, Specimen should be chemically preserved with a fixative such as 95 percent ethanol. Method is by smear and microscopy. Examination of cells obtained by amniocentesis for the presence or absence of sex chromatin is a technique used to determine the infant's sex prior to birth.

88140
Fluorescent staining techniques are used to identify a Barr body in a polymorphonuclear leukocyte. In females one of the two X chromosomes remains tightly coiled. In some nuclei the coiled chromosome is visible as a small dense mass known as a Barr body. In the lobulated nucleus of the polymorphonuclear leukocyte it can be seen as a protrusion, often in the shape of a drumstick.

88141
This test is for the interpretation by a physician of a Papanicolaou (Pap) smear. This code is used in addition to the code for the technical service.

88142-88143
These tests may be identified by the name "thin prep." Specimen collection is by cervical or endocervical scraping or aspiration of vaginal fluid. The physician obtaining the specimen places the specimen in a preservative suspension. At the laboratory, special instruments take the cells in the preservative suspension and "plate-out" a monolayer for screening-the careful review of the specimen for abnormal cells. Report 88142 for manual screening done under physician supervision and 88143 for manual screening followed by manual rescreening, done under physician supervision. System of reporting may be Bethesda or non-Bethesda.

88147-88148
These tests may be identified as a cervical smear, Pap smear, or vaginal cytology. Specimen collection is by cervical or endocervical scraping or aspiration of vaginal fluid. Method is microscopy examination of a spray or liquid fixated smear. Code 88147 should be used to report smears screened by automated system under physician supervision, while 88148 reports automated screening with manual rescreening under physician supervision. System of reporting may be Bethesda or non-Bethesda.

88150-88153
These tests may also be identified as a cervical smear, Pap smear, or vaginal cytology. The specimen cells are collected by scraping or brushing the cervix or endocervix or aspiration of vaginal fluid. The specimen is smeared onto a slide and chemically treated with a preservative. These codes should be reported when any system other than the Bethesda System of evaluating and describing cervical/vaginal cytopathology slides is used. Code selection is based on the screening process used, with manual screening under physician supervision being reported with 88150, manual screening and computer-assisted rescreening under physician supervision with 88152, and manual screening and rescreening under physician supervision with 88153.

88155
This test may also be identified as the maturation index, cytologic estrogen effect, karyopyknotic index, or estrogenic index. Specimen collection is by tongue depressor or wooden spatula of the lateral vaginal wall. Method is microscopy examination of a spray or liquid fixated smear. The test may be used to determine the balance of estrogen and progesterone of the vaginal squamous epithelium.

88160-88162
Specimen collection is by separately reportable percutaneous needle biopsy. Methods include microscopy examination of smears or a centrifuge specimen. These codes report the pathology examination portion of the procedure only. Code 88160 reports screening and interpretation only. Code 88161 reports preparation, screening and interpretation. Code 88162 reports an extended study involving more than five slides and/or multiple stains.

88164-88167
These tests may be identified as a cervical smear, Pap smear, or vaginal cytology. Specimen collection is by scraping or brushing the cervix or endocervix, or aspiration of vaginal fluid. Method is microscopy examination of a spray or liquid coated smear. These codes should be reported when the Bethesda System of evaluating and describing cervical/vaginal cytopathology slides is used. Code selection is based on the screening process used, with manual screening under physician supervision being reported with 88164, manual screening and rescreening under physician supervision with 88165, manual screening and computer-assisted rescreening under physician supervision with 88166, manual screening and computer-assisted rescreening using cell selection and review under physician supervision with 88167.

88172-88173 [88177]
Following fine needle aspiration (a procedure in which fluid or tissue is extracted using a long slender needle), the aspirated cells are often immediately examined microscopically by a physician in order to determine that diagnostic material is present. A preliminary diagnostic assessment may be rendered at that time in order to avoid a repeat operative procedure. Report 88172 for the first evaluation episode (a complete set of cytologic material submitted for evaluation, regardless of the number of needle passes or prepared slides) of each site and 88177 for each separate additional evaluation episode of the same site. Code 88173 reports the final interpretation and report from each anatomic site, regardless of the number of evaluation episodes or needle passes performed during the aspiration procedure.

88174-88175

Specimen collection is by cervical or endocervical scraping or aspiration of vaginal fluid. Report 88174 for automated screening done under physician supervision and 88175 when automated screening is followed by manual rescreening or review under physician supervision.

88182

Flow cytometry allows a single cell to be measured for a variety of characteristics that are determined as the cell flows in a liquid. Information about the cells is gathered by measuring visible and fluorescent light emissions. Specimen collection is by biopsy or needle biopsy for tissue and bone marrow; blood is drawn by venipuncture. To perform DNA or cell cycle analysis, the cells are first stained with a fluorescent dye. Flow analysis is performed to determine a cell's DNA content. Cell cycle analysis performed by cell cytometry can determine a cells position in the cell cycle based on its DNA content.

88184-88185

These codes report the technical component for flow cytometry tests performed to identify specific cell surface, cytoplasmic or nuclear markers. To identify cell surface markers, a fluorescent dye is attached to antibodies or receptor ligands. The cells are subjected to flow cytometry and the amount of the receptor on the surface is detected by the level of fluorescence. Flow cytometry can also be used to detect multiple cell-surface markers simultaneously. Antibodies used in flow cytometry are determined by the presumptive diagnosis. Detection of antigens by flow cytometry allows identification and quantification of cells with specific characteristics that may be indicative of immune deficiencies, malignancies, or other disease processes. Report 88184 for the first marker, and 88185 for each additional marker.

88187-88189

These codes report the interpretation of flow cytometry tests. Flow cytometry results as measured by the detector are typically displayed as dot plots or histograms. The physician must interpret these dot plots and histograms. The physician reports interpretation services based on the number of markers being analyzed. Report 88187 for two to eight markers, 88188 for nine to 15 markers, and 88189 for 16 or more markers.

88230

This code is used to report lymphocyte culture for non-neoplastic disorders, which would include chromosome analysis as well as other cytogenetic studies. Cytogenetics is the branch of genetics that studies cellular (cyto) structure and function as it relates to heredity (genetics). White blood cells, specifically T-lymphocytes, are the most commonly used specimen for chromosome analysis. A peripheral blood specimen is obtained by venipuncture. The blood is separated into its cellular constituents and the white blood cells are extracted. The white blood cells are placed in a tissue culture medium. White blood cells, specifically T-lymphocytes, are stimulated with phytohemagglutinin (PHA) and grown in the tissue culture.

88233

This code is used to report culturing of skin cells or other solid tissue cells for evaluation of nonneoplastic disorders (i.e., chromosome analysis and other cytogenetic studies). Cytogenetics is the branch of genetics that studies cellular (cyto) structure and function as it relates to heredity (genetics). Skin cells may be obtained by buccal smear or separately reportable biopsy. Solid tissue specimen requires separately reportable biopsy. Skin or other solid tissue cells are placed in a tissue culture medium. The cells are stimulated and grown in the tissue culture.

88235

This code is used to report culturing of fetal cells for evaluation of nonneoplastic disorders (i.e., chromosome analysis and other cytogenetic studies). Cytogenetics is the branch of genetics that studies cellular (cyto) structure and function as it relates to heredity (genetics). Fetal cells are normally cultured to detect chromosome abnormalities and sex-linked disorders. A separately reportable amniocentesis or chorionic villus sampling is performed. Culture and growth of an adequate number of fetal cells for analysis may require two to three weeks.

88237

This code is used to report tissue culture only of bone marrow or blood cells for the purpose of evaluating neoplastic, usually malignant, disorders. Many neoplastic disorders have a genetic origin and therefore cytogenetic studies aid in diagnosis and are prognostic indicators. In addition, they may identify individuals at high risk for developing certain cancers. Bone marrow is obtained by separately reportable biopsy. Blood specimen is whole blood. The marrow and blood cells may be separated by cell type. The cells are placed in a tissue culture medium, which stimulates cell growth.

88239

This code is used to report tissue culture only of solid tumor cells for the purpose of evaluating neoplastic, usually malignant, disorders. Many neoplastic disorders have a genetic origin and therefore cytogenetic studies aid in diagnosis and are prognostic indicators. Translocations and deletions of nuclear DNA are especially common in the chromosomes of tumor cells, which makeup is different from that of normal somatic cells. This code reports cell culture prepared from a biopsied or resected solid tumor. The cells are placed in a tissue culture medium, which stimulates cell growth.

88240

Cryopreservation is a technique of freezing and maintaining cells at extremely low temperatures to preserve the genetic and metabolic properties of the cell. Cryopreservation is performed to allow storage of cells for subsequent culture and analysis at a reference laboratory. Report this code for each cell line. A cell line is considered one that holds the potential for indefinite subculture in a lab setting.

88241
Cells frozen by cryopreservation are thawed and expanded (amplified) for study. Report each aliquot separately. An aliquot refers to the equal division of a sample of a substance, with each part related quantitatively to each other and to the sample as a whole.

88245
This cytogenetic study may be requested as a chromosome breakage analysis, sister chromatid exchange (SCE) study, or a chromosome instability test. This test involves evaluation for increased sister chromatid exchange (SCE) of 20 to 25 cells. This exchange refers to the crossing over of genetic information between the sister chromatids. This analysis is specifically for chromosome breakage syndromes, which are characterized by an increased rate of SCE during cell division where exact duplication of the genetic information in each chromatid fails to occur. Instead, genetic information is rearranged between the sister chromatids during cell division. This test would normally use more traditional techniques, such as direct microscopic analysis of cells arrested in metaphase.

88248
This test may be requested by the name of the specific breakage syndrome being evaluated. Examples include Ataxia-telangiectasia (A-T) breakage study, Fanconi anemia (FA) breakage study, Fragile X breakage study, and Xeroderma pigmentosum (XP) chromosome breakage study. It may also be requested simply as a chromosome breakage study or chromosome instability study. Fragile sites along the chromosome that may appear as bent or partially detached fragments characterize chromosome breakage syndromes. The specific location of the fragile site determines the characteristics of the specific syndrome. The syndrome is associated with a moderate degree of intellectual delay. The procedure includes collecting 50 to 100 cells, counting 20, and performing two karyotypes. A karyotype is a visual exam of each chromosome pair from cells arrested in metaphase.

88249
This code reports a specific technique for analysis of breakage syndromes involving clastogen stress. Clastogen is a substance (e.g., chemical or radiation) that causes chromosome breakage when applied to the cell. Some substances that can be used as clastogens include diepoxybutane, mitomycin C, ionizing radiation, and UV radiation. When applied to the cells, these clastogens will identify fragile sites on the chromosome. The location of the fragile site is used to diagnose the specific breakage syndrome. The code includes the scoring of 100 cells.

88261-88262
These codes are reported for chromosome analysis to detect certain inherited disorders or syndromes, excluding breakage syndromes. The chromosomes of individuals with suspected genetic anomalies and neoplastic disorders are analyzed to provide definitive diagnosis. In addition, suspected carriers may be analyzed for recessive traits that may affect, or have affected, their offspring. Code 88261 should be reported for a five-cell count and one karyotype, with banding. Code 88262 should be reported for a 15 to 20-cell count and two karyotypes, with banding. Karyotype is the full chromosome set that genetically defines an individual. Banding refers to the appearance of stripes on stained paired bundles of chromosomes. This test would normally use more traditional techniques, such as direct microscopic analysis of cells arrested in metaphase.

88263
This code is reported for chromosome analysis of 45 cells for the presence of mosaicism. It includes two karyotypes with banding. Mosaicism refers to alterations in chromosomes that do not affect every somatic (non-sex cell) chromosome, but are manifested during embryonic development. The individual is said to have two or more cell lines of different genetic or chromosomal make-up. Karyotype is the full chromosome set that genetically defines an individual. Banding refers to the appearance of stripes on stained paired bundles of chromosomes. This test would normally use more traditional techniques, such as direct microscopic analysis of cells arrested in metaphase.

88264
This test reports chromosome analysis related to malignant neoplasms (cancer). Cancer cytogenetics requires complete analysis (not just counting) of 20-25 cells. Chromosome analysis is performed to identify specific chromosomal anomalies, which can aid in diagnosis and provide prognostic indicators for certain cancers. In addition, identification of aberrant chromosomal bands provides information on the specific genes affected in certain malignancies. Individuals with family histories indicating a high risk for certain types of cancer can be tested to determine whether they carry the aberrant bands.

88267
This is a prenatal technique used to analyze chromosomes from cells of extracted amniotic fluid or chorionic villus for possible genetic abnormalities that can be detected during embryonic development. The code includes a 15-cell count, one karyotype, with banding. Karyotype is the full chromosome set that genetically defines an individual. Banding refers to the appearance of stripes on stained paired bundles of chromosomes. This test would normally use more traditional techniques, such as direct microscopic analysis of cells arrested in metaphase with Giemsa or quinacrine banding techniques.

88269
This is a prenatal technique used to analyze intact chromosomes within the cells of amniotic fluid for possible genetic abnormalities that can be detected during embryonic development. The code includes a cell count from six to 12 colonies, one karyotype, with banding. Karyotype is the full chromosome set that genetically defines an individual. Banding refers to the appearance of stripes on stained paired bundles of chromosomes. By studying the occurrence of different DNA bands in the population, one can calculate the probability of two DNA samples matching one another. Any number of methods may be used, including polymerase chain reaction (PCR), restriction fragment length polymorphism (RFLP), and Northern or Southern blot.

88271
Molecular cytogenetics represents relatively new techniques capable of detecting changes in chromosomes that cannot be detected by traditional microscopic techniques. This code reports the use of a DNA probe to identify chromosomal abnormalities. Fluorescent in situ hybridization (FISH) is one type of DNA probe. It allows chromosomes and genes to be analyzed simultaneously. In situ hybridization involves treating native double-stranded DNA to render it single-stranded. The strand is incubated to allow the strand to recognize complementary bases and to reform as a double-strand (hybridization). When a strand is radioactively marked, it is the "probe." The specificity to which the hybridization takes place is analyzed.

88272-88273
Molecular cytogenetics represent relatively new techniques capable of detecting changes in chromosomes that cannot be detected by traditional microscopic techniques. In situ hybridization is the base pairing of a sequence of DNA to chromosomes on a microscope slide. The technique involves printing thousands of protein-coded DNA (cDNA) clones on a single microscope slide. Fluorescent cDNA probes prepared from any cell or tissue source of interest are paired to provide a large-scale view of gene expression. In situ hybridization is used to determine the consequences of a given genetic alteration on gene expression. Report 88272 when three to five cells are analyzed usually to identify derivatives and markers. Report 88273 when 10 to 30 cells are analyzed usually for the purpose of identifying microdeletions. A microdeletion involves the removal or acquired absence of one or more nucleotides from a gene or chromosome.

88274-88275
Molecular cytogenetics represent relatively new techniques capable of detecting changes in chromosomes that cannot be detected by traditional microscopic techniques. In situ hybridization is the base pairing of a sequence of DNA to chromosomes on a microscope slide. In situ hybridization is used to determine the consequences of a given genetic alteration on gene expression. Report 88274 for in situ hybridization techniques used during interphase (resting phase) of cell division, for analyzing 25 to 99 cells. When 100 to 300 cells are analyzed report 88275.

88280
This code is reported for chromosome analysis to detect certain disorders or syndromes that may be inherited. The chromosomes of individuals with suspected genetic anomalies and neoplastic disorders are analyzed to provide definitive diagnosis. In addition, suspected carriers may be analyzed for recessive traits that may affect, or have affected, their offspring. This code is used for each additional karyotype beyond the number stipulated in other chromosome analysis codes in this same section of CPT 1999. Karyotype is the full chromosome set that genetically defines an individual. The term is also used for the standardized visual maps of chromosomal makeup, a technique used in identifying and organizing abnormalities. This test would usually involve more traditional microscopic techniques.

88283-88285
These codes are used for chromosome analysis to detect certain disorders or syndromes that may be inherited. The chromosomes of individuals with suspected genetic anomalies and neoplastic disorders are analyzed to provide definitive diagnosis. In addition, suspected carriers may be analyzed for recessive traits that may affect, or have affected, their offspring. Code 88283 is used for each additional karyotype specialized banding technique, such as NOR and C-banding. C-banding is a method of identifying banding patterns based on nucleic acid content and staining. Report 88285 for additional cells counted, each study. This test would usually involve more traditional microscopic techniques.

88289
This code is used for chromosome analysis to detect certain disorders or syndromes that may be inherited. The chromosomes of individuals with suspected genetic anomalies and neoplastic disorders are analyzed to provide definitive diagnosis. In addition, suspected carriers may be analyzed for recessive traits that may affect, or have affected, their offspring. This code is used for each additional high resolution study.

88291
This code is used to report physician interpretation and report of complex cytogenetic and molecular cytogenetic tests or when abnormal cytogenetic tests require complex interpretations.

88300
This procedure may be called a gross pathology exam or gross exam of tissue. The exam may not be specifically ordered ahead of time; rather, the tissue is harvested in the course of a surgery and sent for routine lab evaluation. Tissue is submitted in a container labeled with the source, preoperative diagnosis, and patient identification information. Specimens from separate sites must be submitted in

separate containers, each labeled with the tissue source.

88302
This examination may be ordered as a gross and microscopic pathology exam or a gross and microscopic tissue exam. The exam may not be specifically ordered ahead of time; rather, the tissue is harvested in the course of a surgery and sent for routine lab evaluation. Tissue is submitted in a container labeled with the tissue source, preoperative diagnosis, and patient identification information. Specimens from separate sites must be submitted in separate containers, each labeled with the tissue source. This procedure is used to describe examination of tissues presumed normal. It includes both a gross and microscopic examination with the microscopic exam mainly to confirm the tissue is free of disease. Examples of its use might include tissues from a fallopian tube or vas deferens performed in the course of sterilization procedures, newborn foreskin following circumcision, hernia sac, hydrocele sac, etc.

88304-88309
These examinations would be ordered as a gross and microscopic pathology exam or a gross and microscopic tissue exam. Tissue is submitted in a container labeled with the tissue source, preoperative diagnosis, and patient identification information. Specimens from separate sites must be submitted in separate containers, each labeled with the tissue source. Codes 88304-88309 describe levels of service for specimens requiring additional levels of work due to a presumed presence of disease. Code 88304 describes the lowest level of complexity for diseased or abnormal tissue with each subsequent code (88305, 88307, and 88309) describing in ascending order higher levels of complexity and physician work. Specific types of disease and tissue sites are listed for each code in the CPT description.

88311
This procedure is performed in addition to the basic surgical pathology examination (88302-88309) on specimens requiring decalcification for accurate evaluation. When calcium is present in the tissue, the specimen is too hard to be properly sectioned for microscopic evaluation. Using an acid solution, calcareous matter is removed from bone and other tissue (decalcification). The specimen is bathed in a solution to remove calcium ions via an ion exchange. This process may take hours or days depending on the specimen. Decalcification is commonly performed in bone marrow biopsy.

88312-88314
These codes report stains used in the evaluation of some tissue specimens. Depending on the type of specimen and the reason for the pathology examination, different stains may be required to highlight or outline cells for identification. Code 88312 reports Group I stains for microorganisms. Code 88313 reports Group II stains for all other conditions excluding microorganisms, enzyme constituents, immunocytochemistry, and immunohistochemistry. Examples of Group II stains include Ziehl-Neelsen, acid phosphatase stain with and without tartrate, alpha-naphthyl esterase stain with and without fluoride, amyloid, ASD chloroacetate esterase stain, nonspecific esterase, PAS stain, and Sudan black stain. Code 88314 reports histochemical staining on frozen tissue blocks.

88319
This code reports additional histochemistry services performed with basic pathology services, including determinative tests for enzyme constituents, each constituent. An example of a specimen that might require histochemistry for enzyme constituents is a muscle biopsy.

88321-88325
A pathology consultation involves an opinion or advice on the presence or absence of diseased or abnormal tissue provided at the request of another physician. These three codes report consultations and written interpretations on slide or material referred from another facility or source. Report 88321 for a consultation and written report on a slide prepared by another source; 88323 for a consultation and written report on material referred from another source requiring routine preparation of slides by the consultant; and 88325 for a comprehensive consultation with a written report of the consultation that describes the review of records, evaluation of specimens, and may require more complex slide preparation.

88329
The procedure may also be referred to as an intraoperative pathology exam. A pathology consultation involves an opinion or advice on the presence or absence of diseased or abnormal tissue provided at the request of another physician. This code describes a pathology consultation during the course of a surgery, and includes only a gross examination of tissue without concurrent microscopic examination. Intraoperative consultations are performed to assist the surgeon in determining immediate surgical course.

88331-88332
These procedures may also be referred to as an intraoperative pathology exam with frozen section (FS). A pathology consultation involves an opinion or advice on the presence or absence of diseased or abnormal tissue provided at the request of another physician. These codes describe such a pathology consultation during the course of a surgery. The codes include a gross examination of tissue and frozen sections, including a written interpretation of findings. The specimen is immediately frozen in a cold liquid or cold environment (-20 to -70 C) to facilitate sectioning with a microtome. The specimen is sectioned using a cryostat, which is a refrigerated box containing a microtome. Once sectioned, the tissues are placed on a slide, stained, and examined microscopically. Report 88331 for examination of a single block of tissue. Report 88332 for each additional block of tissue from

the same specimen. Intraoperative consultations are performed to assist the surgeon in determining immediate surgical course.

88333-88334
These procedures may also be referred to as intraoperative pathology consultation or intraoperative cytologic examination. During the course of an operation, a specimen is examined cytologically by touch prep where suspicious cells are scraped and smeared onto glass slides for staining and examination, or squash prep where the specimen is minced, placed on a slide, and examined after staining. Report 88333 for the initial site examined and 88334 for each additional site examined.

88342-88344 [88341]
This immunohistochemistry procedure, also referred to as immunostain or peroxidase-antiperoxidase (PAP), identifies specific antigens found in tumor cells. It is used primarily for the diagnosis of poorly differentiated neoplasms. There are several methods of performing immunocytochemistry tests; however, all involve treating the specimen with a tumor specific antibody, incubation, and subsequent washing of the specimen to remove unbound antibody and counterstaining with secondary antibodies to determine the antibody location. The specimen is examined for positive and negative responses. Multiple immunostains are normally performed on each specimen to more specifically identify the suspect neoplasm by providing known positive and negative responses specific to that neoplasm. Report 88342 for the initial single antibody identified; 88341 for each additional single antibody; and 88344 for each multiplex antibody identified.

88346 [88350]
Immunofluorescence study is performed on an initial, single antibody. The technique involves the introduction of fluorescein-tagged antibodies. Antibodies used are dependent upon tissue being examined and the suspected diagnosis, but may include IgG, IgM, IgA, C3, C4, C1q, properdin, fibrin, fibrinogen, and albumin. The specimen is examined under fluorescent microscopy for intensity, pattern, and distribution of immunoglobulins; the antibody introduced attaches to the targeted immunoglobulin. Report 88350 for each additional single antibody stain procedure.

88348
This procedure, also referred to as electron microscopy (EM), transmission electron microscopy, or ultrastructural study, is used primarily for the diagnosis of neoplasms when other techniques have failed to provide a definitive diagnosis. Tissues are prepared and fixed in a plastic polymer. Initially, thick sections (1 micron) are cut and stained to identify best specimen sites for further study. Subsequently, thin sections are cut and prepared with electron dense stain. The specimens are examined using electron microscopy. Code 88348 reports diagnostic EM.

88355-88358
These procedures may also be referred to as histomorphometry. Methodology is by flow cytometry or quantitative image analysis system. Cells are stained and the histologic organization, including structure, composition, and function, is evaluated.

88360-88361
Morphometric analysis may also be referred to as histomorphometry. A quantitative or semiquantitative test is done for tumor immunohistochemistry, such as the Her-2/neu receptor. The HER-2/neu protein is a cell surface growth factor receptor expressed on the cytoplasmic membrane of some epithelial cells. This protein regulates normal cell growth and division. An increased number of HER-2/neu genes in the cell nucleus causes overexpression of the HER-2/neu oncoprotein, which in turn produces growth signals leading to cell transformation and cancer development. Microthin sections of the fixed, paraffin-embedded tissue are mounted on glass slides. Antigen retrieval with citrate buffers or microwaving is done to inhibit peroxidase activity and background staining. Immunostaining is done by adding a dilution containing the primary antibody to the receptor protein and incubating. Counterstaining with secondary antibodies is done to visualize antibody location. Further analysis is done to determine the histologic organization of the tumor and measure its structure, form, and composition, quantitatively or semiquantitatively, manually for 88360 or using computer-assisted technology for 88361. These codes are reported once per specimen for each single antibody stain procedure used to test for a specific protein receptor, such as Her-2/neu, estrogen, or progesterone receptor.

88362
Teased fiber evaluation is a technique used in specialty neuropathology labs. Peripheral nerves are often encased in a myelin sheath. This lipid-like substance is important to nerve function and can be an element in diagnostic evaluation. The technique involves biopsy collection, usually under local anesthetic. Light and electron microscopy are usually employed. Individual nerve fibers are "teased" from surrounding tissues to analyze myelinated nerve fiber size, distribution, and density.

88363
Mutations (changes) in the KRAS gene are often found in certain human cancers and may be predictive of a poor prognosis and limited clinical response to certain therapies. The KRAS protein is involved in cell growth, cell signal pathways, and cell death. This code reports the examination and selection of previously diagnosed tissues for KRAS mutation analysis in tumor types found to harbor KRAS mutations. Specimen may be formalin-fixed, paraffin-embedded block, unstained slides, or fresh snap frozen biopsy.

88365-88366 [88364]
Fluorescence In Situ Hybridization, also known as DNA-to-DNA homology or simply FISH or FISH-IS ™

(Fluorescence In Situ Hybridization—In Suspension), involves isolating and detecting specific nucleotide (mRNA) sequences within morphologically preserved cells and tissues by hybridizing a complementary nucleic acid strand, called a probe, to the sequence of interest within the prepared cells. The cells of interest may be snap-frozen and fixed in paraformaldehyde; left in suspension for fixation, hybridization, and detection; spun out of suspension onto glass slides and fixed with methanol; or fixed in formalin and embedded in paraffin. The probe is first labeled with an easily detectable substance, such as a radioactive isotope, before hybridization. Types of probes used are oligonucleotides, single-stranded DNA, double-stranded DNA, and RNA or riboprobes. The labeled probe strand is added to the prepared cells. The pairing or bonding (hybridization) that occurs between the complementary sequences of nucleotide bases in the probe to the specific mRNA sequences allows the expression of the type of sequence being detected to be seen on the target gene. Report 88365 for the initial single probe stain per specimen; 88364 for each additional single probe stain; and 88366 for each multiplex probe stain.

88367-88369 [88373, 88374, 88377]

Morphometric analysis, also referred to as histomorphometry, is a quantitative or semiquantitative analysis done with in situ hybridization. In situ hybridization involves isolating and detecting specific nucleotide (mRNA) sequences within morphologically preserved cells and tissues by hybridizing a complementary nucleic acid strand, called a probe, to the sequence of interest within the prepared cells. The cells of interest may be snap frozen and fixed in paraformaldehyde, spun out of suspension onto glass slides and fixed with methanol, or formalin fixed embedded in paraffin. The probe is first labeled with an easily detectable substance, such as a radioactive isotope, before hybridization. Types of probes used are oligonucleotides, single-stranded DNA, double-stranded DNA, and RNA or riboprobes. The labeled probe strand is added to the prepared cells. The pairing or bonding (hybridization) that occurs between the complementary sequences of nucleotide bases in the probe to the specific mRNA sequences allows the expression of the type of sequence being detected to be seen on the target gene. Analysis is done to determine the organization, structure, form, and composition within the morphologically preserved cells being studied. Report 88367 for the initial single probe stain, per specimen, using computer-assisted technology; 88373 for each additional single probe stain using computer-assisted technology; and 88374 for each multiplex probe stain using computer-assisted technology. Report 88368 for the initial single probe stain analyzed manually; 88369 for each additional single probe stain analyzed manually; and 88377 for each multiplex probe stain analyzed manually.

88371-88372

Western blot is an immunoassay technique that detects and confirms certain viral antibodies. Protein analysis of tissue involves separation of protein and glycoprotein components by electrophoresis. For certain diagnoses, polyacrylamide gel electrophoresis is used to create substrate bands that are transferred by electrophoretic blotting to a membrane. Patient serum is placed on the substrate strips and any of the targeted antibodies present will bind to the viral antigens. Report 88372 when the protein analysis of tissue by Western blot includes an immunological probe for band identification. The band patterns are visualized by immunohistochemical methods. Either service requires interpretation and written report.

88375

The images captured using an optical endomicroscope during endoscopy are reviewed, interpreted, and a report is generated. The endomicroscope uses laser light to magnify the cells of the mucosa in order to identify the histopathology without a biopsy. This service can be performed during the procedure (real time) or at a later time. This code is reported per endoscopic procedure, not per image.

88380-88381

Laser capture microdissection (LCM) (88380) is a method for procuring pure cells from specific microscopic regions of tissue sections to study developing disease lesions in actual tissue. A transfer film is applied to the surface of the tissue section. Under the microscope, the diagnostic pathologist or researcher views the thin tissue section and chooses microscopic clusters of cells to study. When the cells of choice are in the center of the field of view, a pulsed laser beam activates a spot on the transfer film immediately above the cells of interest. At this location the film melts and fuses with the underlying cells. When the film is removed, the chosen cells are held, while the rest of the tissue is left behind. This allows multiple homogeneous samples within the tissue section to be targeted for analysis. If microdissection is performed utilizing a manual technique (using hand-held tools such as needles or mechanical micromanipulator-based approaches), report 88381.

88387

The physician performs a macroscopic (visual) examination, dissection, and preparation of tissues for analytical studies that are non-microscopic, such as nucleic acid-based molecular studies. Report 88387 for each tissue preparation (e.g., a single lymph node).

88720

Bilirubin is a bile pigment produced through the breakdown of blood components. High bilirubin concentrations in the blood is known as jaundice. Transcutaneous bilirubinometry uses subcutaneous tissue photometry to measure bilirubin concentration, particularly in newborns. The optic head of the photometric analyzer is pressed against the infant's skin and takes several seconds to obtain a measurement.

88738
This test is a quantitative measurement of hemoglobin. One indication is the diagnosis of anemia or polycythemia in order to evaluate the severity of these conditions and to observe the patient's response to treatment. Measurement of hemoglobin by the transcutaneous method eliminates the need to draw blood. Instead, a visible and near-infrared spectroscopic device is used and measurements are obtained by a handheld probe, typically on the forearm.

88740-88741
Carboxyhemoglobin is hemoglobin with carbon monoxide bound to it instead of the normal oxygen. Methemoglobin is hemoglobin that has been altered so that it is unable to carry oxygen. Methemoglobin may be acquired by exposure to certain chemical agents, or it may be due a genetic condition. In vivo measures are noninvasive using visible and near-infrared optical bands.

89049
The Caffeine Halothane Contracture Test (CHCT) is performed on freshly biopsied muscle for diagnosis of malignant hyperthermia (MH) susceptibility. MH is a life-threatening condition resulting from a genetic sensitivity of the skeletal muscles to volatile anesthetics. A muscle biopsy is obtained, usually from the thigh. The specimen is exposed to caffeine and halothane separately and the sustained muscle tension responses are recorded. Comparison of the strength of contracture (sustained muscle tension) for each exposure with previously established standards allows determination of MH susceptibility.

89050-89051
CSF cell count may also be referred to as a CSF analysis or spinal fluid analysis; joint fluid cell count may also be referred to as synovial fluid analysis. In 89050, a manual nucleated blood cell count using a hemacytometer is performed on fluids obtained during a separately reportable spinal puncture or arthrocentesis. In 89051, a differential cell study using manually prepared smears or a cytocentrifuge is performed in addition to the cell count. Depending on the suspected condition, a number of separately reportable additional tests may be performed.

89055
A fecal material leukocyte count is done on a stool sample by direct smear and stain to detect the presence of WBCs and aid in the differential diagnosis of diarrheal disease. Certain conditions are associated with marked fecal leukocyte presence, moderate numbers present, and the absence of fecal leukocytes. Fecal leukocyte absence indicates invasive toxic bacterial infection, giardiasis, or viral infection. Moderate and marked leukocytes indicate antibiotic-associated colitis, shigellosis, amebiasis, and salmonellosis. The methylene blue stain test for fecal polymorphonuclear leukocytes has a high sensitivity for bacterial diarrhea detection but this test does not preempt the use of a culture.

89060
A fluid sample is obtained. A variety of different methods may be used to process the specimen depending on the source. The fluid is analyzed for the presence of crystals using direct light or polarized light microscopy. A newer technique using atomic force microscopy (AFM) may be available in some laboratories.

89125
Prior to obtaining the stool specimen the patient is placed on a diet containing at least 60 gm of fat/day. A random stool specimen is obtained. A small amount of stool is prepared with Sudan III stain and examined microscopically. A random urine sample is obtained. Urine sediment is stained with Sudan III or IV and analyzed using light and polarized microscopy. Respiratory secretions may be obtained by separately reportable bronchoscopy and are stained and analyzed using techniques similar to those for other types of specimens.

89160
An adequate intake of red meat is required for 24-72 hours prior to testing. A stool specimen is obtained. The specimen is mixed with 10 percent solution of eosin in ethanol and stained on a slide for three minutes and cover-slipped. It is analyzed microscopically for rectangular striated muscle fibers.

89190
Two slides are normally obtained. Wright's stain is applied and the specimens are examined microscopically for the presence of eosinophils.

89220
Sputum is obtained for a specimen by using an aerosol-induced technique. This is a separate procedure from the testing of the sputum sample, which is used to study airway inflammation in asthma and other respiratory disorders. Sputum induction is done to collect an adequate sample of secretions from the lower respiratory tract in patients who do not produce sputum spontaneously. This is done by having the patient inhale an aerosol of normal or hypertonic saline. Oral secretions or saliva are not a sputum sample and different protocols have the patient rinse and dry the mouth, spit into a separate cup, or brush his/her teeth and rinse before sample collection to avoid contamination. A nebulizer that provides sufficient output of saline aerosol is used. With patient cooperation, inhalation is done at regular intervals until enough sputum for a sample is expectorated or until the patient feels the urge to cough.

89230
An iontophoresis sweat collection test, also called a chloride sweat test, is done to diagnose cystic fibrosis (CF) in children. Iontophoresis is the topical introduction of ionized drugs into the skin using direct current / positive current is applied to drive positively charged drug molecules into the tissues. Sweat production is stimulated to obtain the sweat sample by placing pads or filter paper soaked in pilocarpine onto

clean skin on the arm or neck. Positive electrodes are strapped over the pads. The circuit is completed by likewise placing negative electrodes over water-soaked pads. Low-voltage electrical current is left on for about five minutes to repel small amounts of pilocarpine into the skin. The electrodes are removed and the skin under the positive electrode is cleansed and dried. Pre-weighed filter paper is placed over the area and secured firmly with cling wrap. The filter paper is removed again after about 30 minutes, placed back in its bottle, and weighed again to calculate the amount of sweat collected. Iontophoresis may be repeated until enough sample is collected; it is then analyzed for chloride and sodium content. People with CF have an increased amount of sodium and chloride (salt) in their sweat. Concentrations greater than 60 mmol/L are consistent with the diagnosis of CF.

89250-89251
Eggs (oocytes) are aspirated transvaginally using ultrasound guidance in a separately reportable procedure. Eggs or previously fertilized embryos are kept in an incubator in a Petri dish culture for less than four days in 89250. Code 89251 is reserved for those instances when co-culture techniques over and above those normally required are performed.

89253
Assisted embryo hatching is performed in selected cases on the day of embryo transfer. A pipette is placed on one side of the embryo to keep it from moving. A very delicate, hollow needle called a hatching needle is placed on the other side of the embryo. An acidic solution is expelled from the needle against the outer shell (zona pellucida) of the embryo. The acidic solution digests a small area of the outer shell. The embryo is washed and replaced in the culture solution in the incubator.

89254
Because the egg (oocyte) is microscopic, only the follicle (fluid filled structure surrounding the egg) can be seen during the ultrasound-guided retrieval. Upon aspiration of the follicle, specially trained personnel use a microscope to search for the oocyte-cumulus complex, which includes the egg and surrounding cumulus cells from the ovary. This is accomplished by pouring the collected fluid into flat dishes and using a microscope to search for eggs.

89255
After the embryos have been cultured for two to six days, three to four healthy embryos are selected for transfer. Selected embryos are loaded into a transfer catheter. In a separately reportable procedure, the catheter is placed in the cervical canal and the embryos are transferred into the uterine cavity.

89257
A separately reportable testicular biopsy with aspiration is performed to obtain sperm. This may be required in cases where azoospermia is due to suspected obstruction to the spermatic ducts or in instances where the patient has had a failed reversal of a vasectomy. This procedure reports microscopic examination of aspirated fluid for the presence of sperm. If sperm are identified, further evaluation services may be performed and would be reported separately.

89258
Embryos not required for current uterine transfer are frozen using a process referred to as cryopreservation. Pre-implantation embryo preservation is a relatively new procedure as compared to sperm preservation (see 89259), but more than two-thirds of the embryos survive the cryopreservation process and can be preserved for an indefinite period of time.

89259
A cryoprotectant, usually glycerol or Dimethyl Sulfoxide (DMSO), is mixed with the semen to reduce damage to sperm during the freezing process. The semen specimen is placed in a vial and frozen in liquid nitrogen at -196 C. This halts all biologic and metabolic processes allowing the sperm to be preserved for many years.

89260
Prior to insemination or further diagnostic studies, the sperm go through a spinning and washing process in a series of solutions. The purpose of this is to separate sperm from seminal fluids, allowing the sperm to go through a process referred to as capacitation. Capacitation is an invisible change mature spermatozoa must undergo to acquire accelerated movement, allowing them to navigate through the uterus and fallopian tube. In addition, this procedure checks the ability of the sperm to swim in a forward progressive fashion. This procedure includes a semen analysis (count, motility, volume and differential).

89261
Prior to insemination or further diagnostic studies, the sperm go through a spinning and washing process in a series of solutions. The purpose of this is to separate sperm from seminal fluids, allowing the sperm to go through a process referred to as capacitation. Capacitation is an invisible change mature spermatozoa must undergo to acquire accelerated movement, allowing them to navigate through the uterus and fallopian tube. This complex prep includes a Percoll gradient and albumin gradient. This procedure includes a semen analysis (count, motility, volume and differential).

89264
A separately reportable testicular biopsy is performed to obtain sperm. A small amount of testicular tissue is taken for microscopic evaluation for the presence of sperm. This test is used only when no other means is available of obtaining a sperm sample because of the possibility of causing further testicular damage.

89268
Insemination requires a sperm cell to be introduced to an egg (oocyte) for fertilization procedures. The sperm is prepared through a washing method, which separates the sperm cells from the seminal fluid. The

washing filters out white blood cells, prostaglandins, and other debris, as well as cells with less motility, to provide the highest concentration of viable sperm. Once the concentrated spermatozoa have been prepared, they are placed in a culture medium with the eggs. If injection is required for fertilization, the protective coating of cells is removed from the egg and the sperm cell is directly injected.

89272
Culture of eggs (oocytes) or embryos usually occurs for 48 to 72 hours. This code describes an extended period of time for the cells to incubate in a culture medium, which will improve the identification of the most viable embryos. It is sometimes necessary to wait up to five days for the embryo to become a blastocyte before implantation due to high risk of multiple gestation or repeated IVF failures.

89280-89281
Assisted oocyte fertilization is done with microtechnique. A single sperm is injected into the egg (oocyte) to enable fertilization when sperm counts are very low or when sperm are non-motile. It requires micromanipulation of the sperm, which is also referred to as microtechnique. The usual method involves intracytoplasmic sperm injection (ICSI). Using ICSI technique, the mature egg is held in place with a holding pipette. A very delicate, sharp, hollow needle is used to immobilize and pick up a single sperm. This needle is inserted through the egg's outer shell (zona pellucida) into the cytoplasm of the egg. The sperm is injected into the cytoplasm and the needle removed. The eggs are checked the next day for evidence of fertilization. Report 89280 for 10 oocytes or less and 89281 for more than 10 oocytes.

89290-89291
Biopsy of an egg (oocyte) polar body or embryo blastomere (an embryo with six to eight cells) is indicated for patients who carry genetic disorders such as Sickle cell anemia, hemophilia, Fragile X syndrome, and others, and for those experiencing difficulty with a successful IVF or ICSI. The process of a biopsy includes inserting a microneedle into a fertilized egg to extract polar bodies of the oocyte, or to extract a single cell from a six to eight cell embryo. Screenings are performed through the process of FISH (fluorescent in-situ hybridization) and PCR (polymerase chain reaction). During FISH, a small amount of DNA is analyzed through staining of fluorochromes. PCR is able to detect gene-sequences or single genes, which may have abnormal mutations. Report 89290 for a biopsy of five or less embryos and 89291 for six or more embryos.

89300-89322
Semen analysis is generally performed in specialized infertility/andrology laboratories. Sexual activity culminating in ejaculation should be avoided for a minimum of 48 hours prior to testing. In 89300, a post coital specimen is obtained using a cervical swab. The test is timed to coincide with ovulation. Semen is tested for the presence (quantity) and/or motility of sperm. In 89310-89322, semen is collected using a condom-like seminal fluid collection device or by masturbation into a sterile container. In 89310, only sperm movement (motility) and number (concentration or count that measures how many million sperm are in each milliliter of fluid) are performed. Code 89320 reports a semen analysis that includes measurement of the ejaculate's volume, number, structure (shape) of sperm, sperm movement (motility), and direction of movement (forward motility). In addition, fluid thickness, acidity, and sugar content may be evaluated. Code 89321 tests only for the presence (quantity) and/or motility of sperm. In 89322, a detailed evaluation of the shape (morphology) is performed utilizing specially stained slides and microscopic examination of the sperm under high power magnification. In order to be considered normal, the sperm must meet a strict set of criteria regarding the shape and size of the head, mid-piece, and tail. A Kruger test is helpful in determining which reproductive techniques and methodologies may be most appropriate and successful. Tests reported with 89300-89322 may be accomplished using a variety of methods including semen function tests and computer-assisted sperm morphology/motility studies.

89325
This procedure tests for antisperm antibodies. A semen sample is placed with immunobeads; alternately, the semen sample may be placed with human or bovine cervical mucus together in a laboratory medium. The sperm antibody may be present in vaginal fluids or the male's blood or semen. Antisperm antibodies bind with the sperm inhibiting movement and their ability to fertilize an egg. The sperm appears clumped together on microscopic examination. Although the sample is sperm, some payers may cover as part of a fertility work-up for either partner.

89329
This test is also called sperm penetration assay (SPA) or hamster zona free ovum (HZFO) and tests the ability of the sperm to penetrate a hamster egg, which has been stripped of the zona pellucida (outer membrane). The patient should abstain from sexual activity culminating in ejaculation for a minimum of 48 hours. Semen is collected postcoitus using a condom-like seminal fluid collection device or by masturbation into a sterile container. Upon receiving the specimen in the laboratory, the sperm is washed and placed in a culture medium along with a single hamster egg. It is examined periodically using phase contrast microscopy. The test measures the ability of sperm to capacitate (invisible change which allows sperm to navigate rapidly forward), acrosome react (structural change fusing the outer membrane of the acrosome with the plasma membrane of the sperm head freeing enzymes in the acrosome which facilitate entry into the ovum), and fuse with the ovum.

89330
Sperm mucus interaction is assessed in vitro. Human or bovine ovulatory mucus is placed in a capillary tube.

Sperm penetration is measured over a period of 90 minutes. Sperm progression measures which sperm have progressed the farthest down the tube. Patient sperm penetration can be compared with fertile sperm specimens using in vitro methods.

89331
Retrograde ejaculation, in which the seminal fluid travels backward into the bladder following ejaculation, is often seen in patients with diabetes, or in men following transurethral surgery at or near the bladder neck, dissection of the retroperitoneal lymph nodes, or spinal cord injuries. The patient may present with low semen volume, motility (movement), and sperm concentration (count). In a urinalysis performed immediately after ejaculation, the specimen is examined under the microscope for the presence of sperm. If detected, the specimen is further processed to evaluate the concentration, motility, and morphology (shape).

89335
Storage of reproductive tissues is cryogenically maintained at an appropriate facility. A cryoprotectant is added to reduce cellular damage and the tissue is placed in vials, straws, or test tubes. The tissue is gradually frozen in the vapor of liquid nitrogen. Once frozen, the tissue is stored in liquid nitrogen at -196 degrees centigrade. Report 89335 for testicular reproductive tissue cryopreservation.

89337
Cryopreservation is a technique of freezing and maintaining cells at extremely low temperatures to preserve the genetic and metabolic properties of the cell. The mature (M-II) oocyte specimens are first preserved in a cryoprotectant solution to reduce cellular damage and the tissue is placed in storage vials. The sample is gradually frozen in liquid nitrogen. Cryopreserved samples are stored at temperatures of -80 to -196 degrees centigrade. The amount of cells being frozen, the source and amount of protective solution used, and the cooling technique may vary. Oocyte cryopreservation (OC) enables patients who may be susceptible to losing ovarian function to preserve reproductive potential through the use of long-term storage of oocytes.

89342-89346
These codes report the long-term maintenance of preserved reproductive tissue samples and fertilized embryos in an appropriate storage facility per year. Report 89342 for embryo(s), 89343 for sperm/semen, 89344 for testicular or ovarian tissue, and 89346 for oocyte(s).

89352-89356
Thawing of cryopreserved tissue requires thawing in different substances for set lengths of time so as to maintain the integrity of the specimen and prevent damage by thawing too quickly. The cryovial is removed from the liquid nitrogen and placed at room temperature until ice crystals have dissolved. A waterbath is prepared at the desired temperature in which the specimen is placed. After the water bath, each specimen is placed in a series of solutions to complete the thawing process. Report 89352 for embryos, 89353 for sperm/semen, 89354 for reproductive testicular/ovarian tissue, and 89356 for oocytes.

Proprietary Laboratory Analysis

0001U-0530U
These services are performed by a single "sole source" laboratory or for laboratory services that are cleared or approved by the Food and Drug Administration (FDA) and licensed and/or marketed to multiple providing laboratories. These services are often referred to as Proprietary Laboratory Analyses or PLA services. Correct code selection is dependent upon the service being provided and the manufacturer of the equipment.

Medicine

90281
This code identifies the immune globulin (Ig), human, for intramuscular use. An immune globulin is a passive immunization agent obtained from donated, pooled human plasma. Passive immunity is achieved for a short period as the antibodies received through the immune globulin are circulated through the body. The recipient's immune system is not stimulated to build its own antibodies. Report this code with the appropriate administration code.

90283
This code identifies the immune globulin (IgIV), human, for intravenous administration. An immune globulin is a passive immunization agent obtained from donated, pooled human plasma. Passive immunity is achieved for a short period as the antibodies received through the immune globulin are circulated through the body. The recipient's immune system is not stimulated to build its own antibodies. Report this code with the appropriate administration code.

90284
This code identifies the human immune globulin for use in subcutaneous infusions (SCIg). An immune globulin is a passive immunization agent obtained from donated pooled human plasma. Passive immunity is achieved for a short period as the antibodies received through the immune globulin are circulated through the body. The recipient's immune system is not stimulated to build its own antibodies. Some patients have insufficient venous access or adverse reactions to intravenous treatments, making them unsuitable candidates for traditional IVIg therapy. Controlled doses of immune globulin are administered over a period of several hours through a small needle placed just under the skin. Report this code with the appropriate administration code.

90287
This code identifies the botulinum antitoxin, equine, administered by any route. The antitoxin is a passive immunizing agent derived from purified serum from previously immunized horses. The antibodies received through the antiserum are circulated through the body and neutralize toxins produced by strains of the botulinum bacteria. Report this code with the appropriate administration code.

90288
This code identifies the botulism immune globulin, human, for intravenous use. This immune globulin is a passive immunization agent that gives protection against Botulism and is obtained from donated, pooled human plasma. Passive immunity is achieved for a short period as the antibodies received through the immune globulin are circulated through the body. The recipient's immune system is not stimulated to build its own antibodies. Report this code with the appropriate administration code.

90291
This code identifies the cytomegalovirus immune globulin (CMV-IgIV), human, for intravenous use. This immune globulin is a passive immunization agent that gives protection against the Cytomegalovirus and is obtained from donated, pooled human plasma. Passive immunity is achieved for a short period as the antibodies received through the immune globulin are circulated through the body. The recipient's immune system is not stimulated to build its own antibodies. Report this code with the appropriate administration code.

90296
This code identifies the diphtheria antitoxin, equine, administered by any route. The antitoxin is a passive immunizing agent derived from purified serum from previously immunized horses. The antibodies received through the antiserum are circulated through the body and neutralize toxins produced by Corynebacterium diphtheriae. Report this code with the appropriate administration code.

90371
This code identifies the hepatitis B immune globulin (HBIg), human, for intramuscular use. This immune globulin is a passive immunization agent that gives protection against Hepatitis B and is obtained from donated, pooled human plasma. Passive immunity is achieved for a short period as the antibodies received through the immune globulin are circulated through the body. The recipient's immune system is not stimulated to build its own antibodies. Report this code with the appropriate administration code.

90375-90377
Code 90375 identifies the rabies immune globulin (RIg), human; 90376 identifies the heat-treated (pasteurized) rabies immune globulin (RIg-HT); and 90377 identifies the heat- and solvent/detergent-treated rabies immune globulin (Rig-HT S/D). All are for intramuscular and/or subcutaneous use. These immune globulins are obtained from donated, pooled human plasma and are passive immunization agents that give protection against rabies when administered immediately after contact with a rabid or possibly rabid animal. Passive immunity is achieved for a short period as the antibodies received through the immune globulin are circulated through the body. The recipient's immune system is not stimulated to build its own antibodies. Report these codes with the appropriate administration code.

90378
Code 90378 identifies the respiratory syncytial virus (RSV) recombinant monoclonal antibody for intramuscular use, 50 mg, each. This humanized monoclonal antibody (IgG) gives protection against the respiratory syncytial virus and is injected once a month during the RSV season. Passive immunity is achieved for a short period as the antibodies received are circulated through the body. The recipient's immune system is not stimulated to build its own antibodies. Report this code with the appropriate administration code.

90380-90381
These codes report a monoclonal antibody injection prepared for seasonal respiratory syncytial virus (RSV). The monoclonal antibodies (IgG) target the RSV virus, inhibiting its replication and reducing the severity and occurrence of RSV infections. It is intended for intramuscular use in neonates and infants younger than 8 months of age who are in their first RSV season and certain at-risk infants and children 8 through 19 months of age before their second RSV season. Report 90380 for administration of the 0.5 mL dosage; 90381 for administration of the 1 mL dosage. These codes report the monoclonal antibody product only and should be reported with the appropriate administration code.

90384-90386
Code 90384 identifies the human Rho(D) immune globulin (RhIg) for intramuscular use, full-dose; 90385 is for a mini-dose. Code 90386 identifies the human Rho(D) immune globulin (RhIgIV) for intravenous use. This immune globulin is a passive immunization agent that gives protection against reactions between blood that is negative for the presence of Rh antigens on the surface of red blood cells to blood that is positive for the presence of Rh antigens on the RBC. Report these codes with the appropriate administration code.

90389
This code identifies a tetanus immune globulin (TIg), human, for intramuscular use. This immune globulin is a passive immunization agent that gives protection against tetanus and is obtained from donated, pooled human plasma. Passive immunity is achieved for a short period as the antibodies received through the immune globulin are circulated through the body. The recipient's immune system is not stimulated to build its own antibodies. Report this code with the appropriate administration code.

90393

This code identifies the vaccinia immune globulin, human, for intramuscular use. This immune globulin is a passive immunization agent that gives protection against vaccinia and is obtained from donated, pooled human plasma. The vaccinia virus causes cutaneous and systemic reactions occurring as a complication of smallpox vaccination. Passive immunity is achieved for a short period as the antibodies received through the immune globulin are circulated through the body. The recipient's immune system is not stimulated to build its own antibodies. Report this code with the appropriate administration code.

90396

This code identifies varicella-zoster immune globulin, human, for intramuscular use. This immune globulin is a passive immunization agent that gives protection against varicella-zoster and is obtained from donated, pooled human plasma. Passive immunity is achieved for a short period as the antibodies received through the immune globulin are circulated through the body. The recipient's immune system is not stimulated to build its own antibodies. Report this code with the appropriate administration code.

90460-90461

The physician or other qualified health care professional instructs the patient or family on the benefits and risks related to the vaccine or toxoid. The physician counsels the patient or family regarding signs and symptoms of adverse effects and when to seek medical attention for any adverse effects. A physician, nurse, or medical assistant administers an immunization by any route to the patient. It may be a single vaccine or a combination vaccine/toxoid in one immunization administration (e.g., diphtheria, pertussis, and tetanus toxoids are in a single DPT immunization). Report 90460 for the first or only vaccine/toxoid component. Report 90461 for each additional component. These codes report immunization administration to patients 18 years of age or younger.

90471-90472

A physician, nurse, or medical assistant administers an injectable (percutaneous, intradermal, subcutaneous, or intramuscular) immunization to the patient. It may be a single vaccine or a combination vaccine/toxoid in one immunization administration (e.g., diphtheria, pertussis, and tetanus toxoids are in a single DPT immunization). Report 90471 for one vaccine and 90472 for each additional vaccine (single or combination vaccine/toxoid).

90473-90474

A physician, nurse, or medical assistant administers an immunization to a patient via an intranasal (e.g., nasal spray) or an oral route (e.g., a liquid that is swallowed). It may be a single vaccine or a combination vaccine/toxoid in one immunization administration (e.g., adenovirus, Rotavirus, typhoid, poliovirus). Report 90473 for one vaccine and 90474 for each additional vaccine (single or combination vaccine/toxoid).

[90480]

This code reports the immunization administration of a single dose vaccine against severe acute respiratory syndrome coronavirus 2, also known as SARS-CoV-2, coronavirus disease, or COVID-19. A vaccine produces active immunization by inducing the immune system to build its own antibodies against specific microorganisms/viruses. The body retains memory of the antibody production pattern for long-term protection. This code includes vaccine risk/benefit counseling, when performed, and can be reported for a patient of any age. This code reports the administration only and should be reported with the appropriate product code.

[91304]

This code reports a recombinant spike protein nanoparticle vaccine against severe acute respiratory syndrome coronavirus 2, also known as SARS-CoV-2, coronavirus disease, or COVID-19. A vaccine produces active immunization by inducing the immune system to build its own antibodies against specific microorganisms/viruses. The body retains memory of the antibody production pattern for long-term protection. This vaccine is intended for intramuscular use in patients ages 12 years and older. It contains a saponin-based adjuvant, a plant glycoside that is designed to enhance the effectiveness of the vaccine. This code is specific to the Novavax 5 mcg/0.5 mL dosage vaccine. This code reports the vaccine product only and should be reported with the appropriate administration code.

[91318]

This code reports a spike protein vaccine against severe acute respiratory syndrome coronavirus 2, also known as SARS-CoV-2, coronavirus disease, or COVID-19. A vaccine produces active immunization by inducing the immune system to build its own antibodies against specific microorganisms/viruses. The body retains memory of the antibody production pattern for long-term protection. Based on messenger RNA (mRNA) that utilizes a lipid nanoparticle (LNP) as a delivery platform, this vaccine is intended for intramuscular use in patients ages 6 months through 4 years. This code is specific to the Pfizer-BioNTech 3 mcg/0.3 mL dosage vaccine that is based on a tris-sucrose buffer. This code reports the vaccine product only and should be reported with the appropriate administration code.

[91319]

This code reports a spike protein vaccine against severe acute respiratory syndrome coronavirus 2, also known as SARS-CoV-2, coronavirus disease, or COVID-19. A vaccine produces active immunization by inducing the immune system to build its own antibodies against specific microorganisms/viruses. The body retains memory of the antibody production pattern for long-term protection. Based on messenger RNA (mRNA) that utilizes a lipid nanoparticle (LNP) as a delivery platform, this vaccine is intended for intramuscular use in patients ages 5 years through 11 years. This code is specific to the Pfizer-BioNTech 10 mcg/0.3 mL dosage vaccine that is based on a tris-sucrose buffer. This code reports the vaccine product only and should be reported with the appropriate administration code.

[91320]

This code reports a spike protein vaccine against severe acute respiratory syndrome coronavirus 2, also known as SARS-CoV-2, coronavirus disease, or COVID-19. A vaccine produces active immunization by inducing the immune system to build its own antibodies against specific microorganisms/viruses. The body retains memory of the antibody production pattern for long-term protection. Based on messenger RNA (mRNA) that utilizes a lipid nanoparticle (LNP) as a delivery platform, this vaccine is intended for intramuscular use in patients ages 12 years and older. This code is specific to the Pfizer-BioNTech 30 mcg/0.3 mL dosage vaccine that is based on a tris-sucrose buffer. This code reports the vaccine product only and should be reported with the appropriate administration code.

[91321]

This code reports a vaccine against severe acute respiratory syndrome coronavirus 2, also known as SARS-CoV-2, coronavirus disease, or COVID-19. A vaccine produces active immunization by inducing the immune system to build its own antibodies against specific microorganisms/viruses. The body retains memory of the antibody production pattern for long-term protection. Based on messenger RNA (mRNA) that utilizes a lipid nanoparticle (LNP) as a delivery platform, this vaccine is intended for intramuscular use in patients ages 6 months through 11 years. This code is specific to the Moderna 25 mcg/0.25 mL dosage vaccine. This code reports the vaccine product only and should be reported with the appropriate administration code.

[91322]

This code reports a vaccine against severe acute respiratory syndrome coronavirus 2, also known as SARS-CoV-2, coronavirus disease, or COVID-19. A vaccine produces active immunization by inducing the immune system to build its own antibodies against specific microorganisms/viruses. The body retains memory of the antibody production pattern for long-term protection. Based on messenger RNA (mRNA) that utilizes a lipid nanoparticle (LNP) as a delivery platform, this vaccine is intended for intramuscular use in patients ages 12 years and older. This code is specific to the Moderna 50 mcg/0.5 mL dosage vaccine. This code reports the vaccine product only and should be reported with the appropriate administration code.

90476, 90477

These codes report live, oral preparations against an adenovirus and contain the actual virus. A vaccine produces active immunization by inducing the immune system to build its own antibodies against specific microorganisms/viruses. The body retains memory of the antibody production pattern for long-term protection. An adenovirus causes diseases of the upper respiratory tract and conjunctivae and is also present in latent infections in normal persons. Types 3, 4, 7, 14, and 21 have been isolated from patients with acute respiratory disease. Use 90476 to report a type 4 adenovirus vaccine and 90477 for a type 7. These codes report the vaccine product only and should be reported with the appropriate administration code.

90581

This code reports a vaccine against anthrax that is prepared for subcutaneous or intramuscular use. A vaccine produces active immunization by inducing the immune system to build its own antibodies against specific microorganisms/viruses. The body retains memory of the antibody production pattern for long-term protection. Cutaneous anthrax is the most common among humans and is caused by the bacteria *Bacillus anthracis* or its spores. It is usually acquired from contact with infected animals or their waste material. The most fatal form of anthrax is inhaled and can cause pneumonia. This code reports the vaccine product only and should be reported with the appropriate administration code.

90585-90586

These vaccines are prepared using Bacillus Calmette-Guerin (BCG) and contain the actual pathogen, a strain of *Mycobacterium bovis*. A vaccine produces active immunization by inducing the immune system to build its own antibodies against specific microorganisms/viruses. The body retains memory of the antibody production pattern for long-term protection. Alternately, vaccines also exist that function as immunotherapy to assist the immune system in seeking out and destroying cancer cells. Report 90585 for the percutaneous vaccine indicated for prevention of tuberculosis, and 90586 for that delivered by intravesical route and indicated for treatment of bladder cancer. These codes report the vaccine product only and should be reported with the appropriate administration codes.

[90589, 90593]

The chikungunya virus (CHIKV) is an arthropod-borne virus primarily transmitted to humans through the bite of Aedes mosquitoes that are infected with *Aedes aegypti* and *Aedes albopictus*. Now identified in over 110 countries in Africa, Asia, Europe, and the Americas, the virus poses a risk of spread to unaffected areas by infected travelers. A vaccine produces active immunization by inducing the immune system to build its own antibodies against specific microorganisms/viruses. The body retains memory of the antibody production pattern for long-term protection. Code 90589 reports a live attenuated or weakened form of the virus that does not cause the disease in healthy patients and is indicated as a single-dose injection for patients ages 18 years and older who are at an increased risk of exposure to CHIKV. Code 90593 reports a CHIKV recombinant vaccine. Both are administered by intramuscular injection; this method allows the vaccine to be absorbed into the bloodstream, providing a strong immune response against the virus. These codes report the vaccine product only and should be reported with the appropriate administration codes.

90587 [90584]
These codes report live quadrivalent dengue vaccines. A vaccine produces active immunization by inducing the immune system to build its own antibodies against specific microorganisms/viruses. The body retains memory of the antibody production pattern for long-term protection. Dengue is an *Aedes aegypti* mosquito-borne flavivirus disease. Also known as the breakbone fever, the disease is extremely painful and can be fatal. Currently, the disease has spread to many of the tropical and subtropical areas of the world. The disease has been identified as being caused by four similar viruses called the Dengue viruses 1-4. Report 90584 for the two-dose schedule and 90587 for the three-dose series. Both are administered subcutaneously. These codes report the vaccine product only and should be reported with the appropriate administration code.

90632-90634
These codes are used to report a hepatitis A vaccine (Hep A) for intramuscular use, prepared in various dosages. The vaccine is prepared from the blood plasma of asymptomatic human carriers of hepatitis caused by the hepatitis A virus or through recombinant DNA technology. Report 90632 for an adult dosage; 90633 for a two-dose schedule for a pediatric/adolescent dosage; and 90634 for a three-dose schedule for pediatric/adolescent dosage. Report these codes with the appropriate administration code.

90636
This code reports a hepatitis A and hepatitis B vaccine (HepA-HepB) for intramuscular use in an adult dosage. The vaccine is prepared from the blood plasma of asymptomatic human carriers of hepatitis caused by the hepatitis A and the hepatitis B virus (HepA-HepB) or through recombinant DNA technology. Report this code with the appropriate administration code.

90647-90648
These codes report vaccines for the prevention of influenza caused by the *Haemophilus influenzae* type b (Hib) bacteria. A vaccine produces active immunization by inducing the immune system to build its own antibodies against specific microorganisms/viruses. The body retains memory of the antibody production pattern for long-term protection. Report 90647 for the PRP-OMP conjugate, which is administered in a three-dose schedule. Report 90648 for the PRP-T conjugate, administered in a four-dose schedule. Both are intended for intramuscular use. These codes report the vaccine product only and should be reported with the appropriate administration code.

90649-90651
These codes report vaccines for human papillomavirus (HPV), a group of viruses that can infect cells on the skin surface or on the inner lining or moist surfaces of such body cavities and organs as the anus, cervix, penis, throat, vagina, and vulva. A vaccine produces active immunization by inducing the immune system to manufacture its own antibodies against specific microorganisms/viruses. The body retains memory of the antibody production pattern for long-term protection. In 90649 and 90650, an HPV vaccine is prepared in a three-dose schedule. The second dose is administered at least one to two months after the first dose and the third dose at least six months after the first dose. In 90651, the dose may be prepared in a two- or three-dose schedule. The vaccine may be bivalent (2vHPV), types 16 and 18; quadrivalent (4vHPV), types 6, 11, 16, and 18; or nonavalent (9vHPV), types 6, 11, 16, 18, 31, 33, 45, 52, and 58; all are intended for intramuscular use. The vaccine immunizes a patient against HPV or assists in producing an immune reaction to the E6 and E7 viral proteins to prevent or destroy the growth of abnormal or cancerous cells. Report 90649 for the quadrivalent vaccine (4vHPV), 90650 for the bivalent vaccine (2vHPV), and 90651 for the nonavalent vaccine (9vHPV). These codes report the vaccine product only and should be reported with the appropriate administration code.

90653
This code reports an inactivated influenza virus suspension vaccine (IIV) of the prevalent strains of influenza combined with a substance designed to enhance effectiveness (adjuvant). A vaccine produces active immunization by inducing the immune system to build its own antibodies against specific microorganisms/viruses. The body retains memory of the antibody production pattern for long-term protection. Provided as a subunit vaccine, it contains only the essential antigens that best stimulate the immune system, rather than the entire pathogen, hence the need for incorporation of an adjuvant. Intended for intramuscular use, this code reports the vaccine product only and should be reported with the appropriate administration code.

90655-90656
These codes report a split virus, preservative free suspension of three (two influenza A and one influenza B) (IIV3) of the most prevalent strains of influenza, prepared for intramuscular injection. A vaccine produces active immunization by inducing the immune system to build its own antibodies against specific microorganisms/viruses. The body retains memory of the antibody production pattern for long-term protection. Report 90655 for a 0.25 mL dose of preservative free, split virus influenza vaccine and 90656 for a 0.50 mL dose. These codes report the vaccine product only and should be reported with the appropriate administration code.

90657-90658
These codes report a split virus suspension of three (two influenza A and one influenza B) (IIV3) of the most prevalent strains of influenza, prepared for intramuscular use. A vaccine produces active

immunization by inducing the immune system to build its own antibodies against specific microorganisms/viruses. The body retains memory of the antibody production pattern for long-term protection. Report 90657 for a 0.25 mL dose and 90658 for a 0.5 mL dose. The vaccine induces active immunity to the highly contagious infection of the respiratory tract caused by a myxovirus and transmitted by airborne droplet infection. These codes report the vaccine product only and should be reported with the appropriate administration code.

90660 [90672]

These codes report a suspension of the prevalent strains of influenza virus, prepared for intranasal use. A vaccine produces active immunization by inducing the immune system to build its own antibodies against specific microorganisms/viruses. The body retains memory of the antibody production pattern for long-term protection. This live vaccination (LAIV3, LAIV4) contains the actual pathogen that has been weakened. Report 90660 when the vaccine contains three strains. Report 90672 when the vaccine is comprised of four strains. These codes report the vaccine product only and should be reported with the appropriate administration code.

90661

This code reports a suspension of the prevalent strain of influenza virus that has been derived from cell cultures, prepared for intramuscular use. A vaccine produces active immunization by inducing the immune system to build its own antibodies against specific microorganisms/viruses. The body retains memory of the antibody production pattern for long-term protection. Cell culture-derived vaccines are those in which the virus is grown in mammalian cells rather than egg-derived. The vaccine provides active immunity to the highly contagious infection of the respiratory tract caused by a myxovirus and transmitted by airborne droplet infection. This vaccine (ccIIV3) is antibiotic-free. This code reports a subunit in a 0.5 mL dose and should be reported with the appropriate administration code.

[90674]

This code reports a suspension of the prevalent strain of influenza virus that has been derived from cell cultures, prepared for intramuscular use. A vaccine produces active immunization by inducing the immune system to build its own antibodies against specific microorganisms/viruses. The body retains memory of the antibody production pattern for long-term protection. Cell culture-derived vaccines are those in which the virus is grown in mammalian cells rather than egg-derived. This vaccine provides active immunity to the highly contagious infection of the respiratory tract caused by a myxovirus and transmitted by airborne droplet infection. This vaccine (ccIIV4) is preservative and antibiotic-free. This code reports a subunit in a 0.5 mL dose and should be reported with the appropriate administration code.

[90756]

This code reports a suspension of the prevalent strain of influenza virus that has been derived from cell cultures, prepared for intramuscular use. A vaccine produces active immunization by inducing the immune system to build its own antibodies against specific microorganisms/viruses. The body retains memory of the antibody production pattern for long-term protection. Cell culture-derived vaccines are those in which the virus is grown in mammalian cells rather than egg-derived. The vaccine provides active immunity to the highly contagious infection of the respiratory tract caused by a myxovirus and transmitted by airborne droplet infection. This vaccine (ccIIV4) is antibiotic-free. This code reports a subunit in a 0.5 mL dose and should be reported with the appropriate administration code.

[90673]

This code reports a trivalent (RIV3) vaccine against the influenza virus that is a suspension derived from recombinant DNA, hemagglutinin (HA) protein only, and prepared for intramuscular use. A vaccine produces active immunization by inducing the immune system to build its own antibodies against specific microorganisms/viruses. The body retains memory of the antibody production pattern for long-term protection. This vaccination is manufactured without the use of the influenza virus and is preservative- and antibiotic-free. This code reports the vaccine product only and should be reported with the appropriate administration code.

90662

This code reports a suspension of the prevalent strain of influenza virus (IIV), prepared for intramuscular use. A vaccine produces active immunization by inducing the immune system to build its own antibodies against specific microorganisms/viruses. The body retains memory of the antibody production pattern for long-term protection. Subvirion (split virus) vaccines do not contain the entire virus; rather, they contain purified portions. Split virus vaccines are believed to cause fewer adverse effects, while maintaining their ability to stimulate an immune response (immunogenicity) comparable to that of whole virus preparations. Due to their decreased rates of side effects, split virus preparations are recommended for use in children younger than 13 years of age but may be administered to patients of any age. This code reports a preservative-free split virus vaccine whose immunogenicity has been enhanced with increased antigens. This code reports the vaccine product only and should be reported with the appropriate administration code.

90664-90668

These codes report pandemic formulations of the influenza virus vaccine. An influenza pandemic is a large-scale eruption of disease that takes place when a new influenza virus emerges in the human population, spreading easily between individuals and resulting in serious illness. A pandemic can rapidly travel across a whole region, a continent, or the world. Unlike seasonal influenza, individuals have little immunity to this virus. A suspension of the live prevalent strain of pandemic influenza virus (LAIV) is prepared for intranasal use in 90664; this live vaccination contains the actual pathogen. Subvirion (split virus) vaccines do not contain the entire virus; rather, they contain purified portions. Split virus vaccines are believed to cause fewer adverse effects in children and young adults, while maintaining its ability to stimulate an immune response (immunogenicity) comparable to that of whole virus preparations. Due to their decreased rates of side effects, only split virus preparations are recommended for children younger than 13 years of age. A suspension of the prevalent strain of pandemic influenza virus (IIV) is prepared for intramuscular use; 90668 reports the split virus vaccine, 90666 reports the preservative-free split-virus version, and 90667 reports the adjuvanted version. These codes identify the vaccine products only and must be reported in addition to the appropriate immunization administration codes.

[90695]

This code reports a cell culture-derived vaccine against the avian influenza virus of the H5N8 subtype that is combined with a substance designed to enhance effectiveness (adjuvant). A vaccine produces active immunization by inducing the immune system to build its own antibodies against specific microorganisms/viruses. The body retains memory of the antibody production pattern for long-term protection. Intended for intramuscular use, this code reports the vaccine product only and should be reported with the appropriate administration code.

90670-90671 [90677, 90684]

Pneumococcal vaccines provide protection against infections of the lungs, blood, brain, and spinal cord caused by various serotypes (valents) of the *Streptococcus pneumoniae* bacteria. A vaccine produces active immunization by inducing the immune system to build its own antibodies against specific microorganisms. The body retains memory of the antibody production pattern for long-term protection. These codes describe active suspension conjugate vaccines for intramuscular use. Report 90670 for supply of the 13 valent (PCV13) vaccine, 90671 for supply of the 15 valent (PCV15) vaccine, 90677 for supply of the 20 valent (PCV20) vaccine, and 90684 for supply of the 21 valent (PCV21) vaccine.

90675-90676

These codes report a vaccine against rabies. A vaccine produces active immunization by inducing the immune system to build its own antibodies against specific microorganisms/viruses. The body retains memory of the antibody production pattern for long-term protection. Code 90675 reports a vaccine for immunization against rabies, and protection against postexposure spread, for intramuscular use; 90676 is for intradermal use. The vaccine is prepared from a suspension of killed rabies virus prepared from duck embryo. These codes report the vaccine product only and should be reported with the appropriate administration code.

90678-90679

Code 90678 reports a nonadjuvanted vaccine for immunization against respiratory syncytial virus (RSV). A vaccine produces active immunization by inducing the immune system to build its own antibodies against specific microorganisms/viruses. The body retains memory of the antibody production pattern for long-term protection. This single-dose bivalent RSV prefusion (preF) vaccine, made up of two proteins selected to optimize protection against RSV A and B strains, is intended for intramuscular use in adults ages 60 years and older. In addition, it is approved for adults in their second or third trimester of pregnancy; antibodies to the RSV antigens are transferred placentally to provide passive immunization that protects infants from birth through 6 months of age. Report 90679 for a single-dose preF recombinant vaccine that includes an adjuvant to strengthen the immune response. The inclusion of an adjuvant enhances the vaccine's effectiveness, ensuring a robust and sustained immune reaction following administration. This vaccine, also intended for intramuscular use, is approved for individuals 60 years of age and older. These codes report the vaccine product only and should be reported with the appropriate administration code.

[90683]

This code reports a vaccine based on messenger RNA (mRNA) technology, enclosed within lipid nanoparticles (LNP), to combat respiratory syncytial virus (RSV), a common respiratory pathogen. A vaccine produces active immunization by inducing the immune system to build its own antibodies against specific microorganisms/viruses. The body retains memory of the antibody production pattern for long-term protection. This vaccine instructs the body's cells to produce prefusion F glycoprotein, which triggers antibodies to recognize and neutralize RSV. It is intended for intramuscular use in patients 60 years of age and older. This code reports the vaccine product only and should be reported with the appropriate administration code.

90680-90681

A rotavirus replicates in the cells of the intestine and causes acute diarrhea, particularly in infants. A vaccine produces active immunization by inducing the immune system to build its own antibodies against specific microorganisms/viruses. The body retains memory of the antibody production pattern for long-term protection. In 90680, vaccine for immunization against a rotavirus (RV5) is prepared for oral use in a three-dose schedule. This live pentavalent vaccine contains the actual virus. Report 90681 for a two-dose oral live attenuated human rotavirus (RV1) vaccine. Report these codes with the appropriate administration code.

90682
This code reports a quadrivalent (RIV4) vaccine against the influenza virus that is derived from recombinant DNA, hemagglutinin (HA) protein only and prepared for intramuscular use. A vaccine produces active immunization by inducing the immune system to build its own antibodies against specific microorganisms/ viruses. The body retains memory of the antibody production pattern for long-term protection. This vaccination is manufactured without the use of the influenza virus and is preservative- and antibiotic-free. This code reports the vaccine product only and should be reported with the appropriate administration code.

90685-90689 [90694]
These codes report a suspension of four (two influenza A and two influenza B) (IIV4) of the most prevalent strains of influenza, prepared for intramuscular injection. A vaccine produces active immunization by inducing the immune system to build its own antibodies against specific microorganisms/viruses. The body retains memory of the antibody production pattern for long-term protection. Report 90685 for a preservative-free, split virus influenza vaccine dose of 0.25 mL and 90686 for a 0.5 mL dose. Report 90687 for a split virus influenza vaccine dose of 0.25 mL that is not preservative-free and 90688 for a 0.5 mL dose. Report 90689 for a preservative-free, inactivated, and adjuvanted quadrivalent influenza vaccine dose of 0.25 mL and 90694 for a 0.5 mL dose. These codes report the vaccine product only and should be reported with the appropriate administration code.

[90637, 90638]
These codes report quadrivalent (qIRV) vaccines that target four strains of the influenza virus. These vaccines are based on messenger RNA (mRNA) technology and are intended for intramuscular use. A vaccine produces active immunization by inducing the immune system to build its own antibodies against specific microorganisms/viruses. The body retains memory of the antibody production pattern for long-term protection. Report 90637 for the 30 mcg/0.5 mL dosage and 90638 for the 60 mcg/0.5 mL dosage. These codes report the vaccine product only and should be reported with the appropriate administration code.

90690
This code reports a typhoid vaccine for immunization against the bacterial infection usually caused by *Salmonella typhi*, prepared for oral use. A vaccine produces active immunization by inducing the immune system to build its own antibodies against specific microorganisms/viruses. The body retains memory of the antibody production pattern for long-term protection. This live vaccine contains the actual pathogen. The bacterial infection is transmitted by contaminated milk, water, and food and causes high fever, diarrhea, and rash. This code reports the vaccine product only and should be reported with the appropriate administration code.

90691
This code reports a typhoid vaccine, Vi capsular polysaccharide form (ViCP), for immunization against the bacterial infection usually caused by *Salmonella typhi*, prepared for intramuscular use. A vaccine produces active immunization by inducing the immune system to build its own antibodies against specific microorganisms/viruses. The body retains memory of the antibody production pattern for long-term protection. The bacterial infection is transmitted by contaminated milk, water, and food and causes high fever, diarrhea, and rash. This code reports the vaccine product only and should be reported with the appropriate administration code.

90696-90700
These codes report a diphtheria, tetanus toxoid, and acellular pertussis vaccine, either alone or in combination with another vaccine, prepared for intramuscular use. A vaccine produces active immunization by inducing the immune system to build its own antibodies against specific microorganisms/ viruses. The body retains memory of these antibody production patterns for long-term protection. Code 90696 describes an intramuscular vaccine for diphtheria, tetanus toxoids, and acellular pertussis (synthetic form), combined with inactivated poliovirus (DTaP-IPV) for administration to children 4 through 6 years of age. Code 90697 reports an intramuscular vaccine for diphtheria, tetanus toxoids, acellular pertussis, and inactivated poliovirus, combined with a *Haemophilus influenza* type b PRP-OMP conjugate vaccine and Hepatitis B vaccine (DTaP-IPV-Hib-HepB). Code 90698 reports the immunization supply of diphtheria, tetanus toxoids, and acellular pertussis (synthetic form), combined with *Haemophilus influenza* type B and inactivated poliovirus vaccine (DTaP-IPV/ Hib) for intramuscular use. Code 90700 describes a vaccine for intramuscular use against diphtheria, tetanus toxoids, and acellular pertussis (DTaP) for administration to children younger than 7 years of age. The DTaP/DTP vaccinations are routine immunizations for children. These codes report the vaccine product only and should be reported with the appropriate administration code.

90702
This code reports toxoids against diphtheria and tetanus (DT), adsorbed for intramuscular use, for administration to individuals younger than age 7. A toxoid stimulates the body's own immune system to produce specific antitoxin antibodies that destroy the toxins secreted by bacteria. This provides immunity that is effective and long lasting. This code reports the toxoid product only and should be reported with the appropriate administration code.

90707
This code reports the combined measles, mumps, and rubella (MMR) vaccine, live, prepared for subcutaneous use. A vaccine produces active immunization by inducing the immune system to build its own antibodies against specific microorganisms/viruses.

The body retains memory of these antibody production patterns for long-term protection. A live vaccine contains the actual pathogens. This code reports the vaccine product only and should be reported with the appropriate administration code.

90710

This code reports a vaccine that combines measles, mumps, rubella, and varicella (MMRV), prepared for subcutaneous use. A vaccine produces active immunization by inducing the immune system to build its own antibodies against specific microorganisms/viruses. The body retains memory of these antibody production patterns for long-term protection. This live vaccine contains the actual pathogens. This code reports the vaccine product only and should be reported with the appropriate administration code.

90713

This code reports an inactivated poliovirus vaccine (IPV), prepared for subcutaneous or intramuscular use. A vaccine produces active immunization by inducing the immune system to manufacture its own antibodies against specific microorganisms/viruses. The body retains memory of these antibody production patterns for long-term protection. This code reports the vaccine product only and should be reported with the appropriate administration code.

[90611]

This code reports a live, preservative-free vaccine indicated for the prevention of smallpox and monkeypox disease in adults 18 years and older who are determined to be at high risk for smallpox or monkeypox infection. A vaccine produces active immunization by stimulating the immune system to build its own antibodies against specific microorganisms/viruses. The body retains memory of these antibody production patterns for long-term protection. This vaccine is made from an attenuated (weakened) virus called vaccinia (a poxvirus similar to smallpox, but less harmful). Two doses, administered 28 days apart, are required of this 0.5 mL dosage, which is indicated for subcutaneous use. This code reports the vaccine product only and should be reported with the appropriate administration code.

90714

This code reports the immunization supply of tetanus and diphtheria toxoids (Td), adsorbed, preservative-free, prepared for intramuscular administration to patients 7 years of age or older. A toxoid stimulates the body's own immune system to produce specific antitoxin antibodies that destroy the toxins secreted by bacteria. This provides immunity that is effective and long lasting. This code reports the toxoid product only and should be reported with the appropriate administration code.

90715

This code reports the immunization supply of tetanus, diphtheria toxoids, and acellular pertussis (synthetic form) vaccine (Tdap), prepared for intramuscular administration to patients 7 years of age or older. A toxoid stimulates the body's own immune system to produce specific antitoxin antibodies that destroy the toxins secreted by bacteria. This provides immunity that is effective and long lasting. A vaccine produces active immunization by inducing the immune system to build its own antibodies against specific microorganisms/viruses. The body retains memory of these antibody production patterns for long-term protection. This code reports the toxoid/vaccine product only and should be reported with the appropriate administration code.

[90626, 90627]

This code reports an inactivated vaccine against tick-borne encephalitis, prepared for intramuscular use. A vaccine produces active immunization by inducing the immune system to build its own antibodies against specific microorganisms/viruses. The body retains memory of these antibody production patterns for long-term protection. Tick-borne encephalitis (TBE), a viral infection of the brain and spine, can be transmitted to humans through the bite of an infected tick or, infrequently, by ingesting unpasteurized milk or milk products from infected animals. Although not currently endemic in the United States, it has been identified in over 35 countries throughout Asia and Europe. This vaccine, developed using a master "seed" virus similar to the natural TBE virus, induces neutralizing antibodies and is intended to prevent TBE in persons 1 year of age and older. Report 90626 for the 0.25 mL dosage and 90627 for the 0.5 mL dosage. This code reports the vaccine product only and should be reported with the appropriate administration code.

[90622]

This code reports a vaccine for smallpox prepared for percutaneous use. A vaccine produces active immunization by stimulating the immune system to build its own antibodies against specific microorganisms/viruses. The body retains memory of these antibody production patterns for long-term protection. Made from a poxvirus similar to, but less harmful than, smallpox (vaccinia), this live vaccine is supplied as a lyophilized (freeze-dried) powder that must be reconstituted with a diluent prior to percutaneous scarification using a prescribed number of jabs with a bifurcated needle. The prescribed dosage of 0.3 mL is indicated for active immunization against smallpox disease for persons 12 months and older determined to be at risk for smallpox infection. Since the monkeypox and smallpox viruses are closely related (both in the orthopox family), this vaccine can provide some protection against monkeypox as well and is also approved by the FDA for use against monkeypox under the expanded access Investigational New Drug (IND) application. This code reports the vaccine product only and should be reported with the appropriate administration code.

90716

This code reports a live varicella virus vaccine (VAR), prepared for subcutaneous use. A vaccine produces active immunization by inducing the immune system

Medicine

to build its own antibodies against specific microorganisms/viruses. The body retains memory of these antibody production patterns for long-term protection. This vaccine contains the actual pathogen. This code reports the vaccine product only and should be reported with the appropriate administration code.

90717
This code reports the live vaccine against yellow fever, prepared for subcutaneous use. A vaccine produces active immunization by inducing the immune system to build its own antibodies against specific microorganisms/viruses. The body retains memory of these antibody production patterns for long-term protection. A live vaccine contains the actual pathogen. This code reports the vaccine product only and should be reported with the appropriate administration code.

90723
This code reports an immunization combining diphtheria and tetanus toxoids, acellular pertussis vaccine, Hepatitis B, and inactivated poliovirus vaccine (DTaP-HepB-IPV), prepared for intramuscular use. A toxoid stimulates the body's own immune system to produce specific antitoxin antibodies that destroy the toxins secreted by microorganisms/viruses. This provides immunity that is effective and long lasting. A vaccine produces active immunization by inducing the immune system to build its own antibodies against specific microorganisms/viruses. The body retains memory of these antibody production patterns for long-term protection. This code reports the toxoid/vaccine product only and should be reported with the appropriate administration code.

[90625]
This code reports the supply of a live cholera vaccine, prepared for oral use. A vaccine produces active immunization by inducing the immune system to build its own antibodies against specific microorganisms/viruses. The body retains memory of these antibody production patterns for long-term protection. This code reports the vaccine product only and should be reported with the appropriate administration code.

90732
This code reports a pneumococcal polysaccharide vaccine, 23-valent (PPSV23), adult or immunosuppressed patient dosage, prepared for subcutaneous or intramuscular administration to patients 2 years of age or older. A vaccine produces active immunization by inducing the immune system to build its own antibodies against specific microorganisms/viruses. The body retains memory of these antibody production patterns for long-term protection. This code reports the vaccine product only and should be reported with the appropriate administration code.

[90644]
This code reports a meningococcal conjugate vaccine (serogroups C & Y) and *Haemophilus influenzae* type b vaccine (Hib-MenCY), prepared for intramuscular use in a four-dose schedule for children 6 weeks to 18 months of age. A vaccine produces active immunization by inducing the immune system to build its own antibodies against specific microorganisms/viruses. The body retains memory of these antibody production patterns for long-term protection. This code reports the vaccine product only and should be reported with the appropriate administration code.

90733
This code reports a meningococcal polysaccharide vaccine, serogroups A, C, Y, and W-135, quadrivalent (MPSV4), prepared for subcutaneous use. A vaccine produces active immunization by inducing the immune system to build its own antibodies against specific microorganisms/viruses. The body retains memory of these antibody production patterns for long-term protection. This code reports the vaccine product only and should be reported with the appropriate administration code.

90734
This code reports the supply of a quadrivalent (serogroups A, C, W, and Y) meningococcal polysaccharide vaccine conjugated to diphtheria toxoid carrier (MenACWY-D) or CRM197 carrier (MenACWY-CRM), prepared for intramuscular use. A vaccine produces active immunization by inducing the immune system to build its own antibodies against specific microorganisms/viruses. The body retains memory of these antibody production patterns for long-term protection. This code reports the vaccine product only and should be reported with the appropriate administration code.

[90619]
This code reports the supply of a quadrivalent (serogroups A, C, W, and Y) meningococcal polysaccharide vaccine conjugated to tetanus toxoid carrier (MenACWY-TT), prepared for intramuscular use. A vaccine produces active immunization by inducing the immune system to build its own antibodies against specific microorganisms/viruses. The body retains memory of these antibody production patterns for long-term protection. This code reports the vaccine product only and should be reported with the appropriate administration code.

[90623]
This code reports a meningococcal pentavalent vaccine, a combination vaccine that protects against multiple strains of meningococcal bacteria, administered via intramuscular injection. A vaccine produces active immunization by inducing the immune system to build its own antibodies against specific microorganisms/viruses. The body retains memory of these antibody production patterns for long-term protection. Tetanus toxoid carrier strains within this vaccine include Men A, C, W, Y, and a specific subtype called MenB-FHbp. It is indicated for individuals 10 through 25 years of age and administered as a two-dose series given six months apart. This code reports the vaccine product only and

should be reported with the appropriate administration code.

[90624]
Meningococcal disease, a bacterial infection caused by *Neisseria meningitidis*, colonizes in the nasopharyngeal mucosal surfaces and is transmitted through direct contact with large-droplet respiratory tract secretions. This code reports a meningococcal pentavalent vaccine, a combination vaccine that protects against five strains of meningococcal bacteria, administered via intramuscular injection. The vaccine consists of Men B-4C recombinant proteins and outer membrane vesicle as well as a diphtheria toxoid carrier conjugated to serogroups A, C, W, and Y. A vaccine produces active immunization by inducing the immune system to build its own antibodies against specific microorganisms/viruses. The body retains memory of these antibody production patterns for long-term protection. This code reports the vaccine product only and should be reported with the appropriate administration code.

[90620, 90621]
These codes report a meningococcal recombinant vaccine, prepared for intramuscular use. A vaccine produces active immunization by inducing the immune system to build its own antibodies against specific microorganisms/viruses. The body retains memory of these antibody production patterns for long-term protection. Report 90620 for a meningococcal recombinant protein and outer membrane vesicle vaccine, serogroup B (MenB-4C). Report 90621 for a meningococcal recombinant lipoprotein vaccine, serogroup B (MenB-FHbp). These codes report the vaccine product only and should be reported with the appropriate administration code.

90736 [90750]
These codes report a zoster vaccine against shingles, prepared for intramuscular use. A vaccine produces active immunization by inducing the immune system to manufacture its own antibodies against specific microorganisms/viruses. The body retains memory of these antibody production patterns for long-term protection. In 90736, a live herpes zoster (HZV) or shingles vaccine for subcutaneous injection is administered. In 90750, a recombinant, subunit, adjuvanted vaccine is administered intramuscularly. Shingles is a reactivation of the herpes zoster virus that causes chickenpox. The virus persists in a dormant state and may reactivate with certain conditions or advancing age that cause or is associated with immune system compromise. This vaccine prevents herpes zoster and postherpetic neuralgia as a result of the dormant virus in sensory nerve cells. These codes report the vaccine product only and should be reported with the appropriate administration code.

90738
This code reports an inactivated Japanese encephalitis virus vaccine, prepared for intramuscular use. A vaccine produces active immunization by inducing the immune system to build its own antibodies against specific microorganisms/viruses. The body retains memory of these antibody production patterns for long-term protection. Japanese encephalitis is a mosquito-borne viral infection and is the foremost cause of viral encephalitis in Asia. This code reports the vaccine product only and should be reported with the appropriate administration code.

90739-90747 [90759]
These codes report the supply of a hepatitis B (HepB) vaccine for intramuscular use, prepared in various dosages. A vaccine produces active immunization by inducing the immune system to build its own antibodies against specific microorganisms/viruses. The body retains memory of these antibody production patterns for long-term protection. Report 90739 for an adult two-dose or four-dose schedule of CpG-adjuvanted vaccine; 90740 for a three-dose schedule for a dialysis or immunosuppressed patient; 90743 for an adolescent two-dose schedule; 90744 for a pediatric/adolescent three-dose schedule; 90746 for an adult three-dose schedule; 90759 for a three-antigen (S, Pre-S1, Pre-S2), 10 mcg dosage, three-dose schedule; and 90747 for a four-dose schedule for a dialysis or immunosuppressed patient. These codes report the vaccine product only and should be reported with the appropriate administration code.

90748
This code reports a combined hepatitis B and *Haemophilus influenzae* type B (Hib-HepB) vaccine, prepared for intramuscular use. A vaccine produces active immunization by inducing the immune system to build its own antibodies against specific microorganisms/viruses. The body retains memory of these antibody production patterns for long-term protection. This code reports the vaccine product only and should be reported with the appropriate administration code.

[90758]
This code reports a vaccine indicated specifically for prevention of disease caused by the Zaire ebolavirus, prepared for intramuscular use; it does not protect against other species of Ebolavirus. Vaccines produce active immunization by inducing the immune system to build its own antibodies against specific microorganisms/viruses. The body retains memory of these antibody production patterns for long-term protection. Ebola virus disease (EVD) is a rare but severe disease in humans, with an average fatality rate of 50 percent. Initially transmitted from wild animals to humans, the virus spreads in the population through human-to-human contact. This code reports the vaccine product only and should be reported with the appropriate administration code.

90785
This code is reported in addition to the code for a primary psychiatric service. It is reported when the patient being treated has certain factors that increase the complexity of treatment rendered. These factors are limited to the following: the need to manage disruptive communication that complicates the

delivery of treatment; complications involving the implementation of a treatment plan due to caregiver behavioral or emotional interference; evidence of a sentinel event with subsequent disclosure to a third party and discussion and/or reporting to the patient(s); or use of play equipment or translator to enable communication when a barrier exists.

90791-90792

A psychiatric diagnostic evaluation is performed, which includes the assessment of the patient's psychosocial history, current mental status, review, and ordering of diagnostic studies followed by appropriate treatment recommendations. In 90792, additional medical services such as physical examination and prescription of pharmaceuticals are provided in addition to the diagnostic evaluation. Interviews and communication with family members or other sources are included in these codes.

90832-90833

Psychotherapy is a variety of treatment techniques in which a physician or other qualified health care provider helps a patient with a mental illness or behavioral disturbance identify and alleviate any emotional disruptions, maladaptive behavioral patterns, and contributing/exacerbating factors. This treatment also involves encouraging personality growth and development through coping techniques and problem-solving skills. Report 90832 for one half hour of face-to-face time spent with the patient without an additional evaluation and management (E/M) service. Report 90833 if a separate E/M service is performed during the same encounter as the 30 minutes of psychotherapy.

90834-90836

Psychotherapy is a variety of treatment techniques in which a physician or other qualified health care provider helps a patient with a mental illness or behavioral disturbance identify and alleviate any emotional disruptions, maladaptive behavioral patterns, and contributing/exacerbating factors. This treatment also involves encouraging personality growth and development through coping techniques and problem-solving skills. Report 90834 for 45 minutes of face-to-face time spent with the patient without an additional evaluation and management (E/M) service. Report 90836 if a separate E/M service is performed during the same encounter as the 45 minutes of psychotherapy.

90837-90838

Psychotherapy is a variety of treatment techniques in which a physician or other qualified health care provider helps a patient with a mental illness or behavioral disturbance identify and alleviate any emotional disruptions, maladaptive behavioral patterns, and contributing/exacerbating factors. This treatment also involves encouraging personality growth and development through coping techniques and problem-solving skills. Report 90837 for one hour of face-to-face time spent with the patient without an additional evaluation and management (E/M) service. Report 90838 if a separate E/M service is performed during the same encounter as the 60 minutes of psychotherapy.

90839-90840

Psychotherapy is a variety of treatment techniques in which a physician or other qualified health care provider helps a patient with a mental illness or behavioral disturbance identify and alleviate any emotional disruptions, maladaptive behavioral patterns, and contributing/exacerbating factors. Report these codes when the psychotherapy is for a patient with a life-threatening or highly complex psychiatric crisis. Code 90839 is used for the first 30 to 74 minutes of intervention and 90840 for each additional 30 minutes. These codes include history, mental status examination, mobilization of resources, and implementation treatment.

90845

The therapist performs psychoanalysis by utilizing methods of intense observation and analytical skills to investigate the patient's past experiences, unconscious motivations, and internal conflicts, as well as contributing medical conditions, to discover how these pilot the patient's current behavior and emotions. The psychiatrist seeks to produce change in maladapted behavior. Psychoanalysis includes reviewing medical notes and making clinical setting arrangements, assisting the patient in further self-awareness, working through barriers, understanding self-observations, and modifying mental behavior and status while continuing to elicit more information and personal exploration. This code also includes follow-up work of documentation, content review, and peer consultation.

90846

The therapist provides 50 minutes of family psychotherapy in a setting where the care provider meets with the patient's family without the patient present. The family is part of the patient evaluation and treatment process. Family dynamics as they relate to the patient's mental status and behavior are a main focus of the sessions. Attention is also given to the impact the patient's condition has on the family, with therapy aimed at improving the interaction between the patient and family members.

90847

The therapist provides 50 minutes of family psychotherapy in a setting where the care provider meets with the patient and the patient's family jointly. The family is part of the patient evaluation and treatment process. Family dynamics as they relate to the patient's mental status and behavior are a main focus of the sessions. Attention is also given to the impact the patient's condition has on the family, with therapy aimed at improving the interaction between the patient and family members. Reviewing records, communicating with other providers, observing and interpreting patterns of behavior and communication between the patient and family members, and decision making regarding treatment, including medication management or any physical exam related to the medication, is included.

90849
Multiple family group psychotherapy provided to a patient and his/her family, as well as other patients and families, altogether. This is usually done in cases involving similar issues and often in settings of group homes, drug treatment facilities, or hospital rehabilitation centers. The session may focus on the issues of the patient's hospitalization or substance abuse problems. This code is reported once for each family group present.

90853
The psychiatric treatment provider conducts psychotherapy for a group of several patients in one session. Group dynamics are explored. Emotional and rational cognitive interactions between individual persons in the group are facilitated and observed. Personal dynamics of any individual patient may be discussed within the group setting. Processes that help patients move toward emotional healing and modification of thought and behavior are used, such as facilitating improved interpersonal exchanges, group support, and reminiscing. The group may be composed of patients with separate and distinct maladaptive disorders or persons sharing some facet of a disorder. This code should be used for group psychotherapy with other patients, and not members of the patients' families.

90863
The patient's medications are managed during a psychiatric service, including the patient's current use of medicines, a medical review of the benefits and treatment progression, management of side effects, and review or change of prescription. This is a pharmacologically related service and is reported in addition to non-crisis related psychotherapy when there is no other evaluation and management service performed during the encounter.

90865
A hypnotic drug known as Amytal or sodium amobarbital is infused into the patient via an intravenous drip for psychiatric diagnostic or psychotherapeutic treatment purposes. Amytal is a hypnotic sedative used for diagnosing dissociative disorders and to treat trauma victims by accessing repressed memories, emotions, or events to facilitate healing. This is often used after other measures have failed and/or when gaining a definitive diagnosis is medically essential. A sodium Amytal interview is often conducted in an inpatient setting, to monitor the effects of the drug. The patient is in a hypnotic state, where memories, as the patient perceives them, are more confidently reviewed. These interviews are often videotaped for later discussion.

90867-90869
Transcranial magnetic stimulation (TMS) is a technique to stimulate the brain by electromagnetic induction with a coil placed on the scalp. For direct stimulation to cortical neurons, a strong magnetic field pulse is generated over the patient's scalp to activate cortical neurons in the brain and to disturb the normal operation of the brain. Report 90867 for the initial treatment session, including cortical mapping, motor threshold determination, delivery, and management. Report 90868 for each subsequent session, including delivery and management only. Report 90869 for a subsequent session in which the motor threshold is re-determined and delivery and management are performed.

90870
The treating clinician initiates a seizure using electroconvulsive therapy (ECT), most often to combat chronic or profound depression, especially psychotic or intractable manic forms and used for people who cannot take antidepressants. The clinician anesthetizes the patient with a barbiturate and a muscle relaxant. Electrodes are placed on the patient's temples and/or forehead and a measured electrical dose is applied for about a second to commence the seizure, typically lasting 30 seconds to a minute. EEG and EKG monitors follow the seizure activity and heart rhythm while the patient sleeps through the therapy. The patient awakens a few minutes later.

90875-90876
The treating clinician gives individual psychophysiological therapy by utilizing biofeedback training together with psychotherapy to modify behavior. The clinician prepares the patient with sensors that read and display skin temperature, blood pressure, muscle tension, or brain wave activity. The patient is taught how certain thought processes, stimuli, and actions affect these physiological responses. The treating clinician works with the patient to learn to recognize and manipulate these responses and to control maladapted physiological functions through relaxation and awareness techniques. Psychotherapy is also rendered using supportive interactions, suggestion, persuasion, reality discussions, re-education, behavior modification techniques, reassurance, and the occasional aid of medication. Individual psychophysiological therapy is performed face to face with the patient. Report 90875 for 30-minute sessions and 90876 for 45-minute sessions.

90880
Hypnosis is used as a modality for psychotherapy. The therapist induces an altered state of consciousness, or focused attention, in the patient. While patients are in this relaxed state of heightened awareness and suggestibility, they can experience changes in the way they feel, think, and behave in response to suggestions directed to them by the hypnotherapist. This modality for psychiatric services helps the therapist to achieve an alteration in the patient's thought and behavior patterns.

90882
The clinician uses this code to report work done with agencies, employers, or institutions on a psychiatric

patient's behalf in order to achieve environmental changes and interventions for managing the patient's medical condition.

90885

The clinician reviews and evaluates the patient's hospital records, other psychiatric reports such as psychometric and projective tests, and other pertinent data for the purpose of gaining a medical diagnosis and insight into the patient's present condition.

90887

The clinician interprets the results of a patient's psychiatric and medical examinations and procedures, as well as any other pertinent recorded data, and spends time explaining the patient's condition to family members and other responsible parties involved with the patient's care and well-being. Advice is also given as to how family members can best assist the patient.

90889

The clinician prepares a report on a patient's mental condition, current psychiatric status, history, treatment regimen, and progress for other providers, agencies, or insurance carriers involved with the patient's care, except for legal or consultative purposes.

90901

Biofeedback trains patients to control their autonomic or involuntary nervous system responses to regulate vital signs such as heart rate, blood pressure, temperature, and muscle tension. Monitors of various types are used to indicate body responses, which the patient learns to associate with related stimuli and also control in serial sessions. This code applies to any of several modalities of biofeedback training. Biofeedback is used for treatment of conditions including high blood pressure, incontinence, Raynaud's syndrome, and anticipatory nausea due to chemotherapy.

90912-90913

Biofeedback trains patients to control their autonomic or involuntary nervous system responses to regulate vital signs, like heartrate, blood pressure, temperature, and muscle tension. This code applies to biofeedback training for monitoring muscles specifically of the anus and/or rectum, perineum, and urethral sphincter. Electromyography, which measures muscle contractions, and/or manometry to measure pressure are included when performed. This particular biofeedback training is done to help the incontinent patient gain control of the related muscles. Report 90912 for the first 15 minutes of one-on-one patient contact by the physician or other qualified health care professional and 90913 for each additional 15 minutes.

90935-90937

Hemodialysis is a process to remove toxins from the blood and to maintain fluid and electrolyte balance when the kidneys no longer function. The procedure involves using a previously placed catheter in an artery or a vein to withdraw the patient's blood, mechanically circulating the blood through a dialysis machine to remove the toxins and wastes, and transfusing the blood back to the patient. Code 90935 applies to one hemodialysis treatment that includes a single physician or other qualified health care provider's evaluation of the patient and 90937 is for a hemodialysis procedure when patient re-evaluation(s) must be done during the procedure, with or without substantial revision of the dialysis prescription.

90940

A hemodialysis access flow study is performed to determine blood flow in a graft or arteriovenous fistula. The health care provider performs the test after approximately 30 minutes of treatment and after turning off ultrafiltration. In the direct dilution method, also known as the urea-based measurement of recirculation, arterial and venous line samples are drawn and the blood rate is reduced to 120 mL/minute. The blood pumped is turned off 10 seconds after reducing the blood flow rate and an arterial line is clamped above the sampling port. Systemic arterial samples are drawn, the line is disconnected, and dialysis is resumed. Measurements of BUN in the arterial, venous, and arterial sample are taken and the percent recirculation is calculated. This code includes the hook-up, measurement, and disconnection.

90945-90947

Dialysis is a process to remove toxins from the blood and to maintain fluid and electrolyte balance when the kidneys no longer function. In peritoneal dialysis, a fluid is introduced into the peritoneal cavity that removes toxins and electrolytes, which passively leach into the fluid. Hemofiltration, similar to hemodialysis, employs passing large volumes of blood over extracorporeal, adsorbent filters that remove waste products from the blood. Other continuous renal replacement therapies may be employed, such as continuous arteriovenous hemofiltration that uses small-volume, low-resistance blood filters that are powered by the patient's own arterial pressure, thus eliminating the need for a mechanical pump. Code 90945 applies to one dialysis procedure, other than hemodialysis, with a single physician or other qualified health care provider's evaluation of the patient. Code 90947 applies to a dialysis procedure, other than hemodialysis, that requires repeated provider evaluations, with or without substantial revision of a dialysis prescription.

90951-90953

These codes apply to all outpatient ESRD-related services provided during a one-month period for patients younger than 2 years of age. These codes include establishing the dialyzing cycle, all outpatient management for each dialysis visit, patient management during the dialysis treatment, any telephone calls, and evaluation and management related to the ESRD, such as assessing the patient's nutritional status, growth, and development and providing parental counseling. Dialysis treatment is not included. Code assignment is based on the number of face-to-face visits by a physician or other qualified health care provider per month. Report

90951 for four or more visits, 90952 for two or three visits, and 90953 for one visit.

90954-90956
These codes apply to all outpatient ESRD-related services provided during a one-month period for patients 2 to 11 years of age. These codes include establishing the dialyzing cycle, all outpatient management for each dialysis visit, patient management during the dialysis treatment, any telephone calls, and evaluation and management related to the ESRD, such as assessing the patient's nutritional status, growth, and development and providing parental counseling. Dialysis treatment is not included. Code assignment is based on the number of face-to-face visits by a physician or other qualified health care provider per month. Report 90954 for four or more visits, 90955 for two or three visits, and 90956 for one visit.

90957-90959
These codes apply to all outpatient ESRD-related services provided during a one-month period for patients 12 to 19 years of age. These codes include establishing the dialyzing cycle, all outpatient management for each dialysis visit, patient management during the dialysis treatment, any telephone calls, and evaluation and management related to the ESRD, such as assessing the patient's nutritional status, growth, and development and providing parental counseling. Dialysis treatment is not included. Code assignment is based on the number of face-to-face visits by a physician or other qualified health care provider per month. Report 90957 for four or more visits, 90958 for two or three visits, and 90959 for one visit.

90960-90962
These codes apply to all outpatient ESRD-related services provided during a one-month period for patients 20 years of age or older. These codes include establishing the dialyzing cycle, all outpatient management for each dialysis visit, patient management during the dialysis treatment, any telephone calls, and evaluation and management related to the ESRD. Dialysis treatment is not included. Code assignment is based on the number of face-to-face visits by a physician or other qualified health care provider per month. Report 90960 for four or more visits, 90961 for two or three visits, and 90962 for one visit.

90963-90966
These codes apply to all ESRD-related physician services provided during a one-month period to home dialysis patients of specified ages. These codes include establishing the dialyzing cycle as well as physician evaluation and management related to the ESRD. Codes 90963-90965 also include assessment of the patient's nutritional status, growth and development, and provision of parental counseling. Code assignment is based on age. Report 90963 for patients younger than 2 years of age, 90964 for patients 2 to 11 years of age, 90965 for patients 12 to 19 years of age, and 90966 for patients over the age of 20.

90967-90970
This code range applies to all ESRD-related services provided to dialysis patients of specified ages who receive dialysis services for less than a full month. These codes are reported per day and are appropriate for use in the following circumstances: home dialysis patients who receive less than a full month of services; patients who are transient; a partial month in which one or more face-to-face visits occurred without a complete assessment; hospitalization of the patient prior to a complete assessment being made; and discontinuance of dialysis due to patient's recovery, receipt of a kidney transplant, or death. For reporting purposes, a month is considered 30 days. Code assignment is based on age. Report 90967 for patients younger than 2 years of age, 90968 for patients 2 to 11 years of age, 90969 for patients 12 to 19 years of age, and 90970 for patients over the age of 20.

90989-90993
The physician or health care provider trains the patient and/or the patient's caregiving helper to perform the dialysis procedure, any mode. Report 90989 when the course is completed; 90993 is reported per training session of the course when it is not completed.

90997
Hemoperfusion is a technique to remove toxins from the blood and to maintain fluid and electrolyte balance when the kidneys no longer function. The physician draws the patient's blood, perfuses the blood through activated charcoal or resin, and transfuses the blood back into the patient using a needle and catheter.

91010-91013
Esophageal motility studies using a manometer are performed to measure the competency of the lower esophageal sphincter and the muscles of the esophagus. The physician inserts a thin tube with pressure sensors (also called a manometer) into the patient's nose or mouth and down into the stomach to perform an esophageal motility study. In 91010, the muscles of the esophagus and/or the gastroesophageal junction, which propel food and water into the stomach, are studied to measure the pressure of the contraction waves and diagnose abnormalities in the esophageal muscles that affect swallowing. The tube is slowly withdrawn and stopped at different points along the esophagus. The patient is directed to swallow a little amount of water at each stopping point and the contraction wave pressure and swallowing action are measured and graphed. Report 91013 in addition to the motility study code when the motility study is combined with stimulation and/or acid or alkali perfusion. This type of study may be administered to attempt to replicate the type of chest pain a patient has been experiencing by diagnosing the pain as noncardiac, due to esophageal reflux. Using a second catheter inserted through the nares, a probe is placed in the distal esophagus and the perfusion substances are introduced. Commonly, these

substances consist of hydrochloric acid and an alternate saline control solution infused one after the other, without the patient being aware of the identity of the solution. The symptoms of chest pain are recorded as the patient identifies them. The patient is again directed to swallow at given intervals in order to record additional pressure measurements. The catheter is removed and the information saved for interpretation.

91020

The physician inserts a tube with sensors into the patient's nose or mouth and down into the stomach to perform a gastric motility study. The muscles of the stomach and the gastroduodenal junction, which propel food and water into the first part of the small intestines, are studied to measure the pressure of the contraction waves and diagnose abnormalities in the muscle that affect digestion. Sensors on the tube measure the amount of pressure generated by the stomach muscles as food is moved into the small intestine. The tighter the muscles contract around the tube, the greater pressure that is sensed. The data is recorded for computer analysis.

91022

The physician inserts a tube with sensors into the patient's nose or mouth and down into the duodenum to perform a duodenal motility study. The muscles of the duodenum and the gastroduodenal junction, which propel food and water into the first part of the small intestines, are studied to measure the pressure of the contraction waves and diagnose abnormalities in the muscle that affect digestion. Sensors on the tube measure the amount of pressure generated by the duodenal muscles as food is moved into the small intestine. The tighter the muscles contract around the tube, the greater pressure that is sensed. The data is recorded for computer analysis.

91030

This code reports a provocative acid perfusion study, also called a Bernstein test, performed on the esophagus, not in conjunction with a motility test. The acid perfusion test is done to try and replicate atypical chest pain the patient has been experiencing and aid in diagnosing the pain as non-cardiac, or due to esophageal reflux/esophagitis. Both hydrochloric acid and an alternate saline control solution are infused one after the other via a nasogastric tube, without the patient being aware of the identity of the solution. The symptoms of chest pain are recorded as the patient identifies them.

91034

The physician performs a gastroesophageal reflux test using esophageal pH electrode placement and recording. This procedure evaluates the proper functioning of the lower esophageal sphincter, the strong muscular ring located at the entrance to the stomach. When this specialized muscle opens at the wrong time, stomach acid will flow back up into the esophagus, causing gastroesophageal reflux. A small, thin probe, or electrode, that measures the pH (acidity) level within the esophagus is affixed at the end of flexible nasal catheter tubing. The catheter is inserted through the nose down to the target area in the esophagus, usually determined by manometry, and connected to a data recorder. The probe records the pH level within the esophagus. Neutral pH is 7. The lower the number, the more acidic the environment. The stomach has a normal pH around 2. The pH recording may be done over the course of a day. The catheter/tubing is taped behind the ear and out of the way under clothing, and connected to a small data recorder that is worn around the waist. This code includes the analysis and interpretation of the recorded results.

91035

The physician performs a gastroesophageal reflux test using mucosal attached telemetry pH electrode placement and recording. A small capsule containing a radiotelemetry pH sensor is inserted endoscopically in the esophagus and temporarily attached to the esophageal wall. The capsule monitors esophageal pH levels over a 48-hour period. This information is transmitted to an external pager-sized receiver worn by the patient that records pH levels. After the 48-hour testing period, the data is downloaded from the receiver to a computer that contains software for analyzing pH levels. The physician provides a written interpretation of the computer analysis. The capsule does not need to be removed as it spontaneously detaches within seven to 10 days and passes through the digestive tract.

91037-91038

The physician performs an esophageal function test with gastroesophageal reflux testing using nasal catheter intraluminal impedance electrode placement and recording. The patient fasts for a minimum of six hours. An impedance probe affixed to flexible nasal catheter tubing is inserted through the nose down to the lower esophageal sphincter following location of the lower sphincter by manometry. The impedance probe contains several electrodes that make up multiple measuring segments each 2 cm in length. The measuring segments are located at intervals above the proximal border of the lower esophageal sphincter. The patient is given a liquid or solid bolus to swallow. As the bolus passes through the esophagus, the average electrical resistance between two adjacent electrodes (impedance) is measured. The electrodes detect esophageal contraction and expansion and movement of the bolus through the esophagus in real time, as well as any gastroesophageal reflux. Esophageal function is evaluated by calculating the bolus transport time (BTT), which is the time it takes the bolus to pass from the proximal measuring segment and exit through the distal measuring segment. Contraction wave velocity (CWV), which is the speed of the contraction wave from the proximal measuring segment to the distal measuring segment, is also evaluated. This test is also referred to as multichannel intraluminal impedance testing or MII. Report 91037 for a recording of one hour or less.

Report 91038 for prolonged recording of greater than one hour, up to 24 hours.

91040

The physician performs a diagnostic esophageal balloon distension study, including provocation, when performed, to evaluate chest pain of undetermined etiology that is suspected to be noncardiac in origin. The patient fasts for a minimum of six hours. A local anesthetic is sprayed into the patient's throat. With the patient in an upright position, a probe is passed through the mouth into the esophagus. The subject is placed supine with the head of the exam table elevated approximately 30 degrees. Manometric pressure recordings are obtained to identify the upper and lower esophageal sphincters. The probe is removed and the physician inserts a balloon into the esophagus. The balloon is moved along the esophagus and inflated multiple times to increasing diameters at selected sites in the esophagus in an attempt to provoke chest pain in the patient. Pain is measured by conscious perception or objective responses to the stimuli. Perception of moderate to severe chest pain with low levels of balloon distension is considered to be positive for noncardiac chest pain.

91065

The hydrogen or methane breath test uses a measurement of these gases in the breath to test for a number of conditions that cause gastrointestinal symptoms. It can be used to diagnose lactase deficiency, fructose intolerance, bacterial overgrowth, or orocecal gastrointestinal (rapid) transit. Bacteria produce gases when they are exposed to unabsorbed food. Regardless of the condition causing the excessive production of gas, some is absorbed into the blood flowing through the wall of the intestine and colon. The blood travels to the lungs where it is released and exhaled in the breath where it can be measured. Prior to hydrogen or methane breath testing, a special diet may be required and individuals must fast for at least 12 hours. At the start of the test, a sample breath is taken. The individual blows into and fills a balloon with a breath of air. The concentration of hydrogen or methane from the sample breath is removed from the balloon and measured. The individual ingests a small amount of the test sugar (lactose, fructose, lactulose). Samples of breath are collected and analyzed every 15 minutes for three to five hours.

91110-91111

Gastrointestinal (GI) tract imaging from inside the lumen of the intestinal tract is done in a noninvasive manner by capsule endoscopy. The patient is required to fast for 10 hours before the procedure. The patient swallows the endoscopic capsule with a glass of water. Color video images from inside the GI tract are recorded as the natural peristaltic movement passes the capsule smoothly and painlessly through the system. Sensors are secured to the patient's abdomen and worn like a belt around the waist, allowing data from the capsule to transmit to a data recorder while the patient goes about daily ambulatory activities. After eight hours, the patient returns the equipment for processing at the computer workstation. The images are reviewed, interpreted, and a report is prepared. Report 91110 when the imaging includes the esophagus through the ileum. Report 91111 when the imaging is of the esophagus only.

[91113]

Colon capsule endoscopy (CCE) is a noninvasive and painless ingestible capsule technique that allows exploration of the colon without the need for sedation and gas insufflation. Imaging of the colon is performed from inside via a very small camera. This camera is encased in a capsule that is swallowed by the patient. As this capsule/camera travels through the colon, many images are captured and delivered to a recorder worn outside the body by the patient. This form of endoscopy allows a visual of areas within the colon that may not otherwise be observed using standard endoscopy. This can aid in detection of cancer, polyps, and other GI tract disorders, as well as helping to evaluate GI bleeds and other obscure symptoms. The images are reviewed, interpreted, and a report is prepared.

91112

Gastrointestinal (GI) transit and pressure measurement are performed via wireless capsule. The patient swallows the capsule with a glass of water. Pressure, pH, and temperature are recorded as the natural peristaltic movement passes the capsule smoothly and painlessly through the system. This information is used to calculate regional transit times, including gastric emptying time, small bowel transit time, colonic transit time, combined small/large bowel transit time, whole gut transit time, pressure contraction patterns from the antrum and duodenum, and motility indices. The data is transmitted from the capsule to a data recorder, worn like a belt around the patient's waist or around the neck, while the patient goes about daily ambulatory activities. The equipment is brought to the provider for processing at the computer workstation. The images are reviewed, interpreted, and a report is prepared.

91117

Colonic motility is measured using various manometric techniques. In one method, a manometric catheter is positioned endoscopically and clipped to the colonic mucosa. A minimum of six hours of continuous recording ensues. Any provocation tests performed are included, as is the interpretation and report.

91120

The physician performs a rectal sensation tone and compliance test using graded balloon distention to evaluate anorectal pathology. Tone tests for relaxation or rigidity in the rectum. Compliance tests the distensibility of the rectum. Sensation tests for fullness and discomfort upon distention. The patient is asked to empty his or her bowels. The patient is placed in left lateral decubitus position with the head lowered 20 degrees. The physician inserts a two-lumen catheter containing a cylindrical bag into the rectum. One lumen is used to inflate the bag; the other is used to measure pressure within the bag. With the distal end of the bag 5 cm from the anal verge, the bag is inflated with air. Inflation is slowly increased and sensation, tone, and compliance monitored. The balloon is deflated when the patient experiences discomfort and urgency lasting more than 30 seconds.

91122
The physician performs anorectal manometry to help in diagnosing constipation and/or incontinence due to myotonic dysfunction or suspected cases of Hirschsprung's Disease. Hirschsprung's Disease is a congenital absence of ganglion nerve cells in the plexus that innervates the colon and/or rectum to relax the internal anorectal sphincter in response to rectal distension. A manometry probe is advanced into the rectum after a digital exam. The probe is slowly withdrawn, taking continuous pressure measurements until the high pressure area of the anal sphincters is located. With the patient relaxed, the "basal anal pressure" is recorded, and highest pressures are recorded as the patient performs a maximum squeeze. The manometry catheter is inserted again with a rectal balloon that is slowly inflated to the patient's first sensation of fullness and the volume is recorded. The anal sphincter response to the rectal distention is also recorded. Another manometry technique using a 3 balloon apparatus may also be employed in which pressure measurements are taken as the external, middle, and internal rectal balloons are inflated and deflated to note threshold levels and sphincter responses.

91132-91133
In electrogastrography (EGG), electrodes are placed on the skin over the stomach at a specific distance from each other and attached to a recording computer. The electrical activity initiated by the distal two-thirds of the stomach (gastric electrical activity or GEA) is recorded and analyzed by the computer. Report 91132 when diagnostic electrogastrography is performed alone. Report 91133 when diagnostic EGG is performed in conjunction with the administration of a drug in an attempt to manipulate conditions and provoke a measurable abnormality.

91200
Liver elastography is a noninvasive procedure for assessing liver stiffness beneficial in determining the amount of fibrosis and scarring of the liver due to damage and may also be used to survey any disorder advancement and help evaluate ongoing therapy. A probe is applied to the skin between the ribs focusing on the liver. The shear wave is mechanically generated causing the probe to discharge pulses that meet the shear wave and bounce back to the probe. This process allows the shear wave to be measured, which leads to values for liver stiffness. This code indicates no imaging; however, interpretation and report is required.

92002
The physician sees a new patient, one who has not been seen within that group practice for at least three years, for intermediate ophthalmological services. The patient's medical history is reviewed, or interval history if more than three years have passed since the patient was seen within that group practice. General medical observations, an external ocular and adnexal examination, and other diagnostic procedures like ophthalmoscopy, biomicroscopy, or tonometry are done. The visit may include mydriasis (the dilation of the patient's pupils). Generally, the patient has an acute condition that does not require a comprehensive service or the patient is being examined for a chronic, but stable, condition (i.e., known cataract).

92004
The physician sees a new patient, one who has not been seen within that group practice for at least three years, for comprehensive ophthalmological services. The physician performs a complete visual system examination, reviews the patient's medical history, or interval history if more than three years have passed since the patient was seen, and performs a general medical observation in addition to external and ophthalmoscopic examinations. Gross visual fields and basic sensorimotor examinations are also done, including biomicroscopy, examination with cycloplegia (temporary immobilization of the ciliary body) or mydriasis (the dilation of pupils), and tonometry. Other examination techniques such as retinoscopy, keratometry, slit lamp viewing, tear testing, corneal staining, corneal sensitivity, fundus examination, and exophthalmometry may also be employed and are included in the comprehensive exam when initiation of diagnostic or treatment programs is dependent upon the examining techniques. It may take more than one patient encounter to complete this service.

92012
The physician sees an established patient for intermediate ophthalmological services. The patient's medical history is reviewed. General medical observations, an external ocular and adnexal examination, and other diagnostic procedures like ophthalmoscopy, biomicroscopy, or tonometry are done when required to continue the diagnostic and treatment regimen. The visit may include mydriasis (the dilation of the patient's pupils). Generally, the patient has an acute condition that does not require a comprehensive service or the patient is being examined for a chronic, but stable, condition (i.e., known cataract).

92014
The physician sees an established patient, one who has been seen by a doctor in that group practice within the last three years, for comprehensive ophthalmological services. The physician performs a complete visual system examination, reviews the patient's medical history, and performs a general medical observation in addition to external and ophthalmoscopic examinations. Gross visual fields and basic sensorimotor examinations are also done, including biomicroscopy, examination with cycloplegia (temporary immobilization of the ciliary body) or

mydriasis (the dilation of pupils), and tonometry. Other examination techniques such as retinoscopy, keratometry, slit lamp viewing, tear testing, corneal staining, corneal sensitivity, fundus examination, and exophthalmometry may also be employed and are included in the comprehensive exam when initiation or continuation of diagnostic or treatment programs is dependent upon the examining techniques. It may take more than one patient encounter to complete the service.

92015

The examiner determines the prescription required for the patient's eyeglasses or contact lenses by evaluating the effectiveness of a series of lenses through which the patient is asked to view an eye chart. This is usually accomplished with a refractor, a device that contains a range of lens powers that can be quickly changed, allowing the patient to compare various combinations when viewing the eye chart. A prescription is issued; no fitting for eyeglasses or contact lenses occurs at this time.

92018-92019

The physician performs an eye exam and evaluation under general anesthesia. The patient may have significant injury or cannot otherwise tolerate the examination while conscious. This exam may include manipulation of the globe to establishing the passive range of motion or another manipulation to help in diagnosing the condition. Report 92018 for a complete examination, such as when gonioscopy (see 92020) is done under anesthesia; and 92019 for a limited examination.

92020

The angle of the anterior chamber of the eye is examined in a gonioscopy to assess for angle closure glaucoma, iris neovascularization, or other injury or disease process in the anterior chamber. Since the cornea's curvature creates internal reflection when the anterior angle structures are viewed directly, a gonioscopic lens is used to observe the angle. Corneal integrity is first determined using fluorescein. The patient is given anesthesia, the goniolens is prepared, and the physician places it on the patient's cornea. The lens puts a concave surface against the cornea, eliminating its refracting surface and allowing the angle to be observed with oblique mirrors. With the illumination lamp and microscope set and the beam oriented parallel to the axis of the mirror, the gonioscopy is accomplished and the angle of the anterior chamber of the eye is examined. The lens is removed, the eye is irrigated, and the cornea is checked again.

92025

This procedure is also known as computer-assisted keratography or videokeratography. A computer images and analyzes the shape of the patient's cornea. The patient is placed facing a light-filled bowl shape. A digital camera resides at the base of the bowl, and the light pattern reflected from the bowl to the cornea is recorded by the camera. The topology of the cornea is then analyzed by the computer software, and reports are produced for physician evaluation.

92060

The examiner utilizes a series of vertical and horizontal prism bars or individual handheld prisms to measure ocular deviation in a sensorimotor examination. Ocular deviations, such as strabismus, are seen when the eyes position themselves to each other on axes different from what is needed. Ocular deviations can occur in the horizontal or vertical plane. The eyes may move in toward each other (convergent) or away from each other (divergent). One eye (monocular) or both eyes (binocular) may be affected. The deviation may be observed to be the same no matter what direction the eyes are looking (concomitant) or to vary depending on where the eyes are looking (nonconcomitant). These deviations can be caused by ocular muscle anomalies, trauma or disease, or neuromuscular damage. The patient is asked to focus on a distant or near object in varying locations. An occluder may be alternately used to cover one eye while testing the other. Multiple measurements are taken and interpreted and a report is prepared.

92065-92066

The physician prescribes exercises to correct ocular problems, most frequently caused by ocular muscle imbalances. The patient is trained to perform these therapeutic exercises to improve vision by gaining the proper binocular cooperation of the eyes one with the other, such as when one eye's vision and movement is neglected to avoid seeing double. These exercises, which are designed to improve the function of the eye muscles, frequently include repetitive tasks with prisms, color cards, or rods, and moving objects progressively closer or further away in different planes. Report 92065 if training is performed by the physician or other qualified health care professional and 92066 if performed under their supervision.

92071-92072

The physician measures the patient's cornea for the fitting of a soft contact lens (also called a collagen shield). During a contact lens fitting, the physician assesses the health of the eyelids, lashes, and cornea. The corneal curvature is determined using an instrument called a keratometer and slit lamp evaluations are used to determine the depth and quality of the tear film. In 92071, the contact lens is for treatment of an ocular surface disorder, such as Stevens-Johnson syndrome. In 92072, the soft contact lens is placed over the cornea to reshape the cornea for management of keratoconus.

92081

A visual field test measures the extent of the field of vision as an eye fixates straight ahead, with standard illumination. Any peripheral vision loss or blind spots are documented. The blind spots are plotted on visual field charts. This code reports a limited examination, such as a tangent screen, Autoplot, arc perimeter, or a single stimulus level automated test, such as Octopus 3 or 7. A tangent screen, for example, is a black screen made of felt mounted on the wall that has meridians, blind spot, and degrees from fixation stitched into it. Fixation is the direction of gaze that allows the object's visual image to fall on the central fovea of the retina, which is the area of most acute vision. With one eye occluded and full distance correction worn, white spots are introduced and the patient is tested at one and/or two meters. The points are transferred from screen to a chart.

92082

A visual field test measures the extent of the field of vision as an eye fixates straight ahead, with standard illumination. Any peripheral vision loss or blind spots are documented. This code describes an intermediate procedure and may involve the use of specialized methods. For example, the Goldmann perimeter may be used with at least two isopters plotted. An isopter is the outer margins of a visual field within which any particular object or stimulus should be seen. A hollow white spherical bowl device is positioned a set distance from the patient and luminous targets that differ in size and intensity are projected onto standardized background illumination, statically or kinetically. The stimulus check is usually static, not moving, when testing inside 30 degrees. This method can test the full limit of peripheral vision and uses internationally standardized testing conditions with fixation always monitored. Fixation is the direction of gaze that allows the object's visual image to fall on the central fovea of the retina, or the area of most acute vision.

92083

A visual field test measures the extent of the field of vision as an eye fixates straight ahead, with standard illumination. Any peripheral vision loss or blind spots are documented. This code describes an extended procedure and may involve the use of specialized methods. The Goldmann perimeter may be used with at least three isopters plotted, plus a static check done within the central 30 degrees. An isopter is the outer margins of a visual field within which any particular object or stimulus should be seen. A hollow white spherical bowl device is positioned a set distance from the patient and luminous targets that differ in size and intensity are projected onto standardized background illumination, statically or kinetically. This method can test the full limit of peripheral vision and uses internationally standardized testing conditions with fixation always monitored. Fixation is the direction of gaze that allows the object's visual image to fall on the central fovea of the retina, or the area of most acute vision.

92100

In a healthy eye's anterior chamber, aqueous humor is continually drained and renewed to maintain a constant overall pressure. Increased pressure from this fluid causes glaucoma and can lead to blindness. Serial tonometry involves multiple pressure checks over the course of a day to monitor significant peaks and acute elevations in intraocular pressure within a 24-hour period (diurnal curve). Different tonography testing equipment and techniques may be used. In Goldmann's applanation tonometry, or the blue-light glaucoma-screening test, the patient is given a drop of fluorescein staining dye and anesthetic. The forehead and chin are supported on a headrest. A slit lamp is positioned until the tonometer probe just touches the cornea and the physician can view a limbal glow, or blue light circle. This applanation method measures the force required to flatten a certain area of the cornea, which is dependent upon the pressure in the eye. The force per area is converted to the intraocular pressure measurement. A portable TonoPen is a device that gives an instant digital measurement when touched to the eye.

92132

Computerized ophthalmic diagnostic imaging of the anterior segment is performed. In one method, optical coherence tomography (OCT) is performed. The patient sits in front of a machine while the eye is scanned. Cross-sectional images of the anterior segment of the eye are produced, including images of the cornea, iris, ciliary body, and lens. Quantitative and qualitative data capture measurements such as the depth and angle of the anterior chamber and thickness of the cornea. Changes of the iris and lens are recorded in response to light and focus changes. This procedure may be performed on one or both eyes; interpretation and report are included.

92133-92134 [92137]

Computerized ophthalmic diagnostic imaging of the posterior segment is performed using various techniques, often as diagnostic measures for glaucoma. One method, the scanning laser glaucoma test (SLGT), analyzes the nerve fiber layer in the posterior portion of the eye using a confocal scanning laser ophthalmoscope and/or polarimetry. During the examination, the patient fixates on a light. A technician aligns and focuses the scanning instrument. The retinal nerve fiber layer (RNFL), which is the only part of the retina that can alter the state of polarized light, is scanned with a low power laser beam that double-passes the RNFL. The instrument measures the change in polarization (retardation) that is directly related to the thickness of the tissue. A computer analyzes the measurements compared to standardized norms. Results are displayed and the data is stored in the computer for use as a comparison for future testing. Optical coherence tomography angiography (OCT-A) may be performed in addition to standard imaging of the retina. OCT-A provides detailed images of the choroidal vasculature and blood flow within the retina. Report 92133 if imaging is performed on the optic nerve; 92134 if performed on the retina; and 92137 when OCT-A is performed in addition to standard imaging of the retina. These codes report unilateral or bilateral procedures and include interpretation and report.

92136

Optical Coherence Biometry (OCB) is an ophthalmic diagnostic test that measures the curvature of the cornea and the depth of the anterior chamber in addition to the axial length of the eye, without ultrasound. This is done to calculate the correct intraocular lens (IOL) power for implantation in order to come as close as possible to the target refraction after surgery. The procedure is non-invasive and uses partial coherence interferometry or birefringent light, as opposed to sound, to perform the imaging. The patient focuses on a small fixation point and the imaging of the eye is achieved with an instrument using light sources at certain wavelengths. When the highest quality axial length display has been found, subsequent measurements are taken and stored in a computer, as well as automatically transferred to an IOL calculator program. This allows immediate and individualized computation of IOL implant options for the patient.

92145

The physician determines corneal hysteresis (CH) by air impulse stimulation. The physician applies force to the cornea by rapid air pulse. The cornea moves inward, reaches the point of being flat (applanation), and then continues in to form a slight concavity. Milliseconds after applanation, the air pump is turned off and the pressure to the eye decreases. As this pressure decreases, the cornea returns to its natural shape while passing through the applanated state. Utilizing an advanced electro-optical system, two intraocular pressure (IOP) measurements are obtained during this process, the first as the cornea moves inward and the second as it returns to its baseline. The difference between these two values is corneal hysteresis. This code reports unilateral or bilateral procedures, including interpretation and report.

92201-92202

The physician performs an extended ophthalmoscopy for evaluation of peripheral retinal disease such as retinal detachment, tear, or tumor in 92201 or for evaluation of glaucoma, macular pathology, or tumor of the optic nerve or macula in 92202. Ophthalmoscopy allows a complete view of the back of the eye. After the pupils have been dilated, views of the retina are seen with the indirect ophthalmoscope. In addition to viewing the vitreous humor, retina, optic nerve, and retinal veins and arteries as in a routine ophthalmoscopy, an extended ophthalmoscopy allows viewing of the optic disk, arteries, veins, retina, choroid, and media. The direct ophthalmoscope allows the highly magnified view of the posterior portion of the retina; an indirect ophthalmoscope gives a broader view that includes the posterior and anterior retina and vitreous. In order to detect lesions that might otherwise go unnoticed, a scleral depression is performed by inserting the tip of a scleral depressor between the globe and the orbit in 92201. This displaces the retina inward, creating an elevation and increasing the contrast between a retinal lesion and the surrounding retinal tissue. An extended ophthalmoscopy can also be performed with a contact lens biomicroscopy, three-mirror lens, or 90-diopter lens. One or both eyes are viewed and the physician provides a detailed drawing of the patient's retinas and their defects in 92201 and of the optic nerve or macula in 92202. These codes include interpretation and report.

92227-92229

Remote imaging procedures are performed for the detection or monitoring of retinal diseases, such as diabetic retinopathy. Since the retina starts to deteriorate very early in diabetic patients who often do not receive eye exams due to such factors as economic status, geography, or distance, early detection and treatment is particularly important. An alternative to the conventional dilated fundus examination, this noninvasive technology uses a digital fundus camera to obtain standard field color and/or monochromatic retinal images, unilaterally or bilaterally. This digital data can be transferred over the internet, where a retinal specialist can diagnose disease or monitor existing disease. Code 92227 includes remote review and report by clinical staff, while 92228 includes remote interpretation and report by a physician or other qualified health care professional. Report 92229 if an autonomous analysis and report is performed at the point-of-care rather than remotely. In this diagnostic procedure, a proprietary camera captures color retinal fundus images of the patient's eyes. The images are then submitted to the cloud for analysis, and screening results are downloaded and a report exported.

92230

Ophthalmoscopy allows a complete view of the back of the eye. This procedure is for detection of abnormalities of retinal blood vessels. The patient's eyes are dilated. The angioscopy begins when a small amount of fluorescein dye is injected into the arm. The dye is transported to the eye through the blood vessels. As the dye traverses the retinal vessels, the retina is viewed through the ophthalmoscope using filters that enhance the fluorescence of the eye.

92235

Ophthalmoscopy allows a complete view of the back of the eye. This procedure is for detection of abnormalities of retinal blood vessels. The patient's eyes are dilated. The angiography begins when a small amount of fluorescein dye is injected into the arm. The dye is transported to the eye through the blood vessels. As the dye traverses the retinal vessels, a motorized camera attached to an ophthalmoscope photographs a sequence, documenting the dye's progress through the vessels of the retina. Both eyes are photographed. The photographs are black and white. The circulation takes seconds, but photography continues in 10- to 30-minute intervals to check for late leakage of recirculating dye. The physician reviews the film and makes a diagnostic evaluation of the patient's retina. Report this service when performed on one or both eyes.

92240

Ophthalmoscopy allows viewing of the eyeball's interior through the pupil. Indocyanine-green (ICG) dye fluoresces through blood and pigment and is used for detecting abnormalities in the vascular choroid, which lies between the retina and sclera. The patient's eyes are dilated. The angioscopy begins when a small amount of ICG is injected into the arm and transported to the eye through the blood vessels. Rapid injection is essential. As the dye transverses the choroid, a motorized camera attached to an ophthalmoscope photographs a sequence, documenting the dye's progress through the choroidal vessels. The photography is generally performed bilaterally, but may be performed unilaterally. Photographs are in black and white. Timing for photography is determined by arm to retinal time. This is estimated at about 10 seconds in young patients and 12 to 18 seconds in older patients. Report this service when performed on one or both eyes.

92242

Ophthalmoscopy allows a complete view of the back of the eye or the eyeball's interior through the pupil. Fluorescein and indocyanine-green (ICG) angiography is performed simultaneously to detect abnormalities of retinal blood vessels or in the vascular choroid, which lies between the retina and sclera. The patient's eyes are dilated. The angiography begins when a small amount of fluorescein and ICG dye are injected into the arm. The dye is transported to the eye through the blood vessels. As the dye traverses the retinal vessels and the choroid, a motorized camera attached to an ophthalmoscope photographs a sequence, documenting the dye's progress through the vessels of the retina and the choroid. The photographs are black and white. Circulation takes seconds but the photography continues in 10- to 30-minute intervals to check for late leakage of recirculating dye. The physician concurrently reviews the film and makes a diagnostic evaluation of the patient's retina and choroid. Report this service when performed on one or both eyes.

92250

Ophthalmoscopy allows a complete view of the back of the eye. The physician or technician aligns the fundus camera, which is attached to an ophthalmoscope, along the patient's optical axis after the patient's pupil has been dilated. The 35 mm camera is, in effect, a large ophthalmoscope that allows viewing of the retina and a light flash system for producing color photographs of the retina. The eyes are dilated to enhance the photographic quality unless unnecessary for image acquisition or clinically contraindicated. Both eyes are photographed. The results are interpreted by the physician.

92260

The physician exerts pressure on the sclera with a spring plunger while observing with an ophthalmoscope the vessels of the optic disc. Ophthalmodynamometry gives a measurement of the relative pressures in the central retinal arteries. It is also an indirect means of assessing carotid artery flow on either side.

92265

The physician or technician applies concentric needle electrodes to the patient's extraocular muscles to record muscle actions. This procedure is mostly applied for research into eye movement.

92270

A normal retina has a predictable electrical response to light. The EOG records metabolic changes in the retinal pigment epithelium by evaluating the retina's response to light. The physician or technician places electrodes on the skin around the eye so that eye movements of both eyes can be recorded separately or together. The EOG is often used in cases where the electroretinography isn't sensitive enough to pick up macular degeneration. The physician interprets the results of the test.

92273-92274

A normal retina has a predictable electrical response to light. To determine if the retina is damaged, the physician places an ocular fitted contact lens electrode on the patient's eye and another electrode on the forehead so that the retina's electrical responses to external stimuli can be recorded under light-adapted conditions. Electroretinography, often abbreviated ERG, is repeated in dark-adapted conditions. The ERG waves are analyzed by the physician. Various techniques may be used based on which area is being targeted. Report 92273 for a full field ERG (flash and flicker). A multifocal ERG targets photoreceptors in a number of separate locations, including the macular, looking for concentrated areas of abnormality and may take more time to complete than a routine ERG. Report 92274 for a multifocal ERG.

92283

This test describes an extended color vision examination involving an anomaloscope or equivalent, which is an instrument used to diagnose abnormalities of color perception in which one-half of a field of color is matched by mixing two other colors.

92284

This diagnostic exam tests the function of the two photoreceptors: the rods and the cones. Rods are most sensitive in dim illumination and are responsible for night vision. The cones are more sensitive in bright illuminations and are responsible for day vision. The eye to be tested is exposed to a bright light and the room is darkened. At 30-second intervals, the light is increased and the effect of the stimulus on the retina is measured by an adaptometer machine. This code includes interpretation and report.

92285

These photos are often referred to as anterior segment photography and are used to document abnormalities of the anterior segment that do not require magnification to be seen in the lids, cornea, anterior chamber, lens, and iris. The physician photographs the eye using a freestanding camera, a camera affixed to a slit lamp, goniophotography, or stereo-photography.

92286
The provider performs microscopy, often called endothelial cell analysis or specular microscopy, to check the integrity and density of the endothelial cells that comprise the innermost layer of the cornea.

92287
The physician performs microscopy to examine the iris. This procedure includes fluorescein angiography, which is for the detection of abnormalities of retinal blood vessels. The angioscopy begins when a small amount of fluorescein dye is injected into the arm. The dye is transported to the eye through the blood vessels. As the dye traverses the vessels in the iris, the iris is viewed through the scope using filters that enhance the fluorescence of the eye. This test is most often used to delineate fine neovascularization of tumors in the anterior segment.

92310
Using a keratometer, the technician determines the patient's corneal curvatures. The lenses are fitted for power, size, curvature, flexibility, and lens type. The fitting includes instruction and training of the wearer and incidental revision of the lens during the training period. This code is to be used for both eyes and for non-aphakic patients.

92311-92312
Using a keratometer, the technician determines the patient's corneal curvature. The lens is fitted for power, size, curvature, flexibility, and lens type. The fitting includes instruction and training of the wearer and incidental revision of the lens during the training period. These codes are to be used for aphakic patients. Report 92311 if one eye is fitted or 92312 for both eyes.

92313
Using a keratometer, the technician determines the patient's corneal curvature. The corneoscleral lens is fitted for power, size, curvature, flexibility, and lens type. The fitting includes instruction and training of the wearer and incidental revision of the lens during the training period.

92314
Using a keratometer, the independent technician determines the patient's corneal curvature. The lens is fitted for power, size, curvature, flexibility, and lens type. The fitting includes instruction and training of the wearer and incidental revision of the lens during the training period. This code is to be used for both eyes and for non-aphakic patients.

92315-92316
Using a keratometer, the independent technician determines the patient's corneal curvature. The lens is fitted for power, size, curvature, flexibility, and lens type. The fitting includes instruction and training of the wearer and incidental revision of the lens during the training period. These codes are to be used for aphakic patients. Report 92315 if one eye is fitted or 92316 for both eyes.

92317
Using a keratometer, the independent technician determines the patient's corneal curvature. The corneoscleral lens is fitted for power, size, curvature, flexibility, and lens type. The fitting includes instruction and training of the wearer and incidental revision of the lens during the training period.

92325
The physician or technician uses a grinder to flatten or polish the contact lens or lens edge to provide a more comfortable fit.

92326
The ophthalmologist meets with the patient to discuss replacement of contact lenses, which may be due to wear and tear of the existing pair, loss, or discomfort. A new prescription is a separately reported service.

92340-92342
The physician or technician measures the patient's anatomical facial characteristics, records the laboratory specifications, and performs the final adjustment of the monofocal (92340), bifocal (92341), or multifocal (92342) spectacles to the visual axes and anatomical topography.

92352-92353
The physician or technician measures the aphakic patient's anatomical facial characteristics, records the laboratory specifications, and performs the final adjustment of the monofocal (92352) or multifocal (92353) spectacles to the visual axes and anatomical topography.

92354
Some low vision aids are simply a convex lens mounted to spectacles. The physician or technician measures the patient's anatomical facial characteristics, records the laboratory specifications, and performs the final adjustment of the monofocal spectacles to the visual axes and anatomical topography.

92355
A focusable Galilean or Keplarian (internal prism) system in a spectacle frame is a popular choice. The fitting of the spectacles is separate from the prescription of the spectacles, which is considered part of the eye exam. The physician measures the anatomical facial characteristics, writes laboratory specifications, and makes the final adjustment of the spectacles to the visual axes and anatomical topography. The supply of materials is a separate component, as is the prescription.

92358
The physician or technician procures or provides a temporary, ready-made contact lens to a patient, whose natural intraocular lens had been previously removed surgically.

92370-92371
The physician or technician repairs or refits a pair of spectacles. Adjustments may be made to the ear or

nosepieces or plastic frames may be heated and bent to better fit the patient, who has natural or artificial intraocular lenses. Report 92370 if the patient is not aphakic and 92371 if the patient is aphakic.

92502
Occasionally, a child or an adult is uncooperative and an otolaryngologic examination cannot be performed until the patient is placed under general anesthesia. At other times, as in the case of a trauma victim, the patient is already anesthetized. At this time a thorough examination of the ear, including otoscopy, nose, and larynx, is completed.

92504
The physician uses an operating binocular microscope to examine the ear and occasionally the nose for direct, detailed visualization.

92507-92508
Under direction of a physician, the patient undergoes developmental programs such as speech therapy, sign language, or lip reading instruction or hearing rehabilitation. In auditory processing disorders, the patient (usually a child) cannot process the information heard due to lack of integration between the ears and the brain, even though hearing may be normal. Central auditory processing disorder (CAPD) is often confused with or functions as an underlying factor to a number of learning disabilities. The treatment program is for the individual in 92507 or in a group setting in 92508.

92511
The examination is performed with the patient lying on his back and under a local anesthetic with topical Lidocaine that is sprayed onto the back of the throat and into the nasal passages. The physician introduces the flexible fiberoptic endoscope through the nose and advances it into the pharynx to determine whether there are any fixed blockages such as a deviated septum, nasal polyps, or enlarged adenoids and tonsils. The physician may position the tip of the endoscope at the level of the hard palate and instruct the patient to perform simple maneuvers that demonstrate airway activity under conditions that promote or prevent collapse. The test may be performed to identify anatomic factors contributing to sleep disorder, stability of the upper airway, and determining treatments.

92512
Nasal function studies are performed for analyzing nasal resistance during breathing. In rhinomanometry, the physician uses a tubular probe to generate and transmit an audible sound signal into the patient's nasal cavity through an anatomically fitted nosepiece. A microphone picks up the sound from the nasal cavity and the data is analyzed by computer to determine area distance in the nasal cavity.

92516
Facial nerve functions studies, such as electroneuronography (ENoG), are used to diagnose facial paralysis disorders, such as Bell's palsy (a unilateral or bilateral facial paralysis due to a viral attack on the facial nerve). These tests include an ENoG or an electromyogram that measure nerve conduction to diagnose degenerative disorders. In an electromyogram, the physician attaches small disc electrodes to the skin surface over the muscle or nerve by inserting small metal needles into the areas. The needle or electrode may be changed as needed for a complete study. An oscilloscope displays and records the data.

92520
Laryngeal studies are performed to evaluate aerodynamic and acoustic testing, including pitch match, phonation, and breath support with phonation. Audio recordings are made and evaluated for pitch, loudness, jitter, and shimmer of speech. Computerized analysis also includes evaluation for extraneous vocal noise and harmonic frequency in addition to airflow (average and peak), vocal efficiency, and subglottal pressure. A report of the findings is provided to the requesting provider.

92521-92524
The physician takes a patient history, including speech and language development, hearing loss, and physical and mental development, and a physical examination is performed. Speech and language evaluations are conducted. Assessment of any deficits is noted and a treatment plan for the patient is made that could involve speech therapy, hearing aids, etc. In auditory processing disorders, the patient (usually children) cannot process the information heard due to a lack of integration between the ears and the brain, even though hearing may be normal. Central auditory processing disorder (CAPD) is often confused with, or functions as, an underlying factor to a number of learning disabilities. In 92521, speech fluency, including stuttering and cluttering, is evaluated. Report 92522 when evaluation of phonics and speech/sound production is performed. Report 92523 when language comprehension is addressed in addition to the evaluation in 92522. Report 92524 for evaluation of voice and resonance.

92526
The treatment of swallowing disorders is aimed at finding the specific cause of the dysfunction to treat the problem, such as anti-reflux medications to decrease stomach acidity or improve esophageal motility. Patients who have had strokes and cannot be treated surgically or by drugs for swallowing dysfunctions may require assistance from a rehabilitation specialist. In severe cases, the physician may elect to insert a feeding tube through the nose or in the stomach through the abdomen.

92531
Nystagmus is uncontrolled rapid movement of the eyeball in a horizontal, vertical, or rotary motion. It can be a symptom of a disturbance in the patient's vestibular system and can be induced to measure the difference between the patient's right and left vestibular functions. The patient's eyes are observed

for spontaneous nystagmus as the patient is asked to look straight ahead, 30 degrees to 45 degrees to the right, and 30 degrees to 45 degrees to the left. No electrodes are used and no recording made.

92532

A positional nystagmus test measures whether the eyes can maintain a static position when the head is in different position, which helps in documenting and quantifying patient complaints of dizziness in certain positions. The test also may be performed as a diagnostic tool to determine if an abnormality is associated with the central nervous system or the peripheral nervous system. The patient is placed in a variety of positions including supine with head extended dorsally, left and right, and sitting in an attempt to induce nystagmus. This is done with the patient's eye open so that eye movements can be observed directly. No recording electrodes are used to record the nystagmus.

92533

Nystagmus is uncontrolled rapid movement of the eyeball in a horizontal, vertical, or rotary motion. It can be a symptom of a disturbance in the patient's vestibular system and can be induced to measure the difference between the patient's right and left vestibular functions. In this test, each ear is separately irrigated with cold water and warm water to create nystagmus in the patient. The physician or audiologist observes the patient to detect any difference between the reaction of the right side and the left side. Four irrigations occur: a warm and cold irrigation for both the right and the left ear.

92534

A rotating drum made of alternating light and dark vertical stripes is placed in front of the patient and the patient is instructed to stare at the drum without focusing on any one stripe. The eyes are observed for nystagmus while the drum is rotated in one direction. The direction of the drum is reversed. No electrodes are used.

92537-92538

Nystagmus is uncontrolled rapid movement of the eyeball in a horizontal, vertical, or rotary motion. It can be a symptom of a disturbance in the patient's vestibular system and can be induced to measure the difference between the patient's right and left vestibular functions. In 92537, each ear is separately irrigated once with cold water and once with warm water to create nystagmus in the patient. Four irrigations occur: a warm and cold irrigation for both the right and the left ear. In 92538, monothermal irrigation is performed, which is one irrigation in each ear for a total of two irrigations. In both cases, ENG recordings are evaluated to detect any difference between the nystagmus of the right side and the left side.

92540

The physician performs a basic vestibular evaluation with recordings, often to evaluate a patient complaint of dizziness. Nystagmus is uncontrolled rapid movement of the eyeball in a horizontal, vertical, or rotary motion. It can be a symptom of a disturbance in the patient's vestibular system and can be induced to measure the difference between the patient's right and left vestibular functions. ENG (electronystagmography) electrodes are placed and the patient is asked to look straight ahead, 30 degrees to 45 degrees to the right, and 30 degrees to 45 degrees to the left. Recordings are made to detect spontaneous nystagmus. In the positional nystagmus test, an ENG recording is made of the rapid eye movements occurring with the patient's head placed in a minimum of four positions (e.g., supine with head extended dorsally, left, right, and sitting). This is often done using infrared video recording systems. An optokinetic nystagmus test is usually done with a rotating drum of alternating light and dark vertical stripes. The drum is placed in front of the patient and the patient is instructed to stare at the drum without focusing on any one stripe. The drum is rotated in one direction and reversed and rotated in the opposite direction. ENG electrodes are used to record nystagmus. In an oscillating tracking test, the patient is asked to follow a swinging object such as a ball on a string. ENG electrodes are in place and a recording is made of the eye tracking the motion. The recording is analyzed for smoothness.

92541

Nystagmus is uncontrolled rapid movement of the eyeball in a horizontal, vertical, or rotary motion. It can be a symptom of a disturbance in the patient's vestibular system and can be induced to measure the difference between the patient's right and left vestibular functions. ENG (electronystagmography) electrodes are placed and the patient is asked to look straight ahead, 30 degrees to 45 degrees to the right, and 30 degrees to 45 degrees to the left. Recordings are made to detect spontaneous nystagmus.

92542

Nystagmus is uncontrolled rapid movement of the eyeball in a horizontal, vertical, or rotary motion and can appear as a symptom of a disturbance in the patient's vestibular system. Nystagmus is measured to determine whether dizziness is due to a disease of the inner ear and whether it affects one or both sides. In the positional nystagmus test, an electronystagmography (ENG) recording is made of the rapid eye movements occurring with the patient's head placed in a variety of positions, e.g., supine with head extended dorsally, left, right, and sitting. This is often done using infrared video recording systems.

92544

Nystagmus is uncontrolled rapid movement of the eyeball in a horizontal, vertical, or rotary motion. It can be a symptom of a disturbance in the patient's vestibular system and can be induced to measure the difference between the patient's right and left vestibular functions. This test is usually done with a rotating drum of alternating light and dark vertical stripes. The drum is placed in front of the patient and the patient is instructed to stare at the drum without focusing on any one stripe. The drum is rotated in one direction and reversed and rotated in the opposite direction. ENG electrodes are used to record nystagmus.

92545
Nystagmus is uncontrolled rapid movement of the eyeball in a horizontal, vertical, or rotary motion. It can be a symptom of a disturbance in the patient's vestibular system and can be induced to measure the difference between the patient's right and left vestibular functions. With ENG electrodes in place, the patient is asked to follow a swinging object such as a ball on a string. A recording is made of the eye tracking the motion. The recording is analyzed for smoothness.

92546
Nystagmus is uncontrolled rapid movement of the eyeball in a horizontal, vertical, or rotary motion. It can be a symptom of a disturbance in the patient's vestibular system and can be induced to measure the difference between the patient's right and left vestibular functions. The patient is placed in a rotary chair with the head positioned at a 30-degree angle and the eyes closed. Electronystagmography (ENG) electrodes are placed on the face near the eyes and the chair is rotated via computer control for 30 to 40 minutes while normal eye movement and involuntary rapid eye movements are recorded. The recording is evaluated to determine whether there is an abnormal labyrinthine response on either side.

92547
ENG electrodes are placed in the periocular area to measure vertical and rotary nystagmus in addition to the primary vestibular evaluation.

92548-92549
A computerized dynamic posturography sensory organization test (CDP-SOT) evaluates a patient's ability to utilize information from the sensory systems (vestibular, visual, and proprioceptive) to achieve and maintain balance and postural control. The patient is placed in the posturography system. The system is made up of a force plate that controls foot support and a visual surround reference that can be controlled. Force transducers measure the vertical and horizontal force output of the patient's feet. The patient's center-of-force is used as an estimate of body sway during testing. The patient is placed in a harness during the test for support and to prevent falls while standing on the plate within the system. Tests performed within the system assess the patient's ability to remain balanced during varying conditions that represent situations similar to those encountered in daily living. The walls of the system as well as the force plate move and testing occurs with eyes open and/or closed. The testing typically takes about 20 minutes and is provided by a qualified technician with results interpreted by a physical therapist to determine a therapy program specific to the patient's needs. Report 92548 for evaluation of six components, including eyes open, eyes closed, visual sway, platform sway, eyes closed platform sway, and platform and visual sway. Report 92549 if the above testing includes a motor control test (MCT) and adaptation test (ADT). The MCT assesses the patient's automatic motor reflex responses and their effectiveness in balance restoration following sudden forward and backward movements of the support surface. The test is useful in identifying impaired motor function and evaluating performance changes following treatment. In one version of an upright motor control test evaluating knee extension and flexion, the patient stands with knees flexed, then lifts the foot of the extremity that is least affected, transferring full weight onto the extremity that is more affected. The patient then attempts to extend the more affected knee. To test extension, the patient stands with knees straight and then lifts the knee of the lower extremity that is more affected toward the chest as rapidly and as high as possible; this is performed three times. These tests are useful in measuring voluntary movement and muscle control in chronic stroke victims. Motor ADT evaluates the performance in repeated movements to determine changes in neuromuscular responses and motor function.

[92517, 92518, 92519]
Vestibular evoked myogenic potential testing (VEMP) is useful in diagnosing superior canal dehiscence syndrome (SCDS), a little-known cause of vertigo and auditory symptoms. Caused by an abnormal opening or dehiscence in the bony roof of the superior semicircular canal in the temporal bone, SCDS may present with excessive sound sensitivity, tinnitus, or dizziness brought on by changes in pressure or sound. This vestibular function test is performed by stimulating one ear repeatedly with pulse or click sounds. Surface EMG responses are then measured over selected muscles, averaging the reaction of the muscle's electrical activity related to each pulse or sound click. In cervical VEMP (cVEMP) (92517), the sound stimulus that is applied to one ear elicits a response within the sternocleidomastoid muscles on the same side (ipsilateral) that can be recorded with surface electrodes and then averaged. In ocular VEMP (oVEMP) (92518), this sound stimulus elicits a response that is greatest when recorded from the opposite (contralateral) inferior oblique muscle by a surface electrode and averaged. Report 92519 if both cVEMP and oVEMP are performed. These codes include interpretation and report.

92550
The audiologist performs tympanometry and reflex threshold measurements. Tympanometry varies the pressure in the external ear canal and identifies the pressure at which maximum sound transmission occurs. This corresponds to current middle ear pressure status. Using an ear probe, the eardrum's resistance to sound transmission is measured in response to pressure changes. The pressures are recorded and compared to normal values. For reflex threshold measurements, the audiologist places a probe in one ear (ipsilateral ear) to measure the impedance of the

middle ear and places an earphone on the patient's opposite ear (contralateral ear). A loud sound is presented in the contralateral or ipsilateral ear and the change in impedance caused by the contraction of the stapedius muscle is measured. The acoustic stapedial reflex threshold test (ASRT) measures response to acoustic stimuli (threshold) using the lowest intensity stimulus to obtain a reliable positive stapedial reflex with an acoustic meter. Among other applications, these measurements are used to diagnose neuro-otologic conditions and/or determine the appropriate treatment or rehabilitation modalities.

92551
Earphones are placed and the patient is asked to respond to tones of different pitches and intensities. This is a limited study using a few different pitches and intensities. If a patient fails to respond appropriately, additional testing is indicated.

92552-92553
Often physicians or technicians can diagnose a cause of hearing loss through tests using an audiometer. Many causes of hearing loss have characteristic threshold curves. In pure tone audiometry, earphones are placed and the patient is asked to respond to tones of different pitches (frequencies) and intensities. The threshold, which is the lowest intensity of the tone that the patient can hear 50 percent of the time, is recorded for a number of frequencies on each ear. Bone thresholds (92553) are obtained in a similar manner except a bone oscillator is used on the mastoid or forehead to conduct the sound instead of tones through earphones. The air and bone thresholds are compared to differentiate between conductive, sensorineural, or mixed hearing losses.

92555-92556
Often physicians or technicians can diagnose a cause of hearing loss through tests using an audiometer. Many causes of hearing loss have characteristic threshold curves unique to that specific diagnosis. In speech audiometry, earphones are placed and the patient is asked to repeat bisyllabic (spondee) words. The softest level at which the patient can correctly repeat 50 percent of the spondee words is called the speech reception threshold. The threshold is recorded for each ear in 92555. This process occurs in 92556, in addition to a discrimination test. There, the word discrimination score is the percentage of spondee words that a patient can repeat correctly at a given intensity level above his or her speech reception threshold. This is also measured for each ear.

92557
Often physicians or technicians can diagnose a cause of hearing loss through tests using an audiometer. Many causes of hearing loss have characteristic threshold curves. In comprehensive audiometry, earphones are placed and the patient is asked to respond to tones of different pitches (frequencies) and intensities. The threshold, which is the lowest intensity of the tone that the patient can hear 50 percent of the time, is recorded for a number of frequencies on each ear. Bone thresholds are obtained in a similar manner except a bone oscillator is used on the mastoid or forehead to conduct the sound instead of tones through earphones. The air and bone thresholds are compared to differentiate between conductive, sensorineural, or mixed hearing losses. With the earphones in place, the patient is also asked to repeat bisyllabic (spondee) words. The softest level at which the patient can correctly repeat 50 percent of the spondee words is called the speech reception threshold. The threshold is recorded for each ear. The word discrimination score is the percentage of spondee words that a patient can repeat correctly at a given intensity level above his or her speech reception threshold. This is also measured for each ear.

92562
Earphones are placed and tones of the same pitch but different intensities are presented to each ear (binaural) or tones of different intensities and pitches are presented to the same ear (monaural). The patient is asked to compare the loudness of the tones. Differences in intensities that are perceived by the patient as the same are measured.

92563
Earphones are placed and a tone is presented to the patient at a volume above the patient's lowest hearing level for that tone. Measurements are made of the time the tone is audible or the increase in volume needed to maintain an audible tone over time. These measurements are compared to established norms and can be reported at different tone frequencies.

92565
This test is for unilateral pseudohypacusis (malingering). It is based on the principle that if two sounds of the same frequency but different intensities are presented simultaneously to both ears, only the louder tone will be heard. Tones are presented to the good ear at a level above that ear's threshold to obtain a response. Tones are presented to the poor ear simultaneously. The intensity of the sound in the poor ear is increased while the intensity presented to the good ear remains the same. The patient will respond until the intensity of the tones in the poor ear exceeds that of the good ear. At that point, the patient will not respond because the patient is not supposed to hear out of the poor ear. However, the patient should still respond, as the intensity of presentation to the good ear has not changed.

92567
Using an ear probe, the eardrum's resistance to sound transmission is measured in response to pressure changes. Tympanometry varies the pressure in the external ear canal and identifies the pressure at which maximum sound transmission occurs. This corresponds to current middle ear pressure status. The pressures are recorded and compared to normal values.

92568

The audiologist places a probe in one ear (ipsilateral ear) to measure the impedance of the middle ear and places an earphone on the patient's opposite ear (contralateral ear). A loud sound is presented in the contralateral or ipsilateral ear and the change in impedance caused by the contraction of the stapedius muscle is measured. The acoustic stapedial reflex threshold test (ASRT) measures response to acoustic stimuli (threshold) using the lowest intensity stimulus to obtain a reliable positive stapedial reflex with an acoustic meter. Among other applications, these measurements are used to diagnose neuro-otologic conditions and/or determine the appropriate treatment or rehabilitation modalities.

92570

The audiologist performs acoustic immittance testing. Using an ear probe, the eardrum's resistance to sound transmission is measured in response to pressure changes. Tympanometry varies the pressure in the external ear canal and identifies the pressure at which maximum sound transmission occurs. This corresponds to current middle ear pressure status. The pressures are recorded and compared to normal values. To measure acoustic reflex threshold testing, the audiologist places a probe in one ear (ipsilateral ear) to measure the impedance of the middle ear and places an earphone on the patient's opposite ear (contralateral ear). A loud sound is presented in the contralateral or ipsilateral ear and the change in impedance caused by the contraction of the stapedius muscle is measured. The acoustic stapedial reflex threshold test (ASRT) measures response to acoustic stimuli (threshold) using the lowest intensity stimulus to obtain a reliable positive stapedial reflex with an acoustic meter. Among other applications, these measurements are used to diagnose neuro-otologic conditions and/or determine the appropriate treatment or rehabilitation modalities. In the acoustic reflex decay test, the audiologist again places a probe to measure impedance in one ear and places an earphone on the other ear. A loud tone is presented to one of the ears and maintained for 10 seconds. The impedance change (acoustic reflex) is measured by the probe. In a normal ear, the reflex persists for 10 seconds. In an abnormal ear, the reflex diminishes at least 50 percent in the first five seconds. The presence or absence of this reflex is important in the diagnosis of middle ear dysfunctions. In neural hearing loss, this reflex adapts or decays. Determining whether it adapts or decays aids in differential diagnosis of sensory and neural hearing loss.

92571

The patient is presented monosyllabic words, which are low pass filtered, allowing only the parts of each word below a certain frequency (pitch) to be presented. A score is given on the number of correct responses. This test is most commonly used to identify central auditory dysfunction.

92572

With the patient wearing earphones, the audiologist presents bisyllabic (spondee) words in groups of two words. The first syllable of the first word is given to one ear (first word ear) and the last syllable of the first word is given to the same ear at the same time the first syllable of the second word is given to the opposite ear (second word ear). The second syllable of the second word is presented alone to the second word ear. The patient is asked to identify the words presented to each ear and a score is given for each ear.

92575

The audiologist places earphones on the patient and presents tones to the patient at different volumes and different frequencies (pitches). The volume at each frequency where the patient responds correctly 50 percent of the time is the threshold at that frequency. The sounds presented through the earphones are air-conduction. The air-conduction thresholds are measured in the presence of noise (masking) through a bone vibrator on the side of the head (bone-conducted masking). The masked and unmasked air-conduction thresholds are compared.

92576

Using earphones, seven-word sentences that do not follow normal rules of grammar are presented to one ear while a taped story is presented to the other ear simultaneously (competition). The patient is scored on the ability to correctly identify the seven-word sentences. This test is principally used for central hearing disorders.

92577

This is a test for unilateral pseudohypacusis (malingering). It is based on the principle that if two sounds of the same frequency and different intensities are presented simultaneously to both ears, only the louder will be heard. Bisyllabic (spondee) words are presented to the good ear at a level above that ear's threshold to respond. Words are presented simultaneously to the poor ear. The intensity of the sound in the poor ear is increased while the intensity presented to the good ear remains the same. The patient will respond until the intensity of the words in the poor ear exceeds that of the good ear. At that point, the patient will not respond because the patient is not supposed to hear out of the poor ear. However, the patient should still respond, as the intensity of presentation to the good ear has not changed.

92579

Visual reinforcement audiometry (VRA) is used to test hearing in infants and in both difficult-to-test children and adults. The process includes case history and otologic examination, typically conducted in a sound booth. Lighted toys are used as reinforcement for response to auditory stimuli. Stimuli may include frequency-specific signals, calibrated noises, or live voice. The results are usually recorded on an audiogram. The interpretation of the testing addresses the type and the severity of hearing loss and any recommendations.

92582
Often physicians or technicians can diagnose a cause of hearing loss through tests using an audiometer. Many causes of hearing loss have characteristic threshold curves. Conditioning play audiometry tests pure tone air and bone conduction and speech thresholds in children. Test sounds can be presented with earphones or sound field testing (pure tone air conduction only). The child is conditioned to perform a simple task (i.e., drop a block in a bucket) when the test sound is heard.

92583
Often physicians or technicians can diagnose a cause of hearing loss through tests using an audiometer. Many causes of hearing loss have characteristic threshold curves. In select picture audiometry, the patient is placed in a booth with or without earphones. The patient is asked to identify different pictures with the instructions given at different intensity levels. A threshold level for speech, which is the intensity level at which the patient responds correctly 50 percent of the time, is obtained.

92584
An electrode is placed through the tympanic membrane into the promontory of the inner ear. The ear is stimulated and recordings are made of the electrical response of the cochlear nerve. This can be done under local, topical, or general anesthesia.

[92650, 92651, 92652, 92653]
In testing auditory evoked potentials (AEPs), electrodes are placed in various locations on the scalp and electrical recordings are made in response to auditory stimulations delivered through earphones. The origin of the electrical response is believed to be from the auditory nerve and brainstem. In 92650, an automated screening is performed with broadband (i.e., frequency nonspecific) stimuli, such as amplitude modulated noise, chirps, or clicks. Broadband stimuli are also used in 92651, which reports a hearing status determination with interpretation and report. Report 92652 for threshold estimation testing using multiple frequencies; this also includes interpretation and report. Code 92653 reports testing to evaluate neural conduction; interpretation and report are included.

[92558]
A probe tip is placed in the ear canal to screen for normal hearing function. The probe tip emits a repeated clicking sound (transient evoked emissions) or two tones at two frequencies (distortion product emissions). The sounds pass through the tympanic membrane, middle ear, and to the inner ear. In the inner ear, the sound is picked up by the hair cells in the cochlea, which in turn bounce the sound back in low intensity sound waves (OAE). These OAEs are recorded and analyzed by computerized equipment.

92587-92588
A probe tip is placed in the ear canal to perform an evaluation of normal hearing function. The probe tip emits two tones at two frequencies (distortion product evoked otoacoustic emissions) or a repeated clicking sound (transient evoked otoacoustic emissions). The sounds pass through the tympanic membrane, middle ear, and to the inner ear. In the inner ear, the sound is picked up by the hair cells in the cochlea, which in turn bounce the sound back in low intensity sound waves (OAE). These OAEs are recorded by computerized equipment. These codes include the provider's interpretation and report based on the recordings. Report 92587 for a limited evaluation to confirm the presence or absence of a hearing disorder using two to three frequencies or transient evoked otoacoustic emission testing. Report 92588 for a comprehensive analysis of the cochlear hair cell's function (mapping) using a minimum of 12 frequencies.

92590-92591
The physician takes a history of hearing loss. The patient's ears are examined. Medical or surgical treatment is offered if possible. The appropriate type of hearing aid is selected to fit the patient's pattern of hearing loss. Report 92590 if one ear is fitted with a hearing aid and 92591 if both ears receive aids.

92592-92593
The audiologist inspects the hearing aid and checks the battery. The aid is cleaned and the power and clarity are checked using a special stethoscope, which attaches to the hearing aid. Report 92592 if a monaural hearing aid is checked and 92593 if both hearing aids are checked.

92594-92595
A printout from a hearing aid analyzer is used to compare the electroacoustical characteristics of a monaural hearing aid with the specifications for that aid in 92594 or a binaural hearing aid with specifications for that aid in 92595.

92596
This test can be performed in one of several ways. One method is to check the speech or pure tone threshold, which is the intensity at which the patient responds correctly 50 percent of the time, with and without ear protection (ear plugs or earphones) while the patient is in a soundproof booth.

92601-92602
A diagnostic analysis of a cochlear implant, including programming, is done post-operatively to fit the previously placed external devices, connect to the implant, and program the stimulator. Cochlear implants are equipped with software that allows for different programming specific to the patient's daily activities. Threshold levels, volume, pulse widths, live-voice speech adjustments, input dynamic range, and frequency shaping templates are evaluated and set according to individual needs. This is done for patients 7 years of age and younger in 92601. For children 7 years of age and younger, speech stimuli are used more frequently to determine the optimal setting. Report 92602 for subsequent modifications or reprogramming.

92603-92604
A diagnostic analysis of a cochlear implant, including programming, is done post-operatively to fit the previously placed external devices, connect to the implant, and program the stimulator. Cochlear implants are equipped with software that allows for different programming specific to the patient's daily activities. Threshold levels, volume, pulse widths, live-voice speech adjustments, input dynamic range, and frequency shaping templates are evaluated and set according to the individual needs. This is done for patients older than 7 years of age in 92603. Patients older than 7 years of age are able to provide significant feedback for fine-tuning adjustment. Report 92604 for subsequent modifications or reprogramming.

[92597]
A voice prosthetic device, such as an amplifier, is used to augment speech for a patient with complete or partial speech loss. This code applies to evaluating the patient for use of and/or fitting the device often by a speech therapist or physician.

92605 [92618]
The assessment for the appropriate non-speech-generating augmentative and alternative communication (AAC) device is highly variable and dependent on the patient's age, ability, and motivation. Motor skills, hearing, vision, cognitive abilities, language comprehension, and general health are evaluated to determine the suitability of a high-tech or low-tech device. Once these are evaluated, an appropriate AAC device is prescribed. Report 92605 for the first hour spent face-to-face with the patient. Report 92618 for each additional 30 minutes.

92606
This code includes therapeutic services associated with the use of non-speech generating devices. Services differ according to the device used. Electronic equipment may require routine maintenance, programming, and mounting systems. Other equipment may require customization (e.g., symbol boards). Non-speech generating devices may require some patient therapeutic, rehabilitation, or occupational training.

92607-92608
The patient is evaluated face to face by a specialist to determine the motor skills, hearing, cognitive abilities, comprehension, natural speech, esophageal and pharyngeal air flow, general health, and patient motivation for prescription of speech-generating augmentative and alternative communication (AAC) device. Once these are evaluated, an appropriate speech-generating device is prescribed. Report 92607 for the first hour and 92608 for each additional 30 minutes.

92609
This code includes therapeutic services associated with the use of speech generating devices. Services differ according to the device used. Electronic equipment may require routine maintenance, programming, or modification. Speech generating devices may require some patient therapeutic, rehabilitation, or occupational training.

92610
The patient is evaluated to determine the oral and pharyngeal swallowing function. Assessment of the oral cavity includes the size, position, resting tone, range of motion and development of the tongue, lips, and palate. Palpation of the thyroid notch or cricoid arch with swallowing is used to determine elevation of the pharynx. Using a curved probe, sensation of the oral cavity may be assessed. An inventory of cranial nerves must also be included.

92611
Motion fluoroscopic examinations are done of the swallowing function by cine or video recording. The patient is seated upright in a normal eating posture. Small amounts of liquid barium and barium-coated foods of varying consistencies, textures, and flavors are administered allowing visualization of the swallowing function by fluoroscopy. The patient is given liquids, pastes, and solid foods that are visually followed from the oral cavity to the pharynx and the cervical esophagus. A portion of this test is usually repeated with the patient in a horizontal position.

92612-92613
A flexible nasopharyngoscope is positioned posterior to the soft palate to allow visualization during swallowing. The patient is given foods of varying consistencies dyed with food coloring to aid visualization of the swallowing function. Liquids, pastes, and solid food are ingested separately and visualized. The procedure is recorded by cine or video. Report 92613 for interpretation and report only.

92614-92615
A flexible laryngoscope is inserted into the nasal passage and advanced just proximal to the test site for laryngeal sensory evaluation. Air pulses of varying degrees in intensity are administered. Vocal fold adduction of the laryngeal adductor reflex is evaluated for vocal fold movement, absence of movement, or swallow initiation and visualized on a video monitor. The procedure is recorded by cine or video. Report 92615 for interpretation and report only.

92616-92617
A flexible nasopharyngoscope is positioned posterior to the soft palate to allow visualization during swallowing. The patient is given foods of varying consistencies dyed with food coloring to aid visualization of the swallowing function. Liquids, pastes, and solid food are ingested separately and visualized. After this portion is complete, laryngeal sensory testing is initiated. A flexible laryngoscope is inserted into the nasal passage and advanced just proximal to the test site. Air pulses of varying degrees in intensity are administered. Vocal fold adduction of the laryngeal adductor reflex is evaluated for vocal fold movement, absence of movement, or swallow

initiation and visualized on a video monitor. The procedure is recorded by cine or video. Report 92617 for interpretation and report only.

92620-92621
The audiologist evaluates central auditory function. Central auditory processes are the auditory mechanisms that are responsible for what the brain does with what the ears hear. Many individuals have no difficulty detecting the presence of sound but have other auditory difficulties related to central auditory processes, such as understanding conversation in noisy environments, following complex directions, and learning new vocabulary words. There are two major categories of tests: behavioral tests and electrophysiologic tests. The behavioral tests can be monotic or dichotic. Monotic tests use a single stimulus presented to one ear at a time or tests in which two stimuli are presented to one ear. Dichotic tests use the same stimulus applied to both ears. Testing may be performed on only one ear (monaural) or both ears simultaneously (binaural). Specific types of tests that can be given include monaural low-redundancy speech tests, dichotic speech tests, temporal patterning tests, and binaural interaction tests. The audiologist selects the appropriate battery of central auditory function tests after evaluating the patient using routine hearing tests. Central auditory function tests are used to differentiate central from peripheral hearing loss and occasionally to identify the site of a lesion in the central nervous system. Report 92620 for the first 60 minutes of the evaluation and 92621 for each additional 15 minutes.

92622-92623
A diagnostic analysis and programming of any type of auditory osseointegrated (bone-anchored) sound processor is performed. Bone conduction implants transfer sound to the inner ear through direct vibration of the skull. Processor attachment, device feedback calibration, device programming, and processor performance are included in the evaluation. Report 92622 for the first 60 minutes and 92623 for each additional 15 minutes thereafter.

92625
The audiologist performs a tinnitus assessment including pitch, loudness, matching, and masking. Subjective tinnitus is an acoustic like sensation, often described as a ringing sound located within the head, for which there is no external cause. Other descriptions of the sound include roaring, hissing, music, crickets, and static-like. A tinnitus assessment is performed to determine the exact nature of the acoustic sensation or sound. First the pitch or frequency of the tinnitus is determined and then the loudness of the sensation or sound. The audiologist tries to reproduce or match the pitch and loudness using sound generators designed for this purpose. The masking process also uses sound generators to identify external sound stimuli that mask the tinnitus. Masking is a procedure that makes the tinnitus less distracting to the patient by use of a controlled noise that covers the noise of the tinnitus.

92626-92627
The patient is seen face to face by a physician or other qualified health care provider for a pre-implant candidacy evaluation or for a post-implant evaluation of a surgically implanted device. The evaluation includes listening inventories and phonetic discrimination testing to determine the patient's level of sound perception and sound discrimination ability. Report 92626 for the first hour and 92627 for each additional 15 minutes.

92630-92633
Auditory rehabilitation is auditory training or therapy conducted by a physician, speech and language therapist, or teacher of the hearing impaired. Pre-lingual hearing loss therapies (92630) remedy hearing impairments that are acquired before the child has acquired language (usually due to trauma or disease) or are congenital in etiology. Post-lingual hearing loss therapies (92633) remedy hearing impairments that occur after the acquisition of speech and language and can be due to disease, medication side effects, or trauma. Post-lingual hearing usually progresses gradually. Rehabilitation goals include maximizing auditory skills and communication abilities. These rehabilitation goals progress from awareness of environmental sound to increasingly higher levels of speech discrimination.

92640
A diagnostic analysis of an auditory brainstem implant, including programming, is done post-operatively to fit the previously placed external devices, connect to the implant, and program the stimulator. Auditory brainstem implants are equipped with software that allows for different programming specific to the patient's daily activities. Threshold levels, volume, pulse widths, live-voice speech adjustments, input dynamic range, and frequency shaping templates are evaluated and set according to individual needs.

92950
Cardiopulmonary arrest occurs when the patient's heart and lungs suddenly stop. In a clinical setting, cardiopulmonary resuscitation, the attempt at restarting the heart and lungs, is usually directed by a physician or another health care provider who is certified in Advanced Cardiac Life Support (ACLS). The patient's lungs are ventilated by mouth-to-mouth breathing or by a bag and mask. The patient's circulation is assisted using external chest compression. An electronic defibrillator may be used to shock the heart into restarting. Medications used to restart the heart include epinephrine and lidocaine.

92953
A temporary pacemaker is placed on the patient's heart to regulate heartbeats considered dangerously irregular. The physician applies electrodes to the chest wall. The electrodes give small electronic shocks through the chest to pace the heart as controlled by the physician.

92960-92961
The physician may administer an electronic shock to the patient's chest to regulate heartbeats considered dangerously irregular. The physician uses a defibrillator machine and places two paddles on the patient's chest and/or back. A measured electric shock is delivered through the chest to the heart to convert the heartbeat to a regular rhythm. Report 92960 for external cardioversion and 92961 when the procedure is performed internally.

92970
In internal circulatory assist, the femoral artery is cannulated and a catheter with balloon or other device is inserted into the aorta. Various devices may be used to assist circulation. This code should be reported for the internal insertion of such a device, but should not be used to report intra-aortic balloon pump (IABP) or implantation of ventricular assist devices that are reported elsewhere.

92971
Devices are placed at the outside of the body to assist circulation. One example of external circulatory assist is Military Anti-Shock Trousers (MAST), which apply counterpressure around the legs and abdomen. The artificial peripheral resistance helps coronary perfusion. In a related procedure, pressure cuffs are used to assist circulation. The patient is placed on a treatment table where their lower extremities are wrapped in a series of three compressive air cuffs, which inflate and deflate in synchronization with the patient's cardiac cycle. During diastole the three sets of air cuffs are inflated sequentially (distal to proximal) compressing the vascular beds within the muscles of the calves, lower thighs, and upper thighs. This action results in an increase in diastolic pressure, generation of retrograde arterial blood flow, and an increase in venous return. The cuffs are deflated simultaneously just prior to systole, which produces a rapid drop in vascular impedance, a decrease in ventricular workload, and an increase in cardiac output. The augmented diastolic pressure and retrograde aortic flow appear to improve myocardial perfusion, while systolic unloading appears to reduce cardiac workload and oxygen requirements. The increased venous return coupled with enhanced systolic flow appears to increase cardiac output.

92986-92990
The physician performs a percutaneous valvuloplasty. The physician makes a small incision in the arm or leg. Two catheters are placed: a central venous catheter and a second catheter threaded up to the heart. The physician inflates a balloon at the tip of the second catheter to open the blocked valve. The catheters are removed. Pressure is placed over the incision for 20 to 30 minutes to stem bleeding. The patient is observed for a period afterward. Report 92986 if the procedure is performed on the aortic valve; 92987 if the procedure is performed on the mitral valve; and 92990 if the procedure is performed on the pulmonary valve.

92997
The purpose of this procedure is to use a balloon to expand a narrowed pulmonary artery. The physician places an introducer sheath in the femoral vein, using percutaneous puncture. The physician places an angioplasty catheter through the introducer sheath into the femoral vein and advances it under fluoroscopic guidance to the right ventricle and out into the main pulmonary artery. The physician advances the angioplasty balloon into the narrowed pulmonary artery, using injections of x-ray contrast material to guide the way. The physician inflates the balloon to expand the pulmonary artery, sometimes using several balloon inflations. The physician removes the catheter and sheath from the femoral vein. Vessel hemostasis is achieved using manual pressure. Pressure is placed on the wound for 20 to 30 minutes to stem bleeding.

92998
Following single vessel percutaneous transluminal pulmonary artery balloon angioplasty (92997), the physician redirects the balloon angioplasty catheter to an additional pulmonary artery. The physician may change to a different sized balloon catheter if the additional pulmonary artery is of different size. The physician inflates the balloon to expand the pulmonary artery, sometimes using several balloon inflations. The physician removes the catheter and sheath from the femoral vein. Pressure is placed on the wound for 20 to 30 minutes to stem bleeding.

[92920, 92921]
The physician makes a small incision in the arm or leg to access the artery for placement of two catheters. A central venous catheter is inserted through the femoral or brachial artery and a second catheter with a balloon tip is threaded up to the heart and into an obstructed native coronary artery. The physician inflates the balloon at the tip of the second catheter to flatten plaque obstructing the artery against the walls of the coronary artery. If sufficient results are not obtained after the first inflation, the physician may reinflate the balloon for a longer period of time or at greater pressure. The catheters are removed. Pressure is placed over the incision for 20 to 30 minutes to stop bleeding. Report 92920 for each angioplasty performed on a single major coronary artery or branch. Report 92921 for each additional branch of the major coronary artery treated during percutaneous coronary intervention.

[92924, 92925]
The physician removes the atherosclerotic plaque blocking a native coronary artery. The physician makes a small incision in the arm or leg to access the artery for placement of two catheters. A central venous catheter is inserted through the femoral or brachial artery and a second catheter threaded up to the coronary artery blockage. The plaque is removed using a rotary cutter introduced through a catheter under radiographic guidance. The blockage may also require subsequent inflation of the balloon on the tip of the second

catheter to flatten any remaining plaque. The catheters are removed. Pressure is placed over the incision for 20 to 30 minutes to stop bleeding. Report 92924 for each atherectomy performed on a single major coronary artery or branch. Report 92925 for each additional branch of the major coronary artery treated during percutaneous coronary intervention.

[92928, 92929]
A stent is used to hold open a blocked or collapsed native artery in the heart. The physician makes a small incision in the arm or leg to access the artery for placement of two catheters. A central venous catheter is inserted through the femoral or brachial artery and a second catheter is threaded up to the affected coronary artery. An obstruction may be treated first by inflating a balloon at the tip of the second catheter (PTCA) to flatten the obstruction. A stent is introduced through a catheter, placed under radiographic guidance, and expanded to fit the lumen of the artery by inflating the balloon on the second catheter. The catheters are removed. Pressure is placed over the incision for 20 to 30 minutes to stop the bleeding. Report 92928 for each stent placement performed on a single major coronary artery or branch. Report 92929 for each additional branch of the major coronary artery stented during percutaneous coronary intervention.

[92933, 92934]
A stent is used to hold open a blocked native coronary artery. The physician makes a small incision in the arm or leg to access the artery for placement of two catheters. A central venous catheter is inserted through the femoral or brachial artery and a second catheter is threaded up to the affected coronary artery. Any obstruction is treated first by using a rotary cutter (atherectomy) to flatten or remove the obstruction. The obstruction may also be treated by inflating a balloon at the tip of the second catheter (PTCA). A stent is introduced through a catheter, placed under radiographic guidance, and expanded to fit the lumen of the artery by inflating the balloon on the second catheter. The catheters are removed. Pressure is placed over the incision for 20 to 30 minutes to stop the bleeding. Report 92933 for each atherectomy with stent placement performed on a single major coronary artery or branch. Report 92934 for each additional branch of the major coronary artery treated with atherectomy and stent during percutaneous coronary intervention.

[92937, 92938]
The use of one or any combination of angioplasty, atherectomy, or stent placement is performed to restore a blocked coronary artery bypass graft (CABG). The physician makes a small incision in the arm or leg to access the artery for placement of two catheters. A central venous catheter is inserted through the femoral or brachial artery and a second catheter is threaded up to the affected graft. The obstruction may be treated by using a rotary cutter (atherectomy) to flatten or remove the obstruction, inflating a balloon at the tip of the second catheter (PTCA), or introducing a stent that is expanded to fit the lumen of the artery. The catheters are removed. Pressure is placed over the incision for 20 to 30 minutes to stop the bleeding. Report 92937 for treatment of the first CABG. Report 92938 for each additional graft treated.

[92941]
The use of one or any combination of angioplasty, atherectomy, or stent placement is performed to restore an acutely blocked coronary artery bypass graft (CABG) or native coronary artery during an acute myocardial infarction. The physician makes a small incision in the arm or leg to access the artery for placement of two catheters. A central venous catheter is inserted through the femoral or brachial artery and a second catheter is threaded up to the affected vessel or graft. The obstruction may be treated by using a rotary cutter (atherectomy) to flatten or remove the obstruction, inflating a balloon at the tip of the second catheter (PTCA), or introducing a stent that is expanded to fit the lumen of the artery. The catheters are removed. Pressure is placed over the incision for 20 to 30 minutes to stop the bleeding.

[92943, 92944]
The use of one or any combination of angioplasty, atherectomy, or stent placement is performed to restore a chronic totally blocked coronary artery bypass graft (CABG) or native coronary artery. The physician makes a small incision in the arm or leg to access the artery for placement of two catheters. A central venous catheter is inserted through the femoral or brachial artery and a second catheter is threaded up to the affected vessel or graft. The obstruction may be treated by using a rotary cutter (atherectomy) to flatten or remove the obstruction, inflating a balloon at the tip of the second catheter (PTCA), or introducing a stent that is expanded to fit the lumen of the artery. The catheters are removed. Pressure is placed over the incision for 20 to 30 minutes to stop the bleeding. Report 92943 for the treatment of the first native artery or CABG. Report 92944 for each additional graft or vessel treated.

[92972]
The physician treats coronary artery calcification, which is known to hinder other percutaneous coronary interventions, with percutaneous transluminal coronary lithotripsy. This procedure is performed in conjunction with other percutaneous transluminal or transcatheter coronary procedures (angioplasty, atherectomy, stent placement, revascularization of bypass graft or occlusion, or thrombolysis). Following femoral or radial access and using a proprietary intravascular lithotripsy (IVL) device, the physician advances the coronary catheter to the target lesion. An integrated balloon is inflated with fluid at a low pressure to contact the arterial wall. IVL is then activated, creating a small bubble within the catheter balloon that rapidly expands and collapses, resulting in shockwaves that travel through the innermost layer of the vessel wall, where it cracks the calcium by creating microfractures.

[92973]
The physician percutaneously removes a blood clot from a native or grafted coronary artery. A double lumen catheter is passed to the area of the clot. A high-pressure saline stream (via a pump) is introduced through a lumen that has multiple jet orifices located at the distal tip. The low-pressure zone created by the jets causes the clot to break up into small pieces and be pushed through the catheter with a force that drives debris from the thrombus through the other lumen (exhaust) and out of the body. The procedure is useful to clear fatty and degenerated arteries and to modify plaques in preparation for more definitive treatment with adjunctive balloon angioplasty or stenting.

[92974]
Using an X-ray machine in a cardiac catheterization laboratory, the physician places the delivery catheter in the coronary artery at the site of the in-stent restenosis (reblockage in the artery). The transfer delivery device is connected to the delivery catheter; the transfer delivery device is used to deliver the radioactive seeds to the location. There are various methods for transcatheter placement, but commonly the methods involve the use of a guiding catheter. The radioactive seeds are positioned at the location for an appropriate length of time to administer radiation to the artery. At the completion of the radiation treatment, the radioactive seeds are returned to the transfer device.

[92975, 92977]
In 92975, the physician places a hollow catheter in the aorta from the arm or leg via a small incision. Using fluoroscopic guidance, the physician advances the catheter tip to the coronary artery to be treated and confirms the presence of thrombus (blood clot) in the artery by injecting contrast material through the catheter into the artery. In 92977, a catheter equipped with an infusion tip is threaded into the vessel. The physician infuses a thrombolytic agent (e.g., urokinase) into the affected artery in order to dissolve the thrombus. The physician may perform contrast injections to assess the size and extent of the thrombus after infusion of the thrombolytic agent. The catheter is removed from the patient's body. Pressure is placed over the incision to stem bleeding. The patient is observed for a period afterward.

[92978, 92979]
Intravascular ultrasound (IVUS) or optical coherence tomography (OCT) may be used for endoluminal imaging during diagnostic evaluation of a coronary vessel or graft. It may also be used before and after a therapeutic intervention on a coronary vessel or graft to assess patency and integrity of the vessel or graft. A needle is inserted through the skin and into a blood vessel. A guidewire is threaded through the needle into a coronary blood vessel or graft. The needle is removed. An intravascular ultrasound catheter is placed over the guidewire. The ultrasound probe is used to obtain images from inside the vessel to assess area and extent of disease prior to interventional therapy, as well as adequacy of therapy after interventional therapy. The ultrasound probe provides a two-dimensional, cross-sectional view of the vessel or graft as the probe is advanced and withdrawn along the area of interest. When the ultrasound examination is complete, the catheter is removed. OCT utilizes light instead of sound to provide cross-sectional images in high resolution within the lumen. Report 92978 for the initial vessel or graft. In 92979, the physician advances the ultrasound catheter into additional vessels or grafts to assess patency and structure. The catheter and guidewire are removed and pressure is applied over the puncture site to stop bleeding.

93000-93010
Multiple electrodes are placed on a patient's chest to record the electrical activity of the heart. A physician interprets the findings. Report 93000 for the combined technical and professional components of an ECG; 93005 for the technical component only; and 93010 for the professional component only.

93015-93018
A continuous recording of electrical activity of the heart is acquired by an assistant supervised by a qualified health care professional while the patient is exercising on a treadmill or bicycle and/or given medicines. The stress on the heart during the test is monitored. Code 93015 includes the test, supervision, and interpretation of the report; 93016 includes only the supervision of the test; 93017 includes performing the test only; and 93018 is reported for the interpretation of a previously performed test.

93024
The purpose of the study is to evaluate for coronary artery spasm. If ergonovine is not available, certain other ergot medications may be infused for the same purpose. Following baseline coronary angiography (coded elsewhere), the physician infuses gradually escalating doses of ergonovine into a peripheral vein, while monitoring for chest discomfort and electrocardiographic changes. Repeat angiography is performed during ergonovine infusion to assess the size of the coronary lumen. If the patient develops symptomatic coronary spasm, the physician may directly infuse vasodilating medications through the intracoronary catheter to relieve the problem.

93025
T-Wave Alternans testing is an electrocardiographic method of measuring the alternating electrical amplitude from beat to beat on an electrocardiogram and is used as a method of evaluating ventricular arrhythmia risk. Microvolt T-wave alternans can be measured during exercise or pharmacologic stress, or during cardiac pacing, using a spectral analytic method with equipment that is able to detect as little as one microvolt of T-wave alternans. In electrode placement for a 12-lead ECG, the health care provider positions the leads on the wrists and ankles or shoulders and groins. Left leg electrodes are placed below the heart (but not on the chest), preferably

below the umbilicus. The sensing electrodes look at the inferior surface of the heart, the left or lateral side of the heart, and at the right side of the heart.

93040
One to three electrodes placed on a patient's chest are used to record electrical activity of the heart. The physician interprets the report.

93041
An assistant records the electrical activity of the heart by placing one to three electrodes on a patient's chest in a predetermined pattern. This code describes the tracing only.

93042
A physician interprets a recording of electrical activities of a patient's heart acquired by placing one to three electrodes on the patient's chest.

93050
Blood pressure pulse wave analysis measures the blood pressure at the heart rather than in the arm as with traditional blood pressure cuffs, as well as providing information regarding the interaction of the heart and blood vessels. The brachial blood pressure is obtained to calibrate the radial pressure waveform. The pressure sensor wand (tonometer) is placed on the wrist where the strongest pulse is present. The pressure waveforms are transmitted and displayed on a data collection screen on a computer. After there is at least 10 seconds of data displayed, the data is captured. The data reflects average central aortic waveform, pressure measurements, and central parameters, as well as reference ranges. The augmentation index can be acquired by direct measurement or acquired pressure waveforms. This index is a percentage of pressure from systolic rise over pressure waves. The nonlinear mathematical transformation can be utilized to differentiate between active and rest blood pressure coinciding with the systolic and diastolic process. This code includes the digitization of the data, as well as the use of nonlinear mathematical transformation to determine pressure, augmentation index, and the provider interpretation and report.

93224-93227
The purpose of this study is to evaluate the patient's ambient heart rhythm during a full daily cycle. The physician or other qualified health care professional instructs the patient in the use of an external electrocardiographic (ECG) recorder, also known as a Holter monitor. A technician places ECG leads on the patient's chest, and the patient wears the recorder for up to 48 hours. During this time, there is continuous rhythm recording and storage. The patient returns the device, and the recorded heart rhythm is played back into digital format by a technician. The technician uses a scanning methodology to classify different ECG waveforms and to generate a report. The generated report describes the overall rhythm and significant arrhythmias. Code 93224 reports the recording, scanning analysis with report, provider review of the data, and the provision of a final interpretation in a report. Code 93225 reports the recording only, which includes connection, recording of data, and disconnection. Code 93226 reports only the scanning analysis with report. Code 93227 reports only the provider review and interpretation.

[93241, 93242, 93243, 93244]
Long-term external electrocardiographic (ECG) recording is a diagnostic procedure that provides continuous rhythm recording of the patient's heart while the patient is engaged in the activities of daily living. The purpose of the study is to evaluate the patient's ambient heart rhythm during a full daily cycle. Rhythm disturbances and waveform abnormalities are detected; information is provided regarding the frequency of these disturbances. The physician or other qualified health care provider instructs the patient in the use of the external ECG recorder. A technician places ECG leads on the patient's chest, and the patient wears the recorder for 48 hours up to seven days. During this time there is continuous rhythm recording and storage. The patient returns the device and the recorded heart rhythm is converted into digital format by a technician. The technician uses a scanning methodology to classify different ECG waveforms and to generate a report. The generated report describes the overall rhythm and significant arrhythmias. Code 93241 reports the recording, scanning analysis with report, provider review of the data, and the provision of a final interpretation in a report. Code 93242 reports the recording only, which includes the connection and initial recording of data. Code 93243 reports only the scanning analysis with report. Code 93244 reports only the provider review and interpretation.

[93245, 93246, 93247, 93248]
Long-term external electrocardiographic (ECG) recording is a diagnostic procedure that provides continuous rhythm recording of the patient's heart while the patient is engaged in the activities of daily living. The purpose of the study is to evaluate the patient's ambient heart rhythm during a full daily cycle. Rhythm disturbances and waveform abnormalities are detected; information is provided regarding the frequency of these disturbances. The physician or other qualified health care provider instructs the patient in the use of the external ECG recorder. A technician places ECG leads on the patient's chest, and the patient wears the recorder for more than seven days up to 15 days. During this time there is continuous rhythm recording and storage. The patient returns the device and the recorded heart rhythm is converted into digital format by a technician. The technician uses a scanning methodology to classify different ECG waveforms and to generate a report. The generated report describes the overall rhythm and significant arrhythmias. Code 93245 reports the recording, scanning analysis with report, provider review of the data, and the provision of a final interpretation in a report. Code 93246 reports the recording only, which includes the connection and

initial recording of data. Code 93247 reports only the scanning analysis with report. Code 93248 reports only the provider review and interpretation.

93228-93229

Mobile cardiovascular telemetry (MCT) uses external electrodes placed on the patient's body to continuously record electrocardiographic rhythm. Data segments are transmitted to a remote surveillance location by phone signal (cellular or landline); this is accomplished automatically and does not require patient intervention. Selected rhythm segments may be triggered for transmission automatically by rapid and slow heart rates or by the patient during a symptomatic episode. Data are analyzed continuously in real time. A remote technician responds to the alerts from the external device, reviewing the data and notifying the physician or other qualified health care professional depending on the stipulated criteria. Report 93228 for provider review and interpretation with report and 93229 for technical support, which includes connection, instructions to the patient for use, attended surveillance, analysis, and transmission of daily and emergent data reports per provider protocol. These codes may be reported only once per 30-day period.

93268-93272

The purpose of this study is to evaluate the patient's ambient heart rhythm during symptoms. The physician or other qualified health care professional instructs the patient in the use of an external rhythm monitor. A technician places ECG leads on the patient's chest, and the monitor uses a symptom-related memory loop mechanism with remote download capability up to 30 days to record the patient's rhythm. During symptoms, the patient activates the monitor by pressing a button. The resulting recording includes ECG activity prior to and during symptoms. The patient uses the device to transmit the recording over the telephone line, allowing a rhythm printout to be generated. The provider reviews and interprets this rhythm strip. Code 93268 reports transmission and provider review and interpretation. Code 93270 reports the recording only (including connection, recording, and disconnection). Code 93271 reports transmission download and analysis. Code 93272 reports only the provider review and interpretation.

93278

Electrodes placed on a patient's chest record the heart's electrical activity. This technique uses signal-averaged electrocardiography (SAECG) and may include a standard electrocardiogram.

[93264]

A pulmonary pressure monitoring system permits ongoing monitoring and measurement of a patient's heartrate as well as systolic, diastolic, and mean pressures in a patient diagnosed with non-rhythm related cardiac conditions (i.e., heart failure). Pulmonary arterial pressure (PAP) readings transmitted from an internally implanted sensor to a wireless electronic unit are subsequently transmitted to an internet-based file server or monitored by a surveillance technician with results sent to an online portal that can be accessed by the patient's treating health care provider. Through accurate monitoring of patients diagnosed with heart failure (HF) for exacerbations, it is possible to minimize the need for additional hospitalizations and the associated complications and allow for early pharmacological intervention. Code 93264 reports the remote monitoring of a wireless pulmonary artery pressure sensor for up to 30 days.

93279-93281

A programming device evaluation is performed in person in order to test the device's function and select the most favorable permanent programmed values. Patients with previously implanted pacemakers require periodic programming device evaluations. This diagnostic procedure includes a face-to-face assessment of all device functions. Components that must be evaluated in order to assign a code from this range include the battery, leads, capture and sensing function, heart rhythm, and programmed parameters. Stored and measured data regarding these components are retrieved using an office, hospital, or emergency room instrument. This information is assessed to discern battery voltage, lead impedance, and settings for rhythm treatment and tachycardia detection, as well as to determine the pacemaker's current programming. If necessary, the sensing value and rate response, upper and lower heart rates, AV intervals, pacing voltage and pulse duration, and diagnostics are adjusted. These codes include physician or other qualified health care professional review, interpretation, and report, and are assigned per procedure. Report 93279 for evaluation of a single-lead pacemaker or leadless system (one in which there is pacing and sensing function in only one chamber of the heart). Report 93280 for evaluation of a dual-lead device (one with pacing and sensing function in only two chambers). Report 93281 for evaluation of a multiple-lead device (one with pacing and sensing function in three or more chambers).

93282-93284

A programming device evaluation is performed in person in order to test the device's function and select the most favorable permanent programmed values. Patients with transvenous implantable defibrillator systems require periodic programming device evaluations. This diagnostic procedure includes a face-to-face assessment of all device functions. Components that must be evaluated in order to assign a code from this range include the battery, leads, programmed parameters, presence or absence of therapy for ventricular tachyarrhythmias, and heart rhythm. Stored and measured data regarding these components are retrieved using an office, hospital, or emergency room instrument. This information is assessed to discern battery voltage, lead impedance, and settings for rhythm treatment and tachycardia detection, as well as to determine the defibrillator's current programming. If necessary, the sensing value and sensor rate response, upper and lower heart rates, AV intervals, pacing voltage and pulse duration, and diagnostics are adjusted. Ventricular tachycardia detection and therapies may also be altered. These codes include physician or other qualified health care professional review, interpretation, and report, and are assigned per procedure. Report 93282 for evaluation of a single-lead system (one in which there is pacing and sensing function in only one chamber of the heart). Report 93283 for evaluation of a dual-lead device (one with pacing and sensing function in only two chambers). Report 93284 for evaluation of a multiple-lead device (one with pacing and sensing function in three or more chambers).

[93260]

A programming device evaluation is performed in person in order to test the device's function and select the most favorable permanent programmed values. Patients with previously placed subcutaneous implantable defibrillator systems require periodic programming device evaluations. This diagnostic procedure includes a face-to-face assessment of all device functions, including analysis, review, and report by a physician or other qualified health care professional. Components that must be evaluated in order to assign a code from this range include the battery, leads, capture and sensing function, heart rhythm, and programmed parameters. Stored and measured data regarding these components are retrieved using an office, hospital, or emergency room instrument. This information is assessed to discern battery voltage, lead impedance, and settings, as well as to determine the system's current programming. If necessary, the parameters are reprogrammed.

93285

A programming device evaluation is performed in person in order to test the device's function and select the most favorable permanent programmed values. Patients with previously placed subcutaneous cardiac rhythm monitor systems require periodic programming device evaluations. This diagnostic procedure includes a face-to-face assessment of all device functions. Components that must be evaluated include heartrate and rhythm during recorded episodes (patient-initiated and device algorithm detected events), as well as programmed parameters. Stored and measured data are retrieved using an office, hospital, or emergency room instrument. This information is assessed to discern current programming and to evaluate specific aspects of the device's function. If necessary, the bradycardia and tachycardia detection criteria are adjusted. This code includes physician or other qualified health care professional review, interpretation, and report, and is assigned per procedure.

93286-93287

A programming device evaluation is performed in person in order to test the device's function and select the most favorable permanent programmed values. Patients with a previously implanted pacemaker or defibrillator systems may require adjustment of the device to patient-specific settings prior to a surgery, test, or procedure. The device system data is interrogated to evaluate the battery, leads, and sensors, as well as the stored patient and system measurements. If necessary, the device is programmed to settings appropriate for the surgery, test, or procedure. A postprocedure evaluation and programming may also be performed, with adjustments as required. Report 93286 for evaluation of a single-, dual-, or multiple-lead implantable pacemaker system or leadless pacemaker system. Report 93287 for evaluation of a single-, dual-, or multiple-lead implantable defibrillator system. Both codes include physician or other qualified health care professional analysis, review, and report.

93288-93292 [93261]

Patients with a previously implanted device, such as a cardiac pacemaker, implantable cardioverter-defibrillator (ICD), implantable cardiovascular monitor (ICM), or implantable loop recorder (ILR), require periodic interrogation device evaluations. This diagnostic procedure includes a face-to-face assessment of all device functions. Components that must be evaluated to assign 93288 include the battery, lead(s), capture and sensing function, heart rhythm, and programmed parameters of a single-, dual-, or multiple-lead pacemaker system. Code 93289 requires evaluation of the battery, lead(s), capture and sensing function, heart rhythm derived elements, presence or absence of therapy for ventricular tachyarrhythmias, and programmed parameters of a single-, dual-, or multiple-lead ICD system. Report 93261 for an interrogation device evaluation of an implantable subcutaneous lead defibrillation system. Code 93290 requires analysis of at least one recorded physiologic cardiovascular data element obtained from internal or external sensors and evaluation of programmed parameters of an ICM. Code 93291 requires evaluation of heart rate and rhythm during recorded episodes (from both patient-initiated and device algorithm detected events), as well as evaluation of programmed parameters of an ILR. Report 93292 for an interrogation device evaluation of a wearable defibrillation system. These codes include physician or other qualified health care professional analysis, review, and report. They also include connection, recording, and disconnection, and are assigned per procedure.

93293

Patients with previously implanted pacemakers require periodic analysis of pacemaker function. A pacemaker may be implanted to control a patient's irregular heartbeat. This code applies to transtelephonic pacemaker monitoring, a form of evaluation in which the patient sends a rhythm strip over the telephone using a transmitter. This transmission is recorded by a receiving location using a receiver/recorder. The rhythm strip is recorded with and without a magnet being applied over the pacemaker and is assessed for heart rate and rhythm, as well as atrial and ventricular capture and sensing (if observed). The pacemaker's battery status is also determined. Code 93293 may be reported for a single, dual, or multiple lead pacemaker system, and includes physician or other qualified health care professional analysis, review, and report. This code should be reported only once per 90-day period.

93294-93296

Patients with a previously implanted device, such as a cardiac pacemaker or implantable defibrillator, require periodic interrogation device evaluations. These codes report remote evaluations only and apply to single-, dual-, multiple-lead or leadless devices. Code 93294 reports the remote evaluation of a pacemaker system with interim physician or other qualified health care professional analysis, review, and report. Components that must be evaluated in order to assign this code include the battery, lead(s), capture and sensing function, heart rhythm, and programmed parameters. Code 93295 reports the remote evaluation of an implantable defibrillator system with interim physician or other qualified health care professional analysis, review, and report. Required evaluation components include the battery, lead(s), capture and sensing function, heart rhythm derived elements, presence or absence of therapy for ventricular tachyarrhythmias, and programmed parameters. Code 93296 reports the acquisition of remote data, transmission receipt and technician review, technical support, and result distribution and applies to pacemaker and defibrillator systems. Codes from this range may be reported only once per 90-day period.

93297-93298

Patients with a previously implanted device, such as an implantable cardiovascular physiologic monitor (ICM) or subcutaneous cardiac rhythm monitor system, require periodic interrogation device evaluations. These codes report remote evaluations only and may be reported once per 30-day period. Report 93297 for the remote evaluation of an ICM, which includes the analysis of at least one recorded physiologic cardiovascular data element obtained from internal or external sensors. Physician or other qualified health care professional analysis, review, and report are also included. Report 93298 for the analysis of recorded heart rhythm data; this code also includes the provider's review and report.

[93150, 93151, 93152, 93153]

Following a specified period (typically one month to permit lead maturation and healing) after the patient undergoes insertion of a phrenic nerve stimulator system for the treatment of moderate to severe central sleep apnea, therapy initiation is undertaken. The system consists of a pulse generator much like a pacemaker, a stimulation electrode, and, when appropriate, a sensing electrode. Respiration sensing is accomplished by the electrodes determining the patient's position at rest/activity to allow for programming of applicable delivery times. This unit assists stable breathing by preventing episodes of apnea followed by rapid breathing. During activation, the device is programmed to automatically begin when the patient is at rest during normal hours of sleep, in a sleeping position, and after lead impedance is measured. Individualized settings, such as therapy start/stop times and stimulation parameters, are determined by testing performed in the office, interviews with the patient about sleep habits, and monitoring the patient's response to overnight stimulation if necessary. Report 93150 for therapy activation of the phrenic nerve stimulator system; this includes all interrogation and programming. Report 93151 for interrogation and programming of at least one parameter of the system; 93152 when interrogation and programming is performed during polysomnography; and 93153 when interrogation of the system is performed without programming.

93303

Transducers are placed on the patient's chest to record an echocardiograph, which uses ultrasound to visualize the heart's function, blood flow, valves, and chambers. This code applies to an evaluation for congenital defects.

93304

Transducers are placed on a patient's chest to record an echocardiograph, which uses ultrasound to visualize the heart's function, blood flow, valves, and chambers. This code applies to a follow-up or a limited evaluation for congenital defects.

93306-93308

This is a noninvasive study that uses ultrasound to visualize the heart's function, blood flow, valves, and chambers. Two-dimensional echocardiography, also referred to as real-time imaging, is performed using multiple transducers or a rotating transducer, and these images are recorded on videotape. Computer reconstruction provides the two-dimensional image of specific planes of the heart. M-mode, when performed, provides additional detail of specific portions of the heart. A stationary ultrasound beam is directed at the area of the heart requiring additional study. Report 93306 for a complete evaluation that includes spectral and color flow Doppler, which provide information regarding intracardiac blood flow and hemodynamics. Report 93307 for a complete evaluation but without spectral or color flow Doppler. Report 93308 for a follow-up or limited study.

93312-93314

Transesophageal echocardiography (TEE) is an invasive technique whereby the transducer is placed at the tip of an endoscope and introduced into the patient's esophagus to record a two-dimensional echocardiograph. This set of codes should be used for TEE used to diagnose cardiac sources of emboli, prosthetic heart valve malfunction, endocarditis, aortic dissection, cardiac tumors, and valvular heart disease excluding congenital heart disease. Code 93312 applies to a complete evaluation including probe placement, image acquisition, and the physician's interpretation. Report 93313 for probe placement only.

Report 93314 for image acquisition, physician interpretation, and report only.

93315-93317
Transesophageal echocardiography (TEE) is an invasive technique whereby the transducer is placed at the tip of an endoscope and introduced into the patient's esophagus to record a two-dimensional echocardiograph. This set of codes should be used for TEE used to diagnose cardiac sources of emboli, prosthetic heart valve malfunction, endocarditis, aortic dissection, cardiac tumors, and valvular heart disease excluding congenital heart disease. The set of codes is specific to evaluations for congenital defects. Report 93315 for a complete evaluation of congenital defects, including probe placement, image acquisition, and the physician's interpretation. Report 93316 for probe placement only. Report 93317 for image acquisition, physician interpretation, and report only.

[93319]
The physician performs 3D echocardiographic imaging/postprocessing during the same procedural episode as transesophageal or transthoracic echocardiography performed to evaluate congenital cardiac abnormalities. Cardiac structures are assessed and may include chambers and valves, interatrial or interventricular septum, or left atrial appendage. Cardiac function may also be assessed at this time.

93318
Transesophageal echocardiography (TEE) is an invasive technique whereby the transducer is placed at the tip of an endoscope and introduced into the patient's esophagus to record a two-dimensional echocardiograph. TEE provides high-quality, real-time images of the beating heart and mediastinal structures. This code reports ongoing hemodynamic monitoring using TEE. TEE may be used to monitor critically ill patients in the intensive care unit as well as patients in certain operative settings. In both the intensive care unit and the operating room, it is used to monitor cardiac function including cardiac preload, contractility, and valve function in patients with acute hemodynamic decompensation. In addition, TEE may also be used to assess and monitor mediastinal, heart, lung, and aortic injury resulting from blunt chest trauma even in patients undergoing other life-saving procedures.

93320-93321
Transducers are placed on a patient's chest to record a Doppler echocardiograph, which uses ultrasound to visualize blood flow velocity, direction, and type of flow in different locations in the heart. Doppler studies can be displayed on a strip chart or video recorder. Report 93320 for a complete evaluation and 93321 for limited or follow-up studies.

93325
The technique for Doppler color flow velocity mapping is similar to that of other echocardiographs with transducers being placed on the patient's chest to record cardiac activity. Color Doppler is two-dimensional Doppler in which the signal is encoded with color to more clearly identify flow direction. List 93325 separately in addition to the code for echocardiography (76825, 76826, 76827, 76828, 93303, 93304, 93308, 93312, 93314, 93315, 93317, 93350, and 93351).

93350-93351, 93352
Transducers are placed on a patient's chest to record a two-dimensional echocardiograph, which uses ultrasound to visualize the heart's function, blood flow, valves, and chambers. In 93350, the echocardiography is completed while the patient is at rest and exercising on a treadmill or stationary bicycle with or without medication and includes M-mode recording, when performed. Code 93351 also includes the performance of continuous electrocardiographic monitoring with supervision by the physician or other qualified health care professional. Code 93352 is assigned as an additional code to report the use of an echocardiographic contrast agent during the stress test and should not be reported more than once per stress echocardiogram. Supply of the contrast agent and/or the drugs used in pharmacologic stress are reported separately in addition to these procedure codes.

[93356]
Myocardial strain imaging, also referred to as echocardiographic strain imaging or deformation (lengthening, shortening, or thickening) imaging, was initially utilized as a feature of Doppler imaging where velocity information is regenerated into strain rate. New technology, known as speckle tracking echocardiography (STE), utilizes image-processing algorithms to track areas of interest. Used in conjunction with two-dimensional or three-dimensional echocardiography for determining the multidirectional components of left ventricular (LV) deformation, these areas contain blocks of 20 to 40 pixels that contain constant patterns referred to as speckles. These markers or fingerprints are helpful in outlining irregularities by comprehensive assessment of regional myocardial function, specifically by discriminating between active and passive myocardial wall movement. Strain rate data assists in early detection of myocardial dysfunction and is beneficial in therapeutic decisions and follow-up of previous cardiac surgery. Report 93356 in addition to applicable codes for echocardiography imaging.

93355
Transesophageal echocardiography (TEE) is an invasive technique whereby the transducer is placed at the tip of an endoscope and introduced into the patient's esophagus as guidance for procedures performed on intracardiac or other great vessels and structures. The transducer sends sound waves to the heart and collects the echoes that bounce back. These echoes become high-quality moving pictures that show up on a computer screen. TEE provides high-quality, real-time images of the beating heart and mediastinal structures. This code reports the guidance during the procedure(s), as well as measurements of the

surrounding structures. It includes probe navigation, image acquisition, and physician's interpretation and report. Diagnostic TEE is included and contrast administration, Doppler, color flow, and 3D images, when performed, are also included.

93451

The physician threads a catheter to the heart, most frequently through an introducing sheath placed percutaneously into the femoral vein. However, the physician may elect to use the subclavian, internal jugular, or antecubital vein instead. The catheter is threaded into the right atrium, through the tricuspid valve into the right ventricle, and across the pulmonary valve into the pulmonary arteries. ECG monitoring for the entirety of the procedure is included, as are intracardiac or intravascular pressure recordings, cardiac output and oxygen saturation measurements, and final evaluation and procedure report. This code applies to catheterizing the heart's right side only.

93452

The physician threads a catheter to the heart, most frequently through an introducing sheath placed percutaneously into the femoral, brachial, or axillary artery using retrograde technique. Using this technique, the catheter passes through the aortic valve into the left ventricle. Intracardiac and intravascular pressures are recorded. Left ventricular injections may be performed for left ventriculography; the physician injects dye through a previously placed catheter threaded through a central line into the left ventricle or atrium to evaluate function with fluoroscopy. Imaging supervision and interpretation, when performed, are included in this code, as is any required repositioning of catheters.

93453

This procedure is performed to evaluate both right and left heart function. To accomplish right heart catheterization, the physician threads a catheter through an introducing sheath placed percutaneously into the femoral, subclavian, internal jugular, or antecubital vein. The catheter is threaded into the right atrium, through the tricuspid valve into the right ventricle, and across the pulmonary valve into the pulmonary arteries. Left heart catheterization is also performed, in this case using retrograde technique. The catheter is inserted through an introducing sheath placed percutaneously into the femoral, brachial, or axillary artery. The catheter is passed through the aortic valve into the left ventricle. Intracardiac and intravascular pressures are recorded. Left ventricular injections may be performed for left ventriculography; the physician injects dye through a previously placed catheter threaded through a central line into the left ventricle or atrium to evaluate function with fluoroscopy. Imaging supervision and interpretation, when performed, are included in this code, as is any required repositioning of catheters.

93454

The physician performs a catheter placement in one or more coronary arteries for coronary angiography, without concomitant left heart catheterization. The physician places an introducer sheath in an artery, typically the femoral artery, using percutaneous puncture. The physician advances an angiography catheter through the introducer sheath into the ascending aorta and advances it, under fluoroscopic guidance, to the opening of the coronary artery. The physician injects radiopaque contrast material through the catheter into the vessel while recording a cineangiogram. The physician removes the catheter and sheath from the femoral artery. Pressure is placed on the wound for 20 to 30 minutes to stem bleeding. This code includes imaging supervision and interpretation, as well as any required repositioning of catheters.

93455

The physician performs a catheter placement in one or more coronary arteries and bypass grafts (i.e., internal mammary, free arterial venous grafts) for coronary and bypass graft angiography, without concomitant left heart catheterization. The physician places an introducer sheath in an artery, typically the femoral artery, using percutaneous puncture. The physician advances an angiography catheter through the introducer sheath into the ascending aorta and advances it, under fluoroscopic guidance, to the opening of the coronary artery or the bypass graft. The physician injects radiopaque contrast material through the catheter into the vessel while recording a cineangiogram. The physician removes the catheter and sheath from the femoral artery. Pressure is placed on the wound for 20 to 30 minutes to stem bleeding. This code includes imaging supervision and interpretation, as well as any required repositioning of catheters.

93456-93457

The physician performs a catheter placement in one or more coronary arteries for coronary angiography, without concomitant left heart catheterization. The physician places an introducer sheath in an artery, typically the femoral artery, using percutaneous puncture. The physician advances an angiography catheter through the introducer sheath into the ascending aorta and advances it, under fluoroscopic guidance, to the opening of the coronary artery. The physician injects radiopaque contrast material through the catheter into the vessel while recording a cineangiogram. The physician removes the catheter and sheath from the femoral artery. Pressure is placed on the wound for 20 to 30 minutes to stem bleeding. These codes include imaging supervision and interpretation, as well as any required repositioning of catheters. Code 93456 includes right heart catheterization, in which the catheter is threaded into the right atrium, through the tricuspid valve into the right ventricle, and across the pulmonary valve into the pulmonary arteries. Code 93457 includes catheter placement in one or more bypass grafts for angiography, in addition to the right heart catheterization. Intracardiac or intravascular pressure recordings are included in these codes, as are cardiac output and oxygen saturation measurements, and final evaluation and procedure report.

93458-93459

The physician places a catheter into one or more coronary arteries for coronary angiography. The physician threads a catheter to the heart, most frequently through an introducing sheath placed percutaneously into the femoral, brachial, or axillary artery using retrograde technique. The catheter passes through the aortic valve into the left ventricle. Intracardiac and intravascular pressures are recorded. Left ventricular injections may be performed for left ventriculography; the physician injects dye through a previously placed catheter threaded through a central line into the left ventricle or atrium to evaluate function with fluoroscopy. Code 93459 includes catheter placement in one or more bypass grafts with bypass graft angiography. The physician removes the catheter and sheath from the femoral artery. Pressure is placed on the wound for 20 to 30 minutes to stem bleeding. These codes include imaging supervision and interpretation, as well as any required repositioning of catheters.

93460-93461

The physician places a catheter in one or more coronary arteries for coronary angiography. In 93460, right and left heart function is evaluated. To accomplish right heart catheterization, the physician threads a catheter through an introducing sheath placed percutaneously into the femoral, subclavian, internal jugular, or antecubital vein. The catheter is threaded into the right atrium, through the tricuspid valve into the right ventricle, and across the pulmonary valve into the pulmonary arteries. Left heart catheterization is also performed, in this case using retrograde technique. The catheter is inserted through an introducing sheath placed percutaneously into the femoral, brachial, or axillary artery. The catheter is passed through the aortic valve into the left ventricle. Intracardiac and intravascular pressures are recorded. Left ventricular injections may be performed for left ventriculography; the physician injects dye through a previously placed catheter threaded through a central line into the left ventricle or atrium to evaluate function with fluoroscopy. Code 93461 includes catheter placement in one or more bypass grafts for angiography. The physician removes the catheter and sheath from the femoral artery. Pressure is placed on the wound for 20 to 30 minutes to stem bleeding. These codes include imaging supervision and interpretation, as well as any required repositioning of catheters.

93462

Transseptal catheterization involves passing a catheter from the right femoral vein into the right atrium. The interatrial wall or septum is punctured and the catheter is passed into the left atrium or left ventricle. When the left atrium is accessed, the catheter may be further advanced through the mitral valve and into the left ventricle. The transapical or direct left ventricular puncture involves using a large bore needle to puncture the chest wall directly into the left ventricular cavity. These methods are used when the patient has had valve replacement and the left heart cannot be accessed any other way.

93463

The physician administers a pharmacologic agent to invoke stress on coronary vessels in order to measure blood flow through and around the heart. This produces the same result as physical exercise. Arteries become enlarged as the body increases physical activity that requires more oxygen. When plaque is present within a vessel, it does not allow for this enlargement. This slows the ability of the oxygenated blood to reach the necessary organs, which can lead to ischemia.

93464

The physician monitors a patient during physiologic exercise (e.g., stationary bicycle) to measure blood flow through and around the heart. During periods of exercise, the arteries become enlarged to allow increased blood flow to supply greater levels of oxygen to the necessary vessels and organs. When plaque is present within a vessel, it does not allow for this enlargement. The oxygenated blood's ability to reach the necessary organs is decreased, which can lead to ischemia. This study is often conducted when narrowing of a coronary artery is discovered during a cardiac catheter procedure.

93503

The physician threads a catheter to the right heart through a central intravenous line often inserted up the femoral vein to take blood samples, pressure and electrical recordings, and/or other tests. This code applies to the insertion of a flow directed catheter, such as the Swan-Ganz device, used for measuring pressure and related parameters.

93505

The physician threads a catheter to the heart through a central intravenous line often inserted up the femoral vein to take tissue samples of the heart's septum.

93563

The physician injects dye into the coronary arteries to evaluate function during congenital heart catheterization procedures. Any required repositioning of catheters or use of automatic power injectors is included in this procedure, as is imaging supervision, interpretation, and report.

93564

The physician injects dye into the coronary arteries to evaluate function during congenital heart catheterization procedures. This code is used when the physician chooses to visualize a specific aortocoronary vessel bypass graft that communicates with other coronary arteries or conduits. Any required repositioning of catheters or use of automatic power injectors is included in this procedure, as is imaging supervision, interpretation, and report.

93565-93566

The physician injects dye into the coronary arteries to evaluate function during heart catheterization procedures. Code 93565 is specific to the visualization of the left atrium or ventricle during catheterization procedures for congenital anomalies, while 93566 reports that associated with the right atrium or ventricle and may be associated with catheterization procedures for congenital or noncongenital indications. These codes do not report the introduction of catheters, but do include any required repositioning of catheters or use of automatic power injectors, as well as radiological supervision, interpretation, and report.

93567

In conjunction with congenital or noncongenital heart catheterization procedures, the physician injects dye into an area of interest to perform an aortogram. Code 93567 is specific to supravalvular ascending aortography, or the visualization of the valves just above the aorta and its branches. The physician repositions the previously placed catheter and attaches it to a power injector, making sure that air is removed from the tubing. After the catheter is positioned (using fluoroscopic guidance to confirm placement) power injection is performed to fill the aorta. Arterial pressures, electrocardiogram, and oxygen saturation are continuously monitored throughout the procedure. Upon injection completion, the injector is detached from the catheter. Note that 93567 does not report the introduction of catheters but does include any required repositioning of catheters or the use of automatic power injectors, as well as radiological supervision, interpretation, and report.

93568-93569 [93573, 93574, 93575]

The physician injects dye into the pulmonary arteries to evaluate function during congenital or noncongenital heart catheterization procedures. Code 93568 is specific to nonselective pulmonary arterial angiography, in which the catheter remains in the vessel originally punctured or advances only to the aorta, at which point dye is injected for visualization of the pulmonary arteries. The physician repositions the previously placed catheter and attaches it to a power injector, making sure that air is removed from the tubing. After the catheter is positioned (using fluoroscopic guidance to confirm placement), power injection is performed to fill the aorta. Arterial pressures, electrocardiogram, and oxygen saturation are continuously monitored throughout the procedure. Upon injection completion, the injector is detached from the catheter. Codes 93569 and 93573 are specific to selective pulmonary arterial angiography, in which the catheter is advanced from the original vessel punctured or from an artery that branches off the aorta. Report 93569 for unilateral visualization of pulmonary arteries in the left or right lung, and 93573 for bilateral visualization of the pulmonary arteries in both the left and right lungs. Report 93574 for selective pulmonary venous angiography of each distinct pulmonary vein during cardiac catheterization and 93575 for selective pulmonary angiography of major aortopulmonary collateral arteries (MAPCAs) arising off the aorta or its systemic branches during cardiac catheterization for congenital heart defects (each distinct vessel). These codes include radiological supervision, interpretation, and report.

93571-93572

The physician measures intravascular Doppler velocity and/or pressure derived fractional flow reserve (FFR) or coronary flow reserve (CFR) during a coronary angiography to determine the hemodynamic significance of a lesion. A guidewire is passed through the coronary vessel or graft, and the baseline flow is measured distal to the lesion. Pharmacologic stress is induced with a bolus or infusion of a radiopharmaceutical agent such as adenosine; velocity blood flow measurements are taken and/or the FFR or CFR is calculated. The guidewire is repositioned in an unaffected artery and measurements are repeated for comparison. Report 93571 for Doppler measurements of the initial vessel; this is an add-on code to be reported with the appropriate primary procedure for the coronary or bypass graft diagnostic or interventional service. Report 93572 for each additional vessel.

93580

A congenital atrial septal defect is closed percutaneously by catheter. This procedure may be performed on infants or adults, usually under moderate sedation. After heparinization in induced, a combined right and left heart catheterization is first undertaken through the existing septal opening. Contrast material is injected for atrial and ventricular angiograms to map the anatomy. Using a specialized catheter, the atrial defect is crossed from the right atrium into the left. The catheter is threaded into the upper left pulmonary vein. A guidewire is inserted, the catheter is removed, and a balloon is threaded over the guidewire into position across the defect and inflated with low pressure. The "stretched" diameter of the defect is measured. Testing is carried out to ensure that the repair will remain hemodynamically stable by occluding the defect temporarily with the balloon while taking right-side pressures and saturation measurements. A dilator and sheath holding the device are advanced over the guidewire and positioned in the left atrium. Positioning is checked using echocardiography or fluoroscopy before releasing the device. The implant is deployed across the atrial opening and positioning is checked again. Any leaks, abnormal placement, or an improperly sized device may require removal of the implant and placement of a second device. The catheters and guidewires are removed.

93581

A congenital ventricular septal defect is closed percutaneously by catheter. The patient is given local anesthesia and the femoral artery and vein are cannulated. A guidewire and catheter are inserted and

Medicine

advanced through the ventricular septum, into the right ventricle, and across the tricuspid valve into the right atrium. A separate venous sheath is placed in the jugular vein to allow passage of a snare catheter. The snare is advanced into the atrium and grasps the free wire or catheter that was threaded through the ventricular septal defect. This provides a through-and-through from the femoral vein to the ventricular septal defect and out the jugular. The jugular end is used to pass a dilator and sheath over the defect for the positioning of the occlusive device into the left ventricle. The sheath must be in the exact position with its tip in the left ventricle for delivery of the occlusive device. If necessary, traction is used at the opposite end to secure the sheath as the dilator is removed. If the sheath is displaced during removal of the dilator, the dilator is reinserted for correct positioning. Once the sheath is in place and the dilator removed, the delivery catheter loaded with an occlusive device is advanced to the center of the right atrium. The device is advanced out of the delivery catheter and into the tip of the sheath. It is gently advanced so that the distal legs are in the left ventricle and the center of the device is in the defect. A slight withdrawing of the sheath causes the distal legs to open within the left ventricle. Further withdrawal of the sheath allows the proximal legs to open in the right ventricle. The occlusion is confirmed with angiography and the delivery system and catheters are removed.

Medicine

93582

A patent ductus arteriosus (PDA) is closed using a transcatheter technique. A small incision is made in an extremity artery (usually the femoral artery). The physician threads a catheter through the arteries and heart to the PDA. A coil or other occlusion device is deployed into the PDA via the catheter. An angiography may be performed to check for patency of the closure device. The catheter is removed and the incision is closed.

93583

Septal reduction therapy, also known as alcohol septal ablation (ASA), is performed to decrease the size of the cardiac septal muscle in patients with hypertrophic cardiomyopathy. A small incision is made in an extremity artery (usually the femoral artery). A catheter is threaded through the arteries to the heart and a coronary angiography is performed to locate the first septal perforator branch of the left anterior descending (LAD) artery. A balloon is inflated within the perforator and contrast is injected to ensure no flow back into the LAD. A slow injection of absolute alcohol is performed until a partial initial response is rendered. The balloon is deflated and an additional coronary angiogram is performed to ensure patency of the LAD. The catheters are removed and the incision is closed.

93590-93592

Percutaneous transcatheter closure of a paravalvular leak (PVL) in the mitral or aortic valve can be achieved by antegrade or retrograde approach. A transesophageal echocardiogram (TEE) for a mitral valve leak or a transthoracic echocardiogram (TTE) for an aortic leak was performed within the previous six months, earlier if the patient was symptomatic. A retrograde transfemoral approach is performed utilizing a catheter and guidewire. Upon crossing the leak, the wire is removed and a stiff wire is inserted along with the device delivery system consisting of a guide catheter or sheath. The wire is removed allowing for advancement and deployment of an occlusion device. In cases where support becomes an issue, a transseptal access and snare may be employed to establish a rail. This entails the snaring of the initial wire within the left atrium or the formation of an apical ventricular rail by left ventricular puncture with the wire crossing the apex. In mitral PVL, if this approach does not achieve the desired results, an antegrade transseptal approach may be used. Upon completion of the procedure for 93590, TEE should indicate fluent leaflets, clear pulmonary veins, and if anterior leak, clear mitral valve. In 93591, the physician must evaluate that the coronary ostia is not covered and leaflets are fluent. For both procedures, the device deployed is dependent upon the defect size. Many closure devices are currently used in these procedures, such as embolization coils, double-umbrella devices, occluders, and plugs approved for other specific defects and may be suitable in most cases. However for PVLs they are limited by size, shape, specific characteristics, and features of delivery system. Report 93592 for each additional occlusion device.

93593-93594

The physician performs a right heart catheterization for congenital cardiac anomalies (regardless of patient's age). The physician investigates congenital cardiac anomalies by measuring pressures, taking blood samples for oximetry, and/or injecting contrast to assess chamber size and function. The physician places an introducer sheath in a vein (typically, the femoral vein) using percutaneous puncture. The physician places a lumen catheter through the introducer sheath into the femoral vein and advances it, under fluoroscopic guidance, to the heart chamber receiving venous circulation. The physician may use the fluid-filled catheter to record intracardiac pressures, withdraw blood samples, or inject radiopaque contrast material. The physician removes the catheter and sheath from the femoral vein. Pressure is placed on the wound for 20 to 30 minutes to stem bleeding. Report 93593 for a procedure performed on a patient with normal native connections (those in which the blood flow pathway follows the expected course through the right and left heart chambers and great vessels) and 93594 for a patient whose native connections are abnormal (those that exist when the blood flow pathway through the heart and great vessels follows alternative connections).

93595

The physician performs a left heart catheterization to evaluate a congenital heart defect. A catheter is threaded to the heart, most frequently through an introducing sheath placed percutaneously into the femoral, brachial, or axillary artery using retrograde technique. Using this technique, the catheter progresses through either normal or abnormal connections into the left ventricle or left atrium. Intracardiac and intravascular pressures are recorded. Left ventriculography or left atrial angiography may be performed and is reported separately; the physician injects dye through a previously placed catheter threaded through a central line into the left ventricle or atrium to evaluate function with fluoroscopy. Imaging guidance used to advance the catheter to the targeted area is included in this code.

93596-93597

The physician performs combined right and left heart catheterization to investigate congenital cardiac anomalies. The physician places an introducer sheath in a vein (typically, the femoral vein) using percutaneous puncture. The physician places a lumen catheter through the introducer sheath into the femoral vein and advances it, under fluoroscopic guidance, to the heart chamber receiving venous circulation. The physician places an introducer sheath in an artery (typically, the femoral artery) using percutaneous puncture. The physician places a lumen catheter through the introducer sheath into the femoral artery and advances it, under fluoroscopic guidance, through the aorta to the heart chamber providing arterial circulation. The physician may use the fluid filled catheters to record intracardiac pressures, withdraw blood samples, or inject radiopaque contrast material. The physician removes the catheters and sheaths from the femoral vessels. Pressure is placed on the wound for 20 to 30 minutes to stem bleeding. Report 93596 for a procedure performed on a patient with normal native connections (those in which the blood flow pathway follows the expected course through the right and left heart chambers and great vessels) and 93597 for a patient whose native connections are abnormal (those that exist when the blood flow pathway through the heart and great vessels follows alternative connections).

[93584, 93585, 93586, 93587, 93588]

The physician performs a venography during a separately reportable procedure to evaluate abnormalities of cardiac anatomy related to an existing congenital heart defect. Venography involves injection of a contrast dye into the venous system to visualize blood flow. An intravenous (IV) line is inserted and guided through a blood vessel, usually in the arm or hand. Contrast material is injected through the catheter into the targeted venous system. As the contrast dye circulates, real-time x-ray images (fluoroscopy) are continuously captured. Acquired images are analyzed to evaluate the area of the congenital heart defect for anatomical abnormalities. The catheter is removed, and pressure is applied to the insertion site to minimize bleeding. Report 93584 for venography involving an anomalous or persistent superior vena cava when it exists as a second contralateral superior vena cava, with native drainage to the heart; 93585 for the azygos/hemiazygos venous system; 93586 for the coronary sinus; 93587 for the venovenous collaterals originating at or above the heart, such as from the innominate vein; and 93588 for the venovenous collaterals originating below the heart, such as from the inferior vena cava. Catheter placement and radiological supervision and interpretation are included in these codes. These are add-on codes and are reported in addition to the primary procedure.

93598

Indicator dilution studies use a technique based on the principle that the volume of a fluid within a container can be determined by adding a known quantity of an indicator to the fluid and measuring the concentration of the indicator after it has completely mixed with the fluid. A time-concentration curve arises and the area of the inscribed curve is calculated. The physician threads a catheter through a central line leading to the heart and dye, such as nontoxic, water-soluble indocyanine green, or a thermal indicator, usually iced saline, is injected. In the thermodilution method, cardiac output is measured by a computer using an equation that incorporates body temperature, injection volume and temperature, time, and other calculated ratios over a denominator of the integral of the change in blood temperature during the cold injection, reflected by the area of the inscribed curve. This procedure is performed during a cardiac catheterization for the evaluation of congenital heart defects.

93600

The physician places a venous sheath, usually in a femoral vein, using standard techniques. The physician advances an electrical catheter through the venous sheath and into the right heart under fluoroscopic guidance. The physician attaches the catheter to an electrical recording device to allow depiction of the intracardiac electrograms obtained from electrodes on the catheter tip. The physician moves the catheter tip to the bundle of His, on the anteroseptal tricuspid annulus, and obtains recordings. Alternatively, the physician may obtain similar recordings by placing a catheter into the left ventricular outflow tract via the aorta.

93602

The physician places a venous sheath, usually in a femoral vein, using standard techniques. The physician advances an electrical catheter through the venous sheath and into the right heart under fluoroscopic guidance. The physician attaches the catheter to an electrical recording device to allow depiction of the intracardiac electrograms obtained from electrodes on the catheter tip. The physician moves the catheter tip to the right atrium and obtains recordings. The physician may obtain left atrial recordings by crossing the interatrial septum. Alternatively, the physician may obtain left atrial recordings by placing an arterial catheter into the aorta and crossing both the aortic and mitral valves in a retrograde fashion.

93603
The physician places a venous sheath, usually in a femoral vein, using standard techniques. The physician advances an electrical catheter through the venous sheath and into the right heart under fluoroscopic guidance. The physician attaches the catheter to an electrical recording device to allow depiction of the intracardiac electrograms obtained from electrodes on the catheter tip. The physician moves the catheter tip to the right ventricle and obtains recordings.

93609
The physician places an appropriate arterial or venous sheath, usually femoral, to allow access to the chamber to be mapped. The physician advances an electrical catheter through the sheath and into the appropriate chamber under fluoroscopic guidance. The physician attaches the catheter to an electrical recording device to allow depiction of the intracardiac electrograms obtained from electrodes on the catheter tip. The physician moves the catheter tip throughout the chamber to be mapped and obtains recordings. The physician compares activation times from different sites in order to identify the origin of the tachycardia.

93610
The physician places a venous sheath, usually in a femoral vein, using standard techniques. The physician advances an electrical catheter through the venous sheath and into the right heart under fluoroscopic guidance. The physician attaches the catheter to an electrical pacing device to allow transmission of pacing impulses through the catheter to the right atrium. The physician may pace the left atrium by placing the catheter in the coronary sinus or by crossing the interatrial septum. Alternatively, the physician may pace the left atrium by placing an arterial catheter into the aorta and crossing both the aortic and mitral valves in a retrograde fashion.

93612
The physician places a venous sheath using standard techniques. The physician advances an electrical catheter through the venous sheath and into the right ventricle under fluoroscopic guidance. The physician attaches the catheter to an electrical pacing device to allow transmission of pacing impulses through the catheter to the right ventricle. Alternatively, the physician may pace the left ventricle by placing the catheter in the right atrium, crossing the intra-atrial septum and mitral valve. Finally, the physician may pace the left ventricle by advancing a catheter through an arterial sheath, via the aorta, across the aortic valve into the left ventricle.

93613
Electrophysiologic studies use electric stimulation and monitoring in the diagnosis of conduction abnormalities that predispose patients to bradyarrhythmias and to determine a patient's chance of developing ventricular and supraventricular tachyarrhythmias. The physician inserts an electrode catheter percutaneously into the right subclavian vein and, under fluoroscopic guidance, positions the electrode catheter at the right ventricular apex, both for recording and stimulating the right atrium and the right ventricle. For mapping, additional electrode catheters are inserted percutaneously from the right femoral artery and advanced to the specific site to be mapped in conjunction with the primary procedure (93620). Ventricular tachycardia is induced by programmed ventricular stimulation from the right and left ventricular apexes. The earliest activation site is determined and the diastolic pressure is recorded on the endocardial activation map during the ventricular tachycardia. Intracardiac electrograms with surface electrocardiograms are simultaneously displayed and recorded on a multichannel oscilloscopic photographic recorder.

93615
The physician places electrodes into the esophagus via an oropharyngeal or nasopharyngeal route. The physician attaches the catheter to an electrical recording device to allow depiction of the esophageal electrograms obtained from electrodes on the catheter tip. The physician moves the catheter tip to the esophageal site that provides the optimal signal and obtains recordings. The physician compares the esophageal and surface electrograms to identify the mechanism of the arrhythmia.

93616
The physician measures the heart's electrical function using a catheter placed into the patient's esophagus. The recording electrode at the end of the probe measures electrical activity of the atrium by pacing with or without recording activity of the ventricle.

93618
The physician places an appropriate arterial or venous sheath, usually femoral, to allow access to the chamber to be studied. The physician advances an electrical catheter through the sheath and into the appropriate chamber under fluoroscopic guidance. The physician attaches the catheter to an electrical pacing device to allow transmission of pacing impulses through the catheter to the heart chamber of interest. The physician stimulates the heart with rapid pacing or programmed electrical stimulation until the arrhythmia is induced.

93619
The physician places three venous sheaths, usually in one or both femoral veins, using standard techniques. The physician advances three electrical catheters through the venous sheaths and into the right heart under fluoroscopic guidance. The physician attaches the three catheters to an electrical recording device to allow depiction of the intracardiac electrograms obtained from electrodes on the catheter tips. The physician moves the tips of the three catheters to the right atrium, the bundle of His, and the right ventricle and obtains recordings.

93620-93621
The electrophysiologist places three venous sheaths, usually in one or both femoral veins, using standard

techniques. Three electrical catheters are threaded through the venous sheaths and into the right heart under fluoroscopic guidance. The catheters are attached to an electrical recording device to allow depiction of the intracardiac electrograms obtained from electrodes on the catheter tips. The physician moves the tips of the catheters to the high right atrium, the bundle of His, and the right ventricle and obtains recordings. The physician then attaches the catheters to an electrical pacing device to allow transmission of pacing impulses through the catheters to the different heart chambers. The physician stimulates the heart with rapid pacing or programmed electrical stimulation in an attempt to induce an arrhythmia. Code 93621 should be reported in addition to 93620 when a fourth catheter is inserted and maneuvered to or through the coronary sinus to the left atrium for additional recording and pacing. If an additional catheter is placed in the left ventricle for pacing and recording, code 93622 should also be reported.

93622

The physician places three central venous sheaths and an arterial sheath using standard techniques. The physician advances four electrical catheters through these sheaths and into the heart under fluoroscopic guidance. The physician attaches the four catheters to an electrical recording device to allow depiction of the intracardiac electrograms obtained from electrodes on the catheter tips. The physician moves the tips of the four catheters to the right atrium, the bundle of His, the right ventricle, and the left ventricle and obtains recordings. The physician may attach the catheters to an electrical pacing device to allow transmission of pacing impulses through the catheters to the different heart chambers. The physician may stimulate the heart with rapid pacing or programmed electrical stimulation in an attempt to induce an arrhythmia.

93623

Following a comprehensive electrophysiological study with or without attempted or actual induction of an arrhythmia, before the electrode catheters are removed, an intravenous drug, such as isoproterenol, is infused. The physician attaches the catheter to an electrical pacing device to allow transmission of pacing impulses through the catheter to the heart chamber of interest. The heart is stimulated using rapid pacing or programmed electrical stimulation in an attempt to induce an arrhythmia. This code is reported in addition to the code for the primary electrophysiological procedure.

93624

Following administration of therapy (antiarrhythmic drugs, surgery, ablation, etc.), the physician places an appropriate arterial or venous sheath, usually femoral, to allow access to the chamber to be studied. Under fluoroscopic guidance, the physician advances an electrical catheter through the sheath and into the appropriate chamber. An intravenous drug, such as isoproterenol, is infused. The physician attaches the catheter to an electrical pacing device to allow transmission of pacing impulses through the catheter to the heart chamber of interest. The physician stimulates the heart with rapid pacing or programmed electrical stimulation in an attempt to induce an arrhythmia.

93631

The purpose of this procedure is to localize the site of tachycardia during open-heart surgery to allow surgical correction of the tachycardia. The physician may place pacing or mapping catheters inside the heart prior to or during surgery using a standard transvenous approach. Additionally, the surgeon will place electrical probes on the outside (epicardium) of the heart in order to allow additional mapping. The physician attaches the catheters and probes to an electrical recording device to allow depiction of the electrograms obtained from electrodes on the catheter and probe tips. The surgeon's electrical probe can be moved around the outside of the heart to allow comparison of electrical activation times from different regions. The physician may attach the catheters to an electrical pacing device to allow transmission of pacing impulses through the catheters to the different heart chambers. The physician may stimulate the heart with rapid pacing or programmed electrical stimulation in an attempt to induce an arrhythmia.

93640

The purpose of this study is to ensure that the cardioverter-defibrillator (ICD) leads are positioned well and working properly, to guarantee proper function of this device in the future. Leads are typically placed in the heart via the subclavian vein, but occasionally defibrillation patches are placed on the epicardium or under the skin. To test the leads, the physician records cardiac electrical signals from the leads and paces the heart through the leads. The physician may test the leads using the actual ICD or by hooking the leads to an external device. The physician uses the leads to pace the heart into an arrhythmia, such as ventricular tachycardia or fibrillation. The ICD or external device detects the arrhythmia and shocks the heart through the ICD leads. The physician may perform this test with several different levels of shock to ensure the ICD can reliably terminate the arrhythmia.

93641

The purpose of this study is to ensure that the cardioverter-defibrillator (ICD) and ICD leads are positioned well and working properly, to guarantee proper function of this device in the future. Leads are typically placed in the heart via the subclavian vein, but occasionally defibrillation patches are placed on the epicardium or under the skin. To test the leads, the physician records cardiac electrical signals from the leads and paces the heart through the leads. The physician attaches the leads to the ICD generator. The physician uses the ICD pulse generator to pace the heart into an arrhythmia, such as ventricular tachycardia or fibrillation. The ICD detects the arrhythmia and shocks the heart through the ICD leads. The physician may perform this test with several different levels of shock to ensure the ICD can reliably terminate the arrhythmia.

93642
The purpose of this study is to ensure that the transvenous pacing cardioverter-defibrillator (ICD) and ICD leads are positioned well and working properly, to guarantee proper function of this device in the future. The physician records cardiac electrical signals from the leads and paces the heart through the leads to determine pacing threshold. The physician uses the ICD pulse generator to pace the heart into an arrhythmia, such as ventricular tachycardia or fibrillation. The ICD detects and terminates the arrhythmia using pacing or shocking the heart through the ICD lead. The physician may reprogram the ICD's treatment parameters to optimize the device function to best treat the patient's arrhythmia.

93644
A study is performed to ensure that the subcutaneous implantable defibrillator system and leads are positioned well and working properly in order to guarantee proper function. The physician records cardiac electrical signals from the leads and paces the heart through the leads to determine pacing threshold. The physician uses the pulse generator to pace the heart into an arrhythmia, such as ventricular tachycardia or fibrillation. The system detects and terminates the arrhythmia using pacing or shocking the heart through the lead. The physician may reprogram the treatment parameters to optimize the device function to best treat the patient's arrhythmia.

93650
The purpose of this procedure is to create complete heart block, usually for control of the ventricular rate during atrial arrhythmias. The physician places a venous sheath, usually in a femoral vein, using standard techniques. The physician advances an electrical catheter through the venous sheath and into the right heart using fluoroscopic guidance. The physician attaches the catheter to an electrical recording device to allow depiction of the intracardiac electrograms obtained from electrodes on the catheter tip. The physician moves the catheter tip to the bundle of His, on the anteroseptal tricuspid annulus, and obtains recordings. Alternatively, the physician may obtain similar recordings by placing a catheter into the left ventricular outflow tract via the aorta. The physician maps the His bundle area and ablates the His bundle by sending cautery (radiofrequency) current through the catheter. The physician may also place a temporary pacing catheter in the right ventricle for this procedure.

93653
Catheter ablation is performed on dual atrioventricular nodal pathways, accessory atrioventricular connections, or other atrial foci causing supraventricular tachycardia (SVT). The physician places three venous sheaths, usually in one or both femoral veins, using standard techniques. The physician advances three electrical catheters through the venous sheaths and into the right heart under fluoroscopic guidance. The three catheters are attached to an electrical recording device to allow depiction of the intracardiac electrograms obtained from electrodes on the catheter tips. The tips of the three catheters are moved to the right atrium, the bundle of His, left atrium and atrial pacing, and the right ventricle and recordings are obtained when clinically indicated. Selective destruction (ablation) of cardiac tissue to correct the SVT is based on the recordings. This code includes the use of three-dimensional mapping software when used.

93654
Catheter ablation is performed on the cardiac tissue causing ventricular tachycardia or ectopy. The physician places three venous sheaths, usually in one or both femoral veins, using standard techniques. The physician advances three electrical catheters through the venous sheaths and into the right heart under fluoroscopic guidance. The three catheters are attached to an electrical recording device to allow depiction of the intracardiac electrograms obtained from electrodes on the catheter tips. The tips of the three catheters are moved to the right atrium, the bundle of His, left atrium and atrial pacing, and the right ventricle and recordings are obtained when clinically indicated. Left ventricle pacing and recording may also be performed. Selective destruction (ablation) of cardiac tissue to correct the tachycardia or ectopy is based on the recordings. This code includes the use of three-dimensional mapping software when used.

93655
After the initial treatment (ablation) for supraventricular or ventricular tachycardia, a postablation evaluation is performed. If there is a new (not previously diagnosed) or different mechanism causing the arrhythmia found on this evaluation, this is recorded and additional cardiac tissue is destroyed via the catheter to correct the newly discovered spontaneous or induced arrhythmia.

93656-93657
During ablation by pulmonary vein isolation, also called pulmonary vein antrum isolation (PVAI), cardiac tissue responsible for the electrical irritability that causes atrial fibrillation is found at the opening of each of the four pulmonary veins that terminate in the left atrium. The physician places three venous sheaths, usually in one or both femoral veins, using standard techniques. Three electrical catheters are advanced through the venous sheaths into the right heart under fluoroscopic guidance and the septum is punctured for access to the left atrium. The physician attaches the three catheters to an electrical recording device to allow depiction of the intracardiac electrograms obtained from electrodes on the catheter tips. The tips of the three catheters are moved to the left atrium and selective destruction (ablation) of the cardiac tissue at the opening of the pulmonary veins is performed to correct the atrial fibrillation. The three catheters may also be maneuvered to the bundle of His and the right

ventricle for pacing and to obtain recording. Report 93656 for the PVAI procedure. This code includes the use of three-dimensional mapping software when employed. Report 93657 when a postablation evaluation is performed after the initial PVAI and a new (not previously diagnosed) or different mechanism causing the atrial fibrillation is found and ablated.

93660

The purpose of this procedure is to evaluate the patient's susceptibility to neurocardiogenic syncope. The physician secures the patient to the tilt table and attaches ECG leads to the chest. The physician also attaches an intermittent blood pressure monitor. The physician tilts the table, with the patient on it, and monitors the patient's symptoms, heart rhythm, and blood pressure. The physician may infuse medication, such as isoproterenol, through a standard intravenous catheter and repeat the tilt test.

93662

During separately reportable electrophysiologic evaluation or intracardiac catheter ablation of arrhythmogenic focus, intracardiac echocardiography (ICE) is performed. ICE uses intravascular ultrasound imaging systems in the cardiac chambers providing direct endocardial visualization. A single rotating transducer that provides a 360-degree field of view in a plane transverse to the long axis of the catheter is introduced through a long vascular sheath. Access is typically via the femoral vein. The transducer is directed to various sites within the heart. During electrophysiologic evaluation, ICE is used to guide placement of mapping and stimulating catheters. During intracardiac ablation procedures, ICE allows for precise anatomic localization of the ablation catheter tip in relation to endocardial structures. Since the focus of some arrhythmias can be anatomically determined, it also allows the ablative procedure to be performed using anatomic landmarks.

93668

An exercise physiologist or nurse supervises rehabilitation exercises in a patient diagnosed with peripheral arterial disease (PAD). Rehabilitation for PAD is provided using a motorized treadmill or a track. The patient is supervised during physical exercise sessions lasting between 45 to 60 minutes in order to achieve symptom-limited claudication. The supervising provider monitors the patient's claudication threshold and other cardiovascular limitations and adjusts the level of activity in order to reduce claudication symptoms and increase exercise tolerance.

93701

Bioimpedance is a noninvasive, continuous measurement of blood flow, respiration, and other cardiopulmonary dynamics, using a patient's thorax as an impedance transducer. The health care provider attaches the patient to the bioimpedance system with solid-gel electrodes placed along the widest dimension of the thorax. The electrical bioimpedance measurement current is passed through the thorax in a direction parallel with the spine between a pair of electrodes placed on the upper neck and a pair of electrodes placed on the upper abdomen. On its way through the thorax, the measurement current seeks the shortest and the most conductive pathway. As a result, the majority of the thoracic electrical bioimpedance (TEB) measurement current flows through the thoracic aorta and superior and inferior vena. The measurement current produces a high-frequency voltage across the impedance of the thorax, sensed by two other pairs of electrodes placed at the beginning of the thorax and the end of the thorax. The sensing electrodes also detect the ECG signal. The heart rate is derived from the R-R intervals of the ECG signal.

93702

Bioimpedance spectroscopy (BIS) is an accurate, reproducible, and noninvasive method that detects alterations in extracellular fluid volume differences between the limbs using a device called an impedance plethysmograph. Skin electrodes are applied to the limb. A small alternating current is passed through the limb via these electrodes, and the impedance (opposition) to the current's flow is measured. This measurement is subsequently converted to fluid levels. Differences in extracellular fluid levels between the limbs can be an early indication of lymphedema (swelling from fluid buildup caused by inadequate functioning of the lymphatic system).

93724

Patients with previously implanted pacemakers require periodic analysis of pacemaker function. This code applies to routine electronic analysis of pacemakers used to control irregularly fast heartbeats (antitachycardial) and includes electrocardiogram, programming, tests, and physician interpretation of the tests.

93740

Temperature gradient studies assess heart or circulatory functions by contrasting temperatures of certain vessels via an intravenous catheter.

93745

The physician or other qualified health care professional performs initial set-up and programming of a wearable cardioverter-defibrillator. A wearable cardioverter-defibrillator is an external device that includes a monitor, electrodes, and an alarm contained in a vest-like garment that is worn 24 hours a day by the patient. The wearable cardioverter-defibrillator is used to detect, monitor, and treat life-threatening tachycardia and fibrillation that can lead to sudden cardiac arrest and death. The wearable cardioverter-defibrillator works by restoring a normal rhythm using low frequency shocks (cardioversion) or by returning a fast, disordered rhythm to normal rhythm by means of high-energy shock(s) (defibrillation). This code reports the initial programming of the system by the provider that includes establishing a baseline ECG. The initial set-up also includes verifying data transmission to a data repository, patient instruction on wearing the device, and patient reporting of events or problems with the device.

93750
Patients with a previously implanted ventricular assist device (VAD) require periodic interrogation of the device. Code 93750 reports a diagnostic procedure that is performed in person and includes a face-to-face assessment of all device functions. Components that must be evaluated include device parameters (alarms, drivelines, and power surges) and a review of the device function (flow/volume status, septum status, and recovery). This code includes physician or other qualified health care professional analysis, review, and report. It also includes device programming, if performed.

93770
Venous blood pressure is measured to assess heart and circulatory system functions. This code applies to the peripheral measurement.

93784-93790
A patient's ambient blood pressure is evaluated during a 24-hour period. A technician attaches the blood pressure monitor to the patient, who wears the monitor continuously for 24 hours. During this period, the device obtains blood pressure measurements and records them on automated report-generating software. Ambulatory blood pressure monitoring (ABPM) may be useful for patients with suspected masked or white coat hypertension. Report 93784 for the complete procedure, including interpretation and report. Report 93786 for the recording only. Report 93788 when a technician scans the data and generates a data summary. Report 93790 for review and interpretation of the data and a subsequent report of the findings.

93792-93793
Home and outpatient international normalized ratio (INR) monitoring is anticoagulant management of warfarin therapy, including ordering, review, and interpretation of new INR test results; patient instructions; and dosage adjustments, as appropriate. In 93792, face-to-face, clinician-directed training is started for the patient and/or caregiver for in-home INR monitoring to include proper use and care of the INR monitoring device, instructions for obtaining blood samples, and reporting INR test results. A documented determination as to the patient's and/or caregiver's ability to adequately perform testing and reporting is also required. Report 93793 for review and interpretation of a new home, office, or lab INR test result with instructions and dosage modifications, as necessary, as well as the scheduling of any additional tests, when performed.

93797-93798
Patients with severe cardiac disease, particularly those who have had myocardial infarctions, surgery on the coronary vessels, and other occlusive coronary artery diseases, often require outpatient rehabilitation. A physician or other qualified health care professional supervises outpatient cardiac rehabilitation in areas of exercise, diet, and related modalities. Report 93798 when continuous electrocardiogram monitoring is provided.

93880
The physician or an assistant performs a Duplex ultrasound scan, which is a combination of real-time and Doppler studies, of the extracranial arteries in the head and neck to evaluate vascular blood flow in relation to blockage. Ultrasound uses high frequency sound waves to provide an image. This code applies to both sides of the head and neck.

93882
The physician or an assistant performs a Duplex ultrasound scan, which is a combination of real-time and Doppler studies, of the extracranial arteries in the head and neck to evaluate vascular blood flow in relation to blockage. Ultrasound uses high frequency sound waves to provide an image. This code applies to a unilateral (one side of the head or neck) or limited study.

93886
The physician or an assistant performs a Doppler ultrasound scan of the intracranial arteries in the head and neck to evaluate vascular blood flow in relation to blockage. This code applies to a complete study of the intracranial arteries.

93888
The physician or an assistant performs a Doppler ultrasound scan of the intracranial arteries in the head and neck to evaluate vascular blood flow in relation to blockage. This code applies to a limited study of the intracranial arteries.

93892-93893
The physician performs a transcranial Doppler (TCD) study of the intracranial arteries for emboli or venous-arterial shunt detection. TCD is a noninvasive ultrasound technology used to evaluate blood flow in the major intracranial arteries. In 93892, emboli detection without intravenous microbubble injection is performed. Intracranial circulating microemboli appear as high intensity transient signals in the TCD waveform. In 93893, venous-arterial shunt detection is performed with intravenous microbubble injection. A venous-arterial shunt is an abnormal connection between the venous and arterial systems. Gas-filled microbubbles are administered intravenously to increase the Doppler signal intensity from the blood for better visualization of the intracranial arteries.

[93896, 93897, 93898]
The physician performs a vasoreactivity study, emboli detection without intravenous microbubble injection, or venous-arterial shunt detection with intravenous microbubble injection on the same day as a complete transcranial Doppler (TCD) study. TCD is a noninvasive ultrasound technology used to evaluate blood flow in the major intracranial arteries. In 93896, the physician performs a vasoreactivity study of the intracranial arteries to identify cerebrovascular disease.

Vasoreactivity, also referred to as vasomotor reactivity, measures changes in blood flow velocity in response to a pharmacologic or other agent. TCD of the intracranial arteries is performed, and flow velocity is measured. A pharmacologic or other agent is administered, and TCD with flow velocity measurement is repeated. Changes in blood flow velocity in the intracranial arteries are compared and analyzed. In 93897, emboli detection without intravenous microbubble injection is performed. Intracranial circulating microemboli appear as high intensity transient signals in the TCD waveform. In 93898, venous-arterial shunt detection is performed with intravenous microbubble injection. A venous-arterial shunt is an abnormal connection between the venous and arterial systems. Gas-filled microbubbles are administered intravenously to increase the Doppler signal intensity from the blood for better visualization of the intracranial arteries. These are add-on codes and are reported in addition to the complete TCD study.

93895

Carotid intima media thickness (IMT) study is a noninvasive assessment performed on the common carotid artery bilaterally. The measurements of the inner two artery layers, the intima and the media, are used as risk factor indicators for atherosclerosis and coronary heart disease. This test is performed by scanning with high-resolution B mode ultrasonography and using computer enhancement and analysis to determine the thickness of the intima and media of the carotid artery. The results evaluate for any thickening or signs of anatomical changes from early atherosclerotic disease.

93922-93923

The physician or assistant physician evaluates the arteries of the arms or legs to check blood flow in relation to blockage. In one method, the physician places a transducer on each leg at a prescribed level and measures the change in blood-handling characteristics during constriction by pneumatic cuffs. The technique is similar to constriction and measuring of tension in the vascular system, but the medium may change. Report 93922 for ultrasound, plethysmography, and oxygen tension measurements in a bilateral evaluation limited to one or two levels. When a unilateral study of one to two levels is performed, report 93922 with modifier 52. This code is also applicable to a unilateral study when three or more levels are recorded or if provocative functional maneuvers are performed. Report 93923 for a complete bilateral study of three or more levels or a single-level study with provocative functional maneuvers.

93924

The physician or assistant evaluates the arteries of the legs to check blood flow in relation to blockage. This code applies to ultrasound and oxygen tension measurements in a bilateral evaluation that occurs before and after a treadmill stress test.

93925-93926

The physician or assistant evaluates the arteries of the legs bilaterally to check blood flow in relation to blockage by use of Duplex ultrasonography, which is a combination of real-time and Doppler studies. Code 93925 refers to a complete bilateral study. Code 93926 applies to studies of one leg or limited areas of both legs.

93930

A diagnostic study is performed on the upper extremity arteries or arterial bypass grafts. A duplex scan involves a two-dimensional ultrasonic scan, which provides a two-dimensional display of the structure. This procedure is a complete bilateral study and is not intended to report unilateral procedures.

93931

A diagnostic study is performed on a specific site or area of the upper extremity arteries. A duplex scan involves a two-dimensional ultrasonic scan, which provides a two-dimensional display of the structure. This reports limited or follow-up ultrasounds.

93970

The physician or assistant performs a Duplex ultrasound scan, which is a combination of real-time and Doppler studies, of the veins in the arms or legs to evaluate vascular blood flow in relation to blockage. This code applies to complete responses to compression and other tests and includes both sides.

93971

The physician or assistant performs a Duplex ultrasound scan, which is a combination of real-time and Doppler studies, of the veins in the arms or legs to evaluate vascular blood flow in relation to blockage. This code applies to complete responses to compression and other tests and includes one side or limited areas of both sides.

93975

The physician or assistant performs a Duplex ultrasound scan, which is a combination of real-time and Doppler studies, of the arteries and veins in the abdominal, pelvic, or genitorectal areas to evaluate vascular blood flow in relation to blockage. This code applies to a complete bilateral evaluation.

93976

The physician or assistant performs a Duplex ultrasound scan, which is a combination of real-time and Doppler studies, of the arteries and veins in the abdominal, pelvic, or genitorectal areas to evaluate vascular blood flow in relation to blockage. This code applies to a limited evaluation.

93978

The physician or assistant performs a Duplex ultrasound scan, which is a combination of real-time and Doppler studies, of the arteries and veins in the aorta, inferior vena cava, or iliac areas to evaluate vascular blood flow in relation to blockage. This code applies to a complete bilateral evaluation.

93979
The physician or assistant performs a Duplex ultrasound scan, which is a combination of real-time and Doppler studies, of the arteries and veins in the aorta, inferior vena cava, or iliac areas to evaluate vascular blood flow in relation to blockage. This code applies to one side or limited areas of the sides.

93980-93981
The physician performs a Duplex ultrasound scan, producing real-time images integrating B-mode two-dimensional structure with Doppler mapping or imaging of motion with time, of the arteries and veins in the penis to evaluate vascular blood flow in and out of the penis in relation to blockages. Report 93980 for a complete evaluation and 93981 for a follow-up or a limited study.

93985-93986
The physician performs a Duplex ultrasound scan, producing real-time images integrating B-mode two-dimensional structure with Doppler mapping or imaging of motion with time for preoperative assessment of vascular blood flow prior to the creation of a hemodialysis access. This assessment includes the arterial inflow and venous outflow. Native arteriovenous fistula (AVF) is the preferred vascular access for hemodialysis patients, lasting longer and having fewer complications than grafts and central venous catheters. The use of the Doppler ultrasound (DUS) in preoperative vascular mapping enables identification of vessels that are most appropriate for fistula construction. Report 93985 for a complete bilateral study and 93986 for a complete unilateral study.

93990
The physician performs a Duplex ultrasound scan, producing real-time images integrating B-mode two-dimensional structure with Doppler mapping or imaging of motion with time, of a hemodialysis access site, including the arterial inflow, body of the access site or device, and venous outflow, to evaluate vascular blood flow in relation to blockage.

94002-94004
A mechanical ventilator is applied with a mask over the nose and mouth or through a tube placed into the trachea for patients requiring help breathing due to a lung disorder. Intermittent positive pressure breathing uses positive pressure during the inspiration phase of breathing. Code 94002 applies to ventilation assistance using adjustments in volume and pressure on the initial day of treatment in a hospital to an inpatient or observation patient and 94003 is reported for ventilation assistance to a hospital inpatient or observation patient provided on subsequent days. Ventilation assistance and management provided to a nursing facility patient is reported with 94004 on a per day basis.

94005
A mechanical ventilator is applied with a mask over the nose and mouth or through a tube placed into the trachea for patients requiring help breathing due to a lung disorder. Intermittent positive pressure breathing uses positive pressure during the inspiration phase of breathing. Code 94005 reports at least 30 minutes of care plan oversight for ventilation assist and management occurring within a calendar month for a patient at home or in assisted living (domiciliary or rest home). The physician reviews lab work and other studies and orders revisions in the care plan as appropriate.

94010
A spirometer in a pulmonary lab is used to measure functions of the lungs including the amount of air contained in the lungs, the rate of expiration, and the volume of air a patient respires. The physician interprets the results of the spirometry and a graphic record is obtained.

94011-94012
A spirometer is an instrument that measures and records the volume of inhaled and exhaled air and is used to assess pulmonary function. This range of codes reports the measurement of spirometric forced expiratory flow in a patient 2 years of age or younger. Patients of this age often require sedation for testing in order to retain relaxed breathing. In one method, the child is positioned on a specialized bed. A technician places a mask over the child's mouth and nose. A loose jacket-type bag is fitted around the chest and upper abdomen. After the child takes a few breaths, the jacket bag inflates, giving the chest a gentle squeeze and forcing the air from the child's lungs. In order to measure lung size, the technician closes the upper portion of the bag and air flow through the mask is briefly discontinued. The resultant change in air pressure allows the computer to measure lung size. Report 94011 for measurements obtained without the use of bronchodilators and 94012 for those obtained before and after the use of a bronchodilator. These codes include laboratory procedures and the interpretation of test results.

94013
This code reports the measurement of lung volumes in children 2 years of age or younger. These measurements are useful in the evaluation of patients with respiratory symptoms and are typically limited to periods of sleep so that maneuvers such as face mask positioning, short occlusions of the airway, and application of an inflatable jacket can be more easily tolerated. Functional residual capacity (FRC) refers to the volume of air contained in the lung at end-tidal expiration and can be determined by gas dilution techniques or whole body plethysmography. Forced vital capacity (FVC) measures the total volume of air exhaled, and expiratory reserve volume (ERV) is the amount of additional air that can be exhaled following normal expiration. This code includes laboratory procedures and interpretation of test results.

94014-94016
A spirometer is an instrument that measures and records the volume of inhaled and exhaled air and is

used to assess pulmonary function. This range of codes is used to report a patient initiated spirometric recording up to a 30-day period. Report 94014 when the procedure includes teaching the patient how to use a spirometer, recording the volume of air exhaled and inhaled, analyzing the data, recalibrating the unit, and a physician or other qualified health care provider's analysis of the pulmonary function. Report 94015 when the procedure involves recording the data (hook-up, continued education, data transmission and capture, trend analysis, and periodic recalibration) without the provider's analysis of the pulmonary function. Report 94016 when the provider reviews and interprets the information only.

94060
A spirometer in a pulmonary lab is used to measure functions of the lungs including the amount of air contained in the lungs, the rate of expiration, and the volume of air a patient respires. The physician performs a bronchodilation responsiveness test by using spirometry completed both before and after administering a bronchodilating medicine to the patient.

94070
A spirometer in a pulmonary lab is used to measure functions of the lungs including the amount of air contained in the lungs, the rate of expiration, and the volume of air a patient respires. This code applies to spirometry conducted multiple times to evaluate bronchospasm provocation after exposing the patient to an agent, such as antigen(s), exercise, cold air, or methacholine. This test usually follows performance of 94010 where reduced airflow is indicated.

94150
This procedure measures the largest volume of air a patient can expire from his lungs. The patient's amount of air inhaled and exhaled is measured and calculated with body size to determine the capacity of the lungs. This test is important for determining the threshold of capacity needed for vitality in patients with compromised respiration. For men, this is typically four to five liters; for women, this is normally three to four liters. It is normally performed as a part of a larger procedure and should only be reported separately when performed alone.

94200
This code applies to measuring maximum breathing capacity or maximal voluntary ventilation (the largest volume of air that a patient can inhale and exhale in 60 seconds). The patient inhales to the maximum vital capacity and exhales into a spirometer. The physician measures the maximal expiratory flow at 50 percent of expired vital capacity and at 75 percent of expired vital capacity.

94375
Pulmonary function testing is performed in a pulmonary lab using helium, nitrogen open circuit, or another method to check lung functions to include residual capacity or residual volume, the volume of air remaining in the lung after a patient exhales. The physician interprets results. This code applies to measuring the respiratory flow volume loop.

94450
Pulmonary function testing is performed in a pulmonary lab using helium, nitrogen open circuit, or another method to check lung functions to include residual capacity or residual volume, the volume of air remaining in the lung after a patient exhales. The physician interprets results. This code applies to a patient's response to low amounts of oxygen.

94452-94453
The physician or other qualified health care provider performs a high altitude simulation test (HAST). This specialized type of oxygenation study is performed on individuals with pulmonary disease who have marginal oxygenation and are considering traveling by airplane and/or going on an excursion to a higher altitude. The test is performed to determine the patient's pulmonary function at higher altitudes and to determine the quantity of supplemental oxygen required for a safe trip at various altitudes. The test is performed at rest and with gradients of activity. The test includes interpretation and written report. Report 94452 if the high altitude simulation test is performed alone. Report 94453 if it is performed with supplemental oxygen titration.

94610
A catheter is inserted into a separately reported endotracheal tube placed in a newborn. The physician or other qualified health care provider administers surfactant in a single bolus or in divided doses through the catheter into the lungs of the patient. Surfactant is usually administered within minutes of birth. Surfactant is formed relatively late in the development of a fetus and is administered to premature infants to prevent or mitigate pulmonary complications.

94617 [94619]
An exercise-induced bronchospasm (EIB) test is performed to diagnose EIB based on the difference in lung function postexercise rather than on symptoms. Bronchospasm, an occurrence that happens when the lungs shrink during exercise, makes it difficult to breathe. The clinician conducts a pre- and post-spirometry test that measures the amount of air a patient inhales and how much air is being exhaled. An EIB test typically involves rapidly increasing the intensity of the exercise, such as cycling or running, over a period of about two to four minutes duration in order to have the patient reach a high rate of breathing dry air via the use of a nasal clip. Exercise is continued until the patient's heartrate is 80 to 90 percent of the predicted maximum or once the patient's breathing reaches 68, 72, or 73 (17.5 to 21 times FEV1). The patient must maintain this level for an additional four to six minutes. Studies have shown that running helps reach these targets faster than any other type of exercise. Measurement of the patient's oxygen level is by pulse oximetry. An electrocardiography (ECG, EKG) is performed to monitor the heart in 94617. Report

94619 when the test is conducted without electrocardiographic recordings.

94618-94621

In 94618, a pulmonary exercise stress test is performed to determine how much air is moving in and out of the lungs during exercise and to establish where breathing problems are occurring, since they may be in the lungs, heart, or circulation. An exercise stress test is done with the patient riding a stationary bike (ergometer) or walking on a treadmill. Heartrate, breathing, and blood pressure are monitored before beginning the exercise. Basic ventilation studies are performed with a spirometer and recording device as the patient breathes through a mouthpiece and connecting tube while a nose clip prevents nasal breathing. Measurement of the patient's oxygen level by pulse oximetry is included, as well as oxygen titration and heartrate, when performed. In 94621, cardiopulmonary exercise testing is performed. Electrodes are placed on the upper body to monitor the heart. Throughout the process, blood samples may be taken to measure oxygen uptake and carbon dioxide waste products in the blood, as well as other tests including minute ventilation and an electrocardiogram (ECG, EKG).

94625-94626

These codes report the professional services provided by the physician or other qualified health care professional for pulmonary rehabilitation performed on an outpatient basis. Report 94625 for each session performed without continuous oximetry monitoring and 94626 for each session performed with continuous oximetry monitoring.

94640

A pressurized or nonpressurized inhalation treatment is administered for therapeutic treatment of an acute obstruction of the airway, preventing the patient from taking in sufficient air on his or her own, or for sputum induction for diagnostic purposes. This is done with an aerosol generator, nebulizer, metered dose inhaler, or intermittent positive pressure breathing (IPPB) device.

94642

An antimicrobial medication called pentamidine is given in cases of pneumocystis carinii pneumonia treatment or prophylaxis in high risk groups. The patient breathes the aerosolized medication into the lungs.

94644-94645

This treatment is often called a nebulized wet aerosol (NWA). A continuous aerosol inhalation treatment is applied for an acute obstruction of the airway that prevents the patient from taking in sufficient air on his or her own. This is done employing an aerosol generator. Report 94644 for the first hour of treatment and 94645 for each additional hour.

94660

A mechanical ventilator is applied with a mask over the nose and mouth or through a tube placed into the trachea for patients requiring help breathing due to a lung disorder. Intermittent positive pressure breathing uses positive pressure during the inspiration phase of breathing. This code applies to initial evaluation or application of continuous positive airway pressure for ventilation assistance with positive pressure during inspiration and exhalation.

94662

A mechanical ventilator is applied with a mask over the nose and mouth or through a tube placed into the trachea for patients requiring help breathing due to a lung disorder. Intermittent negative pressure breathing uses negative pressure during the inspiration phase of breathing. This code applies to subsequent evaluation or application of continuous negative airway pressure for ventilation assistance with negative pressure during inspiration and exhalation.

94664

A demonstration is done for the patient on how to use an aerosol generator, nebulizer, metered dose inhaler, or intermittent positive pressure breathing device (IPPB) and/or the patient's utilization is evaluated.

94667

A respiratory therapist supervised by a physician manipulates the chest wall (cupping, vibration, and percussion) to mobilize secretions and improve breathing for some lung disorders. This code applies to initial evaluation and treatment.

94668

A respiratory therapist supervised by a physician manipulates the chest wall (cupping, vibration, and percussion) to mobilize secretions and improve breathing for some lung disorders. This code applies to subsequent evaluation and treatment.

94669

Mechanical percussion techniques help to clear mucus in the tracheobronchial passages in patients who cannot clear their airways themselves due to a disease process such as cystic fibrosis, emphysema, asthma, etc. An oscillation device is applied to the patient's chest. The device may be a vest or a belt. Pneumatically driven air, mechanical vibrators, and/or direct mechanical compression are applied to the chest wall via the device. Treatment results in an increased expulsion of mucus from the bronchioles and clearing of the airways.

94680-94690

Pulmonary testing is performed to measure the function of the lungs. Code 94680 applies to collecting expired air and evaluating oxygen uptake using direct methods during rest and exercise. Code 94681 applies to collecting expired air and evaluating oxygen uptake, carbon dioxide output, and percentage oxygen extracted. Code 94690 is used to report the collection of expired air and evaluation of oxygen uptake using indirect methods during rest.

94726-94729
Pulmonary function testing of the lungs' volume, airway resistance, and diffusing capacity is performed in multiple ways. In 94726, the lung volume and possibly the airway resistance are evaluated using a variety of methods. In the oldest method, the patient is enclosed in a pressurized small room and the volume of air and air resistance are measured as the patient breathes. In a newer method, two belts with sensors are wrapped around the patient at the rib cage and the abdomen to measure the lung volumes, referred to as respiratory inductance plethysmography. In 94727, lung volumes are tested in a pulmonary lab using helium, nitrogen open circuit, or another method to check lung functions to include residual capacity or residual volume, the volume of air remaining in the lung after a patient exhales. The physician interprets the results. This code applies to the distribution of inspired gas using multiple breath nitrogen washout curves and including alveolar nitrogen or helium equilibration time. In 94728, airway resistance is tested by oscillometry. In one method, the patient breathes into an apparatus called a pneumotachograph. This device uses soundwaves to detect and analyze airway changes. Code 94728 may be reported in addition to gas dilution techniques. In 94729, diffusing capacity is tested. In this test, the patient takes a deep breath, holds it for 10 seconds, and releases the first half. The second half is collected and analyzed for the amount of carbon dioxide it contains.

94760-94762
A sensor is placed on the earlobe or finger to measure oxygen levels in the blood for a pulse oximetry. A light shines through the capillary bed for the measurement. Report 94760 for a single measurement; 94761 for multiple measurements; and 94762 for a continuous overnight measurement.

94772
A pulmonary lab assistant performs pulmonary function testing to measure various aspects of the lungs. A physician interprets the report. This code applies to measuring the circadian respiratory pattern of an infant over a 12- to 24-hour period (pediatric pneumogram).

94774-94777
These codes report clinical services provided for a 30-day period to a pediatric patient who is using an apnea monitor. An apnea monitor is a device designed to detect cessation of breathing, directly through measurement of respiration and/or indirectly through monitoring of physiological signs such as heart rate, pulse, or blood oxygen concentration. Devices typically feature visual and audio alarm systems. Some may provide remote alarm systems, programmed software, or a monitor. An internal and/or hard copy recording system may also be featured. Report 94774 when the service includes hookup, initiation of recording, and disconnection in addition to a report by a physician or other qualified health care provider who reviews the accumulated data; 94775 when the service includes only hookup, initiation of recording, and disconnection; 94776 when only the data is transmitted, downloaded, and analyzed by computer; and 94777 when the provider reviews and reports upon the accumulated data only.

94780-94781
A hospital professional trained in car seat/bed safety and positioning, as well as monitoring for apnea, bradycardia, and oxygen saturations, observes a newborn patient to ensure that a pediatric patient, up to 12 months old, does not have a cardiac or respiratory event. This type of event occurs most often in preterm or low birth weight infants, infants born with hypotonia (e.g., Down syndrome), or infants who undergo congenital cardiac surgery. The newborn is placed in the car seat/bed at a 45-degree angle with the harness clip at chest level. The infant is attached to a monitor that assesses heartrate, respiratory rate, and oxygen saturation. Obstructive apnea monitoring may be performed as well. The infant is constantly observed by clinical staff for 60 to 120 minutes or the amount of time the baby will be in transport home, whichever is longer. This procedure includes the interpretation, recording, and report of the findings. Report 94780 for the first 60 minutes and 94781 for each additional full 30 minutes.

95004
A physician or other qualified health care provider scratches, punctures, or pricks the skin to introduce specific allergy extracts to determine a patient's allergies. The immediate skin reaction is documented. This code includes test interpretation and provider report.

95012
A patient's nitric oxide (NO) level is measured using specialized equipment and under the direct supervision of a clinician. The patient is instructed to exhale, place the testing device in the mouth, and inhale to lung capacity. The clinician monitors the patient to ensure that a steady compliance inhalation and exhalation are performed. The process is repeated and the patient's NO level is determined by the device, which uses the sensitivity of a chemiluminescence gas analyzer and integrated software to measure NO molecules at very low concentrations. This test is commonly used for patients with asthma or other respiratory disorders.

95017-95018
A physician or other qualified health care provider uses any combination of scratches, punctures, pricks, or intradermal injections to determine a patient's allergies. The immediate skin reaction is documented. This code includes the provider's test interpretation and report. The number of tests should be specified. Report 95017 if the allergen being tested is insect venom. Report 95018 if the allergen being tested is drugs or biologicals.

95024
A physician or other qualified health care provider injects suspected allergenic substances into the skin to determine the patient's specific allergies. The immediate skin reaction is documented. This code includes test interpretation and provider report.

95027
A physician or other qualified health care provider uses intracutaneous tests, sequential and incremental, with allergenic extracts for airborne allergens, immediate type reaction, to determine a patient's specific allergies. The number of tests must be specified. This code includes test interpretation and provider report.

95028
A physician injects suspected allergenic substances into a patient to determine the patient's specific allergies. The delayed skin reaction is documented.

95044
A physician applies a patch containing specific allergenic substances to a patient's arm to determine the patient's specific allergies. The reaction is documented.

95052
A physician applies a patch containing specific allergenic substances to a patient's arm and exposes the area to ultraviolet light to determine a patient's specific allergies. The reaction is documented.

95056
A physician exposes an area of the patient's skin to ultraviolet light to determine the patient's allergic reactions. The reaction is documented.

95060
A physician introduces specific allergy extracts to the patient's eye mucus membranes to determine the patient's specific allergic reactions. The reaction is documented.

95065
A physician introduces specific allergy extracts to the patient's mucus membrane in the nose to determine the patient's specific allergic reactions. The reaction is documented.

95070
A physician has the patient inhale histamines, methacholine, or other similar medications in a bronchial provocation test in order to assess airway responsiveness and determine the patient's specific allergens. The reaction is documented.

95076-95079
The physician has a patient ingest specific substances, such as food or drugs, to determine the patient's specific allergies. The reaction is documented. Report 95076 for the first 120 minutes of testing. Report 95079 for each additional 60 minutes of testing.

95115
The health care provider injects small but increasing dosages of a substance to which the patient is allergic for desensitization. This code applies to a single injection of the allergen and does not include the provision of the substance.

95117
The health care provider injects small but increasing dosages of a substance to which the patient is allergic for desensitization. This code applies to two or more injections of the allergen and does not include the provision of the substance.

95120-95125
A physician or other qualified health care provider injects small but increasing dosages of a substance to which the patient is allergic for desensitization. Report 95120 for a single injection of the allergen. Report 95125 for two or more injections of the allergen. Both codes include the provision of the allergen.

95130-95134
A physician or other qualified health care provider injects small but increasing dosages of stinging insect venom to which the patient is allergic for desensitization. Report 95130 for a single venom; 95131 for two venoms; 95132 for three venoms; 95133 for four venoms; and 95134 for five venoms.

95144
This code reports the allergist's preparation and supply of an antigen extract for allergen immunotherapy in a single dosage vial. The antigen is to be administered by another physician. Single dose vials contain one dose to be administered in a single injection.

95145-95170
These codes report the physician's preparation of an antigen for allergen immunotherapy and the provision of the antigen extract itself. These codes also include the providing physician's calculations for the concentration and volume to be used in the dosage based upon the patient's previous skin test results and personal history. These codes do not, however, include the administration of the allergen therapy. The number of doses must be specified and the vial(s) (series of vials from a treatment board or one multiple dose vial) from which the dose may be drawn is irrelevant. Report the code based on the type of antigen prepared. Report 95145 for a dose containing one single stinging insect venom, 95146 for an extract containing two single stinging insect venoms, 95147 for three, 95148 for four, and 95149 for five single stinging insect venoms in one dose extract. Code 95165 reports single or multiple antigens (not stinging insect), and 95170 is for a whole-body extract of a biting insect or other arthropod.

95180
The physician administers small but increasing dosages of a substance that causes the patient's allergic reaction to become less sensitized and thereby develop the patient's tolerance to the substance. This code applies to each hour spent in performing a rapid desensitization procedure to a medication such as insulin, penicillin, or horse serum.

95250-95251 [95249]
The physician or other qualified health care professional monitors glucose levels by continuous recording and storage of glucose values. In 95250, monitoring is performed with a clinician-provided invasive device that monitors glucose levels by insertion of a sensor in the subcutaneous tissue in the lower abdomen or other area. The sensor measures the change in intracellular fluid (ICF) and sends the information from the sensor to a small monitor that stores the data for a minimum of 72 hours. The time intervals at which interstitial glucose is measured are usually every five minutes. After the patient has worn the sensor for a minimum of 72 hours, it is removed and the data from the monitor is downloaded into a computer. Specialized software interprets the data and a technical report is generated. Report 95251 for interpretation and report of the data. When the equipment is furnished by the patient, report 95249.

95803
Actigraphy testing is done continuously for a minimum of three days, including recording, analysis, and interpretation, to study sleep/wake patterns and circadian rhythms. An actigraph device is attached to the patient's wrist, ankle, or trunk. The device contains a movement detector. Movement is sampled several times every second and transduced into an analog electrical form, digitized, and stored for analysis. The data are downloaded to a computer for sleep/wake analysis.

95805
Physiological parameters of a patient asleep in a lab setting are monitored for at least six hours. A physician interprets the results. This code applies to multiple sleep latency testing during periods of napping to assess sleepiness.

95806 [95800, 95801]
Unattended sleep studies are used by physicians in the diagnosis of certain patients with suspected sleep disorders. Without the attendance of a technologist, the test is performed with a portable recording device. Oxygen saturation and cardiorespiratory measurements, including heart rate, respiratory airflow, and respiratory effort (thoracoabdominal movement) are simultaneously recorded during the test reported by 95806. Report 95801 for an unattended sleep study that measures a minimum of heart rate, oxygen saturation, and respiratory analysis by airflow or peripheral arterial tone, and 95800 if these measurements also include sleep time. A physician interprets the results.

95807
Physiological parameters of a patient asleep in a lab setting are monitored for at least six hours. A physician interprets the results. This code applies to testing of several parameters, including ventilation, respiratory effort, ECG or heart rate, oxygen saturation, by a technologist.

95808
Physiological parameters of a patient of any age asleep in a lab setting are monitored for at least six hours for polysomnography studies. In contrast to sleep studies, polysomnography details measurements such as sleep staging with electroencephalogram (EEG), electrooculogram, and submental electromyogram. This code applies to sleep staging with one to three additional measurements, such as respiration, airflow, oximetry, muscle activity, vital signs, and snoring.

95810-95811 [95782, 95783]
Physiological parameters of a pediatric patient asleep in a lab setting are monitored for a minimum of six hours of polysomnography studies in patients 6 years and older or seven hours for patients younger than 6 years. The pediatric patient is attended by a technologist (95810, 95782, respectively) and may require the initiation of continuous positive airway pressure (CPAP) therapy or bilevel ventilation during the study (95811, 95783, respectively). In contrast to sleep studies, polysomnography details measurements such as sleep staging with electroencephalogram (EEG), electrooculogram, and submental electromyogram. These codes include sleep staging with four or more additional measurements, such as respiration, airflow, oximetry, muscle activity, vital signs, and snoring.

95812
Sensors are placed on a patient's head in an electroencephalogram (EEG) to measure and record the brain's electrical activity. Brain waves are captured on paper or electronic medium for study. This code applies to EEG monitoring for 41-60 minutes.

95813
Sensors are placed on a patient's head in an electroencephalogram (EEG) to measure and record the brain's electrical activity. Brainwaves are captured on paper or electronic medium for study. This code applies to EEG monitoring for 61 to 119 minutes and may include hyperventilation and/or photic stimulation.

95816
Sensors are placed on a patient's head in an electroencephalogram (EEG) to measure and record the brain's electrical activity. Brain waves are captured on paper or electronic medium for study. This code applies to a patient awake and drowsy during the EEG.

95819
Sensors are placed on a patient's head in an electroencephalogram (EEG) to measure and record the brain's electrical activity. Brain waves are captured on paper or electronic medium for study. This code applies to a patient intermittently awake and asleep during the EEG.

95822
Sensors are placed on a patient's head in an electroencephalogram (EEG) to measure and record the brain's electrical activity. Brain waves are captured on paper or electronic medium for study. This code

applies to a patient recorded in coma or sleeping during the EEG.

95824
Sensors are placed on a patient's head in an electroencephalogram (EEG) to measure and record the brain's electrical activity. Brain waves are captured on paper or electronic medium for study. This code applies to checking a patient for brain activity and determining whether the patient is brain dead. This involves evaluation by isoelectric encephalogram for a minimum of 30 minutes with no EEG change in response to sound or pain.

95830
The physician or other qualified health care professional places sensors in or near the sphenoid process. Any electroencephalographic (EEG) recording is reported separately.

[95829]
Sensors are placed directly on the brain's surface during surgery in an electrocorticogram to measure and record the brain's electrical activity. Brain waves are captured on paper or electronic medium for study in a separately reported procedure.

[95836]
Electrocorticography (ECoG) describes the intraoperative recording of the brain's electrical activity measured by an electroencephalogram (EEG) using electrode sensors placed on or in the brain. ECoG, as well as electrical stimulation, is often used as a way of indicating the precise position of functional cortical areas in the brain in patients undergoing surgery for epilepsy and can also be used post-surgery to evaluate the thoroughness of the resection procedure and/or pinpoint any remaining areas of epileptiform activity for further examination. Additionally, ECoG has been used for monitoring patients who have undergone resection of other tumors or lesions unrelated to epilepsy as a means of safeguarding the patient from clinical seizures activated by electrical stimulation post discharge from the hospital. Report 95836 only once for unattended ECoG recording, including storage for review and interpretation at a later time during a single 30-day time period. Interpretation and report is included in this service and all dates within the 30-day time period are required to be documented within the report.

95851
Testing determines active and passive range of motion for extremities and joints. This code applies to manually testing each arm or leg or sections of the spine in a separately reported procedure.

95852
Testing determines active and passive range of motion for joints of the hand. This code applies to manually testing the hands.

95857
This test for myasthenia gravis involves injecting a cholinesterase inhibitor (edrophonium chloride) intravascularly. After administration by a physician, eye muscle abnormalities markedly decrease within two minutes in individuals with myasthenia gravis.

95860-95864
Needle electromyography (EMG) records the electrical properties of muscle using an oscilloscope. Recordings, which may be amplified and heard through a loudspeaker, are made during needle insertion, with the muscle at rest, and during contraction. These codes are reported when there are no nerve conduction studies performed in conjunction with these procedures during the same day. Report 95860 when one extremity (arm or leg) is tested; 95861 for tests of two extremities; 95863 for tests of three extremities; and 95864 for tests of four extremities.

95865-95866
Needle electromyography (EMG) records the electrical properties of muscle using an oscilloscope. Recordings, which may be amplified and heard through a loudspeaker, are made during needle insertion with the muscle at rest and during contraction. Internal smooth muscle tissue in the larynx (95865) and hemidiaphragm (95866) are measured by needle placement in muscular organ tissue. Needle placement in the hemidiaphragm may be through the abdominal wall or in the 7th or 8th intercostal space. Ultrasound guidance may be used for needle placement.

95867-95868
Needle electromyography (EMG) records the electrical properties of muscle using an oscilloscope. Recordings, which may be amplified and heard through a loudspeaker, are made during needle insertion, with the muscle at rest, and during contraction. These codes are specific to the 12 nerves that emerge from or enter the cranium. These codes are reported when there are no nerve conduction studies performed in conjunction with these procedures during the same day. Report 95867 for unilateral studies and 95868 for bilateral studies.

95869-95870
Needle electromyography (EMG) records the electrical properties of thoracic paraspinal muscles, excluding T1 or T12 (95869) using an oscilloscope. Recordings, which may be amplified and heard through a loudspeaker, are made during needle insertion, with the muscle at rest, and during contraction. These codes are reported when there are no nerve conduction studies performed in conjunction with these procedures during the same day. Report 95870 for a limited study of muscles in one extremity or non-limb (axial) muscles other than thoracic paraspinal or cranial supplied muscles or sphincters.

95872
Needle electromyography (EMG) records the electrical properties of muscle using an oscilloscope. Recordings, which may be amplified and heard through a loudspeaker, are made during needle insertion, with the muscle at rest, and during contraction. This procedure uses a single fiber electrode to obtain

additional information on specific muscles, including quantitative measurement of jitter, blocking, and/or fiber density.

[95885, 95886]
Needle electromyography (EMG) records the electrical properties of muscle using an oscilloscope. Recordings, which may be amplified and heard through a loudspeaker, are made during needle insertion, with the muscle at rest, and during contraction. Report 95885 per limited study of an extremity and 95886 for a complete (five or more muscles) study of an extremity. Codes 95885-95886 can be reported for a total of four units if all extremities are tested.

[95887]
Needle electromyography (EMG) records the electrical properties of muscle using an oscilloscope. Recordings, which may be amplified and heard through a loudspeaker, are made during needle insertion, with the muscle at rest, and during contraction. This code is specific to the 12 nerves that emerge from or enter the cranium or non-extremity muscles.

95873
Chemodenervation procedures often require not only electromyographic guidance but also an electrical stimulation of the neuromuscular sites to be injected. This stimulation, coupled with the guidance procedures, increases the efficacy of the primary chemodenervation procedure by ensuring precise delivery.

95874
Needle electromyography (EMG) guidance is a component of chemodenervation procedures performed to treat spasticity and myoclonus and dystonia disorders by injection of denervation agents that block the transmission of nerve impulses to muscle tissue. The EMG guidance provides maximum efficiency in delivery of the agents to the affected neuromuscular sites.

95875
This test is useful in the differential diagnosis of metabolic causes of muscle weakness, fatigue, and cramps (e.g., disorders of glycolysis and myoadenylate deaminase) and in the diagnosis of patients complaining of muscle cramps and exercise intolerance. After inflation of a sphygmomanometer (blood pressure) cuff, an intravenous cannula is inserted and a baseline blood sample is drawn from the occluded limb. The patient is exercised and the cuff may be inflated every few seconds for two minutes or the cuff is inflated until a predetermined reading is reached and the limb is then exercised for a specific timeframe. The cuff is deflated and further blood samples are obtained at specific time intervals. These samples are sent to the lab for serum lactate analysis.

95905
Nerve testing uses sensors to measure and record nerve functions including conduction, amplitude, and latency/velocity. Nerves are stimulated with electric shocks along the course of the muscle. The time required to initiate contraction is measured and recorded. Measurements of distal latency (the time required to traverse the segment nearest the muscle) and conduction velocity (the time required for an impulse to travel a measured length of nerve) are also recorded. Code 95905 reports motor and/or sensory nerve conduction tests performed using preconfigured electrode arrays. It includes F-wave study, when performed, as well as interpretation and report. Report 95905 only once for each limb studied.

95907-95913
Three types of nerve conduction studies are represented by these codes: sensory conduction, motor conduction (with or without an F wave test), or an H-reflex test. Electrodes are placed directly over the nerve, in sensory conduction testing, or over the motor point of a specific muscle in motor conduction testing. Electrical stimulation is applied. The latency, amplitude, and conduction velocity of the stimulation are measured. Adjustments to any of the testing elements (stimulus site, recording site, ground site, filtered settings) are made to minimize unintended stimulation of adjacent nerves. A report is generated on site that interprets the numerous test results at each site tested. Each type of study is reported only once regardless of the number of times performed on the same nerve in different areas. Report 95907 for up to two studies; 95908 for three or four studies; 95909 for five or six studies; 95910 for seven or eight studies; 95911 for nine or 10 studies; 95912 for 11 or 12 studies; or 95913 for 13 or more studies.

[95940, 95941]
Continuous intraoperative neurophysiology monitoring (IONM) is performed by a qualified health care provider other than the surgeon or anesthesiologist involved in the surgical procedure. IONM may include various electrophysiologic modalities, such as electroencephalography (EEG), electromyography (EMG), and evoked potentials. The provider must be solely dedicated to monitoring the neurophysiological tests and available to intervene if necessary. Report 95940 for each set of 15 minutes that the monitoring is done from within the operating room in a one-on-one setting. Report 95941 for each hour of monitoring done from a remote or nearby location for one or more overlapping operative sessions.

95919
Pupillometry is a noninvasive diagnostic technique that has been widely employed in the evaluation of many pathological conditions, including intracranial pathology. Pupil reactivity and sensitivity may indicate neurological issues or worsening of neurological status. With the introduction of infrared hand-held cameras, the stimulation and subsequent measurement of pupil reactivity can be measured, creating a more objective and uniform assessment. A pupillometer is made of three components: the light source to stimulate the pupil, an image-capturing device capable of taking measurements of the pupil in real-time, and a data processor that performs the

calculations using the measurements. The device is held in the patient's visual field, the data is interpreted, and a report is generated. The physician or other qualified health care professional provides interpretation and report. This code reports unilateral or bilateral testing.

95921
Utilizing ECG monitoring the patient's autonomic nervous system function is evaluated by performance of at least two of the following tests; deep breathing while timing the inhalation and exhalation with recording and calculation of the longest R-R intervals of each respiration cycle for at least six cycles; recording of ECG during at least three performances of the Valsalva strain including a 30-45 second interval after the strain; or after laying supine for a period of time the patient stands and R-R interval at 15 and 30 seconds is recorded.

95922
To test the sympathetic nervous system's ability to regulate blood pressure, the physician places an electronic blood pressure monitor on the patient. The patient is placed supine and asked to perform the Valsalva maneuver (expelling air against a closed glottis) while blood pressure is checked between heartbeats. The patient is asked to cease the maneuver and is tilted using the table for at least five minutes. Beat by beat blood pressure measurements are taken and evaluated to determine the nervous system's ability to respond to the test.

95923
This test is performed to gauge the damage to the autonomic nerves serving the skin. In the Silastic sweat imprint (method of Minor), the patient lies on the stomach or back. An iodine/castor oil mixture is painted on the area to be tested and left to dry. The area is dusted with powdered starch. The physician injects pilocarpine to stimulate sweating, and remains for 20 to 30 minutes to evaluate the sweating, its amount, and distribution. As the patient sweats, the starch dissolves and reacts with the iodine to produce a dark purple color. Areas not stained indicate impaired sympathetic reactions. The patient is cleaned after the test.

95924
The parasympathetic function and the sympathetic adrenergic function are tested with at least five minutes of passive tilt on the tilt table. To test the parasympathetic function, an ECG is utilized to monitor the patient's autonomic nervous system function during at least two of the following tests: deep breathing while timing the inhalation and exhalation with recording and calculation of the longest R-R intervals of each respiration cycle for at least six cycles; recording of ECG during at least three performances of the Valsalva strain, including a 30 to 45 second interval after the strain; or after laying supine for a period of time, the patient stands and the R-R interval at 15 and 30 seconds is recorded. To test the sympathetic nervous system's ability to regulate blood pressure, the physician places an electronic blood pressure monitor on the patient. The patient is placed supine and asked to perform the Valsalva maneuver (expelling air against a closed glottis) while blood pressure is checked between heartbeats. The patient is asked to cease the maneuver and is tilted using the table for at least five minutes. Beat by beat blood pressure measurements are taken and evaluated to determine the nervous system's ability to respond to the test.

95925-95927 [95938]
The physician uses somatosensory-evoked potential to provide information about the integrity of the peripheral nerves, spinal cord, brain stem, and the cortex. Evoked potentials require low voltages and the placement of electrodes on the scalp near the parts of the nervous system where the signals are generated. The physician may place electrical stimulation at the median nerve of the wrist or the posterior tibial nerve at the ankle, or the physician may stimulate points between these and the central nervous system. Many applications may be necessary to screen background noise to measure the interval between stimulation and the generated response. Report 95925 if the upper limbs are being tested; 95926 for tests of the lower limbs; 95938 if the upper and lower limbs are being tested; and 95927 for tests of the trunk or head.

95928-95929 [95939]
The physician uses transcranial central motor evoked potential to provide information about the integrity of the peripheral nerves, spinal cord, brain stem, and the cortex. Evoked potentials require low voltages and the placement of electrodes on the scalp near the parts of the nervous system where the signals are generated. Following skin preparation with acetone, the physician places electrodes that provide electrical stimulation at selected sites on the scalp. Cutaneous electrodes are also placed at target sites. Common target sites are the finger, forearm, biceps, and/or leg. The physician uses transcranial motor stimulation to test motor response in target muscles. Responses are recorded in target muscles with surface or coaxial electrodes. Transcranial stimulation cannot target specific muscles; however, it does allow stimulation of specific muscle groups. Report 95928 if the upper limbs are being tested; 95929 for tests of the lower limbs; and 95939 for tests of the upper and lower limbs.

95930
The physician uses sensors to measure and record nerve functions such as conduction and amplitude and, in this code, for visual evoked potentials (VEP) to test the central nervous system. This code applies to the checkerboard or flash technique. Supervision and interpretation is included with this procedure.

95933
The physician uses sensors to measure and record nerve functions such as conduction and amplitude. This code applies to testing the blink reflex.

95937
The physician uses sensors to measure and record nerve functions. Muscle responses are recorded after variable rates of nerve stimuli before and after exercise or high-frequency stimuli. The tested body area is often immobilized to prevent artifacts that may impact the collected data. Electromyography is used to record waveforms that represent compound muscle action potential, which can be analyzed for amplitude and configuration change after trains of repetitive nerve stimulation.

95954
The physician or other qualified health care provider places sensors on a patient's head in an electroencephalogram (EEG) to measure and record the brain's electrical activity. This code applies to a patient stimulated by medications or physical activity.

95955
The physician places sensors on a patient's head in an electroencephalogram (EEG) to measure and record the brain's electrical activity. This code applies to an EEG during surgery exclusive of surgery to the brain.

95957
The physician places sensors on a patient's head in an electroencephalogram (EEG) to measure and record the brain's electrical activity. This code applies to computer digital analysis of an EEG as in cases of epilepsy.

95958
The physician places sensors on a patient's head in an electroencephalogram (EEG) to measure and record the brain's electrical activity. This code applies to a Wada activation test to evaluate function of the brain hemispheres.

95961-95962
Sensors record the response of electrodes placed on the brain and stimulated during surgery. The procedure maps the brain's surface to determine the focus of a seizure or other abnormality. Report 95961 for the first hour of physician or other qualified health care provider's attendance and 95962 for each additional hour.

95965-95967
Magnetoencephalography (MEG) provides functional mapping information about how the brain processes sensory stimulation by measuring the associated magnetic fields emanating from the outer surface of the brain. MEG can be used both as a tool for fundamental study of the brain and for assessing patients with specific neurological disorders. The biomagnetometer is commonly housed in a shielded room; the recording device contains magnetic detection coils continuously bathed in liquid helium to superconducting temperatures of -269 degrees Celsius. The spontaneous (95965) or evoked (95966-95967) magnetic fields emanating from the brain induce a current in these coils, which in turn produce a magnetic field in a device called a superconducting quantum interference device (SQUID), which makes images every 1/1000 of a second. MEG identifies where in the brain the electrical current is flowing in response to the stimulus. For example, MEG can be used to determine the millimeters of the brain responsible for fingertip sensation and movement, which can be crucial in surgeries involving neuroresection.

[95700]
An EEG technologist places sensors on a patient's head in an electroencephalogram (EEG) to measure and record the brain's electrical activity. This is a long-term (greater than two hours) continuous recording that captures brainwave activity. Indications include screening of critically ill patients for adverse changes, determination of location or type of seizures, distinguishing seizures from other abnormalities, monitoring of seizure/status epilepticus treatment, or evaluation of a patient's candidacy for epilepsy surgery. This code applies to a minimum eight-channel EEG and reports technical services that may include video, patient/caregiver education, setup, and takedown. Report 95700 once per recording period.

[95705, 95706, 95707]
An EEG technologist places sensors on a patient's head in an electroencephalogram (EEG) to measure and record the brain's electrical activity. This is a long-term (two to 12 hours) continuous recording that captures brainwave activity. Indications include screening of critically ill patients for adverse changes, determination of location or type of seizures, distinguishing seizures from other abnormalities, monitoring of seizure/status epilepticus treatment, or evaluation of a patient's candidacy for epilepsy surgery. No video is utilized. An EEG technologist reviews and provides written documentation of the data. Report 95705 for an unmonitored study; 95706 for a study with intermittent monitoring and maintenance (requiring performance and documentation of real-time review of data by the EEG technologist at least every two hours during the recording period); and 95707 for a study with continuous, real-time monitoring and maintenance. These codes report technical services only.

[95708, 95709, 95710]
An EEG technologist places sensors on a patient's head in an electroencephalogram (EEG) to measure and record the brain's electrical activity. These codes report each increment of 12 to 26 hours of continuous recording that captures brainwave activity. Indications include screening of critically ill patients for adverse changes, determination of location or type of seizures, distinguishing seizures from other abnormalities, monitoring of seizure/status epilepticus treatment, or evaluation of a patient's candidacy for epilepsy surgery. No video is utilized. An EEG technologist reviews and provides written documentation of the data. Report 95708 for an unmonitored study; 95709 for a study with intermittent monitoring and maintenance (requiring performance and documentation of real-time review of data by the EEG technologist at least every two hours during the

recording period); and 95710 for a study with continuous, real-time monitoring and maintenance. These codes report technical services only.

[95711, 95712, 95713]
An EEG technologist places sensors on a patient's head in an electroencephalogram (EEG) to measure and record the brain's electrical activity. This is a long-term (two to 12 hours) continuous recording that captures brainwave activity with the use of video (VEEG). Indications include screening of critically ill patients for adverse changes, determination of location or type of seizures, distinguishing seizures from other abnormalities, monitoring of seizure/status epilepticus treatment, or evaluation of a patient's candidacy for epilepsy surgery. An EEG technologist reviews and provides written documentation of the data. Report 95711 for an unmonitored study; 95712 for a study with intermittent monitoring and maintenance (requiring performance and documentation of real-time review of data by the EEG technologist at least every two hours during the recording period); and 95713 for a study with continuous, real-time monitoring and maintenance. These codes report technical services only.

[95714, 95715, 95716]
An EEG technologist places sensors on a patient's head in an electroencephalogram (EEG) to measure and record the brain's electrical activity. These codes report each increment of 12 to 26 hours of continuous recording that captures brainwave activity with the use of video (VEEG). Indications include screening of critically ill patients for adverse changes, determination of location or type of seizures, distinguishing seizures from other abnormalities, monitoring of seizure/status epilepticus treatment, or evaluation of a patient's candidacy for epilepsy surgery. An EEG technologist reviews and provides written documentation of the data. Report 95714 for an unmonitored study; 95715 for a study with intermittent monitoring and maintenance (requiring performance and documentation of real-time review of data by the EEG technologist at least every two hours during the recording period); and 95716 for a study with continuous, real-time monitoring and maintenance. These codes report technical services only.

[95717, 95718]
A physician or other qualified health care professional places sensors on a patient's head in an electroencephalogram (EEG) to measure and record the brain's electrical activity. This is a long-term (two to 12 hours) continuous recording that captures brainwave activity without the use of video in 95717 and with the use of video (VEEG) in 95718. Indications include screening of critically ill patients for adverse changes, determination of location or type of seizures, distinguishing seizures from other abnormalities, monitoring of seizure/status epilepticus treatment, or evaluation of a patient's candidacy for epilepsy surgery. The physician provides review of recorded events, an analysis of spike and seizure detection, and interpretation and report.

[95719, 95720]
A physician or other qualified health care professional places sensors on a patient's head in an electroencephalogram (EEG) to measure and record the brain's electrical activity. These codes report each increment of 12 to 26 hours of continuous recording that captures brainwave activity without the use of video in 95719 and with the use of video (VEEG) in 95720. Indications include screening of critically ill patients for adverse changes, determination of location or type of seizures, distinguishing seizures from other abnormalities, monitoring of seizure/status epilepticus treatment, or evaluation of a patient's candidacy for epilepsy surgery. The physician provides review of recorded events, an analysis of spike and seizure detection, and interpretation and report after each 24-hour period.

[95721, 95722, 95723, 95724, 95725, 95726]
A physician or other qualified health care professional places sensors on a patient's head in an electroencephalogram (EEG) to measure and record the brain's electrical activity. These codes report a complete study lasting more than 36 hours up to 60 hours without video (95721) or with diagnostic video (VEEG) (95722); greater than 60 hours up to 84 hours without video (95723) or with VEEG (95724); and greater than 84 hours without video (95725) or with VEEG (95726). Indications include screening of critically ill patients for adverse changes, determination of location or type of seizures, distinguishing seizures from other abnormalities, monitoring of seizure/status epilepticus treatment, or evaluation of a patient's candidacy for epilepsy surgery. The physician provides review of recorded events, an analysis of spike and seizure detection, and interpretation and report. The professional interpretation is made following completion and download of the entire study and a single code from this range is reported.

95970
A previously placed neurostimulator pulse generator/transmitter is tested to verify that it is functioning properly. The pulse neurostimulator may be a brain, cranial nerve, spinal cord, peripheral nerve, or sacral nerve device. Functions that may be tested include contact groups, interleaving, amplitude, pulse width, frequency (Hz), on/off cycling, burst, magnet mode, dose lockout, patient selectable parameters, responsive neurostimulation, algorithm detection, closed loop parameters, and passive parameters. This code reports testing without programming of the device.

95971
A previously placed neurostimulator pulse generator/transmitter is tested to verify that it is functioning properly. In this case, a simple spinal cord or peripheral nerve (e.g., sacral nerve) device is tested. A simple device affects only three or fewer of the following: interleaving, amplitude, pulse width, frequency (Hz),

Medicine

on/off cycling, burst, magnet mode, dose lockout, patient selectable parameters, responsive neurostimulation, algorithm detection, closed loop parameters, and passive parameters. Programming of the device by the physician or other qualified health care professional is included in this service.

95972

A previously placed neurostimulator pulse generator/ transmitter is tested to verify that it is functioning properly. In this case, a complex spinal cord or peripheral nerve (e.g., sacral nerve) device is tested. A complex device affects more than three of the following: interleaving, amplitude, pulse width, frequency (Hz), on/off cycling, burst, magnet mode, dose lockout, patient selectable parameters, responsive neurostimulation, algorithm detection, closed loop parameters, and passive parameters. Programming of the device by the physician or other qualified health care professional is included in this service.

95976-95977

A neurostimulator, a device that provides chronic electrical stimulation to the nerves of the central or peripheral nervous system, is implanted in the cranial nerve. The stimulation affects the pulse (amplitude, duration, frequency) to treat, for example, the tremors characteristic of Parkinson's disease. These codes report the electronic analysis and programming of the neurostimulator by a physician or other qualified health care professional performed in an outpatient or inpatient setting, operating suite, or surgical recovery unit. When programming is reported intraoperatively it is separate from the implantation service and may be reported by the implant surgeon or another qualified health care professional. Programming is classified into two categories: simple or complex. Simple programming describes the adjustment of three or fewer parameter(s); complex describes greater than three parameters. When counting parameters, a parameter adjusted two or more times during the course of programming is considered a single parameter. Report 95976 for simple cranial nerve neurostimulator pulse generator/transmitter programming, including nerve interface testing if applicable; for complex programming, report 95977.

[95983, 95984]

A previously placed neurostimulator pulse generator/ transmitter is tested to verify that it is functioning properly. These codes report the electronic analysis of the neurostimulator pulse generator/transmitter by a physician or other qualified health care professional performed in an outpatient or inpatient setting, operating suite, or surgical recovery unit. Some of the elements analyzed during the evaluation include, but are not limited to, contact groups, pulse width, frequency (Hz), closed loop and patient selectable parameters, and on/off cycling. All of the functions that apply may be tested initially or on subsequent occasions. Report 95983 for the first 15 minutes of face-to-face time with the clinician for analysis and programming and 95984 for each additional 15 minutes thereafter. Units of service are reached once the midpoint has passed; face-to-face time of less than eight minutes is not reported.

95980

The physician tests a gastric neurostimulator pulse generator to verify that it is functioning properly. Functions that may be tested include rate, pulse amplitude and duration, configuration of waveform, battery status, electrode selectability, output modulation, cycling, impedance, and patient measurement. This code reports intraoperative testing with programming of the device.

95981

The physician tests a previously placed gastric neurostimulator pulse generator to verify that it is functioning properly. Functions that may be tested include rate, pulse amplitude and duration, configuration of waveform, battery status, electrode selectability, output modulation, cycling, impedance, and patient measurement. This code reports subsequent testing without reprogramming of the device.

95982

The physician tests a previously placed gastric neurostimulator pulse generator to verify that it is functioning properly. Functions that may be tested include rate, pulse amplitude and duration, configuration of waveform, battery status, electrode selectability, output modulation, cycling, impedance, and patient measurement. This code reports subsequent testing with reprogramming of the device.

95990-95991

Refilling and maintenance of an implantable spinal (intrathecal, epidural) or intraventricular (brain) pump or reservoir is done. Implantable pumps or reservoirs are placed in subcutaneous pockets at appropriate sites on the body and hold a long-term supply of the drug or medication being infused into the patient. They are refilled through the skin by a needle placed into the pump device. The patient's specific pump is identified and the required volume amount is checked. The site of the implant is prepped. The refill kit is assembled and a template is positioned over the site. A needle is inserted through the template center hole and into the pump/reservoir, which is filled with more drug infusate. The pump may have electronic analysis performed, including evaluation of reservoir status, alarm status, and drug prescription status. Report 95991 when a physician or other qualified health care provider's skill is required to perform the refill and/or maintenance.

95992

Benign positional vertigo is an inner ear problem caused by crystals (canalith) floating in the fluid of the inner ear. With a change in position, these crystals may stimulate a portion of the inner ear, resulting in short periods of dizziness. The physician treats benign positional vertigo with a series of repositioning movements known as Epley or Semont maneuvers.

The patient is placed in various positions during the maneuver, which may cause temporary dizziness. A neck collar may be worn overnight to assist in keeping the head and neck in the correct position. Report 95992 once for each day of treatment.

96000-96001

Human motion analysis has several applications including biomedical and athletic performance. To conduct a biomedical analysis, patient movements are recorded, digitized, copied on computer, and processed. For example, when calculating net joint moments, the joint center is calculated using a local coordinate system created from body markers. When tracking markers in 3D using video, two or more cameras are used to identify the markers. After all parameters are found (e.g., linear acceleration, angular acceleration, ground reaction forces) and gathered using stereo X-rays or MRI techniques, the resultant net joint forces and movements can be calculated. In 3-D kinematics, joint centers are digitized for the first few frames of the sequence recorded. Linear parameters of movement can be measured to assess horizontal and vertical motion. Also, angular parameters can measure the degrees of movement of the joints to analyze specific joint motion. In 96001, while taking dynamic plantar pressure measurements, data is collected using a pressure sensor platform positioned on a walkway. The patient walks along the walkway so pressure data can be analyzed in areas of the foot (e.g., the heel, metatarsal heads, and the hallux). The peak pressure is determined in all areas and the highest pressure of all sites (i.e., peak pressure foot) is measured. Report 96004 in addition to each of these codes for physician review and interpretation of results, which includes the physician's written report.

96002

Electrodes placed on the muscle belly, parallel to the grain of the muscle fiber, detects an electrical signal that comes from active muscles (the patient is in motion during the test). The strength and pattern of the signal is seen on a computer screen and the data is collected in a software program that is able to run various analyses of the data to create useful reports regarding muscle function. For example, gait analysis allows the clinician to analyze time normal activation patterns separately for stance and swing phases between conditions or against data base values. Report 96002 for a study of one to 12 muscles. Report 96004 in addition to this code for physician review and interpretation of results, which includes the physician's written report.

96004

The physician or other qualified health care provider reviews and interprets computer-based motion analysis, dynamic plantar pressure measurements, and dynamic surface electromyography during walking or other functional activities performed using 96000, 96001, or 96002 to report the primary service.

96020

During a separately reported functional MRI (fMRI), the physician or psychologist administers a series of tests involving language, memory, cognition, movement, and sensation, and reviews the results and reports upon them in a process called functional brain mapping. These reports identify the expected versus observed locations of brain activity documented by the fMRI as the patient performs specific tasks.

96041

A trained genetic counselor performs medical genetics and genetic counseling services. Genetic counselors provide support and guidance when a patient is diagnosed with, or is at risk for, a genetic condition. This may include discussion of treatment options, reproductive decisions, or a recommendation to move forward with genetic testing. Medical and family health histories are reviewed to determine genetic traits or patterns. Counseling may include the patient and family. Report this code for each 30 minutes of total time spent by the genetic counselor on the date of the encounter.

[97151]

The physician or other qualified health care professional spends face-to-face time assessing the patient to identify any impaired social skills, communication deficits, destructive behaviors, and any additional functional limitations resulting from noted maladaptive behaviors. This service includes obtaining a detailed history relative to the patient's behavior, observation of behaviors, administration of standardized and non-standardized testing, focused interviews with the primary guardian or caregiver, and non-face-to-face time reviewing and analyzing the information, scoring/interpreting test results, and the creating a treatment plan and report. The treatment plan may include recommendations for further observational or exposure behavioral follow-up assessments and discussions, including recommendations, with the primary guardian or caregiver. Report this code for each 15 minutes of time provided by the clinician.

[97152]

A single technician administers a behavior identification supporting assessment of a patient with deficient adaptive and maladaptive behaviors or recurring actions or issues related to these behaviors such as communication or social interactions. The technician spends face-to-face time with the patient conducting the assessment, which includes exposure of the patient to a number of social and environmental elements associated with the maladaptive behaviors. Evaluation targeting certain adaptive and maladaptive behaviors includes assessing triggers, events, cues, responses, and consequences associated with the deficient behavior. This code describes assessing and analyzing functional behavior and includes other structured observations, the use of standardized and non-standardized instruments, and procedures that will assist the clinician in establishing the degree of adaptive and maladaptive behaviors or impairments of the patient. This service is performed under the direction of a physician or other qualified health care professional but who is not required to be physically onsite. Report this code for each 15 minutes of face-to-face time provided by the technician.

[97153, 97154]
In 97153, a trained technician or assistant behavior analyst conducts a face-to-face behavior therapy session to a single patient with destructive behavioral concerns, such as harming oneself, damaging property, and aggression or behaviors resulting from recurring actions or issues related to communication or social interactions. A physician or other qualified health care professional, who may or may not be present during the course of the treatment encounter, devises the treatment plan for the technician prior to the patient encounter. For face-to-face services provided to two or more patients, but no more than eight patients, report 97154. Report these codes for each 15 minutes of face-to-face time provided by the technician.

[97155]
The physician or other qualified health care provider conducts a face-to-face behavior therapy session to a single patient with destructive behavioral concerns, such as harming oneself, damaging property, and aggression or behaviors resulting from recurring actions or issues related to communication or social interactions. During the encounter, the provider solves at least one problem with the protocol and may, at the same time, coach a technician or assistant behavior analyst, guardian, and/or caregiver in how to oversee the treatment procedures (modified protocol). The patient must be present during the session, including instructions provided to the technician and/or caregiver. Report this code for each 15 minutes of face-to-face time provided by the clinician.

[97156, 97157]
In 97156, the physician or other qualified health care provider conducts a face-to-face family behavior therapy session for a single patient's guardian and/or caregiver; the patient may or may not be present. During the encounter, the provider helps the guardian and/or caregiver learn how to identify behavioral problems and how to implement treatment strategies to minimize destructive behavioral concerns. Report 97157 when the session involves multiple sets of guardians/caregivers without the patients present. These codes are reported for each 15 minutes of face-to-face time provided by the clinician.

[97158]
The physician or other qualified health care provider conducts a face-to-face group session to assist patients in improving social skills through practice, corrective feedback, and homework assignments, homing in on individual social or behavioral issues. The provider oversees individual needs and makes appropriate adjustments for the group as necessary in real time. This code is reported for groups consisting of no more than eight patients. Report this code for each 15 minutes of face-to-face time provided by the clinician.

96105
The physician or other health care professional administers tests to measure communication problems such as speech and writing in an aphasic patient. This code applies to each hour of testing.

[96125]
A qualified health care professional administers standardized cognitive performance testing to evaluate such factors as the patient's immediate, recent, and remote memory; temporal and spatial orientation; general information recall; problem-solving and abstract reasoning abilities; organizational skills; and auditory processing and retention. This code applies to each hour of testing and includes face-to-face time administering tests to the patient, as well as interpretation and preparation of the report.

96110
The physician or other health care professional performs a developmental screening, such as a developmental milestone survey or a speech and language delay screen. The screening is to determine whether the patient requires additional work up for a developmental disorder or at periodic intervals throughout infancy and adolescent years. This code includes scoring and documentation by standardized instrument.

96112-96113
The physician or other health care professional measures cognitive, motor, social, language, adaptive, and/or cognitive abilities using provider standardized tests (meeting industry standards) via written, oral, or combined format testing. This code applies to testing for developmental disorders and must include the interpretation and report on the findings or a result if generated via automation. Report 96112 for the initial hour of testing, with interpretation and report, and 96113 for each additional 30 minutes.

[96127]
The physician or other health care professional performs a brief assessment of the patient's emotions and behaviors associated with conditions such as depression or attention-deficit/hyperactivity disorder (ADHD) using an inventory or scale method. The screening is used to determine whether the patient requires additional work up or treatment. This code includes scoring and documentation by standardized instrument.

96116-96121
The physician or psychologist evaluates aspects of thinking, reasoning, and judgment to evaluate a patient's neurocognitive abilities. These codes apply to each hour of examination time and must include face-to-face time with the patient and time spent interpreting test results and preparing a report. Report 96116 for the initial hour and 96121 for each additional hour.

96130-96133
The physician or other qualified health care professional evaluates and interprets the results of psychological or neuropsychological testing. Psychological testing in written, oral, computer, or combined formats measures personality, emotions, intellectual functioning, and psychopathology. Report 96130 for the initial hour spent in the evaluation and interpretation of these tests and 96131 for each additional hour. Neuropsychological testing consists of a series of tests in thinking, reasoning, judgment, and memory to evaluate the patient's neurocognitive abilities. Report 96132 for the first hour of evaluation/interpretation and 96133 for each additional hour thereafter. Codes within this range describe the evaluation component, including combining data from different sources, interpreting test results and clinical data, decision-making, and providing a plan of treatment and report, as well as providing interactive feedback with the patient and family members or caregivers. These codes apply to each hour of evaluation and must include face-to-face time with the patient, as well as the time spent integrating and interpreting data; however, the actual test administration and scoring services are not reported by these codes.

96136-96139
A physician, other qualified health care professional, or technician administers and scores two or more psychological or neuropsychological tests by any method. Psychological testing in written, oral, computer, or combined formats measures personality, emotions, intellectual functioning, and psychopathology, while neuropsychological testing consists of a series of tests in thinking, reasoning, judgment, and memory to evaluate the patient's neurocognitive abilities. Report 96136 for the initial 30 minutes of time by a physician or other qualified health care professional and 96137 for each additional 30 minutes. When a technician performs the test administration and scoring, report 96138 for the initial 30 minutes and 96139 for each subsequent 30-minute time period. These codes do not include testing evaluation services, such as the integration of patient data or interpretation of test results.

96146
A psychological or neuropsychological test is administered via a computer providing an automated result, which is interpreted and reported by a qualified health care professional.

96156
A health behavior assessment identifies psychological, behavioral, emotional, cognitive, and relevant social factors that can prevent, treat, or manage physical health problems. The assessment must be associated with the patient's primary diagnosis, which is physical in nature, and focus on factors that could complicate the medical condition and treatment. Assessment is undertaken using a health-focused clinical interview, observation of behavior, and clinical decision-making, and includes evaluation of the patient's response to physical health problems, outlook and coping strategies, and adherence to treatment plans. Preventive medicine counseling and risk factor reduction interventions are not included. Report both health behavior assessment and reassessment with 96156.

96158-96159 [96164, 96165]
These interventional services are prescribed to modify the psychological, behavioral, emotional, cognitive, and social factors relevant to and affecting the patient's physical health problems. Each code applies to a direct, face-to-face intervention and focuses on promoting functional improvement, lessening the psychosocial and psychological obstacles to recovery, and improvement of the patient's coping skills related to the medical conditions. Report 96158 for the initial, 30-minute intervention with the individual/patient only; report 96159 for each additional 15 minutes. Report 96164 for the initial, 30-minute intervention attended by a group of two or more patients; report 96165 for each additional 15 minutes.

[96167, 96168, 96170, 96171]
These interventional services are prescribed to modify the psychological, behavioral, emotional, cognitive, and social factors relevant to and affecting the patient's physical health problems. Each code applies to a direct, face-to-face intervention and focuses on promoting functional improvement, lessening the psychosocial and psychological obstacles to recovery, and improvement of the patient's coping skills related to the medical conditions. Active patient/family engagement and participation is emphasized. Report 96167 for the initial, 30-minute intervention with the family, including the patient; report 96168 for each additional 15 minutes. Report 96170 for the initial, 30-minute intervention attended by the family without the patient's presence; report 96171 for each additional 15 minutes.

96160-96161
A provision in the Patient Protection and Affordable Care Act of 2010 (ACA) established a Medicare Wellness Visit, which included a Health Risk Assessment (HRA) and customized wellness or prevention plan. HRAs are typically completed by a patient or caregiver prior to the encounter with a physician or other qualified health care professional, but can involve the assistance of the clinician and/or staff members. The HRA tool is purposefully designed to be brief, straightforward, and easy to comprehend with questions such as patient demographic information, personal and/or family history, a self-assessment of how the patient interprets his/her health to be, risk factors, biometric measurements, and compliance. Completion of the HRA tool takes approximately 20 minutes and may be done via the internet or on a paper-based document. Assessments that emphasize a patient or caregiver focus may be referred to as HRA plus assessments and as such should be person centered and culturally appropriate in all areas, including, but not limited to, the

assessment instrument, the administration process of the assessment, clinician communication with the patient regarding findings, as well as follow up and monitoring. Additionally, the patient-focused HRA takes into consideration the importance of care support services over and above the health care system; for example, by family members, community support services, or even in the workplace setting where the individual receiving care is not deemed to be a "patient." An emphasis is also placed on cultural competency as means of limited health disparities through respect of the patient's beliefs and understanding the mental and physical ways a patient can experience illness and health and working together to establish a health plan. Another area of patient-focused care involves areas of importance to patients as consumers, such as convenience as well as increasing outcomes that matter to patients; for example, improved quality of life and function. Similarly, caregiver-focused assessment tools serve to identify areas of concern such as stress levels, depression, and the burdens placed on the caregiver. HRAs contribute to the goals of the government to drive health improvements, quality of life, and value for the health care delivery system in the United States. Report 96160 for administration of a patient-focused health risk assessment tool and 96161 for administration of a caregiver-focused assessment tool. Both codes include scoring and documentation of the assessment tool.

96202-96203

The physician or other qualified health care professional provides face-to-face behavior management or modification training to multiple sets of parents, guardians, or caregivers for the patient (who is not present). The physician trains guardians and caregivers with evidence-based strategies and procedures targeted toward the patient's mental or physical health diagnosis and adverse behaviors. The training is intended to equip guardians and caregivers with skills and methods to utilize with the patient with a goal of eliciting more positive behaviors and improved health and well-being. Behavior modification focuses on changing behavioral patterns over the long-term using different motivational methods. Report 96202 for the initial 60 minutes of face-to-face time and 96203 for each additional 15 minutes.

96360-96361

A physician or an assistant under direct physician supervision infuses a hydration solution (prepackaged fluid and electrolytes) for 31 minutes to one hour through an intravenous catheter inserted by needle into a patient's vein or by infusion through an existing indwelling intravascular access catheter or port. Report 96361 for each additional hour beyond the first hour. Intravenous infusion for hydration lasting 30 minutes or less is not reported.

96365-96368

A physician or an assistant under direct physician supervision injects or infuses a therapeutic, prophylactic (preventive), or diagnostic medication other than chemotherapy or other highly complex drugs or biologic agents via intravenous route. Infusions are administered through an intravenous catheter inserted by needle into a patient's vein or by injection or infusion through an existing indwelling intravascular access catheter or port. Report 96365 for the initial hour and 96366 for each additional hour. Report 96367 for each additional sequential infusion of a different substance or drug, up to one hour, and 96368 for each concurrent infusion of substances other than chemotherapy or other highly complex drugs or biologic agents.

96369-96371

A physician or an assistant under direct physician supervision infuses a therapeutic or prophylactic (preventive) medication other than chemotherapy or other highly complex drug or biologic agent via a subcutaneous route. Indications for subcutaneous infusion may include coma, dysphagia, nausea/vomiting, intestinal obstruction, malabsorption, or extreme weakness. Infusions are administered through a needle inserted beneath the skin; common infusion sites include the upper arm, shoulder, abdomen, and thigh. Report 96369 for infusions lasting longer than 15 minutes and up to one hour. This code includes pump set-up and the establishment of subcutaneous infusion sites. Report 96370 for each additional hour and 96371 for an additional pump set-up with the establishment of new subcutaneous infusion sites. Codes 96369 and 96371 should be reported only once per encounter.

96372-96376

The physician or an assistant under direct physician supervision administers a therapeutic, prophylactic, or diagnostic substance by subcutaneous or intramuscular injection (96372), intra-arterial injection (96373), or by push into an intravenous catheter or intravascular access device (96374 for a single or initial substance, 96375 for each additional sequential IV push of a new substance, and 96376 for each additional sequential IV push of the same substance after 30 minutes have elapsed). The push technique involves an infusion of 15 minutes or less, or one in which the physician or supervised assistant is continuously present to administer the injection and observe the patient. Code 96376 may be reported only by facilities.

96377

An on-body injector is applied by a qualified health care provider in order to deliver drug therapy at and for a specified time. The provider pierces the skin and inserts a cannula for drug delivery. The cannula is connected to the device adhered to the outside of the patient's body, typically the abdomen or arm. The device is filled with the appropriate amount of medication and programmed for dose delivery.

[96380, 96381]

These codes report the administration of a monoclonal antibody injection prepared for seasonal respiratory syncytial virus (RSV). The monoclonal antibodies (IgG) target the RSV virus, inhibiting its replication and reducing the severity and occurrence of RSV infections. It is intended for intramuscular use in neonates and infants younger than 8 months of age who are in their first RSV season and certain at-risk infants and children 8 through 19 months of age before their second RSV season. Report 96380 for administration with counseling by a physician or qualified health care professional; 96381 without counseling. These codes report the administration only and should be reported with the appropriate product code.

96401-96402
The physician or supervised assistant prepares and administers non-hormonal medication to combat diseases such as malignant neoplasms or microorganisms. These codes apply to medication injected under the skin (subcutaneous) or into a muscle (intramuscular) often in the arm or leg. Report 96402 for a hormonal medication administered to combat diseases such as malignant neoplasms or microorganisms.

96405-96406
The physician or supervised assistant prepares and administers medication to combat diseases such as malignant neoplasms or microorganisms. Report 96405 when medication is injected directly into the lesion, up to and including seven lesions. Report 96406 when more than seven lesions are treated.

96409-96411
The physician or supervised assistant prepares and administers a chemotherapeutic medication to combat malignant neoplasms or microorganisms. The drug is administered through intravenous (IV) push technique in which the physician or supervised assistant is continuously present to administer the injection and observe the patient or for an infusion of 15 minutes or less. Report 96409 for a single or the initial substance or drug given. Report 96411 for each additional substance or drug given.

96413-96415
The physician or supervised assistant prepares and administers a chemotherapeutic medication to combat malignant neoplasms or microorganisms. These codes describe infusions through catheter tubing placed in a vein. Report 96413 for a single or the initial substance given for up to one hour of service. Report 96415 for each additional hour of service beyond the initial hour.

96416
The physician or supervised assistant prepares and administers a chemotherapeutic medication to combat malignant neoplasms or microorganisms. This code applies to initiating an infusion that will take more than eight hours and requires using an implanted pump or a portable pump to infuse the medication slowly through catheter tubing placed in a vein.

96417
The physician or supervised assistant prepares and administers a chemotherapeutic medication to combat malignant neoplasms or microorganisms. This code applies to initiating a separate additional substance for infusion that is adjunct to the primary chemotherapy infusion service reported by 96413.

96420
The physician or supervised assistant prepares and administers a chemotherapeutic medication to combat malignant neoplasms or microorganisms. The drug is administered by intra-arterial push technique, in which the medication is injected in a timed fashion into the nearest port of a catheter already placed in an artery. Placement of the intra-arterial catheter itself is not included.

96422-96423
The physician or supervised assistant prepares and administers a chemotherapeutic medication to combat malignant neoplasms or microorganisms. The drug is administered through infusion technique, a method in which the medication is allowed to slowly enter the body through a catheter already in place within an artery. Report 96422 for the first hour of intra-arterial infusion and 96423 for each additional hour.

96425
The physician or supervised assistant prepares and administers a chemotherapeutic medication to combat malignant neoplasms or microorganisms. This code applies to initiating an infusion that will take more than eight hours and requires using an implanted pump or a portable pump to infuse the medication very slowly through catheter tubing placed in an artery.

96440
The physician or supervised assistant prepares and administers a chemotherapeutic medication to combat malignant neoplasms or microorganisms. This code applies to medication injected into the lung cavity through a catheter placed into the pleura.

96446
The physician or supervised assistant prepares and administers a chemotherapeutic medication to combat malignant neoplasms or microorganisms. This code applies to medication injected into the peritoneal cavity through an implanted port or catheter.

96450
The physician or supervised assistant prepares and administers a chemotherapeutic medication to combat malignant neoplasms or microorganisms. This code applies to medication injected into the spinal cord through a catheter placed through the space between the lower back bones (lumbar puncture).

96521
The physician or supervised assistant prepares and administers medication to combat diseases such as malignant neoplasms or microorganisms. This code

applies to maintaining or refilling portable pumps used for prolonged infusions.

96522
Refilling and maintenance of an implantable pump or reservoir for systemic drug delivery is done. The implantable pump or reservoir is identified and the required volume amount checked. The site of the implant is prepped. The refill kit is assembled and a template is placed over the appropriate site. A needle is inserted through a template center hole and into the pump/reservoir, which is filled with more drug infusate.

96523
The venous access device is irrigated with an anticoagulant to prevent coagulation at the catheter tip and prepped with alcohol. The anticoagulant in the tubing is withdrawn and flushed with normal saline. A measured amount of anticoagulant is instilled into the tubing.

96542
The physician or supervised assistant prepares and administers a chemotherapeutic medication to combat malignant neoplasms or microorganisms. This code applies to medication infused into the central nervous system through a catheter leading from a subcutaneous reservoir of medication in the brain's subarachnoid or intraventricular space.

96547-96548
A hyperthermic intraperitoneal chemotherapy (HIPEC) procedure is performed to treat certain abdominal malignancies, such as appendix cancer, Wilms' tumor, and soft tissue sarcomas in both pediatric and adult patients. The physician or supervised assistant prepares and administers a chemotherapeutic medication to combat malignant neoplasms. After removing visible tumors in a cytoreductive procedure that is reported separately, heated chemotherapy drugs are circulated in the abdomen to kill any remaining cancer cells. One or more separate incisions in the abdomen may be necessary for access. The incisions are closed with sutures or staples to complete the procedure. Report 96547 for the first hour of the procedure and 96548 for each additional 30 minutes.

96567, 96573-96574
In 96567, photodynamic therapy (PDT) is performed by a provider, other than a physician or other qualified health care provider, by applying a photosensitizing agent, such as 20 percent topical aminolevulinic acid HCl, directly onto the patient's lesions to treat premalignant cells, such as non-hyperkeratotic actinic keratosis and malignant cells. The patient is sent home and scheduled to return within the timeframe required for the light treatment to activate the photosensitive drug. The lesions are irradiated with a photodynamic therapy illuminator for a predetermined amount of minutes. The exposure time does not depend on the number of lesions. The blue light exposure causes a cytotoxic reaction with the topical agent that was applied to the lesions, killing the existing cells and preventing the spread of the suspect or malignant cells. Report 96573 when PDT is provided by a physician or other qualified health care provider. For debridement of premalignant hyperkeratotic lesions performed prior to PDT, report 96574. These codes are reported on a per day basis.

96570-96571
In photodynamic therapy (PDT), the physician injects the photosensitizing agent, such as a porphyrin, into the patient's bloodstream where it is absorbed by cells all over the body. The agent remains in cancer cells for a longer time than it does in normal cells. When the treated cancer cells are exposed to laser light, the photosensitizing agent absorbs the energy from light particles called photons and transfers this energy to surrounding oxygen molecules. This produces an active form of oxygen, toxic free radicals, that destroy the treated cancer cells. Light exposure must be timed so that it occurs when most of the photosensitizing agent has left healthy cells but is still present in the cancer cells. The light source used in the procedure is directed for internal application through a bronchoscope into the lungs for the treatment of lung cancer or through an endoscope into the gastrointestinal tract for the treatment of gastrointestinal tract cancer. Report 96570 for the first 30 minutes and 96571 for each additional 15 minutes. The bronchoscopy and endoscopy procedures for the lung and gastrointestinal tract are reported separately.

96900
The physician uses ultraviolet light to treat skin ailments.

96902
The physician examines by microscope hairs plucked or clipped from a patient's scalp to determine telogen and anagen counts. The physician also looks for structural hair shaft deformities. Results of the test determine if hair loss is result of short-term biological changes, malnutrition, medication, or hereditary.

96904
Whole body integumentary photography, also known as dermatoscopy, epiluminescence microscopy, and skin surface microscopy, is a noninvasive technique of collecting images of skin lesions for identifying features of malignant vs. benign skin changes. Immersion oil is first applied to the skin to remove the natural reflection of light from the skin surface and to render the outermost skin layer transparent. A stereomicroscope is used to visualize the epidermis and the dermal junction. Dermatoscopic images are also recorded, and may be reviewed with the aid of standard or digitized photographs. Digitized images allow computer-aided diagnosis as well as image enhancement for viewing a lesion's distinguishing features. Digitizing also allows the images to be stored and retrieved when following a lesion's progression over time.

96910
The physician uses photosensitive chemicals and light rays to treat skin ailments. This code applies to tar and ultraviolet B rays (Goeckerman treatment) or petrolatum and ultraviolet B rays.

96912
The physician uses photosensitive chemicals and light rays to treat skin ailments. This code applies to psoralens and ultraviolet A rays (PUVA).

96913
The physician uses photosensitive chemicals and light rays to treat skin ailments. This code applies to tar and ultraviolet B rays (Goeckerman treatment) and/or psoralens and ultraviolet A rays (PUVA) used for severe skin problems requiring between four to eight hours of care under a physician's direct supervision.

96920-96922
The physician uses a fiberoptic handpiece to deliver precise and controlled short pulses from a 308-nm excimer laser for the treatment of psoriatic skin lesions. Prior to the start of treatment, the optimal dose is determined by exposing uninvolved skin to the minimal effective amount of targeted UVB. Once this dose is established, mineral oil is applied on the lesion to enhance penetration and reduce scattering. The physician uses the fiberoptic handpiece to irradiate the lesions by using a "painting" motion. The treatment is usually painless and does not require anesthesia. Report 96920 for a total treated area less than 250 sq cm, 96921 for a total area of 250 sq cm to 500 sq cm, and 96922 for an area larger than 500 sq cm.

96931-96936
Reflectance confocal microscopy (RCM) is a unique noninvasive technique that permits examination of the skin "in vivo," or on the living patient versus from a tissue sample under a microscope, rapidly, and in "real time" at a resolution comparable to that of traditional histology. By use of a confocal microscope, near-infrared light from a diode laser is concentrated on a microscopic skin target. As light passes between cellular structures having different refraction indexes, it is naturally reflected, and this reflected light is taken and recomposed into a two-dimensional gray scale image by computer software. By adjusting the focal point on the z-axis of the microscope, images are obtained of different levels within the skin. This technology can be used as a diagnostic tool to investigate benign and malignant tumors of melanocytes and keratinocytes, as well as to study responses to treatments for conditions such as psoriasis, allergic skin reactions, and discoid lupus erythematosus. Report 96931 for image acquisition and interpretation and report, first lesion, and 96934 for each additional lesion. Report 96932 for image acquisition only, first lesion, and 96935 for each additional lesion. Report 96933 for interpretation and report only, first lesion, and 96936 for each additional lesion.

[97161, 97162, 97163, 97164]
Physical therapy evaluation (97161-97163) is a dynamic process in which the physical therapist makes clinical judgments based on data gathered during examination. Examination includes taking a comprehensive history, performing a systems review, and conducting tests and measures. The physical therapist evaluates the examination findings, establishes a physical therapy diagnosis, determines the prognosis, and develops a plan of care that includes goals and expected outcomes, interventions to be used, and anticipated plans for conclusion of care. There are three levels of physical therapy evaluation: low, moderate, and high complexity. The level of evaluation performed is dependent on the degree of clinical decision making and on the severity of the patient's condition. Severity is measured by the number of elements determined present from the following components of the evaluation: body structure and function, activity limitations, and/or participation restrictions. A physical therapy reevaluation (97164) should be reported when the physical therapist reexamines the patient to evaluate progress, and to modify or redirect intervention and/or revise anticipated goals and expected outcomes. Reexamination may be indicated more than once during a plan of care. The physical therapist conducts tests and measures and modifies the plan of care as indicated in support of the medical necessity of skilled intervention. For the purpose of a physical therapy evaluation, body systems are defined as musculoskeletal, neuromuscular, cardiovascular, pulmonary, and integumentary. Body regions are the head, neck, back, lower and upper extremities, and the trunk. A review of the musculoskeletal system comprises assessing gross symmetry, gross range of motion (ROM), gross strength, and the patient's height and weight. For the neuromuscular system, the provider conducts a general assessment of the patient's balance, gait, locomotion, transfers, and transitions as part of their gross coordinated movements, as well as the patient's motor function, including motor control and motor learning. In assessing the cardiovascular and pulmonary body systems, the provider reviews the patient's heart and respiratory rates and blood pressure, and looks for signs of edema. For the integumentary system, the provider reviews the skin's color, texture, and integrity, and whether any scars have formed. In addition to assessing body systems, the physical therapy evaluation should include the general condition of the patient, such as the ability to communicate needs; level of consciousness; being oriented to persons, place, and time; and anticipated emotional and behavioral responses. In addition, the provider should identify which learning or educational needs the patient shows a preference for over another. Body structures are the structural or anatomical parts of the body, such as organs, limbs, and their components, classified according to body systems. Personal factors that exist but do not impact the plan of care should not be considered when selecting the level of evaluation.

Medicine

However, factors that influence how disability is experienced by the individual should be considered. Examples include sex, age, coping styles, social background, education, profession, past and current experience, overall behavior pattern, and character. Coordinating, consulting, and collaborating with other clinicians or agencies regarding the patient's care is rendered as appropriate to the needs of the patient, family, and/or caregivers. Report 97161 for a physical therapy evaluation of low complexity, 97162 for moderate complexity, and 97163 for high complexity. Report 97164 for re-evaluation of an established physical therapist plan of care.

[97165, 97166, 97167, 97168]

The qualified provider evaluates a patient for occupational therapy (OT). The evaluation comprises the following elements: an occupational profile including medical and therapy history, pertinent assessments, and developing a plan of care. There are three levels of evaluation (low, moderate, or high complexity) that providers may report based on documentation of specific elements corresponding to the level of occupational therapy evaluation selected. The performance deficit assessment is conducted to pinpoint areas where the patient is unable to finish an activity due to a lack of skill in one of three categories: physical, cognitive, or psychosocial. An assessment of physical skills is defined to show if the patient is impaired in their balance, mobility, strength, endurance, fine or gross motor coordination, sensation, or dexterity. Deficits noted in the area of cognitive skills refers to the patient's difficulty to attend, perceive, think, comprehend, problem solve, mentally sequence, and learn and recall information. Skills are noted in cases where the individual is involved with task tools/materials, carrying out actions or steps, and changing what they are doing as the result of problems they are encountering. A review of psychosocial skills is determined to show how the individual interacts with other people, their habits and routines, how they adapt or cope with their environment, and how they engage in everyday tasks and social situations. Coordinating, consulting, and collaborating with other clinicians or agencies regarding the individual's care is rendered as appropriate to their needs, family, and/or caregivers. Report 97165 for an OT evaluation of low complexity, 97166 for moderate complexity, and 97167 for high complexity. Report 97168 for a re-evaluation of an established OT plan of care.

[97169, 97170, 97171, 97172]

The physician or other qualified health care professional performs an athletic training evaluation. The evaluations are comprised of elements similar to evaluation and management services and include history, examination, clinical decision making, and developing a plan of care. There are three levels of evaluation: low, moderate, and high complexity. Levels are selected based on the specific elements documented. Physical examinations address a set number of elements determined by the level of evaluation being reported from the following categories: body structures, physical activity, and/or participation deficiencies. For the purposes of an athletic training evaluation, body systems are defined as musculoskeletal, neuromuscular, cardiovascular, pulmonary, and integumentary. Body regions include the head, neck, back, lower and upper extremities, and the trunk. A review of the musculoskeletal system is comprised of assessing gross symmetry, gross range of motion (ROM), gross strength, and the patient's height and weight. For the neuromuscular system, the clinician conducts a general assessment of the patient's balance, gait, locomotion, transfers, and transitions as part of the gross coordinated movements, as well as the patient's motor function, including motor control and motor learning. In assessing the cardiovascular and pulmonary body systems, the provider reviews the patient's heart and respiratory rates, blood pressure, and looks for signs of edema. For the integumentary system, the provider reviews the skin's color, texture, integrity, and whether any scars have formed. In addition to assessing body systems, coordinating, consulting, and collaborating with other clinicians or agencies regarding the patient's care is rendered as appropriate to the needs of the patient, family, and/or caregivers. Report 97169 for an athletic training evaluation of low complexity, 97170 for moderate complexity, and 97171 for high complexity. Report 97172 for re-evaluation of an established athletic training plan of care.

97010

The health care provider applies heat (dry or moist) or cold to one or more body parts with appropriate padding to prevent skin irritation. The patient is given necessary safety instructions. The treatment requires supervision only and typically only one session is reported per day. However, when multiple separate treatment sessions are performed per day, it is appropriate to report each treatment session.

97012

The health care provider applies sustained or intermittent mechanical traction most often to the cervical and/or lumbar spine but can be to any area. The mechanical force produces distraction between the vertebrae or joint thereby relieving pain and increasing tissue flexibility. The treatment requires supervision and typically only one session is reported per day. However, when multiple separate treatment sessions are performed per day, it is appropriate to report each treatment session.

97014

The health care provider applies electrical stimulation to one or more areas in order to stimulate muscle function, enhance healing, and alleviate pain and/or edema. The clinician chooses which type of electrical stimulation is appropriate. The treatment requires supervision and typically only one session is reported per day. However, when multiple separate treatment sessions are performed per day, it is appropriate to report each treatment session.

Medicine

97016
The health care provider applies a vasopneumatic device to treat extremity edema (usually lymphedema). A pressurized sleeve is applied. Girth measurements are taken pre- and posttreatment. Typically only one session is reported per day. However, when multiple separate treatment sessions are performed per day, it is appropriate to report each treatment session.

97018
The health care provider uses a paraffin bath to apply superficial heat to a hand or foot. The body part is repeatedly dipped into the paraffin forming a glove. Use of paraffin facilitates treatment of arthritis and other conditions that cause limitations in joint flexibility. The treatment requires supervision and typically only one session is reported per day. However, when multiple separate treatment sessions are performed per day, it is appropriate to report each session.

97022
The health care provider uses a whirlpool to provide superficial heat and cold in an environment that facilitates range of motion and/or exercise. The provider decides the appropriate water temperature and provides safety instruction. The treatment requires supervision and typically only one session is reported per day. However, when multiple separate treatment sessions are performed per day, it is appropriate to report each session.

97024
The health care provider uses diathermy or microwave as a form of superficial heat for one or more body areas. After application and safety instructions have been provided, the clinician supervises the treatment. Typically only one session is reported per day. However, when multiple separate treatment sessions are performed per day, it is appropriate to report each session.

97026
The health care provider uses infrared light as a form of superficial heat that increases circulation to one or more localized areas. The treatment requires supervision and typically only one session is reported per day. However, when multiple separate treatment sessions are performed per day, it is appropriate to report each session.

97028
The health care provider applies ultraviolet light in the treatment of chronic wounds. Once applied and safety instructions have been provided, the treatment is supervised. Typically only one session is reported per day. However, when multiple separate treatment sessions are performed per day, it is appropriate to report each session.

97032
The health care provider applies electrical stimulation to one or more areas to promote muscle function and/or pain control. This treatment requires direct contact by the provider and is reported in multiple 15-minute units.

[97037]
Low-level laser therapy (LLLT), also known as photobiomodulation therapy, is administered for postoperative pain reduction. LLLT is a noninvasive therapy that utilizes low-intensity lasers to target specific areas of inflammation, swelling, and pain. An LLLT laser or high-intensity light-emitting diodes (LEDs) do not emit heat; therefore, they do not carry the same degree of intensity as a surgical laser. During an LLLT session, a specialized laser device emits gentle, nonthermal light waves that penetrate the skin and interact with cellular structures. This interaction triggers a cascade of biochemical reactions within the body, leading to reduced inflammation and relief from postoperative pain. LLLT may be selected as an optimal method to treat postoperative pain as no pharmaceuticals are needed and side effects are minimal or absent. This code requires constant attendance and is reported in 15-minute units.

97033
The health care provider uses electrical current to administer medication transdermally to one or more areas. Iontophoresis is usually prescribed for soft tissue inflammatory conditions and pain control. This code requires constant attendance by the clinician and is reported in 15-minute units.

97034
A health care provider uses hot and cold baths in a repeated, alternating fashion to stimulate the vasomotor response of a localized body part. This code requires constant attendance and is reported in 15-minute units.

97035
The health care provider applies ultrasound to increase circulation to one or more areas. A water bath or some form of ultrasound lotion must be used as a coupling agent to facilitate the procedure. The delivery of corticosteroid medication via ultrasound is called phonophoresis and is reported using this code. The medication as a supply may or may not be paid by the payer. Ultrasound or phonophoresis requires constant attendance and is reported in 15-minute units.

97036
A Hubbard tank is used when it is necessary to immerse the full body into water. Care of wounds and burns may require use of the Hubbard tank to facilitate tissue cleansing and debridement. This code requires constant attendance of a health care provider and is reported in 15-minute units.

97110
A qualified health care provider is in direct contact with one patient while using techniques specific to therapeutic exercise to one or more body areas to develop strength, endurance, and flexibility. This code requires direct contact by a qualified health care provider with the patient and is reported in 15-minute units.

97112
The qualified health care provider is in direct contact with one patient using neuromuscular techniques to treat one or more body areas that facilitate reeducation of movement, balance, coordination, kinesthetic sense, posture, and proprioception. This code requires direct contact by a qualified health care provider with the patient and is reported in 15-minute units.

97113
A qualified health care provider is in direct contact with one patient using therapeutic exercise techniques with the patient/client in the aquatic environment. This code requires skilled intervention by the qualified health care provider and documentation must support medical necessity of the aquatic environment. This code requires direct contact by a qualified health care provider with the patient and is reported in 15-minute units.

97116
A qualified health care provider trains the patient in specific activities that will facilitate ambulation and stair climbing with or without an assistive device. Proper gait sequencing and safety instructions are included when appropriate. This code requires direct contact by a qualified health care provider with the patient and is reported in 15-minute units.

97124
A health care provider uses massage to provide muscle relaxation, increase localized circulation, soften scar tissue, or mobilize mucous secretions in the lung via tapotement and/or percussion. This code requires direct contact with the health care provider and is reported in 15-minute units, regardless of the number of body parts treated.

97129-97130
A patient with learning disabilities or an individual who has lost cognitive skills because of illness or brain injury is treated on a one-on-one basis by the physician or other qualified health care provider to assist in the development of cognitive skills. The individual often needs to develop compensatory methods of processing and retrieving information when disability, illness, or injury has affected these cognitive processes. Cognitive skill development includes mental exercises that assist the patient in areas such as attention, memory, perception, language, reasoning, planning, problem-solving, executive functioning, and related skills. These codes require direct contact by a qualified health care provider with the patient and are reported in 15-minute units. Report 97129 for the initial 15 minutes and 97130 for each additional 15 minutes. Do not report 97129 more than once a day.

97140
A qualified health care provider performs manual therapy techniques including, but not limited to, soft tissue and joint mobilization, manipulation, manual traction, and/or manual lymphatic drainage to one or more areas. This code requires direct contact by a qualified health care provider with the patient and is reported in 15-minute units.

97150
A qualified health care provider or properly supervised support personnel provides direct contact services to two or more patients at the same time. Services in a group setting could include, but are not limited to, therapeutic exercises, therapeutic activities, aquatic therapy with therapeutic exercises, and neuromuscular reeducation. The patients/clients do not have to be performing the same activity simultaneously; however, the need for skilled intervention must be documented. This code is reported once for each group participant. This code requires constant attendance, but not direct one-to-one contact, by a qualified health care provider with the patient in the group setting.

97530
A qualified health care provider uses dynamic therapeutic activities designed to achieve improved functional performance (e.g., lifting, pulling, bending). This code requires direct contact by a qualified health care provider with the patient and is reported in 15-minute units.

97533
A qualified health care provider works one-on-one with an individual with sensory integration disorders to provide techniques for enhancing sensory processing and adapting to environmental demands. Sensory integration disorders may be the result of a learning disability, illness, or brain injury. Sensory experiences include touch, movement, body awareness, sight, sound, and the pull of gravity. The process of the brain organizing and interpreting this information is called sensory integration. Sensory integration provides a crucial foundation for later, more complex learning and behavior. This code requires direct contact by a qualified health care provider with the patient and is reported in 15-minute units.

97535
A qualified health care provider instructs and trains a patient in self-care and home management activities (e.g., ADL and use of adaptive equipment in the kitchen, bath, and/or car). This code requires direct contact by a qualified health care provider with the patient and is reported in 15-minute units.

97537
A qualified health care provider instructs and trains the patient/client in community/work reintegration activities, including addressing participation restrictions (e.g., work task analysis, money management, shopping, work environment modification, safe accessing of transportation, and the use of available assistive technology devices or adaptive equipment). This code requires direct contact by a qualified health care provider with the patient and is reported in 15-minute units.

97542
A qualified health care provider performs assessments, fitting and adjustments, and instructs and trains the patient in proper wheelchair skills (e.g., propulsion, safety techniques) in his or her home, facility, work, or community environment. This code requires direct contact by a qualified health care provider with the patient and is reported in 15-minute units.

97545-97546
This code is used for a procedure where the injured worker is put through a series of conditioning exercises and job simulation tasks in preparation for return to work. Endurance, strength, and proper body mechanics are emphasized. The patient is also educated in problem-solving skills related to job task performance and employing correct lifting and positioning techniques. Report 97546 for each additional hour after the initial two hours.

97550-97551
Caregiver training is provided without the patient present to teach the caregiver how to facilitate a patient's functional performance in the home or community. The face-to-face training is a structured educational process aimed at equipping the caregiver with the knowledge and skills necessary to support and enhance the independent daily functioning of individuals requiring care. This training encompasses a range of practical strategies and techniques tailored to the specific needs and challenges of the patient, enabling the caregiver to create a safe, conducive, and empowering environment that promotes the patient's well-being, autonomy, and successful engagement in various activities of daily living. Report 97550 for the first 30 minutes of training. Report 97551 for each additional 15 minutes.

97552
Group caregiver training is provided without the patient present to teach caregivers how to facilitate a patient's functional performance in the home or community. Multiple sets of caregivers are present for multiple patients with similar conditions or needs. The face-to-face training is a structured educational process aimed at equipping multiple caregivers with the knowledge and skills necessary to support and enhance the independent daily functioning of individuals requiring care. This training encompasses a range of practical strategies and techniques tailored to the specific needs and challenges of the patient, enabling multiple caregivers to create a safe, conducive, and empowering environment that promotes the patient's well-being, autonomy, and successful engagement in various activities of daily living.

97597-97598
A health care provider performs wound care management by using selective debridement techniques to remove devitalized or necrotic tissue from an open wound. Selective techniques are those in which the provider has complete control over which tissue is removed and which is left behind, and include high-pressure waterjet with or without suction and sharp debridement using scissors, a scalpel, or forceps. Wound assessment, topical applications, instructions regarding ongoing care of the wound, and the possible use of a whirlpool for treatment are included in these codes. Report 97597 for a total wound surface area less than or equal to 20 sq cm and 97598 for each additional 20 sq cm or part thereof.

97602
A health care provider performs wound care management to promote healing using non-selective debridement techniques to remove devitalized tissue. Non-selective debridement techniques are those in which necrotic and healthy tissue are removed. Non-selective techniques, sometimes referred to as mechanical debridement, include wet-to-moist dressings, enzymatic chemicals, autolytic debridement, abrasion, and larval therapy. Wet-to-moist debridement involves allowing a dressing to proceed from wet to moist and manually removing the dressing, which removes the necrotic and healthy tissue. Chemical enzymes are fast acting products that produce slough of necrotic tissue. Autolytic debridement is accomplished using occlusive or semi-occlusive dressings that keep wound fluid in contact with the necrotic tissue. Types of dressing applications used in autolytic debridement include hydrocolloids, hydrogels, and transparent films. Abrasion involves scraping the wound surface with a tongue blade or similar blunt instrument. Larval treatment may include larvae placement on the wound, which in turn feed off the dead tissue and/or application of the larvae digestive excretions allowing for debridement of dead tissue with no damage to viable tissue.

97605-97606
Negative pressure wound therapy (NPWT) is a widely used advanced wound treatment technique. The health care provider performs NPWT via the use of durable medical equipment (DME), such as vacuum assisted drainage collection, to promote healing of a chronic nonhealing wound, including diabetic or pressure (decubitus) ulcers. This procedure includes topical applications to the wound, wound assessment, and patient or caregiver instruction related to ongoing care per session. Negative pressure wound therapy uses controlled application of subatmospheric pressure to a wound. The subatmospheric pressure is generated using an electrical pump. The electrical pump conveys intermittent or continuous subatmospheric pressure by connecting tubing to a specialized wound dressing. The specialized wound dressing includes a porous foam dressing that covers the wound surface and an airtight adhesive dressing that seals the wound and contains the subatmospheric pressure at the wound site. Negative pressure wound therapy promotes healing by increasing local vascularity and oxygenation of the wound bed, evacuating wound fluid thereby reducing edema, and removing exudates and bacteria. Drainage from the wound is collected in a canister. Report 97605 for a

wound(s) with a total surface area less than or equal to 50 sq. cm. Report 97606 for a wound(s) with a total surface area greater than 50 sq. cm.

97607-97608

Negative pressure wound therapy (NPWT) is a widely used advanced wound treatment technique. The health care provider performs NPWT, such as vacuum assisted drainage collection, using disposable, nondurable medical equipment, including the use of an exudate management collection system, to promote healing of a chronic nonhealing wound, including diabetic or pressure (decubitus) ulcers. This procedure includes topical applications to the wound, wound assessment, and patient or caregiver instruction related to ongoing care per session. Negative pressure wound therapy uses controlled application of subatmospheric pressure to a wound. The subatmospheric pressure is generated using an electrical pump. The electrical pump conveys intermittent or continuous subatmospheric pressure through connecting tubing to a specialized wound dressing. The specialized wound dressing includes a porous foam dressing that covers the wound surface and an airtight adhesive dressing that seals the wound and contains the subatmospheric pressure at the wound site. NPWT promotes healing by increasing local vascularity and oxygenation of the wound bed, evacuating wound fluid thereby reducing edema, and removing exudates and bacteria. Drainage from the wound is collected in a canister. Exudate management is the process by which wound care is overseen and is determined based on the wound type and the patient's needs. It involves careful attention and ongoing evaluation of the wound healing process, as well as a focus on the underlying cause of the infection. Report 97607 for a wound(s) with a total surface area less than or equal to 50 sq. cm. Report 97608 for a wound(s) with a total surface area greater than 50 sq. cm.

97610

The physician performs wound treatment utilizing a device that produces low-frequency, ultrasound-generated mist. This noncontact, nonthermal modality promotes wound healing through cellular stimulation. Indicated for acute, chronic, and colonized wounds, as well as burns and ulcers, it provides wound cleansing, bacteria removal, and maintenance debridement of fibrin and tissue exudates. The device uses ultrasound technology to atomize saline, delivering a continuous mist to the treatment site. Multiple passes over the wound are made with the treatment head of the device for a predetermined treatment session. This code includes assessment of the wound, topical applications when performed, and ongoing care instructions. Report this code once per day for the duration of treatment.

97750

The health care provider performs a test of physical performance evaluating function of one or more body areas and evaluates functional capacity. A written report is included. This is in addition to a routine evaluation or re-evaluation (97161-97172). This code can be reported in 15-minute increments.

97755

A health care provider performs an assessment for the suitability and benefits of acquiring any assistive technology device or equipment that will restore, augment, or compensate for existing functional ability in the patient or that will optimize functional tasks and/or maximize the patient's environmental accessibility. This code is reported for one-on-one patient contact time, per 15 minutes, and includes the preparation of a written report.

97760-97763

The health care provider fits and/or trains the patient in the use of an orthotic (97760) device for one or more body parts, including assessment as to the type of orthotic, as appropriate; however, this service does not include fabrication time or cost of materials. Report 97761 for upper or lower extremity prosthetics training only. These codes describe initial encounters. Report 97763 for upper or lower extremity orthotics or prosthetics management and/or training, including evaluating the effectiveness of an existing orthotic or prosthetic device and making recommendations for changes, as appropriate, during a subsequent encounter. Each of these services is reported in 15-minute increments.

97802-97804

A dietetic professional provides medical nutrition therapy assessment or re-assessment and intervention in a face-to-face or group patient setting. After nutritional screening identifies patients at risk, preventive or therapeutic dietary therapy is initiated to induce a positive result in the role nutrition plays in improving health outcomes. Report 97802 for the initial assessment and intervention face-to-face with an individual patient for each 15 minutes of medical nutrition therapy. Report 97803 for re-assessment and intervention with an individual patient for each 15 minutes of medical nutrition therapy. Report 97804 for group medical nutrition therapy provided for two or more individuals, each 30 minutes.

97810-97811

The health care provider applies acupuncture therapy by inserting one or more fine needles into the patient as dictated by acupuncture meridians for the relief of pain. The needles are twirled or manipulated by hand to generate therapeutic stimulation. No electrical stimulation is employed with this procedure. Report 97810 for the initial 15 minutes of personal one-on-one contact with the patient and 97811 for each additional 15 minutes of personal one-on-one contact with the patient, with insertion of needle(s).

97813-97814

The health care provider applies acupuncture therapy by inserting one or more fine needles into the patient as dictated by acupuncture meridians for the relief of pain. The needles are energized by employing a micro-current for electrical stimulation. Report 97813 for the initial 15 minutes of personal one-on-one contact with the patient and 97814 for each additional 15 minutes of personal one-on-one contact with the patient, with insertion of needle(s).

98925-98929

The physician uses these codes to report osteopathic manipulation, unique manual treatments that are used to treat somatic dysfunction and related disorders. Several techniques exist. Body regions included are head, cervical thoracic, lumbar, sacral, pelvic, extremities, rib cage, abdomen, and viscera. Report 98925 if one to two body regions are involved; 98926 if three to four body regions are involved; 98927 if five to six body regions are involved; 98928 if seven to eight body regions are involved; and 98929 if nine body regions are involved.

98940-98943

The chiropractor uses these codes to report the unique manual treatments used to influence joint and neurophysiological function. Several modalities exist. Report 98940 if treatment is spinal, one to two regions; 98941 if treatment is spinal, three to four regions; 98942 if treatment is spinal, five regions; and 98943 if treatment is extraspinal (head, extremities, rib cage, and abdomen), one or more regions.

98960-98962

The qualified health care professional (nonphysician) provides education and training using a standard curriculum. This training is prescribed by a physician to enable the patient to concurrently self-manage established illnesses or diseases with health care providers. Report 98960 for education and training provided for an individual patient for each 30 minutes of service. Report 98961 for a group of two to four patients and 98962 for a group of five to eight patients.

98966-98968

A qualified health care professional (nonphysician) provides telephone assessment and management services to a patient in a non-face-to-face encounter. These episodes of care may be initiated by an established patient or by the patient's guardian. These codes are not reported if the telephone service results in a decision to see the patient within 24 hours or at the next available urgent visit appointment; instead, the phone encounter is regarded as part of the pre-service work of the subsequent face-to-face encounter. These codes are also not reported if the telephone call is in reference to a service performed and reported by the qualified health care professional that occurred within the past seven days or within the postoperative period of a previously completed procedure. This applies both to unsolicited patient follow-up as well as that requested by the health care professional. Report 98966 for telephone services requiring five to 10 minutes of medical discussion, 98967 for telephone services requiring 11 to 20 minutes of medical discussion, and 98968 for telephone services requiring 21 to 30 minutes of medical discussion.

98970-98972

Online digital evaluation and management services are non-face-to-face encounters originating from the established patient to a qualified nonphysician health care professional for evaluation or management of a problem. The patient initiates the digital communication through a Health Insurance Portability and Accountability Act (HIPAA) compliant platform. The service includes all asynchronous (not in real-time) communication with the patient, review of the initial patient query and medical records, personal interaction with clinical staff by the provider related to the patient query, and development of a plan including ordering any necessary prescriptions or tests. The service may include more than one provider responding to the same patient and is only reportable once during seven days for the same encounter. These codes are not reported if the online patient request is related to an E/M service that occurred within the previous seven days or within the global period following a procedure. Report 98970 if the cumulative time during the seven-day period is five to 10 minutes; 98971 for 11 to 20 minutes; and 98972 for 21 or more minutes.

98975-98978

Remote therapeutic monitoring services are performed to assess and evaluate digital monitoring and digital therapy data related to the patient's adherence and response to therapies performed on the respiratory or musculoskeletal system or to cognitive behavioral therapy services. Data may be objective, such as integrated data that is device-generated, or subjective, such as input reported by the patient. These services must be ordered by a physician or other qualified health care provider. The device prescribed must be defined as a medical device by the Food and Drug Administration (FDA) and used for monitoring and therapeutic intervention when necessary. An episode of care begins when the service is initiated and ends once the patient achieves specific treatment goals. Report 98975 for the initial equipment set-up and patient education on devices used for the data collection; this is reported once for each episode of care. Supply of the device for data access or transmissions for monitoring support are reported each 30 days. Report 98976 for devices that monitor the respiratory system, 98977 for devices that monitor the musculoskeletal system, and 98978 for devices that monitor cognitive behavioral therapy. These codes should not be reported for cumulative monitoring of less than 16 days.

98980-98981

The physician or other qualified health care professional (QHP) provides therapeutic monitoring treatment management services remotely to a patient under an individualized treatment plan. The results of remote therapeutic monitoring that has been ordered by a physician or QHP are used in this service, which requires at least one interactive communication with the patient or the patient's caregiver. Report 98980 for the first completed 20 minutes of time spent by the physician or QHP in a calendar month; this is reported once regardless of the number of monitoring modalities performed. Report 98981 for each additional 20 minutes.

99000
This code is adjunct to basic services rendered. This code is reported for the handling and/or conveyance of a specimen from the provider's office to a laboratory.

99001
This code is adjunct to basic services rendered. This code is reported for the handling and/or conveyance of a specimen from the patient in a location other than the provider's office to the laboratory.

99002
This code is adjunct to basic services rendered. The qualified provider reports this code for the handling, conveyance, and/or any other service in connection with the implementation of an order involving devices such as orthotics, protectives, and prosthetics fabricated by an outside laboratory and fitted by the provider.

99024
The physician reports this code to indicate a postoperative follow-up visit, normally included in the surgical package when the physician performs an evaluation and management service for reason(s) that are related to the original procedure.

99026-99027
These codes report the time for hospital mandated on call service provided by the physician and do not include prolonged physician attendance time for standby services or the time spent performing other reportable procedures or services. Report 99026 for each hour of hospital mandated on call service spent in the hospital and 99027 for each hour of hospital mandated on call service spent outside the hospital.

99050
This code is adjunct to basic services rendered. The physician reports this code to indicate services after posted office hours in addition to basic services.

99051
This code is adjunct to basic services rendered. The physician reports this code to indicate services provided during posted evening, weekend, or holiday office hours in addition to basic services.

99053
This code is adjunct to basic services rendered. The physician reports this code to indicate services provided between 10 p.m. and 8 a.m. at a 24-hour facility in addition to basic services.

99056
This code is adjunct to basic services rendered. The physician reports this code to indicate services typically provided in the office that are provided in a different location at the request of a patient.

99058
This code is adjunct to basic services rendered. The physician reports this code to indicate services provided in the office on an emergency basis that disrupt other scheduled office services.

99060
This code is adjunct to basic services rendered. The physician reports this code to indicate services provided on an emergency basis in a location other than the physician's office that disrupt other scheduled office services.

99070, 99072
Code 99070 is adjunct to basic services rendered. The physician or other qualified provider reports this code to indicate supplies and materials provided over and above those usually included with an office visit or services rendered. This code does not include eyeglasses; report the appropriate supply code if eyeglasses are provided. List drugs, trays, supplies, and other materials provided when using this code. Code 99072 reports additional supplies, materials, and clinical staff time necessary to perform safety protocols only during a public health emergency (PHE) due to respiratory-transmitted infectious disease. Examples include cleaning supplies, face shields and surgical masks, pre-visit screenings and instructions, and symptom checks upon patient's arrival to the office. Extra precautions, over and above those usually included in an office visit or other non-facility services, are taken to ensure the safety of patients and health care professionals during in-person interactions while allowing for the provision of evaluation, treatment, or procedural services. Use of this code does not depend on a specific patient diagnosis. It may be reported only once per in-person patient encounter per provider identification number.

99071
This code is adjunct to basic services rendered. The physician or other qualified health care provider reports this code to indicate educational supplies provided at the cost of the provider for the patient's education.

99075
This code is adjunct to basic services rendered. The physician reports this code to indicate medical testimony.

99078
The physician or other qualified health care professional provides educational services to patients in a group setting. The topics vary according to the group but may be related to prenatal care, diet, diabetic instruction, and smoking cessation.

99080
This code is adjunct to basic services rendered. The physician reports this code to indicate reports such as insurance forms, require more than the information in standard communications methods or forms.

99082
This code is adjunct to basic services rendered. The physician reports this code to indicate unusual travel for the purpose of transportation or accompanying the patient.

99100
This code is adjunct to basic services rendered. The physician reports this code to indicate qualifying circumstances regarding anesthesia for a patient younger than 1 year or older than 70 years of age.

99116
This code is adjunct to basic services rendered. The physician reports this code to indicate qualifying circumstances regarding anesthesia complicated by utilization of total body hypothermia.

99135
This code is adjunct to basic services rendered. The physician reports this code to indicate qualifying circumstances regarding anesthesia complicated by utilization of controlled hypotension.

99140
This code is adjunct to basic services rendered. The physician reports this code to indicate qualifying circumstances regarding anesthesia complicated by emergency conditions. Specify emergency conditions encountered when submitting a claim.

99151-99153
A physician or other qualified health care provider administers medication that allows a decreased level of consciousness but does not put the patient completely asleep inducing a state called moderate (conscious) sedation. This allows the patient to breathe without assistance and respond to commands. This type of sedation is used for less invasive procedures and/or as a second medication for pain. These codes report sedation services provided by the same provider performing the primary procedure with the assistance of an independently trained health care professional to assist in monitoring the patient. Report 99151 for the first 15 minutes of intraservice time for sedation services rendered to a patient younger than 5 years of age. Report 99152 for the first 15 minutes of intraservice time for sedation services rendered to a patient age 5 years or older. Report 99153 for each additional 15 minutes of intraservice time.

99155-99157
A physician or other qualified health care provider administers medication that allows a decreased level of consciousness but does not put the patient completely asleep, inducing a state called moderate (conscious) sedation. This allows the patient to breathe without assistance and respond to commands. This type of sedation is used for less invasive procedures and/or as a second medication for pain. These codes report services provided by a qualified provider other than the health care provider performing the diagnostic or therapeutic service that the sedation supports. Report 99155 for the first 15 minutes of intraservice time for sedation services rendered to a patient younger than 5 years of age. Report 99156 for the first 15 minutes of intraservice time for sedation services rendered to a patient age 5 years or older. Report 99157 for each additional 15 minutes of intraservice time.

99170
The physician focuses an endoscope on the anogenital area of a child to magnify and directly observe the condition of living tissues in cases of suspected trauma. This examination allows a more complete examination than a normal physical exam since the colposcope magnifies from six to 40 times.

99172
The patient's visual function is evaluated in this exam with several parts. For visual acuity, the physician asks the patient to stand at a specified distance (20 feet for Snellen eye chart) away from the chart. The patient is instructed to cover the left eye with the left hand or hold a card in front of the lens for those patients wearing eyeglasses. The patient reads the letters on the chart to test the visual acuity of the right eye. The process is repeated for the other eye. Ocular alignment is checked by determining whether the eyes work together in the same direction. The patient is positioned in front of a screen, looking ahead, and the non-tested eye is covered in a field of vision screening. The health care provider flashes objects in various areas in the field of vision and the patient is asked to respond. The patient's response creates a map of the visual field. To test color vision, the patient looks at cards with many different colored dots that make specific shapes. The patient with normal color vision will be able to discern the shapes within the colors. This exam identifies possible vision problems. It does not replace the examination by an ophthalmologist or optometrist and is used as a screening test only.

99173
The physician asks the patient to stand at a specified distance (20 feet for Snellen eye chart) from the chart. The patient is instructed to cover the left eye with the left hand or hold a card in front of the lens for those patients wearing eyeglasses. The patient reads the letters on the screen to test the visual acuity of the right eye. The process is repeated for the other eye. This exam identifies possible vision problems; it does not replace the examination by an ophthalmologist or optometrist and is used as a screening test only.

99174 [99177]
Instrument based ocular screenings are diagnostic eye examinations that use a multitude of ophthalmic devices to perform the exam. Two of the most common types are photoscreening and automated refraction. During photoscreening, a specialized camera or video system obtains images of the pupillary reflexes and red reflexes. Currently there are two types of photoscreening systems available. One type uses a trained evaluator to analyze the data. The second uses a computerized system to interpret the images. Automated refraction uses a highly specialized device composed of a phoropter, controller, eye chart,

autorefractor, and an auto lensmeter to determine a patient's refractive error and prescription for eyeglasses or contacts. Report 99174 for any type of bilateral instrument based ocular screening with remote analysis and report. When performed with on-site analysis, report 99177.

99175
The physician administers ipecac or a similar substance to induce vomiting and observes the patient until the stomach is adequately emptied of poison.

99183
The physician or other qualified health care provider attends and supervises hyperbaric oxygen therapy. Report per session. Report hyperbaric oxygen therapy procedures separately.

99184
Whole body hypothermia or selective head hypothermia may be used to decrease the risk of death or disability in critically ill neonates with birth asphyxia or moderate to severe hypoxic ischemic encephalopathy (HIE). Infants are cooled to an esophageal temperature in the 33 degree range for a specified time period and are then slowly rewarmed. All appropriate patient selection from review of clinical, imaging, and other laboratory data, as well as verification of the esophageal temperature probe's location, evaluating the EEG amplitude, supervising the procedure, and ongoing assessments of the patient during cooling, is included in the reporting of this service. Temperature (rectal and tympanic membrane), blood pressure and full blood count, blood gases and electrolytes, heart rate, and coagulation studies are monitored throughout and following the cooling process. Magnetic resonance imaging (MRI) and neurological assessment of outcome may follow. Selective head hypothermia employs the use of a cooling "cap," a device comprised of soft, water circulating tubes that encircles the child's head, while core body temperature is constantly monitored and kept at safe levels using a radiant warmer. This code should be reported for patients 28 days or younger.

99188
The physician, or other qualified health care provider, uses a small piece of gauze to wipe clean and dry the teeth. Once dry, the topical fluoride is "painted" on the entire surface of each tooth using a small brush. The varnish goes on "tacky" but hardens once saliva from the mouth touches it. Topical fluoride varnish is used to prevent tooth decay by going into the tooth enamel and strengthening the tooth. Use of topical fluoride varnish works to stop the formation of new caries, impede or stop existing tooth decay from worsening, and, in early cases of tooth decay, repairs the tooth completely.

99190-99192
The health care provider assembles and operates a pump with an oxygenator or heat exchanger. Report 99190 to identify each hour; 99191 to report 45 minutes; and 99192 to report 30 minutes.

99195
The health care provider draws blood from the patient to right dramatically imbalanced blood levels (i.e., hemoglobin, potassium salts). The procedure is similar to drawing blood from a donor, but a number of pints may be taken to reduce the imbalance. Blood removal is performed under a physician's direction.

99500
The home health provider may visit patients with prenatal complications from the first month until the birth of the baby in 99500. The home nurse may obtain vaginal-anorectal/cervical cultures, perform a non-stress test and uterine and fetal heart rate monitoring, draw blood for serology (including offering of AFP/HIV testing), and other tests such as glucose screening to check for gestational diabetes.

99501
A home visit for postnatal assessment may include a review of plans for future health maintenance and care, including routine infant immunizations, identification of illness and periodic health evaluations, and linking the family with other sources of support such as social services, parenting classes, and lactation consultants as necessary.

99502
The home health care provider measures vital signs, does a physical examination, and assesses developmental norms in the newborn and discusses feeding and care with the mother. The home health care provider teaches and answers questions regarding childcare and determines if there are any problems requiring a physician's intervention. Postpartum early discharge is defined as six hours to 36 hours after uncomplicated vaginal delivery or 72 hours after uncomplicated cesarean delivery. Specialized nursing helps the family make the transition from hospital to home.

99503
A trained respiratory therapist or other health care professional provides care for patients with temporary or chronic respiratory conditions. The health care professional may provide pulmonary evaluations, patient and family education and counseling, and instruction in self-care. The visit is designed to assist the physician in caring for the patient by avoiding complications, infections, disease progression, and to ultimately reduce hospitalizations. The visit may also include evaluation and monitoring of the equipment used, including diagnostics and calibration of the equipment; changes in medications (e.g., bronchodilator); and/or advice and education about dosage and the use of a particular medication.

99504
A respiratory therapist or other home health care professional visits a patient's home to give mechanical ventilation care. The health care professional instructs the patient and family members on the ventilator

equipment, including checking the machine and the settings. During the home health visit, related equipment or issues, such as oxygen and tracheostomy care (when present), is discussed.

99505
The home health care provider measures vital signs, inspects incisions, assesses mobility and appetite, and determines if there are problems or situations that could require a surgeon's intervention. The provider checks the stoma site and the stoma's function. The home health provider teaches and answers questions the patient may have about the care and maintenance of the colostomy and/or cystostomy. The home health provider also administers medications or draws blood so that the surgeon can continue to monitor the patient's condition. Most patients who have had a colostomy or cystostomy will be seen by a home health provider one or more times after discharge.

99506
The home health provider visits a patient's home to perform an intermuscular injection of medication per a physician's or another valid order. The home health provider brings supplies and medications that are necessary to accomplish the injection to the patient's home, including a syringe, needle, liquid disinfectant, cotton ball, and adhesive tape. The procedure involves inserting the needle, aspiration and slow injection, and at the end of the procedure a cotton ball is placed over the injection site. Adhesive tape is applied over the cotton ball.

99507
The home health provider visits the patient at home for care and maintenance of catheter, such as urinary catheters, and catheters placed for drainage or enteral feeding. Skilled procedures required for the home visit include Foley catheter and suprapubic catheter insertion and management; gastrostomy tube/catheter maintenance and enteral feeding; dressing changes and assessment of catheter-related wounds; management of open or draining wounds, ulcers, or fistulae and drainage tube/catheter management; related suture/staple removal; and urinary incontinence catheter management.

99509
In order to qualify for home assistance with activities of daily living and personal care, the patient must be unable to perform two or more activities of daily living, such as eating, toileting, transferring, bathing, dressing, and continence. When a referral is made, a health care provider visits the home to conduct a comprehensive assessment of the patient's needs. The plan of care is developed in conjunction with the client, physician, and family. Acting as a liaison with the client's physician and other community programs, the case manager responds to all client requests, questions, and concerns and reports frequently on the client's status and progress.

99510
A home health professional makes an initial visit to the home to evaluate specific needs. If home health care would be of benefit, a plan of care is developed based on medical orders from the patient's provider. For example, a plan might specify one or more visits from a therapist. The provider regularly reviews progress reports.

99511
A home health visit includes assistance with dietary management and bowel management/retraining (i.e., use of prescribed medication as well as establishing a habit regimen to treat constipation). The home health caregiver may manually remove the impaction or administer an enema. The amount of fluid administered depends on the age and size of the person receiving the enema. If necessary, a specimen is collected for diagnostic evaluation.

99512
This code reports a home visit for hemodialysis. A home health nurse commonly visits the patient three times a week to provide hemodialysis. Each treatment lasts from two to four hours. Before treatment, access is made to the bloodstream to provide a way for blood to be carried from the patient to the dialysis machine, which filters out wastes and extra fluids and returns the blood back to the patient. The access may be under the skin or outside the body. During treatment, the patient can read, write, sleep, talk, or watch television.

99601-99602
A home health professional visits the patient at home to perform the infusion of a specialty drug per a physician's order. The home health provider brings the supplies and medication required and administers and oversees the infusion. Each infusion takes up to two hours per visit for 99601. Report 99602 for each additional hour.

99605-99607
A pharmacist provides individual management of medication therapy with assessment and intervention. This patient-specific service includes review of pertinent history and profiling of prescription and non-prescription medications. The pharmacist evaluates the medication profile for under- or over-dosing, duplications, and possible drug interactions, and makes recommendations based on the assessment, including communication with the prescriber. Report 99605 for the initial 15-minute individual new patient encounter provided face-to-face by the pharmacist; 99606 for the initial 15-minute individual established patient encounter; and 99607 for each additional 15 minutes spent with the patient.

Evaluation and Management

99202-99205

Providers report these codes for new patients being seen in the doctor's office, a multispecialty group clinic, or other outpatient environment. All require a medically appropriate history and/or examination. Code selection is based on the level of medical decision making (MDM) or total time personally spent by the physician and/or other qualified health care professional(s) on the date of the encounter. Factors to be considered in MDM include the number and complexity of problems addressed during the encounter, amount and complexity of data requiring review and analysis, and the risk of complications and/or morbidity or mortality associated with patient management. The most basic service is represented by 99202, which entails straightforward MDM. If time is used for code selection, a total time of 15 minutes must be met or exceeded on the day of the encounter. Report 99203 for a visit requiring a low level of MDM or meeting or exceeding 30 minutes of total time; 99204 for a visit requiring a moderate level of MDM or meeting or exceeding 45 minutes of total time; and 99205 for a visit requiring a high level of MDM or meeting or exceeding 60 minutes of total time.

99211-99215

Providers report these codes for established patients being seen in the doctor's office, a multispecialty group clinic, or other outpatient environment. All require a medically appropriate history and/or examination excluding the most basic service represented by 99211 that describes an encounter that may not require the presence of a physician or other qualified health care professional. For the remainder of codes within this range, code selection is based on the level of medical decision making (MDM) or total time personally spent by the physician and/or other qualified health care professional(s) on the date of the encounter. Factors to be considered in MDM include the number and complexity of problems addressed during the encounter, amount and complexity of data requiring review and analysis, and the risk of complications and/or morbidity or mortality associated with patient management. Report 99212 for a visit that entails straightforward MDM. If time is used for code selection, a total time of 10 minutes must be met or exceeded on the day of the encounter. Report 99213 for a visit requiring a low level of MDM or meeting or exceeding 20 minutes of total time; 99214 for a moderate level of MDM or meeting or exceeding 30 minutes of total time; and 99215 for a high level of MDM or meeting or exceeding 40 minutes of total time.

[98000, 98001, 98002, 98003]

Providers report these codes for new patients being seen via telehealth using synchronous audio-video as an alternative to an in-person visit. The provider and patient interact from different locations through real-time communication in which they can see and hear each other. All require a medically appropriate history and/or examination. Code selection is based on the level of medical decision making (MDM) or total time personally spent by the physician and/or other qualified health care professional(s) on the date of the encounter. Factors to be considered in MDM include the number and complexity of problems addressed during the encounter, amount and complexity of data requiring review and analysis, and the risk of complications and/or morbidity or mortality associated with patient management. The most basic service is represented by 98000, which entails straightforward MDM. If time is used for code selection, a total time of 15 minutes must be met or exceeded on the day of the encounter. Report 98001 for a visit requiring a low level of MDM or meeting or exceeding 30 minutes of total time; 98002 for a visit requiring a moderate level of MDM or meeting or exceeding 45 minutes of total time; and 98003 for a visit requiring a high level of MDM or meeting or exceeding 60 minutes of total time.

[98004, 98005, 98006, 98007]

Providers report these codes for established patients being seen via telehealth using synchronous audio-video as an alternative to an in-person visit. The provider and patient interact from different locations through real-time communication in which they can see and hear each other. All require a medically appropriate history and/or examination. Code selection is based on the level of medical decision making (MDM) or total time personally spent by the physician and/or other qualified health care professional(s) on the date of the encounter. Factors to be considered in MDM include the number and complexity of problems addressed during the encounter, amount and complexity of data requiring review and analysis, and the risk of complications and/or morbidity or mortality associated with patient management. The most basic service is represented by 98004, which entails straightforward MDM. If time is used for code selection, a total time of 10 minutes must be met or exceeded on the day of the encounter. Report 98005 for a visit requiring a low level of MDM or meeting or exceeding 20 minutes of total time; 98006 for a visit requiring a moderate level of MDM or meeting or exceeding 30 minutes of total time; and 98007 for a visit requiring a high level of MDM or meeting or exceeding 40 minutes of total time.

[98008, 98009, 98010, 98011]

Providers report these codes for new patients being seen via telehealth using synchronous audio as an alternative to an in-person visit. The provider and patient interact from different locations through real-time communication in which they can hear each other. The visit must include more than 10 minutes of medical discussion. Video communication is not required for these services. All require a medically appropriate history and/or examination. Code selection is based on the level of medical decision making (MDM) or total time personally spent by the physician and/or other qualified health care professional(s) on the date of the encounter. Factors to be considered in MDM include the number and complexity of problems addressed during the encounter, amount and complexity of data requiring review and analysis, and the risk of complications and/or morbidity or mortality associated with patient management. The most basic service is represented by 98008, which entails straightforward MDM. If time is used for code selection, a total time of 15 minutes must be met or exceeded on the day of the encounter. Report 98009 for a visit requiring a low level of MDM or meeting or exceeding 30 minutes of total time; 98010 for a visit requiring a moderate level of MDM or meeting or exceeding 45 minutes of total time; and 98011 for a visit requiring a high level of MDM or meeting or exceeding 60 minutes of total time.

[98012, 98013, 98014, 98015]

Providers report these codes for established patients being seen via telehealth using synchronous audio as an alternative to an in-person visit. The provider and patient interact from different locations through real-time communication in which they can hear each other. The visit must include more than 10 minutes of medical discussion. Video communication is not required for these services. All require a medically appropriate history and/or examination. Code selection is based on the level of medical decision making (MDM) or total time personally spent by the physician and/or other qualified health care professional(s) on the date of the encounter. Factors to be considered in MDM include the number and complexity of problems addressed during the encounter, amount and complexity of data requiring review and analysis, and the risk of complications and/or morbidity or mortality associated with patient management. The most basic service is represented by 98012, which entails straightforward MDM. If time is used for code selection, a total time of 10 minutes must be exceeded on the day of the encounter. Report 98013 for a visit requiring a low level of MDM or meeting or exceeding 20 minutes of total time; 98014 for a visit requiring a moderate level of MDM or meeting or exceeding 30 minutes of total time; and 98015 for a visit requiring a high level of MDM or meeting or exceeding 40 minutes of total time.

[98016]

A brief, synchronous service using communication technology is performed by a physician or other qualified health care professional to determine if an office visit or other evaluation and management (E/M) service is needed for an established patient. This virtual check-in or triage service is initiated by the patient. This code requires at least five minutes of real-time medical discussion and should not be reported if the problem discussed is related to an E/M encounter that occurred within the previous seven days or when the problem leads to an E/M encounter or procedure within the following 24 hours or next available appointment opening.

99221-99223

Initial hospital inpatient or observation service codes describe the first encounter with the patient by a physician or qualified clinician. CPT guidelines indicate these services may be reported for the first encounter by the provider of the same specialty/subspecialty of the same group practice. Transition from observation to inpatient status does not qualify as an initial hospital encounter. Codes are reported per day and do not differentiate between new or established patients. Under the initial inpatient or observation care category, there are three levels represented by 99221, 99222, and 99223. All services require a medically appropriate history and/or examination. Code selection is based on the level of medical decision making (MDM) or total time personally spent by the physician and/or other qualified health care professional(s) on the date of the encounter. Factors to be considered in MDM include the number and complexity of problems addressed during the encounter, amount and complexity of data requiring review and analysis, and the risk of complications and/or morbidity or mortality associated with patient management. Report 99221 for a visit that entails straightforward or low MDM. If time is used for code selection, a total time of 40 minutes must be met or exceeded on the day of encounter. Report 99222 for a visit requiring a moderate level of MDM or meeting or exceeding 55 minutes of total time. Report 99223 for a high level of MDM or meeting or exceeding 75 minutes of total time. Note that these codes include services provided to patients in a "partial hospital" setting.

99231-99233

Subsequent hospital inpatient or observation service codes describe visits that occur after the first encounter with a patient by a physician or qualified clinician. Codes are reported per day and do not differentiate between new or established patients. Under the subsequent inpatient or observation care category, there are three levels represented by 99231, 99232, and 99233. All services require a medically appropriate history and/or examination. Code selection is based on the level of medical decision making (MDM) or total time personally spent by the physician and/or other qualified health care professional(s) on the date of the encounter. Factors to be considered in MDM include the number and complexity of problems addressed during the encounter, amount and complexity of data requiring review and analysis, and the risk of complications and/or morbidity or mortality associated with patient management. Report 99231 for a visit that entails straightforward or low MDM. If time is used for code selection, a total time of 25 minutes must be met or exceeded on the day of encounter. Report 99232 for a visit requiring a moderate level of MDM or meeting or exceeding 35 minutes of total time. Report 99233 for a high level of MDM or meeting or exceeding 50 minutes of total time.

99234-99236

Hospital inpatient or observation care services in cases where the patient is admitted and discharged on the same date of service by the supervising or qualified clinician are reported with 99234-99236. Two or more encounters are required on the same date: an admission encounter and a discharge encounter. These codes also require a minimum hospital stay of eight hours. Codes do not differentiate between new or established patients. Under this care category, there are three levels represented by 99234, 99235, and 99236. All services require a medically appropriate history and/or examination. Code selection is based on the level of medical decision making (MDM) or total time personally spent by the physician and/or other qualified health care professional(s) on the date of the encounter. Factors to be considered in MDM include the number and complexity of problems addressed during the encounter, amount and complexity of data requiring review and analysis, and the risk of complications and/or morbidity or mortality associated with patient management. Report 99234 for a visit that entails straightforward or low MDM. If time is used for code selection, a total time of 45 minutes must be met or exceeded on the day of the encounter. Report 99235 for a visit requiring a moderate level of MDM or meeting or exceeding 70 minutes of total time. Report 99236 for a high level of MDM or meeting or exceeding 85 minutes of total time.

99238-99239

Hospital discharge services are time-based codes that, when reported, describe the amount of time spent by the qualified clinician that is responsible for discharge services for inpatient or observation care. These discharge day management codes include all final steps involved in the discharge of a patient from the hospital on a date that differs from the date of admission, including the last patient exam, discussing the hospital stay, instructions for ongoing care as it relates to all pertinent caregivers, as well as preparing the medical discharge records, prescriptions, and/or referrals as applicable. Time reported should be for the total duration of time spent by the provider even when the time spent on that date is not continuous. For a hospital discharge duration of 30 minutes or less, report 99238; for a duration of greater than 30 minutes, report 99239.

99242-99245

Office or other outpatient consultation service codes describe encounters where another qualified clinician's advice or opinion regarding diagnosis and treatment is rendered at the request of the primary treating provider. Consultations may also be requested by another appropriate source (e.g., a third-party payer may request a second opinion). The request for a consultation must be documented in the medical record, as well as a written report of the consultation findings. During a consultation, diagnostic or therapeutic services may be initiated at the same encounter or at a follow-up visit. Office or other outpatient sites include the physician's office, a home or residence, or the emergency department. Consultation codes do not differentiate between new or established patients. All services require a medically appropriate history and/or examination. Code selection is based on the level of medical decision making (MDM) or total time personally spent by the physician and/or other qualified health care professional(s) on the date of the encounter. Factors to be considered in MDM include the number and complexity of problems addressed during the encounter, amount and complexity of data requiring review and analysis, and the risk of complications and/or morbidity or mortality associated with patient management. Report 99242 for a visit that entails straightforward MDM. If time is used for code selection, a total time of 20 minutes must be met or exceeded on the day of the encounter. Report 99243 for a visit requiring a low level of MDM or meeting or exceeding 30 minutes of total time; 99244 for a moderate level of MDM or meeting or exceeding 40 minutes of total time; and 99245 for a high level of MDM or meeting or exceeding 55 minutes of total time.

99252-99255

Inpatient or observation consultation service codes describe encounters with patients admitted to the hospital in inpatient or observation status, those residing in nursing facilities, or to patients in a partial hospital setting where another qualified clinician's advice or opinion regarding diagnosis and treatment is rendered at the request of the primary treating provider. The request for a consultation must be documented in the patient's medical record, as well as a written report of the findings of the consultation to the primary treating physician. During the course of a consultation, diagnostic or therapeutic services may be initiated at the same encounter or at a follow-up visit. Consultation codes do not differentiate between new or established patients. Only one inpatient or observation consultation services code should be reported per admission. Subsequent consultation services during the same hospital stay are reported with subsequent inpatient or observation hospital care codes or subsequent nursing facility care codes. All services require a medically appropriate history and/or examination. Code selection is based on the level of medical decision making (MDM) or total time personally spent by the physician and/or other qualified health care professional(s) on the date of the encounter. Factors to be considered in MDM include the number and complexity of problems addressed during the encounter, amount and complexity of data requiring review and analysis, and the risk of complications and/or morbidity or mortality associated with patient management. Report 99252 for a visit that entails straightforward MDM. If time is used for code selection, a total time of 35 minutes must be met or exceeded on the day of the encounter. Report 99253 for a visit requiring a low level of MDM or meeting or exceeding 45 minutes of total time; 99254 for a moderate level of MDM or meeting or exceeding 60 minutes of total time; and 99255 for a high level of MDM or meeting or exceeding 80 minutes of total time.

99281-99285

Emergency department service codes describe E/M services provided to patients in the emergency department (ED). ED codes are typically reported per day and do not differentiate between new or established patients. Other procedures or services performed in conjunction with the emergency room encounter may be reported separately. Under the emergency department services category, there are five levels represented by 99281-99285. For the lowest level of care, 99281, services can be performed by clinical staff and must be face-to-face. The presence of a physician or qualified clinician is not required, but services are performed under their supervision. There are no time or MDM requirements for 99281. The remaining levels, 99282-99285, require a medically appropriate history and/or examination. Code selection is based on the level of medical decision making (MDM). Factors to be considered in MDM include the number and complexity of problems addressed during the encounter, amount and complexity of data requiring review and analysis, and the risk of complications and/or morbidity or mortality associated with patient management. Time is not listed as a component in the code descriptors for emergency department services as these types of services are provided based on the varying intensity of the patient's condition and may involve emergency providers caring for several patients over an extended period involving multiple encounters, making it difficult for the clinician to accurately detail the amount of time spent face-to-face with the patient. Report 99282 for a visit that entails straightforward MDM; 99283 for a visit requiring a low level of MDM; 99284 for a moderate level of MDM; and 99285 for a high level of MDM.

99288

This code is used to report qualified clinician direction of emergency medical systems (EMS) emergency care or advanced life support in the emergency department (ED). This can involve the clinician communicating via a two-way voice system with emergency medical technicians in an ambulance or with other rescue personnel who are outside of the hospital emergency department. Clinician direction of the performance of medically necessary procedures includes, but is not limited to, telemetry of cardiac rhythm; cardiac and/or pulmonary resuscitation; endotracheal or esophageal obturator airway intubation; administration of intravenous (IV) fluids and/or intramuscular (IM), intra-tracheal, or subcutaneous drugs; and/or electrical conversion of cardiac arrhythmia.

99291-99292

Critical care services are reported by a physician or other qualified health care provider for critically ill or injured patients. Critical illnesses or injuries are defined as those with impairment to one or more vital organ systems with an increased risk of rapid or imminent health deterioration. Critical care services require direct patient/provider involvement with highly complex decision making in order to evaluate, control, and support vital systems functions to treat one or more vital organ system failures and/or to avoid further decline of the patient's condition. Vital organ system failure includes, but is not limited to, failure of the central nervous, circulatory, or respiratory systems; kidneys; liver; shock; and other metabolic processes. Generally, critical care services necessitate the interpretation of many physiologic parameters and/or other applications of advanced technology as available in a critical care unit, pediatric intensive care unit, respiratory care unit, in an emergency facility, patient room or other hospital department; however, in emergent situations, critical care may be provided where these elements are not available. Critical care may be provided so long as the patient's condition continues to warrant the level of care according to the criteria described. Care provided to patients residing in a critical care unit but not fitting the criteria for critical care is reported using other E/M codes, as appropriate. These codes are time based codes, meaning the total time spent must be documented and includes direct patient care bedside or time spent on the patient's floor or unit (reviewing laboratory results or imaging studies and discussing the patient's care with medical staff, time spent with family members, caregivers, or other surrogate decision makers to gather information on the patient's medical history, reviewing the patient's condition or prognosis, and discussing various treatment options or limitations of treatment), as long as the clinician is immediately available and not providing services to any other patient during the same time period. Time spent outside of the patient's unit or floor, including telephone calls, caregiver discussions, or time spent in actions that do not directly contribute to the patient's care rendered in the critical unit are not reported as critical care. Report these codes for attendance of the patient during transport for patients 24 months of age or older to or from a facility. Code 99291 represents the first 30 to 74 minutes of critical care and is reported once per day. Additional time beyond the first 74 minutes is reported in 30 minute increments with 99292.

99304-99306

Initial nursing facility service codes describe the first encounter with a patient by a physician or qualified clinician in nursing facilities and skilled nursing facilities, or for services in a psychiatric residential treatment center and intermediate care facility for patients with intellectual disabilities. Initial nursing facility codes may be reported once per admission, per physician or qualified clinician, per stay. Initial nursing facility codes do not differentiate between new or established patients. Under the initial nursing facility care category, there are three levels represented by 99304, 99305, and 99306. All services require a medically appropriate history and/or examination. Code selection is based on the level of medical decision making (MDM) or total time personally spent by the physician and/or other qualified health care professional(s) on the date of the encounter. Factors to be considered in MDM include the number and complexity of problems addressed during the encounter, amount and complexity of data requiring review and analysis, and the risk of complications and/or morbidity or mortality associated with patient management. Report 99304 for a visit that entails straightforward or low MDM. If time is used for code selection, a total time of 25 minutes must be met or exceeded on the day of the encounter. Report 99305 for a visit requiring a moderate level of MDM or meeting or exceeding 35 minutes of total time. Report 99306 for a high level of MDM or meeting or exceeding 50 minutes of total time. For high MDM, an additional component is recognized for initial nursing facility codes for the number and complexity of problems addressed: multiple morbidities requiring intensive management, for the patient who is at risk of worsening status or hospital admission and requiring frequent evaluations with possible changes to medications and/or treatment.

99307-99310

Subsequent nursing facility care service codes describe visits that occur after the first encounter of the patient's nursing facility admission by the supervising qualified clinician. Codes are reported per day and do not differentiate between new or established patients. All services require a medically appropriate history and/or examination. Code selection is based on the level of medical decision making (MDM) or total time personally spent by the physician and/or other qualified health care professional(s) on the date of the encounter. Factors to be considered in MDM include the number and complexity of problems addressed during the encounter, amount and complexity of data requiring review and analysis, and the risk of complications and/or morbidity or mortality associated with patient management. Report 99307 for a visit that entails straightforward MDM. If time is used for code selection, a total time of 10 minutes must be met or exceeded on the day of the encounter. Report 99308 for a visit requiring a low level of MDM or meeting or exceeding 20 minutes of total time; 99309 for a moderate level of MDM or meeting or exceeding 30 minutes of total time; and 99310 for a high level of MDM or meeting or exceeding 45 minutes of total time.

99315-99316

Nursing facility discharge services are time-based codes that describe the amount of time spent by the clinician during all final steps involved in the discharge of a patient from the nursing facility, including the last patient exam, discussing the nursing facility stay, instructions for ongoing care as it relates to all pertinent caregivers, and preparing the medical discharge records, prescriptions, and/or referrals as applicable. A face-to-face service with the patient or family/caregiver is required and may occur on a date that is prior to the date that the patient leaves the facility. Time reported should be for the total duration of time spent by the provider on the date of the encounter, even when the time spent on that date is not continuous. For a nursing facility discharge duration of 30 minutes or less, report 99315; for a duration of greater than 30 minutes, report 99316. These codes are reported following initial and subsequent nursing facility care codes 99304-99306 and 99307-99310.

99341-99345

Home or residence services codes are reported by providers for E/M services rendered to new patients in a home or residence, including a private residence or temporary lodging. Short-term accommodations such as a hotel, campground, hostel, or cruise ship are included, along with an assisted living facility, group home, custodial care facility, and residential substance abuse treatment facility. All services require a medically appropriate history and/or examination. Code selection is based on the level of medical decision making (MDM) or total time personally spent by the physician and/or other qualified health care professional(s) on the date of the encounter. Travel time is not included when selecting a level based on total time. Factors to be considered in MDM include the number and complexity of problems addressed during the encounter, amount and complexity of data requiring review and analysis, and the risk of complications and/or morbidity or mortality associated with patient management. Report 99341 for a visit that entails straightforward MDM. If time is used for code selection, a total time of 15 minutes must be met or exceeded on the day of the encounter. Report 99342 for a visit requiring a low level of MDM or meeting or exceeding 30 minutes of total time; 99344 for a moderate level of MDM or meeting or exceeding 60 minutes of time; and 99345 for a high level of MDM or meeting or exceeding 75 minutes of total time.

99347-99350

Home or residence services codes are reported by providers for E/M services rendered to established patients in a home or residence, including a private residence or temporary lodging. Short-term accommodations such as a hotel, campground, hostel, or cruise ship are included, along with an assisted living facility, group home, custodial care facility, and residential substance abuse treatment facility. All services require a medically appropriate history and/or examination. Code selection is based on the level of medical decision making (MDM) or total time personally spent by the physician and/or other qualified health care professional(s) on the date of the encounter. Travel time is not included when selecting a level based on total time. Factors to be considered in MDM include the number and complexity of problems addressed during the encounter, amount and complexity of data requiring review and analysis, and the risk of complications and/or morbidity or mortality associated with patient management. Report 99347 for a visit that entails straightforward MDM. If time is used for code selection, a total time of 20 minutes must be met or exceeded on the day of the encounter. Report 99348 for a visit requiring a low level of MDM or meeting or exceeding 30 minutes of total time; 99349 for a moderate level of MDM or meeting or exceeding

40 minutes of time; and 99350 for a high level of MDM or meeting or exceeding 60 minutes of total time.

99358-99359
Prolonged time without direct contact with the patient that is performed by the physician or other qualified clinician on a different day than a related E/M service can be reported with 99358 and 99359. For example, the provider may review records for a patient who received a face-to-face E/M service on a previous date or will receive care on a future date. The reported E/M service does not have to be selected based on time to report these prolonged timed services. Time reported for prolonged care should be for the total duration of time spent by the provider even when the time spent on that date is not continuous. Report 99358 for the first hour of prolonged care without direct patient care that is performed on a different date than the face-to-face E/M service and 99359 for each additional 30 minutes.

[99415, 99416]
Prolonged clinical staff services describe special situations in which the physician's staff provide assistance to a patient beyond the usual time associated with circumstances requiring observation of the patient, such as in cases where the patient was administered a new medication or inhaled drug requiring monitoring to ensure patient safety in the office or outpatient setting. Such cases do not necessitate the clinician being face-to-face with the patient throughout the entire time; observation and monitoring of the patient can be performed by a member of the clinician's staff under the provider's supervision. Report these codes in conjunction with the designated E/M service code, along with any other service provided at the same encounter. Codes in this category should report the total amount of face-to-face time spent with the patient and/or family or caregiver by the clinical staff on the same date of service even if the time is not continuous; time spent rendering other separately reportable services other than the E/M service does not count toward the prolonged services time. Report the first hour of prolonged services on a given date with 99415; for each additional 30 minutes of prolonged services, report 99416.

[99417, 99418]
Prolonged time (with and without direct patient contact combined) that is provided by the physician or other qualified health care professional on the date of an evaluation and management service can be reported with 99417 (outpatient) or 99418 (inpatient or observation). These codes are assigned only when the code for the primary E/M service has been selected based solely on total time, and only after exceeding the required time to report the highest-level of service by at least 15 minutes. For example, when reporting an E/M service for an established patient (99215), code 99417 would not be reported until at least 15 minutes of time beyond 40 minutes has been accumulated (55 minutes) on the day of the encounter. Time spent on procedures that can be reported separately are not included in the prolonged time.

99360
Standby services are those requested of a qualified clinician that involves prolonged attendance without face-to-face contact with the patient (e.g., operative or cesarean/high-risk delivery standby, EEG monitoring, or standby to obtain a frozen section specimen). The clinician on standby is not permitted to provide care or services to other patients during the standby period. This code should not be used to report time spent proctoring another individual nor should it be used if the standby period ends with the standby clinician performing a procedure that is subject to the surgical package. This code encompasses the total duration of time spent on standby on a given date; standby services of less than 30 minutes total duration are not reported separately. A second and subsequent period of standby, after the initial 30 minutes, may be reported contingent that each unit of standby service equates to a full 30 minutes.

99366-99368
A medical team conference is defined as a service where at least three qualified health care professionals from different specialties or disciplines, each of whom provides direct care to the patient, actively engage in the evolution, revision, coordination, and implementation of health care services needed by the patient. The conferences may or may not involve the presence of the patient, family members, community agencies, surrogate decision makers/legal guardians, and/or caregivers. Medical team clinicians should report the time spent in a team conference with the patient and/or family present with the appropriate E/M code, using time as a key controlling factor for selecting a code when counseling and/or coordination of care dominates the service. The individual clinician must be directly involved with rendering face-to-face services outside of the conference visit with other clinicians or agencies. All medical professionals participating on the medical team must document their own individual participation in the team conference, in addition to their contributed information and follow-up treatment recommendations. However, only one individual from the same specialty may report a code from this category at the same encounter. No individuals may report a code from range 99366-99368 if participation in the medical team conference is a part of a facility or organizational service contractually provided by the facility or organization. Team conferences commence upon review of the individual patient case and conclude once the review has come to a conclusion. Record keeping and report generation time is not reportable. The clinician must report all time for which he or she was present. Reportable time is not limited to the time that the clinician is communicating with other team members, the patient, and/or the patient's family. Note that time spent in medical team conferences should not be used toward determining other E/M services such as care plan oversight services,

home, domiciliary, or rest home care plan oversight, prolonged services, psychotherapy, or any other E/M service. Nonphysician qualified health care professionals may report 99366, medical team conference, direct (face-to-face) contact with patient and/or family, when the patient is present for any or all of the medical conference with a duration of at least 30 minutes. This includes such providers as speech-language pathologists, physical therapists, occupational therapists, social workers, and dieticians. Medical conferences of less than 30 minutes duration are not reported. Codes 99367-99368 describe team conferences without direct, face-to-face patient and/or family contact.

99374-99380

Care plan oversight (CPO) services are reported for the primary supervising health care provider's time in reviewing and adjusting treatment plans. These services may include review of multiple modalities; patient status relevant laboratory tests; communication with other health care team members, family members, and/or patient advocates; and developing a new course of action or any adjustments to the current plan. Codes are reported within one calendar month and are classified according to the place of service. The initial service for each location is approximately 15 to 29 minutes in duration; each additional 30 minutes is reported separately. Report 99374-99375 for patients in a home health setting; 99377-99378 for hospice patients; and 99379-99380 for patients residing in a nursing facility. Note that only one clinician is eligible to report CPO services for a specific time period in order to demonstrate the singular or lead role the clinician has with a particular patient.

99381-99387

Initial preventive medicine services are typically well-patient examinations for new patients with code selection dependent upon the patient's age. These services include applicable patient history and examination, guidance/recommendation regarding personal risk factors, and any laboratory and/or diagnostic procedures ordered. Clinicians are not required to report minor or self-limiting problems or complaints noted during the course of the preventive examination when those problems do not require any additional work or necessitate performing the key components of a problem oriented E/M service. Report 99381 for infants younger than 1 year of age; 99382 for children 1 to 4 years of age; 99383 for children 5 to 11 years of age; 99384 for adolescents12 to 17 years of age; 99385 for adult patients 18 to 39 years of age; 99386 for patients 40 to 64 years of age; and 99387 for patients 65 years of age and older.

99391-99397

Periodic comprehensive preventive medicine services are typically well-patient examinations for established patients presenting for reevaluations and/or management of overall health condition with code selection dependent upon the patient's age. These services include applicable patient history and examination, guidance/recommendation regarding personal risk factors, and any laboratory and/or diagnostic procedures ordered. Clinicians are not required to report minor or self-limiting problems or complaints noted during the course of the preventive examination when those problems do not require any additional work or necessitate performing the key components of a problem oriented E/M service. Report 99391 for infants younger than 1 year of age; 99392 for children 1 to 4 years of age; 99393 for children 5 to 11 years of age; 99394 for adolescents12 to 17 years of age; 99395 for adult patients 18 to 39 years of age; 99396 for patients 40 to 64 years of age; and 99397 for patients 65 years of age and older.

99401-99404

Preventive medicine individual counseling services are face-to-face services performed by a qualified clinician in order to foster healthy living and/or avert illness/injury. Risk factor counseling may be utilized in the absence of illness. These services may include counseling/evaluation of family issues, appropriate diet and exercise, high-risk behavior, avoidance of injury, dental issues, and discussion of available laboratory and/or diagnostic results. Report 99401 for encounters lasting 15 minutes; 99402 for 30 minutes; 99403 for 45 minutes; and 99404 for a duration of 60 minutes.

99406-99409

Individual behavior change intervention services are counseling and/or intervention services directed at high-risk behaviors such as tobacco, alcohol, and substance abuse. These services can be reported as treatment of the condition or in relation to the condition that has the potential of causing illness or injury. Additionally, the encounter uses validated instruments to determine the patient's opinion related to behavior change and providing input on a plan to change behavior with appropriate actions and motivation. Report 99406 for smoking and tobacco cessation counseling requiring three to 10 minutes of time and 99407 for counseling requiring more than ten minutes. Report 99408 for alcohol and/or substance abuse screening utilizing such instruments as AUDIT, DAST, and intervention services requiring 15 to 30 minutes; for more than 30 minutes, report 99409.

99411-99412

Preventive medicine group counseling services are face-to-face services performed by a qualified clinician in order to foster healthy living and/or avert illness/injury. Risk factor counseling may be utilized in the absence of illness in a group setting. These services may include counseling/evaluation of family issues, appropriate diet and exercise, high-risk behavior, avoidance of injury, dental issues, and discussion of available laboratory and/or diagnostic results. Report 99411 for encounters of 30 minutes duration and 99412 for encounters lasting 60 minutes.

[99421, 99422, 99423]

Online medical evaluation services are non-face-to-face encounters originating from the established patient to the physician or other qualified health care professional for evaluation or management of a problem. The patient initiates the digital communication through a Health Insurance Portability and Accountability Act (HIPAA) compliant platform. The service includes all asynchronous (not in real-time) communication with the patient, review of the initial patient query and medical records, personal interaction with clinical staff by the provider related to the patient query, and development of a plan including ordering any necessary prescriptions or tests. The service may include more than one provider responding to the same patient and is only reportable once during seven days for the same encounter. These codes are not reported if the online patient request is related to an E/M service that occurred within the previous seven days or within the global period following a procedure. Report 99421 if the cumulative time during the seven-day period is five to 10 minutes; 99422 for 11 to 20 minutes; and 99423 for 21 or more minutes.

99446-99449 [99451, 99452]

Interprofessional telephone/internet/electronic health record consultation services are utilized when the attending qualified clinician requests the input of a physician or qualified clinician with specific knowledge of the condition. This specialist may assist in diagnosis or treatment of the patient without seeing the patient and often occurs when the situation is urgent and/or complex in nature. The patient may be a new or established patient with a new problem or exacerbation of a current problem in the eyes of the consultant; however, the consultant may not have seen the patient within the previous 14 days. This code may not be reported for transfer of care or to schedule a face-to-face with the consultant within the next 14 days or next available appointment opening. This discussion includes appropriate review of medical records, laboratory and radiology results, medication review/tolerance, and pathology results. The consult should account for more than 50 percent of the time in discussion; if more than one discussion is necessary, the time is cumulative with the code reported one time. The patient's medical record should contain a request for consult with an explanation as to the medical necessity of the request and the consultant should provide a verbal and written report to the requesting/treating clinician. These codes are not reportable if the discussion requires less than five minutes of time. Report 99446 for encounters of five to 10 minutes duration; 99447 for 11 to 20 minutes; 99448 for 21 to 30 minutes; and 99449 for encounters of more than 30 minutes duration. Report 99451 for encounters of five or more minutes that include a written report only from the consultant. The attending qualified clinician can report 99452 when 16 to 30 minutes of the clinician's time is spent preparing for or communicating with the consultant; 99452 can only be reported once during a 14-day period.

[99453, 99454]

A physician or other qualified health care professional orders an FDA-defined remote patient monitoring (RPM) device that is used by a patient for the purposes of collecting, monitoring, and reporting health-related data to the provider, including, but not limited to, weight, blood pressure, or pulse oximetry. This technology allows for the gathering of health data from the patient in one location and the electronic transmission of that data to a provider in a different location for review and subsequent recommendations, particularly in patients with ongoing and/or chronic disease processes. Code 99453 reports the work involved with orienting the patient to the RPM process, the initial device set-up, and patient instruction and training for each episode of care. An episode of care is described as starting at the time the RPM device service begins and is complete when the established treatment goal has been reached. Code 99454 reports the supply of the actual device including the daily recordings and program alert transmissions for a 30-day period. These codes should not be reported for monitoring if the duration is less than 16 days.

[99091]

A physician or other qualified health care professional collects and interprets physiologic data. The data (e.g., blood pressure) is stored digitally and may be transmitted by the patient and/or the caregiver to the provider. The report should contain the time it took the provider to acquire the physiologic data, review and interpret the data, and modify any care plan due to the additional data acquisition. A minimum of 30 minutes every 30 days must be spent in the collection and interpretation of data to report this service.

[99473, 99474]

Self-measured blood pressure monitoring (SMBP) has been shown to be an effective approach to lowering blood pressure (BP), improving control in patients with hypertension, and increasing patient compliance with antihypertensive therapy. Also known as out-of-office BP measurement or home BP monitoring, the practice involves the use of devices that have been validated for clinical accuracy. Devices that measure blood pressure over the upper arm remain the most accurate choice compared to other available options, and remain the standard for proper BP measurement over finger, wrist, mobile health, and wearable devices. Report 99473 for patient education/training and device calibration. Report 99474 for separate self-measurements of two readings, one minute apart, twice daily over a 30-day period with a minimum of 12 readings. This includes collection of data reported by the patient and/or caregiver to the physician or other qualified health care professional, with a report of average systolic and diastolic pressures and subsequent communication of a treatment plan to the patient.

[99457, 99458]

The provider or clinical staff utilizes the results obtained from an FDA-defined remote patient physiologic monitoring (RPM) device to oversee the patient's treatment plan. The device is ordered by a physician or other qualified health care provider and used by the patient for the purposes of collecting, monitoring, and reporting health-related data, including, but not limited to, weight, blood pressure, or pulse oximetry. This technology allows for the gathering of health data from the patient in one location and the electronic transmission of that data to a provider in a different location for review and subsequent recommendations, particularly in patients with ongoing and/or chronic disease processes. Report these codes to identify time spent managing care when the patient or the practice does not meet requirements for reporting a more specific service. These codes may be reported simultaneously with chronic care management, principal care management, transitional care management, and behavioral health integration services. Time involved in performing this service should remain separate and distinct from other services and does not count toward the required time for both services in a single month. Live and interactive communication with the patient and/or caregiver is required; data may be patient-reported or device-generated. Report 99457 for the first 20 minutes of clinician time per calendar month and 99458 for each additional 20 minutes.

99450, 99455-99456

Special evaluation and management services are utilized to report encounters where baseline information is obtained for life or disability insurance purposes. These codes do not differentiate between new and/or established patients and do not involve any active treatment for current medical conditions. The basic life examination checks height, weight, and blood pressure with completion of history and required documentation. Blood and urine samples may also be obtained for analysis. The work related examination completes a medical history and examination focused on specific condition, diagnosis, determination of capabilities/impairment, medical treatment planning, and any required documentation completion. Report 99450 for a basic life and/or disability examination; 99455 for a work related or medical disability examination performed by the treating/primary physician; and 99456 for a work related or medical disability examination performed by a provider other than the treating/primary physician.

99460-99463

Newborn care services are reported, per day, for initial examinations of normal newborns during the first 28 days after birth before discharge home. These services include maternal/fetal/newborn history, newborn examination, any orders for diagnostic testing and/or medical treatment, discussion with family, and permanent documentation. Procedures such as circumcision are not included with these codes and should be reported separately, when performed. For initial newborn care services performed in the hospital or birthing center, report 99460; when services are provided in a setting other than the hospital or birthing center, report 99461. Subsequent visits rendered in either setting are reported with 99462. For newborn services provided in the hospital or birthing center where the infant is admitted and discharged on the same date of service, report 99463.

99464-99465

Delivery/birthing room attendance and resuscitation services are reported when special newborn circumstances require additional attendance and/or care. Report 99464 when attendance during delivery is requested by the delivering health care professional with newborn stabilization. Report 99465 for delivery/birthing room resuscitation, including any positive pressure ventilation and/or chest compression when required due to unsatisfactory ventilation or cardiac output.

99466-99467 [99485, 99486]

Pediatric critical care patient transport services report time the physician provides direct or supervisory care of a critically ill/injured patient aged 24 months or younger during interfacility transportation. The timing takes place when the physician acquires initial responsibility for the patient at the first facility and concludes once the receiving facility takes over. For direct patient care, the physician is in contact with the patient during transfer. For supervisory care, the physician is responsible for communication with the transport staff before transfer, at the originating facility, and during transfer to the receiving facility. Additionally, the physician provides instruction on the treatment of the patient to the transport staff who are in direct contact with the patient and provide the care. Several services are included in the care of these patients and are not separately reportable, such as monitoring vital signs, cardiac output evaluation, chest x-rays, pulse oximetry measurement, blood gas, ECGs, intubation, temporary pacing, ventilation oversight, and any required vascular access. Report 99466 for direct patient care during transfer for the first 30 to 74 minutes; report 99467 for each additional 30 minutes. Report 99485 for the initial 30 minutes of supervision of transport, including any interpretation and reports; report 99486 for each additional 30 minutes.

99468-99476

Inpatient neonatal and pediatric critical care services are reported for neonates (28 days of age or younger) and pediatric patients (29 days through less than 6 years of age) beginning with the date of admission to the critical care unit and for all following days that the patient remains in the unit. Codes are only reportable once daily, per patient, by a single provider within the admission range of the specific facility. Several services are included in the care of these patients and are not separately reportable by the provider, such as monitoring vital signs, any required vascular access, ventilation oversight, blood gas, pulse oximetry measurement, evaluation of car seat, blood transfusion, oral/nasogastric tube insertion, suprapubic bladder aspiration and/or bladder catheter placement, and lumbar puncture. Facilities, however, may report these services separately. Report 99468 for initial inpatient neonates; 99469 for subsequent inpatient neonates; 99471 for initial inpatient pediatric patients aged 29 days to 24 months; 99472 for subsequent inpatient pediatric patients aged 29 days to 24 months; 99475 for initial inpatient pediatric patients 2 to 5 years of age; and 99476 for subsequent inpatient pediatric patients 2 to 5 years of age.

99477-99480

Initial and continuing intensive care services are used to report services for children who do not meet the critical care criteria but require attentive observation, regular intercessions, and other intensive care treatment. Codes in this group include those specific to low and very low birth weights and those neonatal patients who may have normal birth weight but require the above mentioned intensive care treatment, such as vital signs and cardiac/respiratory monitoring, body temperature regulation, enteral/parenteral nutrition, laboratory and oxygen testing/adjustments, and full-time oversight by a qualified clinician. Codes are reported once daily, per patient, by a single provider at a specific facility. These codes include the same services defined in the Neonatal and Pediatric Critical Care services. Report 99477 for initial hospital care of neonates 28 days old or younger requiring intensive care; 99478 for subsequent intensive care for infants with very low birth weight (current weight under 1500 grams); 99479 for subsequent intensive care for infants with very low birth weight (current weight 1500 to 2500 grams), and 99480 for subsequent intensive care of the recovering infant (present body weight 2501 to 5000 grams).

99483

Cognitive assessment and care plan services describe a detailed and thorough assessment of a patient who is demonstrating signs and/or symptoms of a cognitive impairment to determine a diagnosis as well as a cause and severity of the impairment. As part of the examination, the clinician assesses a number of factors that could impact cognitive function including, but not limited to, psychosocial, psychoactive medications, depression, chronic pain, infection, tumor, and stroke. In order to report this service, all of the following elements must be documented: assessing activities of daily living (ADL); dementia staging via a standardized instrument (FAST, CDR); review and reconciliation of medication including high-risk medications; screening for neuropsychiatric and behavioral conditions including depression using a standardized instrument; safety evaluation; caregiver identification; developing, updating, or revising an advance care plan; and creating a written care plan to deal with cognitive symptoms, any limitations in function, and referrals to community support services (adult day programs, support groups, rehabilitations) as necessary. Medical decision making for this service needs to include elements such as the patient's prognosis, rehabilitation needs, other personal assistance services such as financial, social, and legal or community-based assistance (meals, transportation), as well as other types of personal assistance services. This service does not differentiate between new or established patient status and the clinician usually spends approximately 60 minutes on the date of the encounter. A single clinician cannot report this code more than once per 180 days.

[99437, 99439, 99490, 99491]

Care management services are defined as those management and support services that are 1) rendered by clinical staff while under the direction of a clinician who may be a physician or other qualified health care professional (QHP) or 2) provided personally by a physician or other QHP to a patient who resides in a personal residence or in an assisted living facility, domiciliary, or rest home. Some components of care management services include the establishment, implementation, monitoring, or revision of the patient's individual care plan; coordination of the care provided by other agencies and professionals; and education afforded to the patient or their caregiver regarding the patient's care plan, condition, and prognosis. Intended to improve coordination of care and patient engagement while reducing hospitalizations and disjointed care, care management services also take into account the patient's other medical conditions, psychosocial needs, and normal activities of daily living (ADL). Chronic care management services are represented by resequenced codes 99490, 99439, 99491, and 99437. Typically, patients receiving this care have a minimum of two and possibly more chronic ongoing or episodic health conditions that are anticipated to last at least one year (or until the patient expires) and that put the patient at increased risk of death, exacerbation, or functional decline. Chronic care management services include the establishment, implementation, revision, or monitoring of a comprehensive care plan. Code 99490 should be reported once per calendar month for the first 20 minutes of clinical staff time when directed by a physician or other QHP; for each additional 20 minutes, report 99439. Code 99439 should not be reported more than twice per calendar month. Code 99491 is also reported once per calendar month and represents the first 30 minutes provided personally by the physician or other QHP involved with care management activities; report 99437 for each additional 30 minutes.

99487-99489

Care management services are defined as those management and support services that are 1) rendered by clinical staff while under the direction of a clinician who may be a physician or other qualified health care professional (QHP) or 2) provided personally by a physician or other QHP to a patient who resides in a personal residence or in an assisted living facility, domiciliary, or rest home. Some components of care management services include the establishment, implementation, monitoring, or revision of the patient's individual care plan; coordination of the care provided by other agencies and professionals; and education afforded to the patient or their caregiver regarding the patient's care plan, condition, and prognosis. Intended to improve

Evaluation and Management

coordination of care and patient engagement while reducing hospitalizations and disjointed care, care management services also consider the patient's other medical conditions, psychosocial needs, and normal activities of daily living (ADL). Complex chronic care management services (99487, 99489) are provided to patients who typically have a minimum of two and possibly more chronic ongoing or episodic health conditions that are anticipated to last at least one year (or until the patient expires) and that put the patient at increased risk of death, exacerbation, or functional decline. Included is the establishment, implementation, revision, or monitoring of a comprehensive care plan that requires moderate or high complexity medical decision making. Code 99487 is reported once per calendar month for the first 60 minutes of clinical staff time when directed by a physician or other QHP; for each additional 30 minutes, report 99489. Code 99489 should not be reported more than twice per calendar month.

[99424, 99425, 99426, 99427]

Principal care management services are provided to patients for a single high-risk disease. There is one complex condition that is chronic and expected to last a minimum of three months that puts the patient at substantial risk of exacerbation, functional decline, hospitalization, or death. The disease-specific care plan related to this condition requires on-going development, monitoring, or revising. Frequent adjustments to the medication regimen are required, or patient comorbidities increase the complexity of the condition's management. Communication and care coordination between those furnishing care is required on an ongoing basis. Report 99424 once per calendar month for the first 30 minutes of care provided personally by a physician or other qualified health care professional (QHP); report 99425 for each additional 30 minutes. Report 99426 once per calendar month for the first 30 minutes of clinical staff time when directed by a physician or other QHP; for each additional 20 minutes, report 99427.

99492-99494

Psychiatric collaborative care management services describe care reported by a qualified clinician overseeing a behavioral health care manager and psychiatric consultant who provide a behavioral health assessment, including establishing, starting, revising, or monitoring a plan of care as well as providing brief interventions to a patient diagnosed with a mental health disorder. The psychiatric consultant contracts directly with the qualified clinician to render the consultation portion of the service. Patients are generally referred to a behavioral health care manager for assistance in receiving treatment for newly diagnosed conditions that have been unresponsive to traditional or standard care provided in a nonpsychiatric environment or who need additional examination and evaluation before a referral to a psychiatric care setting. In 99492, the required elements include outreach and engagement; initial patient assessment that involves the administration of a validated rating scale; development of an individual patient care plan; psychiatric consultant review and modifications, as needed; input of patient data into a registry and tracking of patient progress and follow up; and provision of brief interventions using evidence-based techniques. In 99493, the required elements include tracking patient follow up and progress via registry; weekly caseload participation with a psychiatric consultant; working together and coordinating with the qualified clinician on a regular basis; additional ongoing review of the patient's progress and recommendations for treatment changes, including medications with the psychiatric consultant; provision of brief interventions with the use of evidence-based techniques; monitoring patient outcomes using validated rating scales; and relapse prevention planning. Episodes of care begin when the patient is first directed to the behavioral health care manager and ends when the treatment goals have been reached, the goals were not reached and the patient was referred to another provider for ongoing treatment, or no psychiatric collaborative care management was provided for a period of six consecutive months. These codes do not differentiate between new or established patient status. Report 99492 for the first 70 minutes of initial psychiatric collaborative care management in the first calendar month; 99493 for the first 60 minutes of care in a subsequent month; and 99494 for each additional 30 minutes of initial or subsequent care in a calendar month.

99495-99496

Transitional care management services are reported for patients requiring moderate to high level of medical decision making who are transitioning from an inpatient or observation facility, partial hospital, or a nursing facility to a home or community type setting, including a private residence or temporary lodging. Short-term accommodations such as a hotel, campground, hostel, or cruise ship are included, along with an assisted living facility, custodial care facility, residential substance abuse treatment facility, or a group home that is not licensed as an intermediate care facility for individuals with intellectual disabilities. The start date is the day of discharge and lasts through the following 29 days. These services include one face-to-face encounter in addition to other services performed within the specific timeframe by a physician or qualified clinician or by licensed clinical staff under qualified clinician direction. Initial communication (direct contact, which may include telephonic or electronic means) must occur within two business days of discharge with review of the patient's medication regimen by the date of the initial face-to-face encounter. The date of the first face-to-face encounter and medical decision making drives the code selection. Subsequent evaluation and management services by the same provider may be reported separately. Only one provider may report transitional care management services during the 30 days following discharge. Report 99495 when MDM is of at least a moderate level during the service period, in addition to the face-to-face encounter within 14 days of hospital discharge. Report 99496 when MDM is a high level during the service period and the face-to-face encounter is within seven days of hospital discharge. Note that MDM for transitional care management is determined by the decision making over the entire service period.

99497-99498

Advance care planning services are reported for the discussion and explanation of advanced directives by a qualified clinician. These services are time-based services that do not involve any active management of problems during the course of the face-to-face service between the provider and a patient, family member, or surrogate and may be reported on the same day as another E/M service. Report 99497 for the first 30 minutes of advance care planning and 99498 for each additional 30 minutes.

[99484]

General behavioral health integration care management services are provided by clinical staff, under the direct supervision of a qualified clinician, to a patient with a diagnosed behavioral health condition, including substance use issues, requiring care management services for a minimum of 20 minutes (either face-to-face or non-face-to-face) per calendar month. Specific elements of a treatment plan must be provided and documented, including an initial assessment or follow-up monitoring involving the use of validated rating scales; behavioral health care planning relating to the patient's behavioral or mental health problems with revisions in cases where a patient is not responding to treatment or has a status change; organizing and coordinating all aspects of the patient's mental health care such as therapy, medications, counseling, and/or psychiatric consultations; and continuing ongoing care in conjunction with a designated care team member. The clinician does not need to provide a comprehensive assessment and treatment plan nor is the practice required to have all chronic care management functions. The patient may receive these services in any outpatient setting once certain criteria are established, namely that the clinician maintains a relationship with the patient and clinical staff and that the clinical staff be available to provide the patient with face-to-face services.

[99459]

A pelvic exam is performed in addition to an evaluation and management service in a non-facility setting. The physician places two lubricated and gloved fingers inside the vagina to palpate the cervix, uterus, and ovaries while using the other hand to gently palpate the top of the uterus with pressure on the abdomen, noting the organs' size, shape, and/or any abnormality.

Category III

0042T

Cerebral perfusion analysis is performed to evaluate the blood supply to the brain utilizing computed tomography (CT). A contrast enhancement agent known as a tracer is administered. The blood transports the tracer to the brain, where the tracer perfuses, or fills, the tissue. This perfused tissue appears brighter in the CT image. The rate at which the tissue becomes brighter is proportional to the perfusion rate. A perfusion-weighted image is displayed by the software for the CT scanner, which measures the rate of change.

0054T-0055T

Computer-assisted musculoskeletal navigation techniques are used with many orthopedic procedures, especially for accurate placement of the acetabular component during hip replacement surgery. Preoperative images of patient-specific bone geometry are first obtained for the surgical plan in whatever imaging modality is to be used. The patient-specific surgical plan and images are used during surgery to guide the surgeon by combining these with intraoperative navigation capabilities. Optical targets, or trackers, such as digitizing or LED-equipped probes, are attached to points on the bone anatomy or to surgical tools. An optical camera tracks the position of these for accurate navigation and measurement in relation to any bone or instrument movement as the surgery is performed. The software in these navigational systems matches or "registers" the position of the patient on the operating table to the geometric description of the bony surface derived from the images already used to plan the surgery. Multiple images are simultaneously displayed on the monitor. The "virtual" tool trajectory that corresponds to the tracked tool movements is displayed over the previously saved views in real-time as the surgeon operates. These are add-on codes to be used in addition to the primary procedure. Report 0054T for image-guidance based on fluoroscopic imaging and 0055T for CT/MRI imaging. If CT and MRI are both performed, 0055T is reported only once.

0071T-0072T

Focused ultrasound ablation is a noninvasive surgical technique that uses thermal ablation to destroy uterine leiomyomata. In focused ultrasound ablation the ultrasound beam penetrates through soft tissues causing localized high temperatures for a few seconds at the targeted site, in this case the uterine leiomyomata. This produces thermocoagulation and necrosis of the uterine leiomyomata without damage to overlaying and surrounding tissues. Magnetic resonance (MR) guidance is used in conjunction with focused ultrasound ablation to provide more precise target definition. Since certain MR parameters are also temperature sensitive, MR guidance also allows estimation of optimal thermal doses to the uterine leiomyomata and detection of relatively small temperature elevations in surrounding tissues thereby preventing any irreversible damage to surrounding tissues. Report 0071T for total leiomyomata tissue volume less than 200 cc. Report 0072T for leiomyomata tissue volume equal to or greater than 200 cc.

0075T-0076T

The physician places one or more stents into extracranial vertebral arteries. The procedure may be performed via a percutaneous (through a catheter) or an open approach. A stent delivery system, which may include an embolic capturing device, is loaded into a delivery pod and advanced to the blocked or narrowed artery. The embolic protection device is deployed first, distal to the lesion, so that any emboli are collected as the blood passes through the device. The stent is advanced out of the pod until it expands to open the narrowing. The procedure is performed under radiologic supervision. Report 0075T for the placement of the stent(s) into the initial artery and 0076T for stent placement into each additional vessel. Both codes include radiologic supervision and interpretation.

0095T

The physician removes an artificial disc prosthesis placed during a previous disc arthroplasty by anterior approach. The physician approaches the cervical vertebrae by making an incision through the neck, avoiding the esophagus, trachea, and thyroid. Retractors separate the intervertebral muscles. The implant is located and any adhesions are freed. Distraction is applied to open the intervertebral space and the implant is removed. The area is explored and debrided. When the procedure is complete, the fascia and vertebral muscles are repaired and returned to their anatomical positions, drains are placed, and the wound is closed. Code 0095T must be reported in conjunction with 22864; assign once for each additional cervical interspace.

0098T

The physician revises an artificial disc prosthesis placed during a previous disc arthroplasty through anterior approach. The prosthesis may be migrating from a lack of fixation and require components to be replaced or adjusted. The physician approaches the cervical vertebrae by making an incision through the neck, avoiding the esophagus, trachea, and thyroid. Retractors separate the intervertebral muscles. The implant is located, the area is explored, and any adhesions are freed. Distraction is applied to open the intervertebral space. The arthroplastic disc is removed, and the endplates of the vertebral body are reshaped and prepped for reinsertion. New height, depth, and width dimensions may also be taken with the vertebral body distracted in cases where another, more appropriately sized disc prosthesis is required. The components are reinserted, and the fascia and vertebral muscles are repaired and returned to their anatomical positions. The incision is closed. Code 0098T must be reported in conjunction with 22861; assign once for each additional cervical interspace.

0100T

The physician implants an electronic retinal prosthesis to restore vision through retinal stimulation for patients affected by degenerative conditions of the eye. Under appropriate anesthesia, an incision is made around the whole circumference of the cornea, and the rectus muscles are isolated. The external transmitter (receiver and pulse generator) is placed by extending a receiving coil under the lateral rectus muscle and into the infratemporal quadrant; the electronics case is sutured to the sclera. Using a pars plana approach, a vitrectomy is performed. Three small incisions are made, and an infusion cannula is inserted through one of the openings in the sclera. The posterior hyaloid is stripped from the retina. Membrane peeling may be performed. The intraocular electrode array is inserted through an enlargement of one of the pars plana incisions. The array is positioned over the center of the retina in the area of the fovea centralis and secured with a custom titanium retinal tack. Sutures are placed in the conjunctiva and surgical incisions are closed. Antibiotic ointment and a pressure patch may be applied.

0101T-0102T

Extracorporeal shock wave therapy (ESWT) involves the application of pressure waves that travel through fluid and soft tissue, with effects of the shock wave occurring at sites where there is a change in impedance, such as the bone-soft tissue interface. ESWT, which may also be referred to as acoustic wave therapy, radial pressure wave therapy, or focused shock wave therapy, uses focused ultrasound energy to treat common orthopedic conditions (i.e., plantar calcaneal spurs, epicondylopathic humeri radialis) because of the therapy's stimulatory effect on bone formation. Other potential uses of ESWT include treating bone marrow hypoxia and subperiosteal hemorrhage, increasing regional blood flow, and activating osteogenic factors such as bone morphogenic protein, direct cellular effects, and mechanical effects as a result of strain gradients. Typically performed on an outpatient basis, ESWT is intended as a noninvasive alternative to surgical treatment in certain patients who have failed conventional medical therapy. Report 0101T for extracorporeal shock wave application to the musculoskeletal system; the physician may utilize local anesthesia to numb the targeted area for treatment. Code 0102T requires anesthesia other than local for ESWT performed by a physician on the lateral humeral epicondyle.

[0512T, 0513T]

Extracorporeal shock wave therapy (ESWT) is a noninvasive, low pain, safe treatment for patients suffering from acute and chronic soft tissue wounds, including diabetic and pressure ulcers, burns, and surgical site wounds. This procedure often requires only a local anesthetic (LA), although some studies indicate that ESWT may not be as effective using LA. ESWT is described as a series of sound pulses delivered in two phases, creating temporary pressure into the tissue without any long-term damage. There are various types of shock wave generators that have been developed for ESWT: radial ESWT (i.e., electrohydraulic mode) is the most recognized and consists of a device containing air or gas located within the generator that produces low energy value linear pressure; focused ESWT is created from three different sources, including electromagnetic, electrohydraulic, and piezoelectric that allow pressure pulses to quickly increase and strengthen the sound waves. ESWT works by causing a cellular response improving circulation within even the smallest blood vessels (i.e., microcirculation). The primary difference in these therapies is the frequency (speed) of the sound waves produced and the depth and range of the treatment area. One proprietary system features a handheld wand that attaches to a larger central unit that work together to promote and expedite healing of diabetic foot ulcers. Report 0512T for treatment to the initial wound and 0513T for each additional wound. These codes include topical application and dressing care.

0106T-0107T

Quantitative sensory testing (QST) done with pressure touch or vibration stimuli assesses nerve fiber sensation in a larger diameter and detects sensory loss in cases of diabetes, alcoholism, and drug therapy or evaluates nerve recovery after surgery. When applying vibration stimuli (0107T), described here, a small controller unit with two separate vibrator rods is used. The rods apply the vibration stimulus to the skin while the vibration amplitude is adjusted through the control unit. Report 0106T when similar quantitative sensory testing is done using a device designed to apply touch pressure stimuli at different thresholds to the area being tested.

0108T-0110T

Quantitative sensory testing (QST) done as thermal sensory analysis can diagnose early diabetic neuropathy. A small thermode device capable of heating or cooling is attached to the patient's skin and the extremity is tested with heat or cooling stimuli to assess sensation. The patient's thresholds for warmth, cold, heat-induced pain, or cold-induced pain are quantitatively measured and compared with reference values that are age-matched for the normal population. The test may take up to an hour, depending on the number of sites to be tested. Report 0108T for QST testing and interpretation per extremity using cold stimuli and 0109T for heat-pain stimuli. Use 0110T for QST testing and interpretation per extremity using stimuli other than heat, cold, vibration, or pressure.

0164T

The physician removes an artificial disc prosthesis placed during a previous disc arthroplasty by anterior approach. The physician uses an anterior approach to reach the implant in the lumbar vertebrae by making an incision through the abdomen. Some implants require only minimal access, approximately 7 cm long, for a mini-retroperitoneal approach. Retractors separate the intervertebral muscles. The affected intervertebral implant location is confirmed by separately reportable x-ray. The physician cleans out the intervertebral disc space with a rongeur, removing the cartilaginous material to be replaced in preparation for removing an implant, and removes the implant. With the disc assembly removal complete, the wound is closed and a drain may be placed. Report 0164T for each additional lumbar artificial disc removal after the first, which is reported with 22865.

0165T

The physician revises an artificial disc prosthesis placed during a previous disc arthroplasty through an anterior approach. The prosthesis may be migrating from a lack of fixation and require components to be replaced or adjusted. The lumbar vertebrae are approached by making an incision through the abdomen. Retractors separate the intervertebral muscles. The implant is located, the area is explored, and any adhesions are freed. Distraction is applied to open the intervertebral space. The arthroplastic disc is removed, and the endplates of the vertebral body are reshaped and prepped for reinsertion. New height, depth, and width dimensions may also be taken with the vertebral body distracted in cases where another, more appropriately sized disc prosthesis is required. The components are reinserted, and the fascia and vertebral muscles are repaired and returned to their anatomical positions. The incision is closed. This code reports each additional lumbar interspace and must be reported in conjunction with 22862.

0174T-0175T

Computer-aided detection (CAD) systems are diagnostic tools that assist radiologists in the detection of subtle findings to facilitate early cancer detection. Used as an adjunct to radiographic images of the chest, it analyzes and highlights areas in the image that appear to be solid nodules, alerting the radiologist to the need for additional analysis. The CAD system consists of dedicated computer software and a review workstation. After initial images are obtained, copies are sent to the workstation for user review and also to the processing server for CAD analysis. Areas of irregularity are analyzed and a report generated that points out suspicious areas the radiologist can reassess. Code 0174T reports CAD of chest radiographs with further physician review for interpretation and report performed concurrently with primary interpretation. It is reported in addition to the primary radiology procedure. Code 0175T reports CAD that is performed remotely from the primary interpretation and is not reported in conjunction with the primary procedure.

0184T

The physician excises a rectal tumor using the transanal endoscopic microsurgical (TEMS) approach. Following administration of appropriate anesthesia, the patient is placed in a lithotomy position. Dilation of the rectum is achieved and maintained with constant-flow carbon dioxide insufflation. Using specially designed instruments inserted via a resectoscope, full-thickness excision (including the muscularis propria) of the tumor is achieved.

Dissection and suturing are performed within the rectal cavity.

[0253T, 0671T]

Aqueous drainage devices are employed to treat refractory, primary, open-angle glaucoma. The procedures described here use minimally invasive glaucoma surgery (MIGS), in which the aqueous fluid is drained from the anterior chamber into the Schlemm's canal by shunting or stenting, lowering intraocular pressure (IOP) and decreasing the chances of blindness caused by glaucoma. They use an internal approach that does not disrupt the cornea, no extraocular plate reservoir is utilized, and the procedures are performed without concomitant cataract removal. Typically, the physician makes a small, temporal clear corneal incision using gonioscopy and inspects the angle with a gonioprism to assess the implant location. Viscoelastic may be used to deepen the anterior chamber and to clear any blood from the implantation site. After locating and exposing the scleral spur, the physician introduces the microdelivery system into the anterior chamber and advances it to the desired location. The device is inserted into the targeted location and the inserter is withdrawn. The anterior chamber is flushed and irrigated and may be inflated with balanced saline solution to attain physiologic pressure. In 0671T, one or more drainage devices are inserted into the trabecular meshwork, which is the first layer of tissue regulating aqueous drainage. This is the shortest drainage stent, just penetrating the trabecular meshwork. In 0253T, the stent is inserted into the suprachoroidal space, which is a highly selective part of the ocular anatomy and requires a longer stent.

0198T

The physician tests for glaucoma, a multi-factorial disease that is affected by both intraocular pressure (IOP) and ocular blood flow (OBF). Each time the heart beats, a bolus of blood flows through the ocular choroid, causing IOP to rise and fall with each pulse. Greatest risk to the eye occurs when IOP is high and pulsatile OBF is low, resulting in stress on the retinal neurons near the disc. The physician uses an ocular blood flow tonometer that repeatedly measures the IOP during the cardiac pulse cycle. The tonometer takes multiple readings per second and analyzes the changes in IOP. A computer analyzes the data, calculates the pulsatile OBF, and provides a report of the minimum, average, and maximum values. Code 0198T includes interpretation and report.

0200T-0201T

Percutaneous sacroplasty (sacral augmentation) is a minimally invasive, image-guided procedure performed by a one- or two-sided injection into a sacral insufficiency fracture. A local anesthetic is administered. The radiologist may use imaging techniques, such as CT scanning and fluoroscopy, to guide percutaneous placement of the needle during the procedure and to monitor the injection procedure. Sterile biomaterial such as polymethyl methacrylate is injected from one or both sides into the sacrum and sacral insufficiency fracture and acts as bone cement to reinforce the fractured or collapsed vertebra. The procedure does not restore the original shape to the vertebra, but it does stabilize the bone, preventing further fracture or collapse. Report 0200T for unilateral percutaneous sacroplasty using one or more needles and 0201T for a bilateral procedure using two or more needles. These codes include the use of a balloon or mechanical device, imaging guidance, and bone biopsy, when utilized.

0202T

The physician performs facet joint replacement (facet arthroplasty) of a posterior vertebral joint at a single level of the lumbar spine using fluoroscopic guidance. The paravertebral facet joint consists of the bony surfaces between the vertebrae that articulate with each other. A facet replacement device is inserted in the posterior column of the lumbar spine to restore structure and function. The device replaces all or a portion of a facet joint on a vertebral body. In one method, the physician removes, by partial resection, a posterior vertebral component (facet) and inserts a facet prosthesis. The patient is placed prone and an incision is made overlying the affected vertebra and taken down to the level of the fascia. The fascia is incised and the paravertebral muscles are retracted. The physician removes the affected facet and replaces it with the prosthesis. Facetectomy, laminectomy, foraminotomy, and vertebral column fixation (with or without bone cement injection) may also be performed and are included in this code. Paravertebral muscles are repositioned and the tissue and skin are closed with layered sutures.

0207T [0563T]

The physician evacuates the meibomian glands in order to remove obstruction and restore the natural flow of gland secretions. The outermost layer of the eye is a thin layer made up of lipids (meibum) that are secreted by the meibomian glands located on the upper and lower eyelids. These glands may become occluded or obstructed, resulting in dry eye symptoms. In 0207T, a single-use automated lid unit is utilized, which simultaneously delivers heat to the inner eyelid surface and intermittent pressure to the outer eyelid surface. The physician places the disposable unit around the patient's upper and lower lids, confirming the lid warmer is underneath both eyelids while the eye cup is outside the eyelids. After the proper position is verified, the unit is attached to a separate control system. With the eyelids closed, treatment is initiated and can be monitored (e.g., temperature, pressure status, and treatment time remaining). Once the treatment time is complete, the physician removes and disposes of the unit. Code 0207T is reported once for each affected eye treated. In 0563T, the physician places single-use, disposable devices on the upper and lower exterior eyelids of both eyes. These are attached to wired temple pads, which connect to the control unit. The physician activates the control unit, and targeted thermal energy is delivered to the exterior of the eyelids. The patient may be encouraged to blink throughout the treatment to assist in clearing of the melted meibum. At the conclusion of the 15-minute cycle, the physician removes and disposes of the devices. Topical anesthetic is instilled in both eyes, and the physician manually expresses the meibum from each gland using a disposable gland clearance instrument.

0208T-0209T

Pure tone audiometry is performed using a computer-assisted audiometer. Many causes of hearing loss have characteristic threshold curves. In pure tone audiometry, earphones are placed and the patient is asked to respond to tones of different pitches (frequencies) and intensities. The threshold, which is the lowest intensity of tone the patient can hear 50 percent of the time, is recorded for a number of frequencies on each ear. For pure tone signals, which are single-frequency tones produced electronically and transferred through an earphone or bone conduction vibrator, hearing sensitivity is measured separately in each ear. In one method, noise is masked to the non-test ear when it is determined by the computer that masking is necessary. Through touch-screen operation, the patient self-administers the tests while following verbal and on-screen instructions. Report 0208T for automated audiometry including the air conduction mode only and 0209T for automated audiometry including air and bone conduction modes. The air and bone thresholds are compared to differentiate between conductive, sensorineural, or mixed hearing losses.

0210T-0211T

Automated speech audiometry thresholds are performed using a computer-assisted device. Causes of hearing loss can often be diagnosed through tests using an audiometer. Many causes of hearing loss have characteristic threshold curves unique to that specific diagnosis. In speech audiometry, earphones are placed and the patient is asked to repeat bisyllabic (spondee) words. The softest level at which the patient can correctly repeat 50 percent of the spondee words is called the speech reception threshold. The threshold is recorded for each ear in 0210T. This process occurs in 0211T, in addition to a discrimination test. The word discrimination score is the percentage of spondee words a patient can repeat correctly at a given intensity level above his or her speech reception threshold. This is also measured for each ear.

0212T

Automated comprehensive audiometry threshold evaluation and speech recognition is performed with the use of a computer-assisted device. Causes of hearing loss can often be diagnosed through tests using an audiometer. Many causes of hearing loss have characteristic threshold curves. In comprehensive audiometry, earphones are placed and the patient is asked to respond to tones of different pitches (frequencies) and intensities. The threshold, which is the lowest intensity of tone the patient can hear 50 percent of the time, is recorded for a number of frequencies on each ear. Bone thresholds are obtained in a similar manner except a bone oscillator is used on the mastoid or forehead to conduct the sound instead of tones through earphones. The air and bone thresholds are compared to differentiate between conductive, sensorineural, or mixed hearing losses. With the earphones in place, the patient is also asked to repeat bisyllabic (spondee) words. The softest level at which the patient can correctly repeat 50 percent of the spondee words is called the speech reception threshold. The threshold is recorded for each ear. The word discrimination score is the percentage of spondee words that a patient can repeat correctly at a given intensity level above his or her speech reception threshold. This is also measured for each ear.

0213T-0215T

The physician injects a diagnostic or therapeutic agent into a cervical or thoracic paravertebral facet joint or into the nerves that innervate the joint. Using ultrasound guidance, the physician places a needle in the facet joint and injects the indicated substance, often a long-acting local anesthetic agent that may or may not contain a steroid. The paravertebral facet joints, also called zygapophyseal or "Z" joints, consist of the bony surfaces between the vertebrae that articulate with each other. The injection may be performed on a single level or on multiple levels. Report 0213T for a single level, 0214T for a second level, and 0215T for the third and any additional levels.

0216T-0218T

The physician injects a diagnostic or therapeutic agent into a lumbar or sacral paravertebral facet joint or into the nerves that innervate the joint. Using ultrasound guidance, the physician places a needle in the facet joint and injects the indicated substance, often a long-acting local anesthetic agent that may or may not contain a steroid. The paravertebral facet joints, also called zygapophyseal "Z" joints, consist of the bony surfaces between the vertebrae that articulate with each other. The injection may be performed on a single level or on multiple levels. Report 0216T for a single level, 0217T for a second level, and 0218T for the third and any additional levels.

0219T-0222T

The physician treats facet joint pain caused by degenerative changes or trauma by placing unilateral or bilateral posterior intrafacet implants in the cervical (0219T), thoracic (0220T), or lumbar (0221T) vertebral segments. An alternative to surgical fusion, one operative technique uses an allograft made from bone obtained from both the femur and thigh. Using an open surgical approach or a minimally invasive technique aided by fluoroscopic guidance, the surgeon preps the affected facet surfaces. An allograft dowel with instrumentation is inserted, resulting in expansion and stabilization of the facet joint space. Any bone grafts or synthetic devices used are included in these codes. Report 0222T for each additional vertebral segment.

0232T
The physician injects platelet rich plasma (PRP) into a targeted site. Harvesting and preparation may also be performed using a variety of techniques. In one, venous blood is drawn from the region of the arm in front of the elbow (antecubital vein) using a butterfly needle. The blood is placed into an appropriate container, centrifuged, and separated into platelet poor plasma (PPP), RBC, and PRP. The PPP is extracted and discarded and the PRP is withdrawn for use. The injection site is marked in order to localize the PRP injection; image guidance may be used. Under sterile conditions, the physician injects the PRP directly into the target area, sometimes using lidocaine or Marcaine. If administered to a joint space, calcium chloride and thrombin may also be added in order to provide a gel matrix for the PRP to adhere to. PRP has many indications, including wound care for the treatment of diabetic and venous stasis ulcers, chronic nonhealing tendon injuries, plantar fasciitis, and augmentation and fusion of bone. Studies suggest that PRP can aid in wound and soft tissue healing and can affect narcotic requirements, bone production (osteogenesis), postoperative blood loss, and inflammation.

[0901T]
The physician inserts a bone marrow sampling port to provide an access site for future bone marrow biopsies. The patient is placed supine, and the hip is prepped and draped. Imaging guidance such as CT or fluoroscopy may be used to identify a portal site. Under intravenous sedation (reported separately) and following administration of local anesthesia at the surgical site, an incision is made with dissection through the subcutaneous tissues. The sampling port is guided into the bone using a screwdriver. The skin incision is repaired with a layered closure. This code includes all imaging guidance, when performed.

0234T-0238T
The physician treats a stenosed artery percutaneously or via open surgical incision to relieve a blockage. In the percutaneous approach, a needle punctures the skin at the access site and is followed by a guidewire and an introducer sheath to protect and enclose the opening. A series of catheters and guidewires are inserted until the stenosed area has been traversed. An atherectomy catheter is manipulated to the study area and activated to cut or drill a channel through the plaque lesion and reopen the artery. Contrast medium is injected to fluoroscopically visualize the degree of luminal opening. The process may be repeated with a larger diameter catheter if necessary. In the open surgical approach, the physician creates a femoral cutdown incision to expose one of the femoral arteries. The physician punctures the femoral artery with a large needle and passes a guidewire via the needle into the artery. The physician removes the needle while leaving the guidewire in place, enlarges the arterial opening slightly with a blade, and slides an introducer sheath over the guidewire into the arterial lumen. The physician slides a guidewire through the atherectomy catheter or device and inserts the guidewire/atherectomy catheter combination through the introducer sheath into the stenosed vessel. The atherectomy device is fluoroscopically positioned at the area of stenosis and then activated to remove the stenotic tissue. The physician rechecks the diameter of the lesion by angiography. Several passes with the atherectomy device may be required. The physician removes the atherectomy catheter, guidewire, and introducer sheath, closing the femoral arteriotomy with suture. Report 0234T when the blockage occurs in the renal artery; 0235T in a visceral artery; 0236T in the abdominal aorta; 0237T in the brachiocephalic trunk and branches; and 0238T in the iliac artery.

0263T-0265T
Intramuscular autologous bone marrow cell therapy is performed to treat extreme and end stage peripheral artery disease (PAD). The physician places a large bore needle into the marrow cavity of the sternum, iliac crest, or ribs. The bone marrow is aspirated with a large syringe and placed in a bedside centrifuge to prepare the extracted cells for transplant. Intramuscular bone marrow cell therapy requires significant amounts of bone marrow cells; therefore, multiple harvest sites may be required. The puncture wound(s) is covered with a dressing. The harvested cells are injected into muscle (usually the gastrocnemius); multiple injections are common. Report 0263T when the entire procedure (harvest and transplant) is performed at once. Report 0264T when only the cell preparation and transplant are performed. Report 0265T for a unilateral or bilateral bone marrow cell harvest for use in the procedure at a later date.

0266T-0271T
A carotid sinus baroreflex activation system is implanted for the treatment of advanced heart failure and refractory hypertension. One proprietary stimulation device works by activating the body's baroreceptors (pressure sensors found within the walls of the carotid arteries that regulate heart rate and blood pressure). Consisting of an implantable pulse generator (IPG), a single 2 mm coated carotid sinus lead (electrode), and a wireless programmer system, the device prompts the body's natural reflexes to control blood pressure and the causal elements of heart failure progression. With the patient under general anesthesia, an incision is made on the left or right side of the neck and the soft tissues are dissected until the common carotid artery is located. The electrode, with a 7 mm silicone backer, is sutured to the carotid artery to activate the baroreceptors. An incision is made below the clavicle to form a pocket for the baroreflex activation generator. The wire attached to the electrode is tunneled beneath the skin to the generator pocket and connected to the IPG, which controls the baroreflex activation energy. The physician programs the IPG based on the patient's individual requirements. The IPG is secured within the surgically created pocket. The system is tested, and all incisions are closed routinely. Report 0266T for insertion or replacement of the entire carotid sinus

baroreflex activation system (generator and lead); report 0267T for unilateral lead insertion or replacement; and report 0268T for insertion or replacement of the pulse generator only. Report 0269T for revision or removal of the entire carotid sinus baroreflex activation system (generator and lead); report 0270T for unilateral lead revision or removal; and report 0271T for revision or removal of the pulse generator only. These codes include intraoperative interrogation, programming, and repositioning.

0272T-0273T

The purpose of these studies is to ensure that the carotid sinus baroreflex activation system is positioned well and working properly in order to guarantee proper function of the system in the future. A carotid sinus baroreflex activation system is implanted for refractory hypertension. The baroreflex sends signals to the brain to naturally regulate blood pressure. The insertion of this system allows the signals to be triggered artificially, causing the body to lower blood pressure. There are two components to a baroreflex activation system: a generator, which is positioned in a pocket below the clavicle, and electrodes (leads), one placed on each carotid sinus in the neck. The physician interrogates the device using the wireless programmer and collects and reports information including battery status, lead impedance, pulse amplitude and width, therapy frequency, pathway and burst modes, and therapy start and stop times. This interrogation must be performed in person. Report 0272T for the evaluation and 0273T if programming is performed in addition to the evaluation.

0274T-0275T

The physician performs a minimally invasive procedure to relieve pressure on the nerves of the spinal canal. The decompression is performed under indirect vision. The epidural space is injected with contrast. An incision is made above the vertebra and a cannula is inserted. The ligamentum flavum and small pieces of vertebral lamina are resected and tissue and bone sculpting is performed under radiological guidance. Multiple injections of contrast may be required intraoperatively. These codes include discectomy, facetectomy, and/or foraminotomy performed at the same level(s) during the same operative session. The surgical instruments and cannula are removed and the incision is closed. Report 0274T for a unilateral or bilateral procedure performed on cervical or thoracic vertebra, single or multiple levels. Report 0275T for a unilateral or bilateral procedure performed on lumbar vertebra, single or multiple levels.

0278T

Transcutaneous electrical modulation pain reprocessing (TEMPR) is a process used to treat chronic pain. Electrodes are placed on the skin in the location(s) of the pain. The electrodes transmit a "no-pain" signal to the nerves, signaling to the brain that there is no pain in the affected area. Subsequent treatments may be needed.

0308T

The patient's eye is held open using a lid speculum and an operating microscope is placed over or in front of the eye. The crystalline lens is removed via the surgeon's preferred method of phacoemulsification and aspirated. Alternately, the previously placed intraocular lens is explanted. The anterior chamber and capsular bag are prepped using ophthalmic viscosurgical devices (OVD). The cornea is lifted and the intraocular telescope is inserted, positioned, and sutured into place. The eye is irrigated and any residual OVD is aspirated. A peripheral iridectomy may be performed to reduce the chance of pupillary block. The incisions are closed and checked for leakage.

0329T

A soft, disposable contact lens fitted with a telemetry chip and strain gauge sensor is placed in the patient's eye and intraocular pressure (IOP) is continuously monitored over the course of at least 24 hours. The data is transferred to a computer and analyzed.

0330T

Tear film on the ocular surface is viewed using three imaging technologies to noninvasively investigate changes of tear film in real-time. Optical coherence tomography (OCT) measures tear film thickness. The wavefront sensor helps to objectively measure tear film break-up. The ellipsometer measures the lipid layer and quality of the tear film. The imaging may be performed on one or both eyes. Film interpretation and report is included in this procedure.

0331T-0332T

Myocardial sympathetic innervation imaging is performed to help assess cardiac nerve activity in patients with heart failure. Iodine meta-iodobenzylguanidine (MIBG) is injected intravenously. Planar images are taken at 15 minutes (early) and four hours (late) after injection to test the MIBG concentration levels in the myocardial sympathetic nerve endings. Qualitative and quantitative studies are performed using the average count per pixel and decrease in counts between early and late images. Report 0332T if single-photon emission computed tomography imaging is performed after the early and late planar images.

0333T [0464T]

In 0333T, a diagnostic test is performed to objectively assess the patient's visual acuity. Visual evoked potential (VEP) measures the time it takes for nerves to respond to visual stimuli. Conducting gel and an electroencephalogram (EEG) electrode is applied to the scalp in the occipital region. A strobe light or checkerboard pattern is placed in front of the patient for visual stimuli. Responses from the electrodes are recorded and analyzed. The automated data collection uses an algorithm to calculate the patient's visual acuity or "resolving ability." The clinician completes the test and provides a report. In 0464T, a VEP test is conducted to test for glaucoma. The VEP test measures responses of the eye and optic nerve to light patterns on a screen. The clinician compares the intensity of the response (amplitude) and length of time the patient took to respond (latency) to normal eye values. Patients who have glaucoma may demonstrate difficulty identifying low-contrast patterns or images and often experience a delay in processing those images. The ability to identify these cells can lead to reducing stressors such as lowering the intraocular pressure (IOP) in glaucoma patients and thereby potentially giving the patient a better outcome. Additional testing may be ordered based on the identified visual losses noted in certain areas. VEP responses are often monitored over time and are generally recommended on an annual basis for patients who are at risk for glaucoma, as well as patients already identified as early glaucoma patients. Interpretation and report are included in this service.

0335T [0510T, 0511T]

In 0335T, extra-osseous talotarsal stabilization (EOTTS), also known as arthroereisis or arthrosis, is performed for talotarsal stabilization. The physician makes a small incision in the ankle taking care to avoid damaging any neurovascular structures. A probe is inserted through the sinus tarsi to the sinus canalis to prepare the space and then subsequently removed. A guide pin is inserted. The space is measured for implants using progressively larger sizers over the guide pin until the best fit is found. A sterile implant of the same size is threaded over the guide pin and screwed into place. Intraoperative imaging is performed to ensure correct placement of the implant. A trial implant may be placed and removed prior to the sterile implant to ensure proper fit. The guide pin is removed. The wound is irrigated and closed in layers. Report 0510T for removal only of the sinus tarsi implant and 0511T for removal with reinsertion.

0338T-0339T

A small incision is made over the femoral artery and a catheter with an electrode on the tip is inserted. Using fluoroscopic guidance, the catheter is maneuvered to the renal artery. The catheter is connected to a radiofrequency generator that delivers lower powered, precisely focused bursts of energy to disrupt the surrounding renal nerves and reduce the renal contribution to central blood pressure elevation. Report 0338T for a unilateral procedure and 0339T when performed bilaterally.

0342T

Therapeutic apheresis with selective high-density lipoprotein (HDL) delipidation and plasma reinfusion is a procedure in which plasma is removed from the body by apheresis, processed through a delipidation device, and returned to the patient. This technique may be employed to reduce atherosclerosis development in cardiovascular disease. Vascular access is established. A bag of the patient's blood is collected and the plasma is separated from the rest of the blood constituents. The red blood cells may be returned to the bloodstream. The plasma is treated, removing the cholesterol from HDL (good cholesterol), which results in what is known as pre-beta-HDL. This pre-beta-HDL infused plasma is considered delipidated plasma. The delipidated plasma is infused back into the patient once a week for seven weeks.

0345T

A percutaneous mitral valve repair is performed. The right atrium of the heart is accessed using a catheter inserted in the internal jugular or subclavian vein. The coronary sinus is located and intubated with the compressed device within a sheath. An anchor, which resembles and functions much like a stent, on one end of the device is placed in the great cardiac vein and another is placed at the coronary sinus ostium and expanded, holding them in place. The anchors are connected by a bridge or wire. The bridge is made of dissolvable material that dissipates over time and pulls the anchors together, closing the mitral annulus. If the wire technique is used, the wire is pulled to bring the anchors closer together to shorten the mitral annulus before the anchors are expanded. Coronary compression may be assessed by angiogram and tension of the anchors adjusted. The sheath and catheter are removed and any wounds closed.

0347T

An interstitial device(s) is placed in bone for radiostereometric analysis (RSA). Interstitial devices allow providers to specifically follow the position of an implant, such as a prosthesis, by taking x-rays from different directions. These images are used in the RSA. The provider places these devices into the bone surrounding the prosthesis where they become fixed and can be monitored for migration of a prosthesis part(s).

0348T-0350T

Radiostereometric analysis (RSA) is the method of taking two x-rays from different directions concurrently. X-rays performed in this manner permit a surgeon to use exact measurements to determine how an implant and a joint are interacting. The surgeon inserts very small, seed-like tantalum beads into bone surrounding the implant or prosthesis. Tantalum is the same metal material used in prosthetic implants. Once the beads assimilate into the bone, the physician can use those beads as a reference point to identify any position changes related to the prosthesis. This permits monitoring of the patient's progress, allows for predicting how long a prosthesis may last, and provides data to help improve the design and function of prosthetic implants. Report 0348T for radiostereometric analysis on the spine, 0349T for the upper extremity(ies), and 0350T for the lower extremity(ies).

0351T-0352T

Optical coherence tomography (OCT) is a noninvasive, high-resolution, real-time microscopic optical-imaging technique that provides two- and three-dimensional micro-scale images of tissue structure from bulk tissue sample. This process furnishes improved quality that may be able to distinguish cancer cells from normal cells. When performed at the time of surgical excision, it can allow for immediate detailed information about the tissue sample(s) removed. This process could reduce the amount of additional procedures that may need to be performed without this imaging. Report 0351T for excised tissue from the breast or axillary lymph node, each specimen. Report 0352T for the interpretation and report that is performed immediately or referred.

0353T-0354T

Optical coherence tomography (OCT) is performed on the breast, surgical cavity. OCT is a noninvasive, high-resolution, real-time microscopic optical-imaging technique that provides two- and three-dimensional micro-scale images of tissue structure from bulk tissue sample. This process furnishes improved quality that may be able to distinguish cancer cells from normal cells. When performed at the time of surgical excision, it can allow for immediate detailed information about the tissue sample(s) removed. This process could reduce the amount of additional procedures that may need to be performed without this imaging. Report 0353T when OCT is performed on the surgical cavity, breast, real time intraoperative and 0354T for the interpretation and report, real time or referred.

0358T

Bioelectrical impedance analysis (BIA) is a relatively simple, quick, and noninvasive technique to measure body composition, the measurement of body fat in relation to lean body mass. The provider places electrodes to various parts of the body; often this may be two electrodes on the patient's right hand and right foot. Low level, imperceptible, and painless electrical current is passed through the body. Bioelectrical impedance analysis is a practical method of measuring the degree of resistance to the current as it moves through the water found in muscles and fat tissue. Muscles contain more water than fat; the more water the body has, the easier it is for the current to pass through it. Subsequently, the more fat a patient has, the more difficult it is for the current to pass through. Measurements are taken to determine how much resistance the current meets based on the various types of tissue. BIA provides an estimate of how much body water is present in order to calculate body fat. An interpretation and report are generated after the analysis has been performed.

0362T

An onsite physician or other qualified health care professional, with assistance from two or more technicians, administers a behavior identification supporting assessment of a patient with serious destructive behavioral concerns, such as harming oneself, damaging property, and aggression with injury to others, or behaviors resulting from recurring actions or issues related to communication or social interactions. The technicians spend face-to-face time with the patient conducting the assessment, which includes exposure of the patient to a number of social and environmental elements associated with the maladaptive behaviors conducted in a structured and safe customized environment. Evaluation targeting certain destructive behaviors includes assessing triggers, events, cues, responses, and consequences associated with the destructive behavior(s). This code describes assessing and analyzing functional behavior and includes other structured observations, the use of standardized and non-standardized instruments, and procedures that will assist the clinician in establishing the degree of adaptive and maladaptive behaviors or impairments of the patient. Report only the time of one technician even when two or more technicians are present. Report this code for each 15 minutes of face-to-face time provided by the technician.

0373T

An onsite physician or other qualified health care provider, with assistance from two or more technicians, administers a behavior therapy session for a single patient with serious destructive behavioral concerns, such as harming oneself, damaging property, and aggression or behaviors. During the encounter, two technicians or assistant behavioral analysts spend approximately 15 minutes of face-to-face time in provoking responses from various but specific environmental circumstances the patient may experience or has experienced. The technicians or assistant behavioral analysts record the responses while the provider studies the data and makes appropriate adjustments until specific discharge goals have been met. These services are conducted in controlled and safe settings and may involve the use of protective equipment to ensure the safety of the patient and clinical personnel. Report only the time of one technician even when two or more technicians are present.

0378T-0379T

The physician or other qualified health care provider performs a visual field assessment, which determines where the peripheral vision (e.g., side vision) begins and ends, in addition to how well the patient can see objects in the peripheral vision with full horizontal and vertical range. Visual field assessment is performed one eye at a time, with the opposite (contralateral) eye completely covered to avoid errors. In all testing, the patient must look straight ahead at all times in order to avoid testing the central vision rather than the periphery. This procedure requires thorough instructions and understanding by the patient to achieve accurate results. Typically, this test is utilized to detect disorders affecting vision, including glaucoma and diseases of the retina and optic nerves. These codes include data analysis that is transmitted by the patient to a remote center for evaluation and storage for up to 30 days. Report 0378T when this data is reviewed, interpreted, and a report is provided. Report 0379T for the technical component, including instructions, surveillance, and transmission of data as requested by the health care provider.

0394T-0395T

Conventional high dose rate (HDR) brachytherapy is a very strong form of radiation delivered internally to kill a variety of cancers. It may be used as a primary, standalone treatment or as an adjunct treatment designed to be used after a tumor has been surgically removed to ensure elimination of any remaining cancer cells. This form of brachytherapy is delivered in fewer fractions and at larger doses per fraction, resulting in a treatment duration of four to five days as opposed to the standard five to seven weeks of tumor radiation. Under local anesthesia and utilizing ultrasound guidance, the physician makes a small incision in the skin over the area and inserts a trocar through which a balloon applicator is inserted. The balloon is inflated with sterile water until ultrasound reveals that the cavity is filled and the surgical margin conforms to the applicator. The physician dresses the entrance wound and tapes the applicator shaft to the patient's skin. Details of the treatment plan, formulated using standard treatment planning software, are downloaded into a controller. The x-ray source, which is encased in a sheath, is inserted into the applicator shaft and connected to the controller. The source travels to the distant point of the shaft inside the saline-filled balloon and stops. Radiation treatment is delivered according to the preset treatment plan. Treatments are typically broken down into two fractions per day for five days, for a total of 10 fractions. Following each treatment, the source is removed. The applicator remains inside the breast until the entire treatment regimen is complete, after which it is removed. With this type of treatment, one to 20 catheters are implanted into the tumor site. A computer-controlled machine transfers small radioactive seeds down through each catheter to deliver radiation at multiple depths and varying times. The treatment process can take approximately 10 to 20 minutes. Once the treatment is completed, the seeds are removed to ensure no radioactive material remains in the patient. In 0394T, the physician delivers HDR electronic surface brachytherapy, a process that works without using radioactive isotopes or megavoltage linear accelerators and involves the use of direct a contact applicator and a flexible clamp. Proprietary systems utilize lightweight surface applicators with precision to the tumor while minimizing exposure to healthy tissue. Surface brachytherapy systems lend themselves to establishing a very precise setup and continuous monitoring. In doing so, smaller margins with smaller treatment fields may be possible, which can lead to the possibility of reduced treatment frequencies but at higher doses. A surface applicator may be able to deliver homogenous dose to more than 90 percent of the target area. The radiation oncologist determines the amount of radiation necessary based on the tumor's size, type, and depth as well as the patient's age, history of other treatments, and other criteria. During the procedure, the treatment site is prepped and the use of flexible shield cut to fit around the tumor area and shield healthy adjacent tissue is placed on the patient. A tiny x-ray source is put within the applicator and energized to deliver the radiation. Once the procedure has been completed, the x-ray source is turned off and all equipment is removed. In 0395T, interstitial HDR brachytherapy is used to deliver radiation directly into the diseased tissue, such as in prostate cancer; intracavitary HDR brachytherapy delivers radiation to the tumor area within the cavity that is left after the tumor is removed, such as in the case of breast, cervical, and vaginal cancers.

0397T

Endoscopic retrograde cholangiopancreatography (ERCP) is a diagnostic test performed via a long flexible viewing instrument (duodenoscope) that can be moved and directed around the turns of the stomach and duodenum. The duodenoscope has a thin fiberoptic bundle at the tip that transmits light, as well as a microscopic camera that can project digital video images onto a television screen. The endoscope is designed with an open channel for other instruments to be passed through for biopsies or to insert plastic or metal tubing (stents) to relieve strictures or other obstructions caused by cancer or scarring, as well as to make incisions via electrocautery. Contrast material is injected and x-rays of the bile ducts and the pancreatic duct are taken. Optical endomicroscopy (confocal laser endomicroscopy) involves a very small but strong microscope attached to the end of the scope that allows the physician to see all of the internal structures in precise detail and is frequently used as a tool to diagnose patients with Barrett's esophagus for esophageal cancer much earlier, often without a biopsy due to the high-resolution and detailed imagery, thereby increasing the likelihood of a cure. The procedure is similar in manner to an upper endoscopy. The patient is administered anesthesia, as appropriate, and is placed in the left lateral position. The physician inserts the scope through the mouth and pharynx and into the esophagus with the images being displayed on the screen in real-time with the physician reviewing the images. Note that this code is reported in addition to that for the primary procedure.

0402T

The physician performs collagen cross-linking of the cornea, a treatment intended to prevent progression of keratoconus (a condition in which the cornea thins and weakens) by adding bonds between collagen fibers in the eye. Other indications include the treatment of post-LASIK ectasia. Numbing drops are applied to the eyes, followed by separately reportable riboflavin (vitamin B2) eye drops that enhance light absorption by the cornea. The physician may remove the corneal epithelium prior to administering the riboflavin. This is known as the epi-off technique and provides quicker penetration with the liquid riboflavin. Alternately, the physician may only loosen the corneal epithelium using eye drops or a sponge prior to administering the riboflavin (epi-on technique). The eyes are treated with ultraviolet light. The results of treatment can improve or stabilize the shape of the cornea allowing for better visual acuity and comfort in contact lens wearing.

0403T

A provider conducts a face-to-face intensive behavior change therapy session in a group setting, aimed at diabetes prevention using standard program parameters. Recent studies have shown several behavioral adjustments can be made in order to help prevent diabetes in those at high risk, specifically those patients with minimal physical activity, obesity, and genetic predisposition. Behavioral therapy can address alterations in lifestyle with goals for desired outcomes pertaining to nutrition and exercise while allowing care plan oversight by a trained provider. This code is reported for a minimum of 60 minutes per day of intense therapy.

[0488T]

A lifestyle coach, certified in a nationally recognized training program, conducts an intensive online or other electronically-structured diabetes prevention program with a patient using standard program parameters. Recent studies have shown that several behavioral adjustments can help prevent diabetes in individuals at high risk, specifically those patients with minimal physical activity, obesity, and genetic predisposition. Behavioral therapy can address alterations in lifestyle with goals for desired outcomes pertaining to nutrition, stress, exercise, and weight management while allowing care plan oversight by a trained provider. This code is reported per 30 days of intense therapy. In-person components of the program are included, when performed.

0408T-0411T

Cardiac contractility modulation (CCM) is utilized to improve ventricular pump function and for patients who have normal QRS duration. The device consists of a programmable and rechargeable generator, powered by a lithium battery. The patient is given local anesthesia and the device is implanted within a pocket on the right side of the chest below the collarbone with an electrode fixed on the carotid sinus. One incision allows access to the cervical vagal nerve with another incision made for insertion of the right ventricular electrode. The vagal electrode is connected to the generator via subcutaneous tunnel. This unit includes three standard leads placed transvenously into the right side of the heart: one in the right atrium for sensing and two in the right ventricle for sensing and delivery of impulses. These impulses do not change the cardiac sequence (rhythm), but instead modify contractility by sending high-energy impulses to the myocardium during the refractory period. The unit allows the patient the ability to recharge the battery with an external charger that operates transcutaneously. This is required once a week and typically takes about 90 minutes. Programming and interrogation follows the same process as a pacemaker. Report 0408T for insertion or replacement of the entire system, including evaluation and programming when performed; 0409T for insertion or replacement of the pulse generator only; 0410T for insertion or replacement of the atrial electrode only; and 0411T for insertion or replacement of the ventricular electrode only.

0412T-0413T

In 0412T, the physician removes a cardiac contractility modulation (CCM) system. The pocket is opened. The existing system is disconnected from the wire and removed. In 0413T, the electrodes are removed (atrial or ventricular). Previous insertion incisions may be reopened for removal of electrodes, which are disconnected from the generator as well as the vagal nerve, right atrium, and right ventricle.

0414T

The physician removes and replaces a cardiac contractility modulation (CCM) system generator. The pocket is opened. The existing system is disconnected form the wire and removed. The electrodes remain in position and a new CCM system is inserted into the pocket. The electrodes are connected to the new system and tested. The pocket is closed.

0415T

The physician repositions a previously implanted cardiac contractility modulation transvenous electrode (atrial or ventricular lead). The physician gains access transvenously with imaging guidance and the electrode is repositioned. Depending on the extent of the work, the electrode may require reconnection to the generator, which would be tested for appropriate function. The incisions are closed.

0416T

The physician relocates a cardiac contractility modulation (CCM) system generator due to complications from the original generator placement. The pocket is opened and the generator is removed. A new pocket is formed within the subcutaneous tissue in close proximity of the existing electrodes. The electrodes are brought through a new subcutaneous tunnel into the new pocket. The old pocket is closed. The new or existing generator is inserted into the pocket and the electrodes are attached and tested. The pocket is closed.

0417T-0418T

A programming device evaluation (0417T) or interrogation (0418T) is performed in person in order to test the device's function and select the most favorable permanent programmed values. Patients with previously implanted cardiac contractility modulation (CCM) systems require periodic programming device evaluations. These diagnostic procedures include a face-to-face assessment of all device functions. Components that must be evaluated in order to assign a code from this range include the battery, leads, capture and sensing function, and programmed parameters. Stored and measured data regarding these components are retrieved using an office, hospital, or emergency room instrument. This information is assessed to discern battery voltage, lead impedance, and settings, as well as to determine the device's current programming. In 0417T, if necessary, the sensing value and rate response, upper and lower heart rates, impulses, and diagnostics are adjusted. These codes include physician or other qualified health care professional analysis, review, interpretation, and report, and are assigned per procedure. They also include connection, recording, and disconnection.

0419T-0420T

Neurofibromas are benign soft tissue tumors that develop from the nerve tissue of the peripheral nerve, which are the nerves from the spinal cord that extend into the trunk and extremities. While a patient may present with a single neurofibroma, usually multiple tumors are present. In these cases, the clinician often suspects neurofibromatosis, a genetic condition passed from parent to child. There are two categories of neurofibromatosis: neurofibromatosis type 1 (NF1) and neurofibromatosis type 2 (NF2), which is significantly more severe. Some of the identifying characteristics of NF1 include, but are not limited to, more than one neurofibroma present, learning disabilities, cafe'-au-lait spots, bone deformities, Lisch nodules on the eye, and tumors on the adrenal gland, brain, or spinal cord. These characteristics are also common in type 2, along with a greater likelihood of cataracts and benign ear tumors developing on the vestibulocochlear nerve, often in both ears, which can create balance and hearing problems. Neurofibromas vary in size ranging from a small tumor arising from a skin nerve (cutaneous) to severe enlargement of an extremity, such as in cases of elephantitis arising from a larger nerve. Destruction of neurofibromas is determined by a number of factors, including type, location, and size of the tumor. Destruction of neurofibromas may be performed via straightforward excision using a scalpel, ablation through desiccation, or vaporized via electrosurgery. For patients presenting with a significant amount of neurofibromas, electrodesiccation may be performed. The surgeon utilizes a device to apply an electrical current to the tumor and dries out the tissues the tumor is in contact with. This process allows the surgeon to go into deeper tissue than is possible with other methods. In cases of severe neurofibromatosis, excision and electrodesiccation may be performed in conjunction with each other. For more superficial tumors, fulguration and electrocautery techniques may be used. Another method of destruction may include stereotactic radiosurgery, a minimally invasive technique that destroys the tumors using highly focused beams of radiation resulting in minimal damage to the healthy tissue surrounding the tumor, as well as less side effects than the patient might experience with more traditional surgery. Report 0419T for destruction of 50 or more neurofibromas of the face, head, and neck and 0420T for destruction of 100 or more neurofibromas on the trunk or extremities.

[0714T, 0867T]

The physician treats benign prostatic hyperplasia (BPH) using transperineal laser ablation. Following insertion of a dedicated transrectal ultrasound probe, the physician inserts minute optical fibers percutaneously into the prostate gland. One or two fibers per lobe are typically used, depending on the prostate gland's basal volume. Laser energy is then delivered, which heats and destroys the hyperplastic tissue. Report 0714T for a prostate volume of less than 50 mL; 0867T for a prostate volume of 50 mL or greater. These codes include imaging guidance.

0421T

Transurethral waterjet ablation of the prostate is a minimally invasive procedure that employs an aquablation system to destroy prostatic glandular tissue using a high-speed solution of sodium chloride in water (saline) guided with exact electromechanical control using a real-time transrectal ultrasound image. The surgeon destroys the prostatic tissue by moving along a fixed, predetermined glandular tissue map, while at the same time collecting samples of prostatic tissue to analyze after the procedure has been completed. When needed, control of bleeding (hemostasis) is performed using a low power blue laser beam contained in a water column to cause coagulation. This procedure is performed for patients with symptomatic benign prostatic hyperplasia.

0422T

Tactile breast imaging by computer-aided tactile sensors is a relatively inexpensive, efficient, and uncomplicated technology for evaluation of palpable breast lumps. The physician or other qualified health care provider uses a hand held scan head that is moved over the breast using gentle pressure. A sensor mounted on the scan head and a magnetic position tracker in the handle comprise the other components of the device. While the scan is taking place, a computer digitally displays tactile pressure images and locations on the screen. A tactile map that consists of the spatial average of all the tactile pressures is created in real time. The technology offers an alternative or enhancement to clinical breast examination (CBE) using palpitation because CBE can be difficult for patients to communicate tactile sensations to the provider prohibiting repeatable and consistent examination documentation. Many new methods have been introduced for advancing the quality of breast examinations by relying on the discernible elastic stiffness difference between tumors and normal breast tissue.

0437T

Biosynthetic implants are a fairly recent tool available to surgeons for assisting in ventral hernia repairs in a possible contaminated field, as well as with patients with a significant abdominal wall fascial defect. In these cases, non-biologic or synthetic implants are often preferable to obtaining a tension-free abdominal wall closure. Prosthetic mesh is associated with a higher risk of complications such as infection, fistula, and skin erosion. The concern with these complications has led to the development of alternative materials to attain a tension-free repair in a single operative session even in cases where the patient has a highly contaminated field. Biosynthetic grafts appear to show promise in solving some of these concerns. Essentially a matrix scaffold comprised of collagen and other extracellular components contain fibroblasts that make angiogenesis, which is the natural process in the body of developing new capillary blood vessels for the purposes of healing and reproducing healthy tissue. By their very nature, these implants are more resistant to infections. A number of biosynthetic implants are available and are categorized according to a number of factors, including, but not limited to, species of origin (allogenic, xenogeneic); the specific decellularization process; whether there is cross-linking; the type of collagen used, such as dermis, pericardium, etc.; how the implant is stored; and whether or not it requires rehydration. Note that this code is reported in addition to that for the primary procedure.

0439T

Myocardial contrast perfusion echocardiography is used to examine myocardial microcirculation. Intravenous infusion of contrast containing microbubbles that exist primarily within the vascular space and maintain intravascular characteristics similar to red blood cells is utilized. Injection of contrast into the venous system may also be used since the microbubbles will continue circulating for approximately three to five minutes after injection. Low intensity ultrasound is necessary in order to avoid destroying the microbubbles. The perfusion is analyzed as the microbubbles are destroyed with a burst of high intensity ultrasound and the rate of restoration is evaluated as the microbubbles flow back into myocardial circulation. This evaluation can determine the velocity and peak myocardial signal intensity allowing for quantification of any changes. This imaging provides improved resolution that enables the physician to detect perfusion defects that may not be seen in lower resolution imaging. Note that this code is reported in addition to that for the primary transthoracic echocardiography procedure.

0440T-0442T

Cryoablation of a nerve is performed to relieve chronic nerve pain by damaging the nerve's myelin coating thereby blocking the pain signal to the brain. The patient typically receives conscious sedation during the insertion of the cryoprobe into the nerve causing the pain. With the probe in place, the patient may be further sedated and/or a nerve block is performed with lidocaine. Imaging guidance is utilized to guide the probe placement and verify optimal position. A freezing agent is administered through the probe by way of tubing connecting it to the system distributing liquid nitrogen or argon gas. The system controls the flow of the freezing agent. Upon completion of the procedure, the probe is removed, pressure is applied to stop bleeding, and the skin is bandaged. Report 0440T when an upper extremity distal/peripheral nerve is treated; 0441T when a lower extremity distal/ peripheral nerve is treated; and 0442T when a nerve plexus or other truncal nerve is treated.

0443T

Real-time spectral analysis of prostate tissue by fluorescence spectroscopy is a procedure that uses single or multiple narrowband light sources to identify concentrates of natural fluorophores in prostate tissue, which fluctuates based on a patient's disease state. In addition, it helps to limit the sampling of healthy or benign tissue while targeting only cancerous lesions, which in turn assists in the identification of prostate cancer. Note that this code is reported in addition to 55700, and is reported only once per session.

0444T-0445T

Drug-eluting ocular inserts signify key advances in the treatment and management of eye disease. The inserts are typically sterile, thin, multilayered, drug-impregnated devices of solid or semisolid consistency and are placed by the physician into the cul-de-sac or conjunctival sac. The ocular inserts are designed with a polymeric support and may contain a drug or a drug can be incorporated as dispersion or a solution in the polymeric support at a later time. Drug-eluting ocular inserts offer a number of advantages over traditional treatments such as eye drops because of their ability to have an increased ocular residence as well as having a sustained release of medication into the eye. The insert includes a body portion sized to position within a lachrymal canaliculus of the eyelid. Ocular inserts are categorized according to factors including whether insoluble, soluble, or bioerodible. Release of drugs from the insert is based on the diffusion, osmosis, and bioerosion of the medication. These inserts provide the patient a means of maintaining continuous, sustained therapeutic drug levels with reduced side effects. Types of inserts based on their solubility include diffusion or osmotic inserts and soft contact lenses. Report 0444T for initial placement of an ocular insert, including fitting, training, and insertion, in one or both eyes. Report 0445T for subsequent placement of an ocular insert, including retraining and removal of an existing ocular insert, in one or both eyes.

0446T-0448T

Implantable interstitial glucose sensor devices monitor glucose from interstitial fluid (IF), a solution in the body that surrounds cells, just below the skin's surface. A small sensor is implanted under the skin. Glucose information is transmitted wirelessly to a smart transmitter worn by the patient on the upper arm, above where the sensor has been implanted. One proprietary device uses a distinct fluorescent, glucose-indicating polymer. A light-emitting specialized electronic component called a diode attached to the sensor excites the polymer and the polymer quickly detects a change in the glucose concentration by a change in the light display. The IF glucose measurement is communicated to the transmitter, which calculates the glucose and indicates whether that value is going up or down and at what speed. Additionally, the smart transmitter can relay whether the glucose values exceed preset low and high-target values. When the patient opts to use the smartphone app, data and alerts can also be sent in that manner at the same time to permit real-time tracking of data to assist the patient in monitoring and controlling glucose levels. Sensors can be implanted to provide continuous glucose monitoring (CGM) for a period of up to three months. Report 0446T for initial implantation, including creation of the subcutaneous pocket, insertion of the device, activation, and training; 0447T for removal of the interstitial glucose sensor by incision; and 0448T when the device is removed with creation of a subcutaneous pocket at a different anatomic site and another sensor is implanted and activated.

0449T-0450T

Aqueous drainage devices reduce intraocular pressure (IOP) in the management of primary open angle glaucoma (POAG), the most common type of glaucoma. POAG is associated with a buildup of aqueous fluid pressure within the eye, which can lead to blindness and damage to the optic nerve. Patients often have no pain or discomfort associated with this and no visible abnormality is seen in the anterior chamber despite the aqueous fluid being unable to flow properly. Drainage devices lower IOP by a process of diverting excess fluid from the anterior chamber to the subconjunctival bleb instead of to an extraocular reservoir or another device that is inserted in the eye during cataract surgery and allows the aqueous fluid from the anterior chamber to flow into the Schlemm's canal toward the episcleral drainage system and away from the trabecular meshwork. Report 0449T for initial insertion of an aqueous drainage device and 0450T for insertion of each additional device.

0469T

The physician performs a retinal polarization scan. These scans are a noninvasive method for detecting accurate eye alignment using an approach that changes the polarization of light of nerve fibers (Henle fibers) that encompass the small area of the retina called the fovea. Referred to as retinal birefringence scanning (RBS), this process is able to identify polarization changes that occur as altered polarized light passes through the Henle fibers to the fovea, the area where fixation occurs. RBS is used to help with early detection of visual problems in young children as well as adults with eye-related issues. Polarization scanning has also been used as a diagnostic tool to assist in diagnosing Alzheimer's disease well before symptoms present. The polarized light is able to highlight amyloid protein deposits located behind a patient's retina. These protein deposits have been shown to exist in patients oftentimes decades before experiencing cognitive decline.

0472T-0473T

The physician or other qualified health care provider performs the initial in-person evaluation, interrogation, and programming of an intraocular retinal electrode array, including visual training as well as a review and report. An intraocular retinal electrode array or retinal prosthesis works as a biomedical implant designed to effect visual perception through electrical stimulation of the retina in blind patients or those with severe to profound retinitis pigmentosa. Rods and cones known as photoreceptors in the retina turn light into electrochemical impulses. Those impulses are transmitted through the optic nerve and into the brain and are translated into images. For patients with retinitis pigmentosa, the photoreceptors do not work properly and the transmitted impulses cannot be translated. Proprietary retinal prosthesis systems bypass the nonfunctioning photoreceptors. The prosthesis is surgically implanted in the patient's retina. Glasses containing a tiny video camera are worn by the patient. The video images are transmitted to a video processing unit (VPU) worn by the patient. The video is processed and the data is converted into instructions that are then routed back to the glasses. The instructions are passed on to an antenna located in the prosthesis. Signals are given to the prosthesis and it begins to give off tiny pulses of electricity that pass by the nonworking photoreceptors to trigger remaining retinal cells; those cells in turn send visual data via the optic nerve to the brain resulting in patterns of light. Patients are taught how to understand what these patterns mean using the retinal prosthesis. Report 0473T for subsequent reprogramming services.

0474T

In a minimally invasive surgical procedure, the physician inserts an anterior segment aqueous drainage device into the supraciliary space. An anterior segment aqueous drainage device is used to treat patients with glaucoma who are undergoing cataract surgery. Glaucoma is an eye disease that can damage the optic nerve from rising pressure in the eyes due to an imbalance in production and outflow of ocular fluid. It is the second leading cause of blindness. Typically, the fluids in the eyes help to maintain the shape of the eye with the ocular fluid flowing through the trabecular meshwork before entering the bloodstream. In patients with glaucoma, ocular fluid is not draining to the same degree it is being produced and this causes pressure to build in the eye. The increasing pressure from the buildup of fluid causes damage to the optic nerve and may lead to blindness. The patient undergoes cataract removal under general anesthesia. Once the cataract is removed, a proprietary preloaded deployment device is inserted into the eye to create a diversion or bypass from the front of the eye and the trabecular meshwork allowing more ocular fluid to flow, which avoids an increase in pressure. The procedure is typically performed in the outpatient setting and antibiotic and anti-inflammatory drops are administered following the procedure.

0479T-0480T

In fractional ablative laser fenestration, new openings are created in scar tissue by carbon dioxide ablative fractional laser (CO2AFL) light beams. The physician adjusts the fractional CO2 laser to an appropriate depth in proportion to the scar thickness and, using a low density, passes the laser over the burn scar. The laser light beam splits the single beam into several smaller beams of CO2, which makes holes in the burned scar tissue leaving what is best described as miniature channels. Heat-emitted vaporization begins a process in which the laser treatment totally removes (ablates) some tissue and damage to other scar tissue triggering new wound healing and scar maturation. Intralesional triamcinolone is administered directly into the microchannels. Capillary action resulting from the laser treatment permits the medication to go deep

Category III

into the scar tissue in a more uniform manner. Studies done on this procedure indicate that the remodeling process may lie dormant in the body and through the use of fractional ablative laser fenestration, the process is stimulated to help improve the appearance of burn scars. Report 0479T for the first 100 cm or part thereof or 1 percent of body surface area in infants and children. Report 0480T for each additional 100 cm or each additional 1 percent of body surface area in infants and children.

0481T

The physician injects autologous white blood cell concentrate (autologous protein solution) into any site. Autologous protein solution (APS) is formed from a patient's blood and contains high concentrations of anti-inflammatory cytokines and anabolic growth factors to block inflammation for the treatment of osteoarthritis (OA). The procedure involves one injection of protein harvested directly from a vein in the patient's arm. A proprietary APS self-contained, single use kit is comprised of two different blood processing devices and a single 30 mL vial of Anticoagulant Citrate Dextrose Solution-Formula A (ACD-A). One device is a plastic tube containing a tuned-density buoy that separates cellular and platelet components of whole blood that forms a cellular solution while the second plastic tube contains polyacrylamide absorbent beads that are used to concentrate the cellular solution while further processing and producing the solution to be injected. The physician cleans and preps the patient's injection site using an antiseptic solution. A needle is placed into the intra-articular space using ultrasonic guidance. Joint fluid is aspirated and subsequently discarded. The syringe containing approximately 2.5 mL of solution is attached to a needle and injected into the synovial space of the joint.

0483T-0484T

The physician performs transcatheter mitral valve implantation or replacement (TMVI). Mitral regurgitation (MR) is a condition that may be treated with transcatheter mitral valve implantation or replacement (TMVI/TMVR) in patients who are at high risk for open heart surgery. In 0483T, the procedure is performed via a percutaneous approach and includes a transseptal puncture, when performed. Under general anesthesia, the physician makes an incision over a lower extremity vessel, usually the femoral vein. A catheter with a specially designed prosthesis is maneuvered through the vessels to the heart under fluoroscopic imaging guidance. The catheter is threaded through the inferior vena cava to the right atrium where the interatrial wall or septum is punctured to access the left atrium. When the left atrium is accessed, the catheter is further advanced through the mitral valve and to the left ventricle. A stent-based prosthesis is implanted within the mitral annulus. In 0484T, under general anesthesia, the physician makes a left lateral mini-thoracotomy. The transapical puncture involves using a large bore needle to puncture the chest wall directly into the left ventricular cavity. A small incision is made between ribs (usually the fifth or sixth intercostal space) on the lower left side of the patient's chest to achieve direct access to the heart. A catheter is inserted following the guidewire to the mitral valve. A balloon is inflated to compress the native valve. The self-expanding prosthesis is introduced through the catheter, partially uncovered. Once in the left atrium, the catheter is deployed and secured using polyethylene tether fastened to an epicardial pad. Pledgeted sutures are placed. The tether tension is modified after the prosthesis has been deployed to ensure optimal placement of the device but also to limit movement of it within the annulus. No cardiopulmonary bypass or rapid ventricular pacing is required during the procedure. These procedures include vascular access, catheterization, balloon valvuloplasty, deploying the valve, repositioning the valve as needed, temporary pacemaker insertion for rapid pacing, and access site closure, when performed. Angiography, radiological supervision and interpretation, intraprocedural roadmapping to guide TMVI (e.g., contrast injections, fluoroscopy), left ventriculography (e.g., to assess mitral regurgitation for guidance of TMVI), and completion angiography are also included.

0485T-0486T

The physician performs optical coherence tomography (OCT) of the middle ear. OCT is a noninvasive technology designed to allow physicians to visualize three-dimensional (3-D) images of the eardrum, middle ear bones, and their vibrations. OCT permits better visualization of any potential blockages in the path of the occurring vibrations because it is more readily absorbed by the body and can go deeper into human tissues versus other types of imaging. The technology provides clinicians with another diagnostic tool to aid in easier and faster treatment of middle ear problems. OCT was originally developed and is still currently used for retinal imaging and now has been additionally used in identifying infections such as otitis media or other bacterial colonies, as well as other middle ear conditions that aids in expediting patients to specialists for treatment. OCT handheld imaging devices contain three distinct components: a near-infrared light source (laser), a video camera, and a micro electromechanical (MEMS)-based scanner to direct the light and capture the normal examination of the middle ear in 3D. The physician inserts the laser into the patient's ear and looks at the reflected light returning from various structures located at different depths. The reflections generate an image of the particular tissue being examined that is created from the use of computer algorithms based on the amount of time that it takes for the wavelengths to bounce back from the tissue microstructure. Supervision and interpretation are included in these services. Report 0485T when the exam is performed on one ear and 0486T when the service is performed on both ears.

0489T-0490T

Autologous adipose-derived regenerative cells (ADSC) are living stem cells suctioned from the patient's own fat tissue under the skin by way of a small volume liposuction procedure. Studies have shown that the stem cell frequency in adipose (fat) tissue is 25 hundred times greater than the stem cell frequency in bone marrow. Treatment with these cells mitigates commonly associated transplantation complications such as cell rejection or the transmission of diseases. Additionally, patients do not need to take immunosuppressant drugs. One proprietary cell therapy is a specific type of treatment used for scleroderma. Scleroderma is defined as a rare, chronic connective tissue disease that causes a hardening or tightening of the skin and connective tissues. It is typically classified under autoimmune rheumatic diseases. In 0489T, the process includes harvesting ADSCs, incubating the cells in conjunction with a cell dissociation enzyme, removal of nonviable cells and debris, and determining concentration and dilution of the cells. Report 0490T for multiple injections of the cells into one or both hands.

[0640T, 0859T, 0860T]

Noncontact near-infrared spectroscopy uses specific wavelengths of reflected light to assess oxygenation levels in specific tissue regions and is particularly useful in the management of critical limb ischemia; chronic wounds resulting from circulatory problems, diabetes, or immobilization; and in flap reconstruction procedures. This noninvasive tissue oxygenation measuring system reports an estimated value of oxygen saturation (StO2), relative deoxyhemoglobin (Hb) level, and relative oxyhemoglobin (HbO2) level in superficial tissues. This proprietary device, which consists of a light source, a camera, and a touchscreen PC, displays images of tissue oxygenation of the scanned tissue surface that are color-coded and two-dimensional and reports multispectral measurements for selected areas. Using the LED light source, the skin surface is illuminated by an imaging head that receives returned light, resulting in subtle color changes that occur in hemoglobin when it is oxygenated. Report 0640T for image acquisition and interpretation and report for the first anatomic site for indications other than screening for peripheral arterial disease; 0859T for each additional anatomic site. Report 0860T for image acquisition and interpretation and report for screening for peripheral arterial disease, including provocative maneuvers, of one or both lower extremities.

0494T-0496T

Ex vivo lung perfusion (EVLP) is a leading lung preservation technique that utilizes a lightweight, easy to transport, warm blood perfusion system for living organ transplants. The process permits the cadaver donor lungs to remain in an environment that mirrors the human body rather than in a cold preservation method. The warm, functioning state helps advance the health of the lungs, ensures greater lung function, and provides a more accurate lung transplantation assessment. The lungs continue to function in the normal manner under EVLP. Proprietary technology from different EVLP companies helps ensure that the lungs continue to function outside of the body as they would inside the body, which makes them more suitable for transplantation. Additionally, the transplant surgeon is able to evaluate the lungs and resuscitate and/or improve their function as needed. Most EVLP systems are comprised of a small wireless monitor and a perfusion module unique to the type of transplant organ needed, as well as different solutions to maintain the donor organ. Donor blood is used and the EVLP system provides blood oxygenation, a gas flow, and a pulsatile pumping system within the system. A solution containing nutrients, proteins, and oxygen is infused into the donor blood in order to supplement any missing nutrients or other substances. During an approximately three- to four-hour process, the donor lungs are placed inside a sterile rounded vault that is attached to the system that controls and maintains the proper temperature and humidity levels to keep the organ warmed, maintained, and protected from contamination. Each proprietary system continues to fully assess the lungs functionality and biochemical and metabolic status. The EVLP system is used for organs that may not previously have been used under existing preservation methods because the system enables the surgeon to have the time to evaluate the organ's viability, perform resuscitation, reverse lung injury, and remove excess water, if needed, as well as assist in building up the organ's energy stores and enhance lung function all prior to the transplantation procedure. Once the lungs are deemed suitable, they are transplanted into the patient. Report 0494T for surgical preparation, cannulation, and decannulation (removal of tracheostomy tube) of a cadaver donor lung(s) to an ex vivo organ perfusion system. Report 0495T for initiation and monitoring of EVLP by a physician or other qualified health care professional, first two hours, and 0496T for each additional hour.

[0623T, 0624T, 0625T, 0626T]

Using data from a coronary computed tomographic angiogram (CTA) that is reported separately, the severity of coronary artery disease is assessed by automated quantification/characterization of atherosclerotic plaque. This web-based service uses computerized algorithms to evaluate the degree and severity of disease; the computer-generated findings are then provided to the physician or other qualified health care professional in an interactive format for their final review and report. Report 0624T for data preparation and transmission only; 0625T for the computerized analysis only of data derived from the CTA; 0626T for review of the computerized analysis output to resolve conflicting data and subsequent interpretation and report; and 0623T if all components of the prior listed codes are included. These codes may be reported once per coronary CTA.

[0523T]

Noninvasive 3-dimensional (3-D) fractional flow reserve (FFR) enabled interpretation is performed during a coronary angiography procedure for possible atherosclerotic stenosis as an aid to the physician in making a determination for whether a percutaneous coronary intervention (PCI) is indicated and whether revascularization occurs in each angiography procedure performed. Medically recognized standards generally recommend that revascularization by PCI is to be performed when the patient's stenosis of >50 percent is observed of the left main (LM) stem or proximal left anterior descending (LAD) coronary artery during angiography, the patient has one remaining patent vessel, or the patient suffers from two- or three-vessel disease with a left ventricular ejection fraction of <40 percent. A proprietary FFR platform accurately conveys evidence-based multi-vessel physiologic measurements to enable the physician to confirm whether or not to proceed with intraprocedural PCI therapy.

0505T

The physician bypasses an occlusion or stenosis in the femoral or femoropopliteal arterial segment of the leg by skirting the blocked area using the adjacent femoropopliteal vein as a pathway to place proprietary covered stents. In one method, the physician obtains access to the femoral artery opposite that of the affected limb (contralateral) and advances a guidewire over the aortic bifurcation to the occluded site in the affected femoral artery. A second access is obtained distally on this same side (ipsilateral) in the tibial vein. Proximal and distal anastomoses are created above and below the area of occlusion using a crossing device, a snare cage, and guidewires. Following balloon dilation of both proximal and distal anastomosis sites, stent grafts are inserted and deployed in an overlapping fashion from the popliteal artery into the femoral vein, and from the femoral vein into the femoral artery. Once dilated, the stents create an endograft bypass around the occlusion, utilizing the vein as a conduit. Final angiograms are obtained to verify patency and the incision sites are closed.

[0620T]

The physician performs endovascular venous arterialization of the tibial or peroneal vein with transcatheter placement of one or more intravascular stent grafts in patients suffering from critical limb ischemia. In this chronic condition, there is lack of blood circulation to the foot due to blockages of the arteries in the leg. In one proprietary method, catheters are inserted under ultrasound guidance into the tibial vein at the level of the ankle and into the femoral artery at the level of the groin. Both catheters are advanced simultaneously toward each other; during this time, ultrasound waves are emitted by the arterial catheter toward the receiving venous catheter to assist the physician in determining the most optimal location for channel creation from the artery to the vein. An embedded needle within the arterial ultrasound catheter crosses over and is inserted into the vein, creating the connection between artery and vein. The physician inflates a small angioplasty balloon to allow for the passage of other devices. A valvulotome consisting of a small basket with minute incision hooks is introduced to cut through valves near the bottom of the foot in order to maximize the arterial flow to the vein into the foot. The severed valves are rendered incompetent, allowing oxygenated blood to flow forward and into the foot. Finally, several self-expanding covered metal stents are placed to act as permanent conduits for blood flow to the foot. Catheters are removed, incision sites are closed, and the patient observed. This code includes ultrasound guidance for vascular access, all intraprocedural roadmapping, catheterizations, and imaging guidance necessary to complete the procedure, and all associated radiological supervision and interpretation when performed.

0506T

Heterochromatic Flicker (HF) photometry is a noninvasive, diagnostic test recommended for patients to determine the risk of macular degeneration by measuring the macular pigment optical density (MPOD). MPOD is the depth of the Zeaxanthin, Lutein, and metabolite meso-zeaxanthin in the covering area of the retina called the macula, the primary region for focused vision. In a quiet, darkened examination room, the patient is asked to view and respond to changes detected in light patterns, in one or both eyes, displayed from a small box connected to a computer. Flashes of green wavelengths (non-absorbable) followed by absorbable blue wavelengths (i.e., harmful lighting to photoreceptors from computers, tablets, TV screens, sunlight, etc.) are projected onto the patient's retina. Intervals are so quick that the eye perceives them as a steady light, rather than intermittent flashes; gradually the intervals are increased until the eye perceives a flickering light. The patient is asked to indicate when the change from steady to flickering light is noticed. The computer uses proprietary software that calculates this difference using a mathematical formula to determine the pigment density value. The physician interprets the results and reviews them with the patient.

0507T

Chronic dry eye caused by meibomian gland dysfunction (MGD) is a condition in which a blockage or other abnormality prevents the glands from secreting lipid, the oil that prevents tears from evaporating. MGD can be diagnosed using proprietary systems, such as one comprised of a console with an activator for single use. The physician administers an anesthetic drop to one or both eyes and applies the activator, which employs a proprietary technology transilluminator and near-infrared imaging that warms up the meibum (oil) in the inner lid. The physician applies a gentle and drug-free pressure action to express the glands, releasing the obstructed meibum up and out of the gland. Heat and pressure from the device are regulated using redundant sensors. The procedure takes approximately 12 minutes and may be performed in the physician office. Once the procedure is complete, the physician interprets the results and reviews them with the patient.

0509T
A normal retina has a predictable electrical response to light. To determine if the retina is damaged, the physician places an ocular-fitted contact lens electrode on the patient's eye and another electrode on the forehead so that the retina's electrical responses to external stimuli can be recorded under light-adapted conditions. Electroretinography (ERG) is repeated in dark-adapted conditions. The ERG waves are analyzed by the physician. Various techniques may be used based on the area of the retina being targeted. In a multi-focal pattern electroretinography (mfPERG), a number of regions localized in the retina can be evaluated and tested. The patient covers one eye at a time to view, and focus on, a black and white patterned image that "flips" over and over again rapidly on a screen while a computer records the eye's responses to the images and generates a report for the physician. This test may be used to identify changes that could be an early indicator of glaucoma.

0515T-0517T
The physician inserts a wireless cardiac stimulator for left ventricular pacing. Wireless cardiac stimulator systems include a wireless endocardial left ventricular electrode that is typically implanted in the artery of the left ventricular wall. The electrode is wirelessly powered via ultrasound pulses originating from a transmitter implanted into one of two subcutaneous pockets created on the chest wall. The cardiac stimulator system also includes a pulse generator, which is comprised of two separate elements: a transmitter and a battery. The battery is housed in the other chest wall pocket. The battery and the electrode are connected via a subcutaneously tunneled cable. This system provides biventricular pacing by sensing right ventricular pacing output from a previously placed conventional device (i.e., pacemaker or defibrillator using uni- or biventricular leads) that subsequently transmits an ultrasound pulse to the wireless electrode inserted onto the left ventricle endocardium, resulting in a left ventricular pacing pulse emission. Patients who have both a wireless device and a conventional pacing device require separate programming and interrogation of each device. Report 0515T for insertion of the complete wireless cardiac stimulation system; 0516T for insertion of the electrode only; and 0517T for insertion of the pulse generator only, including both the battery and transmitter. All codes include programming and interrogation and all echocardiography and imaging, when performed.

0518T, 0519T-0520T [0861T]
The physician removes a pulse generator battery and/or transmitter for a wireless cardiac stimulator for left ventricular pacing. Wireless cardiac stimulator systems include a wireless endocardial left ventricular electrode that is typically implanted in the artery of the left ventricular wall. The electrode is wirelessly powered via ultrasound pulses originating from a transmitter implanted into one of two subcutaneous pockets created on the chest wall. The cardiac stimulator system also includes a pulse generator, which is comprised of two separate elements: a transmitter and a battery. The battery is housed in the other chest wall pocket. The battery and the electrode are connected via a subcutaneously tunneled cable. This system provides biventricular pacing by sensing right ventricular pacing output from a previously placed conventional device (i.e., pacemaker or defibrillator using uni- or biventricular leads) that subsequently transmits an ultrasound pulse to the wireless electrode inserted onto the left ventricle endocardium, resulting in a left ventricular pacing pulse emission. Patients who have both a wireless device and a conventional pacing device require separate programming and interrogation of each device. Report 0861T for removal of the pulse generator, including both the battery and transmitter; 0518T for removal of the battery only; 0519T for removal with replacement of the pulse generator, including both battery and transmitter; and 0520T when only the battery component is removed and replaced. Codes 0519T and 0520T include device interrogation and programming.

[0862T, 0863T]
The physician relocates a pulse generator for a wireless cardiac stimulator for left ventricular pacing. Wireless cardiac stimulator systems include a wireless endocardial left ventricular electrode that is typically implanted in the artery of the left ventricular wall. The electrode is wirelessly powered via ultrasound pulses originating from a transmitter implanted into one of two subcutaneous pockets created on the chest wall. The cardiac stimulator system also includes a pulse generator, which is comprised of two separate elements: a transmitter and a battery. The battery is housed in the other chest wall pocket. The battery and the electrode are connected via a subcutaneously tunneled cable. This system provides biventricular pacing by sensing right ventricular pacing output from a previously placed conventional device (i.e., pacemaker or defibrillator using uni- or biventricular leads) that subsequently transmits an ultrasound pulse to the wireless electrode inserted onto the left ventricle endocardium, resulting in a left ventricular pacing pulse emission. Patients who have both a wireless device and a conventional pacing device require separate programming and interrogation of each device. Report 0862T for relocation of the pulse generator battery only; 0863T for the transmitter only. These codes include device interrogation and programming.

0521T-0522T
The physician or other qualified health care provider performs an in-person interrogation or programming device evaluation for a wireless cardiac stimulator for left ventricular pacing. Wireless cardiac stimulator systems include a wireless endocardial left ventricular electrode that is typically implanted in the artery of the left ventricular wall. The electrode is wirelessly powered via ultrasound pulses originating from a transmitter implanted into one of two subcutaneous

pockets created on the chest wall. The cardiac stimulator system also includes a pulse generator, which is comprised of two separate elements: a transmitter and a battery. The battery is housed in the other chest wall pocket. The battery and the electrode are connected via a subcutaneously tunneled cable. This system provides biventricular pacing by sensing right ventricular pacing output from a previously placed conventional device (i.e., pacemaker or defibrillator using uni- or biventricular leads) that subsequently transmits an ultrasound pulse to the wireless electrode inserted onto the left ventricle endocardium, resulting in a left ventricular pacing pulse emission. Patients who have both a wireless device and a conventional pacing device require separate programming and interrogation of each device. Report 0521T for interrogation evaluation, including analysis, review, and report. This code includes connection, recording, and disconnection and is reported per patient encounter. Report 0522T for a programming device evaluation, including analysis, review, and report. This code includes adjustment of the device to test the function and select optimal programmed values.

0524T

Endovascular catheter-directed chemical ablation with balloon isolation (i.e., balloon sclerotherapy) describes treatment of varicose veins in an extremity by incorporating two familiar procedures: sclerotherapy and balloon catheterization as a minimally invasive and cost-effective treatment option. Traditional catheter-based endovenous sclerotherapy can often have negative effects to the overall body system resulting from the combination of air and the sclerosing agent. The physician uses a double lumen balloon catheter as a means of separating or isolating venous blood, allowing the physician to use the minimal amount of sclerosing agent needed while removing the excess amounts and subsequently limiting the potential for systemic risk. Vein occlusion occurs when the physician carefully retracts the expanded balloon containing the captured sclerotherapeutic agent in between.

0525T-0527T

An intracardiac ischemia monitoring system analyzes and records cardiac data to detect ischemic events. If an ischemic event is occurring, the device sends out auditory, visual, and vibrational alerts to the patient to seek medical care immediately. Access to the central caval veins is obtained through the subclavian vein or jugular vein. The vein is penetrated with a large needle and a guidewire is passed through. A fluoroscope is used to guide a standard pacemaker intracardiac lead to the right ventricular apex. A pocket for an implantable device (IMD) that analyzes and records the cardiac data is created and the lead is tested. The lead is connected to the IMD and the subcutaneous pocket is closed. Report 0525T for insertion or replacement of the complete system (electrode and implantable monitor). Report 0526T for insertion or replacement of the electrode only; report 0527T for implantable monitor only. All imaging, including supervision and interpretation, is included in these services.

0528T-0529T

An intracardiac ischemia monitoring system analyzes and records cardiac data to detect ischemic events. If an ischemic event is occurring, the device sends out auditory, visual, and vibrational alerts to the patient to seek medical care immediately. In 0528T, a programming device evaluation is performed in person in order to test the functioning of the device and to select the most favorable permanent programming values. Patients with previously implanted monitoring systems require periodic programming device evaluations. This diagnostic procedure includes a face-to-face assessment of all device functions. Stored and measured data regarding these components are retrieved using an office, hospital, or emergency department instrument. This information is assessed in order to discern lead impedance and settings for detection, as well as to determine the system's current programming. If necessary, sensing values and diagnostics are adjusted. In 0529T, only an in-person device interrogation (extraction of data accumulated in a medical device) is performed, accessing the stored and measured data. Both of these codes include clinician analysis, review, and report.

0530T-0532T

An intracardiac ischemia monitoring system analyzes and records cardiac data to detect ischemic events. If an ischemic event is occurring, the device sends out auditory, visual, and vibrational alerts to the patient to seek medical care immediately. In 0530T, the subcutaneous pocket incision is reopened and the complete system (electrode and implantable monitor) is disconnected from the cardiac lead and removed. The lead is dissected from the scar tissue that has formed around it. Once the lead is completely freed, it is removed. Report 0531T for electrode removal only and 0532T when only the implantable monitor is removed.

0541T-0542T

Magnetocardiography (MCG) is a noninvasive diagnostic tool for detecting ischemia in patients experiencing chest pain without the use of ionizing radiation or mechanical energy. The heart generates electrical activity that creates magnetic fields. The MCG device records these magnetic fields and can generate precise cardiac electric functioning data in real-time. The multichannel device is comprised of a number of sensors placed over the chest but without touching the patient. Once the device is activated, an image is created from the recording of the magnetic field generated by the heart as it goes through the cardiac cycle almost immediately. Ischemia can be detected or ruled out using proprietary analysis processes. The test is very fast, often performed in a span of 10 minutes, and can enhance or be used in place of more invasive and riskier procedures. MCG is considered extremely beneficial in the emergency department setting because it allows patients experiencing chest pain to be evaluated much faster and more effectively to determine if the pain is heart-related. Report 0541T for single study myocardial imaging using MCG, including report. Report 0542T for interpretation and report only.

0543T

This procedure describes treatment for patients with mitral regurgitation, a progressive condition where the mitral valve does not close appropriately resulting in blood leaking back through the mitral valve. The surgeon performs a thoracotomy and places a proprietary system designed for use when the patient's native chordae tendineae (tough, tendinous type strands of the heart) become elongated or rupture from the disease process. The system contains expandable "jaws" that are used to hold the mitral valve leaflet or cusp and an average of three to four artificial chordae are inserted around the edge of the leaflet in order to rehang the prolapsed leaflet. Transesophageal echocardiography (TEE) is used as guidance to reduce the amount of blood leaking back into the mitral valve by varying the lengths of the artificial chordae. Once the appropriate level has been determined, the chordae are fastened to a small piece of absorbent material and attached to the outer layer of the heart wall.

0544T-0545T

The physician performs a transcatheter mitral valve annulus reconstruction with the implantation of an adjustable annulus reconstructive device. A proprietary system is used in these procedures, comprised of three components: the implant catheter (IC) itself, a guide catheter (GC), and a transseptal steerable sheath (TSS). The implant is made of a contraction wire with a covering made of a polyester fabric that is secured along the back annulus of the mitral valve by stainless steel anchors. Once fastened down, the implant is contracted under fluoroscopy and echocardiography imaging in order to reach the optimum constraint and amount of valvular regurgitation. The surgeon accesses the mitral valve using a percutaneous, catheter-delivered approach going through the femoral vein and the inferior vena cava. A transseptal puncture under transesophageal echocardiography (TEE) imaging is performed to identify the interatrial septum over the back middle mitral commissure, the area where the posterior leaflets or cusps are located. A transseptal steerable sheath (TSS) is introduced into the left atrium using a guidewire and the implant delivery system is advanced through the TSS and into the left atrium. It is positioned to line up with the top of the IC near the front lateral trigone using TEE guidance. Anchors are moved through the fabric of the implant and into the annular tissue to ensure the implant is securely fastened. Once secure, the tip of the IC continues to be moved along to each continuous point of anchoring on the commissure. When the last anchor is positioned in the trigone near the posterior medial commissure, the implant is disconnected from the IC with an average of 12 to 17 anchors required based on the length of the implant. Typically, this system and treatment is most often used for patients with functional mitral regurgitation (FMR) and more recently functional tricuspid regurgitation (FTR). Angiography, all radiological supervision and interpretation, intraprocedural road mapping, ventriculography required for device implantation, and adjustment are included. Report 0545T for reconstruction of the tricuspid valve annulus with an implanted adjustable annulus reconstruction device in a similar manner.

[0643T]

Using a proprietary, transcatheter-based structural heart device, the cardiac surgeon, in conjunction with an interventional cardiologist, treats post-myocardial infarction scar tissue on the left ventricle in a beating-heart, minimally invasive procedure. Via a combined right internal jugular transvenous and left lateral mini-thoracotomy approach under fluoroscopic guidance, the physician implants titanium micro-anchor pairs intended to remodel the ventricle in order to reduce wall stress and improve blood flow. The internal (hinged) anchor is placed inside the right ventricle of the heart through the jugular vein, while the external (locking) anchor is placed on the outside of the left ventricle through the thoracoscope, which is inserted via a small incision between two ribs. The anchor pairs are connected by a tether. Once the anchors are in position, the physicians gently pull them toward each other, resulting in the anchor pairs excluding the scar tissue from the healthy tissue on the left ventricle. This isolates the nonfunctioning part of the heart muscle, allowing the remaining healthy tissue to work more effectively. An average of two to three anchor pairs are typically implanted. Left and right heart catheterization and left ventriculography, when performed, are included in this procedure.

0546T

Radiofrequency (RF) spectroscopy is a technology that pinpoints minute electromagnetic differences between normal cells and cancerous cells in real-time. One proprietary system employs RF electromagnetic fields to identify residual cancerous tissue during a partial mastectomy (lumpectomy) procedure. Differences in the tissue sample can be detected in as little as three to five minutes, allowing the surgeon to make an immediate determination of how much more breast tissue to remove during the procedure and reducing the likelihood of more surgery for the patient. This technology has been successfully used during lumpectomy procedures for ductal carcinoma in situ (DCIS) and invasive breast cancers.

0547T

Bone material quality testing is performed by an impact microindenter, a proprietary device used for in vivo measurement of the cortical bone properties. This technology is used to determine how deeply the single-use device tip can "indent" the tibia bone in patients with Paget's disease or other tibia-related conditions. The device was developed after organic superficial bonds were discovered. These bonds act as a type of "glue" and function as a means of preventing "glass-like" fractures because they dispel energy through the bond and strengthen the bone. One key measurable factor of the device evaluates how well the bone is able to resist microindentation, referred to as a Bone Material Strength (BMS) score. The design of the tip of the probe and the amount of pressure applied cause the mineralized collagen fibrils to separate and create microfractures. The deeper the probe indents, the easier the fibrils separate, the more easily the bone fractures, and the lower the BMS score. Software used with the device shows the clinician how many indentations should be made. Assessing the quality of bone allows clinicians to make informed decisions, enhancing the patient's quality of care and, over time, helping patients avoid a fragility fracture.

0552T

Low-level laser therapy (LLLT) is a therapeutic technology used to treat inflammation, swelling, and pain associated with musculoskeletal disorders such as arthritis. LLLT also aids in healing wounds (non-healing leg or pressure ulcers), injuries to soft tissue or joints, and neurological disorders, including shingles and neuropathy using bio-stimulation or photobiomodulation, a photochemical reaction in the cell caused by the LLLT. A LLLT laser or high-intensity light-emitting diodes (LEDs) do not emit heat; therefore, they do not carry the same degree of intensity as a surgical laser. Proprietary devices apply red and near infrared light to the affected area via laser or high-intensity LEDs to lessen oxidative stress and elevate production of adenosine triphosphate (ATP), a key energy source in the body that helps in functions such as muscle contraction and protein production, which in turn enhances the metabolism of cells and lowers inflammation.

0554T-0557T

Bone mineral density (BMD) studies have been used to diagnose osteoporosis, a condition in which the density and quality of the bone is diminished, greatly increasing the patient's risk for a fracture. Studies typically measure the hips and spine for a wide range of reasons. One indication is that hip and spine fractures are greater in patients with osteoporosis and fractures in these areas are generally more serious, require a longer recovery period, cause higher degrees of pain, and potentially increase the possibility of disability. In addition, the bone density of the hip and spine often determine the probability of fractures in other bones. BMD test results are reported using a T score that shows the degree of bone density as compared to a normal healthy adult; the lower the score, the greater the risk of fracture. This procedure describes evaluation of bone strength and fracture risk using finite element analysis (FEA), the central technology used in one proprietary test to conduct a "virtual" stress test for determining breaking strength. This virtual stress test considers the amount of bone mass a patient has, as well as bone size, shape, and internal structure, and provides analysis called Biomechanical Computer Tomography Analysis (BCT), CT-based measurements for BMD and bone strength. A key benefit to this technology is that it enables clinicians to identify patients who may not have osteoporosis per the standard BMD T score scale, but who are still deemed to be at high risk for fractures. Providing the clinician with a T score that combines BMD and the virtual stress test technology represents a more thorough evaluation for determining the presence of osteoporosis than can be found using BMD alone since very low levels of bone strength indicate fragile bones in the same manner that very low levels of BMD at the hip or spine have indicated osteoporosis. Report 0554T for a complete study; 0555T for retrieval and transmission of scan data only; 0556T for assessment of bone strength and fracture risk with BMD; and 0557T for interpretation and report only.

0558T

This code describes biomechanical computed tomography (BCT), a technology incorporating computed tomography (CT) scan image processing, bone biomechanics, and finite element analysis (FEA) to assess bone mineral density (BMD) and bone strength performed using a CT scan the patient previously had done for unrelated reasons as an ancillary analysis to help identify patients at high risk for a hip and spine fracture. This offers a number of benefits, including negating the need for a separate bone mineral density scan as well as being more cost-effective because the clinician is using a previously performed CT imaging study, particularly those of the hip and spine. BCT is provided as an add-on service targeting CT patients with no prior BMD study.

0559T-0560T

These codes describe the creation of three-dimensional (3D) printed models of individually prepared and processed elements of anatomic structures, such as bones, arteries, veins, nerves, ureters, muscles, tendons, ligaments, joints, visceral organs, and the brain. Models may be comprised of one or more distinct parts and incorporate various colors and materials. Uses of 3D-printed anatomic models are continuing to increase for a number of applications including, but not limited to, surgery planning, preparing and practicing for the procedure, training and education of health care professionals, and for patient education. Report 0559T for the first anatomic structure component and 0560T for each additional component.

0561T-0562T

Three-dimensional (3D) printed cutting or drilling guides are patient-specific surgery guides combining individualized imaging information that is used by the surgeon to navigate a procedure. Each guide is a sole, distinctive tool created to be an exact fit to the patient's natural anatomy customized to precisely match every intervention aspect, such as position and angles that mirror the actual surgery. The use of guides saves considerable time and resources; the predictability permitted by the guides allows for greater confidence in the operation room, which subsequently improves patient outcomes. In some cases, the surgery may require the use of a 3D-printed model and cutting or drilling guide for the same patient. Report 0561T for the first anatomic guide and 0562T for each additional anatomic guide.

0565T-0566T
Osteoarthritis of the knees is treated using an intra-articular injection of a substance derived from the patient's own adipose tissue. It is believed that mesenchymal stem cells (MSC) derived from autologous adipose tissue can provide pain relief, functional improvement, and regeneration of knee cartilage. In one method, abdominal liposuction is performed. Adipose tissue is removed by lipoaspiration and processed to isolate, extract, and proliferate the MSCs. Under ultrasound guidance, the cellular suspension is injected into the knee joint. Report 0565T for tissue harvesting and creation of the cellular implant. Report 0566T for injection of the cellular implant into the knee joint.

0569T-0570T
The physician performs a transcatheter tricuspid valve repair utilizing a percutaneous approach. Transcatheter devices currently in clinical testing include annuloplasty devices (suture, direct, or ring), coaptation devices, and heterotopic caval valve implantation. In one repair method, the surgeon accesses the tricuspid valve using a percutaneous, catheter-delivered approach through the left subclavian or axillary vein. An expandable, foam-filled balloon spacer is advanced through a sheath introducer and is stabilized by a rail that is anchored at the right ventricular apex. This device is intended to reduce the regurgitant orifice area by reducing malcoaptation of the tricuspid leaflets. Report 0569T for the initial prosthesis and 0570T for each additional prosthesis used during the same session.

[0646T]
The physician implants or replaces the tricuspid valve with a prosthetic valve using a percutaneous, transcatheter approach; vascular access is typically gained via the jugular or femoral vein. Tricuspid regurgitation occurs when a diseased, damaged, or malfunctioning tricuspid valve fails to close properly, causing blood to flow backward from the right ventricle to the right atrium. Transcatheter tricuspid valve replacement or implantation (TTVR/TTVI) is most often performed on patients with symptomatic tricuspid regurgitation that are high risk or not eligible for traditional open chest surgery. One proprietary device is a bioprosthetic valve created from bovine tissue and polyester fabric. Set inside a flexible metal structure, it can be placed within the patient's own tricuspid valve. The physician gains access to the femoral vein. Under imaging guidance, a catheter with the prosthetic valve is maneuvered through the vessels to the point of placement in the tricuspid valve, where it is deployed. Code 0646T includes right heart catheterization, temporary pacemaker insertion, and selective right ventricular or right atrial angiography, if performed.

0571T-0574T, 0580T [0614T]
The physician inserts an implantable cardioverter-defibrillator system that consists of a subcutaneous pulse generator and at least one substernal electrode. Under appropriate anesthesia, the physician creates a subcutaneous pocket over the lateral ribcage and places the generator. Without entering the pericardial cavity, the electrode is tunneled subcutaneously and placed into the substernal anterior mediastinum, where it performs defibrillation and antitachycardia pacing. This electrode does not perform chronic pacing. All imaging guidance is included, as is the electrophysiological evaluation, which includes evaluation of the defibrillation threshold, arrhythmia induction, evaluation of sensing for termination of arrhythmia, and programming/reprogramming of sensing or therapeutic parameters. Report 0571T for initial insertion of the entire system. Report 0571T along with 0573T and 0580T if the pulse generator and substernal electrodes are removed and subsequently replaced during the same operative episode. Report 0572T for insertion only of the electrode and 0573T for removal only. Report 0573T in conjunction with 0580T if both the pulse generator and electrodes are removed and not replaced. Report 0574T for repositioning of a previously implanted substernal electrode. Report 0580T for removal of the pulse generator only and 0614T if the pulse generator only is concurrently removed and replaced.

0575T-0576T
A physician or other qualified health care provider performs device evaluations of an implantable cardioverter-defibrillator system with substernal electrode. In 0575T, a programming device evaluation is performed, consisting of repetitive adjustments of the device to test function and select optimal permanent programmed values. In 0576T, an interrogation device evaluation is performed, which includes connection, recording, and disconnection per patient encounter. These codes include analysis, review, and report.

0577T
A physician or other qualified health care provider performs an electrophysiologic evaluation of an implantable cardioverter-defibrillator system with substernal electrode. This includes evaluation of defibrillation threshold, arrhythmia induction, evaluation of sensing for arrhythmia termination, and programming or reprogramming of sensing or therapeutic parameters.

0578T-0579T
These codes report remote (up to 90 days) evaluations of a substernal lead implantable cardioverter-defibrillator system. In 0578T, a physician or other qualified health care professional provides interim analysis with review and report. In 0579T, included components are remote data acquisition, receipt of transmissions and technician review,

technical support, and distribution of results. These codes may be reported once per 90 days.

0581T
The physician destroys a malignant breast tumor using percutaneous cryoablation. The patient's skin is cleansed and the ablation site is anesthetized. Imaging guidance may be used to locate the tumor. A small cryoprobe is inserted through a small incision and placed into the tumor. The device initiates ice ball formation by emitting liquid nitrogen, which freezes and destroys the cancerous tissue. Two freezing cycles are undertaken in order to achieve higher cell death. This code reports treatment of one breast.

0582T
The physician performs transurethral destruction of malignant prostate tissue by radiofrequency generated water vapor thermotherapy. The physician inserts an endoscope in the penile urethra. The urethra may be dilated to allow instrument passage. After the endoscope is placed, a radiofrequency generated water vapor thermotherapy stylet is inserted in the urethra and the diseased prostate is treated with steam. The treated prostate is examined for evidence of bleeding, which may be controlled with electrocoagulation. The endoscope and instruments are removed. A urinary catheter is inserted into the bladder and left in place postoperatively.

0583T
Following delivery of an anesthetic with an iontophoresis device, the physician places a tympanostomy tube using a tube delivery system. The tympanic membrane is numbed using an iontophoresis system that employs a small amount of electrical current to aid in the anesthetic's uptake. The physician inserts the automated tube delivery system, quickly creates the myringotomy, and inserts the tube.

0584T-0586T
The physician performs an islet cell transplant in patients with type 1 diabetes, following administration of appropriate anesthesia and sedation. In 0584T, the physician inserts a catheter through a small incision in the patient's abdomen, guides it into the portal vein of the liver under ultrasound guidance, and a solution containing the islet cells is infused into the liver. Report 0585T if the procedure is performed using a laparoscopic approach and 0586T for an open approach. Following transplantation, the beta cells in the islets begin producing and releasing insulin into the patient's bloodstream.

0587T-0588T
In 0587T, the physician implants or replaces an integrated single device neurostimulation system percutaneously (through the skin) for bladder dysfunction. The single device includes an electrode array and a receiver or pulse generator. Under local anesthesia, the device is inserted via a small incision near the vicinity of the neurovascular bundle of the posterior tibial nerve in the lower leg and secured with a small suture. Report 0588T for revision or removal of a neurostimulation device that was initially placed percutaneously for bladder dysfunction. These codes include analysis, programming, and imaging guidance when performed.

0589T-0590T
A physician or qualified health care professional performs an electronic analysis of a previously placed implanted integrated neurostimulation system for bladder dysfunction to verify that it is functioning properly. In 0589T, simple programming of a posterior tibial nerve integrated neurostimulation device is performed. Simple programming includes the adjustment of up to three parameters from the following: contact groups, amplitude, pulse width, frequency [Hz], on/off cycling, burst, dose lockout, patient selectable parameters, responsive neurostimulation, detection algorithms, closed loop parameters, and passive parameters. Report 0590T for complex programming, which includes the adjustment of more than three of these parameters.

0591T-0593T
Health and well-being coaching involves an interpersonal relationship between a patient and an individual who has completed a training program in health/well-being coaching. The content of this program must adhere to standards established by an appropriate national credentialing organization, and the coach must be qualified by education, training, national examination, and, when applicable, licensure/regulation. Training includes communication techniques, behavioral change theory and motivational strategies, and health education/promotion theories. With the face-to-face assistance of a coach, patient-determined goals, learning processes and content education, and self-monitoring behaviors are undertaken to improve and sustain health and well-being. These codes do not report medical nutrition therapy. Report 0591T for the initial assessment of an individual patient and 0592T for a follow-up session of at least 30 minutes. Report 0593T for at least a 30-minute group session that includes two or more individuals.

0594T
Humeral lengthening techniques treat limb length discrepancies, which may be congenital, developmental, or the result of bone disease or trauma. Developed to lengthen the limb gradually without the use of external fixation, a magnet-driven device permits the implant to become longer when manipulated by a hand-held external remote controller (ERC). In one method, the physician inserts an intramedullary lengthening nail via osteotomy of the humeral shaft. Following administration of regional anesthesia, the osteotomy level is identified and marked on the skin. The physician creates multiple drill holes to vent the intramedullary canal at the osteotomy level via a 1 cm anterolateral incision, then marks the proximal humerus entry point on the skin. A wire is inserted percutaneously at the anterolateral border of the acromion to approach the proximal humerus and the position verified fluoroscopically.

After the wire is driven into the center portion of the proximal humerus and its position confirmed, a 3 cm incision is made around the guidewire through the skin and subcutaneous tissues. After the deltoid muscle and rotator cuff are spread, a reamer is placed over the guidewire, a starting hole is created, and the humerus is reamed to the appropriate size to accommodate the implant. Upon completion of the reaming, the physician removes the guidewire, places the nail into the starting hole, and advances it to a point just proximal to the previously drilled vent holes. The osteotomy is then completed with an osteotome and the nail advanced to correct any existing angular deformity. Proximal and distal locking screws are inserted, wounds are irrigated, closed in layers, and dressed. Imaging and management of the device is included.

0596T-0597T

The physician treats permanent urinary retention due to impaired detrusor contractility (IDC) with a replaceable urinary prosthesis that mimics normal urination. This two-component system consists of a urethral insert with an internal valve-pump mechanism and a hand-held rechargeable activator that operates the valve-pump. Approximately one week prior to the insertion procedure, the correct device size is determined using a proprietary sizing tool. On the day of the procedure, the patient is placed in the lithotomy position and the meatus area is cleansed. Analgesic medical lubricant is applied to the external body of the device, after which it is inserted into the urethra using an introducer until the outer flange touches the edge of the meatus. The introducer's plunger is depressed, the device is released, and the introducer is removed. Following insertion, the physician performs a check for leakage and for proper device functioning using the activator. Holding the activator against the lower pubic area just above the urethral opening, the button is depressed to initiate urination. Upon completion of urination, the button is released and the activator is held in place for an additional three seconds until the valve has closed, completing the urination process. Report 0596T for the initial insertion and 0597T for a replacement procedure.

0598T-0599T

The physician uses a proprietary point-of-care handheld portable imaging device to identify the presence, location, and amount of bacteria in a wound. A positive result (104 colony-forming units per gram) can indicate infection. The device produces a safe violet light that causes the bacteria, blood, and tissue in wounds to fluoresce different colors; red fluorescence is indicative of gram-negative and gram-positive species, aerobes, and anaerobes including *E. coli*, *Klebsiella*, and *Staphylococcus*, while cyan fluorescence indicates *Pseudomonas aeruginosa*. The device detects *Acinetobacter*, the *Enterobacteriaceae* family, and *Pseudomonas*, which are considered by the World Health Organization to be "priority pathogens of concern" due to their multi-drug resistance. The physician can also obtain highly accurate wound area measurements, create a digital record of all images, and export the images to electronic health records. A built-in sensor detects optimal lighting conditions. When room lights cannot be turned off and required ambient lighting conditions cannot be met, the device may be used in conjunction with a compatible one-time use polyethylene drape. Report 0598T per session for the first anatomic site and 0599T for each additional anatomic site imaged during the same session.

0600T-0601T

The physician performs tissue ablation of tumors using a surgical method known as irreversible electroporation (IRE). This non-thermal ablation system uses direct current electrical fields to destroy soft tissue tumors by creating minute holes in the tissue's cell membranes. This causes the cell to become porous, resulting in cell death. The patient is placed under general anesthesia. In 0600T, using ultrasound or CT imaging guidance, the physician inserts thin needles percutaneously into precisely targeted locations around the selected tumor. Electrical currents are delivered through the needles and the pulses disrupt the tumor cell membrane without damaging healthy tissues. Report 0601T if performed as an open procedure. These codes report one or more tumors per organ and include imaging guidance.

0602T-0603T

Glomerular filtration rate (GFR) is a test that estimates the amount of blood passing through the glomeruli (the tiny filters in the kidneys that strain waste from the blood). One real-time transdermal measurement system involves a small light sensor being placed on the patient's skin and the administration of a biocompatible fluorescent tracer, such as MB-102 or Relmapirazin. The tracer is removed from the blood solely by GFR, and as it is cleared by the kidney, the measured fluorescence decreases. Algorithms in the device monitor convert these factors into a measured GFR. Intended to measure GFR in patients with normal or impaired renal function, this method can be especially beneficial in those undergoing chemotherapy. Measured GFR levels obtained just prior to drug dosing and at specific times post-infusion may be used to adjust chemotherapy dosage to ensure minimal toxicity while affording maximal efficacy. Report 0602T for transdermal GFR measurement and administration of a single dose of fluorescent pyrazine agent, and 0603T for administration of more than one dose, each 24 hours. Both codes include sensor placement.

0604T-0606T

This proprietary patient-initiated remote optical coherence tomography (OCT) scan is a home-based diagnostic device that allows patients with exudative (wet) age-related macular degeneration (AMD) to perform OCT testing of the retina without requiring technician assistance. This noninvasive imaging technique uses light waves that allow each distinct layer of the retina to be measured and mapped, producing high-resolution retinal images. If retinal fluid is detected, a report that characterizes the quantitative changes is generated and sent to the treating physician, helping to reduce the time from fluid onset to the patient's next treatment. Report 0604T for initial device provision, set-up, and patient education; report 0605T to capture remote surveillance and data analysis each 30 days; and report 0606T to report review and interpretation of the data by the physician or other qualified health care professional each 30 days.

0607T-0608T

This proprietary device uses a "chest patch" sensor and radiofrequency signals to provide continuous external mobile pulmonary fluid monitoring. The noninvasive system, which monitors heart and respiratory rates, lung fluid levels, activity, posture, and EKG data, consists of a chest patch made of copper-based sensors, a microprocessor unit, and a mobile application. Parameters are measured and multiple vital signs are derived from a single measurement at 40 samples per second, making this technology particularly useful for heart failure and hemodialysis patients. Report 0607T for initial set-up and patient education on the use of the equipment and 0608T for data analysis/report transmission to the physician or other qualified health care professional.

0609T-0612T

Determination and localization of discogenic pain of the cervical, thoracic, or lumbar region is made using a proprietary software program along with existing high-field magnetic resonance (MR) technology. In one application, the patient receives an MR spectroscopy scan of the targeted area in the lumbar spine using existing pulse sequences. Utilizing the software program, the data is uploaded to a cloud-based postprocessor where each disc is assessed for degenerative pain biomarker signatures in certain combinations of chemicals such as alanine, carbohydrate, collagen, lactic and propionic acid, and proteoglycan. A report is generated from the cloud postprocessor that contains data to assist the physician in evaluating the chemical composition of a disc relative to other discs; this report is returned to the patient's record in the originating network. This information, combined with other existing patient data, is useful in diagnosing conditions such as degenerative disc disease (DDD) or discogenic pain. Report 0609T for the MR spectroscopy and single voxel data acquisition on biomarkers in at least three discs; report 0610T for transmission of the biomarker data for software analysis; report 0611T for the postprocessing/ analysis of the biomarker data to ascertain the chemical variances between discs; report 0612T for the interpretation and report.

0613T

The interatrial shunt device creates a shunt or "passage" connecting the two atria of the heart. This allows excess blood to flow between the chambers, regulating high pressure in the left atrium and stabilizing left ventricular function without overloading the right heart. The device is typically placed by an interventional cardiologist during a catheterization procedure; right and left heart catheterization, intracardiac echocardiography, and imaging guidance are included in this code when those services are performed in conjunction with the shunt implantation. The patient is placed under general anesthesia. Using a percutaneous approach, the procedure is performed through a transfemoral venous approach under fluoroscopic and transendoscopic echocardiographic (TEE) guidance. The physician places a catheter sheath into the femoral vein and advances the catheter over a guidewire, using fluoroscopic guidance, to the left atrium. The catheter is used to create a transseptal puncture in the intra-atrial septum. The catheter is then withdrawn, leaving the guidewire in place. The device is inserted through an introducer sheath and over the guidewire using a dedicated shunt delivery system designed to deploy the device at the target location across the atrial septum. The device remains in the opening in the septum, allowing blood to flow from the high pressure left side to the lower pressure right side. At the end of the procedure, the guidewire and deployment device are removed. Pressure is placed over the incision for 20 to 30 minutes to stem bleeding. The patient is observed for a period afterward.

0615T

To aid in the testing and diagnosis of a concussion, which is not always detectable with conventional measures such as radiographic imaging, a noninvasive eye-tracking diagnostic procedure is utilized. Analysis of eye movement using non-spatially calibrated tracking assesses brain function using time rather than space. The tracking measures how well the eyes can move and includes an assessment to detect disconjugacy, a condition in which the eyes do not turn together in the same direction; saccades, rapid movements of the eyes with abrupt changes in the point of fixation; and other pupillary dynamics related to a concussion. The subject, using a chin and forehead rest, looks at a monitor on which a short video clip plays repeatedly on an aperture that travels around the edge of the screen. High-resolution binocular eye movements are measured by the testing device, and the pupils are tracked for a specified period for comparison to each other and to a database of control subjects. This code includes interpretation and report.

0619T

The physician treats symptomatic benign prostatic hyperplasia (BPH) with transurethral delivery of therapeutic drugs. In one method, the physician utilizes a proprietary dilation catheter, the end of which has a semi-compliant inflatable double lobe balloon that is coated with the pharmaceutical paclitaxel. The cystourethroscope is introduced into the meatus and the urethra is inspected. The catheter is inserted and exerts radial force to dilate the prostatic urethra, resulting in anterior commissurotomy and localized transfer of the paclitaxel from the drug-coated balloon. The area is observed through the scope and the instruments and cystourethroscope are removed. This code includes transrectal ultrasound and fluoroscopy, when performed.

0621T-0622T

The physician creates multiple laser channels through the trabecular meshwork using a cold (nonthermal) laser system. This microinvasive surgery minimizes tissue fibrosis and helps to bypass the major area of resistance to aqueous outflow, lowering eye pressure in patients with glaucoma. In one method, using gonioscopic or endoscopic visualization, the physician makes a minute clear corneal incision, through which the laser probe is advanced. The probe is navigated through the anterior chamber, which was earlier filled with viscoelastic, and placed in direct contact with the trabecular meshwork. Using a foot pedal system, the physician applies laser energy; typically, 10 microchannels are created over 90 degrees, 500 μm apart, ablating portions of the trabecular meshwork and inner wall of Schlemm's canal. This procedure may be performed alone or in conjunction with cataract surgery. Report 0622T if the procedure is performed with the use of an ophthalmic endoscope and 0621T if performed without.

0627T-0630T

The physician administers a percutaneous injection of a cellular and/or tissue-based product originating from a donor other than the patient (allogeneic) to one or more intervertebral discs. Intervertebral disc diseases are a leading underlying cause of low back pain and disability, with degenerative disc disease and prolapsed intervertebral discs being the two most common. In one method, the physician inserts a needle percutaneously and under imaging guidance into the targeted area of the intervertebral disc. Proprietary allogeneic progenitor cells that were derived from adult human intervertebral disc tissue and biomedically engineered are then injected. Report 0627T for first level lumbar injection under fluoroscopic guidance and 0628T for each additional level. Report 0629T for first level lumbar injection under CT guidance and 0630T for each additional level. These codes report unilateral or bilateral injections.

0631T

Hyperspectral imaging (HSI) technology uses transcutaneous measurements of oxyhemoglobin (HT-Oxy) and deoxyhemoglobin (HT-Deoxy) concentrations by employing wavelengths of visual light that penetrate to 1 to 4 mm below the skin. By analyzing a wide spectrum of light rather than simply assigning primary colors, a two-dimensional, color-coded "oxygen map" is created. This device can be used as a noninvasive screening tool for determining tissue oxygenation and the severity of peripheral vascular disease (PVD) and critical limb ischemia (CLI). Report 0631T for testing, interpretation, per extremity.

0632T

The physician performs transcatheter pulmonary artery (PA) ultrasound ablation of selective nerves that innervate the pulmonary arteries in order to reduce PA pressure in patients with pulmonary arterial hypertension (PAH). One method utilizes a dedicated proprietary catheter that features three ultrasound arrays at the distal tip; these generate high frequency, non-focused ultrasound energy that is delivered through the wall of the pulmonary artery to denervate local nerves that constrict the artery. This procedure is performed during right heart catheterization and may be attempted in the main, right, and left pulmonary arteries, close to the main bifurcation. This code includes the right heart catheterization, angiography of the pulmonary artery, and all imaging guidance.

0633T-0638T

Computed tomography (CT) directs multiple narrow beams of x-rays around a body structure to produce thin, cross-sectional views of anatomical layers (or slices) of the body. Dedicated breast computed tomography (DBCT) is an imaging modality that yields three-dimensional data that can then be recreated into multiple imaging planes. It is not limited by breast density and can be performed without breast compression. In one method, the patient lies prone on a specially designed scan bed that allows for full breast and chest wall access. The noncompressed breast is inserted through the opening of the table and hangs pendant; the bed design allows for one breast at a time to be imaged. Using a cone-beam CT system, the preprogrammed scanner moves and stops at 300 specific positions around the breast as individual images are taken. At the end of the scan, these images are sent to a computer processing workstation, where motion correction software may be utilized. The images are then processed with an algorithm that reconstructs them into a 3D dataset. Report 0633T for unilateral breast CT if no contrast materials are used; 0634T if performed with contrast; and 0635T if performed first without contrast and again following the injection of contrast. Report 0636T for bilateral breast CT without contrast; 0637T for that with contrast; and 0638T if performed first with contrast and again following contrast injection. These codes include 3D rendering if performed.

0639T

A wireless, wearable skin sensor is applied to the patient for continuous or intermittent monitoring of the flow of cerebrospinal fluid (CSF) through an implanted shunt. The accumulation of CSF in the brain can result in a condition known as hydrocephalus. Treatment typically involves implantation of a shunt, a pressure-regulated silicone tube assembly which, unfortunately, frequently malfunctions. This flexible device, which is adhered to the skin surface at the location of the shunt, enables precise measurements of CSF flow and shunt patency by using thermal transport through near-surface skin layers. The device is typically placed at a distal location along the shunt above the clavicle. A handheld ultrasound instrument may be used to provide images of the skin and underlying shunt tubing. Placement of the sensor is guided by palpation and visual examination. A proprietary software application acts as an interface, providing a means to record, store, and display the digital data on a smartphone or tablet. This code includes ultrasound guidance when performed.

0644T
The physician percutaneously removes or debulks intracardiac vegetations, frequently in the treatment of infective endocarditis, using a vacuum or aspiration suction device. Venous access is gained through the right internal jugular vein, the left femoral vein and artery, and the right femoral vein. Heparin is administered. Percutaneous insertion of a cannula into the left femoral vein is achieved to permit blood reinfusion. The right internal jugular vein is dilated using an inflow cannula, dilator, and guidewire. The apparatus is advanced under fluoroscopic guidance to the level of the right atrium; the dilator and guidewire are removed, and the cardiopulmonary bypass circuit is prepared. The proprietary suction system is inserted via the right jugular vein cannula, in this scenario, to the level of the tricuspid valve and the vegetation is aspirated under transesophageal echo guidance using suction in the form of venous extracorporeal bypass. The filtration system allows the aspirated blood to be filtered, removing vegetation. The blood is then reinfused through the left femoral vein. A final echocardiogram is performed to confirm that the infective vegetation has been completely aspirated. Heparin is partially reversed, and the physician removes all catheters and access cannulas. A variation of this procedure may also be used to remove intracardiac masses caused by thrombus.

0645T
The physician implants a coronary sinus reduction (CSR) device using a percutaneous, transcatheter approach in a patient suffering from chronic refractory angina. The device, which creates a focal narrowing and increases coronary venous pressure, consists of a stainless steel mesh pre-mounted on an hourglass-shaped balloon catheter. The physician accesses the right jugular vein percutaneously and advances a diagnostic catheter to the right atrium, where the central venous pressure is recorded. The coronary sinus is selectively engaged and contrast is injected to assess the vessel's anatomy. The physician exchanges a guiding catheter over the wire, positions it distally in the coronary sinus, and advances the reduction device to the targeted implantation site. The guiding catheter is then retracted, exposing the device and allowing the balloon to inflate and the CSR to expand. After the balloon catheter deflates, it is retrieved and a final angiogram is obtained to rule out any complications such as migration or perforation, to evaluate positioning, and to confirm the narrowing.

0647T
The provider places a gastrostomy tube percutaneously, using proprietary magnetic components and ultrasound imaging to guide the placement. Depending on patient status, the procedure may be performed at the bedside or in the interventional radiology (IR) suite. Following appropriate sedation, a proprietary balloon catheter is inserted via the mouth into the stomach. The external magnet component is used to pull the balloon to the anterior stomach wall. The balloon is then filled with saline, which provides a field for safe ultrasound visualization into the stomach. Using this ultrasound guidance, the provider targets the balloon with an introducer needle, inserts the needle percutaneously, and aspirates to verify appropriate placement in the balloon. The proprietary guidewire is then fed through the needle into the balloon. The balloon is deflated, snaring the guidewire, and both are removed through the mouth. A gastrostomy tube is then advanced over the wire, pulled through a dermatotomy in the abdominal wall, and trimmed to the appropriate length. Contrast is injected through the tube to confirm the location within the stomach using a portable x-ray or a fluoroscopic image.

0648T-0649T [0697T, 0698T]
Quantitative magnetic resonance (QMR) is a noninvasive body composition analysis technique. In one application, it is used to help diagnose and treat patients with liver disease by measuring liver tissue characteristics. Used in conjunction with contrast-free abdominal MR images, the proprietary post-processing software aids the physician in assessing patients with diabetes, metabolic syndrome, obesity, and fatty liver who may be at risk of nonalcoholic steatohepatitis (NASH), as well as those with any disease-causing liver inflammation. By using a series of images, it provides metrics for T2*, corrected T1 (cT1) and proton density fat fraction (PDFF) of the liver by measuring liver fat, iron, fibrosis, and inflammation. Report 0648T if this single-organ QMR analysis is obtained without diagnostic MRI examination of the same anatomy during the same session. If obtained with diagnostic MRI of the same anatomy during the same session, report 0649T in addition to the code for the MRI. In another application, this multiparametric, AI-driven MR imaging suite is used in the assessment of multiorgan health and function for patients diagnosed with "long COVID"—effects that last longer than 12 weeks—aiding in the diagnosis and management of cardiac, pancreatic, pulmonary, renal, and splenic diseases. It also allows metabolic profiling of patients with metabolic syndrome and type 2 diabetes. The QMR uses a combination of image formation, MR imagine analysis, and AI in conjunction with a proprietary interface to aid in the diagnosis, treatment planning, and monitoring of the progression disease and can be used by existing diagnostic imaging hardware. Report 0697T if this multiorgan QMR analysis is obtained without diagnostic MRI examination of the same anatomy during the same session. If obtained with diagnostic MRI of the same anatomy during the same session, report 0698T in addition to the code for the MRI.

0650T
Subcutaneous cardiac rhythm monitors provide uninterrupted, long-term cardiac monitoring for those

whose symptoms occur too sporadically to be adequately detected by shorter-term external monitoring methods. Also known as insertable cardiac monitors or implantable loop recorders, these monitors are indicated for adults who exhibit symptoms (e.g., chest pain, dizziness, palpitations, shortness of breath, or syncope) that may indicate a cardiac arrhythmia. They are also indicated for those who are at risk of developing an abnormal heart rhythm. Report 0650T for remote programming of these devices. The physician or other qualified health care professional reviews automatically recorded as well as patient-activated rhythm episodes to assure that arrhythmias are identified accurately, and recording parameters are reviewed and adjusted. Stored and trended historical data are used for comparison to current data measurements and the device function is evaluated for signal strength. Battery life, total memory capacity, and recording capacity parameters are reviewed. Following a thorough examination of all device parameters, a decision is made regarding the adequacy; any changes needed to optimize performance are made and saved in the remote monitoring system.

0651T

The patient undergoes a minimally invasive diagnostic visualization of the esophagus and stomach using a robotically controlled capsule endoscopy system. The proprietary system, which does not require sedation, incorporates a miniaturized wireless endoscope within a single-use capsule that is remotely controlled during the procedure by the physician using magnetic guidance hardware. System components include a controller, which consists of a rotation platform, examination bed, and magnetic head, and a patient console, which consists of the control panel, computer, and software. The physician or nurse activates the capsule locator prior to ingestion. The patient then swallows the ingestible capsule with water prior to beginning the examination. The video camera that is contained within has its own light source and takes pictures of the patient's stomach. A data recorder, which is worn over the clothes during the examination, receives the images captured by the capsule during the procedure, and the component software displays the actual anatomical view and recently captured images. Interpretation and report are included in the procedure.

0652T-0654T

The physician examines the upper gastrointestinal (GI) tract for diagnostic purposes using a transnasal approach as an alternative to conventional transoral esophagogastroduodenoscopy (EGD). Following application of a local topical anesthetic, the physician examines the esophagus, stomach, and duodenum via an ultra-thin flexible endoscope inserted under direct vision through one of the patient's nasal passages. Photo documentation may be obtained of normal landmarks as well as any observed abnormalities. In 0652T, a collection of specimen cells may be obtained by brushing or washing. In 0653T, biopsy forceps are used through the endoscope to obtain one or more samples from the upper GI tract. In 0654T, the physician places a tube or catheter through the endoscope. The endoscope is removed and the patient observed.

0655T

The physician treats prostate cancer (the second most common cancer diagnosed among men in the United States) with transperineal focal laser ablation. Also known as photothermal therapy, laser interstitial therapy, and laser interstitial photocoagulation, focal laser ablation (FLA) destroys tissue using a focused beam of electromagnetic radiation discharged from a laser fiber. In one method, the physician positions the laser fiber into the targeted tumor using a transperineal approach and transrectal imaging guidance. Once the position of the fiber is determined to be correct, a laser light is delivered through the fiber and the temperature of the tissue at the fiber's tip increases, causing coagulative necrosis.

0656T-0657T [0790T]

The physician performs anterior lumbar or thoracolumbar vertebral body tethering, a nonfusion, minimally invasive surgical procedure intended to correct idiopathic scoliosis. Under general anesthesia, the patient is placed in the lateral decubitus (side) position with the spinal convexity side up and the concavity side down. Using a percutaneous endoscopic approach, depending upon the spinal level to be treated, either a video-assisted thoracoscopy is performed through four to five small portal incisions in the hemithorax (thoracic spine) or the endoscope is introduced through small portal incisions on the side of the abdomen (lumbar spine). The lungs may need to be collapsed during the procedure for visualization if the thoracic spine is being treated. Under endoscopic visualization, with CT scan or fluoroscopic guidance, vertebral body titanium screws and anchors are placed in the vertebral bodies on the convexity side. The screws are then connected to the tether device, usually a polyethylene terephthalate flexible cord that secures the instrumentation under the appropriate tension as controlled by the surgeon. When the tether cord is tightened, it compresses the convex side of the spine to help straighten the spine. The scoliotic curve shows an immediate improvement after surgery and continuous improvement as the patient's spine grows, creating a straighter spine. Alternately, the procedure may be carried out with an open approach via anterior thoracotomy. During the surgery, one or both lungs are collapsed, and the parietal pleura is opened over the spine. Screws and anchors are placed in the vertebral bodies and the polyethylene tether is attached and tightened. A chest drainage tube may be placed and set to suction. Report 0656T if up to seven vertebral segments are treated and 0657T if treatment involves eight or more segments. Report 0790T when the tether is replaced, removed, or revised by methods such as augmentation or division; thoracoscopy is included when performed.

0658T
The physician performs electrical impedance spectroscopy (EIS) of one or more skin lesions to obtain an automated melanoma risk score. After the targeted area is cleaned, the lesion is measured using a tool from the proprietary system. The results are analyzed by the system and displayed on the screen component. The classifier produces an EIS score output that reflects the degree of atypia identified. The physician uses this objective information in combination with visual inspection to arrive at an informed clinical decision.

0659T
The physician delivers supersaturated oxygen (SSO2) therapy to a patient suffering a left anterior descending (LAD) ST-elevation myocardial infarction (also known as a widowmaker because of the high mortality rate). Device components of the proprietary system include a console, cartridge, and SSO2 catheter. Immediately following primary percutaneous coronary intervention (PCI) with stenting that is performed within six hours of symptom onset, arterial blood drawn from the existing access site is combined with a highly oxygenated saline solution. The hyperoxemic blood is then delivered by the SSO2 infusion catheter using the femoral access site over a 60-minute period to the affected artery. The pO2 content of the superoxygenated infusion is seven to 10 times higher than that of normal arterial blood, which allows a high rate of oxygen diffusion into the ischemic tissue. Report this code in addition to 92941 for the percutaneous coronary revascularization procedure performed during the acute myocardial infarction.

0660T-0661T
As an alternative to daily eye drop treatment to reduce intraocular pressure in patients with open-angle glaucoma or ocular hypertension, the physician implants a sustained-release drug delivery device in the anterior chamber of the eye. The proprietary titanium implant consists of three parts: a scleral anchor that attaches to the trabecular meshwork, the body of the device that contains the drug, and the elution membrane that controls the drug release. The implant releases an exclusive formulation of travoprost (a prostaglandin analog drug that lowers intraocular pressure by increasing the flow of natural eye fluids out of the eye) inside the anterior chamber; this placement allows minute amounts of the active drug molecule over time. Once all the travoprost is released, the device is removed and replaced. In one method, the surgeon creates a 2.4 mm incision and visualizes the anterior chamber angle using an ab interno approach. The scleral anchor is implanted into the trabecular meshwork and the surgeon nudges the device to ensure that the attachment is secure. Report 0660T for initial implantation and 0661T for removal and reimplantation of the device. The medication is reported separately.

0662T-0663T
Chemotherapy-induced alopecia (hair loss) is one of the most common and distressing side effects of certain cytotoxic drugs. Proprietary devices reduce the temperature of the scalp by a few degrees immediately before, during, and after the administration of chemotherapy. The resulting cooling-induced vasoconstriction causes a reduction in blood flow to the hair follicles, which in turn results in less chemotherapeutic drug being delivered to those follicles. A lightweight silicone cap is placed on the patient's head and connected to a miniature refrigeration system. A special coolant is circulated through the cold cap, lowering scalp temperature. The cap is worn, on average, for approximately 30 minutes pre-infusion and for up to 90 minutes following drug infusion. Report 0662T once per chemotherapy treatment period for the initial measurement and calibration of the cap. Report 0663T once per chemotherapy session in conjunction with the appropriate chemotherapy administration code to reflect the cap's placement, monitoring, and removal.

0664T-0666T
Using an open approach, a healthy uterus from a living or deceased (i.e., brain dead or cadaver) donor is obtained. In one method, using a standard laparotomy technique involving a subumbilical midline incision, the uterus is harvested along with arterial vasculature including the deep uterine artery on either side with a segment of the internal iliac arteries divided just distally to the gluteal artery. The venous vasculature harvested includes one or two deep uterine veins on either side, attached to a segment of the internal iliac vein and/or the proximal parts of the utero-ovarian branch, which is divided before the inlet of the ovarian veins in order to preserve the ovaries in situ. Any bleeding in a living donor is controlled, and the incision is closed by suturing. Report 0664T for a deceased donor and 0665T for a living donor. In an alternate procedure, the uterus is obtained from a living donor using a laparoscopic or robotic technique, reported with 0666T. All codes include perfusing the uterus allograft with cold-preservation solution as well as cold maintenance.

0667T
The physician transplants a uterus obtained from a living or deceased (i.e., brain dead or cadaver) donor into a patient with absolute uterine factor infertility (AUFI). AUFI, a condition in which a woman cannot become pregnant because she either lacks a uterus or the uterus can no longer function correctly, can be congenital or acquired. Uterine transplantation (UTx), an alternative to adoption or surrogacy for those with nonfunctioning or absent uterine factor infertility, entails not only transplantation of the uterus but includes the cervix, a cuff of vagina, the surrounding ligamentous and connective tissues, and the major blood vessels to the level of the internal iliac vessels. In one technique, with the patient under appropriate anesthesia and in a lithotomy position, the physician makes a midline infraumbilical incision and dissects the external iliac artery and vein completely along their length bilaterally. Internal arterial anastomosis is performed using sutures to join the internal iliac artery

patch of the donor graft to the external iliac artery of the recipient. The physician then performs venous anastomosis using the most optimal venous outflow present in the donor graft as determined by backbench inspection; this will be either the uterine or the utero-ovarian vein. Sutures are used to join this vein to the external iliac vein of the recipient. Following allograft reperfusion, the physician performs the anastomosis of the cervix of the donor uterus to the recipient's vaginal vault. A Doppler flow-monitoring probe is placed on one of the donor uterine arteries to monitor the arterial flow. Bleeding is controlled and the infraumbilical incision is closed.

0668T

The surgeon performs a standard backbench preparation of a uterus and attached structures following procurement from a cadaver or living donor. Backbench or back table preparation refers to procedures performed on the donor organ following procurement to prepare the allograft for transplant. After removal from the donor, the graft is inspected for perfusion and vessel quality. A hysteroscopy may be performed. The graft, including all vascular pedicles, is prepared for transplantation. Standard backbench preparation includes dissection and removal of the surrounding soft tissues, as well as any necessary preparation of uterine veins and arteries.

0669T

The physician performs a backbench reconstruction of a cadaver or living donor uterus allograft requiring venous anastomosis prior to transplantation. A vein of a uterus allograft may be unsuitable for anastomosis with that in the intended transplant recipient. Using a vein graft procured from the donor or other source, backbench venous anastomosis is performed on the allograft to create an extension graft. Report 0669T for each venous anastomosis.

0670T

The physician performs a backbench reconstruction of a cadaver or living donor uterus allograft requiring arterial anastomosis prior to transplantation. An artery of a uterus allograft may be unsuitable for anastomosis with that in the intended transplant recipient. Using an artery vein graft procured from the donor or other source, backbench arterial anastomosis is performed on the allograft to create an extension graft. Report 0670T for each arterial anastomosis.

0672T

The physician treats female stress urinary incontinence (SUI) by remodeling the tissues surrounding the bladder neck and proximal urethra. The physician inserts the treatment tip of the proprietary device into the vaginal opening and rotates it. The dual-energy system alternately cools surface tissues and distributes heat to the soft tissues underneath using cryogen-cooled monopolar radiofrequency technology that stimulates the body's natural collagen formation process. The single-session treatment is accomplished in approximately 45 to 60 minutes and requires no anesthesia.

0673T

The physician performs percutaneous laser ablation of one or more benign thyroid nodules. With the patient under conscious sedation, a local anesthetic is injected into the subcutaneous tissue and subcapsular region of the thyroid gland. Using ultrasound guidance, the physician inserts one or more 21G spinal needles into the thyroid nodule and positions the laser fiber through the needle so that the tip is in direct contact with the nodule tissue. Laser treatment is administered with a fixed power protocol (typically 3W to 4W). Total energy delivered for each fiber is frequently in the 1200-2000 J range. In some cases, the laser fibers are retracted one or more times (pull-back technique) and additional energy is administered to address the entire volume of the nodule. Following the procedure, patients may receive a betamethasone injection intramuscularly and are then observed prior to discharge.

0674T-0682T

The physician inserts or replaces a synchronized diaphragmatic stimulation system for augmentation of cardiac function using a standard laparoscopic approach. The system consists of a pulse generator and two or more diaphragmatic leads (electrodes), which deliver synchronized diaphragmatic stimulation (SDS) pulses that cause the muscles of the diaphragm to contract. These contractions are gated to the cardiac cycle and increase intrathoracic pressure, improving both cardiac output and left ventricular function. Under appropriate anesthesia, the physician implants the electrodes in the muscle of the diaphragm using standard laparoscopic technique. The lead wires are tunneled under the skin to the chest area, where the physician has created a subcutaneous pocket for the pulse generator in the pectoral region. The electrodes are connected to the generator and tested prior to pocket closure. Report 0674T for insertion or replacement of the entire SDS system; 0675T for insertion or replacement of the first diaphragmatic lead with connection to an existing pulse generator and 0676T for each additional lead; 0677T for repositioning or relocation of the first diaphragmatic lead with connection to an existing pulse generator and 0678T for each additional lead; and 0679T for the removal of one or more diaphragmatic leads without replacement. Report 0680T for insertion or replacement of the subcutaneous pulse generator only, with connection to the existing leads; 0681T for relocation or repositioning of the pulse generator only, with connection to the existing leads; and 0682T for removal of the pulse generator only. All codes reporting insertion, replacement, or repositioning/relocation include both interrogation and programming by the implant physician when performed.

0683T-0685T

The physician performs an in-person device evaluation of an existing permanent implantable synchronized diaphragmatic stimulation system (SDS). In 0683T, a programming device evaluation is performed in order to test the device's function and select the most favorable permanent programmed values. This involves device adjustments made in a stepwise or iterative fashion. In 0684T, evaluation and programming of SDS parameters are performed prior to or following a surgery, procedure, or test. In 0685T, an interrogation device evaluation is performed that involves connecting, recording, and disconnecting the device; this is reported once per patient encounter. All codes include analysis, review, and report by the physician or other qualified health care professional.

0686T
The physician performs a nonthermal, noninvasive ablation of liver tissue to destroy primary and metastatic tumors. The procedure, known as histotripsy, uses automated external beam therapy that delivers acoustic energy to destroy the tissue. One proprietary platform uses pulsed sound waves to generate "microbubbles" from gases that are naturally present in the targeted liver tissue. The physician plans the treatment by reviewing current MRI and CT data sets to determine the targeted tissue. Using the integrated ultrasound imaging, the physician centers the histotripsy treatment contours onto the target and creates an appropriate treatment volume. The physician then enables the platform to deliver the correct dose of energy to create a "bubble cloud" at distinct points inside the target and creates a personalized treatment plan for each target by setting the energy levels and calculating the time it will take to complete each treatment. In the treatment phase, histotripsy is delivered by the platform to the previously targeted tissue. Using short ultrasound bursts that last for microseconds, acoustic cavitation is generated from the force of the microbubbles and tissue is liquified and destroyed on a subcellular level. Ultrasound imaging is used to guide and monitor the histotripsy procedure in real-time.

0687T-0688T
Amblyopia, also known as lazy eye, is treated using a proprietary computer-based web application. By stimulating the brain's visual cortex, the online digital training program improves vision without the need for invasive surgery and is indicated for patients ages 9 and older. Report 0687T for supply of the device, educational set-up, and the initial session. Report 0688T once per calendar month for an assessment and report by the physician or other qualified health care professional that addresses the patient's performance as well as program data.

0689T-0690T
These codes report the use of nonelastographic ultrasound imaging data and software to analyze tissue characteristics. Performed without (0689T) or with (0690T) diagnostic ultrasound examination of the same anatomy, such as a gland, organ, target structure, or tissue, both codes include interpretation and report.

0691T
Automated analysis using artificial intelligence (AI) technology can accurately detect vertebral fractures on prior CT images containing the spine, such as routine chest or abdomen CTs. The proprietary software tool automatically calculates fracture risk scores by analyzing three bone imaging biomarkers and considering the patient's sex and age. This risk stratification may be predictive of future debilitating osteoporotic vertebral fractures and hip fractures, allowing for earlier interventions and treatment planning for patients at higher risk. Report 0691T for the automated analysis, which includes an assessment of bone density if performed. Data preparation, interpretation, and report are also included.

0692T
Using a proprietary therapeutic ultrafiltration system, also referred to as aquapheresis therapy, excess fluid is removed from patients suffering from fluid overload (hypervolemia). The system is indicated for temporary or extended use in adult and pediatric patients weighing 20 kg or more whose hypervolemia has been unresponsive to medical management such as diuretic therapy. Diagnostic indications include heart failure, fluid overload management in postoperative patients, and management of fluid balance in critically ill pediatric patients. Following central or peripheral venous access, the device mechanically withdraws blood through a catheter, passes it through a hemofilter to remove excess water and sodium, and returns the filtered blood to the patient through the catheter's infusion port.

0693T
Code 0693T reports markerless 3D kinematic and kinetic motion analysis; a comprehensive full body analysis and report is included in this computer-based application.

0694T
Code 0694T reports real-time intraoperative 3-dimensional volumetric imaging and reconstruction of breast or axillary lymph node tissue and includes 3-dimensional specimen orientation with interpretation and report. The code is reported once per specimen.

0695T-0696T
These codes report the electrophysiologic evaluation of pacemaker or pacing cardioverter-defibrillator leads using body surface mapping. Report 0695T when this procedure is performed with the insertion or replacement of pacing electrodes in the cardiac venous system for left ventricular pacing. Report 0696T when this procedure is performed at the time of follow-up interrogation or programming device evaluation.

0699T
An injection of medication is administered to the posterior chamber of the eye (the area between the iris, zonule fibers, and lens).

0700T-0701T
A proprietary handheld fluorescent molecular imaging device provides noninvasive evaluation of a suspicious nevus. Evaluating biological activity originating within

the nevus, the device aids in the identification of moles that have the potential to develop into malignancy. The health care provider applies a topical biocompatible fluorescent biotag to the area of concern and wipes it away. Using the handheld imager positioned over the nevus, white light and fluorescent images are captured. The proprietary software displays and analyzes the images. A probability score is generated to reflect the presence of tissue remodeling that might be suggestive of a progression from benign to atypia. Report 0700T for imaging of the first lesion and 0701T for each additional lesion.

0704T-0706T

Amblyopia, also known as lazy eye, is treated using a proprietary online digital platform. The binocular eye-tracking-based treatment is intended to treat children and aims to replace the eye patch, which has traditionally been the standard treatment. While the child watches any content of choice on the proprietary screen, the image undergoes real-time 3D image processing based on the momentary gaze position. The integrated cloud platform processes data from the system, providing a comprehensive vision summary. The physician can monitor remotely in real-time to measure adherence; feedback is also provided remotely to caregivers and other physicians. Report 0704T for device supply, patient education on equipment use, and initial set-up. Report 0705T for technical support provided by the surveillance center that includes data transmission with analysis; this code is reported each 30 days and requires a minimum of 18 training hours during that time period. Report 0706T once per calendar month for interpretation and report by the physician or other qualified health care professional.

0707T

In a minimally-invasive, fluoroscopically-assisted procedure, the physician fills subchondral bone defects such as bone bruises, bone marrow lesions, microtrabecular fractures, or stress injuries with bone substitute material (BSM). Consisting of an engineered calcium phosphate mineral compound, this bone graft substitute imitates the properties of cancellous bone. During the healing process, the compound resorbs and is replaced with new bone. Sites on which this procedure is typically performed include the foot/ankle, hip, knee, or shoulder. In one scenario, the physician treats an affected knee in which a bone marrow lesion is identified on MRI. Based on the location of the defect, the approach and trajectory are planned. The physician performs arthroscopy of the knee in order to evaluate the extent of the injury to the tibial plateau, aid in targeting the underlying defect, and view and treat other joint structures. Under intraoperative fluoroscopic guidance, the bone defect is localized relative to the MRI findings. The appropriate delivery cannula is drilled to the desired depth in the bone defect and bone substitute material is injected. The arthroscope is used following injection to look for any material that has extravasated into the joint; this is evacuated if any is discovered. The physician leaves the cannula in place until the BSM begins to set. The cannula is then removed and the physician ensures that no excess BSM emerges from the insertion portal. Fluoroscopic imaging is performed to confirm that the BSM is properly placed. Incisions are closed and the patient observed. Imaging guidance and arthroscopic assistance are included in this procedure.

0708T-0709T

The patient receives an intradermal immunotherapy injection for the treatment of cancer, often using a microneedle-based delivery device. Compared to the conventional syringe needle, the smaller size of the microneedle device allows for precise delivery into the dermal layers. Immunotherapy uses an individual's own immune system to fight malignancy. Report 0708T for preparation and initial injection and 0709T for each additional injection.

0710T-0713T

Using software processing of data obtained from CT angiography of noncoronary sites, noninvasive arterial plaque analysis is performed. Report 0710T when analysis includes measurements of the composition and structure of the vessel wall, assessment for lipid-rich necrotic core plaque to calculate the stability of atherosclerotic plaque, data preparation and transmission, data review, interpretation, and report. Report 0711T if analysis is performed with data preparation and transmission only. Report 0712T if analysis is performed with measurements of the vessel wall's composition and structure and assessment for lipid-rich necrotic core plaque to calculate atherosclerotic plaque stability. Report 0713T if analysis is performed with data review, interpretation, and report.

0716T

The health care provider determines coronary artery disease risk scores aided in part by acoustic waveform recordings. Using a computer-aided electronic auscultatory device, the acoustic signals of the heart are acquired, recorded, and analyzed by means of acoustic signal processing algorithms. Recordings from an acoustic sensor are analyzed by the computer to detect certain heart sounds, such as S1, S2, or suspected murmurs, and the results are displayed via a graphic user interface.

0717T-0718T

Adipose-derived regenerative cells (ADRCs) are an alternative source of autologous somatic stem cells for the repair of damaged tissue. Subcutaneous adipose tissues are harvested from the patient by ordinary liposuction technique. Using a proprietary enzyme-based process, the ADRCs are isolated from the fat tissue, washed, and filtered. The final product is injected into the targeted site (the supraspinatus tendon), where it stimulates the repair and regeneration of the damaged tissue in partial thickness rotator cuff tears. Report 0717T for the harvesting, isolation, and preparation of the autologous harvested cells. This code includes incubation with cell dissociation enzymes, filtration, washing, and concentration of ADRCs. Report 0718T for the subsequent unilateral injection under ultrasound guidance of the ADRCs into the patient's supraspinatus tendon.

0719T

As an alternative to lumbar fusion for degenerative lumbar conditions, the physician performs posterior vertebral joint replacement. In lumbar total joint replacement (LTJR), both the disc and facet joints are replaced with a proprietary motion-preserving lumbar device. With the patient in a prone position, the physician performs laminectomy, bilateral facet removal, and complete discectomy. A bilateral transforaminal approach is used to access the disc space. Following complete discectomy, the vertebral endplates are prepared using specialized oscillating rasps. Length and height trials are performed to determine the appropriate implant size, after which the physician works to restore disc height and soft tissue tension by bilateral soft tissue balancing. Two implants are inserted and press-fitted, followed by placement of a retention pedicle screw that allows for specified degrees of flexion and extension across the treated level.

0720T

The physician performs percutaneous electrical nerve field stimulation (PENFS) of the cranial nerves. In one application, a proprietary nonsurgical device targets central pain pathways in the treatment of functional abdominal pain associated with irritable bowel syndrome. Electrodes are applied to specific cranial nerve branches (V, VII, IX, and X) on the external ear. Neurostimulation is administered with alternating frequencies by slight electrical pulses that are transmitted through the electrodes, targeting the brain areas involved with processing pain.

0721T-0722T

Quantitative computed tomography (CT) tissue characterization allows the use of proprietary algorithms with existing patient imaging data to discover early, previously undetected signs of common chronic diseases. These findings can lead to further assessment to identify and establish individualized preventive care pathways for these patients. In one application, an AI-enabled cardiac imaging application detects coronary artery calcium (CAC), which is a known biomarker of cardiovascular disease. With the ability to be integrated into existing radiology workflows, the application helps to recognize and calculate the patient's CAC levels. The patient can then be classified according to their risk of cardiovascular disease and likely need for cardiac work up and treatment. Using routinely ordered non-gated CT scans, the application quantifies the CAC as an incidental finding. Based on the amount of cardiac calcium identified, the application automatically categorizes CT-scanned patients into risk categories. Report 0721T for CT tissue characterization obtained without concurrent CT examination of any structure contained in diagnostic imaging that was previously acquired. If CT tissue characterization is obtained concurrently with diagnostic imaging, report 0722T in addition to the code for the primary procedure.

0723T-0724T

Quantitative magnetic resonance cholangiopancreatography (QMRCP) is a proprietary software service that uses and enhances data obtained from a 3D MRCP. The MRCP allows noninvasive visualization of the biliary tree, gallbladder, and pancreatic ducts, after which the software creates a quantitative model of the pancreatobiliary system. This model permits a more precise and demonstrable portrayal of irregularities such as dilations and strictures by providing measurements such as gallbladder and gross biliary tree volume, as well as cross-sectional diameters of ducts in all areas of the biliary tree. Report 0723T for QMRCP obtained without diagnostic magnetic resonance imaging (MRI) of the same gland, organ, target structure, or tissue performed during the same session. Report 0724T in addition to the code for the primary procedure when QMRCP is obtained with diagnostic MRI of the same anatomy. Both codes include data preparation and transmission, as well as interpretation and report.

0725T-0727T

The physician implants a vestibular device for the treatment of bilateral vestibular hypofunction (BVH) or loss (BVL). This disorder is associated with chronic disequilibrium, postural imbalance, and unsteady gait due to failure of vestibular reflexes that stabilize the eyes, head, and body. Most cases are considered idiopathic, although BVH can be caused by a number of conditions including autoimmune disorders, chronic inflammatory peripheral polyneuropathy, congenital loss, meningitis, neurofibromatosis, ototoxicity, or sequential vestibular neuritis. A vestibular implant translates motion information into electrical signals that are then transmitted to the brain through electrodes that have been implanted near vestibular nerve endings. The system is made up of motion sensors that are affixed to the patient's head, along with a processor and stimulator (the electronic components that provide the translation). With the patient under general anesthesia, the physician makes a U-shaped postauricular incision using a transmastoid approach. Openings are made into the labyrinth, through which the electrode arrays are inserted and bone paste is applied. The receiver/stimulator is fixed with sutures into a bone well and subperiosteal pocket in the postauricular region. Incisions are closed. Report 0725T for vestibular device implantation and 0726T for device removal. Report 0727T for device removal and replacement performed concurrently. All codes report unilateral procedures.

0728T-0729T

A diagnostic analysis of a vestibular implant, including initial (0728T) or subsequent (0729T) programming, is performed postoperatively on a previously placed device designed to treat bilateral vestibular hypofunction (BVH) or loss (BVL). Diagnostic analysis may include programming of implant-related software, connection of software to the implant, and programming of the stimulator. Settings are adjusted to the patient's needs and may include volume, threshold levels, live-voice speech adjustments, pulse widths, input dynamic range, and frequency shaping template.

0730T
The physician performs trabeculotomy by laser technique for the treatment of glaucoma (chronic disorder involving increased pressure in the eye due to fluid buildup). Utilizing optical coherence tomography (OCT), an imaging technique employed to generate a picture of the retina, the physician identifies the drainage system canal and inserts an instrument to open the canal wall to help the fluid inside the eye drain better. The scleral and conjunctival flaps are closed with stitches. This opens a canal that allows for improved outflow of intraocular fluids, reducing the eye's pressure.

0731T
Many diseases present with distinguishing facial characteristics. Facial recognition based on artificial intelligence (AI) permits computers to detect underlying facial patterns to aid in diagnosis and screening of certain diseases based on facial phenotypes (DNA-determined appearance) or deformities using photographs. Advanced technique systems are used to visualize the images in 3D. Facial recognition allows for faster diagnoses of rare genetic disorders that are normally done with blood tests. This code includes analysis with report.

0732T
Intramuscular electroporation (IM/EP) is a vaccine delivery method that improves the ability of DNA vaccines to produce an immune response. Utilizing electrical pulses that are delivered through electrodes in milliseconds, temporary pores are created that allow plasmids to enter the target tissue's cell membrane; this improves cellular uptake of the immunotherapies previously injected at the site of the electrical stimulation. When compared to conventional IM vaccine injection, electroporation reduces the time it takes to reach maximal immune response.

0733T-0734T
Neurological rehabilitation, therapeutic monitoring, and treatment management services using motion capture-based systems (i.e., interactive computer games, video gesture control software, 3D virtual gaming system) are provided remotely. A standardized program is ordered by a physician or other qualified health care professional but supervised by rehabilitation assistants. Patients wear motion sensors and utilize virtual reality and devices to perform targeted functional activities designed by the physical therapist using gesture control. Report 0733T for supply and technical support per 30-day period. Report 0734T for management services provided by the physician or other qualified health care professional per calendar month.

0735T
The radiation oncologist delivers intraoperative radiation therapy (IORT) while the patient is undergoing a craniotomy. A miniature, low energy, isotope-free x-ray source is brought into the operating room at the time the craniotomy is performed to deliver a precise and targeted dose of radiation directly to the craniotomy cavity. The surgeon removes the malignant tumor and awaits the initial pathology report. Once the malignancy is confirmed, the physician prepares the tumor cavity for temporary insertion of a flexible balloon applicator. The radiation oncologist inserts the miniature x-ray source inside a balloon-shaped catheter device and a single dose of radiation is directed at the tumor cavity while medical personnel remain behind a rolling shield. The process takes eight to 12 minutes. Once the treatment is complete, the catheter is withdrawn and the applicator removed. In another method, a proprietary balloon catheter device is utilized for delivery of liquid brachytherapy to the brain following surgical removal of a malignant brain tumor. Radiation is delivered directly to the tissue cavity over a course of three to seven days.

0736T
A health care provider performs colonic lavage to cleanse the colon or large intestine. The patient is seated on a disinfected basin, and a sterile, disposable rectal catheter is inserted approximately 3 cm into the rectum. At least 35 liters of filtered water flows into the bowel using a gravity-fed delivery system, loosening the stool, inducing defecation, and allowing the patient to evacuate the colon.

0737T
The physician implants a xenograft, tissue harvested from a different species (i.e., pigs, cows, or other animals), into a human in need of articular cartilage repair or replacement. Much of the structure and many of the properties of original tissues may be retained through use of xenograft when harvested and processed accordingly. Utilizing a bone burr, the physician prepares the underlying bone bed of the recipient to produce a cancellous bleeding bed. The articular cartilage xenograft may be cut into segments, as repair or replacement of articular cartilage, or may involve the entire articular surface or a portion of the articular surface. The xenograft is implanted and held in place by one or more suture anchors, absorbable pins, screws, or staples. A fibrin clot may also be used to hold the substantially non-immunogenic articular cartilage xenograft in place. The incision is closed.

0738T-0739T
Treatment planning is conducted for magnetic field induction ablation of malignant prostate tissue (0738T). Utilizing data from a previous magnetic resonance imaging (MRI) examination, the physician plans the treatment and determines the targeted tissue. Treatment planning for oncology patients is the process of developing a complete plan for the course of therapy. The optimal way to deliver the treatment to

the malignancy while blocking the dose received by normal tissues must be determined. This requires localizing the tumor, determining its extent of malignancy and the volume to be treated, and choosing the best method of treatment. In 0739T, the physician uses the previously performed treatment plan to guide the ablation procedure. Under appropriate anesthesia, catheters are placed transperineally, and continuous bladder irrigation is initiated. The physician performs ablation of malignant prostate tissue utilizing magnetic field induction using a proprietary technology in which iron nanoparticles are introduced into the prostate cancer lesion via needles inserted through the perineum. The particles are then heated using a magnetic field, which ablates the prostate cancer lesion. All intraprocedural transperineal needle/catheter placement, temperature monitoring, bladder irrigation, thermal dosimetry, and magnetic field nanoparticle activation is included in this code.

0740T-0741T

Diabetes is a growing problem in the United States and abroad. Insulin therapy is extremely effective when used correctly. In 0740T, insulin dosage calculation and titration are obtained utilizing an autonomous algorithm-based system. This technology interprets data and independently generates clinically relevant conclusions without concurrent physician or other QHP involvement. In one proprietary system, a two-user interactive software element is used to calculate the patient's next dose of insulin and to assist in optimizing insulin management. The two-user interactive software is comprised of a Health Care Provider (HCP) software tool and a patient user interface software, which resides on a hand-held device such as a cellular phone or enabled glucose meter; this is used to enter glucose event data and receive recommended insulin doses. The provider utilizes the HCP software to set up the patient software for its intended use, which consists of entering the physician-prescribed, patient-specific starting insulin prescription and sending the information to the patient user software. Insulin instructions include the treatment plan, insulin drug, and doses. Insulin dose may also be calculated via the library, data manually entered via the patient user software, or automatically from the cloud of a linked blood glucose meter. Report 0740T for initial set-up and patient education and 0741T each 30 days for software provision and management, which may include date collection, transmission, and storage.

0742T

The physician performs absolute quantitation of myocardial blood flow (AQMBF) using single-photon emission computed tomography (SPECT), a noninvasive type of nuclear imaging that produces three-dimensional images by using a single or multiple-head camera that rotates around the patient. The specialized cameras take images of the tissue to evaluate blood perfusion and tissue functionality. The provider, as part of an exercise or pharmacologic stress test (and sometimes at rest), injects a radiolabeled tracer that is specific to the target tissue into the bloodstream. Following tracer administration, the patient waits a given amount of time while the tracer circulates and is subsequently taken up by the target tissue. Absolute quantitation of myocardial blood flow (MBF) is the volume of blood transiting through tissue at a certain rate, usually in milliliters per minute per gram of tissue (mL/min/g). The MBF measurement reflects coronary microcirculation and can be used to evaluate for coronary risk factors and myocardial disease.

0743T

Bone mineral density (BMD) studies have been used to diagnose osteoporosis, a condition in which the density and quality of the bone is diminished, greatly increasing the patient's risk for a fracture. Utilizing previously acquired computed tomography scans that have been translated into patient-specific three-dimensional anatomical models, the physician employs finite element analysis, which utilizes bone biomechanical properties, geometry, and loading conditions to assess bone strength and overall fracture risk. This code includes a concurrent vertebral fracture assessment and encompasses all aspects of the service, including retrieval and transmission of the CT data, bone strength/fracture risk assessment, and interpretation and report.

[0749T, 0750T]

Digital X-ray radiogrammetry-bone mineral density (DXR-BMD) analysis calculates bone mineral density using data obtained from a digital x-ray (an advanced form of x-ray inspection in which a digital radiographic image is produced instantly on a computer) and is used to predict fractures and osteoporosis. In 0749T, the physician employs an automated analysis (DXR) to evaluate bone mineral density, bone strength, and fracture risk using the images acquired with the digital X-ray machine. If data from a hand or wrist x-ray performed concurrently for another purpose is also used for the digital DXR-BMD analysis, report the appropriate x-ray code separately. Report 0750T if a single-view digital x-ray of the hand taken specifically for the purpose of DXR-BMD is utilized as a data source.

0744T

The physician uses an open approach to make a 6- to 8-inch incision in the upper thigh to visualize the femoral vein. Clamps are applied to the proximal and distal sites of the target area on the femoral vein. The physician makes a 2 to 3 cm lengthwise incision to open the femoral vein, then inserts a proprietary bioprosthetic valve intended to reduce and eliminate venous reflux, a major cause of deep vein thrombosis (DVT) and chronic venous insufficiency (CVI), into the open femoral vein and sutures the stabilization ring of the valve frame to the wall of the femoral vein. Once the valve is secured in place, the physician sutures the femoral vein and removes the proximal and distal clamps, allowing blood flow to resume through the femoral vein. The patient may require general or regional anesthesia for the procedure. Autogenous or nonautogenous patch graft and duplex ultrasound imaging guidance are included when performed.

0745T-0747T

The physician administers noninvasive radiation therapy (RT) with a proprietary RT system to a target segment of the heart for the purpose of ablating, or scarring, cardiac tissue to correct an arrhythmia, such as ventricular tachycardia. In preparation, the cardiologist or cardiology team conducts testing and imaging (MRI, ECG, PET, or CT) to map precisely where the arrhythmia is originating in the heart. The provider uses this imaging and mapping information to plan and deliver targeted radiation treatment. Prior to radiation administration, the motion of the heart is measured when respiratory motion is a concern or when management of the movement may spare healthy tissue. The patient is brought to the radiation therapy lab and placed supine on the treatment table. The RT system is then used to direct radiation beams to the targeted cardiac site, often using the gray scale to refer to the amount of energy absorbed by the tissue. The patient receives "beam on" therapy for five to seven minutes. In one method, the provider targets the heart with a single dose of stereotactic body radiation therapy (SBRT), which is used commonly in cancer treatment and requires no general anesthesia. Report 0745T for the localization/mapping of the arrhythmia, 0746T for the conversion of this information into a multidimensional radiation treatment plan, and 0747T for the delivery of the radiation therapy directed at the arrhythmia.

0748T

Stem cell therapy is a minimally invasive procedure to treat perianal inflammation and diseased, damaged, or dysfunctional tissue in conditions such as ulcerative colitis and fistulizing Crohn's disease. The physician prepares the area to receive the stem cell product. Excision or debridement of the fistula tract and surrounding areas may be necessary, especially in the presence of a previously positioned seton. After removal, extensive de-epithelization may be performed with a small probe, tracts are cleaned with saline solution to remove devitalized tissue debris, and the internal fistula opening is closed. In one approach, utilizing a needle, mesenchymal stem cells (adult stem cells harvested from bone marrow or fat tissue) are injected around the tissue. In some instances, a half dose may be injected in tissues around the internal orifice while the other half dose is administered through the external orifice. Mesenchymal stem cells have secreting factors called cytokines, which have anti-inflammatory properties and recruit low level immune cells needed to regenerate or repair injured tissue. The surgical procedure is completed with soft massage of the implant area.

0751T-0755T

Digital pathology is a practice in which glass microscope slides are digitally scanned by clinic staff. The digitized images are saved to a computer or cloud-based system, where they can further be viewed, analyzed, and shared. Providers can remotely access digitized pathological images and data for review and diagnosis, in some instances using diagnostic and analysis support from artificial intelligence algorithms. Digital pathology can enhance diagnostic efficiency, prognosis, and prediction of illness. These codes are used to report additional staff work and resource needs associated with the process of scanning and digitizing pathology content. These Category III codes may be reported in addition to the appropriate Category I service code when digitization of glass slides is conducted at the same time. Report 0751T for Level II surgical pathology, gross, and microscopic examination, 0752T for Level III, 0753T for Level IV, 0754T Level V, and 0755T for Level VI.

0756T-0759T

Digital pathology is a practice in which glass microscope slides are digitally scanned by clinic staff. The digitized images are saved to a computer or cloud-based system, where they can further be viewed, analyzed, and shared. Providers can remotely access digitized pathological images and data for review and diagnosis, in some instances using diagnostic and analysis support from artificial intelligence algorithms. Digital pathology can enhance diagnostic efficiency, prognosis, and prediction of illness. These codes are used to report additional staff work and resource needs associated with the process of scanning and digitizing pathology content. These Category III codes include the special stain, interpretation, and report, and may be reported in addition to the appropriate Category I service code when digitization of glass microscopic slides is conducted at the same time. Report 0756T for special stains that are used in group 1 for microorganisms, such as gram positive/negative, methenamine silver, and acid fast. Report 0757T for special stains for group II, which includes all other stains such as thioflavin, fast blue, iron, and trichrome (group II exempts stains for enzyme constituents, stains for microorganisms, and stains for immunocytochemistry and immunohistochemistry). Report 0758T for histochemical stain on frozen section. Report 0759T for specialty stains for group III for enzyme constituents, such as esterase and alkaline phosphatase.

0760T-0762T

Digital pathology is a subfield of pathology in which glass microscopic slides are scanned to produce digitized images and data of pathology samples. The images are managed, shared, and examined from a computer or cloud-based system. Pathologists can then remotely access the digitized data for analysis and provide diagnostic feedback, often with the use of artificial intelligence algorithms. These Category III codes may be reported in addition to the appropriate Category I service code when digitization of glass slides is conducted at the same time. Report 0760T-0762T for each glass microscopic slide specimen that is digitized for immunohistochemistry or immunocytochemistry. Report 0760T for an initial single antibody stain procedure. Report 0761T for each additional single antibody stain procedure. Report 0762T for each multiplex antibody stain procedure.

0763T

Digital pathology is a subfield of pathology in which glass microscopic slides are scanned to produce digitized images and data of pathology samples. The images are managed, shared, and examined from a computer or cloud-based system. Pathologists can then remotely access the digitized data for analysis and provide diagnostic feedback, often with the use of artificial intelligence algorithms. Report 0763T for digitization of glass microscope slides for morphometric analysis and/or tumor immunohistochemistry, which assesses a tissue sample for characteristics such as membrane receptor (estrogen, HER-2/neu) expression. Morphometric analysis, also called histomorphometry, supports prediction of prognosis and development of treatment plan for previously diagnosed malignancies. This code is reported for each specimen and each single antibody stain procedure.

[0827T, 0828T]

Digital pathology is a practice in which glass microscope slides are digitally scanned by clinic staff. The digitized images are saved to a computer or cloud-based system, where they can further be viewed, analyzed, and shared. Providers can remotely access digitized pathological images and data for review and diagnosis, in some instances using diagnostic and analysis support from artificial intelligence algorithms. Digital pathology can enhance diagnostic efficiency, prognosis, and prediction of illness. These codes are used to report additional staff work and resource needs associated with the process of scanning and digitizing pathology content. These Category III codes may be reported in addition to the appropriate Category I service code when digitization of glass slides is conducted at the same time. These codes include slides for cytopathology, fluids, washings, or brushings (except cervical or vaginal). Report 0827T for smears with interpretation and 0828T for simple filter method with interpretation.

[0829T]

Digital pathology is a practice in which glass microscope slides are digitally scanned by clinic staff. The digitized images are saved to a computer or cloud-based system, where they can further be viewed, analyzed, and shared. Providers can remotely access digitized pathological images and data for review and diagnosis, in some instances using diagnostic and analysis support from artificial intelligence algorithms. Digital pathology can enhance diagnostic efficiency, prognosis, and prediction of illness. This code is used to report additional staff work and resource needs associated with the process of scanning and digitizing pathology content. This code may be reported in addition to the appropriate Category I service code when digitization of glass slides is conducted at the same time. Report 0829T for slides for cytopathology, concentration technique (e.g., Saccomanno), smears, and interpretation.

[0830T]

Digital pathology is a practice in which glass microscope slides are digitally scanned by clinic staff. The digitized images are saved to a computer or cloud-based system, where they can further be viewed, analyzed, and shared. Providers can remotely access digitized pathological images and data for review and diagnosis, in some instances using diagnostic and analysis support from artificial intelligence algorithms. Digital pathology can enhance diagnostic efficiency, prognosis, and prediction of illness. This code is used to report additional staff work and resource needs associated with the process of scanning and digitizing pathology content. This code may be reported in addition to the appropriate Category I service code when digitization of glass slides is conducted at the same time. Report 0830T for slides for cytopathology (except cervical or vaginal), selective-cellular enhancement technique such as liquid based slide preparation method, with interpretation.

[0831T]

Digital pathology is a practice in which glass microscope slides are digitally scanned by clinic staff. The digitized images are saved to a computer or cloud-based system, where they can further be viewed, analyzed, and shared. Providers can remotely access digitized pathological images and data for review and diagnosis, in some instances using diagnostic and analysis support from artificial intelligence algorithms. Digital pathology can enhance diagnostic efficiency, prognosis, and prediction of illness. This code is used to report additional staff work and resource needs associated with the process of scanning and digitizing pathology content. This code may be reported in addition to the appropriate Category I service code when digitization of glass slides is conducted at the same time. Report 0831T for slides for cytopathology, cervical or vaginal, that require interpretation by a physician.

[0832T, 0833T, 0834T]

Digital pathology is a practice in which glass microscope slides are digitally scanned by clinic staff. The digitized images are saved to a computer or cloud-based system, where they can further be viewed, analyzed, and shared. Providers can remotely access digitized pathological images and data for review and diagnosis, in some instances using diagnostic and analysis support from artificial intelligence algorithms. Digital pathology can enhance diagnostic efficiency, prognosis, and prediction of illness. These codes are used to report additional staff work and resource needs associated with the process of scanning and digitizing pathology content. These Category III codes may be reported in addition to the appropriate Category I service code when digitization of glass slides is conducted at the same time. These codes include slides for cytopathology, smears, from any other source (meaning non-gynecologic and excluding fluids, washings, or brushings). Report 0832T for screening and interpretation only; 0833T for preparation, screening, and interpretation; and 0834T for an extended study that involves more than five slides and/or multiple stains.

[0835T, 0836T, 0837T]

Digital pathology is a practice in which glass microscope slides are digitally scanned by clinic staff. The digitized images are saved to a computer or cloud-based system, where they can further be viewed, analyzed, and shared. Providers can remotely access digitized pathological images and data for review and diagnosis, in some instances using diagnostic and analysis support from artificial intelligence algorithms. Digital pathology can enhance diagnostic efficiency, prognosis, and prediction of illness. These codes are used to report additional staff work and resource needs associated with the process of scanning and digitizing pathology content. These Category III codes may be reported in addition to the appropriate Category I service code when digitization of glass slides is conducted at the same time. These codes include slides for cytopathology, evaluation of fine needle aspirate. Report 0835T for immediate cytohistologic study to determine adequacy for diagnosis, first evaluation episode, each site and 0836T for each separate additional evaluation episode, same site. Report 0837T for interpretation and report.

[0838T, 0839T, 0840T]

Digital pathology is a practice in which glass microscope slides are digitally scanned by clinic staff. The digitized images are saved to a computer or cloud-based system, where they can further be viewed, analyzed, and shared. Providers can remotely access digitized pathological images and data for review and diagnosis, in some instances using diagnostic and analysis support from artificial intelligence algorithms. Digital pathology can enhance diagnostic efficiency, prognosis, and prediction of illness. These codes are used to report additional staff work and resource needs associated with the process of scanning and digitizing pathology content. These Category III codes may be reported in addition to the appropriate Category I service code when digitization of glass slides is conducted at the same time. These codes include digitization of glass microscope slides for a pathology consultation, which involves an opinion or advice on the presence or absence of diseased or abnormal tissue provided at the request of another physician. Report 0838T for digitization of slides for a consultation and written report on a slide prepared by another source; 0839T for digitization of slides for a consultation and written report on material referred from another source requiring routine preparation of slides by the consultant; and 0840T for digitization of slides for a comprehensive consultation with a written report of the consultation that describes the review of records and evaluation of specimens.

[0841T, 0842T, 0843T, 0844T]

Digital pathology is a practice in which glass microscope slides are digitally scanned by clinic staff. The digitized images are saved to a computer or cloud-based system, where they can further be viewed, analyzed, and shared. Providers can remotely access digitized pathological images and data for review and diagnosis, in some instances using diagnostic and analysis support from artificial intelligence algorithms. Digital pathology can enhance diagnostic efficiency, prognosis, and prediction of illness. These codes are used to report additional staff work and resource needs associated with the process of scanning and digitizing pathology content. These Category III codes may be reported in addition to the appropriate Category I service code when digitization of glass slides is conducted at the same time. These codes include digitization of glass microscope slides for a pathology consultation during surgery. Report 0841T for the first tissue block, with frozen section(s), for a single specimen and 0842T for each additional tissue block with frozen section(s). Report 0843T for cytologic examination such as touch or squash preparation for the initial site and 0844T for cytologic examination of each additional site.

[0845T, 0846T]

Digital pathology is a practice in which glass microscope slides are digitally scanned by clinic staff. The digitized images are saved to a computer or cloud-based system, where they can further be viewed, analyzed, and shared. Providers can remotely access digitized pathological images and data for review and diagnosis, in some instances using diagnostic and analysis support from artificial intelligence algorithms. Digital pathology can enhance diagnostic efficiency, prognosis, and prediction of illness. These codes are used to report additional staff work and resource needs associated with the process of scanning and digitizing pathology content. These Category III codes may be reported in addition to the appropriate Category I service code when digitization of glass slides is conducted at the same time. These codes include slides for immunofluorescence. Report 0845T for the initial single antibody stain procedure and 0846T for each additional single antibody stain procedure. These codes are reported per specimen.

[0847T]

Digital pathology is a practice in which glass microscope slides are digitally scanned by clinic staff. The digitized images are saved to a computer or cloud-based system, where they can further be viewed, analyzed, and shared. Providers can remotely access digitized pathological images and data for review and diagnosis, in some instances using diagnostic and analysis support from artificial intelligence algorithms. Digital pathology can enhance diagnostic efficiency, prognosis, and prediction of illness. This code is used to report additional staff work and resource needs associated with the process of scanning and digitizing pathology content. This code may be reported in addition to the appropriate Category I service code when digitization of glass slides is conducted at the same time. This code includes slides for the examination and selection of previously diagnosed tissues for molecular analysis (e.g., KRAS mutation analysis). Molecular assays may be utilized to identify cancer cells, calculate the percentage of tumor nuclei, or as part of a determination of the most appropriate antineoplastic treatment regimen.

[0848T, 0849T, 0850T]

Digital pathology is a practice in which glass microscope slides are digitally scanned by clinic staff. The digitized images are saved to a computer or cloud-based system, where they can further be viewed, analyzed, and shared. Providers can remotely access digitized pathological images and data for review and diagnosis, in some instances using diagnostic and analysis support from artificial intelligence algorithms. Digital pathology can enhance diagnostic efficiency, prognosis, and prediction of illness. These codes are used to report additional staff work and resource needs associated with the process of scanning and digitizing pathology content. These Category III codes may be reported in addition to the appropriate Category I service code when digitization of glass slides is conducted at the same time. These codes include slides for in situ hybridization (e.g., fluorescence in situ hybridization, FISH). Report 0848T for the initial single probe stain procedure; 0849T for each additional single probe stain procedure; and 0850T for each multiplex probe stain procedure. These codes are reported per specimen.

[0851T, 0852T, 0853T]

Digital pathology is a practice in which glass microscope slides are digitally scanned by clinic staff. The digitized images are saved to a computer or cloud-based system, where they can further be viewed, analyzed, and shared. Providers can remotely access digitized pathological images and data for review and diagnosis, in some instances using diagnostic and analysis support from artificial intelligence algorithms. Digital pathology can enhance diagnostic efficiency, prognosis, and prediction of illness. These codes are used to report additional staff work and resource needs associated with the process of scanning and digitizing pathology content. These Category III codes may be reported in addition to the appropriate Category I service code when digitization of glass slides is conducted at the same time. These codes include slides for morphometric analysis, in situ hybridization such as quantitative or semiquantitative, manual. Report 0851T for the initial single probe stain procedure; 0852T for each additional single probe stain procedure; and 0853T for each multiplex probe stain procedure. These codes are reported per specimen.

[0854T]

Digital pathology is a practice in which glass microscope slides are digitally scanned by clinic staff. The digitized images are saved to a computer or cloud-based system, where they can further be viewed, analyzed, and shared. Providers can remotely access digitized pathological images and data for review and diagnosis, in some instances using diagnostic and analysis support from artificial intelligence algorithms. Digital pathology can enhance diagnostic efficiency, prognosis, and prediction of illness. This code is used to report additional staff work and resource needs associated with the process of scanning and digitizing pathology content. This code may be reported in addition to the appropriate Category I service code when digitization of glass slides is conducted at the same time. This code includes slides for blood smear, peripheral, with interpretation by a physician with a written report.

[0855T]

Digital pathology is a practice in which glass microscope slides are digitally scanned by clinic staff. The digitized images are saved to a computer or cloud-based system, where they can further be viewed, analyzed, and shared. Providers can remotely access digitized pathological images and data for review and diagnosis, in some instances using diagnostic and analysis support from artificial intelligence algorithms. Digital pathology can enhance diagnostic efficiency, prognosis, and prediction of illness. This code is used to report additional staff work and resource needs associated with the process of scanning and digitizing pathology content. This code may be reported in addition to the appropriate Category I service code when digitization of glass slides is conducted at the same time. This code includes slides for bone marrow, smear interpretation.

[0856T]

Digital pathology is a practice in which glass microscope slides are digitally scanned by clinic staff. The digitized images are saved to a computer or cloud-based system, where they can further be viewed, analyzed, and shared. Providers can remotely access digitized pathological images and data for review and diagnosis, in some instances using diagnostic and analysis support from artificial intelligence algorithms. Digital pathology can enhance diagnostic efficiency, prognosis, and prediction of illness. This code is used to report additional staff work and resource needs associated with the process of scanning and digitizing pathology content. This code may be reported in addition to the appropriate Category I service code when digitization of glass slides is conducted at the same time. This code includes slides for diagnostic electron microscopy.

0764T-0765T

Artificial intelligence (AI)-built algorithms can be used to develop risk-based assessment for cardiac dysfunction by analyzing concurrently performed (0764T) or previously performed (0765T) electrocardiograms. The proprietary AI-built algorithms use ECG data to detect signs of cardiovascular dysfunction that might otherwise be missed by human providers. The ECG data is evaluated for many cardiac conditions, including left ventricular dysfunction, hypertrophic cardiomyopathy, pulmonary hypertension, and atherosclerosis. The use of assistive algorithmic assessment in ECG data has the potential to detect cardiac dysfunction years before symptoms appear. ECG algorithmic assessment is also used to enhance proactive cardiac disease management, decrease dependence on more costly and invasive diagnostic testing, and improve patient outcomes.

0766T-0767T

Using a proprietary electromagnetic stimulator, the provider delivers pain management treatment utilizing magnetic pulse technology. Indicated for chronic, recurring nerve pain such as that caused by amputation, localized burn, various forms of injury, or postoperative pain following invasive procedures, the system provides brief, focused pulses that noninvasively stimulate targeted peripheral nerves. The system consists of a magnetic stimulator, a stimulation coil, a liquid cool unit, and a cart. The handheld treatment coil is placed on the skin over areas of damaged nerves, and low-frequency waveforms are delivered transcutaneously. Report 0766T for the first nerve treated and 0767T for each additional nerve. These codes include identification and marking of the injured nerve and treatment location, as well as noninvasive nerve conduction localization when performed.

0770T

Virtual reality (VR) technology can be integrated into several patient therapy modalities as an adjunct therapy and is used to enhance the training or teaching of a therapy-focused skill. Report 0770T in addition to the code for the primary therapy or procedure to capture the practice expense for the software used for VR technology. This code may be reported for each session in which the VR technology is utilized but is not reported more than once per session. No additional therapist time is incurred beyond that which has been reported with the base therapy code.

0771T-0774T

The provider employs virtual reality (VR) procedural dissociation, a recent technology that offers a multi-sensory, immersive, and three-dimensional experience in a patient 5 years of age or older. VR is an altered consciousness that supports and optimizes the patient's comfort, allowing the patient to actively immerse and navigate a virtual world; this increases procedural tolerance and decreases the patient's pain during the associated procedure. VR procedural dissociation is typically presented on a head-mounted display (HMD), and the screens are positioned close to the patient's eyes with full or partial occlusion of their physical surroundings or sound utilizing noise-cancelling headphones. Images are often three-dimensional and continuously adjusted. VR procedural dissociation establishes a computer-generated audio, visual, and proprioceptive immersive environment in which patients respond purposefully to verbal commands and stimuli, either alone or accompanied by light tactile stimulation. VR procedural dissociation does not involve interventions to maintain cardiovascular function, patent airway, or spontaneous ventilation. Report 0771T if performed by the same physician or other qualified health care professional performing the diagnostic or therapeutic service for the initial 15 minutes and 0772T for each additional 15 minutes. Report 0773T if provided by a physician or other qualified health care professional other than the one performing the diagnostic or therapeutic service for the initial 15 minutes and 0774T for each additional 15 minutes.

0776T

The provider administers point-of-care treatment for concussions or mild traumatic brain injury (mTBI) using a proprietary, noninvasive mechanical hypothermic therapy device. Intended to decrease the severity of concussion symptoms by reducing blood temperature before it enters the brain, the device is placed over the carotids and head to provide localized cooling for the head and neck. Monitoring of vital signs and the use of a sport concussion assessment tool 5 (SCAT5) are included. This code reports 30 minutes of treatment time.

0777T

The physician utilizes a real-time pressure-sensing epidural guidance system in which the needle tip measures "exit-pressure" data with a continuous fluid path. The needle is inserted, and the computer monitor displays pulsatile wave form within the epidural space, using the proprietary sensory system.

0778T

The provider conducts a full musculoskeletal and orthopedic assessment to evaluate muscle function and health using a sensor fusion system combining an inertial measurement unit (IMU) and surface mechanomyography (sMMG), a wireless-enabled proprietary technology. The provider applies sensors to the skin, which transmit data that may include dynamic range of motion, movement quality, strength, and functional mobility, equipping providers with information to create an individualized and precise plan of care and to monitor muscle integrity concerning musculoskeletal injury, recovery, and prevention. Data collected are uploaded to a secure cloud-based processing platform, where it is immediately processed and an automated report generated. Note that measurements are obtained in the office setting with the patient physically present; this is not a remote service.

0779T

Gastric and intestinal mechanical and electrical activities (stomach through colon) are recorded noninvasively using cutaneous electrodes on the abdominal skin surface as an aid in the diagnosis/evaluation of various gastrointestinal disorders. Following appropriate skin preparation, electrodes are placed. Electrogastrography (EGG) detects slow gastric activity and provides a record of the gastric myoelectrical activity that precedes contractions. Code 0779T includes study interpretation and report.

0780T

Fecal microbiota transplantation (FMT) is a microbiota-based therapy that shows therapeutic potential in restoring the gut microbiome to a healthy state in recurrent or refractory *Clostridium difficile* infections and other intestinal or extra-intestinal disorders (i.e., inflammatory bowel diseases, irritable bowel syndrome). FMT is predominantly performed with a freshly prepared specimen. Prior to FMT instillation and at the physician's discretion, preparation may consist of fasting, antibiotics, or bowel lavage. The physician instills stool from a healthy donor into the lower gastrointestinal tract of the patient via rectal enema.

0781T-0782T

The physician uses flexible or rigid bronchoscopy to delivery circumferential radiofrequency destruction of the pulmonary nerves, a treatment known as targeted lung denervation (TLD), in patients with COPD and chronic bronchitis. TLD ablates parasympathetic pulmonary nerves running between the lungs and main bronchi, thereby enabling bronchodilation to decrease chronic airway inflammation and COPD exacerbation. Under appropriate anesthesia, the physician introduces a bronchoscope through the nasal or oral cavity. A dual-cooled catheter is placed through the bronchoscope along with an electrode for radiofrequency energy delivery. The physician advances the bronchoscope to the lungs and into the main bronchi (0781T for bilateral mainstem bronchi; 0782T for unilateral mainstem bronchus) where the electrode is activated multiple times, delivering radiofrequency energy until complete circumferential treatment is administered. Fluoroscopic guidance is included in these procedures, when performed.

0783T

Transcutaneous auricular neurostimulation (tAN) is a non-invasive method of delivering nerve stimulation through the ear for the purpose of treating a variety of conditions, including opioid withdrawal symptoms, epilepsy, refractory depression, chronic obesity, and chronic pain. The tAN system has two parts: an earpiece with electrodes that is applied on, around, or just inside the ear and an external pulse generator that delivers neurostimulation. The provider places the earpiece on or around the patient's ear and connects the earpiece to the external pulse generator with a cable. The system delivers mild electrical signals to stimulate cranial nerves (often the vagus and/or trigeminal) to treat the patient's identified condition. The code includes system set-up; setting of parameters to include frequency, session duration, and interval timing; and patient education on system operation.

0784T-0785T

In 0784T, the physician inserts or replaces an electrode array with an integrated neurostimulator percutaneously (through the skin) into the spinal tissue to be stimulated. Under local anesthesia, a small incision is made, and the electrode array is tunneled to the area of the affected nerve using fluoroscopy. Using the same incision site, a subcutaneous pocket is created. After stimulation testing is performed to confirm proper positioning, the rest of the neurostimulator device is introduced into the pocket and anchored in place. The incision is closed in layers. This code includes imaging guidance, when performed. Report 0785T for revision or removal of the electrode array with integrated neurostimulator.

0786T-0787T

In 0786T, the physician inserts or replaces an electrode array with an integrated neurostimulator percutaneously (through the skin) into the sacral tissue to be stimulated. Under local anesthesia, an insulated needle is directed into the foramen. An external power source is connected to the needle using a separate cable. A grounding pad is adhered to the patient, typically to the bottom of the foot. The test stimulation cable is used to determine proper positioning of the needle. An electrode is inserted through the needle, leaving only the integrated neurostimulator and electrode. After confirmatory response testing is performed, a dressing is placed to secure the electrode. This code includes imaging guidance, when performed. Report 0787T for revision or removal of the electrode array with integrated neurostimulator.

0788T-0789T

A physician or qualified health care professional performs an electronic analysis of a previously placed implanted integrated neurostimulation system to verify that it is functioning properly. In 0788T, simple programming of the device is performed. Simple programming includes the adjustment of up to three parameters from the following: contact groups, amplitude, pulse width, frequency [Hz], on/off cycling, burst, dose lockout, patient selectable parameters, responsive neurostimulation, detection algorithms, closed loop parameters, and passive parameters. Report 0789T for complex programming, which includes the adjustment of more than three of these parameters.

0791T

The qualified health care provider trains the patient in specific activities to facilitate ambulation and stair climbing with or without an assistive device using a semi-immersive, or partial, virtual environment. Equipment may include, but is not limited to, treadmill, TV or screen and headphones to create a semi-immersive environment, and safety harness(es). Proper gait sequencing and safety instructions are included when appropriate. This add-on code requires direct contact by a qualified health care provider with the patient and is reported in 15-minute units in addition to the Category I service code for gait training.

0792T

Silver diamine fluoride (SDF) 38% is a topical medication used to relieve dentinal hypersensitivity and treat and prevent dental caries. The provider places the patient in a recumbent position, with the patient's mouth open. Using an application brush, SDF is applied directly to the cavity and affected tooth surface. SDF reacts with the cavity to permanently stain the area nearly black within seconds or over the course of 24 hours. Application time is at least one minute, without use of any compressed air, light-cure, or rinse. Excess SDF is removed with cotton or gauze.

0793T

The physician performs transcatheter pulmonary artery (PA) thermal ablation of selective nerves that innervate the pulmonary arteries to reduce PA pressure in patients with pulmonary arterial hypertension (PAH). Right heart catheterization is conducted under fluoroscopic guidance to measure pulmonary artery hemodynamics. The physician advances a guide catheter through the sheath over a guidewire to the pulmonary artery, followed by a therapeutic radiofrequency catheter. Position is verified using fluoroscopy. Therapeutic radiofrequency energy is applied transmurally to nerve fibers in the main pulmonary artery trunk and its bifurcation, using thermal heat to cause denervation. The guide catheter and radiofrequency catheter may be repositioned to further deliver thermal denervation in the left and right pulmonary arteries. This code includes the right heart catheterization, angiography of the pulmonary artery, and all imaging guidance.

0794T

The physician uses a precision medicine and proprietary artificial intelligence (AI) platform that is built with a curated knowledgebase for the purpose of individually tailoring a patient's cancer treatment. The patient's medical cancer history, including immunohistochemical and pathology results, will have been previously and separately gathered, interpreted, and reported. Algorithmic software will analyze results, rank available drug combinations and monotherapies, and assist the provider in customizing a combination of cancer treatments based upon the patient's unique molecular profile. This code includes time spent submitting the patient's laboratory, molecular, or pathology data by clinical staff, qualified health care professionals, and physicians. Data submission includes original results and interpretations without alteration and should not include genomic sequencing raw data files. Treatment ranking options include potential active clinical trials and FDA-approved drugs, including both on-label and off-label uses for targeted therapies.

0795T-0797T

The physician performs transcatheter insertion of a permanent dual-chamber leadless pacemaker. This system has two pacemakers: one implanted in the right atrium and the other in the right ventricle. Each has its own built-in battery and electrode. The femoral vein is entered using ultrasound guidance, followed by femoral venography for anatomy identification. A guidewire is advanced to the heart via the femoral vein, followed by dilation and upsizing of a femoral sheath. A leadless pacemaker introducer is inserted into the femoral vein, then the guidewire is removed. A delivery catheter is used to feed the leadless pacemaker system through the femoral vein to the inferior vena cava into the right atrium and through the tricuspid valve into the right ventricle via the introducer. Each pacemaker is anchored into the endocardium of its respective chamber with tines or a screw-in helix; a gentle tug conducted under fluoroscopy ensures pacemaker fixation to the chamber wall. The two pacemakers are positioned in accordance with the manufacturer for direct communication prior to release from the catheter. After validation of placement and stabilization of hemodynamics, the physician removes the delivery system and sheath, and sutures the access site closed. The pacemaker's software platform is used for data analysis and programming based on the patient's needs. These codes include imaging guidance and device evaluation, when performed. Report 0795T for insertion of a permanent dual-chamber leadless pacemaker complete system; 0796T for insertion of a right atrial pacemaker component when an existing right ventricular single leadless pacemaker exists to create a dual-chamber leadless pacemaker system; and 0797T for insertion of a right ventricular pacemaker component when it is part of a dual-chamber leadless pacemaker system.

0798T-0800T

The physician performs transcatheter removal of a permanent dual-chamber leadless pacemaker. For one proprietary system, the pacemaker device contains a docking button that facilitates retrieval. Other leadless pacemakers have tines, made specifically for placement positioning and removal. The femoral vein is entered using ultrasound guidance, followed by femoral venography for anatomy identification. A guidewire is advanced to the heart via the femoral vein, followed by dilation and upsizing of a femoral sheath. A pacemaker retrieval introducer is inserted into the femoral vein and the guidewire is removed. The physician inserts a retrieval catheter system that has a single-loop or multiple-loop snare. With continued imaging guidance, the retrieval catheter is advanced to the right atrium and/or right ventricle where the snare is looped around the pacemaker's tines or docking button. Once the pacemaker is securely snared, both the pacemaker and retrieval catheter system are pulled to the edge of a delivery cup, and then further pulled into the retrieval sheath. Both the pacemaker and retrieval system are extracted from the patient's body. The physician removes the delivery system and sheath and sutures the access site closed. Leadless pacemakers may also be removed in a similar snare fashion, but with a steerable sheath, also under fluoroscopic guidance. These codes include imaging guidance and device evaluation, when performed. Report 0798T for removal of a permanent dual-chamber leadless pacemaker complete system; 0799T for removal of a right atrial pacemaker component; and 0800T for removal of a right ventricular pacemaker component when it is part of a dual-chamber leadless pacemaker system.

0801T-0803T

The physician performs transcatheter removal and replacement of one or both components of a permanent dual-chamber leadless pacemaker. The physician removes the old pacemaker by a transcatheter approach through the femoral vein. Imaging guidance is used for insertion of a guidewire, followed by a retrieval catheter system or steerable sheath. The old pacemaker is snared by its tines or docking button and retrieved from the patient's body. A leadless pacemaker introducer is inserted into the femoral vein. A delivery catheter is used to feed the new leadless pacemaker system through the femoral vein to the inferior vena cava into the right atrium and through the tricuspid valve into the right ventricle via the introducer. The pacemaker is positioned in accordance with the manufacturer for direct communication prior to release from the catheter and anchored into the endocardium of its respective chamber. The physician removes the delivery system and sheath and sutures the access site closed. These codes include imaging guidance and device evaluation, when performed. Report 0801T for transcatheter removal and replacement of a permanent dual-chamber leadless pacemaker for an entire system including right atrial and right ventricular pacemaker components; 0802T for transcatheter removal and replacement of a right atrial pacemaker component; and 0803T for transcatheter removal and replacement of a right ventricular pacemaker component when it is part of a dual-chamber leadless pacemaker system.

0804T

A programming device evaluation is performed in person to assess the dual-chamber leadless pacemaker's function and select the most favorable permanent programmed values. The device system data is interrogated to evaluate the battery and hardware, as well as the stored patient and system measurements. If necessary, the device is programmed to settings appropriate for a test or procedure. Postprocedure evaluation and programming may also be performed, with adjustments as required. This code includes physician or other qualified health care professional analysis, review, and report.

0805T-0806T

Caval valve implantation (CAVI) is a type of transcatheter therapy composed of two self-expanding valves that are inserted and advanced percutaneously, then deployed into the inferior and superior vena cava to assist or replace the function of the tricuspid valve in patients with severe tricuspid regurgitation (TR) and heart failure. One proprietary system consists of two bioprosthetic self-expanding nitinol structures with bovine pericardium leaflets, one for the superior vena cava (SVC) and one for the inferior vena cava (IVC), both of which are pre-mounted on a valve delivery system. Sizing selection is based on premeasurements via CT scanning. For this system, three access sites are required: one through the right common femoral vein for system delivery and two through the left common femoral vein for a Swan-Ganz catheter at the right pulmonary artery and a pigtail that assists with control injections and SVC angiography. The physician places a guidewire via percutaneous femoral vein approach with fluoroscopic guidance and advances it to the SVC. A sheath is advanced to the site, after which the guidewire is removed. Fluoroscopy, transesophageal echocardiography, and ventriculography may be used to advance the valve delivery catheter to the vena cava and confirm positioning for deployment. The device's three hooks are released to ensure attachment. The delivery system is re-sheathed and removed from the patient. For deployment of the IVC portion, venography of the hepatic veins may be conducted for deployment reference. The IVC prosthesis is deployed and stabilized, and device hooks are released for further implantation and stabilization. The delivery system is re-sheathed and removed from the patient. Report 0805T if a percutaneous femoral vein approach is used; 0806T for an open femoral approach. These codes include vascular access, placement of access sheath, transseptal puncture, advancement of CAVI delivery system, and positioning and deployment of the device, when performed. Radiological supervision and interpretation and angiography performed for CAVI guidance are not reported separately.

0807T-0808T

The provider uses software to analyze data that measures the patient's pulmonary tissue ventilation from separately obtained cinefluoroscopic images. The software uses algorithms and mathematical models to translate images to quantitative data, which can then be used for diagnosis and treatment planning. Software analysis of the cinefluoroscopic images is done in combination with information that has been obtained from computed tomography (CT) images. Software-analyzed data is used to show pulmonary function changes and regional ventilation, identifying areas of high and low ventilation to help determine overall lung health. Report 0807T when pulmonary tissue ventilation analysis is performed using CT images that were previously acquired. Report 0808T when the CT images are obtained as part of the ventilation analysis. These codes include data preparation and transmission, pulmonary tissue ventilation quantification, review of data, and interpretation and report.

0810T

Subretinal injection allows for delivery of a pharmacological agent, such as a medication for diabetic retinopathy or age-related macular degeneration, into the space between the retinal pigment epithelium (RPE) and photoreceptors. The space is optimal for drug delivery, as the drug comes into direct contact with the plasma membrane of photoreceptors, RPE cells, and subretinal blebs. Preparation may include vitrectomy and pre-bleb creation with retinal elevation at the target site. For manual injection, the delivery needle is attached to high-pressure microdose tubing, which is further primed until the pharmacologic agent drips from the tip of the injection needle without presence of air bubbles. There are three approaches for subretinal injection: transcorneal through the pupil, transscleral through the pars plana or limbus area, and transscleral through the choroid and Bruch's membrane. Using imaging for placement confirmation, the needle is inserted into the vitreous cavity, and the agent is slowly injected under the retina to the point of retinal elevation and detachment of the foveal target zone. The surgical field is inspected for tears or bleeds. This code includes removal of the vitreous and one or more incisions into the retina.

0811T-0812T

In complex uroflowmetry, the physician assesses the rate of emptying of the bladder by electronic equipment. The patient receives a device to be used at home for remote monitoring. The device is placed on the toilet and automatically monitors bladder activity and calculates the frequency, flow, and volume of urine for up to 10 days. The uroflowmetry device is connected to a mobile app; a report is generated for review by the ordering provider at a follow-up visit. Report 0811T for set-up and patient education on use of the equipment and 0812T for supply of the device with automated report generation, up to 10 days.

0813T

In a minimally invasive endoscopic surgery, the physician adjusts the volume in an intragastric bariatric balloon. The endoscope is advanced into the esophagus, stomach, and duodenum with notation of any abnormalities. The previously placed bariatric balloon is identified and the device valve is used to gain access to the inside of the balloon. An adjustment is made with an increase or decrease in volume, as necessary. At the conclusion of the procedure, the endoscope is withdrawn. Light sedation, local, or general anesthesia may be utilized.

0814T

The physician injects calcium-based biodegradable osteoconductive material into the proximal femur to provide stability to a weakened osteoporotic bone to prevent a hip fracture. Under appropriate anesthesia, a small incision is made to gain access to the weakened bone. A guide pin is placed through the center of the femoral neck to guide a canulated drill to the proximal femur. The enhancement site (the area of bone loss) is identified and debrided or irrigated as necessary to create a void. Under fluoroscopic guidance, the calcium-based material is injected to fill the site and is allowed to harden. The cannula is removed, and the incision site is irrigated and closed. This code reports a unilateral procedure and includes all imaging guidance performed.

0815T

Radiofrequency echographic multi-spectrometry (REMS) is an enhanced form of ultrasound technology that is performed to measure bone mineral density (BMD). BMD is evaluated as a screening test for osteoporosis, to evaluate diseases of bone, and to review the responses of bone disease to treatment. Densities can be measured at one or more sites at the hips, pelvis, or spine. REMS uses radiofrequency ultrasound signals instead of ionizing radiation. An ultrasound probe is placed over the targeted bone structure and the transducer depth and focus are adjusted as needed. The physician interprets a report generated by the REMS system that includes comparisons against standard values for bone density and fracture risk.

0816T-0819T

The physician places an integrated neurostimulation system via open approach for bladder dysfunction. The system includes either an electrode array or leadless electrode and a pulse generator or receiver. In 0816T, a small incision is made, and the electrode array is tunneled to the area of the posterior tibial nerve using fluoroscopy. Using the same incision site, a subcutaneous pocket is created. After stimulation testing is performed to confirm proper positioning, the rest of the neurostimulator device is introduced into the pocket and anchored in place. The incision is closed in layers. In 0817T, the incision is made to the level of the subfascial plane over the posterior tibial neurovascular bundle. The neurostimulator device is secured over the bundle after stimulation testing confirms the proper location. The incision is closed in layers. Report 0818T for subcutaneous revision or removal; 0819T for subfascial revision or removal. These codes include analysis, programming, and imaging guidance when performed.

0820T-0822T

A physician or other qualified health care professional (QHP) provides continuous in-person monitoring during psychedelic medication therapy to treat conditions such as treatment resistant depression or post-traumatic stress disorder (PTSD). Examples of psychedelic medications include psilocybin and methylenedioxy-methylamphetamine (MDMA). During a psychedelic therapy session, the patient ingests a dose via capsule. Sessions can last six to eight hours, during which the patient may listen to music or wear an eye mask. Psychological support is available by trained professionals while the patient is experiencing the effects of the drug. Additional involvement such as psychotherapy or crisis intervention by the provider may be necessary. Report 0820T for each hour of in-person time spent with the patient by the physician or QHP providing continuous monitoring; add-on code 0821T for each hour of in-person time spent with the patient by a second physician or QHP, concurrent to the first provider; and add-on code 0822T for each hour of in-person time with the patient by clinical staff, concurrent to the first provider.

0823T-0825T

The physician performs transcatheter insertion, removal, or replacement of a right atrial permanent single-chamber leadless pacemaker. This system includes a pulse generator, electrode, and built-in battery. After accessing the femoral vein, a guidewire is advanced to the heart, followed by dilation and upsizing of a femoral sheath. A leadless pacemaker introducer is inserted into the femoral vein, then the guidewire is removed. A delivery catheter is used to feed the leadless pacemaker system through the femoral vein to the inferior vena cava into the right atrium via the introducer. The pacemaker is anchored into the endocardium of the chamber with tines or a screw-in helix; a gentle tug conducted under fluoroscopy ensures pacemaker fixation to the chamber wall. The pacemaker is positioned in accordance with the manufacturer for direct communication prior to release from the catheter. After validation of placement and stabilization of hemodynamics, the physician removes the delivery system and sheath, and sutures the access site closed. The pacemaker's software platform is used for data analysis and programming based on the patient's needs. These codes include imaging guidance and device evaluation, when performed. Report 0823T for insertion of the pacemaker, 0824T for removal, and 0825T for removal and replacement.

0826T

A programming device evaluation is performed in person for a single-chamber leadless pacemaker to test the device's function and select the most favorable permanent programmed values. Patients with previously implanted pacemakers require periodic programming device evaluations. This diagnostic procedure includes a face-to-face assessment of all device functions. Components that must be evaluated to assign this code include the battery, leads, capture and sensing function, heart rhythm, and programmed parameters. Stored and measured data regarding these components are retrieved using an office, hospital, or emergency room instrument. This information is assessed to discern battery voltage, lead impedance, and settings for rhythm treatment and tachycardia detection, as well as to determine the pacemaker's current programming. If necessary, the sensing value and rate response, upper and lower heart rates, AV intervals, pacing voltage and pulse duration, and diagnostics are adjusted. This code includes physician or other qualified health care professional review, interpretation, and report.

0857T

Opto-acoustic imaging of the breast combines acoustics (sound) and laser optics (light). Pulsed laser light is directed at a breast mass with the use of a transducer, which creates a soundwave that is transmitted as an ultrasound signal. This type of imaging is performed after a separately reportable diagnostic breast ultrasound identifies a solid mass. The purpose of the opto-acoustic imaging is to evaluate the blood concentration and oxygen content within the mass. Malignant tumors tend to be more vascular and have a lower oxygen content. A report is generated that shows the color changes related to blood volume and oxygen, providing a visual color map to assist in the diagnosis of a benign or malignant breast tumor. This code applies to a unilateral study, and imaging of the axilla is included, when performed.

0858T

Transcranial magnetic stimulation (TMS) is a noninvasive study of the brain for evaluation of cortical function. A cap is placed on the patient's head to allow for placement of a stimulating coil. An electric current produces a magnetic field around the coil and into the cortical tissue to stimulate neurons. A resting motor threshold is established with stimulation of increasing intensity over the motor cortex on each side of the brain until a muscle twitch is observed on the opposite side of the body. Evaluation stimulation and recording is performed in two or more cortical areas such as the left or right primary motor cortex or dorsolateral prefrontal cortex. The device software generates an automated report, including quantification of cortical excitability, plasticity, and connectivity with comparison to validated thresholds to evaluate for any structural or functional brain deficits.

0864T

Low-intensity extracorporeal shock wave therapy (Li-ESWT) of the corpus cavernosum can be used for the treatment of erectile dysfunction. The corpora cavernosa are the spongy bodies of the penis, the dual columns of erectile tissue that form the back and sides of the penis. The physician uses a low intensity, unfocused applicator to deliver shock waves to the perineum and shaft and crus of the penis. Moderate pressure may be applied to enhance shock wave penetration toward the prostate. Multiple treatment sessions are often necessary.

0865T-0866T

Artificial intelligence software is used to provide a quantitative analysis of magnetic resonance imaging (MRI) of the brain. Using encryption, a previously interpreted MRI study is prepared and uploaded for analysis. A report is generated that includes information such as detection of lesions, characterization, and quantification. Brain volume quantification for the whole brain or lateral ventricles and/or a severity score may be included. A graph is included to compare the patient to a normative population based on age and gender. The physician or other qualified health care professional interprets the results and prepares a written report. Report 0865T when there is no diagnostic MRI examination of the brain during the same session. Report 0866T in addition to the appropriate MRI code when a diagnostic MRI examination of the brain is performed in conjunction with quantitative analysis.

0868T

High-resolution gastric electrophysiology mapping with simultaneous patient symptom profiling is performed with an electrogastrography (EGG) device intended for use as a noninvasive diagnostic aid, measuring the myoelectrical activity of the stomach at the surface of the abdomen in patients with chronic gastric symptoms. After the patient fasts for at least six hours, an adhesive, single-use electrode array is placed on the abdomen to record gastric activity. A baseline recording is obtained. After the patient consumes a standardized meal in 10 minutes or less, data is obtained continuously for four hours. The patient records symptoms every 15 minutes using a smartphone application. The electrode array is removed, and the data is uploaded into a proprietary computer system. This code includes interpretation of the data with report by the physician or other qualified health care professional.

0869T

The physician places a bone-substitute material in an area that requires hardware fixation augmentation in bone and/or soft tissue. During a repair procedure, often for rotator cuff repair, bone-substitute material is required to reinforce the area where hardware is being anchored. A spinal needle is used percutaneously to identify the appropriate position of the bone substitute delivery system. An outer cannula is drilled into place. The material components are mixed, introduced with the use of an inner cannula, and advanced to the area where augmentation is needed prior to anchor placement. The delivery system is removed. The repair procedure (reported separately) is continued. Imaging guidance is included in this code when performed.

0870T

The physician implants a subcutaneous peritoneal ascites pump system using a percutaneous approach. The pump continuously removes excess fluid in the abdomen related to liver or malignant ascites by moving the fluid through the bladder according to a programmed schedule. A subcutaneous pocket is created with an incision through the skin of the abdomen a few centimeters below the costal margin, and the pump is placed into the pocket. An indwelling catheter is tunneled under the skin to the bladder, and the cuff is fixed to the subcutaneous tissue or fascia with nonresorbable sutures. Another catheter is tunneled to the peritoneal cavity with the cuff inside the rectus muscle. Both catheters are connected to the pump. The incision is repaired with layered closure. This code includes the initial programming of the pump and all imaging, when performed.

0871T-0872T

The physician replaces a subcutaneous peritoneal ascites pump or indwelling bladder and peritoneal catheters. An incision is made to open the previously created subcutaneous pocket in the abdomen. In 0871T, the pump is disconnected from the indwelling bladder and peritoneal catheters and removed. A new pump is placed in the pocket, and the existing catheters are reconnected. The incision is repaired with layered closure. This code includes the initial programming of the pump. In 0872T, only the bladder and peritoneal catheters are replaced. The existing catheters are disconnected from a previously implanted pump, and the cuff of each catheter is unattached from surrounding tissue. A new indwelling catheter is tunneled under the skin to the bladder, and the cuff is fixed to the subcutaneous tissue or fascia with nonresorbable sutures. Another catheter is tunneled to the peritoneal cavity with the cuff inside the rectus muscle. Both catheters are connected to the previously implanted pump. The incision is repaired with layered closure. These codes include all imaging, when performed.

0873T

The physician revises a component of a previously placed peritoneal ascites pump system. This may include the pump and/or the indwelling peritoneal or bladder catheter. For example, catheter migration can occur, which would require the physician to return the catheter to the correct location to avoid leakage. An incision is made to open the previously created subcutaneous pocket in the abdomen. The necessary revision is performed to any component of the pump system. The incision is repaired with layered closure. This code includes the initial programming of the pump and all imaging, when performed.

0874T

The physician removes a peritoneal ascites pump system. An incision is made to open the previously created subcutaneous pocket in the abdomen. The pump is disconnected from the indwelling bladder and peritoneal catheters, and the cuff of each catheter is unattached from surrounding tissue. Each component is removed. The incision is repaired with layered closure.

0875T

The physician or other qualified health care professional performs programming of a subcutaneously implanted peritoneal pump system. The pump continuously removes excess fluid in the abdomen related to liver or malignant ascites by moving the fluid through the bladder. The device is programmed to indicate a certain volume of ascites that should be removed each day using indwelling peritoneal and bladder catheters.

0876T

The technician performs a limited, computer-aided Duplex ultrasound scan, producing real-time images integrating B-mode two-dimensional structure with Doppler mapping or imaging of motion with time, of a hemodialysis fistula. Using a proprietary, automated ultrasound device, data is collected to assess the volume flow rate, diameter, and depth of the body of the fistula to determine if the fistula has matured.

0877T-0880T

A proprietary artificial intelligence technology is used to identify a diagnostic subtype classification of interstitial lung disease, a group of disorders that result in scarring (fibrosis) of the lungs. The data can be used by the physician to identify the appropriate treatment for the individual patient and avoid unnecessary procedures such as a lung biopsy. The patient undergoes a computed tomography (CT) scan of the chest. Data from this test is securely uploaded from the hospital's system to a cloud server. A digital biomarker lab analyzes the data and detects subtle patterns in the images to provide a qualitative classification. This technology is considered augmentative, which means the machine analyzes and/or quantifies the data to produce clinically meaningful output, and a physician or other qualified health care professional provides ar interpretation and report. Report 0877T when analys is obtained without a concurrent CT examination of the data with report by the physician or other qualified health care professional.

0869T

The physician places a bone-substitute material in an area that requires hardware fixation augmentation in bone and/or soft tissue. During a repair procedure, often for rotator cuff repair, bone-substitute material is required to reinforce the area where hardware is being anchored. A spinal needle is used percutaneously to identify the appropriate position of the bone substitute delivery system. An outer cannula is drilled into place. The material components are mixed, introduced with the use of an inner cannula, and advanced to the area where augmentation is needed prior to anchor placement. The delivery system is removed. The repair procedure (reported separately) is continued. Imaging guidance is included in this code when performed.

0870T

The physician implants a subcutaneous peritoneal ascites pump system using a percutaneous approach. The pump continuously removes excess fluid in the abdomen related to liver or malignant ascites by moving the fluid through the bladder according to a programmed schedule. A subcutaneous pocket is created with an incision through the skin of the abdomen a few centimeters below the costal margin, and the pump is placed into the pocket. An indwelling catheter is tunneled under the skin to the bladder, and the cuff is fixed to the subcutaneous tissue or fascia with nonresorbable sutures. Another catheter is tunneled to the peritoneal cavity with the cuff inside the rectus muscle. Both catheters are connected to the pump. The incision is repaired with layered closure. This code includes the initial programming of the pump and all imaging, when performed.

0871T-0872T

The physician replaces a subcutaneous peritoneal ascites pump or indwelling bladder and peritoneal catheters. An incision is made to open the previously created subcutaneous pocket in the abdomen. In 0871T, the pump is disconnected from the indwelling bladder and peritoneal catheters and removed. A new pump is placed in the pocket, and the existing catheters are reconnected. The incision is repaired with layered closure. This code includes the initial programming of the pump. In 0872T, only the bladder and peritoneal catheters are replaced. The existing catheters are disconnected from a previously implanted pump, and the cuff of each catheter is unattached from surrounding tissue. A new indwelling catheter is tunneled under the skin to the bladder, and the cuff is fixed to the subcutaneous tissue or fascia with nonresorbable sutures. Another catheter is tunneled to the peritoneal cavity with the cuff inside the rectus muscle. Both catheters are connected to the previously implanted pump. The incision is repaired with layered closure. These codes include all imaging, when performed.

0873T

The physician revises a component of a previously placed peritoneal ascites pump system. This may include the pump and/or the indwelling peritoneal or bladder catheter. For example, catheter migration can occur, which would require the physician to return the catheter to the correct location to avoid leakage. An incision is made to open the previously created subcutaneous pocket in the abdomen. The necessary revision is performed to any component of the pump system. The incision is repaired with layered closure. This code includes the initial programming of the pump and all imaging, when performed.

0874T

The physician removes a peritoneal ascites pump system. An incision is made to open the previously created subcutaneous pocket in the abdomen. The pump is disconnected from the indwelling bladder and peritoneal catheters, and the cuff of each catheter is unattached from surrounding tissue. Each component is removed. The incision is repaired with layered closure.

0875T

The physician or other qualified health care professional performs programming of a subcutaneously implanted peritoneal pump system. The pump continuously removes excess fluid in the abdomen related to liver or malignant ascites by moving the fluid through the bladder. The device is programmed to indicate a certain volume of ascites that should be removed each day using indwelling peritoneal and bladder catheters.

0876T

The technician performs a limited, computer-aided Duplex ultrasound scan, producing real-time images integrating B-mode two-dimensional structure with Doppler mapping or imaging of motion with time, of a hemodialysis fistula. Using a proprietary, automated ultrasound device, data is collected to assess the volume flow rate, diameter, and depth of the body of the fistula to determine if the fistula has matured.

0877T-0880T

A proprietary artificial intelligence technology is used to identify a diagnostic subtype classification of interstitial lung disease, a group of disorders that result in scarring (fibrosis) of the lungs. The data can be used by the physician to identify the appropriate treatment for the individual patient and avoid unnecessary procedures such as a lung biopsy. The patient undergoes a computed tomography (CT) scan of the chest. Data from this test is securely uploaded from the hospital's system to a cloud server. A digital biomarker lab analyzes the data and detects subtle patterns in the images to provide a qualitative classification. This technology is considered augmentative, which means the machine analyzes and/or quantifies the data to produce clinically meaningful output, and a physician or other qualified health care professional provides an interpretation and report. Report 0877T when analysis is obtained without a concurrent CT examination of any structure that was included in the previously acquired diagnostic imaging; 0878T when there is a concurrent CT examination of the same structure; 0879T for the preparation and transmission of the radiological data; and 0880T for interpretation and report by the physician or other qualified health care professional.

0881T

The physician or licensed clinical staff inserts a device into the patient's mouth to provide temperature cooling to the oral cavity during chemotherapy administration to prevent oral mucositis. The device includes a cooling system with an inner chamber that holds water and an outer chamber that holds a proprietary saline solution. The device is kept in a freezer prior to placement in the oral cavity, acting as an ice pack for the inside of the mouth. The patient is monitored throughout the duration of the encounter to assess tolerance to the cryotherapy. At the end of the treatment, the oral device is removed.

0882T-0883T

The physician promotes peripheral nerve regeneration in an upper extremity using electrical stimulation in addition to a surgical intervention for a nerve injury. Nerve regeneration accelerates axon regrowth and functional recovery of the nerve. A handheld device with an intraoperative lead is used to deliver a controlled burst of electrical stimulation to the nerve near the site of the primary procedure for a minimum of 10 minutes. Report 0882T for the initial nerve and 0883T for each additional nerve in addition to the Category I service code for the primary procedure. These codes include lead placement and removal.

0884T-0886T

The physician treats an esophageal or colonic stricture via an endoscope using a drug coated balloon catheter. After advancing the scope, a guidewire is passed through the stricture. A non-drug coated balloon is passed over the guidewire. After entering the obstructed region, the balloon is briefly inflated several times until the diameter of the stricture is acceptable. After removing the non-drug coated balloon catheter, a paclitaxel-coated balloon catheter is inserted into the predilated channel. The balloon is placed in the proper position, extending slightly beyond the stricture, and left in place approximately one minute for hydration of the drug coating. The balloon is inflated to the appropriate diameter using saline and contrast and held in position for 10 minutes to allow the drug to infiltrate the scar tissue. Fluoroscopy may be used to confirm the position of the balloon and is not reported separately. Once the drug delivery is complete and the balloon is deflated, the balloon and endoscope are removed. Report 0884T when the procedure is performed to treat an esophageal stricture via flexible transoral esophagoscopy; 0885T for treatment of a colonic stricture via flexible colonoscopy; and 0886T for treatment of a colonic stricture via flexible sigmoidoscopy.

0887T

End-tidal (Et) control is an anesthesia semi-closed loop delivery system that automates tasks during administration of an inhaled anesthetic. After a controlled airway is initiated, the anesthesiologist or other qualified anesthesia provider uses Et software to set the end-tidal targets for oxygen (EtO2) and anesthetic agent (EtAA) concentrations. The Et system automatically adjusts to maintain the set targets, eliminating the need for manual control by using breath-by-breath measurements from a respiratory gas module to adjust the gas composition and total flow as necessary. The anesthesia provider uses an interface to adjust expired gas targets and gas flow during the surgical procedure. This code is reported in addition to the primary anesthesia procedure.

0888T

The physician performs a nonthermal, noninvasive ablation of kidney tissue to destroy a primary solid renal tumor. The procedure, known as histotripsy, uses automated external beam therapy that delivers acoustic energy to destroy the tissue. One proprietary platform uses pulsed sound waves to generate "microbubbles" from gases that are naturally present in the targeted kidney tissue. The physician plans the treatment by reviewing current MRI and CT data sets to determine the targeted tissue. Using the integrated ultrasound imaging, the physician centers the histotripsy treatment contours onto the target and creates an appropriate treatment volume. The physician then enables the platform to deliver the correct dose of energy to create a "bubble cloud" at distinct points inside the target and creates a personalized treatment plan for each target by setting the energy levels and calculating the time it will take to complete each treatment. In the treatment phase, histotripsy is delivered by the platform to the previously targeted tissue. Using short ultrasound bursts that last for microseconds, acoustic cavitation is generated from the force of the microbubbles and tissue is liquified and destroyed on a subcellular level. Ultrasound imaging is used to guide and monitor the histotripsy procedure in real-time.

0889T

Accelerated intelligent neuromodulation therapy provides individualized, MRI guided, intermittent theta-burst stimulation (iTBS) for treatment resistant depression. To obtain a personalized target for the patient, the technician extracts data from previously acquired brain MRI scans, both structural and functional. Proprietary software is used to analyze the images and identify the ideal treatment target within the dorsolateral prefrontal cortex. The target area will be the location where the magnetic stimulator is placed during treatment. An analyst reviews the navigation landmarks, treatment target, and the motor threshold starting location. A detailed targeting report is created along with neuronavigation files. A physician reviews and interprets the report, and the patient is scheduled for treatment.

0890T-0891T

Accelerated intelligent neuromodulation therapy provides individualized, MRI guided, intermittent theta-burst stimulation (iTBS) for treatment resistant depression. To begin treatment, a fiducial marker is placed over the targeted area of the brain using a previously obtained neuronavigation file, targeting report, and motor threshold starting point. A stimulating coil is placed over the target. The neurostimulator produces theta-burst stimulation in an accelerated pulse pattern for 10 minutes, followed by a 50-minute break. Stimulation is repeated, typically for a total of 10 sessions with breaks in between. Report 0890T for the first day of treatment; 0891T for each subsequent treatment day.

0892T

Accelerated intelligent neuromodulation therapy provides individualized, MRI guided, intermittent theta-burst stimulation (iTBS) for treatment resistant depression. To begin treatment, a fiducial marker is placed over the targeted area of the brain using a previously obtained neuronavigation file and targeting report. The physician identifies the motor threshold of the stimulating coil by finding the lowest stimulation intensity that results in movement of the muscles in the hand. The stimulating coil is placed over the previously obtained personalized target. Proprietary software calculates the intensity of the treatment based on the identified motor threshold and the location of the coil. The neurostimulator produces theta-burst stimulation in an accelerated pulse pattern for 10 minutes, followed by a 50-minute break. Stimulation is repeated, typically for a total of 10 sessions with breaks in between. This code is reported once per treatment day.

0893T

A gas exchange monitor analyzes exhaled gas samples to determine a patient's cardiorespiratory status. A sensor, or pulse oximeter, is placed on the finger to measure oxygen levels in the blood. A clip is placed on the patient's nose, and the patient is instructed to breathe through a mouthpiece that collects samples of the patient's breath to measure O2 and CO2 gas levels from the lungs. A physician or other qualified health care professional interprets the results from the gas exchange monitor and prepares a written report.

0894T-0896T

Liver normothermic perfusion is a liver preservation technique that utilizes a lightweight, easy to transport, warm blood perfusion system for living organ transplants. The process permits the cadaver donor liver to remain in an environment that mirrors the human body rather than in a cold preservation method. Most normothermic perfusion systems are comprised of a small wireless monitor and a perfusion module unique to the type of transplant organ needed, as well as different solutions to maintain the donor organ. Donor blood is used, and the perfusion system provides blood oxygenation, gas flow, and a pulsatile pumping system. A solution containing nutrients, proteins, and oxygen is infused into the donor blood to supplement any missing nutrients or other substances. After backbench standard preparation, the physician carefully positions and secures cannulae in the hepatic artery, portal vein, and inferior vena cava. The suprahepatic inferior vena cava is sutured. The donor liver is placed inside a sterile, rounded vault that is attached to the system that controls and maintains the proper temperature and humidity levels to keep the organ warmed, maintained, and protected from contamination. Each proprietary system continues to fully assess the liver functionality and biochemical and metabolic status. The cannulae are connected to the perfusion unit. After 15 minutes, a separately reportable glucose reading is obtained using a perfusate sample; this is repeated at least every four hours. The liver is monitored with hourly assessments of elements such as the perfusate temperature and pH; bile production, pH, glucose, and bicarbonate; lactate levels; hemodynamic parameters; and visual inspection. Once the liver is deemed suitable, the cannulae are removed, and the liver is transplanted into the patient. Report 0894T for cannulation prior to connection of the liver allograft to the perfusion system and subsequent decannulation after perfusion is complete. Report 0895T for connection of the liver allograft to the perfusion device with monitoring for the first four hours, and 0896T for each additional hour.

0897T

The patient undergoes a 12-lead electrocardiogram (EKG). Utilizing a proprietary software program, the EKG and relevant clinical parameters are uploaded to a processing platform. Areas of interest are selected from the EKG recording, and maps are generated to identify focal and fibrillation arrhythmias, atrial and ventricular pacing, and beat-by-beat cardiac data in 2D and 3D. This artificial intelligence technology is considered augmentative, which means the machine analyzes and/or quantifies the data to produce clinically meaningful output, and a physician or other qualified health care professional provides an interpretation and report.

0898T

The patient undergoes an image-guided fusion biopsy of the prostate. Utilizing a proprietary software program, the biopsy with pathology data and MRI imaging are uploaded to a secure, cloud-based processing platform. An algorithm is deployed to determine the probability of prostate cancer throughout the prostate. An encapsulation confidence score is generated to indicate the likelihood that the cancer is contained within default margins. The physician is provided with the original MRI image with the cancer estimation map over the top. A viewing tool is used to visualize the tumor in 3D and adjust the margins as needed, which creates a new encapsulation confidence score. Once the physician is satisfied with the location and size of the margins, a treatment plan can be created. This artificial intelligence technology is considered augmentative, which means the machine analyzes and/or quantifies the data to produce clinically meaningful output, and a physician or other qualified health care professional provides an interpretation and report.

0899T-0900T

The patient undergoes contrast cardiac magnetic resonance (CMR) imaging, a radiation-free, noninvasive technique that produces high quality, detailed, three-dimensional imaging of complex congenital heart defects, as well as functional cardiac analysis. Absolute quantitation of myocardial blood flow (MBF) is the volume of blood transiting through tissue at a certain rate, usually in milliliters per minute per gram of tissue (mL/min/g). The MBF measurement reflects coronary microcirculation and can be used to evaluate for coronary risk factors and myocardial disease. Stress MBF, also referred to as hyperemic blood flow, describes the highest amount of blood flow that can be provided to the heart during the topmost period of vasodilation of the heart's vascular bed. Typically, to reach this maximum vasodilation, the patient receives vasodilators or inotropic agents via IV to simulate stress. Utilizing a proprietary software program, the CMR images are uploaded to a processing platform for MBF calculations. Report 0899T for an absolute quantitation of myocardial blood flow determination from an augmentative algorithmic analysis from an artificial intelligence application, which means the machine analyzes and/or quantifies the data to produce clinically meaningful output. Report 0900T for an absolute quantitation of myocardial blood flow estimate from an assistive algorithmic analysis from an artificial intelligence application, which means the machine detects clinically relevant data but does not analyze it or make conclusions. These codes require an interpretation and report by the physician or other qualified health care professional and are reported in addition to the code for the primary procedure.

0902T

Proprietary technology is used to determine the corrected QT interval (QTc) using data from an external electrocardiogram (ECG) device. After selecting the appropriate options in the associated mobile application on a smartphone or tablet, the patient places both thumbs over two electrodes on the top of the ECG device. The electrode on the bottom of the device is held against the left knee or ankle. An ECG recording is captured in less than a minute, and the QT interval is measured. A QT interval represents the time between the start of the Q wave and the end of the T wave on an ECG. A prolonged QT interval can be an indication of a higher risk for ventricular arrythmias or a side effect from certain medications. QTc estimates the QT interval at a standard 60 beats per minute heart rate, allowing the physician to compare the QT intervals over time at different heart rates. This artificial intelligence technology is considered augmentative, which means the machine analyzes and/or quantifies the data to produce clinically meaningful output, and a physician or other qualified health care professional provides an interpretation and report.

0903T-0905T

A 12-lead electrocardiogram (ECG) is generated with reduced leads using artificial intelligence algorithms. The proprietary system consists of an ECG module and a single cable with five electrode connectors. After selecting the appropriate options in the associated mobile application on a smartphone or tablet, electrodes are placed on the chest and limbs by a qualified health care professional or trained personnel. The system provides simultaneous measurements of four channels (leads I, II, V2, V4) with calculations of the remaining limb leads (III, aVR, aVL, aVF). The remaining four precordial leads are synthesized using machine-learning algorithms. Report 0903T for the combined professional and technical components of an ECG, including the tracing and interpretation and report; 0904T for the tracing only; and 0905T for the interpretation and report only.

0906T-0907T

The physician or other qualified health care professional administers concurrent optical and magnetic stimulation (COMS) therapy for the treatment of chronic ulcers of the legs and feet. A proprietary device is placed over the wound for approximately 15 minutes, two or three times per week, over two months. The optical component of the device emits light emitting diodes (LEDs); the magnetic stimulation occurs through coil emitting pulse modulated magnetic fields. The combination of optical and magnetic stimulation promotes tissue regeneration. Report 0906T for the first COMS device application and add-on code 0907T for each additional application. The treatment area is limited to a total wound(s) surface area of 50 sq cm or less per application. These codes include wound assessment and dressing care.

0908T-0910T

The physician places an integrated neurostimulation system via open approach for stimulation of the vagus nerve in 0908T. Following appropriate anesthesia, the physician makes an incision on the left side of the neck over the sternocleidomastoid muscle at the level of C4-C6 and dissects to the area between the subcutaneous fat and the platysma. The physician exposes and retracts the sternocleidomastoid muscle, omohyoid muscle, and strap muscles. Dissection continues until the vagus nerve is exposed, taking care not to damage the jugular vein, carotid artery, and laryngeal nerve. After exposing approximately 3 cm of the vagus nerve, a silicone positioning device is placed under the nerve and allowed to close around the nerve. The integrated neurostimulator device is placed inside the positioning device, which closes around the neurostimulator and is sutured closed. The skin and subcutaneous tissues are closed with layered sutures and skin staples. In 0909T, the physician replaces the integrated neurostimulator system. The physician incises the skin above the positioning device and locates it. Following location, the physician removes the neurostimulator from inside the positioning device and a new neurostimulator is placed inside. The positioning device may also be replaced if necessary. The skin and subcutaneous tissues are closed with sutures and skin staples. In 0910T, the physician removes the integrated neurostimulation system. The physician incises the skin above the positioning device. The neurostimulator device is removed from inside the positioning device. The positioning device is cut into two pieces and each piece is removed. The skin and subcutaneous tissues are closed with sutures and skin staples. Codes 0908T and 0909T include analysis and programming, when performed.

0911T-0912T

The physician or other qualified health care professional performs an electronic analysis of a previously placed integrated neurostimulation system for stimulation of the vagus nerve. Parameters checked may include the dose strength, schedule, or battery charge. Report 0911T for electronic analysis without programming; 0912T for electronic analysis with simple programming such as a change in the dose strength that is saved in the programming application.

0913T-0914T

The physician places a catheter percutaneously (through the skin) for treatment of occlusive disease of the major coronary arteries or branches. An introducer sheath is placed in an artery, typically the femoral artery, using percutaneous puncture. The angiography catheter is advanced through the introducer sheath into the ascending aorta and directed, under fluoroscopic guidance, to the opening of the coronary artery. Following mechanical dilation with a non-drug balloon, a drug-coated balloon is advanced. The balloon's outer surface is coated with a therapeutic drug (paclitaxel) that is delivered directly to the stenosis site. Intravascular ultrasound (IVUS) or optical coherence tomography (OCT) endoluminal imaging may be used during the procedure. For IVUS, a catheter is placed over the guidewire. The ultrasound probe is used to obtain images from inside the vessel to assess area and extent of disease prior to interventional therapy, as well as adequacy of therapy after interventional therapy. The ultrasound probe provides a two-dimensional, cross-sectional view of the vessel or graft as the probe is advanced and withdrawn along the area of interest. When the ultrasound examination is complete, the catheter is removed. In OCT, light is utilized instead of sound to provide cross-sectional images in high resolution within the lumen. Report 0913T for percutaneous transcatheter drug delivery balloon intervention for a single major coronary artery or branch. Report add-on code 0914T in addition to the code for a percutaneous stent or atherectomy intervention when the balloon intervention is performed on a separate target lesion than the target lesion treated during balloon angioplasty, stent placement, or atherectomy. These codes include IVUS and OCT, when performed, and imaging supervision, interpretation, and report.

0915T-0918T

Cardiac contractility modulation-defibrillation (CCM-D) is utilized to improve cardiac output in patients with moderate to severe heart failure. A defibrillator component is included that can provide shock therapy or pacing when an abnormal heart rhythm is detected. The device consists of a programmable and rechargeable generator powered by a lithium battery, a defibrillator lead, and pacemaker lead. Under local anesthesia, dissection is performed directly on top of the fascia in the left pectoral region of the chest to create a subcutaneous pocket. The defibrillator lead is placed in a mid-septum location, while the pacing lead is placed at least 2 cm away on the high septum. Once the leads are placed, they are tested and connected to the pulse generator that is placed in the previously prepared pocket. Sensing and therapeutic parameters are evaluated and programmed as appropriate. The subcutaneous pocket is closed with sutures. Report 0915T for insertion of the pulse generator with dual transvenous leads (pacing and defibrillation); 0916T for insertion of the pulse generator only; 0917T for insertion of a single transvenous lead (pacing or defibrillation) only; and 0918T for dual transvenous leads (pacing and defibrillation) only. These codes include imaging guidance, catheterization, and device evaluation and programming.

0919T-0922T

The physician removes a component of a cardiac contractility modulation-defibrillation (CCM-D) device. In 0919T, only the pulse generator is removed. Under local anesthesia, an incision is made into the previously created subcutaneous pocket. Leads are disconnected and capped. The generator is removed, and the incision is closed with sutures. Report 0920T when only the pacing lead is removed; 0921T when only the defibrillation lead is removed; and 0922T when both the pacing and defibrillation leads are removed.

0923T

The physician removes and replaces a cardiac contractility modulation-defibrillation (CCM-D) pulse generator. Under local anesthesia, an incision is made into the previously created subcutaneous pocket. Leads are disconnected, and the generator is removed. A new pulse generator is inserted into the pocket. Existing leads are connected to the new generator and tested. The incision is closed with sutures.

0924T

The physician repositions one or more previously implanted cardiac contractility modulation-defibrillation (CCM-D) transvenous electrodes/leads due to displacement or abnormal function. An incision is made to access the lead. Fluoroscopy is used to identify the current placement of the lead and reposition it. The lead is secured in place and tested after connection to the pulse generator is verified. The incision is closed with sutures. This code includes fluoroscopic guidance and programming of the sensing and therapeutic parameters.

0925T
The physician relocates the skin pocket for a cardiac contractility modulation-defibrillation (CCM-D) pulse generator due to complications or because the tissue in the area needs to be irradiated. Under local anesthesia, an incision is made into the previously created subcutaneous pocket. Leads are disconnected, and the generator is removed. If a hematoma or abscess is present, it is incised and drained, and this is not reported separately. The pocket is closed with sutures. In a new location, dissection is performed directly on top of the fascia to create a new subcutaneous pocket. The pulse generator is placed in the pocket. Existing leads are connected to the generator and tested. The incision is closed with sutures. This code includes all work associated with the original subcutaneous pocket and creation of a new pocket.

0926T
A programming device evaluation is performed in person to test contractility modulation-defibrillation (CCM-D) device function and select the most favorable permanent programmed values. Patients with previously implanted CCM-D systems require periodic programming device evaluations. This diagnostic procedure includes a face-to-face assessment of all device functions, including sensing and therapeutic parameters. Current settings are analyzed, and the settings may be adjusted to maintain optimal function of the CCM-D device for the individual patient. This code includes the review and report.

0927T-0929T
An interrogation device evaluation is performed for an implantable contractility modulation-defibrillation (CCM-D) system. Interrogation may include testing of the function of the battery, lead(s), capture and sensing function, heart rhythm, and programmed parameters. In 0927T, interrogation is performed in person in a face-to-face assessment. This code includes the analysis, review, report, connection/disconnection, and recording. This code is reported once per patient encounter. In 0928T, a physician or other qualified health care professional provides interim analysis with report for remote device interrogation for a period of up to 90 days. In 0929T, included components are remote data acquisition, receipt of transmissions, technician review, technical support, and distribution of results for remote device interrogation for a period of up to 90 days.

0930T-0931T
A physician or other qualified health care provider performs an electrophysiologic evaluation of contractility modulation-defibrillator (CCM-D) leads. This includes evaluation of a defibrillation threshold including arrhythmia induction with evaluation of sensing and therapy for arrhythmia termination. Report 0930T when the evaluation is performed at the time of the initial implantation or replacement with testing of the CCM-D pulse generator. Report 0931T when the evaluation is performed during a separate encounter from the initial implantation or replacement with testing of the pulse generator.

0932T
Echocardiography image post processing is utilized to detect heart failure with preserved ejection fraction (HFpEF) in adult patients undergoing routine functional cardiovascular assessment using echocardiography. Utilized by an interpreting qualified health care professional (QHP) who determines that the echocardiogram demonstrates a preserved ejection fraction, the noninvasive proprietary device provides information that may be useful in the detection of heart failure. The device is an automated machine learning-based decision support system that takes input from Digital Imaging and Communications in Medicine (DICOM) files of 2D echocardiogram imaging data with an apical four-chamber view. The software employs an artificial intelligence (AI) model to produce an estimate of the absence or presence of HFpEF to the interpreting QHP. The QHP uses this data with other medical information to assist with the diagnosis of the patient. This code reports the interpretation and report of the data produced by the automated machine learning-based decision support system. The echocardiography is performed separately.

0933T
The physician implants a wireless atrial pressure sensor via right heart catheterization. The sensor allows for long-term, remote monitoring of left atrial pressure in patients with symptomatic heart failure. The physician gains access to the femoral vein. Under imaging guidance, a catheter is advanced from the femoral vein into the right atrium. The interatrial wall or septum is punctured, and the catheter is passed into the left atrium. Using a proprietary delivery system, the sensor is advanced to the interatrial septum and deployed. Calibration of the sensor is performed. This code includes all imaging guidance and radiological supervision and interpretation.

0934T
A wireless left atrial pressure sensor allows for long-term, remote monitoring of left atrial pressure (LAP) in patients with symptomatic heart failure. LAP readings are transmitted from a sensor that has been implanted in the interatrial septum. The sensory implant has no battery or leads; the patient wears a portable belt across the chest that powers the implant and transmits real-time LAP data to a cloud-based system. The patient can monitor the readings using a mobile application and adjust diuretics according to a prescribed treatment plan, or the provider can intervene with additional guidance. This code includes remote monitoring of the sensor for a 30-day period; do not report this code for monitoring if the duration is less than 16 days. Analysis of LAP trends with interpretation and report is performed by the physician or other qualified health care professional with any necessary adjustments to treatment paradigm thresholds, diuretics and other medications, or lifestyle recommendations.

0935T

The physician passes a cystourethroscope through the urethra and bladder to treat uncontrolled hypertension with bilateral renal pelvic sympathetic denervation using radiofrequency ablation. Under fluoroscopy, a rigid cystoscope is used to advance a guidewire through the bladder, past the ureteropelvic junction, and into the renal pelvis. A ureteral sheath is passed over the guidewire to enable deployment of a proprietary ablation device with four spherical electrodes. The device is connected to a radiofrequency generator, and electrical energy is dispersed into the renal pelvis for a cycle of two minutes at a temperature of 60 degrees Celsius. The device and sheath are removed and redeployed through the opposite ureter, and a cycle is administered in the opposite kidney. After bilateral ablation is complete, all instruments are removed. This code includes fluoroscopy and all contrast injections.

0936T

Photobiomodulation (PBM) therapy uses low-level light to promote cellular function in the retina for patients with dry age-related macular degeneration (AMD). PBM stimulates mitochondrial function to improve the health of retinal cells. The patient is seated in front of a PBM instrument that sits on a table or desk. Treatment is administered at selected wavelengths to the eye and retinal tissue for approximately four minutes. A series of treatments may be administered over several weeks. Report this code once per treatment session.

0937T-0940T

Long-term external electrocardiographic (ECG) recording is a diagnostic procedure that provides continuous rhythm recording of the patient's heart while the patient is engaged in the activities of daily living. The purpose of the study is to evaluate the patient's ambient heart rhythm during a full daily cycle. Rhythm disturbances and waveform abnormalities are detected; information is provided regarding the frequency of these disturbances. The physician or other qualified health care provider instructs the patient in the use of the external ECG recorder. A technician places ECG leads on the patient's chest, and the patient wears the recorder for more than 15 days up to 30 days. During this time there is continuous rhythm recording and storage. The patient returns the device, and the recorded heart rhythm is converted into digital format by a technician. The technician uses a scanning methodology to classify different ECG waveforms and to generate a report. The generated report describes the overall rhythm and significant arrhythmias. Code 0937T reports the recording, scanning analysis with report, provider review of the data, and the provision of a final interpretation in a report. Code 0938T reports the recording only, which includes the connection and initial recording of data. Code 0939T reports only the scanning analysis with report. Code 0940T reports only the provider review and interpretation.

0941T-0943T

In 0941T, the physician passes a cystourethroscope through the urethra and bladder for placement and expansion of a prostatic urethral scaffold to treat prostate obstruction. The scaffold is used to expand a portion of the urethra that extends through the prostate to allow urine to flow through. A flexible cystoscope is passed into the penis and to the bladder neck with identification of any abnormalities or anatomical considerations that may impact the selection of the appropriate scaffold size. A delivery system balloon is deployed and inflated with release of the expandable scaffold into the prostatic urethra. Adjustments are made to ensure proper positioning before releasing the implant and deflating the balloon. The delivery system and all instruments are removed. In 0942T, the prostatic urethral scaffold is removed and replaced. A sheath is advanced over a flexible cystoscope, and the previously implanted scaffold is removed with the sheath. A new scaffold implant is deployed through the cystoscope using the balloon delivery system. In 0943T, the prostatic urethral scaffold is removed without replacement.

0944T

The physician or other qualified health care professional performs 3D contour simulation of one or more target liver lesions and margins for image-guided percutaneous microwave ablation (MWA). MWA is a minimally invasive procedure that destroys liver lesions with heat using microwaves emitted by an antenna. Ablation margins must be precise to prevent tumor recurrence while minimizing damage to healthy tissues. 3D contouring is performed during the MWA operative session to create a model of the liver to define the ablation zone. Model probe pathways and locations are created along with volumetric calculations of the ablation cavity. Pre- and post-procedure computed tomography (CT) imaging and guidance is performed for post-ablation volume comparisons. Proposed ablation volumes are overlayed onto CT images of the liver to determine the most appropriate MWA treatment plan for the individual patient. 3D contouring is distinct from other types of imaging services performed before or during the procedure. This code should not be reported more than once per microwave ablation session, regardless of the number of lesions ablated.

0945T

Real-time intraoperative assessment is performed during partial mastectomy procedures to detect residual breast cancer. An optical imaging agent (pegulicianine) is injected into the patient prior to surgery, and enzymatic activity in and around the cancer is triggered within two hours. Following tumor removal, the surgeon inserts a handheld probe within the resection cavity. Images are obtained, transmitted, and read by the proprietary patient-calibrated cancer detection software. Any areas identified as being suspicious for remaining cancer are highlighted onscreen for viewing by the surgeon, enabling detection and resection of residual cancerous tissue that might otherwise have been left behind.

0946T

Orthopedic implant movement analysis is used in conjunction with two computed tomography (CT) scans to determine if a joint or extremity implant has moved or become loose over time or to detect pseudoarthrosis, a condition in which the bones have not fused properly after an injury or procedure. This analysis is typically performed for patients with a knee, hip, or spine implant. Two low-dose CT scans with paired views of the extremity or joint are obtained and uploaded into proprietary software for analysis; the CT scans are not reported separately. The physician or other qualified health care professional evaluates the data for the targeted structure and determines if there is a loose implant or pseudoarthrosis. This code includes data acquisition, preparation, and transmission with a written interpretation and report.

0947T

Magnetic resonance image guided low intensity focused ultrasound (MRgFUS) is performed with infusion of microbubbles to temporarily open the blood brain barrier to increase the number of brain tumor biomarkers released into the bloodstream. The biomarkers are analyzed after the procedure to identify disease progression and guide future treatment. The patient's head is shaved and inspected for scars or other lesions that could potentially affect the ultrasound beam. A four-pin stereotactic frame may be placed on the patient's head after administration of a local anesthetic. Positioning of the frame is determined to encompass the center of the brain within the treatment area. After the frame is secured, a silicone membrane containing cooled, degassed water is placed over the patient's head. This membrane allows the ultrasound to travel through. The patient is placed on the MRI table and an MRgFUS helmet is attached. This helmet contains the transducer arrays. Additional cooled, degassed water is added to the space between the patient's head and the helmet. The water is further cooled to a temperature of about 18 degrees Celsius. MR registration images are combined with a pre-procedure MR image. The surgeon views the imaging, evaluating the target, parameters, and treatment plan. An infusion of microbubble resonators is started at 5ul/kg/min and continues for approximately an hour. Blood is collected from an intravenous catheter for subsequent analysis of the released tumor biomarkers. All instruments are removed, and a final MR image is obtained. This code includes stereotactic navigation and frame placement, when performed.